Brain Tumors

To the brave pioneers of brain tumor surgery, to patients with brain tumors and their families, and to our wives, Judy and Margaret, for their support, encouragement and devotion.

For Churchill Livingstone:

Commissioning Editor: Michael Parkinson
Project Editor: Dilys Jones
Copy Editor: Ruth Swan
Indexer: John Sampson
Design Direction: Erik Bigland
Project Controller: Nancy Arnott
Sales Promotion Executive: Duncan Jones

Brain Tumors

An Encyclopedic Approach

Edited by

Andrew H. Kaye MB BS MD FRACS

Professor of Neurosurgery, The University of Melbourne; Director of Neurosurgery and The Melbourne Neuroscience Centre, Royal Melbourne Hospital, Victoria, Australia

Edward R. Laws Jr MD FACS

Professor of Neurosurgery and Professor of Medicine, University of Virginia, Charlottesville, Virginia, USA

CHURCHILL LIVINGSTONE
EDINBURGH HONG KONG LONDON MADRID MELBOURNE NEW YORK AND TOKYO 1995

CHURCHILL LIVINGSTONE
A Division of Harcourt Brace and Company Ltd

First published 1995
Reprinted 1995
Reprinted 1997

ISBN 0-443-04840-1

British Library Cataloguing in Publication Data
A catalogue record for this book is available from the British Library.

Library of Congress Cataloging in Publication Data
A catalogue record for this book is available from the Library of Congress.

The publisher's policy is to use **paper manufactured from sustainable forests**

Produced by Longman Asia Ltd, Hong Kong
NPCC/03

Contents

SECTION 2
Specific brain tumors

PART I
Gliomas

PART II
Neuronal and neuronal precursor tumors

PART III
Nerve sheath tumors

PART IV
Meningeal tumors

PART V
Pineal region tumors

PART VI
Pituitary tumors

PART VII
Skull base tumors

PART VIII
Cerebral lymphoma

PART IX
Tumor-like malformations

PART X
Metastatic brain tumors

Contributors

Ossama Al-Mefty MD
Professor and Chairman, Department of Neurosurgery, University of Arkansas for Medical Sciences, Little Rock, Arkansas, USA

Michael L. J. Apuzzo MD
Edwin M. Todd/Trent H. Wells Jr. Professor, Department of Neurological Surgery and Radiation Oncology, Biology and Physics, University of Southern California School of Medicine; Director of Neurosurgery, Kenneth R. Norris Jr. Cancer Hospital and Research Institute, Los Angeles, California, USA

Mitchel S. Berger MD
Associate Professor of Neurological Surgery, University of Washington School of Medicine, Seattle, Washington, USA

Rajesh K. Bindal BA
Graduate Student, Department of Neurosurgery, The University of Texas, MD Anderson Cancer Center, Houston, Texas, USA

Peter Black MD PhD
Franc D. Ingraham Professor of Neurosurgery, Harvard Medical School; Neurosurgeon-in-Chief, Brigham and Women's Hospital; Neurosurgeon-in-Chief, Children's Hospital; Chief of Neurosurgical Oncology, Dana-Farber Cancer Institute, Boston, Massachusetts, USA

Susan Black MD
Associate Professor of Anesthesiology, University of Chicago, Chicago, Illinois, USA

Jeffrey N. Bruce MD
Assistant Professor, Departments of Neurosurgery and Pathology, College of Physicians and Surgeons of Columbia University, New York, New York, USA

Jan C. Buckner MD
Assistant Professor of Oncology, Department of Medical Oncology, Mayo Clinic and Mayo Foundation, Rochester, Minnesota, USA

Thomas C. Chen MD
Resident in Neurosurgery, Department of Neurosurgery, School of Medicine, University of Southern California, Los Angeles, California, USA

Susan Chang MD
Assistant Clinical Professor, University of California, Neuro-Oncology Service, San Francisco, California, USA

E. Sander Connolly Jr MD
Resident, Department of Neurological Surgery, Columbia University, New York, New York, USA

William T. Couldwell MD PhD
Assistant Professor of Neurological Surgery; Director, Skull Base Surgery, The University of Southern California, Los Angeles, California, USA

H. Alan Crockard MB BCh BAO FRCS (Ed) FRCS (Eng)
Consultant Neurosurgeon, The National Hospital for Neurology and Neurosurgery, London; Honorary Senior Lecturer, Institute of Neurology, London, UK

Roy F. Cucchiara MD
Professor and Chairman of Anesthesiology, University of Florida College of Medicine, Gainesville, Florida, USA

R. Andrew Danks MB BS FRACS
Neurosurgeon, Department of Neurosurgery, Royal Melbourne Hospital, Parkville, Australia

Franco DeMonte MD FRCS (C)
Assistant Professor, Department of Neurosurgery, University of Texas MD Anderson Cancer Center, Houston, Texas; Clinical Assistant Professor, Department of Neurosurgery, Baylor College of Medicine, Houston, Texas, USA

John A. Duncan III
Department of Surgery, Division of Neurosurgery, The Hospital for Sick Children, Toronto, Ontario, Canada

Michael J. Ebersold MD
Associate Professor and Consultant, Department of Neurosurgery, Mayo Clinic, Rochester, Minnesota, USA

Alexandra Flowers MD MS
Clinical Associate, Department of Neurology; Director, Adult Neuro-Oncology, The Cleveland Foundation, Cleveland, Ohio, USA

Robert L. Foote MD
Assistant Professor, Division of Radiation Oncology, Mayo Clinic, Rochester, Minnesota, USA

Kouzou Fukuyama MD
Division of Neurosurgery and the Brain Tumor Research Laboratory, Hospital for Sick Children, University of Toronto, Toronto, Ontario, Canada

Emmanuel Gay MD
Assistant, Chef de Clinique, Service de Neurochirurgie, CHU Grenoble, France

J. Russell Geyer MD
Assistant Professor of Pediatrics, Department of Hematology/Oncology, Children's Hospital, Seattle, Washington, USA

Graham G. Giles PhD
Director, Cancer Epidemiology Center, Anti-Cancer Council of Victoria, Melbourne; Director, Victorian Cancer Registry, Melbourne, Victoria, Australia

Michael F. Gonzales MB BS FRCPA
Consultant Neuropathologist, The Royal Melbourne Hospital, Melbourne; Associate Pathologist, Department of Pathology, The University of Melbourne; Director, Neuropathology Research Laboratory, Royal Melbourne Hospital, Melbourne, Victoria, Australia

Ignacio Gonzales-Gomez MD
Research Scholar, Neuropathology, Department of Pathology and Laboratory Medicine, Children's Hospital of Los Angeles, University of Southern California School of Medicine, Los Angeles, California, USA

Michael D. Green MB BS MD FRACP FACP
Director of Haematology and Medical Oncology, Department of Haematology and Medical Oncology, Western Hospital, Victoria, Australia

Barton L. Guthrie MD
Associate Professor, Division of Neurosurgery, The University of Alabama at Birmingham, Alabama, USA

Georges F. Haddad MD FRCS (C)
Clincal Assistant Professor, American University of Beirut, Medical Center Department of Neurosurgery, Beirut, Lebanon

Griffith Harsh IV MD
Director, Neurosurgical Oncology, Massachusetts General Hospital; Associate Professor of Surgery, Harvard Medical School, Boston, Massachusetts, USA

David R. Hinton MD FRCPC
Associate Professor of Pathology, Neurosurgery and Neurology Neuropathologist, University Hospital, University of Southern California School of Medicine, Los Angeles, California, USA

Harold J. Hoffman MD BSc (med) FRCS (C)
Professor, Department of Surgery, University of Toronto, Toronto; Chief, Division of Neurosurgery, The Hospital for Sick Children, Toronto, Ontario, Canada

Francis G. Johnston MA MB BChir FRCS
Senior Registrar in Neurosurgery, The National Hospital for Nervous Diseases, London

A. B. M. F. Karim MD FRCR PhD
Professor and Chairman, Department of Radiation Oncology, Free University Hospital, Amsterdam, The Netherlands

Andrew H. Kaye MB BS MD FRACS
Professor of Neurosurgery, The University of Melbourne; Director of Neurosurgery and The Melbourne Neuroscience Centre, Royal Melbourne Hospital, Melbourne, Victoria, Australia

Evren Keles MD
Resident in Neurological Surgery, Northwest Neuro-Oncology Research and Therapy Section, Department of Neurological Surgery, University of Washington School of Medicine, Seattle, Washington, USA

John King MB BS MD FRACP
Neurologist, Clinical Neuroscience Centre, Royal Melbourne Hospital, Melbourne, Victoria, Australia

T. T. King MB BS FRCS
Consultant Neurosurgeon, Royal London Hospital, Whitechapel, London, UK

Neil D. Kitchen FRCS
Clinical Research Fellow, Gough Cooper Department of Neurological Surgery, Institute of Neurology, London, UK

John Knightly MD
Neurological Surgery, Division of Neurosciences, National Naval Medical Center, Bethesda, Maryland, USA

John Laidlaw MB BS FRACS
Neurosurgeon, Alfred Hospital, Melbourne, Victoria, Australia

Edward R. Laws Jr MD FACS
Professor of Neurosurgery, Professor of Medicine, University of Virginia, Charlottesville, Virginia, USA

A. Joseph Layon MD
Associate Professor of Anesthesiology and Medicine, University of Florida College of Medicine, Gainesville, Florida, USA

Victor A. Levin MD
Professor and Chairman, Department of Neuro-Oncology, MD Anderson Cancer Center, Houston; Bernard W. Biedenharn Chair in Cancer Research; Director, Brain Tumor Center, MD Anderson Cancer Center, Houston, Texas, USA

M. Beatriz S. Lopes MD
Assistant Professor of Pathology (Neuropathology), Department of Pathology, University of Virginia School of Medicine, Charlottesville, Virginia, USA

J. Gordon McComb MD
Head, Division of Neurosurgery, Children's Hospital of Los Angeles; Professor of Neurosurgery, School of Medicine, University of Southern California, Los Angeles, California, USA

Robert Macfarlane MA BChir MD FRCS
Consultant Neurosurgeon, Addenbrooke's Hospital, Cambridge, UK

Lorenzo Magrassi MD
Fellow in Neurosurgery, Department of Surgery-Neurosurgery, University of Pavia, Italy

John R. Mangiardi MD FACS
Chief of Neurosurgery, Lenox Hill Hospital; Professor of Clinical Neurosurgery, New York University; Chairman, Foundation for Neurosurgical Research, New York, New York, USA

Robert A. Morantz MD FACS
Clinical Associate Professor of Neurological Surgery, University of Kansas School of Medicine, Kansas City, Kansas, USA

Akio Morita MD
Chief Resident Associate, Mayo Clinic, Mayo Graduate School of Medicine, Rochester, Minnesota, USA

Robert G. Ojemann MD
Professor of Surgery, Harvard Medical School, Boston; Visiting Neurosurgeon, Massachusetts General Hospital, Boston, Massachusetts, USA

Kerry D. Olsen MD FACS
Professor and Consultant, Department of Otorhinolaryngology, Head and Neck Surgery, Mayo Clinic, Rochester, Minnesota, USA

Kalmon D. Post MD
Professor and Chairman, Department of Neurosurgery, Mount Sinai School of Medicine, New York, New York, USA

Michael Prados MD FACP
Associate Professor of Neurosurgery, Head of Neuro-Oncology, University of California, San Francisco, California, USA

Lynn M. Quast RN BSN
Nurse Physician Extender, Department of Neurosurgery, Mayo Clinic, Rochester, Minnesota, USA

Craig H. Rabb MD
Clinical Instructor, Department of Neurological Surgery, University of Southern California School of Medicine, Los Angeles, California, USA

Vincent M. Riccardi MD MBA
Director, The Neurofibromatosis Institute, La Crescenta, California, USA

Norbert Roosen Dr med
Co-Director, Experimental Therapeutics Laboratory, Midwest Neuro-Oncology Center; Associate Staff Investigator, Department of Neurological Surgery, Henry Ford Health System, Detroit, Michigan, USA

Mark L. Rosenblum MD
Chairman, Department of Neurological Surgery; Director, Mid-West Neuro-Oncology Center, Henry Ford Health System, Detroit, Michigan, USA

Mark A. Rosenthal MB BS FRACP
Doctoral Fellow, Ludwig Institute for Cancer Research, Melbourne, Australia

James T. Rutka MD PhD FRCSC
Assistant Professor, Division of Neurosurgery, University of Toronto Faculty of Medicine, Toronto, Ontario, Canada

Michael Salcman MD FACS
Clinical Professor of Neurosurgery, George Washington University, School of Medicine, Washington DC; Attending Neurosurgeon, Sinai Hospital, Baltimore, Maryland, USA

Madjid Samii MD PhD
Professor and Chair of Neurosurgery, Medical School Hannover; Director of Neurosurgical Clinic, Nordstadt Hospital, Hannover, Germany

Yutaka Sawamura MD
Instructor, Department of Neurosurgery, University Hospital, Lausanne, Switzerland

Raymond Sawaya MD
Professor and Chairman, Department of Neurosurgery, University of Texas, MD Anderson Cancer Center, Houston, Texas, USA

Bernd W. Scheithauer MD
Professor of Pathology, Mayo Medical School; Consultant in Pathology, Mayo Clinic, Rochester, Minnesota, USA

R. Michael Scott MD
Professor of Surgery, Harvard Medical School, Boston; Director of Pediatric Neurosurgery, The Children's Hospital, Boston, Massachusetts, USA

Laligam N. Sekhar MD FACS
Professor and Chairman, Department of Neurosurgery, George Washington University Medical Center, Washington D.C., USA

Joseph Stachniak MD
Resident, Department of Neurosurgery, University of Florida College of Medicine, Gainesville, Florida, USA

Bennett M. Stein MD
Byron Stookey Professor and Chairman, Department of Neurological Surgery, Columbia University College of Physicians and Surgeons, New York; Director of Service, Neurological Surgery, Columbia-Presbyterian Medical Center, New York, New York, USA

Richard Strauss MD
Assistant Professor, Department of Neurosurgery, Mount Sinai School of Medicine, New York, New York, USA

Marcos Tatagiba MD
Assistant, Neurosurgery Department, Nordstadt Hospital, Hannover, Germany

Kamal Thapar MD
Division of Neurosurgery, Hospital for Sick Children, University of Toronto, Toronto, Ontario, Canada

D. G. T. Thomas FRCP (Glas) FRCSEd
Professor of Neurosurgery, Institute of Neurology, The National Hospital, London, UK

Nicolas de Tribolet MD
Professor and Chairman, Centre Hospitalier Universitaire Vaudois, Department of Neurosurgery, Lausanne, Switzerland

Scott R. VandenBerg MD PhD
Professor of Pathology and Neurological Surgery, Director of Neuropathology, Department of Pathology, University of Virginia School of Medicine, Charlottesville, Virginia, USA

Patrick Y. Wen MD
Assistant Professor of Neurology, Harvard Medical School; Director of Neuro-Oncology, Division of Neurology, Brigham and Women's Hospital, Boston, Massachusetts, USA

Donald C. Wright MD
Professor, Department of Neurological Surgery, George Washington University Medical Center, Washington D.C., USA

Preface

The management of brain tumors is the single most important role of the present day neurosurgeon. The chilling diagnosis of a brain tumor quite reasonably strikes fear into patients, their friends and relatives. The consequences of the diagnosis include the implication of an erosion of the faculties of the mind combined with physical disability and death.

The appropriate diagnosis and management requires the very best skills a neurosurgeon has learned, a culmination of all the knowledge that has been gleaned from his or her first days in medical school to the most recent clinical experience practising the art of neurosurgery, along with the insight that has been obtained into human nature and frailty. Treatment involves the very best of both technical skills and human interaction. Throughout the often protracted management of a patient with a brain tumor the surgeon must constantly strive to utilize the very latest in scientific advancement, whilst maintaining a sympathetic and guiding influence on the patient and the family.

The treatment of brain tumors has expanded rapidly over the past decades. It was the discovery of the cell by Schleiden and Schwann in 1838 and 1839 and the description of neuroglia by Virchow in 1846 that formed the basis for the neuropathology of brain tumors. The concept of cerebral localisation of neurological function developed through the nineteenth century and the first scientifically performed brain tumor operation took place on 25 November 1884 by Rickman Godlee in London. That patient died from the glioma twenty five days after surgery. The subsequent pioneers in brain tumor surgery, including Cushing, Dandy, Keen, Macewen and Horsley demonstrated not only the possibilities of brain tumor surgery, but also at times, the seemingly insurmountable difficulties that had to be overcome for the patient to be treated effectively and safely. The last two decades have, in particular, provided the technological advancement necessary for the understanding of the many varied facets of brain tumors, including their intricate biology, the molecular events that are at the basis of their development, and the equipment necessary for effective treatment. We now know that the ideal management involves a wide range of skills and techniques, utilizing all the best technical and human resources of a hospital and community.

In the past the mystique of brain tumors has, at times, inadvertently restricted the full understanding of these tumors. This book aims to provide a complete coverage of brain tumors, including their biological basis, diagnosis and management techniques. Aiming to be a reference on all the technical facets of brain tumor management, the book describes the present concepts of the treatment and the management of all brain tumors, although we realise that social values vary from region to region and in many countries facilities are less than optimal.

In general, references have been chosen for their general coverage of the topics, ease of access, historical interest, and, in some cases, because they will provide thought provoking alternatives to give a different perspective to the subject.

It is not possible to list and acknowledge all the many people who have helped in the preparation of this volume both knowingly and as the result of their influences on our own neurosurgical practices. We particularly acknowledge our many colleagues, both past and present, who by their influence and example have made this type of book possible.

This work would not have come to fruition without the guidance and stimulation initially from Peter Richardson and then from his colleagues, Michael Parkinson, Dilys Jones and Janice Urquhart at Churchill Livingstone.

We are especially grateful for the encouragement and patience of our wives, Judy and Peggy.

1995

A. K.
E. L.

Basic principles

1. Historical perspective

Andrew H. Kaye Edward R. Laws Jr

The concept of a tumor of the brain is, for most individuals and many physicians as well, one of the most dramatic forms of human illness. Virtually every family has had some exposure to an individual suffering from a tumor of the brain, either within the family proper or within a circle of friends, relatives and acquaintances. Brain tumors occur as the second most common form of malignancy in children and have a dramatic effect on families involved. Among adults, primary tumors of the brain rank from 6th to 8th in frequency of all neoplasms, and tumors metastatic to the brain affect more and more individuals as methods for control of primary cancers become even more effective. The advent of AIDS and immunosuppression associated with organ transplants have led to an increased incidence of lymphomas of the brain.

Primary brain tumors account for about 2% of cancer deaths, but are responsible for 7% of the years of life lost from cancer before the age of 70. They are responsible for 20% of malignant tumors diagnosed before the age of 15. About 30% of deaths are due to cancer in western society, and 1 in 5 of these will have intracranial metastatic deposits at autopsy.

The revolutionary advances that have occurred in the diagnosis of brain tumors have led to an increased detection rate and a major increase in efficacy of surgical management. This is based on the exquisite detail of anatomic relationships afforded by modern imaging techniques. Additionally, there is evidence from epidemiologic studies that brain tumors are becoming increasingly more prevalent, especially as the population ages, and this increase appears to be in excess of the improvement in detection rates.

There has been an explosion in neuroscience related to the molecular biology and genetics of brain tumors which should stimulate major advances in neuro-oncology. The characterization of genes and gene products related to neurofibromatosis has been a major advance. The characterization of other promoter and suppressor genes operative in brain tumor pathogenesis has also occurred and has done much to elucidate basic mechanisms of tumorigenesis. The advent of gene therapy is an exciting therapeutic frontier with major possibilities. Other areas of intense research interest are monoclonal antibodies peculiar to various types of brain tumors and receptors characteristic of certain tumors that may be manipulated for diagnostic and therapeutic purposes.

Despite some earlier reports of surgical success, modern brain tumor surgery is generally thought to have commenced on 25 November 1884, when Rickman Godlee operated on a 25-year-old Scottish farmer named Henderson who had suffered from focal motor epilepsy and a progressive hemiparesis. The operation was performed at the Hospital for Epilepsy and Paralysis, Regent's Park, London (Fig. 1.1), and the patient died 28 days after surgery from meningitis. The patient had been under the care of Hughes Bennett, a neurologist on the staff of that hospital, who had diagnosed that the patient had a brain tumor which involved the cortical substance, was of limited size and was situated in the neighborhood of the upper third of the fissure of Rolando. The tumor proved to be an oligodendroglioma 'about the size of a walnut'. Present at the operation were Hughlings Jackson, David Ferrier, Victor Horsley and perhaps Joseph Lister himself. Rickman Godlee was the nephew of Lister, and Hughes Bennett's father was a well-known Professor of Medicine in Edinburgh who died following a lithotomy in 1875. At autopsy a benign parietal tumor was discovered and it is speculative whether this influenced Hughes Bennett's decision to suggest surgery for his patient.

Modern brain tumor surgery was made possible by three discoveries of the 19th century — anesthesia, asepsis and neurologic localization of cerebral lesions. Rickman Godlee's operation in 1884 was not the first time that a tumor had been removed, but it was the first occasion that a tumor had been localized solely by neurologic methods and antiseptic surgical techniques had been utilized. Previously, tumors of the brain had been removed from time to time when they had spontaneously eroded the skull, or when the skull had been trephined, usually for epilepsy or intractable headache, or where a scar or depressed

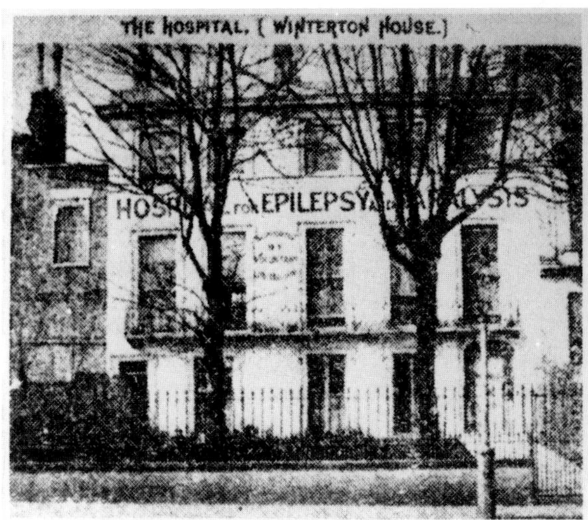

A Mirror

OF

HOSPITAL PRACTICE,

BRITISH AND FOREIGN.

Nulla autem est alia pro certo noscendi via, nisi quamplurimas et morborum et dissectionum historias, tum aliorum tum proprias collectas habere, et inter se comparare.—MORGAGNI De Sed. et Caus. Morb., lib. iv. Prooemium.

HOSPITAL FOR EPILEPSY AND PARALYSIS, REGENT'S PARK.

EXCISION OF A TUMOUR FROM THE BRAIN.

(Under the care of Dr. HUGHES BENNETT and Mr. RICKMAN J. GODLEE.)

DURING the last few weeks several notices have appeared in various medical papers concerning a man at present in the above hospital, from whose brain a tumour has been successfully removed. This operation, performed, we believe, for the first time in the history of medicine, has

Fig. 1.1 The Hospital for Epilepsy and Paralysis, Regent's Park, London, site of the first modern brain tumor operation in 1884. From Spillane J. *Doctrine of the Nerves*. Oxford University Press.

fracture indicated the probable site of a lesion. Archeologists have found skulls with holes bored in them dating from the mesolithic or middle stone age period as well as from neolithic times (Fig. 1.2). There is evidence that patients survived these operations as the holes in the bone are healed by new formation of bone tissue, and the sharp edges of the bored or hacked holes have become rounded off. Trephination was carried out by primitive peoples as late as the beginning of the 20th century. The Serbs of Albania and Montenegro trephined for neuralgia, migraine, psychosis and other maladies using a crude wire saw. In the South Sea Islands of the Pacific, trephining was relatively common, playing an important role in native custom. In the Bismarck Archipelago, the surgical instruments consisted of a tooth of a shark and a sharp shell. It is evident that although there may have been a medical basis to some of the cranial procedures, many were performed for magical rather than medical reasons.

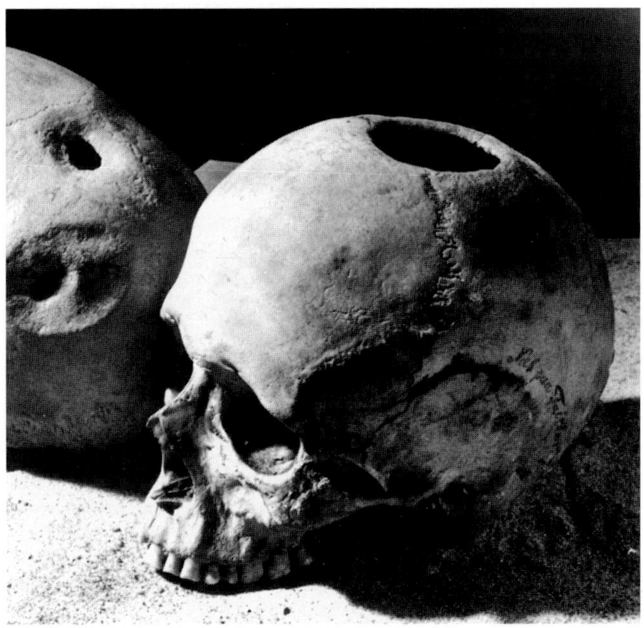

Fig. 1.2 Trephined neolithic skull with evidence of new bone formation, indicating the patient had survived the procedure. From Lyon A S, Petrucelli R J, *Medicine An Illustrated History*. MacMillan, Australia.

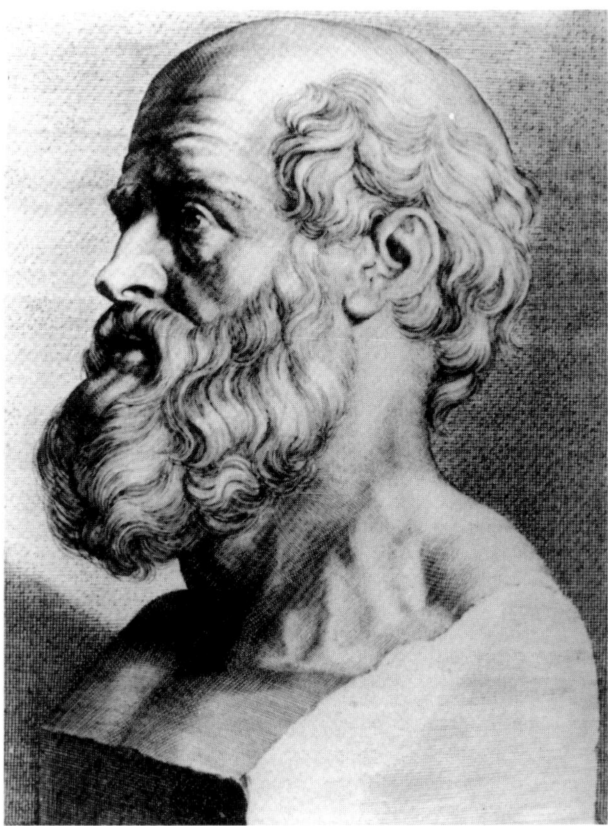

Fig. 1.3 Hippocrates, who described trephination. From *Illustrated History of Surgery*. K. Haeger, Harold Starke.

Hippocrates described trephination in detail, and advised it for headaches, epilepsy, fractures and blindness (Fig. 1.3). The famous 2nd century Chinese neurosurgeon Hua To performed trephination (Fig. 1.4). Hua To's most notorious patient was the warlord Kuan Yun, whose bitter enemy Tsao Tsao consulted Hua To with a headache. Hua To decided to trephine, but the patient thought that Hua To had been bribed by Kuan Yun to murder him. On this suspicion Hua To was summarily executed.

The foundation of modern neurology, which underpins neurosurgical practice, and especially brain tumor surgery, rests on the accomplishments of three men — Galen, Vesalius and Willis. Galen (130–200 AD) was born in Pergamon on the shores of Asia Minor. It was in Pergamon that parchment was first used as a writing material and it was also famous for its medical temple of Asklepios. Often described as the first 'experimental physiologist' Galen became the personal physician to Marcus Aurelius. Many believe that Galen's neurology was the best feature of his medical system. His major works of neurologic interest include *De usu partium*, *De anatomicis administrationibus*, *De locis affectis* and *De facultatibus naturabilus*. Galen described the corpus callosum, ventricles, sympathetic nerves, pituitary, infundibulum and seven pairs of cranial nerves. His anatomy was based on dissection of animals, as at that time autopsy was forbidden. Galen's views dominated European medicine for 1500 years, and although it is a longstanding conventional belief that Galen shackled medical thought, he is unjustly blamed for the blind dependence on his writings, which were sanctified so that any adverse opinion was regarded as heresy.

Andreas Vesalius (1514–1564) (Fig. 1.5), known as the 'founder of anatomy', was appointed to the Chair of Surgery and Anatomy in Padua. His famous *De Fabrica* (*De Humani Coporis fabrica libri septem*) was published in Basle in 1543, when he was only 28. The books are superbly illustrated by Jan Stephan Van Calcar, a favorite disciple of Titian. Book 7, on the brain, surpassed anything previously published and lays the foundations for much of modern neuroanatomy. Vesalius was Harvey Cushing's 'Patron Saint', and Cushing suffered his fatal anginal attack after lifting a heavy Vesalius portfolio.

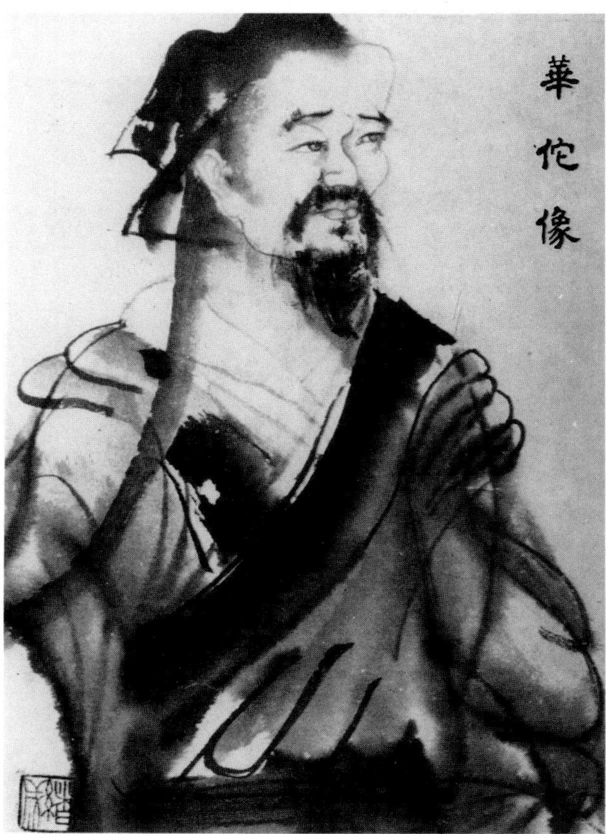

Fig. 1.4 Hua To, the 2nd century Chinese surgeon who practised trephination.

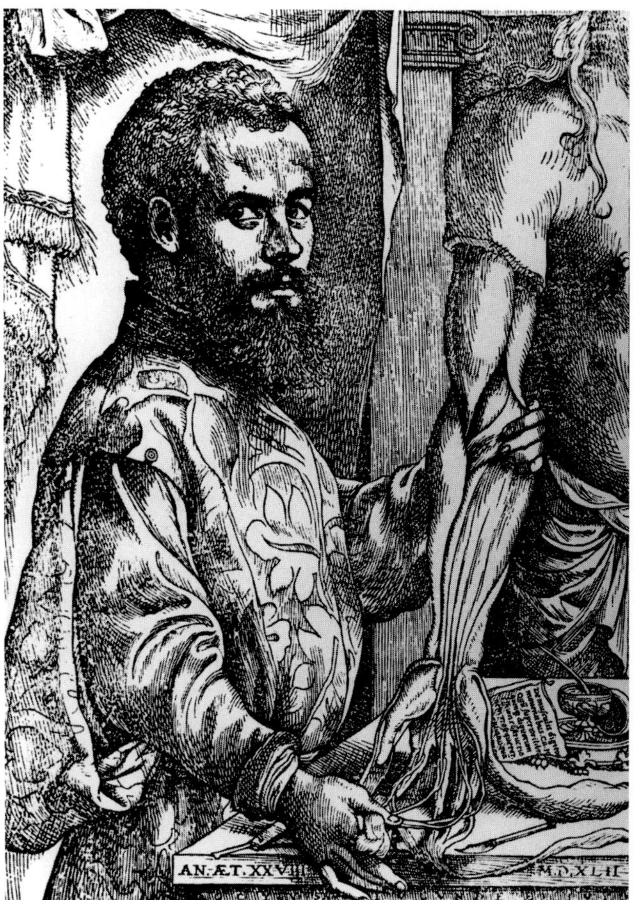

Fig. 1.5 Andreas Vesalius, the 'patron saint' of Harvey Cushing. From Lyon A S, Petrucelli R J, *Medicine An Illustrated History*. Macmillan, Australia.

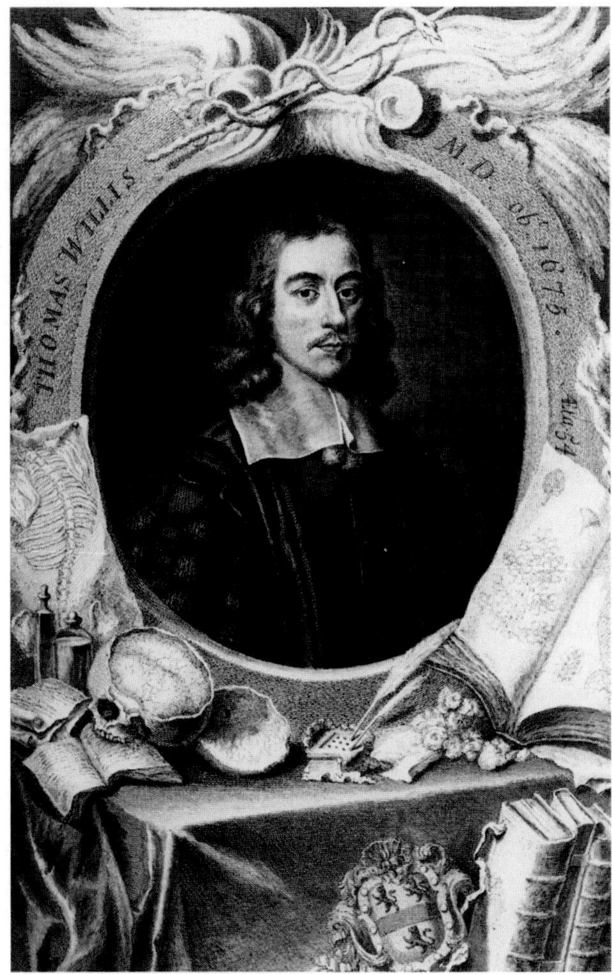

Fig. 1.6 Thomas Willis, a portrait by Vertue, 1742, based on an engraving made in 1666. From Thomas Willis, *Anatomy of the Brain and Nerves*. Classics of Neurology & Neurosurgery, Gryphon Editions.

Thomas Willis (1621–1675) (Fig. 1.6) was the first 'inventor of the nervous system' and coined the word 'neurologie'. He is often described as the 'Harvey of the nervous system'. He was born in the village of Great Bedwyn, Wiltshire, and studied medicine at Oxford, graduating in 1646. He obtained the Chair in Natural Philosophy in Oxford, and his *Cerebri Anatomi* was published in 1664. His contributions to the knowledge of the anatomy of the brain are well established. He suggested such terms as hemisphere, lobe, pyramid, corpus striatum and peduncle; however, many believe that Willis' main contribution was that he realized that neurologic function depended primarily on the brain itself, its stuff and substance and not the hollows within it.

The concept of cerebral localization, which forms the basis of brain tumor surgery, was still in dispute up until the middle of the 19th century. Although these great men and others raised the possibility of some form of cerebral localization, the concept was still doubted by authorities no less brilliant than Brown-Sequard.

Broca's description of two patients with pure motor aphasia, in whom he had defined the pathologic findings, was confirmed by the experimental studies in animals by Fritsch and Hitzig in 1870 in Germany and by Ferrier in 1873 in London. The experimental results were reproduced in a human by Bartholow of Cincinnati in 1874. The opportunity for this remarkable experiment was afforded by a patient whose parietal bones had been destroyed by osteomyelitis caused by an ill-fitting wig that had eroded the skin and bone. Bartholow stimulated the Rolandic areas of the brain by puncturing the dura with an electrode, inducing contralateral, local and spreading contractions and even convulsions.

Suppuration, putrefaction and infection had haunted surgeons up to and during the 19th century and prohibited any realistic possibility of intracranial and especially intradural surgery for brain tumors. Following Pasteur's and Koch's proof of the bacterial origin of putrefaction and a demonstration by Semmelweiss that sepsis could be controlled by hygienic means, hospitals gradually rid themselves of the insanitary practices which fomented infection. Lister (Fig. 1.7), however, deserves the credit for developing the technique to prevent bacterial contamination of wounds during surgical procedures. He introduced carbolic acid 'initially in the form of creosote' on wounds and first reported on the treatment in the Lancet in 1867. This is regarded as the birthdate of

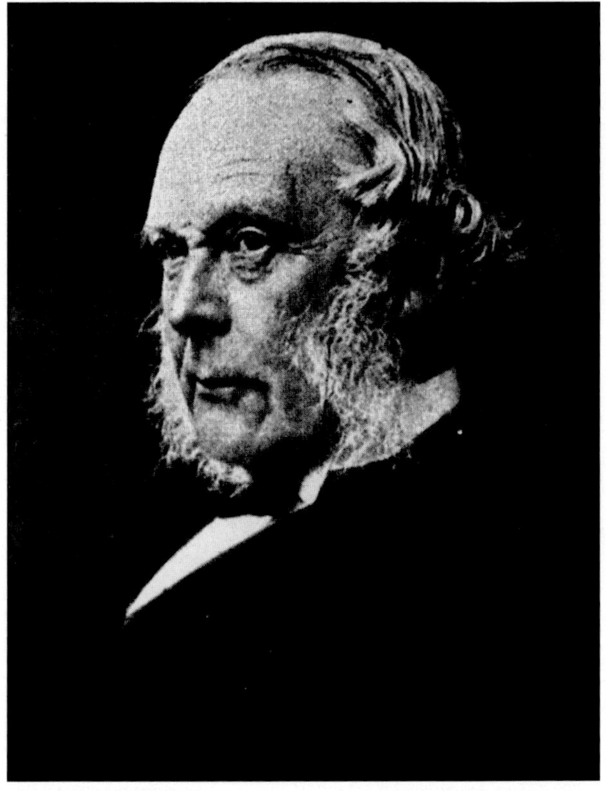

Fig. 1.7 Lord Joseph Lister, who introduced antiseptic techniques in 1867.

antisepsis; intracranial surgery could henceforth be undertaken without the previous high likelihood of infection.

The introduction of anesthesia was a potent influence on surgery in general and neurosurgery in particular. William Morton demonstrated the use of ether on October 16, 1846, which is still celebrated as 'ether day' in the original operating room at the Massachusetts General Hospital in Boston. With the patient asleep it became possible to perform long delicate operations, such as neurosurgical procedures.

An understanding of the pathology of brain tumors was essential before intracranial surgery for these tumors could advance. A new period of rapid advance in knowledge is often consequent upon the discovery of a novel approach or development of a new instrument. The grinding of improved lenses by Amici in 1827 led directly to the development of a well-corrected compound microscope that made possible the recognition of the cell as a basic unit of living matter. Shortly after, Schleidan and Schwann developed the cell theory, and Virchow enunciated the concept that the fundamental changes in human disease can be traced to alterations in cells. Virchow, known during his time as the 'Pope of medicine', was the first to describe the neuroglia and to classify brain tumors, with 'gliomas' as a separate entity (Fig. 1.8).

By the end of the 19th century the development of neurology, neurologic localization of cerebral tumors, anesthesia, antisepsis, and a basic understanding of the histology of brain tumors had laid the groundwork for the earlier operations for cerebral tumors. By 1900, however, the initial enthusiasm over the pioneering operations had waned and at the turn of the century cerebral tumors were only operated on as a last resort. Until the 1920s there was little knowledge of the varied histologic appearance of the gliomas and their correlated clinical course. In an attempt to improve the surgical treatment of brain tumors, and to determine if treatment should vary with the type of tumor, Bailey and Cushing studied the histologic appearance of gliomas and classified them on a histogenetic basis. It was Harvey Cushing (Figs 1.9, 1.10) who introduced the methodical (although at times slow) meticulous technique of Halsted to neurosurgical operations. Macewen, in 1879, was the first to successfully remove an intracranial neoplasm, a meningioma invading the frontal bone, and the first successfully treated meningioma in the United States was removed by W W Keen in December 1887. It was Cushing who coined the term 'meningioma', in 1922, describing the tumor identified by Virchow in 1854 as 'fungus of the dura mater', which he had called a sarcoma.

The improvement in the treatment of patients with brain tumors since the operation by Godlee in November 1884 has been related to the advances in surgical techniques, the introduction of adjuvant therapies, the revolution in imaging brain tumors, and an improved understanding of the biology of these tumors. More recently brain tumor research has concentrated on understanding the pathogenesis of the tumors, investigating the multiple facets of biology of the tumors and studying new treatment methods. Investigations using molecular bio-

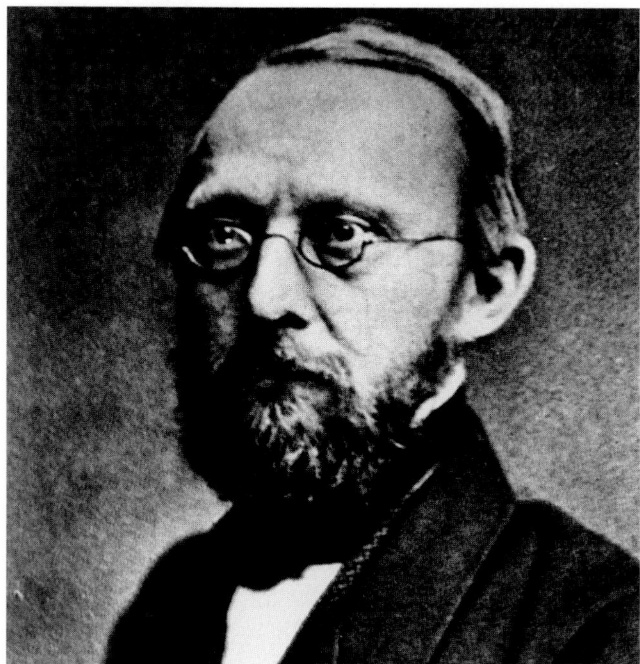

Fig. 1.8 Rudolph Virchow. World Health Organization, Geneva.

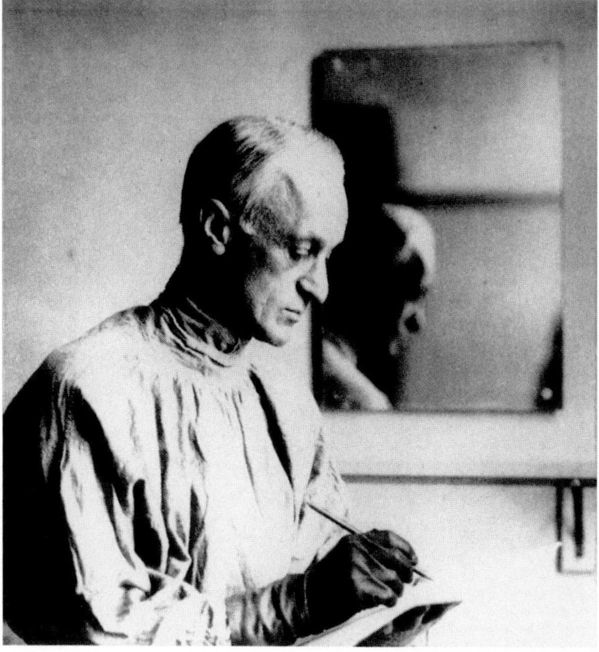

Fig. 1.9 Harvey Cushing. From *A Bibliography of the Writings of Harvey Cushing*. American Association of Neurological Surgeons, Park Ridge, Illinois.

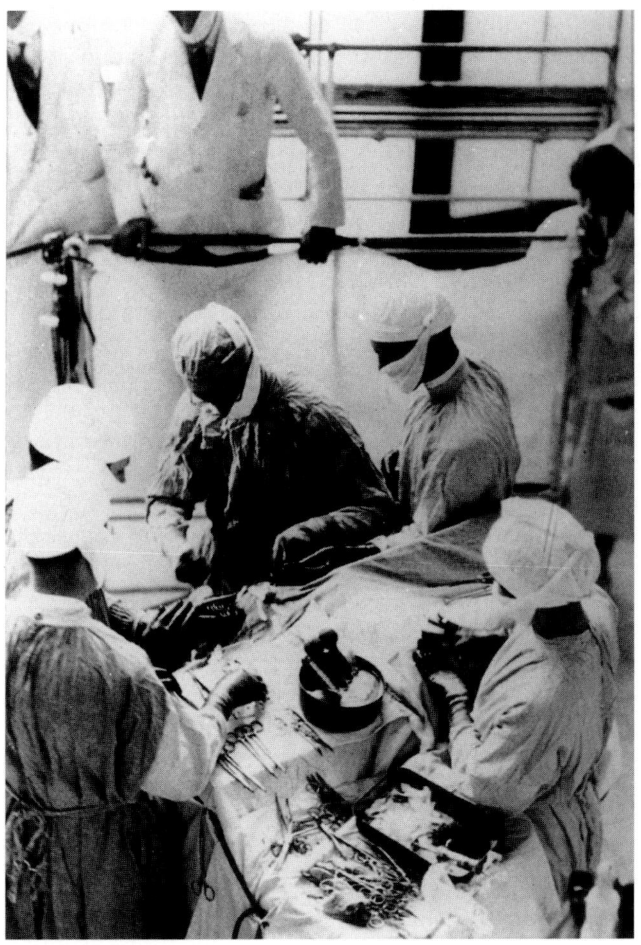

Fig. 1.10 Cushing's 2000th brain tumor operation. From *A Bibliography of the Writings of Harvey Cushing.* American Association of Neurological Surgeons. Park Ridge, Illinois.

logy and cell biology techniques have focused on the intricate and complex orchestra of activities in the normal cells and what disturbances are necessary to produce the cascade of events that results in the development of a tumor cell.

Advances in surgical techniques now usually allow a safe and atraumatic excision of a brain tumor. Standard neurosurgical equipment includes ultrasonic aspiration devices and lasers of a wide range of wavelengths which enable their ablative properties to be tailored to the particular tumor type. Stereotactic equipment has enabled a safer and more accurate exposure of deep intracranial tumors, and when combined with the laser allows a precise excision of deep cerebral tumors in eloquent and dangerous positions. By 1920 radiation therapy was being used for the treatment of cerebral gliomas. This first adjuvant therapy is still the mainstay of treatment for cerebral glioma, the most common type of brain tumor. During this present century many other adjuvant therapies such as chemotherapy, immunotherapy, hyperthermia and photodynamic therapy have been introduced with varying degrees of success. Although in some circumstances the therapy may help control the tumor for a while, none has been shown to be curative. There is now cause for cautious optimism with a better understanding of the pathogenesis and biology of brain tumors, improvements in imaging and surgical techniques, and especially the development of gene therapies.

2. The developing brain and cellular targets for neoplastic transformation

Scott R. VandenBerg

INTRODUCTION

The study of cellular ontogeny within the central nervous system (CNS) provides an important perspective for the study of brain tumors. Such a developmental viewpoint fosters more precise concepts with respect to the cellular lineages that may develop into tumors. In the immature CNS, the focus is on the identification of the diverse progenitor cell populations and the genotypic mechanisms that progressively restrict phenotypic repertoires, i.e. the determination of cell lineages. In the mature nervous system, residual progenitor cells are characterized in terms of proliferative potential and phenotypic plasticity. Closely related to consideration of phenotypic differentiation in the mature CNS is the development of better insights into the physiologically diverse spectrum of distinct macroglial cell populations. Understanding the timing and mechanisms for the creation of cell lineages and the selective differentiation into diverse cell types would permit more precise identification of distinct glial and neuronal cell targets for neoplastic transformation. The current histopathologic strategy for the classification of brain tumors does not consider this important functional diversity. An improvement in the delineation of this diversity should also permit more selective therapeutic approaches aimed at specific physiologic processes.

The second important concept regarding brain tumors, from an ontologic perspective, relates to the complex interplay of the intrinsic genetic regulation and environmental cues that occur during normal and neoplastic development. Particularly significant to tumor cell biology are the extrinsic soluble and matrix-bound signals that affect proliferative activity, differentiation, motility, and cell adhesion during development. Insights into how these are orchestrated in specific cell lineages during development may provide valuable insights for predicting the clinical behavior of tumors and defining additional targets for therapeutic intervention. Despite the potential importance of these insights, one significant caveat must be emphatically stated. The biologic properties of transformed cells and their tumor environments are clearly distinctive from those properties of any normal cellular counterparts within the developing or mature CNS.

The disruption of several key elements of normal CNS development accounts for the differences between normal and neoplastic neurocytogenesis. First, there is an alteration of intrinsic cellular processes that modulate cell proliferation, differentiation and cell death. Second, there is a disruption of the normal, precisely regulated microenvironment that provides important regulatory cues. Third, the association of these perturbed processes generates novel combinations of signals that may have profound effects on biologic activity. Region-specific extrinsic effects in the normal CNS on the expression of either glial or neuronal phenotypes from undifferentiated progenitor cells emphasize the importance of these interactions (Renfranz et al 1991). Thus, a greater potential exists for either heteroplastic phenotypes, such as myofibers in medullobastomas (see Rao et al 1990 for review), or incomplete phenotypic differentiation which is frequent in the neoplastic state. Failure to recognize the fundamental differences between normal ontogeny and neoplastic development can thus easily foster erroneous ideas regarding neoplastic differentiation. Likewise, caution must be recommended in associating certain biochemical factors that appear to be cell lineage-specific during normal development with specific neoplastic cell types. Some features may be more indicative of a particular physiologic state than a specific cellular lineage.

CELLULAR TARGETS OF TRANSFORMATION IN THE IMMATURE BRAIN

Over the past twenty years, studies of experimental tumor induction after exposure in utero to various alkylating agents (Swenberg 1977, Kleihues & Rajewsky 1984, Rajewsky 1985) or after perinatal inoculation of oncogenic viruses (Mukai & Kobayashi 1973) have clearly established fetal cells of various neuroblastic and glial cell lineages as targets for neoplastic transformation. The selective susceptibility of these fetal brain cell targets fostered the idea that neoplastic transformation occurred within the brain during a 'window of vulnerability' for a given cell type (Rubinstein 1985). Inherent in this concept were two ideas. First, the transforming event was most likely to occur during the developmental interval of maximum cell proliferation. Second, actively cycling cells that were already committed to specific lineages could produce tumors with distinct histopathologic and biologic parameters. However, besides proliferative capacity, cells in the developing and reactive brain may have specific genotypic and/or phenotypic states that may confer a greater potential for tumorigenesis. This may be reflected by either a greater vulnerability for neoplastic transformation or a greater biologic advantage after transformation (VandenBerg et al 1987). A recent study using a retrovirus-mediated transfer of the large T antigen of the SV-40 virus into neural transplants provided evidence for such a developmental stage-specific vulnerability for neoplastic transformation of progenitor cell lineages (Eibl et al 1994). Therefore, a better understanding of both the timing and the molecular events associated with the development of 'committed' cell lineages would provide more insight about specific fetal cells as targets for neoplastic transformation and the regulation of their biologic potential(s) after transformation.

During early CNS development, there is a progressive axial restriction of the neural plate and developing neuroepithelium such that distinct topographic fields give rise to the neuroretina, forebrain, midbrain and hindbrain (see Jacobson 1978 for review). The molecular genetic events which determine this axial map are associated with the expression of homeobox-related genes which encode transcription factors for region-specific regulation of gene promoters (Toth et al 1987, Boncinelli et al 1988, Wright et al 1989). As development proceeds, different classes of cells arise within these fields during well-defined time frames and ultimately form specific cell populations with precise cytoarchitectural and functional characteristics. Progenitor cell populations with differing developmental potentials are clearly present within the primitive germinal zones of the CNS (Temple 1990). However, the processes of cellular commitment or determination, i.e. the acquisition of a stable genotypic restriction of cellular phenotype, appear to vary among the different CNS regions (McKay 1989, Anderson 1992). The variation occurs in both the diversity of separate cell lineages which originate from common progenitors and in the cellular intrinsic and extrinsic microenvironments that modulate this diversity. Therefore, tumors which arise within the immature nervous system may be conceptually divided into stem cell or progenitor cell tumors and tumors with more restricted genotypic/phenotypic cell types. The importance of this difference with respect to neuro-oncology would be the markedly different biologic potentials, i.e. how cellular differentiation and the resultant biologic capacities for matrix invasion and proliferation would be regulated.

REGULATION OF NEUROEPITHELIAL DIFFERENTIATION AND NEUROCYTOGENESIS

A multitude of regulatory processes play a role in the early determination of specific neuroepithelial genotypes and the subsequent regulation of phenotypic diversity. Genotypic control resulting in the stable commitment of cellular lineages would putatively need to occur at multiple, often independent, levels, ranging from direct chemical modification of the DNA to more interactive transcriptional controls by cis- and/or trans-activating mechanisms. A comprehensive review of all the processes which could be operative during neurocytogenesis would be beyond the scope of this discussion. However, several putative modes of genotypic regulation for neurocytogenesis merit highlighting.

The first level of potential genetic control would be the higher order of chromatin structural organization with the formation of nucleosomes. This organization is conferred by the association of the DNA with histone core proteins and undoubtedly would cause significant differences in transcriptional activity (see Lemke 1992 for review). However, little is known about the tertiary histone-DNA structures in the dynamic control of tissue or cell specific genotypes, especially in the central nervous system. Direct chemical modification of DNA would be another level of structural regulation that may be operational during the early phases of stable cellular determination. The most well-characterized type of modification is methylation at the 5′-position of the cytosine residues which are contained within CpG-rich regions ('islands') at the 5′ ends of many genes. In addition, this form of DNA modification may, under certain physiologic conditions, predispose the modified cytosines to point mutations. There are several features of DNA methylation which would be fundamental to a putative role in developmental genetic programming: a pattern of methylation can be stably and faithfully maintained in specific cell types; tissue-specific genes are fully methylated in cells that are not actively expressing them; demethylation of particular genes during development is accompanied by active expression; and experimental demethylation is accompanied by differentiation of specific cell types (see Razin & Cedar 1991 for review). However, the importance of DNA methylation is probably associated with the maintenance of static inactivation of genes rather than for regulating gene transcription as a dynamically active process in differentiated cells. An interesting possibility is that tissue-specific gene methylation may confer another level of selectivity as to what factors may interact with an inactive gene to initiate transcription, as opposed to those factors which could mediate expression of an 'activated' demethylated gene (Cedar & Razin 1990). In this context, the relationship between demethylation and the expression of a cell lineage-related transcription factor (MyoD1) (Chen & Jones 1989) is particularly intriguing.

A variety of transcription factors (see Lemke 1992 for review) appear to play more significant regulatory roles than gene methylation in the determination of region- (segmental), tissue-, and lineage-specific cell populations. From the perspective of neural development, the family of homeobox proteins (Wright et al 1989, Lemke et al 1991, Treacy & Rosenfeld 1992), as region-specific transcription factors, and helix-loop-helix (HLH) proteins (Chen & Jones 1989, Galiana et al 1992, 1993) as cell type specific transcription factors, play the most significant roles. Expression of POU domain proteins (POU-specific/POU-homeodomain factors) (Lemke et al 1991, Treacy & Rosenfeld 1992) is especially important during glial differentiation and may be significantly modulated by signal transduction pathways associated with growth factors (Collarini et al 1991). In addition, in a bipotent glial progenitor cell line that was immortalized with the adenovirus E1A gene, growth arrest was accompanied by the expression of novel gene (NPDC-1) for a helix-loop-helix domain protein (Galiana et al 1992). A better understanding of the specific molecular mechanisms by which these transcription factors orchestrate the complex interplay between proliferative activity and the expression of cell lineage specific proteins during differentiation of glial lineages will, undoubtedly, provide an important key to controlling terminal neoplastic differentiation.

Growth factors may regulate the biologic activity of immature neural cells in several different ways. First, the growth factor(s) may stimulate proliferation and induce an overall state of cellular 'activation'. Second, they may regulate the induction of genotypic commitment to specific cell lineages. Third, the factor(s) may maintain cell survival and inhibit the onset of programmed cell death. Within the developing CNS, all three types of actions may occur in various combinations (Noble et al 1992, Raff et al 1993, Rudge 1993). One of the most well-characterized in vitro models of glial progenitor cell differentiation is the explanted O-2A stem cell from the immature rat optic nerve (Barres et al 1992, Noble et al 1992, Wolswijk & Noble 1992). Studies with these progenitor cells have illustrated several salient points about the interactions of primitive and differentiating cell lineages with growth factors. A given growth factor stimulates cellular 'activation' with proliferative activity and increased mobility. Cellular mechanisms can limit this stimulatory effect with a loss of responsiveness and the onset of cell differentiation. Daughter progenitor cells following growth factor-stimulated proliferation may have different responses to growth factors while retaining a progenitor state, and multiple extracellular signals may be necessary for long-term survival of certain differentiated lineages (Barres et al 1993). Combination of growth factors may yield cellular responses that none alone may evoke (McKinnon et al 1993) and cellular responses to growth factors in culture are not equivalent to biologic behavior in vivo (Fulton et al 1991, de los Monteros et al 1993). Additional levels of biologic complexity modulate growth factor activities, including interactions with soluble or matrix binding molecules (Gonias 1992, Lee et al 1992, Webb et al 1992, Calissano et al 1993, Clemmons et al 1993) and secretion in inactive forms that must first interact with proteases for biologic activity (Webb et al 1992). During CNS development and following neoplastic transformation, all these processes are operative and play important roles in mediating both the paracrine and autocrine effects of growth factors and cytokines.

RETINAL DEVELOPMENT AND THE RETINOBLASTOMA

The retinoblastoma, the most common of the pediatric intraocular tumors, is the only multipotential stem cell tumor of the CNS for which the genetic basis of neoplastic transformation is well known. The transforming event occurs within the immature retina when both alleles of the rb tumor suppressor gene are inactivated within a single cell (Gallie et al 1990, Gennett & Cavenee 1990). Although the tumor commonly exhibits fields of poorly differentiated small cells with scant, ill-defined cytoplasm, the majority of tumors contain the more typical rosettes associated with either primitive neuroblastic or neurosensory differentiation (Fig. 2.1). Less common are the more

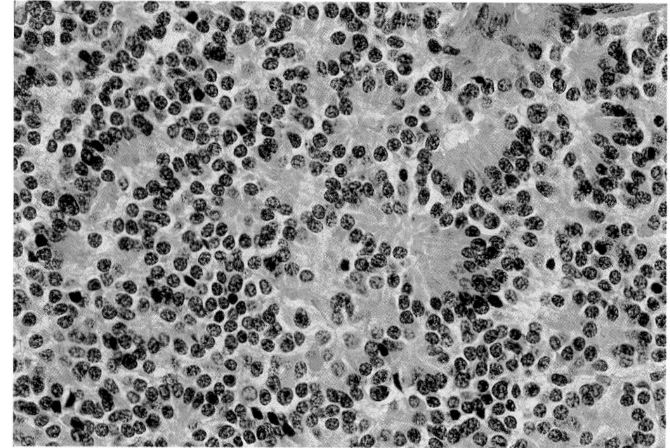

Fig. 2.1 Retinoblastoma. The histopathologic appearance of these tumors is often a combination of patternless sheets of primitive cells admixed with the typical rosettes which are illustrated in this microscopic field. Although the formation of these structures implies an early stage of cellular differentiation, the expression of either photosensory phenotypes or neuronal intermediate filaments is not specifically localized to these structures. H&E.

highly differentiated 'fleurettes', which manifest photosensory phenotypic differentiation. Although the presence of these structures with more cytoarchitectural differentiation generally does not have any predictive value for the clinical behavior of these tumors, rare tumors that are entirely composed of rosettes and have an overall reduced cellularity appear to have a reduced malignant potential. These neoplasms have been designated as 'retinocytomas' (Margo et al 1983) to distinguish their different clinical behavior.

The retinoblastoma, as a tumor arising after transformation of an immature progenitor cell in the inner retinal neuroepithelium, clearly gives rise to phenotypes that are associated with the selective regional determination of retinal cell lineages (Gonzalez-Fernandez et al 1992). The normal development of the retina involves multiple topographic considerations. One of the earliest events is the formation of the inner, primitive neuroretinal epithelium and an outer, pigmented epithelium. These two progenitor fields arise when the primitive, germinal neuroepithelium of the forebrain forms the inner and outer layers of the optic cup. This appears to be accompanied by the differential expression of a paired box- and homeobox-containing gene in the neuroretinal epithelium (Martin et al 1992). The prospective neuroretina appears to exert inductive control over the development of the pigmented cells in the outer layer (Buse et al 1993). Although in vitro culture studies have demonstrated various degrees of plasticity in the formation of both non-neoplastic (Buse & de Groot 1991, Buse et al 1993) and neoplastic (see Gonzalez-Fernandez et al 1992 for review) neuroretinal and pigmented epithelial derivatives, examination of retinoblastomas in situ strongly suggests that these tumors arise from a loss of normal rb function in a primitive neuroretinal cell rather than from a generally pluripotential neuroepithelial cell. An immature neuroretinal cell, as the putative target for neoplastic transformation, would normally maintain the potential for selective divergent differentiation (Fig. 2.2) (Turner & Cepko 1987, Holt et al 1988, Wetts & Fraser 1988). Although there is relatively minimal horizontal dispersion of the radially arrayed progenitor cells in primitive neuroretina (Price 1989), there is no divergence of progenitor cells to produce distinct glial and neuronal/neurosensory clones. In contrast to other germinal matrix zones in the forebrain, a diverse array of phenotypes (photoreceptor, neurons, and Müller cells) are generated from retinal progenitor cells following the final mitotic cycle (Turner & Cepko 1987, Holt et al 1988, Wetts & Fraser 1988).

The expression of photoreceptor (Figs 2.3–2.5) and Müller cell (retinal glia) (Figs 2.6 and 2.7) associated proteins in retinoblastomas clearly demonstrates the unique regional derivation of these tumors (Turner & Cepko 1987, Holt et al 1988, Wetts & Fraser 1988, Price 1989, Gonzalez-Fernandez et al 1992) and is particularly valuable in the study of specific cell types in retinoblastomas. Interphotoreceptor retinoid binding protein (IRBP), cone and rod opsins have strictly defined temporal patterns of expression during normal retinal differentiation. The expression of IRBP occurs very early during neuroretinal development and is normally upregulated before opsin (Gonzalez-Fernandez & Healy 1990, Liou et al 1991, Hauswirth et al 1992, Gonzalez-Fernandez et al 1993). In a series of 22 retinoblastomas (Gonzalez-Fernandez et al 1992), IRBP was detected in over half the tumors (Fig. 2.3) while nearly 70% of the tumors which contained immunoreactive cone (Fig. 2.4) or rod opsin (Fig. 2.5) also demonstrated IRBP. Overall, rod opsin expression was far more restricted in the neoplastic cells than either IRBP or cone opsin. This differential expression of cone and rod

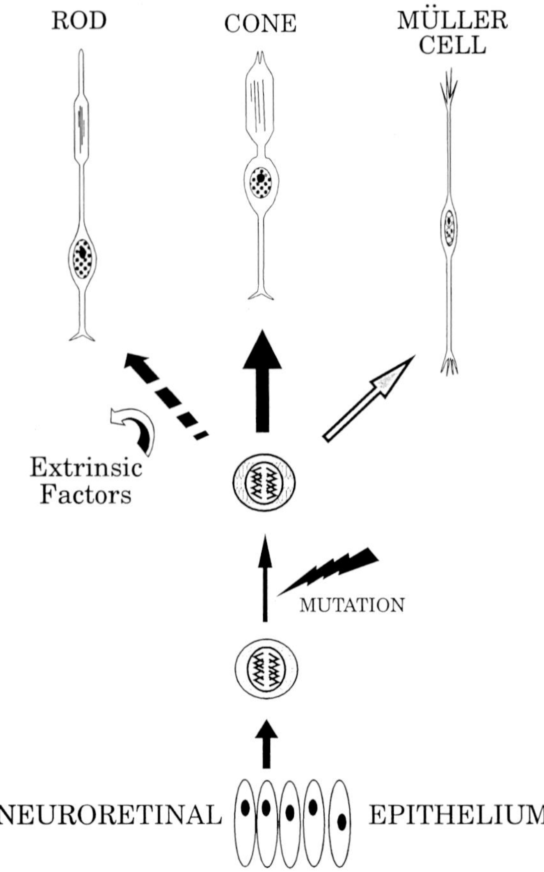

Fig. 2.2 Model of retinoblastoma cytogenesis. Divergent phenotypic restriction normally occurs late (following the last mitotic cycle) in the neuroretinal progenitor cell population. The probable target cell in which the *rb* mutation occurs is a multipotential neuroretinal cell which has not entered its final mitotic cycle. Therefore, both groups of intrinsic neuroretinal cells (neurosensory with IRBP/opsin expression and Müller glia with CRA1BP expression) can arise from the transformed progenitor cells. The cone phenotype would be the most probable neurosensory phenotype since it does not appear to be dependent on the extrinsic signals. Alternatively, rod phenotypic expression is dependent on the presence of normal extrinsic signals that would be frequently disrupted in the tumor environment. (Other neuronal phenotypes that would arise from the transformed progenitors are omitted from this scheme for clarity.)

neoplastic cellular phenotypes corresponds to the normal predominance of cone over rod phenotypes wherein cone differentiation appears to result from a 'default' mechanism (Adler & Hatlee 1989, Raymond 1991). This suggests that this regional property of lineage determination by positional extrinsic signals from the microenvironment, rather than by early autonomous commitment of specific cell lineages, persists even after neoplastic transformation (Fig. 2.2). In addition, the magnitude and diversity of microenvironmental effects also appear to be markedly affected by both the cellular position and the stage of differentiation (Reh & Kljavin 1989, Sparrow et al 1990, Watanbe & Raff 1990). Such differences also clearly emphasize the discrepancies and potential caveats arising

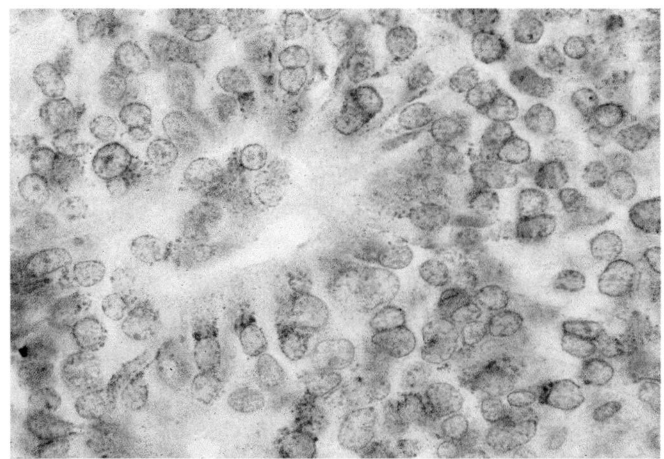

Fig. 2.3 Retinoblastoma. Interphotoreceptor retinoid binding protein (IRBP) is the earliest photoreceptor-associated protein demonstrated in retinoblastoma. Its cytoplasmic localization tends to be polarized in the cell. In rosettes and fleurettes, IRBP is particularly present in the apical cell border. IRBP (RB 504) avidin-biotin immunoperoxidase.

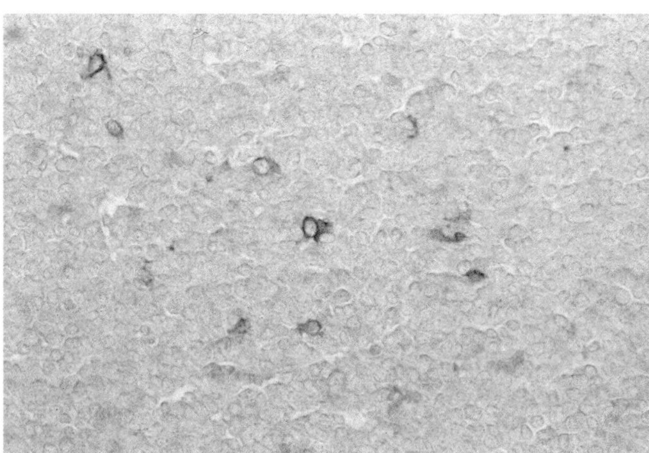

A

B

Fig. 2.4 Retinoblastoma. Cone opsin can be identified within the more amorphous cellular groups of the retinoblastomas **A**. However, the most specific localization of cone opsin is in cytoplasmic processes which protrude into the lumen of fleurettes **B**. Cone opsin (CERN 874) avidin-biotin immunoperoxidase.

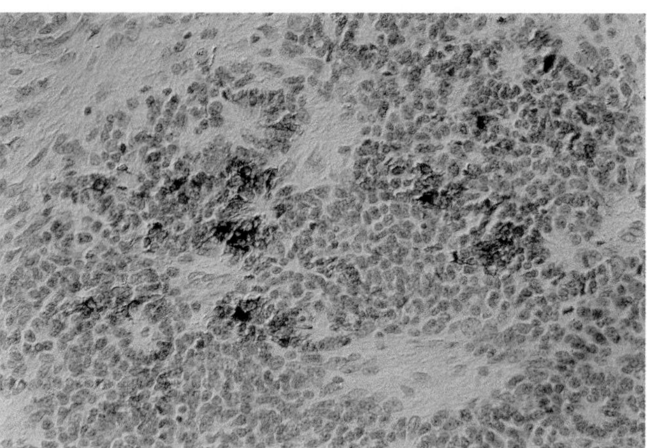

Fig. 2.5 Retinoblastoma. Rod opsin is less commonly present in retinoblastomas than cone opsin (see also Fig. 2.2). Rod opsin is localized in both the cells that form rosettes and in cells within the more amorphous areas of the tumor. Rod opsin (CERN JS85) avidin-biotin immunoperoxidase.

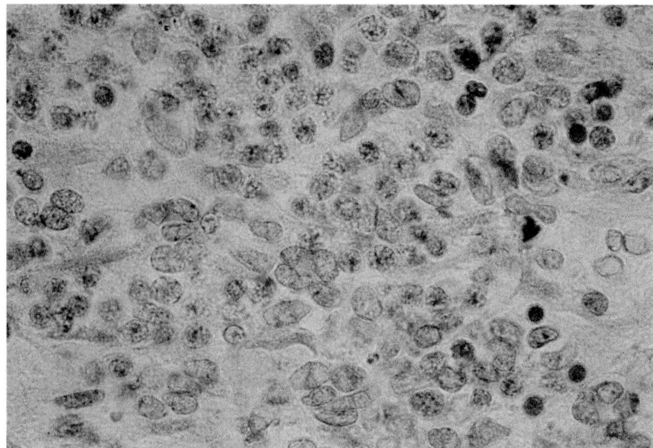

Fig. 2.6 Retinoblastoma. Intrinsic glial cell (Müller cell) differentiation within retinoblastomas is accompanied by the presence of cellular retinaldehyde binding protein (CRA1BP) in tumor cells. Unlike the photoreceptor-associated proteins (IRBP, cone and rod opsins), CRA1BP is never localized within neoplastic specialized photosensory structures. CRA1BP avidin-biotin immunoperoxidase.

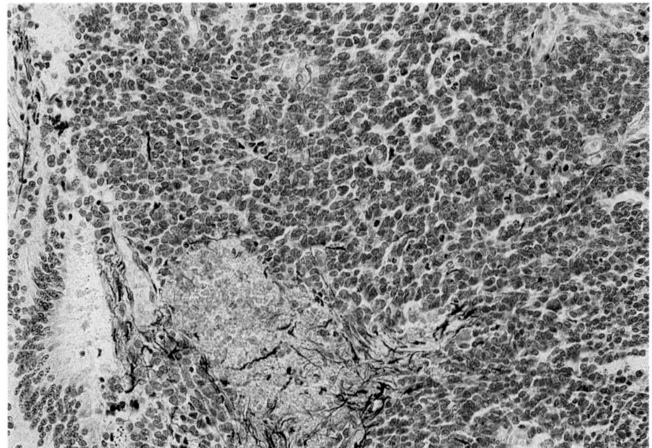

Fig. 2.7 Retinoblastoma. Astroglial cells within retinoblastomas are restricted to reactive stromal cells that are frequently located adjacent to blood vessels or in residual, entrapped retina. GFAP avidin-biotin immunoperoxidase.

from the data derived from in vivo and in vitro studies of cell differentiation in both neoplastic and non-neoplastic cell populations.

CEREBRAL HEMISPHERIC DEVELOPMENT AND NEOPLASTIC TRANSFORMATION

With respect to the forebrain region, identification of the potential targets for neoplastic transformation would require distinguishing the progenitor cell pools, the histogenetic potentials and the final dispersion of cell lineages that arise within the ventricular/periventricular germinal zone. Despite the relatively homogeneous cytoarchitecture of the primitive cells, region-specific and single-cell heterogeneity with respect to histogenetic potential appear to develop early (Temple 1990). This early establishment of specific developmental potentials has been well-documented by various experimental approaches in the avian and rodent brain (Hayes & McKay 1993, Yamada et al 1993). Although the dorsal forebrain does not have the same degree of segment-specific patterning as the hindbrain (Fishell et al 1993), there is still a relative restriction to the nonradial clonal dispersion of progenitor cell populations (Fishell et al 1993, Walsh & Cepko 1993). This regional specificity would potentially contribute to the generation of different subsets of neuronal and glial lineages (Butt 1991, Kettenmann et al 1991, Levison & Goldman 1993, Luskin et al 1993, Marriott & Wilkin 1993, Steindler 1993). As oncogenic targets, these may differ dramatically with respect to cell surface receptors and responsiveness to the microenvironment, secretion of growth factors and neuroregulators, modification of the extracellular matrix, motility, and proliferative potential.

Within the primitive neuroepithelial matrix, there would be, hypothetically, several types of clonal progenitors. The first type would be a pluripotential neural progenitor cell with the capacity to polarize and form epithelial structures. These cells could give rise to progeny along both neuronal and macroglial lines, including formation of ependyma. This progenitor population would necessarily exist for only a relatively short duration of CNS development and most likely would undergo asymmetric divisions, giving rise to proliferative, primitive lineages of ependymal, macroglial, and neuronal cells. A second putative type of progenitor would also be multipotential and produce both neuronal and macroglial lineages (Temple 1990, Cameron & Rakic 1991, Price et al 1991). The principal distinction between the first and second type of stem cell would be the loss, in the second type, of the capacity to form a polarized neuroepithelium and undergo ependymal differentiation. A third type of progenitor would be restricted to the formation of different neuronal or glial lineages (Cameron & Rakic 1991, Luskin et al 1993).

Experimental data for the hypothetical distinction between pluripotential neuroepithelial stem cells and multipotential neural progenitors were provided by in vivo studies of an experimental mouse teratocarcinoma (OTT-6050) from which two distinctive types of primitive, transplantable neural stem cell populations were derived (VandenBerg et al 1981a,b). In the first type, the neural stem cells produced a primitive neuroepithelium resembling ventricular germinal matrix from which the migrating cells displayed either neuronal or glial differentiation. Ependymal differentiation occurred in the more mature neoplastic neuroepithelium. In contrast, the second type of neural stem cell lost the ability to constitute a polarized neuroepithelium and formed only amorphous groups of cells without neuroepithelial structures. Although the developmental potential for either astrocytic or neuronal differentiation was retained, no ependymal differentiation occurred in vivo. With respect to the second and third types of progenitor cells in the forebrain, there is recent experimental evidence for both types in mammalian CNS, especially in the septal and hippocampal regions (Temple 1990, Renfranz et al 1990, Marvin & McKay 1992). One notable group of studies was based on the immortalization of rat embryonic day 16 hippocampal cells by the tsU19 double mutant allele of the SV-40 T antigen (Renfranz et al 1991, Hayes & McKay 1993). Clonal cultures of these immortalized cells retained a primitive neuronal phenotype until transplanted into a postnatal hippocampus wherein both granule cell differentiation and astroglial differentiation occurred. Experiments using these immortalized hippocampal progenitors have also clearly emphasized the importance of the extrinsic microenvironment for both inducing cellular differentiation and determining specific neuronal and glial subsets of cells. When these primitive cells were transplanted in the cerebellum, they developed into Bergmann-like astrocytes and internal granule cell neurons, instead of astrocytes and hippocampal granule cell neurons. However, the relative numbers of specific progenitor lineages that are committed to various cell types are unknown.

Characterization of the relatively homogeneous appearing progenitors of specific cell lineages and of the early stages of cellular differentiation within the ventricular/periventricular germinal zone and migrating cell populations of the forebrain has been somewhat problematic. Most studies have been limited primarily to the immunohistochemical detection of cytoskeletal proteins, including epitopes from several classes of intermediate filaments (IF) and tubulins (Lee et al 1990, Cameron & Rakic 1991), and a variety of cell membrane-associated epitopes, including G_{D3} ganglioside, galactocerebroside, chondroitin sulfate proteoglycan, and 'A2B5' (Eisenbarth et al 1979, Friedman et al 1989, Knott & Pikington 1990, Levine et al 1993). The intermediate filaments that are expressed in association with the multipotential and proliferative progenitor cells are principally restricted to class VI (nestin) (Hockfield & McKay 1985, Lendahl et al 1990) and III (vimentin) (see Cameron & Rakic 1991 for review) IFs. In the primitive neuroepithelial germinal matrix, nestin appears to be down-regulated earlier than vimentin (Tohyama et al 1992), which is still abundant in the ventricular neuroepithelial matrix at 26 weeks gestation (Figs 2.8, 2.9). In contrast, proliferative lineages with glial and neuronal genotypic restriction down-regulate these IFs and up-regulate the expression of class III β-tubulin (Fig. 2.10) and glial fibrillary acidic protein (GFAP), respectively (Fig. 2.11). Previous studies with the primitive and maturing neuroepithelial component of a spontane-

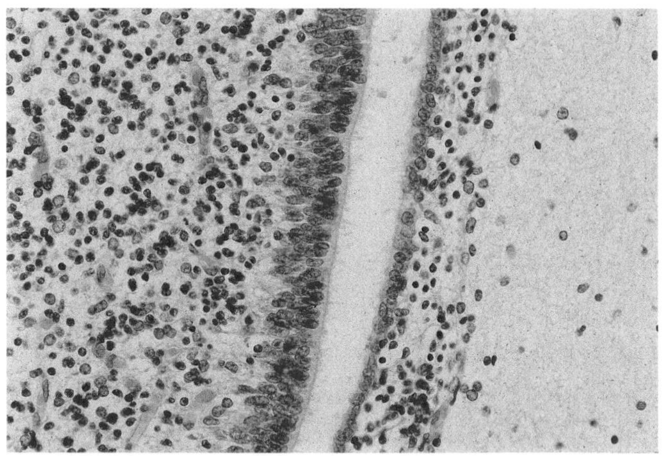

Fig. 2.8 Human 26-week fetal lateral ventricular matrix. The residual neuroepithelium of the germinal matrix in a 26-week fetus exhibits pseudostratified cells with a prominent subventricular zone constituted by immature neural cells. H&E

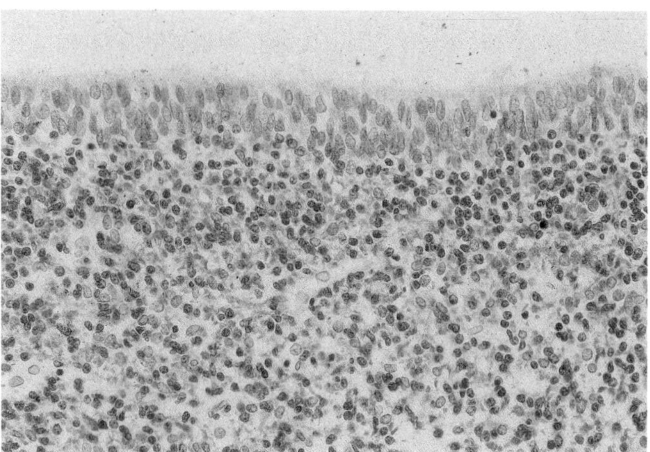

Fig. 2.10 Human 26-week fetal lateral ventricular matrix. Abundant immunoreactivity for class III β-tubulin is localized in primitive neuroblasts and neurites within the subventricular zone. Note that the pseudostratified cell layer is not immunoreactive for this neuron-associated protein. TUJ1 avidin-biotin immunoperoxidase.

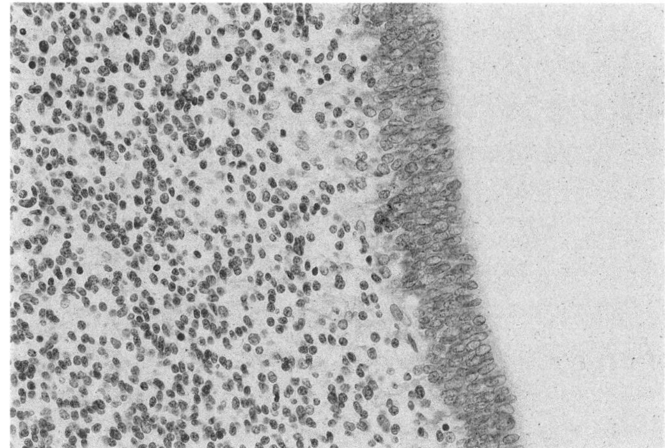

Fig. 2.9 Human 26-week fetal lateral ventricular matrix. The primitive pseudostratified cell layer is strongly immunoreactive for the intermediate filament protein vimentin. A similar pattern of immunoreactivity is present in the epithelial formations of medulloepitheliomas (see Fig. 2.13). Vimentin avidin-biotin immunoperoxidase.

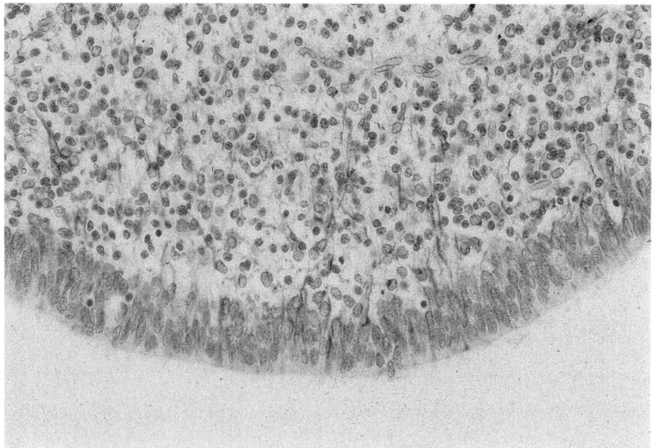

Fig. 2.11 Human 26-week fetal lateral ventricular matrix. GFAP immunohistochemistry highlights glial elements present within the pseudostratified neuroepithelium and thick processes of astrocytes within the subependymal zone. GFAP avidin-biotin immunoperoxidase.

ous murine ovarian teratoma (Caccamo et al 1989) have demonstrated that both vimentin and class III β-tubulin immunoreactive cells were associated with the primitive neuroepithelial matrix that would correspond to the ventricular/periventricular germinal zone during normal development. Although class III β-tubulin immunoreactive cells were occasionally within the primitive neuroepithelium, most immunoreactivity was localized within more unorganized cell populations which were adjacent to the neuroepithelial structures. In addition, neuroregulators with growth factor activity were also demonstrated within cells in the primitive neuroepithelial matrix (Shiurba et al 1991).

From a developmental perspective, the parenchymal tumors that arise within the human forebrain may be divided into three major groups. The first group would be those tumors which most commonly arise during the neonatal or early pediatric period and are composed primarily of primitive or poorly differentiated cells. The second category would be those neoplasms that also arise in the early pediatric stage and have a primitive cell population which, however, is not predominant. In contrast to the first group with predominantly primitive cells, these tumors often display distinctive cellular differentiation. The third group would be those tumors that most commonly arise in the late pediatric or early adult periods without a primitive cell component but with such a unique combination of clinicopathologic features as to suggest distinct oncogenic targets and/or progenitor cell populations within a maturing or mature brain.

The first group of tumors, predominantly composed of primitive cell populations, is relatively uncommon in the forebrain region. Within this group of tumors are neoplasms which putatively arise from transformation of pluripotential neuroepithelial progenitors as well as progenitors with more restricted potential for either neuronal or glial lineage formation (see Ch. 8). These include medulloepithelioma, cerebral neuroblastomas and ganglioneuroblastomas, and ependymoblastomas. While the medulloepithelioma commonly displays multipotential cellular lineages, the neuroblastomas, ganglioneuroblastomas and ependymoblastomas appear to be significantly more restricted to neuronal and ependymal lineages, respectively. In addition, tumors with extremely primitive phenotypes that may have variable evidence for neuronal and/or glial differentiation, analogous to the cerebellar medulloblastoma, have been described under the designation of PNET (Kleihues et al 1993). These tumors most probably manifest the biologic potential of the primitive neural progenitors of the forebrain that give rise to both glial and neuronal lineages. Therefore, forebrain neoplasms generally appear to manifest similar spectra of biologic potentials as the various types of progenitor cells and derivative lineages which arise in the developing brain.

With respect to the first hypothetical type of CNS progenitor, the medulloepithelioma, intriguingly, appears to display a somewhat analogous histogenetic potential to the pluripotential neuroepithelial stem cell. This very rare tumor occurs early in the pediatric period, usually within the cerebral hemispheres (see Ch. 8 for review). The hallmark histopathologic feature of these neoplasms is the mitotically active, pseudostratified columnar epithelium, often arranged in ribbons of tubules or papillary rosettes with variable interposition of delicate stromal elements and more amorphous groups of primitive cells. The epithelial structures recall the primitive neuroepithelium of the ventricular germinal matrix (Fig. 2.12). Analogous to this normal developing neuroepithelium, many cells are vimentin immunoreactive (Fig. 2.13). Neuroblastic/neuronal (Fig. 2.14), astroglial (Fig. 2.15) and/or ependymal cell populations are either intimately admixed with the tubules or present in more well-demarcated fields in about

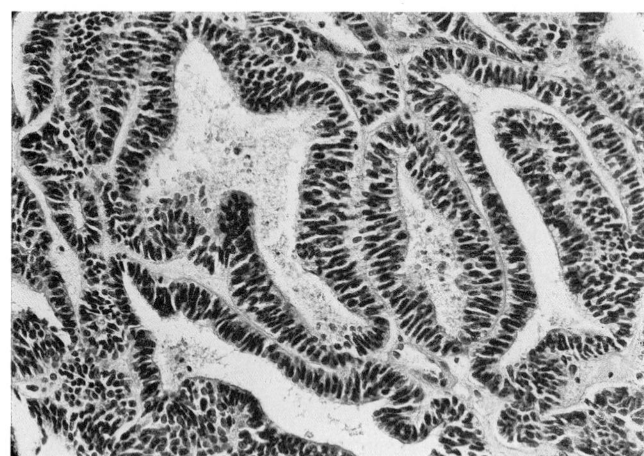

Fig. 2.12 Medulloepithelioma. Medulloepithelioma recalls the structure of the primitive neuroepithelium due to the tubular and ribbon-like formations lined by mitotically active, pseudostratified cells. Other areas of the tumors typically display more amorphous collections of differentiating primitive neural cells. H&E.

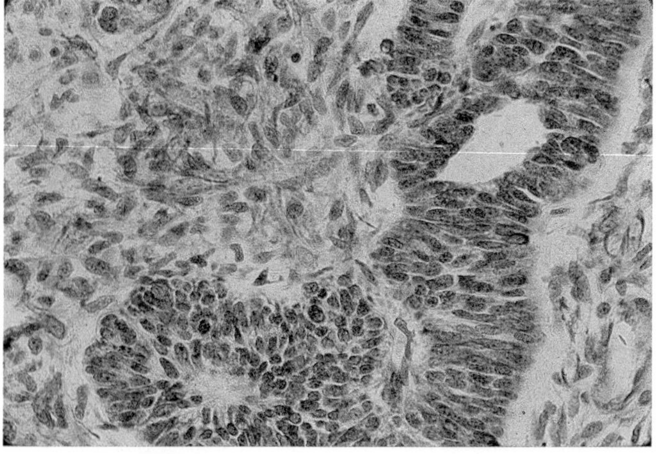

Fig. 2.13 Medulloepithelioma. The great majority of tumor cells composing the neuroepithelium and the adjacent regions demonstrate strong immunoreactivity for vimentin. Vimentin avidin-biotin immunoperoxidase.

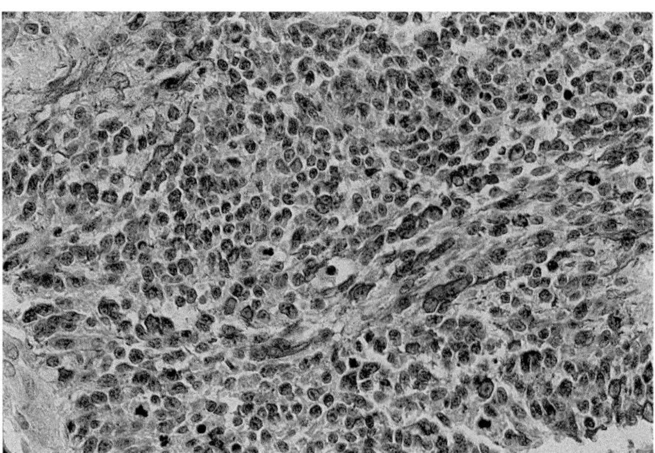

Fig. 2.14 Medulloepithelioma. Immunoreactivity for neuron-associated class III β-tubulin demonstrates neuroblastic differentiation of the primitive tumor cells that are intermixed within the amorphous zones separating the neuroepithelial arrangements. In contrast, this neuronal epitope is rarely present in the neuroepithelial structures. TUJ1 avidin-biotin immunoperoxidase.

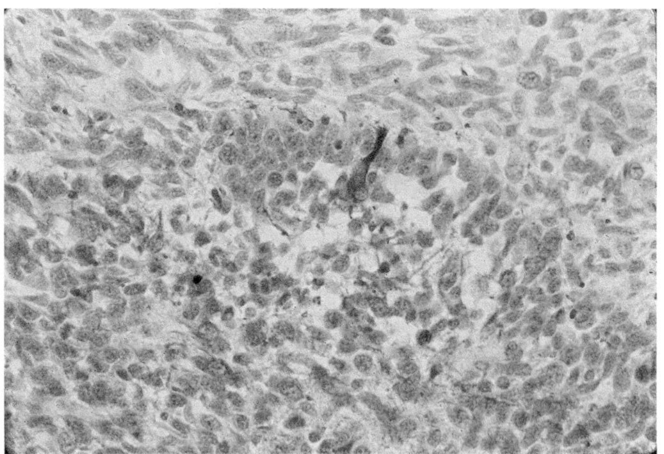

Fig. 2.15 Medulloepithelioma. Glial differentiation is recognized in primitive neural cells of the solid areas of medulloepitheliomas. The tubular structures do not display GFAP immunoreactivity. GFAP avidin-biotin immunoperoxidase.

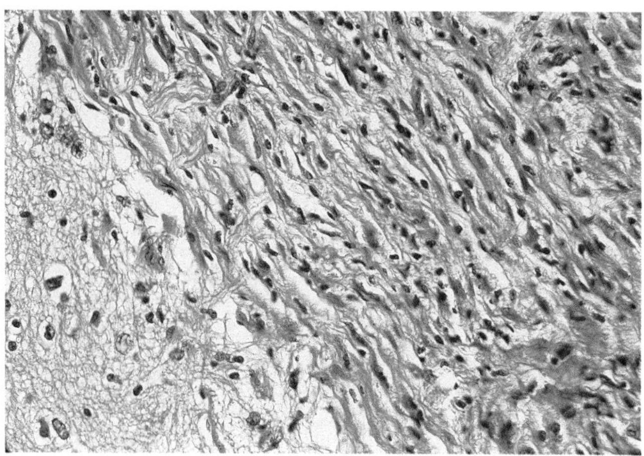

A

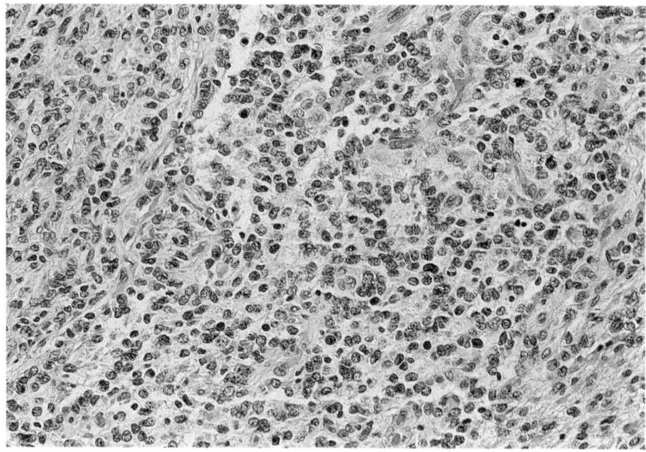

B

Fig. 2.16 Desmoplastic infantile ganglioglioma (DIG). Heterogeneous populations of glial and neuronal elements are intermixed within a prominent desmoplastic stroma in these tumors **A**. A more primitive neuroepithelial cell population is also frequently observed **B**. H&E.

half of the tumors (Russell & Rubinstein 1989). Early ependymal differentiation occurs within the neuroepithelium to form rosettes with abundant proliferative cells that resemble the analogous structures in ependymoblastomas. Similar to the neuroregulators in the primitive neuroepithelial component of the experimental mouse ovarian teratomas (Caccamo et al 1989), immunoreactivity for growth factors that are known to have biologic activity on CNS progenitor cell populations (insulin-like growth factor I and basic fibroblastic growth factor) is abundant in this primitive epithelium (Shiurba et al 1991).

The second group of tumors, those with a significant but not preponderant primitive cell population, is composed of the desmoplastic infantile ganglioglioma (Fig. 2.16A, B) and the desmoplastic cerebral astrocytoma of infancy (VandenBerg 1993). These are rare neoplasms arising in the cerebral hemispheres within the first two years of life. The histogenetic potential of the former reflects bipotential neuronal (Figs 2.17A,B,2.18) and glial (Figs 2.18, 2.19) progenitor cells as putative oncogenic targets while the latter, appearing quite similar in its histopathologic features, is restricted along an astroglial lineage. One distinctive feature of the neoplastic astroglial lineage in both neoplasms is the production of a basal lamina, often associated with normal subpial astrocytes. A second feature is that the neuronal component seldom achieves the cytoarchitectural maturation that is common in the gangliogliomas (Fig. 2.21), which are more common in the mature brain. Therefore the progenitor cell populations, as targets for neoplastic transformation in both tumors, most likely share a common lineage with subpial astroglia and may be related to the potential foci of perinatal and early postnatal neurocytogenesis which might persist in the cerebral subpial zones (Brun 1965).

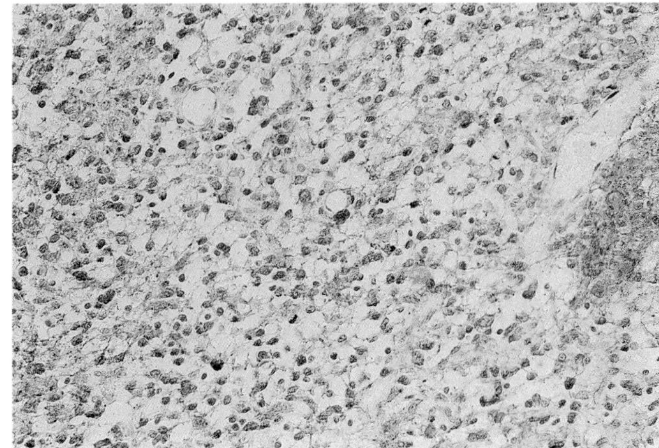

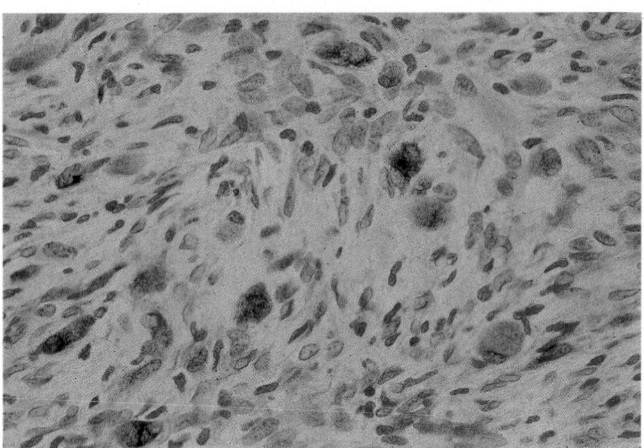

Fig. 2.17 Desmoplastic infantile ganglioglioma (DIG). The neuronal elements of the DIG are immunoreactive for neuron-associated epitopes such as synaptophysin **A** in the more cellular areas and for class III β-tubulin **B** in the larger cells. TUJ1, SY38 avidin-biotin immunoperoxidase.

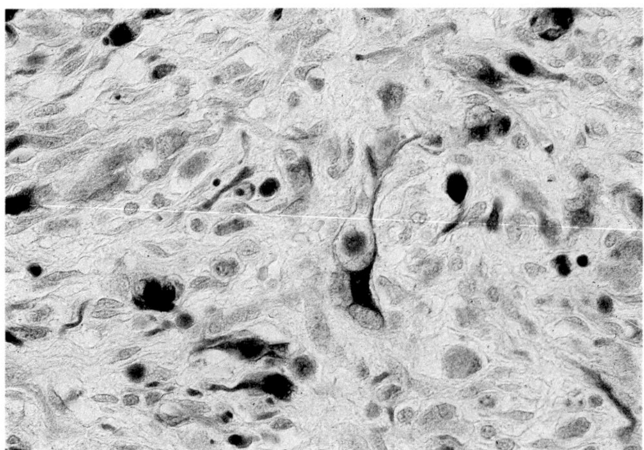

Fig. 2.18 Desmoplastic infantile ganglioglioma (DIG). Double-labeling for GFAP (dark purple) and neurofilament protein (NF-M/H) (red-brown) demonstrates the distinctive populations of neoplastic glial and neuronal cells. Despite the putative bipotential progenitors in the primitive cell population, cells coexpressing both glial and neuronal markers are not seen in the DIG. GFAP/NFT$_{P}$1A3 double immunoperoxidase.

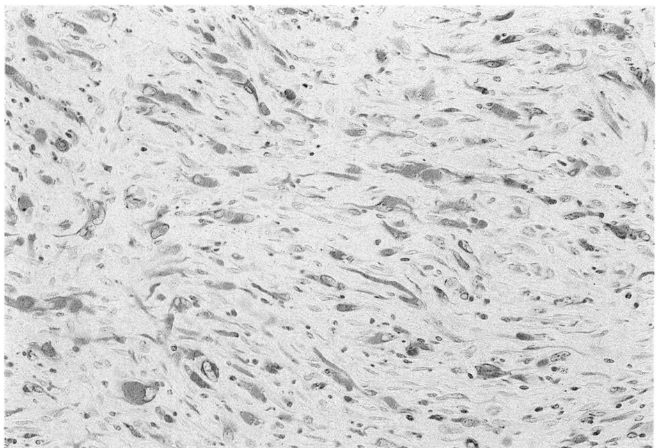

Fig. 2.19 Desmoplastic infantile ganglioglioma (DIG). GFAP immunohistochemistry highlights the neoplastic astrocytes with well-developed processes within the moderately desmoplastic stroma. GFAP avidin-biotin immunoperoxidase.

The experimental data from immortalized supratentorial progenitor cells in rats certainly suggest that region-specific extrinsic factors may have significant effects on the hierarchical commitment of undifferentiated cells to glial and neuronal lineages and in the expression of specific phenotypes of either a glial or neuronal cell type (Renfranz et al 1991, Mehler et al 1993). Such studies may explain the capacity for unipotential or bipotential differentiation from the same group of transformed progenitor cells and could account for the common features between the two types of infantile desmoplastic tumors, differing primarily in the degree of divergent cytogenesis.

The last group of forebrain tumors which display relatively unique developmental potentials are those tumors which usually arise in the late pediatric or young adult periods and are composed of distinctive neuronal or glial phenotypes. With respect to neuronal lineages, the central neurocytoma is a neoplasm that has several important features. These tumors are uncommon; the majority arise in association with the lateral ventricles and, to a lesser extent, the third ventricle (see Hassoun et al 1993). This association with the periventricular regions of the forebrain provocatively suggests that these tumors may arise from distinct populations of cells in the adjacent subventricular zones. Second, although these tumors are composed of a rather homogenous population of small cells with variable, but not significant mitotic activity, they usually behave clinically like a well-differentiated cellular phenotype. Immunohistochemical (Fig. 2.20) and ultrastructural studies have unequivocally demonstrated that the majority of cells composing central neurocytomas are neurons with features that suggest cytoarchitectural maturity. These include synaptic terminals, often with clear and dense core vesicles, and abundant profiles of cellular processes with parallel arrays of microtubules (see Ch. 8 for discussion). Nevertheless, neoplastic neurons with a

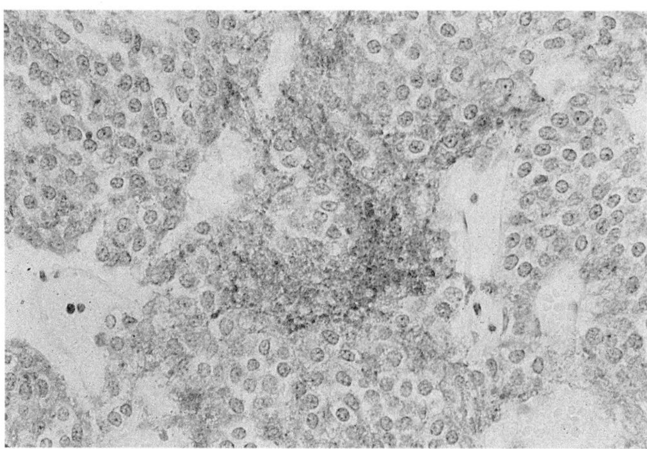

Fig. 2.20 Central neurocytoma. The neuronal nature of central neurocytomas is confirmed by immunohistochemistry for neuronal-associated proteins including synaptophysin. SY38 avidin-biotin immunoperoxidase.

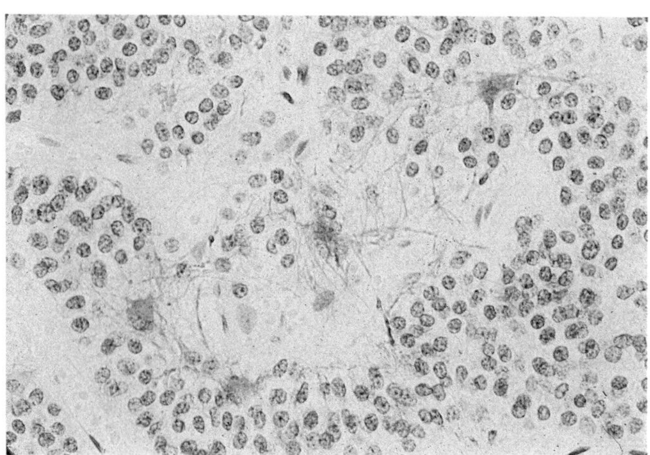

Fig. 2.22 Central neurocytoma. The presence of GFAP-immunoreactive astrocytes is most frequently restricted to reactive stromal cells, which may be present throughout the tumor. GFAP avidin-biotin immunoperoxidase.

ganglionic morphology, similar to the neuronal elements of typical gangliogliomas (Fig. 2.21), are not present in these tumors. This distinctive neuronal phenotype suggests that the neuronal lineages of the central neurocytoma are more analogous to the small interneurons which populate the striatum and thalamus. The third intriguing aspect of these tumors with respect to their putative oncogenic targets, is the rare occurrence of tumor cells with GFAP immunoreactivity in cases which appear to have a more aggressive biologic behavior (von Deimling et al 1990). In most tumors, the only GFAP-immunoreactive cells within the neoplasm are reactive, stromal astrocytes (Fig. 2.22) which contrast with the more abundant, relatively delicate, neoplastic astrocytes in most gangliogliomas (Fig. 2.23).

There are two principal types of glial neoplasms with

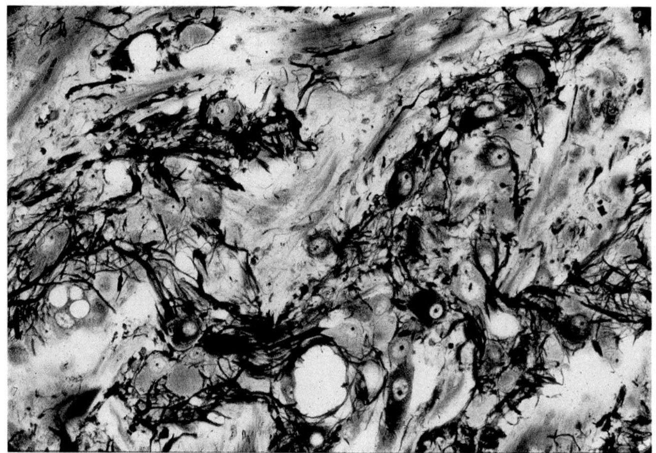

Fig. 2.21 Ganglioglioma. Neuronal diversity is highlighted in the comparison between the large, often bizarre, pyramidal-type ganglion cells which frequently comprise the majority of neuronal cell types in gangliogliomas and the small, interneuron-like cells of the central neurocytomas. Modified Bielshowsky silver stain.

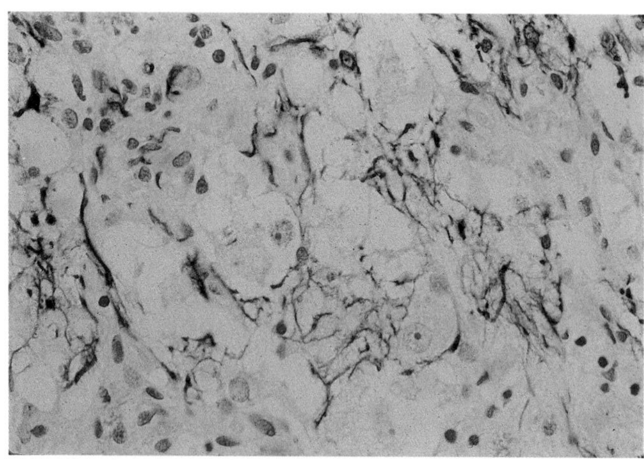

Fig. 2.23 Ganglioglioma. In contrast to the central neurocytoma, the glial component of the ganglioglioma is usually prominent and neoplastic. The astroglial element of these tumors is readily demonstrated by GFAP immunohistochemistry which highlights the admixture of glia and neuronal tumor cells. GFAP immunoperoxidase.

distinctive developmental potentials that occur in the setting of the late pediatric and young adult forebrain. The first is the pilocytic astrocytoma, with a peak incidence around the end of the first decade in children (see Ch. 8). Within the forebrain, these tumors are characteristically located in the midline structures within the hypothalamus, third ventricular region, the thalamus and optic pathways (Forsyth et al 1993). One of the hallmark features of these tumors is relatively indolent growth with a low mitotic rate while inducing the degree of microvascular hyperplasia associated with malignant gliomas. Despite this low growth rate, the tumor cells apparently retain a capacity to effectively invade the adjacent leptomeninges or nerve tracts, with only limited capacity to infiltrate the adjacent brain (Clark et al 1985, Mishima et al 1992, Forsyth et al 1993). This unique invasive behavior implicates a selective alteration of the tumor cell interactions with neural and non-neural extracellular matrix which may be modulated, in part, by the abundance of proteinase inhibitors of the serpin class, such as α_1-antitrypsin and α_1-antichymotrypsin in the tumors (Friedberg et al 1991). The tumor cell populations manifest two forms of distinctive cytoarchitecture with bipolar, highly fibrillated glial cells, recalling features of radial glia, and more stellate cells with short processes, recalling type 1 astrocytes. The fibrillated processes of pilocytic astrocytomas are strongly immunoreactive for both GFAP and vimentin, a characteristic shared with fetal radial glia (Pixley & DeVellis 1984, Schiffer et al 1986, Wilkinson et al 1990).

The second type of glioma with a distinctive developmental potential is the pleomorphic xanthoastrocytoma (PXA). These are characteristically superficial cerebral tumors that occur most commonly in children and young adults (see Ch. 8). Hallmark features of the tumors are a propensity for quite dramatic, but focal leptomeningeal invasion (VandenBerg 1992) with limited capacity for brain invasion. However, in contrast to the pilocytic astrocytomas, there is marked cellular heterogeneity, a more variable growth potential, and a distinctive extracellular matrix with the presence of a pericellular basal lamina (Weldon-Linne et al 1983, Kepes et al 1989) similar to that described in subpial astrocytes (Russell & Rubinstein 1989, Whittle et al 1989). Accordingly, a histogenic relationship between pleomorphic xanthoastrocytomas and this specific astrocytic phenotype has been proposed (Russell & Rubinstein 1989, Whittle et al 1989).

In addition to the neoplasms with relatively well-defined glial or neuronal phenotypes that manifest distinctive developmental features, there are two types of tumors arising within either children or young adults that have a more complex histogenesis, but a benign growth potential. The first type is the subependymal giant cell astrocytoma (SEGA), which typically occurs during the first two decades of life, most frequently in association with tuberous sclerosis (see Ch. 8). The heterogenous tumor cells have negligible capacity for infiltration of adjacent brain and a low proliferative activity. The tumor cells display a wide spectrum of cytoarchitecture from small spindle cells, intermediate size polygonal cells and giant, ganglion-like cells. The majority of tumor cells are astroglial; however, a number of tumor cells may demonstrate both glial and neuron-associated epitopes, including class III β-tubulin, high molecular weight neurofilament proteins and several classes of neurotransmitter substances (Altermatt et al 1993). These tumors may also exhibit ultrastructural features suggestive of neuronal differentiation such as microtubules, dense core granules and occasional synapse formation, similar to the hamartomatous lesions (tubers) of tuberous sclerosis. Since divergent glioneuronal differentiation occurs within tubers, the subependymal giant cell astrocytomas may develop from neoplastic transformation of the same cellular lineages that develop into these hamartomatous lesions in association with a genetic lesion on chromosome 9 (Haines & Short 1993).

The second type of complex glioneuronal neoplasm is the dysembryoplastic neuroepithelial tumor (DNET). These are rare tumors that usually arise in children and young adults with a characteristic long history of a complex partial seizure disorder (Daumas-Duport 1993). Typically, the tumors arise in the temporal lobe and are restricted to the cortex, with a dysplastic disorganization in the adjacent brain. Immunohistochemical studies have demonstrated the glioneuronal nature of these tumors. The neoplastic glia lineages appear to have both astrocytic and oligodendroglial phenotypes. The neuronal component is composed of both more mature, ganglionic cells and a more immature population of cells with a neurocytic appearance (Hirose et al 1994).

The occurrence of tumors with distinctive, often complex histogenetic potentials in the young, but mature forebrain implies the persistence of certain types of neural progenitor cells. Within the forebrain, there appear to be approximately three potential loci for neural progenitor cells in the postnatal mammalian brain: the subventricular zone, the hippocampal dentate fascia, and the cortical subpial layer (Brun 1965, Kaplan & Hinds 1977, Lewis 1981). With respect to putative progenitors in the subpial zone, it is intriguing to consider the desmoplastic infantile astrocytomas and gangliogliomas as arising from these oncogenic targets. The occurrence of these rare tumors only in infants, the primitive cell component and variably divergent differentiation all implicate an origin from a postnatal progenitor cell. Consistent involvement of the superficial leptomeninges and the production of an astroglial basal lamina suggest the possibility of a subpial origin.

The most well-characterized locus is the subventricular zone, particularly in the region of the lateral ventricles in rodents. Recent studies have enumerated several classes of progenitors with respect to the development of neuronal and multiple glial lineages, including the putative O-2A^{adult} progenitors (Levison & Goldman 1993, Lois & Alvarez-Buylla 1993). Although the ultimate histogenetic in vivo potential of the various lineages is not known, it is tempting to speculate that the small neuronal phenotypes that compose central neurocytomas are transformed interneuronal lineages arising from a subventricular progenitor pool. The small percentage of central neurocytomas with an apparent component of neoplastic astrocytes may arise from bipotential progenitors in this zone. The lower frequency of the tumors with divergent neuronal and glial elements may reflect a small number of progenitors with a divergent biologic potential or the fact that development of the neoplastic astrocytic lineages from these progenitors requires more extrinsic factors which are variably present (Temple 1990). With respect to the subependymal giant cell astrocytomas, persistence of progenitors with both divergent and restricted developmental potentials with the tuberous sclerosis genotype may contribute to the unique admixture of neuroglial phenotypes within these tumors.

CEREBELLAR DEVELOPMENT AND NEOPLASTIC TRANSFORMATION

In the cerebellum, there is a regional predilection for two types of neuroepithelial tumors, both more frequent in children (please see Ch. 8). These neoplasms exhibit two dissimilar histogenetic potentials. The first, as the most common primitive tumor in the central nervous system, is the medulloblastoma. It comprises approximately one quarter of all intracranial tumors in children, with a peak incidence near the end of the first decade (Russell & Rubinstein 1989). In contrast, the pilocytic astrocytoma as the second type with a unique set of biologic and histopathologic features, is one of the more indolent astrocytic neoplasms in the CNS. The markedly different biologic potentials of these two types of cerebellar tumors clearly reflect two distinct cellular targets for neoplastic transformation. The medulloblastomas appear to arise within a primitive or progenitor cell population. In contrast, the pilocytic astrocytomas develop from a more differentiated progenitor, analogous to the putative oncogenic target in the forebrain. Recent studies in rodents indicate the presence of glial progenitors in the postnatal cerebellum from which these tumors may develop (Levine et al 1993, Levison & Goldman 1993).

In the early stages of CNS development, the cerebellar progenitor cells arise from two major germinal zones and generate distinct populations of the neural cells that compose the mature cerebellum (see Jacobson 1978 for review). The first is the periventricular germinal matrix in the cerebellar plate over the fourth ventricle which forms the typical ventricular, intermediate and marginal layers during the first 3–8 weeks of development. This zone contains progenitors with divergent potential that will differentiate into several neuronal types (Purkinje and Golgi II neurons) and into the macroglia of the region. In addition, there appears to be parasagittal compartmentalization of the Purkinje cell lineages which arise from these periventricular progenitors during development (Leclerc et al 1992). Although both neuronal and glial differentiation begins relatively early (8–10 weeks gestation — Yachnis et al 1993), experimental studies in the rodent would suggest that, in contrast to the subdivision of Purkinje cells, the bipotential glial progenitors are diffusely dispersed from the periventricular germinal matrix (not the external granular layer) and appear to persist beyond the neonatal period (Levine et al 1993). Although the major portion of these glial progenitors appeared to progressively undergo oligodendroglial differentiation, in vitro studies also demonstrated the potential of these cells to differentiate into type 2 astrocytic lineages (Levine et al 1993). It is tempting to speculate about a relationship between the pool of glial progenitors in the maturing cerebellum and the pilocytic astrocytomas which arise at this site.

The cells which compose the second 'germinal' zone, the external granular layer (EGL), arise in a location remote from where the cells will subsequently form the external granular layer. They originate in a well-defined component of the proliferative subventricular zone (cerebellar portion of the rhombic lip), and migrate over the external surface to populate the external granular layer from the first 10–14 weeks of gestation (Rakic & Sidman 1970). This 'fetal' layer (Fig. 2.24) is clearly present in the perinatal period, but it does not persist normally beyond the first year (Kadin et al 1970). Neuronal histogenesis from these cells (granular, stellate, and basket neurons) has been clearly documented, but the significance of the external granular layer to cerebellar gliogenesis is uncertain. However, more recent experimental studies have suggested that cells which are putatively derived from the neonatal EGL have the potential for Bergmann gliogenesis (see below). Although the EGL, as a putative source of medulloblastomas, may last longer than 12 months (Stevenson & Echlin 1934), it is not clear that these small numbers of cells would necessarily have the same developmental plasticity as the fetal or neonatal EGL. One key observation with respect to oncogenic targets within the fetal EGL, however, is the report by Kadin et al (1970) of a neonatal midline medulloblastoma with striking continuity with the EGL. In this case, there was multifocal proliferation of the EGL as irregular extensions into the molecular layer which linked regions of normal EGL to definitive tumor.

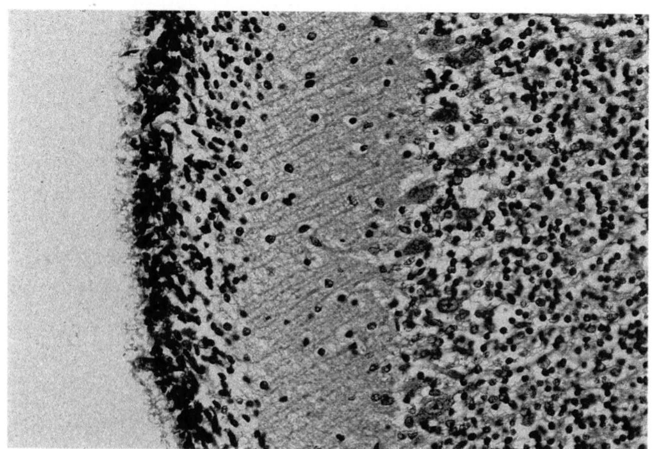

Fig. 2.24 Human cerebellum in late gestation. Human cerebellar cortex at 35 weeks gestation readily demonstrates a prominent superficial external granular layer, Purkinje cell layer and internal granular layer. The external granular layer persists into the first postnatal year as a thin rim of subpial cells. H&E.

Other groups of primitive cells, whose histogenetic potential is completely unknown, have also been described in the human cerebellum during the first postnatal year. The first group is composed of small foci of embryonal cells which are situated in proximity to the germinal zone of the posterior medullary velum (Raaf & Kernohan 1944). The second group are the nests of primitive 'matrix cells', located within the deep cerebellar nuclei, which appear to persist during the first four months (Jellinger 1972, Friede 1973). Given these locations, which were documented in carefully studied postmortem cases, these cellular rests would appear to be derived from the periventricular germinal matrix rather than the external granular layer. It is therefore tempting to speculate that these cells, as oncogenic targets, may have a distinctive potential for divergent differentiation (both neuronal and glial) similar to the periventricular matrix cells that contribute to the cerebellum.

An elegant experimental approach to the study of lineage development and cellular differentiation in the cerebellum has been the use of immortalized rodent cell lines derived from neonatal or early postnatal cerebella. Immortalization by either transfection with a temperature-sensitive allele (tsA58) of the SV-40 T antigen (Hayes & McKay 1993 for review) or with a dominant oncogene v-*myc* (Snyder et al 1992) successfully establishes the proliferative and primitive cellular phenotype. These types of studies exhibited two important results. First, these cell lines (from either neonatal mouse or 4 days postnatal rat) manifested either stable astrocytic or neuronal phenotypes when implanted into the superficial cerebellar regions of neonatal hosts. Second, both types of immortalized, primitive lines with significant proliferative activity in cell culture appeared to lose the abnormal proliferative phenotype and normally differentiate within the environment of the normal host cerebella.

The importance of the tissue environment for the stable modulation of biologic potential of primitive neural cells recalls earlier studies of the mouse C1300 neuroblastoma and teratocarcinoma cells which showed that malignant tumor cells may revert stably to a non-neoplastic phenotype in an appropriate tissue environment (Podesta et al 1984). The fact that these same immortalized cerebellar cells underwent only a scant degree of differentiation in culture (Snyder et al 1992, Hayes & McKay 1993) emphasizes the importance of extrinsic signals and the use of in vivo models for studying the process of neoplastic differentiation. These studies provide the most unequivocal evidence to date for the existence of progenitor cells with potential for divergent differentiation in the neonatal cerebellum. However, both the origin of the progenitors from either the EGL or the periventricular matrix and the quantitative assessment of the different neuronal and glial lineages that develop remain to be determined. It is also notable that no features of astrocytic and neuronal differentiation within the same maturing progenitor cells appeared in vivo.

Most studies of neuronal and glial ontogeny during cerebellar neurocytogenesis have relied on the differential expression of cytoskeletal proteins (Tohyama et al 1992, 1993, Katsetos et al 1993, Yachnis et al 1993), and/or specific morphologic criteria (Rakic & Sidman 1970). As in the forebrain, the immunohistochemical detection of intermediate filament (IF) classes has permitted the relatively selective detection of both primitive progenitor cell populations and cell lineages which manifest either neuronal or astroglial features. The IF proteins that appear in the earliest phases of primitive progenitor cell differentiation are nestin (Tohyama et al 1992, 1993, Yachnis et al 1993) and vimentin (Houle & Fedoroff 1983). These proteins are down-regulated as neurocytogenesis proceeds, with the expression of either neuronal (neurofilament NF-M/H — Tohyama et al 1992, 1993, Yachnis et al 1993) or astrocytic (glial fibrillary acidic protein, GFAP) phenotypes (Cameron & Rakic 1991). However, selective recognition of specific types of primitive cells, particularly within the neuroblastic populations, has been problematic. Katsetos et al (1993), in a study of 40 fetal and postnatal cerebella, demonstrated that immature neuronal derivatives of the ventricular germinal matrix were calbindin-D_{28k} immunoreactive while the neuroblasts of the external granular layer were not immunoreactive. In contrast, the primitive neuroblasts originating in the external granular layer expressed a neuronal class III β-tubulin isotype (TUJ1) that was not expressed in neurons derived from the ventricular germinal matrix (Purkinje and Golgi II cells) until late in neurocytogenesis.

Immunohistochemical studies of medulloblastomas clearly showed evidence for limited cellular differentiation, despite the high cellularity, proliferative activity and biologically aggressive nature that mark these tumors (see Ch. 8). A biologic potential for both neuronal and glial differentiation exists in this tumor group (Molenaar et al 1989, Russell & Rubinstein 1989) and such a potential is consistent with cerebellar progenitor cells as the oncogenic target. However, the histogenetic potential of medulloblastomas is complex and probably reflects a heterogenous category of tumors, somewhat analogous to the major classes of primitive progenitor cells that arise during normal development. Although both neuronal and glial phenotypes occur in medulloblastomas, the incidence of neuronal differentiation appears to be greater (Fig. 2.25) (Kleihues et al 1989, Trojanowski et al 1992). The more common expression of class III β-tubulin immunoreactivity in medulloblastomas, in contrast to the relatively uncommon calbindin-D_{28k} immunoreactivity (< 6%), suggests a putative origin of the tumor cells from external granular layer cells (Katsetos et al 1991). Even in medulloblastomas that exhibit ganglionic differentiation, no calbindin-D_{28k} immunoreactivity could be demonstrated

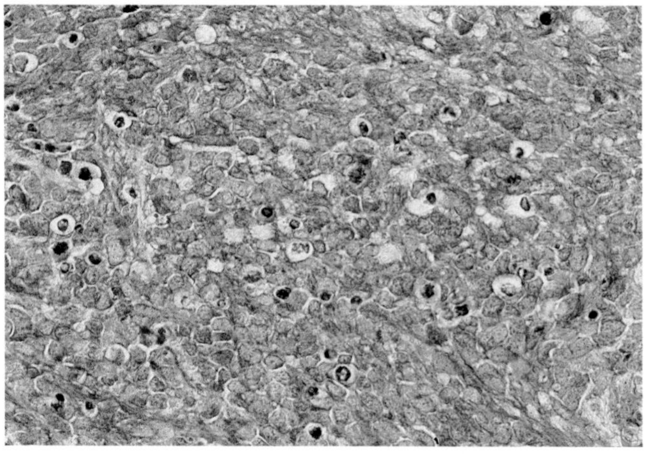

A

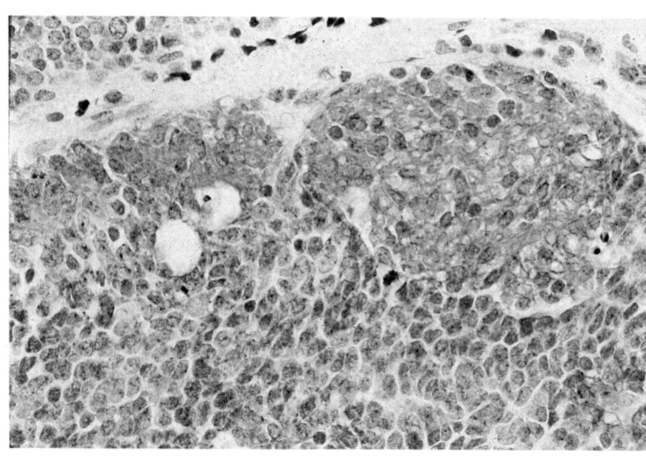

B

Fig. 2.25 Medulloblastoma. Immunohistochemistry for neuron-associated protein, such as the class III β-tubulin, can document neuroblastic cell populations within medulloblastomas. This type of differentiation with the primitive cell populations can be extensive **A** or highly focal **B**. TUJ1 avidin-biotin immunoperoxidase.

(data not shown), whereas the ganglionic cells from a cerebellar ganglioglioma readily expressed calbindin-D_{28k} (Fig. 2.26). Such differences may distinguish a neoplasm arising from the progenitor compartment of the ventricular germinal matrix.

In contrast to neuroblastomas of the forebrain, in which relatively small numbers of cases have precluded any systematic study for immunohistochemically distinct neuronal subtypes, a number of medulloblastoma variants have been described (Russell & Rubinstein 1989). In addition to the more common occurrence of neuron/neurosecretory-associated cytoskeletal epitopes (Molenaar et al 1989, Russell & Rubinstein 1989), approximately 33–50% of medulloblastomas in some series express photoreceptor-associated proteins (opsin and S-Ag — Korf et al 1987, Bonnin & Perentes 1988). The significance of differentiation in these neuronal variants with respect to biologic behavior and therapeutic potential remains undefined. Another variant of the medulloblastoma with a primitive neuronal phenotype that does have a distinctly aggressive behavior is the 'large cell' medulloblastoma which, on the basis of a small number of cases, appears to have early cerebrospinal fluid dissemination (Giangaspero et al 1992).

Another distinctive feature of cellular differentiation in medulloblastomas occurs in the desmoplastic variant,

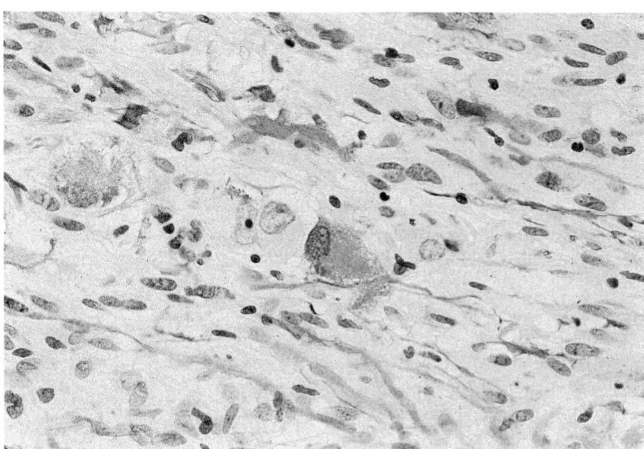

Fig. 2.26 Cerebellar ganglioglioma. Neoplastic neurons may display selective neuronal phenotypes associated with the specific region in which the tumors arise. In this example of a mature cerebellar ganglioglioma, the ganglion cells express calbindin-D_{28k}, a membrane-associated calcium binding protein which is selectively expressed in the cerebellum by Purkinje cells and other neurons derived from the ventricular germinal matrix. Calbindin-D_{28k}, avidin-biotin immunoperoxidase.

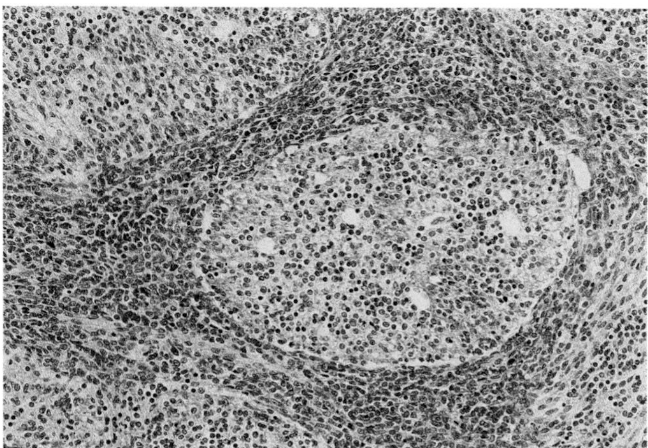

Fig. 2.27 Desmoplastic medulloblastoma. Desmoplastic medulloblastomas exhibit a more stereotyped form of focal cellular differentiation with the biphasic formation of central nodules with increased differentiation which are surrounded by more primitive cells. The islands of more differentiated cells usually demonstrate neuronal differentiation with the presence of neurofilament (NF-M/H) epitopes. SMI33 avidin-biotin immunoperoxidase.

which comprises about 10–12% of cases in some series (Burger et al 1987, Kleihues et al 1989). The tumors are marked by a biphasic histologic architecture with a follicular arrangement of tumor cells (Figs 2.27, 2.28). Highly cellular sheets and trabeculae of typical tumor cells encompass islands of lower cellularity and cells with finely fibrillated processes. The highly cellular periphery commonly has the highest number of cells which are immunoreactive for Ki-67 epitopes, which are detectable in actively proliferating cells (Fig. 2.28). This histologic pattern is particularly well highlighted by reticulin deposition only in the peripheral cellular areas. The reticulin-free 'islands' prominently demonstrate the greatest degree of phenotypic differentiation, usually neuronal (Katsetos et al 1989). It is interesting to note that the characteristic architectural pattern of the desmoplastic variant is not always preserved in the recurrent tumor.

In contrast to the use of specific types of levels of 'differentiation' or 'cytologic maturity' for evaluating the biologic potential of these predominantly neuroblastic tumors, a recent study of the *bcl*-2 oncogene protein shows the potential of another approach for evaluating the biologic potential of these primitive tumors (Swanson 1994). *bcl*-2 is an inner membrane protein of mitochondria that blocks the progression of programmed cell death (apoptosis) (Hockenbery et al 1990). Therefore, this approach encompasses the general concept of controlling apoptosis and the requirement for extrinsic trophic factors to support tumor cell survival. In a series of 34 tumors, preliminary data suggest that medulloblastomas in which *bcl*-2 immunoreactivity was present in >5% of the cells had a significantly worse prognosis with respect to tumor recurrence or mortality. The relationship of *bcl*-2 expression, as detected by immunohistochemistry, to the presence of cellular differentiation in individual medulloblastomas is apparently complex. In desmoplastic medulloblastomas, a variant that typically has neuroblastic differentiation, one half of the tumors were *bcl*-2 immunoreactive. However, the immunoreactivity was apparently distributed in the more proliferative, poorly differentiated cells peripheral to the differentiating 'islands' (see above). Further characterization of *bcl*-2 expression with respect to the cellular phenotypes (neuronal or glial) and tumor growth kinetics, including the rate of proliferation and cell death, remains to be better defined.

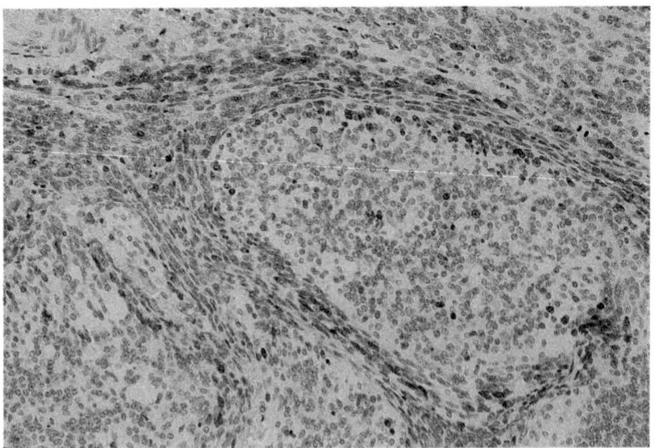

Fig. 2.28 Desmoplastic medulloblastoma. The highly cellular trabeculae of tumor cells which demarcate the islands of cellular differentiation show higher labeling indices of Ki-67 in comparison with the more differentiated areas which correspond to neuronal differentiated zones. MIB 1 avidin-biotin immunoperoxidase.

Although apoptosis may affect a variety of cell types, it may be particularly important where it normally plays a key regulatory role in the control of cell number during development, as in selected neuroblastic and glial cell populations (Jacobson 1978, Raff et al 1993) and during physiologic differentiation with hemopoiesis (Koury 1992). For neuronal and oligodendroglial glial phenotypes, specific growth factors — such as platelet-derived growth factor (PDGF), insulin-like growth factors (IGFs), ciliary neurotropic factor (CNTF) and the neurotrophins (e.g. NGF, NT-3) — prevent the onset of apoptosis (Jacobson 1978, Raff et al 1993) and may play a similar role following neoplastic transformation. In peripheral neuroblastomas, *bcl*-2 levels appear to be regulated during cellular differentiation (Hanada et al 1993) and recent studies suggest that its expression portends a poor prognosis (Castle et al 1993). A recent report suggested that apoptosis may be an important process in the biologic behavior of medulloblastomas (Schiffer et al 1994). Such an interaction of growth factors, cellular differentiation and apoptosis suggests that potentially useful analytical approaches would be aimed at determining growth factor responsiveness rather than the growth factor content of medulloblastomas. Therefore, identification of neuroblastic lineages which are susceptible to selective regulation of apoptosis would be important. Future therapeutic approaches to medulloblastomas may involve pharmacologic manipulation of *bcl*-2 expression as a mechanism for modifying sensitivity to growth factors or chemotherapeutic agents.

The interpretation of neoplastic astrocytic differentiation in medulloblastomas is problematic. Even when strict criteria are used to eliminate the expected component of 'stromal' astrocytes (Fig. 2.29A) (Coffin et al 1983, Schindler & Gullotta 1983, Kleihues et al 1989), at least 10% of cases appear to have neoplastic cells with GFAP immunoreactivity (Fig. 2.29B). The most compelling evidence for neoplastic astrocytic differentiation in medulloblastomas comes from two different sources. First, tumor cells within distant leptomeningeal metastases can have unequivocal GFAP-immunoreactivity (Fig. 2.29C). Second, studies of cultures with cell lines derived from medulloblastomas have demonstrated divergent neuronal and glial phenotypic differentiation (Bigner 1989). More

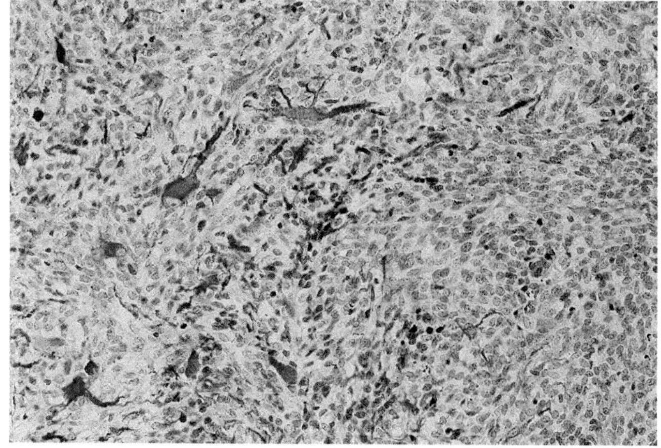

A

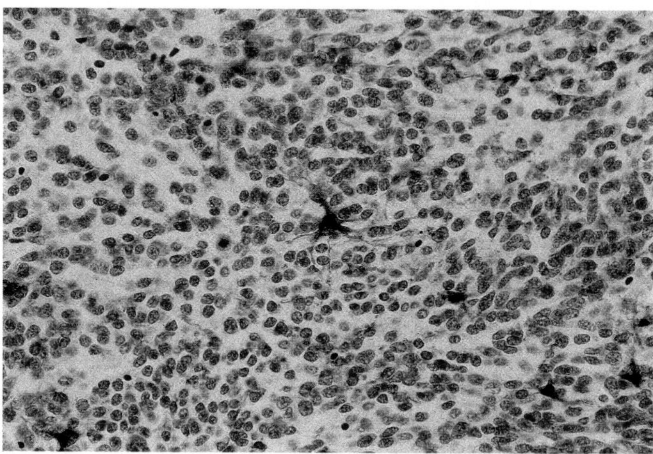

B

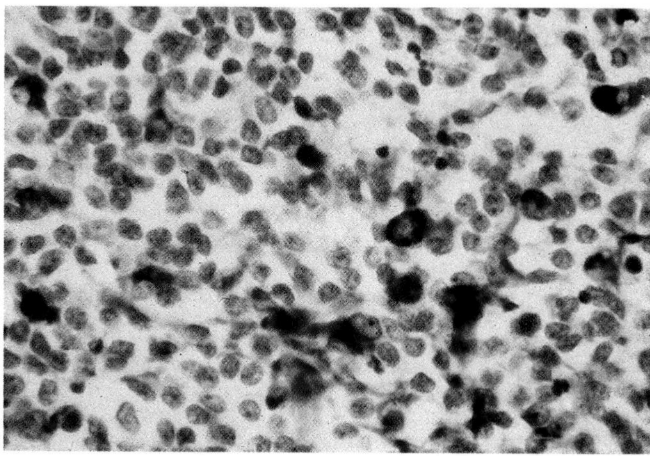

C

Fig. 2.29 Medulloblastoma. Reactive stromal astrocytes are commonly identified in these medulloblastomas by the typical cytoarchitecture **A**. Neoplastic astroglial differentiation in medulloblastomas is present in approximately 10% of the tumors and can be highlighted by GFAP immunoreactivity in often bizarre cells **B**. GFAP immunoreactivity in a leptomeningeal metastatic implant of a medulloblastoma is definitive evidence for neoplastic glial differentiation **C**. GFAP avidin-biotin immunoperoxidase.

recent studies have demonstrated that treatment of cultured medulloblastoma cell lines with a glial maturation factor (GMF-β) can induce expression of GFAP mRNA and immunoreactive protein over a 72-hour period (Keles et al 1993). These data strongly emphasize the importance of extrinsic factors on the growth and differentiation of medulloblastomas. The factors for astroglial differentiation within medulloblastomas in vivo may not be as common as for the neuronal lineages. Alternatively, the differentiation of neuroblastic lineages may be more independent of extrinsic factors.

DIVERSITY OF ASTROGLIAL PHENOTYPES

Aside from astrocytic tumors within the forebrain and cerebellum that are defined presently by unique combinations of clinicopathologic features, studies of glial lineages from the developing and mature brain (Denis-Donini et al 1984, Hansson 1988, Butt 1991, Miller & Szigeti 1991, Ransom 1991, Young 1991, Noble et al 1992, Vayasse & Goldman 1992, Levine et al 1993, Levison & Goldman 1993, Marriott & Wilkin 1993, Steindler 1993) would suggest that the current histopathologic classification of astroglial neoplasms may not indicate accurately the potential for regional physiologic heterogeneity. This diversity, which may be developmentally regulated in a stage-specific manner, is reflected partially by the secretion of specific glial glycoconjugates (Steindler 1993) and the differential migration of transplanted neonatal astrocytes (Hatton et al 1993). These region-specific properties would have the potential to differentially affect tumor cell infiltration of the surrounding brain following transformation. This heterogeneity may also be modified by local cellular interactions (Chamak et al 1987, Beyer et al 1990, Cockram 1990). Another region-specific property that would potentially affect biologic activity following transformation is the developmental and lineage-associated heterogeneity of functional substance P (SP)receptors (Marriott & Wilkin 1993). This heterogeneity suggests that receptors for other neuropeptides/neuroregulators, as potent biologic effectors, may also be lineage- and region-specific.

FUTURE DIRECTIONS IN DEVELOPMENTAL NEURO-ONCOLOGY

The future of developmental neuro-oncology has exciting promise, with several key avenues presently in their early stages. First, investigative work using transfected cells should permit a more precise understanding of the molecular mechanisms in the development of cellular lineages and the regulation of phenotypic plasticity. Second, transgenetic experiments that will determine the mechanisms by which progenitor cells switch to lineage-specific terminal differentiation should lead to a better delineation of oncogenic targets within the developing and mature CNS. Third, further studies on the paracrine and autocrine roles of growth factors and their intracellular signaling pathways according to the cell lineage and stage of differentiation should permit more insight into the extrinsic factors which affect the biologic potentials of immature neoplastic phenotypes. Finally, recognition of the physiologic diversity in transformed glial cells should encourage the development of new diagnostic concepts that are more orientated to therapeutic control of biologic behavior. Collectively these experimental strategies should facilitate more precise, lineage-specific therapeutic attacks on the fundamental cellular processes of proliferation, differentiation, and cell death in brain tumors.

REFERENCES

Adler R, Hatlee M 1989 Plasticity and differentiation of embryonic retina cells after terminal mitosis. Science 243: 391–393

Altermatt H J, Lopes M B S, Scheithauer B W, VandenBerg S R 1993 The immunochemistry of subependymal giant cell astrocytoma (SEGA) in tuberous sclerosis (TS) (abstract). Journal of Neuropathology and Experimental Neurology 52: 326

Anderson D J 1992 Molecular control of neural development. In: Hall Z W (ed) An introduction to molecular neurobiology. Sinauer Associates, Sunderland, Ma, pp 355–387

Barres B A, Hart I K, Coles H S R, Burne J F, Voyvodic J T, Richardson W D, Raff M C 1992 Cell death and control of cell survival in the oligodendrocyte lineage. Cell 70: 32–46

Barres B A, Schmid R, Sendnter M, Raff M C 1993 Multiple extracellular signals are required for long-term oligodendrocyte survival. Development 118: 283–295

Beyer C, Epp B, Fassberg J, Reisert I, Pilgrim C 1990 Region- and sex-related differences in maturation of astrocytes in dissociated cell cultures of embryonic rat brain. Glia 3: 55–64

Bigner D D 1989 Phenotypic analysis of medulloblastoma with monoclonal antibodies. In: Fields W S (ed) Primary brain tumors. A review of histologic classification. Springer Verlag, New York. pp 70–78

Boncinelli E, Somma R, Acampora D, Pannese M, D'Esposito M, Simeone A 1988 Organization of human homeobox genes. Human Reproduction 3: 880–886

Bonnin J M, Perentes E 1988 Retinal S-antigen immunoreactivity in medulloblastomas. Acta Neuropathologica 76: 204–207

Brun A 1965 The subpial granular layer of the foetal cerebral cortex in man. Its ontogeny and significance in congenital cortical malformations. Acta Pathologica et Microbiologica Scandinavica Suppl 179

Burger P C, Grahmann F C, Bliestle A, Kleihues P 1987 Differentiation in the medulloblastoma. A histological and immunohistochemical study. Acta Neuropathologica 73: 115–123

Buse E, de Groot H 1991 Generation of development patterns in the neuroepithelium of the developing mammalian eye: the pigment epithelium of the eye. Neuroscience Letters 126: 63–66

Buse E, Eichmann T, deGroot H, Leker A 1993 Differentiation of the mammalian retinal pigment epithelium in vitro: influence of presumptive retinal neuroepithelium and head mesenchyme. Anatomy and Embryology (Berl) 187: 259–268

Butt A M 1991 Macroglial cell types, lineage, and morphology in the CNS. Annals of the New York Academy of Sciences 633: 90–99

Caccamo D V, Herman M M, Frankfurter A, Katsetos C D, Collins V P, Rubinstein L J 1989 An immunohistological study of neuropeptides and neuronal cytoskeletal proteins in the neuroepithelial component of a spontaneous murine ovarian teratoma. American Journal of Pathology 135: 801–813

Calissano P, Ciotti M T, Battistini L, Zona C, Angelini A, Merlo D, Mercanti D 1993 Recombinant human insulin-like growth factor I exerts a trophic action and confers glutamate sensitivity on glutamate-resistant cerebellar granule cells. Proceedings of the National Academy of Science USA 90: 8752–8756

Cameron R S, Rakic P 1991 Glial cell lineage in the cerebral cortex: A review and synthesis. Glia 4: 124–137

Castle V P, Heidelberger K P, Bromberg J, Ou X, Dole M, Nunoz G 1993 Expression of the apoptosis-suppressing protein *bcl*-2, in neuroblastoma is associated with unfavorable histology and N-*myc* amplification. American Journal of Pathology 143: 1543–1550

Cedar H, Razin A 1990 DNA methylation and development. Biochimica et Biophysica Acta 1049: 1–8

Chamak B A, Fellows J, Glowinski J, Prochiantz A 1987 MaP2 expression and neurite outgrowth and branching are co-regulated through region-specific neuro-astroglial interactions. Journal of Neuroscience 7: 3163–3170

Chen J, Jones P 1989 Determination genes. Current Opinion in Cell Biology 1: 1075–1080

Clark G B, Henry J M, McKeever P E 1985 Cerebral pilocytic astrocytoma. Cancer 56: 1128–1133

Clemmons D R, Jones J I, Busby W H, Wright G 1993 Role of insulin-like growth binding proteins in modifying IGF actions. Annals of the New York Academy of Sciences 662: 10–21

Cockram C S 1990 Growth factors, astrocytes and astrocytomas. Seminars in Developmental Biology 1: 421–435

Coffin C M, Mukai K, Dehner L P 1983 Glial differentiation in medulloblastomas. Histogenetic insight, glial reaction, or invasion of brain? American Journal of Surgical Pathology 7: 555–565

Collarini E J, Pringle N, Mudhar H et al 1991 Growth factors and transcription factors in oligodendroglial development. Journal of Cell Science (suppl) 15: 117–123

Daumas-Duport C 1993 Dysembryoplastic neuroepithelial tumors. Brain Pathology 3: 283–295

de los Monteros A E, Zhang M, de Vellis J 1993 O2A progenitor cells transplanted into the neonatal rat brain develop into oligodendrocytes but not astrocytes. Proceedings of the National Academy of Science 90: 50–54

Denis-Donini S, Glowinski J, Prochiantz A 1984 Glial heterogeneity may define the three-dimensional shape of mouse mesencephalic dopaminergic neurones. Nature 307: 641–643

Eibl R H, Kleihues P, Jat P S, Wiestler O D 1994 A model for primitive neuroectodermal tumors in transgenic neural transplants harboring the SV40 large T antigen. American Journal of Pathology 144: 556–564

Eisenbarth G S, Walsh F S, Nirenberg M 1979 Monoclonal antibody to a plasma membrane antigen of neurons. Proceedings of the National Academy of Science 76: 4913–4917

Fishell G, Mason C A, Hatten M E 1993 Dispersion of neural progenitors within the germinal zones of the forebrain. Nature 362: 636–638

Forsyth P A, Shaw E G, Scheithauer B W, O'Fallon J R, Layton D D, Katzmann J A 1993 Supratentorial pilocytic astrocytomas. A clinicopathologic, prognostic and flow cytometric study of 51 patients. Cancer 72: 1335–1342

Friedberg E, Katsetos C D, Reidy et al 1991 Immunolocalization of protease inhibitors α-1-antitrypsin and α-1-antichymotrypsin in eosinophilic granular bodies of cerebral juvenile pilocytic astrocytomas. Journal of Neuropathology and Experimental Neurology 50: 293

Friede R L 1973 Dating the development of the human cerebellum. Acta Neuropathologica 23: 48–53

Friedman B, Hockfield S, Black J A, Woodruff K A, Waxman S G 1989 In situ demonstration of mature oligodendrocytes and their processes: an immunocytochemical study with a new monoclonal antibody, rip. Glia 2: 380–390

Fulton B P, Burne J F, Raff M C 1991 Glial cells in the rat optic nerve. Annals of the New York Academy of Sciences 633: 27–34

Galiana E, Bernard R, Borde I, Rouget P, Evrard C 1992 Proliferation and differentiation properties of bipotent glial progenitor cell lines immortalized with the adenovirus E1A gene. Annual Review of Neuroscience 15: 139–165

Galiana E, Bernard R, Borde I, Roget P, Evrard C 1993 Proliferation and differentiation properties of bipotent glial progenitor cell lines immortalized with the adenovirus E1A gene. Journal of Neuroscience Research 36: 133–146

Gallie B L, Squire J A, Goddard A et al 1990 Biology of disease. Mechanism of oncogenesis in retinoblastoma. Laboratory Investigation 62: 394–408

Gennett I N, Cavenee W K 1990 Molecular genetics in the pathology and diagnosis of retinoblastoma. Brain Pathology 1: 25–32

Giangaspero F, Rigobello L, Badiali M et al 1992 Large-cell medulloblastomas: A distinct variant with highly aggressive behavior. American Journal of Surgical Pathology 16: 687–693

Gonias S L 1992 α_2-macroglobulin: a protein at the interface of fibrinolysis and cellular growth regulation. Experimental Hematology 20: 302–311

Gonzalez-Fernandez F, Healy J I 1990 Early expression of the gene for interphotoreceptor retinol-binding protein during photoreceptor differentiation suggests a critical role for the interphotoreceptor matrix in retinal development. Journal Cell Biology 111: 2775–2784

Gonzalez-Fernandez F, Lopes M B S, Garcia-Fernandez J M, Foster R G, De Grip W J, Newman S, VandenBerg S R 1992 Expression of developmentally-defined retinal phenotypes in the histogenesis of retinoblastoma. American Journal of Pathology 141: 363–375

Gonzalez-Fernandez F, Van Niel E, Edmonds C et al 1993 Differential expression of interphotoreceptor retinoid-binding protein, opsin, cellular retinaldehyde-binding protein, and basic fibroblast growth factor. Experimental Eye Research 56: 411–427

Haines J L, Short M P 1993 Tuberous sclerosis: hamartomas, subependymal giant cell astrocytomas, and other central nervous system tumors. In: Levine A J, Schmidek H H (eds) Molecular genetics of nervous system tumors. Wiley-Liss, New York, pp 303–310

Hanada M, Krjewski S, Tanaka et al 1993 Regulation of Bel-2 oncoprotein levels with differentiation of human neuroblastoma cells. Cancer Research 53: 4978–4986

Hansson E 1988 Astroglia from defined brain regions as studied with primary cultures. Progress in Neurobiology 30: 369–397

Hassoun J, Söylemezoglu F, Gambarelli D, Figarella-Branger D, con Ammon K, Kleihues P 1993 Central neurocytoma: a synopsis of clinical and histological features. Brain Pathology 3: 297–306

Hatton J D, Nguyen M H, U H S 1993 Differential migration of astrocytes grafted into the developing rat brain. Glia 9: 113–119

Hauswirth W W, Langerijt A V D, Timmers A M, Adamus G, Ulshafer R J 1992 Early expression and localization of rhodopsin and interphotoreceptor retinoid-binding protein (IRBP) in the developing fetal bovine retina. Experimental Eye Research 54: 661–670

Hayes T, McKay R D G 1993 Differentiation of cell types in the central nervous system. In: Levine A J, Schmidek H H (eds) Molecular genetics of nervous system tumors. Wiley-Liss, New York, pp 37–48

Hirose T, Scheithauer B S, Lopes M B, VandenBerg S R 1994 Dysembryoplastic neuroepithelial tumor (DNT): an immunohistochemical and ultrastructural study. Journal of Neuropathology and Experimental Neurology 53: 184–195

Hockenbery D, Nunoz G, Miliman C, Schreiber R D, Korsmeyer S J 1990 Bcl-2 is an inner mitochondrial membrane protein that blocks programmed cell death. Nature 348: 334–336

Hockfield S, McKay R D G 1985 Identification of major cell classes in the developing mammalian nervous system. Journal of Neuroscience 5: 3310–3328

Holt C D, Bertsch T W, Ellis H M 1988 Cellular determination in the *Xenopus* retina is independent of lineage and birth date. Neuron 1: 15–26

Houle J, Fedoroff S 1983 Temporal relationship between the appearance of vimentin and neural tube development. Developmental Brain Research 9: 189–195

Jacobson M 1978 Developmental biology, 2nd edn. Plenum Press, New York, pp 10–16, 76–88

Jellinger K 1972 Embryonal cell nests in human cerebellar nuclei. Zeitschift fur Anatomie und Entwicklungsgeschichte 138: 145–154

Kadin M E, Rubinstein L J, Nelson J S 1970 Neonatal cerebellar medulloblastoma originating from the fetal external granular layer. Journal of Neuropathogy and Experimental Neurology 29: 583–600

Kaplan M S, Hinds J W 1977 Neurogenesis in the adult rat: electron microscopic analysis of light radioautographs. Science 197: 1092–1094

Katsetos C D, Herman M M, Frankfurter A et al 1989 Cerebellar desmoplastic medulloblastomas. A further immunohistochemical characterization of the reticulin-free pale islands. Archives of Pathology and Laboratory Medicine 113: 1019–1029

Katsetos C D, Frankfurter A, Christakos S et al 1991 Differential expression of neuronal class III β-tubulin isotype and calbindin D28 in the developing human cerebellar cortex and cerebellar neuroblastomas ("medulloblastomas"). Journal of Neuropathology and Experimental Neurology 50: 293

Katsetos C D, Frankfurter A, Christakos S, Mancall E L, Vlachos I N, Urich H 1993 Differential localization of class III, beta-tubulin isotype and calbindin-D28k defines distinct neuronal types in the developing human cerebellar cortex. Journal of Neuropathology and Experimental Neurology 52: 655–666

Keles G E, Berger M S, Schofield D, Bothwell M 1993 Nerve growth factor receptor expression in medulloblastomas and the potential role of nerve growth factor as a differentiating agent in medulloblastoma cell lines. Neurosurgery 32: 274–280

Kepes J J, Rubinstein L J, Ansbacher L, Schreiber D J 1989 Histopathological features of recurrent pleomorphic xanthoastrocytomas: Further corroboration of the glial nature of this neoplasm. Acta Neuropathologica 78: 585–593

Kettenmann H, Blankenfield G V, Trotter J 1991 Physiological properties of oligodendrocytes during development. Annals of the New York Academy of Sciences 633: 64–77

Kleihues P, Rajewsky M F 1984 Chemical neuro-oncogenesis: role of structural DNA modifications. DNA repair and neural target cell population. Program of Experimental Tumor Research 27: 1–16

Kleihues P, Aguzzi A, Shibata T, Wiestler O D 1989 Immunohistochemical assessment of differentiation and DNA replication in human brain tumors. In: Fields W S (ed) Primary brain tumors. A review of histologic classification. Springer Verlag, New York, pp 123–132

Kleihues P, Burger P C, Scheithauer B W 1993 Histological typing of tumours of the central nervous system, 2nd edn. Springer-Verlag, Berlin

Knott J C A, Pikington G J 1990 A2B5 surface ganglioside binding distinguishes between two GFAP-positive clones from a human glioma-derived line. Neuroscience Letters 118: 52–56

Korf H W, Czerwionka M, Reiner J, Schachenmayr W, Schalken J J, de Grip W, Gery I 1987 Immunocytochemical evidence of molecular photoreceptor markers in cerebellar medulloblastomas. Cancer 60: 1763–1766

Koury M J 1992 Programmed cell death (apoptosis) in hematopoiesis. Experimental Hematology 20: 391–394

Leclerc N, Schwarting G A, Herrup K, Hawkes R, Yamamoto M 1992 Compartmentation in mammalian cerebellum: Zebrin II and P-path antibodies define three classes of sagittally organized bands of Purkinje cells. Proceedings of the National Academy of Sciences 89: 5006–5010

Lee M K, Tuttle J B, Rebhun L I, Cleveland D W, Frankfurter A 1990 The expression and posttranslational modification of a neuron-specific β-tubulin isotype during chick embryogenesis. Cell Motility and Cytoskeleton 17: 118–132

Lee W-H, Javedan S, Bondy C A 1992 Coordinate expression of insulin-like growth factor system components by neurons and neuroglia during retinal and cerebellar development. Journal of Neuroscience 12: 4737–4744

Lemke G 1992 Gene regulation in the nervous system. In: Hall Z W (ed) An introduction to molecular neurobiology. Sinauer Associates, Sunderland, Ma, pp 313–354

Lemke G, Kuhn R, Monuki E S, Weinmaster G 1991 Expression and activity of the transcription factor SCIP during glial differentiation and myelination. Annals of the New York Academy of Sciences 633: 189–195

Lendahl U, Zimmerman L B, McKay R D G 1990 CNS stem cells express a new class of intermediate filament protein. Cell 60: 585–595
Levine J M, Stincone F, Lee Y-S 1993 Development and differentiation of glial precursor cells in the rat cerebellum. Glia 7: 307–321
Levison S W, Goldman J E 1993 Astrocyte origins. In: Murphy S (ed) Astrocytes: pharmacology and function. Academic Press, San Diego, CA, pp 1–22
Lewis P D 1981 Cell proliferation in the postnatal nervous system and its relationship to the origin of gliomas. Seminars in Neurology 1: 181–187
Liou G I, Geng L, Baehr W 1991 Interphotoreceptor retinoid-binding protein: biochemistry and molecular biology. In: Chader G J, Farber D (eds) Molecular biology of the retina: basic and clinically relevant studies. Alan R Liss, New York, pp 115–137
Lois C, Alvarez-Buylla A 1993 Proliferating subventricular zone cells in the adult mammalian forebrain can differentiate into neurons and glia. Proceedings of the National Academy of Sciences 90: 2074–2077
Luskin M B, Parnavelas J G, Barfield J A 1993 Neurons, astrocytes and oligodendrocytes of the rat cerebral cortex originate from separate progenitor cells: an ultrastructural analysis of clonally related cells. Journal of Neuroscience 13: 1730–1750
McKay R D G 1989 The origins of cellular diversity in the mammalian central nervous system. Cell 58: 815–821
McKinnon R D, Smith C, Behar T, Smith T, Dubois-Dalcq M 1993 Distinct effects of bFGF and PDGF on oligodendrocyte progenitor cells. Glia 7: 245–254
Margo C, Hydayat A, Kopelman J, Zimmerman L E 1983 Retinocytoma: A benign variant of retinoblastoma. Archives of Ophthalmology 101: 1519–1531
Marriott D R, Wilkin G P Substance p receptors on O-2A progenitor cells and type-2 astrocytes in vitro. Journal of Neurochemistry 61: 826–834
Martin P, Carriere C, Dozier et al 1992 Characterization of a paired box- and homeobox-containing quail gene (Pax-QNR) expressed in the neuroretina. Oncogene 7: 1721–1728
Marvin M, McKay R 1992 Multipotential stem cells in the vertebrate CNS. Cell Biology 3: 401–411
Mehler M F, Rozental R, Dougherty M, Spray D C, Kessler J A 1993 Cytokine regulation of neuronal differentiation of hippocampal progenitor cells. Nature 362: 62–65
Miller R H, Szigeti V 1991 Clonal analysis of astrocyte diversity in neonatal rat spinal cord cultures. Development 113: 933
Mishima K, Nakamura M, Nakamura H, Nakamura O, Funata N, Shitara N 1992 Leptomeningeal dissemination of cerebellar pilocytic astrocytoma. Journal of Neurosurgery 77: 788–791
Molenaar W M, Jansson D S, Gould V E et al 1989 Molecular markers of primitive neuroectodermal tumors and other pediatric central nervous system tumors. Laboratory Investigation 61: 635–643
Mukai N, Kobayashi S 1973 Primary brain and spinal cord tumors induced by human adenovirus type 12 in hamsters. Journal of Neuropathology and Experimental Neurology 32: 523–541
Noble M, Wren D, Wolswijk G 1992 The O2-A adult progenitor cell: a glial stem cell of the adult central nervous system. Seminars in Cell Biology 3: 413–422
Pixley S K R, DeVellis J 1984 Transition between immature radial glia and mature astrocytes studied with a monoclonal antibody to vimentin. Development Brain Research 15: 201–209
Podesta A H, Mullins J, Pierce G B, Wells R S 1984 The neurula stage mouse embryo in control neuroblastoma. Proceedings of the National Academy of Science USA 81: 7608–7611
Price J 1989 Cell lineage and lineage markers. Current Opinion in Cell Biology 1: 1071–1074
Price J, Williams B, Moore R, Read J, Grove E 1991 Analysis of cell lineage in the rat cerebral cortex. Annals of the New York Academy of Sciences 633: 56–63
Raaf J, Kernohan J 1944 Relation of abnormal collections of cells in posterior medullary velum of cerebellum to origin of medulloblastoma. Archives of Neurology and Psychiatry 52: 163–169
Raff M C, Barres B A, Burne J F, Coles H S, Ishizaki Y, Jacobson M D 1993 Programmed cell death and the control of cell survival: Lessons from the nervous system. Science 262: 695
Rajewsky M F 1985 Chemical carcinogenesis in the developing nervous system. In: Snati L, Zardi L (eds) Theories and models in cellular transformation. Academic Press, London, pp 156–171
Rakic P, Sidman R L 1970 Histogenesis of cortical layers in human cerebellum, particularly the lamina dissecans. Journal of Comparative Neurology 139: 473–500
Ransom B R 1991 Vertebrate glial classification, lineage, and heterogeneity. Annals of the New York Academy of Sciences 633: 19–34
Rao C, Friedlander M E, Klein E, Anzil A P, Sher J H 1990 Medullomyoblastoma in an adult. Cancer 65: 157–163
Raymond P A 1991 Cell determination and positional cues in the teleost retina: development of photoreceptors and horizontal cells. In: Lam D M-K, Shatz C J (eds) Development of the visual system. MIT, Cambridge, pp 59–78
Razin A, Cedar H 1991 DNA methylation and gene expression. Microbiological Reviews 55: 451–458
Reh T, Kljavin I J 1989 Age of differentiation determines rat retinal germinal phenotype: Induction of differentiation by dissociation. Journal of Neuroscience 9: 4179–4189
Renfranz P J, Cunningham M G, McKay R D G 1991 Regio-specific differentiation of the hippocampal stem cell line hib5 upon implantation into the developing mammalian brain. Cell 66: 713–729
Rubinstein L J 1985 Embryonal central neuroepithelial tumors and their differentiating potential. Journal of Neurosurgery 62: 795–805
Rudge J S 1993 Astrocyte-derived neurotrophic factors. In: Murphy S (ed) Astrocytes: pharmacology and function. Academic Press, San Diego, CA, pp 267–305
Russell D S, Rubinstein L J 1989 Pathology of tumours of the nervous system, 5th edn. Edward Arnold, London
Schiffer D, Giordana M T, Mauro A, Migheli A, Germano I, Giaccone G 1986 Immunohistochemical demonstration of vimentin in human cerebral tumors. Acta Neuropathologica 70: 209–219
Schiffer D, Cavalla P, Chio A, Giordana M T, Marino S, Mauro A, Migheli A 1994 Tumor cell proliferation and apoptosis in medulloblastoma. Acta Neuropathologica 87: 362–370
Schindler E, Gullotta F 1983 Glial fibrillary acidic protein in medulloblastomas and other embryonic CNS tumours of children. Virchows Archives [A] 398: 263–275
Shiurba R A, Buffinger N S, Spencer E M, Urich H 1991 Basic fibroblastic growth factor and somatomedin c in human medulloepithelioma. Cancer 68: 798–808
Snyder E Y, Deitcher D L, Walsh C, Arnold-Aldea S, Hartwieg E A, Cepko C L 1992 Multipotential neural cell lines can engraft and participate in development of mouse cerebellum. Cell 68: 33–51
Sparrow J R, Hicks J D, Barnstable C J 1990 Cell commitment and differentiation in explants of embryonic rat neural retina. Comparison with the developmental potential of dissociated retina. Developmental Brain Research 51: 69–84
Steindler D A 1993 Glial boundaries in the developing nervous system. Annual Review of Neuroscience 16: 445–470
Stevenson L, Echlin R 1934 The nature and origin of some tumors of the cerebellum (medulloblastoma). Archives of Neurology and Psychiatry 31: 93–109
Swanson P E 1994 *bcl*-2 oncopeptide immunoreactivity in medulloblastoma. Modern Pathology 7: 140A
Swenberg J A 1977 Chemical- and virus-induced brain tumors. Modern concepts in brain tumor therapy: Laboratory and clinical investigations. National Cancer Institute Monograph 46: 3–10
Temple S 1990 Characteristics of cells that give rise to the central nervous system. Journal of Cell Science 97: 213–218
Tohyama T, Lee V M-Y, Rorke L B, Marvin M, McKay R D G, Trojanowski J Q 1992 Nestin expression in embryonic human neuroepithelium and in human neuroepithelial tumor cells. Laboratory Investigation 66: 303–313
Tohyama T, Lee V M-Y, Rorke L B, Marvin M, McKay R D G, Trojanowski J Q 1993 Monoclonal antibodies to a rat nestin fusion protein recognize a 22kDa polypeptide in subsets of fetal and adult human central nervous system neurons and in primitive neuroectodermal tumor cells. American Journal of Pathology 143: 258–268
Toth L E, Slawin K L, Pintar J E, Nguyen-Huu M C 1987 Region-specific expression of mouse homeobox gene in the embryonic

mesoderm and central nervous system. Proceedings of the National Academy of Science 84: 6790–6794

Treacy M N, Rosenfeld M G 1992 Expression of a family of POU-domain protein regulatory genes during development of the central nervous system. Annual Reviews of Neuroscience 15: 139–165

Trojanowski J Q, Tohyama T, Lee V M-Y 1992 Medulloblastomas and related primitive neuroectodermal brain tumors of childhood recapitulate molecular milestones in the maturation of neuroblasts. Molecular and Chemical Neuropathology 17: 121–135

Turner D L, Cepko C L 1987 A common progenitor for neurons and glia persists in rat retina late in development. Nature 328: 131–136

VandenBerg S R 1992 Current diagnostic concepts of astrocytic tumors. Journal of Neuropathology and Experimental Neurology 51: 644–657

VandenBerg S R 1993 Desmoplastic infantile ganglioglioma and desmoplastic cerebral astrocytoma of infancy. Brain Pathology 3: 275–281

VandenBerg S R, Chatel M, Griffiths O M, DeArmond S J, Pappas C, Herman M M 1981a Neural differentiation in the OTT-6050 mouse teratoma: production of a tumor fraction restricted to stem cells and neural cells after centrifugal elutriation. Virchows Archives of Pathology [A] 392: 281–294

VandenBerg S R, Hess J R, Herman M M, DeArmond S J, Halks-Miller M, Rubinstein L J 1981b Neural differentiation in the OTT-6050 mouse teratoma: production of a tumor fraction showing melanogenesis in neuroepithelial cells after centrifugal elutriation. Virchows Archives of Pathology [A] 392: 295–308

VandenBerg S R, Herman M M, Rubinstein L J 1987 Embryonal central neuroepithelial tumors: Current concepts and future challenges. Cancer and Metastasis Reviews 5: 343–364

Vayasse P J J, Goldman J E 1992 A distinct type of GD3+, flat astrocyte in rat CNS cultures. Journal of Neuroscience 12: 330–337

von Deimling A, Janzer R, Kleihues P, Wiestler O D 1990 Patterns of differentiation in central neurocytoma: an immunohistochemical study of eleven biopsies. Acta Neuropathologica 79: 473–479

Walsh C, Cepko C L 1993 Clonal dispersion in proliferative layers of developing cerebral cortex. Nature 362: 632–635

Watanbe T, Raff M C 1990 Rod photoreceptor development in vitro. Intrinsic properties of proliferating neuroepithelial cells change as development proceeds in the rat retina. Neuron 2: 461–467

Webb D J, LaMarre J, Gonias S L 1992 Effect of human α-thrombin on the transforming growth factor-β1-binding activity of human α_2-macroglobulin. Seminars in Thrombosis and Hemostasis 18: 305–310

Weldon-Linne G M, Victor T A, Groothuis D R, Vick N A 1983 Pleomorphic xanthoastrocytoma: ultrastructural and immunohistochemical study of a case with a rapidly fatal outcome following surgery. Cancer 52: 2055–2063

Wetts R, Fraser S E 1988 Multipotent precursors can give rise to all major cell types in the frog retina. Science 239: 1142–1145

Whittle I R, Gordon A, Misra B K et al 1989 Pleomorphic xanthoastrocytoma: report of four cases. Journal of Neurosurgery 70: 463–468

Wilkinson M, Hume R, Strange R, Bell J E 1990 Glial and neuronal differentiation in the human fetal brain 9–23 weeks of gestation. Neuropathology and Applied Neurobiology 16: 193–204

Wolswijk G, Noble M J 1992 Cooperation between PDGF and FGF converts slowly dividing O-2A progenitor cells to rapidly dividing cells. Cell Biology 118: 889–900

Wright C V E, Cho K W Y, Oliver G, DeRobertis E M 1989 Vertebrate homeodomain proteins: families of region-specific transcription factors. Trends in Biochemical Sciences 14: 52–56

Yachnis A T, Rorke L B, Lee V M-Y, Trojanowski J Q 1993 Expression of neuronal and glial polypeptides during histogenesis of the human cerebellar cortex including observations on the dentate nucleus. Journal of Comparative Neurology 334: 356–369

Yamada T, Pfaff S L, Edlund T, Jessell T M 1993 Control of cell pattern in the neural tube: motor neuron induction by diffusion factors from notochord and floor plate. Cell 73: 673–686

Young J Z 1991 The concept of neuroglia. Annals of the New York Academy of Sciences 633: 1–18

3. Classification and pathogenesis of brain tumors

Michael F. Gonzales

INTRODUCTION

Formulation of an enduring and widely accepted classification schema of central nervous system (CNS) tumors has been problematic because of their peculiar biology and variety. Present schemata have evolved from the early histogenetic formulations of Bailey & Cushing and Penfield, but reflect the more accurate determination of cell lineage that has become possible with the raising of monoclonal and polyclonal antibodies against a variety of cell markers. Undoubtedly, new data uncovered by molecular genetic techniques will, in a similar way, shape future classifications. The evolution of modern classifications has also been influenced by the accumulation of survival data indicating that splitting of some tumors into confusing subcategories is not justified. For the same reason, however, new types of tumors such as the dysembryoplastic neuroepithelial tumor (DNET), have also been recognized.

CLASSIFICATION AND GRADING SCHEMATA OF CNS TUMORS — HISTORICAL ASPECTS

The first macroscopic descriptions of brain tumors were published by Cruveilhier in 1829. In 1836, Bressler described a number of brain tumors and categorized them macroscopically as fatty, fleshy and bony tumors, medullary sarcomas, melanoses, cystic tumors and hydatids (cited in Leestma 1980). Then, in 1860, Virchow described the neuroglia (literally 'nerve glue') as the interstitial matrix of the brain in which individual cells are suspended. Most of the subsequent advances in understanding the pathology of brain tumors in the remainder of the 19th century can be attributed to Virchow. He was the first to attempt a correlation of the macroscopic and microscopic features of CNS tumors and the first to use the term 'glioma'. The gliomas were described as slowly growing, poorly circumscribed lesions which diffusely infiltrated but did not destroy the brain parenchyma. In contrast, the sarcomas were clearly demarcated from adjacent brain, grew rapidly, exerting what is now recognized as mass effect on adjacent brain, and were frequently hemorrhagic and necrotic. Golgi, in 1884, proposed a narrower definition of 'gliomas' as only tumors composed of fibrous cells. He regarded these as benign tumors. Later, in 1900, Virchow re-interpreted tumors of the dura which we now recognize as meningiomas. He called these 'psammomas' because they contained the concentrically laminated, calcified structures known as psammoma bodies and separated them from dural sarcomas.

Using the heavy metal impregnation techniques perfected by Cajal (1913) and del Rio-Hortega (1919) to demonstrate the morphology of the different cells in the brain, Bailey & Cushing, in 1926, published their schema for classifying gliomas (Fig. 3.1). This schema was based on an hypothesis for CNS histogenesis from primitive medullary epithelium or, as it would now be termed, primitive neuroectoderm, via glial and neuronal precursors and proposed 14 tumor types. The development of each type was suggested to result from developmental arrest at a particular histogenetic stage (Ribbert 1918) and therefore tumors could be classified by correlating the morphological features of their cells with those of normal cells at each defined stage of histogenesis. Though useful because it directed attention to the process of differentiation, Bailey & Cushing's classification suffered from its essentially hypothetical nature and the realization that cells at each of the proposed stages of histogenesis are difficult to recognize morphologically. An important contribution was later made by Cox (1933), who suggested that incorporated, non-neoplastic cells may take on morphological features similar to those of cells at the different stages of histogenesis proposed by Bailey & Cushing. For these reasons, neuropathologists found this classification difficult to apply with acceptable uniformity.

The Bailey & Cushing schema, however, dominated thinking about the gliomas until 1949 when Kernohan and his colleagues put forward a much simpler classification. Kernohan had long believed that glial tumors develop from terminally differentiated cells and that

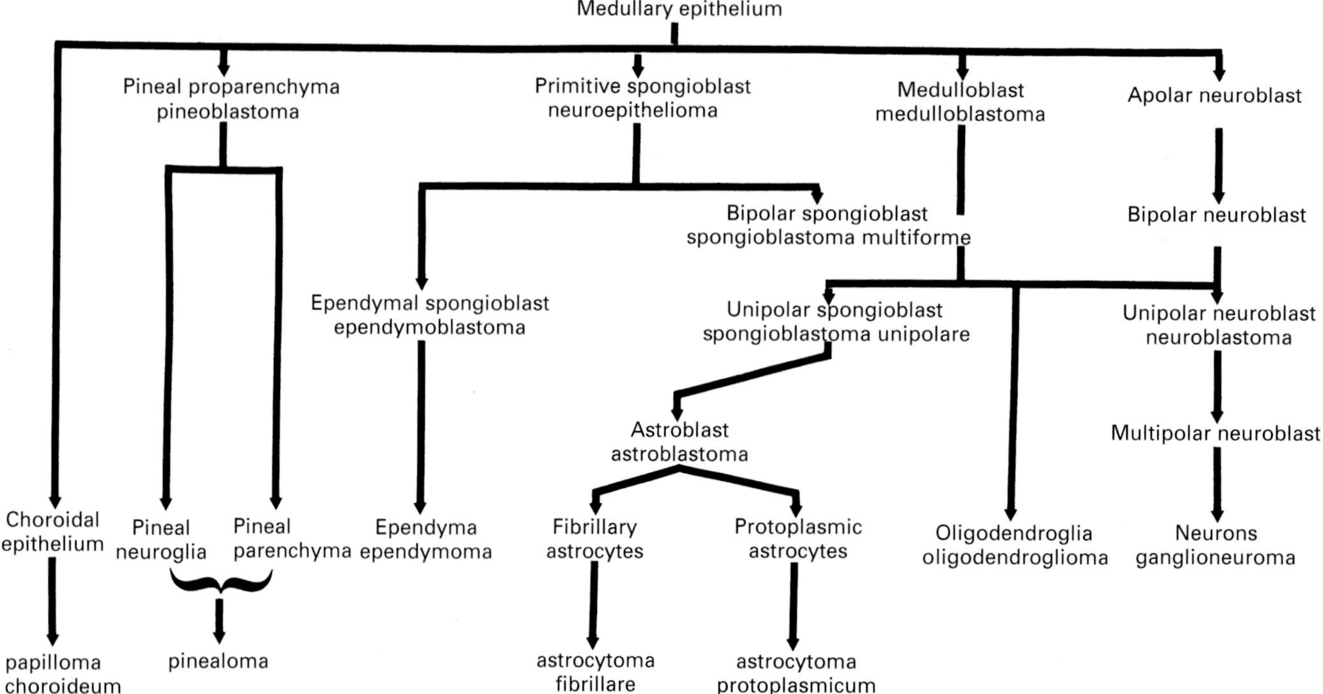

Fig. 3.1 Bailey and Cushing schema for the classification of gliomas (Bailey & Cushing 1926)

different histopathologic appearances do not represent separate tumor types but rather different degrees of dedifferentiation of one tumor type. Thus he dispensed with the confusing histogenetic terminology of Bailey & Cushing and reduced the number of categories of glial tumors from 14 to five — astrocytoma, ependymoma, oligodendroglioma, neuro-astrocytoma and medulloblastoma. He also recognized that mixed glial tumors, in particular oligo-astrocytomas, could occur but did not include these as a separate category. Most importantly, however, Kernohan re-introduced the idea, previously put forward by Tooth in 1912, that the biologic behavior of these tumors could be reckoned from their histopathologic features and proposed a four-tier grading system for astrocytomas and ependymomas. This was based on increasing anaplasia and decreasing differentiation with increasing grade of tumor, similar to the principles for grading carcinoma previously established by Broders (1925).

Introduction of the Kernohan grading system for glial tumors marked the beginning of an era in which attention was directed more at formulating an acceptable grading schema and less at refining different classifications based on histogenesis. The major reason for this shift in emphasis was an increasing awareness amongst neuropathologists, neurosurgeons and neuro-oncologists that a meaningful classification schema of CNS tumors should give some indication of biologic behavior and provide a basis for the development of treatment protocols. Several problems were encountered in applying the Kernohan grading system because many criteria, particularly the assessment of anaplasia and cellularity, are subjective and prone to interobserver variation. This subjectivity gave rise to meaningless, indeterminate gradings such as grade 1–2 and 2–3. Another problem was that necrosis was included by Kernohan as a feature of both astrocytoma grade III and grade IV. Separation of these two grades was based on the denser cellularity, more severe anaplasia and higher mitotic count in grade IV compared with grade III. A communication accompanying the publication of Kernohan's classification and grading schema reported postoperative survival data for 161 patients with astrocytomas graded according to the Kernohan system. These showed a significantly longer mean postoperative survival period and better 3-year survival rate for grade III compared with grade IV (Svien et al 1949). However, there was not a significant difference in the 3-year survival rates for grade II and grade III. These data suggested that a three-tier system of grading might be more appropriate than the more widely used four-tier system.

A system proposing three grades — astrocytoma, astrocytoma with anaplastic foci and glioblastoma multiforme — was put forward in 1950 by Ringertz. In this system, separation between the grades on histologic criteria was much clearer, with the presence of necrosis defining glioblastoma multiforme. Despite the simplicity of its application, the three-tier system did not gain wide acceptance until the mid 1980s, when it was again proposed as a preferable schema to four-tier systems and was promoted for the grading of ependymomas and oligodendrogliomas as well as astrocytic tumors.

The association of necrosis with aggressive biologic behavior and reduced postoperative survival was highlighted in a number of reports of astrocytomas graded by the Ringertz schema (Burger & Vollmer 1980, Nelson et al 1983, Burger et al 1985, Fulling & Garcia 1985, Garcia et al 1985). However, with the publication of survival statistics, it became apparent that there was a wide range in the postoperative survival periods of patients with tumors graded astrocytoma with anaplastic foci or, as this grade has become known, anaplastic astrocytoma (Fulling & Garcia 1985). This led to closer scrutiny of grading schemata by some neuropathologists and movement towards developing a system of grading based on specific histopathologic features in an attempt to determine which were significant indicators of biologic behavior and prognosis. These efforts were embodied in a grading schema proposed by Daumas-Duport & Szikla in 1981 and later supported by survival data (Daumas-Duport et al 1988a). In applying this system, tumors are assessed according to the presence or absence of four morphologic features — nuclear atypia, mitoses, endothelial cell proliferation and necrosis — and graded according to this feature score. Grade 1 tumors have none of the features, grade 2 tumors have 1 feature, grade 3 tumors have 2 features, and grade 4 tumors have 3 or 4 features. In their 1988 publication, Daumas-Duport and her colleagues reported the results of applying their grading schema to 287 astrocytic tumors. Their data showed that the feature score system clearly identified four distinct grades of malignancy, with median survivals of 4 years for grade 2, 1.6 years for grade 3, and 0.7 years for grade 4 tumors respectively. They also reported 94% concordance in grading between different observers. Despite its advantages over the four-tier grading system of Kernohan, the Daumas-Duport system has not yet gained wide acceptance and is presently followed in only a few North American centers.

Several other grading schemata have been developed in North American and European neuro-oncology centers, all supported by local survival data. However, internationally, the Kernohan and Ringertz formulations and, to a slightly lesser extent, the Daumas-Duport system remain the key schemata for the grading of glial tumors.

FORMULATION OF THE WHO CLASSIFICATION OF CNS TUMORS

In 1976, the World Health Organization commissioned a group of eminent neuropathologists to formulate a new classification schema of central nervous system tumors. Their aim was to develop a classification of all central nervous system tumors, not only of the gliomas. This was published three years later (Zulch 1979). Revision of that original classification was undertaken between 1989 and 1990 and has been published in provisional form (Kepes 1990 — Table 3.1). As in the original schema, the revised classification divides tumors according to cell or tissue of origin. Nine categories are recognized — neuroepithelial tumors, tumors of cranial and spinal nerves, tumors of the meninges, hemopoietic tumors, germ cell tumors, cysts and tumor-like lesions, anterior pituitary tumors, local extensions of regional tumors, and metastatic tumors. The categories of unclassified tumors, vascular malformations and vascular tumors in the 1979 schema are no longer included. Capillary hemangioblastoma and monstrocellular sarcoma, regarded as vascular tumors in the 1979 schema, have been reclassified. Hemangioblastoma is now regarded as a mesenchymal, non-meningothelial tumor, but of uncertain histogenesis, while monstrocellular sarcoma is included in tumors of neuroepithelial origin as a subtype of glioblastoma multiforme.

Proposed revision of the 1979 WHO classification of CNS tumors (Kepes 1990)

I. Tumors of neuroepithelial tissue

Nine subcategories of tumors of neuroepithelial tissue are proposed — astrocytic, oligodendroglial, ependymal and mixed glial tumors, choroid plexus tumors, neuroepithelial tumors of uncertain histogenesis, neuronal and mixed neuronal-glial tumors, pineal tumors and embryonal tumors.

A. Astrocytic tumors. The first three categories of astrocytic tumors — astrocytoma, anaplastic astrocytoma and glioblastoma multiforme — reflect the incorporation of a grading schema into the revised classification. The features distinguishing these three categories are essentially degrees of cellularity and anaplasia, with mitotic figures and endothelial cell proliferation being additional features of anaplastic astrocytoma and glioblastoma multiforme. As in the three-tier grading schema, necrosis is stressed as the defining feature of glioblastoma multiforme. Fibrillary, protoplasmic, gemistocytic and mixed astrocytomas are listed as histologic variants of ordinary astrocytoma while giant cell glioblastoma and gliosarcoma are included as histologic variants of glioblastoma multiforme. The suggestion inherent in including protoplasmic and gemistocytic astrocytomas as histologic variants only of ordinary astrocytoma is somewhat misleading as both of these patterns can be seen in anaplastic astrocytomas and glioblastomas multiforme.

Pilocytic astrocytoma, pleomorphic xanthoastrocytoma and subependymal giant cell astrocytoma are correctly separated from the more common types of astrocytoma. Each is histopathologically distinct. Survival data have shown that pilocytic and subependymal giant cell astrocytomas are non-aggressive tumors (Chow et al 1988, Wallner et al 1988). Although these two tumors are readily identified by their distinctive histopathologic features, their benign behavior is not linked to these features and

Table 3.1 World Health Organization proposed new classification of CNS tumors

I. Tumors of neuroepithelial tissue
   A. Astrocytic tumors
      1. Astrocytoma
         Variants: fibrillary, protoplasmic, gemistocytic, mixed
      2. Anaplastic (malignant) astrocytoma
      3. Glioblastoma
         Variants: giant cell glioblastoma, gliosarcoma
      4. Pilocytic astrocytoma
      5. Pleomorphic xanthoastrocytoma
      6. Subependymal giant cell astrocytoma
   B. Oligodendroglial tumors
      1. Oligodendroglioma
      2. Anaplastic (malignant) oligodendroglioma
   C. Ependymal tumors
      1. Ependymoma
         Variants: cellular papillary, epithelial, clear cell, mixed
      2. Anaplastic (malignant) ependymoma
      3. Myxopapillary ependymoma
      4. Subependymoma
   D. Mixed gliomas
      1. Mixed oligo-astrocytoma
      2. Anaplastic (malignant) oligo-astrocytoma
      3. Others
   E. Choroid plexus tumors
      1. Choroid plexus papilloma
      2. Choroid plexus carcinoma
   F. Neuroepithelial tumors of uncertain origin
      1. Astroblastoma
      2. Polar spongioblastoma
      3. Gliomatosis cerebri
   G. Neuronal and mixed neuronal-glial tumors
      1. Gangliocytoma
      2. Dysplastic gangliocytoma of the cerebellum (Lhermitte-Duclos)
      3. Desmoplastic infantile ganglioglioma
      4. Dysembryoplastic neuroepithelial tumor
      5. Ganglioglioma
      6. Anaplastic (malignant) ganglioglioma
   H. Pineal tumors
      1. Pineocytoma
      2. Pineoblastoma
      3. Mixed pineocytoma/pineoblastoma
   I. Embryonal tumors
      1. Medulloepithelioma
      2. Neuroblastoma
         Variant: ganglioneuroblastoma
      3. Ependymoblastoma
      4. Retinoblastoma
      5. Primitive neuroectodermal tumors (PNET)
         with multipotential differentiation — neuronal, astrocytic, ependymal, muscle, melanocytic, etc.
         a. Medulloblastoma
            Variants: desmoplastic, medullomyoblastoma, melanocytic medulloblastoma
         b. Cerebral (supratentorial) and spinal PNETs

II. Tumors of cranial and spinal nerves
   A. Schwannoma (syn: neurilemmoma, neurinoma)
      Variants: cellular, plexiform, melanotic
   B. Neurofibroma
      Variants: circumscribed (solitary), plexiform, mixed neurofibroma/schwannoma
   C. Malignant peripheral nerve sheath tumor (MPNST)
      (syn: neurogenic sarcoma, anaplastic neurofibroma, malignant schwannoma)
      Variants: epithelioid, MPNST with divergent mesenchymal and/or epithelial differentiation, melanotic

III. Tumors of the meninges
   A. Tumors of meningothelial cells
      1. Meningioma
         Histologic types:
         a. Meningothelial (syncytial)
         b. Transitional/mixed
         c. Fibrous (fibroblastic)
         d. Psammomatous
         e. Angiomatous
         f. Microcystic
         g. Secretory
         h. Clear cell
         i. Chordoid
         j. Lymphoplasmacyte-rich
         k. Metaplastic variants (xanthomatous, myxoid, osseous, chondroid)
      2. Atypical meningioma
      3. Anaplastic (malignant) meningioma
      Variants: of a–k above, papillary
   B. Mesenchymal, non-meningothelial tumors
      Benign:
      1. Osteocartilagenous tumors
      2. Lipoma
      3. Fibrous histiocytoma
      4. Others
      Malignant
      1. Mesenchymal chondrosarcoma
      2. Malignant fibrous histiocytoma
      3. Rhabdomyosarcoma
      4. Meningeal sarcomatosis
      5. Others
   C. Primary melanocytic lesions
      1. Diffuse melanosis
      2. Melanocytoma
      3. Malignant melanoma
      Variant: meningeal melanomatosis
   D. Tumors of uncertain origin
      1. Hemangiopericytoma
      2. Capillary hemangioblastoma

IV. Hemopoietic neoplasms
   1. Malignant lymphomas
   2. Plasmacytoma
   3. Granulocytic sarcoma
   4. Others

V. Germ cell tumors
   1. Germinoma
   2. Embryonal carcinoma
   3. Yolk sac tumor (endodermal sinus tumor)
   4. Choriocarcinoma
   5. Teratoma
      Variants: immature, teratoma with malignant transformation
   6. Mixed germ cell tumors

VI. Cysts and tumor-like lesions
   A. Rathke's cleft cyst
   B. Epidermoid cyst
   C. Dermoid cyst
   D. Colloid cyst of the third ventricle
   E. Enterogenous cyst (syn: neuroenteric cyst)
   F. Neuroglial cyst
   G. Other cysts
   H. Lipoma
   I. Granular cell tumor (syn: choristoma, pituicytoma)
   J. Hypothalamic neuronal hamartoma
   K. Nasal glial heterotopias

VII. Tumors of the anterior pituitary
   A. Pituitary adenoma
   B. Pituitary carcinoma

VIII. Local extensions from regional tumors
   A. Craniopharyngioma
      Variants: adamantinomatous, squamous papillary
   B. Paraganglioma (syn: chemodectoma)
   C. Chordoma
      Variant: chondroid chordoma
   D. Chondroma
   E. Chondrosarcoma
   F. Adenoid cystic carcinoma (syn: cylindroma)
   G. Others

IX. Metastatic tumors

they are not graded. Pilocytic astrocytomas are commonly midline tumors, occurring in the optic chiasm, third ventricle and brainstem. Cystic pilocytic tumors are also seen in the cerebellar and cerebral hemispheres in both children and adults (Palma & Guidetti 1985). Pleomorphic xanthoastrocytoma, when first reported (Kepes et al 1979), was also regarded as an astrocytoma subtype with a favorable prognosis. However, with wider recognition of this subtype and longer follow-up, the view has been reached that the majority are associated with prolonged survival but that some may behave aggressively, in the mold of glioblastoma multiforme (Weldon-Linne et al 1983, Kepes et al 1989).

B. Oligodendroglial tumors. Two categories of oligodendroglial tumors — oligodendroglioma and anaplastic or malignant oligodendroglioma — are distinguished. This is in line with the 1979 classification and refutes schemata that have attempted to grade oligodendrogliomas on the basis of their histopathologic features (Smith et al 1983, Mork et al 1986).

C. Ependymal tumors. Four categories of ependymal tumors are delineated — ependymoma, anaplastic or malignant ependymoma, myxopapillary ependymoma and subependymoma. Several histologic variants of ordinary ependymoma are also listed — cellular, papillary, epithelial, clear cell (Kawano et al 1989) and mixed. Myxopapillary ependymoma and subependymoma are now placed in separate subcategories rather than being listed as histologic variants of ordinary ependymoma as in the 1979 schema. The rationale for this modification is the very specific anatomic relationship of myxopapillary ependymomas of the filum terminale of the spinal cord and the characteristic histopathologic features of subependymomas combined with their benign behavior compared with ordinary ependymomas and their association with tuberous sclerosis. As with oligodendrogliomas, the schema resists grading of ependymomas on histopathologic features.

D. Mixed gliomas. Mixed tumors were recognized in the original classification but were listed under oligodendroglial tumors. The revised classification places them in a category in their own right with subtypes of mixed oligo-astrocytoma, anaplastic (malignant) oligo-astrocytoma and others.

E. Choroid plexus tumors. This represents a new separate category of neuroepithelial tumors having been previously linked with ependymal tumors. Two subcategories — choroid plexus papilloma and carcinoma — are distinguished.

F. Neuroepithelial tumors of uncertain origin. The three tumors listed in this category — astroblastoma, polar spongioblastoma and gliomatosis cerebri — have always proven difficult to classify satisfactorily. In the 1979 schema, astroblastoma was classified as a subtype of astrocytoma while polar spongioblastoma and gliomatosis cerebri were placed in the poorly differentiated and embryonal tumor category. Since the original histogenetic classification of Bailey & Cushing, there has been disagreement over whether polar spongioblasts and astroblasts in fact exist, or whether this terminology describes architectural arrangements of cells in some tumors. Rubinstein & Herman (1989) argued for the existence of astroblasts and suggested that, like ependymal cells, they differentiate from radial glia, otherwise known as tanicytes. The nature of polar spongioblasts is less clear. These are spindle cells with bipolar processes that, in tumors, are arranged in palisades. Russell & Cairns (1947) regarded 'true' polar spongioblastomas as poorly differentiated astrocytomas. The palisading that had previously been regarded as characteristic of these tumors was later described in some oligodendrogliomas (Russell & Rubinstein 1989) and cerebral neuroblastomas (Ojeda et al 1987). The majority of neuropathologists regard gliomatosis cerebri as a diffuse infiltration of the brain by neoplastic astrocytes.

G. Neuronal and mixed neuronal-glial tumors. There are six categories of neuronal and mixed neuronal-glial tumors. Gangliocytoma, ganglioglioma and anaplastic (malignant) ganglioglioma have been retained from the 1979 schema, and dysplastic gangliocytoma of the cerebellum (Lhermitte-Duclos), desmoplastic infantile ganglioglioma and dysembryoplastic neuroepithelial tumor are added, the last two tumors having been described since 1979.

The spectrum of gangliocytoma is expanded to include the since-described central neurocytoma. This is a histologically distinctive tumor occurring almost exclusively in the ventricles. Because of similar histopathologic features, neurocytomas were probably designated as oligodendrogliomas before the demonstration of neuronal lineage by immunohistochemistry and electron microscopy (Hassoun et al 1982, Townsend & Seaman 1986). Neuroblastoma and ganglioneuroblastoma have been reclassified as embryonal tumors. Although categorized in the revised schema as a neoplasm, dysplastic gangliocytoma of the cerebellum is regarded by the majority of neuropathologists as a malformative or hamartomatous lesion (Ambler et al 1969). This assessment is supported by their benign behavior and histopathologic features — enlarged cerebellar folia with disrupted cortical architecture, well-developed myelinated fibers forming an outer layer and abnormal neurons resembling Purkinje cells forming an inner layer.

Desmoplastic infantile gangliogliomas (DIG) are supratentorial tumors of the frontal and parietal regions that occur almost exclusively in infants (VandenBerg et al 1987). They are usually very large with pronounced contrast enhancement. The histologic features are dominated by fibrous astrocytes and pronounced desmoplasia. Neurons are also present but occasionally may be inconspicuous. Long tumor-free survival periods have been reported in patients with DIGs and, where they have been subtotally resected, no evidence of tumor progression has been detected.

Dysembryoplastic neuroepithelial tumors (DNET) are regarded as hamartomatous lesions. When first reported (Daumas-Duport et al 1988b) they were noted to have an association with intractable complex partial seizures in young patients. Macroscopically, they are multinodular lesions often confined to an expanded cortex. The majority occur in the temporal and frontal lobes. Cellular heterogeneity with astrocytic, oligodendroglial and neuronal elements is a characteristic microscopic feature. Follow-up studies have confirmed the benign nature of DNETs. Because of the localized nature of these lesions, complete surgical resection is frequently achieved and there is no indication for postoperative radiotherapy.

Gangliogliomas display a wide variation in the content of ganglion cell and glial components. Part of the definition of a ganglioglioma is that the ganglion cells should be seen to be participating in the neoplastic process. This is often difficult to assess, particularly in examples in which the ganglion cells are predominant as they usually appear histologically benign. The behavior of this type of ganglioglioma is benign, and it has been suggested to be a variety of neuronal hamartoma. In anaplastic or malignant gangliogliomas, ganglion cells have atypical features, in particular, multi-nucleation but, probably more important, the glial cell component is predominant and frequently has the features of anaplastic astrocytoma. Some neuropathologists regard the presence of anaplastic astrocytoma to be the determinant of tumor behavior and prognosis and disregard the ganglion cell component, particularly if it is quantitatively less than the glial cell component.

H. Pineal tumors. Pineal tumors, as a category of neuroepithelial tumors is retained and, as in the 1979 schema, these are subdivided into pineocytoma and pineoblastoma. Mixed pineocytoma/pineoblastoma, however, is an additional subcategory.

I. Embryonal tumors. This category has been considerably altered in content. Glioblastoma, polar spongioblastoma and gliomatosis cerebri have been reclassified as subtypes of astrocytoma and neuroepithelial tumors of uncertain origin respectively. Neuroblastoma, retinoblastoma and ependymoblastoma have been added, together with the extremely controversial primitive neuroectodermal tumour (PNET). As in the 1979 schema, medulloepithelioma and medulloblastoma remain in this category, with the latter regarded as a subtype of PNET. The category of primitive neuroectodermal tumor encompasses a range of tumors that can be subdivided into three main types: those showing predominantly neuroblastic and/or neuronal differentiation, those containing neuroblastic and, to a lesser extent, glial components, and those that appear to be truly undifferentiated. Medulloblastoma, with its variants of desmoplastic, myoblastomatous and melanocytic, best fits the first of these categories. Immunoreactivity for glial fibrillary acidic protein (GFAP) can be demonstrated in a number of medulloblastomas. These are examples of the second subtype of PNET. Cerebral and spinal forms of PNETs are also recognized.

II. Tumors of cranial and spinal nerves

Three major categories of peripheral nerve tumors are listed: schwannoma (syn: neurilemmoma, neurinoma), neurofibroma and malignant peripheral nerve sheath tumor (syn: malignant schwannoma, anaplastic neurofibroma, neurogenic sarcoma). This is essentially the same breakdown of cranial and spinal nerve tumors as in the 1979 schema. Cellular, plexiform and melanotic schwannomas are now recognized as histologic variants. Variants of neurofibroma include circumscribed (solitary), plexiform and mixed neurofibroma/schwannoma. Three subtypes of malignant peripheral nerve sheath tumor are listed: epithelioid, malignant peripheral nerve sheath tumor with divergent mesenchymal and/or epithelial differentiation and melanotic.

III. Tumors of the meninges

This category of CNS tumors has also undergone significant reorganization in the revised classification. Four subcategories are recognized: tumors of meningothelial cells, mesenchymal, non-meningothelial tumors, primary melanocytic lesions, and tumors of uncertain origin. The subcategory of meningothelial cell tumors encompasses conventional meningiomas and their atypical and malignant counterparts. Eleven histologic subtypes of conventional, atypical and malignant meningioma are listed, with papillary meningioma an additional histologic subtype of malignant meningioma.

Many neuropathologists would argue that there is little to be gained from subtyping meningiomas into eleven categories by histologic pattern because there are no data suggesting that any one of these histological subtypes behaves differently from any other. However, systemic effects, related to dysglobulinemia and bone marrow plasmacytosis, have been reported in patients with meningiomas that contain prominent infiltrates of lymphocytes and plasma cells (Horten et al 1979). A syndrome of growth retardation, elevated erythrocyte sedimentation rate and hypochromic anemia has also been reported in young children with the chordoid type of meningioma (Kepes et al 1988). These show areas of myxoid degeneration and lymphoplasmacytic infiltration that is sometimes the dominant histopathologic feature.

In assessing meningiomas histopathologically, the significant features that relate to biologic behavior are degree of cellularity, presence of appreciable numbers of mitotic figures, foci of micronecrosis that cannot be ascribed to pre-operative embolization, and invasion of underlying brain. The last two features, in particular, are associated with increased frequency of local recurrence and reduced postoperative survival (McLean et al 1993). Invasion of underlying brain is widely accepted as the criterion of malignancy in meningiomas.

A significant alteration in the revised schema has been the discarding of the terms 'hemangioblastic' and 'hemangiopericytic' meningioma. These were formerly classified as subtypes of angioblastic meningioma, a term which has also been discarded. Supratentorial tumors with dural attachment and histopathologic features identical to cerebellar capillary hemangioblastoma are now categorized as tumors of uncertain origin, as is meningeal hemangiopericytoma. The term 'angiomatous' meningioma is preserved and refers to a meningioma with any of the other ten listed histologic patterns that also contains a prominent vascular component. This component can take several forms — capillary, sinusoidal or hyalinized pseudoarteriolar. In some meningiomas, vascular spaces may be the predominant feature causing potential confusion with vascular malformations.

Benign tumors in the second subcategory of meningeal tumors — mesenchymal non-meningothelial tumors — include osteocartilagenous tumors, lipomas and fibrous histiocytomas. Of these, lipomas are the most commonly encountered. Malignant mesenchymal, non-meningothelial tumors comprise mesenchymal chondrosarcoma, malignant fibrous histiocytoma, rhabdomyosarcoma and meningeal sarcomatosis. Compared to the 1979 classification, mesenchymal chondrosarcoma and rhabdomyosarcoma have been added while polymorphic cell sarcoma has been discarded. Malignant fibrous histiocytoma incorporates the malignant fibroxanthoma of the 1979 schema while fibrosarcoma would now be included under other sarcomas. Diffuse melanosis has been added to the subcategory of primary melanocytic lesions and the old term of meningeal melanomatosis is now listed as a variant of primary malignant melanoma of the meninges.

Because an origin from meningothelial cells has not been demonstrated, hemangiopericytic and hemangioblastic tumors have been reclassified as tumors of the meninges but of uncertain origin. There is still disagreement among neuropathologists concerning the histogenesis of meningeal hemangiopericytomas. Controversy has arisen predominantly because some meningiomas comprise both typical meningothelial areas and areas with the histologic features of hemangiopericytoma. Despite the ongoing debate about histogenesis, there is agreement that tumors designated as hemangiopericytomas behave more aggressively than conventional meningiomas, with a high frequency of local recurrence and progression to poorly differentiated sarcomas.

Similar, though less spirited debate, has occurred over the histogenesis of capillary hemangioblastomas. The majority are cerebellar tumors, but some occur supratentorially and can be demonstrated to have a dural or pial attachment. The lineage of the stromal cells of this tumor remains uncertain. Immunoreactivity for a number of neuroendocrine markers, in particular synaptophysin, substance P and neuropeptide Y, has suggested a neuronal lineage (Becker et al 1989). Immunoreactivity for glial fibrillary acidic protein has been interpreted as indicating incorporation of a few reactive astrocytes among tumor cells.

IV. Hemopoietic tumors

Hemopoietic neoplasms are subdivided into primary malignant lymphoma, plasmacytoma, granulocytic sarcoma, and others. Of these, primary malignant lymphoma has become pre-eminent because of a significant increase in frequency in the past decade (Adams & Howatson 1990). An important subgroup are those that occur in immunocompromised patients as a result of human immunodeficiency virus (HIV) infection (So et al 1986). Primary CNS lymphoma is included in the complications of HIV infection that define acquired immunodeficiency syndrome (AIDS). The majority of primary CNS lymphomas are non-Hodgkin's tumors of B-cell lineage and either intermediate or high grade by the criteria of the International Working Formulation (National Cancer Institute 1982). A number of primary T-cell lymphomas have been reported, some centered on the meninges (Grove & Vyberg 1993). Plasmacytomas usually occur in vertebrae and skull bones and very occasionally may involve the choroid plexus. Granulocytic sarcoma, previously known as chloroma, is regarded as a manifestation of a systemic myeloproliferative disorder. Tumors known collectively as Langerhans cell histiocytosis (previous terminology: histiocytosis X, eosinophilic granuloma), which are usually lesions of skull bones, but which may involve dura mater, and lymphomatoid granulomatosis which is an aggressive, tumefactive, granulomatous process that is destructive of blood vessels and surrounding tissue, are included under 'other' hemopoietic neoplasms.

V. Germ cell tumors

Other than the addition of yolk sac and mixed germ cell tumors, the classification of germ cell tumors of the CNS follows the original WHO schema and is based on the WHO classification of gonadal germ cell tumors. Subcategories of teratoma, immature and teratoma with malignant transformation, are added to the revised classification. The most common germ cell tumor in the CNS is the pineal germinoma. However, because germ cell tumors may occur in other sites, in particular the sella region and anterior third ventricle (germinoma), choroid (embryonal carcinoma and yolk sac tumor), and basal ganglia (teratomas), they have been allotted a category in their own right.

VI. Cysts and tumor-like lesions

This category comprises six varieties of cysts — Rathke's cleft, epidermoid, dermoid, colloid cyst of the third ventricle, enterogenous and neuroglial cysts — and four solid lesions — lipoma (separate from those occurring in the meninges — category IIIB-2), granular cell tumor (syn: choristoma), hypothalamic neuronal hamartoma and nasal glial heterotopias. The only change to this category from the 1979 schema is that craniopharyngioma has been reclassified under local extensions from regional tumors.

There has been much debate among neuropathologists concerning the histogenesis of the cells lining colloid cysts of the third ventricle. These have traditionally been regarded as arising from paraphyseal tissue in the region of the roof of the anterior third ventricle (Kappess 1955). Immunohistochemical studies have reported reactivity for markers of choroid plexus epithelium (Shuangshoti et al 1966, Shuangshoti & Netsky 1966) and gastrointestinal epithelium (Mackenzie & Gilbert 1991). The lining cells of some colloid cysts can also show ultrastructural features of ependyma (Coxe & Luse 1964).

Granular cell tumors occur predominantly in the region of the pituitary infundibulum, display intense reactivity for S-100 protein, and have been suggested to be derived from Schwann cells, despite the origin from muscle cells that was implied in the designation 'granular cell myoblastoma' by which they were originally known (Burston et al 1962). The granularity of their cytoplasm results from accumulation of material in lysosomal vesicles, the membranes of which react with lysosomal markers.

Hypothalamic neuronal hamartoma has histopathologic features and biologic behavior comparable with some of the benign tumors in the category of neuronal and mixed neuronal-glial tumors. Nevertheless it is classified as a tumor-like lesion. Neuronal hamartomas can occur at several sites in the CNS and a general subcategory of neuronal hamartoma may have been more appropriate rather than emphasizing one site.

Other lesions that might have been considered for inclusion in this category are meningio-angiomatosis (Halper et al 1986, Bertoni et al 1990) and the tumefactive collections of histiocytes that are seen in CNS Whipple's disease (Wroe et al 1991). Each of these has clinical and radiologic features that closely simulate tumors. Some lesions of infectious etiology also closely mimic tumors. Of particular importance are abscesses resulting from CNS infection by *Toxoplasma gondii* and the demyelinating lesions of progressive multifocal leukoencephalopathy (PML) associated with JC virus infection. Both of these infections occur most frequently in immunocompromised patients, especially those with HIV infection and, in this setting, must be considered with primary CNS lymphoma in the differential diagnosis of an intra-axial mass lesion (Gonzales & Davis 1988).

VII. Tumors of the anterior pituitary

Only two subcategories of anterior pituitary tumors are listed — adenoma and carcinoma. The 1979 schema divided adenomas into acidophil, basophil, mixed acidophil-basophil and chromophobe subtypes. This classification, which reflects the tinctorial properties of pituitary cells, has been superseded by a functional classification based on immunoreactivity for pituitary hormones and ultrastructural features (Scheithauer 1984). Despite the widespread adoption of the functional classification of pituitary adenomas by pathologists, it has not been included in the revised WHO schema. Acceptable histopathologic criteria for the diagnosis of pituitary carcinoma remain elusive, and examples of craniospinal seeding and extracranial metastases from seemingly benign pituitary adenomas continue to be reported (Scheithauer et al 1985).

VIII. Local extensions of regional tumors

The major alterations to this category have been the addition of craniopharyngioma, with variants of adamantinomatous and squamous papillary, and the discarding of olfactory neuroblastoma (esthesioneuroblastoma). Despite the separation of craniopharyngioma from pituitary tumors in the revised schema, most pathologists regard craniopharyngiomas and pituitary tumors together as tumors of the sella region. Chordoma and the chondroid tumors, chondroma and chondrosarcoma, can be readily grouped together and are pre-eminent in the radiologic and pathologic differential diagnosis of mass lesions in the region of the spheno-occipital syndesmosis, particularly if these are destructive of bone.

In addition to adenoid cystic carcinoma, which usually arises from salivary gland tissue, squamous and adenocarcinomas of sinus mucosa should also be included in this category of local extensions from regional tumors (see Ch. 43). These are frequently seen in woodworkers and can extend into the anterior cranial fossa.

IX. Metastatic tumors

No subcategorization of metastatic tumor has been attempted. This is probably justified on the grounds that a great variety of tumors can metastasize to the CNS. The majority of metastases have their origin in carcinomas of the lung and breast. Of the remaining metastatic brain tumors, a significant number are derived from cutaneous malignant melanomas. The unusual occurrence of metastasis to a primary CNS tumor has also been reported (Farnsworth 1972).

PROBLEMS IN CLASSIFYING CHILDHOOD BRAIN TUMORS

Despite the relative consensus in terminology reached in the 1979 WHO classification of brain tumors and the 1990 revised schema, brain tumors of childhood pose a special problem. Many pediatric neuropathologists routinely deal with complex CNS tumors for which no particular name seems appropriate. Furthermore, the association between individual histopathologic features and biologic behavior of childhood glial tumors is less clear compared with those in adults. Grading schemata based on adult tumors are therefore difficult to apply to childhood tumors. Anatomic location also appears to be a significant factor in biologic behavior. Astrocytomas of the cerebellum, for example, have a much more favorable prognosis than histologically equivalent tumors in the cerebral hemispheres. To address these problems, an adaptation of the 1979 WHO classification of brain tumors, applicable to childhood tumors, was proposed in 1985 (Rorke et al 1985). This schema emphasizes the mixed nature of many childhood glial and neuronal tumors and the influence of anatomic location on tumor behavior. The nosologic problems inherent in the designation primitive neuroectodermal tumor (PNET) are addressed by dividing these lesions into three subcategories: primitive neuroectodermal tumor, not otherwise specified (NOS); PNET with astrocytes, ependymal cells, oligodendroglia, neuronal cells, melanocytes, mesenchymal cells or mixed cellular elements; and medulloepithelioma. Medulloblastoma of the cerebellum and pineoblastoma are regarded as the prototypes of PNET-NOS. Medulloepithelioma is further subdivided into medulloepithelioma NOS, which has a distinctive histologic appearance of structures resembling primitive neural tubes, and medulloepithelioma with astrocytes, ependymal cells, oligodendrocytes, neuronal cells, melanocytes or mesenchymal cells and mixed cellular elements.

PATHOGENESIS OF CENTRAL NERVOUS SYSTEM TUMORS

An intriguing characteristic of CNS tumors, in particular the glial tumors, is their phenotypic variety. Advances in molecular-genetic techniques have disclosed an equally complex genotypic profile. This phenotypic and genotypic heterogeneity indicates that no single factor is responsible for the pathogenesis of CNS tumors but rather a number of influences, operating in an interactive way, contribute to the induction and progression of these tumors. These can be broadly categorized as genetic or environmental. While it has been postulated that some are more influential than others in tumorigenesis, development of a neoplasm appears to be the end result of the cumulative effects of these influences on the cell genome.

Genetic factors influencing the pathogenesis of CNS tumors

A number of epidemiologic studies have indicated that a family history of cancer carries an increased risk of tumor development. Approximately 15% of patients with CNS tumors have a family history of cancer (Mahaley et al 1989). These data have drawn attention to genetic factors in the pathogenesis of CNS tumors. Expansion in the repertoire of molecular-genetic laboratory techniques in the past decade has identified an increasing number and variety of alterations in the genome of tumor cells and the formulation of two interrelated concepts of oncogenesis. These have been invoked to explain the pathogenesis of CNS as well as other tumors.

The first of these proposes that initiation and progression of a tumor is partly the result of inappropriate expression of genes encoding proteins that influence cell differentiation and proliferation. These 'over-active' genes have been termed oncogenes and they are counterparts of normal cellular genes, known as proto-oncogenes (Varmus 1984). Oncogenes and their related proto-oncogenes encode proteins that participate in the signal transduction and second messenger systems that modulate cell metabolism and proliferation. These oncoproteins include growth factors and growth factor receptors such as platelet-derived growth factor (PDGF) and epidermal growth factor receptor (EGFR), tyrosine-specific protein kinases, guanine-binding proteins (G-proteins), guanine triphosphatases (GTPases), and DNA-binding proteins (Table 3.2). A much broader spectrum of activated oncogenes has been found in cell lines derived from CNS tumors, in

Table 3.2 CNS tumor-associated oncogenes and their products

Oncogene	Biologic activity of oncogene product	CNS tumor
c-erb-B1	Truncated form of normal epidermal growth factor receptor which lacks the extracellular EGF-binding domain, allowing continuous activity of the intracytoplasmic tyrosine kinase domain	Astrocytoma Meningioma
c-sis	Platelet-derived growth factor — promotes angiogenesis	Astrocytoma Meningioma
c-erb-B1 *src* *ros*	Tyrosine-specific kinases	Astrocytoma
c-Ha-ras *c-Ki-ras* *N-ras*	G-protein binding, inactivation of GTPase	Astrocytoma Neuroblastoma
c-myc	DNA-binding	Astrocytoma Medulloblastoma
N-myc		Neuroblastoma
c-fos		Astrocytoma

particular from high grade gliomas, than has been found in biopsy material (Ross 1992). Oncogenes may be activated by gene amplification, point mutation, translocation or removal of the counterbalancing influence of other genes. In some animal tumors, oncogene activation also results from insertion of retroviral sequences. The association between activation of some oncogenes and CNS tumors is well-established (for reviews see Schmideck 1987, Akbasak & Sunar-Akbasak 1992 and Ross 1992), in particular over-expression of the *c-erb-B1*, *c-myc* and *ras* oncogenes in astrocytic gliomas. The activation of several oncogenes in the same tumor has also been shown to be associated with histologic grade of astrocytoma, and this phenomenon may be important in progression of astrocytomas from low and intermediate grades of malignancy to high grade (Orian et al 1992). It is also becoming clear that in low grade and anaplastic astrocytomas, over-expression of a number of oncogenes does not occur in all tumor cells but in clones of tumor cells (Orian et al 1992). At the time of histopathologic diagnosis and grading, these may be found to be in a minority but are probably the cells responsible for tumor progression.

In terms of gene alterations underlying altered expression and the effects of mutations on protein structure, the best characterized oncogene product is EGFR, encoded by the *c-erb-B1* proto-oncogene. The gene is located on chromosome 7. Two alterations contribute to activation — deletion mutations (Yamazaki et al 1988) and gene amplification which promotes over-expression (Wong et al 1987). Deletion mutations usually occur in the portion of the *c-erb-B1* gene that encodes the extracellular ligand-binding domain. This results in the expression of a truncated EGFR protein, lacking this domain. Despite this alteration, the cytoplasmic tyrosine-kinase domain is continuously activated and thus an autocrine mechanism, driving second messenger systems, is established. Increased expression of *c-erb-B1* is thought to be related to clones of cells in high grade astrocytomas that contain multiple copies of chromosome 7 (Shapiro et al 1981).

The mechanism of activation of the *c-sis* proto-oncogene, located on chromosome 22, is less clear. Alterations to chromosome 22 are a common feature of high grade glial tumors but amplification and re-arrangement of the *c-sis* gene are uncommon (Nister et al 1988). Receptors for PDGF have been identified on normal glial cells and cells cultured from glial tumors (Heldin et al 1981, Heldin et al 1987). The proto-oncogene for PDGF receptor has been identified as *c-kit* on the long arm of chromosome 4 at 4q11–12 (d'Auriol et al 1988). Messenger RNAs for both PDGF and PDGF receptor have been found in high grade astrocytomas, signal for PDGF receptor mRNA being particularly dense over the nuclei of proliferating endothelial cells (Nister et al 1988, Hermanson et al 1992). This suggests an autocrine activation of second messenger systems in tumor astrocytes and a paracrine mechanism in endothelial cells.

Besides PDGF, other growth factors that have been identified in CNS tumors include basic fibroblast growth factor (Murphy et al 1968), transforming growth factor β_2, which is identical to glioblastoma-derived T-cell suppressor factor (Kuppner et al 1988, Samuels-Pakalvis 1988), a factor similar to the alpha chain of PDGF which is also derived from glioblastomas (Nister et al 1986), and a PDGF-like factor which has been designated vascular endothelial growth factor (VEGF). These factors are thought to influence the kinetics of the cell cycle; FGF, in particular, has been shown to promote entry of G_O cells into the cycle (Kniss & Bury 1988). Vascular endothelial growth factor is a potent promoter of angiogenesis. It is induced by hypoxia (Shweiki et al 1992) and is highly expressed by glioblastoma cells surrounding areas of necrosis (Plate et al 1992). Expression of high affinity receptors for VEGF is also seen in endothelial cells of vessels, both within glioblastomas and in the immediately adjacent brain (Plate et al 1992). The growth-promoting effects of these factors may also be modulated by cytokines and immunoregulatory molecules such as tumor necrosis factor alpha (TNF-α) and interleukin 6 (IL-6), expressed by monocyte/macrophages, microglial cells and lymphocytes that are frequently admixed with tumor cells (Schneider et al 1992).

The second concept of oncogenesis concerns a group of genes that function to negatively regulate the biologic activities of proto-oncogenes. These have been termed tumor suppressor genes (TSGs). Several putative TSGs have been identified and their mechanism of action characterized (for review see Marshall 1991). Molecular-genetic studies in patients with retinoblastoma provided the first evidence that inactivation of some genes is involved in the pathogenesis of human tumors (Francke 1978, Cavanee et al 1983). Two forms of retinoblastoma can occur — sporadic and inherited. In the latter form, a mutation on the long arm of chromosome 13, at 13q14, is inherited in an autosomal dominant fashion and is present in all cells. The development of a tumor, however, requires a second mutation. This second mutation results in what has been termed loss of heterozygosity, i.e. the cells become homozygous for loss of the gene at 13q14 or, in other words, both alleles are inactivated. This has become known as the 'two-hit' theory of tumorigenesis (Klein 1987). Sporadic retinoblastomas are thought to occur when two such mutations occur, at different time points, in retinal cells only, probably as a result of environmental influences. Other central nervous system tumors in which loss of heterozygosity has been identified include astrocytoma, meningioma, hemangioblastoma, in particular those occurring as part of the von Hippel-Lindau syndrome, pituitary adenoma in multiple endocrine neoplasia syndrome type 1 (MEN 1), schwannoma (benign and malignant) and neurofibromata in patients with Von Recklinghausen's neurofibromatosis (NF-1) and those with bilateral acoustic tumors (NF-2) (Seizinger & Breakfield

Table 3.3 Chromosomal deletions and loci of loss of heterozygosity (LOH) in CNS tumors

Tumor	Chromosomal deletions/ loci of LOH
Astrocytoma	#10, #13, 17p, #22
Glioblastoma multiforme	#10, 17p
Medulloblastoma	17q
Retinoblastoma	13q14
Meningioma	#22, 22q12.3-qter
Hemangioblastoma (von Hippel-Lindau)	3p
Pituitary adenoma (MEN-1)	11q
Acoustic nerve tumors (NF-2)	22q
Neurofibromata (NF-1)	17q

(# — denotes loss of whole chromosome)

1990). Table 3.3 summarizes chromosomal deletions and loci of loss of genetic material that have been identified in CNS tumors. In some tumors, only part of a chromosome is lost, e.g. 17p, 13q14, while in others whole chromosomes may be lost, e.g. deletions of chromosomes 10, 13 and 22 in some astrocytomas (Bigner & Vogelstein 1990).

Loss of some genetic material from almost all chromosomes has been identified in the cells of anaplastic astrocytomas and glioblastomas multiforme (Fults et al 1990). Loss of heterozygosity on chromosomes 10 and 17 in combination with mutations in another putative suppressor gene, p53, have been implicated in progression of anaplastic astrocytoma to glioblastoma multiforme (Fults et al 1992). The discovery that loss of genetic material appears to be a factor in the pathogenesis of tumors has raised expectations that some forms of cancer will, in the future, be treated by replacement of deleted or mutated genes. There is already experimental data suggesting that tumor phenotype can be blocked by the introduction of normal chromosomes into tumor cell lines (Weissman et al 1987). Combined analyses of loss of heterozygosity and oncogene activation have identified subsets of glioblastoma multiforme (von Deimling et al 1993). Amplification of the EGFR gene occurs more commonly in glioblastomas that also show loss of portions of chromosome 10 but not chromosome 17. Glioblastomas with loss of 17p infrequently show EGFR amplification. Patients with the latter subset are also significantly younger. To date, however, there are no data indicating a significant difference in survival between patients with these subsets.

Mutations in the p53 gene are now recognized as the most common gene alteration in human cancers. The gene is located on the short arm of chromosome 17, at 17p13. Wild-type p53 encodes a 393-amino-acid phosphoprotein that binds to specific DNA sequences (Kern et al 1991) and regulates proliferation of cells by controlling their entry into the S phase of the cell cycle. It is also a potent inhibitor of oncogene-induced cell transformation (Milner 1991). Because of these biologic activities it has been included in the category of tumor suppressor genes. Mutations are clustered in four highly conserved regions spanning exons 5–9 and result in a prolonged half-life of the mutated p53 oncoprotein which complexes with wild-type p53. As a result of complexing, wild-type p53 protein can no longer exert its negative regulatory effect on cell proliferation. Prolongation of the half-life of mutated p53 oncoprotein may also result from complexing with the 70 kD relative mass heat shock protein (Finlay et al 1988). In vitro studies have demonstrated a link with oncogenes in that mutated p53, isolated from tumor cell lines, co-operates with the *ras* oncogene in transforming other cells (Parada et al 1984).

Mutations in the p53 gene have been clearly documented in astrocytic tumors and meningiomas (Mashiyama et al 1991). This can be a single event or can occur in combination with loss of other portions of chromosome 17 and/or chromosome 10. The combined alterations of p53 mutation and further loss of genetic material from chromosomes 10 and 17 have been proposed to contribute to progression of astrocytomas (Sidransky et al 1992, Fults et al 1992). Although the majority of astrocytomas show mutations, accumulation of wild-type p53 protein in the cells of some astrocytic tumors has also been demonstrated by immunohistochemical techniques (Louis et al 1993). This finding suggests that interference with the normal metabolism of wild-type p53 protein, with prolongation of its half-life, may have a stimulatory effect on cell transformation and proliferation comparable with mutated p53. Allelic loss at a second locus on chromosome 17, separate from the p53 locus, has also been implicated in primitive neuroectodermal tumors of childhood (Biegel et al 1992).

Environmental factors in the pathogenesis of CNS tumors

There are two major categories of environmental factors that are thought to contribute to the pathogenesis of CNS tumors — chemicals and viruses. Although a link between industrial chemicals and CNS tumors was suggested by a number of early epidemiologic studies (Selikoff & Hammond 1982), this was not confirmed in later investigations and the only evidence for direct tumor induction by chemicals has come from animal studies. Evidence for viral induction of CNS tumors in humans is more compelling and experimental studies in laboratory animals have convincingly demonstrated a causative link between some viruses and CNS tumors in susceptible species.

A. Chemically-induced CNS tumors

Epidemiologic studies. In the late 1970s and early 1980s, epidemiologic studies, in particular, in North America and Sweden reported a higher than expected frequency of CNS tumors among workers in the petrochemical and rubber industries (Selikoff & Hammond 1982). Chemicals to which workers in these industries were exposed, and which have been shown to induce CNS tumors in laboratory animals, include aromatic hydrocarbons, hydrazines, bis (chloromethyl) ether, vinyl chloride and acrylonitrile. Workers in some of these industries were also concurrently exposed to ionizing radiation. Follow-up studies in Sweden, however, did not confirm an increased risk with industrial exposure to these agents (McLaughlin et al 1987).

Chemical induction of CNS tumors in animals. Chemical induction of CNS tumors in small laboratory animals was first reported in 1939 by Seligman and Shear and, since that time, this has been a useful paradigm for studying the biology of high grade neuroglial tumors. The commonly utilized compounds include the N-nitrosoureas, the triazenes, the hydrazines and the aromatic hydrocarbons and their derivatives. These agents have been administered by a variety of routes including direct injection into the brain or ventricles. Transplacental induction of tumors has also been achieved with the nitrosoureas. These have been found to be particularly effective inducers of CNS tumors because of their tropism for neural tissue. Following transplacental induction by ethyl-nitrosourea, high grade glial tumors appear in offspring at 300 days. The mechanism of action of the nitrosoureas and other alkylating agents is thought to be the induction of unrepaired damage to DNA leading to point mutations. Further molecular-genetic investigations of gene alterations in CNS tumors induced by nitrosourea compounds led to the identification of the *c-erb-B2* or *HER-neu* oncogene (Schechter et al 1984), supporting induction of point mutations as the likely mechanism of action. However, despite a large body of epidemiologic and animal experimental data, whether any of these compounds is causally related to human brain tumors remains questionable.

B. Oncogenic viruses and brain tumors

The evidence for induction of human CNS tumors by oncogenic viruses is stronger than for chemical induction. There have been several reports of high grade astrocytomas in patients with progressive multifocal leukoencephalopathy, a demyelinating disorder which follows infection of oligodendrocytes and astrocytes by the JC subtype of human papovavirus (Sima et al 1983). Epstein-Barr virus has also been identified in tumor cells in primary CNS lymphoma, both in patients with as well as those without human immunodeficiency virus infection (Geddes et al 1992). Data regarding direct induction of CNS tumors by oncogenic viruses have come exclusively from animal studies. Both DNA and RNA viruses have been shown to be capable of inducing tumors after intracerebral inoculation into susceptible species of laboratory animals. Of the DNA viruses, adenovirus and SV-40, another of the papovaviruses, are particularly effective inducers of neoplasia. Human adenovirus type 12 has a particular affinity for primitive neuroectoderm and induces tumors resembling neuroblastoma, medulloblastoma and medulloepithelioma in the brain and retinoblastoma after intraocular inoculation. SV-40 induces highly malignant sarcomatous tumors, while development of multiple cerebellar medulloblastomas has followed inoculation of JC virus. In recent years these techniques have been refined and tumors induced in mice by the introduction of early sequences of SV-40 and adenovirus into the genome by transgenic technology (Kelly et al 1986).

Several avian and murine retroviruses have been known for some time to be capable of inducing CNS tumors (for review see Bigner & Pegram 1976). The mechanism by which these viruses induce tumors was clarified with the identification of oncogenes. The majority of oncogenes that have been identified to date show sequence homology with retroviruses isolated from animal tumors (Varmus 1984), suggesting that activation of oncogenes may occur by insertion of retroviral sequences. To date, however, this has not been confirmed in transgenic experiments.

Other factors

For some time, hormones have been implicated in the growth and progression of some CNS tumors, in particular meningioma. The overall higher incidence of meningiomas in females and enlargement and rapid growth of meningiomas in the region of the tuberculum sellae and sphenoidal ridge during pregnancy have been recognized for some time (Bickerstaff et al 1958). The demonstration of estrogen, progesterone and androgen receptors in biopsy material from meningiomas (Donnell et al 1979, Schnegg et al 1981) supported the hypothesis that hormones promote tumor growth and raised hopes that hormone treatment might control the growth of aggressive meningiomas. However, such treatment has not been proven to significantly alter the biological behavior of receptor-positive meningiomas.

A variety of other factors — alcohol, tobacco, radiation (in particular, electromagnetic fields) and trauma — have, at different times, been suggested to contribute to the development of CNS tumors. Most data come from epidemiologic studies and are discussed in detail in Chapter 4.

REFERENCES

Adams J H, Howatson A G 1990 Cerebral lymphomas: a review of 70 cases. Journal of Clinical Pathology 43: 544–547

Akbasak A, Sunar-Akbasak B 1992 Oncogenes: cause or consequence in the development of glial tumours. Journal of the Neurological Sciences 111: 119–133

Ambler M, Pogacar S, Sidman R 1969 Lhermitte-Duclos disease

(granule cell hypertrophy of the cerebellum). Pathological analysis of the first familial cases. Journal of Neuropathology and Experimental Neurology 28: 622–630

Bailey P, Cushing H 1926 A classification of tumors of the glioma group on a histogenetic basis. J B Lippincott, Philadelphia, pp 146–167

Becker N, Paulus W, Roggendorf W 1989 Histogenesis of stromal cells in cerebellar haemangioblastoma. An immunohistochemical study. American Journal of Pathology 134: 271–275

Bertoni F, Unni K, Dahlin D C, Beabout J W, Onofrio B M 1990 Calcifying pseudoneoplasm of the neural axis. Journal of Neurosurgery 72: 42–48

Bickerstaff E R, Small J M, Guest I A 1958 The relapsing course of certain meningiomas in relation to pregnancy and menstruation. Journal of Neurology, Neurosurgery and Psychiatry 21: 89–91

Biegel J A, Burk C D, Barr F G, Emanuel B S 1992 Evidence for a tumour related locus distinct from p53 in pediatric primitive neuroectodermal tumours. Cancer Research 52: 3391–3395

Bigner D D, Pegram C N 1976 Virus induced experimental brain tumors and putative associations of viruses with human brain tumors: a review. Advances in Neurology 15: 57–83

Bigner S H, Vogelstein B 1990 Cytogenetics and molecular genetics of malignant gliomas and medulloblastoma. Brain Pathology 1: 12–18

Broders A C 1925 The grading of carcinoma. Minn Medicine 8: 726–730

Burger P C, Vollmer R T 1980 Histological factors of prognostic significance in glioblastoma multiforme. Cancer 46: 1179–1186

Burger P C, Vogel F S, Green S B, Strike T A 1985 Glioblastoma multiforme and anaplastic astrocytoma. Pathologic criteria and prognostic implications. Cancer 56: 1106–1111

Burston J, John R, Spencer H 1962 'Myoblastoma' of the neurohypophysis. Journal of Pathology and Bacteriology 83: 455–461

Cajal S R 1913 Sobre un nuevo proceder de impregnacion de la neuroglia y sus resultados en los centros nerviosos del hombre y animales. Trab Lab Invest Biol Univ Madrid 14: 155–162

Cavanee W K, Dryja T P, Phillips R A et al 1983 Expression of recessive alleles by chromosome mechanisms in retinoblastoma. Nature 305: 779–784

Chow C W, Klug G L, Lewis E A 1988 Subependymal giant cell astrocytoma in children. Journal of Neurosurgery 68: 880–883

Cox L B 1933 The cytology of the glioma group; with special reference to the inclusion of cells derived from the invaded tissue. The American Journal of Pathology 9: 839–898

Coxe W S, Luse S A 1964 Colloid cyst of the third ventricle. An electron microscopic study. Journal of Neuropathology and Experimental Neurology 23: 431–444

Cruveilhier J C 1829 Anatomie pathologique du corps humain. Bailiere, Paris

Daumas-Duport C, Szikla G 1981 Delimitation et configuration spatiale des gliomas cerebraux: Donnees histologiques, incidences therapeutiques. Neurochirurgie 27: 273–284

Daumas-Duport C, Scheithauer B W, O'Fallon J, Kelly P 1988a Grading of astrocytomas. A simple and reproducible method. Cancer 62: 2152–2165

Daumas-Duport C, Scheithauer B W, Chodkiewicz J-P et al 1988b Dysembryoplastic neuroepithelial tumour (DNET): A surgically curable tumour of young subjects with intractable partial seizures. Report of 39 cases. Neurosurgery 23: 545–556

d'Auriol L, Mattei M G, Andre C, Galibert F 1988 Localization of the human *c-kit* proto-oncogene on the q11-q12 region of chromosome 4. Human Genetics 78: 374–376

Donnell M S, Meyer G A, Donegan W L 1979 Estrogen-receptor protein in intracranial meningiomas. Journal of Neurosurgery 50: 499–502

Farnsworth J 1972 Regressing melanoma metastasizing to an oligodendroglioma. Pathology 4: 253–257

Finlay C A, Hinds P W, Tan T-H, Eliyahu D, Oren M, Levine A J 1988 Activating mutations for transformation by p53 produce a gene product that forms an hsc70-p53 complex with an altered half-life. Molecular Cellular Biology 8: 531–539

Francke U 1978 Retinoblastoma and chromosome 13. Birth Defects 12: 131–137

Fulling K H, Garcia D M 1985 Anaplastic astrocytomas of the adult cerebrum. Prognostic value of histological features. Cancer 55: 928–931

Fults D, Pedone C A, Thomas G A, White R 1990 Allelotype of human malignant astrocytoma. Cancer Research 50: 5784–5799

Fults D, Brockmeyer D, Tullous M W, Pedone C A, Cawthorn R M 1992 *p53* mutation and loss of heterozygosity on chromosomes 17 and 10 during human astrocytoma progression. Cancer Research 52: 674–679

Garcia D M, Fulling K H, Marks J E 1985 The value of radiation therapy in addition to surgery for astrocytomas of the adult cerebrum. Cancer 55: 919–927

Geddes J F, Bhattacharjee M B, Savage F, Scaravilli F, McLaughlin J E 1992 Primary cerebral lymphoma: a study of 47 cases probed for Epstein-Barr virus genome. Journal of Clinical Pathology 45: 587–590

Golgi C 1884 Uber die gliome des gehirns (Untersuchungen uber den feineren bau des nervensustems). Fischer, Jena

Gonzales M F, Davis R L 1988 Neuropathology of acquired immunodeficiency syndrome. Neuropathology and Applied Neurobiology 14: 345–363

Grove A, Vyberg M 1993 Primary leptomeningeal T-cell lymphoma: a case and a review of primary T-cell lymphoma of the central nervous system. Clinical Neuropathology 12: 7–12

Halper J, Scheithauer B W, Okasaki H, Laws E R Jr 1986 Meningio-angiomatosis; a report of six cases with special reference to the occurrence of neurofibrillary tangles. Journal of Neuropathology and Experimental Neurology 45: 426–432

Hassoun J, Gambrelli D, Grisoli F 1982 Central neurocytoma: an electron-microscopic study of two cases. Acta Neuropathologica (Berlin) 56: 151–156

Heldin C H, Westermark B, Wasteson A 1981 Specific receptor for platelet derived growth factor on cells derived from connective tissue and glia. Proceedings of the National Academy of Science USA 78: 3664–3668

Heldin C H, Betsholtz C, Claesson-Wels L, Westermark B 1987 Subversion of growth regulatory pathways in malignant transformation. Biochemistry Biophysics Acta 907: 219–244

Hermanson M, Funa K, Hartman M, Claesson-Welsh L, Heldin C H, Westermark B, Nister M 1992 Platelet-derived growth factor and its receptors in human glioma tissue: expression of messenger RNA and protein suggests the presence of autocrine and paracrine loops. Cancer Research 52: 3213–3219

Horten B C, Urich H, Stefoski D 1979 Meningioma with conspicuous plasma cell and lymphocytic components: A report of five cases. Cancer 43: 258–264

Kappess J A 1955 The development of the paraphysis cerebri in man with comments on its relationship to the intercolumnar tubercle and its significance for the origin of cystic tumours of the third ventricle. Journal of Comparative Neurology 102: 425–509

Kawano N, Yada K, Yagashita S 1989 Clear cell ependymoma. A histologic variant with diagnostic implications. Virchow Archives Pathologic Anatomica 415: 467–472

Kelly F, Kellerman O, Mechali F, Gaillard J, Babinet C 1986 Expression of SV40 oncogenes in F9 embryonal carcinoma cells, in transgenic mice and transgenic embryos. In: Botchan M, Grodicker T, Sharp P A (eds) DNA tumor viruses. Control of gene expression and replication. Cold Spring Harbour Laboratory, pp 363–372

Kepes J J 1990 Review of the WHO's proposed new classification of brain tumors. Proceedings of the XIth International Congress of Neuropathology, Kyoto, September 2–8, 1990. Japanese Society of Neuropathology, Kyoto, Japan

Kepes J J, Rubinstein L J, Eng L F 1979 Pleomorphic xanthoastrocytoma: A distinctive meningocerebral glioma in young subjects with relatively favorable prognosis. A study of 12 cases. Cancer 44: 1839–1852

Kepes J J, Chen W X Y, Connors M H, Vogel F S 1988 'Chordoid' meningeal tumors in young individuals with peritumoural lymphoplasmacellular infiltrates. Report of seven cases. Cancer 62: 391–406

Kepes J J, Rubinstein L J, Ansbacher L, Schreiber D J 1989 Histopathological features of recurrent pleomorphic xanthoastrocytomas: further corroboration of the glial nature of this neoplasm. A study of 3 cases. Acta Neuropathologica (Berlin) 78: 585–593

Kern S, Kinzler K W, Bruskin A, Jarosz D, Friedman P, Prives C, Vogelstein B 1991 Identification of p53 as a sequence-specific DNA-binding protein. Science 252: 1708–1711

Kernohan J W, Mabon R F, Svien H J, Adson A W 1949 A simplified classification of gliomas. Proceedings of the Staff Meetings of the Mayo Clinic 24: 71–74

Klein G 1987 The approaching era of tumor suppressor genes. Science 238: 1539–1545

Kniss D A, Burry R W 1988 Serum and fibroblast growth factor stimulate quiescent astrocytes to re-enter the cell cycle. Brain Research 439: 281–288

Kuppner M C, Hamou M F, Bodmer S, Fontana A, de Tribolet N 1988 The glioblastoma-derived T-cell suppressor factor/transforming growth factor $beta_2$ inhibits the generation of lymphokine-activated killer (LAK) cells. International Journal of Cancer 42: 562–567

Leestma J E 1980. In: Scarpelli D G (ed) Brain tumours. American Journal of Pathology Teaching Monograph Series. American Association of Pathologists, Maryland, p 243

Louis D N, von Demling A, Chung R Y et al 1993 Comparative study of p53 gene and protein alterations in human astrocytic tumours. Journal of Neuropathology and Experimental Neurology 52: 31–38

McLaughlin J K, Malker H S R, Blot W J et al 1987 Occupational risks of intracranial gliomas in Sweden. Journal of the National Cancer Institute 78: 253–257

McLean C A, Jolley D, Cukier E, Giles G, Gonzales M F 1993 Atypical and malignant meningiomas: importance of micronecrosis as a prognostic indicator. Histopathology (in press)

Mackenzie I R A, Gilbert J J 1991 Cysts of the neuroaxis of endodermal origin. Journal of Neurology, Neurosurgery and Psychiatry 54: 572–575

Mahaley M S Jr, Mettlin C, Natarajan N, Laws E R Jr, Peace B B 1989 National survey of patterns of care for brain-tumor patients. Journal of Neurosurgery 71: 826–836

Marshall C J 1991 Tumor suppressor genes. Cell 64: 313–326

Mashiyama S, Murakami Y, Yoshimoto T, Sekiya T, Hayashi K 1991 Detection of p53 gene mutations in human brain tumors by single-strand conformation polymorphism analysis of polymerase chain reaction products. Oncogene 6: 1313–1318

Milner J 1991 The role of p53 in normal control of cell proliferation. Current Opinion in Cell Biology 3: 282–286

Mork S J, Halvorsen T B, Lindegaard K-F, Eide G E 1986 Oligodendrogliomas. Histologic evaluation and prognosis. Journal of Neuropathology and Experimental Neurology 45: 65–78

Murphy P R, Sato Y, Sato R, Friesen H G 1988 Regulation of multiple basic fibroblast growth factor messenger ribonucleic acid transcripts by protein kinase C activators. Molecular Endocrinology 2: 1196–1201

National Cancer Institute 1982 NCI-sponsored study of classification of non-Hodgkin's lymphoma and description of a Working Formulation for Clinical Usage. The non-Hodgkin's Lymphoma Pathologic Classification Project. Cancer 49: 2112–2135

Nelson J S, Tsukada Y, Schoenfeld D 1983 Necrosis as a prognosis criteria in malignant supratentorial astrocytic gliomas. Cancer 52: 550–554

Nister M, Heldin C-H, Westermark B 1986 Clonal variation in the production of a platelet-derived growth factor-like protein and expression of corresponding receptors in a human malignant glioma. Cancer Research 46: 332–337

Nister M, Libermann T A, Betsholtz C 1988 Expression of messenger RNA's for platelet derived growth factor and transforming growth factor-alpha and their receptors in human malignant glioma cell lines. Cancer Research 48: 3910–3918

Ojeda V J, Spagnolo D V, Vaughan R J 1987 Palisades in primary cerebral neuroblastoma. A light and electron microscopic study of an adult case. American Journal of Surgical Pathology 4: 316–322

Orian J M, Vasilopoulos K, Yoshida S, Kaye A H, Gonzales M F 1992 Overexpression of multiple oncogenes related to histological grade of astrocytic glioma. British Journal of Cancer 66: 106–112

Palma L, Guidetti B 1985 Cystic pilocytic astrocytomas of the cerebral hemispheres. Surgical experience with 51 cases and long-term results. Journal of Neurosurgery 62: 811–815

Parada L F, Land H, Weinberg R A, Wolf D, Rotter V 1984 Co-operation between gene encoding p53 tumour antigen and *ras* in cellular transformation. Nature 312: 649–651

Penfield W 1931 The classification of gliomas and neuroglia cell types. Archives of Neurology and Psychiatry 26: 745–753

Plate K H, Breier G, Weich H A, Risau W 1992 Vascular endothelial growth factor is a potential tumour angiogenesis factor in human gliomas *in vitro*. Nature 359: 845–848

Ribbert H 1918 Uber das spongioblastom und das gliom. Virchows Archives 225: 195–213

Ringertz N 1950 Grading of gliomas. Acta Pathologica Microbiologica Scandinavica 27: 51–65

de Rio-Hortega P 1919 El tercer elemento de los centros nerviosos. I. La microglia. II. Intervencion de la microglia en los procesos patologicas. III. Naturaleza probable de la microglia. Boletin de la Sociedad Espanola de Biologia 9: 69–120

Rorke L B, Gilles F H, Davis R L, Becker L E 1985 Revision of the World Health Organization classification of brain tumors for childhood brain tumors. Cancer 56: 1869–1886

Ross D A 1992 Molecular genetics of tumours of the central nervous system. In: Crockard A, Hayward R, Hoff J T (eds) Neurosurgery: The scientific basis of clinical practice, 2nd edn. Blackwell Scientific Publications, Oxford, vol 2, pp 556–570

Rubinstein L J, Herman M M 1989 The astroblastoma and its possible cytogenic relationship to the tanicyte. An electronmicroscopic, immunohistochemical, tissue- and organ-culture study. Acta Neuropathologica (Berlin) 78: 427–483

Russell D S, Cairns H 1947 Polar spongioblastomas. Archives of Histology and Pathology 3: 423–441

Russell D S, Rubinstein L J 1989 Pathology of tumors of the nervous system, 5th edn. Williams & Wilkins, Baltimore, p 176

Samuels-Pakalvis V 1988 TGF-beta-like activity in CNS tumours. Journal of Neurosurgery 69: 806–807

Schechter A L, Stern D F, Vaidyanathan L, Decker S J, Drebin J A, Greene M I, Weinberg R A 1984 The *neu* oncogene: an *erb-B*-related gene encoding a 185,000 M_r tumour antigen. Science 312: 513–516

Scheithauer B W 1984 Surgical pathology of the pituitary: The adenomas. Parts I & II. In: Sommers S C, Rosen P P (eds) Pathology Annual, Part I & Part II. Appleton-Century-Crofts, Norwalk, Connecticut, pp 317–374 & 269–330

Scheithauer B W, Randall R V, Laws E R Jr 1985 Prolactin cell carcinoma of the pituitary. Clinicopathologic, immunohistochemical, and ultrastructural study of a case with cranial and extracranial metastases. Cancer 55: 598–604

Schmidek H H 1987 The molecular genetics of nervous system tumors. Journal of Neurosurgery 67: 1–16

Schnegg J F, Gomez F, LeMarchand-Beraud T, de Tribolet N 1981 Presence of sex steroid hormone receptors in meningioma tissue. Surgical Neurology 15: 415–418

Schneider J, Hofman F H, Apuzzo M L J, Hinton D R 1992 Cytokines and immunoregulatory molecules in malignant glial neoplasms. Journal of Neurosurgery 77: 265–273

Seizinger B R, Breakfield X O 1990 The role of tumour suppressor genes in neural tumours. Trends in Neurosciences 13: 3–6

Seligman A M, Shear M J 1939 Studies in carcinogenesis. VIII. Experimental production of brain tumours in mice with methylcholanthrene. American Journal of Cancer 37: 364–399

Selikoff I J, Hammond E C 1982 Brain tumors in the chemical industry. Annals of the New York Academy of Sciences 381: 1–363

Shapiro J R, Yung W-K A, Shapiro W R 1981 Isolation, karyotype, and clonal growth of heterogeneous subpopulations of human malignant gliomas. Cancer Research 41: 2349–2359

Shuangshoti S, Netsky M G 1966 Neuroepithelial (colloid) cysts of the nervous system. Further observation on pathogenesis, location, incidence and histochemistry. Neurology 16: 887–903

Shuangshoti A, Roberts M P, Netsky M G 1965. Neuroepithelial (colloid) cysts. Archives of Pathology 80: 214–224

Shweiki D, Itin A, Soffer D, Keshet E 1992 Vascular endothelial growth factor induced by hypoxia may mediate hypoxia-initiated angiogenesis. Nature 359: 843–845

Sidransky D, Mikkelson T, Schwechheimer K, Rosenblum M L, Cavanee W, Vogelstein B 1992 Clonal expansion of p53 mutant cells is associated with brain tumour progression. Nature 355: 846–847

Sima A A F, Finklestein S D, McLachlan D R 1983 Multiple malignant astrocytomas in a patient with spontaneous progressive multifocal leucoencephalopathy. Annals of Neurology 14: 183–188

Smith M T, Ludwig C L, Godfrey A D, Armbrustmacher V W 1983 Grading of oligodendrogliomas. Cancer 52: 2107–2114

So Y T, Beckstead J H, Davis R L 1986 Primary central nervous system lymphoma in acquired immunodeficiency syndrome: A clinical and pathological study. Annals of Neurology 20: 566–572

Svien H J, Mabon R F, Kernohan J W, Adson A W 1949 Astrocytomas. Proceedings of the Staff Meetings of the Mayo Clinic 24: 54–63

Tooth H H 1912 Some observations on the growth and survival period of intracranial tumors based on the review of 500 cases, with special reference to the pathology of gliomata. Brain 35: 61–108

Townsend J J, Seaman J P 1986 Central neurocytoma — a rare benign intraventricular tumour. Acta Neuropathologica (Berlin) 71: 167–170

VandenBerg S R, May E E, Rubinstein L J, Herman M M 1987 Desmoplastic supratentorial neuroepithelial tumors of infancy with divergent differentiation potential ("desmoplastic infantile ganglioglioma"). A report of 11 cases of a distinctive embryonal tumor with favourable prognosis. Journal of Neurosurgery 66: 58–71

Varmus H E 1984 The molecular genetics of cellular oncogenes. Annual Review of Genetics 18: 553–612

Virchow R 1860 Cellular pathology. Translated from the second German edition (A. Hirschwald) by Chance F. London

Virchow R 1890 Das Psammom. Virchows Archives Anatomical Pathology 160: 32

von Deimling A, von Ammon K, Schoenfeld D, Wiestler O D, Seizinger B R, Louis D N 1993 Subsets of glioblastoma multiforme defined by molecular genetic analysis. Brain Pathology 3: 19–26

Wallner K E, Gonzales M F, Edwards M S B, Wara W M, Sheline G E 1988 Treatment results of juvenile pilocytic astrocytoma. Journal of Neurosurgery 69: 171–176

Weissman B E, Saxon P J, Pasquale S R, Jones G R, Geise A G, Stanbridge E J 1987 Introduction of normal human chromosome 11 into Wilms' tumor cell line controls tumourigenic expression. Science 236: 175–180

Weldon-Linne C, Victor T A, Groothius D R, Vick N A 1983 Pleomorphic xanthoastrocytoma: Ultrastructural and immunohistochemical study of a case with a rapidly fatal outcome after surgery. Cancer 52: 2055–2063

Wong A J, Bigner S H, Bigner D D 1987 Increased expression of the epidermal growth factor receptor gene in malignant gliomas is invariably associated with gene amplification. Proceedings of the National Academy of Science USA 84: 6899–6903

Wroe S J, Pures M, Harding B, Youl B D, Shorvon S 1991 Whipple's disease confined to the CNS presenting with multiple intracerebral mass lesions. Journal of Neurology, Neurosurgery and Psychiatry 54: 989–992

Yamazaki H, Fukui Y, Ueyama Y 1988 Amplification of the structurally and functionally altered epidermal growth factor receptor gene (*c-erb-B*) in human brain tumors. Molecular Cell Biology 8: 1816–1820

Zulch K J 1979 Histologic classification of tumours of the central nervous system. International Classification of Tumours, No 21

4. Epidemiology of brain tumors and factors in prognosis

Graham G. Giles Michael F. Gonzales

INTRODUCTION

Primary tumors of the brain and spinal cord (CNS tumor) account for less than 2% of malignancies diagnosed in Australia (Giles et al 1987) but they are responsible for 7% of the years of life lost from cancer before age 70 (Holman et al 1987). They are important in childhood, accounting for 20% of malignant tumors diagnosed before the age of 15. Little is known of the cause(s) of CNS tumors and, although both genetic and environmental factors are suspected, nothing can be done to prevent them. The epidemiology of CNS tumors has been reviewed by Gold (1980) and Schoenberg (1982). This chapter adds epidemiologic findings published in the last decade, particularly for neuroepithelial CNS tumors.

There are three principal difficulties in describing the epidemiology of CNS tumors: obtaining histologic confirmation of all diagnoses, accurately discerning primary tumors from metastatic disease, and distinguishing malignant from benign tumors. Added to these is a fourth difficulty related to etiological research, notably case-control studies that rely on interviews to collect information about potentially important past exposures to causative agents.

A proportion of CNS tumors are inoperable and in these cases no biopsy material is available for histologic examination. In some cases when tumor material is obtained a clear histologic diagnosis cannot be established (Zulch 1979). Lack of histologic verification increases the probability of including metastatic and benign tumors with primary malignant tumors. This becomes a problem both when examining differences between populations and when studying etiology. Metastatic disease obviously differs etiologically from primary tumors but so too might benign tumors. The proportion of cases which are either benign or metastatic varies from place to place and over time, and this complicates the comparison and interpretation of trends.

There are numerous epidemiologic surveys which describe CNS tumor trends over time and differences in incidence between populations. Sometimes these surveys suggest clues to be followed up in interview studies. Most studies of CNS tumors based on interviews have been retrospective case-control designs in which information has been obtained from cases and unaffected controls concerning relevant aspects of their past life. Case-control studies are very prone to biases which can profoundly affect the validity of their results. In the case of malignant CNS tumors, recall bias is especially pertinent because of possible mental deficits due to the tumor and its treatment, in particular post-operative irradiation. In addition, the rapid progression to fatal outcome of some CNS tumors precludes a proportion of cases from being interviewed. These problems are sometimes overcome by interviewing proxy respondents such as spouses, but differences in quality of information obtained from cases and controls remain a concern when interpreting the findings.

Epidemiologic study has been influenced by the histologic diversity of CNS tumors and by the number of different classification systems that have been used in different parts of the world at different times (Armstrong et al 1990). Without review of pathology, epidemiologic studies of CNS tumors are likely to suffer from the effects of misclassification. The heterogeneity of histologic diagnoses suggests multiple etiologies and a requirement for increased diagnostic specificity in future epidemiologic investigations. Table 4.1 shows incidence rates of the major types of CNS tumors classified according to the WHO schema (see Table 3.1, p. 34). Although rates can be obtained by age and sex for many of these subtypes from several series, they must be viewed in the context of the caveats discussed above. Hospital series benefit from pathology slide review but suffer from selection bias while population series may be complete but are not usually subject to pathologic confirmation of diagnosis. It is important in assessing such data to obtain details of histologic verification and review. Epidemiologic studies of specific histologic subtypes are rare, CNS tumors being investigated either as one entity or at best being grouped into gliomas or meningiomas. Epidemiologic studies have also suffered from poor statistical power because of the small numbers of cases recruited.

Table 4.1 The incidence of CNS malignancies by histologic type and age group, Victoria, Australia 1982–1991. Source: Victorian Cancer Registry, unpublished data

	Age 0–14 years				Age 15 + years				Total	
	Male		*Female*		*Male*		*Female*		*Male*	*Female*
	N	%	N	%	N	%	N	%	Rate	Rate
Glioblastoma multiforme	6	4.20	0	0.00	658	34.50	462	23.80	2.80	1.83
Astrocytoma	61	42.40	58	47.20	311	16.30	216	11.10	1.73	1.29
Medulloblastoma	35	24.30	8	6.50	16	0.80	13	0.70	0.31	0.12
Oligodendroglioma	1	0.70	0	0.00	32	1.70	21	1.10	0.14	0.09
Ependymoma	8	5.60	12	9.80	22	1.20	17	0.90	0.15	0.16
Other glioma	7	4.90	13	10.60	99	5.20	73	3.80	0.46	0.38
Meningioma	5	3.50	4	3.30	297	15.60	661	34.00	1.27	2.69
Nerve sheath tumor	1	0.70	1	0.80	79	4.10	82	4.20	0.35	0.35
Other specified type	8	5.60	7	5.70	33	1.70	39	2.00	0.20	0.21
Unspecified type	1	0.70	0	0.00	9	0.50	2	0.10	0.05	0.01
Not microscopically confirmed	11	7.60	20	16.30	352	18.40	359	18.50	1.47	1.28
Total	144		123		1908		1945		8.91	8.40

TRENDS

CNS tumors vary in incidence by age, sex, ethnic group, country, and also over time. How much of this variation is due to either artefactual influences or etiologic differences has been the subject of much debate. The diagnosis of CNS tumors has been facilitated by advances in imaging technology made during this century. Access to medical technology, therefore, might explain some of the observed variation between different populations and within the same population between subgroups, defined, for example, by age, socioeconomic status or ethnic background. The problem lies with inoperable, image-detected tumors which are seldom verified histologically. The inclusion of these tumors can significantly affect apparent incidence levels and make comparisons difficult if not impossible.

Trends by age and sex

Population-based incidence statistics are routinely obtained from cancer registries. Some cancer registries deliberately include tumors of benign or uncertain behavior in their incidence reporting (Kaye et al 1993). Most, however, attempt to restrict data collection to malignant primary tumors, though the extent to which they are successful probably varies depending on the degree of histologic verification and the specificity of pathologists' reports. Examples of age-standardized incidence rates for total CNS tumors are given in Figure 4.1. Age-standardized incidence rates for the principal histologic types of CNS tumors are given in Table 4.1. It is difficult to make exact comparisons because of the different criteria for tumor inclusion, and it is not easy to compare histology-specific rates because of differences in nomenclature. Artefactual increases in rates are likely to be strongest in elderly populations. For this reason, the cumulative rates chosen to illustrate trends in Table 4.2 have been truncated at age 65.

Table 4.2 CNS tumors cumulative rates percent to age 65 in the five volumes of *Cancer Incidence in Five Continents*. Source: Muir et al 1987, Stukonis 1978

	Vol I	Vol II	Vol III	Vol IV	Vol V
Males					
Israel (Jews born Israel)	n.a.	0.62	0.80	0.70	0.68
Sweden	0.54	0.62	0.64	0.60	0.63
Israel (Jews born Eur, Amer)	n.a.	0.89	0.80	0.70	0.72
Los Angeles (whites)	n.a.	n.a.	n.a.	0.40	0.62
Denmark	0.53	0.60	0.54	0.50	0.60
Los Angeles (blacks)	n.a.	n.a.	n.a.	0.30	0.42
Connecticut (whites)	0.40	0.43	0.42	0.50	0.46
New Zealand (Maori)	n.a	0.22	0.20	0.60	0.59
New Zealand (non-Maori)	n.a.	0.49	0.50	0.50	0.51
California (Alameda, whites)	n.a.	0.42	0.40	0.40	0.46
Australia (NSW)	n.a.	n.a.	n.a.	0.40	0.46
Hawaii (Hawaiian)	0.21	0.19	0.30	0.20	0.24
Los Angeles (Japanese)	n.a.	n.a.	n.a.	0.20	0.21
Hawaii (whites)	0.28	0.40	0.37	0.50	0.43
UK (Birmingham)	0.44	0.45	0.46	0.50	0.44
China (Shanghai)	n.a.	n.a.	n.a.	0.30	0.27
Singapore (Chinese)	0.10	0.15	0.10	0.10	0.12
Colombia (Cali)	0.23	0.34	0.33	0.20	0.28
Hawaii (Japanese)	0.18	0.24	0.24	0.10	0.17
Japan (Miyagi)	0.02	0.20	0.09	0.10	0.15
India (Bombay)	n.a	0.08	0.10	0.10	0.14
Females					
Israel (Jews born Israel)	n.a.	0.71	0.80	0.60	0.95
Sweden	0.52	0.61	0.62	0.60	0.63
Israel (Jews born Eur, Amer)	n.a.	0.79	0.80	0.60	0.62
Los Angeles (whites)	n.a.	n.a.	n.a.	0.30	0.55
Denmark	0.44	0.50	0.50	0.40	0.56
Los Angeles (blacks)	n.a.	n.a.	n.a.	0.20	0.40
Connecticut (whites)	0.28	0.34	0.27	0.30	0.32
New Zealand (Maori)	n.a	0.24	0.20	0.30	0.30
New Zealand (non-Maori)	n.a.	0.34	0.30	0.30	0.34
California (Alameda, whites)	n.a.	0.42	0.40	0.40	0.30
Australia (NSW)	n.a.	n.a.	n.a.	0.30	0.30
Hawaii (Hawaiian)	0.34	0.32	0.16	0.30	0.32
Los Angeles (Japanese)	n.a.	n.a.	n.a.	0.10	0.25
Hawaii (whites)	0.18	0.20	0.46	0.20	0.23
UK (Birmingham)	0.31	0.34	0.33	0.40	0.36
China (Shanghai)	n.a.	n.a.	n.a.	0.20	0.21
Singapore (Chinese)	0.07	0.12	0.10	0.10	0.06
Colombia (Cali)	0.12	0.15	0.13	0.20	0.14
Hawaii (Japanese)	0.06	0.07	0.11	0.10	0.11
Japan (Miyagi)	0.03	0.18	0.05	0.10	0.12
India (Bombay)	n.a.	0.07	0.10	0.10	0.10

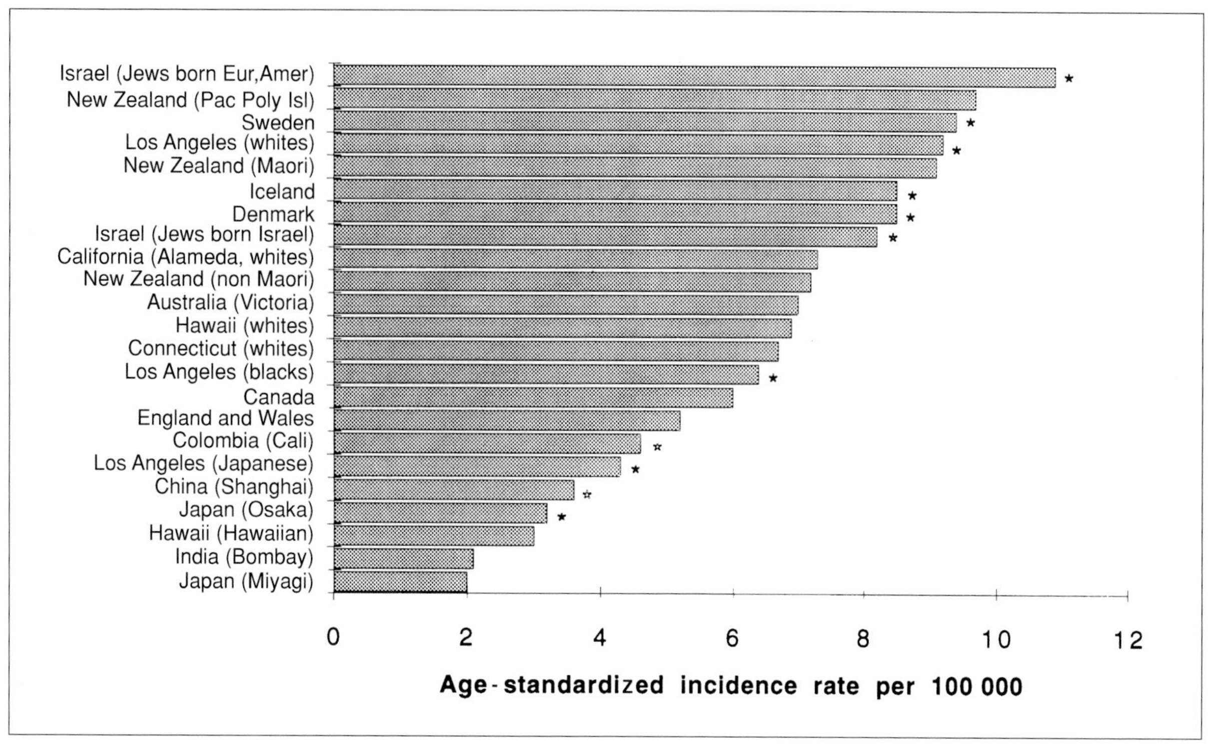

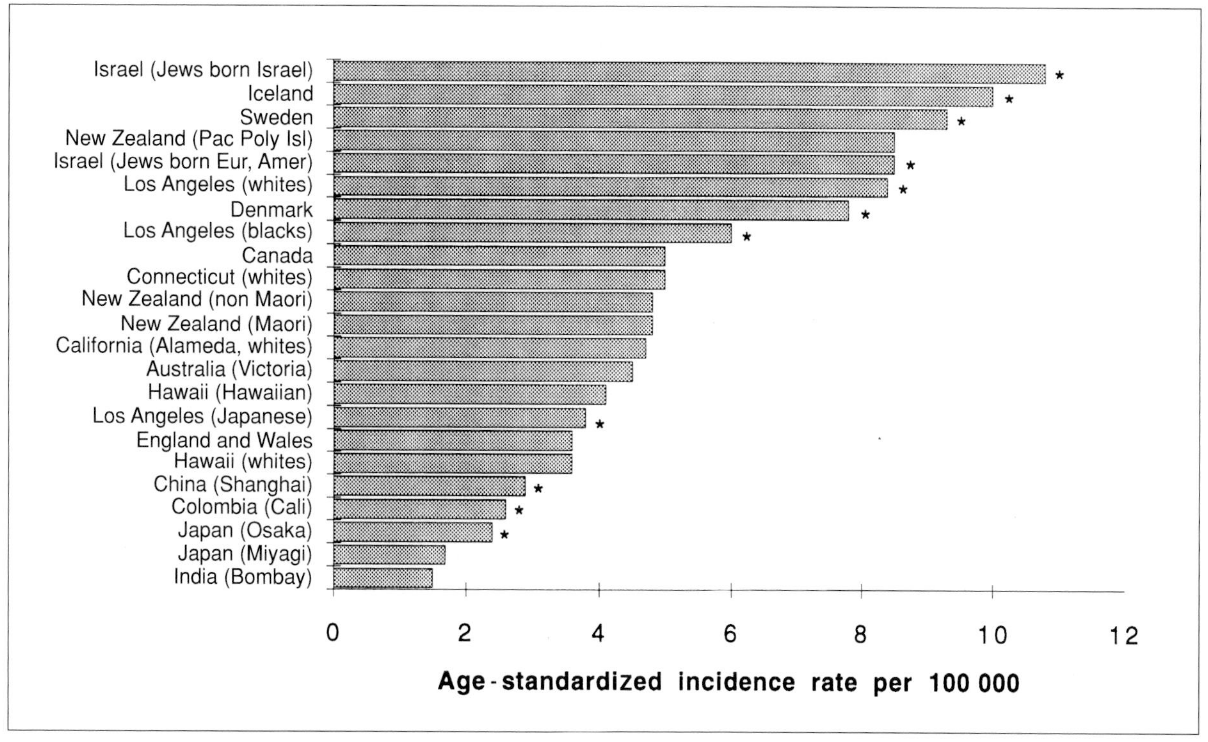

Fig. 4.1 Age-standardized malignant CNS tumor incidence in males and females. Source: Muir et al 1987. *Note*: those countries marked with * include benign and unspecified CNS tumors in their data.

The distribution of CNS tumor incidence with age is characterized by a peak in childhood, an exponential rise from the early twenties until age 70 years, followed by a decline with increasing age thereafter, rates in men being higher than those in women at all ages. Age incidence curves are illustrated (Fig. 4.2) for CNS tumors in selected populations (Muir et al 1987). It is apparent that rates in Sweden differ from other white Western populations in respect to their lack of decline after the age of 70 years. The Swedish pattern is also observed in other high risk populations such as Israeli Jews (Whelan et al 1990). Both these registries include tumors of benign and uncertain behavior, and are based in populations with high levels of medical services and high autopsy rates.

Given the potential for artefactual influences, the age-specific incidence of CNS tumors is remarkably consistent between populations. Velema & Walker (1987) examined age- and sex-specific incidence rates in the age range 35–65 years in 51 populations. The modeled slope of the age incidence curve on a log–log scale was found to be 2.6 for both sexes. There were no significant deviations from this model. Although the age curves had the same slope they were at different levels in different populations (highest in Israel and lowest in Asia) and were thought to reflect differences in exposure or susceptibility to etiological factors. The slope was the same in registries that included only malignant tumors as in registries that included tumors of benign and uncertain behavior, their inclusion merely increasing the level of incidence. The slope of 2.6 was somewhat less than slopes of 4–5 commonly observed for epithelial tumors, and close to a slope of 2.7 observed for soft tissue sarcomas (Cook et al 1969). According to the multi-stage theory (Armitage & Doll 1954), this implies that fewer events are required for the malignant transformation of glial cells compared to epithelial cells. In Moolgavkar's two-stage model (Moolgavkar et al 1980), the slope of the curve is dependent on the growth characteristics of the cells and the level of the curve is related to the probability of cell transformation. This model suggests that the difference in slope indicates differences in growth characteristics between glial and epithelial tissues.

Histologic types also vary in their incidence by age and sex (Fig. 4.3). CNS tumors in childhood (0–14 years) differ from those in adults, particularly in regard to the distribution of histologic types and intracranial location (Lacayo & Farmer 1991). In children medulloblastomas and astrocytomas are more common than other types, whereas in adults gliomas and meningiomas are more common. In children the majority (70%) of tumors are located below the tentorium compared to only 30% in adults (Rubinstein 1972). Table 4.3 contains rates for the principal histologic types of CNS tumors in childhood from selected cancer registries (Parkin et al 1988). There are some clear differences between the distributions in some populations, the most striking being the increased proportion of medulloblastoma in New Zealand Maoris which may indicate a genetic predisposition to this tumor. Differences between white and black children in the US, however, were found to be influenced by differential trends in histologic confirmation and in the proportion of unspecified tumors (Bunin 1987).

Velema & Percy (1987) examined the age curves of malignant CNS tumors by histologic type in adults similarly to the analysis of all CNS tumors by geographic location (Velema & Walker 1987). They discovered that the slopes of the incidence curves in the 35–64-year age range differed significantly by histologic type. The slope increased from 0.4 for ependymomas, to 1.0 for oligodendrogliomas, 1.7 for astrocytomas, 2.8 for meningiomas, and 3.9 for glioblastomas. These data suggest a different carcinogenic mechanism for glioblastoma compared with other CNS tumors. The steeper slope suggests that it may take more cellular events to transform a glial cell to a glioblastoma than is required for a lower grade tumor.

Socioeconomic status (SES) might explain some of the variation in CNS tumor incidence and mortality between populations. People of higher SES generally have better access to health care and are medically investigated more often than people of lower SES. In England and Wales the standardized mortality ratios (SMRs) for males and females aged between 15 and 64 years in social class I were 108 and 137 respectively, compared to SMRs of 92 and 100 for males and females of social class V (Logan 1982). Proportionally more deaths occurred over age 55 in persons from social class I compared to social class V. Under the age of 55 years the proportions of deaths by social class were very similar. Positive associations with SES have also been observed in males in the US (Preston-Martin 1989) but not in Australia (Williams et al 1991).

Trends over time

There is a continuing debate (Desmeules et al 1992) concerning the validity of increasing trends in CNS tumors. Long-term trends are commonly available from mortality statistics, which are subject to all the known shortcomings of death certificates (Garfinkel & Sarokhan 1982, Bahemuka et al 1988). Some longstanding population-based cancer registries such as Connecticut have been able to model age–period–cohort trends in incidence (Roush et al 1987). There is recent evidence that incidence might be increasing in the elderly in the United States (Grieg et al 1990), but this has been questioned (Boyle et al 1990, Modan et al 1992) as a diagnostic artefact related to the advent of CT scanning, given the low levels of histologic verification in the elderly. Similar increases have not been observed in other countries with long-established cancer registries such as Denmark or in Sweden (Ahlbom & Rodvall 1989), but have been seen

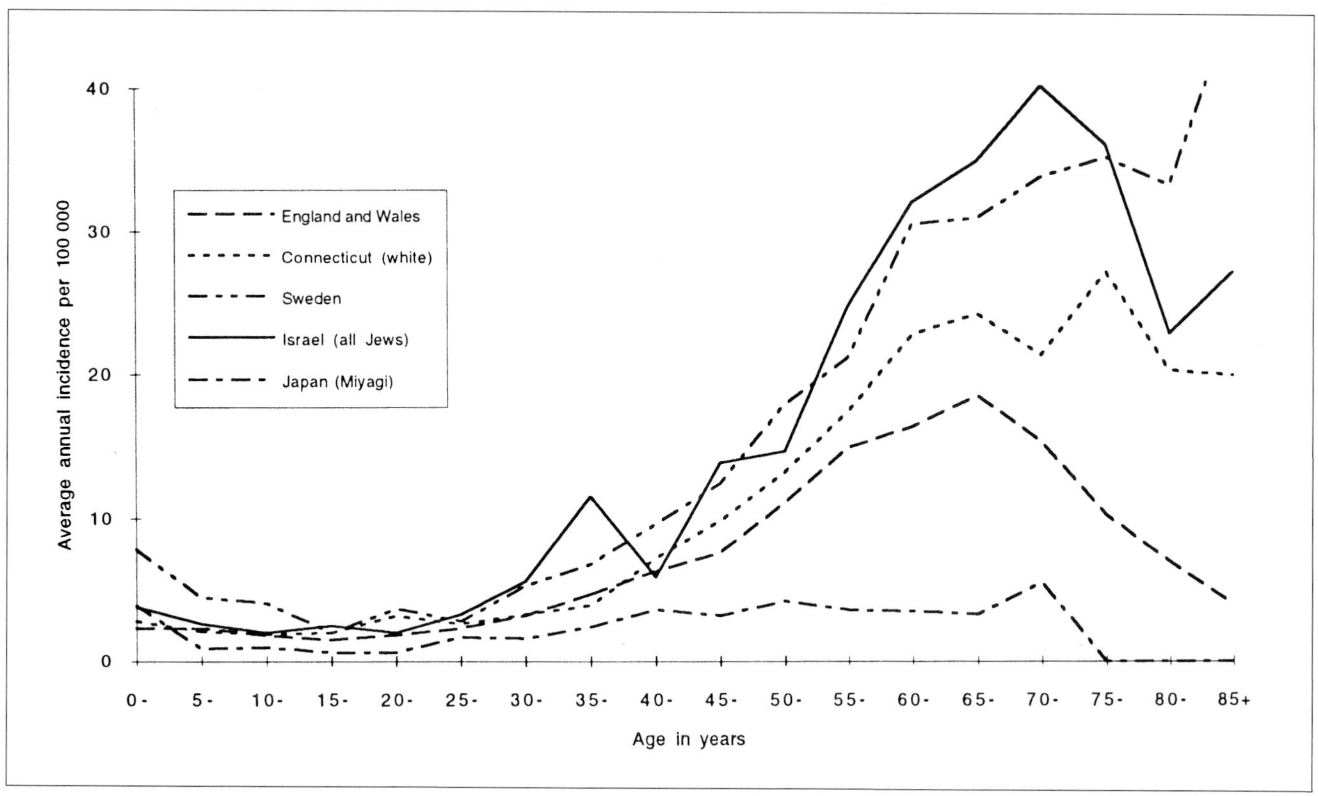

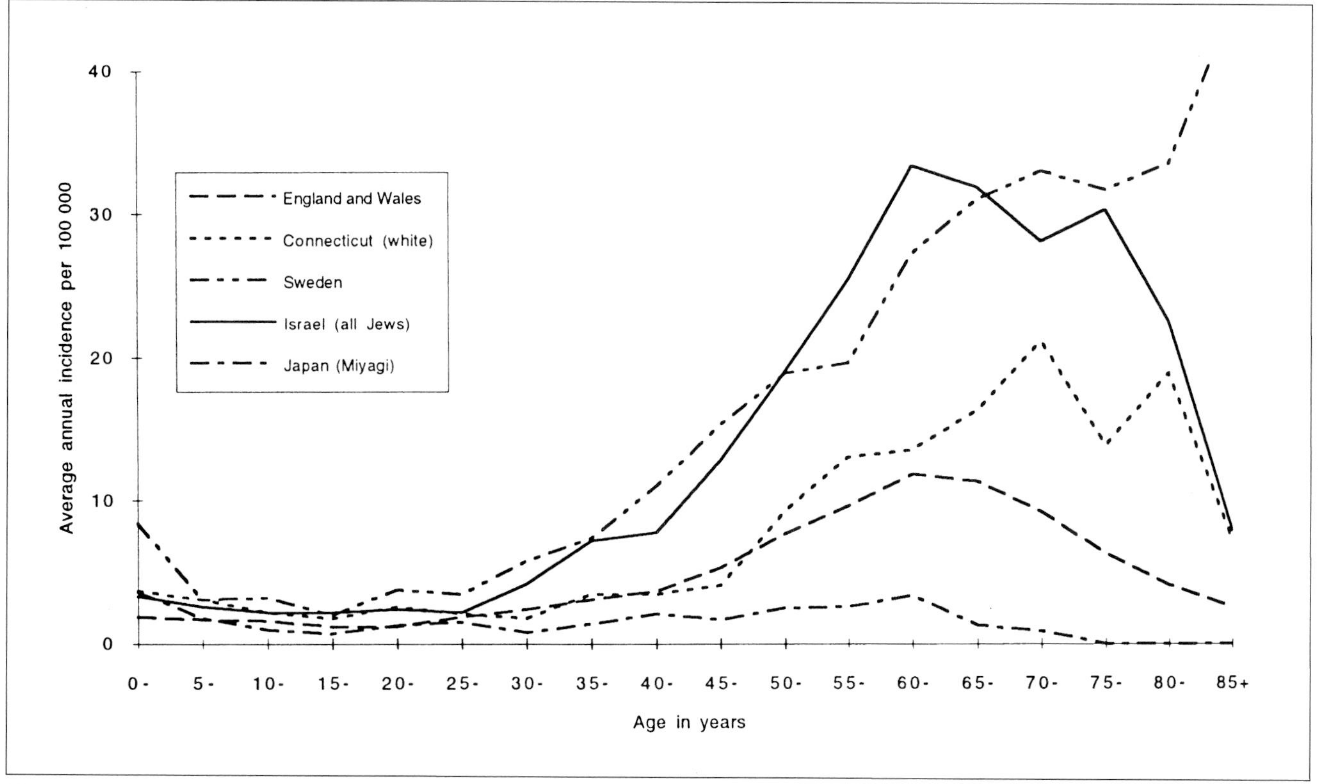

Fig. 4.2 Age-specific incidence rates for malignant CNS tumors in men and women. *Note*: Sweden and Israel include benign and unspecified tumors in their data.

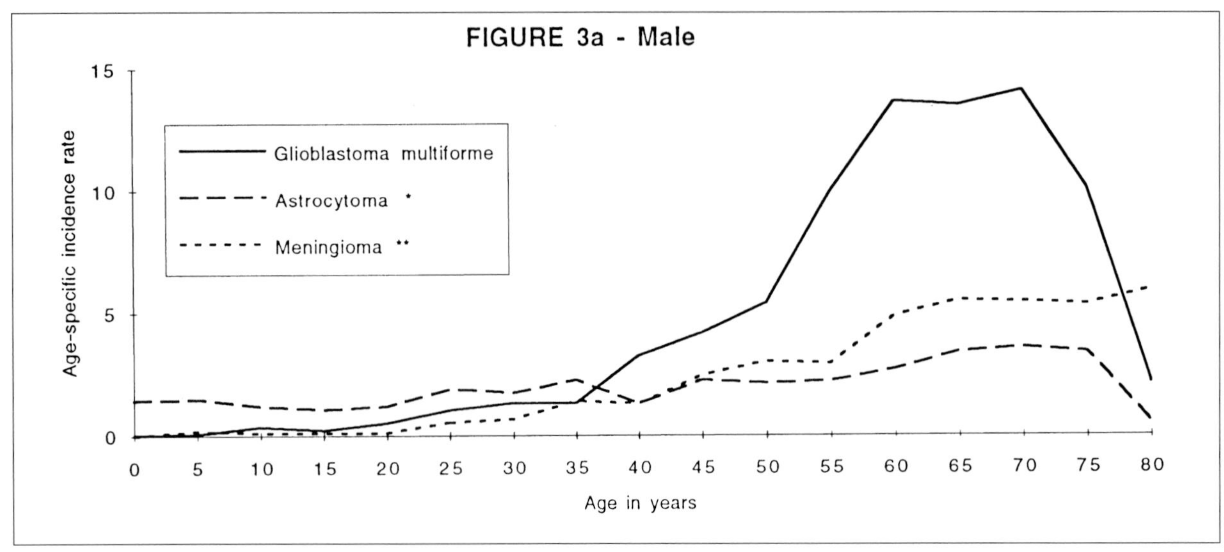

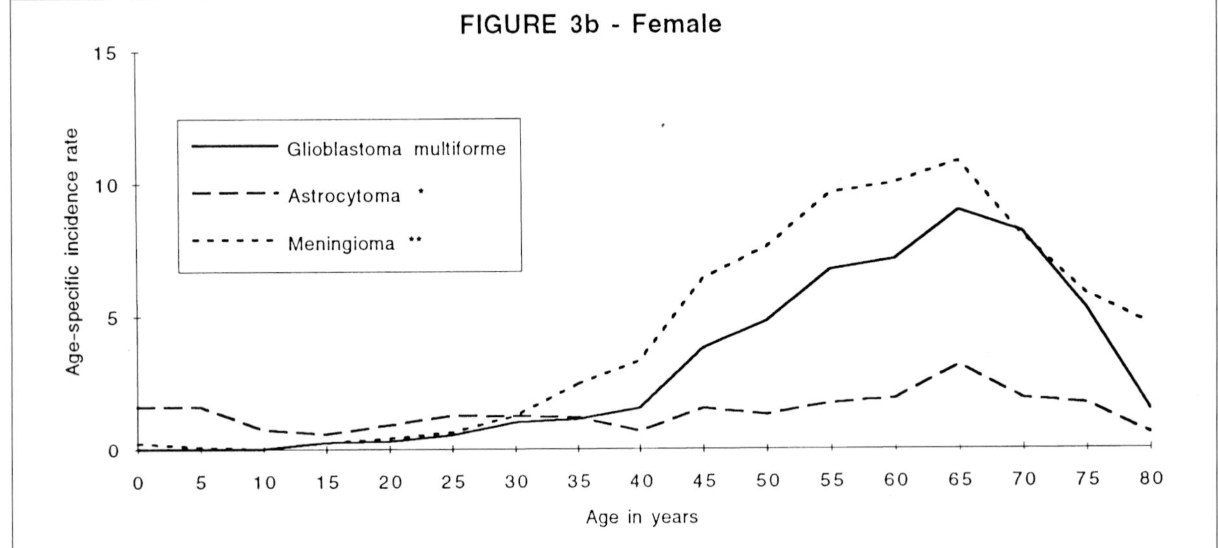

Note: * Anaplastic and well differentiated ** includes benign meningioma

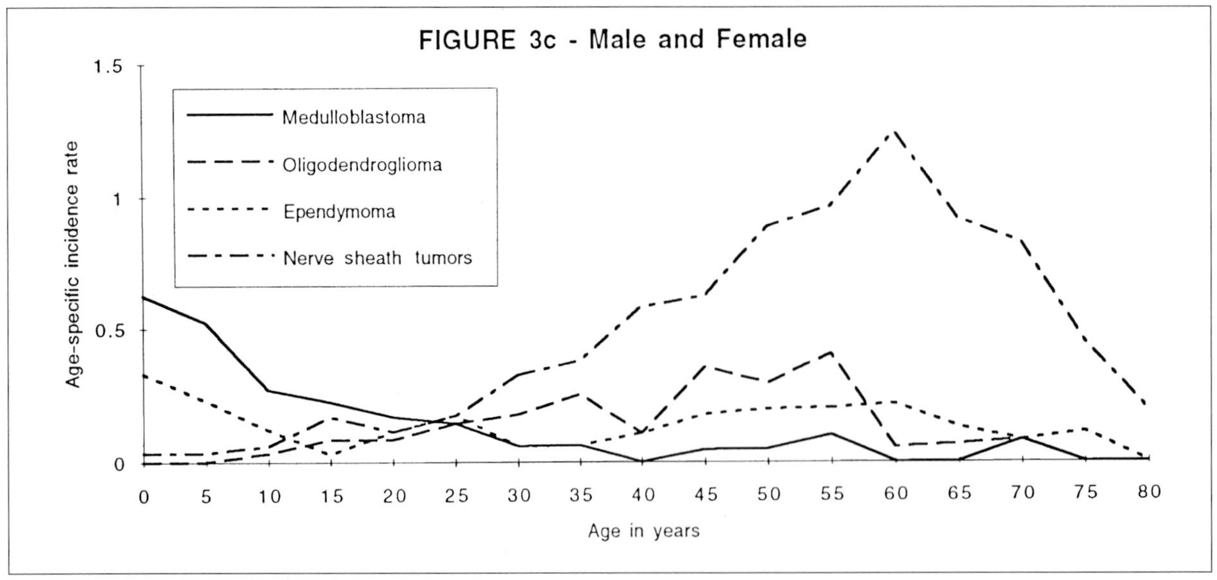

Fig. 4.3 Victoria 1982–1991: age-specific incidence rates by histologic type. Source: Victorian Cancer Registry 1993.

Table 4.3 CNS tumor incidence in children aged 0–14 by histologic type. Source: Parkin et al 1988

	Astrocytoma	Ependymoma	Medulloblastoma	Total
US SEER White	12.3	2.4	5.7	24.9
US SEER Black	9.1	2.1	5.0	22.0
Colombia (Cali)	5.7	0.8	2.7	16.8
Israel (Jews)	8.0	2.1	5.7	23.9
China (Shanghai)	2.7	0.6	1.7	19.9
Singapore (Chinese)	3.8	0.8	1.7	11.7
India (Bombay)	2.9	0.5	1.5	7.7
Japan (Miyagi)	2.8	0.5	2.5	9.5
Japan (Osaka)	2.9	1.6	2.3	24.1
Denmark	11.4	4.9	4.4	30.9
Sweden	15.7	4.3	6.4	33.7
England & Wales	8.9	3.2	4.9	24.4
Australia (NSW)	10.3	3.2	5.6	24.5
New Zealand (Maori)	4.1	2.6	10.3	24.6
New Zealand (non-Maori)	9.6	1.2	6.5	24.7

in others (Helseth et al 1988a). The lack of increase at younger ages also suggests a detection artefact in the elderly. Such artefacts have been shown previously in comparisons of US incidence series (Walker et al 1985).

Table 4.2 contains cumulative incidence rates percent to age 65 for CNS tumors from selected cancer registries in the first five volumes of *Cancer Incidence in Five Continents* (Stukonis 1978, Muir et al 1987) which together cover the period from the 1950s to 1982. The cumulative rate percent is a directly age-standardized rate which closely approximates actuarial estimates of risk (Day 1987). The rates have been truncated to age 65 to discount the effect of over-zealous investigation of the elderly (Peto 1981). All rates included in the table are observed to be less than 1%, and although some variation is present, there is little evidence of increasing trends over time. Many of the registries include tumors of benign and uncertain behavior (denoted by asterisks in the table) and therefore appear to have higher than average rates. Registries following this practice, however, do not provide much evidence of an increase in CNS tumor incidence in those aged under 65 years.

Trends by place and ethnicity

CNS tumors vary in incidence from population to population. Incidence rates standardized to the world population are illustrated in Figure 4.1 for males and females separately. Some of the variation in rates shown in the figure is due to detection artefacts linked with the availability of, and access to, medical technology. Interestingly, Japan, which has comparable technological development to Western industrialized countries, has rates of CNS cancer which are a third or less of those observed in the USA. The incidence in other Asian countries is also low. A substantial proportion of the incidence recorded by many registries is due to either the deliberate inclusion of tumors of benign and uncertain behavior, or failure to exclude them. As already noted in regard to Table 4.2, the exclusion of cases older than 65 years does not remove all of the variation between populations. Geographic variation in childhood CNS tumors is greater than for other childhood malignancies (Breslow & Langholz 1983). There may, therefore, exist real differences between populations due to genetic or environmental factors.

Incidence in ethnic subpopulations reported to *Cancer Incidence in Five Continents* is given in Table 4.4 (Muir et al 1987). Some ethnic groups such as New Zealand Maoris and New Zealand Pacific Polynesian Islanders have higher incidence rates than the 'white' New Zealanders. This contrasts with the US, where black Americans have lower rates than whites. Jews living in Israel and Jewish populations in the US have elevated rates (MacMahon 1960, Newill 1961, Muir et al 1987, Steinitz et al 1989). Asians tend to have low rates. Jewish migrants to Israel from Europe, America, Africa and Asia have higher incidence rates than Jews born in Israel (Steinitz et al 1989), but much of this excess occurs in the elderly and may be a consequence of increased screening.

Migrants to Australia have been the subject of investigation in regard to cancer mortality and incidence. Early analysis of mortality data from 1961–1972 showed elevated rates of malignant CNS tumors in adult males from Poland and Africa, and in adult females from Austria and Yugoslavia. There were no clear patterns with duration of residence, and childhood CNS cancer mortality rates were not statistically different to those for the Australian-born (Armstrong et al 1983). An analysis of Canadian mortality data for 1970–1973 showed excess mortality risk for immigrants from Britain, Germany, Italy, and Holland (Neutel et al 1989). The increased risk was higher in males than in females and was not apparent in the second generation. Australian malignant CNS tumor mortality data for 1979–1988 have been analysed

Table 4.4 Ethnic variation in CNS tumor incidence (truncated rates — ages 35–64). Source: Muir et al 1987

	Males	Females
US White Alameda	10.3	6.8
US White Bay Area	9.5	7.7
US White Los Angeles	13.7	12.1
US White Connecticut	10.0	6.2
US White New Orleans	7.4	4.4
US White Detroit	8.8	6.3
US Black Alameda	4.9	3.8
US Black Bay Area	5.1	5.4
US Black Los Angeles	9.4	9.4
US Black Connecticut	7.7	3.7
US Black New Orleans	4.0	4.2
US Black Detroit	5.8	3.7
US Chinese Bay Area	2.3	4.4
US Chinese Los Angeles	6.1	8.0
US Chinese Hawaii	10.1	—
Singapore Chinese	2.5	0.9
China Shanghai	5.8	4.7
China Tianjin	7.6	5.5
Hong Kong	2.7	2.4
US Japanese Bay Area	8.2	3.9
US Japanese Los Angeles	2.5	3.9
US Japanese Hawaii	3.2	2.0
Japan Miyagi	3.1	2.0
Japan Osaka	3.6	2.7
US Filipino Bay Area	1.7	2.4
US Filipino Los Angeles	2.6	9.8
Phillipines Rizal	2.2	1.5
US Amerindians New Mexico	1.5	—

by country of birth and are presented in the form of age-standardized mortality rate ratios in Figure 4.4 (Giles et al 1993a). Males from the British Isles and Northern Europe have ratios greater than one, and migrants from Asia tend to have low rate ratios. None of the rate ratios are significantly different to those in the Australian-born.

McCredie et al (1990) reviewed CNS tumor incidence by ethnic group in New South Wales and found no statistically significant differences in males but a significantly lower rate in female migrants from Asia. Malignant CNS tumor incidence in Victoria between 1982 and 1987 showed significantly elevated rates in male migrants from Southern Europe and in females from Europe (other than Southern Europe or the British Isles), while rates were significantly lower in female migrants from the Middle East and Asia (Giles et al 1992). These differences are consistent with differences in incidence rates between Australia and the migrants' countries of origin.

Rural residence has been shown to be associated with increased risk of gliomas in some studies (Choi et al 1970a, Musicco et al 1982, Mills et al 1989), but not all (Burch et al 1987). This association has been hypothesized to be related to agricultural exposures e.g. to zoonotic viruses and pesticides. Childhood CNS tumors have been associated with farm residence (Gold et al 1979).

Trends in survival

Survival statistics for specific histologic types of CNS tumor tend to be available for series of patients from specialist centres or from clinical trials and may not represent the experience of the majority of patients. Survival in patients from population-based series is usually only available for all CNS tumors combined and rarely for specific histologic types. Many survival analyses are adjusted using life tables and are reported as relative survival. Relative survival proportions are more comparable between populations than crude proportions, especially when cases tend to occur at older ages, when death from other causes becomes common.

Overall survival from CNS tumors has been comparatively poor, with only small gains being made in recent decades. In the United States, overall 5-year survival proportions for CNS tumors have improved from 18% in 1960–63 to 24% in 1981–86 (Boring et al 1991). In South Australia the average 5-year survival proportion between 1977 and 1990 was 21%, but was better for younger people, with 56% of males and 52% of females aged under 40 years surviving 5 years from diagnosis (Bonett et al 1991). Relative 5-year survival proportions for all gliomas diagnosed at all ages in Finland improved between 1953–68 (21%), 1969–78 (31%) and 1979–88 (36%) (Kallio et al 1991). A US-based national survey of patterns of care in 1980 and 1985 gave actuarial 5-year survival proportions by age and by Karnofsky ratings (Mahaley et al 1989). For patients in the 1980 survey the 5-year survival proportions averaged 5.7% for glioblastoma, 33.5% for astrocytoma, 91.6% for meningioma and 60.9% for medulloblastoma. Survival curves for CNS malignancies diagnosed in Victoria between 1982 and 1991 are illustrated in Figure 4.5. The relative survival proportion for all CNS tumors was 21%, identical to that reported in South Australia. Relative survival proportions for the principal histologic types of tumor in Victoria are given in Table 4.5. The relative survival proportions for CNS tumors not histologically confirmed, but for which there was clinical and imaging evidence, were expectably low.

Survival differs by age group, childhood CNS tumors generally having a better prognosis than those occurring in adults. In Australia between 1978 and 1982 the 5-year survival proportions for children were: astrocytoma 73%, medulloblastoma 43%, and ependymoma 44% (Australian Paediatric Cancer Registry 1989). Survival proportions for childhood CNS tumors in Victoria improved between 1970–79 and 1980–89 (Giles et al 1993b). Although 5-year survival from astrocytoma (70% to 80%) and medulloblastoma (50% to 53%) both increased between these two time periods, only survival from ependymoma increased significantly (37% to 59%). Children in England and Wales diagnosed during 1971–74 obtained 5-year

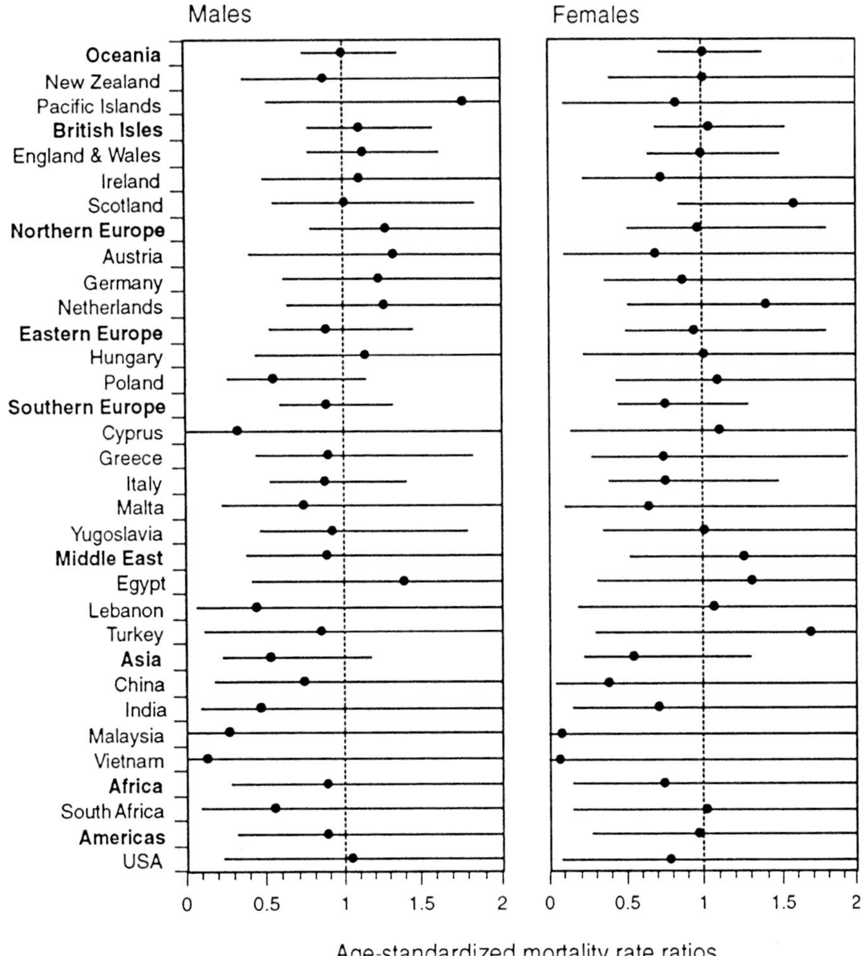

Fig. 4.4 Mortality from CNS tumors in migrants to Australia 1979–1988. Source: Giles et al 1993a. *Note*: the vertical dotted lines are equivalent to the rates in the Australian-born which are 5.2 per 100 000 in males and 3.5 per 100 000 in females.

survival proportions of 56% for astrocytoma, 24% for medulloblastoma and 36% for ependymoma (Office of Population Censuses and Surveys 1981). Astrocytomas in childhood are commonly of lower grade than in adults, and this improves prognosis. Kibirige et al (1988), reviewing astrocytomas from the Manchester Children's Tumour Registry, observed higher 5-year survival proportions for children with juvenile astrocytomas (75%) compared with children having higher grade, adult astrocytomas (15%).

HOST FACTORS

A variety of items relating to personal characteristics or medical history, including immunologic status, family history and genetic factors, have been associated with CNS tumor risk. Common epidemiologic measures of strength of association include odds ratios (OR) which are estimated from case-control studies and which approximate the relative risk (RR) obtained from cohort studies. They estimate the degree to which the factor or attribute under consideration increases tumor risk in comparison to a reference population or control group.

Medical history

Maternal and reproductive factors have been associated with CNS tumors. These findings tend to be isolated reports from small studies which require corroboration. Positive associations have been reported with a prior history of abortion (Choi et al 1970b), increased maternal age (Selvin & Garfinkel 1972), first birth and high birthweight (Gold et al 1979). The occurrence of CNS tumors during pregnancy has been reviewed by Roelvink et al (1987), who conclude that some CNS tumors are hormone sensitive and may respond to the changing hormonal milieu during pregnancy (many CNS tumors have been shown to possess hormone receptors). The relationship(s) are not established and may prove to be provocative rather than causal. Interestingly, meningio-

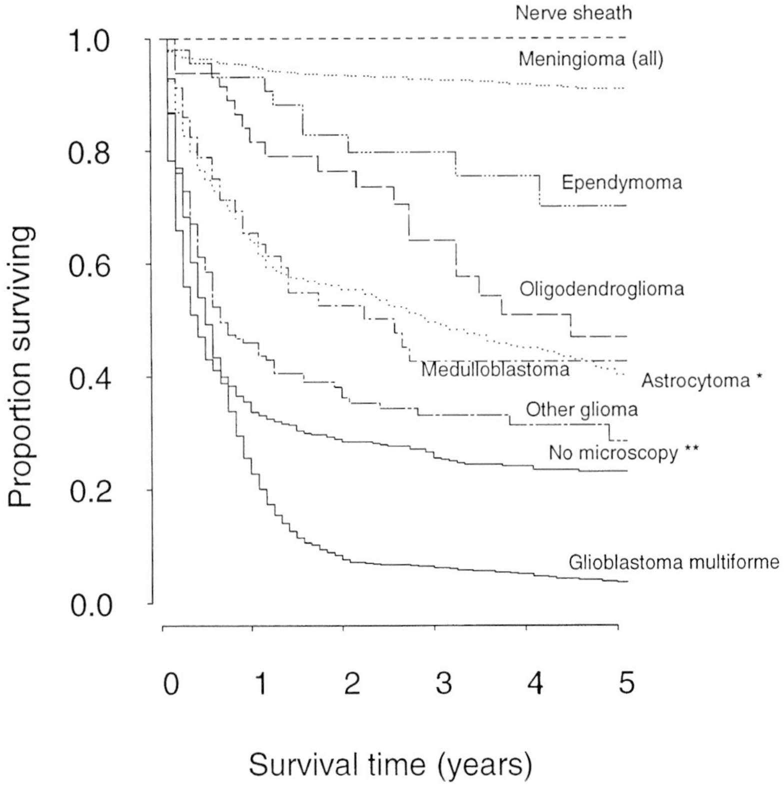

Fig. 4.5 Survival from malignant CNS tumors in Victoria 1982–1991. Source: Victorian Cancer Registry 1993. *Note*: * = anaplastic or well differentiated; ** = presence of tumor ascertained on clinical and/or radiologic data only.

Table 4.5 Five-year relative survival from malignant CNS tumors in Victoria, 1982–1991. Source: Giles et al 1993b

Histology	Survival %
Glioblastoma	4
Astrocytoma	43
Medulloblastoma	41
Oligodendroglioma	47
Ependymoma	59
Other glioma	30
Meningioma (malignant)	50
Other	29
Unspecified	28
No microscopy	21

mas, which occur more often in women than men, have been associated with a prior history of breast cancer (Schoenberg et al 1975, Smith et al 1978) a hormone-dependent malignancy. Schlehofer et al (1992b) found that menopausal women had a much reduced risk of meningioma which decreased further in women who had had a bilateral oophorectomy prior to menopause. Menopausal women were at increased risk of gliomas and acoustic neuromas unless menopause had been surgically induced. These findings support a role for female hormones in CNS tumor development.

Several intercurrent diseases and chronic conditions have also been investigated in regard to their potential influence on CNS tumor risk, including hypertension, stroke, diabetes, epilepsy, and cranial trauma. Hypertension was not associated with either glioma or meningioma risk in Seventh-Day Adventists (Mills et al 1989). Stroke was found to be associated with risk (OR 6.26) of meningioma in women (Mills et al 1989) and with glioblastoma (Dobkin 1985). Diabetes has been associated with both increased risk (Mills et al 1989) and decreased risk of glioma (Aronson & Aronson 1965). Epilepsy (or its treatment) has been associated with excess risk of CNS tumors (Clemmesen et al 1974) but the two are totally confounded. The role of trauma has been a contentious issue but is now considered not to be causal in relation to glioma (Hochberg et al 1990, Schlehofer et al 1992a); however, reports suggest an increased risk of meningioma associated with a history of head injury (Schoenberg 1991). Tonsillectomy has been positively associated with glioma in one study (Mills et al 1989) and either null or negatively associated with glioma in two others (Gold et al 1979, Preston-Martin et al 1982). The association of allergy with CNS tumor risk has been the subject of debate (Vena et al 1985, McWhorter 1988). A history of allergy has been consistently associated with decreased risk of CNS tumor in recent studies (Hochberg et al 1990, Schlehofer et al 1992a), including an OR of 0.5 for glioma (Ryan et al 1992).

Multiple primary tumors following primary brain tumors have been investigated in Connecticut and Denmark cancer registries. In Connecticut residents diagnosed between 1935 and 1982, significant excesses of melanoma and acute non-lymphocytic leukemia were observed (Tucker et al 1985). In Denmark between 1943 and 1984 the RRs of second primaries were kidney 3.2, bone 6.9, connective tissue 4.9, melanoma (females only) 2.5, secondary brain tumors 2.0, CLL (males only) 3.2 (Osterlind et al 1985). The association between breast cancer and subsequent meningioma has already been referred to (Schoenberg et al 1975).

Genetics and familial clustering

As in many other malignancies, familial clustering has been observed with CNS tumors. The literature is based largely on case reports and it is difficult to determine whether such instances are related to genetic or environmental factors shared by family members. In his review, Tijssen (1985) pointed to the concordance of histology and age at diagnosis in 8 pairs of monozygotic twins; the occurrence of similar neuroglial tumors in (often consecutive) siblings; the decreased age at onset in the children of families with both parents and children affected with neuroglial tumors; the dominance of glioblastoma and medulloblastoma in familial CNS tumors; and the occurrence of familial meningioma in several generations, probably associated with neurofibromatosis (Sorensen et al 1985). Hirayama (1989) found that, of 168 Japanese children with CNS tumors, 8 had a family history of CNS tumors compared to 3.6 expected. Mahaley et al (1989) reported a family history of 16% in the patterns of care survey. Farwell & Flannery (1984) reported increased RRs for CNS tumors in the families of children with CNS neoplasms. The RR for CNS tumors in siblings was 8 and for parents 5. When the analysis was limited to children with medulloblastomas, the RR of CNS tumors in siblings increased to 30.

Certain hereditary and congenital diseases are known to carry an increased risk of CNS tumors. They include neurofibromatosis (Blatt et al 1986), Bourneville's disease, Li-Fraumeni tumor syndrome (also known as the SBLA syndrome) (Lynch et al 1989), ataxia telangiectasia (Swift et al 1986), Gorlin syndrome and Turcot syndrome (Bolande 1989). An excess risk of CNS tumors in persons with blood group A has not been substantiated (Yates & Pearce 1960, Choi et al 1970b). Several cytogenetic studies of CNS tumors have shown abnormalities, especially the loss or translocation of parts of chromosome 22 in familial meningioma and acoustic neuroma, and gains on chromosome 7 or losses on 9 or 10 in gliomas, and disturbances involving chromosomes 1, 6, 17, 19 in other CNS tumors (Zang & Singer 1967, Bigner et al 1984, Bolger et al 1985, Seizinger et al 1986, Black 1991a,b).

The genetic epidemiology of CNS tumors is entering an exciting phase. The loss of tumor suppressor genes seems to be a fundamental mechanism in the development of several type of CNS tumors (Seizinger 1991). Another mechanism is the activation of proto-oncogenes and growth factors (Harley 1988, Akbasak & Sunar-Akbasak 1992). For example, amplification of the proto-oncogene for epidermal growth factor receptor has been reported in 25–50% of glioblastomas and 9% of astrocytomas (Bigner et al 1988, Helseth et al 1988b). Epidemiology should play a role in identifying which individual attributes and environmental exposures (particularly the role of viruses) increase susceptibility to, and the probability of, these molecular genetic events.

ENVIRONMENTAL FACTORS

The literature contains many instances of associations between environmental agents and increased risk of CNS tumors. Given the number of studies, their low statistical power, and the number of multiple comparisons made, it is to be expected that many of these will have been chance associations (Ahlbom 1990). Isolated reports and contradictory findings, therefore, have to be viewed with a degree of scepticism. There are also methodological problems with a number of the published studies. Consistent reports from different studies are few, and taken together, the established risk factors for CNS tumors can explain only a small proportion of their incidence.

Radiation

The relationship between ionizing radiation and CNS tumors has not been investigated to the same extent as that with leukemia and certain other cancers because the brain was for some time considered to be relatively resistant to radiation carcinogenesis (National Research Council 1980). Evidence is growing that diagnostic and therapeutic exposures in utero (Bithell & Stewart 1975, Monson & MacMahon 1984), childhood (Ron et al 1988), and adult life (Preston-Martin et al 1983) might increase CNS tumor risk. Atomic bomb survivor data are inconsistent and show either null or modest risks (Seyama et al 1979, Darby et al 1985). However, Japanese have a low susceptibility to CNS tumors and may respond differently to radiation exposure. Children irradiated for tinea capitis have been shown to have increased incidence of CNS tumors, especially meningiomas (RR 9.5), gliomas (RR 2.6), and nerve sheath tumors (RR 18.8) (Ron et al 1988). The increased risk after exposures of between 1 and 2 Gy indicates the possibility of late effects from low dose radiotherapy in childhood. In adults, high dose radiation to the head has been shown to increase the risk of meningioma (Munk et al 1969) and dental X-rays have also been shown to increase the risk of meningioma, especially in women, but not glioma (Preston-Martin et al

1980, Preston-Martin et al 1983, Preston-Martin et al 1985, Ryan et al 1992). Increased risks in dentists and dental nurses have been observed in Sweden (Ahlbom et al 1986). Glioblastoma multiforme and ependymomas have been induced in primates given high dose radiation (Kent & Pickering 1958, Traynor & Casey 1971, Haymaker et al 1972, Krupp 1976). Case reports in humans have been reviewed by Salvati et al (1990).

The role of non-ionizing radiation in the etiology of human CNS tumors is controversial. These forms of radiation do not have tumor-initiating properties and are thought to have promoting effects, if any (Poole & Trichopoulos 1991). It has been suggested that residential magnetic fields may relate to the development of CNS tumors in children (Wertheimer & Leeper 1979). Several studies of residential and occupational magnetic field exposures have followed (Easterly 1981, Ahlbom 1988, Coleman & Beral 1988, Savitz et al 1988). Apart from one study (Feychting & Ahlbom 1992), these have recently been reviewed (National Radiation Protection Board 1992). Generally, the evidence is at best suggestive. The strongest association has been, not with any direct measurement of magnetic fields, but with the configuration of primary and secondary electrical distribution lines outside the residence (wire code) used as an indicator of hypothesized magnetic field levels inside the home, or with time-averaged estimates of magnetic fields. Positive associations have been seen in regard to primary CNS tumors. The National Radiation Protection Board's review gave pooled estimates of the ORs from studies of measured fields to be 1.85 (0.91–3.77); from distance studies to be 1.09 (0.50–2.37); and for wire coding studies to be 2.04 (1.11–3.76) (National Radiation Protection Board 1992). Feychting & Ahlbom (1992) failed to find any significant associations between EMF exposures and CNS tumors in children.

Most studies of magnetic fields and childhood tumor have suffered from problems of selection and recall bias, lack of control of confounders and poor statistical power. The study by Feychting & Ahlbom (1992) made some progress in that it was free of bias and was able to look at some potential confounders (SES and traffic pollution showed no effect). Further studies would benefit from increased disease specificity and a more restricted age group, focusing on ages when residential magnetic fields are the main source of magnetic field exposure. Apart from these design characteristics, the other major problem has been magnetic field exposure assessment. At present no firm conclusions can be drawn concerning the possible relationship between magnetic fields and childhood and CNS tumors.

Infection

The role of infection in CNS tumor etiology is unclear. Isolated reports have usually been countered by lack of associations in other studies. Associations between TB and glioma have been reported (Ward et al 1973, MacPherson 1976). It has been suggested that the development of both TB and glioma might be related to an impaired immune system. A positive reaction to a TB test was associated with an increased but statistically insignificant OR of 1.46 for glioma, and an OR of 1.49 for meningioma in Seventh-Day Adventists (Mills et al 1989). *Toxoplasma gondii* infection, which has a predilection for neural tissue, has been related in one study to astrocytoma (Schuman et al 1967). However, no association between *T. gondii* antibodies and glioma was seen in a recent Australian study which, to the contrary, showed an association (OR 2.06) with meningioma (Ryan et al 1993). Bithell et al (1973) found an association between maternal chickenpox infection and medulloblastoma but this finding has not been replicated (Adelstein & Donovan 1972, Gold 1980). There have also been reports of astrocytomas in patients with multiple sclerosis (Reagan & Freiman 1973). Associations with sick pets and with farm residence have also been reported (Gold et al 1979).

C-type viruses resembling animal leukemia/sarcoma viruses have been detected in human CNS tumors (Yohn 1972). DNA from BK virus, a human papovavirus, has also been detected in human CNS tumors (Corallini et al 1987) and there has been a single report of multifocal high grade astrocytoma in a patient with progressive multifocal leukoencephalopathy related to JC virus infection (Sima et al 1983). Footprints of Simian Virus 40 (a contaminant of polio vaccine given to millions of people between 1955 and 1962) have been detected in human CNS tumors but the question of causation has yet to be proved. Since the HIV epidemic a few cases of cerebral Kaposi's sarcoma have been reported (Charman et al 1988), as well as increases in cerebral lymphomas (Biggar et al 1987). The significance of the ubiquitous presence of EBV in cerebral lymphomas occurring in HIV/AIDS patients is currently unresolved (Morgello 1992).

CNS tumors, particularly sarcomas, have been induced in animals by several oncogenic viruses including Rous Sarcoma Virus, adenovirus type 12, chicken-embryo-lethal-orphan virus, Simian Virus 40, JC papovavirus, and both murine and avian sarcoma viruses (Pitts et al 1983, Tracy et al 1985, Kornbluth et al 1986). Evidence is accumulating that viruses may play a role in CNS carcinogenesis by gene rearrangement and amplification of normal proto-oncogenes (Charman et al 1988).

Occupation

The excess of glioma in males has suggested that occupational exposures might be related to their occurrence (Moss 1985, Kessler & Brandt-Rauf 1987). As with other tumors, the study of occupation and brain tumor has not been without its problems. In their review of brain tumors and occupational risk factors, Thomas & Waxweiler (1986) complained of diagnostic non-specificity, the paucity of case-control studies, the reliance on mortality studies and the statistical inevitability of finding associations in studies which involve multiple comparisons. Furthermore, studies relating CNS tumors to occupation tended to be based largely on descriptions of job titles rather than on exposures to specific agents such as vinyl chloride (Waxweiler et al 1976). Occupations in the electrical and electronics, oil refining, rubber, airplane manufacture, machining, farming and pharmaceutical and chemical industries had been associated with increased CNS tumor risk. The culpable agents were suspected to be various chemicals (Thomas et al 1987b) including benzene and other organic solvents, lubricating oils, acrylonitrile, vinyl chloride, formaldehyde, polycyclic aromatic hydrocarbons, phenol and phenolic compounds, and both ionizing and non-ionizing radiation.

Occupational status in certain white collar professions has also been associated with increased risk, e.g. artists, laboratory professionals, veterinarians and embalmers. Some common exposures to carcinogenic agents were suspected in these professions. Elevated risk in high status jobs also raised the issue of diagnostic sensitivity bias (Greenwald et al 1981), i.e. increased diagnosis in high status groups because of increased access to and use of medical screening. Reif et al (1989) in new Zealand found significantly elevated risks for statisticians, mathematicians and systems analysts (OR 3.72), clergymen (OR 3.8), and electrical engineers (OR 4.06), which were only slightly reduced when compared with other workers in the professional and technical category. An increased risk of CNS tumors in dentists has been demonstrated by Ahlbom et al (1986). An increased risk was also observed for social science professionals in Missouri (Brownson et al 1990). McLaughlin et al (1987) demonstrated increased risks in professional groups in Sweden (medical professionals, biologists, agricultural research scientists, dentists) where there is universal access to free medical care, a medical setting in which there should be no bias due to over-diagnosis in persons from more privileged sections of society.

There has been a sustained interest in electrical workers and their exposure to electromagnetic fields (EMF) (Lin et al 1985, Thomas et al 1987a, Speers et al 1988, Loomis & Savitz 1990, Schlehofer et al 1990). In their review of EMF and tumor, Poole & Trichopoulos (1991) point out similar deficiencies to Thomas & Waxweiler (1986): of the 17 case-control studies that examined occupational exposures to EMF only 5 were sufficiently large and well designed to ascertain exposure to EMF more completely than using routine data from tumor registration or death certification. The available cohort studies tended not to suggest an appreciable association between occupational EMF exposure and CNS tumors. Floderus et al (1992) examined occupational exposure to (measured) EMF in a case-control study and found an RR of 2.8 in the highest exposure category. This excess risk was mainly attributed to cases under age 40 and showed no difference between low grade and high grade astrocytomas. Ryan et al (1992) demonstrated in a case-control study an increased risk of glioma among women who were occupationally exposed to cathode ray tubes, but failed to confirm elevated risks for all workers in electrical or electronics industries.

Employment in the oil refining industry has sometimes shown increased CNS tumor risk and sometimes no risk. No excess risk of CNS tumors was found if tumors of benign and uncertain behavior were included in calculating SMRs (Wong et al 1986), nor was excess risk of histologically confirmed glioma observed in men employed in petroleum refineries in Sweden (McLaughlin et al 1987). Magnani et al (1987), in a death certificate based case-control study, identified increased risk (OR 2.9) in men employed in petroleum refining as process operators. In their review, which included 10 refinery cohort studies in the US, the International Agency for Research on Cancer Working Group on the Evaluation of Carcinogenic Risks to Humans (International Agency for Research on Cancer 1989) concluded that, of the elevated risks reported, only one was statistically significant, and was limited to workers of short duration of employment.

Farming and farm residence has been associated with increased risk of CNS tumor. Farmers may come into contact with a variety of chemical agents and zoonotic viruses but there is no firm evidence inculpating any specific exposure (Blair et al 1985). In New Zealand (Reif et al 1989) the farming risk was found to be strongest for livestock farmers (OR 2.59). One report of higher levels of organochlorine compounds in the adipose tissue of glioblastoma cases compared to controls indicates a possible carcinogenic role for pesticide exposure (Unger & Olsen 1980). Organochlorine exposure has been observed to be higher in woodworkers with glioma compared to woodworker controls (Cordier et al 1988). Men employed in agricultural crop production in Missouri had an OR of 1.5 for CNS tumors of several cell types (Brownson et al 1990).

Other occupations which have been shown to be associated with glioma in males include potters, kilnsmen and glass workers, welders and metal cutters, and employment in the machinery and electronics industries, cellulose plants, brick and tile making, petroleum and coal industries, and coffee shops (McLaughlin et al 1989). A study in New Zealand found significant risks of malignant brain tumor in males employed as textile workers (weavers), plumbers, and sheet and structural metal workers (Reif et al 1989). Speers et al (1988) found increased risk of glioma death in truck drivers (OR 6.65) and utility workers (OR 13.1). Brownson et al (1990) detected an OR of 2.8 for men employed in printing and publishing, and an

OR of 2.5 for brickmasons and tilesetters. A retrospective cohort study of cosmetologists detected a standardized incidence ratio of 168 for CNS tumors in females, which increased to 299 with 35 or more years of follow-up (Teta et al 1984). In the same study, 4 CNS tumors were found in males compared with 1.9 expected. The authors considered an occupational risk to be unlikely, especially in the older beauticians who would have been exposed to fewer chemicals and dyes than their younger counterparts. A possible carcinogenic role for formaldehyde has been postulated following the detection of increased mortality from CNS tumors in embalmers (Walrath & Fraumeni 1983), subsequently supported by increased incidence in anatomists and pathologists (Harrington & Oakes 1984, Stroup et al 1986).

Studies of parental (usually paternal) occupational exposures in regard to the risk of tumor in children have been reviewed (Arundel & Kinnier-Wilson 1986, Savitz & Chen 1990). Some studies have specifically examined CNS tumors (Peters et al 1981, Peters & Preston-Martin 1982, Olshan et al 1986, Johnson et al 1987, Nasca et al 1988, Wilkins & Koutras 1988, Johnson & Spitz 1989, Wilkins & Sinks 1990) but some studies have included neuroblastomas with CNS tumors. Savitz & Chen (1990) summarized the findings of studies of CNS tumors as follows: inconsistent associations with motor vehicle-related occupations, an unreplicated OR of 4.4 for machine repairmen, elevated risks for painters in three of four studies, consistently elevated ORs associated with occupations in chemical and petroleum industries and electrical occupations. Occupational and industrial exposures to ionizing radiation were consistent with ORs of 2.0. Savitz & Chen (1990) noted isolated reports of associations with metal-related occupations, farming, construction, aircraft industry, and printing.

A variety of chemical carcinogens, including N-nitroso compounds, polycyclic aromatic hydrocarbons, acrylonitrile and vinyl chloride, have been shown to cause brain tumors in experimental animals (Maltoni et al 1977, Maltoni et al 1982, Swenburg 1982, Ward & Rice 1982, Zeller et al 1982, Zimmerman 1982). Rice & Ward (1982) indicated that the age dependence of chemically induced CNS tumors in experimental animals was greatest in prenatal life. Transplacental CNS carcinogenesis has been observed to occur, particularly in regard to exposure to nitrosoureas (Druckrey 1973).

Diet

Associations between diet and CNS tumors in humans remain hypothetical. International correlations have been shown between CNS tumors and per capita consumption of total fat, animal protein, and fats and oils (Armstrong & Doll 1975). However, these correlations could easily be due to international differences in technological development and ethnic differences in susceptibility. It is believed that the consumption, and endogenous production, of N-nitroso compounds and their precursors might increase brain tumor risk (Preston-Martin 1990). On the other hand, the consumption of orange juice and vitamin supplements (which contain antioxidant substances such as ascorbic acid which inhibit endogenous nitrosation activity) has been associated with reduced risk of childhood CNS tumors (Preston-Martin et al 1984, Howe et al 1989). Most dietary epidemiologic studies of CNS tumors, however, have used poor measures of intake and have been too small to detect significant risks. Burch et al (1987) suggested a protective effect of fruit but not vegetables. Preston-Martin et al (1989b) suggested that citrus fruits were protective of meningioma but the OR was not statistically significant. A prospective study of Seventh-Day Adventists (Mills et al 1989) showed discrepant and non-significant associations with dietary items. A case-control study in Germany (Boeing et al 1993) detected an increased glioma risk associated with the consumption of ham, processed pork and fried bacon, but no association with endogenous N-nitrosation, or with the intake of vitamin C, or fruit and vegetables. In an Australian study, no increase in risk of glioma or meningioma in adults was found with the regular consumption of foods rich in N-nitroso precursors, nor were any decreases in risk associated with the regular use of foods and supplements containing endogenous nitrosation inhibitors (Ryan et al 1992).

Alcohol

The evidence linking alcoholic beverages with CNS tumors is sparse and inconsistent, and largely negative. Choi et al (1970b) found fewer CNS tumor cases had ever drunk alcohol compared to controls. Brain tumor risk has been associated in one study with increased consumption of wine (Burch et al 1987). This finding was not supported by Preston-Martin et al (1989b) who found no association with alcohol intake. Ryan et al (1992) found decreased risks for glioma and meningioma with all forms of alcohol consumption, a significant reduction in risk (OR 0.58) being observed for glioma and wine consumption. Boeing et al (1993) found no associations between lifetime alcoholic beverage consumption either for total alcohol or for single beverages. Howe et al (1989) found a significant positive association between childhood CNS tumors and the mother drinking beer in pregnancy.

Tobacco

Associations have been shown between passive smoking and childhood CNS tumors (Gold et al 1979, Preston-Martin et al 1982). In a cohort study in Japan (Hirayama 1985), non-smoking wives of men who smoked more than

20 cigarettes a day were shown to have a rate of brain tumor almost five times (95% confidence interval 1.72 to 14.11) that of women married to non-smokers. Ryan et al (1992) found no associations with glioma but direct and passive smoking increases the risk for meningioma, especially in women. Burch et al (1987) showed increasing risk of CNS tumors with increasing consumption of 'plain cigarettes'. No association was found in a cohort of SDAs (Mills et al 1989). Choi et al (1970b) did not show any risk of CNS tumors associated with smoking, and neither did Brownson et al (1990). The passive smoking findings are difficult to interpret given the lack of direct association between smoking and CNS tumors (Hirayama 1985).

Drugs

Clemmesen et al (1974) first raised the question of anticonvulsants causing brain tumor among epileptics who were long-term users. An increased risk of childhood brain tumor was shown in mothers who had used barbiturates during pregnancy (Gold et al 1979) but this was not supported by a later study (Preston-Martin et al 1982). A review of the evidence (MacMahon 1985) concluded that there was no effect on CNS tumors in humans. A recent study of Danish epileptics confirmed an excess risk of CNS tumors after diagnosis of epilepsy which then declined with further follow-up, indicating that epilepsy, rather than the phenobarbitol used to treat it, was associated with the CNS tumor (Olsen et al 1989).

Mills et al (1989) showed increased but statistically non-significant risks for meningioma associated with the regular use of analgesics and tranquilizers. Increased risk of glioma was also associated with the regular use of tranquilizers. Preston-Martin et al (1982) showed increased risk of childhood CNS tumors in children whose mother took antihistamines or diuretics during pregnancy. These findings were not confirmed in a later study of adult CNS tumors (Ryan et al 1992).

Other associations

Some studies have indicated a relationship between raised serum cholesterol and increased risk of CNS tumors (Davey-Smith & Shipley 1989). This has been refuted in a large cohort study in Finland (Knekt et al 1991). Extremely loud noise has been shown to be a risk factor for acoustic neuroma (vestibular schwannoma) (Preston-Martin et al 1989a). A relative risk of 1.7 for childhood brain tumors has been shown with residential proximity to traffic densities of more than 500 vehicles a day (Savitz & Feingold 1989). A suspected agent is benzene from car exhaust.

NON-NEUROEPITHELIAL TUMORS

Renal transplant patients have long been known to be at increased risk of CNS lymphoma (Hoover & Fraumeni 1973). The incidence of CNS lymphomas has increased since the HIV/AIDS epidemic produced large numbers of immune compromised people. There is evidence, however, that CNS lymphoma was increasing prior to this time and that the increase is unrelated to trends in organ transplantation (Eby et al 1988).

The annual incidence of pituitary tumors is said to be approximately 1 per 100 000 population (Schoenberg 1991). Little is known of the epidemiology of pituitary tumors. They appear to occur more often in black Americans than in whites (Heshmat et al 1976).

Different histologic types of tumor occur in the pineal region, pinealomas being very rare. The incidence of pineal tumors in Japan is up to 9 times higher than elsewhere and the regional variation of pineal tumors within Japan is very marked (Hirayama 1989). Such strong geographic variation suggests that an environmental factor is involved in etiology, or that genetic factors are specific to a geographically discrete population.

METASTATIC TUMORS

Most epidemiologic studies of CNS tumors have concentrated on primary tumors, and data regarding metastases are limited. An annual incidence rate of 8.3 per 100 000 was found in one North American study between 1973 and 1974 (Walker et al 1985). Rates of 11 per 100 000 and 5.4 per 100 000 were previously reported in another North American study (Percy et al 1972) and a British study (Brewis et al 1966), respectively. In the study of Walker et al (1985) metastases were more common in men (9.7 versus 7.1 per 100 000). The rate was less than 1 per 100 000 before the age of 35 years and increased to >30 per 100 000 after the age of 60 years. The most common primary site was the lung. Among women, metastases from breast were equal in frequency to metastases from lung. Metastases from cutaneous malignant melanoma were the third commonest secondary neoplasm.

FUTURE PROSPECTS FOR EPIDEMIOLOGY

Although the epidemiology of CNS tumors remains poorly understood, there is little need for any more studies, particularly case-control studies, similar to those that have been conducted over the past two decades. The pooled results of a recent multi-centered case-control study coordinated by the SEARCH program of the International Agency for Research on Cancer have yet to be published. Findings from some of the individual centers, however, have already been reported (Preston-Martin 1990, Schlehofer et al 1990, Ryan et al 1992, Boeing et al 1993), but their contribution to our understanding of the epidemiology of CNS tumors is not likely to be very large; the studies are small, the measurement of exposures is poor and the strengths of the associations are weak. The combined analysis of these studies will probably represent what is maximally achievable using conventional case-control designs. The future for epidemiologic studies of CNS tumors is in research that embraces molecular biology in the search for accurate and specific markers of susceptibility and exposure to carcinogenic agents in specific histologic subtypes of CNS tumor.

FACTORS IN PROGNOSIS

Of the primary CNS tumors, considerations of biological behavior, response to treatment and prognosis are most appropriate for the gliomas as these are the most frequently encountered tumor type. These considerations are also particularly important in astrocytic tumors because the majority of these are aggressive in their behavior. A number of factors influencing tumor behavior have been identified. There are considerable data indicating that histologic grade, patient age, duration of symptoms and neurologic performance at presentation (Karnofsky score), tumor site, and completeness of resection have a significant bearing on prognosis, and the important influences of inherited and acquired gene alterations are being increasingly recognized.

Histologic features

James Kernohan, in 1949, pioneered the link between histopathologic features of gliomas and patient survival through the introduction of a grading system (Kernohan et al 1949). A number of other grading systems have since been introduced, all with the common purpose of determining which histologic features have prognostic value (see Ch. 3). There has been general agreement that necrosis in a glial tumor, irrespective of other features, indicates aggressive biological behavior and shorter post-operative survival (Nelson et al 1983, Fulling & Garcia 1985, Burger et al 1987). Feature score systems of grading, rather than emphasizing one particular feature such as necrosis, consider the influence of a number of specified features on prognosis — nuclear atypia, mitoses, endothelial cell proliferation and necrosis. These systems propose that the length of the post-operative survival period is inversely proportional to the number of these features detected in a particular tumor (Daumas-Duport et al 1988). Histologic grade has also been shown to be predictive of survival in oligodendrogliomas (Shaw et al 1992), while an association between histologic features and survival is less clearly established for ependymomas (Ross & Rubinstein 1989).

The influence of individual histopathologic features on prognosis in low, intermediate and high grade astrocytomas is a separate issue from the recognition that there are histologic subtypes of glial tumors that are associated with prolonged post-operative survival. Pre-eminent amongst these are pilocytic and subependymal giant cell astrocytomas, subependymoma and myxopapillary ependymoma. Despite the prolonged survival associated with these tumors, it remains unclear whether they can be regarded as benign (Scheithauer 1978, Davis & Barnard 1985, Shaw et al 1989).

Patient age

Rate versus age plots for glial tumors consistently show a peak at approximately 10 years and a second, higher peak at 60–65 years. Gliomas occurring before the age of 10 years and after the age of 45 years are generally more undifferentiated and malignant on histopathologic criteria and are associated with more aggressive behavior and shorter mean post-operative survival periods than those occurring between these ages (Burger & Green 1987). A correlation between age and survival has been consistently shown for astrocytomas of all grades. After age 10, longer survival is associated with a younger age at presentation.

Duration of symptoms and neurologic performance at presentation

A history of recent onset and progression of symptoms and poor neurologic performance at presentation are associated with shorter survival and correlate with histopathologic features of malignancy and aggressive tumor behavior. Progression of symptoms and poor neurologic performance both reflect mass effect resulting from rapid enlargement of a high grade tumor combined with vasogenic edema in the immediately surrounding parenchyma. Neurologic performance may also be impaired by a diffusely infiltrating glioma, and complications such as hemorrhage into a tumor may also account for a sudden deterioration in neurologic status.

Tumor site

The influence of tumor site appears to have a bearing on prognosis in childhood gliomas. In particular, astrocytomas of the cerebellum in children are associated with prolonged survival compared with histologically similar supratentorial tumors (Rorke et al 1985). High grade astrocytomas are uncommon in the cerebellum in adults and so the majority of cerebellar astrocytomas are associated with long post-operative survival. Occasionally, patients with supratentorial high grade astrocytomas and long-term survival have been reported (Salford et al 1988). The influence of tumor site, however, is probably linked to histologic type. The majority of cerebellar astrocytomas are of pilocytic type, which are known to behave non-aggressively (Wallner et al 1988).

Gene alterations

Recently established profiles of gene alterations in astrocytic gliomas indicate an association between biological behavior, activation of oncogenes and inactivation of putative tumor suppressor genes (see Ch. 3). Activation of multiple oncogenes in the same tumor appears to influence progression (Orian et al 1992), while loss of heterozygosity at certain loci on chromosomes 10 and 17 together with mutations of the *p53* gene have been linked to the progression of anaplastic astrocytoma to glioblastoma multiforme (Fults et al 1992). Reports of these alterations have come from only small series of tumors and no detailed follow-up data have been published. Determination of whether these alterations influence prognosis will require prospective survival studies.

Meningiomas

The vast majority of meningiomas are benign tumors. Atypical and malignant meningiomas are associated with local recurrence and progression. There has been disagreement among pathologists regarding the criteria for anaplastic and malignant meningiomas. Particular difficulty has been encountered in assessing invasion of the underlying brain, the major feature that has been used in designating a meningioma as malignant. Recent survival studies have indicated that the division into atypical and malignant may not be useful and that the presence of multiple foci of necrosis is the best predictor of local recurrence and reduced survival (McLean et al 1993).

REFERENCES

Adelstein A M, Donovan J W 1972 Malignant disease in children whose mothers had chickenpox, mumps or rubella in pregnancy. British Medical Journal 4: 629–631

Ahlbom A 1988 A review of the epidemiologic literature on magnetic fields and cancer. Scandinavian Journal of Work and Environmental Health 14: 337–343

Ahlbom A 1990 Some notes on brain tumor epidemiology. Annals of the New York Academy of Science 609: 179–185

Ahlbom A, Rodvall Y 1989 Brain cancer trends. Lancet 1: 1272

Ahlbom A, Norell S, Rodvall Y, Nylander M 1986 Dentists, dental nurses, and brain cancers. British Medical Journal 292: 662

Akbasak A, Sunar-Akbasak B 1992 Oncogenes: cause or consequence in the development of gliomas. Journal of Neurological Science 111: 119–133

Armitage P, Doll R 1954 The age distribution of cancer and a multistage theory of carcinogenesis. British Journal of Cancer 8: 1–12

Armstrong B K, Doll R 1975 Environmental factors and cancer incidence and mortality in different countries, with special reference to dietary practices. International Journal of Cancer 15: 617–631

Armstrong B K, Woodings T L, Stenhouse N S, McCall M G 1983 Mortality from cancer in migrants to Australia — 1962 to 1971. University of Western Australia, Perth

Armstrong D D, Almes M J, Buffler P, Frankowski R, McGarry P 1990 A cluster classification for histologic diagnoses of CNS tumors in an epidemiologic study. Neuroepidemiology 9: 2–16

Aronson S M, Aronson B E 1965 Central nervous system in diabetes: lowered frequency of certain intracranial neoplasms. Archives of Neurology 12: 390–398

Arundel S E, Kinnier-Wilson L M 1986 Parental occupations and cancer: a review of the literature. Journal of Epidemiology and Community Health 40: 30–36

Australian Paediatric Cancer Registry 1989 Childhood cancer incidence and survival, Australia 1978 to 1984. Australian Paediatric Cancer Registry, Brisbane

Bahemuka M, Massey E W, Schoenburg B S 1988 International mortality from primary nervous system neoplasms: distribution and trends. International Journal of Epidemiology 17: 33–38

Biggar R J, Horm J, Goedert K, Melbye M 1987 Cancer in a group at risk of acquired immunodeficiency syndrome (AIDS) through 1984. American Journal of Epidemiology 126: 578–586

Bigner S H, Mark J, Mahaley M, Bigner D D 1984 Pattern of the early, gross chromosomal changes in malignant human gliomas. Hereditas 101: 103–113

Bigner S H, Burger P C, Wong A J et al 1988 Gene amplification in malignant human gliomas: clinical and histopathological aspects. Journal of Neuropathology and Experimental Neurology 47: 191–205

Bithell J F, Stewart A M 1975 Pre-natal irradiation and childhood malignancy: a review of British data from the Oxford Survey. British Journal of Cancer 31: 271–287

Bithell J F, Draper J C, Gorbach P D 1973 Association between malignant disease in children and maternal virus infections. British Medical Journal 1: 706–708

Black P M 1991a Medical progress: brain tumors (first of two parts). New England Journal of Medicine 324: 1471–1476

Black P M 1991b Medical progress: brain tumors (second of two parts). New England Journal of Medicine 324: 1555–1564

Blair A, Malker H, Cantor K P, Burmeister L, Wiklund K 1985 Cancer among farmers: a review. Scandinavian Journal of Work and Environmental Health 11: 397–407

Blatt J, Jaffe R, Deutsch M, Adkins J C 1986 Neurofibromatosis and childhood cancers. Cancer 57: 1225–1229

Boeing H, Schlehofer B, Bletiner M, Wahrendorf J 1993 Dietary carcinogens and the risk for glioma and meningioma in Germany. International Journal of Cancer 53: 561–565

Bolande R P 1989 Teratogenesis and oncogenesis: a developmental spectrum. In: Lynch H T, Hirayama T (eds) Genetic epidemiology of cancer. CRC Press, Boca Raton, Florida, pp 55–68

Bolger G B, Stamberg J, Kirsch I R, Hollis G F, Schwarz D F, Thomas G H 1985 Chromosome translocation T (14 22) and oncogenic (c-sis) variant in a pedigree with familial meningioma. New England Journal of Medicine 312: 564–567

Bonett A, Dickman P, Roder D, Gibberd R, Hakulinen T 1991 Survival of cancer patients in South Australia 1977–1990. Lutheran Publishing House, Adelaide

Boring C C, Squires T S, Tong T 1991 Cancer Statistics 1991. CA 41: 19–36

Boyle P, Maisonneuve P, Saracci R, Muir C 1990 Is the increased incidence of primary malignant brain tumors in the elderly real? Journal of the National Cancer Institute 82: 1594–1596

Breslow N E, Langholz B 1983 Childhood cancer incidence: geographic and temporal variations. International Journal of Cancer 32: 703–716

Brewis M, Poskanzer D C, Rolland C, Miller H 1966 Neurological disease in an English city. Acta Neurologica Scandinavica 24 (suppl 42): 1–89

Brownson R C, Reif J S, Chang J C, Davis J R 1990 An analysis of occupational risks for brain cancer. American Journal of Public Health 80: 169–172

Bunin G 1987 Racial patterns of childhood brain cancer by histologic type. Journal of the National Cancer Institute 78: 875–880

Burch J D, Craib K J P, Choi B C K et al 1987 An exploratory case-control study of brain cancers in adults. Journal of the National Cancer Institute 78: 601–609

Burger P C, Vogel F S, Green S B 1987 Glioblastoma multiforme and anaplastic astrocytoma. Pathologic criteria and prognostic implications. Cancer 56: 1106–1111

Burger P G, Green S B 1987 Patient age, histological features and length of survival in patients with glioblastoma multiforme. Cancer 59: 1617–1625

Charman H P, Lowenstein D H, Kyung G C, Dearmond S J, Wilson C B 1988 Primary cerebral angiosarcoma. Journal of Neurosurgery 68: 806–810

Choi N W, Schuman L M, Gullen W H 1970a Epidemiology of primary central nervous system neoplasms. I Mortality from primary central nervous system neoplasms in Minnesota. American Journal of Epidemiology 91: 238–259

Choi N W, Schuman L M, Gullen W H 1970b Epidemiology of primary central nervous system neoplasms. II Case-control study. American Journal of Epidemiology 91: 467–485

Clemmesen J, Fuglsang-Fredricksen V, Plum C 1974 Are anti-convulsants oncogenic? Lancet i: 705–707

Coleman M P, Beral V 1988 A review of epidemiological studies of health effect of living near or working with electricity generating or transmission equipment. International Journal of Epidemiology 17: 1–5

Cook P J, Doll R, Fellingham S A 1969 A mathematical model for the age distribution of cancer in man. International Journal of Cancer 4: 93–112

Corallini A, Pagnani M, Viadana P et al 1987 Association of BK virus with human brain tumors and tumors of pancreatic islets. International Journal of Cancer 39: 60–67

Cordier S, Poisson M, Gerin M, Varin J, Conso F, Hemon D 1988 Gliomas and exposure to wood preservatives. British Journal of Industrial Medicine 45: 705–709

Darby S C, Nakashima E, Kato H 1985 A parallel analysis of cancer mortality among atomic bomb survivors and patients with ankylosing spondylitis given x-ray therapy. Journal of the National Cancer Institute 75: 1–21

Daumas-Duport C, Scheithauer B W, O'Fallon J, Kelly P 1988 Grading of astrocytomas. A simple and reproducible method. Cancer 62: 2152–2165

Davey-Smith G, Shipley M J 1989 Plasma cholesterol concentration and primary brain tumours. British Medical Journal 299: 26–27

Davis C D, Barnard R O 1985 Malignant behaviour of myxo-papillary ependymoma. Journal of Neurosurgery 62: 925–929

Day N E 1987 Cumulative rate and cumulative risk. In: Muir C, Waterhouse J, Mack T, Powell J, Whelan S (eds) Cancer incidence in five continents, vol V. IARC Scientific Publication No 88. International Agency for Research on Cancer, Lyon, pp 787–789

Desmeules M, Mikkelsen T, Mao Y 1992 Increasing incidence of primary malignant brain tumors: influence of diagnostic methods. Journal of the National Cancer Institute 84: 442–445

Dobkin B H 1985 Stroke associated with glioblastoma. Bulletin of Clinical Neuroscience 50: 111–118

Druckrey H 1973 Chemical structure and action in transplacental carcinogenesis and teratogenesis. In: Tomatis L, Mohr U (eds) Transplacental carcinogenesis. IARC Scientific Publication No 4. International Agency for Research on Cancer, Lyon, pp 29–44

Easterly C E 1981 Cancer link to magnetic field exposure: a hypothesis. American Journal of Epidemiology 114: 169–174

Eby N L, Grufferman S, Flanelly C M, Schold S C, Vogel S, Burger P C 1988 Increasing incidence of primary brain lymphoma in the US. Cancer 62: 2461–2465

Farwell J, Flannery J T 1984 Cancer in relatives of children with central nervous system neoplasms. New England Journal of Medicine 311: 349–353

Feychting M, Ahlbom A 1992 Magnetic fields and cancer in people residing near Swedish high voltage power lines. Karolinska Institute, Stockholm

Floderus B, Persson T, Stenlund C et al 1992 Occupational exposure to electromagnetic fields in relation to leukaemia and brain cancers. A case-control study. National Institute of Occupational Health, Sweden

Fulling K H, Garcia D M 1985 Anaplastic astrocytoma of the adult cerebrum. Prognostic value of histological features. Cancer 55: 928–931

Fults D, Brockmeyer D, Tullous M W, Pedone C A, Cawthorn R M 1992 *p53* mutation and loss of heterozygosity on chromosomes 17 and 10 during astrocytoma progression. Cancer Research 52: 674–679

Garfinkel L, Sarokhan B 1982 Trends in brain tumor mortality and morbidity in the United States. Annals of the New York Academy of Science 381: 1–5

Giles G G, Armstrong B K, Smith L N 1987 Cancer in Australia 1982. Australian Institute of Health and Australasian Association of Cancer Registries, Canberra

Giles G G, Farrugia H, Silver B, Staples M 1992 Cancer in Victoria 1982–1987 Anti-Cancer Council of Victoria, Melbourne

Giles G G, Jelfs P, Kliewer E 1993a Cancer mortality in migrants to Australia 1979 to 1988. Australian Institute of Health and Welfare, Canberra

Giles G G, Thursfield V, Staples M et al 1993b Incidence and survival from childhood cancers in Victoria 1970–79 and 1980–89. Anti-Cancer Council of Victoria, Melbourne

Gold E, Gordis L, Tonascia J, Szklo M 1979 Risk factors for brain tumors in children. American Journal of Epidemiology 109: 303–319

Gold E B 1980 Epidemiology of brain tumors. In: Lilienfeld A M (ed) Reviews in cancer epidemiology, vol 1. Elsevier, North Holland, pp 245–292

Greenwald P, Friedlander B R, Lawrence C E, Hearne T, Earle K 1981 Diagnostic sensitivity bias — an epidemiologic explanation for an apparent brain tumor excess. Journal of Occupational Medicine 23: 690–694

Grieg N H, Ries R Y, Rapoport S I 1990 Increasing annual incidence of primary malignant brain tumors in the elderly. Journal of the National Cancer Institute 82: 1621–1624

Harley M R 1988 Proto-oncogenes in the nervous system. Neuron 1: 175–182

Harrington J M, Oakes D 1983 Mortality study of British Pathologists 1974–80. British Journal of Industrial Medicine 41: 188–191

Haymaker W, Rubinstein L, Miguel J 1972 Brain tumours in irradiated monkeys. Acta Neuropathol 20: 267–277

Helseth A, Langmark F, Mork S J 1988a Neoplasms of the central nervous system in Norway, II descriptive epidemiology of intracranial neoplasms. APMIS 96: 1066–1074

Helseth A, Unsgaard G, Dalen A et al 1988b Amplification of the EGF-receptor gene in biopsy specimens from human intracranial tumours. British Journal of Neurosurgery 2: 217–225

Heshmat M Y, Kovi J, Simpson C et al 1976 Neoplasms of the central nervous system: incidence and population selectivity in the Washington DC metropolitan area. Cancer 38: 2135–2142

Hirayama T 1985 Passive smoking — a new target for epidemiology. Tokai J Exp Clin Med 10: 287–293

Hirayama T 1989 Family history and childhood malignancies with special reference to genetic environmental interaction. In: Lynch H T, Hirayama T (eds) Genetic epidemiology of cancer. CRC Press, Boca Raton, Florida, pp 111–118

Hochberg F, Toniolo P, Cole P 1990 Non-occupational risk indicators of glioblastoma in adults. Journal of Neuro-Oncology 8: 55–60

Holman C D J, Hatton W M, Armstrong B K, English D R 1987 Cancer mortality trends in Australia, vol II 1910–1984. Health Department of Western Australia, Perth

Hoover R, Fraumeni J F 1973 Risk of cancer in renal-transplant patients. Lancet 2: 55–57

Howe G R, Burch D, Chiarelli A M et al 1989 An exploratory case-control study of brain tumors in children. Cancer Research 49: 4349–4352

International Agency for Research on Cancer 1989 Occupational exposures in petroleum refining; crude oil and major petroleum fuels. IARC Monographs on the evaluation of carcinogenic risks to humans. Vol 45. International Agency for Research on Cancer, Lyon

Johnson C C, Spitz M R 1989 Childhood nervous system tumours: an assessment of risk associated with paternal occupations involving use, repair, or manufacture of electrical and electronic equipment. International Journal of Epidemiology 18: 756–762

Johnson C C, Annegers J F, Frankowski R F, Spitz M R, Buffler P A 1987 Childhood nervous system tumours: an evaluation of the association with paternal occupational exposure to hydrocarbons. American Journal of Epidemiology 126: 605–613

Kallio M, Sankila R, Jaaskelainen J, Karjalainen S, Hakulinen T 1991 A population-based study on the incidence and survival rates of 3857 glioma patients diagnosed from 1953 to 1984. Cancer 68: 1394–1400

Kaye A, Giles G G, Gonzales M 1993 Primary CNS tumours in Australia: a profile of clinical practice from the Australian Brain Tumour Register. Australia and New Zealand Journal of Surgery 63: 33–38

Kent S P, Pickering J E 1958 Neoplasms in monkeys (Macaca mulatta): spontaneous and irradiation induced. Cancer 35: 138–145

Kernohan J W, Mabon R F, Svien H J, Adson A W 1949 A simplified classification of gliomas. Proceedings of the Staff Meetings of the Mayo Clinic 24: 71–74

Kessler E, Brandt-Rauf P W 1987 Occupational cancers of the nervous system. Seminars in Occupational Medicine 2: 311–314

Kibirige M S, Birch J M, Campbell R H A, Gattamaneni H R, Blair V 1988 A review of astrocytoma in childhood. Pediatric Hematology and Oncology 6: 319–329

Knekt P, Reunanen A, Teppo L 1991 Serum cholesterol concentration and risk of primary brain tumours. British Medical Journal 302: 90

Kornbluth S, Cross F R, Harbison M et al 1986 Transformation of chick embryo fibroblasts and tumor induction by the middle T antigen of polyomavirus carried in an avian retroviral vector. Molecular Cell Biology 6: 1545–1551

Krupp J M 1976 Nine years mortality experience in proton-exposed Macaca mulatta. Radiation Research 67: 244–251

Lacayo A, Farmer P M 1991 Brain tumors in children: a review. Annals of Clinical and Laboratory Science 21: 26–35

Lin R S, Dischinger P C, Conde J, Farrell K P 1985 Occupational exposure to electromagnetic fields and the occurrence of brain tumors. Journal of Occupational Medicine 27: 413–419

Logan W P D 1982 Cancer mortality by occupation and social class 1851–1971. HMSO, London

Loomis D P, Savitz D A 1990 Mortality from brain cancer and leukaemia among electrical workers. British Journal of Industrial Medicine 47: 633–638

Lynch H T, Marcus J M, Watson P, Conway T, Fitzsimmons M L, Lynch J F 1989 Genetic epidemiology of breast cancer. In: Lynch H T, Hirayama T (eds) Genetic epidemiology of cancer. CRC Press, Boca Raton, Florida, pp 289–332

McCredie M, Coates M S, Ford J M 1990 Cancer incidence in migrants to New South Wales. International Journal of Cancer 46: 228–322

McLaughlin J K, Malker H S R, Blot W J et al 1987 Occupational risks for intracranial gliomas in Sweden. Journal of the National Cancer Institute 78: 253–257

McLean C A, Jolley D, Cukier E, Giles G, Gonzales M F 1993 Atypical and malignant meningiomas: importance of micronecrosis as a prognostic indicator. Histopathology (in press)

MacMahon B 1960 The ethnic distribution of cancer mortality in New York City, 1955. Acta Unio Internat Contra Cancrum 16: 53–57

MacMahon B 1985 Phenobarbital: epidemiological evidence. In: Wald N J, Doll R (eds) Interpretation of negative epidemiological evidence for carcinogenicity. IARC Scientific Publication No 65. International Agency for Research on Cancer, Lyon, pp 153–158

MacPherson P 1976 Association between previous tuberculosis infection and glioma. British Medical Journal 2: 1112

McWhorter W P 1988 Allergy and risk of cancer. A prospective study using NHANES1 follow-up data. Cancer 62: 451–455

Magnani C, Coggon D, Osmond C, Acheso E D 1987 Occupation and five cancers: a case-control study using death certificates. British Journal of Industrial Medicine 44: 769–776

Mahaley M S, Mettlin C, Natarajan N, Laws E R, Peace B B 1989 National survey of patterns of care for brain-tumor patients. Journal of Neurosurgery 71: 826–836

Maltoni C A, Ciliberti A, Di Maio V 1977 Carcinogenicity bioassays on rats of acrylonitrile administered by inhalation and by ingestion. La Medicina del Lavoro 68: 401–411

Maltoni C, Ciliberti A, Carretti D 1982 Experimental contributions in identifying brain potential carcinogens in the petrochemical industry. Annals of the New York Academy of Science 381: 216–249

Mills P K, Preston-Martin S, Annegers J F, Beeson W L, Phillips R L, Fraser G E 1989 Risk factors for tumors of the brain and cranial meninges in Seventh-Day Adventists. Neuroepidemiology 8: 266–275

Modan B, Wagener D K, Feldman J J, Rosenberg H M, Feinleib M 1992 Increased mortality from brain tumors: a combined outcome of diagnostic technology and change of attitude toward the elderly. American Journal of Epidemiology 135: 1349–1357

Monson R R, MacMahon B 1984 Pre-natal X-ray exposure and cancer in children. In: Boice J D, Fraumeni J F (eds) Radiation carcinogenesis: epidemiology and biological significance. Raven Press, New York, pp 97–105

Moolgavkar S H, Day N E, Stevens R G 1980 Two-stage model for carcinogenesis: epidemiology of breast cancer in females. Journal of the National Cancer Institute 65: 559–569

Morgello S 1992 Epstein-Barr and Human Immunodeficiency Viruses in Acquired Immunodeficiency Syndrome-related primary central nervous system lymphoma. American Journal of Pathology 141: 441–450

Moss A R 1985 Occupational exposure and brain tumors. Journal of Toxicology and Environmental Health 16: 703–711

Muir C, Waterhouse J, Mack T, Powell J, Whelan S (eds) 1987 Cancer incidence in five continents, vol V. IARC Scientific Publications No 88. International Agency for Research on Cancer, Lyon

Munk J, Peyser R, Gruszkiewicz J 1969 Radiation induced intracranial meningiomas. Clinical Radiology 20: 90–94

Musicco M, Filippini G, Bordo B et al 1982 Gliomas and occupational exposure to carcinogens. American Journal of Epidemiology 116: 789–790

Nasca P C, Baptiste M S, MacCubbin et al 1988 An epidemiologic case-control study of central nervous system tumors in children and parental occupational exposures. American Journal of Epidemiology 128: 1256–1265

National Radiological Protection Board 1992 Electromagnetic fields and the risk of cancer. Report of an advisory group on non-ionising radiation. Documents of the NRPB 3 (1)

National Research Council 1980 The effects on populations of exposure to low levels of ionizing radiation. National Academy of Sciences, Committee on the biological effects of ionizing radiation, Washington DC

Nelson J S, Tsukada Y, Schoenfeld D, Fulling K, Lamarche J, Peress N 1983 Necrosis as a prognostic criterion in malignant supratentorial astrocytic gliomas. Cancer 52: 550–554

Neutel C I, Quinn A, Brancker A 1989 Brain tumour mortality in immigrants. International Journal of Epidemiology 18: 60–66

Newill V A 1961 Distribution of cancer mortality among ethnic subgroups of the white population of New York city. Journal of the National Cancer Institute 26: 405–417

Office of Population Censuses and Surveys 1981 Cancer statistics: incidence, survival and mortality in England and Wales. Studies on medical and population subjects No 43. HMSO, London

Olsen J H, Boice J D, Jensen J P A, Fraumeni J F 1989 Cancer among epileptic patients exposed to anticonvulsant drugs. Journal of the National Cancer Institute 81: 804–808

Olshan A F, Breslow N E, Daling J R et al 1986 Childhood brain tumors and paternal occupation in the aerospace industry. Journal of the National Cancer Institute 77: 17–19

Orian J M, Vasilopoulos K, Yoshida S, Kaye A H, Gonzales M F 1992 Overexpression of multiple oncogenes related to histological grade of astrocytic glioma. British Journal of Cancer 66: 106–112

Osterlind A, Olsen J H, Lynge E, Ewertz M 1985 Second cancer following cutaneous melanoma and cancers of the brain, thyroid, connective tissue, bone, and eye in Denmark. National Cancer Institute Monographs 68: 361–388

Parkin D M, Stiller C A, Draper G J et al 1988 International incidence of childhood cancer. IARC Scientific Publications No 87. International Agency for Research on Cancer, Lyon

Percy A K, Elveback L R, Okazaki H, Kurland L T 1972 Neoplasms of the central nervous system: epidemiological considerations. Neurology (Minneapolis) 22: 40–48

Peters J M, Preston-Martin S 1984 Childhood tumors and parental occupational exposures. Teratogenesis, carcinogenesis and mutagenesis 4: 137–148

Peters J M, Preston-Martin S, Yu M C 1981 Brain tumors in children and occupational exposure of parents. Science 213: 235–237

Peto R 1981 Trends in U.S. Cancer Onset Rates. In: Peto R, Schneiderman M (eds) Quantification of occupational cancer, Banbury Report 9. Cold Spring Harbor Laboratory, Cold Spring Harbor, New York, pp 269–284

Pitts O M, Powers J M, Hoffman P M 1983 Vascular neoplasms induced in rodent central nervous system by murine sarcoma viruses. Lab Invest 49: 171–182

Poole C, Trichopoulos D 1991 Extremely low-frequency electric and magnetic fields and cancer. Cancer Causes Control 2: 267–276
Preston-Martin S 1989 Descriptive epidemiology of tumors of the brain, cranial nerves and cranial meninges in Los Angeles County. Neuroepidemiology 8: 283–295
Preston-Martin S 1990 A case-control study of brain tumors in men in Los Angeles County: investigation of N-nitroso compound exposures. In: O'Neill I K, Chen S H, Bartsch H (eds) Relevance to human cancer of N-nitroso compounds, tobacco smoke and mycotoxins. IARC Scientific Publications No 105. International Agency for Research on Cancer, Lyon, pp 221–227
Preston-Martin S, Paganini-Hill A, Henderson B E, Pike M C, Wood C 1980 Case-control study of intracranial meningiomas in women in Los Angeles County. Journal of the National Cancer Institute 65: 67–73
Preston-Martin S, Yu M C, Henderson B E, Roberts C 1982 N-nitroso compounds and childhood brain tumors. Cancer Research 42: 5240–5245
Preston-Martin S, Yu M C, Henderson B E, Benton B 1983 Risk factors for meningiomas in men. Journal of the National Cancer Institute 70: 863–866
Preston-Martin S, Henderson B E, Yu M C 1984 Epidemiology of intracranial meningiomas: Los Angeles County, California. Neuroepidemiology 2: 164–178
Preston-Martin S, Henderson B E, Bernstein L 1985 Medical and dental X-rays as risk factors for recently diagnosed tumors of the head. National Cancer Institute Monograph 69: 175–179
Preston-Martin S, Thomas D C, Henderson B E, Wright W E 1989a Noise in the aetiology of acoustic neuromas in men in Los Angeles County, 1978–1985. British Journal of Cancer 59: 783–786
Preston-Martin S, Mack W, Henderson B E 1989b Risk factors for gliomas and meningiomas in men in Los Angeles County. Cancer Research 49: 6137–6143
Reagan T J, Freiman I S 1973 Multiple cerebral gliomas in multiple sclerosis. Journal of Neurology, Neurosurgery and Psychiatry 36: 523–528
Reif J S, Pearce N, Fraser J 1989 Occupational risks for brain cancer: a New Zealand cancer registry-based study. Journal of Occupational Medicine 31: 863–867
Rice J M, Ward J M 1982 Age dependence of susceptibility to carcinogenesis in the nervous system. Annals of the New York Academy of Science 381: 274–289
Roelvink C A, Kamphorst W, van Alphen M A, Rao B R 1987 Pregnancy-related primary brain and spinal tumors. Archives of Neurology 44: 209–215
Ron E, Modan B, Boice J D et al 1988 Tumors of the brain and central nervous system after radiotherapy in childhood. New England Journal of Medicine 319: 1033–1039
Rorke L B, Gilles F H, Davis R L, Becker L E 1985 Revision of the World Health Organization classification of brain tumors for childhood brain tumors. Cancer 56: 1869–1886
Ross G W, Rubinstein L J 1989 Lack of histopathological correlation of malignant ependymomas with postoperative survival. Journal of Neurosurgery 70: 31–36
Roush G C, Holford T R, Schymura M J, White C 1987 Cancer risk and incidence trends: the Connecticut perspective. Hemisphere, Washington, pp 335–359
Rubinstein L J 1972 Tumors of the central nervous system. Atlas of tumor pathology, second series, fascicle 6. Armed Forces Institute of Pathology, Washington
Ryan P, Lee M W, North B, McMichael A J 1992 Risk factors for tumors of the brain and meninges: results from the Adelaide adult brain tumour study. International Journal of Cancer 51: 20–27
Ryan P, Hurley S F, Johnson A M et al 1993 Tumours of the brain and possession of antibodies to Toxoplasma gondii: results from two Australian case-control studies. (in press)
Salford L G, Brun A, Nirfalk S 1988 Ten-year survival among patients with supratentorial astrocytomas grade III and IV. Journal of Neurosurgery 69: 506–509
Salvati M, Artico M, Caruso R, Rocchi G, Orlando E R, Nucci F 1990 A report on radiation-induced gliomas. Cancer 67: 392–397
Savitz D, Chen J 1990 Parental occupation and childhood cancer: review of epidemiologic studies. Environmental Health Perspectives 88: 325–337
Savitz D A, Feingold L 1989 Association of childhood cancer with residential traffic density. Scandinavian Journal of Work and Environmental Health 15: 360–363
Savitz D, Wachtel H A, Barnes F, John E M, Tvrdik J G 1988 Case control study of childhood cancer and exposure to 60 Hz magnetic fields. American Journal of Epidemiology 128: 21–38
Scheithauer B W 1978 Symptomatic subependymoma. Report of 21 cases with review of the literature. Journal of Neurosurgery 49: 689–696
Schlehofer B, Kunze F, Sachsenhemer W, Blettner M, Niehof D, Wahrendorf J 1990 Occupational risk factors for brain tumours: results from a population based case-control study in Germany. Cancer Causes Control 1: 209–215
Schlehofer B, Blettner M, Becker N, Martinsohn C, Wahrendorf J 1992a Medical risk factors and the development of brain tumors. Cancer 69: 2541–2547
Schlehofer B, Blettner M, Wahrendorf J 1992b Association between brain tumors and menopausal status. Journal of the National Cancer Institute 84: 1346–1349
Schoenberg B S 1982 Nervous system. In: Schottenfeld D, Fraumeni J F (eds) Cancer epidemiology and prevention. Saunders, Baltimore
Schoenberg B S 1991 Epidemiology of primary intracranial neoplasms: disease distribution and risk factors. In: Salcman M (ed) Neurobiology of brain tumors. Williams & Wilkins, Baltimore, pp 3–18
Schoenberg B S, Christine B W, Whisnant J P 1975 Nervous system neoplasms and primary malignancies of other sites. The unique association between meningiomas and breast cancer. Neurology 25: 705–712
Schuman L M, Choi N M, Gullen W H 1967 Relationship of central nervous system neoplasms to Toxoplasma gondii infection. American Journal of Public Health 57: 848–856
Seizinger B R 1991 Antioncogenes and the development of tumors in the human nervous system. Cancer 70: 1782–1787
Seizinger B R, Martuza R L, Gusella J F 1986 Loss of genes on chromosome 22 in tumorigenesis of acoustic neuroma. Nature 322: 644–647
Selvin S, Garfinkel J 1972 The relationship between paternal age and birth order with the percentage of low birth-weight infants. Human Biology 44: 501–510
Seyama S, Ishimaru T, Iiyima S, Mori K 1979 Primary intracranial tumors among atomic bomb survivors and controls, Hiroshima and Nagasaki, 1961–75. Radiation Effects Research Foundation technical report 15–79. Radiation Effects Research Foundation, Hiroshima
Shaw E G, Daumas-Duport C, Scheithauer B W et al 1989 Radiation therapy in the management of low grade supratentorial astrocytomas. Journal of Neurosurgery 70: 853–861
Shaw E G, Scheithauer B W, O'Fallon J R, Tazelaar H D, Davis D H 1992 Oligodendrogliomas: the Mayo Clinic experience. Journal of Neurosurgery 76: 428–434
Sima A A F, Finklestein S D, McLachlan D R 1983 Multiple malignant astrocytomas in a patient with spontaneous progressive multifocal leucoencephalopathy. Annals of Neurology 14: 183–188
Smith F P, Slavik M, McDonald J S 1978 Association of breast cancer with meningioma. Cancer 42: 1992–1994
Sorensen S A, Mulvihill J J, Nielsen A 1985 Malignancy in neurofibromatosis. In: Muller H, Weber W (eds) Familial cancer. Karger, Basel, pp 119–120
Speers M A, Dobbins J G, Miller V S 1988 Occupational exposures and brain cancer mortality: a preliminary study of East Texas residents. American Journal of Industrial Medicine 13: 629–638
Steinitz R, Parkin D M, Young J L, Bieber C A, Katz L (eds) 1989 Cancer incidence in Jewish migrants to Israel 1961–1981. IARC Scientific Publications No 98. International Agency for Research on Cancer, Lyon
Stroup N E, Blair A, Erikson G E 1986 Brain cancer and other causes of death in anatomists. Journal of the National Cancer Institute 77: 1217–1224
Stukonis M K 1978 Cancer incidence cumulative rates — international comparison. IARC technical report No 78/002. International Agency for Research on Cancer, Lyon
Swenburg J A 1982 Current approaches to the experimental

investigation of chemicals in relation to cancer of the brain. Annals of the New York Academy of Science 381: 43–49

Swift M, Morrell D, Cromartie E, Chambelin A B, Skolnick M H, Bishop D T 1986 The incidence and gene frequency of ataxia-telangiectasia in the United States. American Journal of Human Genetics 39: 573–583

Teta M J, Walrath J, Meigs J W, Flannery J T 1984 Cancer incidence among cosmetologists. Journal of the National Cancer Institute 72: 1051–1057

Thomas T L, Waxweiler R J 1986 Brain tumours and occupational risk factors: a review. Scandinavian Journal of Work and Environmental Health 12: 1–15

Thomas T L, Stolley P D, Stemhagen A et al 1987a Brain tumor mortality risk among men with electrical and electronics jobs: a case-control study. Journal of the National Cancer Institute 79: 233–238

Thomas T L, Stewart P A, Stemhagen A et al 1987b Risk of astrocytic brain tumours associated with occupational chemical exposures. Scandinavian Journal of Work and Environmental Health 13: 417–423

Tijssen C C 1985 Genetic aspects of brain tumours — tumors of neuroepithelial and meningial tissue. In: Muller H, Weber W (eds) Familial cancer. Karger, Basel, pp 98–102

Tracy S E, Woda B A, Robinson H L 1985 Induction of angiosarcoma by a c-erbB transducing virus. Journal of Virology 54: 304–310

Traynor J L, Casey H W 1971 Five year follow up of primates exposed to 55 mev proton. Radiation Research 47: 143–148

Tucker M A, Boice J D, Hoffman D A 1985 Second cancer following cutaneous melanoma and cancers of the brain, thyroid, connective tissue, bone, and eye in Connecticut. National Cancer Institute Monographs 68: 161–190

Unger M, Olsen J 1980 Organochlorine compounds in the adipose tissue of deceased patients with and without cancer. Environmental Research 23: 257–263

Velema J P, Percy C L 1987 Age curves of nervous system tumor incidence in adults: variation of shape by histologic type. Journal of the National Cancer Institute 79: 623–629

Velema J P, Walker A M 1987 The age curve of nervous system tumour incidence in adults: common shape but changing levels by sex, race and geographical location. International Journal of Epidemiology 16: 177–183

Vena J E, Bona J R, Byers T E, Middleton E, Swanson M K, Graham S 1985 Allergy-related diseases and cancer: an inverse association. American Journal of Epidemiology 122: 66–74

Walker A E, Robins M, Weinfeld F D 1985 Epidemiology of brain tumors: the national survey of intracranial neoplasms. Neurology 35: 219–226

Wallner K E, Gonzales M F, Edwards M S B, Wara W M, Sheline G E 1988 Treatment results of juvenile pilocytic astrocytoma. Journal of Neurosurgery 69: 171–176

Walrath J, Fraumeni J F 1983 Mortality patterns among embalmers. International Journal of Cancer 31: 407–411

Ward D, Mattison M L, Finn R 1973 Association between previous tuberculosis infection and cerebral glioma. British Medical Journal 1: 83–84

Ward J, Rice J M 1982 Review of naturally occurring and chemically induced tumors of the central and peripheral nervous systems in mice and rats in the national Toxicology Program/NCI Carcinogenesis Testing Program. Annals of the New York Academy of Science 381: 265–273

Waxweiler R G, Stringer W, Wagoner J K et al 1976 Neoplastic risk among workers exposed to vinyl chloride. Annals of the New York Academy of Science 271: 40–48

Wertheimer N, Leeper E 1979 Electrical wiring configurations and childhood cancer. American Journal of Epidemiology 109: 273

Whelan S L, Parkin D M, Masuyer E 1990 Patterns of cancer in five continents. IARC Scientific Publication No 102. International Agency for Research on Cancer, Lyon

Wilkins J R, Koutras R A 1988 Paternal occupation and brain cancer in offspring: a mortality based case control study. American Journal of Industrial Medicine 14: 299–318

Wilkins J R, Sinks T 1990 Parental occupation and intracranial neoplasms of childhood: results of a case-control interview study. American Journal of Epidemiology 132: 275–292

Williams J W, Clifford C, Hopper J L, Giles G G 1991 Socioeconomic status and cancer mortality and incidence in Melbourne. European Journal of Cancer 27: 917–921

Wong O, Morgan R W, Bailey W J, Swencicki R E, Claxton K, Kheifets L 1986 An epidemiological study of petroleum refinery employees. British Journal of Industrial Medicine 43: 6–17

Yates P O, Pearce K M 1960 Recent change in blood group distribution of astrocytomas. Lancet 1: 194–195

Yohn D S 1972 Oncogenic viruses: expectations and applications in neuropathology. Progress in Experimental Tumor Research 17: 74–92

Zang K D, Singer H 1967 Chromosomal constitution of meningiomas. Nature 216: 84–85

Zeller W J, Ivankovic S, Habs M, Schmahl D 1982 Experimental chemical production of brain tumors. Annals of the New York Academy of Science 381: 250–263

Zimmerman H M 1982 Production of brain tumors with aromatic hydrocarbons. Annals of the New York Academy of Science 381: 320–324

Zulch K J 1979 Histological typing of tumours of the central nervous system. World Health Organization, Geneva

5. Neurogenetics and the molecular biology of human brain tumors

Kamal Thapar Kouzou Fukuyama James T. Rutka

INTRODUCTION

Ten years ago, it would have been impossible to write this chapter. The application of the techniques in molecular biology to the study of human brain tumors has had a profound impact on increasing our knowledge of the fundamental cellular and genetic changes that occur in these tumors. Whereas a decade ago a chapter on the biology of human brain tumors would have included sections on the tumor cell cycle, karyotypic and phenotypic analyses of brain tumors, and intrinsic chemo- and radio-sensitivities of brain tumor cells, today it is very difficult to confine, in the space of a single book chapter, the enormous advances that have taken place concerning the molecular genetics of human brain tumors.

In the mid 80s, there was understandably a flurry of activity in the field of oncogenes and growth factors as possible agents involved in brain tumor initiation and progression. While an understanding of these so-called 'cancer-causing genes', and the growth-promoting peptides that many of them encode for, continues to be essential and is described at some length in this chapter, detailed genetic analyses of many of the neurogenetic syndromes such as neurofibromatosis (NF) types 1 and 2 have led to the important finding that the sequential loss of genetic material also plays a significant role in tumorigenesis.

In this chapter, we review some of the neurogenetic syndromes (NF-1, NF-2, tuberous sclerosis, von Hippel Lindau, and Turcot syndrome) and emphasize the salient features of the molecular genetics of each. The concept of the tumor suppressor gene is developed here and expanded later in the text in the section concerning the special case of the p53 gene in human brain tumors. We describe the major and latest cytogenetic aberrations that have been reported in human brain tumors; techniques such as restriction fragment polymorphism (RFLP) analysis, chromosome walking, and interphase cytogenetics which have provided an enormous amount of informative data about human brain tumors are defined. We summarize our current knowledge of oncogenes, growth factors and cell cycle genes such as the cyclins as agents capable of stimulating the passage of a cell through the cell cycle. As the highly invasive potential of malignant glioma cells continues to thwart effective local therapies, we present a special section on molecular models of glioma cell invasion. And, we provide a synopsis of the multi-step theory of carcinogenesis as proposed by Fearon & Vogelstein (1990), but modified by Mikkelsen et al (1991) and others to account for the molecular genetic changes that are relevant in the pathogenesis of the human glioma.

It has been argued previously, and perhaps cogently, that clinical application of the knowledge obtained in the last decade has not kept pace with our expanding molecular genetic database. We conclude this chapter, however, with a description of recent successful applications of the techniques in molecular biology to treat experimental brain tumors. Preliminary data with 'gene therapy' for experimental brain tumors look very promising, and it is with great anticipation that we look forward to this next decade and the results of gene therapy trials in patients harboring malignant brain tumors.

NEUROGENETIC SYNDROMES

Neurofibromatosis type 1 (NF-1)

NF-1 (previously known as von Recklinghausen's disease and peripheral NF) is the most common form of neurofibromatosis. Occurring without predilection for sex or race and with an approximate frequency of 1 in every 4000 live births, NF-1 is more prevalent than any of the other phakomatoses and is also among the most common of any autosomal dominant heritable human condition (Menon et al 1990). An unexplained peculiarity of the NF-1 genetic locus is its unexplained high spontaneous mutation rate, which is estimated at approximately 1 in 10 000 gametes per generation (Crowe et al 1956). The clinical implication of such genetic instability, which exceeds that of any known human gene, is that almost

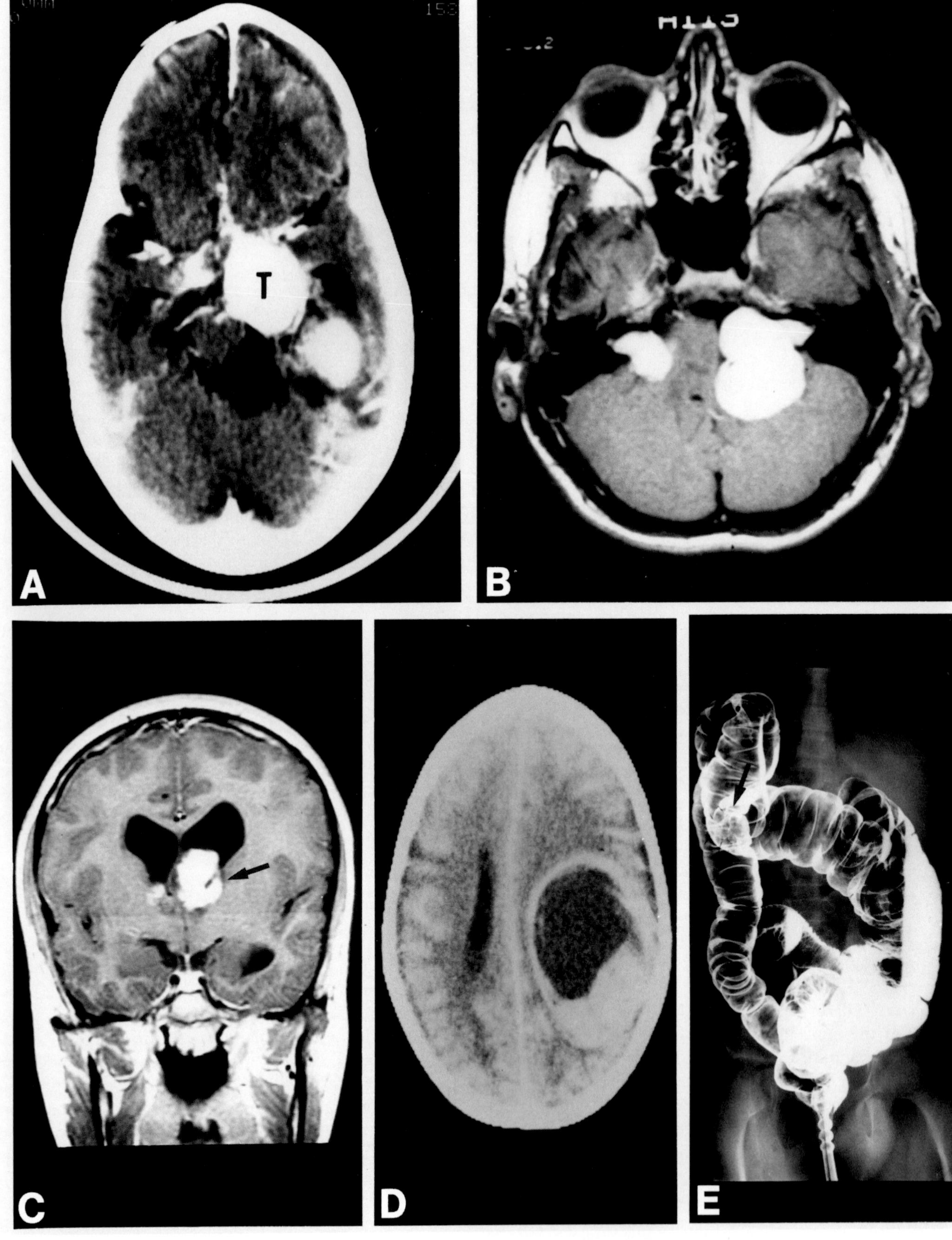
T
A
B
C
D
E

Fig. 5.1 Neurogenetically-linked syndromes with CNS tumor formation.
A. Contrast-enhanced CT scan demonstrating an optic glioma in a young male with NF-1 who presented with visual failure and macrocephaly. A large mass lesion is seen arising from the left optic tract (T), compressing the brainstem and extending posteriorly along the optic radiation. The large lesion was excised surgically, and in follow-up at 2 years, there has been no new growth of tumor. An optic glioma is one of the clinical and radiographic hallmarks of a patient with NF-1.
B. Gadolinium-enhanced axial MRI scan demonstrating bilateral acoustic neurinomas (vestibular schwannomas) in a 14-year-old male with NF-2 who presented with left hearing loss. The acoustic neurinoma on the left is much larger than that on the right, and is compressing the brainstem. Treatment was directed toward excising the larger symptomatic left acoustic neurinoma. He is being followed closely for signs of right hearing loss, and is learning sign language. There continues to be considerable controversy over the best management of the second, asymptomatic acoustic neurinoma in these patients.
C. Gadolinium-enhanced coronal MRI scan demonstrating a large left enhancing lateral ventricular tumor (arrow) taking origin from the region of the caudate nucleus in a 14-year-old female with headaches and papilledema. The tumor is obstructing the interventricular foramen of Monro, and the third ventricle is small. The child was taken to surgery and a transcallosal approach to the left lateral ventricle was undertaken, and the lesion was completely excised. The pathology was subependymal giant cell astrocytoma. She did not require a VP shunt, and is well 2 years after follow-up without evidence of regrowth of tumor.
D & E. Patient with Turcot syndrome. At age 5 years, he developed seizures and a right hemiparesis. A contrast-enhanced CT scan showed a large left cystic parietal brain tumor **D**. A left parietal craniotomy was performed and the tumor was radically excised. He received post-operative radiation therapy, and there has been no evidence of tumor regrowth on subsequent CT scans. At age 11 years, he developed rectal bleeding which was investigated with a double contrast barium enema **E**. A large polyp was identified in the ascending colon (arrow) requiring laparotomy and excision. At present, he is well without evidence of CNS or GI symptomatology some 7 years after treatment.

50% of NF-1 cases are due to spontaneous mutation of the NF-1 gene, and can therefore be considered somatic in origin and, thus, without a familial basis (Riccardi 1991). Regardless of the origin of the NF-1 mutation, germline versus somatic (i.e. hereditary versus sporadic), the disorder is characterized by 100% *penetrance*, which is to say that virtually all patients with the gene defect will have phenotypic (clinical) evidence of the disease. Alternatively, the *expressivity* of the NF-1 mutation is variable, in that clinical severity of the disease (mild, moderate or severe) is unpredictable and can vary among affected individuals, even within familial cohorts.

Clinical manifestations

The clinical features of NF-1 are protean, and characterized by abnormalities affecting tissues derived primarily, but not exclusively, from the neural crest. Multiple café-au-lait spots, multiple cutaneous neurofibromas, axillary freckling, Lisch nodules (iris hamartomas), dysplastic bony lesions (sphenoidal dysplasia, congenital pseudoarthrosis or cortical thinning of long bones, especially tibial) and gliomas of the optic nerve and hypothalamus are considered to be the principal abnormalities. Hamartomatous, heterotopic and dysplastic cerebral lesions are increasingly recognized in association with NF-1, and are the presumed pathological basis for the frequent finding of 'bright spots' on T2-weighted MR brain images of these patients (Mulvihill et al 1990). Less common features of NF-1 include cerebrovascular abnormalities, dural ectasia, architectural abnormalities such as macrocephaly and aqueductal stenosis, and numerous extra-neural abnormalities, including colonic ganglioneuromas and juvenile chronic myelogenous leukemias. A detailed survey of the numerous neural and extra-neural manifestations of NF-1 are described in a recent monograph (Riccardi 1991).

From a neuro-oncological standpoint, NF-1 is associated with a variety of central and peripheral nervous system tumors. Of the CNS tumors, optic nerve gliomas are most commonly associated with NF-1, occurring in approximately 15% of affected individuals, and usually evident by 10 years of age (Fig. 5.1A). Less commonly, low grade gliomas of the hypothalamus, cerebellum, brainstem or spinal cord may also occur. Other CNS tumor types (ependymomas, meningiomas, and primitive neuroectodermal tumors) are said to occur with increased frequency with NF-1, but because the various forms of neurofibromatosis were not reliably distinguished in earlier literature, accurate frequency figures are not available (Riccardi 1991). Peripheral neurofibromas are the hallmark of NF-1, and typically arise from distal cutaneous nerve endings (cutaneous neurofibromas), peripheral nerves (plexiform neurofibromas) and less commonly from cranial nerves. Cutaneous neurofibromas are primarily a cosmetic problem, sometimes causing pain and itching. Only rarely do they undergo malignant transformation. The plexiform neurofibromas can involve any peripheral nerve or plexus, typically arising in sensory or sympathetic fascicles. If symptomatic, their principal feature is pain, particularly in lesions that are rapidly growing, traumatized, or undergoing malignant degeneration. The incidence of the latter, that is the development of fibrosarcoma, is the most worrisome feature of NF-1, though fortunately one which occurs in less than 5% of all patients (Martuza & Rouleau 1990).

Neurofibromas involving spinal roots are a common feature of NF-1, and although frequently small, multiple and asymptomatic, they can also be the source of radicular symptoms or spinal cord compression. It is important to emphasize that true schwannomas of cranial, spinal or peripheral nerves are not features of NF-1, and despite the ongoing tendency to use the terms schwannoma and neurofibroma interchangeably, they are distinct entities from the standpoints of histopathology, clonality, cytogenetic constitution, tendency for malignant degeneration, ease of resection, and occurrence in the two principal forms of neurofibromatosis. In almost 1000 cases of carefully classified NF-1, Riccardi (1991) did not identify a single case of a schwannoma in association with NF-1.

Table 5.1 Genotypic and phenotypic comparisons of NF-1 and NF-2. After Pulst 1990, Mulvihill et al 1990, and Riccardi 1991.

Characteristic	NF-1	NF-2
Incidence	1:4000	1:100 000
Inheritance	autodominant	autodominant
Chromosomal locus	17q11.2	22q11.2*
Gene isolated and cloned	yes	no
Mutation rate	high	uncertain
Penetrance	high	high
Expressivity	variable	not variable WRT bilateral VIII nerve schwannomas
Age of onset	1st decade	2nd–3rd decade
Intellectual deficit	> 25%	usually none
Café-au-lait spots		
> 1	90%	40%
> 6	75%	0%
Cutaneous neurofibroma	frequent	few
Lisch nodules	> 90%	absent**
Juvenile lens opacities	absent	> 85%
Tumors:		
Acoustic neurinoma	rarely found	approaches 100% (bilateral)
Optic nerve glioma	15%	absent
Meningioma	few	> 50% (30% multiple)
Spinal neurofibroma	common	absent
Spinal schwannoma	absent	common

*NF-2 locus delineated to 22q, between markers D22S1 and D22S28 (Rouleau et al 1990)

**Single case of Lisch nodule in NF-2 patient described (Charles et al 1989)

The diagnostic criteria for NF-1, as defined by a recent consensus conference sponsored by the National Institutes of Health, are listed in Table 5.1 (Mulvihill et al 1990). Even though this diagnostic scheme reflects the existing operational definition of NF-1, several caveats warrant emphasis. Firstly, the proposed criteria are the minimal criteria necessary for diagnosis, and are not all-encompassing with respect to the broad spectrum of pathologic findings occurring in this disorder. Furthermore, the sensitivity and specificity of these criteria have yet to be formally tested on a prospective basis. Because these criteria were formulated prior to the isolation of the NF-1 gene, they have not been subject to definitive molecular correlation. Finally, these criteria are more reliable in adults than in children, because penetrance of the NF-1 gene is age dependent, and full penetrance of the gene may not be evident until puberty. Despite these limitations, the proposed criteria are useful in distinguishing the two principal forms of NF.

Molecular biology and pathogenesis of NF-1

Although many of the pathophysiological details concerning NF-1 remain obscure, an important advance in understanding this condition arrived with the recognition, isolation and cloning of the gene responsible for NF-1 (Menon et al 1990, Marchuk et al 1991). Analogous to other hereditary cancer syndromes, affected individuals with NF-1 have a normal copy of the NF-1 gene and an inherited mutated version of the NF-1 gene (Riccardi 1991). For unclear reasons, the mutated version of the gene is most commonly of paternal origin. Because the NF-1 gene appears to function as a tumor suppressor gene (see Tumor Suppressor Genes below), loss, mutation, or inactivation of the remaining normal allele in neural crest tissues is hypothesized as being prerequisite to the development of the neoplastic and other clinical stigmata of NF-1 (Fig. 5.2).

The locus for the gene causing NF-1 was first bracketed to a proximal region of the long arm of chromosome 17 by means of genetic linkage studies (Seizinger et al 1987c). Subsequent physical mapping of the NF-1 gene, facilitated by the analysis of NF-1 translocation breakpoint regions, permitted precise delineation of the NF-1 locus to 17q11.2 (Wallace et al 1990). The NF-1 gene spans more than 300 kb of genomic DNA, consists of more than 49 exons, and embedded within one of its intronic domains are three other discrete genes (OMPG, EV12B and EV12A) which, intriguingly, are transcribed only in the opposite orientation (O'Connell et al 1990, Cawthorn et al 1991, Viskochil et al 1991). Therefore the NF-1 gene is one of the larger and more complex of the human genes so far characterized.

The NF-1 gene product has been termed 'neurofibromin' and is predicted to be a peptide of 2818 amino acids, having a molecular mass of 327 Kd. Although this protein awaits further characterization, some aspects of its putative function are beginning to emerge. Antibodies directed against neurofibromin have been localized to cytoplasmic microtubules, suggesting that neurofibromin maintains some essential cytoskeletal associated function (Guttmann & Collins 1992). Sequence analysis of the NF-1 gene predicts that neurofibromin is composed, in part, of a catalytic domain with striking sequence homology to the mammalian GTPase-activating proteins (GAP) (Xu et al 1990). The GAP protein family are an important class of regulatory peptides, which are most notable for their ability to promote signal transduction in association with the protein product of the *ras* proto-oncogene (p21-*ras*) (see Oncogenes below). p21-*ras* is considered an important positive regulator of cell proliferation, and can exist in either a GTP-bound active state, or a GDP-bound inactive state. When activated, p21-*ras* initiates a series of events, ultimately leading to cell proliferation. The activation of p21-*ras* results in an uncontrolled proliferative signal and has therefore been implicated as a mechanism of tumorigenesis in a variety of human malignancies (Bishop 1991). Normally, p21-*ras* mediated cell proliferation is regulated by GAP, which hydrolyzes the GTP of activated p21-*ras*, returning it to the inactive resting state, and thus terminating the proliferative signal. The finding that the neurofibromin molecule is endowed with a catalytic domain homologous to mammalian GAP, suggests

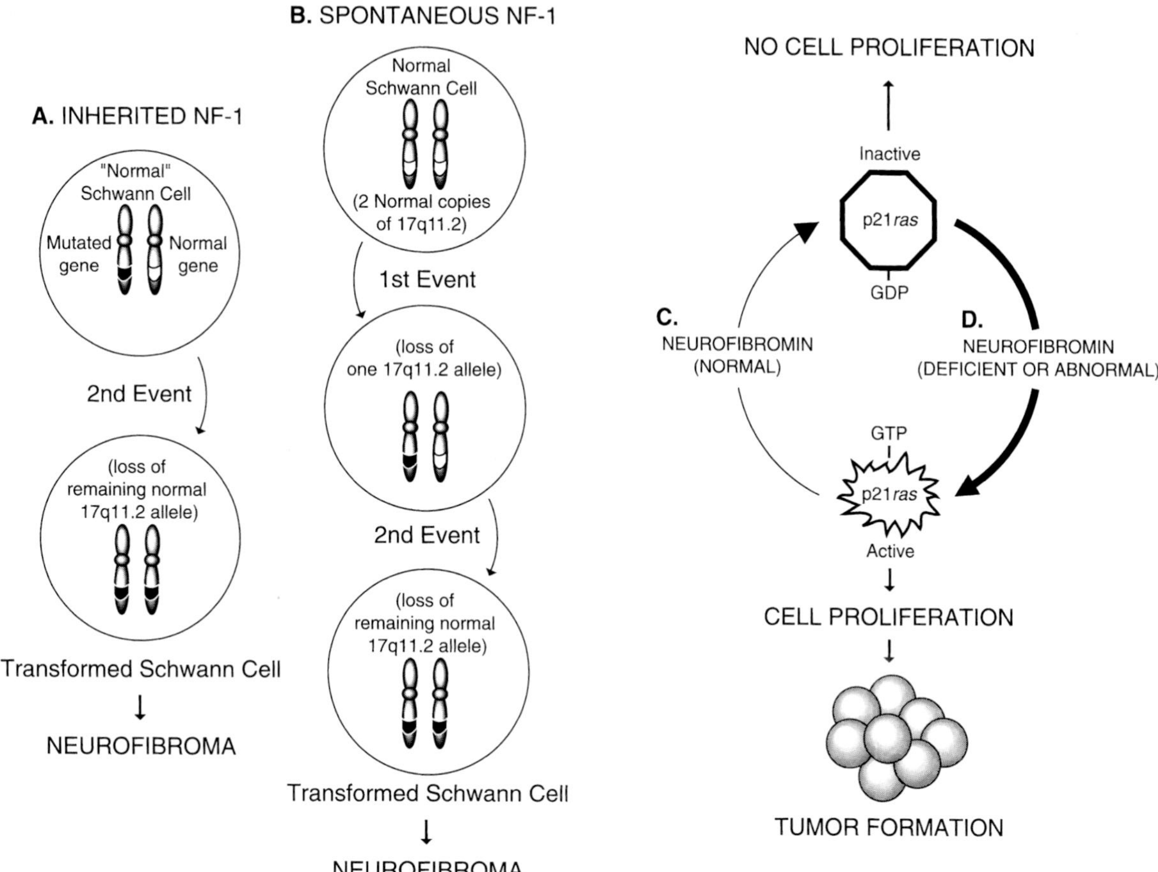

Fig. 5.2 **A,B**. The Knudson (two-step) hypothesis as applied to tumor formation in NF-1, illustrating that tumor formation occurs only after both copies of the NF-1 tumor suppressor gene have been inactivated (deleted, mutated or rearranged). **A**. In the inherited form of NF-1, each somatic cell of affected individuals contains a germline mutation of one NF-1 gene. In susceptible neural crest tissues (i.e. Schwann cells), a second event is necessary to inactivate the remaining normal NF-1 gene, before transformation and tumor formation ensue. **B**. In the spontaneous form of NF-1 all cells begin with a normal genomic constitution. Two distinct events, which sequentially inactivate each copy of the NF-1 gene, are required for transformation and tumor formation. **C,D**. Proposed interaction of the NF-1 gene product, neurofibromin, with protein p21*ras* in the regulation of cell proliferation. **C**. Neurofibromin, endowed with a GAP-related domain, is thought to maintain p21*ras* in a GDP-bound inactive state, thus down regulating signals for cell proliferation. **D**. When neurofibromin is abnormal or absent, as would occur in NF-1, where both NF-1 genes have been inactivated, there is no down regulation of p21*ras* activity. p21*ras* remains in the active state, resulting in unrestrained proliferative signals which contribute to tumor formation.

that one physiologic function of neurofibromin is to maintain p21-*ras* in the inactive state. That neurofibromin is presumably altered or absent in NF-1, suggests that one mechanism of tumor formation in NF-1 may be the result of deficient down regulation of activated p21-*ras* (Guttmann & Collins 1992).

Because the entire NF-1 gene sequence has only recently been determined, the nature of the mutations responsible for NF-1 has been studied on a preliminary basis only. These have ranged from single base pair rearrangements to kilo- and megabase deletions. Except for the case of huge megabase deletions, in which affected NF-1 patients also suffer from mental retardation (presumably reflecting loss of other genes in addition to the NF-1 locus), no correlation between the site and nature of the mutation and the phenotypic severity of the disease has yet been determined. Furthermore, the absence of a consistent mutational pattern of the NF-1 gene has rendered DNA and prenatal diagnosis of NF-1 problematic. Because of the large size of the NF-1 gene, and the high rate of spontaneous mutations, nonspecific strategies to screen for mutations diagnostic of NF-1 would be laborious. Therefore it is unlikely that DNA analysis will be a clinically applicable tool for either the pre- or postnatal diagnosis of NF-1 in the immediate future. In the meantime, prenatal diagnosis and genetic counselling for NF-1 will continue to be done indirectly, by genetic linkage analysis (Pulst 1990, Guttmann & Collins 1992).

Neurofibromatosis type 2 (NF-2)

NF-2 (previously known as central or bilateral acoustic neurofibromatosis) is an autosomal dominant disorder which, beyond a few superficial similarities, is genetically and phenotypically distinct from NF-1. Occurring across all ethnic boundaries, NF-2 is approximately 25 times less frequent than NF-1, having an incidence of approximately 1 case in 100 000 live births (Martuza & Eldridge 1988).

Clinical manifestations

The hallmark of NF-2 is the development of bilateral vestibular schwannomas, which are present in the vast majority of patients (Fig. 5.1B, Table 5.1). With respect to this single feature, the expressivity of NF-2 is considerably less variable than NF-1, although both disorders share almost equal penetrance. Symptoms of NF-2 generally develop later than those of NF-1, usually within the second or third decade. NF-2 patients are also more susceptible to a variety and multiplicity of CNS tumors, including cranial and spinal meningiomas, schwannomas of other cranial and spinal nerves, and occasionally ependymomas and astrocytomas. Meningiomas in NF-2 tend to be multiple, though large en-plaque lesions are also commonly seen. Most ependymomas and astrocytomas arising in association with NF-2 are intraspinal, although brainstem and cerebellar astrocytomas have also been occasionally reported. Optic nerve gliomas are, however, very rare and distinctly unusual features in NF-2. The hamartomas frequently seen in NF-1 are likewise absent in NF-2. Café-au-lait spots and cutaneous neurofibromas can also be seen in NF-2, although they tend to be much less numerous and considerably less obvious than the diffuse presentation typical of NF-1. Ophthalmologic findings in NF-2 are generally restricted to posterior capsular lens opacities, which are seen in 85% of NF-2 patients (Mulvihill et al 1990). These cataracts are frequently bilateral, and result in progressive visual loss. Lisch nodules are almost never a feature of NF-2 and the literature to date describes their occurrence in only one NF-2 patient (Charles et al 1989). Learning disabilities, skeletal and other architectural abnormalities are again rarely features of NF-2. A comparison of the genotypic and phenotypic features of NF-1 and NF-2 is presented in Table 5.2.

In the absence of bilateral acoustic neurinomas (vestibular schwannomas), it can be difficult to arrive at a definitive diagnosis of NF-2. The clinician should therefore be suspicious of a diagnosis of NF-2 in the following clinical settings: (i) any patient with a first degree relative with NF-2; (ii) any patient with a unilateral acoustic schwannoma presenting prior to the age of 30; (iii) any child with a meningioma or a schwann cell tumor; (iv) any patient with multiple neurologic tumors (especially meningiomas). In such settings, all patients should have formal audiologic testing (brainstem auditory evoked response and acoustic reflex studies). If such studies point to a retrocochlear pathology or are inconclusive, gadolinum enhanced MR imaging is indicated (Martuza & Eldridge 1988).

Table 5.2 Diagnostic criteria for neurofibromatosis. Taken from Mulvihill et al 1990.

NF-1: Two or more of the following:
1. Six or more café-au-lait macules, each greater than 5 mm in diameter in prepubertal persons and over 15 mm in diameter in postpubertal persons.
2. Two or more neurofibromas of any type or one plexiform neurofibroma.
3. Freckling in the axillary or inguinal regions.
4. Optic glioma.
5. Two or more Lisch nodules (iris hamartomas).
6. A distinctive osseous lesion such as sphenoid dysplasia or thinning of long bone cortex with or without pseudoarthrosis.
7. A first degree relative (parent, sibling, or offspring) with NF-1 by the above criteria.

NF-2: One of the following:
1. Bilateral eighth nerve tumors seen with magnetic resonance imaging or computerized tomography.
2. A first degree relative with NF-2 and either a unilateral eighth nerve tumor or two of the following:
   — neurofibroma
   — meningioma
   — glioma
   — schwannoma
   — juvenile posterior subcapsular lenticular opacity.

Molecular biology and pathogenesis of NF-2

In contrast to NF-1, in which genetic linkage studies were seminal in identification of its 17q locus, the isolation of the gene responsible for NF-2 was the product of cytogenetic analysis of sporadic meningiomas and schwannomas. The finding that approximately 44% of these tumors shared nonrandom losses of part or all of one copy of chromosome 22 (loss of constitutional heterozygosity) strongly implicated a gene at that site as being either permissive to, or responsible for the development of these tumors (Seizinger et al 1986, 1987b). Similar studies of meningiomas and schwannomas from NF-2 patients revealed consistent losses on the long arm of chromosome 22 (Seizinger et al 1987b). Linkage analysis of a large NF-2 family has since confirmed that the inherited gene responsible for NF-2 is indeed on 22q, and the combination of these data, with those derived from tumor studies has further delineated the NF-2 gene locus to a particular site in the chromosome band 22q11.2 (Rouleau et al 1990). Recent investigations have now led to the cloning and sequencing of the NF-2 gene locus (Rouleau et al 1993, Trofatter et al 1993).

Insofar as the mechanism of action of the NF-1 gene is still a matter of speculation, there is consensus that the genesis of NF-2 and its constituent tumors are mediated by the loss of a tumor suppressor gene at the 22q11.2 locus. NF-2 affected individuals are predisposed to tumor development because each of their somatic cells contains an inactivating germline mutation of the 22q11.2 locus tumor suppressor gene. A second genetic event, such as one occurring with mutation, translocation or deletion of the remaining tumor suppressor gene on the other

22q11.2 allele, would therefore eliminate the tumor suppressive capabilities of the affected cell. When such an event occurs within Schwann or arachnoid cells of the NF-2 individual, the involved cell is liberated from suppressive pressures and the ensuing clonal proliferation results in tumor formation (see Tumor Suppressor Genes below).

The presymptomatic diagnosis of NF-2 gene carriers has, until recently, not been considered possible. In contrast to the large numbers of families with NF-1, there are relatively few NF-2 families. In fact, most of the available genetic linkage data in NF-2 has been derived from a single family, so the issue of genetic heterogeneity (i.e. that more than one gene at different loci can produce NF-2) remained to be excluded. A recent and comprehensive study of 12 NF-2 families has since concluded that NF-2 is indeed a homogeneous condition, occurring as the result of a mutated gene at a single and common locus, and thus a condition for which linkage analysis is a valid form of screening (Narod et al 1992). Polymorphic DNA markers which are closely linked to the NF-2 locus can therefore be used to screen and detect affected presymptomatic individuals. A prospective analysis of such screening should be forthcoming, and if proven effective, will be of immense benefit in distinguishing which asymptomatic patients of NF-2 families carry the defect.

Tuberous sclerosis

Initially described by Bourneville in 1880, tuberous sclerosis is an autosomal dominant disorder of cellular differentiation affecting the brain, skin, heart, kidneys, and other organs. It has an incidence of about one in 10 000 births. It is transmitted as a single gene defect with a penetrance of approximately 80%. Because of the high new mutation rate of the tuberous sclerosis gene, many cases are sporadic. As with NF-1, there is variable expression of the clinical manifestations among patients with tuberous sclerosis.

Clinical manifestations

In 1908, Voght described the clinical triad of sebaceous adenomata, mental retardation, and seizures, which are common in the patient with tuberous sclerosis. In addition to sebaceous adenomata about the face, tuberous sclerosis is characterized by a number of dermatologic manifestations such as subepidermal fibrosis (or shagreen patch), subungual angiofibromas, and ash-leaf spots. Hamartomas are frequently found in the kidney, liver, and the lungs. About half of all cardiac rhabdomyomas are due to tuberous sclerosis (Martuza 1985).

Seizures are thought to be caused by the development of a number of gliotic cortical plaques — also known as 'tubers' — which may also be responsible in part for the neurocognitive decline that is evident in early childhood. Hydrocephalus may develop in some patients when a subependymal tumor occludes the interventricular foramen of Monro (Fig. 5.1C).

Molecular biology and pathogenesis of tuberous sclerosis

The report of the linkage of tuberous sclerosis to the ABO blood group locus on chromosome 9 in 1987 provided the first hope that the gene for this disorder could be identified, cloned and sequenced. At present, however, there are at least two distinct genetic phenotypes for tuberous sclerosis: one linked to chromosome 9q34 (Haines et al 1991), and another linked to markers on chromosome 11q (Kandt et al 1991). Other genetic phenotypes may also be relevant pending further analysis. The analyses of pooled linkage data in tuberous sclerosis genetic studies have consistently revealed genetic heterogeneity. Based on our knowledge of the molecular genetics of tuberous sclerosis, the pathogenesis of this disorder may be analogous to that of NF. That is, a yet to be characterized tumor suppressor gene on chromosome 9q34 (or 11q) is deleted from one chromosome and is followed by a mutation of the corresponding gene on the other chromosome to give rise to the various phenotypic manifestations of the disorder in the characteristic target tissues. Further identification and sequencing of the genes linked to tuberous sclerosis will undoubtedly provide more information about the pathogenesis of this disorder.

Von Hippel-Lindau disease (VHL)

VHL is a devastating disorder associated with various forms of cancer in multiple organ systems (Seizinger 1991). VHL has been found in white, black and Asian populations; it has high penetrance but variable expressivity. An individual harboring the VHL gene defect is susceptible to any one of a number of lesions in any combination. The disorder usually becomes manifest between ages 15 and 50 years.

Clinical manifestations

In VHL, multiple hemangioblastomas are found along the neuraxis in association with certain visceral manifestations. Typically, capillary hemangioblastomas are found within the cerebellum, retina and spinal cord; rarely are they found in the supratentorial compartment. The retinal lesions are present in over 50% of patients with VHL. Cysts of the kidney, epididymis, pancreas and liver are common. Other tumors of the pancreas and liver, phaeochromocytomas, and renal cell carcinomas are well described. Renal cell carcinomas are a particularly frequent cause of death in VHL. In comparison to their sporadic counterparts, familial renal cell carcinomas in VHL are usually bilateral and multifocal and develop at an earlier age (Hudson et al 1986).

Molecular biology and pathogenesis of VHL

The linkage of the VHL gene to chromosome 3p was deduced initially from the pedigrees of patients with hereditary renal cell carcinomas which demonstrated translocations involving chromosome 3p (Cohen et al 1979, Pathak et al 1982), and from karyotypic studies of sporadic renal cell carcinomas which showed chromosome 3p deletions (King 1987, Zbar 1987). These data suggested that the chromosome 3p locus contained a tumor suppressor gene whose loss or inactivation leads to renal cell carcinoma. Seizinger et al (1988) proved conclusively that the VHL gene maps to region 3p25-p26, and is bracketed to a relatively small region of approximately 10 cM near the tip of the short arm of chromosome 3. Analyses of more than 30 VHL families have not shown evidence for genetic heterogeneity, suggesting that VHL is caused by a single gene mutation of 3p25-26. Typically, the tumors of patients with VHL will show loss of the normal (wild-type) copy of the VHL gene with a mutated copy of the retained VHL gene, again supporting the recessive mechanism of tumorigenesis. In future studies, the characterization of the human VHL gene by chromosomal walking or jumping studies will have important implications not only for patients with VHL, but also for a much larger number of cancer patients afflicted with the sporadic counterpart of VHL tumors, such as renal cell carcinoma (Seizinger 1991).

Turcot syndrome

Turcot syndrome is a rare, inheritable condition in which there is an association between multiple adenomatous gastrointestinal polyps and neuroepithelial tumors of the CNS (glioma-polyposis syndrome) (Turcot et al 1959). Since the original description of the condition by Turcot, in 1959, there has been controversy over its mode of inheritance. Many investigators maintain that Turcot syndrome is a phenotypic variant of familial adenomatous polyposis (FAP) — an autosomal dominantly inherited condition in which multiple gastrointestinal polyps form, giving rise to a marked predisposition to early development of colonic adenocarcinomas among affected individuals. The molecular genetics of FAP have been studied, and the gene for FAP has been localized to 5q21-q22 (Groden et al 1991). Others maintain, however, that Turcot syndrome is phenotypically distinct from FAP, being inherited in an autosomal recessive fashion (Tops et al 1992).

The permissible neuroepithelial CNS tumors in Turcot syndrome include astrocytoma, glioblastoma multiforme, and medulloblastoma. We have had the occasion to treat one child with Turcot syndrome at the Hospital for Sick Children (Fig. 5.1D & E). The availability of tumor tissue from both the gastrointestinal tract and the brain of these patients should permit a continued search for the Turcot syndrome gene.

Familial clustering of brain tumors

With the exception of CNS tumors occurring in the predisposing contexts of the phakomatoses and Li-Fraumeni syndrome, and pituitary tumors arising in the context of multiple endocrine neoplasia (MEN) type 1, most intracranial tumors are considered to be sporadic events, without heritable predisposition. Although this appears to be true for the overwhelming majority of CNS tumors, familial aggregation of certain nervous system tumors (glioma, and very rarely, meningioma, and medulloblastoma) has been the subject of ongoing epidemiologic interest (Ikizler et al 1992, Tops et al 1992). Such unexplained familial clustering is not unique to CNS neoplasia, for familial aggregation has been reported for virtually every form of human cancer, and it is generally held that first degree relatives of a cancer patient have a two- to threefold increased risk for developing that tumor (Li 1990).

That gliomas 'run' in families has been the subject of numerous historical and isolated case reports; only recently, however, has the frequency of this phenomenon been methodically approximated. In a recent study of 178 consecutive, newly diagnosed glioma patients without evidence of NF or other predisposing condition, 6.7% of newly diagnosed patients had a blood relative with a positive and pathologically verifiable history of a glial tumor (Ikizler et al 1992). That such a phenomenon could occur by chance alone was generously estimated at 4%, suggesting that the observed familial clustering of gliomas was probably not random, and invoking the influence of some genetic, environmental or other factor. Similar conclusions were reached by Lossignol et al (1990) who observed that 9.4% of patients with anaplastic astrocytoma had at least one first degree relative with an astrocytic tumor. Despite the compelling nature of these reports, familial association alone does not constitute genetic susceptibility. Therefore molecular strategies will be essential in determining whether a germline susceptibility actually exists in these 'glioma families' and, if so, its nature of transmission.

Of the remaining CNS tumors, familial association is an absolute rarity. In the case of meningioma, almost all familial cases occur in the context of NF-2. Ferante et al (1987), in their review of family members of over 1300 operated meningioma patients, found only 1 case of a meningioma in a family member. In an earlier study, Hauge & Harvald (1960) reviewed 1552 family members of 155 meningioma patients, finding only 2 new cases. A rare condition known as Bannayan syndrome (macrocephaly, short stature, and vascular hamartomas), when familial, has been associated with increased risk of meningioma (Hochberg & Gabbai 1990). Because meningiomas can also be asymptomatic, the actual familial incidence is probably higher than reported above, yet is still an exceedingly rare phenomenon. Familial medulloblastoma, usually amongst siblings, has been periodically reported in the literature, but is rare (Hung et al 1990).

THE MOLECULAR BIOLOGY OF HUMAN BRAIN TUMORS

Chromosomal aberrations in human CNS tumors

The earliest and most graphic evidence in support of the concept that cancer represents the successive cellular accumulation of genetic alterations derives from studies depicting the myriad of chromosomal aberrations expressed by cancer cells. Cytogenetic studies of such aberrations have contributed significantly to our understanding of various aspects of tumor biology. This has been especially true in tumors of the CNS, where nonrandom, numerical and structural chromosomal alterations have proven both common and informative to the process and progression of nervous system neoplasia (James et al 1990, Mikkelsen et al 1991, Rasheed & Bigner 1991).

In considering chromosomal alterations in CNS tumors, it is important, but sometimes difficult, to differentiate primary (i.e. etiologic) chromosomal changes from secondary epigenetic chromosomal alterations occurring as the result of genetic instability inherent to cancer cells. It is generally accepted, however, that nonrandom chromosomal changes probably have etiologic significance, and are not simply phenomena of genetic instability. These nonrandom changes can be either numerical or structural, with the latter being most common in CNS tumors. Structural aberrations can take the form of chromosomal deletions, chromosomal rearrangements, or gene amplification, with the latter being represented by the acquisition of double minute chromosomes (DMs — see below) and homogeneously staining regions (HSRs). With the development of chromosomal banding techniques, it is possible to identify the commonest cytogenetic alterations in a variety of nervous system tumors. Genotypic alterations can, however, occur in the absence of gross chromosomal aberrations, requiring restriction fragment length polymorphism (RFLP) analysis (see Tumor Suppressor Gene section) for their identification. Data obtained from both these techniques are reviewed, as applied to the genesis of the principal forms of CNS neoplasia.

Gliomas

Consistent with the existing multi-step paradigm of human carcinogenesis, there appears to be a predictable, preferential and progressive rise in both the number and nature of cytogenetic aberrations acquired by human gliomas during their evolution to increasing grades of histologic and biologic malignancy. Cytogenetic aberrancy in human gliomas can therefore be considered a function of histologic grade, where incremental patterns of cytogenetic atypia are closely mirrored by gradations in malignancy (Bigner et al 1990a, Rasheed & Bigner 1991). Therefore, in contrast to low grade astrocytomas, where there are subtle, if any karyotypic abnormalities, glioblastoma multiforme (GBM) represents the most extreme expression of cytogenetic deviation. Current concepts of malignant progression in astrocytomas suggest that the staged evolution from low grade astrocytoma to anaplastic astrocytoma, and later to GBM, is driven by the successive accumulation of specific cytogenetic insults which are temporally related (see Multi-step Theory below). As a group, though, the most common cytogenetic abnormalities in gliomas are gains or structural alterations of chromosome 7, and losses of chromosome 10, 22, and the sex chromosomes. The most frequently rearranged chromosomes are chromosomes 1>9>7>>>3, and 11 (Bigner et al 1986, Martuza et al 1988, Bigner et al 1990a). Insofar as these changes are common and multiple in GBM, are variably present in anaplastic astrocytomas, and are, for the most part, absent in low grade astrocytomas, their oncologic significance is best considered in the context of histologic grade.

In the more than 100 GBM karyotypes so far published, the most frequent nonrandom deviations involve gains of one or more entire copies of chromosome 7 (80% of cases), losses of chromosome 10 (60% of cases), deletions or rearrangement involving 9p (35% of cases), and the acquisition of DM chromosomes (33% of cases) (Rasheed & Bigner 1991). Subsequent RFLP analysis, while confirming these gross alterations, has also revealed a number of nonrandom subchromosomal alterations. Loss of heterozygosity (LOH — see Tumor Suppressor Gene section below) involving alleles on chromosome 17 (22% of cases); on chromosome 22 (19% of cases); and on chromosome 13 (14% of cases) have been demonstrated with some regularity (James et al 1988), whereas allelic losses of 5p, 11p, 14q and 15p have been less frequently observed (Fults et al 1990).

The aforementioned cytogenetic alterations result in either the augmentation or loss of genetic information, suggesting that both these mechanisms are operative in the genesis of glioblastoma. With respect to the former, the role of polysomy of chromosome 7 in tumorigenesis remains speculative. It is intriguing, however, that chromosome 7 is the locus for two oncologically important proteins: the epidermal growth factor receptor (EGFR) and the platelet-derived growth factor alpha chain (PDGF-α), both of which have been implicated as autocrine mediators of tumorigenesis in gliomas and their cell lines (see

Growth Factors below) (Guha 1991). A more efficient, selective, and possibly more important means to accomplish genomic amplification involves the formation of DM chromosomes, which are present in up to 30% of glioblastomas (Bigner et al 1988a,b). DMs are small, spherical, usually paired chromosome-like structures that lack a centromere and contain repetitive DNA sequences in chromatin form. In the case of glioblastoma, DMs often represent multiple copies of the EGFR gene. EGFR gene amplification appears to be a late event in the progression of astrocytomas — found in 40% of GBMs, and only exceptionally in gliomas of lesser grade (James et al 1990, Fuller & Bigner 1992). In a small percentage of GBMs, DMs represent amplification of other oncogenes such as N-*myc* or *gli* (Fuller & Bigner 1992). The implication of oncogene activation and amplification is discussed below (see Oncogenes section).

That chromosomal or allelic deletions are almost universal cytogenetic findings in GBMs underscores the importance of selective genomic loss as a contributing mechanism to the genesis of this neoplasm. An example of such is the loss of chromosome 10 loci, specifically 10q, which on the combined basis of RFLP and karyotypic analysis is said to occur in up to 80% of glioblastomas (James et al 1988, Fujimoto et al 1989, Bigner et al 1990a). Because 10q losses are restricted almost exclusively to GBMs, and are conspicuously absent in tumors of lesser grade, several authors have ascribed tumor suppressive properties to this locus (see Tumor Suppressor Genes below) (James et al 1990, Mikkelsen et al 1991, Rasheed & Bigner 1991). Further support that a 'glioma suppressor gene' resides at the 10q locus has been obtained from chromosome transfer studies, where partial reversion of tumor phenotype was demonstrated upon transfer of chromosome 10 into a glioblastoma cell line (Steck et al 1991). It is probably more than coincidental that losses of 10q and pericentromeric regions of chromosome 10 have also been implicated in the development of prostate cancer (Carter et al 1990), and melanocytic neoplasia (Parmiter et al 1988).

Allelic deletion of 9p appears to be a relatively common event restricted to gliomas of intermediate or high grade (James et al 1988, 1990), and allelic losses of 13q loci have been demonstrated in approximately 14% of gliomas (James et al 1988). Unlike the other aberrations so far discussed, 13q losses occur in all grades of gliomas, suggesting an early event in their progression (James et al 1990). The 13q locus (specifically 13q14) is of considerable biologic significance, because it is the site of the retinoblastoma (Rb) gene, the best studied and prototypical example of a tumor suppressor gene in human cancer (Friend et al 1986). In one study, 44% of GBMs demonstrated allelic deletions of the Rb gene (Venter et al 1991).

Deletions of 17p have been identified in roughly 22% of human gliomas, being present with similar frequency in low, intermediate and high grade lesions (James et al 1988). Such a uniform distribution of 17p deletions among the various glioma grades suggests that this is an event early in the progression of astrocytic tumors. The significance of 17p aberrations for gliomas in particular, and human cancer in general, will be described in the section on Tumor Suppressor Genes and the special case of the p53 gene. The role of p53 mutations in CNS tumors is reviewed in detail below (see Tumor Suppressor Genes).

Meningiomas

Meningiomas were among the first of any solid human tumor to which a nonrandom chromosomal aberration was consistently ascribed (Fig. 5.3) (Zang & Singer 1967). In fact, in the more than 25 years since the initial description of a consistent group G chromosome loss in meningiomas, several hundred published meningioma karyotypes have confirmed the missing locus to be chromosome 22. As reviewed by Bigner et al (1990a), the reported frequency of complete or partial loss of chromosome 22 in meningiomas varies from 60–90% of cases. More recently, Arnoldus et al using the technique of interphase cytogenetics, demonstrated that 70% of 30 meningiomas studied had consistent losses of 22q (Arnoldus et al 1992). Additional chromosomal aberrations identified included losses of chromosome 11 and 18, and gains of chromosome 6, 7, 17, and the X chromosome. It was of interest that meningiomas demonstrating 22q loss and one or more of these other aberrations were frequently atypical histologically or recurrent clinically. The presence of these more complicated karyotypic abnormalities in recurrent meningiomas has been known for some time, although they have not been useful as markers in predicting recurrence (Bigner et al 1990). This is probably due to the fact that the completeness of surgical resection is a more important factor in forestalling recurrence than is the intrinsic biological aggressiveness of the tumor.

Since loss of chromosome 22 (specifically 22q) is so consistently and frequently a feature of meningiomas, the possibility of a meningioma related tumor suppressor gene residing at that locus has been proposed (Seizinger et al 1987a, Schneider et al 1992). The recent application of RFLP analysis, while confirming the chromosome 22 losses seen karyotypically, has further delineated the precise locus of this putative suppressor gene. Dumanski et al (1990) have demonstrated partial or complete losses of chromosome 22 in 63% of meningiomas and have ascribed locus 22q12.3-qter to meningiomas. It is of interest that despite the association of meningiomas with NF-2, and the presumed proximity of their loci on 22q, the above study has demonstrated that both these disorders derive from clearly distinct loci.

Those meningiomas with cytogenetically non-demon-

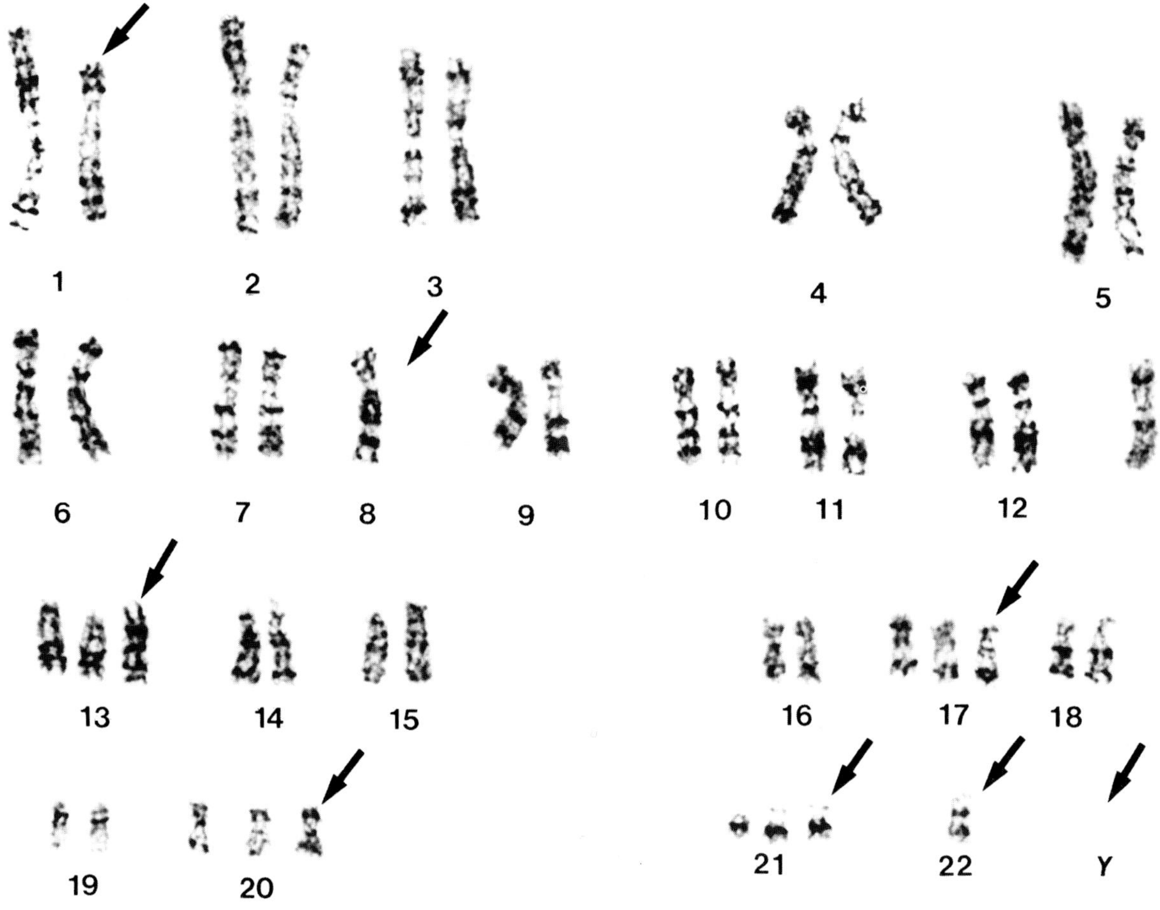

Fig. 5.3 Cytogenetic analysis of pediatric brain tumor. Solid Giemsa staining and G-banding were performed on 20 cells. The karyotype is 47,X, del 1p(32),–8,+13,+17,+20,+21,–22,–Y. A consistent structural abnormality was noted in the form of del 1p(32) (first arrow). Losses and gains of various chromosomes are also noted by arrows. Monosomy 22 was noted in all cells analyzed. The tumor proved histopathologically to be a meningioma, in which monosomy 22 is well described. Cytogenetic analysis and figure courtesy of Dr J Squire, Hospital for Sick Children

strable chromosome 22 deletions may still possess small mutations (such as a point mutation) within the 22q12.3-qter locus which are important in tumorigenesis but are too small to be detected by routine RFLP technology. Therefore, the current opinion of meningioma tumorigenesis conforms well to the two-step Knudson hypothesis, in which sequential loss of both 22q tumor suppressor genes is requisite to tumor induction.

Medulloblastoma

With less than 50 banded karyotypes of medulloblastoma reported in the literature, the cytogenetics of this tumor type have only recently been catalogued. The most notable and consistently occurring cytogenetic aberration in medulloblastomas is the formation of an isochromosome 17q [i(17q)], identifiable in approximately one third of cases (Griffith et al 1988, Beigel et al 1989, Bigner et al 1990a). An isochromosome is the chromosomal structure which results when centromeric separation during mitosis inappropriately occurs in the wrong plane, separating two arms of a chromosome instead of the two chromatids. Additional, but less frequent nonrandom chromosomal alterations in medulloblastoma include other structural and numerical abnormalities of chromosome 17, deletions and translocations involving chromosomes 6, 5, 6q, 16q, 11, 10q, and the sex chromosomes. Gains of chromosome 1 and 7 have also been identified (Griffith et al 1988, Beigel et al 1989, Bigner et al 1990a).

Of the above mentioned aberrations, the most uniform finding has been allelic loss of 17p. Identified by RFLP analysis in almost 50% of medulloblastomas, certain consistently deleted 17p loci are thought to house a tumor suppressor gene(s) important to the genesis of this tumor. The precise site of the medulloblastoma related suppressor gene is unknown; however, it has been narrowed down to two discrete regions of 17p: a proximal site at 17p12 and a distal site at 17p13-pter. Interestingly, these two regions flank the p53 gene locus (Biegel et al 1992, Cogen et al 1992) (see Tumor Suppressor Genes below).

An attempt to predict clinical outcome on the basis of 17p deletion patterns has met with some preliminary success. In a small group of patients, Cogen noted that the combined presence of both proximal and distal 17p deletions was a negative prognostic factor for medulloblastoma patients, particularly in those designated as 'good risk' by clinical parameters (Cogen 1991).

Approximately 10–20% of medulloblastomas contain DM chromosomes. Bigner et al have demonstrated that the amplified gene thought to constitute these DMs is c-*myc* (Bigner et al 1990b). The issue of gene amplification in medulloblastomas is considered in detail below (see Oncogenes p. 81).

Tumor suppressor genes

The special case of the p53 gene

The p53 gene is one of the best characterized tumor suppressor genes, and is frequently altered in a variety of tumor types (Nigro et al 1989, Hollstein et al 1991, Levine et al 1991). The p53 gene product was originally detected in the nucleus of normal mammalian cells as an associated protein of the SV-40 large T antigen and in various transformed cells and was associated with a number of viral oncoproteins: the E1B protein of adenovirus types 2 and 5, the E6 protein of papilloma virus type 16, and the large T antigen of the JC virus. Initially, the p53 gene was thought to be an oncogene capable of transforming somatic cells in conjunction with an activated *ras* gene; however, subsequent gene transfection experiments have shown that the normal (or wild-type) p53 gene suppresses cellular transformation (Finlay et al 1989, Mercer et al 1990).

Typically, a tumor suppressor gene product loses its function when both copies of the gene (that is, maternally and paternally derived alleles) are altered (Fig. 5.2). Some mutant p53 products, however, aggregate in tetrameric or oligomeric forms which can inactivate the normal p53 gene product. Therefore, in contrast to other tumor suppressor genes, a mutation of the p53 gene in a single allele may lead to the production of a mutant protein which acts in a dominant fashion to compete with the normal p53 product.

The human p53 protein is comprised of 393 amino acids, the first 80 amino acids within the amino-terminus being acidic, and the following 80 amino acids being rich in proline. In the carboxy-terminus, the p53 protein has a basic domain which can bind to DNA. The p53 protein thus has features similar to many general transcription factors. In fact the fusion of the normal p53 and the yeast GAL-4 proteins acts as a transcriptional activator (Raycroft et al 1989, Fields & Jang 1991). The expression of the normal p53 gene by certain viral promoters has also been shown to trans-repress promoters of other genes, such as IL-6, c-*fos*, c-*jun*, beta actin, multiple drug resistance gene-1, and p53 itself (Ginsberg et al 1991, Santhanam et al 1991, Chin et al 1992). Apparently, the mutant p53 product is less active in trans-repressing other genes than is the normal p53 product. Moreover, another group reported that the normal p53 product might regulate gene transcription in a sequence-specific manner (at sites on the DNA where there are two direct TGCCT sequences), and compete with the mutant type p53 (Kern et al 1991). Their hypothesis can also explain the 'dominant-negative' action of the p53 product.

The function of the normal p53 gene and gene product is still unclear. The half-life of the normal p53 product is short (5–20 min), but can become greater than 24 h after binding to the SV-40 large T antigen. Mutant p53 products also have prolonged half-lives. p53 levels increase in G1/S phases of the cell cycle. Transformed cells transfected with the normal p53 gene show growth arrest in G1. In addition, it has been reported that the expression of the normal p53 gene causes apoptosis, a process of programmed cell death which is blocked by IL-6 (Yonish-Rouach et al 1991). A recent report suggests that the normal p53 product significantly represses some late G1/S phase genes such as c-*fos*, c-*jun*, or c-*myc* (Lin et al 1991). As a result, the normal p53 gene and product are believed to suppress transition of a cell from G1 to S phases of the cell cycle.

In general, we now believe that most malignant tumors are derived from the accumulation of multiple genetic alterations. These alterations include the amplification of some oncogenes and the loss of certain tumor suppressor genes. With molecular biological techniques, a number of specific DNA markers have been generated to detect polymorphisms in the human genome. When DNA is cut with restriction enzymes, these specific DNA markers can be used to identify polymorphisms in the cut fragments — so-called RFLPs. RFLP analysis can detect loss of genetic material, whether gross or subtle, among paternal and maternal alleles. Loss of an allele from one chromosome is called LOH, and is thought to be important in the process of human tumorigenesis.

Many human cancers show LOHs on specific chromosomes whereas other somatic cells from the same patient typically do not. Examples include LOHs in retinoblastoma on chromosome 13, in Wilms tumor on chromosome 11, and colorectal cancers on chromosomes 17,5, and 18. These LOHs are presumed evidence for the inactivation of putative tumor suppressor genes located around the indicated chromosomes. Some tumor suppressor genes, such as RB, WT-1, DCC, MCC, and FAP genes, have been isolated and sequenced within the lost alleles.

The p53 gene is located on the short arm of chromosome 17 (17p13.1). The p53 gene has four conserved domains (codon 132–143, codon 174–179, codon 236–

248, and codon 272–281) which are thought to play important roles in the tumor suppressing function of the p53 gene. The LOH on chromosome 17, as detected by RFLP analysis in a variety of tumors, has been found within the p53 gene locus, and is thought to relate to the inactivation of the p53 gene. LOHs have also been detected within the p53 gene locus in a variety of human glial tumors. As a result, it has been postulated that p53 gene mutations may play a role in the genesis of glial neoplasms. In fact, most glioma cell lines express an excess amount of p53, and some of them harbor p53 mutations (Fig. 5.4). p53 gene mutations have also been detected in 10–30% of glioma specimens (Mashiyama et al 1991, Tabuchi et al 1991). Primary cultured tumor cells or glioma xenografts have a higher incidence of p53 mutations which might relate to selection of cell types following in vitro propagation of tumor cells. A recent report suggests that GBM patients whose tumors show p53 mutations are distinguished by an earlier age of onset (31 years) and by longer survival

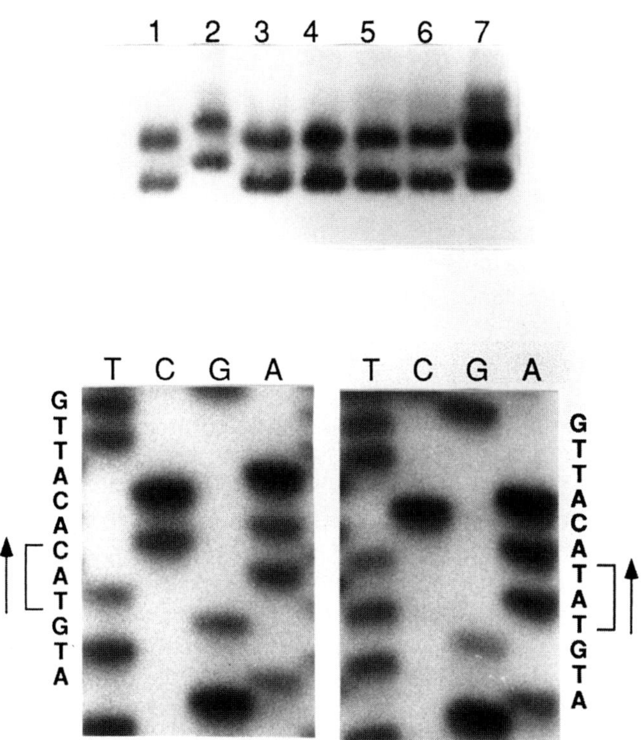

Fig. 5.4 Polymerase chain reaction-single strand conformation polymorphism (PCR-SSCP) analysis and DNA sequence of exon 7 of the p53 gene. The PCR products of exon 7 of the p53 gene were electrophoresed in an 8% polyacrylamide gel after heat denaturing. **Top panel** Lane 2 shows altered mobility of DNA fragments in a human malignant glioma (T98G), suggesting a conformation polymorphism in exon 7 in this tumor, but not in the other tumors. **Bottom panel, right** A point mutation was found in exon 7 of malignant glioma T98G by DNA sequence analysis. A transition from G to A was detected at codon 237 in T98G in contrast to the normal (wild-type) sequence (**bottom panel, left**). This point mutation caused an amino acid substitution from methionine to isoleucine (ATG to ATA). Lane 1: U87MG, 2: T98G, 3: 118MG, 4: A172, 5: U251MG, 6: U373MG, 7: KMG4.

(Chung et al 1990). Interestingly, most p53 mutations described in the different tumor types have been reported within the conserved domains.

It is still unclear whether the p53 mutation is an early or late event in the pathogenesis of glial neoplasms. Sidransky et al (1991) reported that p53 mutations were identified during the progression of astrocytomas from low grade to high grade neoplasms. Others have reported the incidence of p53 mutations to be the same in low grade and high grade gliomas suggesting that p53 mutations did not affect the growth rate, pathological grade, or clinical progression of the tumor. While p53 mutations may be important for certain glial neoplasms, the majority of gliomas do not demonstrate such mutations. Saxena et al (1992) have recently shown evidence for the involvement of a second putative tumor suppressor gene on chromosome 17 distinct from the p53 locus which could be involved in glial tumorigenesis. Interestingly, approximately 50% of human medulloblastomas have been reported to show gene rearrangements on chromosome 17. In medulloblastoma, however, the p53 gene does not appear to be mutated (Saylors et al 1991). It is speculated that a tumor suppressor gene other than p53 on the short arm of chromosome 17 is involved in the pathogenesis of the medulloblastoma.

Germline mutations have been detected in the families of patients with the Li-Fraumeni syndrome — a familial cancer syndrome in which family members develop tumors involving diverse organs, such as breast, soft tissues, brain, bone, blood and adrenal cortex (Srivastava et al 1991, Malkin et al 1992). Most of the patients with this syndrome develop tumors at an unusually early age and at multiple sites. In these studies, germline mutations in the p53 gene were transmitted through several generations and predisposed members to cancer. The Li-Fraumeni syndrome is characterized by autosomal dominant inheritance, and may well explain how the dominant-negative action of the p53 product functions in families with germline mutations. A case of an ependymoma has also been reported in a Li-Fraumeni family carrying a germline mutation in the p53 gene (Metzger et al 1990).

Activation and expression of oncogenes in CNS tumors

Seminal to contemporary paradigms of oncogenesis is the premise that a cellular balance exists between positive and negative growth regulatory mechanisms, the disruption of which leads to the transformed phenotype. Enhanced positive regulation by oncogenes has emerged as a potentially important mechanism mediating the tumorigenic process. The degree to which dominantly acting oncogenes contribute to the genesis of human cancer varies considerably among different tumor types. While N-*myc* oncogene amplification in neuroblastoma represents the most convincing example of the close relationship between oncogenes and tumor progression (Brodeur 1990), the situation is considerably less clear for tumors of the CNS. To date, neither a causal nor a permissive role of any one oncogene has been *definitively* ascribed to any particular CNS tumor. Nevertheless, activation and expression of several oncogenes have been demonstrated in sufficient numbers of CNS tumors that their potential tumorigenic roles in the CNS, if only by association, cannot be ignored. As oncogenes represent a subject of increasingly broad scope, only those aspects of oncogene biology immediately relevant to CNS tumors is presented. A more in-depth coverage of the subject is presented in several recent reviews (Freeman et al 1990, Miller et al 1990, Bishop 1991).

Strictly defined, an oncogene is any DNA sequence which encodes a protein capable of transforming cells in culture or inducing cancer in animals. Because a basic understanding of the terminology, evolutionary significance, and carcinogenic implications of oncogenes is critical at this juncture, their origins and methods of discovery are briefly reviewed here.

Cellular oncogenes (c-*onc*) are known as proto-oncogenes and are present in the genome of every human cell. Although the normal physiological role of most human proto-oncogenes has yet to be elucidated, it is generally held that they subserve functions essential to normal growth and differentiation of the organism. Proto-oncogenes can be mutated by a variety of genetic mechanisms such as point mutations, translocations, deletions, or amplifications (Bishop 1983, Gordon 1985). The mutated or altered form of a proto-oncogene is known as an oncogene, and overexpression of an oncogene is thought to play an important role in the genesis of human cancers. Interestingly, oncogenes were first appreciated during the characterization of acute transforming retroviruses. These retroviruses (v-*onc*) carry 'captured' normal cellular genes that have been altered so as to induce tumor formation in a variety of animals.

Although more than 50 oncogenes have so far been identified, the mechanism by which they exert tumorigenic influences is still speculative. Existing data do suggest, however, that most oncogene products interact with cell growth regulatory systems, and can therefore be functionally considered as either growth factors, growth factor receptors, intracellular transducers or nuclear transcription factors (Oncogene class I–IV, respectively). The spectrum of CNS tumors in which oncogenes have been activated, amplified or overexpressed is presented in Table 5.3. The cumulative data presented suggest that gene amplification is the dominant mechanism of proto-oncogene activation in CNS tumors. Although gene rearrangement is seen considerably less often, the number of studies directed at identifying rearrangements and point mutations have been comparatively few.

Class I oncogenes (growth factors)

Oncogenes only rarely arise from genes encoding growth factors. Derived from the simian sarcoma virus (SSV), v-*sis* is both the prototypical and only naturally occurring growth factor oncogene. The significance of v-*sis* activation in CNS tumors is unclear. However, two indirect lines of evidence suggest that it may be relevant to the genesis of gliomas: firstly, primates injected intracranially with SSV will develop gliomas morphologically similar to those naturally occurring in man (Deinhardt 1980); and secondly the oncogenic protein encoded by v-*sis* is structurally and functionally related to PDGF-B (Robbins et al 1983), a peptide whose gene is frequently overexpressed in human gliomas (Guha 1991). This relationship is reviewed in detail below (see Growth Factors). Despite the regularity with which the normal cellular homologue of v-*sis* — PDGF-B — is overexpressed in gliomas, only a single case of v-*sis* amplification was found in the glioma literature (Fujimoto et al 1989b).

Class II oncogenes (transmembrane receptors)

Proto-oncogenes of this class encode membrane receptor proteins whose function is to bind specific ligands (usually growth factors or hormones) and initiate transduction of regulatory signals from the extracellular environment to the cytoplasm. These signals are frequently those for normal growth and proliferation. Oncogenic versions of these genes mediate their tumorigenic effect by encoding for aberrant receptor proteins which can become, and remain, activated in the absence of ligand binding (constitutive activation), resulting in the transduction of proliferative signals in the absence of a normal regulatory stimulus.

The prototypical example of this class pertaining to the CNS is the EGFR gene, which is the cellular homologue of v-*erb*B oncogene derived from the avian erythroblastoma virus. Activation of the EGFR proto-oncogene in glial tumors is accomplished primarily by gene amplification, although gene rearrangements have become increasingly recognized (Fuller & Bigner 1992). The EGFR gene is the most commonly activated proto-oncogene in human glial tumors. Amplification of the EGFR gene has been identified in approximately 40% of malignant gliomas, and has been found almost exclusively in GBMs (Wong et al 1987, James et al 1990, Fuller & Bigner 1992). EGFR amplification is thought to induce cellular transformation through autocrine pathway mechanisms, mediated by EGF and TGF-alpha (see Growth Factors below). The presence or degree of EGFR amplification does not appear to have prognostic significance, as GBMs exhibiting EGFR amplification have not been found to behave differently from those without amplification (Bigner et al 1988a, Diedrich et al 1991). A significant finding con-

Table 5.3 Proto-oncogene/oncogene analysis in primary biopsies of human CNS tumors. Modified from Rutka et al 1990.

Tumor type	Probe	Aberration	Reference
Astrocytoma	c-*erb* B (EGFR)	A	Diedrich et al 1991
	c-*myc*	EE	Fujimoto et al 1989b
	v-*fos*	EE	Fujimoto et al 1989b
	v-*sis*	EE	Fujimoto et al 1988
	p53	mutation	Cogen 1991
Anaplastic astrocytoma	c-*erb* B (EGFR)	A, RA	Wong et al 1987, Diedrich et al 1991
	N-*myc*	A	Garson et al 1985
	c-*sis* (PDGF)	EE	Maxwell et al 1990a
	p53	mutation	Cogen 1991
Glioblastoma multiforme	c-*erb* B (EGFR)	A, RA, EE	Libermann et al 1985, Wong et al 1987, Diedrich et al 1991
	gli	A, EE	Kinzler et al 1987
	N-*myc*	A, EE	Wong et al 1987, Fujimoto et al 1989b
	v-*myc*	EE	Fujimoto et al 1988
	v-*sis*	A, EE	Fujimoto et al 1989b
	c-*sis* (PDGF)	EE	Maxwell et al 1990a
	v-*fos*	EE	Fujimoto et al 1989b
	N-*ras*	A, EE	Sauceda et al 1988
	Ha-*ras*	rare alleles	Diedrich et al 1988
	c-*mos*	rare alleles	Diedrich et al 1988
	Rb gene	deletion	Venter et al 1991
	p53 gene	point mutation	Nigro et al 1989
Oligodendroglioma	c-*erb* B (EGFR)	A, RA	Diedrich et al 1991
	Ha-*ras*	rare alleles	Diedrich et al 1988
	c-*mos*	rare alleles	Diedrich et al 1988
Ependymoma	c-*erb* B (EGFR)	A	Diedrich et al 1991
	v-*fos*	EE	Fujimoto et al 1989b
	Ha-*ras*	rare alleles	Diedrich et al 1988
	c-*mos*	rare alleles	Diedrich et al 1988
Medulloblastoma	c-*erb* B (EGFR)	A	Wasson et al 1990
	N-*myc*	A, RA	Sauceda et al 1988, Rouah et al 1989
	c-*myc*	A, EE	MacGregor & Ziff 1990, Raffel et al 1990
	v-*myc*	EE	Fujimoto et al 1988
	N-*ras*	point mutation	Iolascon et al 1991
	p53 gene	mutation	Cogen et al 1992
Meningioma	c-*sis* (PDGF)	EE	Maxwell et al 1990a, Riva & Larizza 1992
	c-*myc*	A	Sauceda et al 1988
	c-*fos*	EE	Riva & Larizza 1992
	N-*myc*	A, RA	Sauceda et al 1988
	Ha-*ras*	rare alleles	Diedrich et al 1988
	c-*mos*	rare alleles	Diedrich et al 1988
Acoustic schwannoma	c-*fos*	EE	Riva & Larizza 1992
Pituitary adenoma:			
Prolactinoma	v-*fos*	A	U et al 1988
Prolactinoma	H-*ras*	point mutation	Karga et al 1992
GH-producing adenomas	*gsp*	point mutation	Landis et al 1990

Abbreviations: A = gene amplification; RA = gene rearrangement; EE = enhanced gene expression

cerning EGFR amplification in gliomas is that approximately 50% of tumors exhibiting amplification are also accompanied by EGFR gene rearrangement (Fuller & Bigner 1992). The product of such rearrangements is a truncated EGFR with deletions of the extracellular (receptor binding) domain.

That such mutant EGFRs can become constitutively activated has recently been shown in human gliomas, and is regarded as being a transforming mechanism equivalent to that observed for v-*erb*B (Yamazaki et al 1990). Humphrey et al (1990) have identified an 802 base pair deletion of the EGFR gene, and subsequently developed a monoclonal antibody which selectively recognizes the mutant EGFR encoded by this form of deletion. This novel tumor specific antibody can be used to deliver selectively radioisotopes, chemotherapeutic agents and other toxins directly to tumor cells, thereby opening a variety of promising therapeutic avenues. Despite the frequency with which EGFR amplification and rearrangement is observed in malignant gliomas, it is rarely a feature of other CNS tumor types.

Other common oncogenes of this class such as c-*erb*B2

(*neu*) and c-*mos* have only exceptionally been represented in human gliomas (Wu & Chikaraishi 1990), and therefore are not considered important to the development of most CNS tumors.

Class III oncogenes (intracellular transducers)

Of the various intracranial tumors, only pituitary tumors appear to be targets for this class of oncogenes. The recent discovery that a subgroup of growth hormone (GH)-producing pituitary adenomas exhibited aberrant signal transduction pathways led to the identification of a new oncogene termed *gsp* (Landis et al 1989). Somatotroph proliferation and GH secretion are regulated by GTP binding proteins analogous to the p21*ras* proteins (Fig. 5.5). In a recent report by Landis et al (1990), *gsp* mutations were identified in 40% of GH-producing adenomas. In comparison to those with the wild-type G_s alpha chain, tumors with *gsp* mutations were smaller, had lower basal GH levels, and retained GH suppressibility. The authors felt that patients with this subgroup of GH-producing adenomas enjoyed a more indolent course than those exhibiting the wild-type G_s alpha chain.

Oncogenic mutations of *ras*, the prototypical class III oncogene frequently activated in a variety of tumors originating systemically (pancreatic, colon, lung, leukemia), have only sporadically been demonstrated in pituitary tumors and malignant gliomas (Diedrich et al 1988, Karga et al 1992).

Class IV oncogenes (nuclear transcription factors)

Oncogenes of this class (*myc, jun, fos, gli*) encode nuclear-associated proteins which regulate gene transcription. Of these, only the *myc* family and *gli* oncogenes appear to have any regular association with CNS tumors, although the others have been identified sporadically. Medulloblastoma is the principal CNS tumor in which amplification

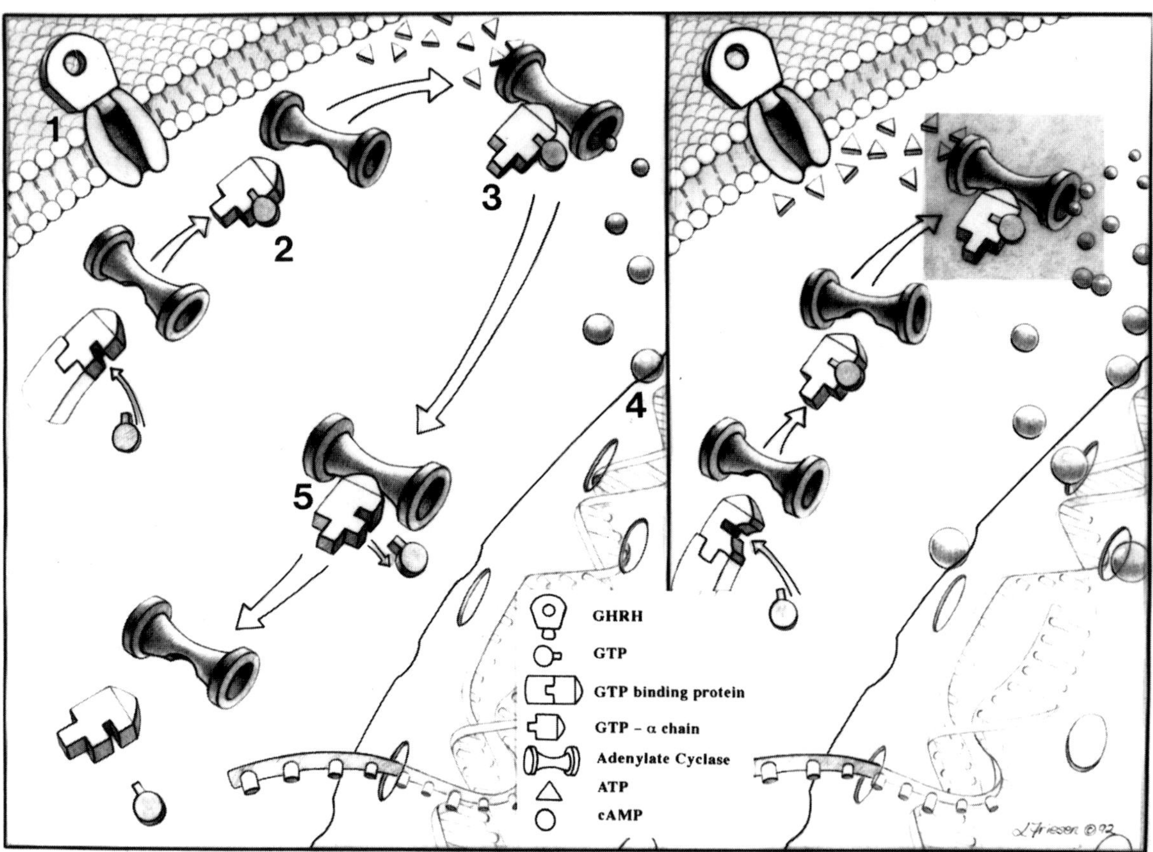

Fig. 5.5 Proposed molecular basis for somatotroph proliferation and GH secretion in the normal state and in tumors with *gsp* oncogenic mutation. **Left panel**: Under normal conditions, binding of GHRH takes place to the somatotroph membrane receptor (**1**); dissociation of the alpha chain of the GTP-binding protein (G_s) occurs and there is GTP binding (**2**); activation of adenylate cyclase and production of cAMP takes place (**3**); cAMP as the second messenger initiates a series of downstream events leading to GH gene transcription and somatotroph proliferation (**4**); the alpha chain regulates the degree of adenylate cyclase activation with intrinsic GTPase activity which hydrolyzes the bound GTP and returns G_s to the resting inactive state, thus 'turning off' the signal for proliferation and GH secretion. **Right panel**: With a *gsp* oncogenic mutation the mutated version of the alpha chain has deficient GTPase activity and cannot 'turn itself off'; GTP remains bound, constitutively activating adenylate cyclase (shaded area). Large amounts of cAMP accumulate, leading to a deregulated and perpetual signal for somatotroph proliferation and GH secretion.

of the *myc* gene family has been consistently, albeit infrequently, described. In their review of the subject, Fuller & Bigner (1992) determined that the cumulative incidence of c-*myc* and N-*myc* amplification in medulloblastomas was 8% and 4% respectively. In contradistinction to the relationship of N-*myc* and neuroblastoma, where the degree of amplification of the former serves as a prognostic marker of the latter, the same has yet to be shown for either c-*myc* or N-*myc* in medulloblastoma. N-*myc* and c-*myc* amplification have also been identified in isolated cases of malignant glioma and their cell lines (Fig. 5.6).

Kinzler et al (1987, 1988) identified an amplified and highly expressed gene from a malignant glioma cell line. This newly identified gene, called *gli*, is localized to chromosome 12, encodes a 'zinc finger' family DNA-binding protein, and is thought to have transcriptional capabilities. Although the precise function of the *gli* protein is unknown, its presence in amplified form in a minority of GBM biopsies (2–4%) implies that it may provide a selective growth advantage to a subset of glial tumors.

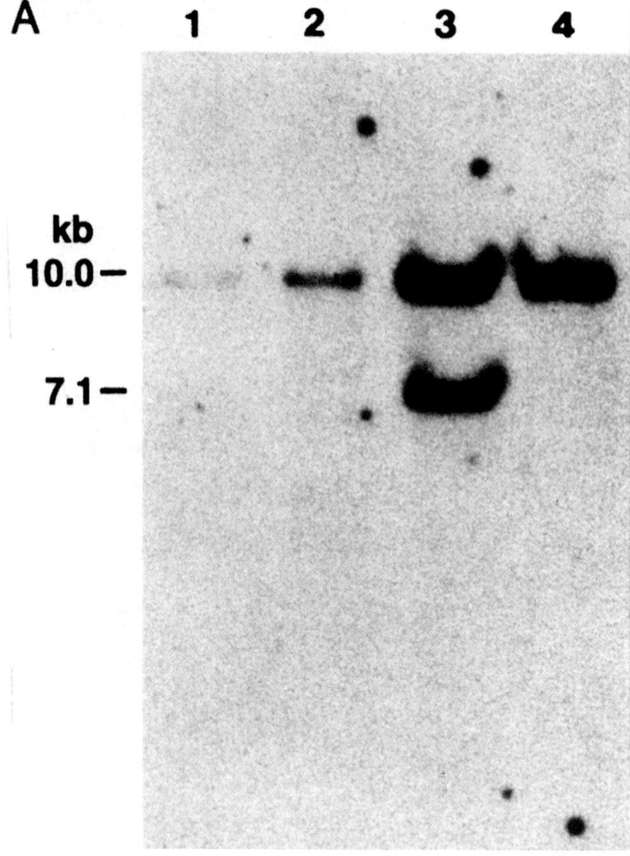

Fig. 5.6 Evidence for amplification, rearrangement and expression of the c-*myc* oncogene in a human malignant glioma cell line. Southern blot analysis of DNA from glioma cells digested with *Hind* III using a c-*myc* gene probe. **Lane 1**, normal human lymphocytes; **lane 2**, Hut23, a human lung cancer cell line with c-*myc* gene amplified 5-fold; **lane 3**, human malignant glioma, SF-188 MG; **lane 4**, NCI-417, a human small cell carcinoma cell line with c-*myc* gene amplified 20-fold. DNA samples (5 μg) were loaded into each lane. There are two DNA fragments, 10.0 and 7.1 kb, present in the human malignant glioma, instead of a single normal 10.0 kb fragment. Each of these two fragments demonstrates a 25-fold amplification of the c-*myc* probe per haploid genome. Because of the two separate fragments, a genetic rearrangement has accompanied the amplification. This is one of the few examples of an amplifed and rearranged c-*myc* oncogene in human CNS tumors. Reproduced with permission from Trent et al 1986.

From the preceding discussion, it is clear that the number of oncogenes implicated in the genesis of CNS tumors significantly outnumbers the established facts pertaining to their exact biological roles and mechanisms of action. Despite these conceptual limitations of existing knowledge, it is clear that oncogene activation is a molecular correlate in only a minority of CNS tumors studied to date.

Growth factors

Emerging more than a decade ago was a new hypothesis, implicating the production and autocrine action of growth factors as central events in the genesis and maintenance of malignancy (Sporn & Roberts 1985). Growth factors are soluble peptides which act in part by their ability to bind to specific cell surface receptors in target cells. This binding is believed to elicit a signal which is transduced across the cell membrane to effect a response from a cellular or nuclear target. Many critical cellular functions such as mitogenesis, angiogenesis, and gene transcription are thought to be regulated by such growth factor-mediated signal transduction systems. Normal cellular proliferation is disrupted and transformation may ensue when the growth factor cascade is altered by, for example, overexpression of a particular growth factor or growth factor receptor. The hypothesis that growth factors, growth factor receptors, and their biochemically active secondary and tertiary messages are involved in malignant cell growth is rapidly gaining substance. The oncogenic potential of growth factors has been further reinforced by the demonstration that the protein products of many oncogenes bear striking structural and functional homology to several growth factors.

Growth factors appear to mediate their physiologic and pathologic effects through one of several basic mechanisms. In order of increasing oncologic importance, these mechanisms can be distinguished as being endocrine, paracrine or autocrine in nature (Fig. 5.7). The endocrine action of growth factors, that is, the release of a blood-borne growth factor which affects receptor-bearing cells remote from the site of secretion, is largely a physiologic process and only exceptionally results in neoplastic change in the CNS. The neuro-oncologically relevant example of such pertains to a minority of pituitary tumors thought to be promoted by overstimulation of hypothalamic trophic factors (Thapar et al 1993).

Paracrine stimulation is a more local phenomenon, induced by the release of a growth factor from one cell, which diffuses and acts upon an adjacent receptor-bearing

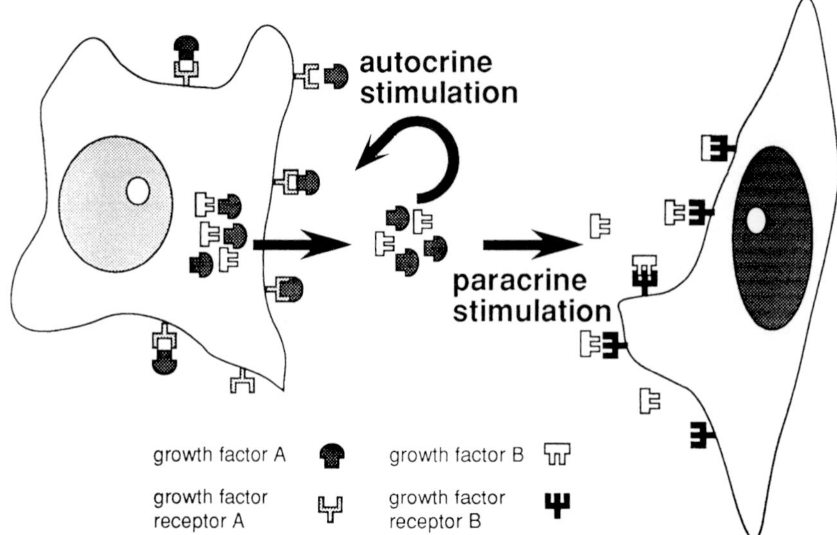

Fig. 5.7 Possible roles for the induction of CNS tumor formation by growth factors. The autocrine hypothesis of CNS tumor formation states that a tumor cell secretes a growth factor (or soluble polypeptide) for which it also has a specific growth factor receptor. The secreted growth factor then binds back to the receptor on the cell of origin creating a signal which is transduced across the cell membrane. This signal is then converted into secondary and tertiary events which ultimately lead to a mitogenic response. By way of contrast, the paracrine hypothesis states that a tumor cell secretes a growth factor which acts at a distance (by diffusion) on a similar or different cell type which bears the specific growth factor receptor. The distant cell is then stimulated to pass more quickly through the cell cycle.

cell. Such a mechanism has been implicated in the genesis of certain mixed tumors which arise from embryologically different tissues. In the case of gliosarcoma, a mixed tumor composed of both glial and mesenchymal elements, it is generally agreed that sarcomatous transformation is a secondary event, occurring in a pre-existing glioma. It has therefore been postulated that transformed glial cells liberate a growth factor, which then induces transformation of neighboring mesenchymal cells in a paracrine fashion (Rutka et al 1986, 1989).

Possibly the most important and widely implicated tumorigenic mechanism of growth factor action is autocrine stimulation (Sporn & Roberts 1985). The autocrine hypothesis of carcinogenesis refers to the situation whereby a cell secretes a particular growth factor for which it also has a membrane receptor. The secreted growth factor then binds to, and acts upon its cell of origin. In this way, growth factors can both initiate and be a product of transformation, establishing self-perpetuating, positive-feedback loops, with unregulated cell proliferation. Such a mechanism has been implicated in the genesis of certain malignant astrocytomas, which both produce and possess receptors for several mitogenic growth factors. Although a dominant theme in tumorigenesis, autocrine secretion also appears to occur in physiologic processes requiring rapid cell growth, such as wound healing, regeneration, and embryogenesis.

The major types of tumor-derived endogenous growth factors so far characterized include: transforming growth factor (TGF)s alpha and beta; monolayer mitogens (PDGF and EGF); insulin-like growth factors (IGF-I and IGF-II); bombesin; and the angiogenic, heparin-binding growth factors such as fibroblast growth factor (FGF), and endothelial cell growth factor (ECGF). The brain appears to be an abundant reservoir of these growth factors which are thought to play important roles in neuroembryogenesis and differentiation. However, the following discussion reviews only those factors and growth factor receptors specifically implicated in CNS tumorigenesis.

Platelet-derived growth factor and receptor

PDGF is a dimeric protein composed of two chains, designated as A and B chains. Each chain derives from a different chromosome (7 and 22 respectively), and each endows the PDGF molecule with different functional properties (Guha 1991). Existing in either a homodimeric form (AA or BB), or in a heterodimeric form (AB), PDGF has been ascribed numerous tentative roles, though its precise function in the CNS or elsewhere is not definitively known. Some proposed CNS-related functions of PDGF include a role in astrocytic proliferation during fetal CNS development (Yeh et al 1991) and in glial scar formation following brain injury (Takamiya et al 1986). The most pertinent aspect of PDGF biology, however, concerns its potential contribution to glial tumorigenesis (see also Oncogenes). Although PDGF alone has established mitogenic potential, the presence of its receptor is necessary for transformation. Many gliomas overexpress PDGF genes, PDGF-like growth factor genes and, less often, PDGF receptors (Nister & Westermark 1986, Nister et al 1988, Maxwell et al 1990a). Using in-situ hybridization, PDGF-B and the PDGF receptor have been localized to areas of hyperplastic endothelium. Such cellular co-localization of both PDGF and its receptor mRNAs to areas of vascular proliferation within malignant glioma tissue argues strongly for a PDGF-mediated autocrine activation of endothelial cells in these tumors (Hermansson et al 1988, Maxwell et al 1990b).

Epidermal growth factor and receptor

EGF is a small single-chained peptide which has, as yet, no definable function in either the adult or developing human CNS. Although EGF has long been known to be a glial mitogen (Leutz & Schachner 1981), neuro-oncologic interest in EGF is minor in comparison to that of its receptor. As discussed above (see Oncogenes), the EGFR has gained importance because it is a cellular homologue of a viral oncoprotein (v-*erb*B) (Downard et al 1984), and because of its frequent presence in amplified and overexpressed form in up to 40% of malignant gliomas. Activation of the EGFR, by virtue of its intrinsic tyrosine kinase activity, is thought to initiate a series of downstream events culminating in cell proliferation. The identification of a mutant EGFR which is constitutively activated is one mechanism by which EGFR aberrations contribute to glial tumorigenesis. Alternatively, in cases where the EGFR is overexpressed, but not constitutively activated, ligand binding is necessary to initiate the process (Westphal & Herrman 1989). Although EGF would appear to be the logical ligand for EGFR binding, EGF is so infrequently expressed in glial tissue (normal and neoplastic), that EGFR activation has been relegated to another growth factor, TGF-α (see below). In fact, no causal relationship between the inappropriate secretion of EGF and a human malignancy has been established (Westphal & Herrman 1989).

Transforming growth factors

The isolation of the transforming growth factors from conditioned medium of retroviral-transformed rodent cells established the principle that tumor cells often release potent growth factors into their environment. TGF-α and TGF-β, though common in name and origin, are entirely different structurally and functionally. TGF-α is a potent mitogen which shares some structural affinity with EGF, binds to the EGFR with equal affinity, and stimulates tyrosine kinase specific activity leading to cellular transformation. TGF-α is frequently expressed in malignant gliomas, suggesting that it is the primary ligand which binds to the EGFR in gliomas. That both TGF-α and EGFR are frequently highly expressed in gliomas illustrates the possibility that autocrine growth stimulation may be important in the pathogenesis of these tumors (Nister et al 1988, Ekstrand et al 1991).

In contrast to the potent mitogenic activity uniformly ascribed to TGF-α, TGF-β interactions appear more complex, being mitogenic in some circumstances, and inhibitory in others (Ryken et al 1992). Its role in the genesis of most intracranial tumors awaits further studies. However, preliminary evidence in the pituitary suggests that TGF-β is intimately involved in the hormonal and growth regulation of gonadotropic cells. Since these cells give rise to a significant proportion of 'non-functioning' pituitary tumors, functional inactivation of TGF-beta or its binding sites has been proposed as an etiologic mechanism for formation of this pituitary tumor type (Thapar et al 1993).

Insulin-like growth factors I and II

IGF-I and IGF-II are known glial mitogens thought to be important in normal neural maturation and development. IGF-I (somatomedin C), because of its role in growth hormone regulation, is best known as a marker of active acromegaly. The observation of elevated IGF-I levels in patients with growth hormone-producing pituitary tumors, and their normalization after successful treatment of the tumor, has rendered this growth factor a useful diagnostic marker of residual or recurrent disease. With regard to tumorigenesis, IGF-I autocrine stimulation has been implicated in the development of a variety of tumor types, including gliomas and meningiomas. Antoniades et al (1992) studied the gene and protein expression of IGF-I, IGF-II, and their corresponding receptor mRNAs in meningiomas, gliomas, and control brain and meningeal tissue. Both tumor types clearly demonstrated an increase in both the gene and protein expression of IGF-I and IGF-II and their receptor mRNAs compared to control tissue. The possibility of an autocrine loop was evident. It appears that the IGFs are probably more important to the growth of an established tumor than to its initiation.

Angiogenic growth factors

The local induction of angiogenesis remains an essential feature of tumor development, progression and metastasis. The process is well illustrated in malignant astrocytomas in which increasing biological malignancy is accompanied by an increasingly exuberant neovascularity. Beginning with proliferation and migration of host capillary endothelial cells, the process of angiogenesis is thought to be a paracrine phenomenon mediated by the release of several tumor-derived angiogenic growth factors. The most important of these include acidic fibroblast (aFGF), basic FGF, and the transforming growth factors previously discussed. Maxwell et al (1991) demonstrated enhanced aFGF gene and protein expression in the majority of malignant gliomas tested, but only minimal expression in the normal brain. In the same study, similar but less exaggerated overexpression was identified for TGF-α and the EGFR gene. bFGF has been found in astrocytomas, ependymomas, and meningiomas by immunohistochemistry (Paulus et al 1990, Takahashi et al 1990, Zagzag et al 1990). In astrocytic tumors, the degree of bFGF expression correlates well with the degree of anaplasia, being highest in GBM. In addition to being identified in tumor cells, bFGF was also identified within endothelial cells of tumor capillaries. Interestingly, this endothelial cell immunoreactivity was restricted primarily to intra- and peritumor vessels, and was not identified in capillaries remote to the tumor. The above findings strongly implicate the FGFs as important mediators of the neovascularization occurring in astrocytic tumors.

Molecular biology of the cell cycle

Whatever the mechanisms proposed for tumor induction, be they activation of proto-oncogenes, loss of tumor suppressor genes, stimulation of growth factor-mediated autocrine loops, or aberrant immune surveillance, the final common pathway for all is the cell cycle, the disruption of which constitutes the most essential, unifying and irrevocable feature of tumorigenesis. That the cell cycle is the eventual substrate upon which all oncogenic influences must ultimately converge has long been appreciated. Only recently, however, has interest in cell cycle research been rekindled, generating enthusiasm in an entirely new field in cancer research. Much of this rejuvenated interest derives from the discovery of novel families of key regulatory proteins (cyclins and cdc (cell division cycle) proteins and others) which not only 'drive' the cell cycle but, in the process, initiate an interactive cascade of events which can be modulated by tumor suppressor gene products (Rb and p53), and possibly oncoproteins and growth factors (Moses et al 1970, Sager 1992). Thus, not unexpectedly, the cell cycle is proving to be a unifying and interactive substrate for those entities currently considered important to tumorigenesis. Some of these cell cycle-specific regulatory proteins have already been used to practical advantage as markers of tumor proliferation (Ki-67 and PCNA). Insofar as many aspects of cell cycle regulation are still within the initial phases of discovery, only a preliminary scheme of the process can be presented. Nevertheless, it will provide some basic familiarity with the emerging concepts likely to dominate neuro-oncology for the foreseeable future.

The cell cycle is the interval between two consecutive mitoses. It can be considered a series of discrete phases which occur sequentially: G1 phase (the gap between previous nuclear division and the beginning of DNA synthesis); S phase (period of DNA synthesis); G2 phase (the gap between DNA duplication and nuclear division); and the M phase (the period of mitosis, during which cytokinesis generates two daughter cells). Some cells such as mature neurons are nonreplicating, and are therefore designated as quiescent (G_0 phase). The biochemical nature of the cell cycle as currently understood, though deduced primarily from experiments in unicellular organisms, appears essentially similar in humans. Despite a billion years of evolution, the principal regulatory proteins governing cell cycle progression in these prokaryotes and lower eukaryotes are functionally and structurally homologous to those so far identified in man.

In the simplest terms, progression through the cell cycle can be viewed as a series of dedicated decisions committing the cell to move from one regulatory state to the next. There appear to be two principal regulatory cascades, both representing critical decision points within the cycle (Kirschner 1992, Pines 1992). The first occurs in late G1, when the cell becomes committed to initiate DNA replication, and has been designated as START. The second checkpoint occurs at the G2–M interface, when the cell becomes committed to enter mitosis. Progression through the cycle is governed by the assembly and subsequent activation of a maturation promoting factor (MPF). The MPF complex is composed of two parts: the protein-serine kinase *cdc*2 and cyclin. Although these terms referred initially to yeast proteins, several human homologues of *cdc*2 and at least 5 versions of human cyclin (cyclins A, B, C, D, and E) have been identified to date (Hunter & Pines 1991). Cyclin confers the regulatory control over this complex, as *cdc*2 concentrations remain constant throughout the cell cycle, whereas cyclin accumulates during G1–M phase, and is rapidly degraded following cell division. The MPF complex becomes activated by dephosphorylation. The activity of MPF is further subject to a cascade of different regulatory influences at each of the transition points (G1–S and G2–M). Activated MPF is critical to the progression of the cell cycle, mediating such processes as chromatin condensation, nuclear envelope breakdown and assembly of the mitotic spindles. Once cytokinesis has been completed, cyclin is degraded and the MPF complex is phosphorylated and disassembled. The entire process is meticulously governed by several levels of regulation, a network of feedback mechanisms, and a host of regulatory proteins, the details of which are only superficially understood.

The intuitive notion that perturbations in cell cycle regulation could contribute to transformation is rapidly being appreciated. This is especially true of the cyclins, which, to date, appear to be the most culpable of the various cell cycle constituents to harbor oncologic potential. The human cyclin A gene is the genomic integration site of the hepatitis B virus, implicating cyclin A in the transformation of hepatocellular carcinoma. A group D cyclin (PRAD1) is grossly overexpressed in parathyroid tumors, is inducible by growth factor stimulation, and is also one of the amplified sequences commonly identified in breast cancer (Hunter & Pines 1991). Despite these and other associations, the transforming potential of these cyclins remains to be established.

The elucidation of the biochemical pathways underlying cell cycle progression has led to the identification of two important antigens, which have gained increasingly wide usage as immunohistochemical proliferation markers: Ki-67 and PCNA (proliferating cell nuclear antigen). Ki-67 is a nuclear associated antigen of uncertain proliferative function, detectable only in cycling cells (G1 to M phase) (Gerdes et al 1984). The value of Ki-67 as a proliferative marker has been evaluated in a variety of CNS and pituitary tumor types (Burger et al 1989, Deckert et al 1989, Knosp et al 1989). Tumor growth fraction, as determined by Ki-67 labeling index, appears to compare favorably with earlier methods of proliferative assessment (BUdR and flow cytometry) (Nishizaki et al 1989, Riley 1992). Consistent trends in the Ki-67 labelling index have been identified, correlating well with both the grade and prognosis in glial tumors (i.e. the percentage of labeled cells being lowest in low grade astrocytomas, higher in intermediate grade lesions, and highest in GBM) (Deckert et al 1989). The applicability of Ki-67 is especially relevant to tumors of the pituitary which frequently lack any histologic or ultrastructural markers of biological behavior. Preliminary studies in the pituitary have demonstrated that Ki-67 labeling is doubled in invasive tumors compared to non-invasive lesions (Knosp et al 1989).

PCNA is a member of the cyclin family, being a critical accessory nuclear protein which complexes with DNA polymerase delta and is essential to DNA replication (Bravo et al 1987). Accordingly, its presence is generally restricted to the late G1 and S phase. Because antibodies to PCNA have only recently become commercially available, data concerning the utility of PCNA as a proliferative marker for CNS tumors are limited (Garcia et al 1989). At the Hospital for Sick Children, PCNA and Ki-67 labeling indices in choroid plexus papillomas and choroid plexus carcinomas were recently determined, and were shown to be more reliable and accurate markers of tumor biology than was the mitotic index (Fig. 5.8).

Glioma cell invasion

For reasons which are poorly understood, most primary brain tumors do not metastasize systemically (Cerame et al 1985). Rather, spread of tumor occurs locally through extensions of infiltrating tumor cells into normal brain, or, more rarely, through CSF dissemination along the neuraxis (Rutka et al 1987, 1988). The highly invasive potential of malignant glioma cells enables them to penetrate normal brain barriers, rendering complete surgical extirpation difficult, focal radiation ineffective, and relapse or recurrence at the primary site commonplace. Attempts to understand the mechanisms underlying glioma cell invasion have justifiably become of foremost importance in recent times so that novel treatment strategies may be determined to control tumor growth. Clues to the process of glioma cell invasion have been ascertained through an increased understanding of the key roles played by the extracellular matrix (ECM), proteases, and cell adhesion molecules (CAMs).

The ECM is the naturally occurring substrate upon which cells migrate, proliferate, and differentiate in vivo (Gospodarowicz et al 1978, Reid & Jefferson 1984). The ECM functions as a biological adhesive that maintains the normal cytoarchitecture of different tissues and defines the key spatial relationships among dissimilar cell types. A loss of coordination and an alteration in the interactions between mesenchymal cells and epithelial cells separated by an ECM are thought to be fundamental steps in the development and progression of cancer. Though less well characterized than the ECM of other tissue types, the ECM of the CNS is comprised of various collagenous and non-collagenous glycoproteins, glycosaminoglycans and proteoglycans (Hay 1981). The ECM has been shown to either inhibit or facilitate glioma growth and invasion, depending on the types of ECM and tumor cells used. A molecular model of the ECM in the CNS has been proposed, and interested readers may refer to a number of key review articles in this field (Carbonetto 1984, Rutka et al 1988).

The invading glioma cell has been compared to the highly migratory undifferentiated pseudostratified and columnar epithelial cells which move away from the ventricular zone of the primitive neural tube during neuroembryogenesis. The migration of these embryonic cells requires fundamental communication between these neuroblasts and their extracellular environment. It has been proposed that macromolecules of the ECM of the CNS are actively involved in directing the migration of neuroblasts away from the primitive germinal matrix (Lander et al 1982). In addition, these migrating cells have been considered rich in secretion of proteases which are capable of digesting ECM macromolecules to arrive at their final destination.

Proteases are important in the remodeling of the ECM during development, growth, and tissue repair (Murphy & Reynolds 1985, Peterson 1985). Uncontrolled degradation of the ECM has been implicated in the pathogenesis of many diseases and in tumor invasion and metastasis (Thorgeirsson et al 1985, Goldfarb & Liotta 1986). For example, the dissolution of basement membrane barriers facilitates the migration, penetration, and hematogenous dissemination of tumor cells. Since gliomas are locally invasive neoplasms requiring proteases to degrade ECM barriers in the CNS, we have tested a variety of glioma cell

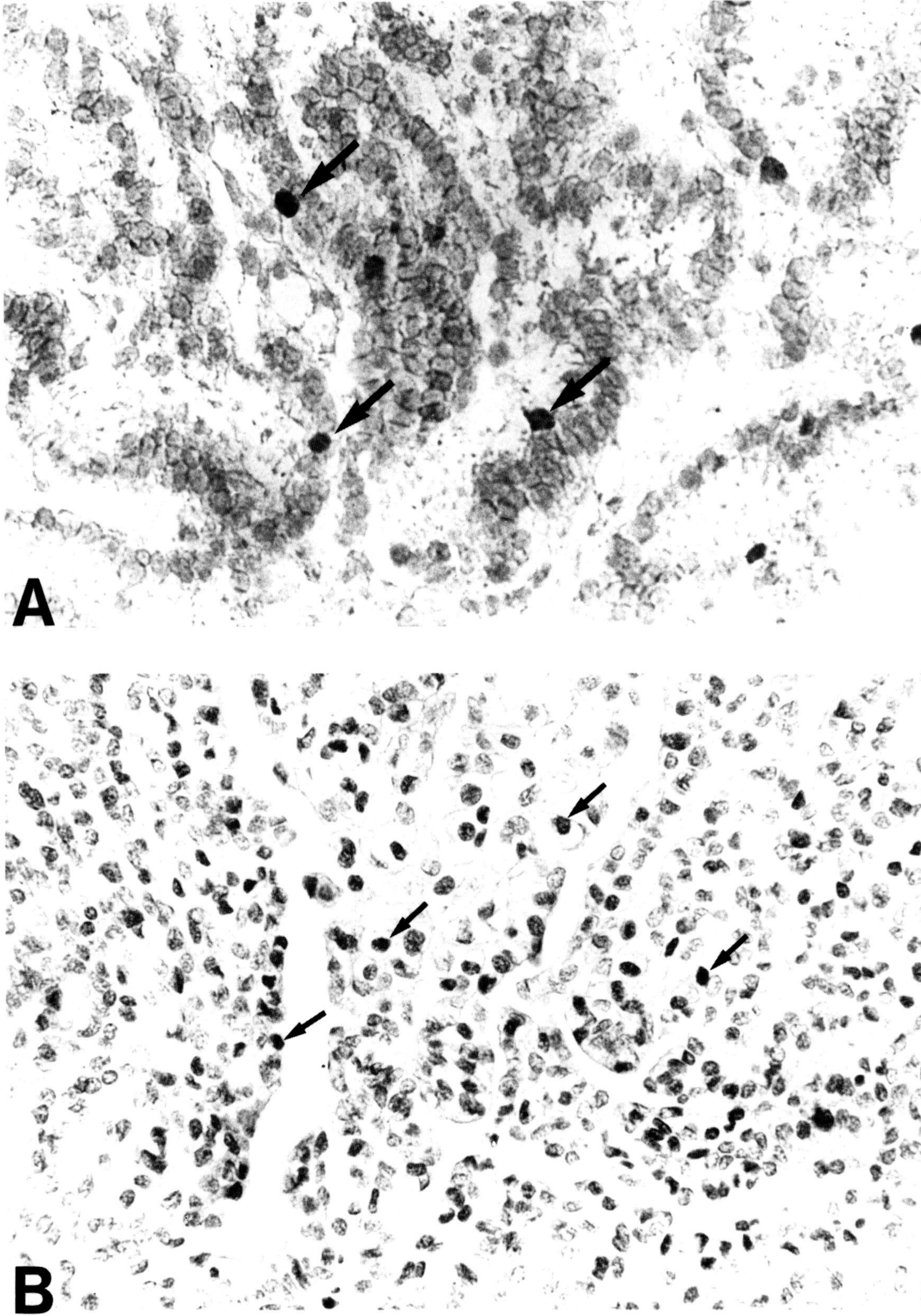

Fig. 5.8 Tumor cell growth fraction estimation with PCNA monoclonal antibody in choroid plexus tumors. **A**. Choroid plexus papilloma immunostained with PCNA monoclonal antibody showing rare immunoreactive tumor cell nuclei (arrows). The growth fraction of a series of 18 choroid plexus papillomas was 0.5%. **B**. Choroid plexus carcinoma immunostained with PCNA monoclonal antibody showing numerous immunoreactive tumor cell nuclei (arrows). The growth fraction of a series of 9 choroid plexus carcinomas was 9%. The development of PCNA and Ki-67 monoclonal antibodies has facilitated estimation of proliferative indices and growth rate of several CNS tumors. Immunohistochemistry, both × 350. Photographs courtesy of Dr Warren Mason.

lines for their ability to secrete metalloproteases (Apodaca et al 1990). All gliomas tested were found to secrete a number of metalloproteases of varying molecular weights which were further characterized as collagenases and gelatinases (Apodaca et al 1990). The levels of proteases secreted by human glioma cell lines have correlated with invasive potential as measured in an in vitro invasion model system (Rosenblum M, personal communication).

Interestingly, many glioma cell lines simultaneously secrete inhibitors of metalloproteases (Rutka 1991). The best characterized of these inhibitors include the tissue inhibitors of metalloproteases (TIMPs) — TIMP-1 and TIMP-2 (Stetler-Stevenson et al 1989). We have recently characterized a number of brain tumor specimens for their expression of TIMP-1 and TIMP-2 mRNAs (Fig. 5.9). The expression of TIMPs may help regulate glioma cell invasion. The down regulation of TIMP mRNA levels by expression of antisense TIMP mRNA in Swiss 3T3 fibroblasts, a normally noninvasive cell line, results in cells that are invasive in an amnion invasion assay and that are both tumorigenic and metastatic when injected into athymic mice (Khokha et al 1989).

Many CNS cell types are characterized by their expression of homophilic receptors known as CAMs that regulate cell:cell interactions (Edelman & Crossin 1991). In general, CAMs fall into three groups: molecules related to the immunoglobulin (Ig) superfamily that have calcium-independent binding (examples include N-CAM, I-CAM, contactin, CEA, and DCC); molecules of a calcium-dependent binding family (known as cadherins); and molecules with no known structural relationship to either of the previous two. All known CAMs are large intrinsic cell-surface glycoproteins that are mobile in the plane of the membrane (Gall & Edelman 1981, Pollerberg et al 1986). A given cell has multiple different CAMs on its surface which must rearrange in the plane of the membrane to form appropriate specific homophilic attachments. The known CAMs are specified by single genes, many of which have been cloned, sequenced and ascribed to a chromosomal localization.

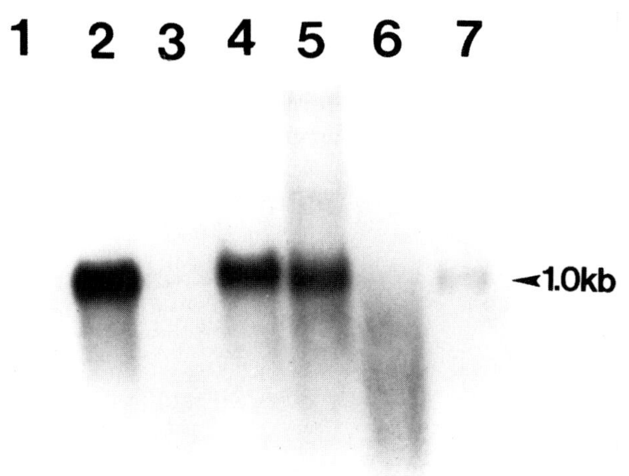

Fig. 5.9 Northern hybridization analysis of TIMP-1 mRNA expression in a series of human brain tumors. There was no discernible TIMP-1 level in two PNETs (lanes 1 and 3), and in one gliosarcoma (lane 6). A strong 1.0 kb TIMP-1 message was found in an anaplastic astrocytoma (lane 2), a meningioma (lane 4), and a low grade astrocytoma (lane 5). A faint TIMP-1 message was detected in another low grade astrocytoma from the cerebellum. These preliminary data suggest that lower grade CNS tumors may produce proportionately more TIMPs than higher grade tumors as one mechanism to prevent their invasiveness.

Various in vitro and in vivo experiments have shown that interference with CAM binding or synthesis results in perturbation of morphology. Work with neural retinal cells transformed with temperature-sensitive mutants of the Rous sarcoma virus has led to the hypothesis that CAM expression may be inversely correlated with the transformation state of certain cells and possibly with their metastatic potential (Brackenbury et al 1984). Although loss of CAM expression in cell lines can be correlated with decreased aggregation, increased motility, and increased invasiveness, this correlation does not apply to all CAMs since many studies have shown that different CAMs are expressed differently in a variety of tumors. N-CAM expression has been observed in neuroblastoma. Several molecules identified in connection with tumor formation have been found to be homologous to N-CAM. These include the CEA, MUC-18, and a gene deleted in colon carcinoma (DCC). It has been postulated that the function of the DCC gene product is as a tumor suppressor, the loss of which forms the final step in a multi-step cascade of carcinogenesis and metastasis (Fearon & Vogelstein 1990, Fearon et al 1990).

We are just beginning to understand how the balance between the secretion of proteases and their corresponding inhibitors in glioma cells is swayed in favor of proteolysis, and how alterations in cell:matrix and cell:cell interactions result in increased glioma invasion. It is hoped that the clues provided by the molecular models described in this section will be used in the future to devise new methods to modulate astrocytoma growth and invasion.

Multi-step theory of tumorigenesis for human gliomas

The proclivity for human neoplasms to evolve to higher states of biological aggressiveness represents an eventuality common to many forms of human cancer. This concept of malignant progression appears especially applicable to human gliomas, where longitudinal studies of low grade gliomas have repeatedly demonstrated that more than 50% of such lesions, however treated, will ultimately progress to lesions of higher grade (Guthrie & Laws 1990). Furthermore the phenomenon of tumor heterogeneity, whereby histological specimens of glioma tissue frequently show regional morphologic variations in histologic grade, provides additional evidence of the dynamic nature of oncogenic processes operative in individual tumors. Both these clinical and pathological aspects of glioma biology have been accommodated by a tentative model of malignant progression deduced from the pattern of cytogenetic aberrations discussed above (see Chromosomal Aberrations section) (James et al 1990, Mikkelsen et al 1991, Rasheed & Bigner 1991).

From the foregoing discussion, there appear to be a minimum of six molecular genetic events which frequently occur and accumulate during the malignant evolution of gliomas. As illustrated in Figure 5.10, the earliest of these involves loss of 17p (possibly the p53 gene), loss of 13q (possibly the Rb gene), and partial or complete loss of chromosome 22, all of which have been identified in low grade gliomas. The transition of low grade glioma to anaplastic astrocytoma is thought to be facilitated by loss of 9p (possibly the interferon alpha and beta genes). Subsequent evolution to GBM is thought to be the result of deletions of 10q ('glioma suppressor gene') and amplification of the EGFR gene, aberrations almost exclusive to this advanced grade of glioma. Although this model accounts for the cytogenetic alterations tested in various grades of morphologic malignancy, the number of accumulated genetic events is probably more important to malignant progression than is their temporal occurrence. In that this model is derived within the limitations of existing knowledge, it is necessarily simplistic, and while it may not represent a unifying mechanism for the genesis and progression of all gliomas, it does provide a rudimentary

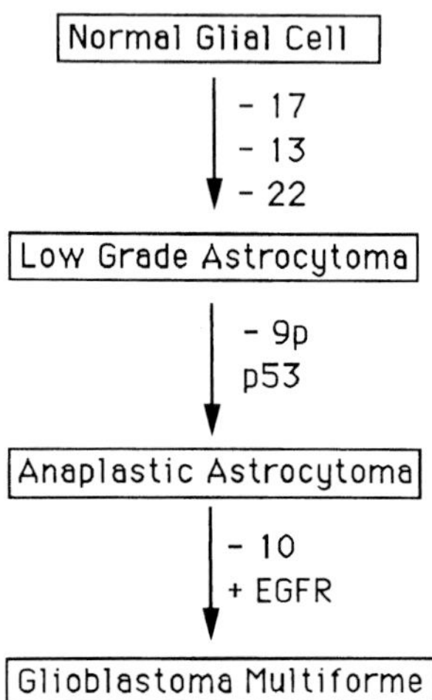

Fig. 5.10 Proposed multi-step theory of the pathogenesis of the human glioma. Though not proven, early steps initiating a heritable change in cellular DNA transforming a normal glial cell to a low grade precursor would include the loss of 17p (possibly the p53 gene), loss of 13q (possibly the Rb gene), and partial or complete loss of chromosome 22. All of these cytogenetic aberrancies are common to low grade gliomas. The transition of low grade glioma to anaplastic astrocytoma is thought to be facilitated by loss of 9p. Subsequent evolution to GBM is thought to be the result of deletions of 10q ('glioma suppressor gene') and amplification of the EGFR gene. These latter two aberrations are almost exclusive to this advanced grade of glioma. After Mikkelsen et al 1991.

framework of the events currently considered important in the evolution of glial tumors.

CONCLUSION

Impact of molecular biology on future therapies

Gene therapy

Until recently, the prospect that human brain tumor cells could be manipulated in such a manner to permit high level expression of heterologous or 'foreign' genes was considered impossible. The ability to transfer and express genetic material in human brain tumors, however, has become possible through great strides in molecular biology. We are on the verge now of applying gene therapy strategies to patients harboring malignant brain tumors.

Gene therapy may be defined as the introduction of a known gene encoding for a beneficial host protein for which the host is deficient, or a gene which controls the expression of an abnormally expressed protein. In standard procedures, cells are extracted from a patient who lacks normal copies of a particular gene. The gene is then introduced into the cells via a vector (often a virus), and the cells carrying the normal gene are then re-injected into the patient. The first human gene therapy trial was begun in 1990, and involved the transfer of the adenosine deaminase (ADA) gene into lymphocytes of a patient having an otherwise lethal defect in this enzyme which produces immune deficiency.

The fundamental components of a mammalian gene are described in detail in Figure 5.11. The process of heterologous DNA transfer is known as 'transfection'. There are two general methods for introducing genetic information into mammalian cells: (1) by direct DNA transfer, and (2) by virus infection. By direct DNA transfer, the gene of interest may be introduced into human brain tumor cells by microcellular injection, calcium phosphate and liposome transfection, or electroporation (Levinson 1990). An example of a genetic 'construct' which permits efficient gene transfer and expression in vitro is shown in Figure 5.12. While these techniques of direct DNA transfer have worked effectively to answer specific questions about gene function in vitro, unfortunately they are not directly applicable to intact organisms, or to in vivo model systems.

For this reason, a number of groups are now studying the effect of gene transfection by virus infection in human brain tumors (Martuza et al 1991, Culver et al 1992). Properties of viruses which make them advantageous over other gene transfer strategies are that they are efficient at carrying genes into cells, they may be cell or tissue specific, they may be cytolytic with a latency period, they may reproduce efficiently in the cell, and the viral genome can be defined and genetically engineered. Martuza et al (1991) have used a thymidine kinase-negative mutant

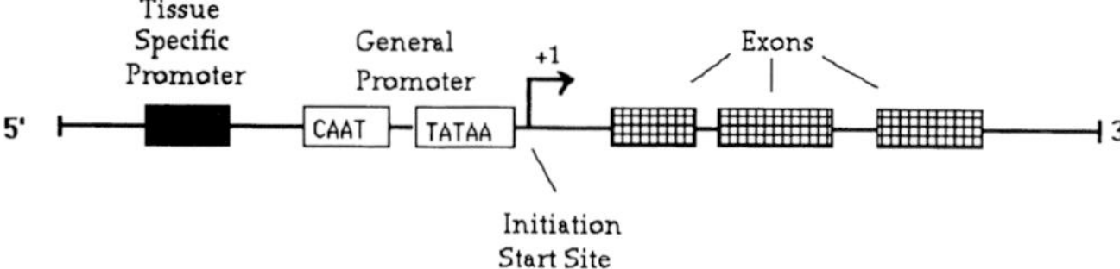

Fig. 5.11 Representative model of a mammalian gene. All genes studied have nucleotide arrangements giving 5′ to 3′ directionality. Most mammalian genes are composed of coding and regulatory sequences (separated above by the initiation start site). The coding sequences are comprised of exons and introns. Exons represent those coding sequences that will be transcribed and will appear as sequence information in mature RNA species (messenger RNA, ribosomal RNA, and transfer RNA). Introns are found between the exons and act as interrupting sequences that are removed when the DNA is transcribed to RNA. The regulatory region of a gene contains general and tissue specific promoter sequences that regulate gene transcription by RNA polymerase II. Tissue specific promoters often provide unique sequence information to direct gene transcription in specific tissues. For example, the glial fibrillary acidic protein (GFAP) promoter directs expression of the GFAP gene in human glial cells; this promoter is presumably inactivated by mechanisms which are not clear in other tissues so that GFAP is not expressed in, say, the lungs or liver. The general promoter sequences are frequently characterized by nucleotide sequences known as the TATA box and the CAAT box. The TATA box is usually located about 25 bp 'upstream' (i.e. to the left or 5′ end) of the initiation start site, and is responsible for the selection of the exact initiation site of a gene. An understanding of the basic mechanisms of gene regulation is important to remember when considering how the neoplastic process can affect the transcription of certain genes.

of herpes simplex virus 1 (HSV) that was attenuated for neurovirulence to transfect U-87 MG human glioma cells. They showed that this genetically engineered virus mutant caused growth inhibition of astrocytoma cells in vitro and prolonged survival of nude mice bearing tumors.

In another related study, Culver et al (1992) used a retroviral-based vector carrying the herpes simplex thymidine kinase gene to transfect murine fibroblasts. The murine fibroblasts were then stereotactically implanted into cerebral gliomas growing in rats. The fibroblasts continued to make copies of the retroviral vector which infected nearby tumor cells. The infected tumor cells produced thymidine kinase, and became targets for antiviral therapy with the drug ganciclovir (Culver et al 1992). Interestingly, in this study, in addition to killing the tumor cells known to have the herpes gene in them, ganciclovir killed other tumor cells in their vicinity, providing a profound 'bystander effect' on tumor growth. Rats bearing gliomas treated with ganciclovir demonstrated complete macroscopic and microscopic regression of tumor, and had lengthened survivals over controls.

Based on the success of these gene transfection trials in animals, approval has been given for the Phase I study of the MRI-guided stereotactic implantation of retroviral constructs into human brain tumors (Stone 1992). While this technique looks extremely promising, some caveats to be aware of include the infection of noncancerous cells through helper virus contamination, immunologic intolerance of the xenografted murine viral packaging cells, and

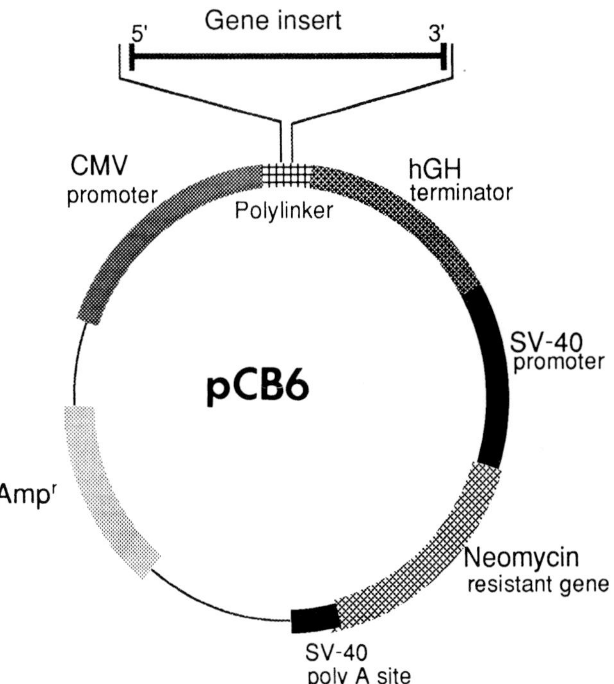

Fig. 5.12 Example of genetically engineered mammalian expression vector (called pCB6) used to transfer foreign or new DNA into target cells. The gene of interest (labeled as 'Gene insert') containing the necessary coding sequence can be inserted into the polylinker site of the vector. This new construct (construct = vector plus insert) can then be transferred into targeted mammalian cells by techniques mentioned in the text. The construct may then integrate into the mammalian genome. The cytomegalovirus (CMV) promoter will use host enzymes to transcribe the inserted gene sequence which will be terminated by the growth hormone (GH) terminator sequence. Selection for only those cells expressing the inserted gene may be accomplished by exposing the cells to neomycin. The construct contains a neomycin resistance gene under control of the SV-40 virus promoter sequence, and terminated by the SV-40 polyA site. The construct also contains a gene for ampicillin resistance which can be used to isolate large quantities of the construct in *E. coli* bacteria.

the possibility that a germline mutagenic event is created when a foreign gene is randomly inserted into the human genome.

The treatment of human brain tumors by gene transfer has now moved from the theoretical to the practical realm. An era of 'molecular surgery' has clearly dawned for the patient with a malignant brain tumor. A decade hence we fully anticipate that the treatment of the patient with a brain tumor will be more successful, largely because of our increased understanding of the molecular genetics underlying the process of carcinogenesis, and our ability to reverse some of the characteristic genetic lesions in a brain tumor.

Acknowledgement

This chapter was possible through grants from the National Cancer Institute of Canada, and Lunenfeld Foundation (JTR). Dr Rutka is recipient of a career scientist award from the Ontario Ministry of Health.

REFERENCES

Antoniades H N, Galanopoulous T, Neville-Golden J, Maxwell M 1992 Expression of insulin-like growth factors I and II and their receptor mRNAs in primary human astrocytomas and meningiomas; In vivo studies using in situ hybridization and immunohistochemistry. International Journal of Cancer 50: 215–222

Apodaca G, Rutka J T, Bouhana K et al 1990 Expression of metalloproteinases and metalloproteinase inhibitors by fetal astrocytes and glioma cells. Cancer Research 50: 2322–2329

Arnoldus E P, Wolters L B, Voormolen J H et al 1992 Interphase cytogenetics: a new tool for the study of genetic changes in brain tumors. Journal of Neurosurgery 76: 997–1003

Beigel J A, Rorke L B, Packer R J et al 1989 Isochromosome 17q in primitive neuroectodermal tumors of the central nervous system. Genes Chrom Cancer 1: 139–147

Biegel J A, Burk C D, Barr F G, Emanuel B S 1992 Evidence for a 17p tumor related loci distinct from p53 in pediatric primitive neuroectodermal tumors. Cancer Research 52: 3391–3395

Bigner S H, Mark J, Bullard D E et al 1986 Chromosomal evolution in malignant human gliomas starts with specific and usually numeric deviations. Cancer Genetics and Cytogenetics 22: 121

Bigner S H, Burger P C, Wong A J et al 1988a Gene amplification in malignant human gliomas: clinical and histopathologic aspects. Journal of Neuropathology and Experimental Neurology 47: 191–205

Bigner S H, Mark J, Burger P et al 1988b Specific chromosome abnormalities in malignant human gliomas. Cancer Research 48: 405–411

Bigner S, Mark J, Bigner D 1990a Cytogenetics of human brain tumors. Cancer Genetics and Cytogenetics 47: 141–154

Bigner S H, Freidman B, Vogelstein W J et al 1990b Amplification of the c-*myc* gene in human medulloblastoma cell lines and xenografts. Cancer Research 50: 2347–2350

Bishop J M 1983 Cellular oncogens and retroviruses. Ann Rev Biochem 52: 301–354

Bishop J M 1991 Molecular themes in oncogenesis. Cell 64: 235–248

Brackenbury R, Greenberg M E, Edelman G M 1984 Phenotypic changes and loss of N-CAM-mediated adhesion in transformed embryonic chicken retinal cells. Journal of Cell Biology 99: 1944–1954

Bravo R, Frank R, Blundell, MacDonald-Bravo H 1987 Cyclin/PCNA is the auxiliary protein of DNA polymerase-δ. Nature 326: 515–517

Brodeur G M 1990 Neuroblastoma: clinical applications of molecular parameters. Brain Pathology 1: 47–54

Burger P C, Shibata T, Kleiheus P 1989 The use of the monoclonal antibody Ki-67 in the identification of proliferating cells: application to surgical neuropathology. American Journal of Surgery and Pathology 10: 611–617

Carbonetto S 1984 The extracellular matrix of the nervous system. Trends in Neuroscience 7: 382–387

Carter B S, Ewing C M, Ward W S et al 1990 Allelic loss of chromosomes 16q and 10q in human prostate cancer. Proceedings of the National Academy of Sciences of the USA 87: 8751–8755

Cawthorn R M, Andersen L B, Buchberg A et al 1991 cDNA sequence and genomic structure of EV12B, a gene lying within an intron of the neurofibromatosis type 1 gene. Genomics 9: 446–460

Cerame M A, Guthikonda M, Kohli C M 1985 Extraneural metastases in gliosarcoma: A case report and review of the literature. Neurosurgery 17: 413–418

Charles S J, Moore A T, Yates J R W et al 1989 Lisch nodules in neurofibromatosis type 2. Archives of Ophthalmology 107: 1571

Chin K V, Ueda K, Pastan I et al 1992 Modulation of activity of the promoter of the human MDR1 gene by Ras and p53. Science 255: 459–462

Chung R Y, Whaley J M, Anderson K M et al 1990 p53 gene mutations in human glioblastoma associated with early age of onset and better survival. Proc AACR 31: 6a

Cogen P H 1991 Prognostic significance of molecular genetic markers in childhood brain tumors. Pediatric Neurosurgery 17: 245–250

Cogen P H, Daneshvar L, Metzger A K et al 1992 Involvement of multiple chromosome 17p loci in medulloblastoma tumorigenesis. American Journal of Human Genetics 50: 584–589

Cohen A J, Li F P, Berg S et al 1979 Hereditary renal cell carcinoma associated with a chromosomal translocation. NEJM 301: 592–595

Crowe F W, Schull W J, Neel J V 1956 A clinical, pathological, and genetic study of multiple neurofibromatosis. Charles C Thomas, Springfield, Ill, pp 1–181

Culver K W, Ram Z, Wallbridge S, Ishii H, Oldfield E H, Blaese R M 1992 In vivo gene transfer with retroviral vector-producer cells for treatment of experimental brain tumors. Science 256: 1550–1552

Deckert M, Reifenberger G, Wechsler W 1989 Determination of the proliferative potential of human brain tumors using the monoclonal antibody Ki-67. Cancer Research and Clinical Oncology 115: 179–188

Deinhardt F 1980 In: Klein G (ed) Biology of primate retroviruses: Viral oncology. Raven Press, New York, pp 357–398

Diedrich U, Eckermann O, Schmidtke J 1988 Rare Ha-*ras* and c-*mos* alleles in patients with intracranial tumors. Neurology 38: 587–589

Diedrich U, Soja S, Behnke J et al 1991 Amplification of the c-erb B oncogene is associated with malignancy in primary tumors of neuroepithelial tissue. Journal of Neurology 238: 221–224

Downard J, Yarden Y, Mayes E et al 1984 Close similarity of the epidermal growth factor receptor and the v-*erb*- B oncogene protein sequences. Nature 307: 521–527

Dumanski J P, Rouleau G A, Nordenskjold M, Collins V P 1990 Molecular genetic analysis of chromosome 22 in 81 cases of meningioma. Cancer Res 50: 5863–5867

Edelman G M, Crossin K L 1991 Cell adhesion molecules: Implications for molecular histology. Ann Rev Biochem 60: 155–190

Ekstrand A J, James C D, Cavenee B et al 1991 Genes for epidermal growth factor receptor, transforming growth factor alpha, and epidermal growth factor and their expression in human gliomas in vivo. Cancer Res. 51: 2164–2172

Fearon E R, Vogelstein B 1990 A genetic model for colorectal tumorigenesis. Cell 61: 759–767

Fearon E R, Cho K R, Nigro J M et al 1990 Identification of a chromosome 18q gene which is altered in colorectal carcinomas. Science 247: 49–56

Ferrante L, Acqui M, Mastronardi L et al 1987 Familial meningiomas, report of two cases. J Neurosurg Sci 31: 145–151

Fields S, Jang S K 1991 Presence of a potent transcription activating sequence in the p53 protein. Science 249: 1046–1049

Finlay C A, Hinds P W, Levine A J 1989 The p53 proto-oncogene can act as a suppressor of transformation. Cell 57: 1083–1093

Freeman C S, Martin M R, Marks C L 1990 An overview of tumor biology. Cancer Invest 8: 71–90

Friend S H, Bernards R, Rogelj S et al 1986 A human cDNA segment with properties of the gene that predisposes to retinoblastoma and osteosarcoma. Nature 323: 643–646

Fujimoto M, Weaker F, Herbert D et al 1988 Expression of three viral oncogenes (v-sis, v-myc, v-fos) in primary human brain tumors of neuroectodermal origin. Neurology 38: 289–293

Fujimoto M, Fults D W, Thomas G A et al 1989a Loss of heterozygosity on chromosome 10 in human glioblastoma multiforme. Genomics 4: 210–214

Fujimoto M, Sheridan Z, Sharp F et al 1989b Proto-onocogene analysis in brain tumors. J. Neurosurg 70: 910–915

Fuller G N, Bigner S H 1992 Amplified cellular oncogenes in neoplasms of the human central nervous system. Mutation Research 276: 299–306

Fults D, Pedone C A, Thomas G A et al 1990 Allelotype of human malignant astrocytoma. Cancer Research 50: 5784–5789

Gall W E, Edelman G M 1981 Lateral diffusion of surface molecules in animal cells and tissues. Science 213: 903–905

Garcia R L, Coltrera M D, Gown A M 1989 Analysis of proliferative grade using anti-PCNA/cyclin monoclonal antibodies in fixed, embedded tissues. Comparison with flow cytometric analysis. American Journal of Pathology 134; 4: 733–739

Garson J A, McIntryre P G, Kemshed J T 1985 N-*myc* amplification in malignant astrocytoma. Lancet 2: 718–719

Gerdes J, Lemke H, Baisch H et al 1984 Cell cycle analysis of a cell proliferation-associated human nuclear antigen defined by the monoclonal antibody Ki-67. Journal of Immunology 133: 1710–1715

Ginsberg D, Mechta F, Yaniv M et al 1991 Wild-type p53 can down-modulate the activity of various promoters. Proceedings of the National Academy of Sciences of the USA 88: 9979–9983

Goldfarb R H, Liotta L A 1986 Proteolytic enzymes in cancer invasion and metastasis. Sem Throm Hemost 12: 294–307

Gordon H 1985 Oncogenes. Mayo Clinic Proceedings 60: 697–713

Gospodarowicz D, Greenburg G, Birdwell C R 1978 Determination of cellular shape by the extracellular matrix and its correlation with the control of cellular growth. Cancer Research 38: 4155–4171

Griffith C A, Hawkins A L, Packer R J et al 1988 Chromosome abnormalities in pediatric brain tumors. Cancer Research 48: 175–180

Groden J, Thliveris A, Samowitz W et al 1991 Identification and characterization of the familial adenomatous polyposis coli gene. Cell 66: 589–600

Guha A 1991 Platelet-derived growth factor: A general review with emphasis on astrocytomas. Pediatric Neurosurgery 17: 14–20

Guthrie B L, Laws E R 1990 Supratentorial low-grade gliomas. Neurosurgery Clinics of North America 1: 37–48

Guttmann D H, Collins F S 1991 Recent progress toward understanding the molecular biology of von Recklinghausen neurofibromatosis. Ann Neurol 31: 555–561

Haines J L, Short M P, Kwiatkowski D J et al 1991 Localization of one gene for tuberous sclerosis within 9q32-9q34, and further evidence for heterogeneity. American Journal of Human Genetics 49: 764–772

Hauge M, Harvald B 1960 Studies in the etiology of intracranial tumors. Acta Psychiatr Neurol Scand 35: 163–170

Hay E D 1981 The extracellular matrix. Journal of Cell Biology. 91: 205–226

Hermansson M, Nister M, Betsholtz C et al 1988 Endothelial cell hyperplasia in human glioblastoma: Coexpression of mRNA for PDGF B chain and PDGF receptor suggest autocrine growth stimulation. Proceedings of the National Academy of Sciences of the USA 87: 7748–7752

Hochberg F H, Gabbai A A 1990 Risk factors in the development of glioblastoma and other brain tumors. In: Wilkins R H, Rengachary S S (eds) Neurosurgery update I. McGraw Hill, New York, p 236

Hollstein M, Sidranski D, Vogelstein B et al 1991 p53 mutations in human cancers. Science 253: 49–53

Humphrey P A, Wong A J, Vogelstein B et al 1990 Anti-synthetic peptide antibody reacting at the fusion junction of deletion-mutant epidermal growth factor receptors in human glioblastomas. Proceedings of the National Academy of Sciences of the USA 87: 4207–4211

Hung K L, Wu C M, Huang J S, How S W 1990 Familial medulloblastoma in siblings: report in one family and review of the literature. Surg Neurol 33: 341–346

Hunter T, Pines J 1991 Cylins and cancer. Cell 66: 1071–1074

Huson S M, Harper P S, Hourihan M D et al 1986 Cerebellar hemangioblastoma and von Hippel-Lindau disease. Brain 109: 1297–1301

Ikizler Y, van Meyel D J, Ramsay G L et al 1992 Gliomas in families. Canadian Journal of Neurological Science 19: 492–497

Iolascon A, Lania A, Dadiali M et al 1991 Analysis of N-*ras* gene mutations in medulloblastomas by polymerase chain reaction and oligonucleotide probes in formalin fixed, paraffin embedded tissues. Medical and Pediatric Oncology 19; 4: 240–245

James C, Mikkelsen T, Cavenee W, Collins V 1990 Molecular genetic aspects of glial tumor evolution. Cancer Surveys 9: 631–644

James C D, Carlbom E, Dumanski J P et al 1988 Clonal genomic alterations in gliomas malignancy stages. Cancer Research 48: 5546–5551

Kandt R S, Pericak-Vance M A, Hung W Y et al 1991 Linkage studies in tuberous sclerosis Chromosome 9?, 11? or maybe 14! Annals of the New York Academy of Science 615: 284–297

Karga H J, Alexander K M, Hedley-White E T et al 1992 *Ras* mutations in human pituitary tumors. J. Clin Endocrinol Metab 74: 914–919

Kern S E, Pietenpol J A, Thiagalingam S et al 1991 Oncogenic forms of p53 inhibit p53-regulated gene expression. Science 256: 827–830

Khokha R, Waterhouse P, Yagel S et al 1989 Antisense RNA-induced reduction in murine TIMP levels confers oncogenicity on Swiss 3T3 cells. Science 243: 947–950

King C R 1987 Proximal 3p deletion in renal cell carcinoma cells from a patient with von Hippel-Lindau disease. Cancer Genetics and Cytogenetics 27: 345–348

Kinzler K W, Bigner S H, Bigner D D et al 1987 Identification of an amplified, highly expressed gene in a malignant glioma. Science 236: 70–73

Kinzler K W, Ruppert J M, Bigner S H et al 1988 The GLI gene is a member of the Kruppel family of since finger proteins. Nature 332: 371–374

Kirschner M W 1992 The biochemical nature of the cell cycle. In: Devita V, Hellman S, Rosenberg S A (eds) Important advances in oncology 1992. J D Lippincott, Philadelphia, pp 3–15

Knosp E, Kitz K, Perneczky A 1989 Proliferative activity in pituitary adenomas: Measurement by monoclonal antibody Ki-67. Neurosurgery 25; 6: 927–930

Lander A D, Fujii D K, Gospodarowicz D et al 1982 Characterization of a factor that promotes neurite outgrowth: Evidence linking activity to a heparan sulfate proteoglycan. Journal of Cell Biology 94: 574–585

Landis C A, Masters S B, Spada A et al 1989 GTPase inhibiting mutation activate the alpha chain of Gs and stimulate adenyl cyclase in human pituitary tumors. Nature 340: 692–696

Landis C A, Harsh G, Lyons J et al 1990 Clinical characteristics of acromegalic patients whose pituitary tumors contain mutant Gs protein. J Clin Endocrinol Metab 71: 1416–1420

Leutz A, Schachner M 1981 Epidermal growth factor stimulates DNA synthesis of astrocytes in primary cerebellar cultures. Cell Tissue Research 220: 393–404

Levine A J, Momand J, Finlay C A 1991 The p53 tumor suppressor gene. Nature 351: 453–456

Levinson A D 1990 Expression of heterologous genes in mammalian cells. In: Goeddel D (ed) Methods in enzymology, vol 185. Academic Press, Toronto, pp 485–595

Li F P 1990 Familial cancer syndromes and clusters. Current Problems in Cancer 14: 77

Libermann, T A, Nusbaum H R, Razon N et al 1985 Amplification, enhanced expression and possibly rearrangement of the EGF receptor gene in primary human brain tumors of glial origin. Nature (London) 313: 144–147

Lin D, Shields M T, Ullrich S J et al 1992 Growth arrest induced by wild-type p53 protein blocks cells prior to or near the restriction point in late G1 phase. Proceedings of the National Academy of Sciences of the USA 89: 9210–9214

Lossignol D, Grossman S A, Sheidler C R et al 1990 Familial clustering of malignant astrocytomas. Journal of Neuro-oncology 9: 139–145

McDowell J R 1990 Familial meningioma. Neurology 40: 312–314

MacGregor D D, Ziff E B 1990 Elevated c-*myc* expression in childhood medulloblastoma. Pediatric Research 28: 36–68

Malkin D, Li F P, Strong L C et al 1992 Germ line p53 mutations in a familial syndrome of breast cancer, sarcomas, and other neoplasms. Science 250: 1233–1238

Marchuk D A, Saulino A M, Tavakkol R et al 1991 cDNA cloning of the type 1 neurofibromatosis gene: complete sequence of the NF1 gene product. Genomics 11: 931–940

Martuza R L 1985 Neurofibromatosis and other phakomatoses. In: Wilkins R H, Rengachary S S (eds) Neurosurgery. McGraw Hill, Toronto, pp 511–522

Martuza R L, Eldridge R 1988 Neurofibromatosis 2 (Bilateral acoustic neurofibromatosis). New England Journal of Medicine 11: 684–688

Martuza R L, Rouleau G 1990 Genetic aspects of neurosurgical problems. In: Youmans J R (ed) Neurological surgery, 3rd edn, vol 2. WB Saunders, Philadelphia, pp 1061–1080

Martuza R L, Seizinger B R, Jacoby L B, Rouleau G A, Gusella J F 1988 The molecular biology of human glial tumors. TINS 112: 22–27

Martuza R L, Malick A, Markert J M et al 1991 Experimental therapy of human glioma by means of a genetically engineered virus mutant. Science 252: 854–856

Mashiyama S, Murakami Y, Yoshimoto T et al 1991 Detection of p53 gene mutations in human brain tumors by single-strand conformation polymorphism analysis of polymerase chain reaction products. Oncogene 6: 1313–1318

Maxwell M, Naber S P, Wolf H J et al 1990a Coexpression of platelet-derived growth factor (PDGF) and PDGF receptor gene by primary human astrocytomas may contribute to their development and maintenance. Journal of Clinical Investigation 85: 131–140

Maxwell M, Galanpoulos T, Hedley-White E T et al 1990b Human meningiomas co-express platelet-derived growth factor (PDGF) and PDGF-receptor genes and their protein products. International Journal of Cancer 46: 16–21

Maxwell M, Naber S P, Wolf H J et al 1991 Expression of angiogenic growth factor genes in primary human astrocytomas may contribute to their growth and progression. Cancer Research 51: 1345–1351

Menon A G, Gusella J F, Seizinger B R 1990 Progress towards the isolation and characterization of the genes causing neurofibromatosis. Cancer Surveys 4: 689–702

Mercer W E, Shields M T, Amin M et al 1990 Negative regulation in a glioblastoma tumor cell line that conditionally expresses human wild-type p53. Proceedings of the National Academy of Sciences of the USA 87: 6616–6170

Metzger A K, Sheffield V C, Duyk G et al 1990 Identification of a germ-line mutation in the p53 gene in a patient with an intracranial ependymoma. Proceedings of the National Academy of Sciences of the USA 88: 7825–7829

Mikkelsen T, Cairncross J, Cavenee W 1991 Genetics of the malignant progression of astrocytomas. Journal of Cell Biochemistry 46: 3–8

Miller D M, Blume S, Borst M et al 1990 Oncogenes, malignant transformation and modern medicine. American Journal of Medical Science 300: 59–69

Moses H, Yang E, Pietenpol J A 1990 TGF-beta1 stimulation and inhibition of cell proliferation: New mechanistic insights. Cell 63: 245–247

Mulvihill J J, Parry D M, Sherman J L et al 1990 Neurofibromatosis 1 (Recklinghausen disease) and neurofibromatosis 2 (bilateral acoustic neurofibromatosis): an update. Annals of Internal Medicine 113: 39–52

Murphy G, Reynolds J J 1985 Progress towards understanding the resorption of connective tissues. Bioessays 2: 55–60

Narod S A, Parry D M, Parboosingh J et al 1992 Neurofibromatosis type 2 appears to be a genetically homogeneous disease. American Journal of Human Genetics 51: 486–496

Nigro J M, Baker S J, Preisinger A C et al 1989 Mutations in the p53 gene occur in diverse human tumor types. Nature 342: 705–708

Nishizaki T, Orita T, Furutani Y et al 1989 Flow cytometric DNA analysis and immunohistochemical measurement of Ki-67 and BUdR labelling indices in human brain tumors. Journal of Neurosurgery 70: 379–384

Nister M, Westermark B 1986 Clonal variations in the production of a PDGF-like protein and expression of corresponding receptors in human malignant gliomas. Cancer Research 46: 332–340

Nister M, Libermann T A, Betsholtz C et al 1988 Expression of messenger RNAs for PDGF and TGF-alpha and their receptors in human malignant glioma cell lines. Cancer Research 48: 3910–3918

O'Connell P, Viskochil D, Buchberg A et al 1990 The human homolog of murine EVI2 lies between two von Recklinghausen neurofibromatosis translocations. Genomics 7: 547–554

Parmiter A H, Balaban G, Clark W H et al 1988 Possible involvement of chromosome region 10q24-q26 in early stages of melanocytic neoplasia. Cancer Genetics and Cytogenetics 30: 313–317

Pathak S L, Strong L C, Ferrell R E et al 1982 Familial renal cell carcinoma with a 3;11 translocation limited to tumor cells. Science 217: 939–949

Paulus W, Grothe C, Sensenbrenner M et al 1990 Localization of basic fibroblast growth factor, a mitogen and angiogenic factor in human brain tumors. Acta Neuropathol 79: 418–423

Peterson P H 1985 On the role of proteases, their inhibitors and the extracellular matrix in promoting neurite outgrowth. Journal of Physiology (London) 80: 207–211

Pines J 1992 Cell proliferation and control. Current Opinion in Cell Biology 4: 144–148

Pollerberg G E, Schachner M, Davoust J 1986 Differentiation state-dependent surface mobilities of 2 forms of the neural cell adhesion molecule. Nature 324: 462–465

Pulst S M 1990 Prenatal diagnosis of the neurofibromatoses. Clinics in Perinatology 4: 829–843

Raffel C, Gilles F E, Weingberg K I 1990 Reduction to homozygosity and gene amplification in central nervous system primitive neuroectodermal tumors of childhood. Cancer Research 50: 587–591

Rasheed B K A, Bigner S H 1991 Genetic alterations in glioma and medulloblastoma. Cancer and Metastasis Reviews 10: 289–299

Raycroft L, Wu H, Lozano G 1989 Transcriptional activation by wild-type but not transforming mutants of the p53 anti-oncogene. Science 249: 1049–105

Reid L M, Jefferson D M 1984 Cell culture studies using extracts of ECM to study growth and differentiation in mammalian cells. In: Mather J P (ed) Mammalian cell culture. Plenum, New York, pp 239–280

Riccardi V M 1991 Neurofibromatosis: Phenotype, natural history, and pathogenesis, 2nd edn. Johns Hopkins University Press, Baltimore, pp 1–450

Riley R S 1992 Cellular proliferation markers in the evaluation of human cancer. Clinics in Laboratory Medicine 12: 2

Riva P, Larizza T 1992 Expression of c-*sis* and c-*fos* genes in human meningiomas and neurinomas. International Journal of Cancer 51: 873–877

Robbins K, Antoniades H, Deharve S et al 1982 Structural and immunological similarities between simian sarcoma virus gene product(s) and human PDGF. Nature 305: 605–608

Rouah E, Wilson R, Armstrong D et al 1989 N-*myc* amplification and neuronal differentiation in human primitive neuroectodermal tumors of the central nervous system. Cancer Research 49: 1797–1801

Rouleau G A, Seizinger B R, Wertelecki W et al 1990 Flanking markers bracket the neurofibromatosis 2 (NF 2) gene in chromosome 22. American Journal of Human Genetics 46: 323–328

Rouleau G A, Merel P, Lutchman M et al 1993 Alteration in a new gene encoding a putative membrane – organizing protein causes neurofibromatosis type 2. Nature 363: 515–518

Rutka J T 1991 The extracellular matrix: Cues from the microcellular environment which can inhibit or facilitate glioma cell growth. In: Tabuchi K (ed) Biological aspects of brain tumors. Springer-Verlag, Tokyo, pp 73–86

Rutka J T, Giblin J R, Hoifodt H K et al 1986 Establishment and characterization of a cell line from a human gliosarcoma. Cancer Research 46: 5893–5902

Rutka J T, Dougherty D V, Giblin J R et al 1987 Growth of a medulloblastoma on normal leptomeningeal cells in culture: Interaction of tumor cells and normal cells. Neurosurgery 21: 872–878

Rutka J T, Apodaca G, Stern R, Rosenblum M 1988 The extracellular matrix of the central and peripheral nervous system. Structure and function. Journal of Neurosurgery 69: 155–170

Rutka J T, Rosenblum M L, Stern R et al 1989 Isolation and partial purification of growth factors with TGF-like activity from human gliomas. Journal of Neurosurgery 71: 875

Rutka J T, Trent J M, Rosenblum M L 1990 Molecular probes in neuro-oncology: A review. Cancer Investigation 8: 425–438

Ryken T C, Traynelis V C, Lim R 1992 Interaction of acidic fibroblast growth factor and transforming growth factor beta in normal and transformed glia *in vitro*. Journal of Neurosurgery 76: 850–855

Sager R 1992 Tumor suppressor genes in the cell cycle. Current Opinion in Cell Biology 4: 155–160

Santhanam U, Ray A, Sehgal P 1991 Repression of the interleukin 6 gene promoter by p53 and the retinoblastoma susceptibility gene product. Proceedings of the National Academy of Sciences of the USA 88: 7605–7609

Sauceda R, Ocadiz R, Gutierrez A et al 1988 Novel combination of c-*myc*, N-*myc*, and N-*ras* oncogene alteration in brain tumors. Molecular Brain Research 3: 123–132

Saxena A, Clark C, Robertson J T et al 1992 Evidence for the involvement of a potential second tumor suppressor gene on chromosome 17 distinct from p53 in malignant astrocytomas. Cancer Research 52: 6716–6721

Saylors R L, Sidransky D, Friedman H S et al 1991 Infrequent p53 gene mutations in medulloblastomas. Cancer Research 51: 4721–4723

Schneider G, Luta S, Henn W et al 1992 Search for putative suppressor genes in meningioma: significance of chromosome 22. Human Genetics 88: 576–582

Seizinger B R 1991 Toward the isolation of the primary genetic defect in von Hippel-Lindau disease. Annals of the New York Academy of Science 615: 332–337

Seizinger B R, Martuza R L, Gusella J F 1986 Loss of genes on chromosome 22 in tumorigenesis of human acoustic neuroma. Nature 322: 644–647

Seizinger B R, de la Monte S, Atkins L et al 1987a Molecular genetic approach to human meningiomas: Loss of genes of chromosome 22. Proceedings of the National Academy of Sciences of the USA 84: 5419–5423

Seizinger B R, Rouleau G, Ozelius L J et al 1987b Common pathogenetic mechanism for three tumor types in bilateral acoustic neurofibromatosis. Science 236: 317–319

Seizinger B R, Rouleau G A, Ozelius L J et al 1987c Genetic linkage of von Recklinghausen neurofibromatosis to the nerve growth factor receptor gene. Cell 49: 589–594

Seizinger B R, Rouleau G A, Ozelius L J et al 1988 von Hippel Lindau disease maps to the region on chromosome 3 associated with renal cell carcinoma. Nature 332: 269–270

Sidransky D, Mikkelsen T, Schwechheimer K et al 1991 Clonal expression of the p53 mutant cells is associated with brain tumor progression. Nature 355: 846–847

Sporn M B, Roberts A B 1985 Autocrine growth factors and cancer. Nature 313: 745–747

Srivastava S, Zou Z, Pirollo K et al 1991 Germ-line transmission of a mutated p53 gene in a cancer-prone family with Li-Fraumeni syndrome. Nature 348: 747–749

Steck P A, Pershouse M A, Hadi A et al 1991 Partial reversion of tumorigenic phenotype of human glioblastoma cells (LG-11) by microcell-mediated transfer of chromosome 10. Proc AACR 32: 1691a

Stetler-Stevenson W G, Krutzch H C, Liotta L A 1989 Tissue inhibitor of metalloproteinase (TIMP-2). A new member of the metalloproteinase inhibitor family. Journal of Biology and Chemistry 264: 17374–17378

Stone R 1992 Molecular surgery for human brain tumors. Science (News and Comment) 256: 1513

Tabuchi K, Fukuyama K, Mineta T et al 1991 Alterations and expression of the p53 gene in human neuroepithelial tumors. Neurol. Med. Chir. (Tokyo) 32: 725–732

Takahashi J A, Mori H, Fujimoto M et al 1990 Gene expression of fibroblast growth factors in human gliomas and meningiomas: Demonstration of cellular source of basic fibroblast growth factor mRNA and peptide in tumor tissues. Proceedings of the National Academy of Sciences of the USA 87: 5710–5714

Takamiya Y, Koshaka S, Toya S et al 1986 Possible association of PDGF with the appearance of reactive astrocytes following brain injury in situ. Brain Research 383: 305–309

Thapar K, Kovacs K, Laws E R et al 1993 Pituitary adenomas: Current concepts in classification, histopathology and molecular biology. The Endocrinologist (in press)

Thorgeirsson U P, Turpeenniemi-Hujanen T, Liotta L A 1985 Cancer cells, components of basement membranes, and proteolytic enzymes. International Review of Experimental Pathology 27: 203–234

Tops C M, Vasen H F, van-Berge-Henegouwen G et al 1992 Genetic evidence that Turcot syndrome is not allelic to familial adenomatous polyposis. American Journal of Medical Genetics 43: 888–893

Trent J et al 1986 Evidence for rearrangement, amplification, and expression of c-myc in a human glioblastoma. PNAS 83: 470–473

Trofatter J A, MacCollin M M, Rutter J L et al 1993 A novel moesin$_{-1}$ radixin-like gene is a candidate for the neurofibromatosis^{2} tumor suppressor. Cell 72: 791–796

Turcot J, Despres J P, St. Pierre F 1959 Malignant tumors of the CNS associated with familial polyposis of the colon: report of two cases. Diseases of the Colon and Rectum 2: 465–468

U H S, Kelley P, Lee W H 1988 Abnormalities of the human growth hormone gene and protooncogenes in some human pituitary tumors. Molecular Endocrinology 2: 85–89

Venter D J, Bevan K L, Ludwig R L et al 1991 Retinoblastoma gene deletions in human glioblastomas. Oncogene 6: 445–448

Viskochil D, Cawthon R, O'Connell P et al 1991 The gene encoding the oligodendrocyte myelin glycoprotein is embedded within the neurofibromatosis type 1 gene. Molecular Cell Biology 11: 906–912

Wallace M R, Marchuk D A, Andersen L B et al 1990 Type 1 neurofibromatosis gene: identification of a large transcript disrupted in three NF1 patients. Science 249: 181–186

Wasson J C, Saylors R L, Zeltzer P et al 1990 Oncogene amplification in pediatric brain tumors. Cancer Research 50: 2987–2990

Westphal M, Herrman H D 1989 Growth factor biology and oncogene activation in human gliomas and their implications for specific therapeutic concepts. Neurosurgery 25: 681–694

Wong A J, Bigner S H, Bigner D D et al 1987 Increased expression of the epidermal growth factor receptor gene in malignant gliomas is invariably associated with gene amplification. Proceedings of the National Academy of Sciences of the USA 84: 6899–6903

Wu J K, Chikaraishi D M 1990 Differential expression of *mos* oncogene in primary human astrocytomas and astrocytoma cell lines. Cancer Research 50: 3032–3035

Xu G, O'Connel P, Viskochil D et al 1990 The neurofibromatosis type 1 gene encodes a protein related to GAP. Cell 62: 599–608

Yamazaki H, Ohba N, Tamaoki N et al 1990 A deletion mutation within the ligand binding domain is responsible for activation of epidermal growth factor receptor gene in human brain tumors. Japanese Journal of Cancer Research 81: 773–779

Yeh H, Ruit K, Wang Y et al 1991 PDGF-A chain is expressed in mammalian neurons during development and in maturity. Cell 64: 209–216

Yonish-Rouach E, Resnitzky D, Lotem J et al 1991 Wild-type p53 induces apoptosis of myeloid leukemic cells that is inhibited by interleukin-6. Nature 352: 345–347

Zagzag D, Miller D C, Sato Y et al 1990 Immunohistochemical localization of basic fibroblast growth factor in astrocytoma. Cancer Research 50: 7393–7398

Zang K D, Singer H 1967 Chromosomal constitution of meningiomas. Nature 216: 84–85

Zbar B 1987 Loss of alleles of loci on the short arm of chromosome 3 in renal cell carcinoma. Nature 327: 721–724

6. Biochemistry and metabolism of brain tumors

John R. Mangiardi

INTRODUCTION

This chapter will outline the basic biochemical attributes of the malignant neural crest tumors, the malignant astrocytoma in particular. Because of the polyclonal character of the malignant astrocytoma, biochemical studies have been understandably hampered by the phenotypic diversity of the multiple cell lines within a single tumor. Also, due to the variable character of the in vivo malignant tumor, with its 20% growth fraction, large percentage of tumor in G_0 phase of the cell cycle, and the sometimes larger fraction of frankly necrotic tumor, initial studies done in the 60s and 70s were frustrating and nonspecific. Over time, however, some common factors have become obvious with the development of cell and animal culture techniques, oncogene product identification, and cell surface receptor technology, as well as in vivo imaging techniques such as MR spectroscopy, positron emission tomography, and single photon emission tomography (SPECT) (Brooks 1990, Wang 1992).

The process of anaplasia includes *survival mechanisms* that allow a neoplasm to compete successfully with its host. These include: (1) utilization of various *primitive enzyme systems* that give the tumor energy management and growth advantages over the host, (2) *tumor versus host products*, such as tissue lytic enzymes, immune system suppressors, growth factors, autocrine factors, and other tumor poisons, (3) *extracellular matrix modifications*, including chemical makeup, pH and oxygen tension levels, and alterations in tissue perfusion, (4) *cell membrane alterations*, including cytostructural variation, antigenic changes, receptor site and second messenger system enhancements, and cellular transport system modifications, and *autoinduction*, a process whereby the cell guarantees its own unrestrained growth and replication.

THE MALIGNANT CELL (Fig. 6.1)

Anaplasia refers to a process of malignant change ('disordered change') which may occur in any tissue type. When a primitive tissue type undergoes malignant change, an anaplastic primitive tumor develops. By the same token, an anaplastic tumor of a more mature tissue type, such as the malignant astrocytoma, arises from the tissue of the same type (the astrocyte).

Tumors of more primitive tumor types may undergo *maturation*, becoming anaplastic neoplasms of more mature tissue types. For example, the medulloblastoma may develop, in time, areas of both astrocytoma and ganglioglioma, thus mimicking along malignant lines the ontogeny of the medulloblast along glial and neuronal cell lines.

The concept of *dedifferentiation* probably does not apply to the primary brain tumors. In other words, an anaplastic tumor of a mature tumor type does not revert to an anaplastic tumor of a more primitive tumor type. One of the survival mechanisms of anaplastic tumors is the utilization of various primitive enzyme systems to attain a competitive advantage over the host. This mechanism, which is limited to the loss of suppression of a small number of genes, is often confused with dedifferentiation, which refers to a global return to an ontologically earlier status of the entire genome. Understanding the mechanisms whereby specific gene suppression is reversed would allow for a better understanding of the biochemical processes involved.

THE CELL MEMBRANE

Numerous changes in the cell membrane occur with anaplasia. Early studies focused on the relative concentrations of the various components of the cell membrane and other membranous structures of the cell. The complex gangliosides are the characteristic membrane components of brain tissue. The physiology of both the cell membrane and subcellular membranes is in part a function of the relative content of the various phospholipids. Therefore, the changes in the complex lipids that occur after neoplastic transformation of the cell result in significant

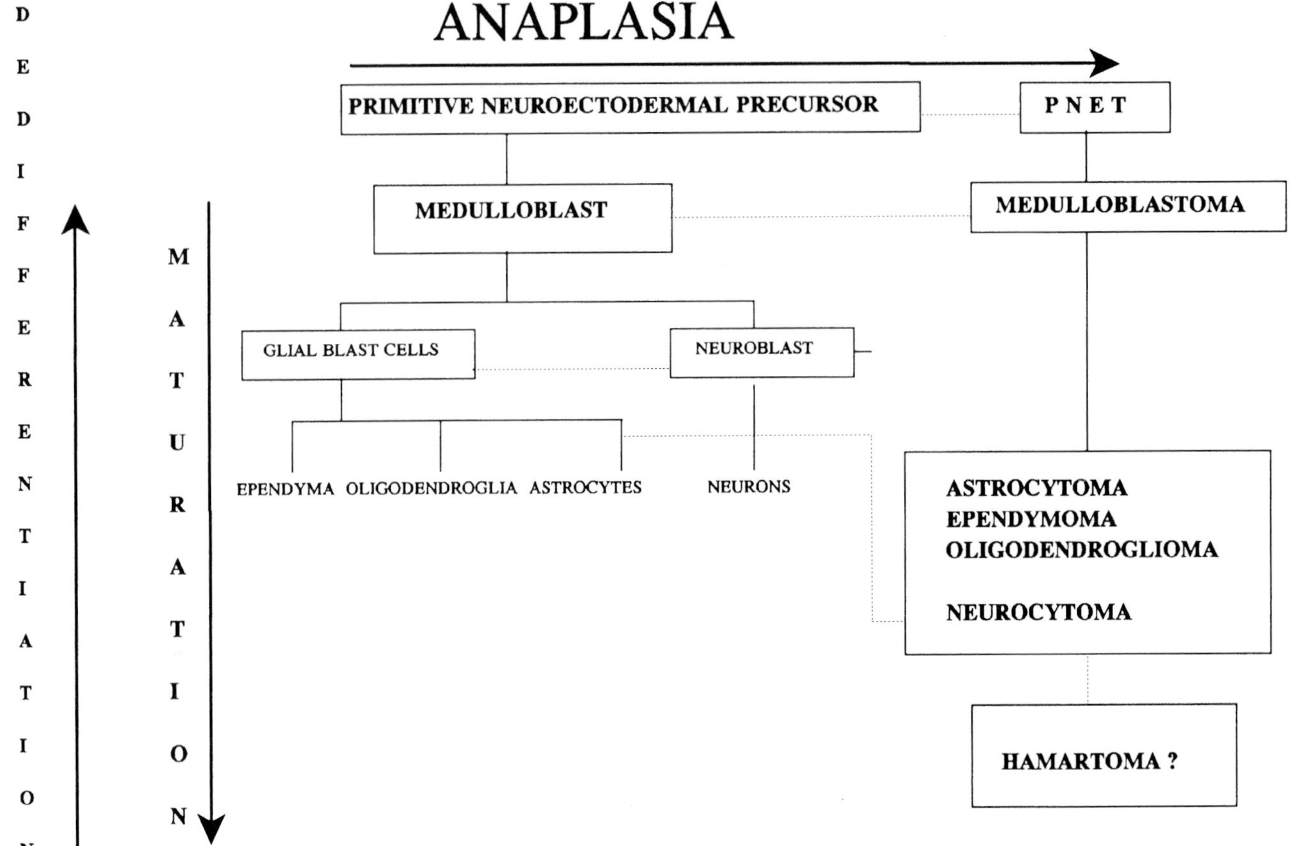

Fig. 6.1 The malignant cell.

alterations of function. It is probable that the changes of glycosphingolipid and other glycolipid concentrations in the cell membrane are responsible for the *loss of contact inhibition* characteristic of malignant cell growth. Such alterations are probably also responsible for the variable antigenic character of malignant cells, as well as receptor site, ionic channel, and transmembrane transport system variations found (Couldwell et al 1992).

The changes in membrane gangliosides affect the various functions of both the cellular (contact inhibition and cell adhesion, molecular and pinocytotic transport, cytostructure, ionic channels, receptors, growth factor activity, second messenger production) and subcellular (lysosomes, endoplasmic reticulum, mitochondria, peroxisomes, nucleus) membranes. These changes are in part a function of the relative content of the various phospholipids that make up the gangliosides. Not surprisingly, there are both quantitative (decreased phosphatidylethanolamine and glycosphingolipid; increased phosphatidylcholine, sphingomyelin, GM2, GD2, GD3, LM1 and LD1) and qualitative (simplified pattern of complex gangliosides, higher ratio of protein to phospholipid, presence of the primitive chondroitin sulfate proteoglycan NG2, and the embryonal intermediate filament cytoskeleton protein known as IFAP 300 kD) characteristics of tumor cell membranes that are strikingly different than normal adult brain. Notably, there is similarity to the membranes of fetal brain.

Glioma specific antigens

Various antigenic determinants have been identified with glial tumors, including the S-100 protein, glial fibrillary acid protein (GFAP), α_2-glycoprotein, 14-3-2 protein, myelin basic protein, and the diacylganglioside GD2. GFAP is an intracytoplasmic cytostructural protein that is present in normal glia, and occurs in decreasing quantities with increasing anaplasia. The possibility of therapeutic intervention with monoclonal antibody systems has sparked interest in the search for unique cellular antigens in malignant gliomas. However, almost all of these surface antigens are nonspecific. There is a correlation with fetal antigens, and with other tissues of neuroectodermal origin. The most difficult problem presented by the malignant glial tumors has been their polyclonicity, sometimes over 1000 clones/tumor, that leads to great variability in cell surface characteristics. What is clear is that the chimeral quality of antigens presented to the host defense system by the malignant astrocytoma is certainly confounding.

Receptor sites for the various growth factors have antigenic properties. They have been demonstrated to have enough specificity to allow for experimental therapeutic trials of antibodies directed toward these receptors.

Receptor site changes

As tumor cells proliferate they secrete autocrine growth factors to which they themselves respond (see below). The number and expression of these receptor sites appear to be enhanced with the production of growth factors.

Another receptor that is expressed in tumor but not normal brain tissue is transferrin receptor. The role of iron in tumor cell growth is outlined below.

The benzodiazepine receptors occur in two types — a CNS type located on neurons and associated with the GABA receptor, and a peripheral type found outside the CNS. Peripheral type benzodiazepine receptors have been found in significant quantity both in animal cell lines and in human malignant glioma tissue. There may be a relationship between benzodiazepine activity and tumor cell mitochondrial reproduction. Antisense benzodiazepine ligands have been shown to inhibit mitochondrial DNA polymerase in cultured glioma cell lines.

Ionic channel changes

Because the method of glucose metabolism utilized by malignant neuroectodermal neoplasms results in the production of large amounts of lactate (see below), the hydrogen ion transport system is enhanced to prevent intracellular acidification from occurring.

Zinc is an important trace element for the function of the metalloenzymes. The concentrations of copper and zinc, as well as the ratio of Cu/Zn, are increased in malignant gliomas. With increased growth activity the requirements for enzymatic trace element cofactors increase. Zinc is particularly important for enzymes such as alkylguanine-DNA-acyltransferase that are targeted for depletion with chemotherapeutic combinations such as BCNU and streptozotocin. It is probable that the ionic transport systems for these trace elements are enhanced.

Iron is managed in the normal cell by a tightly regulated system involving iron uptake, transport, storage and utilization by such molecules as transferrin, hemin, ferritin, ferritin repressor protein, catalase, and ribonucleotide reductase. Free iron is cytotoxic, as it induces membrane lipid peroxidation, subsequent disruption of subcellular organelles and degradation of amino acids and deoxyribose.

Transferrin presents the iron molecule to the tumor cell surface where it attaches to specific transferrin receptors. Iron is then pinocytotically absorbed. Alternatively it may be carried into the cytosol directly by hemin, which freely permeates the cell membrane. Once inside the cell, the iron is transferred to ferritin, where it remains in storage. It is then competitively moved off the ferritin molecule by various enzymes for use as a cofactor. One such enzyme is catalase, responsible for the catalysis of hydrogen peroxide. Iron is also a cofactor for another enzyme that is especially important in the rapidly reproducing cell, ribonucleotide reductase.

The number of transferrin receptors is increased in malignant neuroectodermal tumor cells. Cultured tumor cells, like normal cells, respond to increased intracellular iron by increasing their content of ferritin.

Calcium enters the cell by way of a variety of channels, including voltage-dependent and NMDR. Calcium is extremely important for certain enzymes of the protein kinase cascade. This is particularly true for protein kinase C (type A), which is virtually calcium dependent. Thus increased cytosol calcium levels are a prerequisite for neuroectodermal tumor growth because of the large correlation between PKC activity and cell growth.

ENERGY METABOLISM (Mangiardi & Yodice 1990)

One way to view the organization of the cell is from the point of view of energy metabolism. All cells have as their primary concern the acquisition of substrate to be transformed into high energy phosphate compounds, such as ATP and creatine phosphate, which are used to power the machinery of metabolism. This process is biochemically the simplest biologic function of the cell. The various products of energy metabolism are then incorporated into the more complex structural elements of the cell, namely lipids, proteins, polysaccharides, and nucleic acids. These in turn are variously combined to form the membranes, cytostructure, cytosol, and subcellular organelles of the cell. The environment created by these structural elements allows for the final end product of metabolic flow and most complex of cellular functions, replication.

Of the various organs of the body the brain is unique in that it depends solely upon glucose as its source of energy (Fig. 6.2). In essence, the brain is an 'end organ' vis a vis substrate, depending solely upon the supply of glucose (or ketone bodies during starvation) presented by the cerebral vasculature. Substrate supply is then a function of cerebral blood flow. Storage components such as fats, polysaccharides, and even glycogen are not maintained, and the enzyme systems for their breakdown to glucose are not active.

The best measure of metabolic sufficiency of tissue is its level of ATP. A surplus of ATP is a good biochemical indicator that a cell has established a supply of energy satisfactory to meet intrinsic metabolic demands. In the case of the malignant astrocytoma, energy storage and release is adequate not only to satisfy the basal metabolic requirements of an already established neoplasm, but also to allow for tumor growth. The mean ATP and total adenylate levels in this tumor are higher than in normal brain.

In the normal brain, energy (in the form of ATP) is

BRAIN CELLS	OTHER CELLS
• GLUCOSE	• GLUCOSE • FATS • PROTEINS • STARCH

Fig. 6.2 Sources of energy.

generated from oxidative phosphorylation in the presence of adequate oxygen (Fig. 6.3). Glucose is used as substrate and is metabolized via the glycolytic pathway to coenzyme A (acetyl-CoA). This in turn enters the Krebs cycle, where nicotinamide adenine dinucleotide (NADH) is produced. This metabolite is then utilized by the electron transport chain as it consumes oxygen to form a total of 36 moles of ATP in the process of oxidative phosphorylation. When oxygen is in short supply, normal tissues may temporarily survive by shifting to anaerobic glycolysis. In this process the glycolytic pathway leads to the formation of lactic acid rather than acetyl-CoA, resulting in the production of 2 moles of ATP. When oxygen becomes available again, the tissue shifts back again to the production of acetyl-CoA and the use of oxidative phosphorylation.

The malignant glioma relies upon glycolysis rather than respiration for the production of ATP. Lactate production continues even when oxygen is present; oxygen consumption is markedly reduced; and although only 2 moles of ATP are produced for each mole of glucose consumed, adequate stores of ATP are maintained. Although originally referred to as *fermentation* by Warburg (1930), this mode of ATP production has come to be known as *aerobic glycolysis* because of the persistence of glycolytic lactic acid production despite adequate oxygen supply (Fig. 6.4). Aerobic glycolysis then becomes a strategy for tumor survival whether oxygen is present or not. Only a satisfactory glucose supply is necessary, and tumor viability is maintained even under ischemic conditions.

A consequence of aerobic glycolysis (Fig. 6.5) is that the metabolic activity of these tumors must be assessed by glucose uptake rather than by oxygen consumption. This

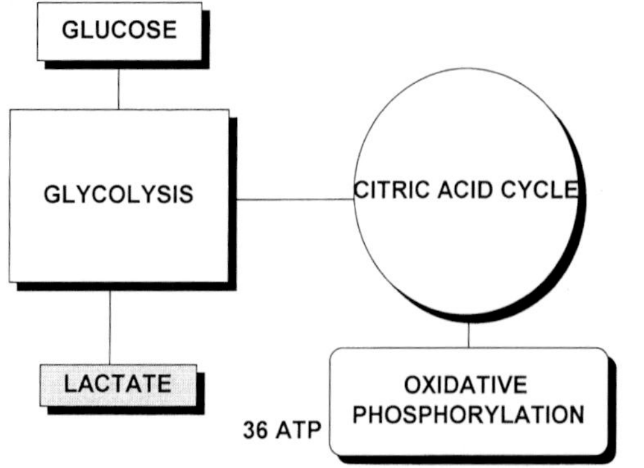

Fig. 6.3 Generation of energy (ATP) by oxidative phosphorylation in the normal brain.

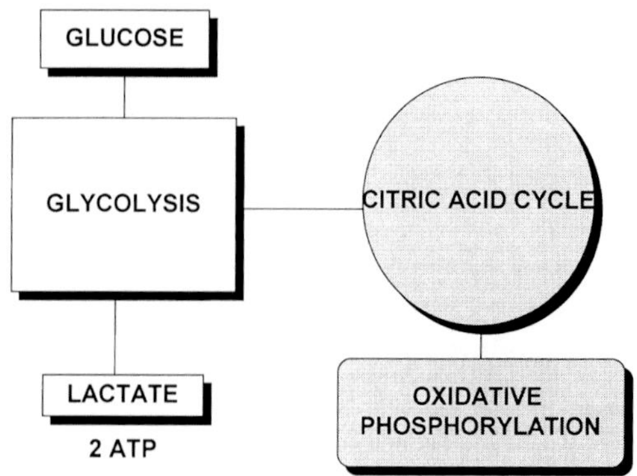

Fig. 6.4 Generation of ATP by aerobic glycolysis in malignant glioma.

has been demonstrated both in vitro and in vivo (using the deoxyglucose methods of positron emission tomography) where cerebral glucose uptake and consumption by tumor are over 300% that of normal brain, while respiration studies demonstrate that oxygen consumption is dramatically reduced. Studies of the enzymes of the citric acid cycle and of oxidative phosphorylation disclose that these pathways have limited activity, suggesting that there is a 'turning off' of certain enzymes, resulting in the accumulation of pyruvate rather than acetyl-CoA, leading to the increased production of lactic acid. Moreover, both the citric acid cycle and the respiratory chain enzymes are located in mitochondria. As important as the reduction in enzymatic activity of these enzymes is the observation that malignant neuroectodermal tumors have far fewer mitochondria than do normal cells. This quantitative reduction in the enzymes of mitochondrial energy production may be even more significant than any quantitative changes in activity.

The glycolytic pathway

The three rate-limiting enzymes of the glycolytic pathway are hexokinase, phosphofructokinase, and pyruvate kinase. Of these, phosphofructokinase is the primary determinant of the rate of glycolysis. It is inhibited by both ATP and citrate, resulting in a slowing in the uptake of glucose. Inhibition of phosphofructokinase leads to the accumulation of glucose-6-phosphate, which, in turn, inhibits hexokinase. Pyruvate kinase, like phosphofructokinase, is inhibited by excess ATP. When measured experimentally, the activities of the initial rate-limiting enzymes of glycoly-

Oxygen consumption:	90% reduction
Glucose uptake:	300% increase
Mitochondria:	80% reduction
TCA enzyme activity:	depressed
Oxidative phosphorylation enzyme activity:	depressed

Fig. 6.5 Consequences of aerobic glycolysis.

sis are reduced, while those of the distal enzymes of the pathway are increased. The activity of lactate dehydrogenase is equivalent to that of normal brain. The combination of a depressed citric acid cycle (with the consequent increase in pyruvate availability), and increased distal glycolytic enzyme activity, results in a marked increase in lactate production. This in turn places an increased load on the acid ion transport system and finally results in the increased extracellular acid equivalent levels found in these tumors.

The enzymes of glycolysis in malignant neuroectodermal tumors are different from those in normal tissue in that they exist in a more primitive form. For example, pyruvate kinase is a tetramer. It may exist as different isoenzymes made up of either K or M subunits, or as a hybrid of both. The K type is dominant in fetal life while the M type prevails in mature tissues. In the glioblastoma, the K type predominates. Hexokinase also exists in different isomeric forms. Normal brain contains only type I hexokinase, while fetal brain contains only type II. Again, it is the primitive type II isoenzyme that is found in malignant gliomas. Lactic dehydrogenase (LDH) is a tetrameric enzyme that is composed of 2 subunit types, H (heart) and M (muscle). The H subunit is found in aerobic tissues with high metabolic rates, such as heart and normal brain. The M subunit is found in tissues that tend to accumulate lactic acid, such as skeletal muscle. In the malignant astrocytoma there is a shift to the production of the M subunit, in keeping with the dependence of this tumor upon aerobic glycolysis. Thus, the isoenzyme LDH_5 (which contains only M subunits) is almost 5 times that of normal brain.

It will be interesting to compare the primitive neuroectodermal tumors (PNET) to fetal brain tissues regarding their energy management strategy. It is teleologically important to understand that both have in common stunningly simple requirements for survival, enabling them to flourish in the face of adversities of all but one kind, lack of glucose.

Pentose shunt

While the major energy production pathways of the cell appear to be 'turned off', the pentose phosphate shunt pathway is apparently 'turned on' (Fig. 6.6). This alternative pathway for glucose metabolism generates energy in the normal cell in the form of reducing elements such as NADPH. It also produces ribulose-5-phosphate (P-5-P), the precursor of phosphoribosylpyrophosphate (PRPP), the substrate for both pyrimidine and purine biosynthesis. The first step in this pathway shunts glucose-6-phosphate from the glycolytic pathway, which exists in increased quantity in tumor tissue. The activity of PRPP synthetase is also probably increased.

It is likely that the pentose shunt is more active in tumors because of increased forward demand for nucleic acid building blocks for the replicating cell. Of interest is the observation that 6-aminonicotinamide, an inhibitor of the pentose shunt, has powerful cytotoxic capability in in vitro human malignant glioma cell lines.

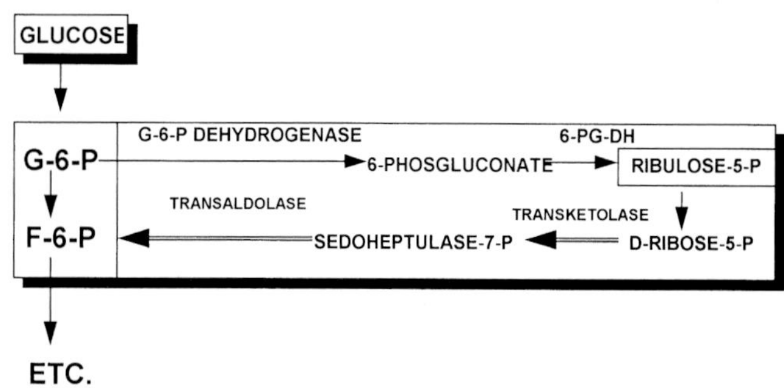

Fig. 6.6 The pentose phosphate shunt pathway.

Citric acid cycle and oxidative phosphorylation

As mentioned above, there is a marked decrease in the number of mitochondria found in malignant neuroectodermal cells. In the mitochondria that do exist, the activities of many of the enzymes of the citric acid cycle (such as citrate synthetase and malate dehydrogenase), and the oxidative phosphorylation chain (such as cytochrome oxidase) are markedly decreased when compared to normal brain.

The net result of this is that: (1) NADH (the energy product of the citric acid cycle that serves as the source of hydrogen atoms that contribute their electrons to the respiratory chain) is not produced, (2) oxygen is not consumed, and (3) pyruvate accumulation occurs, forcing the formation of abnormal levels of lactic acid.

Acetyl-coenzyme A

In the metabolism of the normal cell, acetyl-CoA has a pivotal role involving multiple pathways, both catabolic and anabolic (Fig. 6.7). It represents the major energy metabolite of the cell, and is produced during the catabolism of polysaccharides, fats and proteins. Energy production is guaranteed when a mole of acetyl-CoA has been committed to the Krebs cycle. Each time this happens, 11 moles of ATP are produced. It can be metabolized when necessary to ketone bodies during starvation for further use as an energy source.

Since the citric acid cycle and oxidative phosphorylation are not functioning in these tumors, the catabolic utilization of acetyl-CoA must be limited.

METABOLISM OF STRUCTURAL COMPONENTS

Lipids

The lipids have four major functions:

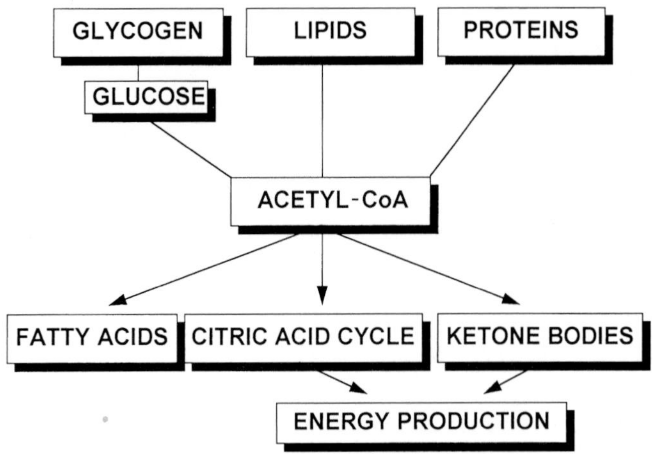

Fig. 6.7 Role of acetyl-CoA in the metabolism of the normal cell.

1. Fatty acids are the major energy storage source in normal cells as triacylglycerols, which are metabolized to acetyl-CoA and taken up by the citric acid cycle. (As mentioned above, the brain is an end organ insofar as energy stores are concerned, and triacylglycerols are not utilized as an energy source.) They are also the basic anabolic unit of the complex lipids (Fig. 6.8).

2. The complex lipids constitute the major structural components of cell and subcellular membranes.

3. Specialized lipids such as prostaglandins, leukotrienes and the steroids are powerful physiologic modulators.

4. The abnormal products of lipid auto-oxidation are the lipid hydroperoxides and are responsible for free radical damage after various cellular insults.

Fatty acids and sterols

On the anabolic side, acetyl-CoA is the major building block of the fatty acids and sterols (such as cholesterol). The coenzyme is produced from three different metabolic sources, (1) from glycolysis (pyruvate) via the lactate dehydrogenase reaction, (2) from the beta oxidation of fatty acids, and (3) from the deamination/oxidation of amino acids. As simple sugars are the building blocks of polysaccharides, acetyl-CoA is the basic component of fatty acids, and in turn the complex lipids of the cell's cytostructure.

The fatty acids are synthesized by a process that begins when the control enzyme of fatty acid anabolism, acetyl-CoA carboxylase, incorporates dissolved bicarbonate to form malonyl-CoA. Thereafter, sequential addition of 2 carbon units from acetyl-CoA by the enzyme fatty acid-synthetase leads to the formation of the 16-carbon straight chain, palmitic acid, from which most other fatty acids are formed. These fatty acids are then incorporated into the triacylglycerols and the complex membrane lipids.

The synthesis of sterols also begins with acetyl-CoA (Fig. 6.9), which is twice condensed to form hydroxymethylglutaryl-CoA (HMG-CoA). This in turn is catalyzed by the rate limiting enzyme HMG-CoA reductase to form mevalonic acid. This is then metabolized by a number of steps to desmosterol, the immediate precursor of cholesterol, the major sterol of the malignant astrocytoma (95%). Brain tumors contain 2 to 3 times more free fatty acids, sterol esters, and glycerol esters than normal brain. Desmosterol, not found in appreciable amounts in normal brain, may account for up 5% of the total sterol content in malignant tumors. Also, tumors have the capacity to incorporate acetate-^{14}C into cholesterol, while normal brain does not. (Therapeutic interference with cholesterol synthesis, however, does little to alter tumor growth in the clinical setting.)

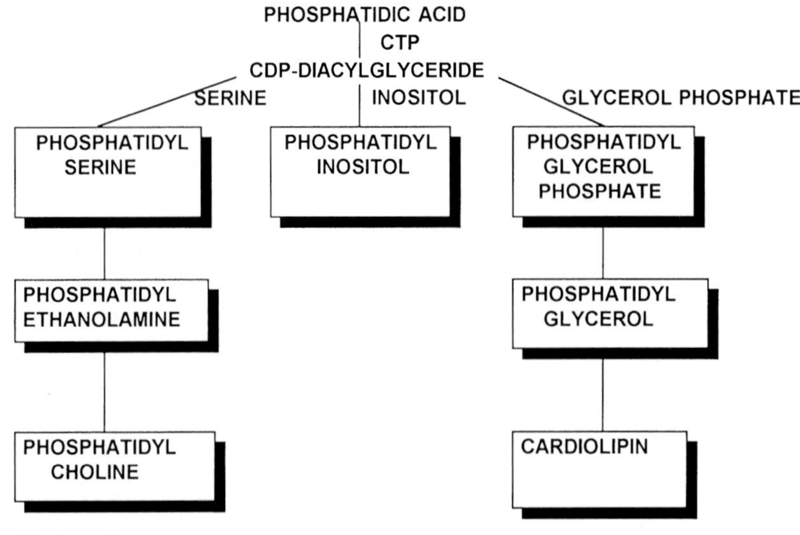

Fig. 6.8 Complex lipids.

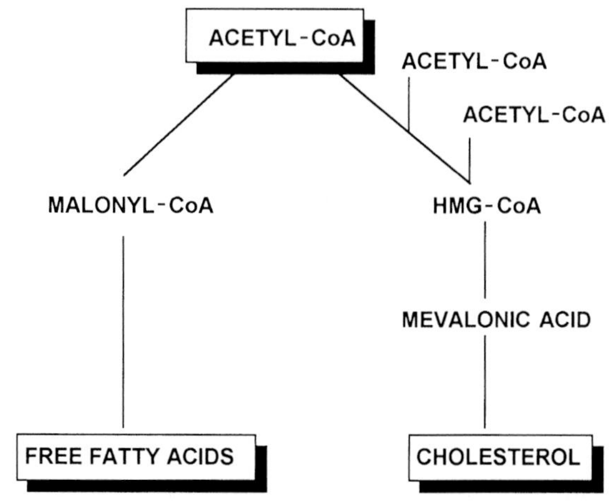

Fig. 6.9 Synthesis of sterols.

Complex lipids

The complex lipids are anabolically formed from fatty acids that are linked to become phosphatidic acid and then CDP-diacylglyceride. From there, the various complex structural membrane lipids are formed. The relative changes in content and type of complex gangliosides are noted above.

An important enzyme (choline acetyltransferase) in the synthesis of the complex lipids is responsible for choline uptake. This enzyme exists in two forms — the high-affinity type found in normal neurons that is responsible for the production of the neurotransmitter acetylcholine, and the low-affinity type that is involved in the general metabolism of choline throughout the brain. Malignant glioma cells have only neuronal high-affinity type, while the low-affinity type is lacking, again mimicking the situation found in fetal neuroectodermal cells.

Arachidonic acid metabolism (Fig. 6.10)

Arachidonic acid is derived from membrane phospholipids by the action of the enzyme phospholipase A_2, and is abundant in normal brain tissue. In high-grade astrocytomas there is a change in the arachidonic metabolite profile, and an overall increase in arachidonic metabolism corresponding to the degree of anaplasia of a tumor. The biochemical basis of the vasogenic brain edema seen around malignant brain neoplasms may be a tumor versus host event caused by arachidonic acid metabolites.

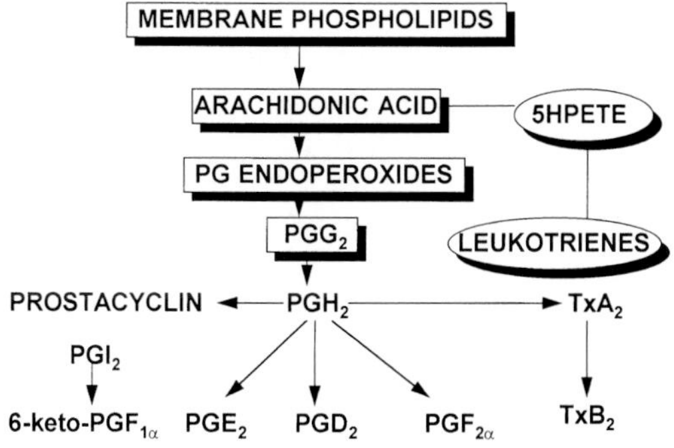

Fig. 6.10 Arachidonic acid metabolism.

Arachidonic acid may then be metabolized to either the prostaglandins, prostacyclins, or thromboxanes by the enzyme cyclo-oxygenase, or to the leukotrienes by the enzyme lipo-oxygenase.

Changes noted in malignant astrocytomas include a 250% increase in thromboxane B_2, an increase in TxA_2, and decreases in the levels of PGD_2 and PGI_2. TxA_2 may be associated with tumor initiation, while the prostaglandins PGD_2 and PGI_2 may have antineoplastic properties. PGE_2 is also produced in quantity, and acts as a suppressant of LAK cell cytokine production.

The leukotrienes are powerfully vasoactive hydroxylipids (LTB4) and peptolipids (LTC4, LTD4, and LTE4). LTC4 levels correlate well with the amount of vasogenic edema seen around malignant tumors. The leukotrienes are particularly interesting because selective intra-arterial infusion of tumor specific LTs may be used to open the blood-brain barrier around tumor and not whole brain (thus providing an advantage over mannitol), allowing for focal delivery of lipid-insoluble chemotherapeutic agents to tumor alone.

Lipid oxidation products

The lipid peroxides are formed as a result of the autooxidation of fatty acids after various cellular insults including radiation, nitrogen oxides, hydrogen peroxide, and the various products of oxygen metabolism (singlet oxygen, superoxide anion, hydroxy radical) that occur after the tissue oxidation seen after stress, trauma and ischemia. The cascade of events (voltage-dependent ionic channel opening, excitatory amino acid release (glutamate), N-methyl-d-aspartate (NMDA)-receptor channel opening, massive calcium influx and potassium release, and finally intracellular acidosis, lipolysis, proteolysis and protein phosphorylation) that causes free radical damage to cellular membranes has been studied in normal glia, but not in the glial tumors. Most tissues produce superoxide dismutase (SOD), an endogenous free radical 'scavenger' that provides protection from tissue peroxidation when it occurs.

The clinical importance of free radical production by tumors is based upon the fact that the mechanisms of therapeutic effect of radiation and some chemotherapeutic agents are the result of free radical damage to growing neoplastic cells. It is likely that the malignant neuroectodermal tumors may be relatively free of damage by lipid peroxidation products, especially when growing in an oxygen-free environment where peroxidation cannot occur. This, in part, accounts for the resistance of tumors to radiation. At the same time, the activity of SOD in malignant gliomas has been shown to be decreased in some animal models, suggesting that tumor cells might be particularly sensitive to free radical damage when induced by such agents as radiation sensitizers and high tissue oxygen tension.

Intracellular pH and tumor perfusion

Because a growing tumor is not homogeneous in terms of metabolic supply and phase of the growth cycle, differences in the metabolic state are reflected by local variations in intracellular pH. In regions with high blood flow and glucose supply, ATP levels are sufficient to maintain the intracellular sodium gradient through the Na^+/K^+-ATPase exchange pump, which in turn allows hydrogen ions generated by glycolysis to be transported out to the extracellular space by the Na^+/H^+ antiporter system. This creates a slightly alkaline intracellular pH despite the high concentrations of lactate produced during aerobic glycolysis. This is referred to as 'lactoalkalosis'. This has been demonstrated in animal models with in vitro techniques, and in vivo with phosphorous magnetic resonance spectroscopy (Yoshikazu et al 1992).

The opposite is true in areas of perfusion and substrate insufficiency. Here the sodium gradient is lost, cytotoxic edema ensues, and intracellular hydrogen ions accumulate with the failure of hydrogen ion exchange.

GROWTH FACTORS, THE PROTEIN KINASE CASCADE, AND MITOGENIC SIGNAL TRANSDUCTION

There is an integrated network of regulatory pathways, mediated by phosphorylation-dephosphorylating protein kinases, that allows diverse cellular events to be controlled by external physiological stimuli such as neuronal input, hormones and polypeptide growth factors (Westphal & Herrman 1989, Aaronson 1991, Boyle 1992, Wang 1992, Feng et al 1993). This receptor-driven 'second messenger' system has been expanded (Fig. 6.11) to include: (1) transmembrane proteins (surface receptor and ligand, membrane component, and intracellular tyrosine kinase catalytic portion), (2) the second messengers themselves (e.g. cyclic AMP, cGMP, ceramide, diacylglycerol, calcium (?)), that are formed respectively by (3) particular members from a group of catalytic proteins called the SH2-SH3 ('src homology' DNA domain regions 2 & 3) phosphotyrosine binding proteins, (4) the intracellular protein kinase cascade (including protein kinase A and C), and (5) the intranuclear cdc kinase/cyclin family of protein kinases that results in regulation of mitotic activity. The field of protein kinase study has exploded in the past few years as molecular biologic studies have revealed certain oncogenes (such as *ras, raf, erb* B, and the *src* DNA domain regions) to be specific for some of the protein kinases. The possibility of controlling tumor cell growth both through gene manipulation, anti-growth factor agents, and the inhibitors of the various protein kinases has been enticing.

- GROWTH FACTORS
- RECEPTORS (cell membrane, exterior)
- TYROSINE KINASES (cell membrane, interior)
- PROTEIN KINASE CASCADE (cytoplasm)
- cdc-Kinase/CYCLIN CYCLE (nucleus)

Fig. 6.11 Growth factors — how do they work?

Autocrine growth factors and their cell surface receptors

Growth factors are polypeptides that are normally involved in both enhancement and suppression of cell growth and proliferation. One of the strategies used by tumors involves 'autoinduction' or 'autocrine feedback', a process whereby a cell secretes a hormone-like substance that stimulates its own cell surface receptors for growth factors. Tumors thus escape the normal system of growth regulation both by this process and by the enhancement in the number of receptors found on the cell surface.

In neuroectodermal tumors, the cell surface receptors at the start of the mitogenic protein kinase cascade are responsive to a number of polypeptide growth factors, including platelet-derived growth factor (PDGF), epidermal growth factor (EGF), fibroblast growth factor, insulin-like growth factors (IGFs), and transforming growth factor (TGF).

EGF is a 53 amino acid polypeptide. The receptor for this growth factor is a membrane-bound 185 kilodalton glycoprotein. In the malignant glial cell this receptor is different both in structure and activity when compared to the normal cell. EGF is coded for by *erb-b*, an amplified oncogene.

TGF in its alpha form has been found to be a growth factor in malignant gliomas. It is a 50 amino acid polypeptide derived from a 160 amino acid precursor that is similar to that of EGF. In fact, TGF-α competes with EGF for the same tyrosine kinase cell surface receptor.

PDGF is produced by a number of cell types and is found in abundance around malignant glioma cells in the extracellular matrix. This protein exists as a dimer and exists in three states, α-A, β-A, and β-B. The beta chain of this protein is one of the tumor 'autocrine' products that causes increased proliferation of the tumor. It is encoded for by the *sis* oncogene.

There are two IGFs, IGF-I and IGF-II, present in normal brain. IGF-I is identical to somatomedin C, and is an effector of skeletal growth under the control of growth hormone. Its cell surface receptor is a tyrosine kinase in the adult. The level of IGF-I in and around astrocytoma cells increases with tumor grade and approaches that found around fetal cells. IGF-II is a fetal growth factor that plays a role during development. Its receptor lacks kinase activity. Both growth factors increase mitogenic activity in malignant glioma cell lines.

FGF is both a mitogen and a powerful angiogenesis factor. It is encoded for by a group of oncogenes that includes FGF-5, hst1-/K FGF, hst2/FGF-6 and int-2. RNA expression for the basic FGF gene has been found in almost 95% of glioma tissues. FGF belongs to a group of acidic proteins with a size of approximately 16 000 daltons. In normal cells FGF and TFG-βs act antagonistically as a biologic 'switch' that controls cell growth and differentiation. However, this antagonism appears to be lost in transformed cells.

Endothelin (ET) is a 21 amino acid polypeptide, originally derived from endothelial cells, that acts as an endogenous agonist for voltage-dependent calcium channels, and is vasoactive. It may function as a modulator of other growth factors by interfering with calcium metabolism, and does appear to have growth factor capabilities of its own.

Growth factor receptors and the tyrosine kinases

The various growth factor receptors have been divided into five classes (Figs 6.12, 6.13) according to their protein makeup and receptor size. Class I includes the EGF group of receptors and TGF, which are large (170–185 kD), and are rich in cysteine. Class II includes the insulin family of receptors. Class III includes the PDGF receptors, and class IV includes the FGF; both have immunoglobulin-like repeating units. Class V, again a cysteine-rich receptor, may include ET.

- Epidermal Growth Factor (EGF)
- Insulin-like Growth Factors (IGFs I–IV)
- Platelet-derived Growth Factor (PDGF)
- Transforming Growth Factor (TGF-α, -β)
- Endothelin (ET)

Fig. 6.12 Growth factors.

I	II	III	IV	V
RECEPTORS				
EGF	INSULIN	PDGF	FGF-1–4	Endothelin?
TGF-α	IGF	CSF-1		
	BDNF			
	NGF			
TYROSINE KINASES				
EGF-R	met	PDGfr	FGFR-1–4/flg,bek	eph
HER-2/neu	IGF-Ir	CSF-1R/fms		elk
erb B	Trk, trkB			eck
N-myc				
C-myc				

Fig. 6.13 Receptor classes I–IV.

Once a particular growth factor binds to its receptor, the dimerization of two, or many, receptors follows. The immediate result of receptor dimerization is the activation of the intracellular tyrosine kinase portion of the transmembranous receptor protein. The tyrosine kinase then becomes ready to start the relay of mitogenic signal transmission by picking up the high energy phosphate baton in a process called *autophosphorylation* (Fig. 6.14).

As there are five classes of cell surface receptors, there are five different types of intracellular tyrosine kinase, since each end of these complex membrane proteins is linked by a transmembranous portion. Each type of tyrosine kinase passes a high energy phosphate group to a tyrosine residue of a particular intracellular protein (via phosphorylation) referred to as *SH2-SH3 containing proteins*, to produce the various 'second messengers'. They all appear to share a common polypeptide sequence that is coded for by *src*-homology regions 2 or 3. Thus far, these enzymes include GTPase, cAMP kinase, phospholipase C, phosphoinositol kinase, the *src* family of protein tyrosine kinases, serine-threonine protein kinase, and (the feedback regulator of tyrosine kinase activity) phosphotyrosine phosphatase (Fig. 6.15).

Second messenger production by SH-kinases

Well-known 'second messengers' (Fig. 6.16) include cAMP, the ceramides, diacylglycerol and possibly calcium. In most cases the number of steps between messenger production and stimulation of the intranuclear cdc kinase/cyclin system (responsible for DNA synthesis and mitosis) is not known.

The protein kinase cascade and protein kinase C

The number of steps in the protein kinase cascade probably varies according to the receptor/tyrosine kinase

- Growth factor lands on its receptor
- Surface receptor/transmembrane portion/intracellular tyrosine kinase complex dimerization
- Autophosphorylation of tyrosine kinases
- Ready to pass high energy phosphate baton to the protein kinase cascade

Fig. 6.14 Receptor/tyrosine kinase activation.

- p21 ras-GTPase activating protein
- phospholipase C-γ
- phosphatidylinositol-3-kinase
- c-Raf serine-threonine protein kinase
- the src-family of protein kinases
- Negative feedback via phosphotyrosine phosphatase (a src kinase)

Fig. 6.15 The SH-2 family of proteins.

- cAMP
- cGMP
- ceramide
- diacylglycerol
- Calcium ?

Fig. 6.16 Second messengers or cofactors?

class at the start of each series. It is likely that the number varies between three and five or six. One series begins with the EGF receptor class, phosphorylation of the SH-2 enzyme phospholipase C-γ, enzymatic degradation of adjacent, cell-membrane-bound phosphatidylinositol to diacylglycerol and inositol triphosphate, 'second messenger' activation of protein kinase C by diacylglycerol and calcium channel opening by inositol triphosphate, and finally the phosphorylation of serine and threonine kinases in the kinase cascade.

The cAMP-dependent protein kinases exist in three isoenzyme forms. Type I is found in adults, type II in fetal cells, and type III in malignant astrocytomas. Only the type III isoenzyme (which is similar to the fetal type II) is active in the astrocytoma. It is activated both by cAMP and cGMP. In tumors cGMP appears to be a tumor promoter, while cAMP acts as a tumor inhibitor.

Each series of protein kinase cascade appears to involve the PKCs. There are two families of protein kinases, PKA and PKC. In neuroectodermal tumors the PKC isoenzymes appear to play a pivotal role in the kinase cascade toward cell growth. Some PKCs are phospholipid dependent and are activated by diacylglycerol in the presence of increased intracellular calcium. When activated they cause the phosphorylation of more distal members of the protein kinase cascade. The PKC family of isoenzymes occurs in three subtypes, α, β, and γ. Protein kinase C-α appears to play an important role in facilitating clonal expansion in transformed astrocytes.

The actual initiation of DNA synthesis and the regulation of mitosis occur under the control of the cdc2-family of protein kinases and their regulator molecules known as the cyclins. This cell cycle 'program' (Fig. 6.17) is turned on when the extranuclear mitogenic signals are received via the protein kinase cascade. The transducers of these signals are the cdc2/G1 cyclin complexes which, when phosphorylated, enter the program and commit the cell to mitosis and DNA synthesis. Cd2kinase/M-cyclins control the flow of mitosis, while the cdk/S-cyclins allow for the institution of DNA synthesis. In some tumors (e.g. hepatomas and parathyroid adenomas) the overexpression of cyclins may be responsible for the activation of the cell-cycle control 'program' in an unlimited way. Alternatively, the unrestrained activation of the G1 phase cyclins by the continual mitogenic stimulation of the autocrine protein kinase cascade is responsible for neuroepithelial tumor cell proliferation.

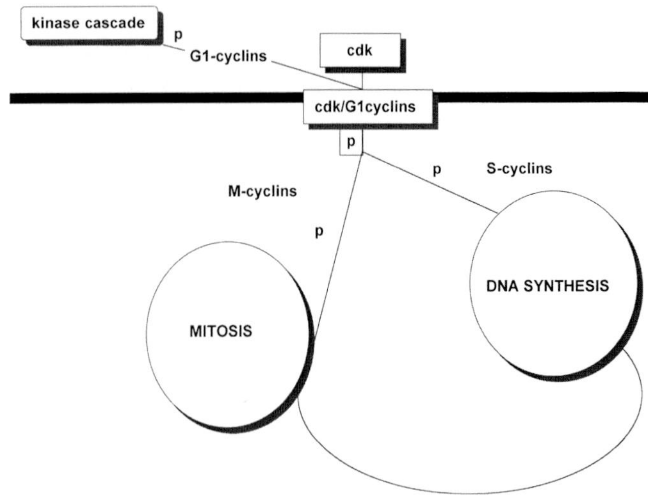

Fig. 6.17 Cell cycle 'program'.

Modulation of the growth factor/kinase/cyclin system (Fig. 6.18)

Control of tumor cell growth may occur in any of a number of ways, including calcium ion concentration control by inositol triphosphate or ET, antagonism between FGF and the TGF-βs, inhibitors of the 'start' message in the G1-cyclin system, and the various products produced by tumor suppressor genes.

DNA and RNA metabolism (Fig. 6.19)

In contrast to mature neuroectodermal cells with little or no nucleic acid metabolic activity, the synthesis of purines, pyrimidines, and subsequently RNA and DNA in

- ET controls cytoplasmic Ca^{++} Concentration
- FGF and TGF-βs are antagonists
- Phosphotyrosine phosphatase
- G1 cyclin inhibitors ?
- Suppressor gene products

Fig. 6.18 Modulation of growth.

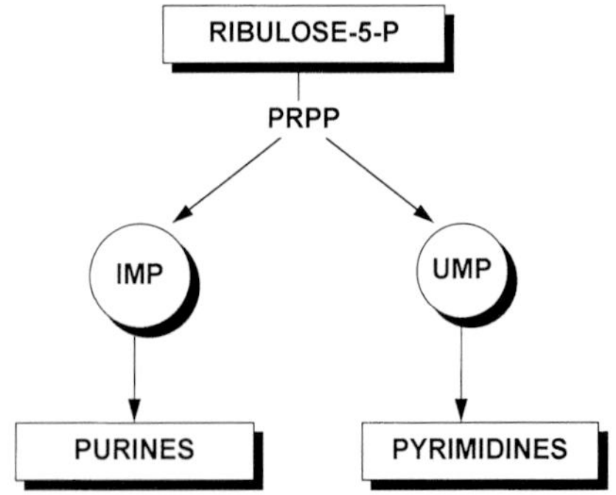

Fig. 6.19 DNA and RNA metabolism.

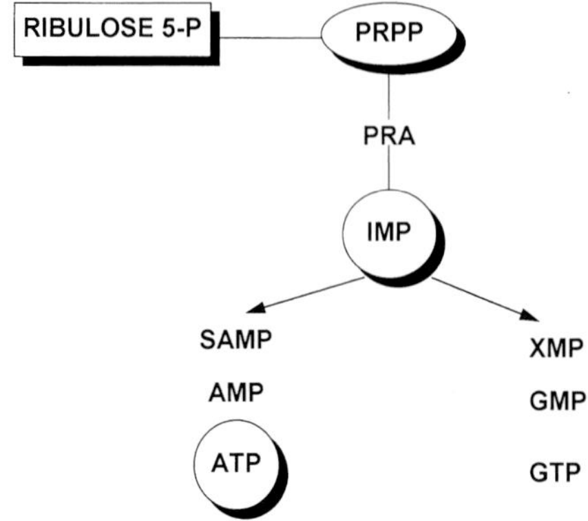

Fig. 6.20 Purine synthesis.

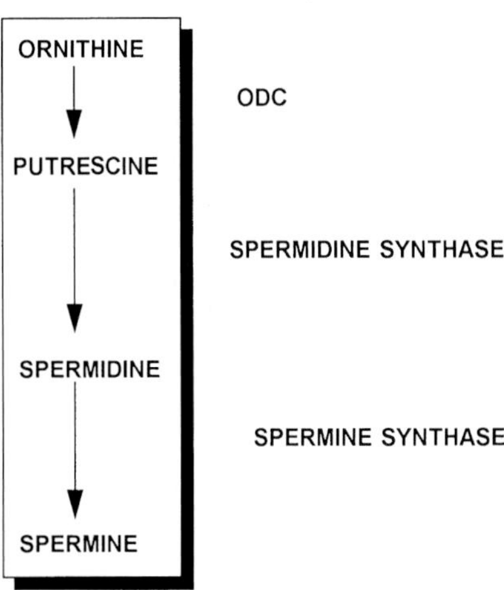

Fig. 6.21 Polyamines.

the malignant astrocytoma occurs at a brisk pace. This activity is initiated when phosphorylation of ribonucleotide synthetic enzymes occurs at the hand of the cdk-kinase/S-phase cyclin portion of the intranuclear kinase/cyclin system.

Purine synthesis (Fig. 6.20) begins with the transformation of phosphoribosylpyrophosphate (PRPP) into phosphoribosylamine (PRA) by the action of the enzyme amidotransferase. This is further metabolized to inosine monophosphate (IMP), the precursor of AMP (via adenylsuccinate synthetase) and GMP (via IMP dehydrogenase). These are then phosphorylated to become ATP and GTP respectively.

Pyrimidine synthesis of UTP and CTP begins with the formation of carbamoyl phosphate from glutamine and CO_2. The action of aspartate transcarbamoylase (a fetal enzyme in the brain) then results in the formation of carbamoylaspartic acid. Further steps lead to the synthesis of UMP, which is metabolized to UTP. UTP may then be converted to CTP.

There are 'salvage' pathways for nucleotide synthesis wherein DNA nuclease breakdown mononucleotides may be recycled after hydrolysis to free bases. These salvage enzymes (e.g. deoxycytidine deaminase) are also fetal-like in normal brain.

The enzyme RNA polymerase incorporates deoxyribonucleotides into RNA during transcription. Although present in normal glia, the RNA polymerase found in the astrocytoma is different in that it can be inhibited by rifampicin.

DNA polymerase activity has been measured by 3H-thymidine uptake, flow cytometry, and bromodeoxyuridine incorporation studies.

Polyamines (Fig. 6.21)

The polyamines are ubiquitous cellular compounds that mediate aggregation and catenation of nucleic acids during cellular division. Understandably, their production is increased in growing neoplastic cells. They are formed from the synthetic combination of amines. The amines are extracellular effectors and neurotransmitters, and include histamine, choline, ornithine, and the catecholamines norepinephrine and epinephrine. The polyamines include the compounds putrescine, spermine and spermidine. Putrescine is formed from ornithine by the rate-limiting enzyme ornithine decarboxylase (ODC), an enzyme that is active during embryonal life in the normal cell. ODC activity is highest in grade IV astrocytomas and in medulloblastomas. The enzyme adenosylmethionine decarboxylase (AMD) is indirectly involved with the conversion of putrescine to spermidine, and is found in adult tissue. It is found in astrocytomas, but is lacking in the more primitive medulloblastoma. Spermine and spermidine act as substrates for copper metabolism in the pyridoxine phosphate oxidase reaction.

TUMOR VERSUS HOST PRODUCTS

For a transformed cell to survive it must evade and overcome the elaborate defense machinery of the host, including the immune surveillance system, its cytokine system (macrophage-produced peptide tumor necrosis factor (TNF or cachectin), lymphocyte-produced interleukins, macrophage chemoattractant protein or granulocyte-macrophage colony stimulating factor GM-CSF, and various interferons), and the lysosymes of activated killer (LAK) cells. It must also lose the character of contact inhibition, acquire the ability to gather vascular supply to itself, and actively invade surrounding tissues.

Immune system suppressors (Couldwell et al 1991, Roszman et al 1991)

Another strategy utilized by human malignant gliomas is to secrete products that cause immunosuppression of the host, allowing the transformed cell to escape the immune surveillance system. This is particularly true for the cell-mediated axis of the immune system, where patients are noted to have depressed activity and production of killer cells, and suppression of cytotoxic T lymphocytes.

Lymphokine-activated killer (LAK) cells are produced as a host versus tumor response to most neoplasms. The lytic sequence of killer cells occurs in four stages including binding, programming for lysis, secretion of lytic factors, and the killer cell independent stage. Among the lytic factors produced are the cytokines. The production of the cytokine tumor necrosis factor (TNF), lymphotoxin (LT) and interferon-γ is markedly suppressed. One glioblastoma-derived T-cell suppressor factor is the 12.4 kilodalton polypeptide TGF-β2, which acts as a cell growth inhibitor in normal tissue (where TGF-βs are secreted as biologically inactive forms bound to TGF-β binding protein, latency associated peptide, and α_2-macroglobulin prior to becoming active). Another suppressor of cytokine production is PGE_2, a prostaglandin secreted by malignant glioma cells.

Tumor infiltration by macrophages has been observed in pathologic specimens. Granulocyte-macrophage colony stimulating factor (GM-CSF) has not been found in tumor cell lines in vivo, suggesting that another chemoattractant may be responsible, or they are produced by tumor infiltrating lymphocytes as cytokine.

Tumor angiogenesis factors

TGF-alpha and beta, and FGF, among their other functions, play a role in the neovascularization of malignant glioma in the presence of tumor-secreted endothelial cell chemotactic factor. Tumor angiogenesis appears to be a three-staged orchestrated event that includes (1) release of proteases and initial stimulation of endothelial cell production after secretion of endothelial cell chemotactic factor, (2) digestion of the vascular basement membrane and the release of angiogenesis factors, (3) vascular remodeling with endothelial cell proliferation and later growth of tumor cells toward the normal blood vessel. One of the endothelial cell growth factors is vascular permeability factor (VPF). It also increases microvascular permeability, possibly through the generation of nitric oxide (also called endothelial derived relaxing factor) from endothelial cell contained L-arginine. VPF may, along with the leukotrienes, be responsible for tumor induced brain edema.

Lytic enzymes

As the malignant neuroepithelial tumor grows it releases numerous lytic products from lysosomes that allow for effective tumor invasion of host tissues. These include lytic enzymes that are responsible for the frank digestion of surrounding structures, including vascular structures, cellular cytostructure, basement membranes, extracellular matrix, and other extracellular proteins. This strategy allows for the tumor to overcome barriers to neoplastic expansion, invading surrounding tissue planes and penetrating vascular walls as a preliminary stage to tumor angiogenesis. The proteins of cell surfaces and basement membranes include glycoproteins, and collagens, laminin and heparin sulfate proteoglycans respectively, while those of the extracellular matrix include mucopolysaccharides, collagen and fibronectin. The proteases secreted by malignant astrocytomas include α_1-antitrypsin, tissue plasminogen activator, urokinase, plasminogen activator, type IV collagenase, cysteine protease and other metalloproteases such as gelatinase. Not only do these enzymes disrupt the local host environment through digestion, but they also cause local hemorrhage and systemic coagulopathies.

The extracellular matrix (Rutka et al 1988)

The extracellular matrix represents the field of play for tumor cells. The ECM is composed of proteoglycans, glycoproteins, glycosaminoglycans, and collagens, and contains fibronectin, laminin and types I and IV collagen. These proteins are among the recognition molecules for fetal and transformed neuroepithelial cellular migration, adhesion and neoplastic invasion. The ECM is important for the expression and storage of growth factors, serving both as a chemotactic genetic induction medium and as a slow release reservoir.

Proteoglycans consist of a core protein and are modified by the addition of glycosaminoglycan side chains such as heparan sulfate and chondroitin sulfate. The proteoglycans interact with the actin-based cytoskeleton of the cell during migration and cellular adhesion.

Laminin is associated with the development and regeneration of neuroectodermal tissues, and is the preferred substrate for growth of astrocytes and neurons. It is secreted by injured cells along the basal lamina of the glia limitans and the perivascular space.

Fibronectin is found only in fetal and transformed tissue. It behaves as a latticework along which neuroectodermal cells travel during development as they migrate toward their preprogrammed destination in tissue. It is apparently produced by the transformed cell as well and may serve to direct the invasive radiation of tumor into the surrounding tissues.

Modification of the ECM by malignant gliomas occurs in two ways: (1) synthesis and secretion of glycosaminoglycans and primitive adhesion proteins, and (2) enzymatic digestion of various ECM proteins, including thrombolysis of blood products (e.g. fibrin) found in the ECM. This results in changes in cell–cell and cell–matrix interactions, chemotaxis, and cellular migration, as well as electrolyte, water and protein content. The major modification consists of changes in the concentrations of the glycosaminoglycans heparin sulfate and dermatan sulfate, and matrix degradation by proteases such as the metalloproteases (e.g. type IV collagenase). ECM modification aids the loss of contact inhibition that allows tumor cells to freely migrate and invade surrounding tissues.

Another major modification of the ECM that occurs is that of increased water secondary to vasogenic (leukotrienes) and possibly ionic edema (transmembrane ion exchange). This allows for the bulk flow of cellular products and of exchanged ions away from the tumor into the surrounding tissues.

pH levels, and tumor perfusion

Extracellular pH varies in a manner similar to intracellular pH depending upon the metabolic sufficiency of the tumor tissue as determined by local blood perfusion. When the cell is well supplied metabolically, the transmembrane hydrogen ion exchange system is functioning well to maintain an alkaline intracellular environment in the face of lactic acid production during aerobic glycolysis. The resultant decrease in extracellular pH has been responsible for some confusion in the literature, leading some researchers to conclude that high intracellular lactate is responsible for 'damaging' tumor tissue acidosis. (Interestingly, the same conclusion has been made for ischemic tissue, leading anesthesiologists to avoid glucose solutions during surgery with potential for brain ischemia.)

SPECIFIC TUMORS

Meningioma (Schrell et al 1990)

Meningiomas are mesodermal tumors that arise from arachnoid cap cells located in the pachionian granulations of the meninges. That meningiomas are more prevalent in females is well known. As in the fibroid tumor of the uterus, cell surface receptors for both estrogen and progesterone are present. A high percentage of meningiomas are progesterone receptor positive even in the absence of estrogen receptors. The relationship between meningioma cell growth and these receptors has been studied in vitro. Clinical control of meningioma growth has not yet been convincingly demonstrated with anti-progesterone compounds.

While the thromboxanes are present in increased quantities in malignant gliomas, the meningiomas have lower levels of TxA_2 and elevated levels of PGI_2 and PGD_2.

Pineal tumors

The pineocyte is a neuroectodermally derived cell that ontologically develops along its own path. The mature cell is endocrine-like in that it is aligned around a duct and has short cellular extensions containing processes that are seen on silver staining. The pineal gland is the organ responsible for the day/night modulation of the hypothalamic axis hormones. In lower animals the pineal acts as the 'third' eye and is responsible for the translation of day/night and seasonal information, and in turn is responsible for variations in behavior, circadian changes in hormonal levels, migration, hibernation, and estrus cycles. It receives information about ambient light levels by way of a circuitous route that includes the retina — optic nerve and tract — super optic nucleus — hypothalamus — sympathetic nervous system — nervii conari — pineal gland. This information is then processed by the pineal gland, acting as a neuroendocrine transducer, transforming light information into melatonin output. Melatonin is produced from the tryptophan metabolite N-acetylserotonin by the enzyme hydroxy-O-methyl transferase (HIOMT), an enzyme that is unique to the pineal gland. Melatonin acts as a neural modulating hormone, traveling by both CSF and hematogenous routes. It plays a significant role in regulation of the hypothalamic-pituitary-hormonal axis, control of the sleep-wake cycle, and as a modulator of circadian rhythms in the human.

The pineal region tumors of pineocyte origin are probably the pineocytoma and pineoblastoma. The teratomas, germinomas, and astrocytomas arise from other cell types. HIOMT might serve as a cytologic marker for the pineal origin tumors. Interestingly, these tumors produce lower than normal levels of melatonin, and thus its use as an indicator of tumor growth is not of value.

PNET and medulloblastoma

The primitive neuroectodermal tumors appear to have in common with the malignant glial series of tumors the utilization of primitive enzyme and structural systems to gain advantage over the host. Of interest is the observation that these neoplasms may mature along neoplastic lines, mimicking normal ontogeny. The medulloblastoma, for example, may mature into both astrocytoma and neuronal cell tumor. It may also express both glial and neuronal cytoskeleton proteins prior to maturation.

Neurocytoma (primary cerebral neuroblastoma)

Primitive neural crest cells, called neuroblasts, are thought to be the origin of the neurocytoma of the brain, and the peripheral neuroblastoma. As primitive cells, they retain the potential for maturation along neuronal cell lines, producing one of the various neurotransmitters according to the direction of maturation of a particular neuroblast. Peripheral neuroblastomas typically produce norepinephrine. Studies done in primary cerebral neuroblastoma have disclosed production of serotonin in at least one case, and dopamine in another.

REFERENCES

Aaronson S A 1991 Growth factors and cancer. Science 254: 1146–1153

Boyle W J 1992 Growth factors and tyrosine kinase receptors during development and cancer. Current Opinion in Oncology 4: 156–162

Braverman S, Helson C, Abraham N, Helson L 1993 Sequential addition of deferoxamine and hemin inhibits glioma tumor cell growth. International Journal of Oncology 2: 97–103

Brooks D J 1990 In vivo metabolism of human cerebral tumors. In: Primary malignant brain tumors. Johns Hopkins University Press, Baltimore, pp 122–134

Couldwell W T, de Tribolet N, Antel J P et al 1992 Adhesion molecules and malignant glioma: implications for tumorigenesis. Journal of Neurosurgery 76: 782–791

Couldwell W T, Dore-Duffy P, Apuzzo M L et al 1991 Malignant glioma modulation of immune function: relative contribution of different soluble factors. Journal of Neuroimmunology 33: 89–96

Feng G, Hui C, Pawson T 1993 SH2-containing phosphotyrosine phosphatase as a target of protein-tyrosine kinases. Science 259: 1607–1614

Mangiardi J R, Yodice P 1990 Metabolism of the malignant astrocytoma. Neurosurgery 26: 1–19

Roszman T, Elliott L, Brooks W 1991 Modulation of T-cell function by gliomas. Immunology Today 12: 370–374

Rutka J T, Apodaca G, Stern R 1988 The extracellular matrix of the central and peripheral nervous systems: structure and function. Journal of Neurosurgery 69: 155–165

Schrell U M H, Adams E F, Fahlbusch R et al 1990 Hormonal dependency of cerebral meningiomas. Journal of Neurosurgery 73: 743–755

Sutton L N, Wang Z, Gusnard D et al 1992 Proton magnetic spectroscopy of pediatric brain tumors. Neurosurgery 31: 195–202

Victor J V, Wolf A 1937 Metabolism of brain tumors. Proceedings of the Association for Research into Nervous and Mental Disorders 16: 44–58

Wang Y J J 1992 Oncoprotein phosphorylation and cell cycle control. Biochemica et Biophysica Acta 1114: 179–192

Warburg O 1930 The metabolism of tumors. Arnold Constable, London, pp 75–327

Westphal M, Herrman H D 1989 Growth factor biology and oncogene activation in human gliomas and their implications for specific therapeutic concepts. Neurosurgery 25: 681–694

Yoshikazu O, Kloiber O, Konstantin H 1992 Regional metabolism in experimental brain tumors in cats: relationship with acid/base, water, and electrolyte homeostasis. Journal of Neurosurgery 31: 917–926

7. Immunobiology of brain tumors and implications for immunotherapy

Yutaka Sawamura Nicolas de Tribolet

INTRODUCTION

Although new surgical techniques allow a more radical elimination of a brain tumor mass, infiltrating tumor cells remain the most important source of tumor recurrence. These disseminated cells may be particularly appropriate targets for immunotherapy (Lampson et al 1992). In spite of copious efforts in many institutes, studies of immunotherapy for brain tumors are still in the early stages of development. Thus far, preliminary clinical trials have not yielded convincing therapeutic benefit.

Host immunity and tumor biology are important cofactors in brain tumor immunotherapy. Much of the research on brain tumor immunobiology has centered upon evaluation of tumor cell antigenicity and cell-mediated immune responses. Research using monoclonal antibodies to determine the presence of brain-tumor associated antigens and of cytokine interactions between the host immune system and brain tumors is producing evidence. It should be noted that a host versus tumor reaction occurs at the site of tumor growth and that the cell-mediated immune system may have a central role for possible control of neoplastic growth. There has also been, however, an increasing awareness of the ways in which a brain tumor could evade host immune reactions.

During the past decade, new immunotherapeutic approaches have become available as a result of developments in genetic engineering and cell culture technology. Appropriate monoclonal antibodies may be used as carriers for chemotherapeutic and radiotherapeutic agents. The cellular immune system can be manipulated by either administration of exogenous biological response modifiers or by the transfer of activated killer lymphocytes.

The human immune system is, however, extremely complex, multi-faceted and highly specific. The unique nature of the host–tumor relationship in each individual patient makes the development and clinical study of immunotherapy very difficult. The response of animals to chemotherapy, radiation and surgery is generally predictive of their effect in human patients; this is nevertheless not the case with immunotherapy. Many immunotherapeutic agents are inactive in other species, and animal models do not mimic the biology of human patients with cancer (Osband & Ross 1990). Advances in immunotherapy especially require accumulation of clinical data derived from patients who are treated with the immunotherapy.

Nevertheless the reported evidence from animal models and clinical experience has indicated that immunotherapy will have its greatest effect in healthy patients with the smallest tumor burden, or in an adjuvant setting where there is a high likelihood of tumor recurrence but no evident disease at the time of treatment. Clinical studies of immunotherapy in end-stage patients with large tumor burdens carry the danger of yielding false-negative results for therapeutic agents that might be active if they were tried in the proper clinical setting (Osband & Ross 1990).

In this chapter, ideas for potential therapeutic manipulation of host-tumor immune interactions will be reviewed. We are including a brief introduction describing some of the basic concepts of immunology, which are also illustrated in Figure 7.1.

One function of the immune system is to recognize foreign structures and trigger a series of reactions which eventually lead to their elimination. Effector function must therefore be tightly linked to recognition mechanisms in order to be focused on specific target molecules on foreign, infected or transformed cells and to avoid damage to normal cells. Antigen presenting cells (APC) possess the capacity to mediate antigen capture and processing as well as to secrete monokines such as interleukin 1 (IL-1) and tumor necrosis factor (TNF). IL-1 stimulates lymphokine release from T cells and stimulates IL-2 receptor expression on T cells. TNF modulates the expression of major histocompatibility complex (MHC) class I antigens and is capable of inducing necrosis of cells including tumor cells.

T cells recognize an antigen only after the antigen is

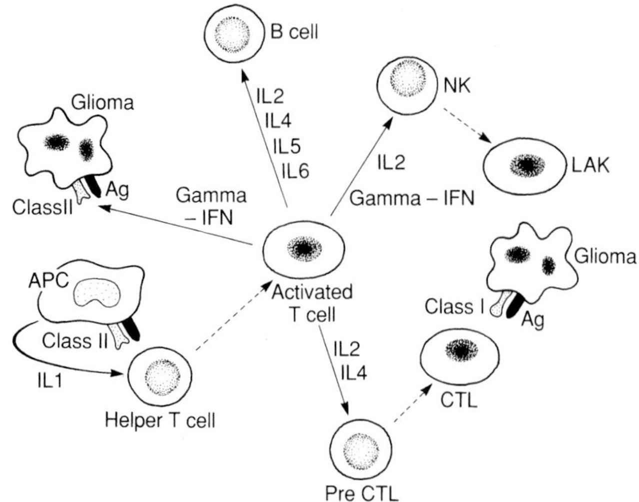

Fig. 7.1 Interaction of immunocompetent cells and cytokines.

displayed on the surface of an APC in physical association with a MHC class II molecule. Activated T cells, in particular helper T cells, synthesize and secrete a number of lymphokines including IL-2, IL-3, IL-4, IL-5 and interferon-γ (IFN-γ) which can stimulate B cells as well as effector T cells. As a consequence of this activation, specific effector function of either T cells or B cells can be induced and amplified. Although antigens trigger only certain T and B cells by interacting with their surface antigen receptor and immunoglobulin, respectively, the lymphokines produced in response to activation are independent of the specific antigen initiating the immune response. IL-2 binds to specific receptors on activated T and B cells, giving rise to the expansion of the activated clone. Finally antigen-specific cytotoxic T lymphocytes (CTL) recognize and kill the target tumor cells expressing the antigen in association with MHC class I molecules.

On the other hand it has become evident in recent years that some effector functions of killer lymphocytes are non-specific. For example, natural killer (NK) cells display cytotoxicity toward certain tumor cell types independently of MHC expression, and lymphokine activated killer (LAK) cells, generated by culturing peripheral blood lymphocytes with IL-2, are non-antigen-specific killer cells supposedly capable of killing tumor targets in a non-MHC-restricted manner. NK cells normally exist in the organism whereas LAK cells can only be generated in vitro or in vivo by stimulation with high doses of IL-2. The mechanisms by which LAK cells mediate cytotoxicity are still poorly understood.

THE IMMUNE SYSTEM IN THE CNS (CENTRAL NERVOUS SYSTEM)

There is no lymphatic system in the CNS, as is the case in the anterior chamber of the eye, the thyroid and the testicle. There are, however, resting mononuclear cells called resident microglia. Microglia appear to arise from monocytes in the developing brain (Thomas 1992). Microglia in the brain express some macrophage markers such as OX-42 and are phagocytic in culture. In normal adult brain tissue, ramified microglia with down-regulated macrophage functional properties appear to activate and convert into active macrophages/microglia (Thomas 1992). It has been suggested that the activated microglia in the CNS may function in antigen presentation and lymphocyte activation for CNS immune responses similar to tissue macrophages in other organs. The expression of MHC (major histocompatibility complex) class I and class II antigens has also been demonstrated on microglia. Furthermore they can secrete various factors such as interferon-γ, TNF-α (tumor necrosis factor α), IL-1 (interleukin 1), IL-6, and GM-CSF (granulocyte-macrophage colony stimulating factor). IL-3 and GM-CSF are likely to be potent growth factors for microglia. Microglia derived from brain cortex of mice were shown to lyse human tumor cell lines expressing EGF (epidermal growth factor) receptors in the presence of a monoclonal anti-EGF receptor antibody (MAb 425) (Sutter et al 1991).

Histologically, there is an accumulation of monocyte/macrophage lineage cells which may come from the blood circulation, but the number and function of microglia in malignant brain tumors is still unknown.

In normal brain vessels, adjacent endothelial cells are joined by continuous bands of tight junctions, no fenestrations are present, and the density of endothelial vesicles is very low. These vascular structures, in combination with astrocytes, constitute the blood-brain barrier which shields the brain to a certain extent from systemic humoral and cellular immunity. Immunoglobulins and cytokines such as IL-2, TNF or interferons would not be expected to effectively permeate the blood-brain barrier. As a result of tumor-induced endothelial changes, however, the blood vessels lose their blood-brain barrier properties and become abnormal. The large pores in the altered vascular walls provide a pathway both for extravasation of larger molecules, including serum proteins, and conversely for many factors secreted by tumor cells, except for a part of the tumor periphery where the barrier is intact.

BRAIN TUMOR IMMUNOBIOLOGY

There are two sorts of cellular immune responses against neoplastic cells, i.e. MHC-restricted and non-MHC-restricted responses.

An efficient MHC-restricted cellular immune response against brain tumors requires that: (1) antigenic determinants are preferentially expressed on tumor cells; (2) these antigens must bind MHC molecules; (3) peripheral T cells must recognize the presented antigens; (4) presented antigens must be able to stimulate both helper T-cell and cytotoxic T-cell responses; and (5) effector cells must reach the tumor site and cause tumor destruction (Lotze & Finn 1990). Clearly, therefore, antigen presentation of tumor cells recognized by host immune competent cells is the first critical issue of brain tumor immunology.

Tumor-associated antigens

The central question in tumor immunology is whether tumor cells demonstrate differences from their normal cellular counterparts that can be recognized by the host immune system. A number of tumor-associated antigens on brain tumor cells which are, however, mostly shared by histogenetically related tumors, have been found and characterized (Carrel et al 1982, de Muralt et al 1985, Fischer et al 1988). Neuroectodermal antigens, for instance Mel-14 antigen, form a major component of the surface antigens found on glioma cells. They have been detected on gliomas, melanomas, and neuroblastomas as well as fetal brain cells and endothelial cells within gliomas. Glial tumor-associated antigens, such as tenascin, are primarily displayed on gliomas. Monoclonal antibodies directed to the glial antigens have some additional minor specificity for other non-neuroectodermal tissues and reactive astrocytes; however, the immunogenicity of these brain tumor associated antigens is weak in humans.

The coexpression of certain MHC class II antigens (particularly HLA-DR) with tumor-associated antigens is necessary to elicit an MHC-restricted immune response; a putative tumor antigen can be immunogenic only if it is recognized together with the self MHC molecule by antigen presenting cells. MHC class I (particularly HLA-A) expression is required on the target cells for the lytic action of effector cells to take place. Although normal resting brain astrocytes do not exhibit MHC class II antigens, it is noteworthy that some activated astrocytes and astrocytic tumor cells as well as hyperplastic tumor endothelial cells can express HLA-DR (de Tribolet et al 1984, Frank et al 1986). MHC class II and class I expression can be induced and enhanced by interferon-γ or TNF on a number of glioma cell lines. In contrast, TGF-β_2 (transforming growth factor β_2) secreted by glioma cells produces a partial but significant decrease of constitutive and interferon-γ-induced HLA-DR antigen expression on glioma cells.

Astrocytic tumor cells express CD10 (CALLA — common acute lymphocytic leukemia antigen) and CD57 antigens. The expression of these lymphoid differentiation antigens as well as the secretion of some cytokines by glioma cells implicates common functional properties shared by immune competent cells and glial cells. Recently it has been found that CD10 is a membrane-bound enzyme identical to neutral endopeptidase (Monod et al 1992) which can catabolize the IL-1 molecule.

The immune defense system recognizes cell abnormalities at the molecular level as non-self determinants. Recently, some mutant molecules produced by glial tumor cells have been found, e.g. mutant (altered) p53 tumor suppressor gene product and mutant EGF receptor. Expression of the mutant p53 protein in gliomas is detectable by murine monoclonal antibodies in immunohistology and is highly positive in astrocytic cells (Bruner et al 1991). Growth factor receptors are altered and/or growth factors themselves are abnormally produced. The most commonly amplified cellular oncogene in glioblastomas is the EGF receptor gene, which is amplified in about one third of glioblastomas (Fullar & Bigner 1992). The EGF receptor gene has been shown to be structurally altered in a number of glioblastomas (Libermann et al 1985). Murine antibodies specific for the mutant EGF receptor have been produced. It is not yet clear whether these mutant proteins can act as an immunogenic tumor-specific antigen.

It must be considered, however, that the antigenicity and immunogenicity of malignant brain tumors is low, or might even be absent. Consequently, they may not always be susceptible to attack by immune-based therapies.

Humoral immune response

The presence of limited anti-glioma activity was reported within the sera of a small number of patients harboring gliomas. Some patients with malignant gliomas have immune complexes in their sera; the survival of these patients was reported to be shorter than that observed in those who did not have such complexes. Furthermore, elevated immunoglobulin levels in the cerebrospinal fluid in certain patients with either malignant or benign gliomas were reported. In certain glioma tissues populations of B cells are present, but their ability to produce anti-glioma antibodies capable of participating in complement-dependent or antibody-dependent cell-mediated cytotoxic responses is doubtful. It is of interest to mention that IL-6, which promotes immunoglobulin production by activated B cells, can be secreted by glioma cells (van Meir et al 1990) and brain macrophages in vivo.

Circulating antibodies specific for p53 protein have been found in the sera of lung and breast cancer patients (Davidoff et al 1992, Winter et al 1992). Since mutation and overexpression of the p53 gene have also been demonstrated in human gliomas, the development of anti-p53 antibodies may represent an interesting model system for studying humoral immune responses against mutant oncogene products (Winter et al 1992) in brain tumor patients.

Monoclonal antibodies

A monoclonal antibody which is specific for one single

structure on malignant brain tumors can be produced in large quantities either from ascites or in vitro culture of murine hybridoma with a high degree of purity. Brain tumor-associated antigens detected by practically available monoclonal antibodies, which have been well characterized, are often a part of 'self' antigens rather than tumor-specific antigens; most monoclonal antibodies against brain tumors cross-react with some normal tissues. This does not matter from an immunotherapeutic point of view if a glioma antigen, which may exhibit therapeutically functional specificity, is also expressed by other tumors, since distinction from the host's normal tissue is the essential requirement.

Monoclonal antibody 81C6 defines tenascin, the glioma mesenchymal extracellular matrix (GMEM) antigen, on the basement membrane of glioblastomas and is associated with the proliferative endothelium of hyperplastic vessels (Lee et al 1988, Schuster et al 1991). Tenascin is present on most glioma and fibroblast cell lines, some human cancer cell lines, fetal and adult spleen, liver, adult kidney and mesenchymal cells, but not on normal adult brain. UJ13A recognizes all neuroectodermal tumors except melanomas and also reacts with fetal brain, peripheral nerves, adrenal medulla, adult thyroid epithelium, fetal kidney tubules, and primary cultures of fetal myoblasts. Me1-14 reacts with an antigen found on a large number of melanoma cell lines and other neuroectodermal tumors including gliomas. Cross-reactivity is not detected with the normal adult tissues tested.

Murine antibodies specific for mutant proteins produced by human neoplastic cells have been produced and provide stimulating new potential avenues for tumor targeting therapy (Fullar & Bigner 1992). For instance, the monoclonal antibody 425 binds to an abnormal protein determinant on the external domain of the EGF receptor.

A variety of potentially toxic molecules can be linked to these monoclonal antibodies. Immunotoxins comprise a new class of cell-type specific cytotoxic heteroconjugates which consist of a monoclonal antibody linked to a protein toxin such as the A chain of ricin (Johnson et al 1989). Another possibility is the antibody-drug conjugate aiming at high drug delivery to the target cells and reducing the adverse effects on normal cells. Monoclonal antibodies can also act as carriers for radionuclides. This method has been widely investigated and may be the most promising among monoclonal-antibody directed therapies for brain tumor patients (Wikstrand et al 1987, Lee et al 1988). Antibody-carrying radionuclides, as opposed to antibody-carrying toxins or chemotherapeutic agents, can destroy antigen-negative cells adjacent to antigen-positive cells binding the antibody.

The major obstacles inherent in current monoclonal antibody therapy are cross-reactivity with normal tissues, impermeability of the blood-brain barrier, and immunogenicity of murine-derived monoclonal antibodies (Moseley et al 1992).

After administration to a patient, the monoclonal antibody is diluted in the circulating blood, where it can bind to normal cells with cross-reactivity and to pre-existing human anti-mouse antibodies (antiglobulin response). After a second infusion of the monoclonal antibody the level of circulating anti-mouse antibody is much higher and there is an increased risk of anaphylactic reaction. Some tumor-associated antigens are shed from the tumor in the blood. Furthermore, in certain cases the radiolabeled antibody can be trapped rapidly in the reticuloendothelial system, especially in the liver, therefore reducing the tumor uptake.

To resolve the problem inherent in using murine monoclonal antibodies, there has been an effort to develop human monoclonal antibodies. A human monoclonal antibody, CLN-IgG, was produced from a human-human hybridoma derived from lymphocytes of a patient with cervical carcinoma. CLN-IgG reacts with various human glioma cells, but not with normal adult brain tissue. Antigen recognized by CLN-IgG was rarely detected in tumor cyst fluid, sera, or cerebrospinal fluid of glioma patients (Kokunai et al 1990).

Another point to be taken into consideration is that the blood–tumor tissue transport rate is influenced by the regional blood flow, the vascular permeability of the substance, the extent of vascularization, arterio-venous shunts, and the extracellular fluid circulation. In particular, the delivery of the antibody could be partially or completely blocked by a low blood flow. Since whole immunoglobulin crosses capillary passively, the smaller size of antibody fragments may enter the tumor more efficiently. A higher specific localization in the tumor tissue by the $F(ab')_2$ fragments of monoclonal antibody and a substantially higher radiation dose to the tumor than to normal tissue have been demonstrated in rodent models (Colapinto et al 1988).

Prior to the delivery of a therapeutic dose of isotopes conjugated with monoclonal antibody, imaging of patients for dosimetry is of critical importance (Foon 1989). It has been demonstrated that tumor samples obtained at operation after injection of isotope-labeled monoclonal antibody contained levels of radioactivity which were clearly insufficient for therapeutic use (Moseley et al 1987, Behnke et al 1988). This finding in preclinical studies has led some to question the feasibility of using radiolabeled monoclonal antibodies for tumor therapy, reasoning that adequate radiation doses cannot be achieved in the tumor without unacceptable radiation exposure to normal tissues.

Despite the limitations mentioned above, several experimental clinical trials have been attempted for brain tumor patients (Brady et al 1988). The efficacy of these trials is questionable.

An attractive way of using monoclonal antibody for antibody-guided irradiation is via the intrathecal route for neoplastic meningitis. Under these conditions the neoplastic cells grow in the subarachnoid space, thus being more accessible to monoclonal antibody than those in the solid mass. Some remissions using the intrathecal application of radiolabeled monoclonal antibodies in patients who suffered from neoplastic meningitis secondary to pineal tumors or melanomas have been reported (Coakham et al 1988). The major toxicity associated with the intrathecal administration of radio-labeled monoclonal antibodies was bone-marrow suppression (Moseley et al 1992). The human monoclonal antibody, CLN-IgG, has also been under early clinical trial by intracranial administration.

Cell-mediated immune response

It has been repeatedly emphasized that the systemic cellular immune response in patients with a malignant brain tumor is significantly depressed according to the following evidence: impaired blastogenic response of peripheral blood lymphocytes (PBL), inhibitory effect of patients' sera on T-cell responsiveness to mitogens, suppressed NK (natural killer) cell activity, reduced IL-2 production and IL-2 receptor expression of mitogen-stimulated T cells.

It should be stated that a reaction of the host immune system against tumor tissue occurs predominantly at the site of tumor growth. Human brain tumors show variable levels of leukocyte infiltration at the time of biopsy or autopsy (Rossi et al 1989). Although controversial, a number of reports have suggested that an increasing degree of lymphocyte infiltration in brain neoplasms may have some relevance to a better prognosis (Paine et al 1986). Mononuclear cell infiltration is most pronounced at the tumor periphery. It has recently been reported that leukocytes may have access to disseminating tumor cells within the brain parenchyma (Lampson et al 1992).

The mononuclear cells found in malignant brain tumor tissue have been identified as being mostly T cells with a predominance of the CD8+ subset and macrophages. NK-cell and B-cell infiltrations have also been reported.

An adhesion molecule (ICAM-1 — intercellular adhesion molecule 1) is expressed on intratumoral endothelial cells and can be enhanced by interferon-γ, IL-1, or TNF (Kuppner et al 1990). T cells have the cell surface receptor (LFA-1 — lymphocyte associated antigen 1) for ICAM-1. An adhesion between the T cells and the brain endothelial cells can be induced. The T cells may then pass through the altered blood-brain barrier into tumor tissue. In the brain parenchyma, inflammatory cells may accumulate in response to secondary or disseminated signals, rather than recognition of the tumor cells per se (Stewart et al 1988). IL-8, a chemoattractant for T cells as well as neutrophils, may lead the lymphocyte infiltration. IL-8 is produced by glioma cells and is found in glioma tissue and cerebrospinal fluid of patients (van Meir et al 1992).

A novel chemotactic factor (MCP-1 — human monocyte chemoattractant protein 1), recently characterized as a secretory product of glioblastoma cells (Yoshimura et al 1991), may attract monocytes from the blood circulation. Within the tumor tissue, blood-derived monocytes and brain microglia may increase in cell numbers as a result of tumor-derived growth factors such as GM-CSF (Frei et al 1992).

A tumor antigen in combination with products of the MHC may stimulate T cells through specific T-cell receptors. This important question concerning the immunogenicity of brain-tumor antigens recognized by T cells has yet to be resolved. Recently the predominant role of particular T-cell receptors in human tumor immunity was reported, for instance Vα2 predominantly expressed by anti-melanoma T-cell clones. Some specific T-cell populations may be directed to antigenic determinants in melanoma cells (Nitta et al 1992). If so, certain human cancer cells may express the specific antigen that stimulates T lymphocytes expressing a limited repertoire of T-cell receptors. A predominant expression of the Vα2 T-cell receptor gene in glioma-infiltrating lymphocytes has also been observed (Nitta et al 1992).

On the other hand, lymphoid cells in a population of CD3– or CD3+ lymphocytes can mediate tumor lysis in a non-MHC-restricted manner. The target molecule(s) on brain tumor cells for this non-MHC-restricted lysis are unknown. Binding of immune complexes on Fc receptors in association with various lymphokine messages may generate cytotoxicity of the effector lymphocytes. It has been demonstrated that interleukin 2 can activate peripheral blood lymphocytes obtained from glioma patients to lyse their autologous glioma cells in vitro (Jacobs et al 1986). These effector cells are known as LAK (lymphokine-activated killer) cells.

Maturation and activation of the glioma-derived tumor-infiltrating lymphocytes (TILs) can be generated after in vitro exposure to IL-2. The in vitro expanded TILs are capable of killing autologous glioma cells and additionally a panel of human cancer cell lines (Miescher et al 1988, Sawamura et al 1989a). However lymphocyte infiltration in glial tumors is scarce and the number of TIL isolated from gliomas is extremely low, in comparison with that found in metastatic brain tumors or in cancers of other organs. Furthermore, T cells isolated from brain tumors have been shown to be small, nonblastic and negative for activation antigens. The suppression of glioma-infiltrating precursors by the glioma cells in situ is more profound than that of TIL in the cancers of other organs.

Among various types of primary brain tumors, intracranial germinoma in particular, may give us an example of the cellular immune reaction against brain neoplasms. It is histologically characterized by the presence of two types of cells: large neoplastic cells and small lymphoid cells. This tumor shows varying amounts of rich lymphocytic infiltration, with or without a granulomatous reaction in the stroma. It has been suggested that there is an association between this stromal reaction and a favorable prognosis. T cells (CD3+CD4+ or CD3+CD8+) are the predominant cell type of lymphoid cells. Germinoma-derived lymphocytes are very responsive to IL-2 stimulation in vitro, in contrast to glioma-derived lymphocytes, showing marked DNA synthesis, and are able to lyse a panel of NK-resistant target cells (Sawamura et al 1989b).

Adoptive immunotherapy

Various immune effectors have been identified with a potential to inhibit tumor cell growth. These include CTLs, NK cells, LAK cells (lymphokine-activated killer cells), and macrophages, which can acquire nonspecific tumoricidal activity upon activation or kill tumor cells by an antibody-dependent mechanism (Herberman 1985, Khavari 1987, Rosenberg 1988, Tepper et al 1989).

As mentioned above, glioma patients' PBL (peripheral blood lymphocytes) can be activated by in vitro culture in the presence of IL-2 (Jacobs et al 1986). The activated PBL, so-called LAK cells, become capable of killing autologous glioma cells and allogeneic glioma cells. All normal brain cells are presumably LAK-resistant. The antitumor effector cells in LAK-cell culture are reported to be large granular lymphocytes. For clinical application, at least 10^9 up to 10^{11} LAK cells are required for local immunotherapy against malignant brain tumors. LAK cells are transferred to patients by a direct injection into residual tumor tissue during a craniotomy or administered into the tumor cavity post-operatively through a subcutaneous reservoir.

Although glioma patients are known to have an impaired cell-mediated immune response, it is possible to activate PBL derived from patients who have been treated by chemotherapy, irradiation or corticosteroid administration after surgery (McVicar et al 1992).

Adoptive immunotherapy, where LAK cells are transferred to patients with malignant brain tumors in combination with IL-2, has been reported in several preliminary clinical trials (Yoshida et al 1988, Barba et al 1989, Merchant et al 1989). The therapy does not yet appear to have a significant impact on patient survival and a majority of the reported remissions were transient. Although the local adoptive immunotherapy caused no irreversible toxicity, numerous reversible side-effects have been observed including frequent fever, nausea, vomiting, headache, fatiguability and occasional mild somnolence. In addition, an intracranial injection of large amounts of LAK cells with IL-2 caused cerebral edema, increased intracranial pressure and hydrocephalus. The mechanisms of the adverse effects can be explained by endothelial injury induced by LAK cells or increased vascular permeability by IL-2.

The in situ activity of the transferred LAK cells is totally obscure. Since effector cells must physically bind to target tumor cells to kill, successful adoptive immunotherapy presumably depends on the accumulation of transferred effector cells at the site of tumor growth. Regarding the distribution pattern of LAK cells, these transferred cells remained localized at the injection site and did not appear to migrate preferentially to the peripheral site of tumor growth. It is thus supposed that one of the major limitations of therapy with LAK cells is their inability to actively infiltrate the tumor tissue.

Another approach to adoptive immunotherapy is to expand tumor-specific T lymphocytes (CTL) with IL-2 in vitro. In many animal models the therapeutic efficacy of the CTL has been repeatedly emphasized. The existence of brain tumor-specific killer cells present in patients' PBL was suggested in early reports, and attempts to sensitize patient's PBL in vitro against autologous tumor cells have also been made. The specificity of CTL clones against autologous tumor cells is, however, doubtful. One should remember that a single human solid tumor is composed of a heterogeneous population of cells with respect to susceptibility to lysis by autologous CTL clones. This implies that a therapeutic modality must be capable of activating the overall immune response to the heterogeneous tumor cells rather than being directed to a single tumor clone.

Adoptive immunotherapy using autologous TILs in place of LAK cells has already been administered to cancer patients. The TILs have been expected to include CTL populations (Miescher et al 1988). TILs in human malignant gliomas can be isolated from a surgical specimen and expanded by an in vitro culture system with a substantial increase in cell numbers (Sawamura et al 1989a). The expanding glioma-derived TILs consist of T cells, approximately 90%, including both CD4+ and CD8+ subpopulations. NK cells are also observed in the TIL culture; however, a definitive benefit of glioma-derived TIL over LAK cells as transferred effector cells has not been found.

No publication has clearly demonstrated a beneficial effect mediated by adoptive immunotherapy for malignant cerebral gliomas. Until a totally new direction can be achieved, assuring a proper substrate of reduced tumor burden as well as absolute demonstration of cell delivery and migration to and through affected areas, this form of adoptive immunotherapy should be abandoned (Apuzzo 1991).

Suppressive modulation of the host-immune system by gliomas

Augmentation of immunity requires induction of increased effector function, and also requires concomitant

Table 7.1 Theoretical immunomodulation by malignant gliomas

Factor	Possible mechanism
TGF-β2	Suppression of: (1) IL-2 receptor expression on lymphocytes, (2) IL-2-dependent proliferation and activation of lymphocytes, (3) IL-1-dependent lymphocyte proliferation, (4) immunoglobulin production by B cells.
PGE_2	Suppression of: (1) IL-2 production and IL-2 receptor expression on lymphocytes, (2) CTL, NK cell, and B-cell activation, (3) cell-mediated cytotoxicity, (4) expression of MHC class II molecules.
IL-10	(1) Inhibition of IL-1, interferon-γ, TNF and IL-6 synthesis by activated monocytes, (2) synergism with TGF-β2 to inhibit macrophage cytotoxic activity and macrophage accessory-cell function by down-regulating class II MHC expression.
IL-6	(1) Activation and final differentiation of B cells, (2) activation of NK cells, (3) generation of CTL.
IL-8	Chemoattractant for neutrophils and T cells.
MCP-1	Chemoattractant for macrophages.

abatement of suppressor activities. One of the key functional parameters of an immune regulation is the local production of cytokines. Human brain tumors can secrete a variety of immunoregulatory (suppressive) factors, as summarized in Table 7.1, and this inhibitory role is thought to provide the means for tumor self-defense. For instance, the TILs derived from gliomas have a strikingly reduced proliferative potential (Miescher et al 1988) and this implicates an immune suppression by glioma cells. Human malignant glioma cells produce TGF-β2, IL-10 and PGE_2 (prostaglandin E_2), which may be responsible for the immunosuppression observed in glioma patients (Fontana et al 1982, de Martin et al 1987, Miescher et al 1988).

Human glioblastoma cells secrete the active form of TGF-β2 (Constam et al 1992) which can be detected in the cerebrospinal fluid of the patients. TGF-β2 has immunosuppressive effects on multiple immune functions such as: IL-2-dependent proliferation and IL-2 receptor expression on stimulated T cells and NK cells, IL-1-dependent lymphocyte proliferation, immunoglobulin production and B-cell proliferation. Increasing concentrations of IL-2 can partially overcome the suppressive activity of TGF-β2 on IL-2-dependent proliferation of lymphocytes (Kuppner et al 1988). TNF abrogates the inhibition of cytotoxic T-cell development by TGF-β2.

IL-10 is referred to as cytokine synthesis inhibitory factor (CSIF). IL-10 inhibits synthesis of IL-1, interferon-α, TNF and IL-6 by activated monocytes. In contrast to TGF-β2, however, IL-10 does not inhibit IL-2-induced proliferation or activation of peripheral blood lymphocytes, but synergizes with TGF-β2 to inhibit macrophage cytotoxic activity and macrophage accessory-cell function by down-regulating class II MHC expression.

PGE_2 also exerts profound suppressive effects on a variety of immune functions such as: IL-2 production and IL-2 receptor expression on lymphocytes, activation of CTL, NK cell, LAK cell and macrophage-mediated cytotoxicity, activation and proliferation of B cells, and expression of MHC class II molecules on the cell surface of macrophages.

In addition, glioblastoma cell lines secrete some plasminogen activator, plasminogen-activator inhibitor and α_1-antitrypsin, which were found to inhibit cytotoxic activities of lymphocytes. Certain glioma cell lines produce a mucopolysaccharide coat on their cell surface which impairs activation of lymphocytes and hinders direct interaction of glioma cells with other cells. Ganglioside composition of human gliomas correlate with their histological grade. The degree of malignancy is associated with an increasing expression of certain gangliosides. Gangliosides inhibit IL-2-stimulated proliferation of T cells, binding of IL-2 to the high affinity IL-2 receptor, function of the CD4 molecule, and the accessory cell function and IL-1 production by monocytes.

Cytokine production by gliomas

On the other hand, human glioma cells have an ability to secrete other cytokines in vitro, such as IL-1, IL-6, IL-8, IL-10, and GM-CSF (van Meir et al 1990, 1992, Frei et al 1992); their production can be enhanced by IL-1 or TNF stimulation. TNF itself may be produced by certain glioma cell lines. Interferon-α/β-like activities in glioma cell culture supernatants have also been suggested. The mechanism of production and secretion of these cytokines by in situ neoplastic cells, however, remains unclear. An immunohistochemical study demonstrated that in malignant gliomas, TNF and IL-6, although weakly present in neoplastic cells, are most prominent in infiltrating macrophages and in those regions of the tumors that include little TGF-β2 protein (Schneider et al 1992).

Most glioblastoma cell lines naturally produce IL-6, which can be increased by IL-1 or TNF stimulation. A significant degree of IL-6 bioactivity is detected in patients' cerebrospinal fluid and tumor cysts (van Meir et al 1990). IL-6 controls the final maturation of B cells into antibody-producing cells and stimulates immunoglobulin synthesis. The elevated levels of serum acute proteins and immune complexes found in glioblastoma patients might be the result of this secretion (van Meir et al 1990). IL-6 can also stimulate the activation of NK cells and the generation of cytotoxic T-lymphocytes. IL-6 bioactivity in vivo may participate in the activation of T cells.

Glioma cell lines constitutively produce the 77 amino acid form of IL-8 which is enhanced by IL-1 or TNF stimulation (van Meir et al 1992, Tada et al 1993). The cerebrospinal fluid obtained from glioma patients, but not from meningioma, contains IL-8 protein and its activity. Although IL-8 is a powerful chemoattractant, especially for neutrophils, there is no evidence of neutrophilia in glioma patients' CNS. IL-8 may require additional factor(s) to induce neutrophilia (Tada et al 1993).

Human glioma cell lines produce GM-CSF naturally or when stimulated with TNF or IL-1. There is, however, no evidence for GM-CSF production by glioma cells in vivo; fresh tumor samples lack the mRNA and the protein is not detectable in the cerebrospinal fluid of the patients (Frei et al 1992). Furthermore, even after an intratumoral injection of TNF, GM-CSF cannot be detected in the patients' body fluids (Tada et al 1993). This absence of GM-CSF in vivo might be explained by the presence of tumor-derived inhibitory factors, such as TGF-β2 and PGE_2, which suppress GM-CSF production by glioblastoma cells. Human glioma cells do not express significant GM-CSF receptors on their membrane and do not respond to a stimulation of exogenous GM-CSF.

Malignant glioma cells may be able to produce TNF both in vitro after stimulation and in vivo (Bethea et al 1992, Schneider et al 1992). IL-1β may be a potent inducer of TNF production by malignant glioma cells (Bethea et al 1992); however, TNF cannot be detected in the cerebrospinal fluid of the patients. An intracranial administration of exogenous TNF into gliomas may elicit substantial biological responses in the CNS (Tada et al 1993); it is therefore not likely that a significant amount of TNF is produced spontaneously in human glioma tissue.

IL-1α and IL-1β proteins have been suspected to be produced by stimulated glioblastoma cells in vitro. Cerebrospinal fluid of glioma patients contains neither IL-1β protein nor its bioactivity; interestingly, the cerebrospinal fluid samples obtained from the patients who were treated with TNF intralesionally contained IL-1β (Tada et al 1993). A rodent model has demonstrated that systemic treatment with recombinant IL-1β inhibited growth of a malignant glioma inducing leukocyte infiltration in the tumor tissue, but with remarkable IL-1β toxicity at effective dose (Rice & Merchant 1992).

Biological response modification

Non-specific immunomodulators

Adjuvant immunotherapy with immunomodulating agents is an attempt to enhance or stimulate the suboptimal immune response of patients with brain malignancies. Early attempts used immunization with mycobacteria, either bacille de Calmette-Guerin (BCG) or *Corynebacterium parvum*; however there was no significant prolongation of patients' survival. Similar disappointing results were reported with immunomodulatory drugs such as levamisole, OK-432 (lyophilized powder of *Streptococcus pyogenes* preparation) or PS-K (protein-bound polysaccharide Kureha form *Basidiomycetes*). It was reported that OK-432 possesses various immunopharmacological activities, such as augmentation of cytotoxic activity and stimulation of cytokine production of various lymphocytes and macrophages. According to an early report of a cooperative study using OK-432 with chemoradiation therapy including ACNU and vincristine, the survival of glioma patients receiving OK-432 was significantly longer than that of controls. In contrast, another cooperative study showed that survival rates of glioma patients treated with or without OK-432 were similar, and that there was no clinical effect of OK-432 (Shibata et al 1987).

Cytokines

Recent advances in genetic engineering enabled us to use a large amount of bioactive molecules such as recombinant cytokines for brain tumor immunotherapy. TNF and interferons possess direct tumor cytotoxicity and they have a capacity for immune modulation. Besides the direct cytotoxic/cytostatic effects on tumor cells, multiple indirect processes are possibly involved in the regulation of tumors in vivo, even if the tumor is resistant to a given cytokine in vitro. These include the potent immunomodulatory effects in recruiting and activating leukocytes, the augmentation of expression of cell surface molecules, and inducing the production of other intermediate cytokines.

Three major types of human interferons have been identified — interferon-α, interferon-β and interferon-γ. Numerous studies have shown that human interferon-α and interferon-β can inhibit the growth of human neuroectodermal tumors in murine models. In vitro studies have suggested that interferon-α and -β exhibit a direct antiproliferative activity on human glioma cell lines. A similar growth inhibitory effect of interferon-β has been reported on human glioma xenografts in nude mice. Interferon-α and -β can induce enhancement of host effector functions, such as NK and macrophage cytotoxicities, and modulation of surface antigens on the tumor cell membrane.

Several types of interferons such as human lymphoblastoid interferon-α, fibroblast interferon-β, recombinant interferon-α, recombinant interferon-β and recombinant interferon-γ are now available for clinical use (Nagai 1988). Clinical studies using interferon-α or interferon-β have been performed for malignant brain tumor patients. The interferons were administered daily in doses ranging from 1.0 to 9.0 × 10^6 units/body weight locally, intravenously, or intramuscularly, and were continued for approximately 4 weeks or longer (Nagai 1988). The trials reported 14–28% response rates (significant tumor volume reduction) in glioma patients. The efficacy via the local (intratumoral or intrathecal) route was reported to be similar to that of systemic administration. The overall results in a number of clinical reports have been equivocal and interferons given as single agents have not effected a major impact in the therapy of brain tumors. A controlled phase III study has not yet been carried out; furthermore, the mechanisms of interferon-mediated antitumor effects in humans remain obscure.

Transient side effects of interferon-β occurred in 60–100% of patients, including fever, headache, lassitude, chills, seizures, hypotension, nausea and vomiting. Suppression of hemopoietic function and liver dysfunction were mild and generally returned to normal without withdrawal of the medication; however, in certain cases bone marrow suppression was sufficiently profound to interrupt the therapy.

The receptor (type 2) for interferon-γ differs from the receptor (type 1) for interferon-α and interferon-β. Interferon-γ has limited direct anti-glioma cytotoxicity in vitro in comparison with interferon-α or interferon-β. Interferon-γ is, however, a potent regulator of cell gene expression, structure, and function. Manipulation of the enhancement of tumor antigenicity and of host effector cytotoxicity is another potential area. A rat model has demonstrated that intracerebral injections of interferon-γ caused multiple immunological effects (Sethna & Lampson 1991); among them was the observation that lymphocytes and other inflammatory cells were recruited to the injection site — CD4+ T cells into the perivascular space, OX-42+ monocytes/macrophages into brain parenchyma and possibly NK cells also. Interferon-γ caused increased MHC expression on brain cells: class I antigen on local endothelial and ependymal cells, and class II antigen on microglia, expendymal, and perivascular cells throughout both hemispheres of the brain.

A clinical trial of interferon-γ in glioma patients has been reported with disappointing results (Mahaley et al 1988), and the side effects of interferon-γ are generally so severe that clinical trials of interferon-γ alone have been interrupted. Current trials of interferon therapy are directed to combination with other types of immunotherapy or chemotherapeutic agents. Interferon-γ at a proper low dose in order to enhance tumor immunogenicity might be utilized in combination with the other immunotherapeutic approaches.

TNF was originally thought to have direct cytocidal effects on human cancer cells. In contrast to previous expectations that TNF was able to kill certain glioma cell lines or to inhibit the growth of primary cultures from human malignant brain tumors (Helseth et al 1989, Rutka et al 1988), TNF in fact produced only few antiproliferative effects (Zuber et al 1988). The vast majority of human glioma cells, especially at low dose, are resistant to TNF cytotoxic activity. Low dose TNF accumulates certain glioma cells in the G_0/G_1 phase and suppresses DNA synthesis. Its in vitro immunomodulatory properties are activation of macrophages, and enhancement of HLA-ABC expression and of certain tumor-associated antigens on human glioma cells (Zuber et al 1988). TNF stimulates glioma cells to produce IL-6, IL-8, GM-CSF, PGE_2, and manganous superoxide dismutase. It is particularly interesting that TNF has inverse regulatory roles against TGF-β2 produced by glioma cells.

It has been shown that in a rodent glioma model, TNF increased blood-brain barrier permeability in and around the tumor, neutrophilic infiltration into the area of glioma, and hemorrhagic necrosis of tumor vessels (Kido et al 1991). TNF preferentially affects newly-formed vasculature of the tumor and has little effect on the integrity of normal cerebral vessels. The intravenous TNF injection induced adherence of neutrophils and monocytes only to the tumor vessels, not to normal ones (Kido et al 1991).

Certain phase I trials in advanced cancer patients reported toxicity over a broad range of doses, while antitumor activity was minimal. Current clinical studies of TNF for malignant glioma patients consist of local administration either through the intracranial or intracarotid route. The intracranial administration of TNF induces remarkable local neutrophil migration followed by T helper cells and macrophages. Secondary increases in the levels of IL-1β, IL-6, IL-8, and prostaglandin-E2 in the patient's cerebrospinal fluid occur several hours after the TNF injection (Tada et al 1993).

IL-2 is a cytokine produced by activated T cells that activates a variety of lymphocyte populations and induces lymphocyte proliferation. IL-2-activated NK cells and T cells can mediate cytotoxicity against a panel of malignant brain tumors. Thus it was supposed that IL-2 should enhance tumor cell lysis by immune effector cells infiltrating brain tumor tissue.

A huge amount of intravenous IL-2, more than 10^6 units of IL-2 every 8 hours, is required to achieve an adequate dose (3–6 units/ml) in the CSF (Saris et al 1988), which can activate LAK-precursor lymphocytes and/or maintain LAK cells in the CSF. Systemic IL-2 therapy as a single agent for cancer patients did not result in tumor regression in spite of serious toxicity. Furthermore, patients with intracranial metastasis have been excluded from the protocol of systemic IL-2 therapy because of the risk of brain edema and poor results in pilot studies. In addition, an intravenous high-dose IL-2 therapy elicits mental status changes (confusion, disorientation, or lethargy) in approximately one third of patients, and may last days or weeks.

IL-2 has been utilized locally to augment the effect of intracranially transferred LAK cells. In preliminary clinical studies, when IL-2 was injected into the peritumoral area of glioma patients either during or after surgery, no irreversible toxicity was reported (Jacobs et al 1986). In contrast, transient adverse effects were frequent including headache, moderate grade fever, nausea, chill, mild confusion or occasional dysesthesia in lower limbs after either intratumoral or intrathecal injection of IL-2, when doses ranged from 10^3 to 2×10^4 units.

Drug delivery into brain tumors is limited by the intact blood-brain barrier, especially at the tumor periphery. An intracerebral injection of IL-2 causes a temporary breakdown of the blood-brain barrier. This effect of IL-2 on brain endothelial cells may enhance drug penetration into peritumoral areas with an intact blood-brain barrier (Watts & Merchant 1992).

Novel approaches improving delivery of biological response modifiers

Cytokines exert their effects, which are highly pleiotropic, indirectly via mobilization of host-mediated defenses or a modification of the production of tumor cell growth factors. Administration of cytokines to a tumor-bearing host is hampered by the potential short half-life of the factor and the need to obtain it in quantities sufficient to achieve effective dose levels, usually with remarkable adverse effects. To overcome them, some novel means of utilizing gene technology have been proposed.

IL-4 is a multifunctional cytokine produced by helper T cells and has a broad range of activities on B and T cells. An IL-4 gene was transfected into murine tumor lines of various histologic types, including glioma, to produce IL-4 proteins. By measuring the ability of transfectants to form tumors alone and when mixed with nontransfected tumor cells, a potent antitumor effect of IL-4 in vivo was demonstrated. This antitumor effect seemed to be mediated by an inflammatory infiltrate composed of eosinophils and macrophages (Tepper et al 1989).

A mouse interferon-γ gene was transfected to murine cytotoxic T lymphocytes specific against a murine glioma line. Exogenous expression of the interferon-γ gene was demonstrated to be able to augment the cell killing of the cytotoxic T lymphocytes both in vitro and in vivo (Miyatake et al 1990).

A human interferon-β gene inserted into a eukaryotic expression vector was entrapped in liposomes. Liposome-mediated transfection of the gene into cultured glioma cells was performed and resulted in the secretion of interferon-β by the cells. Gene therapy of malignant gliomas with specific delivery of the human interferon-β gene into glioma cells by the use of such liposomes has been proposed (Mizuno et al 1991).

CONCLUSION

The effectiveness of surgical removal and radiation therapy as the treatment for malignant brain tumors is limited, chemotherapy adding very little. Biological therapy should be considered as a fourth modality of brain tumor treatment. Although there has been little practical success in the development of immunotherapy, the research efforts enabled us to gain some more insight into the ways in which immune responses to the tumors can be modulated. The idea of biological response modification in complex and sequential form is quite elegant; however, it should be applied in the context of the entire spectrum of scientific and clinical knowledge of the problem of malignant cerebral gliomas.

REFERENCES

Apuzzo M L 1991 Adoptive immunotherapy of primary brain tumors; Comment. Neurosurgery 28: 23

Barba D, Saris S C, Holder R N, Rosenberg S A, Oldfield E H 1989 Intratumoral LAK cell and interleukin-2 therapy of human gliomas. Journal of Neurosurgery 70: 175–182

Behnke J, Coakham H B, Mach J P, Carrel S, de Tribolet N 1988 Monoclonal antibodies in the diagnosis and therapy of brain tumors. In: Kornblith P L, Walker M D (eds) Advances in neuro-oncology. Futura, Mount Kisco, N Y, pp 249–285

Bethea J R, Chung I Y, Sparacio G Y, Benveniste E N 1992 Interleukin-1 beta induction of tumor necrosis factor-alpha gene expression in human astroglial cells. Journal of Neuroimmunology 36: 179–191

Brady L W, Woo D V, Karlsson U, Steplewski Z, Rackover M, Koprowski H 1988 Radioimmunotherapy of human gliomas using I-125 labeled monoclonal antibody to epidermal growth factor receptor. Proceedings of ASCO 7: 83

Bruner J M, Saya H, Moser R P 1991 Immunohistochemical detection of p53 in human gliomas. Mod Pathol 4: 671–674

Carrel S, de Tribolet N, Mach J P 1982 Expression of neuroectodermal antigens common to melanomas, gliomas and neuroblastomas. I. Identification by monoclonal anti-melanoma and anti-glioma antibodies. Acta Neuropathol 57: 158–164

Coakham H B, Richardson R B, Davies A G, Bourne S P, Eckert H, Kemshead J T 1988 Neoplastic meningitis from a pineal tumor treated by antibody-guided irradiation via the intrathecal route. British Journal of Neurosurgery 2: 299

Colapinto E V, Humphrey P A, Zalutsky M R et al 1988 Comparative localization of murine monoclonal antibody Mel-14 F(ab')2 fragment and whole IgG2a in human glioma xenografts. Cancer Research 48: 5701–5707

Constam D B, Philipp J, Malipiero U V, ten Dijke P, Schachner M, Fontana A 1992 Differential expression of transforming growth factor-beta 1, -beta 2, and -beta 3 by glioblastoma cells, astrocytes, and microglia. Journal of Immunology 148: 1404–1410

Davidoff A M, Iglehart J D, Marks J R 1992 Immune response to p53 is dependent upon p53/HSP70 complexes in breast cancers. Proceedings of the National Academy of Sciences of the USA 89: 3439–3442

de Martin R, Haendler B, Hofer-Warbinek R et al 1987 Complementary DNA for human glioblastoma-derived T cell suppressor factor, a novel member of the transforming growth factor-β gene family. EMBO 6: 3673–3677

de Muralt B, de Tribolet N, Diserens A C, Stavrou D, Mach J P, Carrel S 1985 Phenotyping of 60 cultured human gliomas and 34 other neuroectodermal tumors by means of monoclonal antibodies against glioma, melanoma and HLA-DR antigen. European Journal of Cancer and Clinical Oncology 21: 207–216

de Tribolet N, Hamou M F, Mach J P, Carrel S, Schreyer M 1984 Demonstration of HLA-DR antigens in normal human brain. Journal of Neurological and Neurosurgical Psychiatry 47: 417–418

Fischer D K, Chen T L, Narayan R K 1988 Immunological and biochemical strategies for the identification of brain tumor-associated antigens. Journal of Neurosurgery 68: 165–180

Fontana A, Kristensen F, Dubs R, Gemsa D, Weber E 1982 Production of prostaglandin E and an interleukin 1-like factor by cultured astrocytes and C6 glioma cells. Journal of Immunology 129: 2413–2419

Foon K A 1989 Perspective in cancer research. Biological response modifiers: The new immunotherapy. Cancer Research 49: 1621–1639

Frank E, Pulver M, de Tribolet N 1986 Expression of class II major histocompatibility antigens on reactive astrocytes and endothelial cells within the gliosis surrounding metastasis and abscesses. Journal of Neuroimmunology 12: 29–36

Frei K, Piani D, Malipiero U V, van Meir E, de Tribolet N, Fontana A 1992 Granulocyte-macrophage colony-stimulating factor (GM-CSF) production by glioblastoma cells. Despite the presence of inducing signals GM-CSF is not expressed in vivo. I Immunol 148: 3140–3146

Fullar G N, Bigner S H 1992 Amplified cellular oncogene in neoplasms of the human central nervous system. Mutation Research 276: 299–306

Helseth E, Torp S, Dalen A, Unsgaard G 1989 Effects of interferon-gamma and tumor necrosis factor-alpha on clonogenic growth of cell lines and primary cultures from human malignant gliomas and brain metastases. APMIS 97: 569–574

Herberman R B 1985 Multiple functions of natural killer cells, including immunoregulation as well as resistance to tumor growth. Concepts in Immunopathology 1: 96–132

Jacobs S K, Wilson D J, Kornblith P L, Grimm E A 1986 Interleukin 2 or autologous lymphokine-activated killer cell treatment of malignant glioma: Phase I trial. Cancer Research 46: 2101–2104

Johnson V G, Wrobel C, Wilson D et al 1989 Improved tumor-specific immunotoxins in the treatment of CNS and leptomeningeal neoplasia. Journal of Neurosurgery 70: 240–248

Khavari P 1987 Cytotoxic cellular mediators of the immune response to neoplasia: a review. Yale Journal of Biology and Medicine 60: 409–419

Kido G, Wright J L, Merchant R E 1991 Acute effects of human recombinant tumor necrosis factor-α on the cerebral vasculature of the rat in both normal brain and in an experimental glioma model. Journal of Neurooncology 10: 95–109

Kokunai T, Tamaki N, Matsumoto S 1990 Antigen related to cell proliferation in malignant gliomas recognized by a human monoclonal antibody. Journal of Neurosurgery 73: 901–908

Kuppner M C, Hamou M F, Bodmer S, Fontana A, Tribolet N 1988 The glioblastoma-derived T-cell suppressor factor/transforming growth factor beta2 inhibits the generation of lymphokine-activated killer (LAK) cells. International Journal of Cancer 42: 562–567

Kuppner M C, van Meir E, Hamou M F, de Tribolet N 1990 Cytokine regulation of intercellular adhesion molecule-1 (ICAM-1) expression on human glioblastoma cells. Clinical and Experimental Immunology 81: 142–148

Lampson L A, Wen P, Roman V A, Horris J M, Sarid J A 1992 Disseminating tumor cells and their interactions with leukocytes visualized in the brain. Cancer Research 52: 1018–1025

Lee Y, Bullard D E, Humphrey P A et al 1988 Treatment of intracranial human glioma xenografts with ^{131}I-labeled anti-tenascin monoclonal antibody 81C6. Cancer Research 48: 2904–2910

Libermann T A, Nusbaum H R, Razon N et al 1985 Amplification, enhanced expression and possible rearrangement of EGFR gene in human brain tumor. Nature 313: 144–147

Lotze M T, Finn O J 1990 Recent advances in cellular immunology: implications for immunity to cancer. Immunology Today 11: 190–193

Mahaley M S, Bertsch L, Cush S, Gillespie G Y 1988 Systematic gamma-interferon therapy for recurrent gliomas. Journal of Neurosurgery 69: 826–829

McVicar D W, Davis D F, Merchant R E 1992 In vitro analysis of the proliferative potential of T cells from patients with brain tumor: glioma-associated immunosuppression unrelated to intrinsic cellular defect. Journal of Neurosurgery 76: 251–260

Merchant R E, Merchant L H, Cook S H S, McVicar D W, Young H F 1989 Intratumoral infusion of lymphokine-activated killer (LAK) cells and recombinant interleukin-2 (IL-2) for the treatment of patients with malignant brain tumor. Neurosurgery 23: 725–732

Miescher S, Whiteside T L, de Tribolet N, von Fliedner V 1988 In situ characterization, colonogenic potential, and antitumor cytolytic activity of T lymphocytes infiltrating human brain cancers. Journal of Neurosurgery 68: 438–448

Miyatake S, Nishihara K, Kikuchi H, Yamashita J, Namba Y, Hanaoka M, Watanabe Y 1990 Efficient tumor suppression by glioma-specific murine cytotoxic T lymphocytes transfected with interferon-gamma gene. Journal of the National Cancer Institute 82: 217–220

Mizuno M, Yoshida J, Sugita K et al 1991 Growth inhibition of glioma cells transfected with the human beta-interferon gene by liposomes coupled with a monoclonal antibody. Cancer Research 50: 7826–7829

Monod L, Hamou A C, Ronco P, Verroust P, de Tribolet N 1992 Expression of cALLa/NEP on gliomas: a possible marker of malignancy. Acta Neurochirurgica (Wien) 114: 3–7

Moseley R P, Zalutsky M R, Coakham H B, Coleman R E, Bigner D D 1987 Distribution of 131I 81C6 monoclonal antibody (Mab) administered via carotid artery in patients with glioma. Journal of Nuclear Medicine 28: 603–604

Moseley R P, Papanastassiou V, Zalutsky M R et al 1992 Immunoreactivity, pharmacokinetics and bone marrow dosimetry of intrathecal radioimmunoconjugates. International Journal of Cancer 52: 38–43

Nagai M 1988 Clinical use of interferons in the treatment of malignant brain tumor. In: Revel M (ed) Clinical aspects of interferons. Kluwer Academic Publishers, Boston, pp 183–194

Nitta T, Sato K, Okumura K, Steinman L 1992 An analysis of T-cell-receptor variable-region genes in tumor-infiltrating lymphocytes within malignant tumors. International Journal of Cancer 49: 545–550

Osband M L, Ross S 1990 Problems in the investigational study and clinical use of cancer immunotherapy. Immunology Today 11: 193–195

Paine J T, Handa H, Yamazaki T, Yamashita J, Miyatake S 1986 Immunohistochemical analysis of infiltrating lymphocytes in central nervous system tumors. Neurosurgery 18: 766–772

Rice C D, Merchant R E 1992 Systemic treatment with murine recombinant interleukin-1 beta inhibits the growth and progression of malignant glioma in the rat. Journal of Neurooncology 13: 43–55

Rosenberg S A 1988 Immunotherapy of cancer using interleukin 2: current status and future prospects. Immunology Today 9: 58–62

Rossi M L, Jones N R, Candy E et al 1989 The mononuclear cell infiltrate compared with survival in high-grade astrocytomas. Acta Neuropathol 78: 189–193

Rutka J T, Giblin J R, Berens M E et al 1988 The effects of human recombinant tumor necrosis factor on glioma-derived cell lines: cellular proliferation, cytotoxicity, morphological and radioreceptor studies. International Journal of Cancer 41: 573–582

Saris S C, Rosenberg S A, Friedman R B, Rubin J T, Barba D, Oldfield E H 1988 Penetration of recombinant interleukin-2 across the blood-cerebrospinal fluid barrier. Journal of Neurosurgery 69: 29–34

Sawamura Y, Hosokawa M, Kuppner M C et al 1989a Antitumor activity and surface phenotypes of human glioma-infiltrating lymphocytes after in vitro expansion in the presence of interleukin 2. Cancer Research 49: 1843–1849

Sawamura Y, Hamou M F, Kuppner M, de Tribolet N 1989b Immunohistochemical and in vitro functional analysis of pineal-germinoma infiltrating lymphocytes: Report of a case. Neurosurgery 25: 454–457

Schneider J, Hofman F M, Apuzzo M L, Hinton D R 1992 Cytokines and immunoregulatory molecules in malignant glial neoplasms. Journal of Neurosurgery 77: 265–273

Schuster J M, Garg P K, Bigner D D, Zalutsky M R 1991 Improved therapeutic efficacy of a monoclonal antibody radioiodinated using N-succinimidyl-3-(tri-n-butylstannyl)benzoate. Cancer Research 51: 4164–4169

Sethna M P, Lampson L A 1991 Immune modulation within the brain: recruitment of inflammatory cells and increased major histocompatibility antigen expression following intracerebral injection of interferon-gamma. Journal of Neuroimmunology 34: 121–132

Shibata S, Mori K, Moriyama T, Tanaka K, Moroki T 1987 Randomized controlled study of the effect of adjuvant immunotherapy with Picibanil on 51 malignant gliomas. Surgical Neurology 27: 259–263

Stewart C C, Stevenson A P, Hibbs J 1988 Effector mechanisms for macrophage-induced cytostasis and cytolysis of tumor cells. In: Heppner G H, Fulton A M (eds) Macrophages and cancer. CRC Press, Boca Raton, FL, pp 39–59

Sutter A, Hekmat A, Luchenbach G A 1991 Antibody-mediated tumor cytotoxicity of microglia. Pathobiology 59: 254–258

Tada M, Sawamura Y, Sakuma S et al 1993 Cellular and cytokine responses in the human central nervous system to intracranial administration of tumor necrosis factor-a for the treatment of malignant gliomas. Cancer Immunology and Immunotherapy (in press)

Tepper R I, Pattengale P K, Leder P 1989 Murine interleukin-4 displays potent anti-tumor activity in vitro. Cell 57: 503–512

Thomas W E 1992 Brain macrophages: evaluation of microglia and their functions. Brain Res Brain Res Rev 17: 61–74

van Meir E, Sawamura Y, Diserens A C, Hamou M F, de Tribolet N 1990 Human glioblastoma cells release interleukin 6 in vivo and in vitro. Cancer Research 50: 6683–6688

van Meir E, Ceska M, Effenberger F et al 1992 Interleukin-8 is produced in neoplastic and infectious diseases of the human central nervous system. Cancer Research 52: 4297–4305

Watts R G, Merchant R E 1992 Cerebrovascular effects and tumor kinetics after a single intratumoral injection of human recombinant interleukin-2 alone or in combination with intravenous chemotherapy in a rat model of glioma. Neurosurgery 31: 89–98

Wikstrand C J, McLendon R E, Carrel S et al 1987 Comparative localization of glioma-reactive monoclonal antibodies in vivo in an athymic mouse human glioma xenograft model. Journal of Neuroimmunology 15: 37–56

Winter S F, Minna J D, Johnson B E, Takahashi T, Gazdar A F, Carbone D P 1992 Development of antibodies against p53 in lung cancer patients appears to be dependent on the type of p53 mutation. Cancer Research 52: 4168–4174

Yoshida S, Tanaka R, Takai N, Ono K 1988 Local administration of autologous lymphokine-activated killer cells and recombinant interleukin 2 to patients with malignant brain tumors. Cancer Research 48: 5011–5016

Yoshimura T, Takeya M, Takahashi K, Kuratsu J, Leonard E J 1991 Production and characterization of mouse monoclonal antibodies against human monocyte chemoattractant protein-1. Journal of Immunology 147: 2229–2233

Zuber P, Accolla R S, Carrel S, Diserens A C, de Tribolet N 1988 Effects of recombinant human tumor necrosis factor-α on the surface phenotype and the growth of human malignant glioma cell lines. International Journal of Cancer 42: 780–786

8. Histopathology, immunochemistry and ultrastructure of brain tumors

M. Beatriz S. Lopes   Scott R. VandenBerg   Bernd W. Scheithauer

INTRODUCTION

During the past decade, the histopathologic evaluation of tumors arising in the nervous system has been dramatically affected by increasing numbers of special morphologic procedures, especially immunohistochemistry and ultrastructural immunocytochemistry. With respect to cytoskeletal proteins, membrane proteins, growth factors, oncogenes and growth kinetics, these techniques have provided the neuro-oncologist with a greater understanding of tumor histogenesis. Accordingly, a revised classification system for tumors of the nervous system was formulated by a WHO working group (Kleihues et al 1993a — see Appendix 3). Clinical neuro-oncology has also had a significant impact on the practice of diagnostic neuropathology. Advances in neuroimaging techniques, and the expanded use of stereotactic biopsies now require neuropathologists to evaluate diminutive tissue fragments, often obtained from heterogeneous neoplasms. In these circumstances, definition of key histopathologic features for the classification of brain tumors is crucial.

The histologic subtypes and varied distribution of CNS tumors in children and adults reflect the unique histogenesis of the nervous system. Although the CNS is derived from an essentially epithelial structure, the complex morphogenesis that culminates in the mature brain precludes the persistence of a single well-defined, evenly distributed population of mitotic stem cells to serve as a reserve population for continued cell renewal. This property, combined with a relatively limited window of vulnerability to carcinogen exposure (Kriek et al 1984), accounts for the relatively infrequent occurrence of tumors in the adult brain (Rubinstein 1972). Nonetheless, the frequency of specific types of tumors may be increasing due to yet undefined etiologies (O'Sullivan et al 1991, Desmeules et al 1992). In contrast, the nervous system is the second most common site of primary tumors in the pediatric population, one where in approximately two thirds are infratentorial. The variance is likely a reflection of the different populations of biologically distinct cell target sites for neoplastic transformation. It is most dramatically illustrated by medulloblastoma and glioblastoma, the most frequently occurring of malignant tumors. Another age-related dissimilarity is the prevalence of the more circumscribed, relatively benign, astrocytic tumors in adolescents and young adults. These age-, histogenetic, and site-related distinctions serve as important reminders that the histopathologic diagnosis of tumors of the central nervous system cannot be accurately assessed in the absence of clinical data.

This chapter will focus upon recent revisions in the WHO classification of tumors of the central nervous system (Kleihues et al 1993a). Categories significantly revised include the neuroepithelial tumors and those of the meninges. In addition, we will discuss tumors of cranial and spinal nerves with emphasis upon their occurrence in the setting of the neurofibromatoses. This review will stress the distinctive cytologic and histopathologic properties of these tumors as well as their salient clinical features.

TUMORS OF NEUROEPITHELIAL TISSUE

1. Astrocytic tumors

The WHO classification (Kleihues et al 1993a) separates the astrocytic tumors into two major categories: the diffusely infiltrating astrocytomas and the relatively more circumscribed, specialized variants of astrocytoma (pilocytic astrocytoma, pleomorphic xanthoastrocytoma, and subependymal giant cell astrocytoma). The first group is composed of astrocytic tumors which generally infiltrate diffusely beyond the macroscopically apparent brain-tumor interface and undergo anaplastic progression with significant frequency. In contrast, the second group of astrocytomas comprises tumors which grow in a relatively circumscribed pattern, show more limited infiltration of adjacent brain, and infrequently undergo anaplastic progression.

Astrocytic tumors of the diffuse type are classified on the basis of increasing anaplasia. Several grading systems have been developed over the years in an attempt to correlate histology and prognosis. We will briefly discuss these systems but will utilize the WHO grading system in this chapter. Therefore, the tumors will be designated accordingly as astrocytoma (WHO grade II), anaplastic astrocytoma (WHO grade III) and glioblastoma multiforme (WHO grade IV).

A. Grading of astrocytic tumors

The method of grading diffusely infiltrating astrocytomas along the spectrum from well-differentiated lesions to glioblastomas varies among different laboratories. Extensive discussion regarding the different grading systems is presented elsewhere (Daumas-Duport et al 1988a, Davis 1989, VandenBerg 1992, Kleihues et al 1993b). Most current systems of grading use three-tiered systems similar to the WHO designations of astrocytoma (grade II), anaplastic astrocytoma (grade III), and glioblastoma (grade IV) (Kleihues et al 1993a). As regards specific criteria for grading, according to the WHO scheme, tumors with nuclear atypia alone are considered grade II; those which in addition demonstrate mitotic activity are grade III; and neoplasms showing atypia, mitoses, endothelial proliferation and/or necrosis are considered grade IV. This grading system basically represents a simplification of the St Anne-Mayo system (Daumas-Duport et al 1988a), wherein grades are determined by combinations of these same morphologic criteria (atypia, mitoses, endothelial proliferation, necrosis). Accordingly, tumors with a single feature (usually nuclear and/or cytoplasmic atypia) were designated grade 2, those with two criteria (usually atypia and mitotic activity) grade 3, and those with three or four features grade 4. There is also no implicit hierarchy of grading features in this grading system. These features, however, have been somewhat weighted by experience, such that in very small biopsies the presence of atypia combined with endothelial/pericytic proliferation without any observed mitoses or necrosis would still be highly suggestive of an astrocytoma grade 4. The multiple sampling of targets in conjunction with stereotactic techniques significantly increases the precision of this grading system (Daumas-Duport 1992). The application of the St Anne-Mayo system demonstrated strong interobserver reproducibility and a high degree of correlation between the histologic ranking and survival curves in two large series (Daumas-Duport et al 1988a, Kim et al 1991).

B. Astrocytoma (WHO grade II)

Three major variants of diffusely infiltrating astrocytomas are histopathologically recognized: the *fibrillary astrocytoma,* the *gemistocytic astrocytoma* and the *protoplasmic astrocytoma.* This subclassification of astrocytic tumors tends to correlate the morphology of the neoplastic astrocytes to the basic astroglial forms recognized in the normal and reactive brain, i.e. fibrillary, protoplasmic, and gemistocytic astrocytes. Although this subdivision of astrocytoma variants is based upon the predominant 'cell type' present in a given tumor, they are often found to be intermixed in the same neoplasm. Among these variants, *fibrillary* tumors are the most common. *Gemistocytic astrocytoma,* the second most common variant, accounts for no more than 20% of astrocytomas (Krouwer et al 1991), and is commonly defined as a tumor with greater than 60% of gemistocytes (Krouwer et al 1991); however, cells with gemistocytic characteristics are commonly observed in astrocytomas of all grades (Fig. 8.1A). In one well-

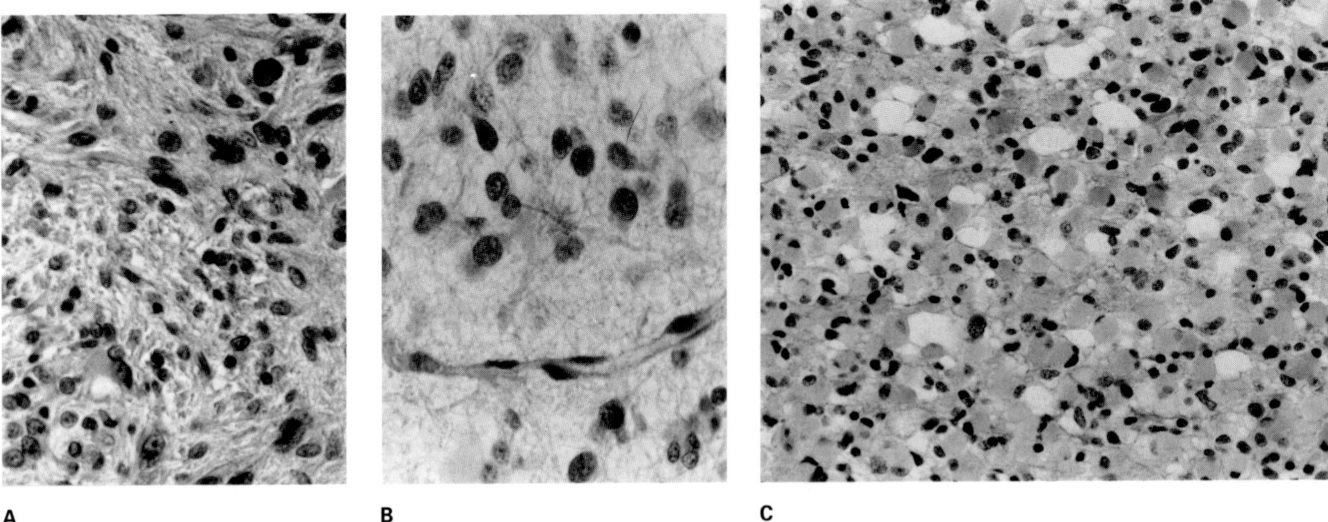

Fig. 8.1 Astrocytoma. **A, B**. Diffuse infiltrating astrocytomas (WHO grade II) display variable degrees of cellularity and cellular atypia in a fibrillary matrix. The majority of the tumors demonstrate mixed populations of fibrillary and gemistocytic astrocytes **B**. Delicate vessels are present. **C**. Gemistocytic astrocytomas are composed of a majority of cells with abundant, round cytoplasm and commonly eccentric nuclei. **A–C** H&E.

documented series of cases, astrocytomas composed of greater than 20% gemistocytes were considered more aggressive than more fibrillary tumors of similar grade (Krouwer et al 1991). *Protoplasmic astrocytomas* are the least frequently occurring variant, representing less than 1% of diffusely infiltrative astrocytic tumors (Russell & Rubinstein 1989).

On gross examination, the consistency of astrocytomas depends upon the predominant component of the tumor. Protoplasmic astrocytomas appear as gelatinous masses because of the frequent presence of microcystic degeneration. In contrast, the high proportion of fibrillary astrocytes in fibrillary astrocytomas confers firmness to the tumor specimen. Intraoperative smears of astrocytomas usually demonstrate a variably abundant fibrillary matrix formed by the cytoplasmic tumor cell processes. Given their marked variation in cytology, the cytoplasm of astrocytoma cells may range from those with a barely discernable perinuclear rim of cytoplasm to cells that are more fusiform or markedly elongated (Fig. 8.1A,B). Gemistocytic astrocytomas are composed of round to slightly angulated cells with abundant, well-defined eosinophilic cytoplasm and eccentric nuclei (Fig. 8.1C). The tumor cells often have shorter, less conspicuous processes compared to the prominent radiating processes of reactive astrocytes. Protoplasmic astrocytomas have a matrix composed of poorly fibrillated processes, and the tumor cells tend to have a more stellate geometry with short, delicate processes.

Regardless of the predominant cell type, grade 2 astrocytomas exhibit mild atypia, and the degree of cellularity varies from near normal to marked. By definition, mitoses, endothelial proliferation, and necrosis are lacking. Such tumors are equivalent to grade 2 astrocytomas in the St Anne-Mayo scheme.

Fibrillar glial processes can be highlighted by phosphotungstic acid hematoxylin (PTAH) stain but, for diagnostic purposes, the far more specific immunohistochemical demonstration of glial fibrillary acidic protein (GFAP) is in more common use. GFAP is the major constituent of intermediate filaments in normal, reactive and neoplastic astrocytes. Immature oligodendrocytes and anaplastic oligodendrogliomas, reactive and neoplastic ependyma, and choroid plexus epithelium may also show variable GFAP immunoreactivity. The relatively frequent expression of this intermediate filament protein is of diagnostic importance as it serves as a marker of glial differentiation. In astrocytomas, the relative expression of GFAP appears to be related to cellular differentiation and to proliferative potential (Rutka & Smith 1993). An exception is the protoplasmic astrocytoma, which demonstrates minimal or no GFAP immunoreactivity (Perentes & Rubinstein 1987, Russell & Rubinstein 1989).

Vimentin is an intermediate filament protein with a relatively wide cellular distribution, being particularly abundant in normal and neoplastic mesenchymal tissues. During development, it is transiently expressed by astrocytes (Kennedy & Fok-Seang 1986). In astrocytomas, vimentin is usually present, with distribution similar to GFAP, albeit with less prominence (Schiffer et al 1986). A number of other proteins may also be expressed in astrocytic tumors; these include S-100 protein (Perentes & Rubinstein 1987), Leu-7 (Perentes & Rubinstein 1986), and neuron-specific enolase (γγenolase, NSE) (Perentes & Rubinstein 1987). It is important to note that these proteins are of restricted diagnostic utility, particularly in distinguishing astrocytomas from other neuroepithelial tumors.

C. *Anaplastic astrocytoma (WHO grade III)*

All types of diffusely infiltrating astrocytomas, among which fibrillary tumors are most frequent, have a variable capacity for progression to anaplastic astrocytomas. Although anaplastic progression is anticipated in up to 80% of such tumors (Scherer 1940, Russell & Rubinstein 1989), the latent period to progression is quite variable. In recurrent astrocytomas, the frequency of progression to a higher grade than was observed in the original tumor is approximately 50–75% (Russell & Rubinstein 1989). Anaplastic astrocytomas may also arise de novo, without an intermediate phase of anaplastic progression from lower grade tumor. As in grade II astrocytomas, anaplastic astrocytomas exhibit considerable variation in morphologic cellularity as well as in heterogeneity. As a rule, cellularity is greater, atypia is more conspicuous, and mitotic figures are present (Fig. 8.2). Such tumors are the equivalent to those of St Anne-Mayo grade 3.

D. *Glioblastoma multiforme (WHO grade IV)*

Glioblastomas represent 15–20% of all intracranial tumors and approximately 50% of gliomas in adults (Burger et al 1991). In most series, a significant number arise in anaplastic progression from astrocytomas and anaplastic astrocytomas (Muller et al 1977, Laws et al 1984, Dropcho et al 1987). Less frequently, glioblastomas arise de novo, being unaccompanied by a lower grade precursor lesion. Glioblastomas may also occur in pediatric groups (Itoh et al 1987), and it is in this population that they must be differentiated from embryonal tumors (see below). A particular subgroup of glioblastomas, one with mutations in the conserved region of the p53 gene, appears selectively to affect women and the young (Louis et al 1993).

Glioblastomas have neuroimaging and macroscopic features which reflect the aggressive nature of the lesion. Salient features include an expansive lesion on CT or MRI, with features of contrast enhancement and variable, often central, lack of enhancement. Whereas the latter

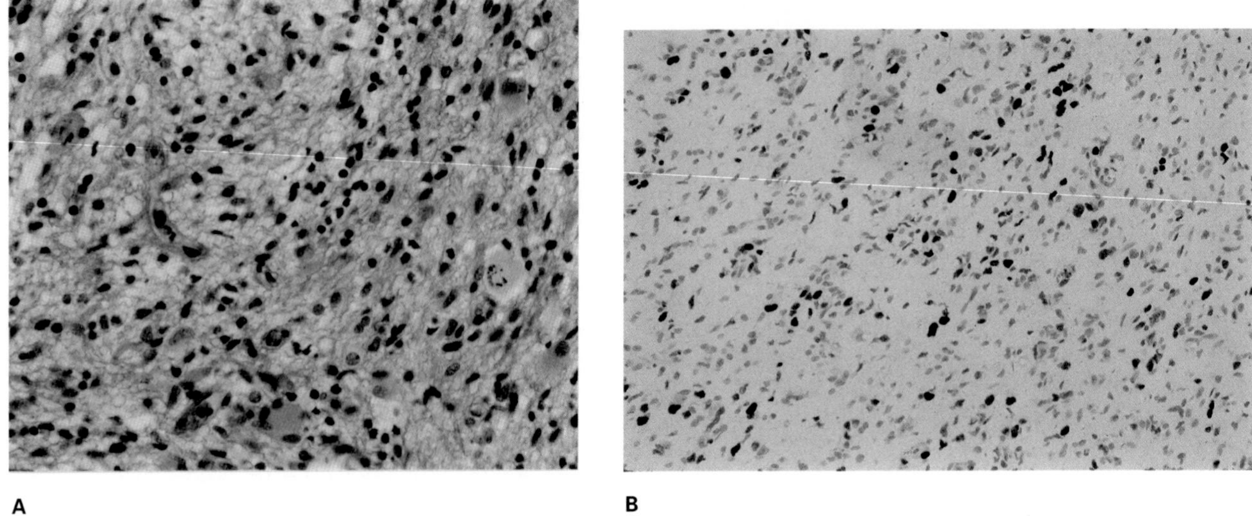

Fig. 8.2 Anaplastic astrocytoma. **A**. Hypercellularity, cellular atypia and high mitotic activity are features of anaplastic astrocytomas (WHO grade III). H&E. **B**. Ki-67 immunohistochemistry shows moderate elevated labeling indices. Ki-67 (MIB-1) avidin biotin-immunoperoxidase.

represents necrosis, the zone of enhancement corresponds to hypercellular, often solid tumor with neovascularization (Earnest et al 1988). The heterogeneous signal frequently noted on T2-weighted MRI images correlates with areas of hypercellularity and vascularity alternating with zones of necrosis or lower cellularity. Despite the rather circumscribed neuroimaging and gross appearance of the glioblastomas, diffuse infiltration of the surrounding brain parenchyma by isolated, single cells or small clusters of neoplastic cells is an almost invariable finding. The extent of parenchymal infiltration is highly variable, as has been demonstrated by detailed mapping studies of glioblastomas (Burger & Kleihues 1989). Indeed, it may range from a few millimeters to many centimeters. Spreading of the tumor cells along fiber tracts may be particularly extensive, a classic example being extension across the corpus callosum to the opposite hemisphere ('butterfly' pattern).

Histologically, glioblastomas exhibit marked cellular heterogeneity. Cytoplasmic and nuclear pleomorphism may be minimal or striking. Such tumors range from closely packed lesions consisting largely of small cells with scant cytoplasm and round to oval, variably hyperchromatic nuclei, to tumors consisting largely of bizarre, multinucleated giant cells (Fig. 8.3A–C). Most tumors exhibit a mixed pattern. Mitotic figures, including atypical forms, are often readily identified, but vary considerably within different portions of the tumor. Glioblastomas are distinguished from astrocytomas of grade III by the presence within the former of either endothelial proliferation or necrosis. Micronecrosis or broad geographic zones of necrosis, when surrounded by dense palisades of tumor cells, are attributable to true tumoral necrosis in that palisading is generally lacking in radiation necrosis. In recurrent tumors, the presence of intrinsic tumoral necrosis should be distinguished from the effects of prior treatment, particularly radiation therapy. Endothelial proliferation and necrosis need not be specifically related; they may be present in the same microscopic field or they may be widely segmented. As defined in the present WHO scheme, glioblastomas correspond to astrocytomas of St Anne-Mayo grade 4. Other histopathologic features that may be present in glioblastomas are cytoplasmic lipidization, stromal mucin accumulation, myxoid change, and desmoplasia in areas of meningeal, particularly dural, invasion (Kepes et al 1984, Russell & Rubinstein 1989).

Two distinct histopathologic subvariants of glioblastomas are recognized in the WHO classification. The first of these, *giant cell glioblastoma*, appears to have distinctive neuroradiologic and, to a lesser extent, clinical features. They have a slight predilection for the temporal lobe (Margetts & Kalyan-Raman 1989), and both on neuroimaging and gross examination appear remarkably circumscribed. Affected patients may frequently exceed the median survival time for those with more ordinary glioblastomas (Russell & Rubinstein 1989, Margetts & Kalyan-Raman, 1989). Histologically, giant cell glioblastomas in large part are composed of huge, bizarre, multinucleated giant cells with abundant eosinophilic cytoplasm and large vesicular nuclei (Fig. 8.3D). The frequent presence of more ordinary fibrillary cells or small astrocytes confirms the essentially astrocytic nature of these tumors. A variable histologic feature is an increase in reticulin fibers, one most conspicuous in relation to blood vessels and areas of necrosis. The giant cells are S-100 protein-positive but often lack significant immunoreactivity for GFAP, the latter being more prominent in the fusiform cells.

Gliosarcoma, or Feigin tumor, is the second principal variant of glioblastoma. The derivation of the sarcomatous element is usually thought to be malignant transforma-

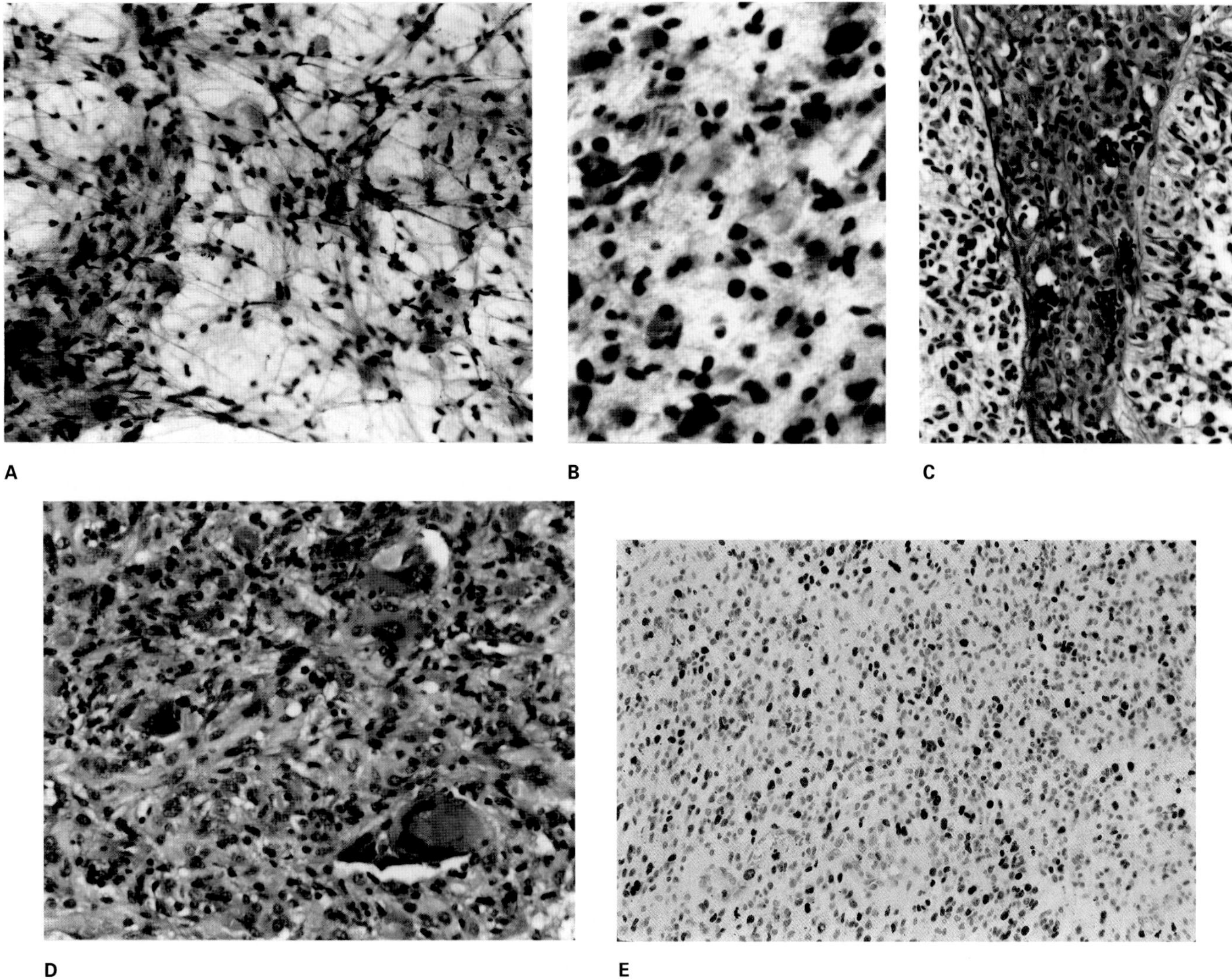

Fig. 8.3 Glioblastoma multiforme. **A**. Marked cellular pleomorphism and atypia can be readily appreciated in glioblastoma smears. The characteristic fibrillary matrix of astrocytomas is highlighted in smears. **B**, **C**. Cellular atypia, high mitotic activity, exuberant endothelial proliferation and necrosis constitute the histopathologic features of glioblastomas. **D**. Multinucleated giant cells with abundant cytoplasm and bizarre nuclei are the predominant feature of giant cell glioblastomas. **A–D** H&E. **E**. The Ki-67 labeling index is remarkably high in glioblastomas. Compare this picture with anaplastic astrocytoma. Ki-67 (MIB-1) avidin biotin-immunoperoxidase.

tion, either of the mesenchymal elements accompanying hyperplastic microvasculature or of those within adjacent meninges. Although endothelial and pericytic proliferation is a significant feature of all glioblastomas, the frequency of sarcomatous transformation in these tumors ranges from only 2–8% (Morantz et al 1976, Meis et al 1991). The ratio of glial to sarcomatous components is highly variable, both within individual tumors and in the group as a whole. The relative proportions of the two cell populations are such that the glial component tends over time to become minor. As a result, the lesion may eventuate in a primarily sarcomatous proliferation. As a rule, the two components can readily be distinguished on the basis of their morphologic features and special stains, such as reticulin and PTAH preparations, and by immunohistochemistry for GFAP which is reactive in the neoplastic glial component. Reticulin and collagen stains serve to highlight the sarcomatous component, which in most cases resembles either fibrosarcoma or malignant fibrous histiocytoma. Osteocartilaginous and rhabdomyoblastic elements may also rarely be present (Barnard et al 1986, Hayashi et al 1993). Immunohistochemical and ultrastructural studies suggest that the sarcomatous elements are likely derived from undifferentiated mesenchymal cells of the vascular adventitia which have a capacity for differentiating along endothelial, smooth muscle and pericytic cell lines (Grant et al 1989, Ho 1990, Ng & Poon 1990, Haddad et al 1991, Miller et al 1991). Because of the capacity for neoplastic astroglia to produce basal lamina and to elaborate extracellular matrix of the kind associated with mesenchymal differentiation, it may be an oversimplification to assume that the 'sarcomatous' element is invariably derived from nonglial cells (Paulus et al 1993).

E. Cytogenetic alterations in astrocytic tumors

The process of anaplastic progression in astrocytic tumors is reflected in genetic events. Mutations of the tumor suppressor gene p53 seem to represent the earliest detectable genetic alteration occurring in diffusely infiltrative astrocytomas (von Deimling et al 1992a, Louis et al 1993). Indeed, their progression to glioblastoma may be related to a clonal expansion of cells carrying a p53 mutation (Sidranski et al 1992). Such cells can be identified in approximately 30% of astrocytomas of all grades (Frankel et al 1992, Fults et al 1992, Louis et al 1993).

Genetic abnormalities, other than those affecting the p53 gene, are found in diffusely infiltrating astrocytomas. Allelic deletions have been demonstrated on chromosomes 9p, 10, 13, 17p, 19q and 22 (see Collins & James 1993 for review). Loss of heterozygosity on chromosome 17p occurs in approximately 30% of astrocytomas. Independent of tumor grade, it is frequently associated with point mutations in the p53 tumor suppressor gene (Frankel et al 1992, Fults et al 1992, von Deimling et al 1992a). In contrast, chromosome 10 deletions are found primarily in anaplastic astrocytoma and glioblastoma (Fults et al 1992).

A tentative subclassification of glioblastomas, one based upon their molecular genetic profile, has been recently proposed (von Deimling et al 1993). One subtype is characterized by deletions on the short arm of chromosome 17 and the absence of EGFR gene amplification. This type of glioblastoma occurs primarily in younger patients, and may have as its origin malignant transformation of lower grade astrocytomas. The other subset is identified by deletions on chromosome 10 and EGFR gene amplification without apparent deletions on chromosome 17. This second subtype of glioblastoma apparently arises de novo in an older patient population, is unassociated with an antecedent low grade astrocytoma, and invariably has a poor prognosis.

F. Immunohistochemical markers of proliferation

Special studies to estimate growth potential of diffusely infiltrative astrocytic neoplasms have been applied in routine diagnostic neuropathology. Cell cycle-associated nuclear proteins have been primarily utilized for this purpose. These proteins include proliferating cell nuclear antigen (PCNA) and the family of nuclear proteins identified by the Ki-67 epitope.

PCNA is a 36 kD cofactor of DNA-polymerase δ which is apparently synthesized at a greater rate in early S-phase and accumulates in the nucleus during S-phase. The amount and distribution of this protein apparently diminishes when the cell enters a noncycling phase (Celis & Celis 1985, Bravo et al 1987). These decreases are relative, however, and are more qualitative than quantitative. As a result, correlation of immunoreactive protein levels with proliferative activity is imprecise. The thresholds for 'positive' immunoreactivity must be determined not only for specific cell type, but also for methods of tissue processing and for variations related to the specific antibody used (Galand & Degraef 1989, Allegranza et al 1991, Louis et al 1991, Schiffer et al 1993). In summary, caution is advised with regard to interpretation of 'positive' immunoreactivity for PCNA. Not only is precise standardization required in each laboratory but processing of the tissue sections should be performed in batches with samples of known immunoreactivity.

The monoclonal antibody Ki-67 recognizes an epitope which is associated with a specific category of cell cycle-associated, non-histone nuclear proteins which appear to be necessary to the maintenance of the proliferative state (Schlüter et al 1993). The Ki-67 epitope is strictly associated with cell proliferation (G_1, S, G_2, and mitosis) and is absent in quiescent (G_O phase) cells (Gerdes et al 1983, 1984). Until recently, Ki-67 immunohistochemistry could only be applied to frozen sections. A recently introduced, commercially available, monoclonal antibody (MIB-1) is now available, and reacts with the Ki-67 epitope in routinely processed, paraffin-embedded material (Cattoretti et al 1992, Gerdes et al 1992, Sawhney & Hall 1992, Karamitopoulou et al 1993). Because of the simplicity of the procedure and the highly reliable staining results, the application of MIB-1 staining is rapidly becoming the most common method for determining tumor proliferative indices in neuropathology laboratories.

The evaluation of growth fraction by labeling indices of these proteins appears to correlate well with the histopathologic grade of astrocytomas (Figs 8.2B, 8.3E) (Burger et al 1986, Giangaspero et al 1987, Patsouris et al 1988, Reifenberger et al 1989, Louis et al 1991, Schröder et al 1991, Karamitopoulou et al 1993). Nonetheless, as is the case with simple H&E sections, heterogeneity in diffuse infiltrative astrocytic tumors leads to false interpretation of labeling results in limited samples (Coons & Johnson 1993).

An excellent method for the evaluation of growth fraction in astrocytomas is the in vivo (perioperative) labeling of cells in S-phase with bromodeoxyuridine (BUdR) (Hoshino et al 1988, Nishizaki et al 1988, 1989, Labrousse et al 1991). Its incorporation with subsequent immunohistochemical labeling of BUdR-containing cells in the resected tumor specimen permits an accurate assessment of tumor proliferation. This in situ method is applicable only in centers with appropriate resources and commitment to the technique. Although a few studies using in vitro BUdR labeling of resected tumor tissue

(Nishizaki et al 1988) suggest that this method has potential for diagnostic use, the feasibility of this approach for routine diagnosis has yet to be established.

G. Pilocytic astrocytoma (WHO grade I)

Pilocytic astrocytomas occur most frequently in children and young adults, their peak incidence being in the second decade. In adult patients, such tumors tend to appear one decade earlier (mean 22 years) than do diffusely infiltrative cerebral astrocytomas (Garcia & Fulling 1985). Pilocytic astrocytomas arise at all levels of the neuraxis; however, these tumors are characteristically located in the midline structures, e.g. cerebellum, third ventricular region, optic pathways, brainstem, and spinal cord. Although supratentorial pilocytic astrocytomas show a tendency to involve the temporo-parietal region, thalamus, hypothalamus or third ventricle, they may also arise in the fronto-parietal lobes (Forsyth et al 1993). Pilocytic astrocytomas comprise a large proportion (58%) of spinal astrocytomas, a site at which they tend to occur in an older population (Minehan et al 1993). Compared to the diffusely infiltrating astrocytomas previously discussed, pilocytic astrocytomas are less biologically aggressive, relatively well-circumscribed tumors, which displace rather than infiltrate the surrounding brain. As a result, they have a more favorable prognosis (Clark et al 1985, Forsyth et al 1993).

Although pilocytic astrocytomas are often macroscopically circumscribed, some degree of parenchymal infiltration and of invasion of leptomeninges is common, particularly in cerebellar examples (Tomlinson et al 1992). Even distant, cerebrospinal metastases have been reported (Obana et al 1991). It is important to emphasize that such behavior does not indicate anaplastic progression (Mishima et al 1992). Despite the rather indolent behavior and low proliferative potential of pilocytic astrocytomas, they can recur. This is particularly true of tumors found in unfavorable locations, and ones that are subtotally resected (Brown et al 1992).

Macroscopic features common to these tumors include the formation of a cyst associated with a solid mural nodule. Microscopically, pilocytic astrocytomas typically show a biphasic pattern of growth consisting of bipolar, highly fibrillated or piloid cells accompanied by Rosenthal fibers (Fig. 8.4B) and a loose knit microcystic component made up of stellate cells resembling protoplasmic astrocytes often associated with granular bodies or protein droplets (Fig. 8.4A). GFAP immunohistochemistry highlights the often dense fibrillated elements and is highly variable in microcystic areas. Vimentin, on the other hand, is demonstrable in both components (Schiffer et al 1986). Cellular atypia, replete with nuclear cytoplasmic inclusions as well as multinucleated cells may be present and is considered degenerative in nature. Glomeruloid microvascular proliferation is relatively common, but does not imply malignant transformation.

Histologic malignancy is rare in pilocytic astrocytomas. Brisk mitotic activity may be the most useful indicator of anaplastic progression, a process rarely seen to occur in these tumors (Schwartz & Ghatak 1991). In a recent series of 107 pilocytic astrocytomas of the cerebellum

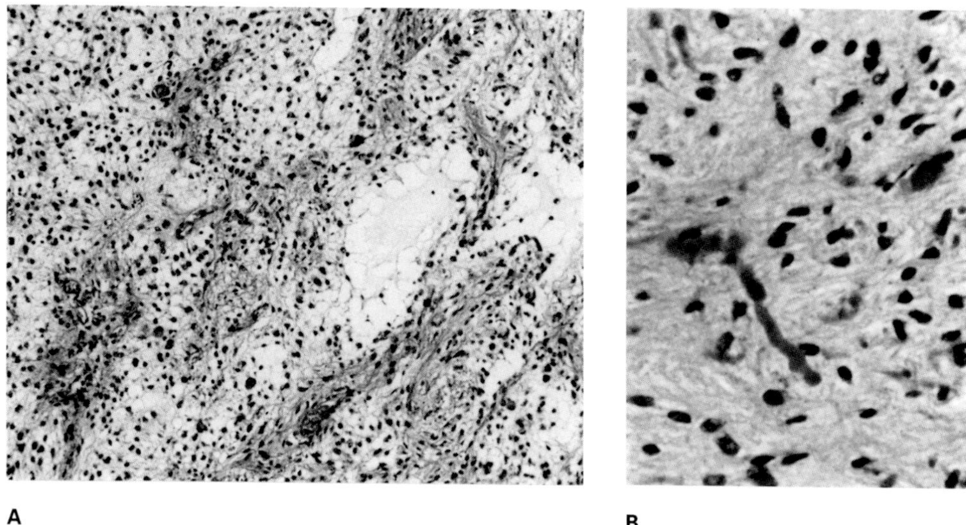

Fig. 8.4 Pilocytic astrocytoma.
A, B. A characteristic biphasic pattern is present in pilocytic astrocytomas. **A**. Stellate cells compose a loose-textured tissue often associated with microcystic changes **B**. Bipolar, piloid cells arranged in bundles are often associated with Rosenthal fibers **A, B** H&E.

(Tomlinson et al 1992), anaplastic progression occurred in only 0.9% of cases; these tumors had relatively high fractions of S-phase cells on DNA flow cytometry. The prognosis of such tumors is still favorable relative to that of diffuse infiltrative astrocytomas with similar features of malignancy (Tomlinson et al 1992).

H. Pleomorphic xanthoastrocytoma (WHO grade II–III)

The pleomorphic xanthoastrocytoma (PXA) is a superficially situated cerebral tumor that occurs most often in children or young adults (Kepes et al 1979, Pasquier et al 1985, Kawano 1991). Given its predilection for involvement of the temporal lobe, it is not surprising that an association with seizures is reported in up to 78% of the cases (Kawano 1991). The tumors are generally somewhat circumscribed masses exhibiting frequent leptomeningeal involvement and underlying cyst formation. As a rule, the dura is uninvolved (Kepes et al 1979, Strom & Skullerud 1983, Kawano 1991). Although a well-defined macroscopic border with the subjacent brain is generally present, focal microscopic infiltration of brain parenchyma is apparent when multiple microsections are carefully examined. Infiltration of Virchow-Robin spaces may be observed but is not, of itself, indicative of a worse prognosis (VandenBerg 1992).

The histopathologic appearance of pleomorphic xanthoastrocytoma is somewhat stereotypic. Most exhibit moderate cellularity and pleomorphism, the cells ranging from spindle cells intermixed with plump or polygonal cells to multinucleated giant cells (Fig. 8.5A). Nuclei are pleomorphic, exhibit great variety of shape and size, and are commonly hyperchromatic. Nuclear cytoplasmic inclusions are commonly seen. Cytoplasmic lipidization, especially of giant cells, may be conspicuous but is highly variable. Mitoses, when present, are not numerous. Necrosis and endothelial proliferation are absent. Focal chronic inflammation is frequent. Cytofluorometric analysis demonstrates a low percentage of S-phase cells, consistent with a low frequency of mitotic figures (Hosokawa et al 1991). The astroglial character of the cells is demonstrated by GFAP immunohistochemistry, although not all cells are GFAP immunoreactive, particularly giant cells (Fig. 8.5C).

A characteristic feature of PXA is its variable texture, ranging from firm to indistinguishable from the adjacent brain. This variation in texture often contributes to the impression that the tumor is well demarcated. The increased firmness of many tumors is due in part to the presence of an extracellular matrix, visualized on reticulin staining and occasionally on collagen stains (Fig. 8.5B), delineating clusters of cells or surrounding individual tumor cells. Although a stroma may be present in any portion of the tumor, it is most conspicuous in areas of

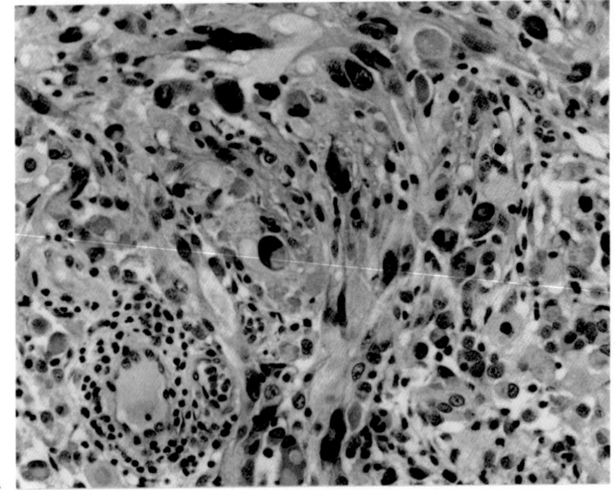
A

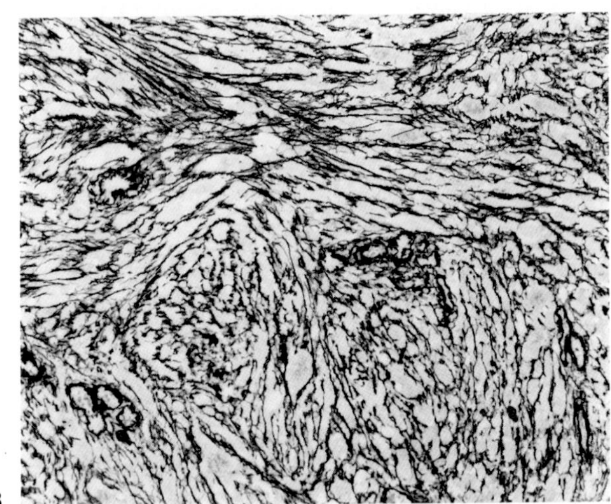
B

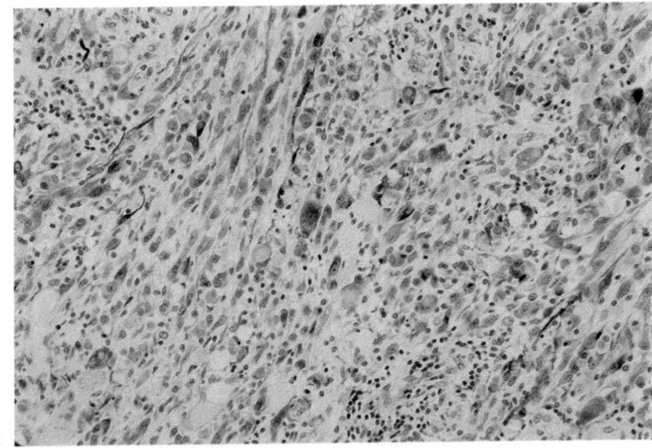
C

Fig. 8.5 Pleomorphic xanthoastrocytoma. **A.** Marked cellular heterogeneity, moderate cellular pleomorphism and xanthomatous changes are present in the PXA. H&E. **B.** The characteristic intercellular reticulin stroma defines fascicles of cells and surrounds individual tumor cells. Gordon and Sweet's reticulin. **C.** The astroglial nature of PXA is demonstrated by GFAP immunohistochemistry, although GFAP can be rather irregular in tumor cells. GFAP avidin biotin-immunoperoxidase.

leptomeningeal involvement. Ultrastructural studies demonstrate a pericellular basal lamina (Weldon-Linne et al 1983, Kepes et al 1989), similar to that described surrounding subpial astrocytes (Russell & Rubinstein 1989, Whittle et al 1989). Consequently, a histogenetic relationship between PXA and this special subpial phenotype of astrocytes has been suggested by some authors (Kepes et al 1979, Russell & Rubinstein 1989, Whittle et al 1989). A number of cases without prominent reticulin staining, but with otherwise typical features of PXA, have been also described (Kawano 1991).

The biologic behavior of PXA and its potential for anaplastic progression remain uncertain. Although the initial description of the entity suggested that PXA should be considered a low grade neoplasm (Kepes et al 1979), a number of cases have recurred and exhibited anaplastic progression (Weldon-Linne et al 1983, Kepes et al 1989, Daita et al 1991). The process appears to be significantly less frequent than for diffuse infiltrative astrocytomas. Nonetheless, when compared to the other more circumscribed, prognostically favorable variants of astrocytomas, i.e. pilocytic and subependymal giant cell astrocytomas, PXA should be generally considered a tumor with a significant potential for aggressive biologic behavior. Accordingly, these tumors are designated as grade II–III by the WHO classification (Kleihues et al 1993a). The histopathologic features of the infiltrating margin may be an important clue to the potential for recurrence and anaplastic progression (Weldon-Linne et al 1983, Kepes et al 1989, Daita et al 1991).

I. Subependymal giant cell astrocytoma (WHO grade I)

Subependymal giant cell astrocytoma (SEGA) typically occurs in the first two decades of life, mostly in the setting of tuberous sclerosis. Despite opinion to the contrary (Shepherd et al 1991), a small number of similar tumors may occur in patients without this phakomatosis. The tumors most commonly arise in the wall of the lateral ventricles at the level of the basal ganglia. Extension into the third ventricle region may also be seen. SEGAs are typically circumscribed, solid nodules, well demarcated from the adjacent parenchyma. Calcifications are often present.

Histologically, the cells comprising subependymal giant cell astrocytomas are heterogeneous, exhibiting a broad range of astroglial phenotypes (Fig. 8.6A). Three principal cell types may be seen enmeshed in a variably fibrillated matrix: small spindle cells, intermediate size polygonal or 'gemistocytic' cells, and giant, ganglion-like cells. In all cell types the nuclei have a finely granular chromatin pattern with distinct nucleoli. The majority of tumor cells demonstrate variable immunoreactivity for GFAP (Fig. 8.6B) and S-100 protein, thus confirming the essentially astroglial nature of this tumor. A number of tumors, however, demonstrate both glial and neuronal-associated epitopes such as class III β-tubulin, high molecular weight neurofilament proteins, and neurotransmitter substances (Altermatt et al 1993). These tumors may also exhibit ultrastructural features suggestive of neuronal differentiation, such as microtubules, occasional dense core granules, and rare synapse formation. These features are similar to those seen in tubers, the hamartomatous cortical lesions of tuberous sclerosis. Divergent glioneuronal differentiation is a hallmark feature of tubers and subependymal giant cell astrocytomas.

Subependymal giant cell astrocytomas may demonstrate considerable cellular pleomorphism, occasional mitotic figures and, rarely, necrosis. These features are not indicative of clinically meaningful anaplastic progres-

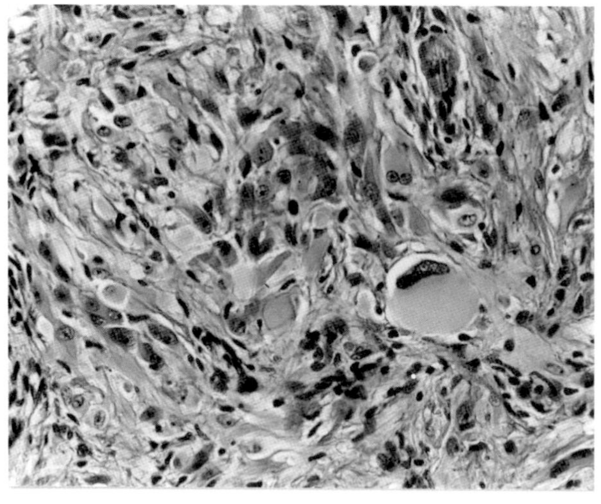
A

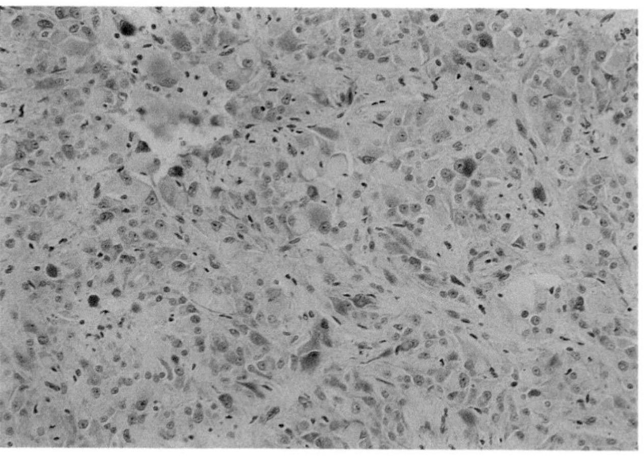
B

Fig. 8.6 Subependymal giant cell astrocytoma. **A**. Cellular heterogeneity is typical for SEGA, with spindle, polygonal and ganglion-like cells. H&E. **B**. The majority of tumor cells display variable immunoreactivity for GFAP. GFAP avidin biotin-immunoperoxidase ×500.

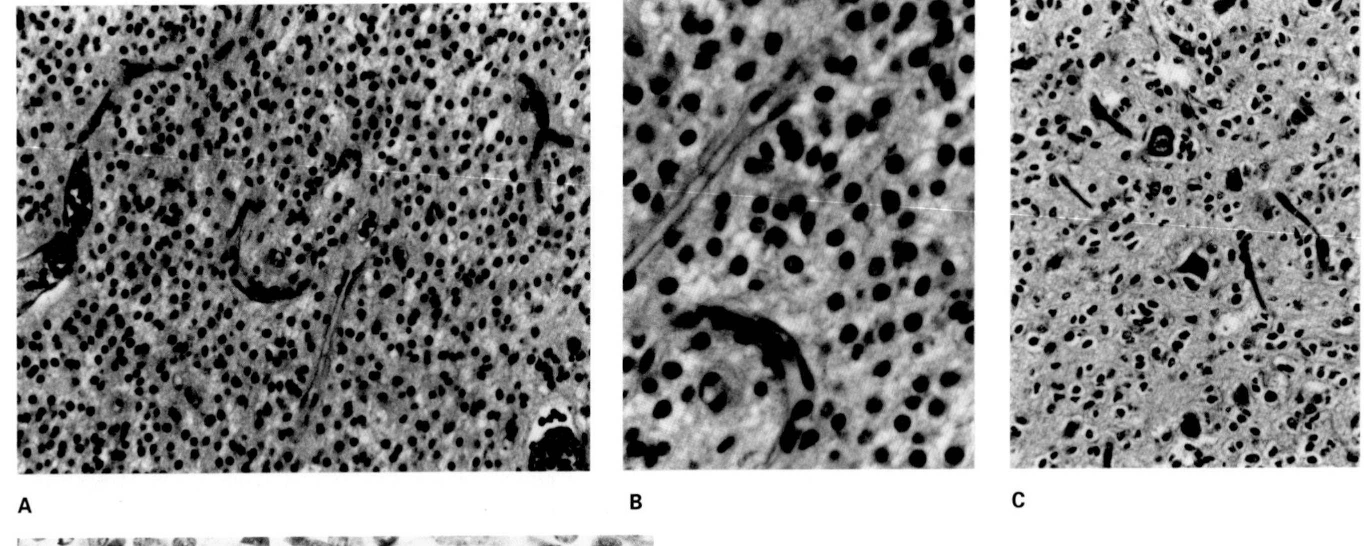

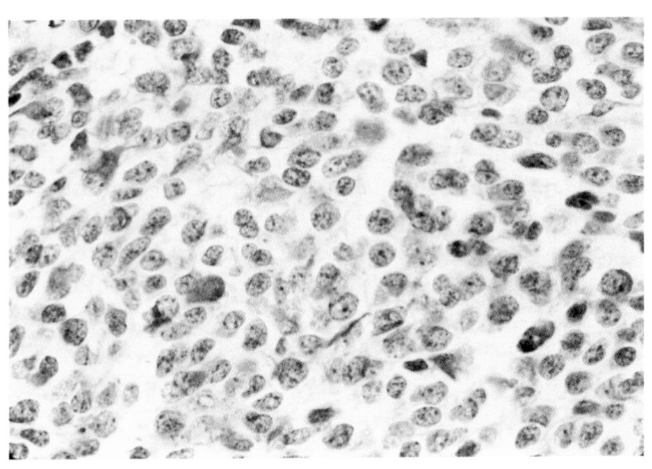

Fig. 8.7 Oligodendroglioma. **A**. Oligodendrogliomas display a uniform cell population with round nuclei and perinuclear halos. Delicate blood vessels are conspicuously present. **B**. Delicate chromatin distribution and slight lobulated nuclei contours are typical of oligodendrogliomas. **C**. Diffuse infiltration of the cerebral cortex with perineuronal satellitosis is frequently seen in oligodendrogliomas. **A–C** H&E. **D**. GFAP immunoreactivity is present in 'gliofibrillary' oligodendrocytes. These GFAP-positive cells should be differentiated from reactive, stromal astrocytes. GFAP avidin biotin-immunoperoxidase.

sion (Shepherd et al 1991). As a matter of fact, those rare examples of SEGA that do recur have not been reported to show malignant transformation (Halmagyi et al 1979).

2. Oligodendroglial tumors

A. Oligodendroglioma (WHO grade II)

This underdiagnosed lesion represents approximately 30% of intracranial gliomas. Although they occur at any age, the majority of tumors arise in adults, with a peak incidence in the fourth and fifth decades (Mørk et al 1985, Zülch 1986). Oligodendrogliomas most frequently occur in the frontotemporal region but actually arise in any region of the neuraxis in relative proportion to its volume of white matter. Macroscopically, oligodendrogliomas are soft and translucent. Grossly apparent foci of calcification are the exception. Tumor cells have poorly defined cytoplasm and are loosely cohesive within a poorly-fibrillated matrix. The nuclei are typically round to slightly lobulated with a more fine chromatin pattern than astrocytes (Fig. 8.7A–C). The tumor cells may be arranged in a broad spectrum of histologic patterns. Most common is a diffuse or a pseudolobulated pattern, resulting from division of the tumor into lobules circumscribed in part by delicate, often acutely branching vessels, a pattern loosely termed the 'chicken wire' pattern. Other cellular arrangements include uninterrupted diffuse or nodular growth, as well as parallel rows of cells forming palisades. Intercellular microcyst formation due to stromal mucin accumulation is common, particularly in low grade tumors. Reactive astrocytes are frequently found scattered throughout the tumor, preferentially around blood vessels. Mitotic figures may be present in small numbers. Capillaries may be prominent but bona fide endothelial proliferation is generally limited to anaplastic oligodendroglioma.

The majority of proteins and antigenic markers that characterize mature oligodendrocytes and oligodendrocytic cells during brain development are inconstantly expressed in neoplastic oligodendrocytes. Their variable expression is further complicated by the frequent loss of epitopes of these markers after routine tissue processing. Consequently, no specific immunocytochemical marker of oligodendroglial differentiation is available for the purpose of tumor classification. It is of note that the characterization of oligodendrogliomas with markers of mature and developing oligodendrocytes has yielded mixed results. For instance, myelin basic protein (MBP) and proteolipid protein (PLP) constitute up to 80% of all CNS myelin proteins (Less & Brostoff 1984). Nonetheless, immunoreactivity for MBP has on one occasion been reported in neoplastic oligodendrocytes (Figols et al 1985), some authors finding no reactivity (Nakagawa et al 1986). Furthermore, myelin-associated glycoprotein (MAG), a protein present in myelin in smaller quantities than is MBP, has been demonstrated in a limited number of oligodendrogliomas (Perentes & Rubinstein 1987). Two major series of oligodendroglial tumors reporting the immunohistochemical detection of galactocerebroside (GalC), a major oligodendroglial-specific glycolipid of myelin (Norton & Cammer 1984), have also reported variable results. It is of interest that Kennedy et al (1987), in a study of 7 oligodendrogliomas and 4 mixed oligo-astrocytomas, could not demonstrate GalC expression. In contrast, de la Monte (1989) described it in 27 of 28 oligodendroglial tumors; all mixed oligo-astrocytomas of this series exhibited GalC in both the oligodendrocytic and astrocytic components. Leu-7, a marker of natural killer cells also designated HNK-1 (Abo & Balch 1981), which recognizes a carbohydrate epitope associated with myelin (McGarry et al 1983, Sato et al 1983) has been demonstrated in the majority of oligodendrogliomas (Perentes & Rubinstein 1986). Unfortunately, this surface antigen is not particularly useful for definitively discriminating oligodendrogliomas from other gliomas.

Because the majority of oligodendroglioma cells do not express vimentin (Jagadha et al 1986), and anaplastic oligodendrogliomas are more likely to do so (Cruz-Sanchez et al 1991), we exploit this property for diagnostic purposes. Neoplastic oligodendrocytes with a more prominent, globoid cell body, so-called 'gliofibrillary oligodendrocytes' (Herpers & Budka 1984, Wondrusch et al 1991, Kros et al 1992), commonly exhibit intense GFAP immunoreactivity (Fig. 8.7D) (Kros et al 1990). Such cells are present in a significant proportion of oligodendrogliomas (Herpers & Budka 1984, Nakagawa et al 1986). The GFAP immunoreactivity of these, as well as 'minigemistocytes', oligodendrocytes with even more abundant cytoplasm, must be distinguished from bona fide mixed oligo-astrocytoma. The latter exhibit obvious fibrillary astrocytic or fully developed gemistocytic elements.

The finding of GFAP immunoreactivity in neoplastic oligodendrogliomas may be analogous to the transient expression of GFAP in immature oligodendrocytes prior to normal myelinogenesis (Choi & Kim 1984). The histogenesis of such GFAP-immunoreactive cells is still unclear. One possibility is that the tumors represent a subset of oligodendrogliomas wherein oligodendroglial progenitors, neoplastic counterparts of O-2A cells, persist and give rise to a GFAP-immunoreactive phenotype. Studies suggest that oligodendrocytes and type-2 astrocytes arise from a common progenitor cell in rodents designated O-2A, which is 'A2B5' immunoreactive (Raff et al 1983). In examining 28 oligodendrogliomas, de la Monte (1989) demonstrated a high percentage of A2B5 immunoreactive cells, most of which also coexpressed GalC, thus suggesting that neoplastic GFAP-immunoreactive oligodendrocytes within oligodendrogliomas may originate from O-2A-like progenitor cells. Unfortunately, an attempt to reclassify gliomas on the basis of the antigenic scheme developed in the in vitro rodent model was not successful. Expression of 'cell-specific' epitopes appeared to be more 'promiscuous' in human neoplastic cell populations (see Noble et al 1991 for review). Another explanation for GFAP immunoreactivity in oligodendrocytes may be that it represents cross-reactivity of common polypeptide sequences, which are also present in cytokeratins (Kashima et al 1993). Regardless of the question of cellular lineage and cross-reactivity, GFAP-immunoreactive cells tend to increase in number with anaplastic progression of oligodendrogliomas (Herpers & Budka 1984, Kros et al 1990).

B. *Anaplastic oligodendroglioma (WHO grade III)*

Anaplastic oligodendrogliomas are characterized by the presence of histopathologic features similar to those associated with anaplasia in the diffuse infiltrative astrocytomas. These include cellularity, often high, widespread nuclear atypia and pleomorphism, a brisk mitotic index, endothelial proliferation and necrosis (Fig. 8.8A,B) (Smith et al 1983, Mørk et al 1985, Burger 1989). No general agreement has been reached as to what constitutes the most important criteria for 'anaplastic oligodendroglioma'. Tumors exhibiting the cytology of oligodendroglioma but the vascularity and necrosis typical of glioblastoma are regarded as grade 4 oligodendrogliomas, not glioblastoma. The latter is, by definition, an astrocytic neoplasm.

3. Ependymal tumors

A. *Ependymoma* (WHO grade II)

Ependymomas represent approximately 10% of brain tumors and 6% of intracranial gliomas (Russell & Rubinstein 1989). They occur in any age population, but constitute a higher percentage of gliomas in childhood and adolescence than in adults (Yates et al 1979). They typically arise in the vicinity of the ventricles, the fourth ventricle being the most frequent site, followed by the aqueduct and the spinal cord. In children and adolescents, ependymomas tend to be intracranial, a high pro-

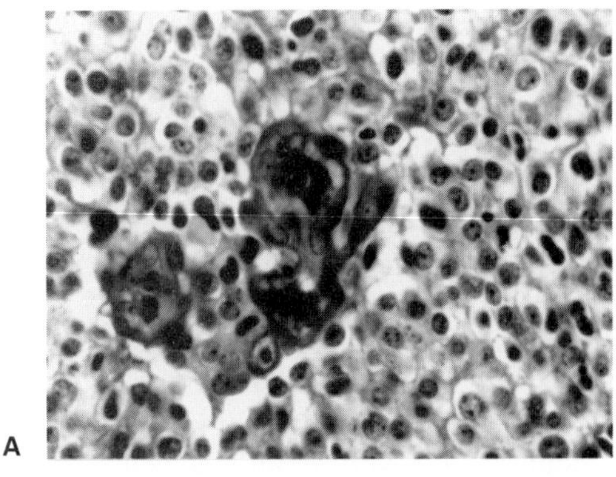

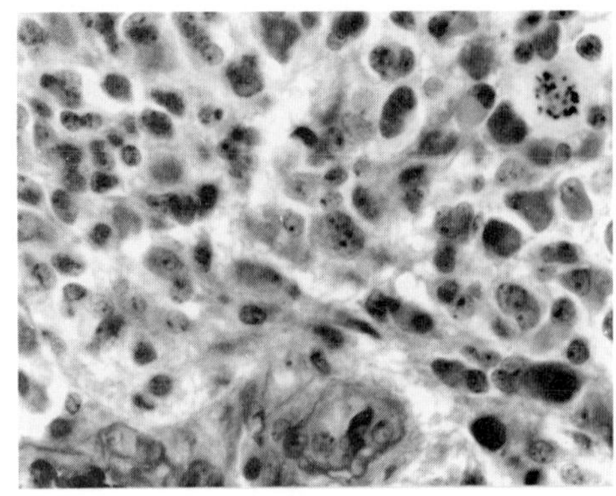

Fig. 8.8 Anaplastic oligodendroglioma. **A, B**. Hypercellularity, cellular pleomorphism, mitotic figures and endothelial proliferation are characteristics of anaplastic oligodendrogliomas. The characteristic round nuclei of the cells are retained by the anaplastic tumors **A**. Many cells, however, display a glassy, eosinophilic cytoplasm similar to 'gemistocytic' cells **B**. **A, B** H&E.

portion arising in the fourth ventricle, whereas in adults they represent over 60% of spinal cord gliomas (Salazar et al 1983).

Macroscopically, ependymomas are well demarcated, their macroscopically 'pushing borders' affording a plane of resection. Despite a sharp parenchymal interface, a small proportion gain access to the ventricular space and undergo subarachnoid spread. This is particularly true of fourth ventricular ependymomas, which show a tendency to expand into surrounding cisterns and may come to encase the cervical spinal cord. Cystic degeneration and calcifications are common features of ependymoma.

A characteristic, albeit infrequently observed, histologic feature of ependymomas is the tendency of their polarized cells to encircle an extracellular space to form a lumen (*ependymal rosettes*). Although typical of these tumors, 'true' ependymal rosettes and epithelial-lined tubules are much less common than are so-called *pseudorosettes*, wherein the processes of cells radiate toward a central blood vessel (Fig. 8.9A). Aside from forming true rosettes and pseudorosettes, cells of ependymomas vary from patently glial to epithelial appearing. Cellularity varies but most ependymomas are of the 'cellular' type. In distinctly glial appearing tumors, the elongate cell processes that contribute to the fibrillary matrix (Fig. 8.9B) can be highlighted by PTAH staining or by immunostains for GFAP or vimentin (Fig. 8.9D). The often clustered nuclei vary in appearance from those with delicate, 'open' chromatin to those that are somewhat hyperchromatic. Distinct nucleoli are a helpful diagnostic feature of ependymomas. Nuclear atypia and even small foci of necrosis may be present without indicating anaplastic change (see below). Mitoses are absent to infrequent.

The WHO classification recognizes three histologic variants of ependymomas: *cellular, papillary* and *clear cell*. These tumors have basically the same clinical outcome, but their recognition as variants of ependymoma is important in distinguishing them from anaplastic gliomas, choroid plexus tumors and oligodendrogliomas, respectively. *Cellular* ependymomas vary considerably in pattern and cytology. Some are patternless and exhibit little in the way of rosetting. The *papillary* variant tends to show dehiscence of sheets to form papillae; as a result, such tumors may mimic choroid plexus tumors. The ependymal nature of such tumors is most easily confirmed by their immunoreactivity for GFAP and lack of cytokeratin staining. The *clear cell* variant (Fig. 8.9C) shows a distinct honeycomb appearance due to perinuclear halo formation within the crowded cells. Pseudorosettes may be uncommon. Such tumors present a problem in differential diagnosis with oligodendrogliomas. The proper diagnosis is suggested by other ependymal features such as sharp demarcation, and contrast enhancement on CT and MRI. Routine histochemical and immunostains, even for GFAP, may not permit their identification, particularly in a small biopsy. The ultrastructural finding of intercellular microvilli and cilia containing spaces as well as junctional complexes, is diagnostic of ependymoma (Kawano et al 1989).

B. Anaplastic ependymoma (WHO grade III)

Anaplastic progression of ependymomas can occur in most sites, but is very uncommon in the ependymomas of the spinal cord (Russell & Rubinstein 1989). Anaplastic ependymomas are histologically recognized by their increased cellularity, varying degree of cellular/nuclear atypia, brisk mitotic activity, and by the frequent presence of endothelial proliferation. The correlation between histopathologic features of such tumors and the clinical outcome of patients with anaplastic ependymomas is not well defined. A prognostic factor of particular significance in supratentorial examples is the mitotic index (Schiffer et al 1991). This observation is indirectly confirmed by tumor growth fraction measurements, either by BUdR uptake (Asai et al 1992) or Ki-67 immunohistochemistry (Schröder et al 1993). By both methods, high labeling indices correlate with high histologic grade and early tumor recurrence. A recent study of pediatric ependymomas indicates that progression relates closely to a set

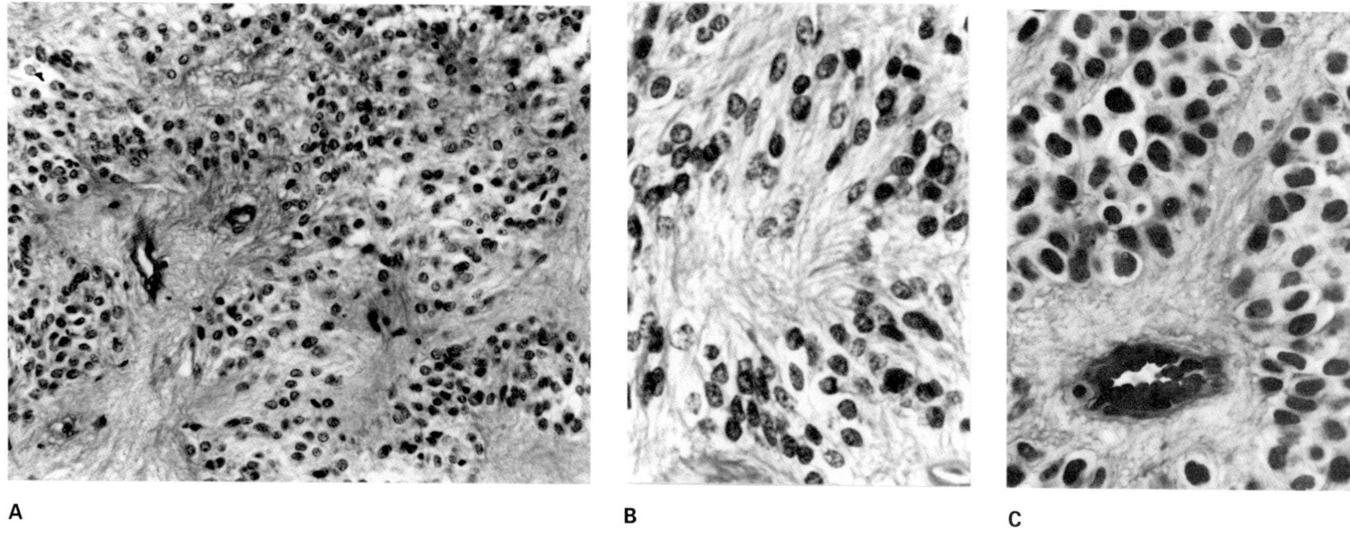

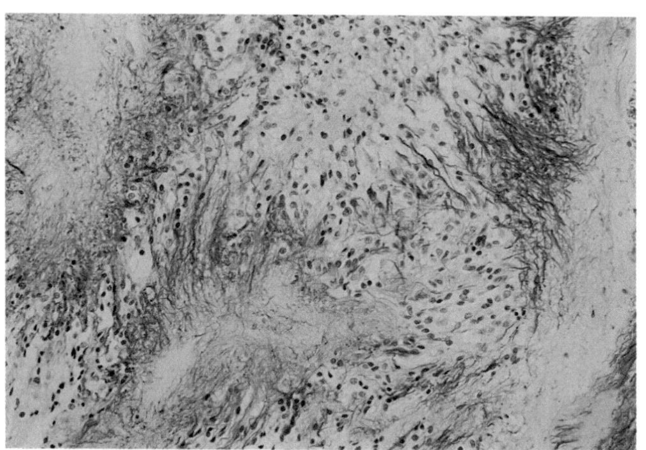

Fig. 8.9 Ependymoma. **A**. Low power fields of ependymomas show the classic perivascular pseudorosettes. Note the uniformity of the round nuclei. **B**. Perivascular pseudorosettes and ependymal rosettes are hallmarks of ependymomas. **C**. Ependymomas with clear cell areas can resemble oligodendrogliomas because of the perinuclear halos and nuclear uniformity. **A–C** H&E. **D**. Fibrillary processes of neoplastic ependymal cells are strongly immunoreactive for GFAP. GFAP avidin biotin-immunoperoxidase.

of clinicopathologic parameters, particularly age, DNA ploidy and histologic grade (Keating et al 1993).

An important distinction should be drawn between the anaplastic ependymomas and the ependymoblastomas. The latter, an embryonal neoplasm (see below), represents a highly malignant, often bulky tumor which usually arises in the supratentorial region of infants and children under the age of five years. In contrast to ependymomas, ependymoblastomas aggressively invade surrounding structures and show a distinct tendency to craniospinal seeding.

C. Myxopapillary ependymoma (WHO grade I)

The myxopapillary ependymoma is a slow-growing, distinct variant of ependymoma which commonly occurs in the cauda equina of adults (Morantz et al 1979, Sonneland et al 1985, Pulitzer et al 1988). The tumors are either discrete, sausage-shaped masses arising from the filum terminale, compressing spinal nerve roots of the cauda equina, or are found locally disseminated at first surgery. Infrequently, myxopapillary ependymomas present as extradural lesions in the presacral space or in retrosacral soft tissue. Such ectopic tumors presumably arise from ependymal rests (Morantz et al 1979, Pulitzer et al 1988). Although the majority of the tumors are biologically benign and slow-growing, local recurrences are common. Spreading within the neuraxis is far more common than the rare extraneural metastases (Patterson et al 1961, Rubinstein & Logan 1970, Sonneland et al 1985). The prognosis of this unique ependymoma variant is related to its resectability. Only a minority are found to be an intact bag-like lesion at the time of surgery. Every effort should be made to resect such lesions intact. Puncture or gutting of the tumor in situ facilitates recurrence and diminished likelihood of cure (Sonneland et al 1985).

Histologically, most myxopapillary ependymomas are composed, in part, of papillary arrangements of elongated fibrillary cells, the processes of which extend to blood vessels surrounded by a mucinous or hyalinized stroma. Mucin may also accompany neoplastic cells not in contact with vessels and is therefore a product of the neoplasm rather than simply a stromal response. Electron microscopy has confirmed the ependymal nature of these lesions, revealing cytoplasmic intermediate filaments, pockets of microvilli often associated with numerous cellular interdigitations and abundant basal lamina (Rawlinson et al 1973, Specht et al 1986). The presence of glial fibrils, verified by PTAH stain and immunohistochemistry for GFAP, distinguishes this tumor from the schwannomas and from paragangliomas which also occur in this region (Sonneland et al 1986).

D. Subependymoma (WHO grade I)

Subependymomas are well-circumscribed, generally asymptomatic nodules located in the walls of the fourth (66–70% of cases) and lateral ventricles (Scheithauer 1978, Lombardi et al 1991). The septum pellucidum, foramen of Monro and, less commonly, spinal cord may also be affected by these tumors (Pagni et al 1992). Although the majority are incidental findings at post mortem, symptomatic subependymomas occur with some frequency, usually in older adults, and present either with increased intracranial pressure due to obstruction of CSF flow or with spontaneous tumoral hemorrhage.

Histologically, subependymomas exhibit features of both ependymal and astrocytic differentiation. Hypocellular and composed of a dense fibrillary matrix, the tumor's low power architecture is characterized by clusters of cells surrounded by skeins of fibrillar processes. Ependymal features such as pseudorosettes are not uncommon, whereas true rosettes are rare. Astrocytic appearing cells, elongated to somewhat gemistocytic, may also be focally present. The association of astrocytic and ependymal features has also been confirmed by electron microscopic and tissue culture studies (Fu et al 1974, Azzarelli et al 1977). Microcystic degeneration and microcalcification are common, as is vascular hyalinization and hemosiderin deposition suggestive of prior, often subclinical, hemorrhage. Nuclear atypia and limited mitotic activity may be present, but is of no prognostic significance. Tumor location and surgical factors relative to the degree of attempted resection, particularly with respect to tumors situated on the floor of the fourth ventricle, are the most important prognostic factors (Lombardi et al 1991).

4. Mixed gliomas

Arriving at a consensus with regard to what constitutes 'mixed' gliomas has been a longstanding problem. Tumors composed of admixtures of neoplastic glial elements are, therefore, one of the challenges of diagnostic neuropathology in the 1990s. Techniques developed in the last decades, particularly electron microscopy and immunohistochemistry, have brought about the notion that such tumors, usually ones composed of astrocytes and oligodendroglia, less frequently ones with ependymal components, are not rare. Their recognition and proper classification are, however, problematic. There is at present no accepted definition of mixed gliomas; even the percentage of the various cellular components varies among different laboratories. Furthermore, the principal cells composing such lesions, particularly neoplastic oligodendroglia, vary considerably in terms of their morphology. Not only does the relative proportion of the different cells pose a problem, but their relationship within any one tumor varies from diffuse admixtures to geographically discrete populations. Attempting to set guidelines, some workers have defined mixed tumors as gliomas in which the minor cell type exceeds 30% (Hurtt et al 1992). Tumor heterogeneity also frustrates the diagnosis of mixed gliomas and adequate tissue sampling is necessary. Thus, the array of special techniques currently available for the study of mixed tumors often cannot be applied, particularly to non-representative samples or to stereotactic biopsies. Lastly, the features which indicate anaplastic progression vary among different components of gliomas, certain cells such as gemistocytic astrocytes being more likely to undergo anaplastic transformation. This aspect is especially significant in oligo-astrocytomas wherein the morphologic criteria for anaplasia are not equivalent in the two glial populations. Progression also alters the histopathologic character of the tumor from one point to another.

A. Mixed oligo-astrocytoma (WHO grade II)

These mixed gliomas are composed of oligodendrocytes and a significant population of neoplastic astrocytes. The predominant component is often oligodendroglial (Rubinstein 1972), but proportions do vary considerably. The two neoplastic cell populations may be focally or diffusely distributed. Mixed oligo-astrocytomas must be distinguished from oligodendrogliomas which contain varying numbers of reactive astrocytes. In addition, the simple detection of GFAP immunoreactivity in 'gliofibrillary' or 'minigemistocytic' oligodendrocytes should not be overinterpreted as indicative of an astrocytic component.

The histogenesis of mixed oligo-astrocytomas remains unclear. They may arise from 'transitional' cells, with characteristics intermediate between mature oligodendrocytes and astrocytes (Herpers & Budka 1984), or from transformed precursor cells analogous to the O-2A progenitor cells described in the rodent optic nerve (see Oligodendrogliomas). Recent experimental studies have demonstrated the presence of such true progenitor cells in the adult rat brain (Wren et al 1992), capable of generating both oligodendrocytes and type-2 astrocytes. Although this information is derived principally from rodent tissue in culture (Miller et al 1989, Lillien & Raff 1990), the demonstration of such progenitor cells in the adult nervous system may shed light upon the histogenesis of oligodendrogliomas and mixed oligo-astrocytomas (Bishop & de la Monte 1989). Yet another possibility, that one glial component induces neoplastic transformation in a second histogenetically distinct cell line, cannot simply be dismissed.

B. Malignant oligo-astrocytoma (WHO grade III)

The frequency with which oligo-astrocytomas undergo anaplastic progression is unknown. It is generally agreed upon that the astrocytic component is more susceptible to anaplastic change (Muller et al 1977, Russell & Rubinstein 1989). The histopathologic features of the anaplastic elements of these tumors are similar to those previously described for anaplastic astrocytomas and oligodendrogliomas.

5. Choroid plexus tumors

A. Choroid plexus papilloma (WHO grade I)

Choroid plexus papillomas comprise only 2.0% of intracranial gliomas (Zülch 1986). In children, most arise in the lateral ventricles (Laurence 1979, Russell & Rubinstein 1989) whereas in adults the fourth ventricle is the most commonly affected site (Russell & Rubinstein 1989). Clinical symptoms are often due to increased intracranial pressure, either secondary to obstruction of the CSF pathways or to increased production of CSF.

Grossly, choroid plexus papillomas are demarcated and resemble a cauliflower. Calcification is common and varies considerably. Their histopathologic appearance is one of a benign, papillary neoplasm composed of a single, often pseudostratified layer of columnar epithelium surrounding a delicate fibrovascular core (Fig. 8.10A). In contrast to normal choroid plexus epithelium, papillomas are hypercellular and exhibit some degree of cellular pleomorphism. Oncocytic and xanthomatous changes may be present (Kepes 1983, Bonnin et al 1987). As a rule, mitotic figures are inconspicuous, and necrosis and invasion of the adjacent parenchyma are minimal. When prominent, combinations of these features indicate malignant transformation and an increased likelihood of recurrence and cerebrospinal spread (Masuzawa et al 1981, Russell & Rubinstein 1989, Paulus & Jänisch 1990). Symptomatic subarachnoid seeding is very uncommon (Wolfson & Brown 1977, McGirr et al 1988).

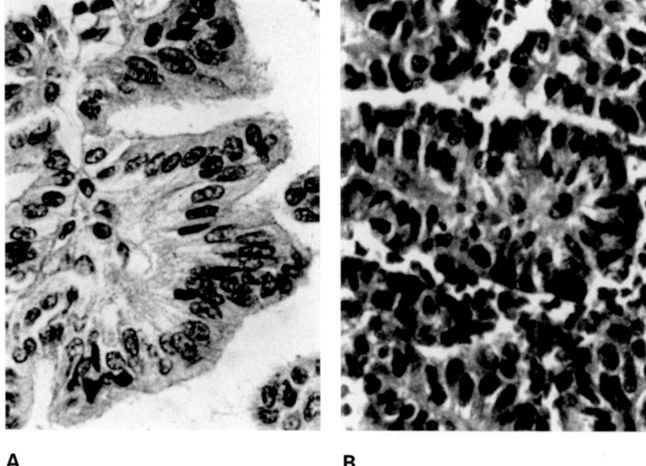

Fig. 8.10 Choroid plexus tumors. **A**. Papillomas demonstrate papillary structures composed of single or multiple layers of columnar epithelium surrounding a delicate fibrovascular core. **B**. Although the papillary structures are still present, carcinomas exhibit a high degree of cellular pleomorphism and mitotic figures. **A**, **B** H&E.

The differential diagnosis of choroid plexus papilloma includes the papillary variant of ependymoma. GFAP cannot distinguish papillomas from ependymomas because the majority of choroid plexus papillomas are to some extent GFAP positive (Rubinstein & Brucher 1981, Taratuto et al 1983, Miettinen et al 1986, Lopes et al 1989). Immunoreactivity for cytokeratin and transthyretin (TTR), both common to papillomas, may be useful for this purpose (Paulus & Jänisch 1990, Albrecht et al 1991), although TTR has been reported to occur in ependymomas (Kaneko et al 1990). Ultrastructural examination is helpful in that, like normal choroid plexus, papillomas exhibit apical junctional complexes replete with tight junctions rather than the extensive zonulae adherens seen in ependymomas.

B. Choroid plexus carcinoma (WHO grade III–IV)

Malignant transformation in choroid plexus papillomas is an uncommon event, occurring in less than 20% of cases (Laurence 1979). Carcinomas are most likely to arise within the lateral ventricles, particularly in young children. Unlike the papillomas, choroid plexus carcinomas are more often frankly invasive. In addition, subarachnoid spread and CSF dissemination are far more common. Metastasis outside the neuraxis is a rare event (Vraa-Jensen 1950). Carcinomas tend to have a less obviously papillary architecture, the cells often being arranged in cellular, patternless sheets (Fig. 8.10B). Marked cytologic atypia, brisk mitotic activity, and extensive necrosis are usually present. The differential diagnosis includes metastatic adenocarcinoma, especially in those rare cases affecting adults.

Transthyretin (TTR) immunoreactivity does not discriminate choroid plexus tumors from metastates, particularly papillary carcinomas (Liddle et al 1985, Albrecht et al 1991). The absence of epithelial membrane antigen (EMA) staining as well as other epithelial, non-cytokeratin HEA 125 and Ber EP4, in the presence of vimentin, S-100 protein, and GFAP antigens may facilitate the differential diagnosis with metastatic adenocarcinomas (Gottschalk et al 1993). It has been suggested that TTR may be of use in monitoring recurrence in confirmed cases of choroid plexus carcinoma (Paulus & Jänisch 1990). In children and adolescents, other neoplasms to be considered in the differential diagnosis include teratocarcinoma and embryonal carcinoma.

6. Neuronal and mixed neuronal-glial tumors

6.1. Neuronal tumors

A. Gangliocytomas (WHO grade I). Gangliocytomas

are slow-growing, well-circumscribed lesions which generally arise in the temporal lobes of children and young adults. Their nature, whether malformative or neoplastic, is unsettled. Less common than gangliogliomas, they also differ clinically from the latter in that most show no association with a chronic seizure disorder (see below). Gangliocytomas are composed of mature neurons in a paucicellular stroma. Their differential diagnosis includes cortical dysplasia and hamartomatous lesions. Unlike cortical dysplasia, the ganglion cells of gangliocytomas show greater pleomorphism, including the presence of bizarre and multinucleate forms. Silver impregnation techniques and neurofilament immunohistochemistry reveal the presence of abnormal neuritic processes. Unlike gangliogliomas (see below), a neoplastic glial component is not present. Gangliocytomas possess no potential for anaplastic progression.

B. Dysplastic gangliocytoma of the cerebellum (WHO grade I). Lhermitte-Duclos disease can be considered a special variant of gangliocytoma, one affecting the cerebellum. It too shows features of hamartoma and neoplasia. The lesion generally manifests in early life with megaencephaly, becoming more obviously symptomatic during the second and third decades, at which time mass effect becomes apparent. MR imaging shows a peculiar, focal, laminar thickening of cerebellar folia (Milbouw et al 1988, Reeder et al 1988, Ashley et al 1990).

Dysplastic gangliocytoma consists of hypertrophy of abnormal neurons, superficially resembling Purkinje cells, in association with large myelinated fibers forming parallel structures beneath the pia. The granular layer, when present, is often reduced in thickness. The underlying white matter typically shows a decrease in myelination. Studies of the abnormal neurons differ in their findings. Some report the expression of synaptic and surface membrane proteins related to Purkinje cell lineage (Shiruba et al 1988, Russell & Rubinstein 1989, Faillot et al 1990), whereas others suggest that the cells are related to granular cell neurons (Reznik & Schoenen 1983, Yachnis et al 1988). It is likely that the neuronal proliferation arises from a cytogenetically more heterogeneous group of cells. Like other gangliocytomas, these show no tendency to anaplastic progression. Nonetheless, recurrences have been reported following subtotal resection (Banerjee & Gleathil 1979, Marano et al 1988).

C. Central neurocytoma (WHO grade I). Central neurocytomas are rare supratentorial, intraventricular tumors of neuronal type which affect young adults and are associated with a favorable prognosis following surgical resection alone (von Deimling et al 1990). They typically present as well-demarcated, often calcified masses projecting into the lateral ventricles, usually in the region of the foramen of Monro. Large tumors may show extension into the third ventricle (Hessler et al 1992). A detailed review of 127 published cases has been recently reported (Hassoun et al 1993).

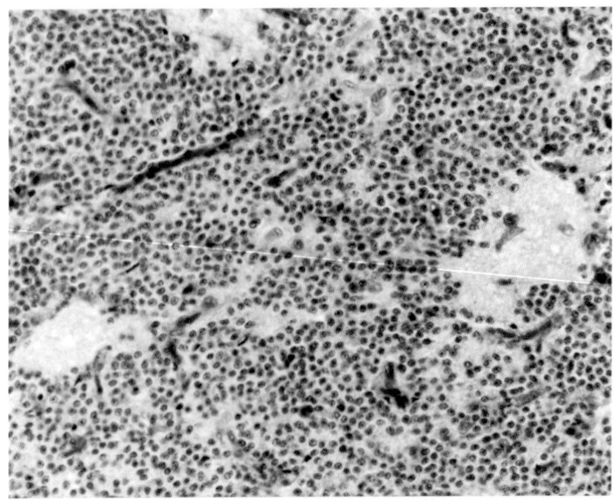

Fig. 8.11 Central neurocytoma. Central neurocytomas characteristically consist of homogeneous cell populations with ill-defined borders and a fine fibrillary matrix, specially recognized in the anuclear areas. H&E.

The histopathologic features of central neurocytomas are relatively typical (Fig. 8.11). The tumor is composed of a homogeneous population of small uniform cells with ill-defined cytoplasm, round to slightly lobulated nuclei and a conspicuously fibrillated matrix. The cells are arranged in moderately cellular areas alternating with anuclear islands composed of a dense fibrillary matrix. Delicate blood vessels form a branching network in a pattern analogous to oligodendrogliomas. A small number of neurocytomas show mitotic activity, nuclear atypia, endothelial proliferation and even microfoci of necrosis; although these changes may be associated with a less favorable outcome, they are less well correlated with prognosis than in glial neoplasms (von Deimling et al 1990, 1991, Söwlemezogou et al 1994). Tumors resembling neurocytomas rarely occur at other sites, such as the hypothalamus; their prognosis may not be as favorable as typical neurocytomas which readily lend themselves to resection.

Ultrastructural features of neurocytoma emphasize their high degree of neuronal maturation, including clear and dense-core vesicles, cellular processes with parallel arrays of microtubules, and the formation of synapses (Hassoun et al 1982, Townsend & Seaman 1986, Nishio et al 1988; von Deimling et al 1990, Kubota et al 1991, Hessler et al 1992). Its neuronal nature is also confirmed by immunohistochemistry for neuronal-associated proteins and synaptophysin (von Deimling et al 1990, Hessler et al 1992). GFAP immunoreactivity has been described in two tumors, the suggestion being made that its presence is associated with aggressive behavior (von Deimling et al 1990). More often, however, GFAP is restricted to reactive stromal astrocytes (Hessler et al 1992).

6.2. Mixed neuronal glial tumors

A. Gangliogliomas (WHO grade I–II). Representing approximately 1% of all brain tumors (Kalyan-Raman & Olivero 1987) and 4–5% of pediatric CNS neoplasms (Sutton et al 1983), gangliogliomas are the most common of mixed neuronal-glial tumors. Most arise in the temporal lobe, although any site of the neuraxis may be affected. The majority of the patients have an associated history of seizures. Indeed, gangliogliomas may represent up to 20% of lesions in temporal lobectomies performed for refractory seizures (Berger et al 1993, Jay et al 1993).

Grossly, gangliogliomas are relatively well-demarcated and frequently show cystic change and focal calcification. Histologically, they demonstrate a variable admixture of abnormal neuronal and glial cells (Fig. 8.12A,B). The glial component is usually astrocytic, although oligodendrocytes may be present in occasional cases (Allegranza et al 1990). Immunohistochemistry for GFAP and for neuronal-associated cytoskeletal proteins (Fig. 8.12C,D) aids in the distinction of bizarre glial cells and neurons. Histochemical stains, including silver impregnation techniques and stains for Nissl substance, are helpful for demonstrating neoplastic neurons. The latter show dysmorphism, binucleation being of particular diagnostic significance. At the ultrastructural level, synapses, dense-core vesicles and microtubules containing processes are also present (Takahashi et al 1987). The stromal component of gangliogliomas varies from purely glial to fibrovascular, the latter being reticulin- and occasionally collagen-rich. The perivascular lymphocytic infiltration is common and

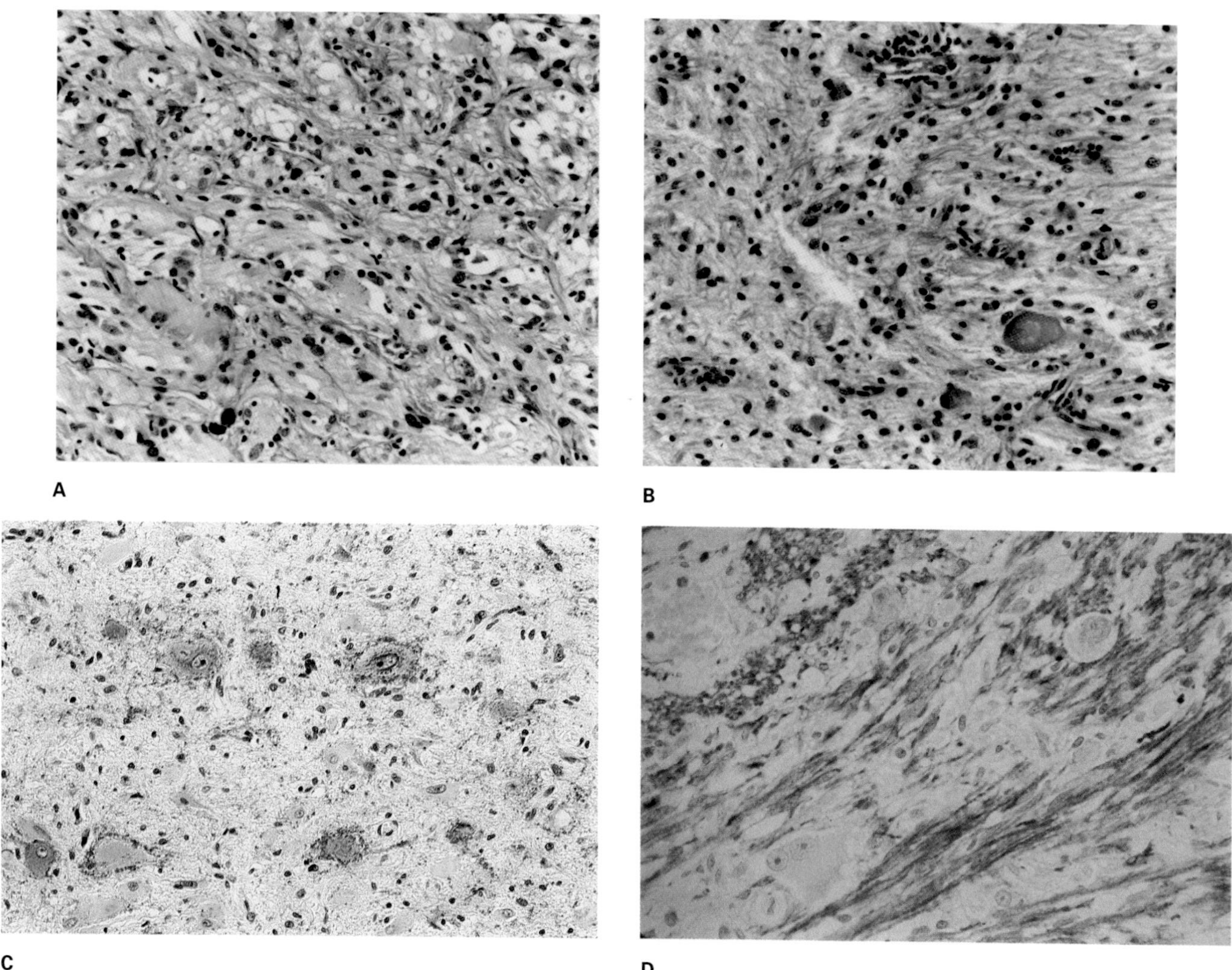

Fig. 8.12 Ganglioglioma. **A, B**. Mixed population of abnormal ganglionic cells and neoplastic astrocytes, often enmeshed in a fibrillary matrix. **B**. Lymphocytic infiltrate and prominent vasculature are common features of gangliogliomas. **A, B** H&E. **C**. Synaptophysin immunohistochemistry highlights the ganglionic elements within the fibrillary glial matrix. Synaptophysin avidin biotin-immunoperoxidase. **D**. The glial component of these tumors is readily identified by GFAP immunohistochemistry. GFAP avidin biotin-immunoperoxidase.

should not be misinterpreted as evidence of neuroblastic differentiation. On occasion the glomeruloid capillaries or hyalinized vessels may be sufficiently abundant as to resemble a vascular malformation.

It is the glial component, usually astrocytic in nature, that contributes the potential for recurrence and anaplastic progression. Nonetheless, malignant transformation is rare (Russell & Rubinstein 1989). Anaplastic transformation may be clinically suspected in patients with a recent exacerbation of chronic seizure activity and radiologic features suggestive of progression. The histologic appearance of such lesions is similar to that of anaplastic astrocytomas and may ultimately resemble glioblastoma. Similar malignant transformation may also occur within oligodendroglial elements of a ganglioglioma (Allegranza et al 1990).

B. Desmoplastic infantile ganglioglioma (WHO grade I). A rare variant of the mixed neuronal-glial neoplasms, occurring almost exclusively during infancy, desmoplastic infantile ganglioglioma (DIG) typically presents as a massive supratentorial tumor with a cystic component. Most arise in the frontal or parietal lobes and are grossly well-demarcated masses. Nonetheless, on microscopic examination, the interface between the tumor and surrounding brain is often infiltrative in nature. The most conspicuous feature of DIG is its remarkable desmoplastic stroma, which confers an occasionally woody firmness. This aspect is most apparent in the leptomeningeal component or at the interface with involved dura.

Histologically, DIGs exhibit an admixture of neoplastic astrocytes and eosinophilic globoid cells which, despite their superficial resemblance to astrocytes, represent neurons infiltrating the desmoplastic stroma (Fig. 8.13A,B). In addition, a minority of DIGs show a minor, more primitive neuroepithelial cell population (VandenBerg 1991, 1993). Mitoses and limited foci of necrosis occur mainly in association with such primitive elements and are not indicative of anaplastic progression. An important clinical feature of these tumors is their association with a favorable clinical outcome following complete or even subtotal surgical resection (Gambarelli et al 1982, VandenBerg et al 1987, Ng et al 1990, VandenBerg 1991, 1993).

Tumors with similar clinical and pathologic features, but limited to astrocytic differentiation, have been termed 'desmoplastic cerebral astrocytomas of infancy' (Taratuto et al 1984, De Chadarévian et al 1990). The histogenetic relationship between these two desmoplastic tumors of infancy is unclear. For a detailed discussion of the subject see VandenBerg (1993).

C. Dysembryoplastic neuroepithelial tumor (WHO grade I). The dysembryoplastic neuroepithelial tumor (DNT) is a rare lesion, usually arising in children and young adults with longstanding complex partial seizures. The entity was first described in a clinicopathologic report of 39 cases (Daumas-Duport et al 1988b). A detailed review of DNT has more recently been published (Daumas-Duport 1993). The lesion exhibits a morphologic spectrum with common clinical manifestations (Daumas-Duport 1993). DNTs are characteristically multinodular, intracortical and show a predilection for the temporal lobes. Microscopically, the nodules are most often composed of oligodendrocyte-like cells but in some cases astrocytes, particularly pilocytic astrocytes, may be prominent. The internodular cortex typically contains a diffuse proliferation of oligodendrocytes, within which neurons appear to float in a mucoid matrix (Fig. 8.14). Typically, the cortex surrounding DNT displays variable degrees of disorganization (cortical dysplasia). Cellular atypia is not a typical

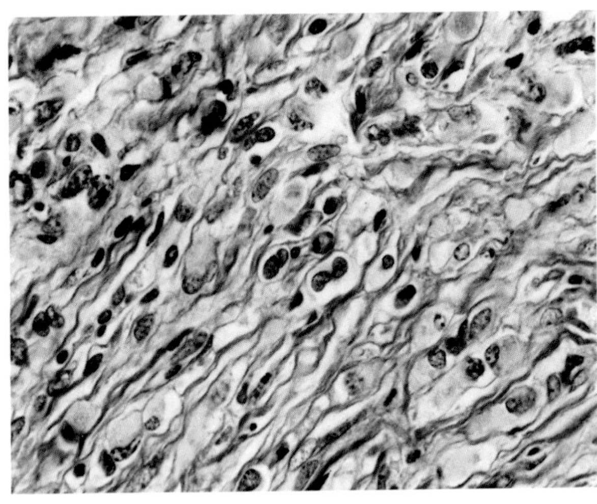

A

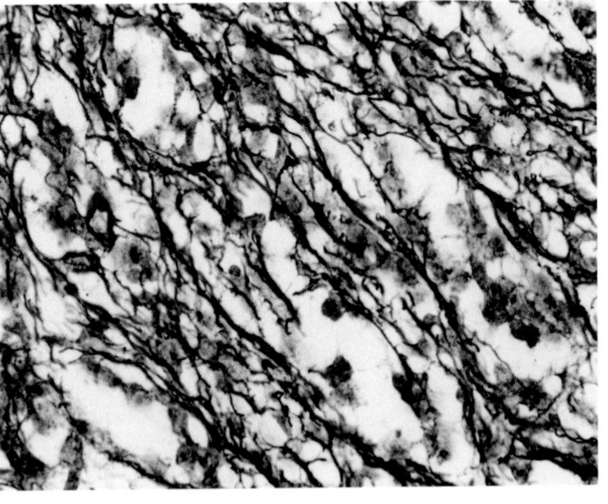

B

Fig. 8.13 Desmoplastic infantile ganglioglioma. **A**. Heterogeneous populations of neuroepithelial cells arranged in small clusters or single cells intermixed within a prominent stroma are the hallmark of these tumors. H&E. **B**. Reticulin stain accentuates the desmoplastic stroma of these tumors. Gordon and Sweet's reticulin.

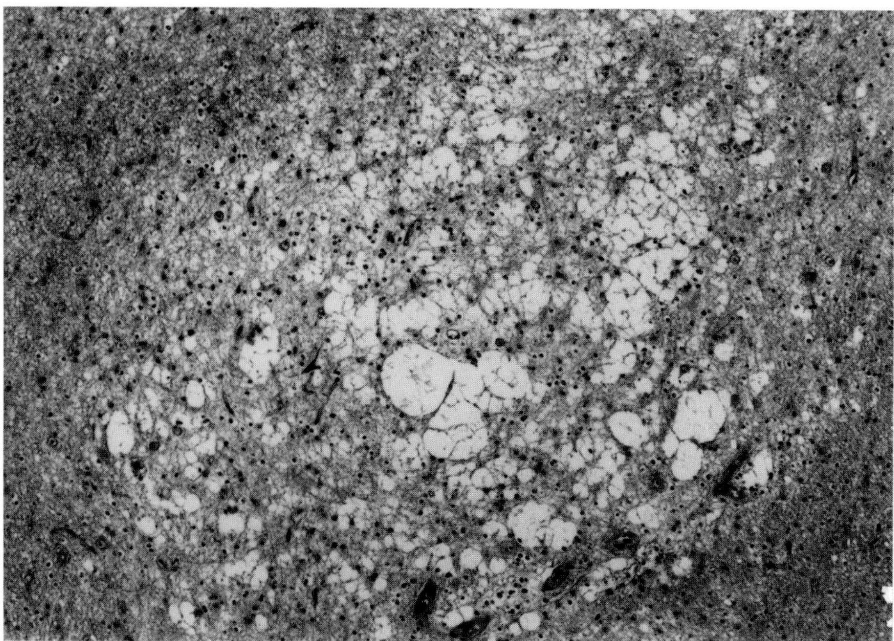

Fig. 8.14 Dysembryoplastic neuroepithelial tumor. Multiple intracortical nodules are a principal diagnostic component of DNT. The nodules are basically composed of oligodendrocytes, with a few astrocytes and neurons intermixed in an abundant extracellular mucoid matrix. H&E.

feature of DNT, but rare mitotic figures may be observed. Immunohistochemical studies have confirmed the glioneuronal nature of these lesions. Not only are mature, occasionally dysmorphic neurons an essential component, but a recent detailed immunochemical and ultrastructural study of DNT suggests that the oligodendrocyte-like cells are capable of divergent glioneuronal differentiation (Hirose et al 1994).

Considering the varied morphology of these lesions, some aspects of which are best appreciated at lower power magnification, adequate sampling is very important for diagnosis. Most often, nonrepresentative or minute specimens mimic mixed oligoastrocytomas. The distinction of DNT from gliomas is extremely important since they are associated with a favorable prognosis following even subtotal resection (Daumas-Duport et al 1988b). Radiation and chemotherapy play no role in the treatment of DNT.

7. Pineal parenchymal tumors

Pineal parenchymal neoplasms constitute less than 1% of all intracranial tumors (Zülch 1986) and represent approximately 15–30% of the pineal region tumors (Herrick & Rubinstein 1979, Herrick 1984, Scheithauer 1985). A review of clinical, histopathologic and therapeutic aspects of 30 cases of pineal parenchymal tumors has been recently published (Schild et al 1993). Although tumors of pineal parenchymal cells exhibit a morphologic spectrum, varying both in histologic grade and clinical behavior, the current WHO classification includes three basic lesions. At one end of the spectrum is the pineoblastoma, a highly malignant, small cell neoplasm with a propensity for invasive growth and cerebrospinal dissemination. At the opposite end is the well-differentiated pineocytoma, the cytologic features of which are similar to those of normal pineocytes; a conspicuous, diagnostically helpful feature is the presence of pineocytomatous rosettes. Such tumors usually compress rather than invade surrounding brain, and exhibit no significant tendency to spread within the neuraxis. An intermediate group, the so-called 'mixed' pineocytoma/pineoblastoma, includes neoplasms which are either intermediate in their cytoarchitectural features, or show a combination of patterns of pineocytoma-blastoma features. The behavior of tumor in the 'mixed' category is less predictable (Schild et al 1993).

A. Pineocytoma (WHO grade II)

Although pineocytomas most commonly occur in adults (Schild et al 1993), some series report a wide range of patient age at diagnosis (11–78 years) (Herrick & Rubinstein 1979, Vaquero et al 1990). Pineocytomas are typically well-demarcated masses which, as previously noted, compress adjacent parenchyma and show little tendency to infiltration. Microscopically, they are moderately cellular neoplasms which, when adequately sampled, show the formation of diagnostic 'pineocytomatous rosettes' consisting of a circular arrangement of cytologically uniform cells, the processes of which form a central, delicately fibrillated zone (Borit et al 1980) (Fig. 8.15). Silver carbonate impregnation for pineocyte processes (DeGirolami & Zvaigne 1973) demonstrates delicate,

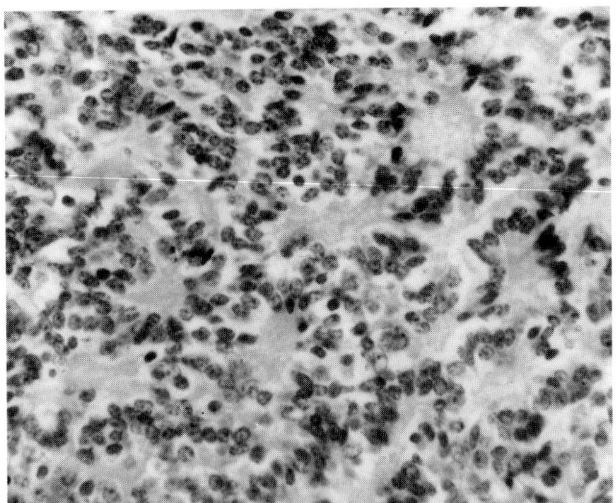

Fig. 8.15 Pineocytoma. Pineocytomas typically show groups of uniform cells surrounding delicate anuclear areas forming the so-called 'pineocytomatous rosettes'. H&E.

argyrophilic processes within the centers of the rosettes. Occasional giant cells may be seen but, as a rule, mitoses are absent or rare. Neither of these features correlates with clinical behavior. Calcification may occasionally be prominent.

Pineocytomas express neuronal-associated proteins, neurofilament protein and synaptophysin being present in virtually all optimally fixed specimens. Retinal S-antigen (S-Ag) has also been demonstrated in pineocytomas (Korf et al 1986, Perentes et al 1986, Rushing et al 1991), a feature no doubt related to the transient photosensory differentiation occurring in pineocytes during development (Reiter 1981). Ultrastructural features of pineocytomas include the presence of tangled microtubule-containing processes, 9+0 neurosensory cilia, intermediate filament bundles, centrioles, dense-core and clear vesicles, as well as well-developed annulate lamellae (Kline et al 1979, Markesbery et al 1981, Hassoun et al 1983, 1984, Hassoun & Gambarelli 1989) — all features of normal pineocytic/neurosensory cells.

B. *Pineoblastoma* (WHO grade IV)

Pineoblastomas are the most primitive of the pineal parenchymal tumors and account for approximately 3–17% of pineal region tumors in children (D'Andrea et al 1987, Edwards et al 1988). In contrast to pineocytomas, they preferentially occur in the first decade of life (Russell & Rubinstein 1989), with a male to female ratio of 2:1. Macroscopically, pineoblastomas are poorly demarcated masses, showing a high tendency to invade the adjacent brain and to seed the neuraxis. Necrosis is common but calcification is generally scant.

Pineoblastomas are highly cellular neoplasms composed of small, poorly differentiated cells with round to oval, hyperchromatic nuclei containing coarse chromatin. The cells are arranged in patternless sheets, but Homer Wright rosettes may be present. Silver carbonate impregnation may demonstrate small cell processes. Their ultrastructural features are those of a poorly differentiated neuroepithelial neoplasm, occasionally with a distinct photosensory phenotype (Kline et al 1979, Markesbery et al 1981, Min et al 1990). Pineal parenchymal tumors, especially pineoblastomas, exhibit highly variable and incomplete photosensory differentiation. In some instances it is morphologically inapparent, being limited to the immunochemical expression of photosensory retinal S-antigen (S-Ag) (Perentes et al 1986). In others it is evidenced by the presence of Flexner-Wintersteiner rosettes and fleurettes (Stefanko & Manschot 1979, Sobel et al 1981, Russell & Rubinstein 1989). The presence of photosensory proteins in pineal parenchymal tumors not only reflects a biochemical relationship between the retina and the pineal, but also suggests a link between the two embryonal tumors, namely retinoblastomas and pineoblastomas. That the latter exists is underscored by the occurrence of the so-called 'trilateral' retinoblastoma (Johnson et al 1985).

C. *Mixed pineocytoma/pineoblastoma* (WHO grade III)

A significant number of pineal parenchymal tumors are morphologically intermediate between pineocytoma and pineoblastoma. Termed 'mixed pineocytoma/pineoblastoma', such tumors pose a problem, both in terms of classification and treatment. Their clinical behavior is relatively unpredictable, but they are usually more aggressive than the well-differentiated pineocytoma, some showing not only local infiltration but distant cerebrospinal spread. The precise frequency of these tumors has not been established, given the lack of a uniform definition, some being reported as 'malignant pineocytomas', other as 'pineocytomas without neuronal differentiation' (Herrick & Rubinstein 1979).

Histologically, the majority of the tumors exhibit morphologic features intermediate between pineocytomas and pineoblastomas. Most show moderate cellularity. The formation of cell processes is often less conspicuous than in pineocytoma and, as a rule, pineocytomatous rosettes are absent. Cytologic atypia is variable and mitotic activity is present. Foci of necrosis may be observed. Mixed tumors exhibiting distinct pineocytomatous and blastic components are rare. Like pineoblastomas, mixed pineal tumors may show photosensory differentiation as evidenced by the expression of interphotoreceptor retinoid-binding protein (IRBP) (Lopes et al 1993). The finding of a neuroretinal protein in a neoplasm of the pineal region is diagnostically useful and distinguishes pineal parenchymal neoplasms from other neuroepithelial tumors, particularly central neurocytomas and ependymomas.

8. Embryonal tumors (WHO grade IV)

The embryonal tumors are a group of clinically aggressive neoplasms that usually occur during the first decade of life. Regardless of their subtype, they share the common histologic features of high cellularity, brisk mitotic activity, and a tendency to at least focal necrosis. Most show a distinct tendency to leptomeningeal invasion and subsequent spread within the cerebrospinal pathways. The umbrella term *embryonal* is not intended to indicate that these tumors are composed of cells in every way equivalent to the immature cells of the normal developing nervous system. Instead the term suggests that these tumors arise as the result of transformation of fetal cell targets. It is reasonable to assume that these target cell populations are composed of both primitive progenitor cells and immature neuroepithelial cells with more restricted genotypic/phenotypic potential.

Although embryonal tumors share some common histopathologic features with anaplastic tumors occurring in adults, they are distinct, both in clinical and pathologic terms. This is particularly true of their respective transforming events and the cellular targets for transformation (Bigner et al 1990, Bigner & Vogelstein 1990, Wasson et al 1990, Thomas & Raffel 1991). Various cell populations of the immature nervous system, with different capacities for differentiation, represent vulnerable targets for neoplastic transformation (Kleihues et al 1990). Of these, some are capable of divergent glial-neuronal differentiation (see Ch. 2). The current classification of embryonal tumors takes this potential for variety into consideration, recognizing a number of embryonal tumors showing relatively defined differentiation. The latter include cerebral neuroblastoma, ependymoblastoma, and retinoblastoma — tumors which exhibit differentiation along neuronal, ependymal and retinal cell lines, respectively. A very rare embryonal neoplasm which merits separate consideration is the medulloepithelioma. In contrast to the previously mentioned tumors, this neoplasm has the greatest cytogenetic potential, exhibiting not only glioneuronal but mesenchymal differentiation as well.

The designation of primitive neuroectodermal tumor (PNET) promotes the concept that primitive tumors arising in the pediatric CNS are derived from primitive neuroepithelial progenitor cells, distributed throughout the neuraxis and displaying similar histopathologic features as well as biologic behavior. Implicit in this concept is the notion that the potential for divergent phenotypic differentiation in a PNET is the result of transformation of an undifferentiated neuroepithelial cell (Gould et al 1990). Pluripotential differentiation could take place if neoplastic transformation occurs in a committed but not fully differentiated stem cell with a pluripotent capacity of differentiation (Schmidek 1993). The PNET concept thus excludes the possibility that neoplastic differentiation in embryonal tumors may be a reflection of transformation of a more 'stable' cell with an already restricted genotype. Currently, the use of the term PNET for classification purposes is limited to medulloblastoma and to neoplasms indistinguishable from medulloblastomas but located at other sites within the central nervous system.

A. *Medulloblastoma* (WHO grade IV)

This most common of embryonal tumors has been the subject of an exhaustive clinicopathologic review (Tomlinson et al 1992a,b). It comprises approximately 25% of all intracranial tumors in children (Zülch 1986). Its peak incidence is near the end of the first decade, there being a slight male predilection. The majority of medulloblastomas are located in the cerebellar vermis, although hemispheric examples are not uncommon, particularly in the adult (Russell & Rubinstein 1989). Macroscopically, the tumors are soft, and appear rather demarcated from the adjacent brain. Necrosis may be microfocal or confluent; massive necrosis is infrequent. The desmoplastic variant of medulloblastoma may be remarkably firm in consistency.

Medulloblastomas are highly cellular neoplasms, composed of relatively small cells with scant cytoplasm and ill-defined cell borders (Fig. 8.16A). The nuclei vary in chromatin pattern and shape although in most cases they are hyperchromatic and are angular to ovoid in shape. Mitoses are scant to frequent. Endothelial/pericytic proliferation is rarely observed. Neuroblastic differentiation as evidenced by the presence of Homer Wright (neuroblastic) rosettes may be present in approximately 40% (Kleihues et al 1989). A neoplastic ganglionic component is present in about 7% of the cases with neuroblastic differentiation. Immunoreactivity for neuronal-associated proteins, such as class III β-tubulin, neurofilament epitopes and synaptophysin, is often present not only in obviously neuroblastic areas, but also in tumors without cytologic evidence of differentiation. In contrast, the issue of astroglial differentiation in medulloblastomas is more problematic. Using conventional fixation and tissue processing, approximately 10% of medulloblastomas contain tumor cells showing GFAP immunoreactivity (Coffin et al 1983, Schindler & Gullotta 1983, Kleihues et al 1989). The figure is much higher when special processing is used (Gould et al 1990). Divergent neuronal and glial differentiation is also noted in medulloblastoma cell lines including DAOY, D-283 MED and D-341 MED (He et al 1989).

The desmoplastic variant of medulloblastoma constitutes 10–12% of cases (Burger et al 1987, Kleihues et al 1989) and is distinctive for its often biphasic architecture (Fig. 8.16B). This pattern consists of highly cellular sheets and trabeculae of tumor cells interspersed with

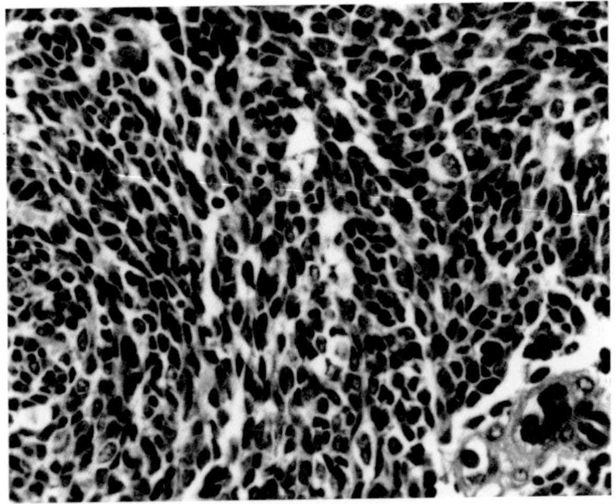

A

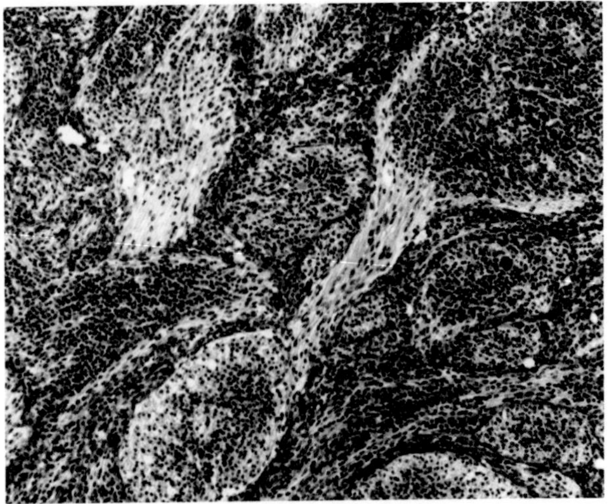

B

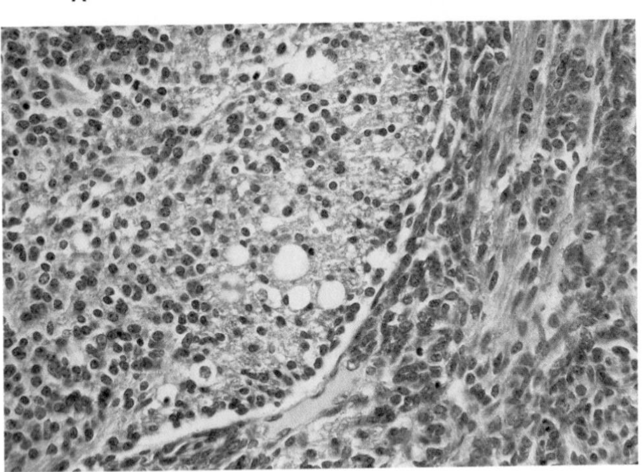

C

Fig. 8.16 Medulloblastoma. **A**. Medulloblastomas are highly cellular neoplasms composed of primitive cells in a fine fibrillated matrix. **B**. The desmoplastic variant exhibits a lobular pattern with islands of more differentiated cells. **A**, **B** H&E. **C**. The reticulin-free areas usually demonstrate neuronal differentiation, here demonstrated by immunoreactivity for neuronal-associated class III β-tubulin. TUJ1 avidin biotin-immunoperoxidase.

hypocellular islands composed of cells with a more differentiated appearance. This 'follicular' architecture is highlighted on reticulin stain wherein areas of dense cellularity are enmeshed in reticulin and follicles are free of staining. Follicles do contain cells with more advanced differentiation, as evidenced by the formation of delicate processes. In addition, neuronal-associated β-tubulin (Katsetos et al 1989), neurofilament (Katsetos et al 1989) (Fig. 8.16C) and synaptophysin reactive cells are also seen within the follicles, thus suggesting advanced neuronal differentiation. Indirect evidence for differentiation within reticulin-free follicles is their lower labeling index of Ki-67 preparations, a finding suggesting the emergence of post-mitotic neuronal cells.

Other less frequent variants of medulloblastoma show striated muscle cell differentiation, hence the term *medullomyoblastoma* (Rao et al 1990). Yet others exhibit pigmentation of epithelial-appearing cells in papillary arrangements, a picture likened to melanotic neuroectodermal tumor of infancy (Russell & Rubinstein 1989). A set of medulloblastomas composed basically of large cells with large vesicular nuclei and prominent nucleoli has also been described; such tumors are highly aggressive and often undergo early CSF dissemination despite adjuvant therapy (Giangaspero et al 1992).

The broad repertoire of differentiation exhibited by medulloblastomas may reflect an innate heterogeneity of these tumors. In addition to the spectrum of neuroepithelial differentiation referred to above, medulloblastomas may demonstrate photosensory differentiation, as suggested by the presence of retinal S-antigen (Korf et al 1987, Bonnin & Perentes 1988), rod opsin (Korf et al 1987, Czerwionka et al 1989, Kramm et al 1991), and IRBP (Korf et al 1992). These observations suggest a link between medulloblastomas and other more differentiated embryonal tumors, including neuroblastomas, retinoblastomas, and pineoblastomas.

B. *Neuroblastoma* (WHO grade IV)

Neuroblastomas are rare embryonal neoplasms occurring with greater frequency in children, particularly early in the first decade. Although they may arise in any part of the neuraxis, including the brainstem and spinal cord, the majority of neuroblastomas are supratentorial in location, showing a predilection for the frontoparietal regions (Horten & Rubinstein 1976, Berger et al 1983, Bennett & Rubinstein 1984). In general, they are massive, multicystic and show a discrete border with the adjacent brain. In some, a variably desmoplastic stroma confers a firmer texture and a somewhat lobulated appearance.

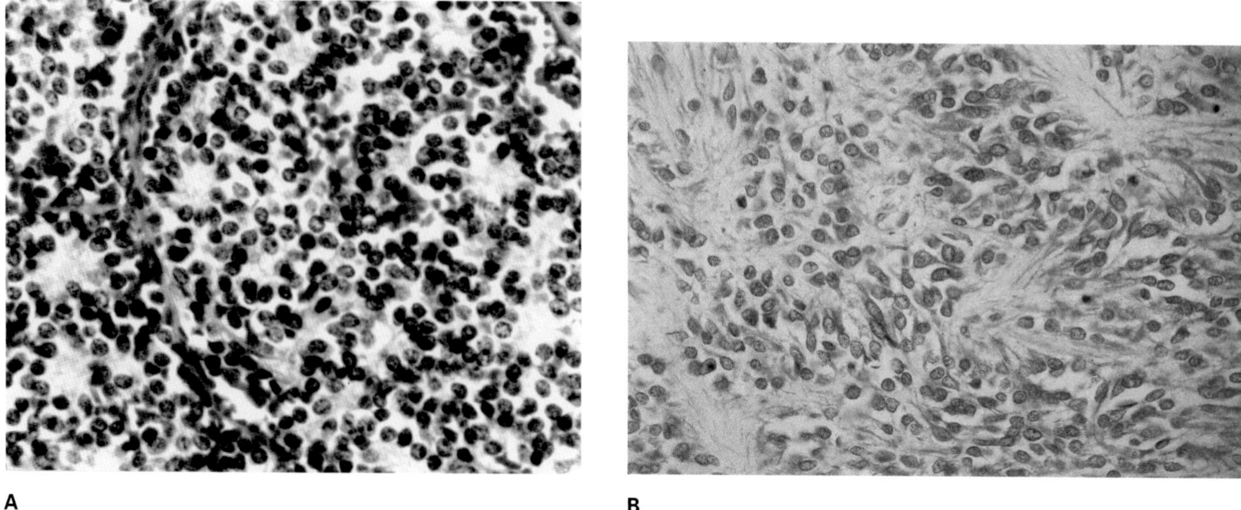

Fig. 8.17 Neuroblastoma. **A**. Monotonous sheets of poorly differentiated small cells are intermixed with the characteristic Homer Wright (neuroblastic) rosettes. H&E. **B**. Delicate cellular processes (neurites), here highlighted by the neuronal-associated class III β-tubulin, form the fibrillated matrix of these tumors. TUJ1 avidin biotin-immunoperoxidase.

Histologically, central neuroblastomas are highly cellular tumors composed of small cells with poorly defined cytoplasm, round to ovoid nuclei and hyperchromatic nuclei (Fig. 8.17A). Neuronal maturation is evidenced by cells with more abundant cytoplasm, conspicuous processes, and vesicular nuclei. The cells tend to be arranged in monotonous sheets, the intercellular spaces containing varying numbers of cell processes (neurites). Characteristic Homer Wright or neuroblastic rosettes, the centers of which are formed of entangled cellular processes, are present in varying number. Neurites may be detected by silver impregnation methods and immunohistochemistry for synaptophysin and neuron-associated cytoskeletal proteins (Fig. 8.17B). Ultrastructural features of neuroblastic differentiation include microtubule-containing cell processes, neurosecretory granules or vesicles, and occasional synapses (Russell & Rubinstein 1989). Differentiation to ganglion cells may be focally seen in approximately 50% of cases, but is never abundant (Bennett & Rubinstein 1984). Advanced neuronal maturation is apparent not only on electron microscopy (Russell & Rubinstein 1989), but is also evidenced on immunostain preparations by the presence of neuronal proteins associated with cell maturation, including middle and high molecular weight neurofilament proteins.

C. Ependymoblastoma (WHO grade IV)

This rare ependymal tumor usually presents in young children, the median age in one series being 2 years (Mørk & Rubinstein 1985). Nearly all reported examples have been massive supratentorial tumors. Their relationship to the ventricular system may be hard to assess given their large size. The tumors tend to be macroscopically discrete masses, although microscopic infiltration of surrounding brain and leptomeninges may be seen.

Microscopically, ependymoblastomas are highly cellular and are composed of small, poorly differentiated cells arranged in patternless sheets punctuated by ependymoblastic rosettes and tubules (Fig. 8.18). In contrast to the ordinary ependymal rosettes, those of ependymoblastoma are pseudostratified and show frequent juxtaluminal mitoses. Well-developed perivascular rosettes of the type seen in ependymomas are rare. The ultrastructural finding of luminal cytoplasmic specialization, including microvilli, 9+2 cilia, and complex zonulae adherens-type junctions, is clear evidence of ependymal differentiation (Langford 1986). GFAP immunohistochemistry (Cruz-Sanchez et al

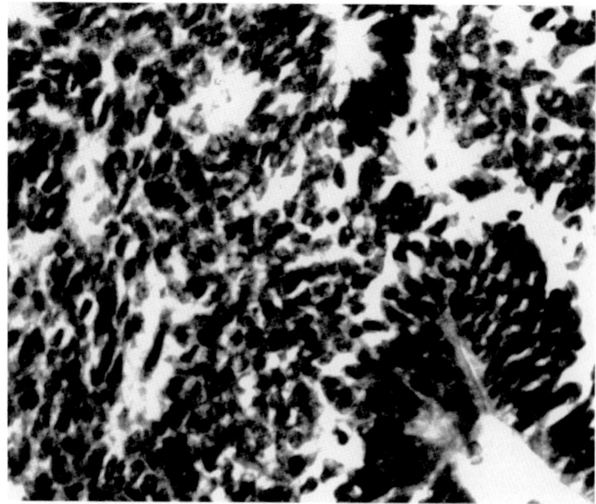

Fig. 8.18 Ependymoblastoma. Multilayer ependymoblastic rosettes constitute the primary histopathologic feature of the highly cellular ependymoblastomas. H&E.

1988, Pigott et al 1990) further defines the glial character of these tumors, highlighting groups of primitive polygonal cells and, particularly, the cell processes situated around blood vessels.

For therapeutic and prognostic purposes, ependymoblastomas should be distinguished from anaplastic ependymomas. Ependymoblastomas are tumors of early childhood whereas anaplastic ependymomas are typically found in adults. Their histologic distinction is based upon the PNET-like appearance of ependymoblastomas, their multilayered true rosettes, and the absence of well-developed pseudorosettes. Ependymoblastomas also seldom show the degree of cytoplasmic or nuclear pleomorphism characteristic of anaplastic ependymomas. Furthermore, endothelial proliferation, an often conspicuous feature of anaplastic ependymomas, is generally absent in ependymoblastomas. Although necrosis may be present in both tumors, geographic necrosis with pseudopalisading is found primarily in anaplastic ependymomas.

D. *Retinoblastoma* (WHO grade IV)

Retinoblastoma is the most common intraocular tumor of childhood, and the only embryonal tumor for which a specific genetic basis of neoplastic transformation has been demonstrated. The transforming event occurs in the immature retina when both alleles of the *Rb* tumor suppressor gene on chromosome 13 are inactivated by mutation and chromosomal loss (Gallie et al 1990, Gennett & Cavenee 1990). Retinoblastomas may be familial or sporadic in occurrence. The histopathologic picture is similar in both forms of retinoblastomas, the tumors being composed of amorphous sheets of poorly differentiated small cells with varying proportions of specialized cell arrangements, these being the Flexner-Wintersteiner (photosensory) and Homer Wright (neuroblastic) rosettes. A small number of tumors may also exhibit particularly well-developed photosensory structures termed *fleurettes*. Marked mitotic activity and extensive areas of necrosis can be seen. In larger tumors, infiltration of the optic nerve and of choroid vessels is often present.

The expression of neuronal-associated proteins, including neurofilament isotypes (Kivelä et al 1986, Perentes et al 1987, Kleinert 1991), synaptophysin (Kivelä et al 1989, Katsetos et al 1991), neuronal-associated β-tubulin, and microtubule-associated tubulin-2 (MAP2) (Katsetos et al 1991), has been demonstrated in these tumors. Photoreceptor proteins including retinal S-antigen (see Donoso et al 1989 for review), IRBP, and rod/cone opsins (Gonzalez-Fernandez et al 1992) have been demonstrated by immunohistochemistry, but these substances show no preferential localization to rosettes or fleurettes. GFAP immunoreactivity in retinoblastomas is confined to reactive 'stromal' astrocytes associated with blood vessels or lying at the interface between the retina and the infiltrating tumor (Gonzalez-Fernandez et al 1992). Rare tumors with numerous fleurettes and low cellularity have been designated 'retinocytomas', and appear to have a more benign behavior (Margo et al 1983).

The histogenesis of retinoblastomas is still not completely understood. A recent study in 22 cases suggests that retinoblastomas have a histogenetic potential analogous to that of the immature retinal neuroepithelium but restricted to photosensory (cone and rod) as well as Müller cell lineages (Gonzalez-Fernandez et al 1992).

E. *Medulloepithelioma* (WHO grade IV)

This very rare tumor usually affects children in the first decade of life. In the approximately 25 cases described to date (Caccamo et al 1989, Russell & Rubinstein 1989), the cerebral hemispheres are most frequently affected. The hallmark histopathologic feature of these neoplasms is the formation of primitive epithelium resembling that of the embryonic neural tube. It consists of mitotically active, pseudostratified columnar epithelium, often arranged in ribbons, tubules, or even papillae delimited by a PAS-positive basement membrane.

Ultrastructural studies of two tumors have demonstrated a paucity of cytoplasmic organelles, moderately developed juxtaluminal zonulae adherens, and a conspicuous lack of apical differentiation (Pollak & Friede 1977, Troost et al 1990). By immunohistochemistry, strong vimentin immunoreactivity is present in the epithelial structures, but only occasionally is there expression of neuroblastic or glial cytoskeletal proteins, e.g. class III β-tubulin and GFAP, respectively (Caccamo et al 1989). In contrast, glial and neuronal differentiation can readily be demonstrated within the differentiating components present in many tumors (Caccamo et al 1989). These findings are remarkably similar to those noted during the formation and differentiation of the embryonic neural tube (Cameron & Rakic 1991). Not only can medulloepitheliomas show the full spectrum of glioneuronal differentiation but some also exhibit specialized mesenchymal elements.

TUMORS OF CRANIAL AND SPINAL NERVES

The two principal lesions of this group are the schwannoma and the neurofibroma. Schwann cells are the exclusive constituent of the former whereas neurofibromas also consist in part of perineurial cells and fibroblasts. Both tumors exhibit distinct histopathologic patterns and clinical associations. Schwannomas usually present as solitary masses involving cranial and spinal nerve roots rather than peripheral nerves. Neurofibromas, in contrast, are often multiple and usually involve large or small peripheral nerves.

Schwannomas and neurofibromas may occur either sporadically or as part of the spectrum of neurofibromatosis (NF). Both NF-1 (von Recklinghausen's disease or 'peripheral' neurofibromatosis) and NF-2 ('central' neurofibromatosis) are associated with the development of nerve sheath tumors. Schwannomas are more a part of NF-2 than of NF-1. Bilateral 'acoustic' (vestibular) schwannomas are characteristic of NF-2. Intraspinal schwannomas are more often sporadic or associated with NF-2 than with NF-1 (Halliday et al 1991). In contrast, neurofibromas are the principal nerve sheath tumors in NF-1, a setting wherein they affect peripheral nerves and far outnumber the schwannomas.

1. **Schwannoma** (WHO grade I)

Intracranial and intraspinal schwannomas are usually slow-growing tumors occurring in adults. A female predominance is reported in the intracranial examples (Russell & Rubinstein 1989). Schwannomas characteristically involve sensory nerves, including the posterior spinal roots. Intracranial examples usually involve the vestibular nerve, followed much less frequently by the trigeminal and vagal nerves. Intracranial parenchymal schwannomas, unrelated to a major cranial nerve, may also occur (Casadei et al 1993). Small perivascular nerves are presumed to be the origin for these tumors.

Macroscopically, schwannomas are well-circumscribed, encapsulated lesions which largely displace the parent nerve. Unlike neurofibromas, the nerve of origin can often be identified. Vestibular schwannomas involve the cerebellopontine angle and expand the internal auditory meatus, whereas spinal examples tend to grow through the intervertebral foramina, the result being the typical 'dumbbell' configuration evident on neuroimaging. At cut surface, most are predominantly solid, but cystic and hemorrhagic degeneration may be seen, particularly in large tumors.

Histopathologically, schwannomas exhibit two main patterns, termed Antoni A and Antoni B (Fig. 8.19A), both of which are often present. The Antoni A pattern consists of fascicles of fusiform cells with elongate nuclei. Such cells are often arranged in a palisading pattern. A particularly localized arrangement of such palisades is termed the 'Verocay body'. Both nuclear palisading and Verocay bodies are a common feature of spinal schwannomas. Rich pericellular reticulin staining is characteristic of Antoni A tissue. At the ultrastructural level this finding corresponds to the presence of pericellular basement membrane and intercellular basement membrane-like material (Erlandson 1985). By immunohistochemistry, the basement membranes are strongly reactive for laminin (Miettinen et al 1983, Leivo et al 1989) and type IV collagen. The Antoni B tissue is less cellular and is characterized by multipolar cells with round nuclei arranged in a loose pattern. Cytoplasmic vacuolation and nuclear pleomorphism also typify Antoni B tissue. Reticulin fibers are scant and irregularly distributed. Collagen fibrils are commonly seen on ultrastructure (Erlandson 1985).

Hyalinized blood vessels are usually a prominent feature in schwannomas, some showing sinusoidal dilatations assuming cavernous proportions (Fig. 8.19B). Thrombosis may also be seen. Spontaneous hemorrhages with necrosis are not uncommon, and may be accompanied by infiltration of macrophages and hemosiderin deposition. Other degenerative changes such as enlargement and hyperchromasia of the nuclei and hypercellularity are common, having no prognostic significance.

Nerve sheath tumors share a number of immunohistochemical features and they will be discussed together.

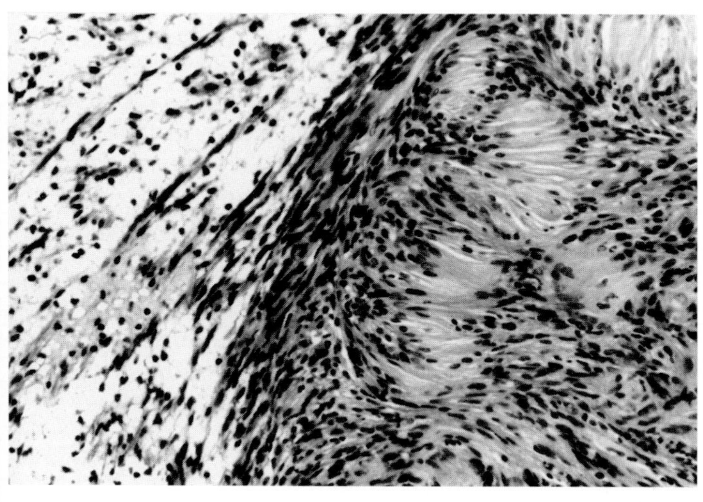

A

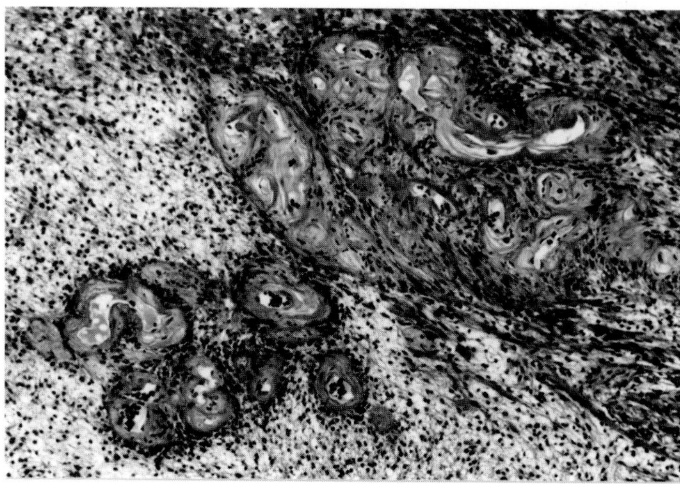

B

Fig. 8.19 Schwannoma. **A.** Spindle cells arranged in fascicles and Verocay bodies are features of the Antoni A type of tissue (right), whereas Antoni B (left) displays a loose texture in the tumor. **B.** Numerous blood vessels with hyalinized walls are usually present in schwannomas. **A, B** H&E.

Schwannomas are diffusely immunoreactive for S-100 protein (Rubinstein 1988). In contrast, neurofibromas show more variable, less pronounced staining, a not unexpected finding given the mixed composition of these tumors (see below) (Hirose et al 1986). Leu-7 (HNK-1) epitope is present in about half of the nerve sheath tumors (Perentes & Rubinstein 1986). The presence of myelin basic protein (MBP) has also been reported in both schwannomas and neurofibromas, albeit in a small proportion of cases (Mogollon et al 1984, Penneys et al 1984). The application of S-100 protein and Leu-7 stains aids in the distinction of schwannomas and neurofibromas from other soft tissue tumors (Russell & Rubinstein 1989). Epithelial membrane antigen (EMA), a marker for perineurial cells (Pinkus & Kurtin 1985, Theaker et al 1987), is occasionally detected in neurofibromas (Perentes et al 1988). Vimentin is the predominant intermediate filament protein in nerve sheath neoplasms (Gould et al 1986, Gray et al 1989). Its ubiquitous nature makes its identification irrelevant to diagnosis. For reasons not yet ascertained, immunoreactivity for GFAP has been demonstrated in both schwannomas and neurofibromas, as well as in malignant peripheral nerve sheath tumors (MPNST) (Gould et al 1986, Stanton et al 1987, Gray et al 1989). It appears that the actual protein present in these cells differs slightly from the form of GFAP found in glial cells (Stanton et al 1987).

Cellular schwannoma. This subtype of schwannoma is characterized by high cellularity, predominance of Antoni A tissue, and the presence of variable mitotic activity (Woodruff et al 1981). Although they may be mistaken for malignant peripheral nerve sheath tumors (MPNST), cellular schwannomas are associated with an excellent prognosis (Woodruff et al 1981, White et al 1990, Scheithauer et al 1993). These tumors exhibit typical architectural features of an ordinary schwannoma, including encapsulation, vascular hyalinization, dense pericellular reticulin staining, strong generalized S-100 protein immunoreactivity and ultrastructural features of advanced Schwann cell differentiation (White et al 1990). The presence of these features distinguishes cellular schwannomas from MPNST (see below). Even the finding of hypercellularity and mitotic activity is not to be considered evidence of anaplastic change. Nonetheless, it is of note that tumors paravertebral, sacral or intracranial in location show a significant frequency of recurrence compared to peripherally situated tumors (Casadei et al 1993).

2. **Neurofibroma** (WHO grade I)

Neurofibromas are divided into two major groups, the intraneural and the diffusely infiltrative, often cutaneous, tumors. Whereas the nerve of origin is often inapparent in diffuse tumors, intraneural examples often affect larger, readily recognized nerves. The latter may be either solitary, fusiform tumors or, less frequently, are multinodular and involve numerous branches. Such so-called 'plexiform' neurofibromas are pathognomonic of NF-1. Intraneural neurofibromas frequently involve cervical, brachial and lumbosacral nerves (Burger et al 1991). Intraspinal neurofibromas are frequently associated with NF-1 (Halliday et al 1991).

Compared to schwannomas, neurofibromas tend to be soft, almost gelatinous in consistency, and are somewhat translucent in appearance. Both solitary and plexiform types demonstrate similar histopathologic features, being composed in large part of spindle-shaped, wavy Schwann cells arranged in loose bundles within a matrix rich in collagen and mucopolysaccharides which gives the lesions their translucent appearance. Varying proportions of perineurial cells and fibroblasts are also present. Myelinated and nonmyelinated nerve fibers may be found within neurofibromas. Their presence facilitates the distinction of neurofibromas from schwannomas, wherein nerve fibers tend to be displaced rather than incorporated into the lesion. Silver stains for axons, myelin preparations and immunohistochemistry for neuronal-associated proteins are helpful to assess the presence of nerve fibers.

Ultrastructural studies indicate that Schwann cells are the principal component of the neurofibromas, followed in frequency by the perineurial cells and fibroblasts (Enzinger & Weiss 1988). Immunohistochemical studies have occasionally detected the presence of perineurial cells with anti-EMA antibodies (Perentes et al 1987, Theaker et al 1988).

In contrast to schwannomas, neurofibromas show a distinct tendency to undergo malignant transformation. This is particularly relevant to plexiform neurofibromas, wherein its frequency is 5–10% (Burger et al 1991). Malignant transformation should be clinically suspected on the basis of rapid enlargement of pre-existing neurofibroma, pain, or a change in neurologic symptoms (Ducatman et al 1986). From the histopathologic standpoint, tumors showing hypercellularity, nuclear atypia, and more than an occasional mitotic figure are considered to show anaplastic transformation. The process may be focal or extensive; thorough examination of the specimen is required in that limited or nonrepresentative biopsy often fails to show the sarcoma.

3. **Malignant peripheral nerve sheath tumors (MPNST), neurogenic sarcoma, neurofibrosarcoma** (WHO grade III–IV)

Malignant peripheral nerve sheath tumors are, in almost all instances, malignant counterparts of neurofibroma. Anaplastic transformation of schwannomas is an extremely rare event. The overall incidence of MPNST is 0.001% in the general population and 4.6% among patients with NF-1 (Ducatman et al 1986). In the setting of NF-1, the highest incidence of these tumors is observed in children and young adults (Ducatman et al 1986, Matsui et al 1993, Wanebo et al 1993). MPNST may occur de novo but more frequently arises by malignant transformation of a pre-existing neurofibroma. Actually, in a great number of the MPNST (61% of the cases reported from the Mayo Clinic series — Ducatman et al 1986), a co-existent neurofibromatous component can be demonstrated with thorough sampling. The association is more evident in patients with NF-1 than in those with sporadic MPNST (81% versus 60%, respectively) (Ducatman et al 1986). Radiation-induced tumors have been reported both in patients with and without NF-1 (Ducatman & Scheithauer 1983, Ducatman et al 1986, Wanebo et al 1993). Overexpression of p53 has been described in approximately one half of MPNST. Its presence appears to be associated with the malignant progression of neurofibromas to MPNST (Halling et al 1993).

The distribution of the MPNST is similar to that of solitary and plexiform neurofibromas, favored sites being the head and neck, trunk and proximal limbs. Tumors in NF-1 are more often centrally located (Ducatman et al 1986). Intracranial examples are extremely rare; the few cases reported have involved the trigeminal or, more rarely, the vestibular nerve (Russell & Rubinstein 1989). A single intraparenchymal example has also been reported (Stefanko et al 1986).

Grossly, the configuration of MPNST closely resembles that of neurofibromas, ranging from well-circumscribed fusiform or globular enlargement of a nerve to a lesion unassociated with an obvious nerve and showing more infiltrative soft tissue extension. The texture of tumor often varies, depending upon the presence or absence of necrosis. Histologically, MPNST shows a range of cytologic and histologic appearances. The majority consist of fascicles of spindle cells, sometimes arranged in a herringbone or storiform pattern. Cytoarchitectural features suggestive of schwannian differentiation, including cells with a wavy configuration, may also be present. Most tumors are highly cellular, display nuclear/cellular pleomorphism, and show abundant mitotic activity. Microvasculature proliferation and areas of necrosis are frequent. Necrosis may be of a geographic type accompanied by peripheral palisading.

Heterologous differentiation may be seen in approximately 15% of cases, including skeletal muscle, bone, cartilage, epithelial and neuroendocrine elements (Ducatman & Scheithauer 1984, Enzinger & Weiss 1988, Meis et al 1992). A small number of MPNST may be basically composed of lobules or groups of plump cells with round vesicular nuclei and prominent nucleoli. These 'epithelioid' lesions are often termed 'malignant epithelioid schwannoma' in that they superficially resemble carcinoma or amelanotic melanoma. Areas of more typical MPNST are also frequently present. Strong S-100 protein immunoreactivity (Robey et al 1987, Wick et al 1987, Chu & Shmookler 1988) and lack of reactivity for cytokeratins (Wick et al 1987) help to differentiate such tumors from carcinomas. It is of note that epithelioid MPNST may demonstrate immunoreactivity for HMB-45, a marker of melanoma cells (Burger et al 1991), thus complicating the differential diagnosis with melanoma. In such instances, laminin or collagen IV immunostain as well as the ultrastructural demonstration of basement membrane is of assistance. Tumors presenting divergent differentiation behave no differently from ordinary MPNST (Ducatman et al 1986).

TUMOR OF THE MENINGES

1. Tumors of meningothelial cells

A. Meningioma (WHO grade I)

Meningiomas are tumors composed of or derived from the arachnoidal cells (Kepes 1982, Russell & Rubinstein 1989). They account for about 15% of all intracranial tumors (Russell & Rubinstein 1989), and about 25% of intraspinal tumors (Slooff et al 1964). In general, meningiomas become clinically evident in mid-life, being rare in childhood. A marked female predominance (3:1) is seen in adults, whereas in childhood and old age, no sex predilection is evident (Pascual-Castroviejo 1990). Multiple meningiomas occur in up to 8% of cases (Nakasu et al 1987), and are particularly frequent in the setting of NF-2 (Russell & Rubinstein 1989). Other genetic abnormalities have also been described in affected families (Smidt et al 1990). Loss of heterozygosity for loci on chromosome 22 is present in 40–80% of sporadic tumors (Zankl & Zang 1972, Zang 1982, Dumanski et al 1990, Poulsgard et al 1990), the genetic defect being localized to 22q12.3 (Lekanne Deprez et al 1991). In tumors displaying varying degrees of anaplasia, an increased frequency of other complex structural and numerical chromosome abnormalities may be seen (Casartelli et al 1989, Vagner-Capodano et al 1993).

Most meningiomas are well-demarcated, dura-based globular masses with a thin capsule. An exception — the flat, carpet-like or 'en plaque' meningioma — typically occurs at the skull base, particularly lying over the sphenoid ridge. Meningiomas grow slowly, compress the brain and erode adjacent structures. Invasion of the dura and bone occurs with regularity, the latter prompting variable degrees of hyperostosis.

Meningiomas are subdivided into three histopathologic categories according to their aggressiveness and malignant potential — *meningioma, atypical meningioma* and *anaplastic (malignant) meningioma.* Numerous histologic variants of meningioma have been included in the new WHO classification (Scheithauer 1990, Kleihues et al 1993a),

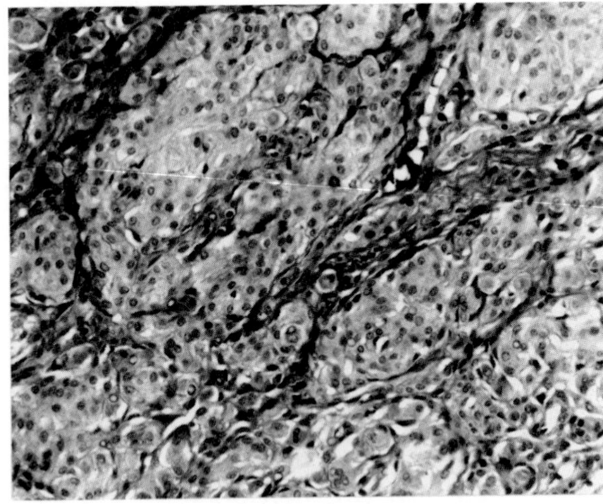

A

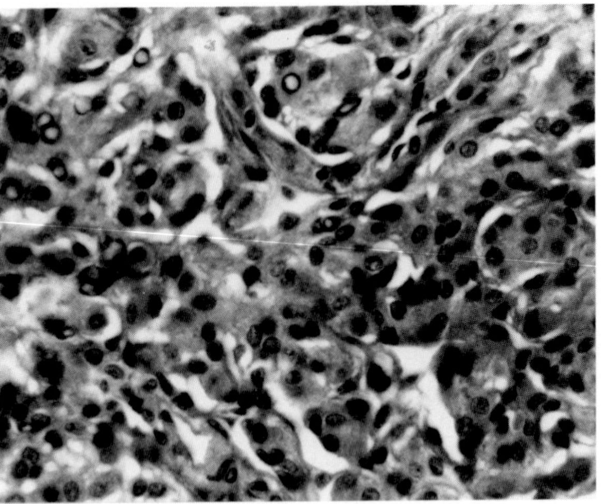

B

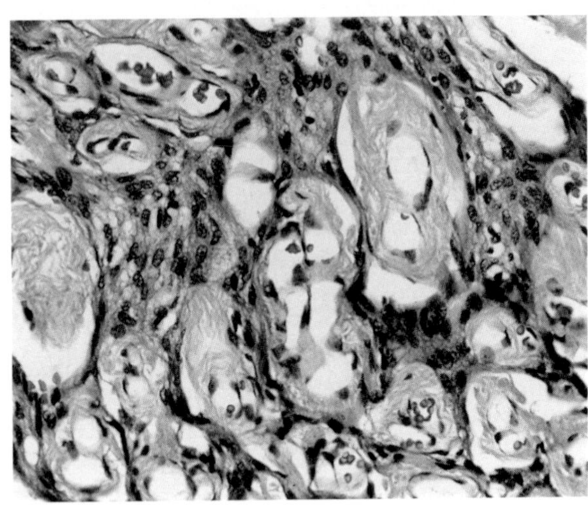

C

Fig. 8.20 Meningioma. **A, B**. Meningothelial meningiomas exhibit the syncytial arrangement of cells and whorl formations. The delicate chromatin pattern and regular nuclei are characteristic of meningiomas **B**. Intranuclear pseudoinclusions are commonly seen in these tumors. **B, C**. Angiomatous meningiomas display numerous blood vessels intermixed with nests of meningothelial cells. **A–C** H&E.

reflecting the capacity of meningothelium to exhibit a mesenchymal or epithelial phenotype. Although the majority of these variants show similar biologic behavior, the importance of their recognition resides in the fact that some are associated with systemic manifestations, such as Castleman's disease with the chordoid variant (Kepes et al 1988), and polyclonal gammopathies with lymphoplasmacyte-rich tumors (Horten et al 1979), etc.

The *meningotheliomatous* (syncytial) variant of meningioma is most frequent (Fig. 8.20A,B). Such tumors are characterized by plump epithelioid cells with poorly defined cell borders forming sheets, lobules and occasional whorls around vessels and other stromal elements. The cells contain nuclei with finely distributed chromatin and inconspicuous nucleoli. Nuclear cytoplasmic invaginations are frequent, the result being 'intranuclear pseudoinclusion' formation (Fig. 8.20B). At the ultrastructural level, meningothelial cells show a tendency to form membrane interdigitations and to display desmosomes and hemidesmosomes (Kepes 1982). The *transitional* meningioma possesses not only syncytial-appearing but spindle-shaped cells with a greater tendency to whorl formation. Psammoma bodies are a common feature of this variant.

Fibroblastic, angiomatous (Fig. 8.20C) and *metaplastic* variants constitute the 'mesenchymal' end of the meningioma spectrum. They possess a variable degree of reticulin and are collagen-rich (Russell & Rubinstein 1989); extracellular matrix proteins, such as laminin, fibronectin, and collagen types IV and V are found. The 'epithelial' phenotype of meningiomas is expressed by the *microcystic, secretory, clear cell* (glycogen-rich), *chordoid* and *papillary* variants. PAS-positive inclusions are commonly found in the secretory variant, the intracytoplasmic lumina within which they lie being lined by microvilli (Radley et al 1989). Clear cell meningiomas are glycogen-rich, often posterior fossa or spinal in location, and behave in an aggressive manner which includes spinal seeding (Zorludemir et al 1994).

Meningiomas display immunohistochemical properties consistent with both the mesenchymal and epithelial nature of the arachnoidal cells. The major intermediate filament, present in virtually almost 100% of the cases, is vimentin (Schnitt & Vogel 1986, Russell & Rubinstein 1989). S-100 protein is variably demonstrated in 20–50% of the cases, particularly in the fibroblastic variants (Schnitt & Vogel 1986, Artlich & Schmidt 1990). Cytokeratin and epithelial membrane antigen (EMA) are present in various degrees in approximately 5–20% of the meningiomas, but are found with greatest frequency

(40%) in epithelial variants (Schnitt & Vogel 1986, Meis et al 1986, Theaker et al 1987).

B. Atypical meningioma (WHO grade II)

The new WHO classification recognizes a form of meningioma with biologic behavior intermediate between the typical meningioma and the anaplastic (malignant) meningioma. Although these tumors lack histopathologic features clearly associated with malignancy, they show an increased tendency to recurrence and locally aggressive behavior (Jellinger & Slowik 1975, de la Monte et al 1986, Jääskeläinen et al 1986, Jellinger 1989, Chen & Liu 1990). Important histopathologic features of such atypical tumors include hypercellularity, increased mitotic activity, diffuse or sheet-like growth, increased nuclear pleomorphism with nucleolar prominence, and the presence of micronecrosis. These features may be present in any histologic variant of meningioma and may be focal in a given tumor. Thus careful examination of multiple tissue sections is necessary in evaluating meningiomas. The presence of a focal papillary pattern is associated with an increased likelihood of recurrence (Chen & Liu 1990) (see Papillary meningiomas, below).

One of the most valuable parameters for predicting recurrence appears to be a quantitative assessment of mitotic activity, at least 5 mitotic figures in 10 high power fields being a commonly accepted number (Maier et al 1992) as well as proliferative activity indices by flow cytometric or immunohistochemical methods. Determination of tumor kinetics with the assessment of BUdR uptake, immunohistochemistry for Ki-67 antigen (MIB-1), and flow cytometric measurement of S-phase fraction are of value in identifying tumors which are likely to recur (Cho et al 1986, May et al 1989, Lee et al 1990). Labeling indices above 1% appear to distinguish atypical meningiomas (Lee et al 1990). The AgNOR technique has also been successfully used to distinguish tumors with a significant potential for recurrence (Orita et al 1990).

C. Anaplastic (malignant) meningioma (WHO grade III)

In this category are included meningiomas with frankly anaplastic features, including marked nuclear and cellular pleomorphism, abundant mitotic activity, and obvious necrosis (Fig. 8.21A, B). The evaluation of malignant potential often cannot be based on histopathologic evidence alone. Not all clinically malignant tumors, including those exhibiting brain invasion or metastasis, show histologic anaplasia. Brain invasion (Fig. 8.21C, D) is considered an indicator of malignancy, regardless of the presence or absence of histologic anaplasia. A careful study of the tumor-brain interface is mandatory in any meningioma, not only at surgery but by histologic study of the periphery of large tumor fragments.

D. Papillary meningioma (WHO grade III)

This rare malignant variant of meningiomas affects primarily children and young adults (Deen et al 1982), and has a high tendency to regional and brain invasion, recurrence, and even distant metastasis (Ludwin et al 1975, Pasquier et al 1986). Histologically, such tumors are highly cellular and composed of epithelial-like cells arranged in papillary structures around blood vessels. 'Epithelial' ribbons may also be seen, a pattern simulating metastatic adenocarcinoma (Kepes et al 1983). The perivascular cells present thin processes which on ultrastructure contain bundles of 10 nm filaments (Piatt et al 1986). Such processes may be PTAH positive, thus mimicking fibrils of glial neoplasms. In contrast to gliomas, however, GFAP immunoreactivity is invariably absent. The papillary pattern is predominant in only a minority of tumors, most demonstrating areas of more recognizable meningioma. High mitotic activity and evidence of brain invasion are commonly seen.

2. Mesenchymal, nonmeningothelial tumors

Several mesenchymal neoplasms may arise in the meninges. Although very uncommon, the benign tumors in this category include chondroma, osteochondroma, osteoma and lipoma. Among the sarcomas, those most frequent are hemangiopericytoma, chondrosarcoma, malignant fibrous histiocytoma and rhabdomyosarcoma. In general, these tumors display similar features to their counterparts outside the CNS. It is of particular importance to discuss the hemangiopericytoma since it was, until recently, considered an 'angioblastic' variant of meningiomas. Because of the histopathologic, immunophenotypic and ultrastructural similarities between these tumors and the soft tissue hemangiopericytomas, the dura-based tumors are now grouped under the mesenchymal, nonmeningothelial, tumors in the new WHO classification.

A. Hemangiopericytoma (WHO grade II–III)

Hemangiopericytomas of the meninges account for about 1–7% of all meningeal tumors. They are remarkably aggressive neoplasms exhibiting a high rate of recurrence and metastasis (Guthrie et al 1989, Jellinger & Paulus 1991, Mena et al 1991). The majority arise in adults and show a slight male predominance. As previously discussed, the histogenesis of these tumors has been the subject of longstanding controversy among neuropathologists. Although meningeal hemangiopericytomas are regarded as being identical to those of soft tissue

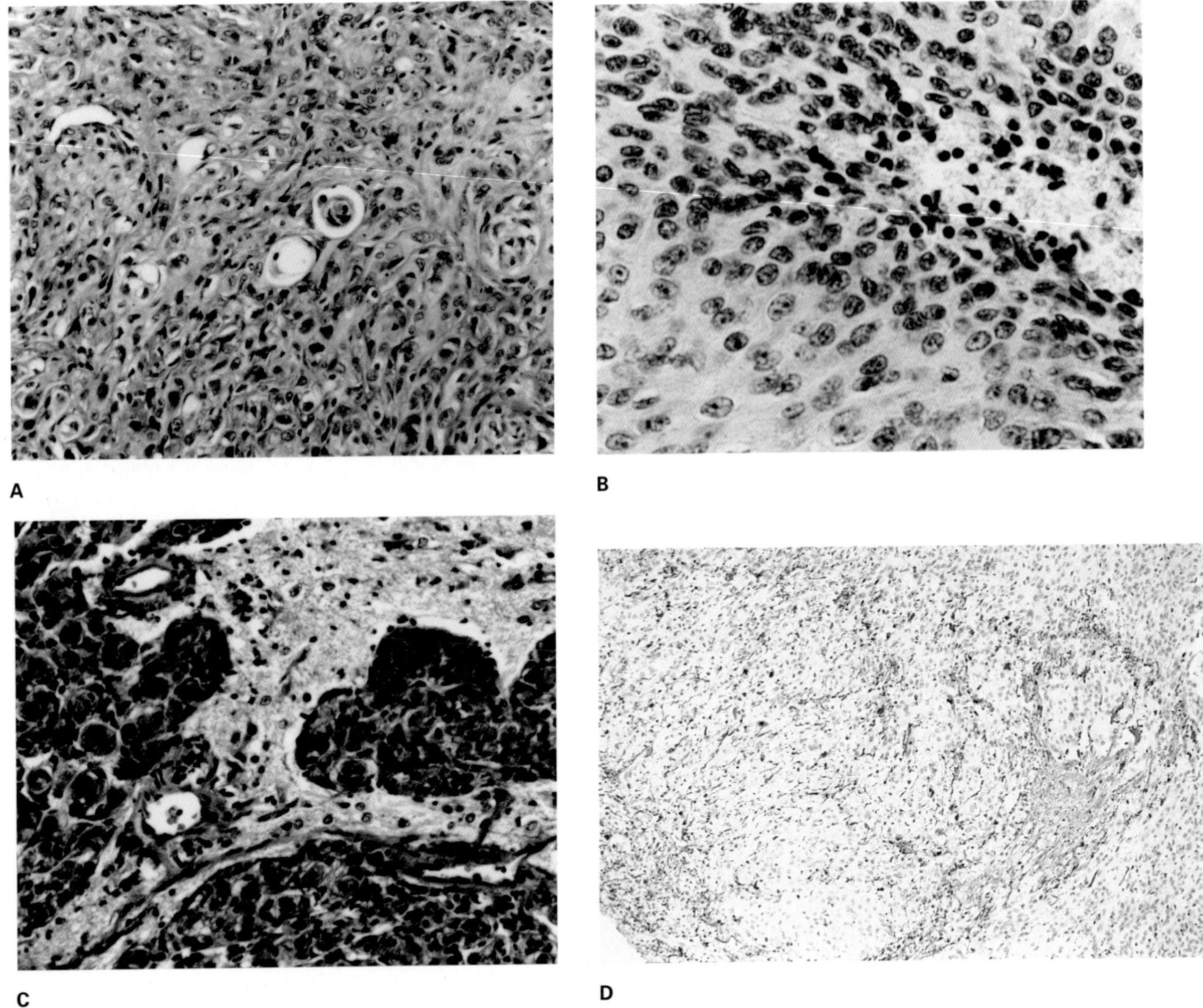

Fig. 8.21 Anaplastic meningioma. A. Hypercellularity, cellular atypia and loss of growth pattern are features of anaplastic meningiomas. B. Nuclear pleomorphism and prominent nucleoli, associated with areas of necrosis, are present in these tumors. C. Brain invasion is definitive evidence for the aggressive biological behavior of meningiomas. A–C H&E. D. GFAP immunohistochemistry demonstrating included reactive brain in an invasive, malignant meningioma. GFAP avidin biotin-immunoperoxidase.

(Scheithauer 1990, Burger et al 1991), some still consider them to be at one end of the spectrum for meningiomas (Horten et al 1977, Holden et al 1987, Nakamura et al 1987, Russell & Rubinstein 1989, Winek et al 1989, D'Amore et al 1990, Theunissen et al 1990). Recent ultrastructural (Dardick et al 1989) and cytogenetic studies (Hereth et al 1994) show dural hemangiopericytomas to be entirely distinct from meningothelial neoplasms.

Histologically, these tumors show the features of hemangiopericytomas of soft tissue. They are highly cellular neoplasms composed of small plump to spindle cells, with ill-defined cytoplasmic borders, their oval to somewhat elongated nuclei being crowded (Fig. 8.22A). A delicate cleft-like vascular network likened to a 'staghorn' pattern is typically present but is not diagnostic of this lesion. Reticulin deposition (Fig. 8.22B) is usually present around individual tumors. Mitotic activity is quite variable. Immunohistochemical studies show vimentin reactivity but, unlike meningiomas, EMA, S-100 protein and cytokeratin are lacking (Nakamura et al 1987, Winek et al 1989, D'Amore et al 1990, Theunissen et al 1990).

3. Tumors of uncertain histogenesis

A. Hemangioblastoma (WHO grade I)

Capillary hemangioblastomas represent less than 2.5% of all intracranial tumors (Zülch 1986), and are mostly found in adults, with a peak of incidence in the fourth decade (Russell & Rubinstein 1989). Their classic loca-

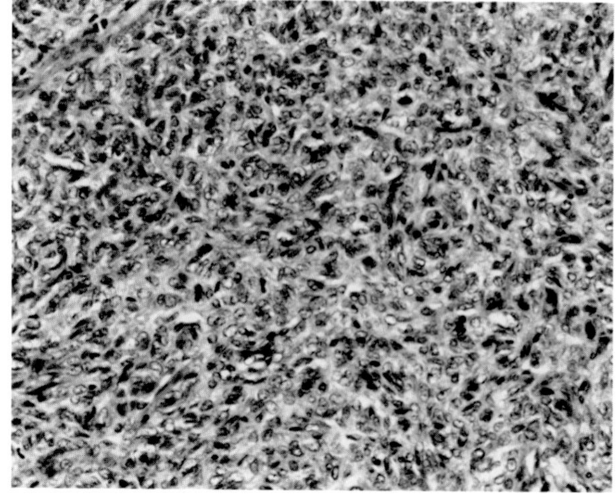

A

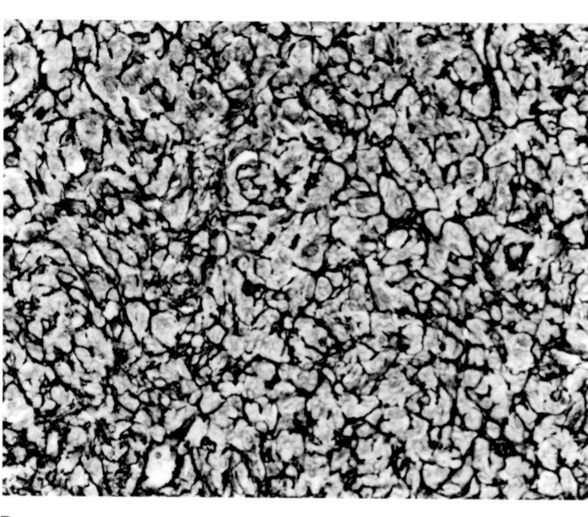

B

Fig. 8.22 Hemangiopericytoma. **A**. Hemangiopericytomas are highly cellular neoplasms composed of short plump spindle cells with moderate pleomorphism. H&E. **B**. A branching vascular network is easily demonstrated by reticulin stains. Gordon and Sweet's reticulin.

tion is the cerebellum, but they also occur in the brainstem and spinal cord (Nakamura et al 1985, Sanford & Smith 1986). Supratentorial examples are rare, and the majority are associated with von Hippel-Lindau disease (Russell & Rubinstein 1989).

Hemangioblastomas are well-circumscribed, cystic lesions composed of one or occasionally more mural nodules. Histologically, they are characterized by an anastomosing network of delicate vessels that separate groups of large polygonal stromal cells, with lipid-laden cytoplasm and hyperchromatic nuclei. The various endothelial, pericytic and stromal cells are readily identified in smear preparations. The origin of the stromal cells is not completely understood. Intense immunoreactivity for vimentin and neuron-specific enolase (NSE) is a constant finding, but the presence of NSE does not indicate a neuroepithelial origin. The lack of EMA immunohistochemistry, on the other hand, is helpful in distinguishing hemangioblastomas from metastatic renal cell carcinoma (Mills et al 1990).

Hemangioblastomas are typically well-circumscribed tumors that nearly always abut the leptomeninges. Although invasion of the adjacent parenchyma is uncommon, an exuberant astrogliosis with Rosenthal fiber formation is frequently seen in the surrounding parenchyma. This special pattern may result in an erroneous diagnosis of pilocytic astrocytoma in small biopsies or on smear preparations.

CONCLUSION

Neuropathological advances continue to shed light on brain tumor biology. Further studies based on exciting advances in molecular biology will be even more helpful in guiding diagnosis and therapy.

REFERENCES

Abo T, Balch T A 1981 Differentiation antigen of human NK and K cells identified by a monoclonal antibody (HNK-1). Journal of Immunology 127: 1024–1029

Albrecht S, Rouah E, Becker L E, Bruner J 1991 Immunoreactivity for transthyretin in choroid plexus neoplasms and brain metastases (abstract). Journal of Neuropathology and Experimental Neurology 50: 366

Allegranza A, Pileri S, Frank G, Ferracini R 1990 Cerebral ganglioglioma with anaplastic oligodendroglial component. Histopathology 17: 439–441

Allegranza A, Girlando S, Arrigoni G L et al 1991 Proliferating cell nuclear antigen expression in central nervous system neoplasms. Virchows Archives [A] 419: 417–423

Altermatt H J, Lopes M B S, Scheithauer B W, VandenBerg S R 1993 The immunochemistry of subependymal giant cell astrocytoma (SEGA) in tuberous sclerosis (TS) (abstract). Journal of Neuropathology and Experimental Neurology 52: 326

Artlich A, Schmidt D 1990 Immunohistochemical profile of meningiomas and their histological subtypes. Human Pathology 21: 843–849

Asai A, Hoshino T, Edwards M S B, Davis R L 1992 Predicting the recurrence of ependymomas from the bromodeoxyuridine labeling index. Child's Nervous System 8: 273–278

Ashley D G, Zee C-S, Chandrasoma P T, Segall H D 1990 Lhermitte-Duclos disease: CT and MR findings. Journal of Computerized Assisted Tomography 14: 984–987

Azzarelli B, Rekate H L, Roessman U 1977 Subependymoma: a case report with ultrastructural study. Acta Neuropathologica 40: 279–282

Banerjee A K, Gleathill C A 1979 Lhermitte-Duclos disease (diffuse cerebellar hypertrophy): prolonged post-operative survival. Irish Journal of Medicine Sciences 148: 97–99

Barnard R O, Bradford R, Scott T, Thomas D G T 1986 Gliomyosarcoma. Report of a case of rhabdomyosarcoma arising in a malignant glioma. Acta Neuropathologica 69: 23–27

Bennett J P Jr, Rubinstein L J 1984 The biologic behavior of primary cerebral neuroblastoma: a reappraisal of the clinical course in a series of 70 cases. Annals of Neurology 16: 21–27

Berger M S, Edwards M S B, Wilson C B 1983 Primary cerebral neuroblastoma. Follow-up analysis of eleven cases. In: Concepts in pediatric surgery, vol 3. American Society for Pediatric Neurosurgery. S Karger, Basel, pp 35–43

Berger M S, Ghatan S, Haglund M M, Dobbins J, Ojemann G A 1993 Low-grade gliomas associated with intractable epilepsy: seizure outcome utilizing electrocorticography during tumor resection. Journal of Neurosurgery 79: 62–69

Bigner S H, Vogelstein B 1990 Cytogenetics and molecular genetics of malignant gliomas and medulloblastoma. Brain Pathology 1: 12–18

Bigner S H, Mark J, Bigner D D 1990 Cytogenetics of human brain tumors. Cancer Genetics and Cytogenetics 47: 141–154

Bishop M, de la Monte S M 1989 Dual lineage of astrocytomas. American Journal of Pathology 135: 517–527

Bonnin J M, Perentes E 1988 Retinal S-antigen immunoreactivity in medulloblastomas. Acta Neuropathologica 76: 204–207

Bonnin J M, Colon L E, Morawetz R B 1987 Focal glial differentiation and oncocytic transformation in choroid plexus papilloma. Acta Neuropathologica 72: 277–280

Borit A, Blackwood W, Mair W G P 1980 The separation of pineocytoma from pineoblastoma. Cancer 45: 1408–1418

Bravo R, Frank R, Blundell P A, MacDonald-Bravo H 1987 Cyclin/PCNA is the auxiliary protein of DNA polymerase-δ. Nature 326: 515–517

Brown M T, Friedman H S, Oakes J, Boyko O B, Hockenberger B, Schold S C Jr 1992 Chemotherapy for pilocytic astrocytoma. Cancer 71: 3165–3172

Burger P C 1989 The grading of astrocytomas and oligodendrogliomas. In: Field W S (ed) Primary brain tumors. A review of histologic classification. Springer Verlag, New York, pp 171–180

Burger P C, Kleihues P 1989 Cytologic composition of the untreated glioblastoma with implications for evaluation of needle biopsies. Cancer 63: 2014–2023

Burger P C, Shibata T, Kleihues P 1986 The use of the monoclonal antibody Ki-67 in the identification of proliferating cells: application to surgical neuropathology. American Journal of Surgical Pathology 10: 611–617

Burger P C, Grahmann F C, Bliestle A, Kleihues P 1987 Differentiation in the medulloblastoma. A histological and immunohistochemical study. Acta Neuropathology 73: 115–123

Burger P C, Scheithauer B W, Vogel F S 1991 Surgical pathology of the nervous system and its coverings, 3rd edn. Churchill Livingstone, New York

Caccamo D V, Herman M M, Rubinstein L J 1989 An immunohistochemical study of the primitive and maturing elements of human cerebral medulloepitheliomas. Acta Neuropathologica 79: 248–254

Cameron R S, Rakic P 1991 Glial cell lineage in the cerebral cortex: a review and synthesis. Glia 4: 124–137

Casadei G P, Komori T, Scheithauer B W, Miller G M, Parisi J E, Kelly P J 1993 Intracranial parenchymal schwannoma. A clinicopathological and neuroimaging study of nine cases. Journal of Neurosurgery 79: 217–222

Casartelli C, Rogatto S R, Barbieri Neto J 1989 Karyotypic evolution of human meningioma — progression through malignancy. Cancer Genetics and Cytogenetics 40: 33–45

Cattoretti G, Becker M H G, Key G, Duchrow M, Schlüter C, Galle J, Gerdes J 1992 Monoclonal antibodies against recombinant parts of the Ki-67 antigen (MIB 1 and MIB 3) detect proliferating cells in microwave-processed formalin-fixed paraffin sections. Journal of Pathology 168: 357–363

Celis J E, Celis A 1985 Cell cycle-dependent variations in the distribution of the nuclear protein cyclin proliferating cell nuclear antigen in cultured cells: Subdivision of S phase. Proceedings of the National Academy of Sciences USA 82: 3262–3266

Chen W Y, Liu H C 1990 Atypical (anaplastic) meningioma: relationship between histologic features and recurrence — a clinicopathologic study. Clinical Neuropathology 9: 74–81

Cho K G, Hoshino T, Nagashima T et al 1986 Prediction of tumor-doubling time in recurrent meningiomas: cell kinetic studies with bromodeoxyuridine labeling. Journal of Neurosurgery 65: 790–794

Choi B H, Kim R C 1984 Expression of glial fibrillary acidic protein in immature oligodendroglia. Science 223: 407–408

Chu T-A, Shmookler B M 1988 Malignant epithelioid schwannoma: a light microscopic and immunohistochemical study. Journal of Surgical Oncology 39: 68–72

Clark G B, Henry J M, McKeever P E 1985 Cerebral pylocytic astrocytoma. Cancer 56: 1128–1133

Coffin C M, Mukai K, Dehner L P 1983 Glial differentiation in medulloblastomas. Histogenetic insight, glial reaction, or invasion of brain? American Journal of Surgical Pathology 7: 555–565

Collins V P, James C D 1993 Gene and chromosomal alterations associated with the development of human gliomas. FASEB Journal 7: 926–930

Coons S W, Johnson P C 1993 Regional heterogeneity in the proliferative activity of human gliomas as measured by the Ki-67 labeling index. Journal of Neuropathology and Experimental Neurology 52: 609–618

Cruz-Sanchez F F, Haustein J, Rossie M L et al 1988 Ependymoblastoma: a histological, immunohistochemical and ultrastructural study of five cases. Histopathology 12: 17–27

Cruz-Sanchez F F, Rossi M L, Buller J R, Carboni P Jr, Fineron P W 1991 Oligodendrogliomas: a clinical, histological, immunocytochemical and lectin-binding study. Histopathology 19: 361–367

Czerwionka M, Korf H W, Hoffman O, Busch H, Schachenmayr W 1989 Differentiation in medulloblastomas: correlation between the immunocytochemical demonstration of photoreceptor markers (S-antigen, rod-opsin) and the survival rate in 66 patients. Acta Neuropathologica 78: 629–636

D'Amore E S G, Manivel J C, Sung J H 1990 Soft-tissue and meningeal hemangiopericytomas: An immunohistochemical and ultrastructural study. Human Pathology 21: 414–423

D'Andrea A D, Packer R J, Rorke L B et al 1987 Pineocytomas of childhood: a reappraisal of natural history and response to therapy. Cancer 59: 1353–1357

Daita G, Yonemasu Y, Muraoka S et al 1991 A case of anaplastic astrocytoma transformed from pleomorphic xanthoastrocytoma. Brain Tumor Pathology 8: 63–66

Dardick I, Hammar S P, Scheithauer B W 1989 Ultrastructural spectrum of hemangiopericytoma: a comparative study of fetal, adult and neoplastic pericytes. Ultrastructural Pathology 13: 111–154

Daumas-Duport C 1992 Histological grading of gliomas. Current Opinion in Neurology and Neurosurgery 5: 924–931

Daumas-Duport C 1993 Dysembryoplastic neuroepithelial tumours. Brain Pathology 3: 283–295

Daumas-Duport C, Scheithauer B W, O'Fallon J, Kelly P 1988a Grading of astrocytomas. A simple and reproducible method. Cancer 62: 2152–2165

Daumas-Duport C, Scheithauer B W, Chodkiewicz J-P et al 1988b Dysembryoplastic neuroepithelial tumor: A surgically curable tumor of young patients with intractable partial seizures: Report of thirty-nine cases. Neurosurgery 23: 545–556

Davis R L 1989 Grading of gliomas. In: Fields W S (ed) Primary brain tumors. A review of histologic classification. Springer Verlag, New York, pp 150–158

De Chadarévian J-P, Pattisapu J V, Faerber E N 1990 Desmoplastic cerebral astrocytoma of infancy. Light microscopy, immunocytochemistry, and ultrastructure. Cancer 66: 173–179

Deen H G Jr, Scheithauer B W, Ebersold M J 1982 Clinical and pathological study of meningiomas of the first two decades of life. Journal of Neurosurgery 56: 317–322

De Girolami U, Zvaigzne O 1973 Modification of the Achúcarro-Hortega pineal stain for paraffin-embedded formalin-fixed tissue. Stain Technology 48: 48–50

de la Monte S M 1989 Uniform lineage of oligodendrogliomas. American Journal of Pathology 153: 529–540

de la Monte S M, Flickinger J, Linggood R M 1986 Histopathologic features predicting recurrence of meningiomas following subtotal resection. American Journal of Surgical Pathology 10: 836–843

Desmeules M, Mikkelsen T, Mao Y 1992 Increasing incidence of primary malignant brain tumors: influence of diagnostic methods. Journal of the National Cancer Institute 84: 442–445

Donoso L A, Shields C L, Lee E Y-H P 1989 Immunohistochemistry of retinoblastoma. A review. Ophthalmic Paediatrics Genetics 10: 3–32

Dropcho E J, Wisoff J H, Walker R W, Allen J C 1987 Supratentorial malignant gliomas in childhood: A review of fifty cases. Annals of Neurology 22: 355–364

Ducatman B S, Scheithauer B W 1983 Post-irradiation neurofibrosarcoma. Cancer 51: 1028–1033

Ducatman B S, Scheithauer B W 1984 Malignant peripheral nerve sheath tumors with divergent differentiation. Cancer 54: 1049–1057

Ducatman B S, Scheithauer B W, Piepgras D G, Reiman H M, Ilstrup D M 1986 Malignant peripheral nerve sheath tumors. A clinicopathological study of 120 cases. Cancer 57: 2006–2021

Dumanski J P, Rouleau G A, Nordenskjöld M, Collins V P 1990 Molecular genetic analysis of chromosome 22 in 81 cases of meningioma. Cancer Research 50: 5863–5867

Earnest F IVth, Kelly P J, Scheithauer B W et al 1988 Cerebral astrocytomas: histopathologic correlation of MR and CT contrast enhancement with stereotactic biopsy. Radiology 166: 823–827

Edwards M S B, Hudgins R J, Wilson C B et al 1988 Pineal region tumors in children. Journal of Neurosurgery 68: 689–697

Enzinger F M, Weiss S W 1988 Soft tissue tumors, 2nd edn. CV Mosby, St Louis, pp 719–780

Erlandson R A 1985 Peripheral nerve sheath tumors. Ultrastructural Pathology 9: 113–122

Faillot T, Sichez J-P, Brault J-L et al 1990 Lhermitte-Duclos disease (dysplastic gangliocytoma of the cerebellum). Report of a case and review of the literature. Acta Neurochirurgica 105: 44–49

Figols J, Iglesias-Rozas J R, Kazner E 1985 Myelin basic protein (MBP) in human gliomas: a study of twenty-five cases. Clinical Neuropathology 4: 116–120

Forsyth P A, Shaw E G, Scheithauer B W, O'Fallon J R, Layton D D, Katzmann J A 1993 Supratentorial pilocytic astrocytomas. A clinicopathologic, prognostic and flow cytometric study of 51 patients. Cancer 72: 1335–1342

Frankel R H, Bayonna W, Koslow M, Newcomb E W 1992 p53 mutations in human malignant gliomas: comparison of loss of heterozygosity with mutation frequency. Cancer Research 52: 1427–1433

Fu Y-S, Chen A T L, Kay S, Young H F 1974 Is subependymoma (subependymal glomerate astrocytoma) an astrocytoma or ependymoma? A comparative ultrastructural and tissue culture study. Cancer 34: 1992–2008

Fults D, Brockmeyer D, Tullous M W, Pedone C A, Cawthon R M 1992 p53 mutation and loss of heterozygosity on chromosome 17 and 10 during human astrocytoma progression. Cancer Research 52: 674–679

Galand P, Degraef C 1989 Cyclin/PCNA immunostaining as an alternative to tritiated thymidine pulse labelling for marking S phase cells in paraffin sections from animal and human tissues. Cell Tissue Kinetics 22: 383–392

Gallie B L, Squire J A, Goddard A et al 1990 Biology of disease. Mechanism of oncogenesis in retinoblastoma. Laboratory Investigation 62: 394–408

Gambarelli D, Hassoun J, Choux M et al 1982 Complex cerebral tumor with evidence of neuronal, glial and Schwann cell differentiation: A histologic immunocytochemical and ultrastructural study. Cancer 49: 1420–1428

Garcia D M, Fulling K H 1985 Juvenile pilocytic astrocytoma of the cerebrum in adults. A distinctive neoplasm with favorable prognosis. Journal of Neurosurgery 63: 382–386

Gennett I N, Cavenee W K 1990 Molecular genetics in the pathology and diagnosis of retinoblastoma. Brain Pathology 1: 25–32

Gerdes J, Schwab U, Lemke H, Stein H 1983 Production of a mouse monoclonal antibody reactive with a human nuclear antigen associated with cell proliferation. International Journal of Cancer 31: 13–20

Gerdes J, Lemke H, Baisch H et al 1984 Cell cycle analysis of a cell proliferation-associated human nuclear antigen defined by the monoclonal antibody Ki-67. Journal of Immunology 133: 1710–1715

Gerdes J, Becker M H G, Key G, Cattoretto G 1992 Immunohistochemical detection of tumour growth fraction (Ki-67 antigen) in formalin-fixed and routinely processed tissues. Journal of Pathology 168: 85–87

Giangaspero F, Doglioni C, Rivano M T et al 1987 Growth factor in human brain tumors defined by the monoclonal antibody Ki-67. Acta Neuropathologica 74: 179–182

Giangaspero F, Rigobello L, Badiali et al 1992 Large-cell medulloblastomas. A distinctive variant with highly aggressive behavior. American Journal of Surgical Pathology 16: 687–693

Gonzalez-Fernandez F, Lopes M B S, Garcia-Fernandez J M et al 1992 Expression of developmentally-defined retinal phenotypes in the histogenesis of retinoblastoma. American Journal of Pathology 141: 363–375

Gottschalk J, Jautzke G, Paulus W, Goebel S, Cervos-Navarro J 1993 The use of immunomorphology to differentiate choroid plexus tumors from metastatic carcinomas. Cancer 72: 1343–1349

Gould V E, Moll R, Moll I, Lee I, Schwechheimer K, Franke W W 1986 The intermediate filament complement of the spectrum of nerve sheath neoplasms. Laboratory Investigation 55: 463–474

Gould V E, Rorke L B, Jansson D S et al 1990 Primitive neuroectodermal tumors of the central nervous system express neuroendocrine markers and may express all classes of intermediate filaments. Human Pathology 21: 245–252

Grant J W, Steart P V, Aguzzi A et al 1989 Gliosarcoma: An immunohistochemical study. Acta Neuropathologica 79: 305–309

Gray M H, Rosenberg A E, Dickersin G R, Bhan A K 1989 Glial fibrillary acidic protein and keratin expression by benign and malignant nerve sheath tumors. Human Pathology 20: 1089–1096

Guthrie B L, Ebersold M J, Scheithauer B W, Shaw E G 1989 Meningeal hemangiopericytoma: histopathological features, treatment, and long-term follow-up of 44 cases. Neurosurgery 25: 514–522

Haddad S F, Moore S A, Schelper R L, Goeken J 1991 Smooth muscle cells can comprise the sarcomatous component of gliosarcomas (abstract). Journal of Neuropathology and Experimental Neurology 50: 291

Halliday A L, Sobel R A, Martuza R L 1991 Benign spinal nerve sheath tumors: their occurrence sporadically and in neurofibromatosis types 1 and 2. Journal of Neurosurgery 74: 248–253

Halling K C, Ziesmer S C, Roche P C, Scheithauer B W, Nascimento A G 1993 p53 expression in neurofibrosarcomas (malignant schwannomas) and neurofibromas (abstract). American Journal of Clinical Pathology 100: 329

Halmagyi G M, Bignold L P, Allsop J L 1979 Recurrent subependymal giant-cell astrocytoma in the absence of tuberous sclerosis. Journal of Neurosurgery 50: 106–109

Hassoun J, Gambarelli D 1989 Pinealomas: need for an ultrastructural diagnosis. In: Fields W S (ed) Primary brain tumors. A review of histologic classification. Springer Verlag, New York, pp 82–85

Hassoun J, Gambarelli D, Grisoli F et al 1982 Central neurocytoma: an electron-microscopic study of two cases. Acta Neuropathologica 56: 151–156

Hassoun J, Gambarelli D, Peragut J C, Toga M 1983 Specific ultrastructural markers of human pinealomas: a study of four cases. Acta Neuropathologica 62: 31–40

Hassoun J, Devictor B, Gambarelli D et al 1984 Paired twisted filaments: a new ultrastructural marker of human pinealomas? Acta Neuropathologica 65: 163–165

Hassoun J, Söylemezoglu F, Gambarelli D, Figarella-Branger D, con Ammon K, Kleihues P 1993 Central neurocytoma: a synopsis of clinical and histological features. Brain Pathology 3: 297–306

Hayashi H, Ohara N, Jeon H J, Akagi S, Takahashi K, Akagi T, Namba S 1993 Gliosarcoma with features of chondroblastic osteosarcoma. Cancer 72: 850–855

He X, Skapek S X, Wikstrand C J et al 1989 Phenotypic analysis of four human medulloblastoma cell lines and transplantable xenografts. Journal of Neuropathology and Experimental Neurology 48: 48–68

Hereth S, Stelberger P, Doll R, Parisi J E, Scheithauer B W, Jenkins R B 1994 Cytogenetic studies of four hemangiopericytomas. Cancer Genetics and Cytogenetics (in press)

Herpers M J H M, Budka H 1984 Glial fibrillary acidic protein (GFAP) in oligodendroglial tumors: gliofibrillary oligodendroglioma and transitional oligoastrocytoma as subtypes of oligodendroglioma. Acta Neuropathologica 64: 265–272

Herrick M K 1984 Pathology of pineal tumors. In: Neuwelt E A (ed) Diagnosis and treatment of pineal region tumors. Williams & Wilkins, Baltimore, pp 31–60

Herrick M K, Rubinstein L J 1979 The cytological differentiating potential of pineal parenchymal neoplasms (true pinealomas): a clinicopathologic study of 28 tumours. Brain 102: 289–320

Hessler R B, Lopes M B S, Frankfurter A, Reidy J, VandenBerg S R 1992 Cytoskeletal immunohistochemistry of central neurocytomas. American Journal of Surgical Pathology 16: 1031–1038

Hirose T, Sano T, Kizawa K 1986 Ultrastructural localization of S-100 protein in neurofibroma. Acta Neuropathologica 69: 103–110

Hirose T, Scheithauer B W, Lopes M B, VandenBerg S R 1994 Dysembryoplastic neuroepithelial tumor (DNT): an immunohistochemical and ultrastructural study. Journal of Neuropathology and Experimental Neurology 53: 184–195

Ho K-L 1990 Histogenesis of sarcomatous component of the gliosarcoma: an ultrastructural study. Acta Neuropathologica 81: 178–188

Holden J, Dolman C L, Churg A 1987 Immunohistochemistry of meningiomas including the angioblastic type. Journal of Neuropathology and Experimental Neurology 46: 50–56

Horten B C, Rubinstein L J 1976 Primary cerebral neuroblastoma. A clinicopathologic study of 35 cases. Brain 99: 735–756

Horten B C, Urich H, Rubinstein L J, Montague S R 1977 The angioblastic meningioma: a reappraisal of a nosological problem. Journal of Neurologic Sciences 31: 387–410

Horten B C, Urich H, Stefoski D 1979 Meningiomas with conspicuous plasma cell-lymphocytic components. Cancer 43: 258–264

Hoshino T, Rodriquez L A, Cho K G et al 1988 Prognostic implications of the proliferative potential low-grade astrocytomas. Journal of Neurosurgery 69: 839–842

Hosokawa Y, Tsuchihashi Y, Okabe H et al 1991 Pleomorphic xanthastrocytoma. Ultrastructural, immunohistochemical, and DNA cytofluorometric study of a case. Cancer 68: 853–859

Hurtt M R, Moosy J, Donovan-Peluso M, Locker J 1992 Amplification of epidermal growth factor receptor gene in gliomas: histopathology and prognosis. Journal of Neuropathology and Experimental Neurology 51: 84–90

Itoh Y, Kowada M, Mineura K, Kojima H 1987 Congenital glioblastoma of the cerebellum with cytofluorometric deoxyribonucleic acid analysis. Surgical Neurology 27: 163–167

Jääskeläinen J, Haltia M, Servo A 1986 Atypical and anaplastic meningiomas: radiology, surgery, radiotherapy, and outcome. Surgical Neurology 25: 233–242

Jagadha V, Halliday W C, Becker L E 1986 Glial fibrillary acidic protein (GFAP) in oligodendrogliomas: a reflection of transient GFAP expression by immature oligodendroglia. Canadian Journal of Neurologic Sciences 13: 307–311

Jay V, Becker L E, Otsubo H, Hwang P A, Hoffman H J, Harwood-Nash D 1993 Pathology of temporal lobectomy for refractory seizures in children. Review of 20 cases including some unique malformative lesions. Journal of Neurosurgery 79: 53–61

Jellinger K L 1989 Biologic behavior of meningiomas. In: Fields W S (ed) Primary brain tumors. A review of histologic classification. Springer Verlag, New York, pp 231–238

Jellinger K, Paulus W 1991 Mesenchymal, non-meningothelial tumors of the central nervous system. Brain Pathology 1: 79–87

Jellinger K, Slowik F 1975 Histological subtypes and prognostic problems in meningiomas. Journal of Neurology 208: 279–298

Johnson D L, Chandra R, Fisher W S, Hammock M K, McKeown C A 1985 Trilateral retinoblastoma: ocular and pineal retinoblastomas. Journal of Neurosurgery 63: 367–370

Kalyan-Raman U P, Olivero W C 1987 Ganglioglioma: A correlative clinicopathological and radiological study of ten surgically treated cases with follow-up. Neurosurgery 20: 428–433

Kaneko Y, Takeshita I, Matsushima T, Iwaki T, Tashima T, Fukui M 1990 Immunohistochemical study of ependymal neoplasms: histological subtypes and glial and epithelial characteristics. Virchows Archives [A] 417: 97–103

Karamitopoulou E, Perentes E, Diamantis I 1993 Ki-67 immunoreactivity in human central nervous system tumors. A retrospective study with MIB 1 monoclonal antibody (abstract). Journal of Neuropathology and Experimental Neurology 52: 290

Kashima T, Tiu S N, Merrill J E, Vinters H V, Dawson G, Campagnoni A T 1993 Expression of oligodendrocyte-associated genes in cell lines derived from human gliomas and neuroblastomas. Cancer Research 53: 170–175

Katsetos C D, Herman M M, Frankfurter A et al 1989 Cerebellar desmoplastic medulloblastomas. A further immunohistochemical characterization of the reticulin-free pale islands. Archives of Pathology and Laboratory Medicine 113: 1019–1029

Katsetos C D, Frankfurter A, Christakos S et al 1991 Differential expression of neuronal class III β-tubulin isotype and calbindin D28K in the developing human cerebellar cortex and cerebellar neuroblastomas ("medulloblastomas"). Journal of Neuropathology and Experimental Neurology 50: 293

Kawano N 1991 Pleomorphic xanthoastrocytoma (PXA) in Japan: its clinico-pathologic features and diagnostic clues. Brain Tumor Pathology 8: 5–10

Kawano N, Yada K, Yagishita S 1989 Clear cell ependymoma. A histological variant with diagnostic implications. Virchows Archives [A] 415: 467–472

Keating G, Scheithauer B W, Groover R V et al 1993 Pediatric ependymomas: the relation of histologic and flow cytometric parameters to prognosis (abstract). Modern Pathology 6: 128

Kennedy P G E, Fok-Seang J 1986 Studies on the development, antigenic phenotype and function of human glial cells in tissue culture. Brain 109: 1261–1277

Kennedy P G E, Watkins B A, Thomas D G T, Noble M D 1987 Antigenic expression by cells derived from human glioma does not correlate with morphological classification. Neuropathology and Applied Neurobiology 13: 327–347

Kepes J J 1982 Meningiomas. Biology, pathology, and differential diagnosis. Masson, New York

Kepes J J 1983 Oncocytic transformation of choroid plexus epithelium. Acta Neuropathologica 62: 145–148

Kepes J J, Rubinstein L J, Eng L F 1979 Pleomorphic xanthoastrocytoma: A distinctive meningocerebral glioma of young subjects with relatively favorable prognosis; a study of 12 cases. Cancer 44: 1839–1852

Kepes J J, Goldware S, Leoni R 1983 Meningioma with pseudoglandular pattern. Journal of Neuropathology and Experimental Neurology 42: 61–68

Kepes J J, Rubinstein L J, Chiang H 1984 The role of astrocytes in the formation of cartilage in gliomas. An immunohistochemical study of four cases. American Journal of Pathology 117: 471–483

Kepes J J, Chen W Y-K, Connors M H, Vogel F S 1988 "Chordoid" meningeal tumors in young individuals with peritumoral lymphoplasmacellular infiltrates causing systemic manifestation of Castleman Syndrome. A report of seven cases. Cancer 62: 391–406

Kepes J J, Rubinstein L J, Ansbacher L, Schreiber D J 1989 Histopathological features of recurrent pleomorphic xanthoastrocytomas: Further corroboration of the glial nature of this neoplasm. Acta Neuropathologica 78: 585–593

Kim T S, Halliday A L, Hedley-Whyte E T, Convery K 1991 Correlates of survival and the Daumas-Duport grading system for astrocytomas. Journal of Neurosurgery 74: 27–37

Kivelä T, Tarkkanen A, Virtanen I 1986 Intermediate filaments in the human retina and retinoblastoma. An immunohistochemical study of vimentin, glial fibrillary acidic protein, and neurofilaments. Investigative Ophthalmology and Visual Science 27: 1075–1084

Kivelä T, Tarkkanen A, Virtanen I 1989 Synaptophysin in the human retina and retinoblastoma. An immunohistochemical and Western blotting study. Investigative Ophthalmology and Visual Science 30: 212–219

Kleihues P, Aguzzi A, Shibata T, Wiestler O D 1989 Immunohistochemical assessment of differentiation and DNA replication in human brain tumors. In: Fields W S (ed) Primary brain tumors. A review of histologic classification. New York, Springer Verlag, pp 123–132

Kleihues P, Aguzzi A, Wiestler O D 1990 Cellular and molecular aspects of neurocarcinogenesis. Toxicology Pathology 18: 193–203

Kleihues P, Burger P C, Scheithauer B W 1993a Histological typing of tumours of the central nervous system, 2nd edn. Springer-Verlag, Berlin

Kleihues P, Burger P C, Scheithauer B W 1993b The new WHO classification of brain tumours. Brain Pathology 3: 255–268

Kleinert K 1991 Immunohistochemical characterization of primitive neuroectodermal tumors and their possible relationship to the stepwise ontogenetic development of the central nervous system. 2. Tumor studies. Acta Neuropathologica 82: 508–515

Kline K T, Damjanov I, Katz S M, Schmidek H 1979 Pineoblastoma: an electron microscopic study. Cancer 44: 1692–1699

Korf H W, Klein D C, Zigler J S et al 1986 S-antigen-like immunoreactivity in a human pineocytoma. Acta Neuropathologica 69: 165–167

Korf H W, Czerwionka M, Reiner J, Schachenmayr W, Schalken J J, de Grip W, Gery I 1987 Immunocytochemical evidence of molecular photoreceptor markers in cerebellar medulloblastomas. Cancer 60: 1763–1766

Korf H W, Korf B, Schachenmayr W, Chader G J, Wiggert B 1992 Immunocytochemical demonstration of interphotoreceptor retinoid-binding protein in cerebellar medulloblastoma. Acta Neuropathologica 83: 482–487

Kramm C M, Korf H W, Czerwionka M, Schachenmayr W, de Grip W J 1991 Photoreceptor differentiation in cerebellar medulloblastoma: evidence for a functional photopigment and authentic S-antigen (arrestin). Acta Neuropathologica 81: 296–302

Kriek E, Engelsen L D, Scherer E, Westra J G 1984 Formation of DNA modifications by chemical carcinogens identification, localization and quantification. Biochimica et Biophysica Acta 738: 181–201

Kros J M, Van Eden C G, Stefanko S Z, Waayer-Van Batenburg M, van der Kwast Th H 1990 Prognostic implications of glial fibrillary acidic protein containing cell types in oligodendrogliomas. Cancer 66: 1204–1212

Kros J M, de Jong A A, van der Kwast Th H 1992 Ultrastructural characterization of transitional cells in oligodendrogliomas. Journal of Neuropathology and Experimental Neurology 51: 186–193

Krouwer H G J, Davis R L, Silver R, Prados M 1991 Gemistocytic astrocytomas: a reappraisal. Journal of Neurosurgery 74: 399–406

Kubota T, Hayashi M, Kawano H et al 1991 Central neurocytoma: immunohistochemical and ultrastructural study. Acta Neuropathologica 81: 418–427

Labrousse F, Daumas-Duport C, Batorski L, Hoshino T 1991 Histological grading and bromodeoxyuridine labeling index of astrocytomas. Comparative study in a series of 60 cases. Journal of Neurosurgery 75: 202–205

Langford L A 1986 The ultrastructure of the ependymoblastoma. Acta Neuropathologica 71: 136–141

Laurence K M 1979 The biology of choroid plexus papilloma in infancy and childhood. Acta Neurochirurgica 50: 79–90

Laws E R Jr, Taylor W F, Clifton M B, Okazaki H 1984 Neurosurgical management of low-grade astrocytoma of the cerebral hemispheres. Journal of Neurosurgery 61: 665–673

Lee K S, Hoshino T, Rodriguez L A et al 1990 Bromodeoxyuridine labeling study of intracranial meningiomas: proliferative potential and recurrence. Acta Neuropathologica 80: 311–317

Leivo I, Engvall E, Laurila P, Miettinen M 1989 Distribution of merosin, a laminin-related tissue-specific basement membrane protein, in human schwann cell neoplasms. Laboratory Investigation 61: 426–432

Lekanne Deprez R H, Groen N A, Van Biezen N A et al 1991 A t(4;22) in a meningioma points to the localization of a putative tumor-suppressor gene. American Journal of Genetics 48: 783–790

Less M B, Brostoff S W 1984 Proteins of myelin. In: Morell P (ed) Myelin, 2nd edn. Plenum Press, New York, pp 197–224

Liddle C N, Reid W A, Kennedy J S, Miller I D, Horne C H W 1985 Immunolocalization of prealbumin: distribution in normal human tissue. Journal of Pathology 146: 107–113

Lillien L E, Raff M C 1990 Differentiation signals in the CNS: type-2 astrocyte development in vitro as a model system. Neuron 5: 111–119

Lombardi D, Scheithauer B W, Meyer F B et al 1991 Symptomatic subependymoma: a clinicopathological and flow cytometric study. Journal of Neurosurgery 75: 583–588

Lopes M B S, Rosemberg S, Cardoso de Almeida P C, Pestana C B 1989 Glial fibrillary acidic protein and cytokeratin in choroid plexus tumors: an immunohistochemical study. Pathology Research and Practice 185: 339–341

Lopes M B S, Gonzalez-Fernandez F, Scheithauer B W, VandenBerg S R 1993 Differential expression of retinal proteins in a pineal parenchymal tumor. Journal of Neuropathology and Experimental Neurology 52: 516–524

Louis D N, Edgerton S, Thor A D, Hedley-Whyte E T 1991 Proliferating cell nuclear antigen and Ki-67 immunohistochemistry in brain tumors: a comparative study. Acta Neuropathologica 81: 675–679

Louis D N, von Deimling A, Chung R Y et al 1993 Comparative study of p53 gene and protein alterations in human astrocytic tumors. Journal of Neuropathology and Experimental Neurology 52: 31–38

Ludwin S K, Rubinstein L J, Russell D S 1975 Papillary meningioma: A malignant variant of meningioma. Cancer 36: 1363–1373

McGarry R C, Helfand S L, Qaurles R H et al 1983 Recognition of myelin-associated glycoprotein by the monoclonal antibody HNK-1. Nature 306: 376–378

McGirr S J, Ebersold M J, Scheithauer B W 1988 Choroid plexus papillomas: long term follow-up of a surgically treated series. Journal of Neurosurgery 69: 843–849

Maier H, Ofner D, Hittmair A, Kitz K, Budka H 1992 Classic, atypical, and anaplastic meningioma: Three histopathological subtypes of relevance. Journal of Neurosurgery 77: 616–623

Marano S R, Johnson P C, Spetzler R F 1988 Recurrent Lhermitte-Duclos disease in a child. Journal of Neurosurgery 69: 599–603

Margetts J C, Kalyan-Raman U P 1989 Giant-celled glioblastoma of brain: a clinico-pathological and radiological study of ten cases (including immunohistochemistry and ultrastructure). Cancer 63: 524–531

Margo C, Hydayat A, Kopelman J, Zimmerman L E 1983 Retinocytoma: A benign variant of retinoblastoma. Archives of Ophthalmology 101: 1519–1531

Markesbery W R, Haugh R M, Young A B 1981 Ultrastructure of pineal parenchymal neoplasms. Acta Neuropathologica 55: 143–149

Masuzawa T, Shimabukuro H, Yoshimizu N, Sato F 1981 Ultrastructure of disseminated choroid plexus papilloma. Acta Neuropathologica 54: 321–324

Matsui I, Tanimura M, Kobayashi N, Sawada T, Nagahara N, Akatsuka J 1993 Neurofibromatosis type 1 and childhood cancer. Cancer 72: 2746–2754

May P L, Broome J C, Lawry J et al 1989 The prediction of recurrence in meningiomas. A flow cytometric study of paraffin-embedded archival material. Journal of Neurosurgery 71: 347–351

Meis J M, Ordóñez N G, Bruner J M 1986 Meningiomas: An immunohistochemical study of 50 cases. Archives of Pathology and Laboratory Medicine 110: 934–937

Meis J M, Martz K L, Nelson J S 1991 Mixed glioblastoma multiforme and sarcoma. A clinicopathologic study of 26 radiation therapy oncology group cases. Cancer 67: 2342–2349

Meis J M, Enzinger F M, Martz K L, Neal J A 1992 Malignant peripheral nerve sheath tumors (malignant schwannomas) in children. American Journal of Surgical Pathology 16: 694–707

Mena H, Ribas J L, Pezeshkpour G H, Cowan D N, Parisi J E 1991 Hemangiopericytoma of the central nervous system: a review of 94 cases. Human Pathology 22: 84–91

Miettinen M, Foidart J M, Ekblom P 1983 Immunohistochemical demonstration of laminin, the major glycoprotein of basement membranes, as an aid in the diagnosis of soft tissue tumors. American Journal of Clinical Pathology 79: 306–311

Miettinen M, Clark R, Virtanen I 1986 Intermediate filament proteins in choroid plexus and ependyma and their tumors. American Journal of Pathology 123: 231–240

Milbouw G, Born J D, Martin D et al 1988 Clinical and radiological aspects of dysplastic gangliocytoma (Lhermitte-Duclos disease): A report of two cases with review of the literature. Neurosurgery 22: 124–128

Miller L L, Ostrow P T, Chau R 1991 Characterization of gliosarcomas by image analysis of superimposed serial sections (abstract). Journal of Neuropathology and Experimental Neurology 50: 365

Miller R H, French-Constant C, Raff M C 1989 The macroglial cells of the rat optic nerve. Annals Review Neurosciences 12: 517–534

Mills S E, Ross G W, Perentes E, Nakagawa Y, Scheithauer B W 1990 Cerebellar hemangioblastoma: immunohistochemical distinction from metastatic renal cell carcinoma. Surgical Pathology 3: 121–132

Min K W, Scheithauer B W, Brumbach R A 1990 Pineal parenchymal tumors: an ultrastructural study (abstract). Journal of Neuropathology and Experimental Neurology 49: 342

Minehan K, Scheithauer B, Shaw E, Onofrio B 1993 Astrocytic tumors of the spinal cord (abstract). Journal of Neuropathology and Experimental Neurology 52: 289

Mishima K, Nakamura M, Nakamura H, Nakamura O, Funata N, Shitara N 1992 Leptomeningeal dissemination of cerebellar pilocytic astrocytoma. Journal of Neurosurgery 77: 788–791

Mogollon R, Penneys N, Albores-Saavedra J et al 1984 Malignant schwannoma presenting as a skin mass: Confirmation by the demonstration of myelin basic protein within tumor cells. Cancer 53: 1190–1193

Morantz R A, Feigin I, Ransohoff J III 1976 Clinical and pathological study of 24 cases of gliosarcoma. Journal of Neurosurgery 45: 398–408

Morantz R A, Kepes J J, Batnitzky S, Masterson B J 1979 Extraspinal ependymomas: report of three cases. Journal of Neurosurgery 51: 383–391

Mørk S J, Rubinstein L J 1985 Ependymoblastoma. A reappraisal of a rare embryonal tumor. Cancer 55: 1536–1542

Mørk S J, Lindegaad K-F, Halvorsen T B et al 1985 Oligodendroglioma: incidence and biological behavior in a defined population. Journal of Neurosurgery 63: 881–889

Muller W, Afra D, Schroder R 1977 Supratentorial recurrences of gliomas: morphological studies in relation to time intervals with 544 astrocytomas. Acta Neurochirurgica 37: 75–91

Nakagawa Y, Perentes E, Rubinstein L J 1986 Immunohistochemical characterization of oligodendrogliomas: an analysis of multiple markers. Acta Neuropathologica 72: 15–22

Nakamura M, Inoue H K, Ono N, Kunimine H, Tamada J 1987 Analysis of hemangiopericytic meningiomas by immunohistochemistry, electron microscopy and cell culture. Journal of Neuropathology and Experimental Neurology 46: 57–71

Nakamura N, Sekino H, Taguchi Y, Fuse T 1985 Successful total extirpation of hemangioblastoma originating in the medulla oblongata. Surgical Neurology 24: 87–94

Nakasu S, Hirano A, Shimura T, Llena J F 1987 Incidental meningiomas in autopsy study. Surgical Neurology 27: 319–322

Ng T H K, Poon W S 1990 Gliosarcoma of the posterior fossa with features of a malignant fibrous histiocytoma. Cancer 65: 1161–1166

Ng T H K, Furg C F, Ma L T 1990 The pathological spectrum of desmoplastic infantile gangliogliomas. Histopathology 16: 235–241

Nishio S, Tashima T, Takeshita I, Fukui M 1988 Intraventricular neurocytoma—clinicopathological features of six cases. Journal of Neurosurgery 68: 665–670

Nishizaki T, Orita T, Saiki M, Furutani Y, Aoki H 1988 Cell kinetics studies of human brain tumors by *in vitro* labeling using anti-BUdR monoclonal antibody. Journal of Neurosurgery 69: 371–374

Nishizaki T, Orita T, Furutani Y, Ykeyama Y, Aoki H, Sasaki K 1989 Flow-cytometric DNA analysis and immunohistochemical measurement of Ki-67 and BUdR labeling indices in human brain tumors. Journal of Neurosurgery 70: 379–384

Noble M, Ataliotis P, Barnett S C et al 1991 Development, regeneration and neoplasia of glial cells in the central nervous system. Annals New York Academy Sciences 633: 35–47

Norton W T, Cammer W 1984 Isolation and characterization of myelin. In: Morell P (ed) Myelin, 2nd edn. Plenum Press, New York, pp 147–195

Obana W G, Cogen P H, Davis R L, Edwards M S B 1991 Metastatic juvenile pilocytic astrocytoma. Journal of Neurosurgery 75: 972–975

O'Sullivan M G, Whittle I R, Gregor A, Ironside J W 1991 Increasing incidence of CNS primary lymphoma in south-east Scotland. Lancet 338: 895–896

Orita T, Kajiwara K, Nishizaki T et al 1990 Nucleolar organizer regions in meningioma. Neurosurgery 26: 43–46

Pagni C A, Canavero S, Giordana M T, Mascalchi M, Arnetoli G 1992 Spinal intramedullary subependymomas: case report and review of the literature. Neurosurgery 30: 115–117

Pascual-Castroviejo I 1990 Tumors of the meninges and roots. In: Pascual-Castroviejo I (ed) Spinal tumors in children and adolescents. Raven Press, New York, pp 101–109

Pasquier B, Kojder I, Labat F et al 1985 Le xanthoastrocytome du sujet jeune. Annale Pathologie 5: 29–43

Pasquier B, Gasnier F, Pasquier D, Keddari E, Morens A, Couderc P 1986 Papillary meningioma. Clinicopathologic study of seven cases and review of the literature. Cancer 58: 299–305

Patsouris E, Stocker U, Kallmeyer V, Keiditsch E, Mehraein P, Stavrou D 1988 Relationship between Ki-67 positive cells, growth rate and histological type of human intracranial tumors. Anticancer Research 8: 537–544

Patterson R H Jr, Campbell W G Jr, Parsons H 1961 Ependymoma of the cauda equina with multiple visceral metastases: report of a case. Journal of Neurosurgery 18: 145–150

Paulus W, Jänisch W 1990 Clinicopathologic correlations in epithelial choroid plexus neoplasms: a study of 52 cases. Acta Neuropathologica 80: 635–641

Paulus W, Bayas A, Ott G, Roggendorf W 1993 Interphase cytogenetics of glioblastoma and gliosarcoma: glial versus mesenchymal elements (abstract). Journal of Neuropathology and Experimental Neurology 52: 267

Penneys N S, Mogollon R, Kowalczyk A et al 1984 A survey of cutaneous neural lesions for the presence of myelin basic protein: An immunohistochemical study. Archives of Dermatology 120: 210–213

Perentes E, Rubinstein L J 1986 Immunohistochemical recognition of human neuro-epithelial tumors by anti-Leu 7 (HNK-1) monoclonal antibody. Acta Neuropathologica 69: 227–233

Perentes E, Rubinstein L J 1987 Recent applications of immunoperoxidase histochemistry in human neuro-oncology. Archives of Pathology and Laboratory Medicine 111: 796–812

Perentes E, Rubinstein L J, Herman M M, Donoso L A 1986 S-antigen immunoreactivity in human pineal glands and pineal parenchymal tumors. A monoclonal antibody study. Acta Neuropathologica 71: 224–227

Perentes E, Herbort C P, Rubinstein L J, Herman M M, Uffer S, Donoso L A, Collins V P 1987 Immunohistochemical characterization of human retinoblastomas in situ with multiple markers. American Journal of Ophthalmology 103: 647–658

Piatt J H Jr, Campbell G A, Oakes W J 1986 Papillary meningioma involving the oculomotor nerve in an infant: case report. Journal of Neurosurgery 64: 808–812

Pigott T J D, Punt J A G, Lowe J S et al 1990 The clinical, radiological and histopathological features of cerebral primitive neuroectodermal tumours. British Journal of Neurosurgery 4: 287–298

Pinkus G S, Kurtin P J 1985 Epithelial membrane antigen — a diagnostic discriminant in surgical pathology: immunohistochemical profile in epithelial, mesenchymal, and hematopoietic neoplasms using paraffin sections and monoclonal antibodies. Human Pathology 16: 929–940

Pollak A, Friede R L 1977 Fine structure of medulloepithelioma. Journal of Neuropathology and Experimental Neurology 36: 721–725

Poulsgard L, Schröder H D, Rønne M 1990 Cytogenetic studies of 11 meningiomas and their clinical significance. II. Anticancer Research 10: 535–538

Pulitzer D R, Martin P C, Collins P C, Ralph D R 1988 Subcutaneous sacrococcygeal ("myxopapillary") ependymal rests. American Journal of Surgical Pathology 12: 672–677

Radley M G, Di Sant'Agnese P A, Eskin T A, Wilbur D C 1989 Epithelial differentiation in meningiomas. An immunohistochemical, histochemical and ultrastructural study — with review of literature. American Journal of Clinical Pathology 92: 266–272

Raff M C, Miller R H, Noble M 1983 A glial progenitor cell that develops *in vitro* into an astrocyte or an oligodendrocyte depending on culture medium. Nature 303: 390–396

Rao C, Friedlander M E, Klein E et al 1990 Medullomyoblastoma in an adult. Cancer 65: 157–163

Rawlinson D G, Herman M M, Rubinstein L J 1973 The fine structure of a myxopapillary ependymoma of the filum terminale. Acta Neuropathologica 25: 1–13

Reeder R F, Saunders R L, Roberts D W et al 1988 Magnetic resonance imaging in the diagnosis and treatment of Lhermitte-Duclos disease (dysplastic gangliocytoma of the cerebellum). Neurosurgery 23: 240–245

Reifenberger G, Prior R, Deckert M, Wechsler W 1989 Epidermal growth factor receptor expression and growth fraction in human tumours of the nervous system. Virchows Archives [A] 414: 147–155

Reiter R J 1981 The pineal gland. Vol I — Anatomy and biochemistry. CRC Press, New York, pp 121–154

Reznik M, Schoenen J 1983 Lhermitte-Duclos disease. Acta Neuropathologica 59: 88–94

Robey S S, deMent S H, Eaton K K, Aoun H 1987 Malignant epithelioid peripheral nerve sheath tumor arising in a benign schwannoma. Surgical Neurology 28: 441–446

Rubinstein L J 1972 Tumors of the central nervous system. Atlas of tumor pathology (fascicle 6). Armed Forces Institute of Pathology, Washington, DC

Rubinstein L J 1988 Diagnostic markers in human neurooncology. Annals of the New York Academy of Sciences 540: 78–90

Rubinstein L J, Brucher J M 1981 Ependymal differentiation in choroid plexus papillomas. Acta Neuropathologica 53: 29–33

Rubinstein L J, Logan W J 1970 Extraneural metastases in ependymoma of the cauda equina. Journal of Neurology, Neurosurgery and Psychiatry 33: 763–770

Rushing E J, Mena H, Ribas J L 1991 Primary pineal parenchymal lesions: a review of 53 cases (abstract). Journal of Neuropathology and Experimental Neurology 50: 364

Russell D S, Rubinstein L J 1989 Pathology of tumours of the nervous system, 5th edn. Edward Arnold, London

Rutka J T, Smith S L 1993 Transfection of human astrocytoma cells with glial fibrillary acidic protein complementary DNA: analysis of expression, proliferation and tumorigenicity. Cancer Research 53: 3624–3631

Salazar O M, Castro-Vita H, VanHoutte P et al 1983 Improved survival in cases of intracranial ependymoma after radiation therapy: late report and recommendations. Journal of Neurosurgery 59: 652–659

Sanford R A, Smith R A 1986 Hemangioblastoma of the cervicomedullary junction: report of three cases. Journal of Neurosurgery 64: 317–321

Sato S, Baba H, Tanaka M et al 1983 Antigenic determinant shared between myelin-associated glycoprotein from human brain and natural killer cells. Biomedical Research 4: 489–494

Sawhney N, Hall P A 1992 Ki-67 — structure, function and new antibodies. Editorial. Journal of Pathology 168: 161–162

Scheithauer B W 1978 Symptomatic subependymoma: report of 21 cases with review of the literature. Journal of Neurosurgery 49: 689–696

Scheithauer B W 1985 Neuropathology of pineal region tumors. Clinical Neurosurgery 32: 351–383

Scheithauer B W 1990 Tumors of the meninges: proposed modifications of the World Health Organization classification. Acta Neuropathologica 80: 343–354

Scheithauer B W, Casadei G P, Manfrini M, Wood M B 1993 Cellular schwannoma: a clinicopathologic study of 56 cases (abstract). Journal of Neuropathology and Experimental Neurology 52: 329

Scherer H J 1940 Cerebral astrocytomas and their derivatives. American Journal of Cancer 40: 159–198

Schiffer D, Giordana M T, Mauro A et al 1986 Immunohistochemical demonstration of vimentin in human cerebral tumors. Acta Neuropathologica 70: 209–219

Schiffer D, Chiò A, Giordana M T et al 1991 Histologic prognostic factors in ependymoma. Child's Nervous System 7: 177–182

Schiffer D, Chiò A, Giordana M T et al 1993 Proliferating cell nuclear antigen expression in brain tumors and its prognostic role in ependymomas: an immunohistochemical study. Acta Neuropathologica 85: 495–502

Schild S E, Scheithauer B W, Schomberg P J et al 1993 Pineal parenchymal tumors. Clinical, pathological and therapeutic aspects. Cancer 72: 870–880

Schindler E, Gullotta F 1983 Glial fibrillary acidic protein in medulloblastomas and other embryonic CNS tumours of children. Virchows Archives [A] 398: 263–275

Schlüter C, Duchrow M, Wohlenberg C, Becker M H G, Key G, Flad H-D, Gerdes J 1993 The cell proliferation-associated antigen of antibody Ki-67: a very large, ubiquitous nuclear protein with numerous repeated elements, representing a new kind of cell cycle-maintaining protein. Journal Cell Biology 123: 513–522

Schmidek H H 1993 Some current concepts regarding medulloblastomas. In: Levine A J, Schmidek H H (eds) Molecular genetics of nervous system tumors. Wiley-Liss, New York, pp 283–286

Schnitt S J, Vogel H 1986 Meningiomas: Diagnostic value of immunoperoxidase staining for epithelial membrane antigen. American Journal of Surgical Pathology 10: 640–649

Schröder R, Bien K, Kott R, Meyers I, Vossing R 1991 The relationship between Ki-67 labeling index and mitotic index in gliomas and meningiomas: Demonstration of the variability of the intermitotic cycle time. Acta Neuropathologica 82: 389–394

Schröder R, Ploner C, Ernestus R I 1993 The growth potential of ependymomas with varying grades of malignancy measured by the Ki-67 labelling index and mitotic index. Neurosurgery Review 16: 145–150

Schwartz A N, Ghatak N R 1990 Malignant transformation of benign cerebellar astrocytoma. Cancer 56: 333–336

Shepherd C W, Scheithauer B W, Gomez M R et al 1991 Subependymal giant cell astrocytoma: a clinical, pathological, and flow cytometric study. Neurosurgery 28: 864–868

Shiruba R A, Gessaga E C, Eng L F et al 1988 Lhermitte-Duclos disease: An immunohistochemical study of the cerebellar cortex. Acta Neuropathologica 75: 474–480

Sidranski D, Mikkelsen T, Schwechheimer K, Rosenblum M L, Cavanee W, Vogelstein B 1992 Clonal expansion of p53 mutant cells is associated with brain tumour progression. Nature 355: 846–847

Slooff J L, Kernohan J W, MacCarty C S 1964 Primary intramedullary tumors of the spinal cord and filum terminale. WB Saunders, Philadelphia

Smidt M, Kirsch I, Ratner L 1990 Deletion of Alu sequences in the fifth c-sis intron in individuals with meningiomas. Journal of Clinical Investigation 86: 1151–1157

Smith M T, Ludwig C L, Godfrey A D, Armbrustmacher V W 1983 Grading of oligodendrogliomas. Cancer 52: 2107–2114

Sobel R A, Trice J E, Nielsen S L, Ellis W G 1981 Pineoblastoma with ganglionic and glial differentiation: report of two cases. Acta Neuropathologica 55: 243–246

Sonneland P R L, Scheithauer B W, Onofrio B M 1985 Myxopapillary ependymoma: a clinicopathologic and immunocytochemical study of 77 cases. Cancer 56: 883–893

Sonneland P R L, Scheithauer B W, LeChago J, Crawford B G, Onofrio B M 1986 Paraganglioma of the cauda equina region. Clinicopathologic study of 31 cases with special reference to immunocytology and ultrastructure. Cancer 58: 1720–1735

Söwlemezogou F, Kleihues P, Scheithauer B W 1994 Atypical central neurocytoma. Brain Pathology (in press)

Specht C S, Smith T W, DeGirolami U, Price J M 1986 Myxopapillary ependymoma of the filum terminale: a light and electron microscopic study. Cancer 58: 310–317

Stanton C, Perentes E, Collins V P, Rubinstein L J 1987 GFA protein reactivity in nerve sheath tumors: a polyvalent and monoclonal antibody study. Journal of Neuropathology and Experimental Neurology 46: 634–643

Stefanko S Z, Manschot W A 1979 Pinealoblastoma with retinomatous differentiation. Brain 102: 321–332

Stefanko S Z, Vuzevski V D, Maas A I R et al 1986 Intracerebral malignant schwannoma. Acta Neuropathologica 71: 321–325

Strom E H, Skullerud K 1983 Pleomorphic xanthoastrocytoma: report of 5 cases. Clinical Neuropathology 2: 188–191

Sutton L N, Packer R J, Rorke L B et al 1983 Cerebral gangliogliomas during childhood. Neurosurgery 13: 124–128

Takahashi H, Ikuta F, Tsuchida T, Tanaka R 1987 Ultrastructural alterations of neuronal cells in a brain stem ganglioglioma. Acta Neuropathologica 74: 307–312

Taratuto A L, Molina H, Monges J 1983 Choroid plexus tumors in infancy and childhood. Focal ependymal differentiation. An immunoperoxidase study. Acta Neuropathologica 59: 304–308

Taratuto A L, Monges J, Lylyk P, Leiguarda R 1984 Superficial cerebral astrocytoma attached to dura. Report of six cases in infants. Cancer 54: 2505–2512

Theaker J M, Gatter K C, Esiri M M, Fleming K A 1987 Epithelial membrane antigen and cytokeratin expression by meningiomas: an immunohistological study. Journal of Clinical Pathology 39: 435–439

Theaker J M, Gatter K C, Puddle J 1988 Epithelial membrane antigen expression by the perineurium of peripheral nerve and in peripheral nerve tumours. Histopathology 13: 171–179

Theunissen P H M H, Baerts M D-T, Blaauw G 1990 Histogenesis of intracranial haemangiopericytoma and haemangioblastoma. An immunohistochemical study. Acta Neuropathologica 80: 68–71

Thomas G A, Raffel C 1991 Loss of heterozygosity on 6q, 16q and 17p in human central nervous system primitive neuroectodermal tumors. Cancer Research 51: 639–643

Tomlinson F H, Scheithauer B W, Hayostek C H, Parisi J E, Meyer F B, Shaw E G 1992 Atypia and malignancy in pilocytic astrocytoma of the cerebellum: a clinicopathologic and flow cytometric study (abstract). Journal of Neuropathology and Experimental Pathology 51: 331

Tomlinson F H, Scheithauer B W, Meyer F B, Smithson W A, Shaw E G, Miller G M, Groover R V 1992a Medulloblastoma: I. Clinical, diagnostic, and therapeutic overview. Journal of Child Neurology 7: 142–155

Tomlinson F H, Scheithauer B W, Jenkins R B 1992b Medulloblastoma: II. A pathobiologic overview. Journal of Child Neurology 7: 240–252

Townsend J J, Seaman J P 1986 Central neurocytoma — a rare benign intraventricular tumor. Acta Neuropathologica 71: 167–170

Troost D, Jansen G H, Dingemans K P 1990 Cerebral medulloepithelioma — electron microscopy and immunohistochemistry. Acta Neuropathologica 80: 103–107

Vagner-Capodano A M, Grisoli F, Gambarelli D, Sedan R, Oellet W, De Victor B 1993 Correlation between cytogenetic and histopathological findings in 75 human meningiomas. Neurosurgery 32: 892–900

VandenBerg S R 1991 Desmoplastic infantile ganglioglioma: A clinicopathologic review of sixteen cases. Brain Tumor Pathology 8: 25–31

VandenBerg S R 1992 Current diagnostic concepts of astrocytic tumors. Journal of Neuropathology and Experimental Neurology 51: 644–657

VandenBerg S R 1993 Desmoplastic infantile ganglioglioma and desmoplastic cerebral astrocytoma of infancy. Brain Pathology 3: 275–281

VandenBerg S R, May E E, Rubinstein L J et al 1987 Desmoplastic supratentorial neuroepithelial tumors of infancy with divergent differentiation potential ("desmoplastic infantile gangliogliomas"). Report on 11 cases of a distinctive embryonal tumor with favorable prognosis. Journal of Neurosurgery 66: 58–71

Vaquero J, Ramiro J, Martínez R et al 1990 Clinicopathological experience with pineocytomas: Report of five surgically treated cases. Neurosurgery 27: 612–619

von Deimling A, Janzer R, Kleihues P, Wiestler O D 1990 Patterns of differentiation in central neurocytoma: an immunohistochemical study of eleven biopsies. Acta Neuropathologica 79: 473–479

von Deimling A, Kleihues P, Saremaslani P, Yasargil G M, Spoerri O, Südhof C, Wiestler O D 1991 Histogenesis and differentiation potential of central neurocytomas. Laboratory Investigation 64: 585–591

von Deimling A, Eibl R H, Ohgaki H et al 1992a p53 mutations are associated with 17p allelic loss in grade II and grade III astrocytoma. Cancer Research 52: 2987–2990

von Deimling A, Louis D N, von Ammon K et al 1992b Association of epidermal growth factor receptor gene amplification with loss of chromosome 10 in human glioblastoma multiforme. Journal of Neurosurgery 77: 295–301

von Deimling A, von Ammon K, Schoenfeld A, Wiestler O D, Seizinger B R, Louis D N 1993 Subsets of glioblastoma multiforme defined by molecular genetic analysis. Brain Pathology 3: 19–26

Vraa-Jensen G 1950 Papilloma of the choroid plexus with pulmonary metastases. Acta Psychiatric Neurology 25: 299–306

Wanebo J E, Malik J M, VandenBerg S R, Wanebo H J, Driesen N, Persing J A 1993 Malignant peripheral nerve sheath tumors. A clinicopathologic study of 28 cases. Cancer 71: 1247–1253

Wasson J C, Saylors R L, Zeltzer P et al 1990 Oncogene amplification in pediatric tumors. Cancer Research 50: 2987–2990

Weldon-Linne G M, Victor T A, Groothuis D R, Vick N A 1983 Pleomorphic xanthoastrocytoma: ultrastructural and immunohistochemical study of a case with a rapidly fatal outcome following surgery. Cancer 52: 2055–2063

White W, Shiu M H, Rosenblum M K, Erlandson R A, Woodruff J M 1990 Cellular schwannoma. A clinicopathological study of 57 patients and 58 tumors. Cancer 66: 1266–1275

Whittle I R, Gordon A, Misra B K et al 1989 Pleomorphic xanthoastrocytoma: report of four cases. Journal of Neurosurgery 70: 463–468

Wick M R, Swanson P E, Scheithauer B W, Manivel J C 1987 Malignant peripheral nerve sheath tumor. An immunohistochemical study of 62 cases. American Journal of Clinical Pathology 87: 425–433

Winek R R, Scheithauer B W, Wick M R 1989 Meningioma, meningeal hemangiopericytoma (angioblastic meningioma), peripheral hemangiopericytoma and acoustic schwannoma. A comparative immunohistochemical study. American Journal of Surgical Pathology 13: 251–261

Wolfson W L, Brown W J 1977 Disseminated choroid plexus papilloma: an ultrastructural study. Archives of Pathology and Laboratory Medicine 101: 366–368

Wondrusch E, Huemer M, Budka H 1991 Production of glial fibrillary acidic protein (GFAP) by neoplastic oligodendrocytes: gliofibrillary oligodendroglioma and transitional oligoastrocytoma revisited. Brain Tumor Pathology 8: 11–15

Woodruff J M, Godwin T A, Erlandson R A, Susin M, Martini N 1981 Cellular schwannoma. A variety of schwannoma sometimes mistaken for a malignant tumor. American Journal of Surgical Pathology 5: 733–744

Wren D, Wolwijk G, Noble M 1992 In vitro analysis of the origin and maintenance of O-2A^{adult} progenitor cells. Journal of Cell Biology 116: 167–176

Yachnis A T, Trojanowski J Q, Memmo M, Schlaepfer W W 1988 Expression of neurofilament proteins in the hypertrophic granule cells of Lhermitte-Duclos disease: An explanation for the mass effect and the myelination of parallel fibers in the disease state. Journal of Neuropathology and Experimental Neurology 47: 206–216

Yates A J, Becker L E, Sachs L A 1979 Brain tumors in childhood. Child's Brain 5: 31–39

Zang K D 1982 Cytological and cytogenetical studies on human meningioma. Cancer Genetics and Cytogenetics 6: 249–274

Zankle H, Zang K D 1972 Cytological and cytogenical studies on brain tumors. IV. Identification of the missing G chromosome in human meningiomas as no. 22 by fluorescence technique. Humangenetik 14: 167–169

Zorludemir S, Scheithauer B W, Hirose T, Van Houten C 1994 Clear cell meningioma: a clinicopathologic, histochemical, proliferation marker, flow cytometric, and ultrastructural study. Abstract # 818. United States and Canadian Academy of Pathology Meeting, March, San Francisco

Zülch K J 1986 Brain tumors. Their biology and pathology, 3rd edn. Springer-Verlag, Berlin

9. Brain edema, increased intracranial pressure, vascular effects, and other epiphenomena of human brain tumors

Kamal Thapar James T. Rutka Edward R. Laws Jr

INTRODUCTION

Brain tumors are a heterogeneous group, comprised of neoplasms having varied cellular origins and diverse biologic profiles. Yet despite this vast morphologic and biologic diversity, brain tumors do have a number of important features in common. Their ability to disrupt the blood-brain barrier, induce cerebral edema, increase intracranial pressure, and generate seizures are unifying features shared by virtually all brain tumors, regardless of histologic type or biologic constitution. It is these areas of common ground that are the prime focus of this chapter.

As a necessary first step in understanding these and other phenomena of brain tumors, we begin with a discussion of the blood-brain barrier and how its structural and subcellular disruption by tumoral microvasculature leads to the formation of cerebral edema. Since tumor-associated edema remains so important a source of brain tumor morbidity and mortality, we discuss its pathophysiology in detail, as well as the established and emerging therapies available for its control. Many of the clinical effects of brain tumors ultimately derive from elevations in ICP, so this important phenomenon is also reviewed. Using the Monro–Kellie doctrine to illustrate the special vulnerability and unique constraints of the intracranial environment, intracranial pressure dynamics, pressure waves, and herniation phenomena as they relate to brain tumors are all discussed.

Given their highly localized and non-metastasizing nature, there is a natural tendency to overlook some of the systemic effects of brain tumors, specifically those relating to the immune and hematologic systems. Alterations of the former are of some conceptual relevance in understanding the true nature of brain tumors, particularly malignant gliomas. Alterations in the latter are of very real practical concern, given the high prevalence of thromboembolic complications in brain tumor patients. Thus, current knowledge of both these phenomena is briefly reviewed.

THE BLOOD-BRAIN BARRIER

Central to the understanding of many pathophysiologic phenomena accompanying brain tumors is a basic appreciation of the blood-brain barrier. This dynamic regulatory interface, separating brain from body, has been the subject of much speculation and debate for more than a century. The 'barrier' concept stemmed from the observation that vital dyes, when injected intravenously, permeated all body tissues except the brain (Ehrlich 1885). When delivered directly into the CSF, however, these same dyes would readily enter brain parenchyma, but would be restricted therein, being excluded from the vascular compartment and, thus, the rest of the body (Goldman 1913). These experiments established that permeability barriers existed between the blood and the brain as well as between the blood and the CSF, but that no permeability barrier separated brain and CSF. Subsequent ultrastructural studies conclusively established the brain endothelial cell as the anatomic site of the blood-brain barrier (Reese & Karnovsky 1967). Since that time, the blood-brain barrier has been an area of active study. Many of the early and recent developments in the field have been summarized in a number of recent reviews (Bradbury 1985, Cornfield 1985, Goldstein & Betz 1986, Neuwelt 1989a,b, Johansson 1990, Salcman & Broadwell 1991, Fishman 1992).

Despite the occasional tendency to think of it as such, the blood-brain barrier is not a brick wall. Instead it is a complex regulatory interface which is part structural, part biochemical, part enzymatic, part pharmacologic, part electrical, and part immunologic. Given this multifaceted functional configuration, the blood-brain barrier is capable of selectively expediting the passage of certain substances, while absolutely denying access to others. The most essential anatomic substrate of the blood-brain barrier, one which accounts for this selective permeability, is the capillary endothelial cell. These endothelial cells have several anatomic properties which readily distinguish them from

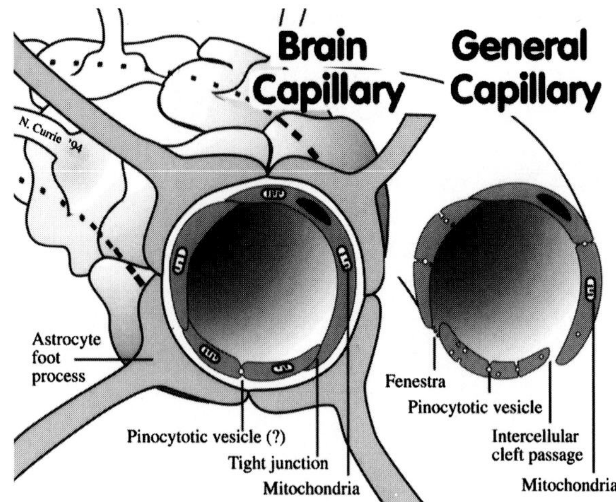

Fig. 9.1 Morphologic differences between endothelia of brain capillaries and systemic capillaries. Note the absence of fenestrae and intercellular clefts in cerebral capillaries, as well as a paucity of pinocytotic vesicles. Reflecting their reliance on energy-dependent transport, mitochondria are abundant in cerebral endothelia. Tumor capillaries assume many of the morphologic features present in systemic capillaries (see text).

general systemic capillaries (Fig. 9.1). Firstly, unlike endothelial cells of extracerebral capillaries, these are nonfenestrated. They also lack intracellular clefts, such that they are closed circumferentially by belts of *tight junctions*. These tight junctions have high electrical impedance and low permeability to polar solutes, thus providing an electrochemical barrier as well as an anatomic one. A third feature is an absolute paucity of pinocytotic vesicles, a transport vehicle found in great abundance within extracerebral endothelial cells. The near absence of such vesicles in cerebral capillaries likely accounts for the relative exclusion of plasma proteins from the CSF. The fourth feature is a marked abundance of mitochondria in cerebral endothelial cells; they have 3–5 times the mitochondrial content of systemic endothelial cells. Such high mitochondrial density presumably reflects the high energy demands of cerebral endothelial cells in order to maintain energy-dependent transport mechanisms. The final, and perhaps most curious feature of cerebral endothelia is their circumferential enclosure by astrocytic foot processes. Although anatomically dramatic, such astrocytic encasement of capillaries is not regarded as a physical component of the blood-brain barrier. Aside from possible contributions to the structural integrity of cerebral capillaries, the function of astrocytic foot processes remains speculative.

The passage of substances through the blood-brain barrier is accomplished by a variety of transport systems, including passive and facilitative diffusion, multiple different types of carrier-mediated transport, various poorly characterized forms of transendothelial passage, and possibly even vesicular transport, although this latter route remains both enigmatic and controversial (Broadwell 1993).

The pharmacologic characteristics of the solute to be transported are of foremost importance in determining blood-brain barrier permeability. As a rule, one of the most decisive factors is lipid solubility; the more lipid soluble a compound is, the more readily it traverses the blood-brain barrier. Additional factors favoring the transport of substances across the blood-brain barrier include low molecular weight, lack of a protein-bound state, and a nonpolar or noninonized state at physiologic pH (reviewed in Pardridge 1988).

A second component of the blood-brain barrier separates blood from CSF, and has therefore been termed the blood-CSF barrier. Located in the choroid plexus, the blood-CSF barrier is functionally similar to the blood-brain barrier, however there are a few important differences. Firstly, the anatomic site of the barrier is the *epithelial* cell of the choroid plexus, not the capillary endothelial cell of the choroid plexus. Here, tight junctions are present between epithelial cells. Choroid plexus capillary endothelial cells, like 'leaky' extracerebral endothelia, possess a full complement of fenestrations, intracellular clefts, and pinocytotic vesicles. In general, the permeability properties of the choroid epithelial cells are similar to those of brain capillary endothelium. A detailed physiologic discussion of the blood-CSF barrier has been provided by Fishman (1992).

Although the blood-brain barrier spans the entire length of the CNS in a virtually uninterrupted fashion, its absence has been conspicuously noted in several areas. The neurohypophysis, median eminence, subforniceal organ, pineal gland, and area postrema are all devoid of a blood-brain barrier.

Brain tumors and the blood-brain barrier

Given their locally destructive nature, their induction of exuberant neoangiogenesis, and their rapid uptake of radiographic contrast agents, brain tumors tend to conjure the impression that they are also a source of local blood-brain barrier 'loss'. Perhaps to the disappointment of the chemotherapist, the blood-brain barrier, even in the face of seemingly dramatic local perturbation, does retain some semblance of functionality. Thus, in the setting of brain tumors, it is customary to speak of blood-brain barrier breakdown, rather than its absolute loss per se.

First demonstrated by brain scintiscanning, and now routinely with contrast-enhanced CT and MR imaging, local disruption of the blood-brain barrier is acknowledged as a common accompaniment to brain tumors. Important insights into the nature of this permeability defect were provided by several investigators who studied the capillary ultrastructure of human brain tumors, primarily malignant gliomas (Luse 1960, Nystrom 1960, Long

1970). The earlier reports demonstrated that brain tumor capillaries suffered from a variety of ultrastructural abnormalities, and that tumor capillaries became progressively atypical with increasing malignancy. It was the comprehensive ultrastructural study of Long (1970), however, which provided the most convincing morphologic evidence that alterations in capillary endothelium are the underlying cause of barrier disruption in tumors. In his analysis of 19 malignant brain tumors, of which 13 were malignant gliomas, he reported on the striking presence of open intercellular 'tight' junctions which provided free communication between the vessel lumen, basement membrane, and the extracellular space. Wide gap junctions, increased numbers of endothelial vesicles, endothelial proliferation, atypical endothelial cell shapes, defects in capillary basement membranes, and abnormalities of the glial investiture were also noted. In a subsequent study of capillary ultrastructure among meningiomas and schwannomas, the loss of tight junctions and the presence of gap junctions, capillary fenestrations, and increased pinocytotic vesicles were noted (Long 1973). Similar observations were also made in brain metastases, with the additional feature that tumor capillaries retained the morphologic features of capillaries in the tissue of origin (Long 1979).

On the basis of the foregoing observations, it is now generally accepted that opening of 'tight' junctions, and the presence of capillary fenestrations, gap junctions, and increased pinocytotic vesicles are the basis for barrier permeability in brain tumors (Grieg 1989). Of these, it has been suggested that opening of 'tight' junctions is mechanistically the most important (Bar-Sella et al 1979). Not surprisingly, opening of tight junctions is also one of the more important underlying objectives in the therapeutic manipulation of blood-brain barrier permeability. All these permeability mechanisms are important, however, particularly in the formation of tumor-associated edema, wherein each serves as an anatomic conduit for extravasation of fluid.

An important question is whether or not disruption of the blood-brain barrier is confined to the pathologic margins of the tumor, or whether it extends beyond into peritumoral brain. This has obvious implications for the development of peritumoral edema. In two of the aforementioned studies by Long, in which peritumoral brain was specifically analyzed, there was no morphologic evidence that peritumoral capillaries suffered from increased permeability (Long 1970, 1979). Although the issue is not definitively settled, one ultrastructural study of peritumoral capillaries in 'normal' brain has documented various structural abnormalities that would be consistent with a permeability breach (Stewart et al 1987). The authors suggested that structural abnormalities in peritumoral capillaries may be the consequence of unidentified 'inducing factors' liberated by the tumor.

BRAIN EDEMA

Brain edema is one of the most important factors contributing to the morbidity and mortality associated with brain tumors. In addition to being a common accompaniment to many brain tumors, brain edema may significantly complicate the recovery of patients in the postoperative period. The potentially lethal aspect of tumor-associated edema is especially well illustrated by the precipitous and almost ten-fold decline in brain tumor operative mortality rates which coincided with the introduction of steroid therapy in the early 1960s (Jelsma & Bucy 1967). Still, tumor-associated edema remains a common and ongoing problem for many patients with brain tumors, and its nature and pathophysiology must be thoroughly understood by all physicians caring for such patients.

Brain edema: definition and classification

Despite the confusion which stems from the use of imprecise terms as 'brain swelling', 'brain congestion', 'brain engorgement' and others in referring to the phenomenon of brain edema, the latter is, in fact, a precisely defined entity. Strictly defined, brain edema is an increase in brain volume resulting from an increase in water and sodium content. With this fundamental biochemical definition in mind, several distinct forms of brain edema have been recognized. Much like the clinical condition of pitting edema of the ankles, brain edema may be the end result of multiple and very different pathophysiological mechanisms. Much of our current understanding of the various forms of brain edema can be attributed to the landmark studies of Igor Klatzo, conducted almost three decades ago. On the basis of both experimental and neuropathological observations, he distinguished brain edema as being either *vasogenic* or *cytotoxic* in nature, a classification which continues to be widely quoted and accepted (Klatzo 1967). To these, a third category of *hydrocephalic or interstitial* edema has since been added (Fishman 1975). Each type of edema arises from different mechanisms and becomes manifest in different clinical settings. In the case of vasogenic edema, of which tumor-associated edema is the prototypal example, increased capillary permeability is the responsible factor. In cytotoxic edema, now more appropriately termed cellular edema, the primary target is the intracellular metabolic machinery (e.g. ATP-dependent sodium pumps) and/or metabolic substrates. In the interstitial form of edema, neither vascular permeability nor cellular metabolism is perturbed; instead, it is the generation of a transependymal pressure gradient forcing CSF from the ventricular to the extracellular space which underlies edema formation. From the standpoint of tumor-associated edema, vasogenic edema is the dominant form, although in certain clinical situations it may be secondarily complicated by elements of cellular or interstitial edema.

Vasogenic edema

Vasogenic brain edema is the most frequent form of brain edema, commonly encountered in proximity to brain tumors, inflammatory lesions (abscesses, encephalitis), infarcts, intracerebral hemorrhages, and contusions (see Fig. 9.4, p. 171). Although these lesions are pathologically diverse, the feature shared by all is local disruption of the blood-brain barrier. As originally proposed by Klatzo, subsequently validated by ultrastructural and tracer experiments, and most recently re-affirmed by contrast-enhanced CT and MR imaging, focal disruption of the blood-brain barrier is an absolute prerequisite to the development of vasogenic edema. The increased capillary permeability afforded by such disruption leads to the extravasation of a protein-rich filtrate of plasma; its accumulation and permeation within the extracellular space of the brain constitutes vasogenic edema. Thus the development of vasogenic edema requires three elements:

(i) increased capillary permeability;
(ii) a pressure gradient from vascular to extracellular compartments; and
(iii) retention of fluid in the extracellular space.

Increased capillary permeability

One of the earliest misconceptions regarding tumor-associated edema was the notion that edema fluid was a secretory product of the tumor, actively exuded by tumor tissue and eventually percolating into adjacent brain. Prompted by his astute observation that cystic meningiomas were accompanied by a disproportionately large amount of edema relative to their size, Cushing incorrectly implied that the secretory mechanisms responsible for cyst fluid accumulation may be the same as those responsible for peritumoral edema. That edema fluid actually originated from plasma, and was not a secretory by-product of tumor tissue per se, was demonstrated by a series of elegant experiments using the cold injury model of vasogenic edema, a model which most closely simulates the edema surrounding a discrete cerebral metastasis. The chemical composition of edema fluid surrounding the cold injury was shown to be a filtrate of plasma, replete with albumin and other plasma proteins of various types (Gazendam et al 1979). Moreover, using the same model, Arabi & Long (1979) conclusively demonstrated the importance of a damaged, but functional vascular bed in the production and propagation of vasogenic edema. They observed that edema emanating from a cortical freezing lesion could be prevented or abruptly terminated by complete microexcision of the cold lesion. Moreover, even if the excised injured brain was immediately reinserted into brain, no recurrence of edema was evident. These experiments established the pivotal role of the damaged vascular bed in generating vasogenic edema. The continuous delivery of plasma and associated proteins to a damaged vascular bed is, therefore, an essential requirement to edema formation.

Given the all-important role of blood-brain barrier disruption in the genesis of vasogenic edema, the latter has been aptly termed 'open-barrier edema'. How the blood-brain barrier becomes disrupted remains an area of ongoing study, although several mechanisms have been elucidated. Ultrastructural studies have documented the presence of defects in endothelial tight junctions, increased numbers of pinocytotic vesicles, increased vesicular transport, and an increase in nonpinocytotic transendothelial flow in various underlying conditions associated with vasogenic edema (reviewed by Fishman 1992) (Fig. 9.2). In the case of brain tumors, anatomic evidence of barrier disruption is more clear cut. As mentioned previously, brain tumor capillaries contain defective tight junctions, fenestrations, and, less consistently, increased numbers of pinocytotic vesicles, all providing adequate conduits for extravasation of fluid and protein macromolecules. Furthermore, defects in capillary permeability are not merely confined within the gross margins of the tumor, but extend some distance into peritumoral brain tissue (Stewart et al 1987). As mentioned, the ultrastructural documentation of defective tight junctions and increased vesicular transport in peritumoral capillaries reflects a potential inductive effect of tumor cells or their secretory products on the permeability of adjacent microvasculature. This may explain the extension/presence of edema at subcortical sites distant from the actual tumor, as commonly occurs in metastases, for example.

It has been suggested that structural defects of the

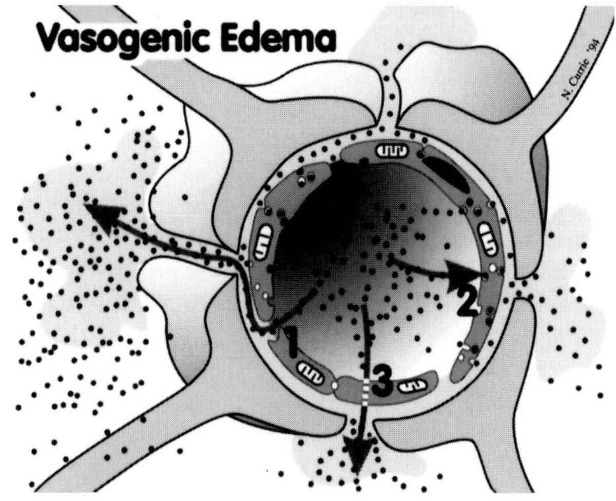

Fig. 9.2 Alterations in the capillary permeability which underlies vasogenic edema are of three principal types: **1**, opening of 'tight' junctions; **2**, an increase in pinocytotic transport, particularly of plasma proteins; and **3**, an increase in nonpinocytotic transendothelial passage by simple diffusion, carrier-mediated transport, and possibly other poorly characterized mechanisms. Note the accumulation and retention of fluid within the extracellular space; swelling of astroglial or neuronal elements is not a feature of this type of edema.

blood-brain barrier alone, though clearly a critical component of tumor-associated edema, are only part of the overall process contributing to increased capillary permeability and vasogenic edema (Pappius 1989). Moreover, the prompt therapeutic effectiveness of steroids in ameliorating tumor-associated edema argues cogently for the presence of additional nonstructural permeability mechanisms underlying the development of vasogenic edema. That being the case, there has been increasing interest in characterizing certain chemical mediators which may accentuate capillary permeability and thus contribute to vasogenic edema. The list of candidate permeability factors is now extensive, including members of the kallikrein-kininogen-kinin system, biogenic amines, arachidonic acid, prostaglandins, leukotrienes, eicosanoids, platelet-activating factor, free radicals, and the glioma-derived vascular permeability factor (VPF). VPF (also known as vascular endothelial growth factor) is a recently described 36–46 kD dimeric glycoprotein secreted by human gliomas which is about 1000 times more potent than histamine in inducing capillary permeability, and may play a significant role in enhancing edema formation (Connolly 1991, Goldman et al 1993).

Recently, prompted by the correlation which appears to exist between the degree of peritumoral macrophage infiltration and the amount of peritumoral edema, attention has also been directed toward a possible role for various macrophage secretory products. These secretory products, comprising some of the chemical mediators mentioned above, further include various inflammatory enzymes such as myeloperoxidase, acid hydrolases, alkaline phosphatase, and lysozyme. Multiple roles have been proposed for these biologic, chemical, and enzymatic mediators, including a direct permeability effect on endothelial cells, alteration of morphologic and permeability characteristics of peritumoral microvaculature, and induction of vesicular transport. At the present time, however, the list of candidate permeability factors significantly outnumbers the established facts pertaining to their precise mechanisms of permeability enhancement. Thus, a discussion of these factors is beyond the scope of this chapter; the reader is referred to a number of reviews on the subject (Baethmann et al 1988, Joo & Klatzo 1989, Del Maestro et al 1990, Wahl et al 1990, Joo 1993).

Deserving of special mention, however, are those biologic mediators related to the arachidonic acid cascade. Although their role as permeability enhancers in vasogenic edema is still far from settled, these mediators have a particular theoretical appeal, engendered by the hope that pharmacologic blockade of the arachidonic acid cascade harbors therapeutic potential as a form of anti-edema therapy. Alternatively, therapeutic exploitation of their permeability characteristics also holds promise as a means of selective blood-tumor barrier disruption for the effective delivery of antineoplastic agents. Since lipids comprise a significant proportion of brain tissue, particularly of white matter, a reasonable expectation is that these mediators are involved in pathologic processes occurring therein, including cerebral edema. In fact, the concentration of free fatty acids has been shown to be increased in peritumoral edema, presumably by way of membrane breakdown (Baethman et al 1980). Arachidonic acid, the most significant of these fatty acids, is a major membrane component of cells and subcellular organelles in both normal and neoplastic brain tissue. During a variety of metabolic and pathologic events, arachidonic acid may be liberated from its phospholipid-bound state, under the actions of phospholipase A_2 (an enzyme also known to be inhibited by corticosteroids) and phospholipase C. Once released, free arachidonic acid has been shown dramatically and nonspecifically to increase brain capillary permeability, a phenomenon well documented in a rat brain model (Chan & Fishman 1984). Aside from these direct effects on capillary permeability, the role of arachidonic acid as a mediator of tumor-associated edema is further substantiated by the effects of arachidonic acid metabolites, many of which are even more robust permeability enhancers than is arachidonic acid itself. Oxidative metabolism of arachidonic acid produces prostaglandins and leukotrienes via the cyclo-oxygenase and lipoxygenase pathways, respectively. In addition, the action of these and other metabolic pathways on arachidonic acid leads to the formation of free superoxide and hydroxyl radicals, as well as lipid peroxides. From the standpoint of cerebral edema, free radicals and leukotrienes appear to be of most importance. Free radicals, given their capacity to uncouple oxidative phosphorylation and interfere with cellular energy metabolism, are probably far more relevant mediators in the setting of cytotoxic edema. Their role in vasogenic edema is a secondary one, deriving primarily from their activation of phospholipases which, in turn, increase the amount of available free arachidonic acid. This forms a self-perpetuating cycle which not only potentiates the permeability effects of arachidonic acid, but also provides substrate for the formation of leukotrienes, the arachidonic acid derivative receiving greatest attention in the context of peritumoral edema (Fishman 1992).

The subject of numerous recent reports, leukotrienes have generated considerable interest as potential mediators of vasogenic edema. The presence of one particular leukotriene species, leukotriene C4, has been demonstrated in human brain tumors and surrounding peritumoral tissue (Black et al 1986). More importantly, the concentration of leukotriene C4 was positively and significantly correlated with the amount of peritumoral edema. In this study, meningiomas had the lowest amount of peritumoral edema and also the lowest leukotriene C4 content, intermediate amounts of edema and leukotriene C4 were present in gliomas, and the highest levels of both were present in metastatic tumors. This clear correlation between tissue leukotriene C4 content and the amount of peritumoral edema implicates the permeability effects of the former in underlying the development of the latter. Whereas leukotrienes are generally well known for their potent permeability enhancement of systemic capillaries, a similar effect on brain capillaries is normally quenched by the presence of degrading enzymes inherent in the blood-brain barrier. γ-glutamyl transpeptidase, the most important of these inactivating enzymes, has been found to be deficient in the capillaries of various experimental brain tumors (Black et al 1990). If corroborated in human tumors, this finding would explain the apparent accumulation of leukotriene C4 therein, and further substantiate its role in the development of peritumoral edema.

Given the selective permeability effects ascribed to leukotriene C4 on neoplastic brain capillaries, an emerging area of related interest concerns the therapeutic use of this agent in selectively opening the blood-tumor barrier for the delivery of antineoplastic agents. To date, the reports have been conflicting. Chio and colleagues, superfusing rats bearing experimental glial (RG-2) tumors with various leukotrienes, documented a selective 3.5-fold increase in blood-tumor permeability, but no change in the permeability of normal brain (Chio et al 1992). Others, using a cold-injury model of vasogenic edema, could not demonstrate any permeability effect of leukotrienes (Unterberg et al 1991).

Pressure gradients from vascular to extracellular compartments

Once capillary permeability has been breached, the development of peritumoral edema requires the presence of a pressure gradient forcing fluids and proteins from the vascular compartment to the extracellular space. Such a gradient is both hydrostatic and osmotic in nature, and its strength, together with the surface area of barrier breakdown, are the basic physical determinants governing the rate of edema formation. Aside from its physiologic relevance, recognition of this gradient is important only insofar as there are conditions known to affect it adversely, thus aggravating the rate of edema formation. Arterial hypertension and hyponatremia are two such *treatable* examples, both of which are commonly seen in brain tumor patients, particularly in the postoperative period. Severe hyponatremia may also be a source of cellular edema (discussed below).

Retention of fluid within the extracellular compartment

Having accessed the extracellular space, edema fluid is propelled by bulk flow, often great distances beyond the actual pathologic margins of the tumor. The distribution of tumor-associated edema within the hemisphere is characteristic, tending to occur almost exclusively within white matter. Such dramatic differences in affinity for white over gray matter have been ascribed to differences in tissue architecture. The morphology of white matter consists of parallel bundles of fibers with a surrounding loose extracellular space, an arrangement readily accepting of extravasated fluid. Gray matter, in addition to having a much higher cell density, is enmeshed by an interwoven network of connecting fibers which offers high resistance to the front of edema fluid, thus redirecting it below to the more compliant white matter. In vasogenic edema, the extravasated fluid is, by definition, wholly restricted to the extracellular space.

While there is a tendency to view vasogenic edema as the product of unidirectional flow, it is in fact a far more dynamic process, wherein fluid formation and fluid resorption occur simultaneously. One estimate suggests that the rate of fluid formation around a malignant brain tumor is in the order of 14–78 ml per day (Reulen et al 1990). To accommodate this excess volume, several mechanisms of edema fluid absorption have been proposed. Transependymal retrograde flow into the ventricle is likely to be an important mechanism, being reputed to clear as much as 90 ml/day. A second mechanism relates to uptake and phagocytosis of protein and other macromolecules by astrocytes, resulting in an erosion of the osmotic gradient in the extracellular space. Removal of fluid along the perivascular spaces with reabsorption of fluid into brain capillaries has also been proposed (Reulen et al 1990).

The special case of meningiomas and peritumoral edema

From the standpoint of peritumoral edema, meningiomas are unique lesions. Despite their typically benign constitution, their overall slow growth rate, their extracerebral location, and the impermeable leptomeningeal barrier which separates them from brain parenchyma, at least half of all meningiomas are still capable of inducing peritumoral edema (Smith et al 1981, Gilbert et al 1983). How this occurs remains very much an enigma, although several hypotheses have been proposed. One possibility is that meningiomas induce edema in a fashion similar to intrinsic brain tumors, by the same permeability mechanisms discussed above. Although meningiomas have been shown to possess alterations in capillary structure similar to those found in glial tumors, this alone should not produce peritumoral edema unless the tumor physically penetrates brain substance. This is, of course, an uncommon occurrence, but one in which there is a direct correlation with the amount of peritumoral edema (Go et al 1988). For most meningiomas, however, the intervening leptomeningeal barrier renders them anatomically isolated from the cortex; the arachnoid is impermeable to fluids and the pia mater is largely impermeable to protein macromolecules. Moreover, were abnormally permeable capillaries the source of extravasated fluid and the leptomeninges impermeable, one would expect an extracerebral accumulation of edema fluid, but this does not occur. Thus, if 'leaky' tumor vessels are indeed the source of meningioma-associated edema, one must necessarily assume a functional breach of the leptomeningeal barrier. Failure to make this assumption not only violates this theory, but also seriously undermines the plausibility of alternate theories discussed below.

A second hypothesis is that edema is produced in response to the tumor's mass effect. Whereas some studies have shown a trend of increasing edema with increased tumor size and surface area (Gilbert et al 1983), others have not (Smith et al 1981). In clinical practice, one is often impressed by the unpredictable relationship between tumor size and peritumoral edema; large meningiomas may be unassociated with edema whereas small meningiomas may generate massive, holo-hemispheric edema. It is generally accepted that rate of meningioma growth is probably a more reliable predictor of peritumoral edema than absolute tumor size per se. The same argument has been used to explain the disproportionately large amount of edema which typically accompanies metastatic tumors. Mitotic activity, increased cellularity, and necrosis are the generic measures of proliferative capacity, providing some estimate of a tumor's rate of growth. Peritumoral edema has been demonstrated in more than 90% of meningiomas exhibiting these histologic features, and was marked in approximately 70% of cases. In tumors without these features of morphologic aggressiveness, only half of all meningiomas had marked edema (Vassilouthis & Ambrose 1979). Flow cytometric analyses of meningiomas have also shown a positive correlation between the amount of peritumoral edema and the proliferative capacity of the tumor, as determined by the number of cycling cells in G_2 and S phases (Crone et al 1988).

The third commonly invoked mechanism of edema formation around meningiomas relates to venous occlusion. Hypothetically, occlusion of draining cortical veins or venous sinuses as the result of compression or invasion, respectively, would be a source of peritumoral edema. The resultant increase in cerebral venous pressure would result in transudation of fluid, although the fluid would *not* be the protein-rich exudate typical of classic vasogenic edema. Although this concept is mechanistically attractive, it is at odds with what is known of collateral recruitment in the setting of progressive venous occlusion. Moreover, various clinical studies addressing this issue have shown that peritumoral edema can be severe in the presence of angiographically patent sinuses and draining veins, yet it may be absent in the presence of total sinus occlusion (reviewed in Lindley et al 1991).

Finally, peritumoral edema surrounding meningiomas may be the result of various chemical and biologic mediators. Any or all of the mediators mentioned in the foregoing discussion may have a role in inducing edema with meningiomas. One recent study positively correlated levels of tumor prostaglandins with the amount of peritumoral edema in meningiomas (Constantini et al 1993).

A substantial body of clinicopathologic data now exists detailing the association of various clinical parameters with peritumoral edema in meningiomas. For example, there is some evidence to suggest that meningiomas arising at different intracranial sites induce varying degrees of peritumoral edema. Meningiomas located along the sphenoid ridge, convexity, and frontal-basal regions, as well as those situated parasagittally, appear most prone to evoke significant amounts of edema. Alternatively, suprasellar, intraventricular, and posterior fossa meningiomas are said to produce the least (Bradac et al 1986). In other studies, however, tumor location correlated little with either the presence or the amount of surrounding edema (Smith et al 1981).

The histologic subtype appears to be loosely associated with the amount of peritumoral edema. Whereas meningotheliomatous and transitional subtypes are said to induce more edema than fibroblastic and psammomatous subtypes (Bradac et al 1986), the most consistent correlation is seen with angioblastic meningiomas or those with a hemangiopericytic component. Virtually all tumors in the latter two categories are accompanied by significant edema (Smith et al 1981, Bradac et al 1986). Not surprisingly, malignant meningiomas (i.e. those tumors with histologically evident brain invasion) are associated with moderate to severe edema in 83% of cases (Gilbert et al 1983).

The relationship between tumor vascularity and peritumoral edema, despite its obvious theoretical importance, remains to be settled. In some studies, the vascularity of the tumor, as determined by histology or angiography, seems to be correlated with the amount of peritumoral edema (Smith et al 1981, Stevens et al 1983); however, this has not been a uniform finding (Gilbert et al 1983, Maiuri et al 1987).

A final consideration relates to the recent correlations between the sex steroid receptor status of meningiomas and the amount of peritumoral edema. In two reports, the presence of progesterone receptors correlated perfectly with the presence of peritumoral edema (i.e. 100% of progesterone-positive tumors had peritumoral edema, whereas none of the progesterone receptor-negative tumors had any edema) (Maiuri et al 1987, Benzel & Gelder 1988). In a third study, the progesterone receptor status was indeterminate with respect to the presence or absence of edema (Phillipon et al 1984). The relationship between estrogen receptor status and edema formation is inconclusive.

For a more detailed discussion of the link between meningioma-associated edema and clinicopathologic data, the reader is referred to a comprehensive recent review (Lindley et al 1991).

Cellular (cytotoxic) edema

Cellular edema is characterized by acute swelling of all cellular elements of the brain (endothelial cells, astroglial elements, and neurons), with a concomitant reduction in the volume of the brain's extracellular space (Fishman 1992). This form of edema is most commonly seen in the setting of acute cerebral ischemia resulting from cardiac arrest or cerebral trauma; less common causes include acute hypo-osmolality (SIADH), osmotic dysequilibrium syndromes (hemodialysis), and Reye's syndrome. By definition, vascular permeability and the blood-brain barrier remain unimpaired in cellular edema, at least initially. Instead, the primary target is the ATP-dependent sodium-potassium pumps. Their failure results in the intracellular accumulation of sodium, an event which establishes an osmotic gradient and, thus, the secondary intracellular accumulation of water. The edema fluid consists primarily of sodium and water; proteins are not present. Both gray and white matter are affected by this type of edema.

As a rule, cellular edema is not a primary component of tumor-associated edema. In certain situations, however, cellular edema may further complicate the underlying vasogenic edema associated with a brain tumor. This occurs when the mass effects of a tumor cause (i) compression of the local microcirculation or (ii) brain shifts and herniation phenomenon. In both instances, secondary vascular compromise may superimpose an element of cellular edema. Acute hyponatremia, whether the result of SIADH or inappropriate perioperative fluid management, can add an additional cellular insult to the underlying problem of vasogenic edema.

Interstitial 'hydrocephalic' edema

The last of the major forms of brain edema to be characterized, interstitial edema refers to the extracellular accumulation of fluid which occurs in the setting of hydrocephalus. The condition is best illustrated in the context of obstructive hydrocephalus, wherein obstruction

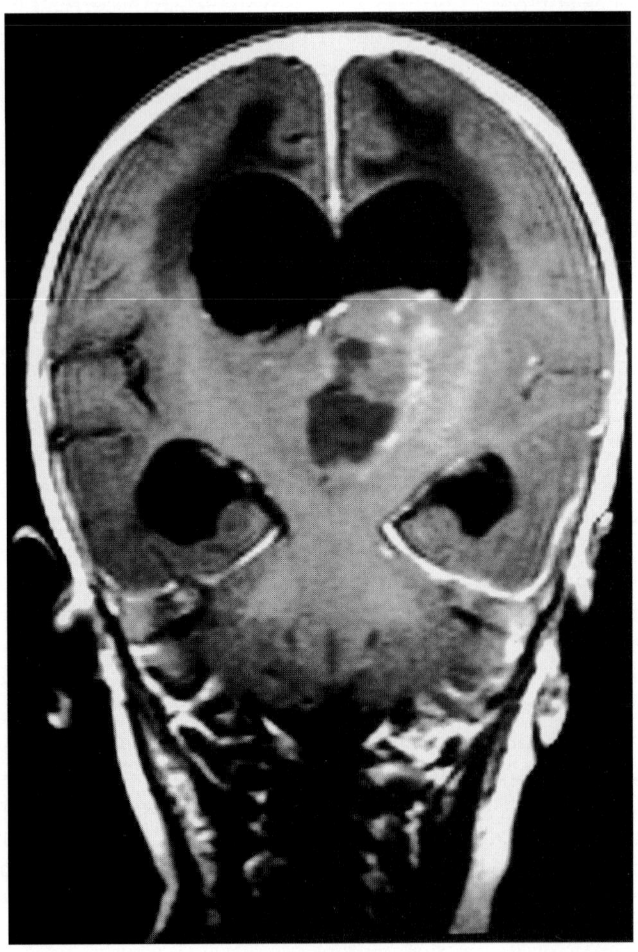

A

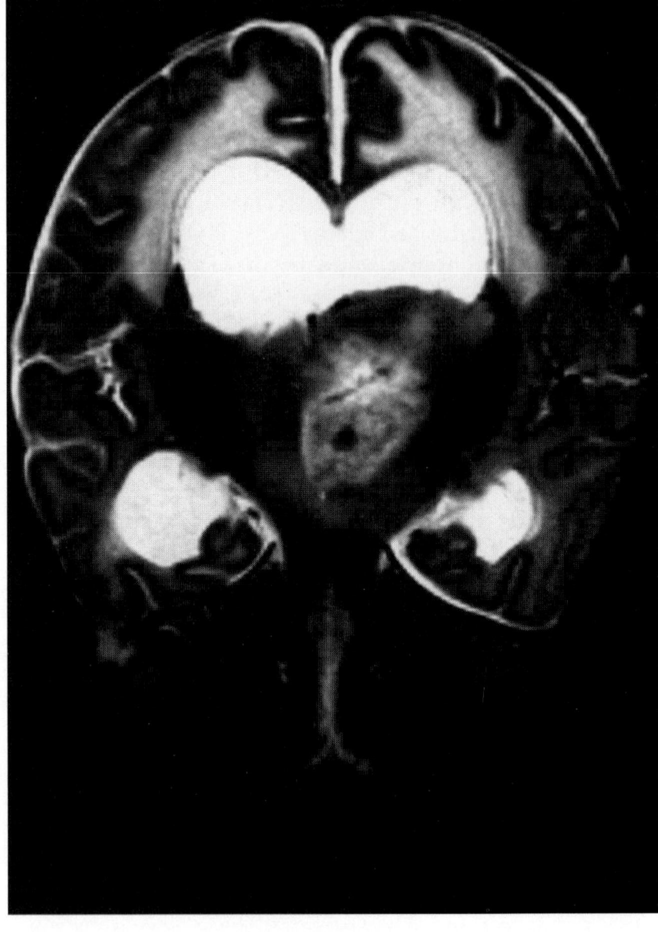

B

Fig. 9.3 Interstitial edema. Coronal MR images of a malignant astrocytoma of the thalamus in a 9-month-old male. On the T1 sequence **A**, the lesion is seen to fill the third ventricle, resulting in marked obstructive hydrocephalus. Note the decreased signal intensity of the periventricular white matter, which is indicative of interstitial edema. The full extent of the edema is best represented on the T2 sequence **B**, where the accumulation of a high signal, CSF-like fluid in the periventricular white matter is the result of transependymal flow.

to CSF flow generates a hydrostatic pressure gradient between the ventricular compartment and the brain parenchyma. What results is transependymal movement of CSF from the ventricles to the extracellular space. Fluid accumulation is most marked in the periventricular white matter, a finding readily visible on CT scanning as periventricular lucencies (Fig. 9.3). The accumulated fluid is similar in composition to CSF. The absence of blood-brain barrier disruption and the presence of normal cellular energy metabolism distinguish interstitial edema from the vasogenic and cellular types, respectively.

Interstitial edema is an occasional accompaniment to brain tumors. Obvious examples are those tumors causing obstructive hydrocephalus such as posterior fossa, pineal region, or intraventricular tumors. Communicating hydrocephalus, as the result of tumors leaking debris into the CSF, can also be the source of interstitial edema. As a rule, restitution of normal CSF flow leads to prompt resolution of interstitial edema.

Clinical aspects of tumor-associated edema

Brain edema may contribute to headache, focal neurologic signs, and depressed levels of consciousness. In some cases, particularly with malignant gliomas, it can be difficult, at least initially, to separate the relative contributions of tumor and edema to the neurologic dysfunction of the patient. That the condition of such patients often improves dramatically with steroid therapy reflects how profound a contribution edema can make.

Tumor-associated edema is readily detectable on CT and MR imaging. With the former, edema appears as an area of low attenuation, typically surrounding a tumor. It can occasionally be difficult to delineate precisely where the tumor stops and the edema begins, a problem most commonly encountered among low grade gliomas. When edema is obvious and marked, its prominence among arborizing fiber tracts of the white matter produces a characteristic pattern, often described as a 'finger-like' configuration. As a result of its high water content, edematous brain displays longer relaxation times and therefore appears bright on proton density and T2-weighted MR scans (Fig. 9.4). T2 sequences are particularly sensitive to the presence of edema and may indicate an underlying neoplasm at a very early stage (Huk et al 1990). The problem of precisely delineating tumor margins from adja-

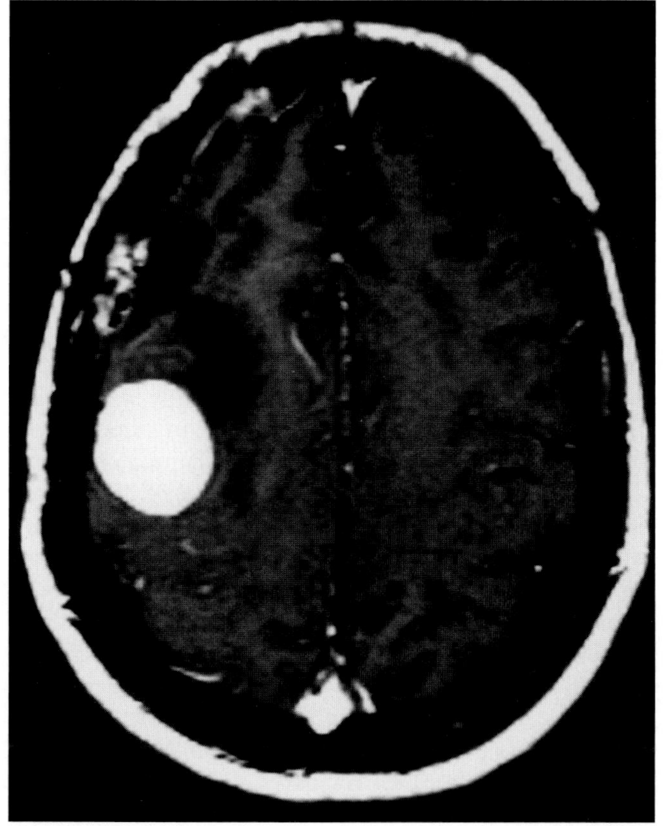

A

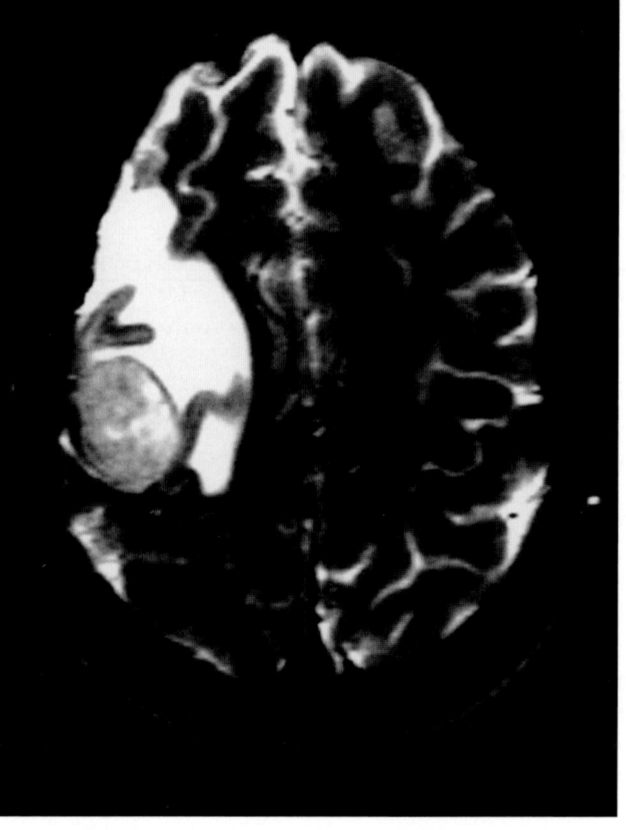

B

Fig. 9.4 Vasogenic edema. Axial MR images of a rare hemispheric astroblastoma in a 16-year-old female. In the T1 sequence **A**, only a small amount of peritumoral edema is visible, appearing as an area of decreased signal intensity. The true extent of the peritumoral edema is better represented by the T2 sequence **B**, wherein peritumoral edema appears as an area of increased signal. In this case, edema is readily distinguishable from tumor on the T2 sequence, however this is not always the case.

cent edema remains, as the area of increased signal on T2 often incorporates both tumor and edema.

The amount of preoperative tumor-associated edema often provides some indication of the potential for edema-related complications postoperatively. It has been shown that intraoperative increases in ICP are most apt to occur in brain tumor patients with large amounts of tumor-associated edema, as determined by preoperative CT scans (Bedford et al 1982). A similar correlation has not been found with other factors such as tumor size or degree of midline shift. Two recent reports clearly documented worsening of tumor-associated edema in patients undergoing operation for supratentorial gliomas. Severe postoperative edema and herniation occurred in 4 of 42 (Ciric et al 1987) and 10 of 213 (Fadul et al 1988) patients. These reports also showed clearly that severe postoperative edema is a far more common occurrence when tumors are partially resected or subjected to open biopsy than when gross 'total' resection is achieved; 12 of the 14 cases of severe edema and herniation in the above reports occurred in partially resected or biopsied tumors. Ciric and colleagues suggested that partial resection aggravates underlying tumor-associated edema by a foreign body-like effect, exerted by residual tumor and necrotic debris. In general, postoperative peritumoral edema peaks at 36–72 hours; a time during which plateau pressure waves have also been documented.

Treatment of tumor-associated edema

Corticosteroids

Since their introduction more than 30 years ago glucocorticoids have served as the mainstay therapy for tumor-associated edema. By providing an effective and consistent means of edema control, steroids not only restore edema-related neurologic deficits but also permit a much safer form of operative therapy. With respect to the latter, steroids have revolutionized the surgical possibilities available; procedures previously unimaginable in the pre-steroid era can now be confidently performed because of the effectiveness of steroids in both minimizing and preventing complications arising from tumor-associated edema.

The rationale for steroid use in tumor-associated edema is largely empiric, for the mechanism by which steroids mediate their anti-edema effects remains very much an enigma. It is generally accepted that the favorable effects of steroids are primarily related to a reduction in the permeability of a disrupted blood-brain barrier. Numerous mechanisms have been proposed to account for such an effect, although the relative importance of each is uncertain (reviewed in Capildeo 1989, Yamada et al 1989). Some of the more prominent ones include: inhibition of phospholipase A_2, the enzyme responsible for arachidonic acid release; stabilization of membrane lysosomes; a direct stabilizing effect on cerebral capillaries; and an improvement in peritumoral microcirculation.

Whatever the mechanism, steroids are effective in reducing peritumoral edema and the response is rapid. Reductions in capillary permeability have been detected experimentally as early as 1 hour after a single dose (Shapiro et al 1990). Prompt clinical responses are also seen. Among brain tumor patients, it is not uncommon for steroids to reverse a hemiparesis or dysphasia, or restore the alertness of a somnolent patient after just a few doses. Different types of brain tumors vary in their clinical response to steroids. Metastases show the most gratifying response; an intermediate response is seen in malignant gliomas and meningiomas, although the response in the latter is frequently inconsistent. This differential response is presumably a reflection of the density of glucocorticoid receptors expressed by these tumors and their peritumoral tissue (Yu et al 1981).

Dexamethasone is the most commonly used steroid for tumor-associated edema. It is usually given in divided doses of 16 mg per day, although in some patients higher doses may be necessary. It must be remembered that steroids are associated with a wide range of adverse side effects, all of which add to patient morbidity. The nature and management of these have been recently reviewed (Bilsky & Posner 1993).

Other measures

For most patients, steroids alone will usually suffice in ameliorating the effects of tumor-associated edema. Occasionally, when peritumoral edema gets out of control and brain herniation is imminent, additional measures of ICP control are necessary. In such emergency situations, only prompt intervention with mannitol, hyperventilation, and tumor resection are likely to revive such patients.

There has been increasing interest recently in additional pharmacologic agents for the treatment of tumor-associated edema. The nonsteroidal anti-inflammatory agents (NSAIDs) and the lazeroids are two types of drugs which have been subjected to preliminary study. Given the potential culpability of the arachidonic cascade in the development of tumor-associated edema, there is a theoretical possibility that blockade of this pathway may be of therapeutic benefit. Ibuprofen, a cyclo-oxygenase inhibitor, is one NSAID which has been subject to both experimental and clinical study. In one preliminary report, ibuprofen improved the Karnofsky performance in 40% of a small series of patients (Del Maestro & Mattar 1988, Del Maestro et al 1990). The lazeroids are experimental non-glucocorticoid steroids with potent inhibition of lipid peroxidation. Their effects on peritumoral edema have been studied in a rat glioma model, with conflicting results. In one study, the lazeroid agent U-74006F did not alter permeability or edema formation (Megyesi et al 1990). In a second study, this agent appeared to reduce tumor size and also to prevent neurologic dysfunction, although permeability parameters were not altered (King et al 1991). If lazeroids do favorably affect brain edema, they appear to do so by mechanisms other than reduction in vascular permeability.

INCREASED INTRACRANIAL PRESSURE

Perhaps no pathophysiologic component of intracranial pathology dominates the attention of the neurosurgeon more than the phenomenon of elevated intracranial pressure (ICP). This is especially germane to brain tumors, for without (and sometimes despite) timely intervention, increased ICP often proves an inevitable and frequently fatal accompaniment to the progressive growth and evolution of many intracranial tumors. Indeed, the high mortality which once characterized early operative attempts at brain tumor removal stemmed, in large measure, from limited understanding of intracranial pressure dynamics and their peri- and intraoperative control. Lessons learned from these early endeavors, together with several decades of experimental discovery and clinical experience, have provided fundamental understanding of the factors regulating intracranial pressure in both normal and pathologic states. Knowledge of intracranial pressure dynamics is essential to the neurosurgeon treating brain tumor patients, for anticipation, avoidance, timely recognition, and appropriate control of elevated ICP remain cornerstones of contemporary brain tumor management.

Intracranial pressure dynamics

The Monro–Kellie doctrine

The intracranial compartment is an environment of special vulnerability. This vulnerability arises because the intracranial contents are housed within the rigid and unyielding confines of a fixed-volume cranial vault. Having a collective total volume of 1400–1700 ml, the three main components of the intracranial space are brain, CSF, and the intracranial blood volume. That a predicted force of almost 10 000 tons would be required to reduce the volume of normal brain by half indicates that these intracranial constituents can, for all practical purposes, be considered noncompressible (Brown 1991). The virtual incompressibility of intracranial contents confined to a cranial cavity of fixed volume is now epitomized as the modified Monro–Kellie doctrine, and serves as the basis for the current volumetric concept of the genesis of intracranial hypertension. This concept proposes that any volumetric addition or change to one of the intracranial constituents (brain, CSF, or cerebrovascular blood volume), must be compensated for by reciprocal and equivalent volume reductions in other constituents. As discussed in detail below, ICP will rise only when these volumetric compensatory mechanisms have become exhausted.

Physiological determinants of intracranial pressure

It is of therapeutic importance to recognize that even in situations in which there is a precipitous rise in ICP, such as those imposed by a rapidly growing glioblastoma and accompanying vasogenic edema, ICP dynamics do not entirely escape physiologic regulatory controls. In other words, and excluding preterminal thresholds of autoregulatory collapse, ICP elevations, even severe ones, are often still responsive to physiologically-based therapeutic maneuvers such as hyperventilation. Thus, a critical component of ICP management relates to the successful manipulation of those physiologic parameters which, in the normal state, determine ICP. In this section, these physiologic determinants of steady state ICP are reviewed.

In the adult, normal ICP is generally accepted as ranging from 5–15 mmHg, whereas in young children the upper limit is significantly lower: 5 mmHg in a 5-year-old child and 3 mmHg in the newborn (Welch 1980). Even in the steady state, ICP is a dynamic pressure, as is evident from the two superimposed frequencies which characterize the normal ICP tracing. The first and slower frequency is synchronous with respiratory excursions; a small reduction in ICP occurs with inspiration and a slight increase occurs with expiration. These changes simply reflect changes in intrathoracic venous pressure which are readily transmitted to the intracranial compartment. Sudden elevations in ICP which accompany coughing, straining, positive end expiratory pressure (PEEP) ventilation, and compression of neck veins are similarly explained on this venous basis. Whereas the ICP elevations associated with such maneuvers are easily tolerated by the normal brain, they may not be in a brain already compromised by a growing tumor. The second baseline fluctuation of ICP is synchronous with the cardiac pulse and is related to distension of the intracranial arterial tree following systole. In states of elevated ICP, including brain tumors, arterial pulsations are seen to increase in magnitude (Langfitt 1975). This finding relates to abnormal intracranial compliance.

In the normal state, intracranial pressure is equally distributed throughout the length of the craniospinal axis and can therefore be considered synonymous with the CSF pressure, as determined by lumbar puncture. A clear requirement for such uniform distribution of ICP is patency and free communication within the CSF space, both within and outside the ventricular system. In the case of many brain tumors, particularly those associated with mass effect, CSF pressure as determined by lumbar puncture frequently does not accurately reflect the true ICP; the latter is often significantly higher. A major conceptual milestone was the recognition that brain tumors and other intracranial mass lesions could generate *pressure gradients* between the supra- and infratentorial compartments, and/or between the intracranial and intraspinal compartments (Smyth & Henderson 1938, Langfitt et al 1964a, b). These gradients arise as the result of intracranial herniations, occluding the subarachnoid space at the level of the tentorial hiatus in the case of the former, and obliterating the subarachnoid space at the foramen magnum in the case of the latter.

As indicated by the Monro–Kellie doctrine, the principal determinants of ICP include the volumes of brain, CSF, and intracranial blood. Brain tissue, the largest component, has an approximate volume of 1400 ml. Intracranial volumes of blood and CSF are often reported to be in the order of 75–150 ml each, although both are highly variable. In the absence of brain pathology, the volume of brain tissue can be considered fixed, thus CSF volume and cerebral blood volume emerge as the most important factors regulating steady state ICP. The relationship between ICP and these two factors has been expressed in the form of an equation, wherein ICP equals the pressure in the sagittal sinus plus the product of the CSF formation rate and the CSF outflow resistance (Marmarou et al 1978):

$$ICP = Pressure_{\text{sagittal sinus}} + (CSF_{\text{formation rate}} \times CSF_{\text{outflow resistance}})$$

Total CSF volume in adults is usually quoted as being 150 ml, almost half of which is said to reside in the intracranial compartment. These data, all old and derived primarily from autopsy and pneumoencephalographic studies, do not reflect the tremendous variation that exists in normal intracranial CSF volume. More recently, data obtained from magnetic resonance imaging suggest that total intracranial CSF volume ranges from 57–286 ml in volunteers aged 18–64 years (Condon et al 1986, 1987). Whatever the absolute volume of CSF in any given patient, the most important aspect of CSF from the standpoint of brain tumors is that it represents a fluid compartment which can be readily mobilized and diminished to accommodate a growing neoplasm and forestall elevations in ICP.

CSF is formed at a relatively constant rate (0.35 ml/min or ~500 ml/day) and is considered an ultrafiltrate of plasma (Fishman 1992). Almost 70% of CSF is secreted by the choroid plexus. The remainder is believed to be secreted by a variety of poorly characterized extrachoroidal sources, of which brain parenchyma may be the most important. After its exit from the ventricular system and transit through the intracranial and spinal subarachnoid spaces, CSF is normally absorbed at a rate equal to its production. Whereas it is generally well accepted that CSF is absorbed into the venous compartment via the arachnoid granulations along the cerebral convexity, the precise mechanism of absorption remains unclear. The rate of CSF production is, under most conditions, fairly constant, being unaffected by changes in cerebral perfusion pressure and cerebral blood flow, or by moderate changes of ICP. Very high levels of ICP, sufficient to cause cerebral ischemia, may reduce CSF production (reviewed in Fishman 1992). It is unclear whether moderate elevations of ICP occurring in a subacute fashion, such as those associated with brain tumors, alter CSF production. On the other hand, CSF absorption is closely linked to elevations in ICP, increasing in a passive manner according to increase in pressure.

Pathogenesis of elevated intracranial pressure

Brain tumors generate ICP elevations by two basic mechanisms. The first, and most common mechanism is simple volumetric addition of tumor tissue to the intracranial compartment. In many instances, the effective size of the tumor mass is supplemented by peritumoral vasogenic edema which, as noted above, can be considerable. Occasionally, the effective mass of the tumor may be further increased by intratumoral hemorrhage, a complication in roughly 4%, of brain tumors (see Vascular phenomena, below). The second mechanism of brain tumor induced ICP elevation is CSF obstruction and resultant hydrocephalus. Sometimes this arises in the setting of a purely intraventricular tumor (e.g. colloid cyst), although a more frequent occurrence is secondary compression and/or distortion of extraventricular or cisternal CSF pathways from an expanding intraparenchymal lesion. Thus, in a proportion of brain tumor patients, both mechanisms may be operative in the development of elevated ICP.

Pressure-volume relationships

Fundamental insight into the dynamics of the ICP elevations generated by brain tumors and other mass lesions evolved primarily as an application of pressure–volume mechanics. Thus, the derivation of the well-known pressure–volume curve which defines the temporal profile of ICP rise in response to an expanding intracranial mass is an important concept which forms the basis of ICP dynamics, as currently understood (Fig. 9.5). Central to the understanding of pressure–volume curves are the interrelated concepts of compliance and elastance. Compliance (dV/dP) is a measure of the distensibility or 'give' available within the intracranial space. Elastance (dP/dV) is the inverse of compliance, referring to the resistance offered to the expansion of an intracranial mass. Both compliance and elastance are measures of the adaptive capacity of the brain to maintain intracranial equilibrium in response to physiologic or pathologic challenges to the system. From an intracranial pressure standpoint, a physiologically favorable state would be one characterized by high compliance

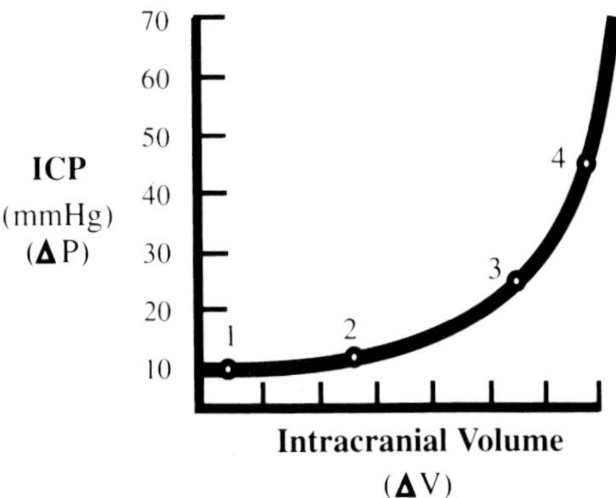

Fig. 9.5 Idealized pressure–volume curve which can be used to characterize changes in ICP which accompany the progressive growth of an intracranial tumor. Brain tumors may cause few early ICP effects because tumor volume is initially well tolerated (point 1); compliance is high, compensatory mechanisms are operating at full efficiency. Eventually (point 2), progressive tumor growth exhausts compensatory mechanisms and compliance declines, thus ICP begins to rise. If treatment is not instituted, the steep portion of the curve is reached (point 3) where compliance is negligibly low and small increments in tumor volume cause large jumps in ICP; established or imminent herniation characterizes this stage. Finally, a point of vasomotor paralysis is reached (point 4), characterized by an ICP which passively rises with systemic arterial pressure.

and low elastance; that is, a large change in volume is accompanied by a small change in pressure. Far less desirable is a state of low compliance and high elastance wherein a small change in volume induces a large change in pressure.

As derived experimentally, using an inflatable balloon in a primate model, and reaffirmed by decades of clinical experience with brain tumors, the ICP response to a progressively enlarging intracranial mass is a staged and exponential one. As depicted by the idealized pressure–volume curve (Fig. 9.5), the ICP response to increasing volume consists of three stages. In the first stage, volumetric addition is well tolerated and is unaccompanied by an increase in ICP; compliance is high and compensatory mechanisms are operating at maximum efficiency. The CSF system has the dominant role in the compensatory response, providing 70% of all spatial compensation (Lofgren & Zwetnow 1973). This is achieved primarily by displacement of CSF from the cranial to the spinal compartment, increased absorption of CSF, and, possibly, reduced production of CSF as well. Vascular factors also have a role in the response. Initially, there is a reduction in cerebral blood volume, a maneuver which, for a time, can be achieved without accompanying reductions in cerebral blood flow. Blood volume within cerebral veins is reduced. With progressive volumetric addition, compensatory reserves eventually approach exhaustion and compliance begins to decline. It is in this transitional phase where ICP first begins to rise in response to further volumetric increments. The rate of ICP rise is initially gradual, but very quickly a stage of decompensation is reached, where additional volume increments elicit exponential rises in ICP; compensatory mechanisms have failed and compliance is negligibly low. This is an extremely vulnerable period for the patient because even the slightest additional increase in volume, such as would occur with temporary vasodilation, will induce ICP elevations of magnitudes sufficient to precipitate a clinical crisis. As the slope of the pressure–volume curve steepens further, a point of no return is reached, characterized by loss of autoregulation, vasomotor paralysis, and an intracranial pressure which passively approaches arterial blood pressure, with cessation of cerebral perfusion and brain death.

Admittedly, the concept of a single idealized pressure–volume curve underlying the genesis of intracranial hypertension is an oversimplification, prompting some to suggest that the true situation is more accurately depicted by series of similarly shaped but different curves which change over time. Nonetheless, the idealized curve does serve as a useful model in explaining many of the clinical phenomena observed in brain tumor patients. The slow initial evolution but rapid late deterioration so characteristic of brain tumor patients is readily explained by this curve. By shifting the curve to the left or right, this model can accommodate tumors of differing growth rates. In the case of a rapidly growing glioblastoma, ICP-related symptoms evolve faster, as reflected by a leftward shirt of the curve and a shorter initial phase of spatial compensation indicating that compensatory mechanisms are promptly overwhelmed by the tumor's rapid growth. The early morning headaches experienced by these patients simply reflect their position on the steep part of the pressure–volume curve, where failing compensatory mechanisms cannot accommodate the hypercarbia, vasodilation, and plateau waves (see below) which accompany REM sleep. The vulnerability of such patients to certain anesthetics, seizures, venous obstruction, or any other maneuver causing additional ICP elevations of any degree, again reflects their precarious position on the pressure–volume curve. Indeed, the catastrophic deterioration of a brain tumor patient, though frequently ascribed to intratumoral hemorrhage, is much more likely to be the result of sudden vasodilation superimposed upon a brain having negligible compensatory reserve.

In the case of meningiomas, which can undergo years of covert growth and assume gigantic proportions before becoming symptomatic, the curve appears shifted to the right and is remarkable for a long initial stage of spatial compensation. The slow growth of such tumors, while providing maximal opportunity for the above-mentioned compensatory mechanisms to operate to their fullest, also exploits another compensatory feature of the brain known as plasticity. The term describes the capacity of the brain to undergo slow deformation over time, particularly obvious with large meningiomas. The sometimes dramatic indentation, compression, and deformation exhibited by the brain as it accommodates a large meningioma is an example of such plasticity. Thus, the favorable pressure–volume dynamics of slow growing tumors are the result of maximal exploitation of compensatory mechanisms, explaining why many such tumors can grow to a large size without necessarily increasing ICP.

Intracranial pressure waves

Periodic pressure fluctuations known as pressure waves further perturb ICP dynamics in states of elevated ICP. As described in the now classic work of Nils Lundberg, pathologic pressure waves are of three types, designated as A, B, and C waves; all have been recorded in brain tumor patients (Lundberg 1960). 'A' waves, also known as plateau waves, are clinically the most significant of the three and are discussed in detail below. B waves are cyclic, highly peaked waves with a frequency of 0.5–2 per minute and unsustained peak pressures of 50 mmHg or so above baseline. Their origin is unclear, but they appear to be related to changes in respiration and/or cerebral vasomotor tone. Despite the high pressures generated by these waves, and despite their documentation in brain tumor patients, particularly in the evening and early morning, their clinical significance remains unclear. Similarly uncertain is the pathophysiologic significance of the C wave, another cyclic fluctuation whose occurrence 4–5 times per minute is thought to be related to the so-called Traube–Hering–Mayer variations in arterial blood pressure.

Unlike pressure waves of the B and C type, whose pathophysiologic contribution to elevated ICP remains somewhat conjectural, plateau waves are well known for their detrimental effects during decompensating states with elevated ICP. Patients with brain tumor, trauma, or hydrocephalus appear especially vulnerable to the development of plateau waves. In its most classic form, the temporal profile of the plateau wave begins with an acute and abrupt elevation of ICP, typically 50–100 mmHg above baseline (Fig. 9.6). This elevated level of ICP is sustained for periods ranging from several minutes to an hour before precipitously returning to near baseline levels. During the height of pressure elevation, a variety of clinical symptoms and signs may occur, including increasing

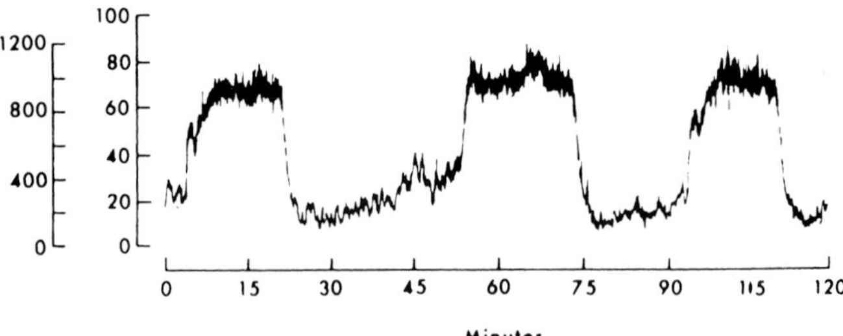

Fig. 9.6 Plateau waves in a patient with a glioblastoma from the original series of Lundberg. During the waves, a rapid increase in signs of cerebral dysfunction was noted. (Reprinted with permission from Fishman 1975; adapted from Lundberg 1960).

headache, nausea, vomiting, facial flushing, confusion, altered consciousness, pupillary dilation, respiratory change, and even frank decerebration. Such symptomatology, though not invariably present, can be considered a manifestation of acute brainstem dysfunction and/or incipient herniation. As a rule, plateau waves are restricted to states of advanced intracranial hypertension, in which compensatory mechanisms are limited and cranial compliance is low. The occurrence of plateau waves is therefore generally regarded as an ominous finding, indicative of a position on the steep portion of the pressure–volume curve and the very real possibility of impending life-threatening decompensation. Moreover, plateau waves tend to occur with greater frequency, increasing amplitude, and longer duration as patients approach death.

Whereas plateau waves may occur spontaneously without obvious cause, in many instances their onset can often be correlated with various physiologic or iatrogenic maneuvers that perturb cerebral vasomotor tone. Rosner & Becker (1984) have suggested that plateau waves may be precipitated by cerebral vasodilation, such as would occur with a reduction in arterial blood pressure. The triggering effect of such a 'vasodilatory cascade' explains why brain tumor patients are so prone to the development of plateau waves during REM sleep, seizures, febrile periods, respiratory obstruction and anesthetic induction. Every effort should be made to anticipate and avoid events known to trigger plateau waves in such patients.

Elevated ICP: clinical features

Despite the direct and detrimental contribution of raised ICP to the clinical course of the brain tumor patient, few signs or symptoms are directly attributable to elevated ICP per se. Much of the symptomatology associated with raised ICP emanates not from the mere presence of intracranial hypertension, but rather from its secondary effects, as mediated by pressure gradients, compartmental shifts, brain herniation, and vascular changes. Interestingly, of the clinical features classically and commonly regarded as the 'generalized manifestations' of increased ICP (headache, vomiting, disturbances of consciousness, papilledema, and abducens palsy), it may be argued that only papilledema is a genuine, *direct* effect of elevated ICP, the others being the result of secondary compression, traction, and/or distortion of various intracranial structures. Nonetheless, all these clinical features, be they direct or indirect effects of elevated ICP, are diagnostically important in recognizing states of intracranial hypertension.

Headache is the initial symptom in about half of all brain tumor patients, and is eventually experienced by the majority of patients at some point during their clinical course. It is caused by traction, distortion, or irritation of pain-sensitive structures within the intracranial compartment, specifically dural coverings and blood vessels. Brain tumor associated headaches often exhibit a number of characteristic features distinguishing them from headaches due to other causes. Of particular importance is their temporal profile. Recent in onset, yet clearly progressive in nature, these headaches often increase in frequency, severity, and duration over a period of weeks to months. Their tendency to become especially prominent in the early morning hours is well known. Impaired compliance further accounts for the exacerbation of such headaches with various Valsalva-type maneuvers which increase jugular venous pressure. Intermittent headaches that have a strong postural component should raise the possibility of an intraventricular tumor.

Although brain tumor patients frequently experience diffuse and bilateral headaches, devoid of localizing value, in some patients the location or laterality of the headache is suggestive of the site or side of the tumor. Supraorbital headache may indicate the presence of an anterior or middle fossa tumor, referring pain from meningeal branches of the trigeminal nerve's first division to the supraorbital group of nerves. Supra- and infratentorial tumors distorting the tentorium have been known to refer pain to the external auditory meatus, via branches of the vagal or glossopharyngeal nerves. Finally, suboccipital and upper cervical pain may be indicative of an inferiorly situated posterior fossa tumor, referring pain via the upper three cervical nerves.

Vomiting is an occasional accompaniment to the headache of brain tumors. It is a far more common occurrence in children than in adults, and more so with infratentorial or fourth ventricular tumors than with supratentorial lesions. In children, vomiting may be especially dramatic, so much so that its sudden occurrence without warning has been aptly described as 'projectile' in nature. The physiologic basis of vomiting in the setting of brain tumors and elevated ICP is poorly understood; only exceptionally is it truly the result of direct involvement of the area postrema or vagal nucleus — from a fourth ventricular ependymoma, for example. Lundberg (1960) noted that vomiting can sometimes terminate pressure waves and ameliorate headache, presumably by way of the hyperventilation which often accompanies vomiting. This phenomenon is also seen clinically.

Alterations in consciousness, including both the level of consciousness and/or its quality, are commonly experienced by the brain tumor patient at some point during the clinical course. It is important to reiterate that alterations in consciousness are not the primary effects of raised ICP. Instead, they represent secondary effects as mediated by brain shifts, herniations, and vascular disturbances, or the primary effect of compressive or destructive tumors involving eloquent brain substance. Brain tumors can induce a wide spectrum of mental status changes, ranging from subtle alterations in personality to states of profound and irretrievable coma. Given these two extremes, it follows that normal consciousness is derived from two components: cognitive content and arousal. Many changes in higher cognitive function (memory loss, intellectual decay, impaired judgment, personality change, language dysfunction, emotional lability, and psychiatric symptoms), can be regarded as focal and site-specific manifestations of a tumor's local compressive and/or destructive effects. Such alterations depend, predictably, upon which eloquent brain areas are immediately involved by tumor and are, for the most part, independent of changes in ICP. Of greater relevance to this discussion are those states of *depressed* consciousness which accompany brain herniation and, thus, are more reliably equated with the presence of raised ICP. Preservation of arousal depends on the integrity of the brainstem reticular activating system and the bilateral cortical structures to which it projects. Because severe bilateral cortical damage rarely occurs in the setting of brain tumors, the depressed consciousness which accompanies them is usually the result of secondary brainstem compression from herniation phenomena. A less common occurrence is direct involvement of the reticular activating system by tumor. The somnolence which accompanies such lesions as thalamic gliomas is an example of this mechanism.

Papilledema is both most common and most reliable sign of elevated ICP. Whereas papilledema is reliable evidence of elevated ICP, its absence provides no guarantee that ICP is normal. Very often, this discrepancy relates to the duration of elevated pressure; sustained ICP elevations over a period of days to weeks are more apt to produce papilledema than are acute elevations. In the pre-CT era, papilledema was a presenting feature in more than half of all patients with intracranial tumors. Even today, despite the earlier diagnosis afforded by contemporary imaging techniques, papilledema is still a regular feature in many such patients. The cardinal ophthalmologic manifestations of papilledema include: elevation of the optic disc, blurred disc margins, obscuration of retinal vessels crossing the disc edge, loss of spontaneous venous pulsations, opacification of the nerve fiber layer, and retinal hemorrhages. From the standpoint of fundoscopy, the distinction between papilledema and other forms of disc swelling of acquired or congenital type can be troublesome. Fluorescein angiography is often helpful in this regard. As a rule, visual acuity is preserved in true papilledema. With the exception of an enlarged blind spot, visual fields should also be preserved unless the tumor involves other components of the visual sensory system.

The pathogenesis of papilledema relates primarily to the transmission of intracranial pressure along the optic nerve sheath with resultant blockade of axoplasmic transport within the optic nerve; accumulation of axoplasm results in swelling of both the optic nerve and nerve head. A secondary contributing factor is increased retinal venous pressure which results in vascular congestion, extravasation of proteinaceous debris, and the formation of extracellular edema within the nerve.

'Cushing's triad' refers to the combination of bradycardia, respiratory slowing, and hypertension with a wide pulse pressure. Both the significance and mechanisms of this triad are subject to ongoing controversy. Most believe this triad to be the result of brain shift and brainstem compression, rather than elevated ICP alone (Fishman 1992).

Brain herniation

As the result of relentless growth and edema formation, brain tumors will assume sufficient critical mass to overwhelm mechanisms of spatial compensation. As a result, intercompartmental brain herniations, brainstem compression, secondary vascular compromise, and eventual brain death will ensue. When considering the various forms of brain herniation, several anatomic relationships deserve special mention. Because the falx cerebri and tentorium cerebelli act as somewhat rigid spacers, the cranial space is a compartmentalized cavity. Communication between the different cranial spaces takes place through the tentorial hiatus. The only available exit from the cranial cavity is the foramen magnum. Given this anatomic arrangement, it follows that various forms of brain herniation can occur. The principal forms of brain herniation, as summarized by Plum & Posner (1980), include: cingulate herniation, uncal (transtentorial) herniation, central (transtentorial) herniation, upward cerebellar herniation, and cerebellar-foramen magnum herniation (Fig. 9.7).

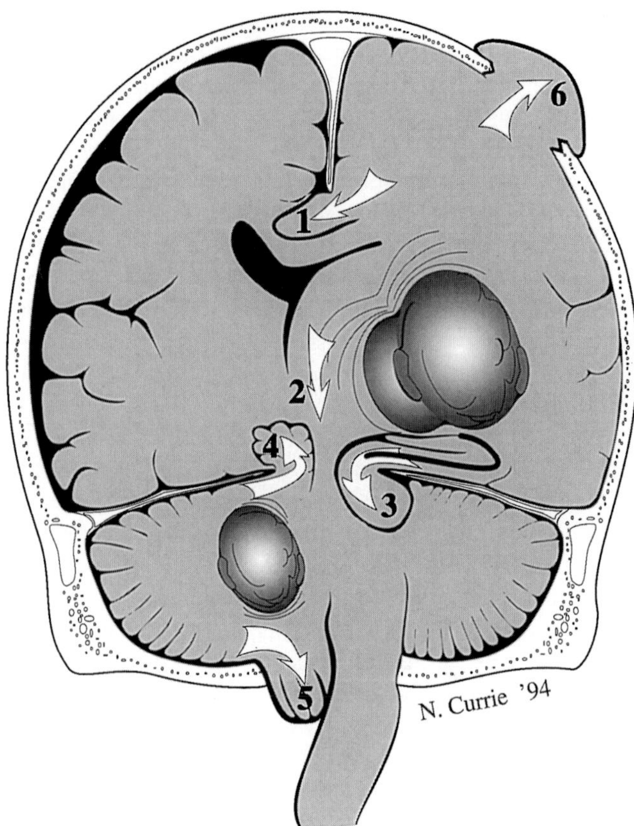

Fig. 9.7 Schematic of various types of herniation phenomena which may accompany brain tumors. **1** Subfalcine or cingulate herniation; **2** central transtentorial herniation; **3** uncal transtentorial herniation; **4** upward cerebellar herniation; **5** cerebellar tonsillar herniation; **6** transcalvarial brain herniation. Note the obliteration of the subarachnoid space in the tumor-containing hemisphere. Loss of free communication within the subarachnoid space is a prerequisite to the development of pressure gradients (see text).

Whereas each of the above-mentioned herniation syndromes has various distinguishing features, several general pathophysiologic features are applicable to all forms of herniation. Firstly, the driving force behind brain herniation at any site is a pressure gradient. The generation of a pressure gradient begins with local obliteration of the subarachnoid space at the herniation site. The resultant loss of free communication within the CSF space prevents pressure equilibration, thus establishing the gradient. Moreover, once a pressure gradient has been established, it is a self-perpetuating process in that further upstream increments in pressure must be borne by a compartment of reduced effective size and lesser compliance. The situation is directly analogous to the case of obstructive hydrocephalus, wherein dramatic and rapid pressure elevations can occur above the obstructing lesion. Furthermore, obliteration of CSF spaces, particularly the perimesencephalic cistern and cisterna magna, provides strong radiologic evidence of a 'tight' brain, with high risk of brain herniation (Teasdale et al 1984). The second general feature of brain herniation concerns vascular changes. Virtually every form of brain herniation leaves in its wake some form of vascular compromise and ischemic damage. Sometimes this is the result of large vessel compromise, as would occur with anterior cerebral artery compression and resultant cortical infarction following subfalcine herniations. In other situations, the microvascular circulation is compromised. The entire phenomenon of brain herniation is a progressive and self-perpetuating process. Secondary injury as the result of ischemic damage, together with swelling of incarcerated or prolapsed brain, fuels the underlying expanding process by adding further edema and congestion.

Cingulate herniation. This form of herniation, although a common radiologic finding in anteriorly situated hemispheric tumors, is the least detrimental of the various herniation syndromes. It refers to the situation where an expanding hemispheric tumor forces the ipsilateral cingulate gyrus underneath the falx to the opposite hemispheric cavity (Fig. 9.7). Accompanying the herniation is compression of the ipsilateral pericallosal and/or callosomarginal arteries and displacement of the internal cerebral vein. Although this form of herniation is often asymptomatic, it may contribute to the early behavioral or cognitive symptoms which sometimes accompany anterior hemispheric tumors. Less often, cingulate herniation may be associated with ischemia and/or infarction in the anterior cerebral artery distribution.

Uncal herniation. One of the most frequent, well known, and clinically significant brain herniation syndromes, uncal herniation is most apt to occur with tumors situated within the temporal lobe or middle fossa, although virtually any supratentorial hemispheric tumor, when sufficiently large, may precipitate uncal herniation. The basic phenomenon is medial and downward displacement of the basal uncal edge and hippocampal gyrus over the free margin of the tentorium, through the tentorial hiatus and into the posterior fossa. As the parahippocampal gyrus and uncus begin their prolapse into the tentorial hiatus, the midbrain becomes narrowed in its transverse axis and the contralateral cerebral peduncle is driven into the opposite tentorial edge, sometimes producing the so-called Kernohan's notch phenomenon (see below). In the process, the ipsilateral third nerve becomes compressed between the posterior cerebral artery and the tentorial edge or the petroclinoid ligament. The resulting third nerve palsy and unilateral pupillary dilation is thus the most consistent early sign of uncal herniation. Because the diencephalon is not consistently the first region compromised by uncal herniation, a decreased level of consciousness is not necessarily an early feature of this syndrome. By the time of established pupillary dilation, however, sufficient brainstem distortion has generally occurred to cause some degree of obtundation, stupor or frank coma. Accompanying each stage of rostral-caudal deterioration are abnormal respiratory patterns of various types (hyperventilation, Cheyne–Stokes respiration).

As a result of the tumor itself, some degree of motor dysfunction is often present prior to the development of uncal herniation. With the onset of herniation and compression of the crus cerebri, pre-existing motor deficits will predictably worsen. The usual pattern is one of increasing contralateral weakness which, in short order, gives rise to decorticate and, later, decerebrate posturing as rostral-caudal compromise proceeds. Whereas motor signs contralateral to the side of the tumor are the rule, motor deficits ipsilateral to the lesion can also occur. Known as the Kernohan's notch phenomenon, this false localizing sign is the result of compression of the contralateral cerebral peduncle against the opposite tentorial edge.

As a result of the inferiorly displaced and edematous brain incarcerated within the tentorial incisura, compression and distortion of arteries can occur. Compression of the posterior cerebral artery may lead to infarction of the thalamus, mesial temporal and occipital lobes. Less frequently, compression of the superior cerebellar artery can lead to cerebellar infarction. The relative immobility of the basilar artery in the face of downward displacement and anteroposterior distortion of the brainstem may disrupt delicate perforating branches of the former, causing brainstem ischemia. A similar mechanism has been proposed to account for small, but devastating hemorrhages (Duret hemorrhages) which occur in the midbrain and lower pons during transtentorial herniation.

Central transtentorial herniation. A symmetrical pattern of brain herniation, characterized by a more orderly and complete pattern of rostral-caudal deterioration, is that of central transtentorial herniation. In the setting of brain tumors, this form of brain herniation is most often seen in response to enlarging hemispheric tumors of the frontal, parietal or occipital lobes, particularly those situated along the frontal or occipital poles and those at the vertex. Of the latter, parasagittal meningiomas, given their tendency for clinically silent growth and large size at diagnosis, may occasionally present with evidence of early central herniation. Bilaterally expanding lesions such as multiple metastatic deposits and midline gliomas, or obstructing third ventricular tumors causing biventricular hydrocephalus, may also give rise to a central herniation syndrome. Among brain tumor patients, the presence of central herniation, at least in its earliest stages, is probably a far more common occurrence than is currently recognized. Somnolence, inattentiveness, or some form of clouded consciousness is evident in as many as 20% of patients.

Diencephalic and midbrain compromise with resultant disruption of the ascending reticular activating system accounts for the early depression of consciousness which typifies this form of herniation. Impaired concentration, drowsiness, and agitation are the early symptoms, eventually replaced by progressive somnolence, obdundation, and, finally, coma. Altered respiratory activity may also be seen at this stage, manifesting as yawns, deep sighs, or periodic breathing of the Cheyne–Stokes type. Decorticate responses frequently emerge with progressive diencephalic failure. As a rule, when central herniation is arrested or relieved by tumor removal or other measures while still at the diencephalic stage, full neurologic recovery is possible because the underlying injury is compressive. With continued herniation, however, irreparable midbrain failure eventually supervenes, as simple compression gives way to secondary ischemic injury and brainstem hemorrhage. Pupils become unresponsive and fixed in midposition, motor responses progress from decorticate to decerebrate to flaccid, brainstem reflexes are lost, and respiratory activity deteriorates from hyperventilation to agonal.

Cerebellar (tonsillar) herniation. The posterior fossa is less tolerant than is the supratentorial compartment to mass effects imposed by tumors growing therein. Given these volumetric constraints, brain herniations caused by infratentorial tumors tend to be more frequent, occur sooner, and evolve more rapidly than those associated with supratentorial tumors. The most common pattern of infratentorial herniation is that of downward protrusion and impaction of the cerebellar tonsils at the level of the foramen magnum. This occurs most commonly with posterior fossa tumors of any type, and less frequently, as a late sequela of central transtentorial herniation from a supratentorial mass. The cerebellar tonsils descend through the foramen magnum, often protruding several centimeters into the cervical canal. Obstructive hydrocephalus, which is virtually always present to some degree, contributes to the pressure gradient and increases the herniation effect. In the most severe cases, the tonsils become so forcibly incarcerated and edematous that they eventually undergo infarction. The crucial consequence of such herniations, however, is medullary compression, an occurrence which can be the source of sudden and unpredictable cardiorespiratory collapse. Indeed, the most dramatic clinical presentation of severe tonsillar impaction is sudden death in a patient who, until just moments before, was lucid, conversing, and following commands. Admittedly, this is a rare occurrence, but nevertheless one which should always be an underlying concern in any patient with a posterior fossa tumor and established tonsillar herniation.

Cerebellar herniation, even when marked, may or may not be evident clinically. In some instances, particularly in children, painful neck stiffness which is aggravated by movement, L'Hermitte's sign, head tilt and even frank torticollis can all signify its presence. In the infant, an arched opisthotonic posture is sometimes a dramatic manifestation of tonsillar impaction. Not uncommonly, however, foraminal impaction may produce few symptoms, being overshadowed by the overt manifestations of cerebellar dysfunction or hydrocephalus which typically accompany many posterior fossa tumors. Still, even in asymptomatic cases, the degree of tonsillar herniation identified at surgery is often impressive. Tonsillar herniation and its clinical effects may be precipitated by an ill-advised lumbar puncture in a patient with increased intracranial pressure.

Upward cerebellar herniation. A second, but less commonly recognized form of cerebellar herniation involves the upward protrusion of cerebellar tissue through the tentorial hiatus. It occurs most often with sizable tumors of the cerebellum, but has also been well described with large acoustic schwannomas (Vastine & Kinney 1927, Cuneo et al 1979). Of particular concern, however, is the well-documented occurrence of upward herniation in response to ventricular drainage or shunting for obstructive hydrocephalus caused by a posterior fossa tumor. One estimate suggests that shunting carries a 3% risk of precipitating such herniations in children with posterior fossa tumors (Albright 1992).

With progressive growth, cerebellar tumors force the apical portion of the cerebellum and vermis, together with the adjacent upper pons, through the tentorial incisura. As a result, the midbrain becomes compressed from below and the pons suffers mechanical distortion. The upward protrusion may also compress the veins of Galen and Rosenthal, raising supratentorial venous pressure. Compression of the the superior cerebellar artery against the tentorial edge may lead to cerebellar infarction, thus further accelerating the process. Finally, kinking of the aqueduct may cause hydrocephalus of the supratentorial ventricular system.

The clinical features of upward herniation are not as clearly defined as they are in other herniation states. When symptomatic, upward herniation is generally an acute event, one characterized by midposition and fixed pupils, absent caloric responses, and decerebrate posturing (Cuneo et al 1979). Another possible manifestation of upward herniation are the so-called 'cerebellar fits', a loosely characterized phenomenon seen in children with posterior fossa tumors. Features include sudden decerebration, opisthotonos, and coma.

Treatment of elevated ICP

The perioperative course of most brain tumor patients will *not* be complicated by elevated ICP. Thus, for the majority of patients, including many with clinical and/or radiologic evidence of raised ICP preoperatively, the combination of corticosteroids and tumor resection will be generally be sufficient for ICP control. In a sizable minority, however, perioperative edema and raised ICP will be a problem, sometimes a life-threatening one.

In one study where ICP was monitored after elective intracranial surgery, patients with malignant gliomas, low grade astrocytomas, and meningiomas had ICP elevations greater than 20 torr in 27.2%, 21.4%, and 17.5%, of cases, respectively (Constantini et al 1988). Other studies further indicate that the temporal profile of ICP elevations differs between astrocytomas and meningiomas. In the case of the former, ICP tends to peak during the first postoperative day, whereas ICP elevations related to meningiomas are maximal at day three (Hase et al 1978). Furthermore, ICP elevations are said to be more sustained with meningiomas, being detectable even one week postoperatively, at a time when most ICP elevations related to astrocytomas have long dissipated (Cunha e Sa & Quest 1993). In some brain tumor patients, hydrocephalus may also contribute to perioperative elevations in ICP. This is particularly true of posterior fossa, pineal region, and intraventricular tumors. As discussed in the preceding section on brain edema, incompletely resected tumors are especially prone to the development of postoperative ICP problems.

Measures to control ICP include corticosteroids, mannitol, diuretics, hyperventilation, and ventricular drainage. Whereas corticosteroids are used perioperatively in virtually all brain tumor patients, the need for additional measures will usually be dictated by the clinical situation at hand. In acutely decompensating patients with established or impending herniation, immediate intervention with mannitol and hyperventilation is often required, followed by prompt removal of the responsible tumor. The need for these measures may also continue into the postoperative period. When hydrocephalus is a complicating factor, such as may occur in posterior fossa or intraventricular tumors, external ventricular drainage serves as an important adjunct for ICP control. In many such tumors, however, restitution of normal CSF flow often accompanies tumor removal, thus obviating the routine need for ventricular drainage.

Finally, adequate seizure control is an important component of both ICP control and the general management of the brain tumor patient. With respect to the former, seizures are accompanied by an increase in cerebral blood flow, an occurrence which may precipitate herniation in the patient whose intracranial pressure dynamics are already severely compromised by the mass and associated edema of a tumor. Thus, effective prophylactic anticonvulsants should be used in all patients with supratentorial tumors. Metabolic derangements known to reduce seizure thresholds, such as hyponatremia, and less often hypoglycemia or hypocalcemia, should be recognized and appropriately corrected. For a more detailed review of ICP management in brain tumor patients, the reader is referred to a comprehensive recent analysis (Bilsky & Posner 1993).

VASCULAR EFFECTS OF BRAIN TUMORS

Since the very earliest descriptions, brain tumors have been well recognized to be a source of cerebrovascular complications. Whilst their occasional tendency to undergo spontaneous hemorrhage is well known, brain tumors may also be a source of cerebral ischemia, mimicking an acute 'completed' stroke syndrome, or even transient ischemic attacks (TIAs). In both situations, such vascular complications may be the source of diagnostic confusion, and the possibility of an underlying brain tumor may be overlooked in favor of more common etiologies. This was especially true in the pre-CT era, when unsuspected tumors accounted for 3% of all acute strokes.

Brain tumors and intracranial hemorrhage

Based on Salcman's recent and comprehensive analysis of the literature, the overall incidence of brain tumor as a cause of acute intracranial hemorrhage is 4.6%. Alternatively, the incidence of hemorrhage within brain tumors is 3.9% (Salcman 1992). If microscopic and/or subclinical hemorrhages are also considered, the overall rate of tumoral hemorrhage approaches 15% (Kondziolka et al 1987). Although hemorrhagic tendencies will vary with histologic type, as a group metastatic tumors are more prone to spontaneous hemorrhage than are primary brain tumors.

Primary brain tumors

Spontaneous hemorrhage has been reported in virtually every histologic type of primary brain tumor. For some tumors (e.g. schwannoma), spontaneous hemorrhage is so exceedingly rare that its occurrence can be dismissed as an anomalous biologic accident. For other tumors (e.g. oligodendrogliomas), however, spontaneous hemorrhage is seen with sufficient regularity that an inherent hemorrhagic tendency cannot be excluded (Table 9.1). Among primary brain tumors, gliomas are the most prone to spontaneous hemorrhage. Glioblastoma, oligodendroglioma, and mixed gliomas have gained particular notoriety as having the highest inherent hemorrhagic tendencies (Kondziolka et al 1987, Salcman 1992). A far less common tumor, the choroid plexus papilloma, also has a distinct predilection for both acute and subclinical hemorrhage.

Intracranial hemorrhage of virtually every type can be attributed to brain tumors. For intrinsic brain tumors, intratumoral hemorrhage is by far the most common pattern, followed in frequency by intraparenchymal clots, subarachnoid hemorrhage, and subdural hematomas. In one series, the respective frequency of each was 67%, 15.5%, 15.5%, and 2% (Wakai et al 1982). Meningiomas, while not regarded as having any unique propensity for spontaneous hemorrhage, do appear to have a unique pattern of bleeding. Subarachnoid hemorrhage appears far more commonly in meningiomas than in intrinsic tumors, accounting for almost a third of all meningioma-associated hemorrhages. Given their extracerebral location, meningiomas are also five times more likely to produce subdural hematomas than are intrinsic neoplasms. Finally, intratumoral hemorrhage appears distinctly uncommon among meningiomas, contrasting with the predominance of this form of hemorrhage among intrinsic tumors. In one study, the distribution of 46 meningioma-associated hemorrhages was as follows: subarachnoid (30.4%); intracerebral (28.3%); intracerebral and extraparenchymal (23.9%); subdural (10.9%); intratumoral (2.2%); and other (6.5%) (Kohli & Crouch 1984). It was also ob-

Table 9.1 Incidence of hemorrhage by primary intracranial tumors. From Salcman (1992)

Tumor	Number of cases	Number bleeding	% Bleeding
Astrocytoma	472	12	2.5
Oligodendroglioma	72	6	8.3
Ependymoma	105	7	6.6
Choroid plexus papilloma	12	2	16.6
Glioblastoma	399	25	6.3
Medulloblastoma	145	2	1.4
Schwannoma	193	0	0
Meningioma	310	4	1.3
Hemangioblastoma	34	0	0
Craniopharyngioma	91	3	3.3
Pituitary adenoma	311	49	15.8

served that convexity, parasagittal, and intraventricular meningiomas were more prone to bleed than those situated elsewhere, as were angioblastic and meningotheliomatous meningiomas, independent of location.

Mechanistically, intratumoral hemorrhages are probably the easiest to understand. The seemingly mundane adage of a 'tumor outrunning its blood supply', however simplistic, is likely an accurate depiction of such events. This notion has also been validated by pathologic studies which routinely reveal areas of central necrosis as being most vulnerable to secondary hemorrhage. Structural failure of tumor vessels is almost certainly an important contributing factor, relevant to all types of tumor-associated hemorrhage. As discussed in preceding sections, the vascular organization of brain tumors is often so mechanically aberrant that one wonders why tumoral hemorrhage is not an even more frequent occurrence. Presumably the product of endothelial proliferation, the microvasculature of malignant gliomas is often disposed in a somewhat chaotic network of tortuous and glomeruloid vessels, replete with conglomerates of retiform capillaries, immature capillary buds, and thin-walled sinusoids (Liwnicz et al 1987). Not only would such angioarchitecture suffer from inherent structural weaknesses, it would also be subject to progressive thrombosis, resulting in tumoral infarction, loss of perivascular support, and eventual secondary hemorrhage. Since peritumoral angiogenesis proceeds from host vessels, peritumoral 'normal' brain will also exhibit alterations in capillary structure, which may be the source of intraparenchymal hemorrhages occurring adjacent to tumors. Structural failure of cerebral vessels has also been implicated as the dominant mechanism underlying tumor-associated subarachnoid hemorrhage (Glass & Abbott 1955). A more obvious, but considerably less frequent cause of subarachnoid hemorrhage relates to direct tumoral erosion and invasion of cerebral vessels, sometimes resulting in aneurysmal change (Cowel et al 1970). In a minority of patients, coagulation abnormalities may be a further confounding factor underlying tumor-related hemorrhage (Kondziolka et al 1987).

For some patients, tumor-associated hemorrhage will be an acute and apoplectic event, presenting with sudden neurologic deficits and progressive decrease in consciousness. In a substantial proportion of patients, however, a subacute presentation has been noted, similar to that of an evolving stroke (Wakai et al 1982, Kondziolka et al 1987). In all patients, the hemorrhage may be the first sign of an underlying tumor. Nowadays, the diagnosis of tumor-associated hemorrhage will be fairly obvious, at least radiologically, as both the hemorrhage and the responsible tumor will be identified on unenhanced and contrast-enhanced CT, respectively. Occasionally, however, there may be little radiologic evidence of an underlying tumor. In such situations, clinical suspicion becomes important. A pre-existing history of headache, seizure, mental status changes, or other neurologic symptoms should be carefully sought. A hemorrhage whose radiographic appearance or location deviates ever so slightly from the typical hypertensive, amyloid, or aneurysmal hemorrhage should always raise suspicions of an underlying tumor. The patient's clinical condition permitting, MRI may be necessary to identify the responsible tumor, or angiography may be needed to exclude a cerebral aneurysm or vascular malformation.

Very often, symptomatic tumor-associated hemorrhages require emergency evacuation. When a tumor is suspected or confirmed as the source of hemorrhage, every effort should be made to remove the tumor as completely as possible; residual tumor is often a source of recurrent or postoperative hemorrhage. If obvious tumor tissue is not encountered during clot removal, the walls of the hematoma cavity should be biopsied in order to exclude histologically an underlying neoplasm.

Pituitary tumors

When all intracranial tumors are considered, pituitary tumors are among the most prone to spontaneous hemorrhage. As an incidental finding, subclinical hemorrhage into a pituitary adenoma is seen with surprising regularity, being discovered radiologically, operatively, or pathologically in as many as 10% of all pituitary adenomas (Mohr & Hardy 1982). Of much greater importance, however, are the 1–2% of pituitary adenomas which undergo symptomatic hemorrhagic infarction, producing the often dramatic clinical syndrome of *pituitary apoplexy*.

Classically defined, pituitary apoplexy refers to the abrupt, and occasionally catastrophic occurrence of acute hemorrhagic infarction of a pituitary adenoma. The clinical syndrome is easily recognized, consisting of acute headache, meningismus, visual impairment, ophthalmoplegia, and alterations in consciousness (Ebersold et al 1983). Without timely intervention, patients are likely to die of subarachnoid hemorrhage or succumb to acute, life-threatening hypopituitarism. There is little consensus in the literature as to which tumor types, if any, are most vulnerable to apoplectic hemorrhage. Some have suggested that hormonally active tumors associated with acromegaly and Cushing's disease are especially prone to apoplexy, whereas other have found large nonfunctioning tumors to bear substantial risk.

The pathophysiologic basis of pituitary apoplexy remains speculative. Ischemic necrosis of a rapidly growing tumor, intrinsic vascular abnormalities peculiar to pituitary tumors, and compression of the superior hypophyseal artery against the sellar diaphragm have all been suggested as mechanisms contributing to apoplectic hemorrhage (Cardoso & Peterson 1984). Predisposing factors loosely associated with apoplexy include bromocriptine therapy, anticoagulation, diabetic ketoacidosis, head trauma, estrogen therapy, and pituitary irradiation. Most cases occur in the absence of any known predisposing condition. Chronologically, pituitary apoplexy begins with infarction of the tumor and the surrounding gland, followed by hemorrhage and edema. This sudden increase in intratumoral pressure and volume causes precipitous expansion of the tumor, followed by mechanical compression of the optic apparatus and of structures within the cavernous sinus. The bulk of the hemorrhage is generally contained within a tense tumor capsule, although extravasation of blood into the subarachnoid space is a frequent occurrence. Obstructive hydrocephalus may further complicate apoplexy in large macroadenomas having a significant suprasellar component. Glandular destruction of varying degree is a regular pathologic feature of apoplexy, accounting for partial, total, transient, or permanent hypopituitarism. The posterior pituitary, having its own blood supply, generally escapes injury. Accordingly, diabetes insipidus is rarely an accompaniment of pituitary apoplexy.

Imaging studies will invariably reveal a sellar region mass, although CT scanning will reveal hemorrhage in only a minority of patients; the presence and extent of hemorrhage are best defined by MR imaging. The diagnosis should be considered in any patient presenting with acute headache and/or meningismus in whom the history or physical exam suggests a hypersecretory state or chronic hypopituitarism. In other patients, historical or clinical findings may be few and the initial picture may be typical of aneurysmal subarachnoid hemorrhage. Although the presence of a sellar mass on imaging studies will generally secure the correct diagnosis, it is worth mentioning that in as many as 4% of pituitary adenomas, a cerebral aneurysm may coexist (Weir 1992). Despite periodic suggestions to the contrary, pituitary apoplexy *is* a surgical emergency in which prompt action can be lifesaving, while maximizing chances for neurologic and visual recovery. The report of Ebersold et al (1983) established that rapid diagnosis of this condition, followed by steroid replacement and early transsphenoidal decompression, constitutes the therapy of choice for pituitary apoplexy. In that series, such an approach provided good to excellent results in 11 of 13 patients.

Metastatic tumors

As mentioned previously, metastatic tumors are generally more prone to undergo spontaneous hemorrhage than are primary tumors (Scott 1975, Salcman 1992). This fact tends to be more evident among clinicopathologic series in which pathologic material was studied, than in surgical surveys of tumor-associated hemorrhage. Among the metastatic tumors most prone to hemorrhage, metastatic melanoma, choriocarcinoma, and renal cell carcinoma are notoriously prominent. At least half of all choriocarcinomas and melanomas metastatic to brain can be expected to bleed (Graus et al 1985, Kondziolka et al 1987). Hemorrhage is also commonly observed in metastatic bronchogenic carcinoma, a fact more likely to be related to its great prevalence, rather than to an inherent hemorrhagic tendency. Like hemorrhages from primary brain tumors, bleeding from metastatic deposits may result in all major types of intracranial hemorrhage. The mechanisms responsible for hemorrhage in brain metastases are probably similar to those described above for primary tumors. An additional, though uncommon mechanism relates to embolic occlusion of cerebral vessels by clumps of tumor cells with resultant hemorrhagic infarction. This phenomenon has been observed in cardiac myxoma and other tumors. In the case of metastases, intercurrent coagulopathy, either primary or iatrogenic, often assumes greater importance.

Brain tumors mimicking cerebral ischemic syndromes

Somewhat less frequent than a hemorrhagic presentation is the occasional tendency for primary brain tumors to mimic ischemic cerebrovascular syndromes. 'Completed' ischemic stroke, stroke in evolution, and even transient ischemic attacks have all been perfectly imitated by an underlying brain tumor (Weissberg & Nice 1977). In one series of 905 patients, almost 3% of all brain tumor patients presented with a 'classic' stroke/TIA syndrome (Kondziolka et al 1987). The ability of brain tumors to masquerade as TIAs has been particularly striking, a phenomenon having received sufficient notoriety to be dubbed 'transient tumor attack' (Ross 1983). Transient symptoms of cerebral ischemia appear most likely to occur with tumors of the skull base, particularly meningiomas (Spallone 1980, Ross 1983). In one series of 210 supratentorial meningiomas, 17 patients presented with transient cerebral symptoms; some of the these probably represented seizure activity, but others appeared to have bona fide signs of anterior circulation TIAs (Daly et al 1961). Gliomas, too, have been known to mimic TIAs. In one lamentable account, an unsuspected glioblastoma so perfectly imitated occlusive extracranial carotid disease that a carotid endarterectomy was performed (Salcman 1990).

The basis by which brain tumors produce ischemic symptoms is unclear. In some symptomatic patients, occlusion of the carotid artery as a result of tumor encasement has been shown to coexist (Launay et al 1977, Spallone 1980). Although the gradual nature of the occlusive process would be expected to produce adequate collateral circulation, in selected instances thrombosis of the vessel and distal embolization are believed to be an underlying mechanism. Direct vascular occlusion aside, the other major mechanism proposed for tumor-related ischemia relates to arterial 'steal' in the region of the tumor with resultant peritumoral ischemia (Ross 1983). Certainly the rich vascularity and slow flow of such tumors might be expected to predispose to a steal phenomenon, however data actually documenting such an occurrence are scarce. Postirradiation arteriopathy may occasionally be a contributing factor in some patients; cerebral infarction has been reported in patients months or even years following radiation therapy for primary brain tumors (Mori et al 1978, Graus et al 1985).

Cerebrovascular complications are more common in patients with cerebral metastases than in patients with primary brain tumors. This is because intercurrent systemic effects such as nonthrombotic bacterial endocarditis and disseminated intravascular coagulation (DIC) may also coexist (Graus et al 1985).

OTHER EPIPHENOMENA OF BRAIN TUMORS

Seizures

Of the various 'epiphenomena' associated with brain tumors, seizures are numerically and diagnostically the most important. Whereas brain tumors account for only 3–5% of all cases of epilepsy, seizures complicate brain tumors in a third to one half of cases (Leblanc & Rasmussen 1974, Cascino 1990). The etiologic association between seizures and brain tumors tends to grow stronger with age. In the pediatric population, seizures are more apt to be the result of perinatal injury or various developmental conditions; tumors are responsible for only 0.5% of seizures in this age group. During middle age, brain tumors emerge as the single most frequent cause of new onset seizures (Penfield et al 1940). Brain tumors remain an important cause of seizures in the elderly, being eclipsed only by cerebrovascular disease, which is prevalent at this age. One study of new onset seizures in the elderly patient established a brain tumor etiology in 11% of patients (Ettinger & Shinnar 1993). Given this age-related etiologic association, it is axiomatic that any adult with new onset seizures be considered to have a brain tumor or other mass until proven otherwise. Additional features of the clinical history suggestive of a neoplastic etiology for seizures include: change in seizure pattern, status epilepticus, resistance to medical control, postictal paralysis, and associated neurologic symptoms (McKeran & Thomas 1980). Understandably, seizures resulting from brain tumor tend to be more often focal than generalized.

The likelihood that a brain tumor will generate seizures depends on a number of tumor-related factors, including location, histology, and rate of growth. Tumors located in the frontal, temporal, or parietal lobe are more likely to cause seizures than those situated in the occipital lobe, basal ganglia, or thalamus. As a rule, infratentorial tumors are not a source of seizures. The periodic accounts of seizures accompanying posterior fossa tumors have been loosely associated with the development of obstructive hydrocephalus and increased ICP, although the mechanism by which these phenomena facilitate seizures is unknown. Because the epileptogenicity of a neoplastic focus seems to be a phenomenon which evolves over time, seizures are more likely to occur in slow-growing 'benign' tumors than in rapidly growing malignant ones. Thus, low grade astrocytomas, oligodendrogliomas, and gangliogliomas are associated with seizures at some time in their course in at least 70% of cases (Ketz 1974, Cascino 1990, Berger et al 1991). Based on early retrospective reviews, the seizure frequency in various types of brain tumors is as follows: oligodendroglioma (75–95%); low grade astrocytoma (65–70%); meningiomas (60–67%); and glioblastomas (37%) (Ketz 1974, Leblanc & Rasmussen 1974). For metastatic tumors, the frequency of seizures is considerably lower. One recent retrospective review of 195 patients with cerebral metastases found that seizure was a presenting feature in only 18% of patients (Cohen et al 1988).

The pathophysiology underlying the generation of seizures by brain tumors remains speculative. One possibility is that brain tumors, like other structural lesions, non-specifically 'irritate' surrounding cortex as the result of mass effect, inflammation, and/or local ischemia. Although the latter two factors may contribute to epileptogenicity (Morris & Estes 1993), mass effect alone does not appear to correlate with the presence of seizures (Berger et al 1991). Disruption of the neurochemical circuitry in peritumoral cortex has also been proposed as an epileptogenic mechanism. Changes in GABA (γ-aminobutyric acid) and somatostatin have been identified in epileptic cortex adjacent to low grade gliomas (Haglund et al 1993).

The subject of brain tumors and epilepsy is reviewed in detail in Chapter 12.

Hematologic phenomena

It is widely known that hematologic abnormalities are commonly seen in cancer patients, manifesting clinically as thrombosis, bleeding, and susceptibility to infection. Far less well appreciated, however, is the fact that hematologic abnormalities may also accompany primary brain tumors, perhaps at a frequency far in excess of that which is currently acknowledged. Admittedly, the overall magnitude of the problem is far greater in the setting of malignancies arising systemically. Still, certain elements of the problem, such as the occurrence of deep vein thrombosis (DVT) in brain tumor patients, are sufficiently relevant that the relationship between brain tumors and hematologic dysfunction warrants some discussion.

It is convenient to categorize tumor-related hematologic disorders as being either thromboembolic or hemorrhagic in nature. A third category relates to infectious complications stemming from disorders of leukocytes. Although this latter problem has not been specifically studied, clinical experience has shown it to be of negligible importance in brain tumor patients, thus it is not discussed further. It should be mentioned, however, that leukocyte function and resistance to infection are both commonly impaired in brain tumor patients as the result of steroid therapy.

Thromboembolic complications

Thromboembolic complications have been generally regarded as an inherent risk of any intracranial procedure, a risk which has seemingly been more often related to the length of the operative procedure or the duration of patient immobility rather than to any specific effect of the underlying pathology. Accumulating evidence, however, suggests that such a view is not entirely valid, and that certain underlying conditions, specifically brain tumors, may dramatically increase the risk of thromboembolic phenomena, independently of other factors. In an early autopsy series of neurosurgical patients, the incidence of fatal postoperative pulmonary embolus was 3% (Wetzel et al 1960). In a second autopsy study focusing specifically on brain tumor patients, the prevalence of pulmonary embolism was 8.4% (Brisman & Mendell 1973). Similarly, the incidence of DVTs among autopsied patients with brain tumor has been shown to be 27.5%, contrasting with the 17% incidence identified in the control neurosurgical group (Kayser-Gatchalian & Kayser 1975).

The issue of which types of brain tumors are most apt to suffer from thromboembolic complications was recently addressed by Sawaya et al (1992) in a prospective study of 46 brain tumor patients. Using ^{125}I-fibrinogen scanning, they demonstrated DVTs in 72% of meningiomas, 60% of glioblastomas, and 20% of brain metastases. Importantly, no statistically significant correlation could be demonstrated between the presence of a DVT and various clinical factors such as length of operation, occurrence in a paretic limb, or ambulatory status. Thus, they concluded that the frequency of thromboembolic complications related specifically to tumor type.

Tumor location has also been proposed as a potential risk factor for thromboembolic complications. Several studies have shown suprasellar tumors to bear substantial risk (Brisman & Mendall 1973, Blabey et al 1975, Sjoberg et al 1976, Sawaya et al 1984, Al-Mefty et al 1985). In one of these reports, patients with suprasellar tumors were five times more likely to suffer pulmonary emboli than those with tumors situated elsewhere (Brisman & Mendall 1973). Not all studies, however, have equated a suprasellar location with increased risk (Constantini et al 1991).

While the foregoing data clearly establish brain tumor patients as being at increased risk for thromboembolic complications, the pathophysiologic basis of this enhanced thrombogenicity remains speculative. Early reports suggested that brain tumor patients suffered from increased platelet adhesiveness, a finding which was subsequently found to be more prominent among malignant brain tumors than benign ones (Nathanson & Savitsky 1952, Millac 1967). More recently, Sawaya & Highsmith (1992) suggested that brain tumors induce a complex prethrombotic state which is reminiscent of chronic disseminated intravascular coagulation (DIC) and believed to result, in part, from tumoral release of thrombogenic substances. Measurable abnormalities in the coagulation profile of brain tumor patients undergoing surgery were also recently documented (Iberti et al 1994). A significant reduction in the bleeding time and activated partial thromboplastin time (aPTT) was observed. The authors also raised the possibility that the common perioperative practice of maintaining brain tumor patients in a fluid-restricted and hyperosmolar state may further contribute to hypercoagulability.

Whatever the underlying mechanism, brain tumor patients are definitely at risk for thromboembolic complications. Thus, the use of prophylactic measures such as pneumatic compression devices should be routinely incorporated into the perioperative management of such patients. Once identified, proximal venous thrombosis warrants therapy, the nature of which includes anticoagulation and/or inferior vena caval filters, depending on the length of time since surgery. The management of thromboembolism in brain tumor patients and other neurosurgical conditions has been recently reviewed (Hamilton et al 1994).

Hypocoagulable states

Whereas the foregoing supports the existence of a hypercoagulable state in brain tumors, there exists the possibility that a tumor-induced hypocoagulable state may also occur. As discussed previously (see Vascular effects), spontaneous hemorrhage in brain tumors has most often been ascribed to the structural fragility of tumor vessels. The extent to which tumor-induced coagulopathy further contributes to both spontaneous and intraoperative hemorrhage is uncertain. There has been recent interest in various tumor-related plasminogen activators which are known to be produced by glial, meningeal, and metastatic brain tumors. Their capacity to disrupt local hemostasis in favor of an enhanced fibrinolytic state has been proposed as one mechanism potentially related to tumoral hemorrhage (reviewed in Sawaya & Highsmith 1988).

Miscellaneous hematologic abnormalities

The liberation of erythropoietin by hemangioblastomas is known to result in polycythemia. Noted in 15–20% of patients with cerebellar hemangioblastomas, paraneoplastic polycythemia occurs more frequently with this tumor than with any other human tumor (Golde et al 1981).

On rare occasions, meningiomas may be associated with polycythemia (Saint-Jean et al 1985), thrombocytosis

(Lartique et al 1987), and altered sedimentation rates (Mignot et al 1978).

Alterations in immunocompetence

In a theoretical sense, cancer can be regarded as disorder of immune surveillance, characterized by the failure of immune mechanisms appropriately to recognize and respond to, and effectively to curtail the proliferation of neoplastic cells. Although the concept is not new, it has gained momentum with the awareness that certain congenital or acquired perturbations of the immune system are associated with an increased risk of malignancy. Moreover, the documentation of impaired immune regulation in patients with cancers of various sorts lends further support to this hypothesis. The same has also been shown to be true of patients harboring gliomas, many of whom exhibit a marked and generalized depression of immune competence affecting both humoral and cellular effector systems. Sophisticated interpretation of these findings, however, continues to be handicapped by the relatively primitive status of contemporary immunology. Still, some understanding of the altered immunity accompanying gliomas has emerged, and this is briefly summarized below. Such knowledge is also important as a prelude to the rational use of immunotherapy, wherein the goal is restoration and/or fortification of defective components of the immune axis.

Because of their role in tumor cell lysis, cell-mediated immune mechanisms assume foremost importance in the context of tumor immunology. Defects in cell-mediated immunity are reflected by an impaired delayed hypersensitivity reaction in response to a number of subcutaneously administered test antigens, such as PPD, *Candida*, and dinitrochlorbenzene. In their landmark studies of cellular immunity, Mahaley et al (1977) documented the presence of defective cell-mediated immunity in malignant gliomas. As revealed by an impaired delayed hypersensitivity reaction to various antigens, the magnitude of cellular anergy was proportional to the presence and extent of anaplasia within the glioma. Moreover, sequential testing revealed that tumor progression was accompanied by a stepwise decline in cellular anergy. Similar defects are not observed in low grade gliomas.

The obvious sequel to the foregoing observations was to determine the role played by T lymphocytes in undermining the cell-mediated response. Malignant glioma patients were shown to have a quantitative defect in T-cell number, as the complement of circulating T-helper cells was shown to be disproportionately reduced by 30% (Roszman et al 1982). Qualitative defects in T-cell function have also been documented. Peripheral blood lymphocytes from patients with malignant gliomas have been studied in vitro for blastogenic responses to T-cell antigens; whereas depressed blastogenic responses were observed in half of all lymphocyte samples from glioblastoma patients, the response was preserved in lymphocytes from patients with low grade gliomas (Young et al 1976). A more recent proposal suggests that T-cell dysfunction in malignant gliomas may result from decreased secretion of interleukin 2 (IL-2) and/or decreased expression of the IL-2 receptor (Elliot et al 1987, Yoshida et al 1987). The latter is an important cytokine which stimulates the proliferation and differentiation of antigen-primed cytotoxic T lymphocytes, one of the principal effectors of tumor cell destruction. A final mechanism accounting for impaired cellular responses in malignant gliomas relates to tumoral secretion of various suppressive factors which would impair proliferation and/or function of T lymphocytes. One such factor is transforming growth factor β_2 (TGF-β_2) (Wrann et al 1987). Known to be a secretory product of glioblastomas, this growth factor is believed to inhibit T-cell proliferation and the generation of cytotoxic T cells via an IL-2-dependent mechanism.

One of the unexplained curiosities of gliomas relates to the frequent finding of a cellular infiltrate composed of lymphocytes and monocytes on histologic sections of gliomas. Such a pattern can be detected in more than half of all malignant glioma specimens (Ridley & Cavannaugh 1971). It was originally proposed that this infiltrate may be a manifestation of host resistance, akin to the better known host versus graft rejection response. Immunotyping of the cells constituting this infiltrate suggested a preponderance of $CD8^+$ T cells (von Hanwher et al 1984). This phenotypic designation refers to cells of the suppressor or cytotoxic types, believed to be essential to tumor immunity. Although clinicopathologic correlations have been drawn between the presence/nature of this infiltrate and various clinical parameters, including survival, these data have neither been entirely consistent nor convincing (Brooks et al 1978, Palma et al 1978, Rossi et al 1989). This infiltrate does have one important and perhaps encouraging aspect. It establishes malignant gliomas as being accessible to effector cells arising in the periphery, which has obvious immunotherapeutic relevance.

REFERENCES

Aarabi B, Long D M 1979 Dynamics of cerebral edema. The role of an intact vascular bed in the production and propagation of vasogenic edema. Journal of Neurosurgery 51: 779–784

Albright A L 1992 Posterior fossa tumors. Neurosurgery Clinics of North America 3: 881–891

Al-Mefty O, Holoubi A, Rifai A, Fox J L 1985 Microsurgical removal of suprasellar meningiomas. Neurosurgery 16: 364–372

Baethmann A, Oettinger W, Rothenfulsser W et al 1980 Brain edema factors: Current state with special reference to plasma constituents and glutamate. Advances in Neurology 28: 171–178

Baethmann A, Maier-Hauff K, Kempski O et al 1988 Mediators of brain edema and secondary brain damage. Critical Care Medicine 16: 972–978

Bar-Sella P, Frost D, Hardoff R et al 1979 Ultrastructural basis for different pertechnetate uptake patterns by various human tumors. Journal of Neurology Neurosurgery and Psychiatry 42: 924–930

Bedford R F, Morris L, Jane J A 1982 Intracranial hypertension during surgery for supratentorial tumor: Correlation with preoperative computed tomography scans. Anesthesia and Analgesia 61: 430–433

Benzel E C, Gelder F B 1988 Correlation between sex hormone binding and peritumoral edema in intracranial meningiomas. Neurosurgery 23: 169–174

Berger M S, Ghatan S, Geyer J R et al 1991 Seizure outcome in children with hemispheric tumors and associated intractable epilepsy: The role of tumor removal combined with seizure foci resection. Pediatric Neurosurgery 17: 185–191

Bhio C C, Baba T, Black K L 1992 Selective blood-tumor barrier disruption by leukotrienes. Journal of Neurosurgery 77: 407–410

Bilsky M, Posner J B 1993 Intensive and postoperative care of intracranial tumors. In: Ropper A H (ed) Neurological and neurosurgical intensive care, 3rd edn. Raven Press, New York, pp 309–329

Blabey R G, Weil R III, Santuli T V 1975 Iliofemoral thrombophlebitis associated with central nervous system pathology. American Journal of Surgery 130: 315–316

Black K L, Hoff J T, McGillicuddy J E, Gebarski S S 1986 Increased leukotriene C4 and vasogenic edema surrounding brain tumors in humans. Annals of Neurology 19: 592–595

Black K L, King W L, Ikezaki K 1990 Selective opening of the blood-tumor barrier by intracarotid infusion of leukotriene C4. Journal of Neurosurgery 72: 912–916

Bradac G B, Ferszt R, Bender A, Schorner W 1986 Peritumoral edema in meningiomas. A radiological and histological study. Neuroradiology 28: 304–312

Bradbury M W B 1985 The blood-brain barrier. Circulation Research 57; 2: 213–222

Brisman R, Mendell J 1973 Thromboembolism and brain tumor. Journal of Neurosurgery 38: 337–338

Broadwell R D 1993 Endothelial cell biology and the enigma of transcytosis through the blood-brain barrier. In: Drewes L R, Betz A L (eds) Frontiers in cerebral vascular biology: Transport and its regulation. Plenum Press, New York, pp 137–141

Brooks W H, Markesbury W R, Gupta G D, Roszman T L 1978 Relationship of lymphocyte invasion and survival of brain tumor patients. Annals of Neurology 4: 249–224

Brown J K 1991 Mechanisms of production of raised intracranial pressure. In: Minns R A (ed) Problems of intracranial pressure in childhood. Mac Keith Press, London, pp 13–35

Capildeo R (ed) 1989 Steroids in diseases of the central nervous system. John Wiley, Chichester, pp 1–306

Cardoso E R, Petersen E W 1984 Pituitary apoplexy: a review. Neurosurgery 14: 363–373

Cascino G D 1990 Epilepsy and brain tumors: Implications for treatment. Epilepsia 3: (suppl) S37–S34

Chan P H, Fishman R A 1984 The role of arachidonic acid in vasogenic brain edema. Federation Proceedings 43: 210–213

Ciric I, Ammirati M, Vick N, Mikheal M 1987 Supratentorial gliomas: Surgical considerations and immediate postoperative results. Neurosurgery 21: 21–26

Cohen N, Strauss G, Lew R et al 1988 Should prophylactic anticonvulsants be administered to patients with newly diagnosed cerebral metastases? A retrospective analysis. Journal of Clinical Oncology 6: 1621–1624

Condon B, Patterson J, Wyper D et al 1986 A quantitative index of ventricular and extraventricular intracranial CSF volumes using MRI. Journal of Computer Assisted Tomography 10: 784–792

Condon B, Patterson J, Jenkins A et al 1987 MR relaxation times of cerebrospinal fluid. Journal of Computer Assisted Tomography 11(2): 203–207

Connolly D T 1991 Vascular permeability factor: a unique regulator of blood vessel function. Journal of Cell Biochemistry 47: 219–223

Constantini S, Cotev S, Rappaport H, Pomeranz S, Shalit M N 1988 Intracranial pressure monitoring after elective intracranial surgery. Journal of Neurosurgery 69: 540–544

Constantini S, Kornowski R, Pomeranz S, Rappaport H 1991 Thromboembolic phenomena in neurosurgical patients operated for primary and metastatic brain tumors. Acta Neurochirurgica (Wein) 109: 93–97

Constantini S, Tamir J, Gomori M J, Shohami 1993 Tumor prostaglandin levels correlated with edema surrounding meningiomas. Neurosurgery 33: 204–211

Cornfield B M 1985 The blood-brain barrier, a dynamic regulatory interface. Molecular Physiology 7: 219–260

Cowel R L, Siqueira E B, George E 1970 Angiographic demonstration of glioma involving the wall of the anterior cerebral artery. Report of a case. Radiology 97: 577–578

Crone K R, Challa V R, Kute T E, Moody D M, Kelly D L Jr 1988 Relationship between flow cytometric features and clinical behavior of meningiomas. Neurosurgery 23: 720–724

Cuneo R A, Caronna J J, Pitts L et al 1979 Syndrome of upward cerebellar herniation. Archives of Neurology 36: 618–623

Cunha E Sa M, Quest D O 1993 Complications in the surgery of meningiomas. In: Post K D, Friedman E, McCormick P (eds) Postoperative complications in intracranial neurosurgery. Thieme Medical Publishers, New York, pp 35–49

Daly D D, Svien H J, Yoss R E 1961 Intermittent cerebral symptoms with meningiomas. Archives of Neurology 5: 287–293

Del Maestro R F, Mattar A G 1988 The influence of ibuprofen on patients with peritumoral edema. Canadian Journal of Neurological Science 15: 227 (abstract)

Del Maestro R F, Megyesi J F, Farrell C L 1990 Mechanisms of tumor-associated edema: A review. Canadian Journal of Neurological Sciences 17: 177–183

Ebersold M J, Laws E R Jr, Scheithauer B W, Randall R V 1983 Pituitary adenomas treated by transphenoidal surgery. A clinicopathological and immunocytochemical study. Journal of Neurosurgery 58: 315–320

Ehrlich P 1885 Das Sauerstoff-Bedurnfniss des Oraganismus. Eine farbenanalytische Studie. Berlin, Hirschwold, (cited by Friedmann 1942)

Elliot L H, Brooks W H, Roszman T L 1987 Role of interleukin-2 (IL-2) and IL-2 receptor expression in the proliferative defect observed in mitogen-stimulated lymphocytes from patients with gliomas. Journal of the National Cancer Institute 78: 919–922

Ettinger A B, Shinnar 1993 New-onset seizures in an elderly hospitalized population. Neurology 43: 489–492

Fadul C, Wood J, Thaler H, Galichich J, Patterson R H, Posner J B 1988 Morbidity and mortality of craniotomy for excision of supratentorial gliomas. Neurology 36: 1374–1379

Fishman R A 1975 Brain edema. New England Journal of Medicine 293: 706–711

Fishman R A 1992 Cerebrospinal fluid diseases of the nervous system, 2nd edn. WB Saunders, Philadelphia, pp 1–431

Friedmann U 1942 Blood-brain barrier. Physiology Reviews 22: 125–145

Gazendam J, Go K G, van Zanten A K 1979 Composition of isolated edema fluid in cold-induced brain edema. Journal of Neurosurgery 51: 70–77

Gilbert J J, Paulseth J E, Coates R K, Malott D 1983 Cerebral edema associated with meningiomas. Neurosurgery 12: 599–605

Glass B, Abbott K H (1955) Subarachnoid hemorrhage consequent to intracranial tumors. Review of the literature and report of seven cases. American Medical Association Archives of Neurology and Psychiatry 73: 369–379

Go K G, Wilmink J T, Molenaar W M 1988 Peritumoral brain edema associated with meningiomas. Neurosurgery 23: 175–179

Golde D W, Hocking W G, Koeffler H P et al 1981 Polycythemia: Mechanisms and management. Annals of Internal Medicine 95: 71–87

Goldman C K, Kim J, Wong W L, King V, Brock T, Gillespie G Y 1993 Epidermal growth factor stimulates vascular endothelial growth factor production by human malignant glioma cells: a model of glioblastoma multiforme pathophysiology. Mol Bio Cell 4: 121–133

Goldmann E E 1913 Vitalfarbung an Zentralnervensystem. Abh Preuss, Akad. Wiss Phys Math 1: 1–60 (cited by Friedmann 1942)

Goldstein G W, Betz A L 1986 The blood-brain barrier. Scientific American 255; 3: 74–83
Graus F, Rogers L R, Posner J B 1985 Cerebrovascular complications in patients with cancer. Medicine 64: 16–35
Grieg N H 1989 Brain tumors and the blood-brain barrier. In: Neuwelt E A (ed) Implications of the blood-brain barrier and its manipulation, vol 2. Plenum Press, New York, pp 77–106
Haglund M M, Berger M S, Kunkel D D et al 1992 Changes in gamma-aminobutyric acid and somatostatin in epileptic cortex associated with low-grade gliomas. Journal of Neurosurgery 77: 209–214
Hamilton M G, Hull R D, Pineo G F 1994 Venous thromboembolism in neurosurgery and neurology patients: A review. Neurosurgery 34: 280–296
Harsh G R, Wilson C B 1990 Neuroepithelial tumors of the adult brain. In: Youmans J R (ed) Neurological surgery, 3rd edn. pp 3046
Huk W J, Gadermann G, Friedmann G 1990 MRI of central nervous system diseases. Springer-Verlag, Berlin, pp 115–116
Iberti T J, Miller M, Abalos A et al 1994 Abnormal coagulation profile in brain tumor patients during surgery. Neurosurgery 34: 389–395
Jelsma R, Bucy P C 1967 The treatment of glioblastoma multiforme of the brain. Journal of Neurosurgery 27: 388–400
Johansson B B 1990 The physiology of the blood-brain barrier. In: Porter J C, Jezova D (eds) Circulating regulatory factors and neuroendocrine function. Plenum Press, New York, pp 25–39
Joo F 1993 Minireview: regulation by second messengers of permeability in the cerebral microvessels. Neurobiology 1: 3–10
Joo F, Klatzo I 1989 Role of cerebral endothelium in brain oedema. Neurological Research 11: 67–75
Kayser-Gatchalian M C, Kayser K 1975 Thrombosis and intracranial tumors. Journal of Neurology 209: 217–224
Ketz E 1974 Brain tumors and epilepsy In: Vinkin P J, Bruyn G W (eds) Handbook of clinical neurology, vol 16. North Holland Publishing, Amsterdam, pp 254–269
King W A, Black K L, Ikezaki K, Conklin S, Becker D P 1991 Tumor-associated neurological dysfunction prevented by lazeroids in rats. Journal of Neurosurgery 74: 112–115
Klatzo I 1967 Neuropathological aspects of brain edema. Journal of Neuropathology and Experimental Neurology 26: 1–14
Kohli C M, Crouch R L 1984 Meningiomas with intracerebral hematoma. Neurosurgery 15: 237–240
Kondziolka D, Bernstein M, Resch L, Tator C H, Flemming J F R, Vanderlinden R G, Schutz H 1987 Significance of hemorrhage into brain tumors: clinicopathological study. Journal of Neurosurgery 67: 852–857
Langfitt T W 1975 Clinical methods for monitoring intracranial pressure and measuring cerebral blood flow. Clinical Neurosurgery 22: 302–320
Langfitt T W, Weinstein J D, Kassell N F, Simone F A 1964a Transmission of increased intracranial pressures. I. Within the craniospinal axis. Journal of Neurosurgery 21: 989–997
Langfitt T W, Weinstein J D, Kassell N F, Gagliardi W 1964b Transmission of increased intracranial pressure. II. Within the supratentorial space. Journal of Neurosurgery 21: 998–1005
Lartique C, Roualdes G, Guilhot F, Maissin F, Deglaire B, Mezc M 1987 Méningiome cérébral associé á une thrombocytose. Presse Med 16: 637
Launay M, Fredy D, Merland J J, Bories 1977 Narrowing and occlusion of arteries by intracranial tumors. Neuroradiology 14: 117–126
Le Blanc F E, Rasmussen T 1974 Cerebral seizures and brain tumors. In: Vinken P J, Bruyn G W (eds) Handbook of clinical neurology, vol 15. The epilepsies. North Holland Publishing, Amsterdam, pp 295–301
Lindley J G, Challa V R, Kelly D L 1991 Meningiomas and brain edema. In: Al-Mefty O (ed) Meningiomas. Raven Press, New York, pp 59–73
Liwnicz B H, Wu S Z, Tew J M 1987 The relationship between the capillary structure and hemorrhage in gliomas. Journal of Neurosurgery 66: 536–541
Lofgren J, Zwetnow N N 1973 Cranial and spinal components of the cerebrospinal pressure-volume curve. Acta Neurologica Scandinavica 49: 575–585
Long D 1970 Capillary ultrastructure and the blood-brain barrier in human malignant brain tumors. Journal of Neurosurgery 32: 127–144
Long D 1973 Vascular ultrastructure in human meningiomas and schwannomas. Journal of Neurosurgery 38: 409–419
Long D 1979 Capillary ultrastructure in human metastatic brain tumors. Journal of Neurosurgery 51: 53–58
Lundberg N 1960 Continuous recording and control of ventricular fluid pressure in neurosurgical practice. Acta Psychiatria et Neurologica Scandinavica 36 (suppl 149): 1–193
Luse S 1960 Electron microscopic studies of brain tumors. Neurology (NY) 18: 881–905
Mahaley M S, Brooks W H, Roszman T L et al 1977 Depressed cell-mediated immunity in patients with primary intracranial tumors. Part 1: Studies of cellular and humoral immune competence of brain-tumor patients. Journal of Neurosurgery 46: 467–476
Maiuri F, Gangemi M, Cirillo S et al 1987 Cerebral edema associated with meningiomas. Surgical Neurology 27: 64–68
Marmarou A, Shulman K, Rosende R M 1978 A nonlinear analysis of the cerebrospinal fluid system and intracranial pressure dynamics. Journal of Neurosurgery 48: 332–334
Megyesi J F, Farrell C L, Del Maestro R F 1990 Investigation of an inhibitor of lipid peroxidation U74006F on tumor growth and protein extravasation on the C6 astrocytoma spheroid implantation glioma model. Journal of Neuro-Oncology 8: 135–137
Mignot B, Hauw J J, Pasquier P, Herve de Sigalony J P, Bricaire F 1978 Perturbations biologiques réversibles, évoluant parallélement a un méningiome récidivant et avec métastases. Sem Hop Paris 54: 1231–1237
Millac P 1967 Platelet stickiness in patients with intracranial tumors. British Medical Journal 4: 25–26
Mohr G, Hardy J 1982 Hemorrhage, necrosis, and apoplexy in pituitary adenomas. Surgical Neurology 18: 181–189
Mori K, Takeuchi J, Ishikawa M, Handa H, Yoyama M, Yamaki T 1978 Occlusive arteriopathy and brain tumor. Journal of Neurosurgery 49: 22–27
Morris H H, Estes M L 1993 Brain tumors and chronic epilepsy. In: Wyllie (ed) The treatment of epilepsy: Principles and practice. Lea & Febiger, Philadelphia, pp 659–666
Nathanson M, Savitsky J P 1952 Platelet adhesive index studies in multiple sclerosis and other neurological disorders. Bulletin of the New York Academy of Medicine 28: 462–468
Neuwelt E A 1989a Implications of the blood-brain barrier and its manipulation, vol 1. Plenum Press, New York, pp 1–403
Neuwelt E A 1989b Implications of the blood-brain barrier and its manipulation, vol 2. Plenum Press, New York, pp 1–633
Nystrom S 1960 Pathological changes in blood vessels of human glioblastoma multiforme. Comparative studies using plastic casting, angiography, light microscopy and electron microscopy with reference to some other brain tumors. Acta Pathol Microbiol Scand 49: 1–185
Palma L, DeLorenzo N, Guidetti B 1978 Lymphocytic infiltrates in primary glioblastomas and recidivous gliomas: incidence, fat and relevance to prognosis in 228 operated cases. Journal of Neurosurgery 49: 854–861
Pappius H M 1989 Cerebral edema and the blood-brain barrier. In: Neuwelt E A (ed) Implications of the blood-brain barrier and its manipulation, vol 1. Plenum Press, New York, pp 293–310
Pardrige W M 1988 Recent advances in blood-brain barrier transport. Annual Review of Pharmacology and Toxicology 28: 25–39
Penfield W, Erickson T C, Tarlov I 1940 Relation of intracranial tumors and symptomatic epilepsy. Archives of Neurology and Psychiatry 44: 300–315
Phillipon J, Foncin J F, Grob R, Srour A, Poisson M, Pertuiset B F 1984 Cerebral edema associated with meningiomas: Possible role of a secretory-excitatory phenomenon. Neurosurgery 14: 295–301
Plum F, Posner J B 1980 The diagnosis of stupor and coma, 3rd edn. F A Davis, Philadelphia, pp 1–176
Reese T S, Karnovsky M J 1967 Fine structural localization of a bloodbrain barrier to exogenous peroxidase. Journal of Cellular Biology 34: 207–217
Reulen H-J, Huber P, Ito U, Groger U 1990 Peritumoral brain edema. Advances in Neurology 52: 307–315
Ridley A, Cavenaugh J B 1971 Lymphocytic infiltration in gliomas: Evidence of possible host resistance. Brain 94: 117–124

Rosner M J, Becker D P 1984 Origin and evolution of plateau waves: experimental observations and a theoretical model. Journal of Neurosurgery 60: 312–324

Ross R T 1983 Transient tumor attacks. Archives of Neurology 40: 633–636

Rossi M L, Jones N R, Candy E et al 1989 The mononuclear cell infiltrate compared with survival in high-grade astrocytomas. Acta Neuropathologica 78: 189–193

Roszman T L, Brooks W H, Elliott L H 1982 Immunobiology of primary intracranial tumors, VI: suppressor cell function and lectin-binding lymphocyte subpopulations in patients with cerebral tumors. Cancer 50: 1273–1279

Saint-Jean O, Boffa G A, Bouchon J P, Verret J 1985 Polyglobuline secondaire avec hyper-erythropoiétinémie. Méningiome sustenoriel. Rev Neurol (Paris) 141: 143–145

Salcman M 1990 Neoplastic emergencies. In: Salcman M (ed) Neurologic emergencies. Raven Press, New York, pp 121

Salcman M 1992 Intracranial hemorrhage caused by brain tumor. In: Kaufman H H (ed) Intracerebral hematomas. Raven Press, New York, pp 95–106

Salcman M, Broadwell R D 1991 The blood brain barrier. In: Salcman M (ed) Neurobiology of brain tumors. Williams & Wilkins, Baltimore, pp 229–249

Sawaya R, Highsmith R 1988 Brain tumors and the fibrinolytic enzyme system. In: Kornblith P L, Walker M D (eds) Advances in neuro-oncology. Futura, Mount Kisco, New York, pp 103–157

Sawaya R, Highsmith R F 1992 Postoperative venous thromboembolism and brain tumors: Part III. Biochemical profile. Journal of Neuro-Oncology 14: 113–118

Sawaya R, DeCourten-Myers G, Copeland B 1984 Massive preoperative pulmonary embolism and suprasellar brain tumor: Case report and review of the literature. Neurosurgery 15: 566–571

Sawaya R, Zuccarrello M, Elkalliny M, Nishiyama H 1992 Postoperative venous thromboembolism and brain tumors: Part I. Clinical profile. Journal of Neuro-Oncology 14: 119–125

Scott M 1975 Spontaneous intracerebral hematoma caused by cerebral neoplasms. Journal of Neurosurgery 43: 338–342

Shapiro W R, Hiesiger E M, Cooney G A et al 1990 Temporal effects of dexamethasone on the blood-to-brain and blood-to-tumor transport of 14C-alpha-aminoiso-butyric acid in rat C6 gliomas. Journal of Neurooncology 8: 197–202

Sjoberg H E, Blomback M, Granberg P O 1976 Thromboembolic complications, heparin treatment and increase in coagulation factors in Cushing's syndrome. Acta Med Scand 199: 95–98

Smith H P, Challa V R, Moody D M, Kelly D R Jr 1981 Biological features of meningiomas that determine the production of cerebral edema. Neurosurgery 8: 428–433

Smyth G E, Henderson W R 1938 Observation on the cerebrospinal fluid pressure on simultaneous ventricular and lumbar punctures. Journal of Neurology and Psychiatry 1: 226–237

Spallone A 1980 Occlusion of the internal carotid artery by intracranial tumors. Surgical Neurology 15: 51–57

Stevens J M, Ruiz J S, Kendall B E 1983 Observations on peritumoral oedema in meningiomas. Part II: Mechanisms of oedema production. Neuroradiology 25: 125–131

Stewart P A, Hayakawa K, Farrell C L, Del Maestro R F 1987 Quantitative study of microvessel ultrastructure in human peritumoral brain tissue: Evidence for a blood-brain barrier defect. Journal of Neurosurgery 67: 697–705

Teasdale E, Cardoso E, Galbraith S, Teasdale G 1984 A new CT scan appearance with raised intracranial pressure in severe diffuse head injury. Journal of Neurology, Neurosurgery, and Psychiatry 47: 600–603

Unterberg A, Schmidt W, Wahl M, Ellis E, Marmarou A, Baethmann A 1991 Evidence against leukotrienes as mediators of brain edema. Journal of Neurosurgery 74: 773–780

Vassilouthis J, Ambrose J 1979 Computerized tomography scanning appearances of intracranial meningiomas. An attempt to predict histological features. Journal of Neurosurgery 50: 320–327

Vastine J H, Kinney K K 1927 The pineal shadow as an aid in the localization of brain tumors. American Journal of Roentgenology 17: 320–324

von Hanwher R I, Hofman F M, Taylor C R, Apuzzo M L J 1984 Mononuclear lymphoid populations infiltrating the microenvironment of primary CNS tumors: characterization of cell subsets with monoclonal antibodies. Journal of Neurosurgery 60: 1138–1147

Wahl M, Unterberg A, Baethmann A, Schilling L 1990 Mediators of vasogenic brain edema. Journal of Basic and Clinical Physiology and Pharmacology 1: 221–233

Wakai S, Yamakowa K, Manaka S, Takakura K 1982 Spontaneous intracranial hemorrhage caused by brain tumor. Its incidence and clinical significance. Neurosurgery 10: 437–444

Weir B 1992 Pituitary tumors and aneurysm: Case report and review of the literature. Neurosurgery 30: 585–591

Weisberg L A, Nice C N 1977 Intracranial tumors simulating the presentation of cerebrovascular syndromes. Early detection with cerebral computed tomography (CCT). American Journal of Medicine 63: 517–524

Welch K 1980 The intracranial pressure in infancy. Journal of Neurosurgery 52: 693–699

Wetzel N, Anderson M C, Shields T W 1960 Pulmonary embolism as a cause of death in neurosurgical patients. Journal of Neurosurgery 17: 664–668

Wrann M, Bodmer S, de Martin R et al 1987 T-cell suppressor factor from human glioblastoma cells is a 12.5 kd protein closely related to transforming growth factor-beta. EMBO Journal 6: 1633–1636

Yamada K, Ushio Y, Hayakawa T 1989 Effects of steroids on the blood brain barrier. In: Neuwelt E A (ed) Implications of the blood-brain barrier and its manipulation, vol 2. Plenum Press, New York, pp 53–76

Yoshida S, Takai N, Tanaka R 1987 Functional analysis of interleukin-2 in immune surveillance against brain tumors. Neurosurgery 21: 627–630

Young H F, Sakalas R, Kaplan A M 1976 Inhibition of cell-mediated immunity in patients with brain tumors. Surgical Neurology 5: 19–23

Yu Z Y, Wrange O, Boethiars J et al 1981 A study of glucocorticoid receptors in intracranial tumors. Journal of Neurosurgery 55: 757–760

10. Clinical, imaging and laboratory diagnosis of brain tumors

Peter Black Patrick Y. Wen

INTRODUCTION

The diagnosis of brain tumors is changing considerably as more sophisticated diagnostic techniques evolve. The physician should be aware of the subtlety of presentation of brain tumors in many patients and the need for efficient and expeditious diagnosis. A single seizure, a loss of interest in usual activities, or a loss of hearing for high frequencies may all be signs of a tumor, and the physician is well advised to have a high index of suspicion in these settings.

In this chapter the clinical, imaging, and laboratory diagnosis of brain tumors will be discussed, followed by a review of the diagnosis of specific tumors.

A. CLINICAL DIAGNOSIS

Patients with brain tumors typically present with headaches, seizures, nonspecific cognitive or personality changes, or focal neurologic signs (Thomas & McKeran 1990, Jaeckle 1991, Wen & Schiff 1993). As a result of the widespread availability of sensitive imaging techniques, such as magnetic resonance imaging (MRI), tumors are being detected at an earlier stage and patients have increasingly subtle clinical symptoms and signs at diagnosis.

Headaches

Headaches are the presenting symptom in approximately 35% of patients with brain tumors and develop during the course of the disease in 70% (McKeran & Thomas 1980). The majority of these headaches are intermittent and nonspecific. They are generally dull, non-throbbing and often indistinguishable from tension headaches (Rushton & Rooke 1962, Forsyth & Posner 1992). The headaches are usually on the same side as the tumor. Supratentorial tumors usually produce headaches with a frontal location since the majority of supratentorial pain-sensitive structures are supplied by the trigeminal nerve. The posterior fossa is innervated by cranial nerves IX and X and upper cervical nerves, and usually produces pain in the occipital region and neck. Occasionally posterior fossa tumors can produce headaches located in the vertex or retro-orbital region (Jaeckle 1991). Certain features of the headache increase the possibility of a tumor. These include headaches that wake the patient at night (10–32%) or are worse on waking and improve over the course of the day (15–36%), headaches exacerbated by postural change, coughing or exercise (20–32%), headaches of recent onset that are different from the patient's usual headaches or are greater in severity, the presence of nausea or vomiting (30–40%), papilledema or focal neurologic signs (Jaeckle 1991, Forsyth & Posner 1992). Patients with these features usually require further evaluation with CT or MRI scanning.

Papilledema

Papilledema is important evidence of increased intracranial pressure transmitted through the optic nerve sheath. The incidence of papilledema in an older series of patients with brain tumors has been reported to be 50–70% (McKeran & Thomas 1980). Advances in neuro-imaging have resulted in many patients being diagnosed at an earlier stage, and the incidence of papilledema in patients with brain tumor today is probably much lower. In a recent review of 100 consecutive patients with malignant gliomas who underwent surgery at Brigham and Women's Hospital, only 8% had papilledema at the time of diagnosis (El-Ouahabi et al, unpublished data). Papilledema tends to be more common in children, in slowly growing tumors and in posterior fossa tumors. It may be associated with symptoms of transient obscuration of vision, especially with postural change.

Seizures

Seizures are the presenting symptom in approximately one third of patients with brain tumors and are present at some stage of the illness in 50–70% of patients (McKeran & Thomas 1980). Approximately half the patients have focal seizures and the other half have generalized seizures. In patients with gliomas, seizures occur in 59% of frontal tumors, 42% of parietal tumors, 35% of temporal tumors and 33% of occipital tumors (Scott & Gibberd 1980). Tumors in subcortical areas such as thalamus and the posterior fossa are much less epileptogenic. Slowly growing tumors and tumors located near the Rolandic fissure are particularly likely to cause seizures. Approximately 10–20% of adult patients with new onset seizures have brain tumors (Dam et al 1985) and these patients should almost always have CT or MRI scanning as part of their evaluation, especially if they also have focal findings on examination or on electroencephalography. Patients with malignant gliomas who present with seizure tend to have a better prognosis (Gehan & Walker 1977).

Altered mental status

Mental status changes are the initial symptom in 15–20% of patients with brain tumors and are frequently present in patients by the time of diagnosis (McKeran & Thomas 1980). These changes may range from subtle problems with concentration, memory, affect, personality, initiative and abstract reasoning to severe cognitive problems and confusion. Changes in mentation are especially common in frontal lobe tumors but will also occur in patients with increased intracranial pressure or gliomatosis cerebri. With increasing intracranial pressure there is also depression of the level of consciousness, resulting in drowsiness and eventually leading to stupor and coma if treatment is not given.

Focal neurologic symptoms and signs

Whereas headaches, seizures and altered mental status may be seen with tumors in many locations, certain clinical features have specific localizing value.

Cortical tumors

Frontal lobe tumors are often clinically silent initially. As the tumor enlarges there may be personality changes such as disinhibition, irritability, impaired judgement and lack of initiative (abulia). In addition there may be hemiparesis, seizures, aphasia, urinary frequency and urgency and gait difficulties. Gaze preference and primitive reflexes, such as forced grasping and snout, may be present. Meningiomas of the olfactory groove may produce anosmia.

Temporal lobe tumors frequently cause seizures. These include simple partial seizures characterized by olfactory and gustatory hallucinations, déjà vu, and feelings of fear and pleasure, and complex partial seizures characterized by impairment of consciousness, repetitive psychomotor movements and automatic behavior. Temporal lobe tumors may also cause memory disturbances, visual field defects (superior quadrantanopsia), and when the dominant temporal lobe is involved, aphasia.

Tumors of the parietal lobe can produce contralateral sensory loss, involving particularly joint position sense, two-point discrimination, stereognosis and graphesthesia, although other modalities are also involved. Lesions in the dominant parietal lobe are associated with aphasia, while lesions in the non-dominant parietal lobe may result in neglect of the contralateral side and the loss of ability to acknowledge deficits (anosognosia). There may also be hemiparesis, homonymous visual defects (or neglect), agnosias, apraxias, sensory seizures, and disturbance of visual spatial ability.

Occipital lobe astrocytomas may cause homonymous hemianopsia, and less commonly visual seizures characterized by lights, colors and formed geometric patterns. Tumors at the parieto-occipital junction may produce visual agnosias such as aprosopagnosia (inability to recognize faces) or Balint's syndrome.

Brainstem tumors

Thalamic tumors may produce contralateral sensory loss, hemiparesis, cognitive impairment and occasionally visual defects and aphasia. Obstructive hydrocephalus occurs commonly and is associated with headache, nausea, vomiting, gait unsteadiness and urinary incontinence.

Brainstem tumors produce cranial neuropathies, weakness, numbness, ataxia and occasionally vertigo, nausea, vomiting and hiccups. As the tumor increases in size there may be compression of the aqueduct or the fourth ventricle producing hydrocephalus.

Pineal region and third ventricular tumors

Pineal tumors present either with symptoms of hydrocephalus resulting from compression of the third ventricle and aqueduct or with symptoms produced by compression of the tectum of the midbrain. Midbrain compression may result in disturbance of extraocular function including Parinaud's syndrome characterized by impairment of upgaze and pupillary light-accommodation reflex disturbance. Occasionally children may present with precocious puberty.

Tumors around the third ventricle may produce hydrocephalus. Valsalva maneuvers and positional changes may increase CSF obstruction and lead to severe headaches and occasionally leg weakness and syncope. Tumors in this region may also produce symptoms resulting from hypothalamic dysfunction, autonomic dysfunction and impaired memory.

Cerebellar tumors

Headaches and ataxia are the two most common symptoms in patients with cerebellar tumors. The headaches may be due to the tumor or from hydrocephalus. They are often occipital and associated with nausea, vomiting and occasionally neck stiffness. Some patients may experience vertigo. Midline cerebellar lesions may produce truncal ataxia while lesions in the cerebellar hemispheres may cause appendicular ataxia, although frequently the findings are relatively subtle. Examination may also show nystagmus, hypotonia and frequently cranial nerve and corticospinal tract signs from brainstem compression. Head tilt away from the lesion may occur with incipient tonsillar herniation.

Cranial nerves

Skull base tumors frequently affect cranial nerves. The pattern of involvement and the presence of accompanying neurologic signs depend on the location of the tumor. Meningiomas of the olfactory groove may produce anosmia. Involvement of the optic nerve by optic nerve gliomas or meningiomas may produce unilateral visual loss and should be distinguished from optic neuritis or other primary optic nerve problems. Visual field defects are common. Bitemporal hemianopia is caused by pituitary adenomas or suprasellar tumors; homonymous hemianopias are caused by intrinsic tumors involving the optic radiations. Extraocular movement weakness may occur with meningiomas of the cavernous sinus or brainstem gliomas. Unilateral sixth nerve palsy is frequently a false localizing sign reflecting increased intracranial pressure. Peripheral facial nerve weakness is uncommon as a tumor finding except with very large acoustic neurinomas (vestibular schwannomas). Hearing loss, on the other hand, is a common finding with acoustic neurinomas, and sensorineural loss should be investigated by MRI. Lower cranial nerve deficits usually result from brainstem or posterior fossa tumors. Multiple cranial nerve palsies occur with neoplastic meningitis, in which tumor deposits coat the cranial nerves.

False localizing signs

Occasionally, when tumors produce increased intracranial pressure, shifting of intracranial structures occurs and results in clinical features suggesting involvement of sites distant from the tumor — false localizing signs. Examples of this include abducens (VIth) nerve palsy resulting from compression of the nerve as it passes forwards over the petrous ligament, and compression of the cerebral peduncle by the free edge of the tentorium cerebelli contralateral to a herniating uncus, producing hemiparesis on the same side as the lesion (Jaeckle 1991).

Differential diagnosis

Clinically, many conditions producing increased intracranial pressure or progressive neurologic deficits may mimic brain tumors. These include subdural hematomas, brain abscesses, hydrocephalus, benign intracranial hypertension, progressive multifocal leukoencephalopathy, multiple sclerosis, vascular malformations, cerebral infarctions, and Alzheimer's disease. Many of these conditions have characteristic radiologic appearances which enable them to be differentiated from brain tumors. However, some of these conditions cannot be distinguished from brain tumors on the basis of their radiologic appearances alone, and a definitive diagnosis often requires biopsy. These conditions include brain abscess and certain inflammatory lesions, demyelinating disease, hamartomas and congenital anomalies. Even when the imaging characteristics of a lesion are very suggestive of a tumor, a biopsy is usually indicated to obtain tissue for precise histologic diagnosis and grading of the tumor since these factors will have a significant influence on treatment.

B. RADIOLOGIC DIAGNOSIS

The introduction of CT scanning and more recently MR imaging have revolutionized the diagnosis and management of brain tumors (Hicks et al 1990, Kingsley 1990, Brody 1991, Barkovitch 1992).

Skull X-rays

Plain skull films are rarely necessary today with the widespread availability of CT and MR imaging. Occasionally they may be useful in demonstrating calcification, bony erosion or hyperostosis.

Plain films may demonstrate calcifications related to tumors. The presence of calcification usually indicates a relatively slow growing tumor. Astrocytomas are the most common calcifying tumor. Although calcifications occur only in approximately 20% of astrocytomas, their overall frequency more than compensates. Other tumors that frequently calcify are oligodendrogliomas, craniopharyngiomas, ependymomas, gangliogliomas and meningiomas. Calcification occurs in 50–60% of oligodendrogliomas, 70–80% of craniopharyngiomas, 50% of ependymomas, 35% of gangliogliomas and about 10% of meningiomas (Segall et al 1990).

Persistent elevation of intracranial pressure can result in erosion of normally calcified structures. In children, erosion of the inner table of the skull may lead to a 'hammered metal' appearance. Pituitary tumors may produce erosion of the clinoid processes and sella turcica. Slow growing tumors such as meningiomas may produce hyperostosis of the adjacent skull.

Tomography was previously used to demonstrate the double floor of the sella in pituitary tumors and enlargement of the internal auditory canal in acoustic tumors but is now rarely used: rather CT with bone windows will demonstrate these changes.

Computed tomography (CT)

Computed tomography remains the most widely used form of neuro-imaging for the diagnosis of brain tumors due to its wider availability and lower cost, although MR imaging is used with increasing frequency. CT scans will detect over 90% of brain tumors. Small tumors (<0.5 cm), tumors adjacent to bone such as pituitary adenomas, clival tumors and acoustic neurinomas (vestibular schwannomas), brainstem tumors and low grade astrocytomas may be missed and are better detected by the more sensitive MRI. CT scans tend to be better tolerated than MRI because of their shorter scanning time and are more sensitive at detecting calcification and bony involvement. Although CT scans are less sensitive than MR scans, the CT appearances of certain tumors may be more specific. For example, small round cell tumors such as medulloblastomas are isodense or hyperdense compared to brain parenchyma before contrast administration, whereas astrocytomas are almost always hypodense. Thus medulloblastomas can frequently be differentiated from cerebellar astrocytomas with the use of CT scanning. MR appearances of tumors tend to be less specific, and making a similar differentiation with MR imaging is often more difficult (Barkovich 1992).

The use of contrast enhancement is indispensable in the evaluation of brain tumors and may help disclose an isodense lesion from the surrounding parenchyma or a hypodense lesion hidden within an area of edema (Segall et al 1990). The introduction of nonionic contrast media has resulted in a four to five-fold reduction in serious contrast reactions. Other recent advances in CT scanning include shorter scan times and increased sensitivity of detectors resulting in decreased radiation dosage.

There is a trend towards increasing use of MRI because of its greater sensitivity. However, some studies suggest that there may be no advantage in using MRI for the detection of metastatic brain tumors (Sze et al 1988) or for the routine management of patients with malignant gliomas (El-Ouahabi et al 1993, unpublished data).

CT findings in specific tumors are discussed below.

Magnetic resonance imaging (MRI)

MRI is a complex, rapidly evolving modality which has assumed an increasingly important role in the diagnosis of brain tumors. The technical aspects of MRI are beyond the scope of this review and the reader is referred to Edelman & Hesselink (1990) for details. Very briefly, the patient is placed in a strong magnetic field which causes the protons in the water molecules of the body to align parallel or anti-parallel with the field. Then a radiofrequency (RF) pulse is introduced which excites these spinning protons, causing them to move out of alignment with the magnetic field. When the RF excitation stops, the protons return to their resting state within the main magnetic field, giving off the RF energy acquired during RF pulsation. The signal is spatially localized by the rapid turning on and off of spatially varying magnetic field gradients. This signal is detected by radioantennae (coils) within the scanner and used to generate the image. Each proton's behavior reflects the chemical microenvironment of that proton. The differences in the behavior of the protons result in differences in the MRI appearances of each tissue (Brody 1991). The amount of signal a tissue produces is dependent on the number of mobile hydrogen protons, the speed with which the tissue is moving, the tissue's T_1 relaxation time (the time needed for the protons within the tissue to return to their original state of magnetization) and the tissue's T_2 relaxation time (the time required for the protons perturbed into coherent oscillation by the radiofrequency pulse to lose this coherence) (Brody 1991). As T_1 and T_2 relaxation times are time dependent, the timing of the RF pulse and the reading of the radiated RF energy change the appearance of the image. The repetition time (TR) describes the time between successive applications of RF pulse sequences. The echo time (TE) describes the delay before the RF energy radiated by the tissue in question is measured. The pulse sequence which is described by the TR and TE and indicates the technique used to administer the RF energy can be chosen to maximize the effect of differences in T_1 or T_2. This gives rise to the description of an MRI image as T_1 or T_2 weighted (Brody 1991).

The standard MRI pulse sequence for anatomic and pathological detail is a spin echo sequence. T_1-weighted images (short TR; short TE) provide better anatomic detail, while T_2-weighted images (long TR; long TE), which are more sensitive to water content, are more sensitive to pathology. The intermediate or proton density images (long TR; short TE) provide improved contrast between lesions and cerebrospinal fluid.

MRI has the advantage of being more sensitive than CT scans, enabling the detection of small tumors that may be missed by CT scans. It provides much greater anatomic detail in multiple planes and is especially useful for visualizing skull base, brainstem, and posterior fossa tumors. MRI is also superior to CT scans in detecting hemorrhage and solid and cystic components within tumors and in demonstrating the relationship of the tumors to intracranial vessels.

As with CT scans the administration of a contrast agent, gadolinium diethylenetriaminepentaacetic acid (Gd-DTPA), to T1-weighted MR scans greatly increases the sensitivity of the test.

MRI is evolving rapidly. Newer imaging sequences are continually being developed, reducing scan times and improving the information obtained from the images. Newer techniques such as magnetic resonance spectroscopy, which allows direct investigation of tumor metabolism, and echoplanar MRI which can scan images in less than 100 milliseconds and provide information on tumor perfusion and diffusion, are currently being evaluated for possible use in separating recurrent tumor from radiation change. Echoplanar MRI may also be useful in helping to differentiate tumor from edema. MR angiography provides a means of displaying blood vessels in the brain in a noninvasive manner. It is being used increasingly in place of conventional angiography, although angiography has better resolution and is still necessary in certain situations (Brody 1991). MRI is also being integrated with advanced image processing techniques to produce three-dimensional definition of brain tumors to aid in surgical planning (Jolesz et al 1993) (Fig. 10.1).

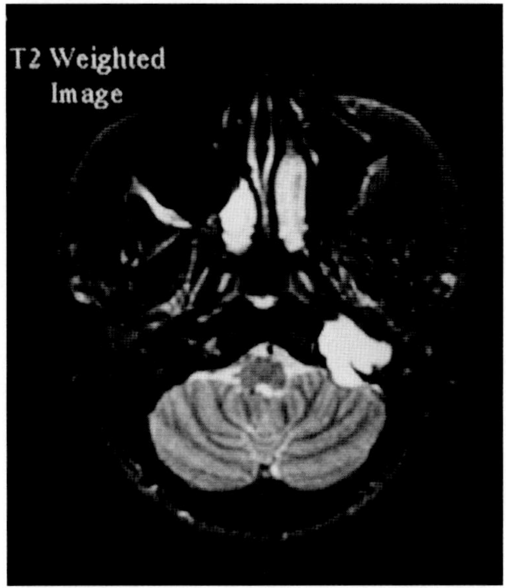

A

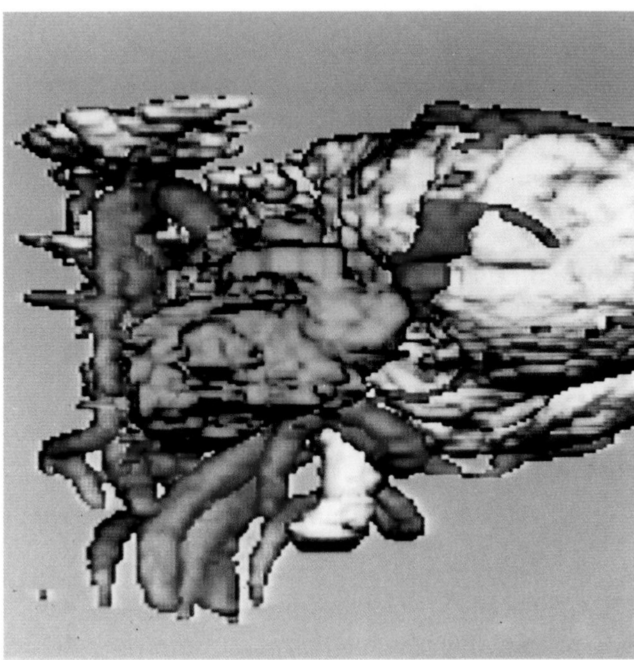

B

Fig. 10.1 **A**. Axial T2-weighted MRI showing hyperintense chondrosarcoma in the left cerebellopontine angle; **B**. three-dimensional MRI reconstruction (right lateral view) showing relationship of the tumor (in green) to the brainstem and surrounding blood vessels.

Angiography

The importance of angiography has diminished significantly with the availability of CT and MR imaging. It is no longer used for the routine diagnosis of brain tumors. Its role is limited to:

1. the preoperative evaluation of the vascular anatomy in certain patients (e.g. sphenoid wing meningioma encircling the carotid artery),
2. the assessment of the patency of venous sinuses in extracerebral tumors (e.g. falx meningioma),
3. use as part of the procedure for embolizing large tumors such as meningiomas, and
4. ruling out the presence of arteriovenous malformations and aneurysms in patients who present with hemorrhage.

However, even for many of these indications MR angiography is increasingly taking the place of conventional angiography.

Positron emission tomography (PET)

PET is a versatile imaging modality that provides dynamic information regarding the metabolism and physiology of the brain and brain tumors (DiChiro 1987, Rozental 1991). Its use is unfortunately limited by its high cost, restricted availability and limited scanner resolution. PET is not used for the routine diagnosis of brain tumors but it can provide important information complementing that obtained by CT and MR scanning. PET with [^{18}F]fluorodeoxyglucose to measure glucose metabolism can be used to noninvasively determine tumor grade in patients with malignant gliomas (DiChiro et al 1985). PET can also be used to differentiate radiation necrosis from recurrent tumor and study the metabolic effects of chemotherapy, radiation therapy and steroids on tumor metabolism (Rozental 1991, Phillips 1992).

Single-photon emission computed tomography (SPECT)

SPECT involves the intravenous administration of radiopharmaceuticals which are taken up by the brain and tumor cells. These radiopharmaceuticals emit photons which are detected by a rotating gamma camera. Standard tomography reconstruction algorithms are then used to generate cross-sectional images of the brain. Although SPECT is not used in the initial diagnosis of brain tumors it is increasingly being used to complement information obtained by CT or MRI scanning. Thallium 201 chloride,

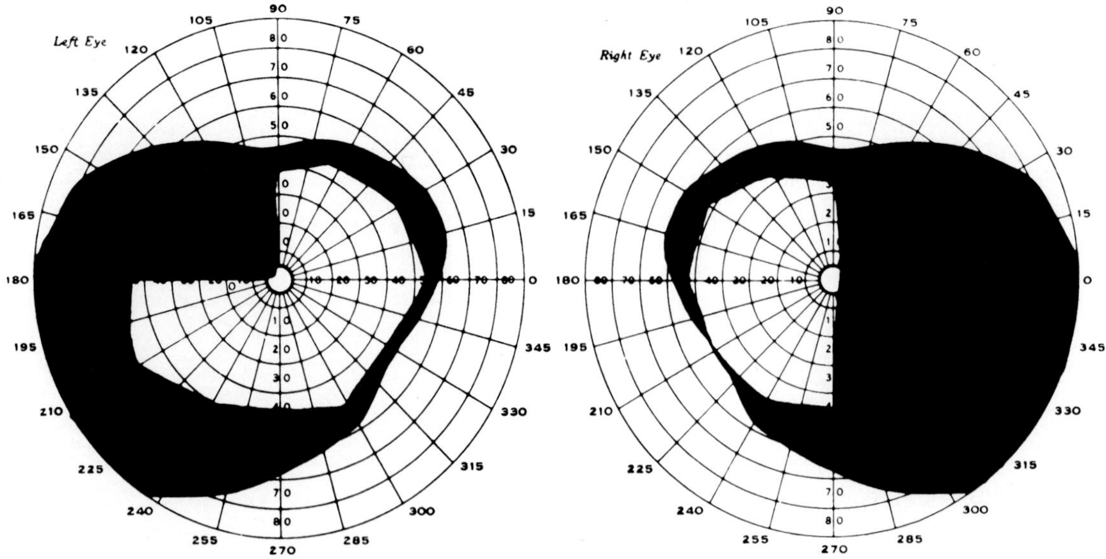

Fig. 10.2 Visual fields showing bitemporal hemianopia in a patient with a chromophobe pituitary adenoma. There is complete loss of vision in the right temporal field, and predominant involvement of the superior quadrant in the left temporal field. Reproduced with permission from Haerer 1992

a potassium analog that is taken up by viable tumor cells, has been used to differentiate low grade from high grade gliomas (Black et al 1989) and to identify residual astrocytoma after radiation therapy (Mountz et al 1988). More recently it has been used in combination with technetium 99m hexamethylpropylene amine oxime (^{201}Tc HMPAO), a blood flow tracer that crosses normal blood-brain barrier, to differentiate radiation necrosis from recurrent glioma (Carvalho et al 1992).

C. LABORATORY DIAGNOSIS

Perimetry

Visual fields can be quantitatively evaluated using a combination of Goldmann kinetic perimetry and static perimetry using Humphries visual fields. Measurement of visual fields is especially important in the evaluation of tumors in the vicinity of the optic chiasm such as pituitary adenomas. Perimetry may be useful in confirming deficits found on examination, detecting subtle changes not found on confrontation, and monitoring the effects of treatment, especially surgery (Fig. 10.2).

Electroencephalography (EEG)

Seizures are the presenting symptom in approximately one-third of patients with brain tumors. The presence of focal slow waves and spikes or frank epileptiform activity on EEG may be the first indication of a focal lesion and the need for cerebral imaging. Large tumors producing mass effect and tumors involving the diencephalon may produce asynchronous generalized slowing. However the EEG is often normal in patients with brain tumors and thus has limited value as a screening test (Fig. 10.3) (Fisher-Williams 1987).

Evoked potentials

Evoked potentials have a role in the diagnosis of certain brain tumors. The brainstem auditory evoked potentials (BSAEP) are abnormal in 92–96% of patients with acoustic neurinomas (vestibular schwannomas) and are a cost effective screening test for patients with a low probability of these tumors (Selters & Brackman 1977, Welling et al 1990). The most useful indications of compression of the auditory nerve are prolongation of the wave I–III and wave I–V interwave latencies. When wave I cannot be visualized, the ear to ear difference and the absolute latency of wave V may be useful (Fig. 10.4). Compression of the anterior visual pathway by tumors can reduce the amplitude of visual evoked potentials (VEP), however these tumors are usually diagnosed by MRI and VEPs are rarely necessary. Evoked potentials also have an important role in monitoring neurologic function during surgical resection of tumors.

Cerebrospinal fluid analysis

Examination of the cerebrospinal fluid (CSF) can be useful in the diagnosis of certain brain tumors and evaluating the extent of leptomeningeal spread. It is important, however, to recognize that lumbar puncture holds definite risks for individuals with increased intracranial pressure and should be avoided in these patients.

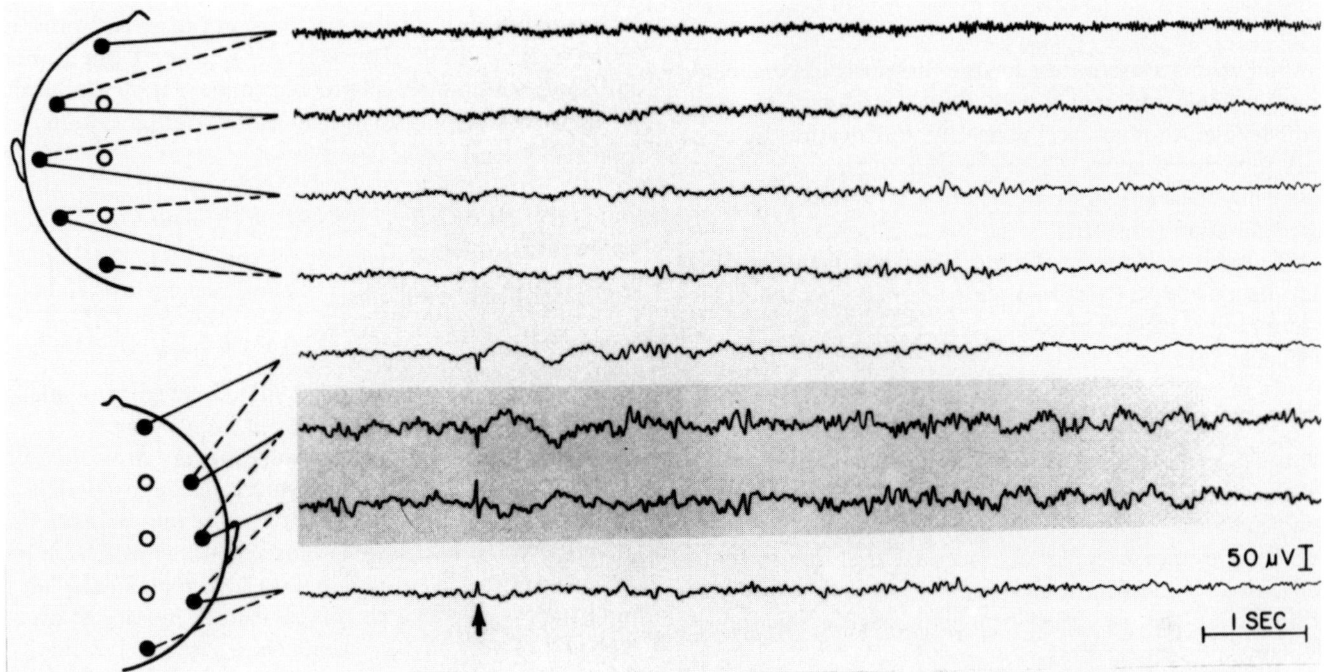

Fig. 10.3 EEG focal slow waves of 1–3 hertz (shaded) appearing continuously in the right temporal region in a patient with a meningioma. Arrow shows a sharp wave in the same region. The EEG from the left hemisphere is normal. Reproduced with permission from Spehlmann 1981

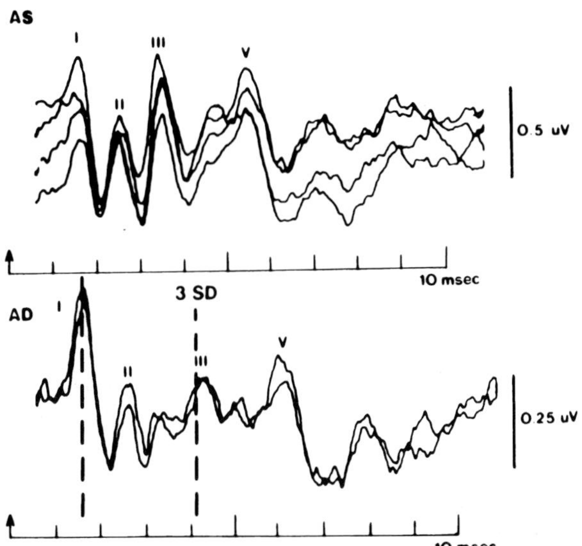

Fig. 10.4 Brainstem auditory evoked potential (BSAEP) from a patient with bilateral acoustic neurinomas. The BSAEP from the right ear (AD) is abnormal and shows a markedly prolonged I–III interpeak latency. The BSAEP from the left ear (AS) is normal despite the presence of a small acoustic neurinoma on CT scan. Reproduced with permission from Chiappa 1983

Examination of the CSF is very useful in patients with primary CNS lymphoma. It helps eliminate infections which are often the main differential diagnosis, and may help make the diagnosis if tumor cells are identified (DeAngelis 1993). A positive cytology may also be helpful in the diagnosis of pineal region tumors which are often difficult to biopsy. Examination of the CSF is important in postoperative staging of patients with medulloblastomas and primitive neuroectodermal tumors since the presence of leptomeningeal disease influences prognosis and treatment (Friedman et al 1991). Cytologic examination of the CSF may also be useful in the diagnosis of neoplastic meningitis in patients with metastatic brain tumors (Grossman & Moynihan 1991) and occasionally in patients with gliomas with leptomeningeal spread. CSF cytology is rarely useful in the initial diagnosis of gliomas.

Germ cell tumors arising in the pineal region may produce biological markers such as α-fetoprotein, β subunit of human chorionic gonadotrophin and placental alkaline phosphatase (Baumgartner & Edwards 1992). The presence of these markers helps in the diagnosis and subsequent follow-up of these germ cell tumors (Table 10.1).

Table 10.1 Tumor markers in patients with pineal tumors

Tumor type	AFP	HCG	PLAP
Germinoma	–	+/–	+
Teratoma	–	–	+/–
Malignant teratoma	+/–	+/–	+/–
Undifferentiated germ cell tumor	+/–	+/–	+/–
Choriocarcinoma	–	+	+/–
Endodermal sinus tumor	+	–	+/–
Embryonal cell tumor	+	+	+/–
Pineocytoma	–	–	–
Pineoblastoma	–	–	–

Key: AFP = α-fetoprotein, HCG = human chorionic gonadotropin, PLAP = placental alkaline phosphatase

Audiometry

Audiometry is a useful test for the diagnosis of cerebellopontine angle tumors. Ninety eight % of patients with acoustic neurinomas have sensorineural hearing loss on pure tone audiometry. The most common pattern is high frequency hearing loss, together with reduced speech discrimination (Fig. 10.5).

Vestibular testing, including electronystagmography, may be positive in patients with cerebellopontine angle tumors but is rarely needed.

Endocrine evaluation

Tumors in the region of the pituitary gland and hypothalamus may be associated with a variety of endocrine abnormalities. Evaluation of the hypothalamic-pituitary axis involves measurement of hormonal levels in the blood and urine, dynamic testing, and occasionally hormonal sampling of venous sinuses to help localize the tumor (Klibanski & Zervas 1991).

Future

The rapid advances in understanding the molecular and cellular biology of brain tumors may eventually lead to more effective laboratory tests for their diagnosis and follow-up. For example, urine and serum levels of the basic fibroblast growth factor (basic-FGF) may correlate with prognosis and disease activity in breast and prostate cancers. Basic-FGF is produced by many brain tumors and studies are under way to determine if it may be useful for the diagnosis and follow-up of these brain tumors.

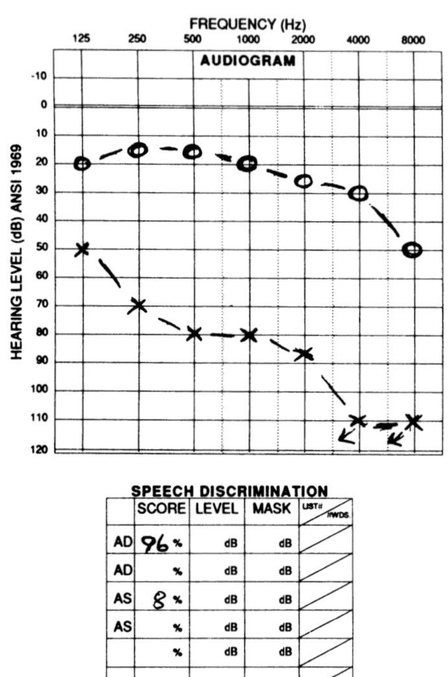

Fig. 10.5 Audiogram of a patient with a left acoustic neurinoma showing significant hearing loss, especially at high frequency in the left ear (x). Hearing in the right ear (0) is relatively normal. The lower panel shows decreased speech discrimination in the right ear.

D. THE PRESENTATION OF SPECIFIC BRAIN TUMORS

Malignant brain tumors

Astrocytomas

Astrocytomas will be included in the category of malignant tumors although some are relatively benign.

Low grade pilocytic astrocytomas. Most histologically benign forms of astrocytoma occur in childhood. The most potentially curable form is the pilocytic cerebellar astrocytoma in children. This accounts for 55% of low grade astrocytomas in childhood (Rekate & Rakfal 1991) and usually presents with clinical features related to hydrocephalus. These include headaches (usually bifrontal or suboccipital), nausea, vomiting, somnolence, papilledema and sixth nerve palsies. Gait unsteadiness or dysmetria may be present but is often subtle. A posterior head tilt may be present with caudal tonsillar herniation. CT or MRI shows a tumor arising within the vermis or cerebellar hemispheres. Typically there is a large cyst with a single enhancing mural nodule, although they can have multiple cysts or be completely solid (Rekate & Rakfal 1991, Barkovitch 1992) (Fig. 10.6).

Other groups of low grade childhood astrocytomas include the optic gliomas, which occur in the optic nerve

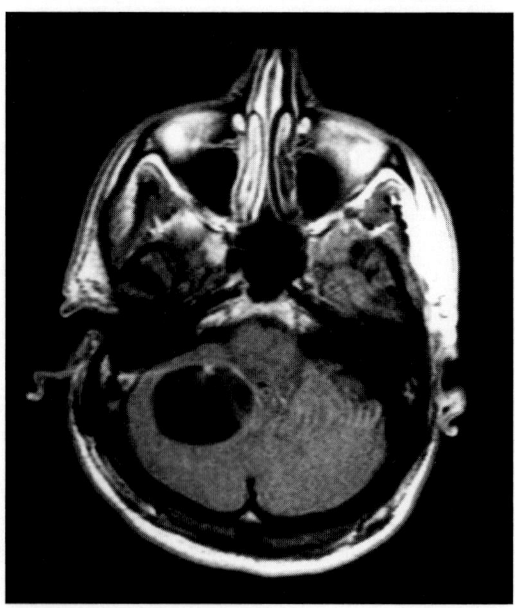

Fig. 10.6 Pilocytic astrocytoma. Post-contrast axial MRI showing large cystic tumor in right cerebellar hemisphere with small enhancing mural nodule.

and chiasm, hypothalamic gliomas, and brainstem gliomas, usually in the pons. In children these neoplasms are characterized pathologically by Rosenthal fibers and only slight hypercellularity. Clinically, they have an indolent course in most cases. They give symptoms referable to their locations: gradual visual loss for optic nerve gliomas (Cohen & Duffner 1991); a syndrome characterized by emaciation, hyperactivity, precocious puberty, and hypotension for hypothalamic gliomas; and for pontine gliomas, cranial nerve palsies, especially involving extraocular movement, together with contralateral corticospinal tract signs and sensory loss (Packer et al 1992). The diagnoses are made by demonstrating symmetrical diffuse enlargement with variable enhancement of the optic nerve and chiasm (Fig. 10.7A,B), hypothalamus, or pons (Fig. 10.8A,B) respectively by CT or MRI. MRI is especially valuable in demonstrating the extent of these tumors and their relationship to surrounding structures.

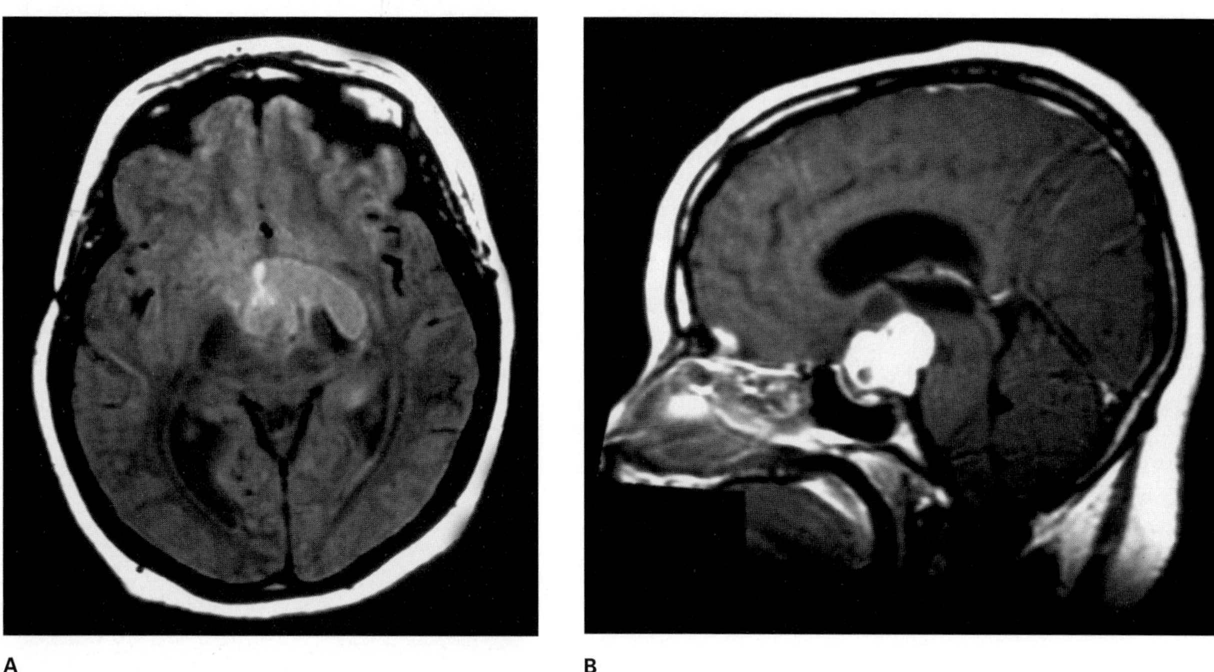

Fig. 10.7 Optic glioma. **A**. Axial MRI scan showing slightly hyperintense left optic glioma involving the chiasm on T1-weighted image. **B**. Sagittal MRI showing the same tumor enhancing densely with contrast.

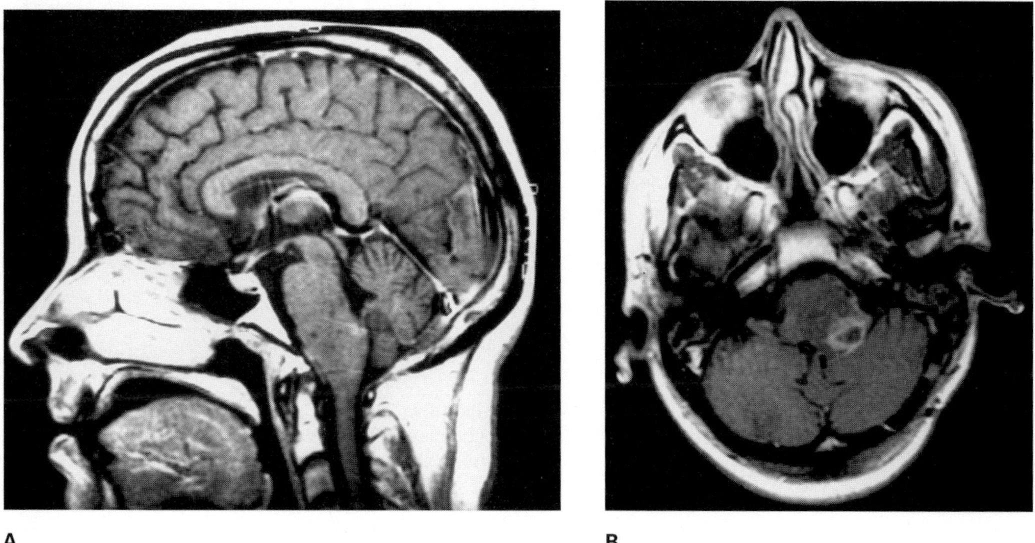

Fig. 10.8 Brainstem glioma. **A**. Parasagittal gadolinium-enhanced MRI showing diffusely enlarged pons and medulla with a small area of enhancement in the medulla. **B**. Axial MRI of the same patient showing enlargement of the brainstem and an area of enhancement to the left of midline.

Diffuse low grade astrocytomas. These usually occur in adults and may present with seizures, headaches or gradually progressive neurologic deficits. Patients may have had these symptoms for a long period of time before the diagnosis is made. Characteristic locations are the frontal or subfrontal regions or the white matter of the hemisphere. The CT scan typically shows a well-circumscribed, non-enhancing, hypodense or isodense lesion, usually with little surrounding edema. MRI is more sensitive than the CT scan and is the most useful test for identifying these lesions and perhaps for establishing their extent; often regions normal by CT will show up as abnormal areas of increased T2 signal and decreased T1 signal on MRI (Fig. 10.9A,B).

Malignant astrocytomas. Malignant astrocytomas (anaplastic astrocytomas and glioblastomas) reach their peak in adults between the ages of 40 and 60. Anaplastic astrocytomas have a median age of 40–50, while glioblastomas occur in a slightly older age group — median age 50–60. There is a slight male preponderance. Both types of malignant gliomas have similar presenting features. These include seizures, headaches, subtle cognitive problems or personality change, and focal neurologic deficits reflecting the location of the tumor such as aphasia, hemiparesis, sensory deficits and visual field loss. In a series of 100 malignant astrocytomas from our institution 35% had only seizures and 30% had only headache as presenting symptoms (El-Ouahabi et al 1993, unpublished data). The headaches are nonspecific and frequently indistinguishable from tension headaches, although advanced cases will have features of increased intracranial pressure. Neurologic signs are present in slightly over half the patients (El-Ouahabi et al 1993, unpublished data). This is less than reported in older series (McKeran & Thomas 1980) and probably reflects the current availability of cerebral imaging and earlier diagnosis of these tumors.

The presentation of malignant astrocytomas can be subtle, and reliance on headache characteristics, specific symptoms or physical signs may lead to delay in diagnosis. A low threshold for early imaging would result in earlier diagnosis of these tumors but must be weighed against the cost effectiveness of performing greater numbers of scans (Weingarten et al 1992).

Malignant astrocytomas have a variable appearance radiographically. In general they tend to be less circumscribed than low grade astrocytomas and surrounded with more edema. On CT scans they appear as hypodense or isodense lesions which enhance variably with contrast. Glioblastomas frequently have a central hypodense area of necrosis surrounded by a thick enhancing rim of tumor. There is often extensive surrounding edema (Fig. 10.10A,B). On MRI these tumors characteristically have low signal intensity on T1-weighted and high signal intensity on T2-weighted images. Tumor cells extend at least as far as the margins of increased T2 signal (Kelly et al 1987). Hemorrhage may be present but calcification is uncommon unless the malignant glioma arose from a preexisting lower grade lesion. These tumors tend to infiltrate along white matter tracts and frequently involve and cross the corpus callosum. Angiography may show increased vascularity and early draining veins but is rarely necessary.

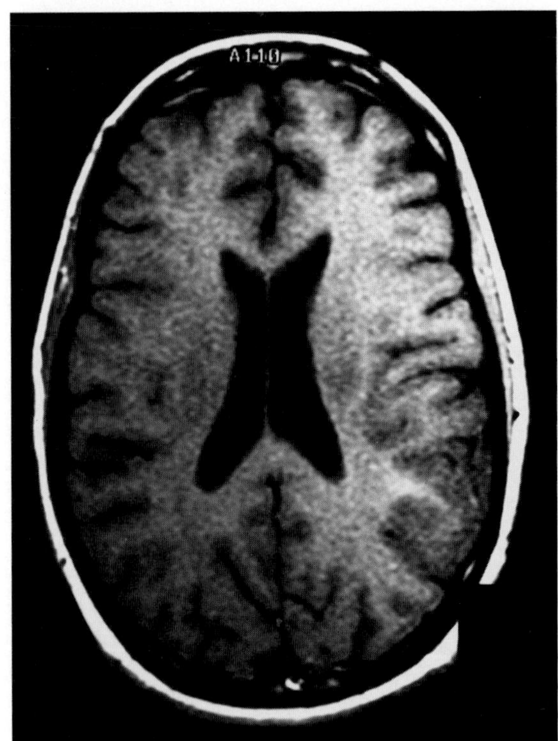

A

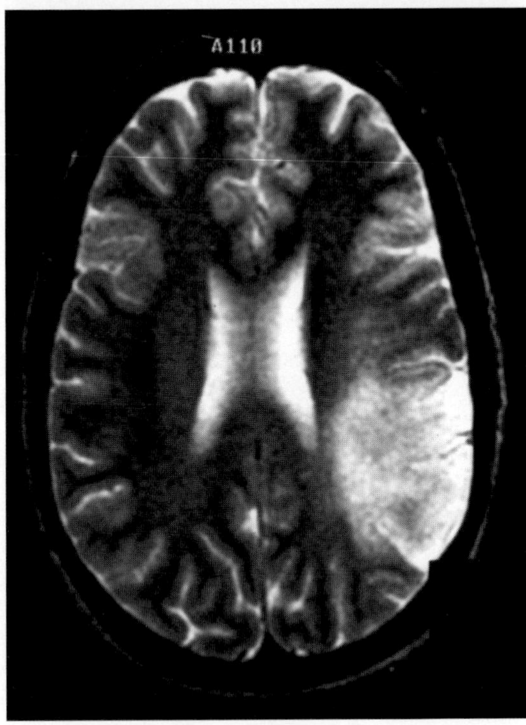

B

Fig. 10.9 Low grade astrocytoma. Axial MRI scans showing slightly hypointense non-enhancing left parietal tumor on T1-weighted images (**A**) and hyperintense tumor on T2-weighted images (**B**).

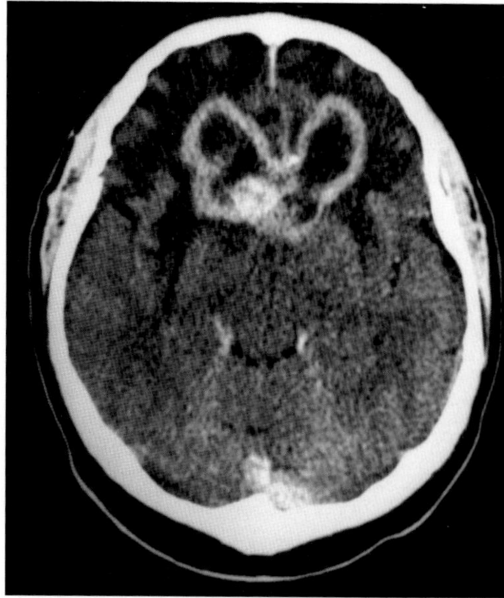

A

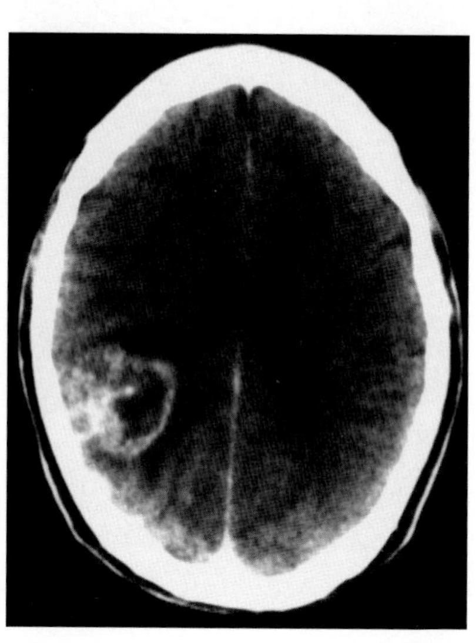

B

Fig. 10.10 Glioblastoma. **A**. Contrast-enhanced CT scan showing a ring enhancing lesion involving the corpus callosum and both frontal lobes with surrounding edema (butterfly glioma). **B**. Post-contrast CT scan showing ring enhancing tumor in right parietal lobe.

Enhancing tumors tend to have a higher histologic grade than non-enhancing tumors but there are frequent exceptions and caution should be used when relating contrast enhancement to malignancy. Approximately 10% of glioblastomas do not enhance and a higher percentage of low grade gliomas show enhancement (Segall et al 1990). Functional imaging techniques such as PET scanning using fluorodeoxyglucose (DiChiro 1987) and thallium 201 SPECT scanning (Black et al 1989) can provide a noninvasive method of evaluating tumor grade.

In recent years the introduction of new treatment modalities, such as stereotactic brachytherapy and radiosurgery, has resulted in an increased incidence of radiation necrosis. These appear as contrast-enhancing lesions with surrounding edema on CT or MRI, indistinguishable from tumor recurrence. However, functional imaging with PET (Doyle et al 1987) and thallium 201/technetium 99m HMPAO SPECT (Carvalho et al 1992) have proved effective in differentiating these radiation changes from tumor recurrence (Fig. 10.11).

Oligodendrogliomas

Oligodendrogliomas account for 5% of primary brain tumors (Shaw et al 1992), and are distinguished pathologically from astrocytomas by the characteristic 'fried

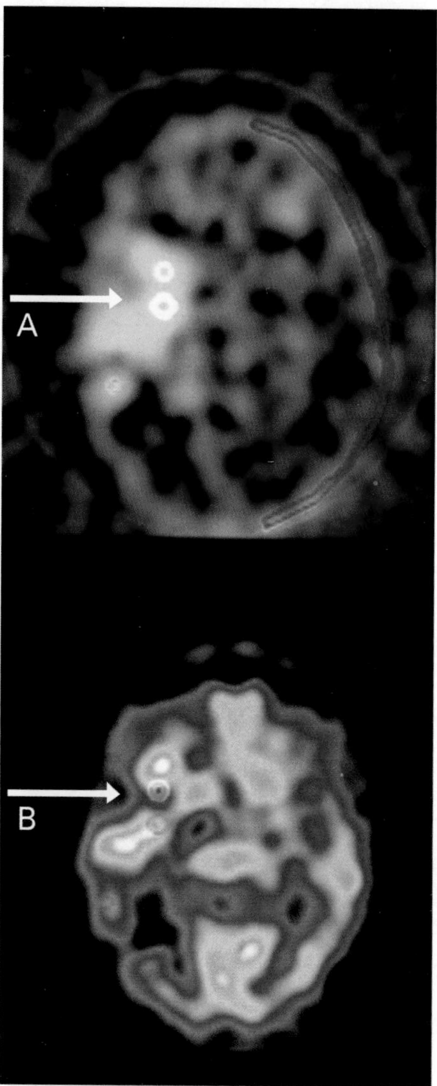

Fig. 10.11 Thallium 201/technetium 99m HMPAO SPECT scan of patient with recurrent glioblastoma. Arrow A shows area of increased thallium 201 uptake in the right frontal lobe. Arrow B shows corresponding area of increased technetium 99m HMPAO uptake indicating presence of perfusion. The combination of increased thallium and technetium uptake suggests tumor recurrence and not radiation necrosis. Radiation necrosis is associated with decreased or moderately increased thallium uptake and decreased technetium uptake.

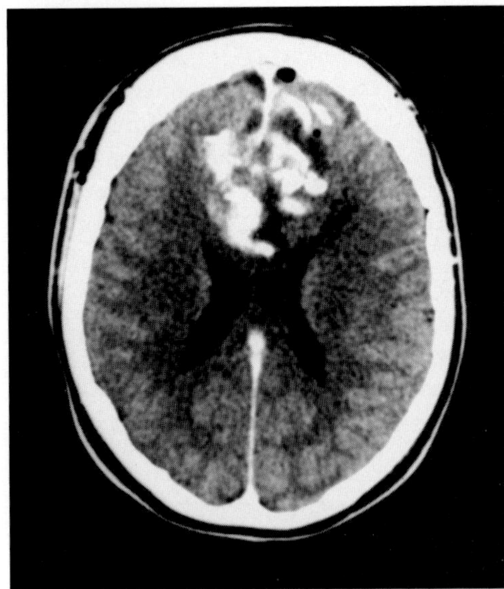

Fig. 10.12 Oligodendroglioma. Enhanced postoperative CT scan showing large residual tumor involving the corpus callosum and both frontal lobes with areas of heavy calcification.

egg' appearance, with a central nucleus surrounded by a 'halo' of empty cytoplasm. They are generally slow growing tumors with a mean age of onset of approximately 40 years. Patients frequently have had symptoms for months or years before diagnosis. Seizures are the most common presenting symptom, but some patients may present with headaches or slowly progressive neurologic deficits. Oligodendrogliomas are usually located in the frontal lobes and appear on CT scans as hypodense lesions often with heavy calcification (50%) (Russell & Rubinstein 1977). Higher grade oligodendrogliomas or those with mixed astrocytic components are more likely to enhance (Fig. 10.12).

Gangliogliomas

Gangliogliomas are rare, slow growing, minimally aggressive tumors occurring in children and young adults. Patients usually present with seizures or headaches. The radiologic appearances are nonspecific and usually consist of a well-circumscribed, variably enhancing mass with one or more cysts (Castillo et al 1990) (Fig. 10.13A,B). Calcification occurs in 35% of these tumors.

Ependymomas

Ependymomas arise from the ventricular lining and are characterized by ciliary bodies on electron microscopy or ependymal rosettes histologically. They occur primarily in children and young adults and present with gait ataxia and hydrocephalus. About 70% of ependymomas occur in the fourth ventricle and often extend through the foramen of Luschka into the cerebello-pontine angle cisterns. A small

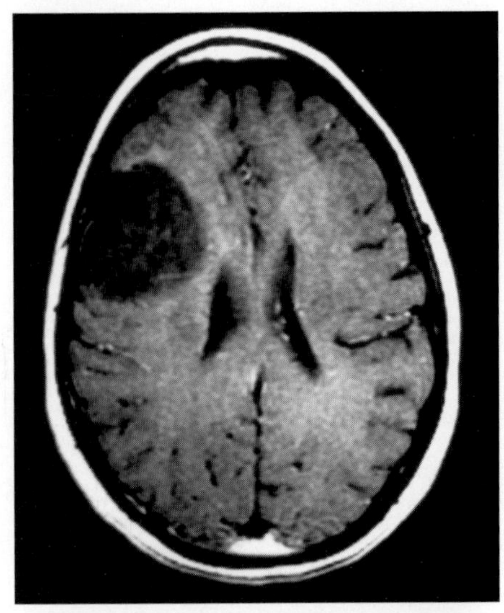

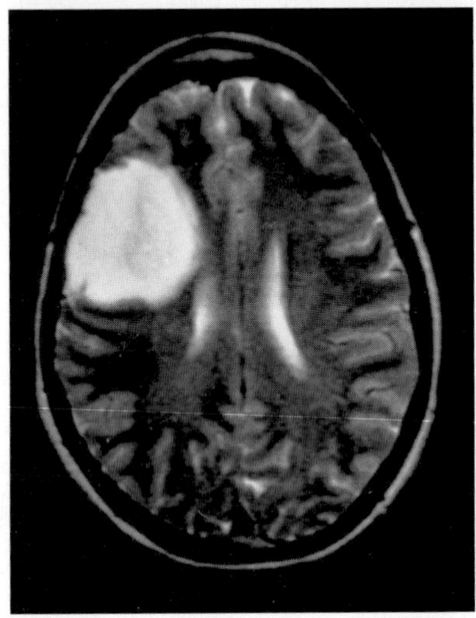

Fig. 10.13 Ganglioglioma. **A**. Post contrast axial T1-weighted MRI showing non-enhancing hypointense frontal tumor. **B**. The same lesion appears hyperintense on T2-weighted MRI.

percentage of ependymomas, especially in the very young, occur supratentorially. They have a variable appearance on CT and MRI imaging. They are often low intensity on T1-weighted images and high intensity on T2-weighted images. Calcification, cysts and hemorrhages are common (Barkovitch 1992). After contrast administration the solid portion of the tumor usually enhances.

Medulloblastoma/primitive neuroectodermal tumors (PNET)

Medulloblastomas/PNET account for approximately 20% of primary brain tumors in children and are the most common type of pediatric brain tumor. They are usually located in the posterior fossa and present with symptoms of headache, nausea, vomiting, and ataxia. They typically appear on CT scans as well-defined hyperdense tumors of the vermis and cerebellar hemisphere which enhance with contrast. Hydrocephalus is present in 90% of patients. The MRI appearance is somewhat variable and nonspecific but it is useful in defining the anatomy (Barkovich 1992). Because these tumors tend to disseminate within the subarachnoid space, gadolinium-enhanced MRI imaging of the spine or CT myelography and examination of the spinal fluid for neoplastic cells should be performed in all patients, together with bone marrow aspiration and bone scans, as part of their postoperative staging (Friedman et al 1991) (Fig. 10.14A,B).

Pineal region tumors

Pineal region tumors account for approximately 1% of brain tumors. They are divided into tumors derived from pineal parenchymal cells (pineocytomas and pineoblastomas) and germ cells (including germinomas, teratomas, embryonal carcinomas, yolk sac tumors and choriocarcinomas). Other lesions in this region include astrocytomas, ependymomas, meningiomas, gangliogliomas, dermoids and epidermoids and pineal cysts.

Patients with these tumors present with symptoms resulting from hydrocephalus, Parinaud's syndrome and other symptoms of brainstem compression, precocious puberty and occasionally ataxia when cerebellar pathways are involved.

The radiologic appearances vary depending on the tumor type. Germinomas are well-defined isodense or

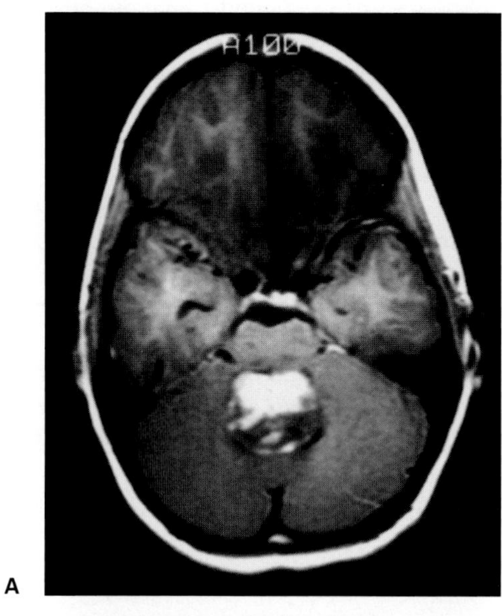

A

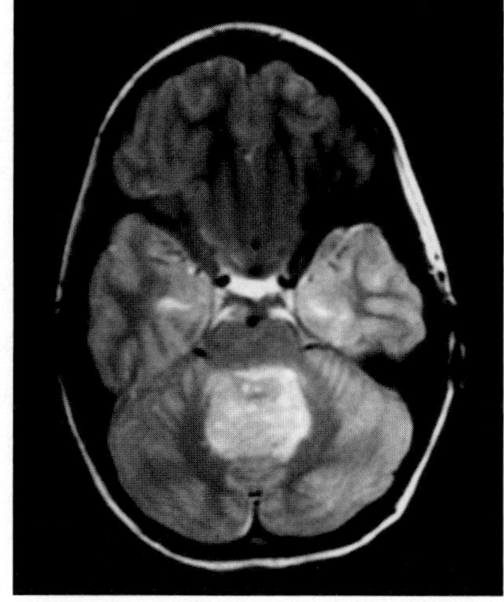

B

Fig. 10.14 Medulloblastoma. **A**. Gadolinium-enhanced axial T1-weighted MRI showing irregularly enhancing tumor in the cerebellar vermis. **B**. Axial T2-weighted MRI of the same patient showing increased signal from the tumor.

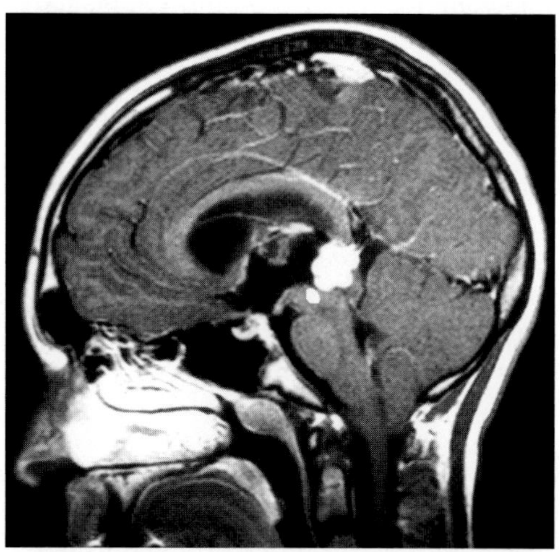

A

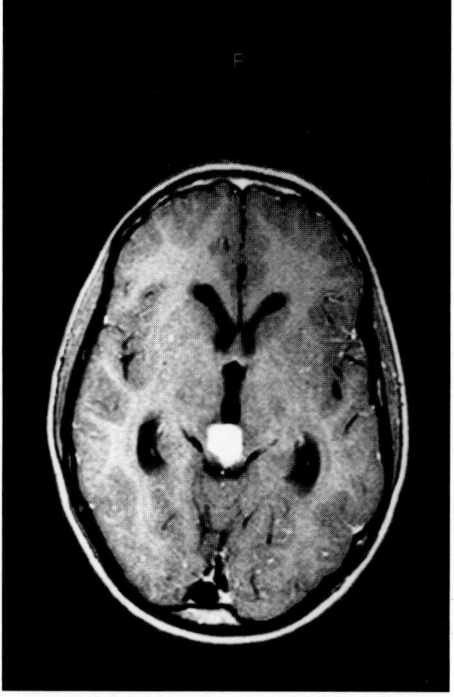

B

Fig. 10.15 Pineal germinoma. Post contrast T1-weighted MRI in the sagittal (**A**) and axial (**B**) planes showing enhancing pineal tumor.

hyperdense lesions which enhance with contrast (Fig. 10.15A,B). Teratomas characteristically have a heterogeneous appearance with solid and cystic areas and often areas of fat and calcification. Pineal parenchymal tumors are lobulated isodense or hyperdense lesions, which enhance markedly with contrast. These tumors often have areas of calcification. The multiplanar capability of MRI delineates pineal tumors better than CT and allows the relationship of the tumor to the surrounding structures to be demonstrated. The malignant pineal tumors may seed along CSF pathways, and gadolinium MRI imaging of the entire neuroaxis is important. When a pineal region mass is demonstrated radiologically, the cerebrospinal fluid should be examined, preoperatively if possible, looking for tumor cells and tumor markers such as α-fetoprotein, human chorionic gonadotropin and placental alkaline phosphatase which are produced by some of the germ cell tumors (Baumgartner & Edwards 1992) (Table 10.1).

Pineal cysts are frequently seen on MR scans as incidental findings. These do not change with time and often have a low intensity center on both T1- and T2-weighted images with an enhancing ring (Mamourian & Towfigi 1986). It is important to differentiate these benign lesions from the malignant pineal tumors.

Primary CNS lymphoma

Primary CNS lymphoma (PCNSL) was formerly a rare tumor accounting for 1% of primary brain tumors. However, the incidence is increasing dramatically and it has been estimated that PCNSL will be the most common primary brain neoplasm by the turn of the decade. The reason for this is partly due to the increased number of PCNSL in patients with AIDS and cardiac and renal transplants, and partly due to a three-fold increase in the incidence of PCNSL in immunocompetent patients from unknown reasons (Eby et al 1988).

The presentation can be nonspecific and diagnosis requires a high index of suspicion, especially in non-immunocompromised patients. In one series 35% of patients had focal neurologic deficits, 24% had personality changes, 15% headaches, 13% seizures, and 8% had visual changes (Hochberg & Miller 1988). Because this is a rapidly growing tumor, symptoms are usually present for a short duration, weeks to a few months, before a diagnosis is made (DeAngelis 1993).

CT and MRI scans visualize intracranial lesions in 95% of patients. The radiologic appearances are usually quite distinctive and the diagnosis may be suspected on the basis of the radiographic appearance alone. Two thirds of patients have solitary lesions initially but these soon become multiple and there is frequently leptomeningeal involvement. The tumor deposits appear as densely enhancing masses with somewhat indistinct margins, often with a periventricular location. There is usually a variable amount of surrounding edema (Fig. 10.16A–C). Immunocompromised patients with PCNSL have a higher incidence of ring enhancement, making it difficult to differentiate from infections such as toxoplasmosis.

In addition to radiologic examination of the brain, patients with PCNSL should have serologic testing for human immunodeficiency virus (HIV), syphilis, toxoplasmosis, slit lamp examination of the eye (involved in 20% of patients) and examination of the cerebrospinal fluid. Bone marrow examination and CT scanning of the chest

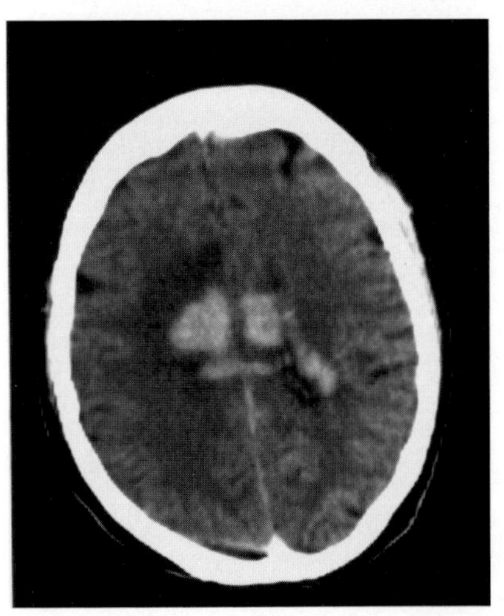
A

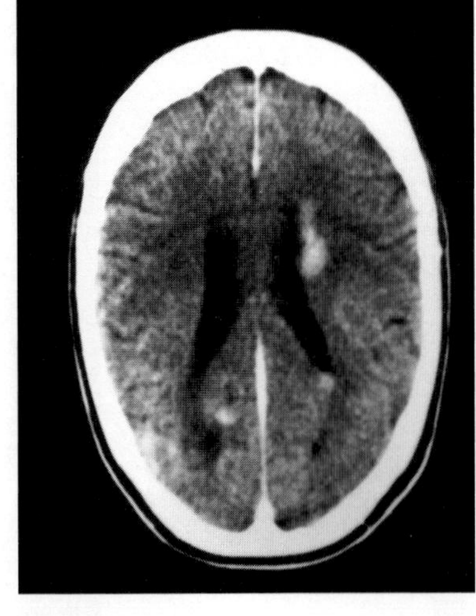
B

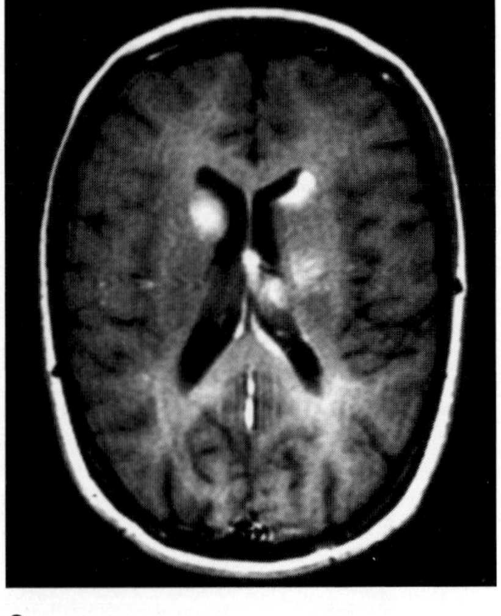
C

Fig. 10.16 Primary CNS lymphoma. **A**. Contrast-enhanced CT scan showing several densely enhancing irregular masses in both hemispheres, corpus callosum and wall of left lateral ventricle, with some surrounding edema. **B**. Contrast-enhanced CT scan showing several enhancing areas of tumor with the typical periventricular location. **C**. Axial gadolinium-enhanced T1-weighted MRI showing the enhancing periventricular lesion with little surrounding edema.

and abdomen are rarely useful as only 5% of patients presenting with brain tumor have systemic lymphoma.

Diagnosis is usually made by biopsy, but examination of the cerebrospinal fluid is often useful, especially if biopsy is felt to be difficult. There may be lymphocytic pleocytosis (50%), elevated protein (85%) (rarely above 150 mg%) and in severe cases low glucose. Cytologic examination may show neoplastic cells although it may be difficult to differentiate these from reactive lymphocytes. In patients where the cytology is equivocal, the finding of a monoclonal B-cell population on immunoperoxidase (Li et al 1986) or the demonstration of clonality of immunoglobulin gene rearrangement may help in establishing the diagnosis (Kumanishi et al 1989).

In immunocompromised patients the main differential diagnosis is from toxoplasmosis. If the patient has toxoplasma antibodies a therapeutic trial with anti-toxoplasma therapy may be helpful in making the diagnosis. PCNSL are very sensitive to the cytolytic effects of steroids in the short term, and occasionally the response to a therapeutic trial with high dose steroids may also be useful in differentiating PCNSL from other tumors.

Brain metastases

Brain metastases occur in approximately 20–30% of all cancer patients. Lung cancer and breast cancer are the most common tumors to the head, accounting for 40% and 20% of all symptomatic cases respectively. The next most frequent causes are melanoma, gastrointestinal cancers and renal cancer. Melanoma has the greatest predilection for the brain, with approximately 40% of patients with systemic disease developing cerebral metastases (Patchell 1991).

Eighty % of metastases are supratentorial. Generally the distribution of metastases in the brain is proportional to the weight and blood flow of that region, although pelvic neoplasms have a predilection for the posterior fossa (Delattre et al 1988). Forty seven % of metastases are single, 53% are multiple; 11% of patients have more than 5 metastases on presentation. Lung cancer and melanoma are more likely to produce multiple lesions.

Metastases present with similar symptoms and signs as primary brain tumors. Headaches are the most common symptom followed by mental status changes and focal neurologic deficits. Seizures are the presenting symptom in approximately 10% of patients. Occasionally they can present with hemorrhage. Melanoma, choriocarcinoma, renal cell, thyroid and lung cancers are the most likely to bleed.

Brain metastases usually appear as contrast-enhancing lesions on CT and MRI scans (>90%). There is often a central hypodense area of necrosis within an enhancing ring. MRI scans may be more sensitive for diagnosing multiple lesions (Fig. 10.17A,B). The radiologic appearances are often indistinguishable from malignant gliomas, although the demonstration of multiple lesions favors the diagnosis of metastasis. Most tumors are hypodense on unenhanced CT scans but melanoma, sarcoma and small cell lung cancer will occasionally appear as hyperdense lesions.

The differential diagnosis includes primary brain tumors (including gliomas and lymphomas), abscesses, vascular lesions (hemorrhages, arteriovenous malformation), radiation necrosis and progressive multifocal leukoencephalopathy.

A

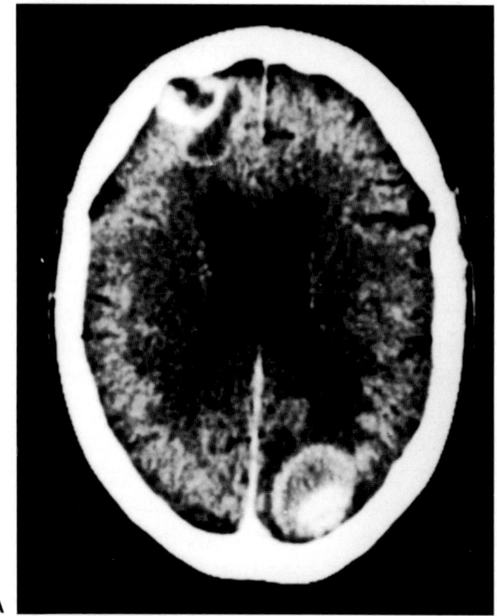

B

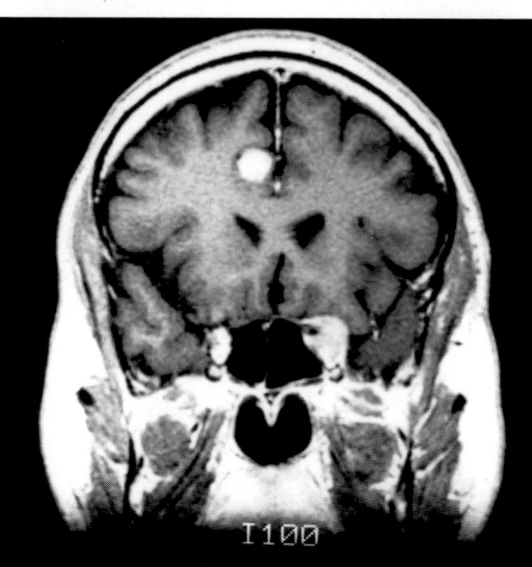

Fig. 10.17 Brain metastases. **A**. Post-contrast CT scan showing large enhancing melanoma metastases in the right frontal and left occipital region. **B**. Coronal enhanced MRI showing right frontal and left cavernous sinus metastases from lung adenocarcinoma.

Bony metastases are characterized by hyperintense lesions on T2 and proton density weighted images that have replaced the lower signal from the diploic space and cortical bone.

Benign brain tumors

Meningiomas

Meningiomas are the most common benign tumors, accounting for 15–20% of all primary brain tumors (Rachlin & Rosenblum 1991). They are most commonly located in the parasagittal region followed by the sphenoid wings, parasellar region, olfactory groove, cerebellopontine angle, and rarely the ventricles. They are more common in women (3:1) and occur in middle age. The most common presentations of intracranial meningiomas are seizures, headaches or gradually increasing neurologic deficits. The deficits depend on tumor location but may include hemiparesis, cortical sensory deficits, incoordination, or personality change. Parasagittal tumors may produce unilateral or bilateral leg weakness if they are against the motor strip, together with urinary incontinence. Subfrontal (17%) and sphenoid ridge (17%) meningiomas are often surprisingly large before producing symptoms. Parasellar meningiomas produce visual symptoms, especially visual field defects. Other less common meningiomas may have characteristic signs and symptoms: optic nerve sheath meningiomas present with monocular blindness, cerebellopontine angle meningiomas with hearing loss, spinal cord meningiomas with spinal cord symptoms, and tentorial notch and intraventricular meningiomas may have almost no symptoms.

The CT scan and MRI are similar in the imaging diagnosis of meningiomas. The usual pattern is an isodense, or hyperdense, homogeneous extra-axial mass with smooth or lobulated clearly demarcated contours which enhance homogeneously and densely with contrast (Zimmerman et al 1985, Spagnoli et al 1986). The tumors frequently have areas of calcification and produce hyperostosis of adjacent bone. These features are better demonstrated by CT scans. There is often an enhancing dural tail extending from the tumor attachment. These may reflect meningeal reaction and do not necessarily indicate tumor extension. MRI is especially useful in assessing arterial encasement and venous sinus invasion. There may be a variable amount of surrounding edema which tends to be greater with parasagittal and sphenoid ridge tumors (Fig. 10.18A–E).

Acoustic neurinomas

Acoustic neurinomas are benign schwannomas arising from the vestibular portion of the eighth nerve. They account for 10% of all brain tumors. Ninety five % of these tumors are unilateral; 5% are bilateral and associated with neurofibromatosis type 2. Hearing loss is an invariable symptom in these lesions, but it may be dismissed for many years as a result of aging or trauma. The hearing loss is usually asymmetric and progressive, but 10% of patients have sudden hearing loss. Other early symptoms include tinnitus and vertigo. With increasing size there may be compression of the facial and trigeminal nerve resulting in facial weakness and numbness. Further enlargement of the tumor produces brainstem and cerebellar compression and leads to ataxia, headaches, diplopia, dysphagia, hemiparesis, and hydrocephalus.

The audiogram shows sensorineural hearing loss in the affected ear in 98% of patients at the time of diagnosis. This is frequently associated with reduced speech discrimination.

The brainstem auditory evoked potentials (BSAEP) are abnormal in 92–96% of patients with acoustic neurinomas (vestibular schwannomas) (Selters & Brackman 1990, Welling et al 1990). The most useful indications of compression of the auditory nerve are prolongation of the wave I–III and wave I–V interwave latencies. When wave I cannot be visualized, the ear-to-ear difference and the absolute latency of wave V may be useful. BSAEPs are a useful cost-effective screening test for patients with a low probability of acoustic neurinomas.

CT scans, together with the use of air contrast, can detect tumors under 1 cm and may show erosion of the internal auditory canal. MRI is much more sensitive and is the imaging modality of choice. The tumors appear hypointense on T1-weighted and hyperintense on T2-weighted scans and usually enhance intensely with gadolinium (Fig. 10.19A,B). With enhanced MRI tumors as small as 3 mm in diameter can be detected (Mafee et al 1988). These small tumors often have normal BSAEP.

The main differential diagnosis is meningioma. Unlike acoustic neurinomas these tumors are not centered on the internal auditory canal, and have a broad base at their attachment to the petrous ridge or tentorial margin.

Electronystagmography and angiography are usually not helpful.

Pituitary adenomas

Pituitary adenomas comprise about 10–15% of symptomatic brain tumors in surgical series. They arise from the anterior lobe of the pituitary gland and may be secretory or non-secretory. Secretory tumors produce endocrine syndromes and tend to present earlier than non-secreting tumors which tend to produce symptoms resulting from compression of adjacent structures.

Endocrine syndromes may reflect increased or decreased function. Five syndromes of increased function have been described with pituitary tumors.

The most common hypersecretion syndrome is hyperprolactinemia. This is caused by prolactinomas, which

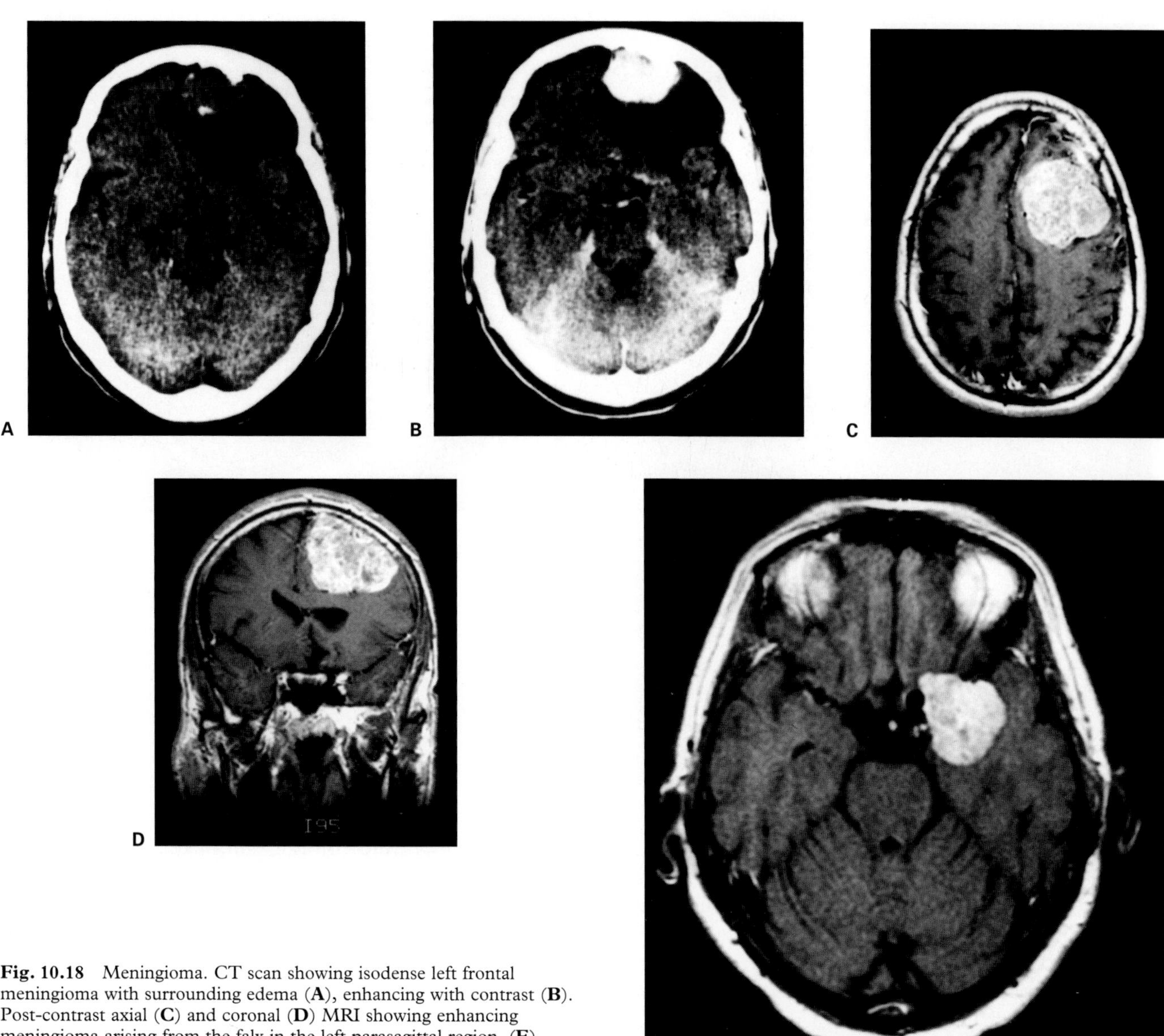

Fig. 10.18 Meningioma. CT scan showing isodense left frontal meningioma with surrounding edema (**A**), enhancing with contrast (**B**). Post-contrast axial (**C**) and coronal (**D**) MRI showing enhancing meningioma arising from the falx in the left parasagittal region. (**E**) Post-contrast axial MRI showing enhancing sphenoid wing meningioma involving carotid artery.

account for 40% of pituitary tumors. In premenopausal women this is associated with amenorrhea, infertility and galactorrhea; in men with impotence and infertility.

Growth hormone hypersecretion is next most common and is characterized by gigantism in children and adolescents and by acromegaly in adults (Melamed 1990). Patients with acromegaly have characteristic appearances including coarsening of facial features, prominent forehead, broad chin and nose, wide spacing of the teeth, and wide phalanges of hands and feet. More important than the skeletal changes in acromegaly are its metabolic abnormalities, which include hypertension, cardiomyopathy and diabetes mellitus.

Cushing's disease — hypersecretion of cortisol from a corticotrophin (ACTH)-producing adenoma — is next in frequency and is potentially life-threatening. The external features typically include truncal obesity, skin striae, capillary fragility, hirsutism and buffalo hump. The syndrome also includes diabetes mellitus, osteoporosis, hypertension and psychiatric abnormalities. Cushing's disease is the result of a pituitary adenoma; Cushing's syndrome is the same clinical picture from any cause including steroid therapy, pituitary adenoma, or an ectopic source of ACTH. Nelson's syndrome is a disorder of ACTH overproduction in response to prior surgical adrenalectomy. It is characterized by skin hyperpigmentation and aggressive pituitary tumor behavior.

Less common is a syndrome of overproduction of glycoprotein hormones (luteinizing hormone (LH), follicle-stimulating hormone (FSH), and thyroid-stimulating

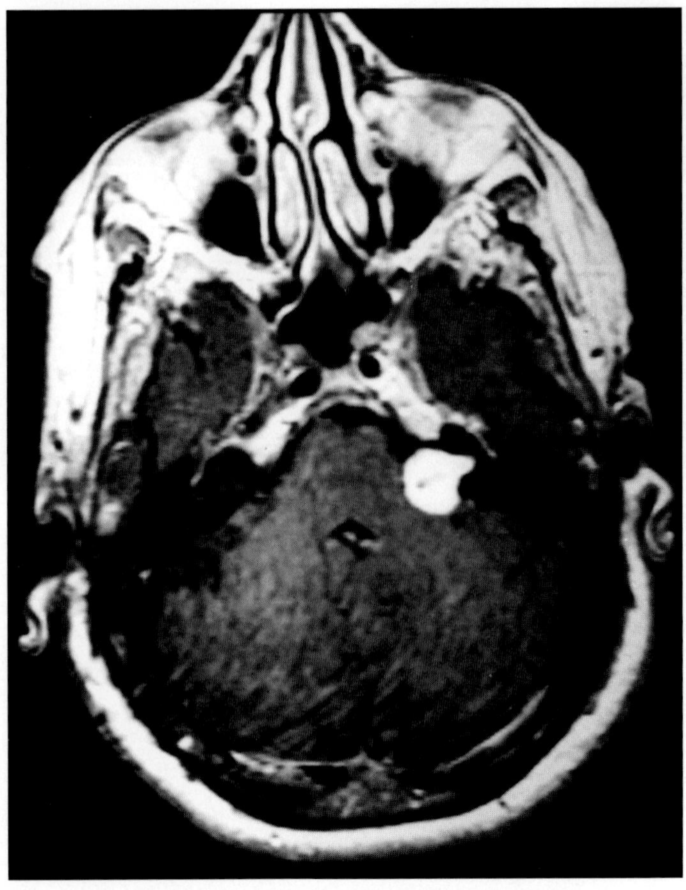

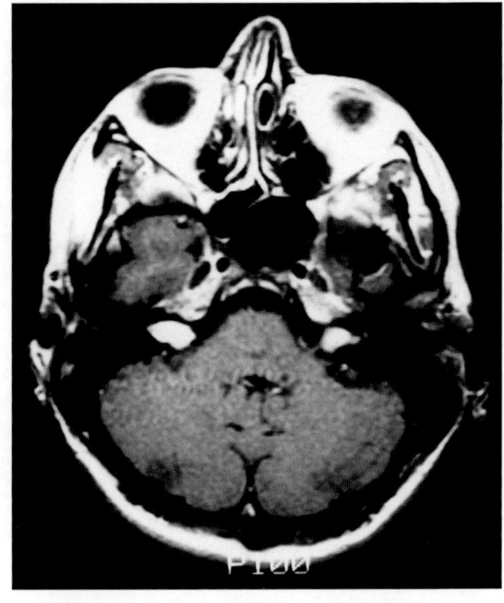

Fig. 10.19 Acoustic neurinoma (vestibular schwannoma). Axial post-contrast MRI scan showing (**A**) 1 cm enhancing tumor in the left cerebellopontine angle, (**B**) bilateral enhancing acoustic neurinomas in a patient with neurofibromatosis type 2.

hormone (TSH)) characterized by the presence of elevated levels of the α subunit of these glycoprotein hormones in the serum. Typically these tumors, which occur in both men and women, do not have a characteristic syndrome of excess hormone production and present with symptoms of mass effect, including headaches, visual loss and hypopituitarism.

Very rarely TSH-secreting adenomas may cause hyperthyroidism.

In addition to syndromes of endocrine hypersecretion there is also a syndrome of hypopituitarism which can be caused by large adenomas. Growth hormone deficiency is most common and in children may result in growth failure. Gonadotrophin deficiency results in amenorrhea and infertility in women, decreased libido and facial hair and testicular atrophy in men. TSH deficiency causes hypothyroidism, and corticotrophin deficiency results in cortisol deficiency with fatigue, weight loss, hypotension and an abnormal response to stress.

The mass effects of a pituitary tumor are diverse. Headaches occur commonly and are thought to result from stretching of the diaphragma sella. They are most often referred to the vertex and to the retro-orbital region but can occur in other areas. They tend to be constant and dull and have no particular distinguishing characteristics. Visual field loss from compression of the optic chiasm is usually bitemporal, but may also be unilateral. If the tumor extends into the third ventricle, obstructive hydrocephalus with headache, nausea, vomiting and obtundation may result. Invasion of the hypothalamus may result in hyperphagia, abnormal temperature regulation, and impairment of consciousness. If the tumor extends laterally into the cavernous sinus, extraocular palsies of the oculomotor, abducens, or trochlear nerves can be present. If it extends into the sphenoid sinus, nosebleeds may occur.

About 1% of patients with pituitary adenomas will present with pituitary apoplexy. This usually involves severe headache, nausea, vomiting, obtundation and visual field loss or extraocular movement palsies from sudden hemorrhagic tumor infarction, but less severe forms also occur. These symptoms may occasionally be confused with subarachnoid hemorrhage from aneurysm rupture.

Evaluation of pituitary tumors includes radiologic, endocrine, and ophthalmologic assessment. On plain skull X-rays the sella turcica may be enlarged or asymmetrical; little else can be gained from them. CT scans, especially with coronal cuts, may show a large iso- or hyperdense tumor that enhances variably. Erosion of the sellar floor may be present. MRI is the imaging modality of choice. Microadenomas (<1 cm diameter) appear as low intensity

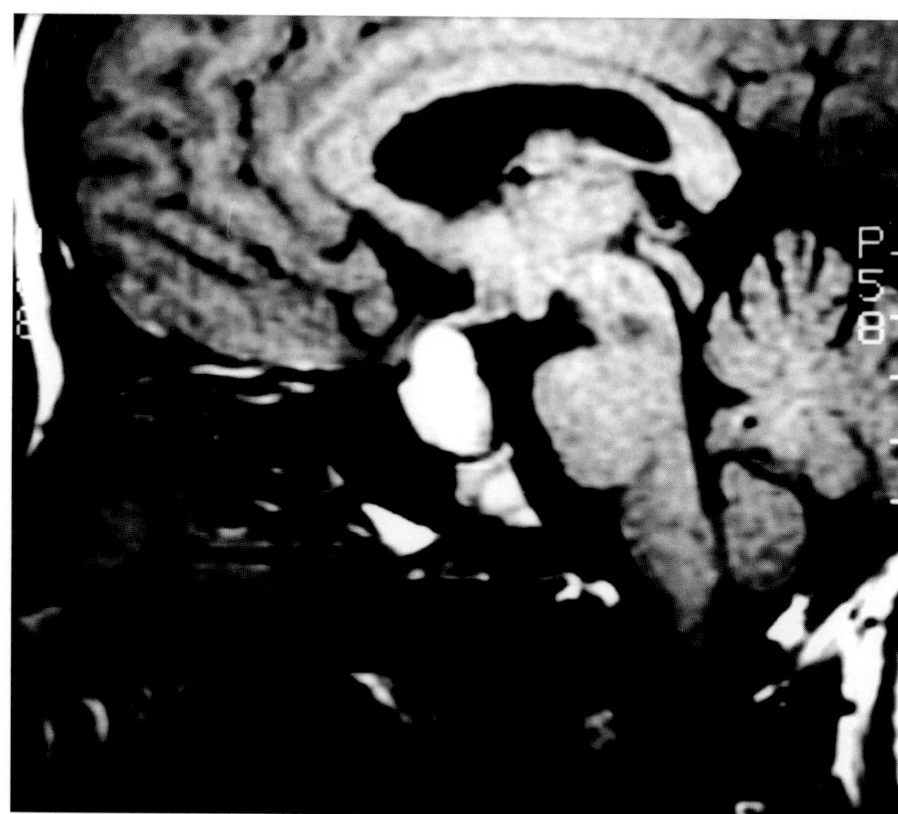

A

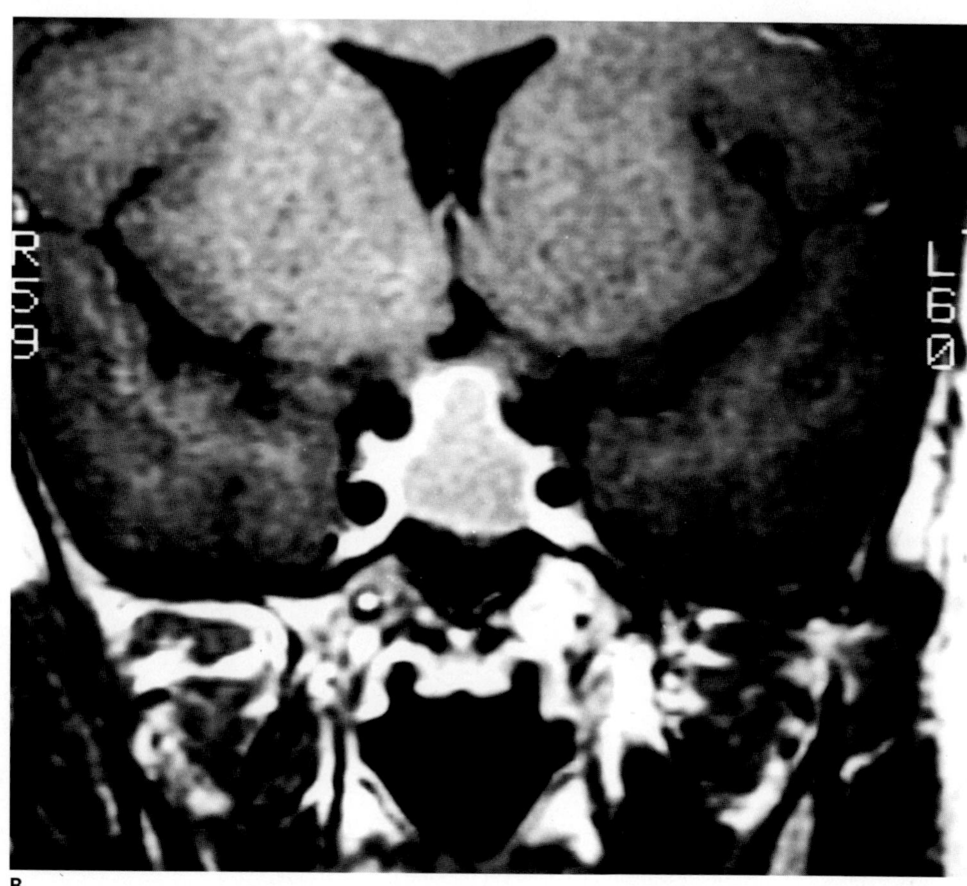

B

Fig. 10.20 Pituitary adenoma.
A. Unenhanced sagittal MRI showing hyperintense pituitary adenoma with suprasellar extension and compression of the optic chiasm. **B**. Coronal contrast-enhanced MRI of the same patient.

lesions on T1-weighted scans (Kurcharczyk et al 1986). Gadolinium enhances the normal gland adjacent to the adenoma and highlights the lesion. Macroadenomas are usually isointense on T1-weighted images and enhance homogeneously with gadolinium. The multiplanar capability of MRI enables the full extent of larger lesions to be visualized. In sagittal reconstruction it will show a tumor's relation to the clivus and brainstem, and in coronal sections its relation to the optic chiasm and cavernous sinus (Fig. 10.20A,B).

Endocrine evaluation of a patient with a suspected pituitary tumor should include baseline prolactin, growth hormone, and 8 a.m. cortisol levels as well as thyroid function tests. If these are normal it may also be worth getting LH, FSH, and the α subunit levels tested since increasing numbers of apparently non-functioning adenomas appear to have glycoprotein hormone production.

In evaluating prolactin, a level above 20 ng/ml is abnormal, but stalk compression effects, stress, medications, renal failure and hypothyroidism can increase prolactin without a tumor. To be certain that a prolactin-producing tumor is present, the level should be over 200 ng/ml. To demonstrate growth hormone excess, a baseline fasting growth hormone level greater than 10 ng/ml is diagnostic. Measurement of a random somatomedin C (insulin-like growth factor 1) and failure of growth hormone secretion to suppress with hypoglycemia in an oral glucose tolerance test are also helpful. To demonstrate overproduction of ACTH by a pituitary adenoma two tests are necessary: first, documenting ACTH elevation by high fasting cortisol or 24-hour urinary corticosteroids; second, documenting that this high level does not suppress with low dose (1 mg) dexamethasone given orally. ACTH production by an ectopic tumor may give high morning cortisols but is associated with the failure of exogenous dexamethasone to suppress levels (Daniels & Martin 1987, Klibanski & Zervas 1991). Measurement of ACTH levels from blood obtained from sampling the petrosal sinuses may be useful in localizing small ACTH-producing tumors (Klibanski & Zervas 1991).

A

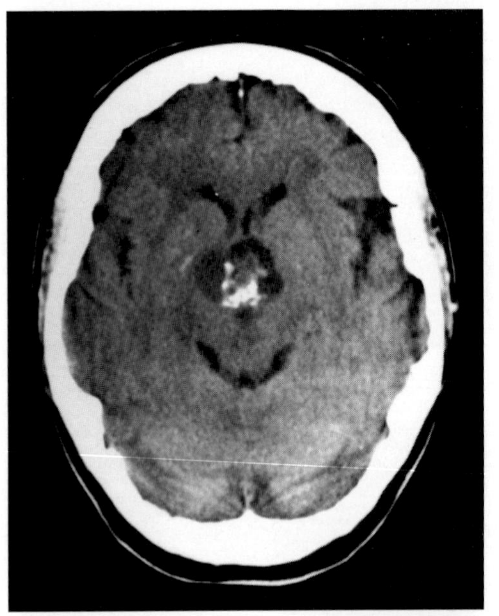

B

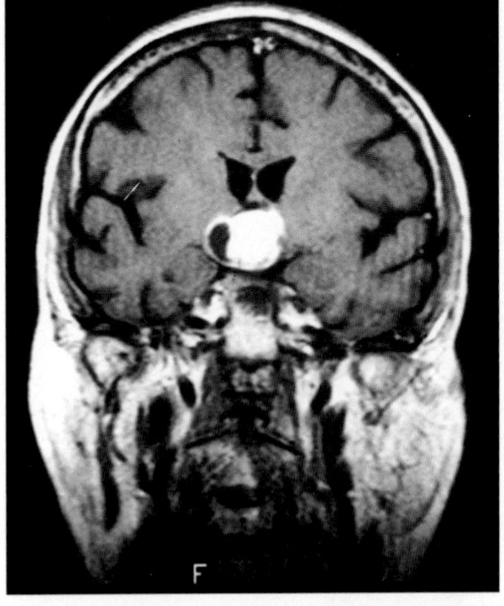

C

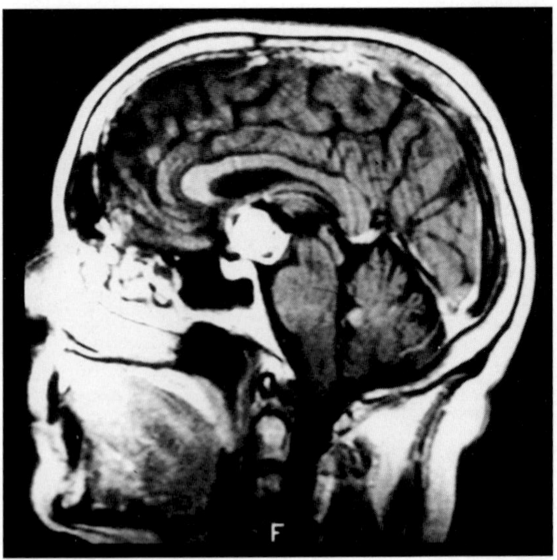

Fig. 10.21 Craniopharyngioma. **A**. Non-enhanced axial CT scan showing irregular suprasellar mass with calcification and cystic components. **B**. Coronal gadolinium-enhanced T1-weighted MRI of the same tumor showing an enhancing solid portion of the tumor together with a hypodense cystic component on the right side of the tumor. **C**. Parasagittal MRI of the same tumor showing the suprasellar location.

Craniopharyngiomas

Craniopharyngiomas constitute 1.2–4% of all brain tumors (Sanford & Muhlbauer 1991) but have inspired a disproportionate interest in the literature, perhaps because they challenge the neurosurgeon's skill to such a degree. They are histologically benign remnants of alimentary epithelium in the region of the hypothalamus. These remnants shed epithelial cells within them to increase slowly in size. Although histologically 'benign' their location may make them act malignant as they recur or continue to grow and compress the hypothalamus and visual apparatus.

Craniopharyngiomas are most commonly found between 5 and 10 years of age with a relatively constant percentage occurring through each decade of life (Sanford & Mulbauer 1991). They typically present with headache, nausea, vomiting, visual disturbances, visual field deficits and endocrinologic and hypothalamic dysfunction. Short stature, hypothyroidism, diabetes insipidus and delayed puberty are the most common endocrinologic abnormalities found at presentation.

Skull X-rays are usually abnormal and may show an enlarged sella turcica and suprasellar calcification. The CT scan typically shows an enhancing rounded, partly calcified cystic mass arising from the sellar or suprasellar region. Calcification is more common in children (80–90%) than in adults (15%) and may appear as chunks of calcium within the solid portion of the tumor or as a circumferential rim. Hydrocephalus is frequently present. MRI is superior to CT in delineating the relationship of the tumor to adjacent anatomic structures but is less effective at identifying tumor calcification (Fig. 10.21A–C). Detailed endocrine testing may demonstrate a variety of pituitary deficiencies and visual field testing may show deficits (Sanford & Muhlbauer 1991).

Choroid plexus papillomas

Choroid plexus papillomas arise from cells of the choroid plexus, usually in the lateral or fourth ventricles. They occur in children and are often associated with increased CSF production leading to hydrocephalus. They have well-defined margins and are isointense with adjacent brain on T1-weighted scans and slightly hyperintense on T2-weighted scans and enhance intensely with gadolinium administration.

Hemangioblastomas

Hemangioblastomas are benign tumors of blood vessels that usually occur in the cerebellum. They may be a part of Von Hippel-Lindau disease when they are associated with retinal angiomas, renal cell carcinoma, pancreatic cysts, pheochromocytoma and polycythemia (Neumann et al 1989). They typically present with headaches, hydrocephalus and ataxia. They appear on CT scans as low density cysts with an enhancing vascular nodule or as a solid vascular mass (Barkovitch 1992). The solid portion may not be visible on CT but may be demonstrated by angiography or MRI (Fig. 10.22A,B).

Epidermoid and dermoid tumors

These contain what appear to be desquamated fragments of epidermis within them.

Epidermoids have a predominantly paramedian location (cerebellopontine angle, parasellar region, ventricular

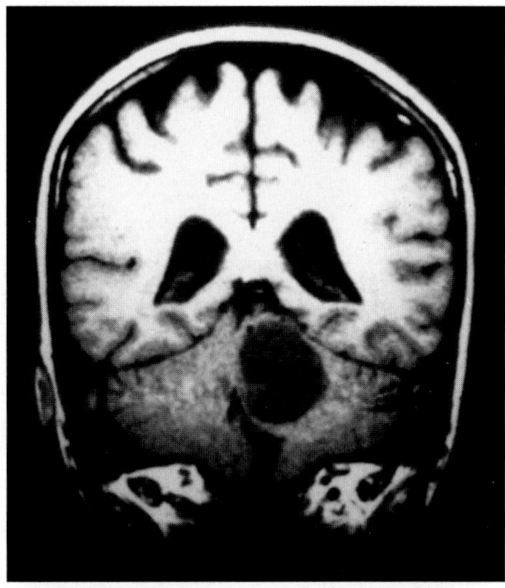

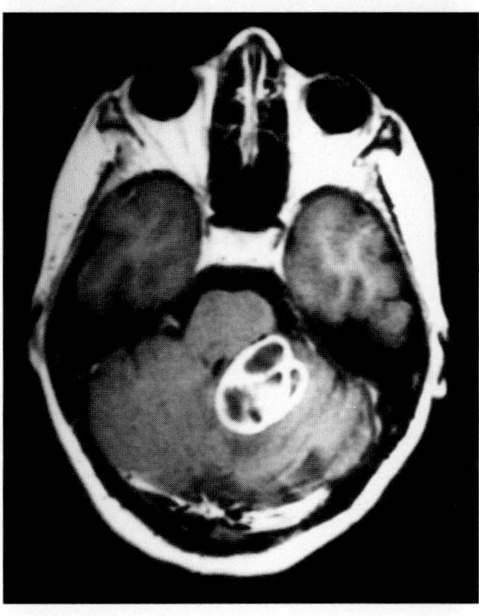

Fig. 10.22 Hemangioblastoma. Hypointense tumor on unenhanced coronal T1-weighted images (**A**) and enhancing left cerebellar tumor with cystic components on axial post-contrast T1-weighted images (**B**). These tumors may also appear as a single cystic lesion with a mural nodule.

system). They may be clinically silent or present in middle age with variable symptoms depending on their location. Suprasellar lesions may cause visual problems or pituitary dysfunction, parasellar lesions may cause seizures, and posterior fossa lesions may cause cranial nerve palsies, ataxia and hemiparesis. They are seen on CT as low attenuation lobulated masses in characteristic locations. The density is identical to CSF, making visualization of these lesions sometimes difficult. On MRI they appear as extra-axial masses with prolonged T1 and T2 values (Barkovitch 1992, Shah & Haines 1992) (Fig. 10.23A,B).

Dermoids have a predominantly midline location (cerebellar vermis). They present in the second decade with ataxia or aseptic meningitis as a result of rupture of the cyst. On CT they appear as fat density midline lesions. On MRI they are identical to lipomas with short T1 and T2 values (Barkovitch 1992, Shah & Haines 1992).

Colloid cysts

Colloid cysts arise from primitive neuorepithelium within the roof of the third ventricle and lend themselves to complete extirpation. They usually present with headaches which may be severe if there is hydrocephalus. They can occasionally cause sudden death. On MRI these cysts appear as smooth, spherical lesions in the third ventricle which are isointense on T1-weighted and hypointense with a hyperintense capsule on T-2 weighted images (Roosen et al 1987). Hydrocephalus is frequently present (Fig. 10.24).

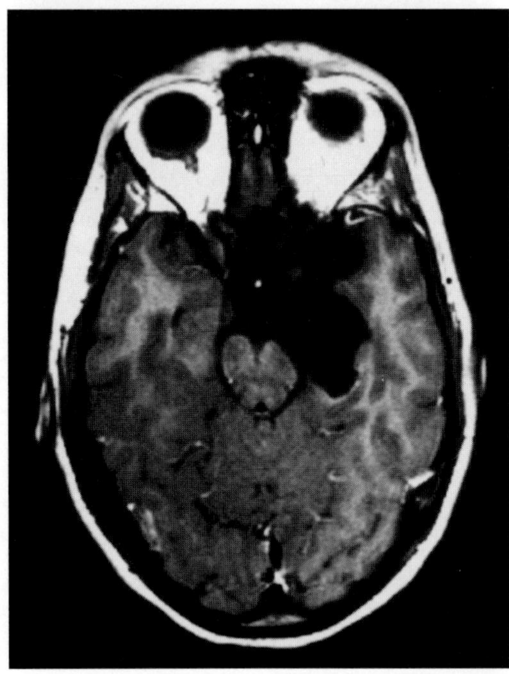

Fig. 10.23 Epidermoid. **A**. Contrast-enhanced CT scan showing irregular non-enhancing hypodense mass on the medial surface of the left anterior temporal lobe extending to the cavernous sinus. The signal intensity is slightly above that of CSF. **B**. T1-weighted image showing the same epidermoid as a hypodense mass.

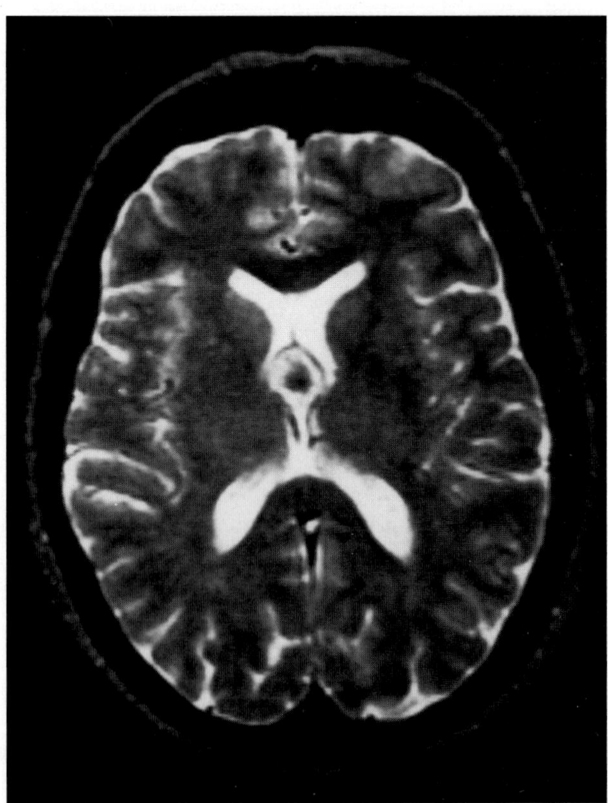

Fig. 10.24 Colloid cyst. Axial T2-weighted MRI showing colloid cyst in the region of the third ventricle.

Arachnoid cysts

Arachnoid cysts are CSF-filled loculations of arachnoid occurring in the temporal lobe, parasagittal region, or cerebellum which may act as intracranial masses. They are smoothly marginated lesions that follow CSF on T1- and T2-weighted images but often have higher than CSF intensity on proton density images. Large arachnoid cysts may cause remodelling of the adjacent skull. If the lesion progresses and causes neurologic deficits excision or shunting may be indicated. Otherwise they may be observed with sequential CT or MRI scans over many years.

SUMMARY

The diagnosis of brain tumors depends on careful clinical evaluation of the patient and judicious use of imaging and laboratory tests. Recent advances in imaging techniques have revolutionized the diagnosis of brain tumors and have allowed patients to be diagnosed at earlier stages of their illness. The challenge for the future lies not only in developing improved methods of diagnosis, however, but also in assuring cost-effective evaluation.

Acknowledgements

We gratefully acknowledge the help of Dr Amir Zamani with providing many of the CT and MRI scans, Dr David Vernick with providing the audiogram and MRI of the acoustic neurinoma, Dr Langham Gleason with providing the three-dimensional MRI reconstruction, and Dr Basem Garada and Dr Leonard Holman with providing the SPECT scan.

REFERENCES

Barkovich A J 1992 Neuroimaging of pediatric brain tumors. Neurosurgery Clinics 3: 739–769

Baumgartner J E, Edwards M S B 1992 Pineal tumors. Neurosurgery Clinics 3: 853–862

Black K L, Hawkins R A, Kim K T et al 1989 Use of thallium-201 SPECT to quantitate malignancy grade of gliomas. Journal of Neurosurgery 71: 342–346

Brody A S 1991 New perspectives in CT and MRI imaging. Neurology Clinics 9: 273–286

Carvalho P A, Schwartz R B, Alexander E et al 1992 Detection of recurrent gliomas with quantitative thallium-201/technetium-99m HMPAO single-photon emission computerized tomography. Journal of Neurosurgery 77: 565–570

Castillo M, Davis P C, Takei et al 1990 Intracranial ganglioglioma: MR, CT, and clinical findings in 18 patients. American Journal of Roentgenology 154: 607–612

Chiappa K H 1983 Evoked potentials in clinical medicine. Raven Press, New York

Cohen M E, Duffner P K 1991 Optic pathway tumors. Neurology Clinics 9: 467–479

Dam A M, Fuglsang-Frederiksen A, Svarre-Olsen U, Dam A 1985 Late onset epilepsy: Etiologies, type of seizure, and value of clinical investigation, EEG and computerized tomography scan. Epilepsia 26: 227–231

Daniels G H, Martin J B 1987 Neuroendocrine regulation and diseases of the anterior pituitary and hypothalamus. In: Braunwald E, Isselbacher K J, Petersdorf R G, Wilson J D, Martin J B, Fauci A S (eds) Harrison's Principles of internal medicine, 11th edn. McGraw-Hill, New York, pp 1694–1718

DeAngelis L M 1993 Primary CNS lymphoma. In: DeVita V T, Hellman S, Rosenberg S A (eds) Principles and practice of oncology update series. Lippincott. In press

Delattre J Y, Krol G, Thaler H T et al 1988 Distribution of brain metastases. Archives of Neurology 45: 741–744

Di Chiro G 1987 Positron Emission Tomography using (^{18}F) Fluorodeoxyglucose in brain tumors. A powerful diagnostic and prognostic tool. Investigative Radiology 22: 360–371

Di Chiro G, Brooks R A, Bairamian D et al 1985 Diagnostic and prognostic value of positron emission tomography using (^{18}F) fluorodeoxyglucose in brain tumors. In: Reivitch M, Alavi A (eds) Positron emission tomography. Alan R Liss, New York, pp 291–309

Doyle W K, Budinger T F, Valk P E et al 1987 Differentiation of cerebral radiation necrosis from tumor recurrence by (^{18}F) FDG and ^{82}Rb positron emission tomography. Journal of Computerized Assisted Tomography 11: 563–570

Eby N L, Grufferman S, Flannelly C M et al 1988 Increasing incidence of primary brain lymphoma in the US. Cancer 62: 2461–2465

Edelman R R, Hesselink J R 1990 Clinical magnetic resonance imaging. WB Saunders, Philadelphia

Fischer-Williams M 1987 Brain tumors and other space-occupying lesions. In: Niedermyer E, Lopes da Silva F (eds) Electroencephalography. Basic principles, clinical applications and related fields, 2nd edn. Urban & Schwarzenberg, Baltimore, pp 229–258

Forsyth P, Posner J B 1992 Headaches in patients with brain tumors: A study of 111 patients. Annals of Neurology 32: 289

Friedman H S, Oakes W J, Bigner S H et al 1991 Medulloblastoma: tumor biological and clinical perspectives. Journal of Neuro-Oncology 11: 1–15

Gehan E A, Walker M D 1977 Prognostic factors for patients with brain tumors. In: Bailar J C, Weisberger E K (eds) Modern concepts in brain tumor therapy: laboratory and clinical investigations. National Cancer Institute Monograph 46: 189–195

Grossman S A, Moynihan T J 1991 Neoplastic meningitis. Neurology Clinics 9: 843–856

Haerer A F 1992 DeJong's Neurologic examination, 5th edn. J B Lippincott, Philadelphia

Hicks R J, Hesselink J R, Wismaer G L et al 1990 Brain: neoplasia. In: Edelman R, Hesselink J R (eds) Clinical magnetic resonance imaging. Ch. 15. W B Saunders, Philadelphia, pp 483–515

Hochberg F H, Miller D C 1988 Primary central nervous system lymphoma. Journal of Neurosurgery 68: 835–853

Jaeckle K A 1991 Clinical presentation and therapy of nervous system tumors. In: Bradley W G, Daroff R B, Fenichel G M, Marsden C D (eds) Neurology in clinical practice. Butterworth-Heinemann, Boston, MA, pp 1008–1030

Jolesz F A, Kikinis R, Cline H E et al 1993 The use of computerized image processing for neurosurgical planning. In: Black P McL, Schoene W, Lampson L A (eds) Astrocytomas. Blackwell, Oxford, pp 50–56

Kelly P J, Daumas-Duport C, Kispert D B et al 1987 Imaging-based stereotaxic serial biopsies in untreated intracranial glial neoplasms. Journal of Neurosurgery 66: 865–874

Kingsley D P E 1990 Neuroradiological imaging of brain tumors. In: Thomas D G T (ed) Neuro-oncology. Primary malignant brain tumors. Johns Hopkins University Press, Baltimore, pp 94–121

Klibanski A, Zervas N T 1991 Diagnosis and management of hormone-secreting pituitary adenomas. New England Journal of Medicine 324: 822–831

Kumanishi T, Washiyama K, Nishiyama A et al 1989 Primary malignant lymphoma of the brain: demonstration of immunoglobulin

gene rearrangements in four cases by the Southern blot hybridization technique. Acta Neuropathologica 79: 23–26
Kucharczyk W, Davis D O, Kelly W M et al 1986 Pituitary adenomas: High resolution MR imaging at 1.5 T. Radiology 161: 761–765
Li C Y, Witzig T E, Phyliky R L et al 1986 Diagnosis of B-cell non-Hodgkin's lymphoma of the central nervous system by immunocytochemical analysis of cerebrospinal fluid lymphocytes. Cancer 57: 737–744
Mafee M F, Valvassori G E, Kumar A et al 1988 Tumors and tumor-like conditions of the middle ear and mastoid: role of CT and MRI. Otolaryngology Clinics of North America 21: 349
Mamourian A C, Towfigi J 1986 Pineal cysts: MR imaging. American Journal of Neuroradiology 7: 1081–1086
McKeran R O, Thomas D G T 1980 The clinical study of gliomas. In: Thomas D G T, Graham D L (eds) Brain tumors: scientific basis, clinical investigation and current therapy. Baltimore, pp 194–230
Melamed S 1990 Acromegaly. New England Journal of Medicine 322: 966–977
Mountz J M, Stafford-Schuck K, McKeever P E et al 1988 Thalium-201 tumor/cardiac ratio estimation of residual astrocytoma. Journal of Neurosurgery 68: 705–709
Neumann H P, Eggert H R, Weigel K et al 1989 Hemangioblastomas of the nervous system: a 10 year study with special reference to von-Hippel-Lindau syndrome. Journal of Neurosurgery 70: 24–30
Packer R J, Nicholson S, Vezina G, Johnson D L 1992 Brainstem gliomas. Neurosurgery Clinics 3: 863–880
Patchell R 1991 Brain metastases. Neurology Clinics 9: 817–824
Phillips P C 1992 Positron emission tomographic studies of transport and metabolism in brain tumors. In: Packer R J, Bleyer W A, Pochedly C (eds) Pediatric neuro-oncology. Harwood Academic Publishers, Philadelphia, PA, pp 91–110
Rachlin J R, Rosenblum M L 1991 Etiology and biology of meningiomas. In: Al-Mefty O (ed). Meningiomas. Raven, New York, pp 22–37
Rekate H L, Rakfal S M 1991 Low grade astrocytomas of childhood. Neurology Clinics 9: 423–440
Roosen N, Gahlen D, Stork W et al 1987 Magnetic resonance imaging of colloid cysts of the third ventricle. Neuroradiology 29: 10–14
Rozental J M 1991 Positron emission tomography (PET) and single photon emission computed tomography (SPECT) of brain tumors. Neurology Clinics 9: 287–305
Rushton J G, Rooke E D 1962 Brain tumor headache. Headache 2: 139–146
Russell D S, Rubinstein L J 1977 Pathology of tumors of the nervous system, 4th edn. Wilkins & Wilkins, Baltimore
Sanford R A, Muhlbauer M S 1991 Craniopharyngioma in children. Neurology Clinics 9: 453–465
Scott G M, Gibberd F B 1980 Epilepsy and other factors in the prognosis of gliomas. Acta Neurologica Scandinavia 61: 227–239
Segall H D, Destian S, Nelson et al 1990 CT and MR imaging in malignant gliomas. In: Apuzzo M L J (ed) Malignant cerebral glioma. American Association of Neurologic Surgeons, Park Ridge, Illinois, pp 63–78
Selters W A, Brackman D E 1977 Acoustic tumor detection with brainstem electric response audiometry. Archives of Otolaryngology 103: 181–187
Shah M V, Haines S J 1992 Pediatric skull, skull base, and meningeal tumors. Neurosurgery Clinics 4: 893–924
Shaw E G, Scheithauer B W, O'Fallon J R et al 1992 Oligodendroglioma: the Mayo Clinic experience. Journal of Neurosurgery 76: 428–434
Spagnoli M V, Goldberg H I, Grossman R I et al 1986 Intracranial meningiomas: High-field MR imaging. Radiology 161: 369–375
Spehlmann R 1981 EEG Primer. Elsevier/North Holland Biomedical Press, Amsterdam
Sze G, Shih J, Krol G et al 1988 Intraparenchymal brain metastases: MR imaging versus contrast-enhanced CT. Radiology 168: 187–194
Thomas D G T, McKeran R O 1990 Clinical manifestations of brain tumors. In: Thomas D G T (ed) Neuro-oncology. Primary malignant brain tumors: Johns Hopkins University Press, Baltimore, pp 94–121
Valk P E, Budinger T F, Levin V A et al 1988 PET of malignant cerebral tumors after interstitial brachytherapy. Demonstration of metabolic activity and correlation with clinical outcome. Journal of Neurosurgery 69: 830–838
Weingarten S, Kleinman M, Elperin L, Larson E B 1992 The effectiveness of cerebral imaging in the diagnosis of chronic headache. Archives of Internal Medicine 152: 2457–2462
Welling D B, Glasscock M E, Woods C I, Jackson C G 1990. Acoustic neuroma: A cost effective approach. Otolaryngology Head Neck Surgery 103: 364–370
Wen P Y, Schiff D 1993 Clinical evaluation of patients with astrocytomas. In: Black P McL, Schoene W, Lampson L A (eds) Astrocytomas. Blackwell, Oxford, pp 26–35
Zimmerman R D, Fleming C A, Saint-Louis C A et al 1985 Magnetic resonance imaging of meningiomas. American Journal of Neuroradiology 6: 149–157

11. Neuro-ophthalmology of brain tumors

John King

Prior to the advent of computerized tomography and magnetic resonance imaging neuro-ophthalmic examination was important in localizing brain tumors for a number of reasons. Firstly the visual sensory pathway passes horizontally through areas noted for a high incidence of tumors, especially the suprasellar area. Secondly the ocular motor pathways dip deep into the brainstem and their integrity is essential for normal ocular movements and balance. Thirdly raised intracranial pressure often presents with visual symptoms and signs. Finally the visual system generally is very sensitive to minor changes in function. These visual symptoms are often the presenting features of an intracranial tumor.

Better imaging has in practical terms reduced the need for detailed clinical assessment but an ability to take a good history and perform an adequate examination is essential for the neurosurgeon. Such skills are also vital in the emergency situation and at the bedside for accurate assessment of the patient. The ordering of appropriate investigations and interpretation of the results are dependent upon a thorough clinical evaluation. For example, slowly progressive visual loss in one eye with signs of an optic nerve lesion is likely to be due to compression of the optic nerve despite negative radiology.

HISTORY AND EXAMINATION

As in many areas of medicine, a neuro-ophthalmic diagnosis is often made on the basis of the history, in particular the pattern of evolution of symptoms. It is often surprising to the clinician how infrequently patients give their histories in a logical sequence.

The neuro-ophthalmic examination can be carried out at the bedside and should be followed by examination of the remainder of the cranial nerves and limbs.

The neuro-ophthalmic assessment involves:

1. history of visual symptoms
2. examination (Table 11.1).

Table 11.1 Examination

Examination	Technique	Additional
Sense of smell		
Visual acuity	Snellen	Reading type Photostress test
Visual fields	Confrontation	Perimetry Amsler grid
Fundi		
Eyelids		
Pupils	Swinging flashlight test	
Eye movements	Saccadic Pursuit	Oculo-cephalic and oculo-vestibular reflexes Bell's phenomenon
Trigeminal nerve	Corneal reflexes Motor and sensory function	

History of visual symptoms

Visual loss may be unilateral or bilateral, sudden or progressive, transient or permanent, and painful or painless. If the visual loss occurs suddenly in one eye the patient is usually aware of the change, whereas slowly progressive loss may go unnoticed. Details of a previous recording of visual acuity such as a school medical or driver's license examination may be useful in dating a decline in vision.

Amblyopia is decreased visual acuity without obvious cause. It is usually associated with strabismus, unequal refractive error or congenital abnormality such as cataract and is thought to be due to failure of development of neural connections with the visual cortex. It is a common cause of visual impairment but is not progressive after 6–8 years of age. A history of a 'lazy eye', reduced acuity from early childhood, and previous evidence of squint or refractive error, together with normal color vision, optic discs, and pupillary responses makes a diagnosis of amblyopia likely.

In monocular visual loss an awareness of a shadow, i.e. a positive scotoma, suggests vitreous or retinal disease, whereas an optic nerve lesion gives a negative scotoma. The blind spot is an example of a negative scotoma.

Where objects look smaller or straight lines are bent or distorted, a macular abnormality should be suspected. The specific visual symptoms of brain tumors affecting discrete areas of the visual and ocular motor pathways will be discussed later.

The sense of smell should always be tested because of the proximity of the olfactory pathway to the optic nerves and chiasm.

Visual acuity

The normal visual acuity using a Snellen chart is 20/20 (6/6 in metric measurements) or better in each eye and failure to achieve this requires explanation. The term '20/20' means the patient sees at 20 feet the line of the Snellen chart that a 'normal' person is expected to see at 20 feet. The acuity in each eye should be recorded and, if the patient has spectacles, they should be worn at the time of testing. Measurements should be made using the Snellen chart, reading type or failing that, even small newsprint which approximates N8 of the reading type. Where the acuity is less than 20/400, counting fingers, hand movements, perception of light or no perception of light (NPL) can be recorded. In the absence of spectacles, a reduced acuity is checked using a pin hole, and although not infallible this simple device eliminates most refractive errors.

If possible the color vision in each eye should be recorded using the Ishihara plates. Covering one eye the patient is asked to read the plates as they are rapidly turned from page to page and the number of plates read correctly should be recorded. A relative inability to read the color plates in one eye in the absence of gross ocular disease indicates an optic nerve lesion. A subtle hemianopic defect may be revealed by failure to identify the one figure of a two figure number which falls in the affected field.

The photostress test is positive in macular disease. The patient's best acuity is recorded in the affected eye, then a bright light is shone in the eye for 10 seconds. The time taken for this eye to return to original acuity is compared with the time taken for the normal eye. In macular disease there is a marked delay in recovery (Glaser et al 1977).

Visual fields

A knowledge of the visual pathways is essential (Fig. 11.1A). At the bedside visual field testing should consist of two parts. The first is a screening test where the patient is asked to fix on the examiner's nose whilst the examiner's hands are held first in the upper and then lower quadrants. Subtle finger movements should be readily detected when the fields are normal and a qualitative difference in the clarity of the examiner's hands may indicate a relative homonymous hemianopia. This test is especially valuable in parietal lobe tumors. The visual field of each eye should then be checked separately by confron-

A

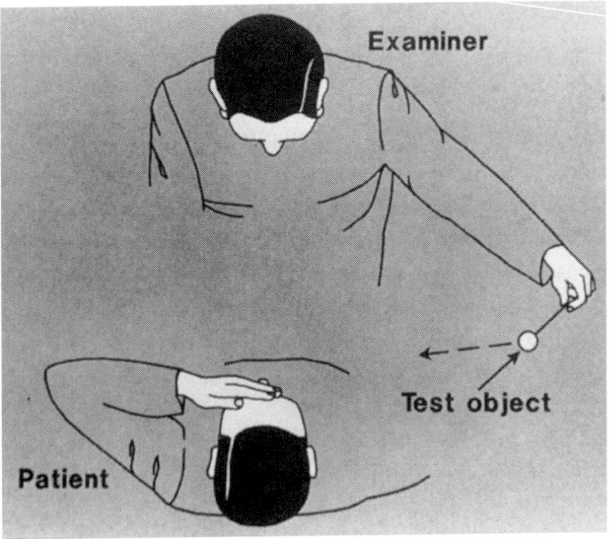

B

Fig. 11.1 **A**. The visual pathways, showing common patterns of field loss. **B**. Visual field testing by confrontation (Kaye 1991).

tation using a red pin (Fig. 11.1B). Where defects are found or where documented fields are necessary for a follow-up, formal perimetry using the Bjerrum, Goldmann or automated perimeters is required. The Amsler grid is valuable for testing the central 10 degrees of vision.

Fundi

Examination of the fundi is essential and all clinicians need to be proficient in the use of an ophthalmoscope. Dilatation of the pupils greatly improves the view of the fundi and should be performed wherever possible.

Eyelids and pupils

Assessment of the eyelids, and degree of ptosis, proptosis and the pupillary size precedes testing eye movements. A relative afferent pupil defect or Marcus Gunn pupil (Gunn 1904) is sought using the swinging flashlight test. With the patient fixing in the distance, a bright flashlight is shone from one pupil to the other. With each eye the light is directed at the pupil long enough to assess the briskness of contraction and the ability to sustain contraction. Normal or physiological pupillary unrest, in which the pupil contracts and dilates, must be distinguished from the afferent pupil defect where the pupil on the side of the optic nerve lesion is unable to sustain contraction (Thompson et al 1981). This important objective sign is usually supported by the patient's observation that the flashlight is less bright in the eye on the side of the optic nerve lesion.

Eye movements

The pursuit movements are best tested at the bedside using a bright light moved in an 'H'-shaped fashion to test the individual yoke muscles of the eyes. Any loss of alignment of the two eyes is noted and it is always worth asking the patient at this stage if double vision is present. The saccadic eye movements are examined by asking the patient to look from the finger of one hand to the thumb of the other held in a horizontal plane and then a vertical plane on either side of fixation. The speed, range and accuracy of the movement of each eye is observed. Doll's head eye movements (oculo-cephalic reflexes) in horizontal and vertical planes are useful in the obtunded patient as a means of checking ocular motor pathways. Iced water caloric testing of the oculo-vestibular reflexes is also useful in checking the integrity of the brainstem.

During examination of the eye movements, an effort is made to look for nystagmus in the primary position and at extremes of horizontal and vertical gaze. The classification of nystagmus is complex and is well covered in several excellent texts (Dell'Osso et al 1990, Newman 1992).

Trigeminal nerve

Testing of the corneal reflexes, facial sensation and power complete the neuro-ophthalmic examination. Although the first six cranial nerves are the major area for abnormal findings, examination of the remaining cranial nerves and the limbs should not be overlooked.

GENERAL (NON-LOCALIZING) SYMPTOMS AND SIGNS OF BRAIN TUMORS

Brain tumors grow in a closed box and therefore produce symptoms and signs from the effects of raised intracranial pressure in addition to direct effects on neighboring structures.

Headache

Headache as a manifestation of raised intracranial pressure is felt bilaterally in the forehead or occiput, is worse when lying down as on waking and also when coughing, straining or bending. The pain is often described as dull, bursting or throbbing. Faced with a history of this type of headache, the important features to seek are the presence of nausea, vomiting, obscurations of vision and diplopia.

Obscurations

Obscurations of vision are a most important symptom of raised intracranial pressure. They are brief episodes of blurring of vision proceeding to complete blindness for no more than a few seconds and precipitated by activities which raise intracranial pressure or lower capillary perfusion pressure in the optic nerve head (Sadun et al 1984). They occur with straining, bending or standing up and can be unilateral or bilateral. Their significance is that they indicate marginal perfusion in the optic nerve head and unless the intracranial pressure is promptly treated, permanent visual loss will ensue. Obscurations are almost always associated with obvious papilledema and tend to occur on the side with the more severe disc swelling, which in turn correlates with the side of the tumor.

Diplopia

Diplopia as a non-localizing symptom associated with raised intracranial pressure is due to unilateral or bilateral abducens palsies. The earliest symptom is often diplopia with horizontal separation of images for distant objects. Later the diplopia may be present to one or both sides. The abducens nerves run a sigmoid course and are tethered at the ponto-medullary junction and the petrous apex. Downward pressure on the brainstem from a supratentorial mass stretches the abducens nerves and renders them liable to ischemia or compression at each end.

Papilledema

Papilledema is the crucial clinical sign of raised intracranial pressure and the term is used synonymously with that disorder. Early papilledema is difficult to detect and requires considerable experience; however, if venous pulsation is present in retinal veins on the optic disc the intracranial pressure is less than 200 millimetres of water (Walsh et al 1969). The absence of venous pulsation does not mean that intracranial pressure is raised since about 20% of normal eyes do not show spontaneous pulsation of veins as they enter the optic disc. The earliest changes in the fundus associated with raised intracranial pressure are blurring and darkening of the nerve fiber layer adjacent to the superior and inferior disc margins (Hoyt & Knight 1973). These changes are due to swelling of axons from obstructed axoplasmic flow in the anterior end of the optic nerve, secondary to ischemia produced by increased intracranial pressure reflected down the subarachnoid space inside the optic nerve sheath. The earliest changes are best seen using a red-free light from the ophthalmoscope (Fig. 11.2).

Swelling of the nerve fiber layer on the disc blurs the disc margins and then nerve fiber layer hemorrhages (flame shaped) and infarcted axons (cotton wool spots) may appear (Fig. 11.3). Venous distension is observed but the details of the veins and arteries on the disc are buried by the swollen axons and hyperemia of the disc surface. The swelling of the optic disc may be surrounded by circumferential retinal folds (Bird & Sanders 1973).

In more chronic papilledema the hemorrhages and nerve fiber infarcts disappear but a telangiectatic mesh of small dilated capillaries appears on the disc surface. The disc takes on a champagne cork or donut appearance. Later, hard exudates resembling small drusen bodies appear. These are thought to be formed from products of axon breakdown. With prolonged raised intracranial pressure the disc swelling becomes paler and less evident

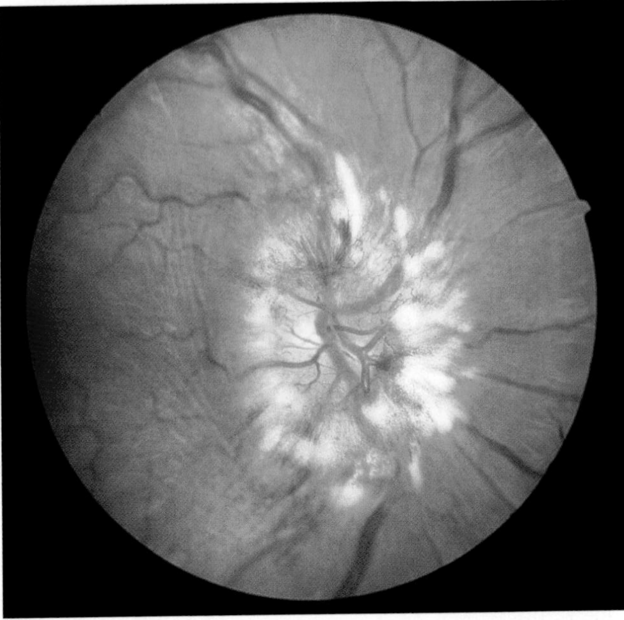

Fig. 11.3 Fundal photograph of acute papilledema with multiple infarcted axons (cotton wool spots), some nerve fiber layer hemorrhages and circumferential retinal folds.

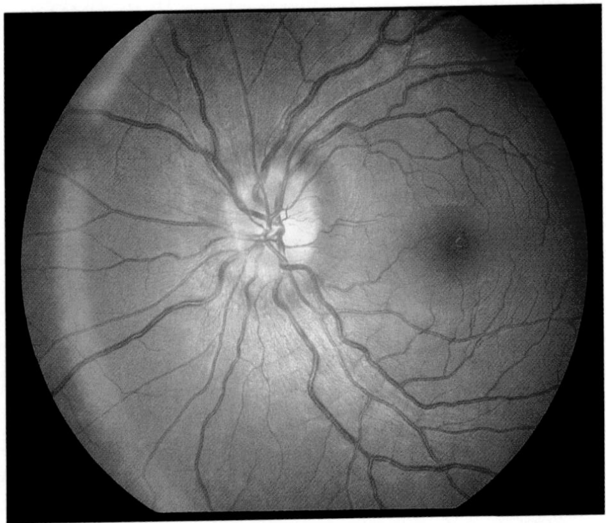

Fig. 11.2 Fundal photograph in early papilledema showing blurring and darkening of the peripapillary nerve fiber layer around the optic disc.

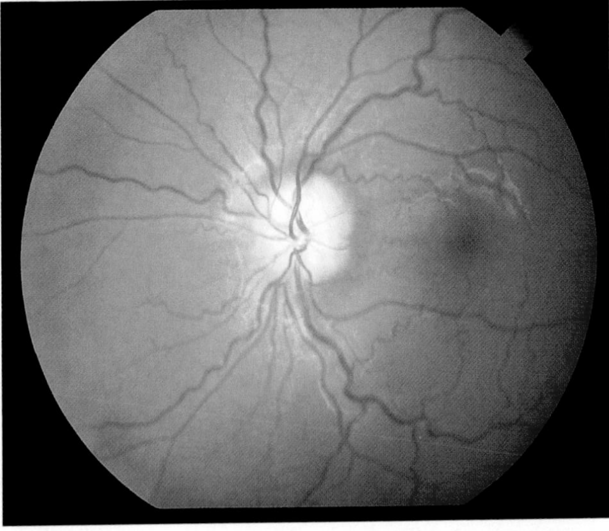

Fig. 11.4 Chronic atrophic papilledema with a pale swollen disc and loss of nerve fibers.

as axons die off (Fig. 11.4). This eventually leads to consecutive optic atrophy which is a pale disc with blurred margins due to gliosis.

TUMORS OF THE OPTIC NERVE

Unilateral optic nerve tumors may be intraorbital, intracanalicular, intracranial, or combinations of the above.

They all present with the complaint of ipsilateral visual loss with poor perception of color and brightness. In some instances where the optic nerve function fails slowly over a long period, the patient may be unaware of the visual impairment until the normal eye is covered inadvertently.

In the presence of a tumor involving the optic nerve the acuity will be reduced and there may be difficulty in reading the Ishihara plates. With extrinsic compression of the optic nerve, the visual field shows a central scotoma with 'breaking through' as the defect increases. This leaves a peripheral crescent of preserved vision. The optic disc will gradually become pale and atrophic with continued compression of the nerve. An afferent pupillary defect accompanies the above findings. If the diagnosis of optic nerve compression is to be made before there is significant irreversible visual loss, it is vital for the clinician to look for the signs above. If there is no obvious explanation for the unilateral visual loss in the fundal examination, it should be presumed that the optic nerve is being compressed somewhere in its course behind the globe.

Signs of an optic nerve lesion:

- Decreased visual acuity
- Impaired color vision
- Central scotoma
- Optic disc pallor
- Afferent pupillary defect.

The two important intraorbital tumors to cause an optic nerve lesion are the perioptic meningioma and the optic nerve glioma. The *perioptic meningioma*, which is much more common in females, shows the features of optic nerve compression but in addition to slowly progressive visual loss the optic disc is swollen, atrophic and may display opto-ciliary shunt vessels (Wright et al 1980, Sibony et al 1984, Sarkies 1987). These are tortuous, dilated veins on the surface of the optic disc (Fig. 11.5) which drain venous blood from the obstructed central retinal vein, via choroidal veins to the ophthalmic veins (Frisen et al 1973). A bulky intraorbital tumor may also produce choroidal folds and eventually proptosis (Fig. 11.6, 11.7). *Optic nerve gliomas* involving the intraorbital optic nerve present in childhood with slowly progressive proptosis and often mild visual loss (Miller et al 1974, Alvord & Lofton 1988). Other stigmata of neurofibromatosis are often present.

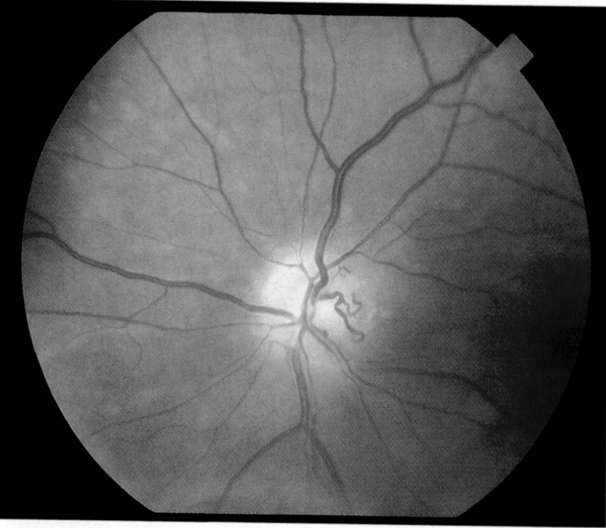

Fig. 11.5 Fundal photograph of a 63-year-old female with a perioptic meningioma. The optic disc is pale and swollen and shows an opto-ciliary shunt vessel.

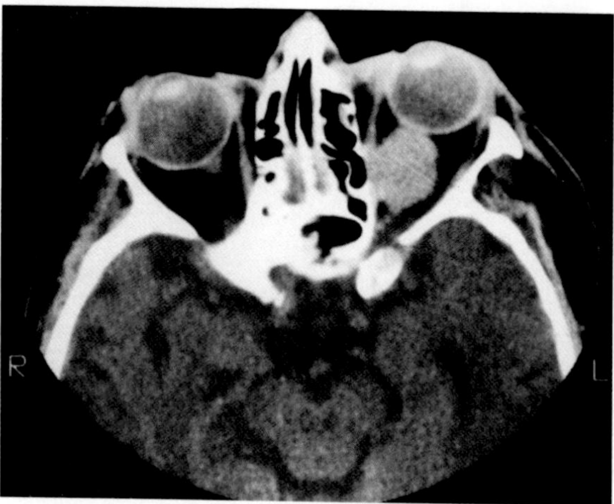

Fig. 11.6 CT of the orbits showing a large perioptic meningioma producing proptosis.

The intracanalicular optic nerve lesion is usually due to a meningioma growing back from a perioptic tumor or forward into the optic canal from the anterior clinoid area. A primary meningioma arising within the optic canal is rare but presents with slowly progressive signs of an optic nerve lesion with negative radiologic investigations (Sanders & Falconer 1964).

The intracranial or prechiasmal optic nerve may be involved by meningioma arising from the posterior optic foramen, the tuberculum sellae or the anterior clinoid process, with no signs other than those of a progressive unilateral optic nerve lesion (Fig. 11.8). Apart from this presentation, also known as the anterior clinoid syndrome, these tumors may show features of chiasmal involvement (Finn & Mount 1974, Gregorius et al 1975). Occasionally a pituitary tumor with suprasellar extension under one

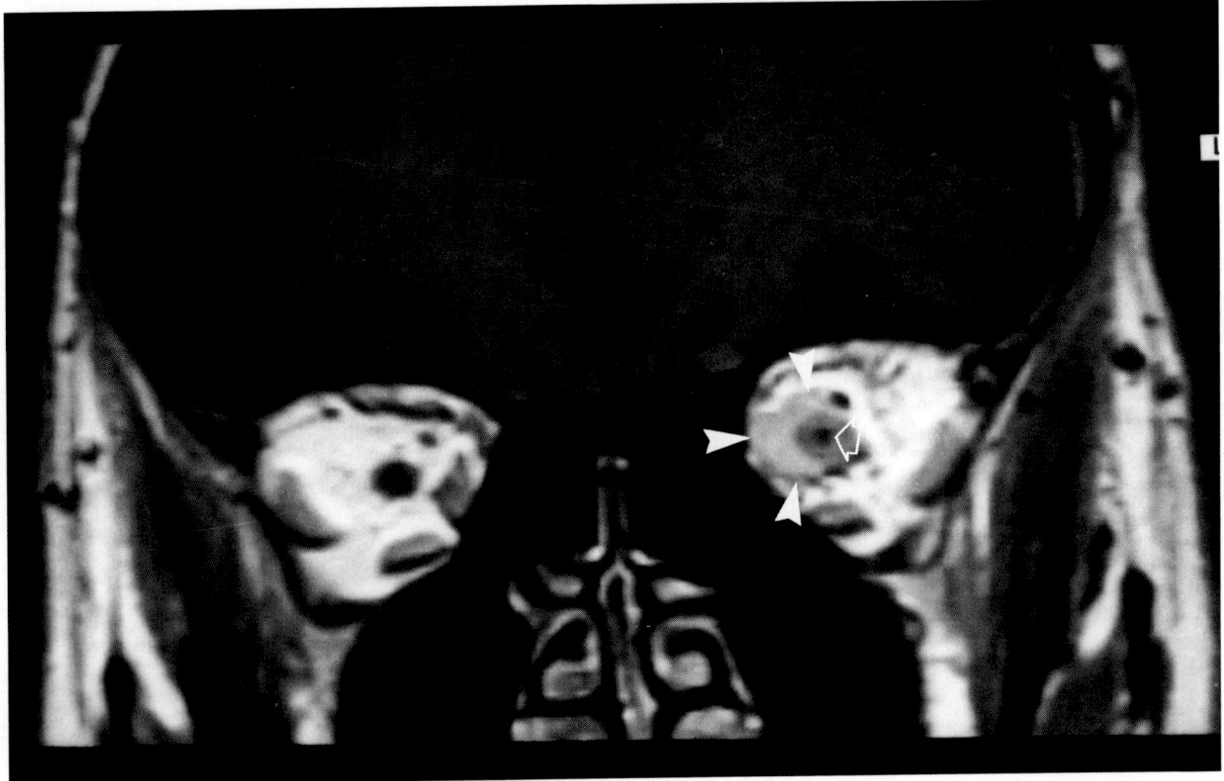

Fig. 11.7 MR coronal post-gadolinium enhanced T1 image showing a perioptic meningioma (white arrows) with two different densities surrounding an atrophic optic nerve (open arrow head).

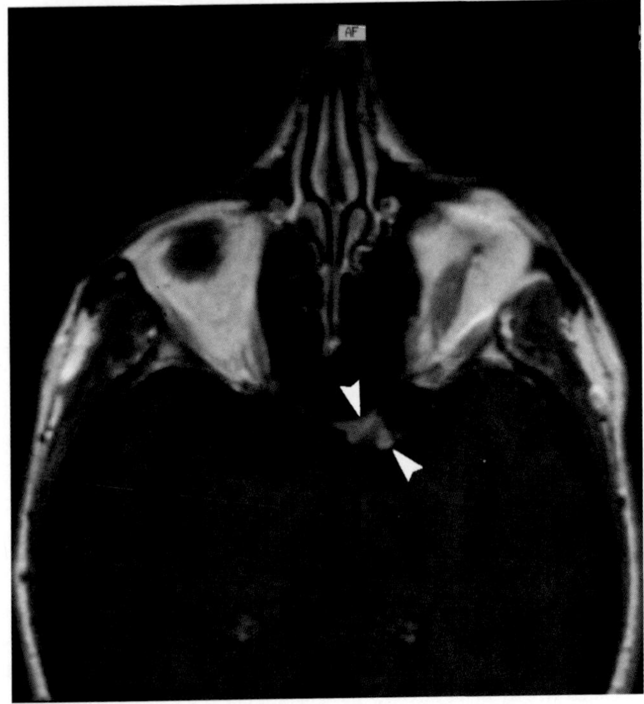

Fig. 11.8 MR axial post-gadolinium enhanced T1 image with a small meningioma involving the prechiasmal optic nerve.

nerve, especially with a prefixed chiasm, can present as a unilateral optic nerve lesion.

Carcinomatous or lymphomatous optic neuropathy is due to meningeal infiltration by neoplastic cells, usually but not always in patients with known metastatic carcinoma or lymphoma. The visual loss is painless, acute or subacute, and usually involves the second eye quite rapidly (Altrocchi et al 1972). The diagnosis is dependent upon demonstrating malignant cells in the CSF in a patient with signs of a progressive optic nerve lesion.

SUPRASELLAR TUMORS

About 25% of all intracranial tumors arise in the chiasmal area, and of the lesions causing chiasmal compression 50% are pituitary adenomas, 25% are craniopharyngiomas and 10% meningiomas (Hollenhorst & Younge 1973).

Involvement of the optic chiasm by suprasellar tumors produces a limited spectrum of important symptoms and signs. The earliest symptom of chiasmal compression by a *pituitary adenoma* is insidious painless visual loss which is often vague and indefinite. Because initial symptoms are transient and attributed to fatigue they are overlooked for lengthy periods.

Post-fixation blindness refers to objects disappearing behind the point of fixation, e.g. the eye of a needle disappears when the patient fixes on the thread, or a word being written disappears if the point of fixation shortens above the tip of the pen (Fig. 11.9) When reading, letters or numbers may be missed. The area beyond fixation projects to the blind nasal retina of both eyes (Nachtigaller & Hoyt 1970).

The hemislide phenomenon is the basis for further symptoms. In chiasmal lesions there is no means of tying or linking the images from both eyes together and consequently the two images slide apart or together, horizontally or vertically. Patients complain of double vision, usually in the primary position (Kirkham 1972). This 'non-paretic diplopia' manifests as two cars on the road ahead, side by side or one on top of the other, or if there is a lesser slide, double pairs of headlights. Another complaint is of the white line on the road dividing into two. Sometimes this phenomenon may cause objects such as buses to elongate or shorten, or one side of a building to seem lower than the other side (Fig. 11.10). These symptoms only occur in the presence of bitemporal field defects, but they often precede the more florid symptoms caused by bitemporal hemianopia. Patients often do not present until they are aware of poor vision in one eye which occurs when there is asymmetric growth of the suprasellar mass under one optic nerve.

The visual loss with chiasmal compression by pituitary adenoma, suprasellar meningioma and craniopharyngioma is usually insidious, however *pituitary apoplexy* may lead to sudden bilateral severe visual loss, even blindness, together with headache, diplopia and disturbed consciousness. This entity — due to hemorrhage or infarction of the pituitary tumor — may also involve the cavernous sinus on one or both sides with the result that there may be external and internal ophthalmoplegia (David et al 1975). Involvement of the oculomotor, trochlear or abducens nerves causing diplopia and ptosis is unusual in uncomplicated pituitary tumors.

In the majority of patients with chiasmal compression by tumors, there is some asymmetry which gives rise to a greater degree of visual loss in one eye. Typically patients will read down the Snellen chart missing the letters in their temporal field for each eye. Similarly, when reading the Ishihara plates, they will miss the figure which falls in the temporal field if a two digit number is presented.

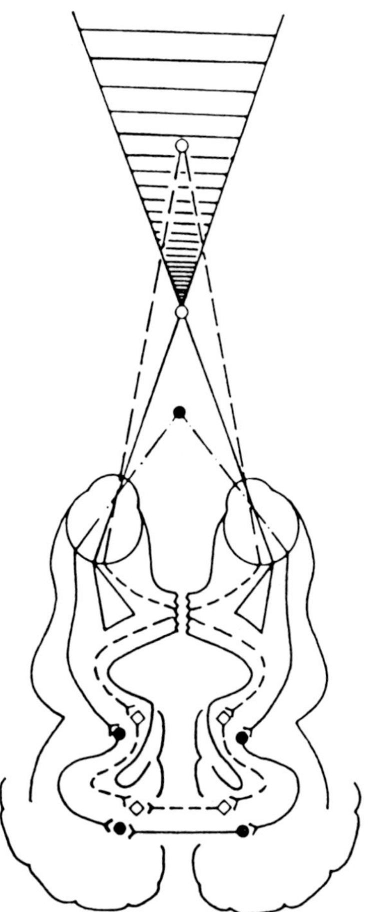

Fig. 11.9 Diagram showing the formation of a blind triangular area of visual field that occurs just beyond fixation in patients with complete bitemporal hemianopia or dense bitemporal hemianopic scotomata. Reproduced from Kirkham (1972) with permission.

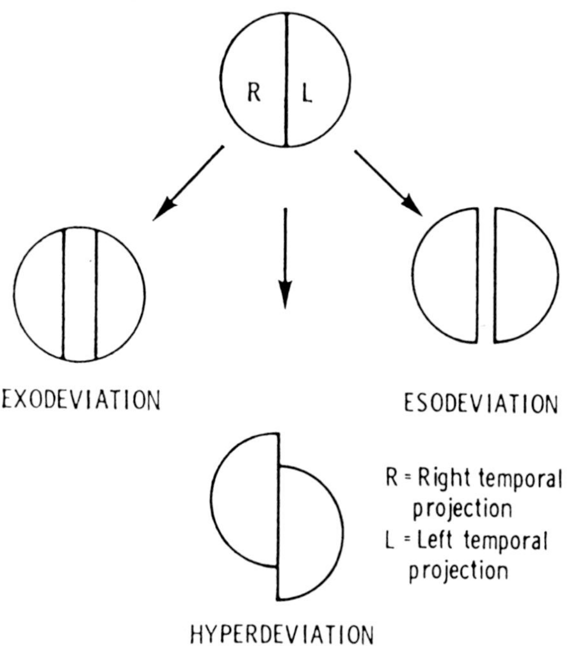

Fig. 11.10 A chiasmal lesion interrupts the physiological linkage between the two half fields and allows intermittent overlap or separation of the two nasal fields. Reproduced from Kirkham (1972) with permission.

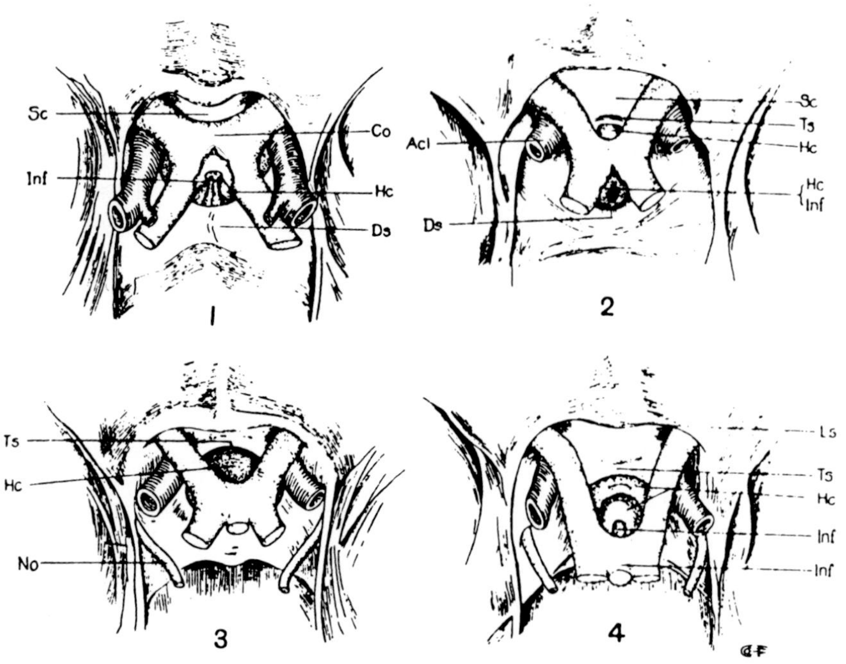

Fig. 11.11 Variations in the position of the optic chiasm: **1** prefixed chiasm, **2** and **3** chiasm over pituitary gland, **4** post-fixed chiasm. Sc = sulcus, Inf = infundibulum, Co = chiasm, Hc = hypophysis, Ds = dorsum sellae, Acl = internal carotid artery, Ts = tuberculum sellae, Ls = limbus sphenoidale, No = third nerve. Reproduced from Whitnall (1932) by permission of Oxford University Press.

Signs of a chiasmal lesion:

- Visual acuity may be reduced in one or both eyes
- Loss of color vision in temporal fields
- Bitemporal hemianopia
- Optic disc pallor with 'bow-tie' atrophy.

The pattern of visual field loss with pituitary tumors depends on the direction of the growth of the tumor and whether the chiasm is pre-fixed (9%) with short optic nerves and chiasm over the tuberculum, the chiasm over the pituitary gland (80%), or post-fixed (11%) with the chiasm over the dorsum sellae (Figs 11.11, 11.12). In the study of 1000 pituitary tumors, bitemporal field defects occurred in 67%, junctional scotoma in 29%, homonymous hemianopia in 7% (Fig. 11.13) and prechiasmal pattern in 2% (Hollenhorst & Younge 1973). The homonymous hemianopic field defect is more likely with a prefixed chiasm; nerve fibre bundle defects, albeit rare, are seen in post-fixed chiasms (Kearns & Rucker 1958).

The bitemporal pattern of field loss characteristically starts in the upper temporal field of each eye and, although asymmetric, gradually descends into the lower temporal field and then into the lower nasal quadrant. In the most advanced cases the patients are left with small islands of preserved vision adjacent to fixation in the upper nasal field.

Suprasellar meningiomas arise from the dura of the tuberculum sellae and rarely from the diaphragma sellae (Fig. 11.14). Cushing's 'syndrome of the chiasm' consisting of bitemporal visual field defects, bilateral optic atrophy and a normal sella turcica on plain radiographs was due to tuberculum sellae meningiomas (Cushing 1930). The major symptoms are painless progressive visual loss and headache (Symon & Rosenstein 1984). The visual field defects are asymmetric as is the visual loss and optic atrophy, but there is usually bilateral involvement (Rosenberg & Miller 1984). Occasionally these tumors can be so large as to cause papilledema.

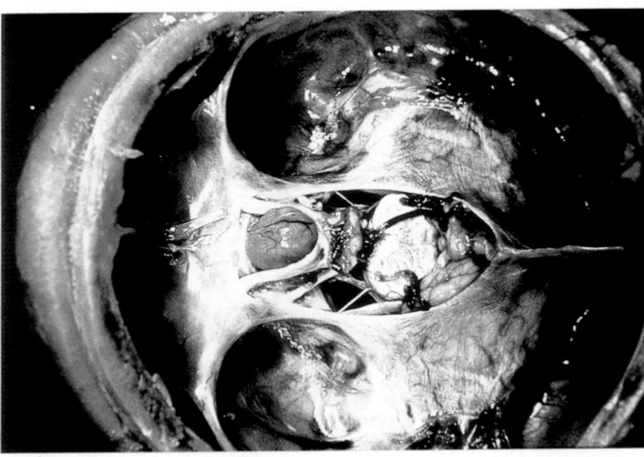

Fig. 11.12 Post-mortem photograph of skull base. A pituitary tumor has grown between post-fixed optic nerves.

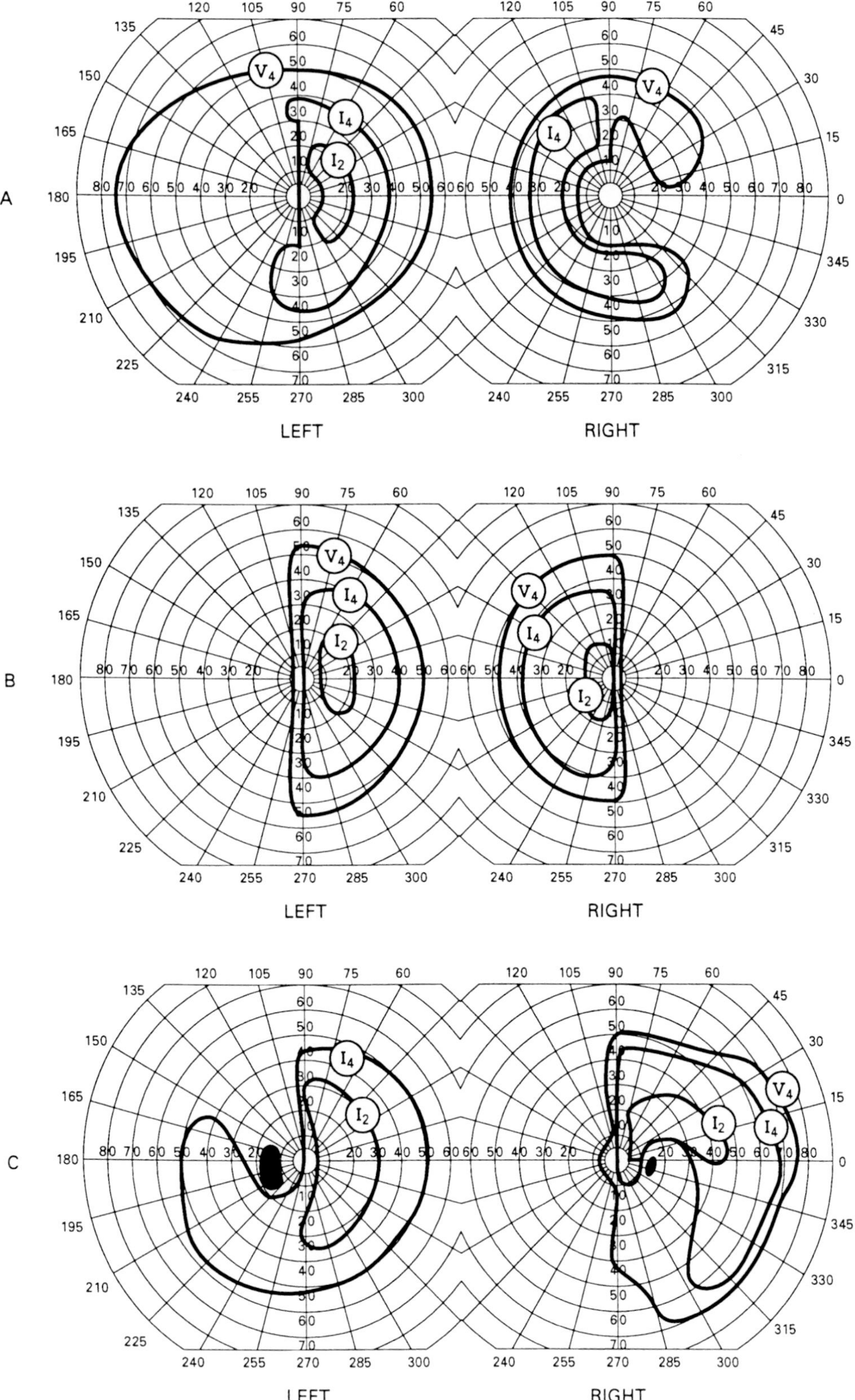

Fig. 11.13 Three forms of visual field loss with chiasmal compression. **A**. Junctional defect: right central scotoma with left temporal hemianopia due to a lesion at junction of right optic nerve and chiasm. **B**. Bitemporal hemianopia: complete defect to largest isopter. **C**. Incongruous homonymous hemianopia: from involvement of right optic tract. Reproduced with permission from Burde et al (1992).

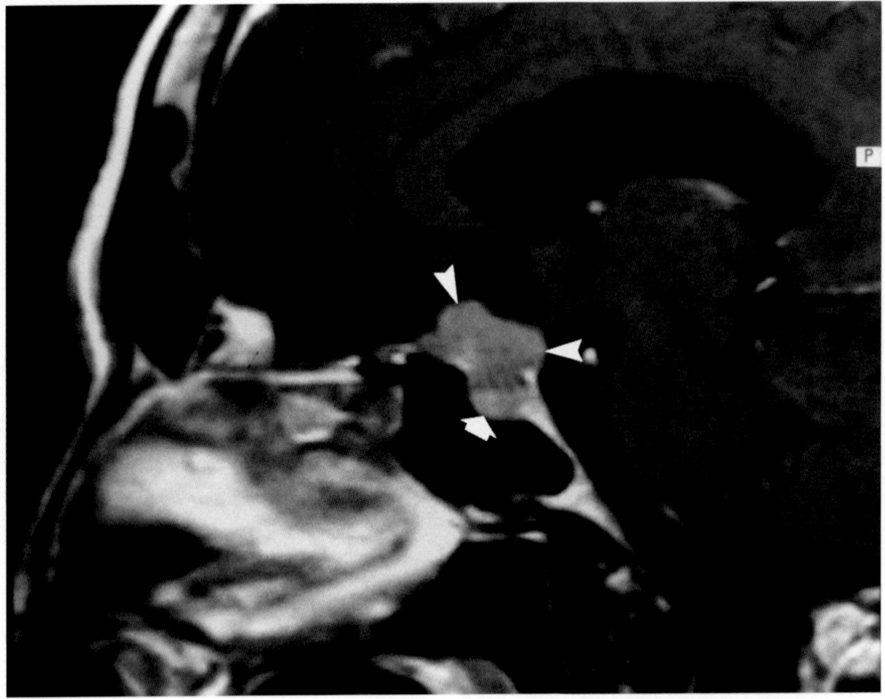

Fig. 11.14 MR sagittal post-gadolinium enhanced T1 image showing suprasellar meningioma. Pituitary gland is seen flattened in the pituitary fossa (broad arrow).

A less common but well-recognized pattern of field loss with suprasellar tumors is the 'junctional' syndrome or anterior chiasmal syndrome. The tumor compresses the medial aspect of the junction between the chiasm and one optic nerve. This leads to visual loss in the ipsilateral eye which may show greater loss in the temporal field but also optic atrophy and an afferent pupil defect. The other eye, which is thought by the patient to be normal, will have a superior temporal field defect due to the involvement of the inferior nasal fibres of the contralateral eye which sweep across the chiasm and briefly enter the distal ipsilateral optic nerve before passing posteriorly.

In rare instances the pituitary tumor may involve the optic tract and produce an optic tract syndrome consisting of a complete or incongruous homonymous hemianopia, a relative afferent pupillary defect in the eye with reduced central acuity or greater visual field loss, or both, and 'hemioptic' optic atrophy (Moyt et al 1972, Savino et al 1978). The reduced acuity and afferent defect indicate that the chiasm is involved as well as the optic tract. This clinical picture can also be produced by craniopharyngiomas and aneurysms. As mentioned above, monocular visual loss due to optic nerve involvement can also occur with pituitary adenoma.

Optic tract syndrome

- Complete or incongruous homonymous hemianopia
- Bilateral optic atrophy — hemioptic type.

With prolonged chiasmal compression optic atrophy begins to appear in both eyes. Initially this takes the form of 'band' or 'bow-tie' atrophy. In each eye the fibres run from the ganglion cells of preserved temporal retina to the optic disc in the superior and inferior arcuate bundles. The fibres to the nasal retina undergo degeneration and they leave areas of pallor of the disc surface in the wedges between 2 and 4 o'clock and 8 and 10 o'clock, hence the name 'bow-tie' atrophy (Fig. 11.15). With time the atrophy becomes more pronounced and the prospects of recovery of vision postoperatively are diminished. Papilledema in a patient with a chiasmal syndrome should raise the possibility of the tumor being a *craniopharyngioma.* In children with this tumor, half will have papilledema in addition to chiasmal and optic tract field defects, however in adults disc swelling is uncommon (Stahnke et al 1984). Because of the infiltrative and extensive growth of craniopharyngiomas, there is a higher incidence of ocular motor nerve palsies (Baskin & Wilson 1986).

Primary gliomas of the chiasm (Fig. 11.16) present in childhood with unilateral or bilateral loss of vision, 'amblyopia', strabismus, optic atrophy or nystagmus (Miller et al 1974).

See-saw nystagmus is a rare sign seen with chiasmal lesions and is thought to be the result of diencephalic dysfunction involving pathways from the zona incerta to the interstitial nucleus of Cajal. It is characterized by intortion and elevation of one eye and extortion and depression of the other eye. The sequence is then reversed to give the see-saw effect.

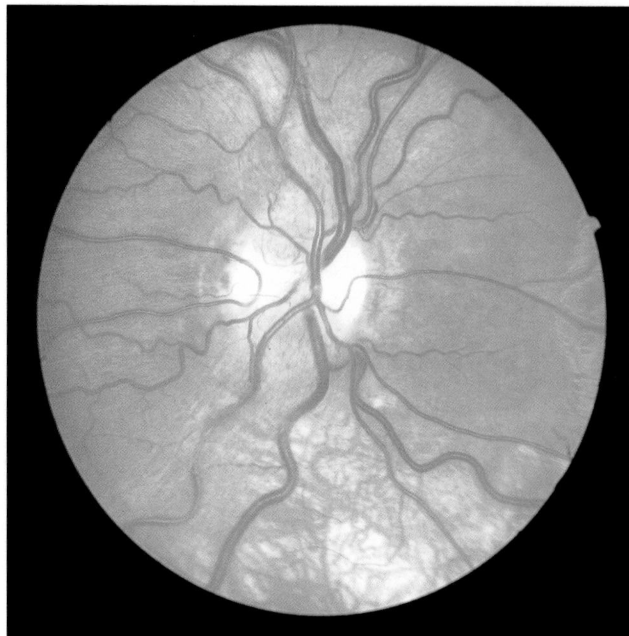

Fig. 11.15 Fundal photograph of a patient with a suprasellar tumor. The optic disc is atrophic in a 'bow-tie' pattern.

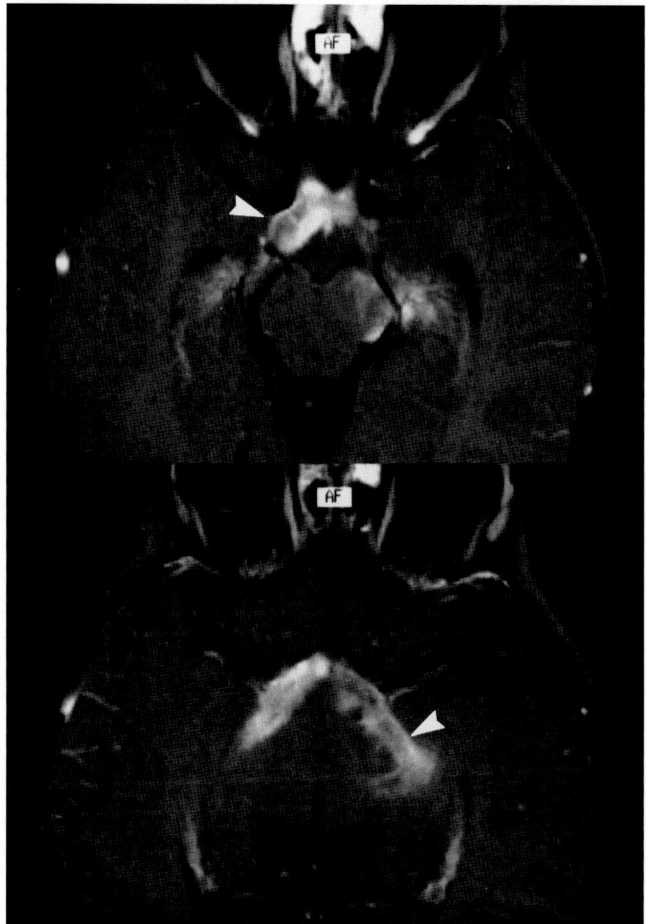

Fig. 11.16 Axial gadolinium-enhanced, fat-saturated T1-weighted image through the level of the chiasm showing an optic chiasmal glioma with minimal involvement of the optic nerves but extensive infiltration of the optic tracts. Tumor is indicated by white arrow heads.

TUMORS INVOLVING THE CAVERNOUS SINUS

Tumors arising in the area of the cavernous sinus produce a slowly progressive constellation of clinical features known as the cavernous sinus syndrome. These are involvement of the oculomotor, trochlear and abducens nerves and ophthalmic and maxillary divisions of the trigeminal nerve, including the oculo-sympathetic nerves. This entity overlaps with the parasellar syndrome (Thomas & Yoss, 1920). Although the typical picture may be associated with an intracavernous carotid aneurysm, a number of tumors, particularly meningioma, nasopharygngeal carcinoma and metastases, present in this manner.

Cavernous sinus syndrome

This consists of variable involvement of the following:

- Oculomotor nerve
- Trochlear nerve
- Trigeminal nerve — ophthalmic division
  — maxillary division
- Abducens nerve
- Oculo-sympathetic nerves

Unlike the intracavernous aneurysm which arises within the cavernous sinus and expands outwards, *meningiomas* usually arise from the dura of the middle fossa near the petrous apex and invade the cavernous sinus from outside (Fig. 11.17).

The major symptoms are diplopia, ptosis, dysesthesia and pain in the upper face. Involvement of the oculomotor nerve gives rise to variable degrees of progressive ophthalmoparesis including ptosis and pupillary changes.

The pupil is usually dilated due to compression of the pupillomotor fibres in the oculomotor nerve. If the oculo-sympathetic fibres arising from the internal carotid artery are also involved the pupil may be mid-dilated (Trobe et al 1978). Aberrant regeneration of the oculomotor nerve can be produced by an intracavernous meningioma in the absence of an acute oculomotor palsy and in this case the dilated pupil will constrict on attempted adduction and the ptosed lid may lift on adduction and downgaze (Schatz et al 1977).

The trochlear nerve is only involved in the cavernous sinus when the other nerves are affected. In the presence of an oculomotor palsy the eye is turned down and out. If intortion of the globe, i.e. clockwise rotation of the right eye or anticlockwise rotation of the left eye, can be demonstrated, the trochlear nerve is intact.

With intracavernous aneurysms, the abducens nerve may show an isolated palsy, but with meningiomas evidence of oculomotor, trochlear, oculo-sympathetic and trigeminal nerve damage is usually present (Jefferson 1953). With meningiomas, the ophthalmic and maxillary divisions may be affected but total impairment of all three

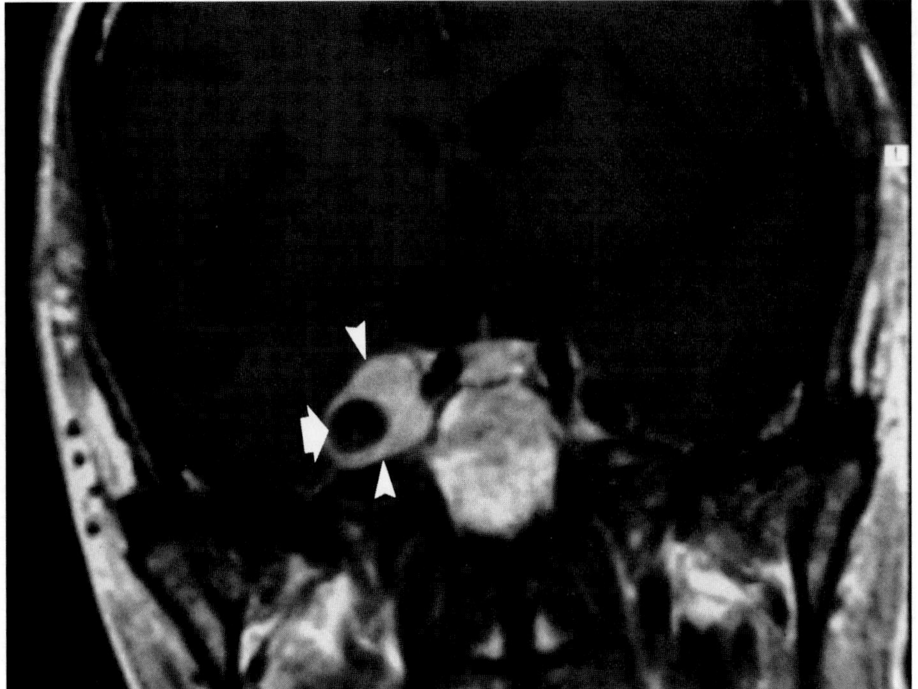

Fig. 11.17 MR coronal post-gadolinium enhanced T1 image of meningioma involving the cavernous sinus. The dark structure enveloped by the tumor is the trigeminal ganglion (broad arrow).

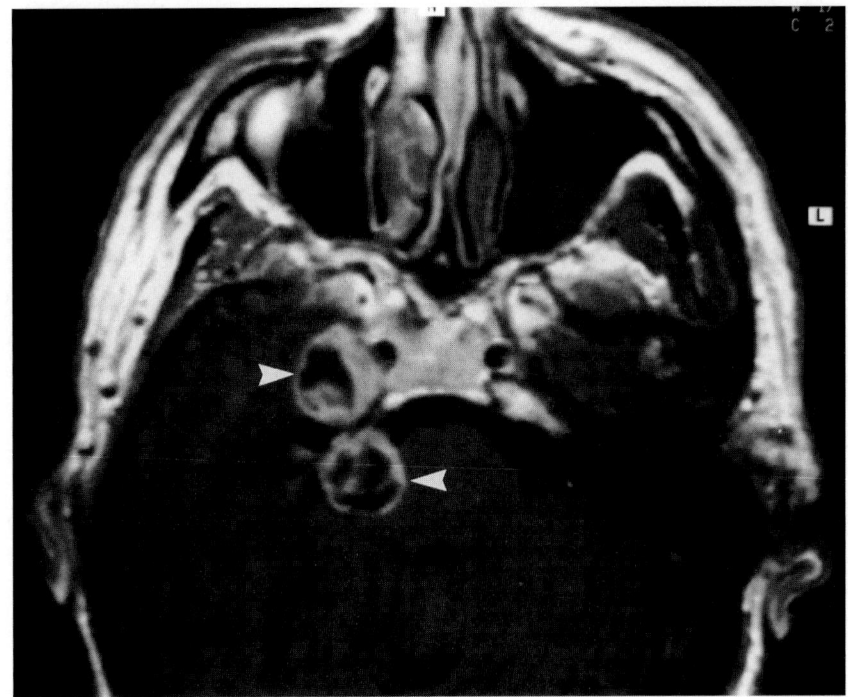

Fig. 11.18 MR axial post-gadolinium enhanced T1 image of a biopsy proven bilobular trigeminal neurinoma.

divisions of the trigeminal nerve suggests a neurinoma of that nerve (Fig. 11.18). Depression of the ipsilateral corneal reflex is always a very significant finding in a patient with an oculomotor nerve palsy. Nasopharyngeal carcinoma needs to be considered in all cases of cavernous sinus syndrome, as should the possibility of metastatic carcinoma from lung, breast and prostate. In addition perineural spread of squamous cell carcinoma from the face along nerves into the cavernous sinus may occur years after dermatological excision (Moore et al 1976).

Table 11.2 Sphenoid wing tumors

Localization	Pterional (outer third)	Alar (middle third)	Clinoidal (inner third)
Presentation	1. Large mass with raised intracranial pressure of epilepsy.	Mass with raised intracranial pressure or epilepsy.	1. Superior orbital fissure syndrome with oculomotor, trochlear, abducens palsies, involvement of ophthalmic division of trigeminal and oculo-sympathetic nerves, proptosis.
	2. Meningioma-en-plaque with ptosis, downward displacement of globe, periorbital and temporal fossa swelling.	May grow medially to present as clinoidal tumor.	2. Anterior clinoid syndrome with ipsilateral progressive optic nerve lesion.

SPHENOID WING TUMORS

Tumors of the sphenoid wing present in three groups (Table 11.2): outer third (pterional), middle third (alar) and inner third (clinoidal). The pterional tumors can become quite large masses before diagnosis and present with features of raised intracranial pressure, including headache and papilledema. Alternatively a meningioma-en-plaque arising in this area causes slowly progressive ptosis and downward displacement of the globe due to marked hyperostosis of the greater wing. In addition there can be mild ptosis with periorbital swelling but preserved vision and eye movements (Fig. 11.19). The temporal fossa may be swollen on the side of the tumor (Cushing & Eisenhardt 1938).

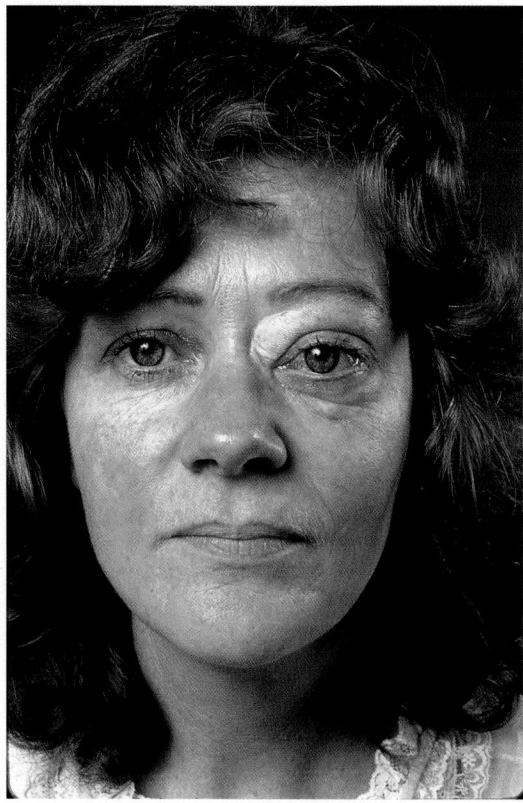

Fig. 11.19 A 40-year-old woman with a left-sided sphenoid wing meningioma-en-plaque. There is a mild ptosis, proptosis and periorbital swelling.

Tumors of the middle third project back into the temporal lobe and often present with seizures. As they enlarge medially, they involve structures in the superior orbital fissure. The middle and inner thirds of the sphenoid ridge are part of the lesser sphenoid wing and the inner third has a close relationship to the clinoid process and the superior orbital fissure. Tumors of this region, principally small meningiomas, present in two groups — the superior orbital fissure syndrome and the anterior clinoid syndrome (Huber 1976a).

The superior orbital fissure syndrome arises from involvement of the nerves which pass through the superior orbital fissure, namely oculomotor, trochlear, abducens, ophthalmic division of the trigeminal nerve and branches of the internal carotid plexus of the sympathetic. Tumors arising in this area may grow back toward the cavernous sinus or forward into the orbit resulting in a variety of clinical features. The commonest manifestations are diplopia and proptosis. The diplopia, which is usually slowly progressive over many years, results from involvement of the oculomotor, trochlear and abducens nerves to variable degrees. Ptosis and internal ophthalmoplegia reflect oculomotor involvement but a mid-dilated pupil can result from an associated oculo-sympathetic palsy, i.e. a superimposed Horner's syndrome.

Proptosis is usually present in 50% of cases but may be mild and cause only a sensation of pressure behind the globe or an awareness of the eye. There is a resistance to pressure over the globe and congestion of conjunctival veins. Occasionally when proptosis is more marked, it may be difficult to decide if the restriction of movement is due to proptosis or ophthalmoplegia. The eye is gradually displaced downward and outward, and periorbital swelling becomes prominent.

The involvement of the ophthalmic branch of the trigeminal nerve is an important sign, manifesting in its earliest stage as a depressed corneal reflex. Patients may complain of facial pain, numbness or dysesthesia in the ophthalmic distribution. The superior orbital fissure syndrome is similar to the cavernous sinus syndrome except for the presence of proptosis.

The anterior clinoid syndrome, commonly due to a small meningioma arising from the inner ridge of the sphenoid wing (Fig. 11.8), consists of unilateral progressive visual loss which may initially pass unnoticed by the patient until the other eye is inadvertently closed. The signs are reduced visual acuity and color vision, a central scotoma, pale disc and an afferent pupillary defect. This tumor gradually enlarges and growth forward will cause anosmia. Growth upward eventually may give rise to increased intracranial pressure and the Foster Kennedy syndrome (Kennedy 1911). This syndrome consists of ipsilateral optic atrophy, contralateral papilledema and anosmia. It was described with olfactory groove meningiomas but can rarely be seen with meningiomas of the inner sphenoid ridge growing forward. If the tumor grows medially, it may resemble the tuberculum sellae meningioma with features of a chiasmal lesion or involvement of the contralateral optic nerve. Because of the involvement of the ipsilateral and contralateral optic nerves, the optic chiasm, optic tract and the ipsilateral temporal lobe, a wide range of field defects is possible. These include a central scotoma, monocular nasal or temporal hemianopia, and quadrantic or homonymous hemianopia due to temporal lobe compression.

Whilst meningiomas are by far the most common cause of the sphenoid ridge syndrome, other tumors may be responsible, namely metastases, dermoids, nasopharyngeal carcinoma, lymphoma, osteochondromas and intraneural spread of squamous cell carcinoma from the face and scalp.

PINEAL AND MIDBRAIN TUMORS

The dorsal midbrain syndrome is a striking combination of neuro-ophthalmic signs which indicates disease of the pineal body or dorsal midbrain. This is also known as Parinaud's syndrome, Koerber-Salus-Elschnig syndrome, Sylvian aqueduct syndrome or pretectal syndrome.

Clinical features of dorsal midbrain syndrome:

- Failure of upward saccades
- Dilated pupils with light — near dissociation
- Defective convergence
- Convergence — retraction nystagmus
- Papilledema
- Loss of upward pursuit eye movements
- Skew deviation
- Trochlear nerve palsy
- Lid retraction
- Loss of downward saccades.

Over 80% of patients with pineal tumors at presentation have features of raised intracranial pressure due to blockage of the Sylvian aqueduct. Thus they have headaches, nausea, vomiting, papilledema and abducens nerve palsies (Packer et al, 1984).

The earliest dorsal midbrain involvement gives rise to failure of upward gaze. Initially there is a saccadic palsy with preserved pursuit and doll's head-eye movements, but later these movements are lost and downward gaze may also be affected. Convergence is often defective and convergence — retraction nystagmus is seen on attempted upgaze or convergence (Gay et al 1963). This synchronous jerking retraction and adduction of the eyes may be evident by observing one eye from the side whilst rotating the optokinetic drum downward. Loss of the pupillary responses to light also occurs early. The pupils are generally both dilated and unresponsive to light but briskly reactive to a near stimulus (Seybold et al 1971). Bilateral lid retraction 'Collier's sign of the posterior commissure' is a sign associated with conjugate upward gaze paralysis (Collier 1927).

The clinical picture is complicated by nuclear and infranuclear involvement of the oculomotor and trochlear nerves and also skew deviation caused by damage to the medial longitudinal fasciculus. This accounts for the complaint of diplopia which would not ordinarily be expected with supranuclear gaze disorders.

The so-called 'ectopic pinealoma' refers to the suprasellar germinoma (Fig. 11.20) Germinomas are the commonest tumors of the pineal body but occasionally they may arise in the midline hypothalamic region, thalamus and basal ganglia. When they arise in the pineal region, patients present with raised intracranial pressure and signs of the dorsal midbrain syndrome. Germinomas arising in the hypothalamus cause diabetes insipidus, or precocious puberty followed by bitemporal hemianopia and bilateral optic atrophy (Kageyama & Belsky 1961).

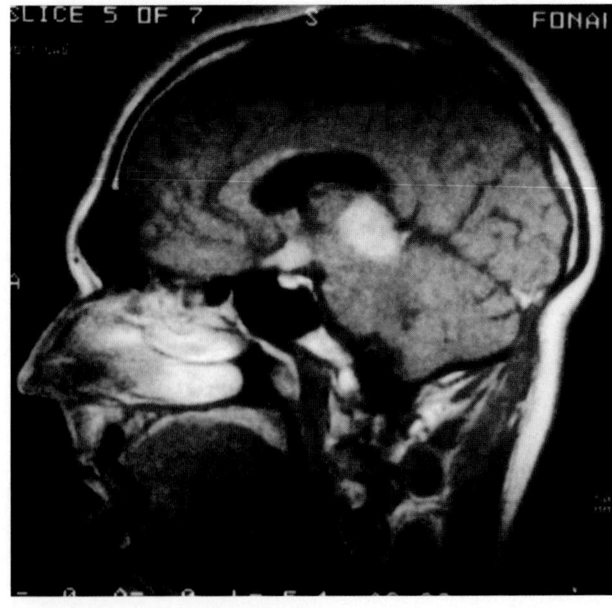

Fig. 11.20 MR sagittal post-gadolinium enhanced T1 image of a 30-year-old male with a pineal germinoma. Tumor is also seen in the hypothalamus and optic chiasm.

TUMORS OF THE THALAMUS AND BASAL GANGLIA

Tumors arising primarily in the thalamus are rare and there are no characteristic neuro-ophthalmic features. With increase in size there will be signs of raised intracranial pressure such as papilledema and abducens nerve palsies. Invasion of the internal capsule, lateral geniculate body and optic tract and radiation will cause contralateral hemiplegia, hemianesthesia and homonymous hemianopia. The more anterior the involvement of the postchiasmal visual pathway, the more incongruous the homonymous hemianopia. With hemianopias due to optic tract lesions optic atrophy can develop as axons die back, but this will not occur with retrogeniculate tumors. Other signs develop if the tumor extends into the midbrain.

Similarly basal ganglia tumors eventually show features of raised intracranial pressure. Other signs are dependent on the invasion of diencephalic and midbrain structures.

TUMORS OF THE BASE OF THE SKULL

Tumors arising from the base of the skull include meningioma, chordoma, nasopharyngeal carcinoma, acoustic and trigeminal neurinomas. In the anterior and middle fossa these tumors arise around the cavernous sinus.

Tumors of the clivus, principally meningiomas and chordomas, present with slowly progressive cranial neuropathies. A progressive abducens nerve palsy is usually very significant even in the absence of radiologic abnormalities (Savino et al 1982, Currie et al 1983). Involvement of the trigeminal nerve will cause increasing numbness and paresthesia of the face or atypical trigeminal neuralgia. In the pre-antibiotic era, an abducens nerve palsy with ipsilateral facial pain and numbness was due to petrous osteitis (Gradenigo's syndrome) but is now more likely the result of a meningioma or nasopharyngeal carcinoma at the petrous apex. Fortunately MR imaging has made identification of such tumors easier in early cases.

TUMORS OF THE CORPUS CALLOSUM

Butterfly gliomas in the anterior aspect of the corpus callosum usually present with behavioral changes such as apathy and hypokinesia similar to frontal lobe tumors; however, raised intracranial pressure will eventually occur. A dorsal midbrain syndrome may result from downward pressure on the upper brainstem.

With large tumors of the splenium, invasion of the dominant occipital lobe will cause alexia without agraphia, but if the angular gyrus is involved, there will be alexia with agraphia. Homonymous field defects are seen when the visual pathway is involved.

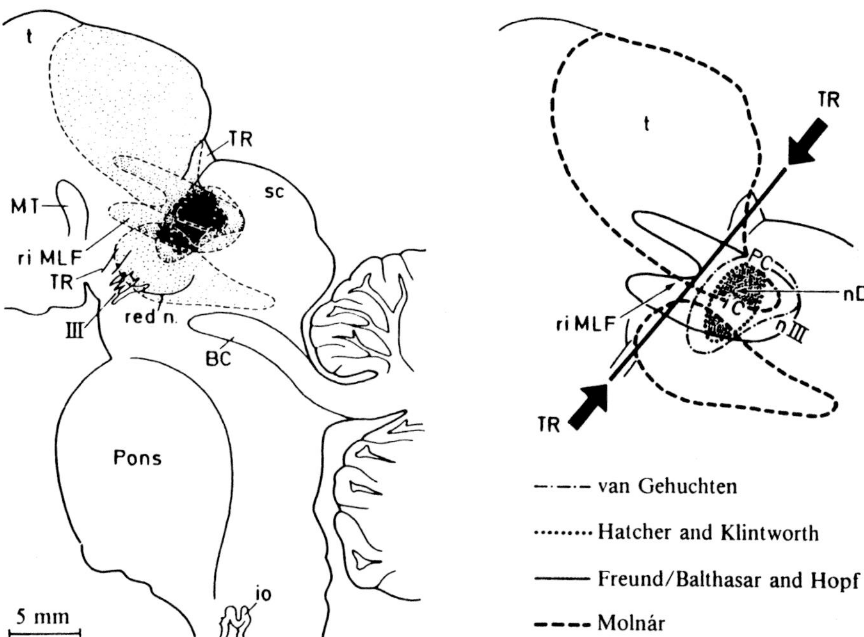

Fig. 11.21 Four lesions giving rise to upward gaze paralysis superimposed on a sagittal section of the human brain. The enlargement of the lesion on the right shows the common areas involved (stippled), including the interstitial nucleus of Cajal (iC), nucleus of Darkschewitsch (nD), and fibers of the posterior commissure (PC). Key to other abbreviations: TR = tractus retroflexus, MT = mammillo-thalamic tract, riMLF = rostral interstitial nucleus of the medial longitudinal fasciculus, III = oculomotor nerve, SC = superior colliculus, nIII = oculomotor nucleus, BC = brachium conjunctivum, io = inferior olive. Reproduced from Büttner-Ennever et al (1982) by permission of Oxford University Press.

TUMORS OF THE BRAINSTEM

Disruption of the ocular motor pathway by brainstem lesions provides a plethora of neuro-ophthalmic signs which aid in localization and diagnosis. These intra-axial lesions are divided into mesencephalic, pontine and medullary syndromes.

Mesencephalic syndrome

Midbrain tumors may closely mimic pineal tumors and can present with the dorsal midbrain syndrome as discussed above. The centre for upward gaze in the dorsal midbrain is in the region of the interstitial nucleus of Cajal, nucleus of Darkschewitsch, and the fibers of the posterior commissure (Fig. 11.21). Downward gaze appears best localized to the rostral interstitial nucleus of the medial longitudinal fasciculus, and the nucleus of Darkschewitsch (Büttner-Ennever et al 1982). Pressure from intrinsic midbrain tumors tends to involve supranuclear, nuclear and infranuclear structures, but also the red nucleus, the brachium conjunctivum, the substantia nigra, and pyramidal tracts.

Oculomotor nuclear lesions generally produce bilateral signs (Daroff 1971). The levator muscles are innervated by a single midline nucleus caudal to the oculomotor complex. A localized lesion in this area would give rise to bilateral ptosis. In tumor cases involvement of the other components of the oculomotor nucleus would be expected to accompany a lesion of the levator nucleus, but in a case described by Keane et al (1984) a metastasis from lung carcinoma involved the rostral oculomotor nucleus on one side and spared the caudal levator nucleus. This resulted in a unilateral oculomotor palsy without ptosis. Whilst the oculomotor nuclear complex lies on each side of the midline, and ipsilateral subnuclei give rise to fibers destined for extraocular muscles of the eye on that side, the superior rectus subnucleus gives rise to some fibers which cross the midline and join the oculomotor fibers arising from the contralateral subnuclei. This anatomic arrangement allows an ipsilateral oculomotor nuclear lesion to give rise to weakness of upgaze in the

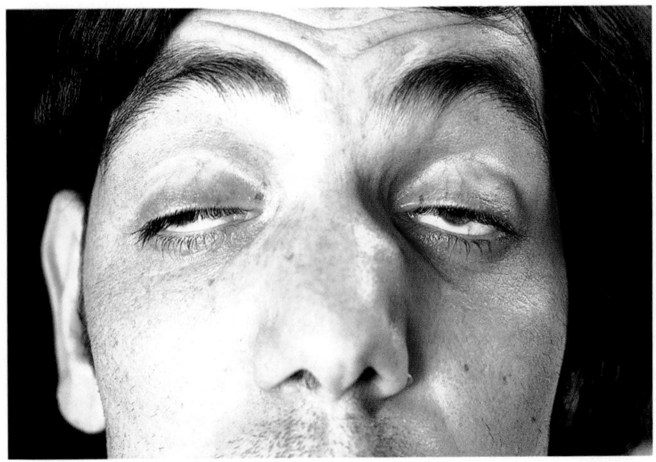

A

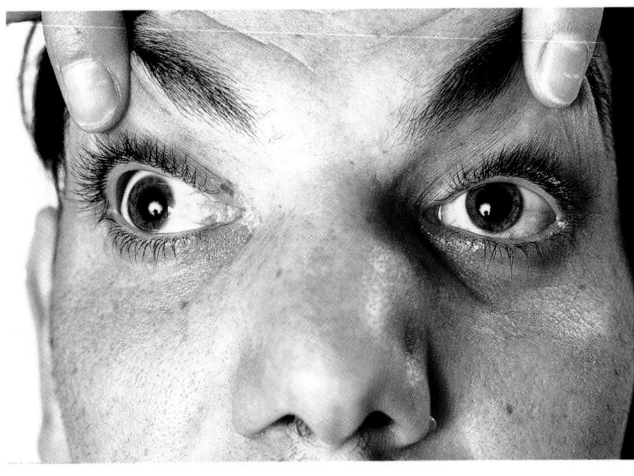

B

C

Fig. 11.22 **A**. A 28-year-old man with metastatic carcinoma involving the oculomotor nucleus. **B**. With eyelids lifted, the patient has dilated pupils and bilateral third nerve palsies. **C**. MRI of midbrain showing metastasis anterior to aqueduct.

contralateral eye as well as the ipsilateral eye. The Edinger-Westphal nucleus occupies a dorsal rostral position in the oculomotor nuclear complex and bilateral pupillary dilatation is likely with lesions of this area. Thus tumors of the oculomotor nucleus give rise to bilateral ptosis, internal and external ophthalmoplegia (Fig. 11.22A–C).

Fascicular lesions of the oculomotor nerve are diagnosed by the accompanying neurologic signs. In children these are usually due to gliomas, whereas in adults metastases are likely. Involvement of the oculomotor nerve fascicle in the area of the brachium conjunctivum produces an ipsilateral oculomotor nerve palsy and cerebellar ataxia. Benedikt's syndrome is ipsilateral oculomotor palsy, contralateral hemipareis and contralateral tremor due to damage to the red nucleus and cerebral peduncle (Liu et al 1992), and Weber's syndrome implies involvement of the oculomotor nerve in the medial end of the cerebral peduncle, giving rise to a contralateral hemiparesis and ipsilateral oculomotor palsy. Peduncular hallucinosis, an entity characterized by vivid and prolonged visual hallucinations and most often seen after vertebral angiography, has been described with tumors of the mesencephalon (Bing & Haymaker 1940). The trochlear nerves arise from a paired group of motor neurons caudal to the oculomotor nucleus and pass dorsally to decussate before emerging from the dorsal brainstem just below the inferior colliculi. Nuclear lesions of the trochlear nerve have been described with astrocytoma (Krohel et al 1982).

Mesencephelic tumors may block the aqueduct of Sylvius and give rise to papilledema with other signs of raised intracranial pressure.

Pontine syndromes

Tumors of the pons can present with either a ventral or dorsal pontine syndrome (Table 11.3).

The ventral pontine syndrome consists of an ipsilateral abducens palsy and a contralateral hemiplegia (Raymond's syndrome). The facial nerve may be involved to give an ipsilateral lower motor neuron facial palsy (Millard–Gubler syndrome).

Table 11.3 Clinical features of pontine syndromes

Ventral pontine syndrome	Dorsal pontine syndrome
Ipsilateral abducens palsy facial palsy (lower) motor neuron) Contralateral hemiplegia	Ipsilateral horizontal gaze palsy abducens palsy facial palsy (lower motor neuron) facial hemianesthesia loss of taste Horner's syndrome ataxia internuclear ophthalmoplegia Contralateral limb hemianesthesia Skew deviation 'One-and-a-half' syndrome

The dorsal pontine syndrome results from tumors involving the pontine tegmentum, and the important structures in this discrete area are the abducens nucleus, pontine paramedian reticular formation (PPRF), facial nucleus and fascicle. The physical signs due to lesions in this area are an ipsilateral horizontal gaze palsy, ipsilateral paralysis of abduction, and ipsilateral lower motor neuron facial weakness. Such patients may also show ipsilateral loss of taste, Horner's syndrome, deafness and facial analgesia (Foville's syndrome).

Some degree of bilateral involvement is likely with tumors of the brainstem. Unilateral destruction of the medial longitudinal fasciculus (MLF) will give an internuclear ophthalmoplegia (INO) or, if both sides are damaged, a bilateral internuclear ophthalmoplegia. If the PPRF and MLF on the same side are destroyed by tumor, a 'one-and-a-half syndrome' results. This consists of an ipsilateral gaze palsy plus an ipsilateral INO, leaving contralateral abduction as the only horizontal eye movement (Wall & Wray 1983).

Horizontal nystagmus, both gaze evoked and gaze paretic, may be seen as well as upbeating nystagmus (Troost et al 1980).

Skew deviation is a vertical misalignment of the visual axes caused by an imbalance of prenuclear inputs. In the absence of neuromuscular disease and restrictive disorders, the occurrence of vertical diplopia that cannot be isolated to a single extraocular muscle or muscles is defined as skew deviation. The vertical misalignment may be constant in all positions of gaze or may vary, in which case the possibility of vertical extraocular muscle palsy must be considered. The associated clinical features may indicate skew deviation if there is involvement of the pathway from the otolith crossing in the medulla and ascending to the midbrain in the MLF with projections to oculomotor and trochlear nuclei and also mesencephalic reticular nuclei (Keane 1975).

The corneal reflex may be depressed in pontine tumors by involvement of either trigeminal nerve, root or sensory nucleus, interneurons or the facial nucleus or fascicle in the brainstem. Apart from facial weakness, myokymia involving the facial musculature can be a sign of pontine malignancy as can spastic paretic facial contracture. Ocular bobbing has been described with hemorrhage into a pontine glioma (Daroff & Waldman 1965) and in metastatic disease of the pons (Walsh & Hoyt 1969). Typical bobbing is where both eyes jerk downward and then slowly drift back to the midposition.

Medullary syndromes

Bulbar and respiratory difficulties together with quadriparesis overshadow the neuro-ophthalmic features of tumors of the medulla.

The abducens nerve leaves the brainstem at the pontomedullary junction and may therefore be involved by tumors of the pons and medulla. Similarly such tumors can cause horizontal gaze palsies. Skew deviation is well recorded with both pontine and medullary tumors involving the MLF. Down-beating nystagmus is characteristic of medullary disease and has been described in the presence of tumors of the medulla as well as a non-metastatic manifestation of tumors (Halmagyi et al 1983). Other types of nystagmus such as horizontal and torsional nystagmus reflect damage to the vestibular nuclei.

CEREBELLOPONTINE ANGLE TUMORS

Cerebellopontine angle syndrome

This syndrome is usually due to an acoustic schwannoma arising from the vestibular nerve. Other tumors presenting in this area are meningioma, epidermoid, pontine glioma and cerebellar astrocytoma.

The earliest symptoms are usually a sense of imbalance rather than vertigo and tinnitus, and slowly progressive deafness which is often overlooked. Visual symptoms are uncommon but may include diplopia due to an abducens palsy and papilledema due to raised intracranial pressure. Neuro-ophthalmic signs are important, with nystagmus being present in over 60–90% of cases. The gaze evoked nystagmus to the side opposite the lesion is fine and rapid whereas to the side of the lesion, the nystagmus is of low frequency and large amplitude, the so-called Brun's nystagmus (Baloh et al 1976).

As the tumor enlarges, vertical nystagmus, rebound nystagmus and centripetal nystagmus are seen.

A depression of the ipsilateral corneal reflex is a valuable early sign of a cerebellopontine angle lesion extending beyond the internal auditory meatus. Facial weakness is surprisingly late considering the proximity of the facial nerve to the tumor.

CEREBELLAR TUMORS

Tumors of the cerebellum, being confined to the posterior fossa, do not produce field defects but give rise to disorders of ocular movement and increased intracranial pressure. Primary tumors of the cerebellum are more commonly seen in children, and 75% of such tumors are astrocytomas and medulloblastomas.

Due to raised intracranial pressure, headache, nausea and vomiting are frequent symptoms in addition to vague dizziness, vertigo, obscurations and neck stiffness. Diplopia is usually caused by an abducens nerve palsy but can be due to skew deviation.

Nystagmus is one of the most frequent signs of cerebellar tumors and is due to both cerebellar and brainstem disease. The commonest form of nystagmus is horizontal jerk nystagmus of central type, arising from lesions of the vestibulo-cerebellar pathways or vestibular nuclei. With this type of nystagmus, the apparent direction of the vertiginous movement is in the direction of the slow phase of the jerk nystagmus, and past pointing and Romberg fall are towards the fast phase. The nystagmus may be spontaneous in the primary position but is more often seen with greater amplitude on gaze to the side of the lesion. The nystagmus from cerebellar tumors may be horizontal or vertical and symmetric or asymmetric in the two eyes. It is not usually horizontal — rotary nystagmus. Vertical gaze nystagmus is a characteristic of cerebellar vermis lesions, especially medulloblastoma.

Positional nystagmus of central type can arise from midline cerebellar tumors. Mild vertigo occurring immediately on head movement associated with nystagmus which shows no latent period nor any habituation, indicates a central rather than peripheral (end-organ) lesion (Baloh et al 1987).

Dissociated nystagmus, in which the direction and amplitude of nystagmus is greater in one eye than the other, is a feature of some cerebellar tumors. Rebound nystagmus is a brief jerk nystagmus which occurs after a patient who has maintained eccentric gaze returns fixation to the primary position. This cerebellar form of nystagmus has been described with a tumor of the flocculus (Yamazaki & Zee 1979).

Cerebellar tumors compressing the brainstem may display a horizontal gaze paresis. Other disorders of eye movement reported with such tumors are ocular dysmetria, ocular flutter, opsoclonus and saccadic pursuit (Daroff et al 1990).

Because an expanding mass in one cerebellar hemisphere rapidly exerts an effect on midline structures, the separation of clinical presentation into lateral and midline cerebellar syndromes is not always helpful. In general, however, the midline tumors — medulloblastomas and solid astrocytomas — present with features of raised intracranial pressure and truncal ataxia, whereas the lateral tumors — cystic astrocytoma and hemangioblastomas — produce unilateral ataxia and less diplopia but still display a high incidence of raised intracranial pressure (Fig. 11.23A–C). Hemangioblastomas are associated with retinal capillary angiomas in 10–40% cases (von Hippel-Lindau disease) and although these angiomas are usually small and asymptomatic, they may be multiple and bilateral (Hardwig & Robertson 1984).

TUMORS OF THE VENTRICLES

Lateral ventricles

Tumors arising in the lateral ventricles present with symptoms and signs of raised intracranial pressure. Such tumors are meningiomas, choroid plexus papillomas, ependymomas and other congenital tumors (Collmann et al 1985).

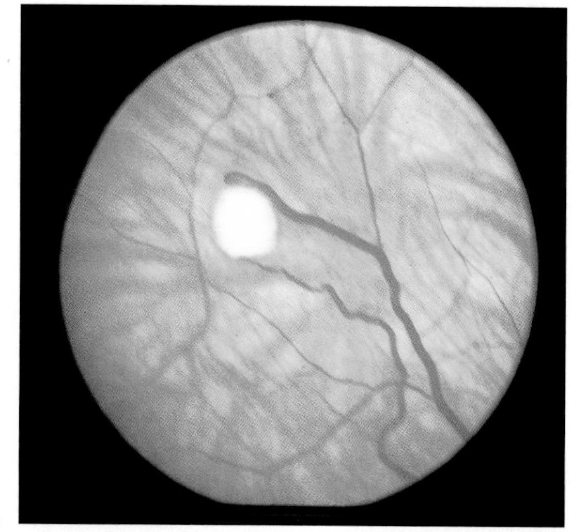

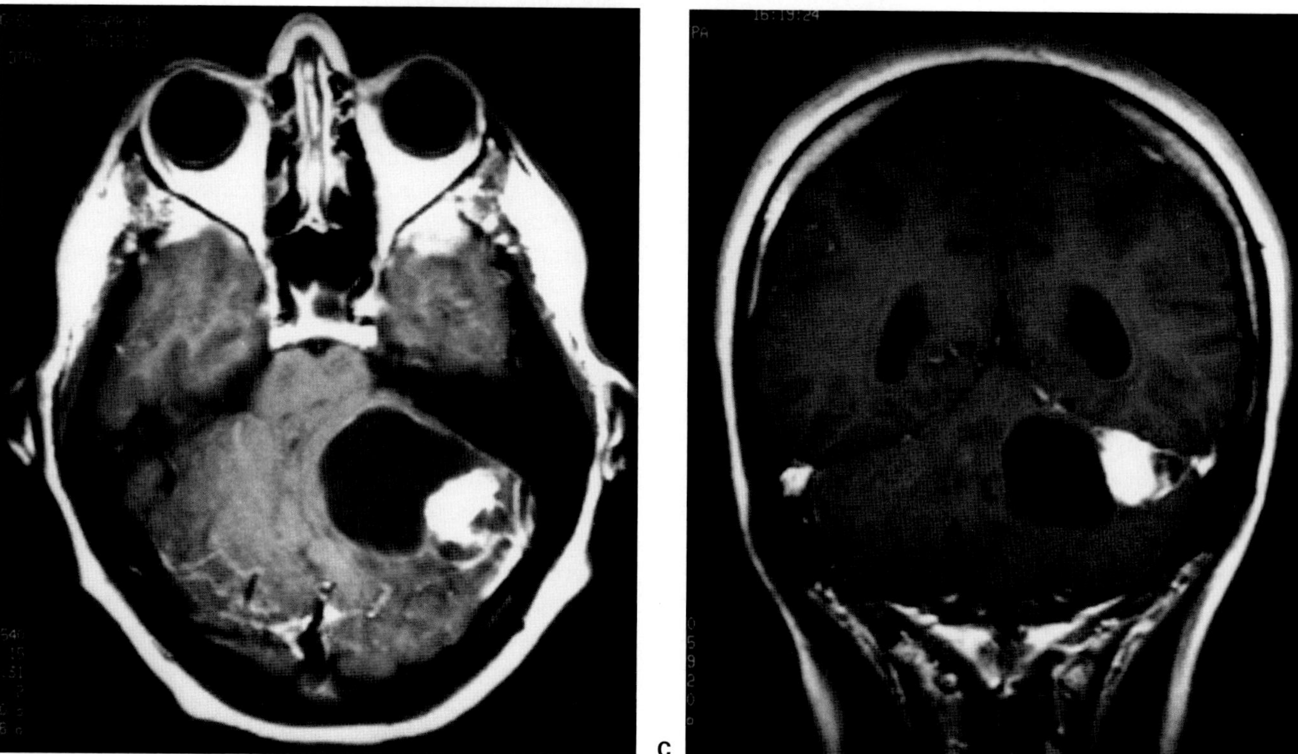

Fig. 11.23 **A**. Fundal photograph of a retinal capillary angioma in a patient with von Hippel-Lindau disease. The angioma is associated with intraretinal extravasation of lipid. **B, C**. Axial and coronal MR post-gadolinium T1 images of patient with cerebellar hemangioblastoma showing typical cyst and tumor nodule.

Third ventricle

Tumors of the third ventricle predominantly present with features of raised intracranial pressure, especially paroxysmal headache, nausea, vomiting and obscurations. The visual fields show asymmetric bitemporal hemianopia starting with inferior temporal field loss. This is due to dilatation of the third ventricle with pressure on the chiasm from above. The extension of the tumor may cause a wide range of field defects including homonymous hemianopia, binasal field defects, arcuate defects and central scotomata (Gradin et al 1983). The obstruction to the cerebrospinal fluid causes gross papilledema which eventually gives way to the chronic atrophic form.

Growth of the tumor upward and backward in the third ventricle can give rise to Parinaud's syndrome. The commonest tumors of the third ventricle are colloid cysts, ependymomas, choroid plexus papillomas and epidermoids.

Fourth ventricle

Ependymomas and choroid plexus papillomas are the common tumors of the fourth ventricle but astrocytomas and medulloblastomas of the cerebellum encroach upon the ventricle.

These tumors present with features of raised intracranial pressure, namely headache, vomiting, obscurations and papilledema. Nystagmus and ataxia may be seen, and gaze paresis and internuclear ophthalmoplegia have been reported.

FRONTAL LOBE TUMORS

Neuro-ophthalmic features of frontal lobe tumors may be dramatic, such as adversive seizures seen with a small tumor in the frontal gaze centre (Wyllie et al 1986), but often the only features may be those of raised intracranial pressure with a large non-dominant frontal tumor. Thus bilateral papilledema together with a personality change toward indifference and apathy may result in visual loss from consecutive atrophy. Visual loss may also result from direct extension downward and backward of frontal tumors to involve the optic nerves and chiasm.

The Foster Kennedy syndrome, which strictly speaking is a triad of optic atrophy, contralateral papilledema and anosmia, is very rarely due to a frontal tumor but is more likely with an olfactory groove meningioma (Bakay 1984).

Whilst a tumor involving the frontal gaze centre almost invariably will result in adversive seizures involving the head and eyes turning to the opposite side, rarely there may be ipsiversive seizures in which the head and eyes deviate to the same side as the tumor. Unlike stroke involving the frontal lobe which can result in conjugate gaze paralysis, this is not seen with tumors.

A frontal lobe tumor may cause contralateral facial weakness which mainly involves the lower face but there is often some weakness of eyelid closure and slower blinking on that side. A failure of voluntary closure of the eyelids bilaterally has been termed 'compulsive eye opening' and 'apraxia of eyelid closure'. This entity has been reported with vascular and degenerative lesions but also with a frontal tumor (Miller 1988).

TEMPORAL LOBE TUMORS

Tumors of the non-dominant temporal lobe can be quite large before producing symptoms of raised intracranial pressure such as headache, nausea, vomiting, obscurations and papilledema. Eventually medial extension of the tumor or herniation of the hippocampus causes oculomotor nerve paresis, and trochlear and abducens palsies can result from brainstem distortion.

Involvement of Meyer's loop by tumor of either temporal lobe gives rise to contralateral superior homonymous quadrantic field defects but usually, by the time the patient is seen, an incomplete homonymous hemianopia is found.

Visual hallucinations, although rare, are a dramatic manifestation of a temporal lobe tumor. They characteristically are complex formed hallucinations with vivid scenes, objects and persons, lasting seconds and not necessarily confined to the contralateral visual field. The visual hallucinations may be distorted (metamorphosia) with objects smaller (micropsia) or objects larger (macropsia). The hallucinations are regarded as epileptic phenomena (Gittinger et al 1982).

PARIETAL LOBE TUMORS

Visual inattention is commonly seen in parietal tumors, especially involving the non-dominant lobe. There is a failure to see a hand movement in the left half field when hand movements are presented in both right and left fields simultaneously. This is known as Oppenheim's test (Oppenheim 1907) which demonstrates a form of neglect, often associated with sensory inattention. It is an early sign of a subtle homonymous hemianopia.

At the same time the patient will often fail to localize accurately objects in the affected field. For example there may be an inability to touch the examiner's finger accurately in that field (defective visual localization). Similarly the 'quality' or clarity of objects in that field is impaired and the patient may be unable to count fingers briefly shown in that field. These features are typically seen in right parietal tumors. With enlargement of such tumors an homonymous hemianopia develops with the inferior quadrant loss being more marked initially. Formal perimetry is difficult with non-dominant parietal lesions due to neglect and motor impersistence.

Cogan (1966) described two signs in parietal lobe lesions which are of interest. Spasticity of conjugate gaze is tonic deviation of the eyes to the side opposite parietal lesions during attempted Bell's phenomenon. Optokinetic nystagmus is absent with rotation of the drum toward the side of the parietal lesion, and this is thought to be due to a defect of ipsilateral pursuit.

Visual hallucinations, more typically related to temporal and occipital tumors, may occur with extensive parietal tumors. Palinopsia or visual perseveration is the persistence of normal images within the homonymous hemianopia. The images persist for several minutes but can last hours, however, the phenomena are usually transitory (Michel & Troost 1980).

A tumor of the left angular gyrus of the parietal lobe may cause alexia, also known as word blindness. The patient is rendered illiterate, as if the significance of words or figures were never learned.

OCCIPITAL LOBE TUMORS

The characteristic features of tumors of the occipital lobe are the visual field defects (Parkinson & Craig 1951). These range from incomplete to complete homonymous hemianopia which are congruous and usually do not spare the macula (Fig. 11.24A,B). Some patients are unaware of their field defect. The 'Riddoch phenomenon' in which a patient sees a moving target, but not a static target in one field, was considered a sign of an occipital lesion but this is not always the case (Riddoch 1915).

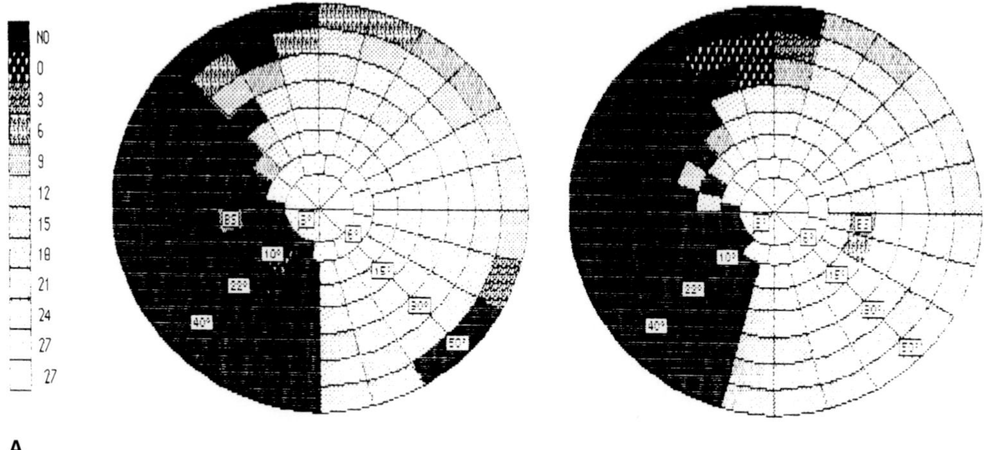

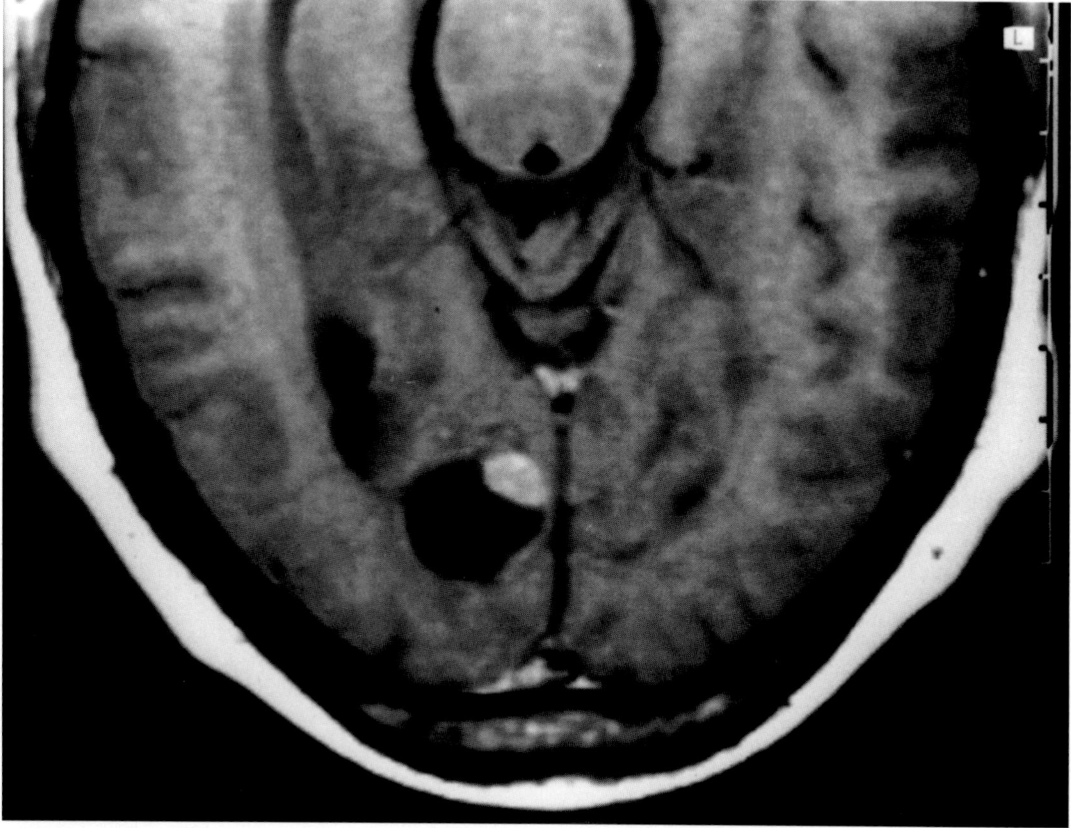

Fig. 11.24 **A**. Automated perimetry in a patient with a right occipital hematoma associated with a nodule of metastatic melanoma. Using a Bjerrum screen the field defect was an incomplete congruous homonymous hemianopia. **B**. MR post-gadolinium enhanced image of a right occipital hematoma with underlying nodule of metastatic melanoma.

The complex perceptual disorders associated with occipital lobe disease are usually due to bilateral involvement of occipito-temporal areas and are thus unlikely with tumors. Visual object agnosia is the failure to recognize a familiar object, despite intact vision and speech, yet the object is readily identified by touch, smell or sound (Trobe & Bouer 1986). This entity has been localized to a left occipito-temporal lesion. It is often associated with prosopagnosia — failure to recognize faces — in which case bilateral occipito-temporal lesions are present. Simultanagnosia is the entity in which individuals cannot see more than one object at once, e.g. they will only pick up one sheep in a farmyard scene. This is also a disorder associated with bilateral damage. An acquired loss of the ability to discriminate between a range of colours is known as central achromotopsia. It is usually associated with bilateral upper quadrantic field defects and prosopagnosia (Green & Lessell 1977).

Visual hallucinations arising in cases of occipital lobe tumors are typically unformed, e.g. flashing lights, colors or zig-zag lines which need to be distinguished from migrainous phenomena. They may appear before a field defect is evident or within the blind hemifield. They represent a form of visual epilepsy whilst other seizures arising from occipital tumors may cause transient cortical blindness. Permanent cortical blindness is rarely due to an occipital tumor (Huber 1976b) since this would require bilateral destruction of the occipital lobes. However, it can occur indirectly by compression of both posterior cerebral arteries at the tentorial notch from a supratentorial tumor exerting downward pressure on the brainstem.

Alexia without agraphia arises when there is a left occipital lesion with an extension into the splenium which interrupts the fibers arising from the right occipital lobe running to the left angular gyrus. Such patients, who have a right homonymous hemianopia, cannot read what they have written. Most cases of this syndrome arise from proximal posterior cerebral artery occlusion but its occurrence with tumor has been reported (Turgman et al 1979).

Acknowledgement

The assistance of Dr Richard O'Sullivan of Melbourne Diagnostic Group (Radiology) in providing the MR illustrations is gratefully acknowledged.

REFERENCES

Altrocchi P A, Reinhardt P M, Eckman P B 1972 Blindness and meningeal carcinomatosis. Archives of Ophthalmology 88: 508–512

Alvord E C, Lofton S 1988 Gliomas of the optic nerve or chiasm: outcome by patient's age, tumor site and treatment. Journal of Neurosurgery 68: 85–98

Baloh R W, Konrad H R, Dirks D et al 1976 Cerebello-pontine angle tumors. Results of quantitative vestibulo-ocular testing. Archives of Neurology 33: 507–512

Baloh R W, Honrubia V, Jacobson K 1987 Benign positional vertigo: clinical and oculographic features in 240 cases. Neurology 37: 371–378

Bakay L 1984 Olfactory meningiomas: the missed diagnosis. Journal of the American Medical Association 251: 53–55

Baskin D S, Wilson C B 1986 Surgical management of craniopharyngiomas: a review of 74 cases. Journal of Neurosurgery 65: 22–27

Bing R, Haymaker W 1940 Compendium of regional diagnosis in lesions of the brain and spinal cord, 11th edn. Mosby, St Louis

Bird A C, Sanders M D 1973 Choroidal folds in association with papilledema. British Journal of Ophthalmology 57: 89–97

Burde, R M, Savino P J, Trobe J D 1992 Clinical decisions in neuro-ophthalmology, 2nd edn, Mosby Year Book, St Louis, p. 27

Büttner-Ennever J A, Buttner U, Cohen B et al 1982 Vertical gaze paralysis and the rostal interstitial nucleus of the medial longitudinal fasciculus. Brain 105: 125–149

Cogan D G 1966 Neurology of the visual system. Charles C Thomas, Springfield, p 254

Collier J 1927 Nuclear ophthalmoplegia: with especial reference to retraction of lids and ptosis and to lesions of the posterior commissure. Brain 50: 488–498

Collmann H, Kazner E, Sprung C 1985 Supratentorial intraventricular tumors in childhood. Acta Neurochirurgica Supplement 35: 75–79

Currie J, Lubin J H, Lessell S 1983 Chronic isolated abducens nerve paresis from tumors at the base of the brain. Archives of Neurology 40: 226–229

Cushing H 1930 The chiasmal syndrome of primary optic atrophy and bitemporal field defects in adults with a normal sella turcica. Archives of Ophthalmology 3: 505–551, 704–735

Cushing H, Eisenhardt L 1938 Meningiomas: their classification, regional behaviour, life history, and surgical end results. Charles C Thomas, Springfield

Daroff R B 1971 Ocular motor manifestations of brainstem and cerebellar dysfunction. In: Smith J L (ed) Neuro-ophthalmology: Symposium of the University of Miami and Bascom Palmer Eye Institute. Huffman, Hallandale, Florida, 5: 104

Daroff R B, Waldman A L 1965 Ocular bobbing. Journal of Neurology, Neurosurgery and Psychiatry 28: 375–377

Daroff R B, Troost B T, Leigh R J 1990 Supranuclear disorders of eye movements. In: Glaser J S (ed) Neuro-ophthalmology, 2nd edn. Lippincott, Philadephia, p 312

David N J, Gargano F P, Glaser J S 1975 Pituitary apoplexy in perspective. In: Glaser J S, Smith J L (eds) Neuro-ophthalmology: Symposium of the University of Miami and the Bascom Palmer Eye Institute, vol 8. Mosby-Year Book, St Louis, pp 140–165

Dell'Osso L F, Daroff R B, Troost B T 1990 Nystagmus and saccadic intrusions and oscillations. In: Glaser J S (ed) Neuro-ophthalmology, 2nd edn. Lippincott, Philadelphia, pp 325–356

Finn J E, Mount L A 1974 Meningiomas of the tuberculum sellae and planum sphenoidale: a review of 83 cases. Archives of Ophthalmology 92: 23–27

Frisen L, Hoyt W F, Tengroth B M 1973 Optociliary veins, disc pallor, and visual loss: a triad of signs indicating spheno-orbital meningiomas. Acta Ophthalmologica 51: 241–249

Gay A J, Brodkey J, Miller J E 1963 Convergence retraction nystagmus: an electromyographic study. Archives of Ophthalmology 70: 456–461

Gittinger J W, Miller N R, Keltner J W et al 1982 Sugarplum fairies. Visual hallucinations. Survey of Ophthalmology 27: 42–48

Glaser J S, Savino P J, Sumers K D et al 1977 The photostress recovery test in the clinical assessment of visual function. American Journal of Ophthalmology 83: 255–260

Gradin W C, Taylon C, Fruin A H 1983 Choroid plexus papilloma of the third ventricle: case report and review of the literature. Neurosurgery 12: 217–220

Green G J, Lessell S 1977 Acquired cerebral dyschromatopsia. Archives of Ophthalmology 95: 121–128

Gregorius F K, Hepler R S, Stein W E 1975 Loss and recovery of vision with suprasellar meningiomas. Journal of Neurosurgery 42: 69–75
Gunn R M 1904 Discussion on retro-ocular neuritis. Lancet 2: 412–413
Halmagyi G M, Rudge P, Gresty M A et al 1983 Downbeating nystagmus: a review of 62 cases. Archives of Neurology 40: 777–784
Hardwig P, Robertson D M 1984 von Hippel-Lindau disease: a familial, often lethal multisystem phakomatosis. Ophthalmology 91: 263–270
Hollenhorst R W, Younge B R 1973 Ocular manifestations produced by adenomas of the pituitary gland: analysis of 1000 cases. In: Kohler P O, Ross G T (eds) Diagnosis and treatment of pituitary tumors. Excerpta Medica, Amsterdam, pp 53–68
Hoyt W F, Rios-Montenegro E N, Behrens M M et al 1972 Homonymous hemioptic hypoplasia. British Journal of Ophthalmology 56: 537–545
Hoyt W F, Knight C L 1973 Comparison of congenital disc blurring and incipient papilledema in red free light: a photographic study. Investigative Ophthalmology 12: 241–247
Huber A 1976a Eye signs and symptoms in brain tumors, 3rd edn. CV Mosby, St Louis, p 248
Huber A 1976b Eye signs and symptoms in brain tumors, 3rd edn. CV Mosby, St Louis, p 193
Jefferson G 1953 The Bowman Lecture: concerning injuries, aneurysms and tumors involving the cavernous sinus. Transactions of the Ophthalmological Society of United Kingdom 73: 117–152
Kageyama N, Belsky R 1961 Ectopic pinealoma in the chiasmal region. Neurology 11: 318–327
Kaye A H 1991 Essential neurosurgery. Churchill Livingstone, Edinburgh
Keane J R 1975 Ocular skew deviation: analysis of 100 cases. Archives of Neurology 32: 185–190
Keane J R, Zaias B, Itabashi H H 1984 Levator sparing oculomotor nerve palsy caused by solitary mid brain metastasis. Archives of Neurology 41: 210–212
Kearns T P, Rucker W C 1958 Arcuate defects in the visual fields due to chromophobe adenoma of the pituitary gland. American Journal of Ophthalmology 45: 505–507
Kennedy F 1991 Retrobulbar neuritis as an exact diagnostic sign of certain tumors and abscesses in the frontal lobes. American Journal of Medical Science 142: 355–368
Kirkham T H 1972 The ocular symptomatology of pituitary tumors. Proceedings of Royal Society of Medicine 65: 517–518
Krohel G B, Mansour A M, Petersen W L et al 1982 Isolated trochlear nerve palsy secondary to juvenile pilocytic astrocytoma. Journal of Clinical Neuro-ophthalmology 1: 119–123
Liu G T, Crenner C W, Logigian E L et al 1992 Midbrain syndromes of Benedikt, Claude and Nothnagel. Neurology 42: 1820–1822
Michel E M, Troost B T 1980 Palinopsia: cerebral localisation with computed tomography. Neurology 30: 887–889
Miller N R 1988 Walsh and Hoyt's Clinical neuro-ophthalmology, 4th edn, vol 3. Williams & Wilkins, Baltimore, p 1238
Miller N R, Iliff W J, Green W R 1974 Evaluation and management of gliomas of the anterior visual pathways. Brain 97: 743–754
Moore C E, Hoyt W F, North J B 1976 Painful ophthalmoplegia following treated squamous cell carcinoma of the forehead. Medical Journal of Australia 1: 657–659
Nachtigaller H, Hoyt W F 1970 Storungen des Seheindruckes bei bitemporaler Hemianopsie und Verschiebung der Sehachsen. Klinische Monatsblatter fur Augenheikunde und augenarztliche Fortbildung 156: 821–834
Newman N M 1992 Neuro-ophthalmology, a practical text. Appleton & Lange, Norwalk, Connecticut, pp 217–225
Olivecrona H 1967 Acoustic tumors. Journal of Neurosurgery 26: 6–13
Oppenheim H 1907 Beitrage zur Diagnostik und Therapie der Geschwulste im Bereich des zentralen Nervensystems. Berlin
Packer R J, Sutton L N, Rosenstock J G et al 1984 Pineal region tumors of childhood. Pediatrics 74: 97–102
Parkinson D, Craig W M 1951 Tumors of the brain, occipital lobe: their signs and symptoms. Canadian Medical Association Journal 64: 111–113
Riddoch G 1915 Dissociation of visual perception due to occipital injuries with special reference to appreciation of movement. Brain 40: 15
Rosenberg L F, Miller N R 1984 Visual results after microsurgical removal of meningiomas involving the anterior visual system. Archives of Ophthalmology 102: 1019–1023
Sadun A A, Currie J N, Lessell S 1984 Transient visual obscurations with elevated optic discs. Annals of Neurology 16: 489–494
Sanders M D, Falconer M A 1964 Optic nerve compression by an intracanalicular meningioma. British Journal of Ophthalmology 48: 13–18
Sarkies N J C 1987 Optic nerve sheath meningiomas: diagnostic features and therapeutic alternatives. Eye 1: 597–602
Savino P J, Paris M, Schatz N J et al 1978 Optic tract syndrome: a review of 21 patients. Archives of Ophthalmology 96: 656–663
Savino P J, Hilliker J M, Casell G H et al 1982 Chronic sixth nerve palsies: are they really harbingers of serious intracranial disease? Archives of Ophthalmology 100: 1442–1444
Schatz N J, Savino P J, Corbett J J 1977 Primary aberrant oculomotor regeneration: a sign of intracavernous meningioma. Archives of Neurology 34: 29–32
Seybold M E, Yoss R E, Hollenhorst R W et al 1971 Pupillary abnormalities associated with tumors of the pineal region. Neurology 21: 232–237
Sibony P A, Krauss H R, Kennerdell J S et al 1984 Optic nerve sheath meningiomas, clinical manifestations. Ophthalmology 91: 1313–1326
Stahnke N, Grubel G, Lagenstein I et al 1984 Long-term follow-up of children with craniopharyngioma. European Journal of Pediatrics 142: 179–185
Symon L, Rosenstein J 1984 Surgical management of suprasellar meningiomas. Part 1: The influence of tumor size, duration of symptoms and microsurgery on surgical outcome in 101 consecutive cases. Journal of Neurosurgery 61: 633–641
Thomas J E, Yoss R E 1920 The parasellar syndrome: problems in determining etiology. Mayo Clinic Proceedings 46: 617–623
Thompson H S, Corbett J J, Cox T A 1981 How to measure the relative afferent pupillary defect. Survey of Ophthalmology 26: 39–42
Trobe J D, Bauer R M 1986 Seeing but not recognising. Survey of Ophthalmology 30: 328–336
Trobe J D, Glaser J S, Post J D 1978 Meningiomas and aneurysms of the cavernous sinus: neuro-ophthalmologic features. Archives of Ophthalmology 96: 457–467
Troost B T, Martinez J, Abel L A et al 1980 Upbeat nystagmus and internuclear ophthalmoplegia with brainstem glioma. Archives of Neurology 37: 453–456
Turgman J, Goldhammer Y, Braham J 1979 Alexia, without agraphia, due to brain tumors, a reversible syndrome. Annals of Neurology 6: 265–268
Wall M, Wray S H 1983 The one-and-a-half syndrome — a unilateral disorder of the pontine tegmentum: a study of 20 cases and a review of the literature. Neurology 33: 971–980
Walsh F B, Hoyt W F 1969 Clinical neuro-ophthalmology, 3rd edn, vol 3. Williams & Wilkins, Baltimore, p 2218
Walsh T J, Garden J, Gallagher B 1969 Obliteration of retinal venous pulsations during elevation of cerebrospinal fluid pressure. American Journal of Ophthalmology 67: 954–956
Whitnall S E 1932 The anatomy of the human orbit, 2nd edn. Oxford University Press, Oxford, p 385
Wright J E, Call N B, Liaricos S 1980 Primary optic nerve meningiomas. British Journal of Ophthalmology 64: 553–558
Wyllie E, Luders H, Morris H H et al 1986 The lateralizing significance of versive head and eye movements during epileptic seizures. Neurology 36: 606–611
Yamazaki A, Zee D S 1979 Rebound nystagmus: EOG analysis of a case with a floccular tumor. British Journal of Ophthalmology 63: 782–786

12. Epilepsy associated with brain tumors

Mitchel S. Berger Evren Keles

INTRODUCTION

Seizures are a common presenting feature in patients with intracranial tumors, especially low grade gliomas (Penfield et al 1940, White et al 1948, Arseni & Petrovici 1971, Rasmussen 1975, Piepmeier 1987, Hirsch et al 1989, Pilcher et al 1993). The incidence of epilepsy associated with brain tumors is approximately 35% when all locations and histological types are considered (Ribaric 1984) (Table 12.1). If one considers the likelihood of a tumor as the etiology of a first time seizure in an individual 15 years of age and older, however, the incidence is approximately 8% (see Table 12.2). Age increases the risk of epilepsy being caused by a tumor, especially in individuals beyond 45 years of age (Table 12.3). The finding of a non-focal neurological examination in combination with a first time seizure reduces the occurrence of an associated tumor to only 4.5% (Sempere et al 1982).

The characteristics of a tumor's growth pattern often influence the incidence of seizures, which are more common for the relatively slow growing tumors, e.g. astrocytomas, oligodendrogliomas, mixed oligoastrocytomas, and gangliogliomas. In a series from the Montreal Neurological Institute, seizures were documented at some time during the clinical course in 48% of 209 patients with hemispheric astrocytomas (Gonzales & Elvidge 1962). In Penfield et al's 1940 series including 230 astrocytomas, 37% of glioblastomas were associated with epileptic activity, which is nearly half as frequent as the low grade gliomas. In addition to glial and neuronal neoplasms, tumors originating from the meninges and vascular structures may also cause intermittent seizure activity at a reduced frequency compared to gliomas. In Gonzales & Elvidge's 1962 study, there was no difference in the age and sex distribution of patients with and without seizures,

Table 12.1 Common tumors associated with epilepsy.

Gliomas
- Oligodendroglioma[1]
- Ganglioglioma[1]
- Astrocytoma[1]
- Mixed oligo-astrocytoma[1]
- Anaplastic astrocytoma
- Glioblastoma multiforme

Metastases
- Lung[2]

Meningioma
- Convexity[3]

[1]Most commonly associated with intractable epilepsy
[2]Most common histology presenting with seizures
[3]Most frequent location associated with seizures

Table 12.2 The causes of a first seizure in adults 15 years of age and older.

Cause	No (%)
Idiopathic	27 (27.6)
Cerebral infarction	23 (23.5)
Alcohol withdrawal	11 (11.2)
CNS infection	9 (9.2)
Tumor	**8 (8.2)**
Vascular malformation	6 (6.1)
Trauma	4 (4.1)
Drug toxicity	3 (3.1)
Subdural hematoma	2 (2)
Hyperglycemia	2 (2)
Uremia	1 (1)
Hyponatremia	1 (1)
Cerebral malformation	1 (1)

Table 12.3 The causes of a first seizure based on age distribution.

Cause	< 45 yrs	> 45yrs
Idiopathic	18 (45%)	9 (15.5%)
Cerebral infarction	1 (2.5%)	22 (37.9%)
Alcohol related	6 (15%)	5 (8.6%)
CNS infection	7 (17.5%)	2 (3.4%)
Tumor	**1 (2.5%)**	**7 (12%)**
Vascular malformation	3 (7.5%)	3 (5.2%)
Trauma	3 (7.5%)	1 (1.7%)
Drug toxicity	0 (0%)	3 (5.2%)
Subdural hematoma	0 (0%)	2 (3.4%)
Hyperglycemia	0 (0%)	2 (3.4%)
Uremia	0 (0%)	1 (1.7%)
Hyponatremia	1 (2.5%)	0 (0%)
Cerebral malformation	0 (0%)	1 (1.7%)

and the frontal lobe was found to be affected in 58% of patients with epilepsy.

In reviewing the literature, there are numerous studies involving patients with medically intractable epilepsy who have structural brain lesions (Falconer & Kennedy 1961, Rasmussen 1975, Spencer et al 1984, Morrell 1985, Drake et al 1987, Berger et al 1990). As a result of recent advances in neuro-imaging techniques, the presence of a tumor is now more frequently observed in patients with epilepsy. In a large series of 1661 patients with seizures, the presence of a brain tumor was detected in 30% of the patients (Wyke 1959), which is similar to a recently published community based study demonstrating that 23.4% of patients who presented with partial seizures were found to have a brain tumor (Manford et al 1992).

The critical factors responsible for the development of epilepsy in this context appear to be associated with the indolent growth pattern and location of the lesion (Penfield et al 1940, Rasmussen 1975, Franceschetti et al 1990). The chronic nature of a mass lesion will often account for the adverse effects of a tumor on the adjacent cortical neurons (Penfield et al 1940), which occur morphologically and biochemically in the form of neurotransmitter alterations (deLanerolle et al 1989, Kim et al 1990). It has also recently been demonstrated that the hyperexcitable cortex surrounding the tumor nidus in low grade gliomas has a significantly decreased population of γ-aminobutyric acid and somatostatin containing neurons, when compared to adjacent non-tumor, non-epileptogenic cortex from the same patient (Haglund et al 1992).

While there may be evidence to support the concept of separate seizure foci surrounding a tumor (Penfield et al 1940, Falconer et al 1962, Gonzales & Elvidge 1962, Morrell 1985) or other structural lesions such as arteriovenous malformations (Rasmussen 1975, Buckingham et al 1989, Yeh et al 1990), controversy exists as to whether it is essential to include these peripheral epileptogenic zones in the surgical resection. It has been shown that resection of the tumor alone may result in good postoperative control of the patient's seizures (Falconer & Kennedy 1961, Falconer et al 1962, Goldring et al 1986, Hirsch et al 1989, Cascino 1990, Franceschetti et al 1990). Yet, in patients with intractable epilepsy associated with low grade glial tumors, resection of the tumor without the use of intraoperative electrocorticography or extraoperative grid monitoring to define epileptogenic foci may often result in only a slightly reduced or unchanged seizure frequency (White et al 1948, Schisano et al 1963, Spencer et al 1984, Goldring et al 1986, Hirsch et al 1989, Cascino 1990, Cascino et al 1990, Franceschetti et al 1990, Awad 1991). In patients achieving good seizure control with lesion removal alone, dependence upon antiepileptic drugs to maintain a patient without further seizure activity appears to be critical in some studies (Hirsch et al 1989, Cascino 1990, Cascino et al 1990, Franceschetti et al 1990), yet unclear in other investigations (Goldring et al 1986).

LOW GRADE GLIOMAS ASSOCIATED WITH INTRACTABLE EPILEPSY

To determine the seizure frequency and control of tumor associated epilepsy following surgery, all adult and pediatric patients at our University with the diagnosis of a low grade glioma who were operated on during the time period from 1980 to 1990 were retrospectively evaluated. Patients with seizures refractory to medical therapy always underwent electrocorticography during tumor removal at our institution, and formed the basis for this evaluation. Patients with low grade gliomas who had occasional seizures or were seizure free on medication did not undergo monitoring during tumor removal and were excluded from this analysis. Subsequently, in this chapter, we will compare the results with a review of the literature concerning the outcome of patients with intractable epilepsy associated with a brain tumor.

Patient characteristics

The patients varied in age between 4 and 73 years (mean, 30 years), with nearly equal numbers of male and female patients. 45 patients with astrocytomas (n = 13), oligodendrogliomas (n = 14), gangliogliomas (n = 9), and mixed oligoastrocytomas (n = 9) comprised our patient population. The most common presenting symptom was intractable seizure activity, and very few patients had focal motor or sensory signs, which, when present, were subtle. Virtually all patients had generalized or partial complex seizures, or a combination of both (Fig. 12.1).

The seizure frequency varied between one per month and greater than 10 seizures per day (mean, 541 seizures/year). The preoperative duration varied from one to 324 months (mean, 86 months). The majority of patients were treated with multiple drug combinations prior to the operative procedure. At the time of surgery, 40 patients had been treated with two or more antiepileptic drugs and had documented therapeutic serum drug concentrations. The remaining 5 patients were treated with only one anticonvulsant which was also maintained in the therapeutic range.

Preoperative scalp electroencephalograms were obtained in 31 patients to determine lateralization and proximity of the seizure focus to the tumor. The EEG correctly localized epileptiform activity to the hemisphere with the tumor in only 22 of these patients (71%).

All patients evaluated for this analysis had preoperative computed tomography (CT) scans and most individuals had a magnetic resonance (MR) imaging study (n = 42). Intravenous contrast agents were used in both or either studies in each case, and minimal contrast enhancement was documented in only a few patients. CT scans showed

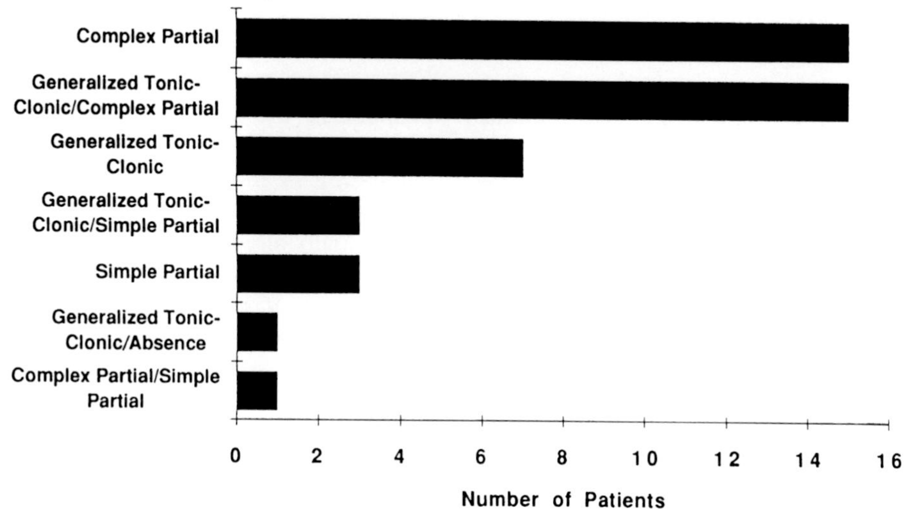

Fig. 12.1 The distribution of seizure type in patients with low grade gliomas and intractable epilepsy.

the typical appearance of a homogeneously hypodense lesion in every instance. MR imaging studies demonstrated a hypointense signal on T1-weighted images in all except 5 patients who had iso- or hyperintense appearing lesions.

There were 12 right-sided tumors, yet in most cases (n = 33) the mass was located in the dominant (left) hemisphere. Cerebral dominance was determined preoperatively by a history of right-handedness when a left hemisphere lesion was detected. Speech lateralization to the left hemisphere was confirmed in every case using language mapping. Right-handed patients with right hemisphere tumors were operated upon while asleep. Patients who were ambidextrous or who had left hemisphere tumors and were left-handed, or, right hemispheric tumors with left-hand preference underwent preoperative language localization using the Wada test (Wada & Rasmussen 1960) to confirm cerebral dominance.

When patients cannot tolerate awake surgery a subdural electrode array is used, which is also applicable when a seizure pattern is complex and electrocorticography is needed to further localize and characterize seizure foci prior to the definitive tumor resection. The subdural electrode arrays are inserted 5–7 days prior to the tumor removal while the patient is under general anesthesia. Extraoperative electrocorticography, language testing and localization of the sensory-motor (Rolandic) cortex is achieved via stimulation mapping through the electrode grid in a telemetry room on the hospital ward.

A seizure focus is defined as an area of epileptic activity located under an electrode contact or within the confines of several electrodes overlying a contiguous cortical region. Non-contiguous epileptic zones are referred to as multiple seizure foci. For example, epileptic discharges originating from the mesial temporal lobe (amygdala, hippocampus, parahippocampal gyrus) without lateral temporal or frontal spike activity indicate a single focus. Epileptic discharges originating from mesial temporal structures and lateral temporal cortical sites associated with a temporal lobe tumor would constitute two, i.e. multiple, seizure foci.

Intraoperative mapping strategies

The techniques of stimulation mapping, including electrocorticography, have been previously detailed (Berger et al 1989, Ojemann et al 1989, Berger et al 1990). Briefly, patients operated upon while awake are mildly sedated if they are anxious (Innovar, 0.5–1 ml), and the scalp is anesthetized with a 0.25% lidocaine-bupivacaine mixture. An alternative approach is to use a propofol (Diprivan) infusion during the bone flap removal which provides a deep sedative state that is reversible in 5–25 minutes. A wide exposure of the cortical surface is essential to map several areas adjacent to and beyond the tumor nidus to detect the seizure focus (foci) and identify speech and Rolandic cortex. A bipolar electrode (5 mm spacing) is used to stimulate the brain utilizing a train of biphasic, square wave pulses (60 Hz, 1 ms, single phase duration). The current will vary from 2–16 mA depending upon the anesthetic condition of the patient and the afterdischarge threshold (see below). Subcortical motor pathways may also be identified using the bipolar electrode when resecting tumor near the internal capsule or cerebral peduncle (Berger et al 1990).

Electrocorticography is performed using an array of carbon-tipped electrodes held in place with a horseshoe apparatus attached to the skull. Subdural strip electrodes are used to record from inferior and mesial temporal lobe, and inferior and interhemispheric frontal lobe. Recordings usually extend over a 10–20 minute period. An intravenous injection of methohexitone (1 mg/kg) may be used to induce epileptiform activity if the interictal record is not informative, yet this is rarely necessary. Following the initial electrocorticography data, a small electrical current (2–8 mA) is applied to the cortex to evoke one or a few afterdischarge potentials, thus establishing the optimal current for blocking language tasks without provoking seizure activity. Following tumor removal, electrocorticography is repeated to ensure that all areas of documented epileptiform activity have been resected prior to termination of the procedure. Epileptic activity that is distant from the resection cavity and occasional, or is located in functional cortex, is not resected.

Localization of seizure foci

Among our 45 patients, 56 seizure foci were detected using electrocorticography. In 6 of the patients, no seizure focus could be identified. Nine seizure foci occupied functional cortex and were not removed. All of the remaining epileptogenic areas were resected and 40 of these were submitted for histologic analysis. Thirty six foci (90%) were not infiltrated with tumor, and the majority of these were characterized as having mild gliosis, especially in the subpial region. In patients harboring predominantly temporal lobe tumors, the vast majority (90%) of the epileptiform discharges originated from mesial temporal lobe structures, i.e. amygdala, uncus, anterior hippocampus, and parahippocampal gyrus. Of those patients with a lateral temporal seizure focus, all but two patients had evidence of additional epileptiform discharges emanating from mesial structures. Patients with frontal or parietal low grade gliomas typically had their seizure foci located directly adjacent to the tumor nidus. In 40 patients, post-resection mapping was performed and 24 persistent seizure foci were identified and resected, except for 9 foci located in functional cortex.

Eighteen patients had two separate (multiple) seizure foci in the following lobes: mesial and lateral temporal (78%), mesial temporal and frontal (6%), and parietal and frontal (17%). Seventeen of these 18 patients (94%) had a seizure frequency of greater than one per week. The duration of the epilepsy was greater than three years in 14 of these 18 patients (78%). There were 21 patients with a single epileptic focus, and of those patients only 12 had a duration of symptoms greater than three years (57%). The difference between these two groups, i.e. single versus multiple seizure foci, in terms of seizure duration was not statistically significant. Five of the remaining 9 patients with a single seizure focus had a preoperative duration of seizures for only 6 months or less, however, the seizure frequency was similar in both groups of patients regardless of whether they had single or multiple seizure foci.

Control of seizure activity

Analyzing the complete group of patients, 41 (91%) are seizure free with a mean follow-up of 50 months. At the present time, 24 patients who have not had any seizure activity are off antiepileptic drugs (mean follow-up, 54 months; mean time off medication, 40 months). Another 17 patients are seizure-free but continue to take antiepileptic drugs at lower doses than preoperatively (mean follow-up, 44 months). Ten of these patients have had one or two seizures at some time in the postoperative period, usually after having their anticonvulsants discontinued (mean time to first postoperative seizure, 38 months; mean time off medication at which first postoperative seizure occurred, 14 months). The remaining 7 of 17 patients (all adults) are on antiepileptic drugs without an explanation at the time of this analysis. In each case, the patients live away from our institution and were primarily under the care of the referring physician who preferred not to taper their medications, although none had seizure activity postoperatively. Therefore, based on our previous experience we would anticipate complete withdrawal of anticonvulsants without subsequent seizure activity.

Four patients in the study group continue to have seizures on anticonvulsants, although with markedly reduced frequency and severity. In one patient, a single seizure focus was identified and found to be unresectable due to its location in functional cortex. In two other cases, diffuse tumor infiltration throughout areas of the Rolandic cortex resulted in a subtotal tumor resection. In both of these circumstances, the residual tumor undercut functional Rolandic cortex which may explain why the seizure pattern has changed from complex to simple partial seizures. The remaining patient was considered a surgical failure because, following the tumor resection, repeat electrocorticography was not performed, thus leaving behind potentially resectable seizure foci.

When comparing the seizure outcome without anticonvulsants between adults and children, we were able to demonstrate that 13 of 32 (41%) adults were seizure-free and off medication (mean follow-up, 50 months; mean time off anticonvulsants, 36 months). If those 7 additional adults are added to this group, assuming they would now be successfully tapered off their medications, then, maximally, 20 of 28 adults (71%) who are seizure-free would be off antiepileptic drugs. The remaining 4 of 32 adults have seizures on medication; however, all 13 pediatric patients, i.e. less than 19 years of age at surgery, no longer have seizures (mean follow-up, 56 months). Eleven of these 13 children (85%) are off medication (mean follow-up, 58 months; mean time off anticonvulsants, 44 months). The difference between seizure control in adults and children who are off antiepileptic drugs in our patient population is statistically significant ($p = 0.016$).

MANAGEMENT OF BRAIN TUMOR PATIENTS WITH EPILEPSY

Seizure focus mapping

Based on our experience, the management of patients

with intractable epilepsy associated with various brain tumors has included identification and resection, when possible, of the seizure focus (foci) in addition to performing an aggressive tumor removal. The use of electrocorticography to improve seizure control in this patient population is not a new concept. Management of patients with intractable epilepsy, however, is clearly different from that of those individuals whose seizures are well-controlled with medication. If the patient is under complete seizure control preoperatively, or has an occasional seizure on medication, we, as others, would not advocate the routine use of intraoperative cortical recordings during the tumor resection. In this circumstance, seizure control with or without the need for postoperative anticonvulsants is often achieved with radical tumor resection alone.

Perhaps the greatest difficulty in interpreting the past literature in regard to seizure control for patients with tumors is whether the need exists for long-term anticonvulsants following surgery. Gonzales & Elvidge (1962) demonstrated an improved seizure outcome when the tumor resection was combined with electrocorticography, yet the status of anticonvulsant requirements was not documented. Similarly, in two studies published by Van Buren et al (1975a,b) in which electrocorticography was used, details regarding seizure control in those particular patients with temporal lobe tumors was not provided. In a patient population including 91 individuals with intractable epilepsy and low grade gliomas who survived long enough to be evaluated, Rasmussen (1975) demonstrated that as many as 79% had either no seizures or a marked reduction with a median follow-up period of seven years. No information was provided regarding the use of medication to achieve that outcome.

Ribaric (1984) reported two patients with excellent seizure control following resection of multiple seizure foci, verified with mapping, yet no description of antiepileptic drug use to attain a seizure-free condition was provided. This work emphasized the finding that multiple seizure foci associated with low grade gliomas commonly occur in patients with a longer history of seizures. This fact also became apparent in our experience, and may further support the need to use electrocorticography during the tumor resection in patients with a longstanding seizure disorder to facilitate localization of multiple epileptogenic foci that might not have been found without the use of intraoperative recordings.

Drake and colleagues (1987) described their experience in children with structural lesions of the temporal lobe using electrocorticography guided removal of seizure foci, and emphasized that epileptogenic activity often originates from the brain adjacent to the tumor. Six of 11 patients were rendered seizure-free with or without anticonvulsants, while the remaining patients required medication to reduce their seizure frequency by half. Although post-resection electrocorticography was used to maximize seizure control, it remains unknown if both mesial structures and lateral temporal lobe cortex were remapped, e.g. following tumor removal, in the Drake study as we did in our own patients.

It has been reported that improved seizure control may be achieved in patients with structural lesions when the extent of the epileptogenic focus resection is complete (Wyllie et al 1987). Using subdural recordings to map areas of seizure activity, Wyllie and colleagues (1987) accomplished excellent results even when a less than total resection of the mass was completed. This implied that multiple seizure foci are often present, thus necessitating extraoperative seizure mapping to augment the tumor resection. Several years later, Awad (1991) reviewed many of the same patients, looking at seizure control as it related to the proximity of the epileptogenic focus to the structural lesion. He also assessed what effect the extent of lesion and focus resection had in controlling the patient's seizures. Indeed, the amount of lesion removed significantly affected postoperative seizure control. Even when the seizure focus was less than completely resected, the seizure outcome was good if the lesion was completely resected. If the lesion removal was subtotal, however, seizure control was improved when a more aggressive focus resection was performed. It should be noted that the patients included in their study required anticonvulsants to maintain their level of postoperative seizure control. Post-resection electrocorticography may have improved their results, since persistent epileptiform activity following tumor resection has been previously shown to be associated with recurrence of seizures (Gloor 1975). Several other authors also utilize a surgical approach that does not include, as part of the resection, multiple recordings, following the initial tumor and seizure focus removal (Ajmone-Marsan & Baldwin 1958, Gibbs et al 1958, Walker et al 1960). Because low grade gliomas are often diffuse and ill-defined, a subtotal tumor resection is usually achieved which further supports the need to independently map and resect single or multiple epileptogenic foci for optimal seizure control.

Radical tumor removal without perioperative seizure mapping

Several published studies do not agree with the use of electrocorticography during the tumor resection to maximize control of epilepsy associated with a tumor. However, in each of these studies, in addition to removing the tumor, brain adjacent to the lesion was also included in the resection strategy. In an earlier study completed by Falconer & Cavanaugh (1959), 9 of 13 patients with intractable epilepsy and a tumor became seizure-free with this approach, but no information was provided regarding the need for continuation of anticonvulsants. The authors concluded that their good results were influenced by removal of brain surrounding the lesion that may have 'interrupted neuronal circuits which were involved in the seizure mechanism'. In another study, Lindsay et al (1984) reported two children with low grade gliomas located in the temporal lobe who became seizure-free following radical temporal lobectomies including the tumor.

Spencer et al (1984) reviewed the status of 19 patients with gliomas who underwent surgery to remove the mass only, versus those patients who had a primary seizure operation in which removal of adjacent mesial temporal or frontal lobe brain tissue was carried out. All patients except four had a follow-up of greater than 6 months. Every patient who underwent the more extensive procedure had greater than 95% reduction in seizure frequency. This is in contrast to only half of those patients with mass resection or biopsy alone who achieved the same results. Although the authors demonstrated better results with 'seizure surgery', they did not recommend the routine use of intraoperative monitoring to improve the seizure outcome. Their patients did not have complete relief of seizure activity and the need for postoperative anticonvulsants was not mentioned.

Sperling et al (1989) reported an example of a minimal tumor resection in the posterior temporal lobe which resulted in complete seizure control because anterior, non-tumor involved temporal lobe structures were resected. This patient still needed antiepileptic drugs to maintain a seizure-free status.

Focal tumor resection without perioperative seizure mapping

Patients with astrocytomas who had preoperative seizures were evaluated by Penfield et al (1940) and White et al (1948) in two separate studies. Although it is not known whether these patients had intractable epilepsy, following tumor removal 85% and 90% of patients, respectively, continued to have seizures. Falconer et al (1962) reported two patients with posterior temporal gliomas who became seizure-free following tumor resection without removal of adjacent temporal lobe structures. Postoperatively, one of these two patients required anticonvulsants to maintain a seizure-free condition. In another study, Schisano et al (1963) reported patients who had epilepsy associated with an astrocytoma, 39% of whom continued to have seizures after resection of the tumor. No information was provided regarding the need for continuation of antiepileptic drugs.

Because of the chronic nature of gangliogliomas, both adults and children are particularly susceptible to the development of seizures. Seizure control, without the use of electrocorticography, following resection of gangliogliomas has been addressed in three series (Sutton et al 1983, Demierre et al 1987, Kalyan-Raman & Olivere 1987). All together, 11 of 25 patients were documented as having medically refractory seizures, and 6 (54%) of these patients were reported to be seizure-free following tumor resection. No information regarding the postoperative use of anticonvulsants was provided in two of the three series, however Sutton et al (1983) indicated that all of their patients remained on medication, although half were seizure-free. In our experience, which includes 9 patients with gangliogliomas, 6 patients were seizure-free without taking anticonvulsants. Two of our patients are seizure-free but must be maintained on antiepileptic drugs, while the remaining patient continues to have seizures at a reduced frequency while taking medication.

In a study conducted by Goldring and colleagues (1986) regarding seizure control in patients with glial tumors who had a 'chronic seizure disorder', mapping of seizure foci was utilized during the tumor removal in only 3 of 40 cases. The frequency of seizures and the number of anticonvulsants used by each patient in this study was not known. Although 82% of these patients were seizure-free following surgery, 7 patients had anterior temporal lobectomies, while in 3 additional patients electrocorticography was used. Another important aspect of this study indicated that 23 patients had temporal lobe tumors which often involved mesial structures, thus implying that lesion resection in this area may have also included portions of the amygdala, hippocampus, and parahippocampal gyrus. In addition, no mention was made regarding the postoperative use of antiepileptic drugs to maintain an 82% seizure-free status.

Computer assisted stereotactic tumor resection, possibly the most precise form of focal tumor resection alone without removing adjacent, potentially epileptogenic brain, results in a reduced seizure frequency in the majority of patients who undergo this procedure (Cascino 1990, Cascino et al 1990). Although this occurred in 86% of the 30 patients with tumors, 97% remained on anticonvulsants to maintain that level of control. The proponents of this method concluded that tumor resection alone in a patient with medically refractory epilepsy is often inadequate, as removal of the seizure focus (foci) adjacent to the lesion cannot be accomplished with their surgical technique, which does not utilize electrocorticography. Continued use of antiepileptic drugs is usually necessary, and in some patients an additional operation may be required for persistent seizure activity.

Boon et al (1991) reported on 50 patients with intractable epilepsy associated with structural lesions including 38 tumors in which long-term follow-up was available. In each case the lesion was removed with a 'variable amount of surrounding brain' and the extent of resection was apparently determined by 'obtaining tumor-free margins'. It was not clear from this study how they quantified adjacent brain resection. Furthermore, the number of margins submitted for analysis and the percentage of those margins with infiltrating tumor were not delineated. No information based on the histological diagnosis of the primary tumor, as it correlated with seizure outcome, was provided. Nonetheless, in the entire group, 83% of the patients were seizure-free without the use of intraoperative mapping, although no data were given regarding the requirement of anticonvulsants to maintain this outcome.

Control of seizures associated with pediatric brain tumors

Blume et al (1982) reported an excellent outcome in seizure control when a 'complete' tumor removal was accomplished. 87% of children who had a complete resection were seizure-free, whereas only 33% of patients with a partial tumor resection had no further seizure activity. Most of the patients in Blume's series still required anticonvulsants at a reduced dose. Three infants with gliomas involving the temporal lobe (two of which were low grade), who presented with intractable seizures, became seizure-free following tumor resection without electrocorticography as reported by Rutledge and colleagues (1987). They all required continuation of the antiepileptic medication to remain seizure-free.

Goldring (1987) reported his experience utilizing the technique of extraoperative recordings from an epidurally implanted electrode array in 40 children with gliomas, most of whom had low grade tumors. Although the patients had 'intractable' seizures, data regarding the frequency or location of the epileptiform discharges in relation to the tumor were not provided. The author stated that the 'presumed epileptogenic cortex adjacent to the lesion' was not resected. Seven patients had an accompanying anterior temporal lobectomy together with the tumor resection, and, in other cases, excision of the cortex to 'gain access' to the tumor was undertaken. It was stated that over 80% of those patients with gliomas who underwent removal of the lesion in the aforementioned context had cessation of their seizures. It is therefore difficult to know how many patients simply had only the tumor removed or whether the resection included adjacent epileptogenic brain. As in other reports, there was no mention of the need for postoperative anticonvulsants.

Hirsch et al (1989), in their study on 42 children with low grade astrocytomas and oligodendrogliomas, evaluated seizure control without the use of intraoperative electrocorticography. Only 32 patients had preoperative seizures, and 20 of these (62%) were classified as intractable. Almost all patients had a 'macroscopically complete' tumor resection without disturbing the surrounding cortex. Although the outcome of intractable seizures was not separately analyzed, 57% of the entire series became seizure-free without medication. An additional 24% of patients required anticonvulsants to remain seizure-free, whereas the remaining 19% continued to have seizures despite the use of antiepileptic drugs.

SUMMARY

The majority of patients with tumor associated epilepsy harbor slow growing, indolent neoplasms such as low grade gliomas and meningiomas. In the majority of cases, including those patients with malignant gliomas or metastases, the seizures are infrequent and easily controlled with one antiepileptic drug. In this setting, removal of the tumor alone usually controls the epilepsy with or without the need for additional anticonvulsants; however, patients with these indolent tumors may have seizure activity that is refractory to medical therapy. Optimal control of the epilepsy without postoperative anticonvulsants in this situation is provided when perioperative, e.g. extraoperative or intraoperative, electrocorticographic mapping of separate seizure foci accompanies the tumor resection. When mapping is not utilized and a radical tumor resection is carried out with adjacent brain, the occurrence of seizures will be lessened but most patients will have to remain on antiepileptic drugs.

Acknowledgement

This work was supported by NIH Grant KO8 NS01253–01, American Cancer Society Professor of Clinical Oncology #071 (M S Berger), NIH Grant T32NS07144–13.

Certain aspects of this Chapter are reproduced from the Journal of Neurosurgery, Vol 79, 1993, with permission of the editor, John A. Jane MD PhD, to whom we are grateful.

REFERENCES

Ajmone-Marsan C, Baldwin M 1958 Electroencephalography. In: Baldwin M, Bailey P (eds) Temporal lobe epilepsy. Charles C. Thomas, Springfield, IL

Arseni C, Petrovici I N 1971 Epilepsy of temporal lobe tumours. European Neurology 5: 201–214

Awad I 1991 Intractable epilepsy and structural lesions of the brain: mapping, resection strategies, and seizures outcome. Epilepsia 32: 179–186

Berger M S, Kincaid J, Ojemann G A et al 1989 Brain mapping techniques to maximize resection, safety, and seizure control in children with brain tumors. Neurosurgery 25: 786–792

Berger M S, Ojemann G A, Lettich E 1990 Neurophysiological monitoring to facilitate resection during astrocytoma surgery. In: Neurosurgery Clinics of North America, WB Saunders, Inc., vol 1, no 1, pp 65–80

Blume W T, Girvin J P, Kaufmann J C 1982 Childhood brain tumors presenting as chronic uncontrolled focal seizure disorders. Ann Neurol 12: 538–541

Boon P A, Williamson P D, Fried I et al 1991 Intracranial, intraaxial, space-occupying lesions in patients with intractable partial seizures: an anatomical, neuropsychological, and surgical correlation. Epilepsia 32: 467–476

Buckingham M J, Crone K R, Ball W S et al 1989 Management of cerebral cavernous angiomas in children presenting with seizures. Child's Nervous System 5: 347–349

Cascino G D 1990 Epilepsy and brain tumors: implications for treatment. Epilepsia 31 (suppl 3): S37–S44

Cascino G D, Kelly P J, Hirschhorn K A et al 1990 Stereotactic resection of intra-axial cerebral lesions in partial epilepsy. Mayo Clinic Proceedings 65: 1053–1060

deLanerolle N C, Kim J H, Robbins R J et al 1989 Hippocampal interneuron loss and plasticity in human temporal lobe epilepsy. Brain Research 49: 387–395

Demierre B, Stichnoth F A, Hori A et al 1987 Intracerebral gangliogliomas. Journal of Neurosurgery 21: 792–797

Drake J, Hoffman H J, Kobayashi J et al 1987 Surgical management of children with temporal lobe epilepsy and mass lesions. Neurosurgery 21: 792–797

Falconer M A, Cavanaugh J B 1959 Clinico-pathological considerations of temporal lobe epilepsy due to small focal lesions. A study of cases submitted to operation. Brain 82: 483–504

Falconer M A, Kennedy W A 1961 Epilepsy due to small focal temporal lesions with bilateral independent spike-discharging foci. A study of seven cases relieved by operation. Journal of Neurology, Neurosurgery and Psychiatry 24: 205–212

Falconer M A, Driver M V, Serafetinides E A 1962 Temporal lobe epilepsy due to distant lesions: two cases relieved by operation. Brain 85: 521–534

Franceschetti S, Binelli S, Casazza M et al 1990 Influence of surgery and antiepileptic drugs on seizures symptomatic of cerebral tumours. Acta Neurochirurgica (Wien) 103: 47–51

Gibbs F A, Amador L, Rich C 1958 Electroencephalographic findings and therapeutic results in surgical treatment of psychomotor epilepsy. In: Baldwin M, Bailey P (eds) Temporal lobe epilepsy. Charles C. Thomas, Springfield, IL

Gloor P 1975 Contributions of electroencephalography and electrocorticography to the neurosurgical treatment of the epilepsies. In: Neurosurgical management of the epilepsies. Advances in neurology, vol 8. Raven Press, New York, pp 59–105

Goldring S 1987 Pediatric epilepsy surgery. Epilepsia 28: S82–102

Golding S, Rich K M, Picker S 1986 Experience with gliomas in patients presenting with a chronic seizure disorder. In: Little J R (ed) Clinical neurosurgery, vol 33. Raven Press, New York, pp 15–42

Gonzales D, Elvidge A R 1962 On the occurrence of epilepsy caused by astrocytoma of the cerebral hemispheres. Journal of Neurosurgery 19: 470–482

Haglund M M, Berger M S, Kunkel D D et al 1992 Changes in GABA and somatostatin in epileptic cortex associated with low-grade gliomas. Journal of Neurosurgery 77: 209–216

Hirsch J F, Rose C S, Pierre-Khan A et al 1989 Benign astrocytic and oligodendrocytic tumors of the cerebral hemispheres in children. Journal of Neurosurgery 70: 568–572

Kalyan-Raman U P, Olivere W C 1987 Gangliogliomas: A correlative clinicopathological and radiological study of ten surgically treated cases with follow-up. Neurosurgery 20: 428–433

Kim J H, Guimaraes P O, Shen M Y et al 1990 Hippocampal neuronal density in temporal lobe epilepsy. Acta Neuropathololologica 80: 41–45

Lindsay J, Ounsted C, Richards P 1984 Long-term outcome in children with temporal lobe seizure. V: Indications and contraindications for neurosurgery. Dev Med & Child Neurol 26: 25–32

Manford M, Hart Y M, Sander J W A S et al 1992 National General Practice Study of Epilepsy (NGPSE): Partial seizure patterns in a general population. Neurology 42: 1911–1917

Morrell F 1985 Secondary epileptogenesis in man. Archives of Neurology 42: 318–335

Ojemann G A, Ojemann J, Lettich E et al 1989 Cortical language localization in left, dominant hemisphere. An electrical stimulation mapping investigation in 117 patients. Journal of Neurosurgery 71: 316–326

Penfield W, Erickson T C, Tarlov I M 1940 Relation of intracranial tumors and symptomatic epilepsy. Archives of Neurology and Psychiatry 44: 300–315

Piepmeier J M 1987 Observations on the current treatment of low-grade astrocytic tumors of the cerebral hemispheres. Journal of Neurosurgery 67: 177–181

Pilcher W H, Silbergeld D L, Berger M S et al 1993 Combined resection of tumor and epileptogenic brain in patients with gangliogliomas: impact upon seizure outcome. Journal of Neurosurgery (in press)

Rasmussen T B 1975 Surgery of epilepsy associated with brain tumors. In: Neurosurgical management of the epilepsies. Advances in neurology, vol 8. Raven Press, New York, pp 227–239

Ribaric I I 1984 Excision of two and three independent and separate ipsilateral potentially epileptogenic cortical areas. Acta Neurochirurgica S33: 145–148

Rutledge S L, Snead O C, Morawetz R et al 1987 Brain tumors presenting as a seizure disorder in infants. Journal of Child Neurology 2: 214–219

Schisano G, Tovi D, Nordenstam H 1963 Spongioblastoma polare of the cerebral hemisphere. Journal of Neurosurgery 20: 241–251

Sempere A P, Villaverde F J, Martinez-Menendez B et al 1982 First seizure in adults: a prospective study from the Emergency Department. Acta Neurologica Scandinavica 86: 134–138

Spencer D D, Spencer S S, Mattson R H et al 1984 Intracerebral masses in patients with intractable partial epilepsy. Neurology 34: 432–436

Sperling M R, Cahan L D, Brown W J 1989 Relief of seizures from a predominantly posterior temporal tumor with anterior temporal lobectomy. Epilepsia 30: 559–563

Sutton L N, Packer R J, Rorke L B 1983 Cerebral gangliomas during childhood. Neurosurgery 13: 124–128

Van Buren J M, Ajmone-Marsan C, Mutsuga N et al 1975a Surgery of temporal lobe epilepsy. In: Purpura D P, Penry J K, Walter R D (eds) Neurosurgical management of the epilepsies. Advances in neurology, vol 8. Raven Press, New York, pp 155–196

Van Buren J M, Ajmone-Marsan C, Mutsuga N 1975b Temporal lobe seizures with additional foci treated by resection. Journal of Neurosurgery 43: 596–607

Wada J, Rasmussen T 1960 Intracarotid injections of sodium amytal for the lateralization of cerebral speech dominance. Journal of Neurosurgery 17: 266–282

Walker A E, Lichtenstein R S, Marshall C 1960 A critical analysis of electroencephalography in temporal lobe epilepsy. Archives of Neurology 2: 172–182

White J C, Liu C T, Mixter W J 1948 Focal epilepsy. A statistical study of its causes and the results of surgical treatment. Epilepsy secondary to intracranial tumors. New England Journal of Medicine 238: 891–899

Wyke B D 1959 The cortical control of movement: A contribution to the surgical physiology of seizures. Epilepsia 1: 4–35

Wyllie E, Luders H, Morris H H et al 1987 Clinical outcome after complete or partial cortical resection for intractable epilepsy. Neurology 37: 1634–1641

Yeh H S, Kashiwagi S, Tew J M et al 1990 Surgical management of epilepsy associated with cerebral arteriovenous malformations. Journal of Neurosurgery 72: 216–223

13. Functional and metabolic imaging of brain tumors

D. G. T. Thomas   N. D. Kitchen

INTRODUCTION

The current neuroradiological techniques of high resolution computed tomography (CT) and magnetic resonance imaging (MRI) can supply elegant anatomic information regarding brain tumor position and extent (Kelly et al 1987, Burger et al 1988) and digital subtraction angiography (DSA) can accurately display tumor vascularity. However, only a limited amount of indirect functional information is, at present, available from such studies (for example, CT and MR contrast enhancement reflecting blood-brain barrier alterations). Furthermore, as the number and sophistication of MR imaging sequences rapidly increase, the significance of the varying image appearances is becoming less certain. These facts have implications both in terms of the scientific understanding underlying the technique, but also clinically, where it is often impossible to differentiate viable and necrotic tumor from edematous or gliotic brain (for example the practical problem following surgical or radiotherapy treatment where both CT (Cairncross et al 1985) and MRI (Elster & Di Persio 1990) can show extensive 'post-treatment' changes which are nonspecific). The functional imaging techniques of positron emission tomography (PET), single positron emission computed tomography (SPECT) and magnetic resonance spectroscopy (MRS), in contrast, are able to demonstrate, and in some instances to quantitate, various aspects of the metabolism of such brain tumors in vivo. The functional data obtained from PET, SPECT and MRS are not only of great scientific interest, but may also have important therapeutic implications. Thus, knowledge regarding tumor blood flow, the rate of tumor growth, the degree of oxygenation, the pH and the selective amino acid, nucleic acid and carbohydrate metabolism of tumors is currently being amassed and evaluated as to clinical significance.

Functional and metabolic imaging of human brain tumors in vivo provides unique scientific information which complements the large amount of in vitro and animal in vivo studies on brain tumor metabolism. Not only will such research yield basic scientific information about different types of tumors but may also aid in the management of the individual patient (Mazziotta 1991). Already functional imaging techniques are being used to detect viable residual tumor following surgical treatment, to detect early recurrences before other imaging techniques, to show how tumor biology responds to treatment in serial studies, to differentiate radiation-induced brain necrosis from tumor and, perhaps most significantly, to help formulate a prognosis for the individual patient (Glantz et al 1991).

COMPUTED TOMOGRAPHY (CT)

The CT enhancement of brain tumors that is seen following the administration of water soluble contrast agents gives a qualitative indication of the vascularity of the tumor and the associated disruption of the blood-brain barrier. In addition, however, CT has been used to quantitate transcapillary transport in human brain tumors. Using a method whereby the Hounsfield Unit values of specified CT voxels were compared with simultaneous arterial samples following the administration of meglumine iothalamate (Conray-60), Groothius et al (1991) demonstrated that the blood-to-tissue transport rates (K_1) varied considerably both between and within astrocytomas, with focal increases up to fifty times those found in normal cortex. The demonstration of the blood-brain barrier disruption by this technique and others (most notably SPECT and PET) is of great clinical interest for a number of reasons, including questions regarding the therapeutic implications regarding delivery of various chemotherapeutic agents administered systemically, the mechanism of the beneficial effects of corticosteroids and the mode of local tumor spread.

POSITRON EMISSION TOMOGRAPHY (PET — Fig. 13.1)

The underlying principle of PET scanning is annihilation coincidence detection (Phelps et al 1975). When a positron-emitting isotope decays it releases a positron which

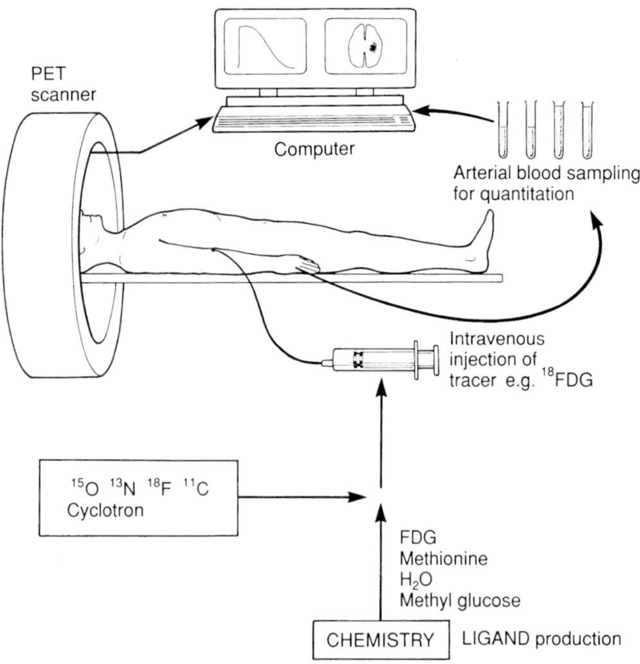

Fig. 13.1 The constituent parts of a PET investigation.

travels up to approximately 2 mm before being captured by an electron, undergoing annihilation and thereby releasing energy in the form of two 511 keV energy gamma rays or 'annihilation photons' at 180 degrees to one another. The circular array of detectors in a PET scanner registers the arrival of these gamma rays as a 'coincident' event. By summation of these coincident events a spatial distribution of the positron-emitting isotope in the plane of the scan can be constructed.

Examples of positron-emitting isotopes which are currently being used to investigate normal and abnormal human physiology include oxygen-15 (^{15}O), nitrogen-13 (^{13}N), fluorine-18 (^{18}F) and carbon-11 (^{11}C). All require to be generated in a cyclotron and have half-lives of 2 minutes, 10 minutes, 20 minutes and 90 minutes respectively. Fluorine is used as a substitute for hydrogen, as no easily usable alternative exists. In some cases however a PET tracer may be made without the need for a cyclotron, for example rubidium-82 (^{82}Rb), produced from the decay of its long-lived parent isotope strontium-82, which has a half-life of 25 days. These isotopes may be used to label organic substrates (ligands) such as amino acids or sugars, thus forming positron-emitting tracers.

Positron emission tomography can be used simply in a qualitative manner, as a tracer imaging device, but also, and more significantly, by comparing regional kinetics with the time course of the systemic tracer in arterial blood, it can be used in a quantitative fashion to measure blood flow, oxygen utilization and pH, as well as glucose and amino acid metabolism. Such quantitation infinitely increases the power of PET as a research tool, though such analysis is complicated and time-consuming and may not be necessary to provide clinically relevant information which may be obtained more simply by qualitative image analysis (DiChiro & Brooks 1988, Glantz et al 1991). Quantitation of the regional concentrations of tracer can be obtained if the attenuation coefficient of each region is known. This is measured by placing a ring source of positron-emitting isotope (usually germanium-68) between the detectors and the region of interest. The photons travel through the body region to the opposite detector. The data from this transmission scan provide the information on tissue attenuation and are used to correct the emission data, allowing absolute values of tracer concentration to be determined.

Positron emission tomography can be used to measure the regional concentration of a tracer molecule in this way. However, to make sense of the data in functional terms a thorough knowledge of the fate of the tracer in the body must be known. PET scanning is not just another imaging technique; many alternative tracer molecules could be used to label abnormal tissue, such as brain tumors, in nonspecific ways. Rather, it is the quantitation and kinetic data provided by the technique which make it such a powerful research tool, and it is in these areas where a large proportion of the ongoing research is taking place. Conversely, where valid models do not yet exist, as is the case for most labelled drugs, the studies can only be qualitative. However this does not necessarily detract from their clinical usefulness in localizing and characterizing lesions.

The current spatial resolution of PET scanning is in the region of 5 mm. However the current generation of PET scanner computer software (as found, for example, on the Siemens 953B scanner at the MRC Cyclotron Unit at the Hammersmith Hospital, London, UK) does allow three-dimensional data acquisition. This feature, in which the lead septa are retracted from the scanner detector ring, allows the detection of random coincidences from all the contralateral detectors and not just via the orthogonal plane. This results in a more complete, but also far more complex, representation of events. It is only with the advent of highly sophisticated computer technology that analysis of the vast amount of data generated using this technique has become possible and meaningful.

Certain technical limitations must be taken into consideration in order to optimize the data obtained from PET. The three principal factors are: first, the spatial resolution of the scanner in relation to the size of the region of interest, secondly the statistics and methods used for the calculation of random coincidences, and thirdly the method of attenuation correction. In practice these constraints favor the measurement of a steady state tracer level with the accumulation of tracer over a period of time in order to allow the statistics to be made as favorable as possible to enhance spatial resolution and signal-to-noise ratio. Furthermore, multiple slices and 3D data acquisitions require increased time to accumulate the data. In addition to these general technical limitations individual tracers require important assumptions to be used in the quantitation algorithms which, depending on the ligand used and its kinetic model, limits the validity of the findings.

With respect to brain tumors the majority of completed PET studies may be divided into those concerned with blood flow and oxygen utilization, glucose metabolism and blood-brain barrier alterations.

a. Blood flow and oxygen utilization

Regional cerebral blood flow (rCBF), regional cerebral arterial oxygen extraction (rOER), and regional cerebral oxygen utilization ($rCMRO_2$) can be measured by asking the subject to inhale in turn $C^{15}O_2$ and $^{15}O_2$ during PET scanning, whilst regional cerebral blood volume (rCBV) can be measured using ^{11}CO or ^{15}CO as tracers (though they actually measure red cell volume and therefore the hematocrit needs to be determined concurrently). More simply, rCBF can be determined by injecting intravenously ^{15}O-labelled water using a steady infusion method. This technique is less invasive and ensures a controlled dose of tracer, but does require special algorithms and has only been in use relatively recently. As $H_2{}^{15}O$ diffuses into the brain its regional tissue concentration reaches equilibrium after 3–5 half-lives (i.e. 6–10 minutes). Thus the tissue $H_2{}^{15}O$ concentration is a balance between diffusion into and diffusion out of the brain, with a proportion lost by decay. The short half-life of ^{15}O prevents tissue $H_2{}^{15}O$ from ever reaching that obtained arterially, but the relationship between the two varies with flow and this can be used to quantitate rCBF.

Results have shown that while the blood flow in gliomas may be highly variable (particularly with the higher grades) and not coupled to blood volume, oxygen extraction and utilization are consistently lower than normal brain tissue (Ito et al 1982, Beaney et al 1985). Furthermore, to date, PET scanning has failed to detect any ischemic areas within brain tumors (where the oxygen extraction approaches 100%) despite the presence of necrosis. These findings are surprising, but are consistent with those obtained with respect to glucose utilization using PET (vide infra). However, PET is a macroscopic investigatory technique and cannot exclude areas of microscopic tumor hypoxia beyond the level of resolution.

Areas of peritumoral edema have been found to have low blood flow and oxygen utilization but with normal levels of arterial oxygen extraction (i.e. 40%), indicating that these areas are not ischemic. Decreased blood flow and oxygen utilization has been found in the cerebral hemisphere contralateral to brain tumors (versus age-matched controls) though such depression of cortical function returns partially to normal on surgical removal of the tumor.

Using PET, dexamethasone has been shown to cause a coupled decrease in blood flow and volume both in the ipsilateral and contralateral cerebral cortex in patients with intrinsic brain tumors, thus causing a rapid decrease in intracranial pressure and improvement in any symptoms of raised intracranial pressure. Radiotherapy has been shown to cause a progressive fall in oxygen utilization and blood flow in the tumor region, but in the contralateral cerebral cortex blood flow rises acutely and then subsequently diminishes. Oxygen utilization, however, in the contralateral brain tissue remains unaltered by radiotherapy.

b. Glucose metabolism

Increased glucose uptake and glycolysis has long been associated with malignancy (Warburg 1930). The analog of glucose ^{18}F-fluoro-2-deoxyglucose (^{18}FDG) is the tracer most widely used to measure regional cerebral glucose utilization in patients with brain tumors (Fig. 13.2). This tracer behaves like glucose and is transported across the blood-brain barrier by the same facilitated transport mechanism (i.e. the hexose carrier) and is then phosphorylated by hexokinase. The resultant metabolite, FDG-6-phosphate, is relatively stable and is effectively trapped within the cells unable to participate in either glycogen or glucose synthesis.

Kinetic models have been developed to relate the distribution of the ^{18}FDG following intravenous injection to the regional glucose uptake and utilization within the brain, and recent evidence suggests that ^{18}FDG uptake into brain tumors is governed principally by phosphorylation and is largely independent of ^{18}FDG transcellular transport (Herholz et al 1992a). However, one difficulty with these models is that they rely upon the 'lumped constant' which relates the relative values of ^{18}FDG and glucose transport across the blood-brain barrier to their relative rates of phosphorylation. The value for the lumped constant in regions of abnormal brain which are infiltrated with brain tumor is uncertain, and may be larger in brain tumors than in normal brain (Gjedde et al 1985). In addition, when the blood-brain barrier breaks down significantly, the higher levels of ^{18}FDG may accumulate in the extracellular space, leading to artefactual rises in concentration. Thus, there remains controversy about the values for the lumped constant, as well as about the individual rate constants for transport, phosphorylation and dephosphorylation embodied in the equations.

In spite of the above reservations ^{18}FDG has been investigated by a number of research groups studying the glucose metabolism of brain tumors and a number of consistent findings of importance have emerged. In patients where both oxygen and glucose uptake have been meas-

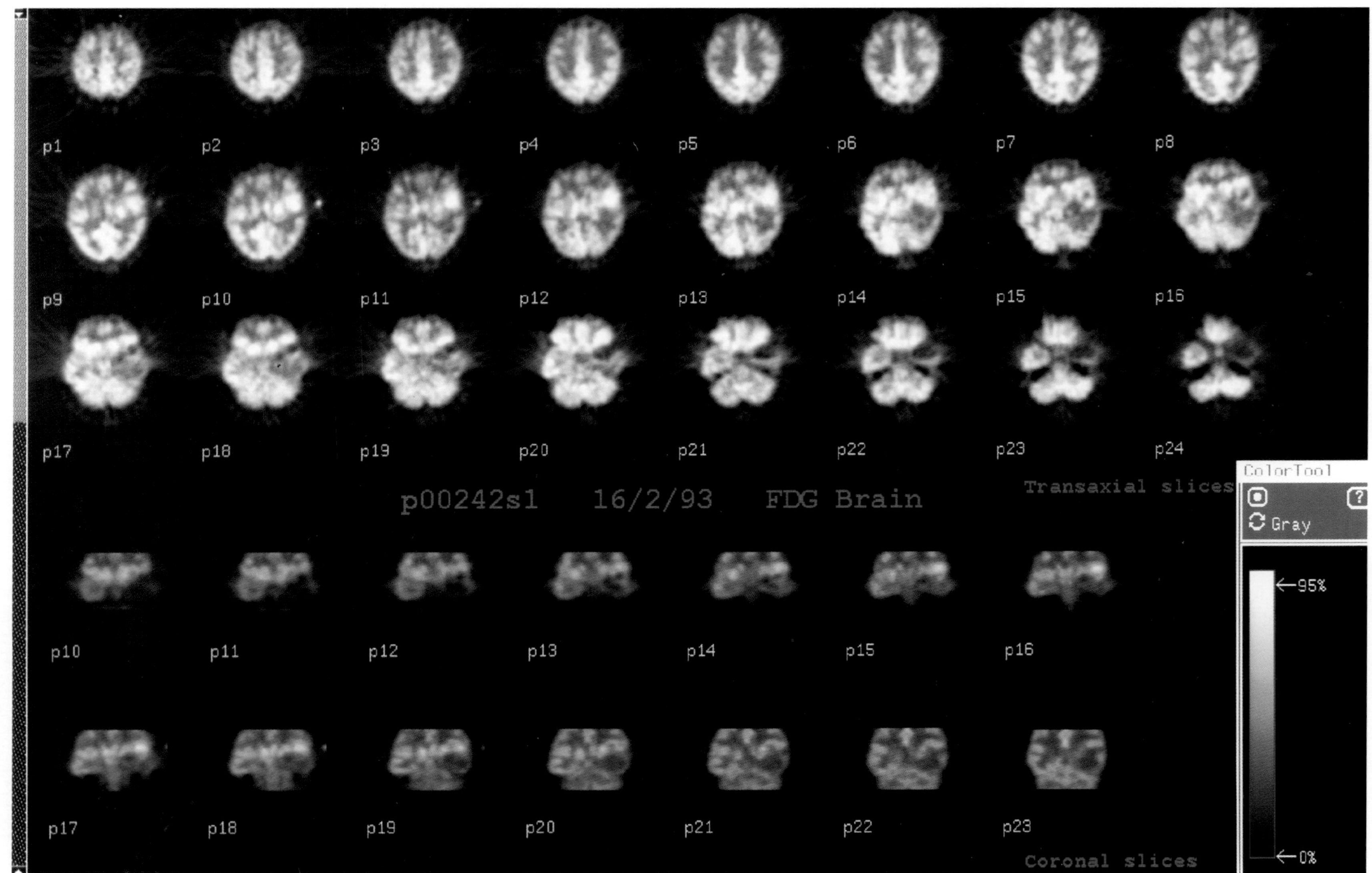

Fig. 13.2 [18]FDG PET scan. Coronal and axial series. In this patient with a right temporal lobe cystic astrocytoma there is an ametabolic area in the region of the cyst. Anteriorly there is an area of increased uptake corresponding to the solid portion of the tumor. Courtesy of The Clinical PET Centre, St Thomas' Hospital, London, UK.

ured, tumor glucose extraction remains similar to normal cortex, while regional oxygen extraction is characteristically depressed, indicating an increased level of non-oxidative metabolism of glucose in the presence of an adequate oxygen supply (Rhodes et al 1983). DiChiro and co-workers found a direct correlation between glucose utilization and grade of primary brain tumors (DiChiro et al 1982) and this finding has been confirmed by more recent studies in an attempt to correlate glucose uptake with prognosis (Patronas et al 1985, DiChiro 1986). However, although the maximal ^{18}FDG uptake may be proportional to grade, the variability in uptake values increases markedly as the tumors become more malignant. Hence ^{18}FDG PET has been found to be most useful in grade 2 gliomas, where low uptake has been shown to be reasonably reliable as a good prognostic indicator. Herholz et al (1992b) used ^{18}FDG PET in 36 patients with WHO grade 2 and 3 tumors and found that 10 out of 11 with a low metabolic index, as defined in the study, as opposed to 4 out of 10 with a high metabolic index survived during a mean follow-up period of 24 months. DiChiro also reliably found depression of ^{18}FDG uptake in areas of peritumoral edema and, in some cases, in the contralateral cerebellar cortex (cerebellar diaschisis). Furthermore, he has used ^{18}FDG PET as an index of meningioma aggressiveness to try and predict the chances of recurrence (DiChiro et al 1987). It is possible that ^{18}FDG uptake in gliomas is proportional to cell number (Herholz, personal communication 1993) and this observation may well explain the discrepancies in the findings between centers with respect to the grade of glioma.

^{18}FDG PET uptake has been used to study the effect of treatment on glioma metabolism (Ogawa et al 1988). Thus, for example after brachytherapy, uptake has been shown to decrease (Fig. 13.3), but this change may take several weeks to occur, and the prognostic significance of the finding is uncertain.

c. Blood-brain barrier studies in brain tumors

Although most tracers used with PET are dependent on blood flow kinetics and tumor uptake across the blood-brain barrier, gallium-68 EDTA, ^{11}C-albumin, ^{11}C-methyl-glucose and rubidium-82 have all been used in PET studies, specifically with the rationale of localizing tumors by the breakdown of the blood-brain barrier (Yamamoto et al 1977, Yen et al 1982, Doyle et al 1987). Indeed there is the possibility of using these tracers of different molecular weights in order to study the subtleties of blood-brain barrier breakdown. Thus, ^{11}C-methyl-glucose gives a measure of facilitated diffusion mechanisms across the endothelium appropriate to normal glucose, rubidium-82 utilizes the same active transport mechanism as potassium, whilst ^{11}C-albumin, a much larger molecule, is transported by pinocytosis.

It has been shown that gliomas have increased ^{11}C-methyl-glucose uptake fractions of up to 30% (mean 22%, range 12–30%) as opposed to around 15% for normal brain (Brooks et al 1986a, Thomas et al 1987). In the contralateral hemisphere glucose influx and efflux are also significantly reduced. Brooks et al (1986) found only 2 out of 7 tumors studied had any increase in ^{11}C-albumin uptake and that, using this technique, the small to large vessel hematocrit ratio (normal 0.7) varied widely from 0.52 to 0.84 and did not correlate with rCBF in the tumor.

The normal brain is highly impermeable to potassium cations (thought to be controlled by ATPases in the endothelial membrane) and ^{82}Rb (which is chemically similar to potassium and has a half-life of 75 seconds) which is also, therefore, normally retained within the cerebral vasculature. It is possible, using a steady state method employing a continuous intravenous infusion of rubidium-82, to use PET to measure blood-brain barrier breakdown (Brooks et al 1984). rCBF and rCBV are measured concurrently, allowing the regional extraction of ^{82}Rb, corrected for the presence of intravascular ^{82}Rb, to be calculated. Using this method, the mean ^{82}Rb extraction in gliomas is 29% ± 13% as compared with 0.5–2% for the normal contralateral cerebral hemisphere. Such increased ^{82}Rb extraction appears to correlate well with CT contrast enhancement, and conversely non-enhancing tumors have ^{82}Rb extraction fractions consistently in the normal range. Interestingly, ^{82}Rb extraction may increase to up to 70% following external beam radiotherapy, although the permeability of normal brain appears to be unaffected. In addition a significant reduction in ^{82}Rb extraction has been found within 72 hours of high dose dexamethasone administration (Jarden et al 1985).

d. Other PET studies in human brain tumors

The labelling of therapeutic drugs to follow their quantitative distribution throughout the brain has formidable methodological problems (Maeda et al 1972, Baron et al 1982), but is being attempted. With respect to neuro-oncology, the kinetics of the cytotoxic BCNU used in the treatment of malignant brain tumors have been studied using PET (Yamamoto et al 1983) and show that initial tumor uptake of ^{11}C-BCNU parallels blood flow after intravenous administration. If mannitol is administered beforehand, increased tumor uptake occurs. However highest tumor concentrations are achieved by selective intra-arterial cannulation.

Amino acid metabolism is highly complex and, as a result, kinetic models of amino acid tracers used in PET are less satisfactory than those used, for example, for

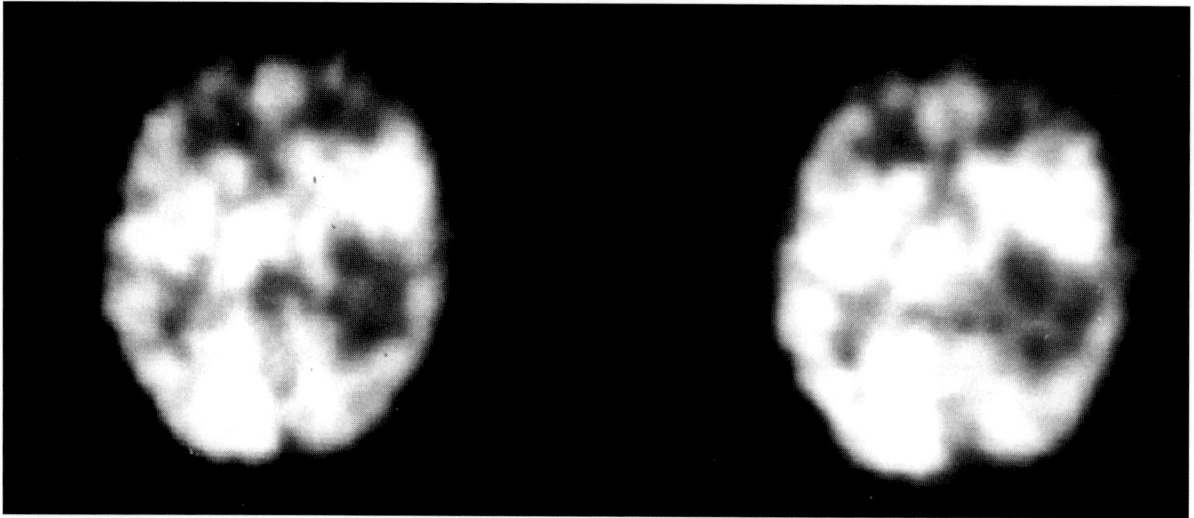

A

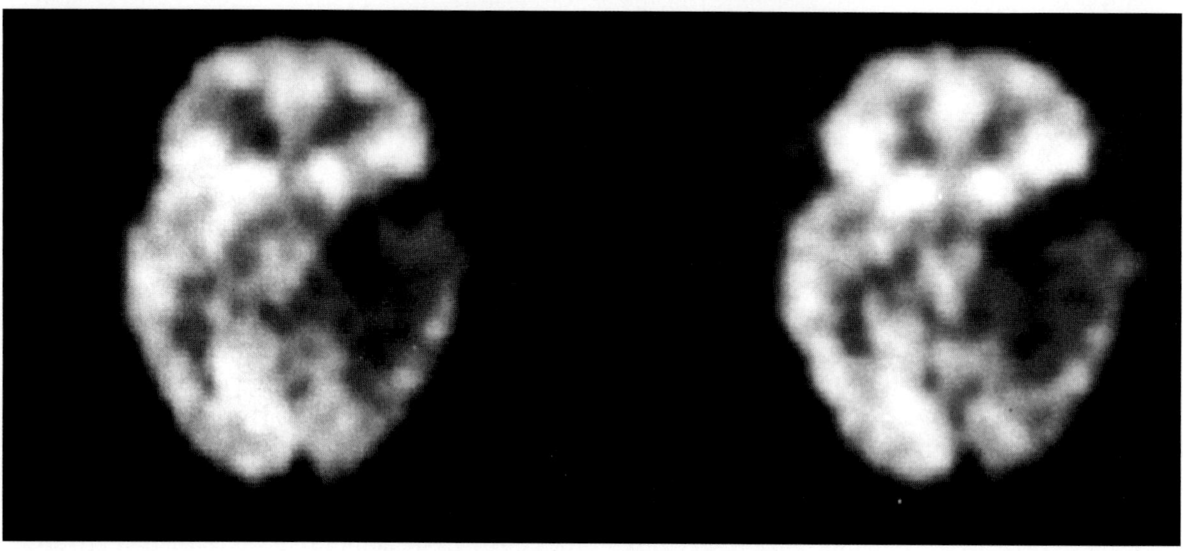

B

Fig. 13.3 ^{18}FDG PET scan. **A**, Pre- and **B**, post-interstitial brachytherapy treatment of a recurrent malignant astrocytoma. On the pre-treatment study there is an area of hypometabolism corresponding to an area of cystic tumor as seen on CT. Anteriorly there is increased uptake of ^{18}FDG by the solid portion of the tumor. It was this latter area that had been treated with brachytherapy using high dose iodine-125 seeds. Decreased uptake is seen in this area in the postoperative study which was performed six weeks following treatment. In addition there has been general improvement in the surrounding cortex and contralateral hemisphere metabolism. Courtesy of The Clinical PET Centre, St Thomas' Hospital, London, UK.

^{18}FDG. ^{11}C-methionine has been the most widely used amino acid tracer (Ericson et al 1985, O'Tuama et al 1990, Shishido et al 1990). The model used assumes that ^{11}C-methionine is either free or incorporated within protein, and that no amino acid metabolism occurs (Bustany et al 1981 & 1986). ^{11}C-Methionine PET has been used to determine the regional protein synthesis rate in brain tumors, for distinguishing tumor recurrence from radionecrosis, and as a highly sensitive means for diagnosing otherwise occult brain tumors (Bergstrom et al 1983). Thus, ^{18}FDG PET studies have been found to be most useful for prognosis in brain tumors. ^{11}C-methionine is perhaps better at determining the anatomic extent of the tumor and differentiating tumor from surrounding brain and from other brain disorders such as radiation changes (O'Tuama 1989). Methionine is a more sensitive flow marker, and has some blood-brain barrier related properties, although final methionine uptake and utilization is liable to be related to tumor cell number.

Other tracers which are currently being employed, and

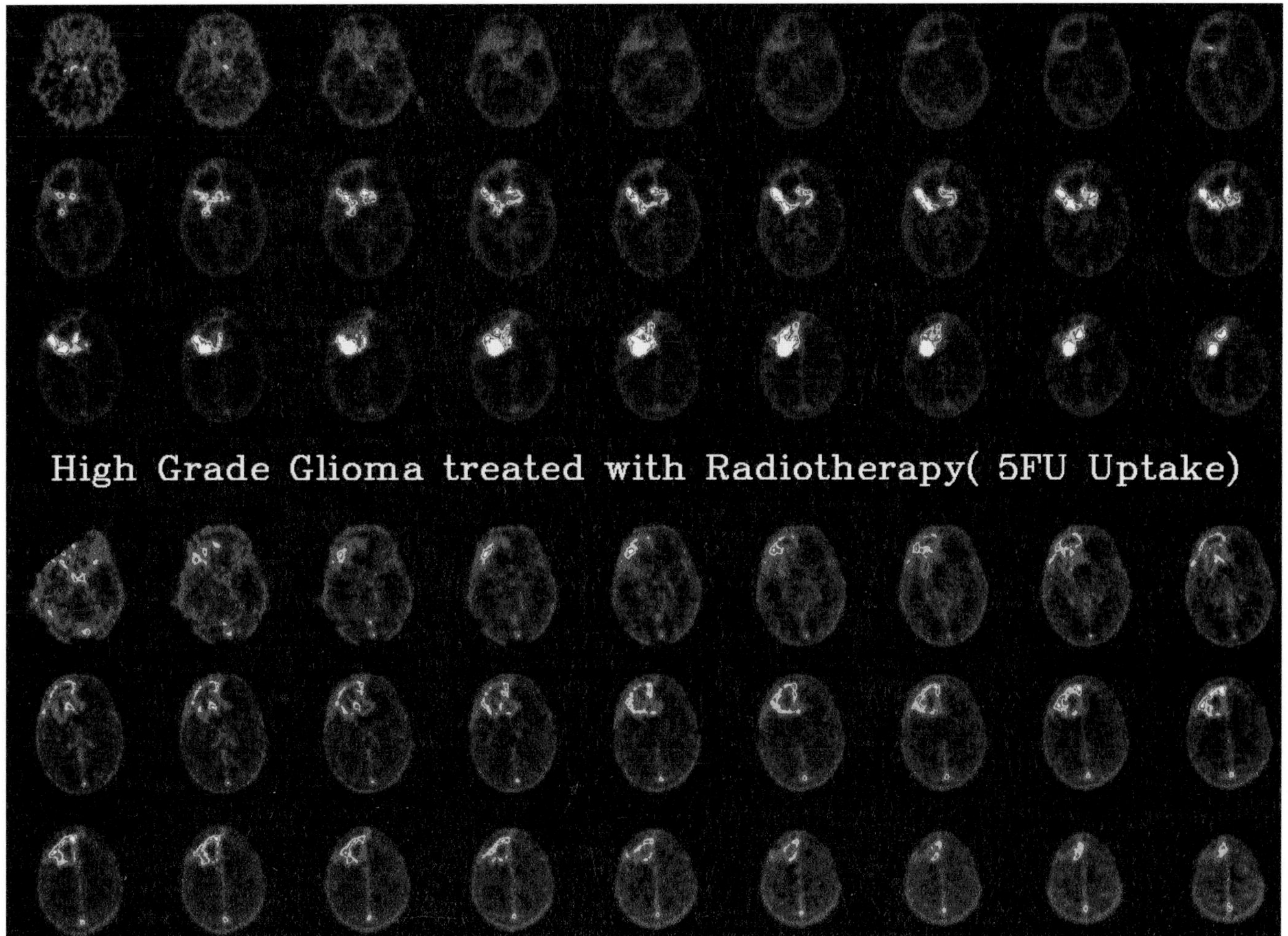

Fig. 13.4 5FU PET scan. Malignant oligodendroglioma. Pre- and post-radiotherapy. Studies taken after debulking surgery. There is residual tumor posteriorly which has responded to radiotherapy as shown by decreased uracil uptake. Courtesy of The MRC Cyclotron Unit, Hammersmith Hospital, London, UK.

their usefulness evaluated, include 5-fluorouracil (Figs 13.4, 13.5), thymidine, valine, leucine, tyrosine and tryptophan (Hubner et al 1982, Phelps et al 1982, Wienhard et al 1991). The tracers valine, tryptophan and uracil do concentrate in tumors, but this may be related as much to blood-brain barrier breakdown as to increased amino-acid metabolism. Conversely the leucine and methionine models rely on an intact blood-brain barrier.

SINGLE PHOTON EMISSION COMPUTED TOMOGRAPHY (SPECT — Fig. 13.6)

SPECT imaging has several distinct advantages over the more sophisticated PET studies in terms of cost, availability and simplicity. Though it is quite clearly a less powerful research tool, these features have ensured that SPECT imaging has become used widely in the clinical situation where the drawbacks of primitive quantitation techniques and slightly poorer resolution are not so obvious.

In SPECT imaging a radioisotope is administered to the patient, either by inhalation or by intravenous injection. It is then carried to the cerebral circulation where it crosses the blood-brain barrier into the brain. A rotating gamma camera and standard CT reconstruction algorithms are then used to detect and display the distribution of the tracer (Holman et al 1990) thus reflecting in some way patterns of rCBF, depending on the tracer used. Some machines employ planar views using a blood flow marker in order to locate the region of interest (Fig. 13.7A–C) which may then be focused on using finer slices and the desired tracer (Fig. 13.7D). The SPECT images produced resemble PET scans except that, in general, SPECT only images blood flow, and ligand quantitation and kinetic studies are not generally possible (although attempts are being made to develop and use labelled amino acid tracers suitable for SPECT — Biersack et al 1989, Langen et al 1991). Some form of semi-quantitative estimation of the image signal is, however, possible and

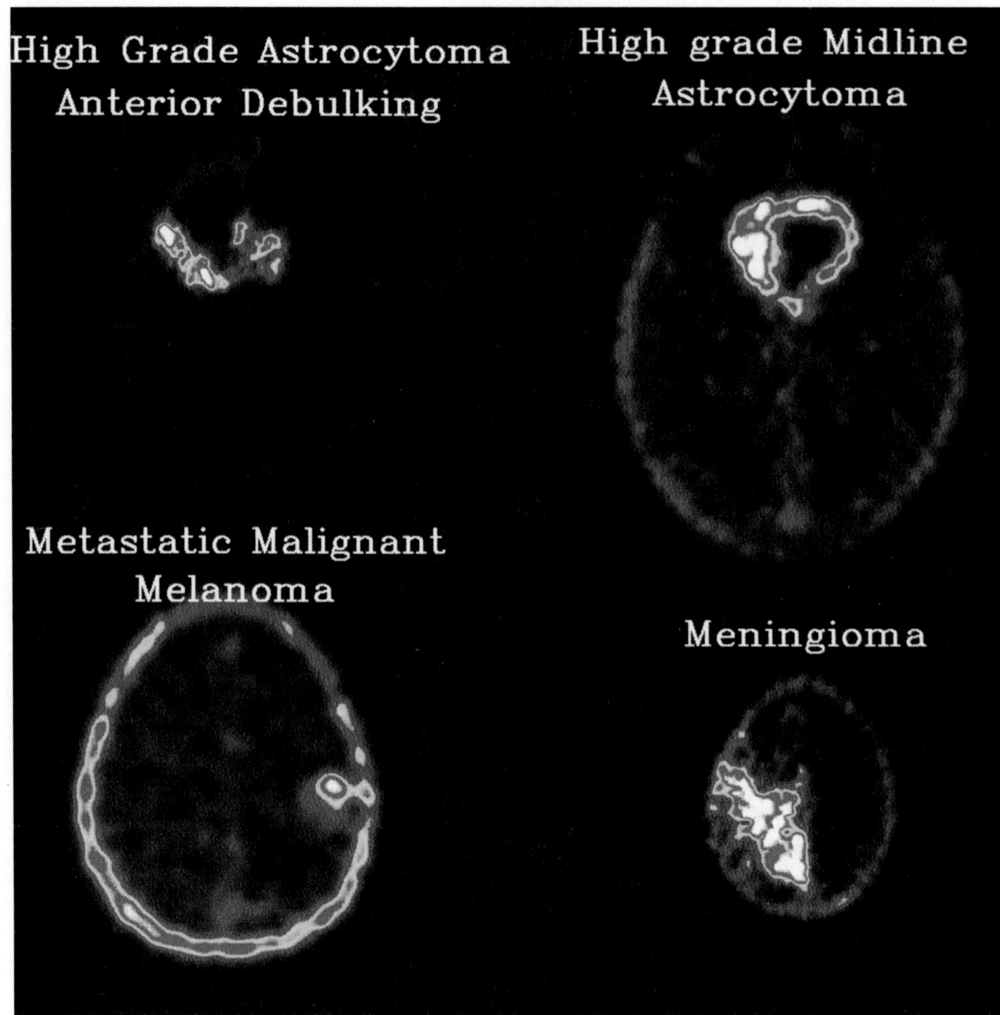

Fig. 13.5 5FU PET scans. Representative images from PET scans performed on patients with various intracranial tumors, demonstrating possible applications. Courtesy of The MRC Cyclotron Unit, Hammersmith Hospital, London, UK.

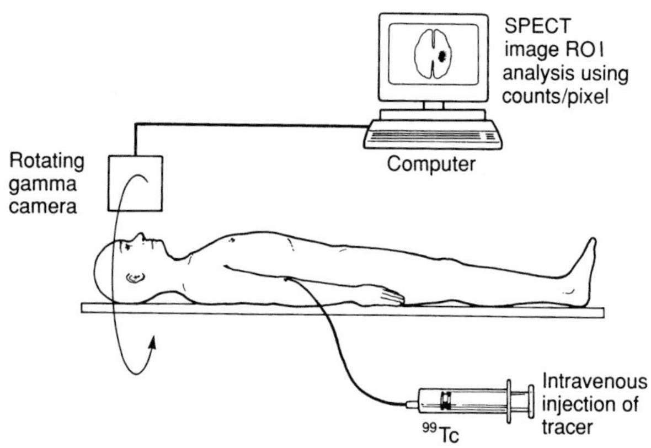

Fig. 13.6 The constituent parts of a SPECT investigation.

clinically useful information may be obtained. This is performed usually by measuring the counts per pixel of a defined region of interest (ROI) and comparing with a reference ROI, such as the contralateral cortex, scalp, cerebellum, or sometimes cardiac activity, though the latter is technically more difficult (Mountz et al 1988). In addition the spatial resolution of SPECT scans is less (in the region of 5–10 mm in modern scanners). With dynamic SPECT (D-SPECT) xenon-133 is inhaled by the subject during scanning and thus the image produced relates to the blood flow during the scan period (Devous et al 1985). Static SPECT uses a tracer which is injected and 'fixed' to the brain for a time after intravenous injection; the scan is done during this time and reflects rCBF at the time of the initial injection.

SPECT scanning uses the traditional radioisotopes utilized in nuclear medicine, namely technetium, gallium, thallium and iodine, which act primarily as blood flow

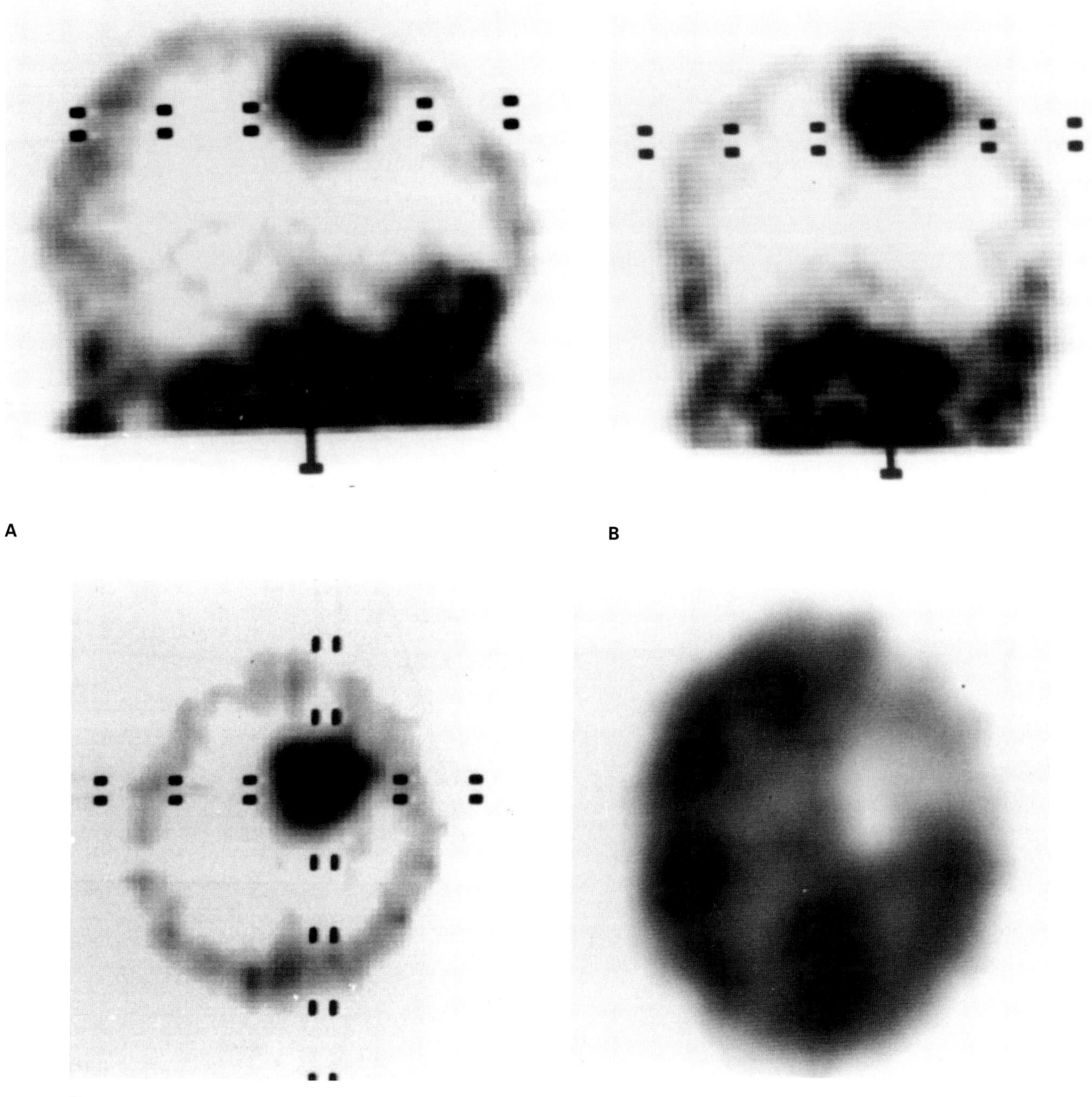

Fig. 13.7 Co-planar HMPAO SPECT images in the **A**, sagittal, **B**, coronal and **C**, axial plane. Orientation in all three planes allows the ROI to be defined before using the desired tracer such as IMP (**D**).

markers (Mut et al 1993). Thallium-201 is taken up as potassium and in this way acts as blood flow tracer (Fig. 13.8). However, once in the brain there is some further metabolism of the tracer involving transmembrane transport into viable tumor cells (Brismar et al 1989). Thallium is highly sensitive for detecting viable tumor (Kaplan et al 1987, Mountz et al 1989, Kim et al 1990), and has even been used to grade astrocytomas (Black et al 1989, Burkard et al 1992). However, the tracer lacks a high degree of specificity (Schwartz et al 1991) and modest increased uptake is seen in a wide range of conditions such as infections and necrosis, probably due to its blood flow tracer properties.

Two isotopes have been developed specifically for SPECT usage, namely ^{123}I iodoamphetamine (IMP) and ^{99}Tc hexamethyl-propylene-amine oxime (HMPAO). Both

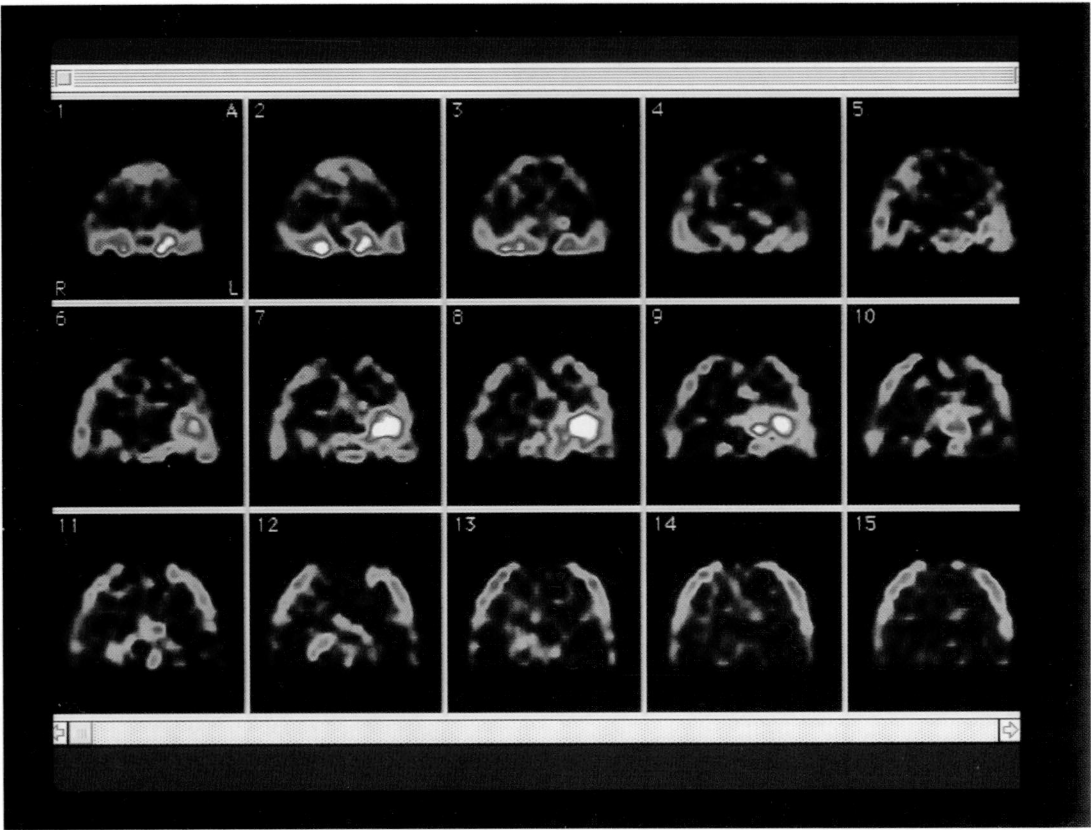

Fig. 13.8 Thallium SPECT study in a patient with a recurrent anaplastic astrocytoma in the left temporo-parietal region. In these late coronal views thallium has accumulated in the tumor, resulting in an increased signal. Courtesy of The Institute of Neurological Sciences, Glasgow, UK.

these substances pass through the blood-brain barrier and provide an image of cerebral perfusion. Once HMPAO, a highly lipophilic oxime, enters the brain its distribution remains fixed for up to six hours; it thus provides a good indicator of rCBF in brain tumors (Fig. 13.9) and has been the tracer most extensively used in this situation since its introduction in 1987 (Neirinckx et al 1987) and indeed positively correlates with rCBF as measured by simultaneous PET. Langen et al (1987) found a correlation coefficient of 0.95 in 10 cases of glioblastoma multiforme when comparing SPECT counts per pixel versus standard PET rCBF quantitation algorithms, though in this study there was a tendency for HMPAO uptake to be relatively higher in areas of low rCBF as measured by PET. HMPAO has been combined with thallium SPECT to enable identification of recurrent gliomas following radiotherapy (Carvalho et al 1991, 1992, Schwartz et al 1991, Zhang et al 1992). In contrast, IMP has not been proven to be especially clinically useful in this situation; once IMP crosses the blood-brain barrier it binds to various nonspecific amine receptors. Thus, although the early images are blood flow dependent, delayed images acquired after 2–3 hours represent metabolically active synapses. As there are relatively few such receptors in brain tumors they have no special affinity for IMP and do not demonstrate increased uptake regardless of tumor type and perfusion (Creutzig et al 1986, see Fig. 13.7D).

MAGNETIC RESONANCE SPECTROSCOPY (MRS — Fig. 13.10)

Magnetic resonance spectroscopy (MRS) is based on the concept that certain atomic nuclei have inherent spin properties. Examples include ^{1}H, ^{19}F, ^{31}P and ^{13}C. In the presence of a static magnetic field these nuclei acquire energy in discrete amounts. The introduction of electromagnetic radiation of the correct frequency, at right angles to the static magnetic field, causes the nuclei to jump to spin states of higher energy levels. The nuclei subsequently drop back to their ground spin states by emitting electromagnetic radiation at a rate determined by the T_1 (spin lattice) and T_2 relaxation times. The emitted radiation is detected by a receiver coil and the range of frequencies and their intensities comprise the MR spectrum.

MRS can be performed both in vitro and in vivo, each technique providing complementary information (Gill et al 1990). In vitro studies can be performed on protein

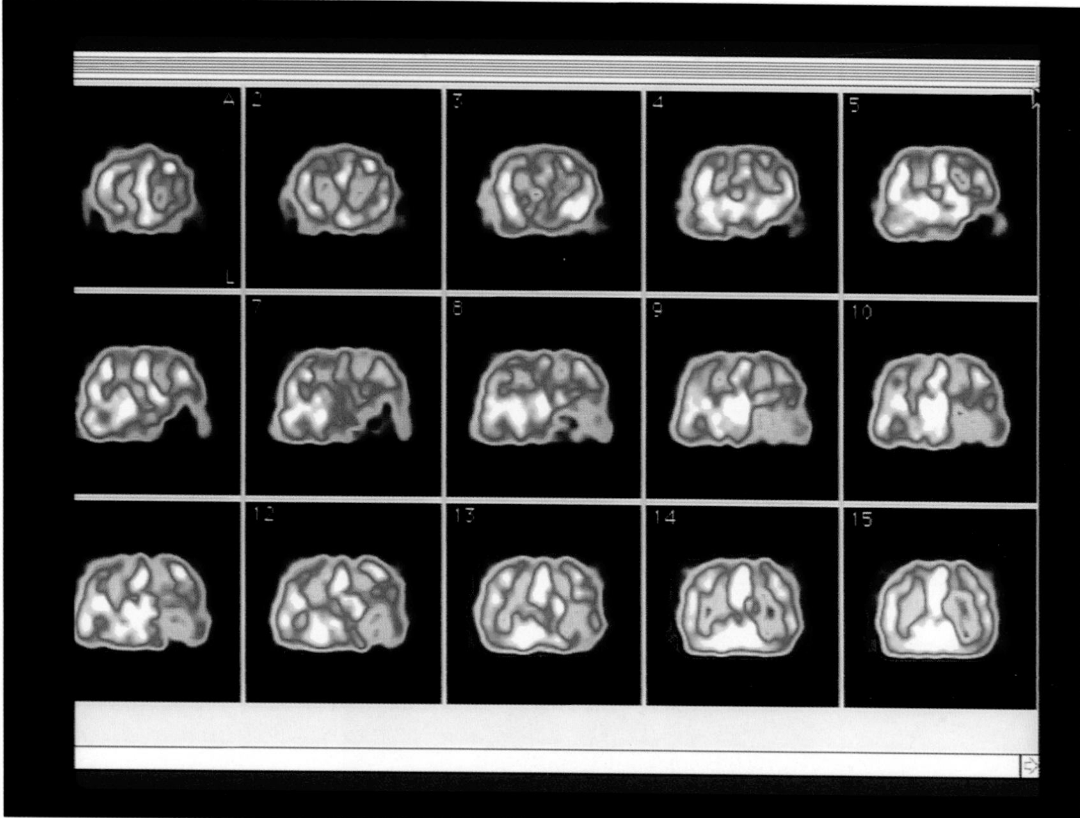

Fig. 13.9 HMPAO SPECT study in the same patient. Coronal series. There is decreased uptake in the region of the tumor. Courtesy of The Institute of Neurological Sciences, Glasgow, UK.

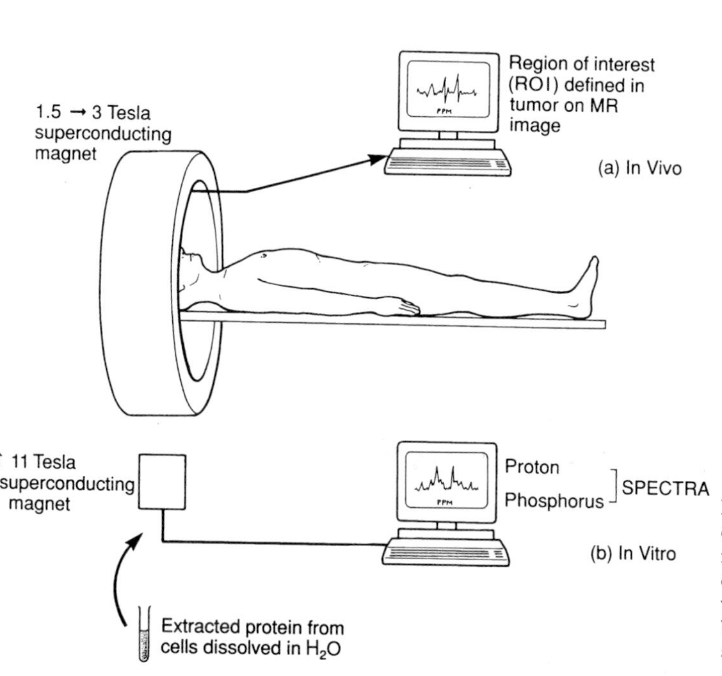

Fig. 13.10 The constituent parts of in vitro and in vivo MRS.

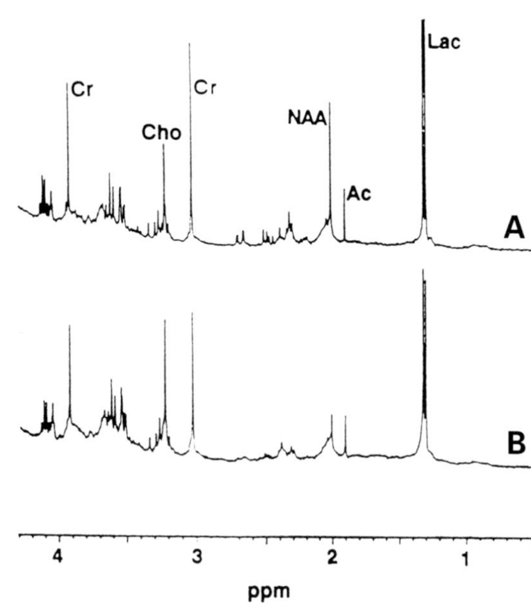

Fig. 13.11 In vitro ^{1}H MRS spectra obtained from perchloric acid extracts of 2 biopsy specimens from the same patient. **A**, Normal white matter; **B**, grade 3 astrocytoma. A great many metabolites are displayed. Lactate (Lac) is greatly elevated relative to the expected in vivo value because of the inevitable anerobic metabolism that occurs between the surgical removal and freezing. Spectrum (**B**) from within an area of tumor shows decreased NAA and increased choline levels. Acetate (Ac) has entered as an impurity during extraction and storage. Reprinted with permission from Gill et al 1990.

derived from tissue extracts of surgical specimens or from tumor cells cultured in vitro. These studies have the significant advantage that they have no time constraints and may be performed over several hours and using very high field magnets (up to 12 Tesla), thus yielding highly resolved spectra which are particularly useful for peak identification and absolute concentration measurements (Fig. 13.11). In contrast, in vivo MRS allows the non-invasive study of human spectra in the living patient. However, there are time and magnetic field strength limits which affect resolution. In addition the defined volume of interest (VOI) for study is relatively large (approximately 10 ml, in a near cubic shape, e.g. $20 \times 20 \times 25$ mm) and is usually defined before the gadolinium-enhanced imaging sequences (as gadolinium interferes with spectral analysis); also, in practice, it is difficult to exclude non-tumorous brain or necrotic tissue from the VOI (Fig. 13.12) and thus the spectra are prone to artefact. For these reasons

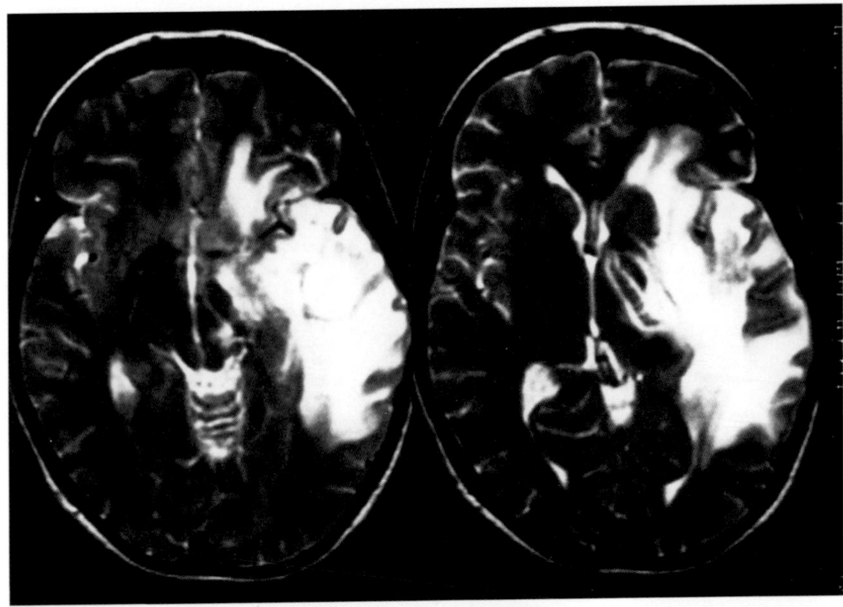
A

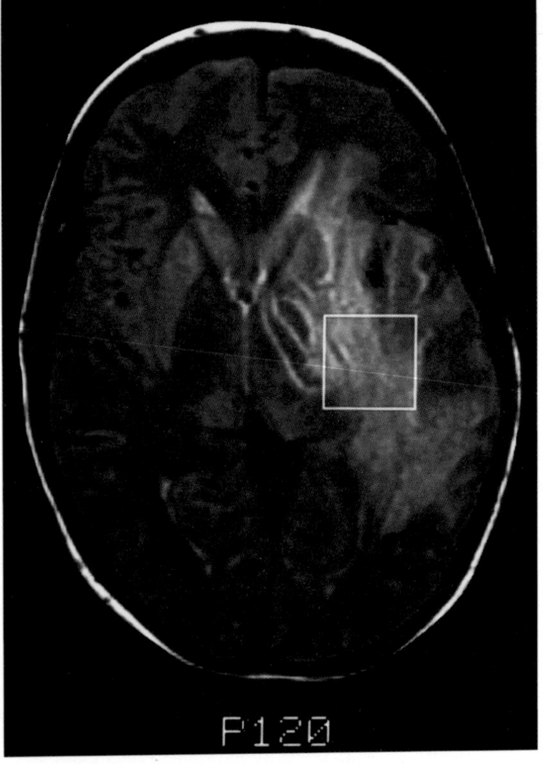

B

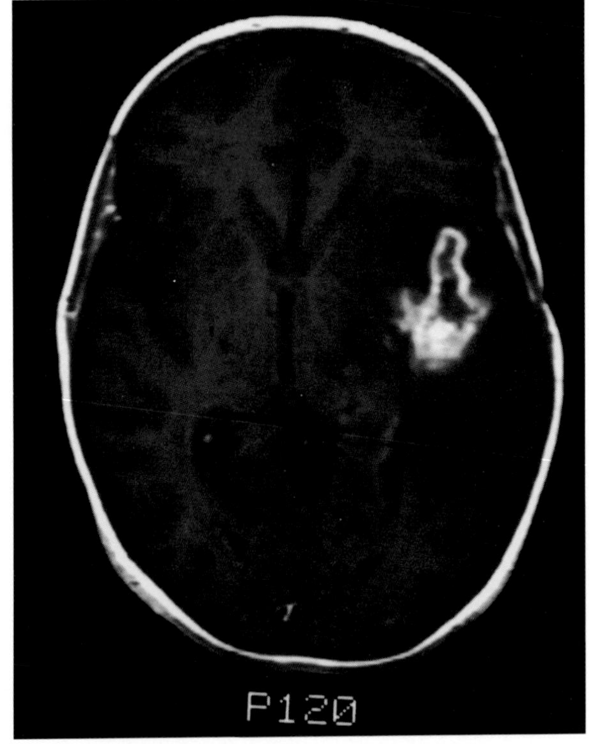

C

Fig. 13.12 In vivo MRS from a left temporal lobe glioma. Imaging sequences: **A**, T2, **B**, proton density with VOI defined for spectroscopy and **C**, post-gadolinium enhancement. The VOI does correlate precisely with the area of gadolinium enhancement and also contains some low signal areas compatible with edematous cortex. Courtesy of the NMR Research Group, Institute of Neurology, London, UK.

concentrations of metabolites are in practice measured relative to creatine and are not absolute. Thus, in vitro MRS provides detailed quantitative information about small areas of tumor whereas in vivo MRS gives more general information regarding the overall metabolism of the lesion. Newer techniques and increasing computer power are allowing the visual display of MRS imaging 'maps', where metabolite levels are shown simultaneously throughout the cerebrum, in a manner similar to the display methods employed in PET (Fulham et al 1992).

^{31}P MRS is the most widely used spectroscopic method in biological studies. Phosphorus has a pK of 6.8 and is therefore an excellent pH probe. Furthermore, phosphorus metabolism is vital to the energy status of the cell and ^{31}P is found in ATP, phosphocreatine and inorganic phosphorus in concentrations high enough for MRS investigation. ^{31}P MR spectroscopy has been used, to a limited extent, to study brain tumors in vivo, and has shown that in the majority of tumor cases the phosphocreatine:ATP ratio was lower than that of normal brain tissue (Oberhaensli et al 1986). The significance of this finding is uncertain, although it is likely to be a result of the altered glycolysis favored by such tumors being less able to generate phosphocreatine than normal tissue. ^{31}P MR spectroscopy has also been used to study the pH of tumors and has agreed with PET studies, demonstrating a tendency for these tumors to be slightly more alkaline than normal brain tissue.

Proton magnetic resonance spectroscopy (^{1}H MRS) permits the in vivo detection of lactate and other metabolites like N-acetyl aspartate (NAA), choline and phosphocreatine in human brain tumors (Bruhn et al 1989, Segebarth et al 1990, Demaerel et al 1991, Fulham et al 1992). ^{1}H is ubiquitous and is the sensitive stable nucleus. However, for useful MRS, a high field magnet (over 4 Tesla) is required for good resolution as the chemical shift is poor. In addition the intense H_2O signal requires selective saturation to prevent swamping of the signals from the metabolites of interest. Suppression of the fat and protein signals is also essential to study small molecules. In ^{1}H MRS of gliomas typical spectral findings are increased choline levels (indicating increased membrane turnover), increased lactate levels (indicating increased anerobic metabolism either in tumor cells or possibly leukocytes; the lactate peak is characteristically a 'doublet'), and markedly decreased NAA, as the neuronal population is replaced with proliferating glial cells. These features are displayed in Figure 13.13. Both the NAA:Cr and the choline:Cr ratios appear to correlate with the histologic grade of astrocytomas, at least to a certain extent (Gill et al 1990), though this is not an invariable finding as extensive necrosis (found in the higher grade tumors) within the VOI decreases choline levels.

Herholz et al (1992c) have analyzed the relationships between MRS-demonstrated lactate concentrations and PET-demonstrated ^{18}FDG uptake levels in 20 patients with histologically proven gliomas. The maximum ^{18}FDG uptake levels (indicating maximum metabolic rates of glucose) were significantly correlated with maximum lactate concentrations. However, spatial analysis revealed that the maximum lactate levels within tumors were not found in the same location as the maximum glucose metabolism, but rather tended to accumulate in areas of necrosis and tumor cysts. Such combined studies give important information regarding the spatial relationship between the two ends of abnormal glucose metabolism found within these tumors. However, further research is required to determine whether ^{1}H MRS markers of non-oxidative glycolysis can have the same prognostic importance as PET studies utilizing ^{18}FDG. The elevated lactate levels that are frequently observed in gliomas could prove useful in assessing treatment response, by the use of serial studies. Furthermore, the important relationship between intratumoral lactate levels and pH requires further research (Paschem et al 1987). Combined proton and phosphorus MRS may offer a means of achieving this.

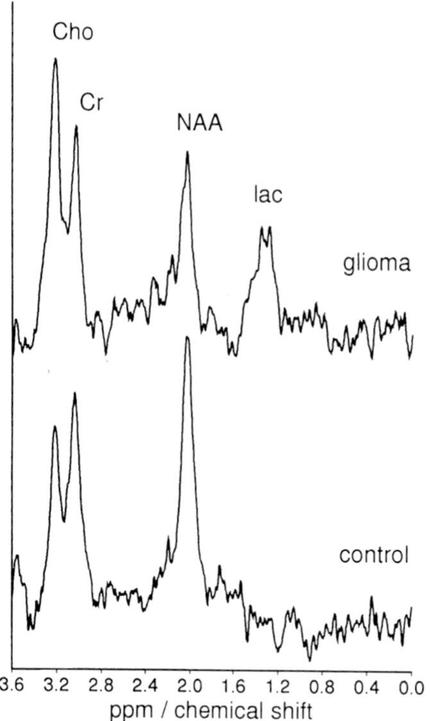

Fig. 13.13 ^{1}H MRS from the same patient as Fig. 13.12. Spectra obtained using sequence of TE 270 ms and TR 3 s. As compared to the age-matched control there is decreased NAA and increased lac and choline levels. The NAA levels are not as low as is sometimes seen in these tumors, probably due to the presence of non-tumorous tissue within the VOI. Cho = choline-containing compounds, Cr = creatine/phosphocreatine; NAA = N-acetylaspartate; lac = lactate. Courtesy of the NMR Research Group, Institute of Neurology, London, UK.

CLINICAL RELEVANCE OF FUNCTIONAL IMAGING IN THE MANAGEMENT OF BRAIN TUMORS

Post-radiotherapy brain swelling and radiation necrosis can have identical appearances to those of recurrent tumor on CT and MRI. In this situation the final diagnosis is often only made on histologic examination after surgical resection of the mass lesion. Functional imaging provides an alternative approach to this problem. ^{11}C-methionine and rubidium-82/^{18}FDG together have been applied diagnostically in this clinical situation (Doyle et al 1987). Rubidium-82, which is a potassium analog, and closely follows blood-brain barrier breakdown (vide supra) is used to identify the locality of the lesion, whilst ^{18}FDG determines the metabolic state of the lesion. Combining ^{82}Rb with ^{18}FDG PET is said to improve the specificity, in that by outlining the blood-brain barrier, the lesion boundaries may be defined and this information combined with glucose utilization as demonstrated by ^{18}FDG uptake.

The techniques of PET and stereotaxis have been combined in some instances with the aim of providing maximal information regarding the site of the stereotactic biopsy and to ensure that representative samples are taken (Von Holst et al 1988, Levivier et al 1992). Both FDG and methionine have been used in this situation. In addition PET has been combined with serial stereotactic biopsy techniques and multimodal image registration in research settings in order to find out more about the tumor edge and tumor infiltration as defined by the various neuroradiologic techniques (MR, CT, PET) and by histopathologic methods (Mosskin et al 1987, Thomas et al 1990). There are limits, however, with using PET in this situation due to the poor spatial resolution.

CONCLUSIONS

The functional imaging techniques described above — PET, SPECT and MRS — are complementary methods for the in vivo investigation of human brain tumor biology. PET remains unsurpassed as a quantitative research tool. However, there are some basic scientific problems with several of the kinetic models used in brain tumor work and it will be important to perform correlative studies with magnetic resonance spectroscopy and with other biochemical methods to validate the methods employed in PET. Both PET (which requires an on-site cyclotron to generate those tracers with short half-lives) and MRS (which requires a high field magnet facility) rely on expensive equipment, are personnel intensive and are highly complex methods best suited to research units in specialized centers. It remains at present the case that, although they provide unique information about human brain tumor biology in vivo, their role in routine patient management is limited.

REFERENCES

Baron J C, Roeda D, Munari C et al 1982 Brain regional pharmacokinetics of C-11-diphenylhydantoin: positron emission tomography in man. In: Raynaud (ed) 3rd World Congress of Nuclear Medicine and Biology, vol 2. Pergamon Press, Oxford, pp 1748–1751

Beaney R P, Brooks D J, Leenders K L et al 1985 Blood flow and oxygen utilisation in the contralateral cerebral cortex of patients with untreated intracranial tumours as studied by positron emission tomography with observations on the effect of decompressive surgery. Journal of Neurology, Neurosurgery and Psychiatry 48: 310–319

Bergstrom M, Collins P, Ehrin E et al 1983 Discrepancies in brain tumour extent as shown by computerised tomography and positron emission tomography using ^{68}Ga-EDTA, ^{11}C-glucose and ^{11}C-methionine. Journal of Computer Assisted Tomography 7: 1062–1066

Biersack H J, Coenen H H, Stocklin G et al 1989 Imaging of brain tumours with L-3-[^{123}I]-iodo-alpha-methyl-tyrosine and SPECT. Journal of Nuclear Medicine 30: 110–112

Black K L, Hawkins R A, Kim K T et al 1989 Use of thallium-201 SPECT to quantitate malignancy grade in gliomas. Journal of Neurosurgery 71: 342–346

Brismar T, Collins V P, Kesselberg M 1989 Thallium-201 uptake relates to membrane potential and potassium permeability in human glioma cells. Brain Research 500: 30–36

Brooks D J, Beaney R P, Lammertsma A A et al 1984 Quantitative measurement of the blood brain barrier permeability using ^{82}Rb and positron emission tomography. Journal of Cerebral Blood Flow and Metabolism 4: 535–545

Brooks D J, Beaney R P, Lammertsma A A et al 1986a Glucose transport across the blood-brain barrier in normal human subjects and patients with cerebral tumours studied using {^{11}C}3-0-Methyl-D-Glucose and positron emission tomography. Journal of Computer Assisted Tomography 6: 230–239

Brooks D J, Beaney R P, Lammertsma A A et al 1986b Studies on regional cerebral haematocrit and blood flow in patients with cerebral tumors using positron emission tomography. Microvascular Research 31: 267–276

Bruhn H, Frahm J, Gyngell M L et al 1989 Noninvasive differentiation of tumours with use of localised H-1 MR spectroscopy in vivo: initial experience in patients with cerebral tumors. Radiology 172: 541–548

Burger P C, Heinz E R, Shibata T et al 1988 Topographic anatomy and CT correlations in the untreated glioblastoma multiforme. Journal of Neurosurgery 68: 698–704

Burkard R, Kaiser K P, Wieler H et al 1992 Contribution of thallium-201 SPECT to the grading of tumorous alterations of the brain. Neurosurgical Review 15: 265–273

Bustany P, Sargent T, Saudubray J M et al 1981 Regional human brain uptake and protein incorporation of ^{11}C-L-Methionine studied in vivo with PET. Journal of Cerebral Blood Flow and Metabolism 1(suppl 1): 17–18

Bustany P, Chatel M, Derlon J M et al 1986 Brain tumour protein synthesis and histological grades: a study by positron emission tomography with C-11-L-methionine. Journal of Neuro-oncology 3: 397–404

Cairncross J G, Pexman J H W, Rathbone M P 1985 Post-surgical contrast enhancement mimicking residual brain tumour. Canadian Journal of Neurological Science 12: 75

Carvalho P A, Schwartz R B, Alexander E III et al 1991 Extracranial metastatic glioblastoma: appearance on thallium-201-chloride/technetium-99m-HMPAO SPECT images. Journal of Nuclear Medicine 32: 322–324

Carvalho P A, Schwartz R B, Alexander E III et al 1992 Detection of recurrent gliomas with quantitative thallium-201/technetium-99m HMPAO single-photon emission computerized tomography. Journal of Neurosurgery 77: 565–570

Creutzig H, Schobom O, Gilow P et al 1986 Cerebral dynamics of N-isopropye-123-I-(para-amphetamine). Journal of Nuclear Medicine 27: 178–183

Demaerel P, Johannik K, van Hecke P et al 1991 Localised ^{1}H NMR spectroscopy in fifty cases of newly diagnosed intracranial tumours. Journal of Computer Assisted Tomography 15: 67–76

Devous M D, Stokely E M, Bonte F J 1985 Quantitative imaging of regional cerebral blood flow by dynamic single photon tomography. In: Holman B L (ed) Radionuclide imaging of the brain. Churchill Livingstone, New York

DiChiro G 1986 Positron emission tomography using {^{18}F} fluorodeoxyglucose on brain tumors. A powerful diagnostic and prognostic tool. Investigations in Radiology 22: 360–371

DiChiro G, Brooks R A 1988 PET quantitation: blessing and curse. Journal of Nuclear Medicine 29: 1603–1604

DiChiro G, De La Paz R L, Brooks R A et al 1982 Glucose utilization of cerebral gliomas measured by ^{18}F Fluorodeoxyglucose and positron emission tomography. Neurology 32: 1323–1329

DiChiro G, Hatazawa J, Katz D A et al 1987 Glucose utilization by intracranial meningiomas as an index of tumor aggressivity and probability of recurrence: a PET study. Radiology 164: 521–526

Doyle W K, Budinger T F, Valk P E et al 1987 Differentiation of cerebral radiation necrosis from tumor recurrence by [^{18}F]FDG and ^{82}Rb positron emission tomography. Journal of Computer Assisted Tomography 11: 563–570

Elster A D, DiPersio D A 1990 Cranial postoperative site: assessment with contrast-enhanced MR imaging. Radiology 174: 93–98

Ericson K, Lilja A, Bergstrom M et al 1985 Positron Emission Tomography with ({11C}methyl)-L-methionine, {11C}D-glucose, and {68Ga}EDTA in supratentorial tumors. Journal of Computer Assisted Tomography 9: 683–689

Fulham M J, Bizzi A, Dietz M J et al 1992 Mapping of brain tumour metabolites with proton MR spectroscopic imaging: clinical relevance. Radiology 185: 675–686

Gill S S, Thomas D G T, Van Bruggen N et al 1990 Proton MR spectroscopy of intracranial tumours: in vivo and in vitro studies. Journal of Computer Assisted Tomography 497–504

Gjedde A, Wienhard K, Heiss W D et al 1985 Comparative regional analysis of 2-fluorodeoxyglucose and methylglucose uptake in brain of four stroke patients. With special reference to the regional estimation of the lumped constant. Journal of Cerebral Blood Flow and Metabolism 5: 163–178

Glantz M J, Hoffman J M, Coleman E et al 1991 Identification of early recurrence of primary central nervous system tumours by {^{18}F}fluorodeoxyglucose positron emission tomography. Annals of Neurology 29: 347–355

Groothius D R, Vriesendorp F J, Kupfer B et al 1991 Quantitative measurements of capillary transport in human brain tumours by computed tomography. Annals of Neurology 30: 581–588

Herholz K, Rudolf J, Heiss W D 1992a FDG transport and phosphorylation in human gliomas measured with dynamic PET. Journal of Neuro-oncology 12: 159–165

Herholz K, Friedrichs B, Jeske J et al 1992b Prognostic significance of positron emission tomography with F-18-fluorodeoxyglucose in gliomas. Journal of Cancer Research and Clinical Oncology 118: 119

Herholz K, Heindel W, Luyten P R et al 1992c In vivo imaging of glucose consumption and lactate concentration in human gliomas. Annals of Neurology 31: 319–327

Holman B L, Carvalho P A, Zimmerman R E et al 1990 Brain perfusion SPECT using an annular single crystal camera: initial clinical experience. Journal of Nuclear Medicine 31: 1456–1461

Hubner K F, Purvis J T, Mahaley S M et al 1982 Brain tumor imaging by positron emission computed tomography using ^{11}C-labelled amino-acids. Journal of Computer Assisted Tomography 6: 544–550

Ito M, Lammertsma A A, Wise R J S et al 1982 Measurement of regional cerebral blood flow and oxygen utilisation in patients with cerebral tumors using ^{15}O and positron emission tomography: analytical techniques and preliminary results. Neuroradiology 23: 63–74

Jarden J O, Dhawan V, Poltorak A et al 1985 Positron emission tomographic measurement of blood-to-brain and blood-to-tumour transport of ^{82}Rb: the effect of dexamethasone and whole-brain radiation therapy. Annals of Neurology 18: 636–646

Kaplan W D, Takvorian T, Morris J H et al 1987 Thallium-201 brain tumour imaging: a comparative study with pathologic correlation. Journal of Nuclear Medicine 28: 47–52

Kelly P J, Daumas-Duport C, Scheithauer B W et al 1987 Stereotactic histologic correlations of CT and MRI-defined abnormalities in patients with glial neoplasms. Mayo Clinic Proceedings 62: 450–459

Kim K T, Black K L, Marciano D et al 1990 Thallium-201 SPECT imaging of brain tumours: methods and results. Journal of Nuclear Medicine 31: 965–969

Langen K J, Hergoz H, Rota E et al 1987 Tomographic studies of rCBF with ^{99}Tc-HMPAO SPECT in comparison with PET in patients with primary brain tumours. Neurosurgical Review 10: 23–24

Langen K J, Roose N, Coenen H H et al 1991 Brain and brain tumor uptake of L-3-[^{123}I] iodo-alpha-methyl-tyrosine: Competition with L-amino-acids. Journal of Nuclear Medicine 32: 1225–1228

Levivier M, Goldman S, Bidaut L M et al 1992 Positron Emission Tomography-guided stereotactic brain biopsy. Neurosurgery 31: 792–797

Maeda T, Kono A, Kojima M 1972 Tumor scanning with ^{57}Co-bleomycin. Radioisotopes (Tokyo) 21: 436–438

Mazziotta J C 1991 The continuing challenge of primary brain tumour management: The contribution of positron emission tomography. Annals of Neurology 29: 345–346

Mosskin M, von Holst H, Bergstrom M et al 1987 Positron emission tomography with 11C-methionine and computed tomography of intracranial tumors compared with histopathologic examination of multiple biopsies. Acta Radiol 28: 673–681

Mountz J M, Stafford-Schuck K, McKeever P E et al 1988 Thallium-201 tumor/cardiac ratio estimation of residual astrocytoma. Journal of Neurosurgery 68: 705–709

Mountz J M, Raymond P A, McKeever P E et al 1989 Specific localization of thallium 201 in human high-grade astrocytoma by microautoradiography. Cancer Research 49: 4053–4056

Mut F, Bianco A, Nunez M et al 1993 Tc-99m isonitrile uptake in a brain metastatic lesion — comparison with Tc-99m DTPA using planar and SPECT imaging. Clinical Nuclear Medicine 18: 143–146

Neirinckx R D, Canning L R, Piper I M et al 1987 Technetium-99m d, 1-HMPAO: a new radiopharmaceutical for SPECT imaging of regional cerebral blood flow perfusion. Journal of Nuclear Medicine 28: 191–202

Oberhaensli R D, Hilton-Jones D, Bore P J et al 1986 Biochemical investigation of human tumours in-vivo with phosphorus-31 magnetic resonance spectroscopy. Lancet ii: 8–11

Ogawa T, Uemura K, Shishido F et al 1988 Changes in cerebral blood flow, oxygen and glucose metabolism following radiochemotherapy of gliomas: a PET study. Journal of Computer Assisted Tomography 12: 290–297

O'Tuama L A 1989 Methionine transport in brain tumors. J Neuropsych Clin Neurosc 1: s37–s44

O'Tuama L A, Phillips P C, Strauss L C et al 1990 Two-phase {11 C}L-methionine PET scanning in diagnosis of childhood brain tumors. Pediatric Neurology 6: 163–170

Paschem W, Djuricic B, Mies G et al 1987 Lactate and pH in the brain: association and dissociation in different pathophysiological states. Journal of Neurochemistry 48: 154–159

Patronas N J, Di Chiro G, Kufta C et al 1985 Prediction of survival in glioma patients by means of positron emission tomography. Journal of Neurosurgery 62: 816–822

Phelps M E, Hoffman E J, Mullani N A 1975 Application of annihilation coincidence detection by transaxial reconstruction tomography. Journal of Nuclear Medicine 16: 210–223

Phelps M E, Mazziotta J C, Huang S C 1982 Study of cerebral function with positron computed tomography. Journal of Cerebral Blood Flow and Metabolism 2: 113–162

Rhodes C G, Wise R J S, Gibbs J M et al 1983 In vivo disturbance of the oxidative metabolism of glucose in human cerebral gliomas. Annals of Neurology 14: 614–626

Schwartz R B, Carvalho P A, Alexander E III et al 1991 Radiation necrosis vs high-grade recurrent glioma: differentiation by using dual-isotope SPECT with ^{201}Tl and ^{99}mTc-HMPAO. AJNR 12: 1187–1192

Segebarth C M, Baleriaux D F, Luyten P R et al 1990 Detection of metabolic heterogeneity in human intracranial tumours in vivo by ^{1}H NMR spectroscopic imaging. Magnetic Resonance Medicine 13: 62–76

Shishido F, Uemura K, Inugami A et al 1990 Value of 11 C-methionine and PET in the diagnosis of low grade gliomas. Kaku Igaku 27: 293–302

Thomas D G T, Brooks D J, Yoshino E et al 1987 Brain tumours and their metabolism. Neurosurgeons 6: 121–127

Thomas D G T, Gill S S, Wilson C B et al 1990 Use of a relocatable frame to integrate positron emission tomography and computed tomography images: application to human malignant brain tumours. Stereotactic Functional Neurosurgery 54 + 55: 388–392

Von Holst H, Ericson K, Bergstrom M et al 1988 Stereotactic positron emission tomography imaging for tumor diagnosis. In: Lunsford D (ed) Modern stereotactic neurosurgery. Martinus Nijhoff, Boston, pp 195–205

Warburg O 1930 The metabolism of tumors. Constable, London

Wienhard K, Herholz K, Coenen H H et al 1991 Increased amino acid transport into brain tumors measured by PET of l-(2-^{18}F)fluorotyrosine. Journal of Nuclear Medicine 32: 1338–1346

Yamamoto Y L, Thompson C J, Meyer E et al 1977 Dynamic positron emission tomography for the study of cerebral hemodynamics in cross section of the head using positron emitting ^{68}Ga-EDTA and ^{77}K. Journal of Computer Assisted Tomography 1: 43–56

Yamamoto Y L, Diksio M, Sako K 1983 Pharmacokinetic and metabolic studies in human malignant glioma. In: Magistratti P L (ed) Functional radionuclide imaging of the brain. Raven Press, New York, pp 327–335

Yen C K, Yano Y, Budinger T F et al 1982 Brain tumour evaluation using Rb-82 and positron emission tomography. Journal of Nuclear Medicine 23: 532–537

Zhang J J, Park C H, Kim S M et al 1992 Dual isotope SPECT in the evaluation of recurrent brain tumour. Clinical Nuclear Medicine 17: 663–664

14. Anesthesia and intensive care management of patients with brain tumors

Roy F. Cucchiara Susan Black Joseph Stachniak A. Joseph Layon

In neurosurgery, the anesthesiologist has a definite impact on making the surgical procedure possible, safe, and even easier. Communication between anesthesiologist and neurosurgeon is essential. This communication must be based on known facts tempered with experience to provide patient safety, the best operating conditions, and high quality anesthesia care. The anesthesiologist must be knowledgeable about the physiology, pathology, and pharmacology of the brain to effectively apply clinical principles in the operating room.

EFFECTS OF ANESTHETIC AGENTS ON CEREBRAL BLOOD FLOW AND CEREBRAL METABOLIC RATE FOR OXYGEN

Inhalation agents

The volatile anesthetic agents are direct cerebral vasodilators that cause an increase in cerebral blood flow (CBF) (Theye & Michenfelder 1968a, Cucchiara et al 1974, Michenfelder & Cucchiara 1974, Newberg et al 1983, Sakabe et al 1983, Todd & Drummond 1984, Eintrei et al 1985, Drummond et al 1986) and also depress cerebral metabolism, decreasing cerebral metabolic rate for oxygen ($CMRO_2$) and glucose (Cucchiara et al 1974, Michenfelder & Cucchiara 1974, Stullken et al 1977, Newberg et al 1983, Sakabe et al 1983, Todd & Drummond 1984). As a result, they are said to 'uncouple' the relationship between CBF and metabolism (Fig. 14.1). A number of studies in both animal models and man have indicated that halothane is the most potent cerebral vasodilator and isoflurane is the least potent cerebral vasodilator of the three commonly used volatile anesthetic drugs (Theye & Michenfelder 1968a, Michenfelder & Cucchiara 1974, Newberg et al 1983, Boarini et al 1984, Todd & Drummond 1984, Eintrei et al 1985, Drummond et al 1986). Enflurane in higher concentrations (1.5 mean alveolar concentration [MAC]) and in combination with hypocapnia has been documented to cause seizure activity that results in a marked increase in both CBF and $CMRO_2$ (Michenfelder & Cucchiara 1974).

Increases in CBF due to volatile anesthetic-induced decreases in cerebrovascular resistance (CVR) lead to increases in cerebral blood volume (CBV) with resultant increases in intracranial pressure (ICP) (Artru 1983). This effect is potentially deleterious in neurosurgical patients with altered intracranial elastance. Halothane-induced increases in CBF and resultant increase in ICP seen in some neurosurgical patients can be prevented by hyperventilation of the lungs prior to the addition of halothane to the inspired gas mixture. However, simultaneous institution of hyperventilation with administration of halothane will not blunt the increases in CBF and ICP caused by halothane (Adams et al 1972). In contrast, increases in CBF and ICP caused by isoflurane in neurosurgical patients are effectively blocked by simultaneous institution of hyperventilation (Adams et al 1981). The combination of isoflurane anesthesia and marked hyperventilation ($PaCO_2$ 20–25 mmHg) has been demonstrated to cause a decrease in CBF (Scheller et al 1986). This decrease in CBF, even during isoflurane-induced hypo-

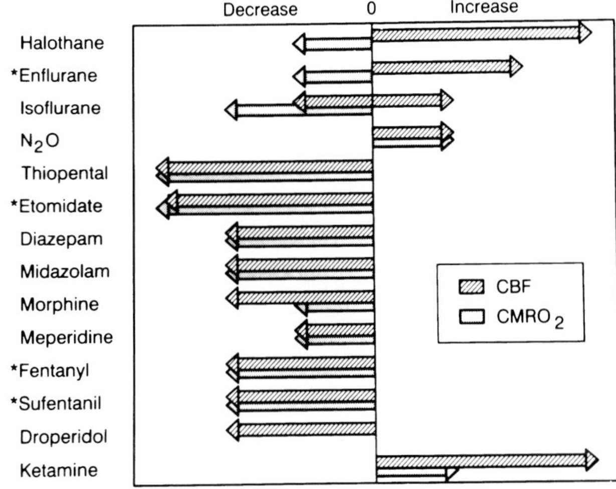

Fig. 14.1 The effects of anesthetic agents on cerebral blood flow and cerebral metabolism. *Agents which have been shown to produce spike activity of EEG.

tension, did not result in adverse effects on the cerebral metabolic balance (Artru 1986).

Volatile anesthetics cause a dose-dependent decrease in $CMRO_2$. This response is nonlinear at concentrations below 1.0 MAC, with the greatest decrease in $CMRO_2$ occurring at the anesthetic concentrations causing a change in the EEG pattern from awake to anesthetized (Stullken et al 1977). The degree of depression of cerebral metabolism varies among halothane, enflurane, and isoflurane. Both enflurane and halothane result in decreases in $CMRO_2$ of 16–30% (Theye & Michenfelder 1968a, Michenfelder & Cucchiara 1974, Sakabe et al 1983); however, with enflurane-induced seizure activity, $CMRO_2$ increases by 48% (Michenfelder & Cucchiara 1974). Isoflurane causes the greatest decrease in $CMRO_2$. In clinically relevant concentrations, 2.0 MAC, isoflurane results in complete suppression of cerebral electrical activity and a decrease of $CMRO_2$ to approximately 50% of control values. This property of isoflurane is unique among the currently available volatile agents (Cucchiara et al 1974, Michenfelder & Theye 1975, Newberg et al 1983, Todd & Drummond 1984).

It has been suggested that the net effect on CBF of a volatile anesthetic agent is a combination of the direct cerebral vasodilation to increase CBF and the indirect decrease in CBF 'coupled' to the decrease in $CMRO_2$. Isoflurane causes the greatest degree of depression of cerebral metabolism opposing the direct vasodilator properties with a net result of little to no change in CBF. In animal studies with maximal depression of cerebral electrical activity by barbiturates prior to the administration of isoflurane and halothane, both agents resulted in equal increases in CBF and decreases in cerebral vascular resistance (Drummond et al 1986). This supports the concept that isoflurane has as potent a direct vasodilator activity as halothane, and that the markedly different effects on CBF in most clinical situations are due to the more potent depressant effect on cerebral metabolism of isoflurane. Caution should be exercised in administering isoflurane to patients whose cerebral metabolism is depressed either by other drugs, such as barbiturates, or by pathologic conditions causing decreases in cerebral function and metabolism, as these patients may exhibit a greater than expected increase in CBF with administration of isoflurane.

The effect of nitrous oxide (N_2O) on cerebral metabolism and blood flow is the subject of much controversy and conflicting reports. In several well-controlled studies using a rat model, N_2O was consistently found to have only minimal effects on both CBF and $CMRO_2$. In these studies, either no effect or clinically insignificant decreases in CBF or $CMRO_2$ were found (Carlsson et al 1976b, Dahlgren et al 1981). In other studies using several different animal models, including dogs, goats, and cats, and in humans, however, N_2O was found to result in small increases in $CMRO_2$ (11–21%) and significant (35–103%) increases in CBF (Theye & Michenfelder 1968b, Phirman & Shapiro 1977, Sakabe et al 1978, Oshita et al 1979, Manohar & Parks 1984, Pelligrino et al 1984). One factor contributing to these conflicting results is the inability to deliver N_2O in concentrations equal to or above 1 MAC. The varying results could be due to the effects of either sympathetic stimulation under light anesthesia or the effects of the different drugs administered to supplement the N_2O anesthesia in different models. Even while taking these factors into consideration and attempting to control for them, however, a species difference between rats and other animal models persists. In rats, N_2O has minimal effects on cerebral metabolism or blood flow, but, in the other animal models, N_2O causes mild increases in $CMRO_2$ and significant increases in CBF. Considering these results, in man, it is likely that N_2O causes significant cerebral vasodilation; however, these effects are easily modulated by other factors, including hyperventilation of the lungs (Adams et al 1972, Adams et al 1981) and vasoconstrictive drugs, such as thiopental, diazepam, and morphine (Phirman & Shapiro 1977, Jobes et al 1977).

Intravenous drugs

Most intravenous drugs cause some degree of cerebral vasoconstriction, decrease in CBF, and a depression of $CMRO_2$, and do not 'uncouple' the relationship of blood flow to metabolism (Fig. 14.1). Thiopental and other barbiturates result in a dose-dependent decrease in CBF and $CMRO_2$, with a maximal decrease in $CMRO_2$ of 50–55% and in CBF of 40–60%. This occurs at a dose adequate to completely suppress cerebral function and results in electrical silence (Cucchiara & Michenfelder 1973, Michenfelder 1974, Kassell et al 1981). Further doses of thiopental beyond that causing an isoelectric EEG result in no further decreases in $CMRO_2$ or CBF (Michenfelder 1974). This suggests that the decrease in $CMRO_2$ requirements by thiopental is due to a decrease in cerebral function. Like the barbiturates, etomidate causes a dose-dependent decrease in CBF or $CMRO_2$, which is maximal at doses sufficient to cause electrical silence. Further increases in etomidate dose cause no further decreases in CBF or $CMRO_2$. $CMRO_2$ decreases by 45–52%, and CBF by 34–77% (Renou et al 1978, Milde et al 1985). Cases of etomidate-induced seizures have been reported, suggesting a potential for increased $CMRO_2$ and CBF in those patients. The benzodiazepines, diazepam and midazolam, both cause dose-dependent decreases in $CMRO_2$ and CBF. The effects of propofol on cerebral hemodynamics are similar to those of other intravenous induction agents. It causes a decrease in CBF and CMR and an increase in CVR to a similar degree as thiopental (Sebel & Lowdon 1989). The decreases in CBF and $CMRO_2$ with diazepam are reported to be 15–40% and 16–40%, respectively (Maekawa et al 1974, Carlsson et al 1976a), and, for midazolam, 33–45% and 45–55%, maintaining a favorable CBF to $CMRO_2$ ratio (Forster et al 1982, Forster et al 1983, Hoffman et al 1986). Opioids increase cerebrovascular resistance and decrease CBF and $CMRO_2$. Intravenous morphine causes a decrease in CBF of 27–55% and a decrease in $CMRO_2$ of 15–30% (Renou et al 1978, Matsumiya & Dohi 1983). Meperidine (2 mg/kg^{-1}) decreases CBF by only 10% and $CMRO_2$ by 13% (Messick & Theye 1969). Fentanyl at high doses decreases CBF by 40–50% and $CMRO_2$ by 18–40% (Michenfelder & Theye 1971, Carlsson et al 1981, Carlsson et al 1982). Sufentanil results in similar decreases in CBF (53%) and $CMRO_2$ (53%) (Keykhah et al 1985). Very high doses of both fentanyl and sufentanil have been demonstrated to result in seizure activity and increases in $CMRO_2$ in animal models (Carlsson et al 1981, Keykhah et al 1985). It is likely that, in clinical doses, opioids cause relatively little decrease in CBF. Droperidol causes a decrease in CBF of 40% and no significant change in $CMRO_2$ (Michenfelder & Theye 1971). Ketamine differs from the other intravenous agents in that it results in an increase in CBF and $CMRO_2$. Ketamine increases CBF by 62–80% with lesser increases in $CMRO_2$ (0–16%) (Dawson et al 1971, Takeshita et al 1972, Hougaard et al 1974).

The osmotic diuretic, mannitol, which is used relatively frequently in neurosurgical patients, results in an early transient increase in CBF during and immediately following mannitol infusion, with CBF returning to control values by 10 min following completion of the infusion in experimental animals (Johnston & Harper 1973).

ELECTROPHYSIOLOGIC NEUROLOGIC TECHNIQUES

Evoked potentials

Intraoperative monitoring of sensory evoked potentials (SEP) allows for continuous assessment of neural pathways at a time when these pathways are at risk of damage during operations on the spine and spinal cord, brainstem, and posterior fossa structures (Raudzens 1982, Grundy 1983). An understanding of the origin of these potentials and the effects of anesthesia and operation is crucial to effective monitoring. It is a goal of monitoring SEP that alterations detected intraoperatively will reliably predict possible embarrassment of neural structures. Effective monitoring implies that equipment utilized is sensitive enough to record such changes, that trained observers can detect alterations in the potentials, and that therapeutic manipulations may subsequently alter outcome if changes are detected. Current experience with SEP monitoring indicates good reliability in predicting and preventing adverse postoperative outcome in most cases, but concerns over the sensitivity of isolated pathways predicting global dysfunction still exist.

Nature of evoked potentials

SEP represent pathways elicited by stimulation of sensory structures. Monitoring of SEP requires computer signal averaging of sensory stimulus-induced events that can be separated from the background EEG. The waves of the evoked potential are plotted as a voltage versus time response, and are felt to represent potentials from specific neural generators. The evoked potential is described in terms of the type of eliciting sensory stimulus (somatosensory, auditory, visual), post-stimulus latency, wave amplitude, and distance separating the neural generators and recording electrodes.

SEP can also be described in terms of monitoring location. For example, the generated somatosensory evoked potential (SSEP) can be monitored with surface electrodes at the level of the peripheral nerve, spinal cord, and cerebral cortex. In addition, the SSEP can be monitored via direct recording from the spine or epidural space. Knowledge of timing of specific events at the spinal and cortical level allows calculation of impulse conduction time through central neuronal pathways.

Types of sensory evoked potentials

SSEP are generated via electrical stimulation of peripheral nerves, usually the median nerve at the wrist or the posterior tibial nerve at the ankle. Repetitive stimuli are required to allow for computer summation of the evoked potential, which represents a sensory impulse in response to the peripheral stimulation. As described previously, the potentials can be monitored at various levels from peripheral nerve to cortical levels, and probably represent a sensory pathway that ascends from peripheral nerve to dorsal spinal columns to thalamus and cortex. A typical scalp-recorded SSEP is shown in Figure 14.2. The early cortical components are typically monitored intraoperatively. These components are sensitive to anesthetics, especially the inhaled drugs, but can still be effectively monitored. The later cortical components are very sensitive to anesthetics and more difficult to monitor.

Brainstem auditory evoked responses (BAER) are elicited via repetitive auditory click stimulation, which is achieved through headphones or ear inserts. The sensory pathway elicited represents transmission through the peripheral eighth cranial nerve through pathways into the brainstem at the level of the medulla, with subsequent relay to the pons, midbrain, and then to the cortex via thalamic pathways. The elicited potential is generally recorded over the scalp, but can be recorded intraoperatively directly from the eighth cranial nerve (Møller &

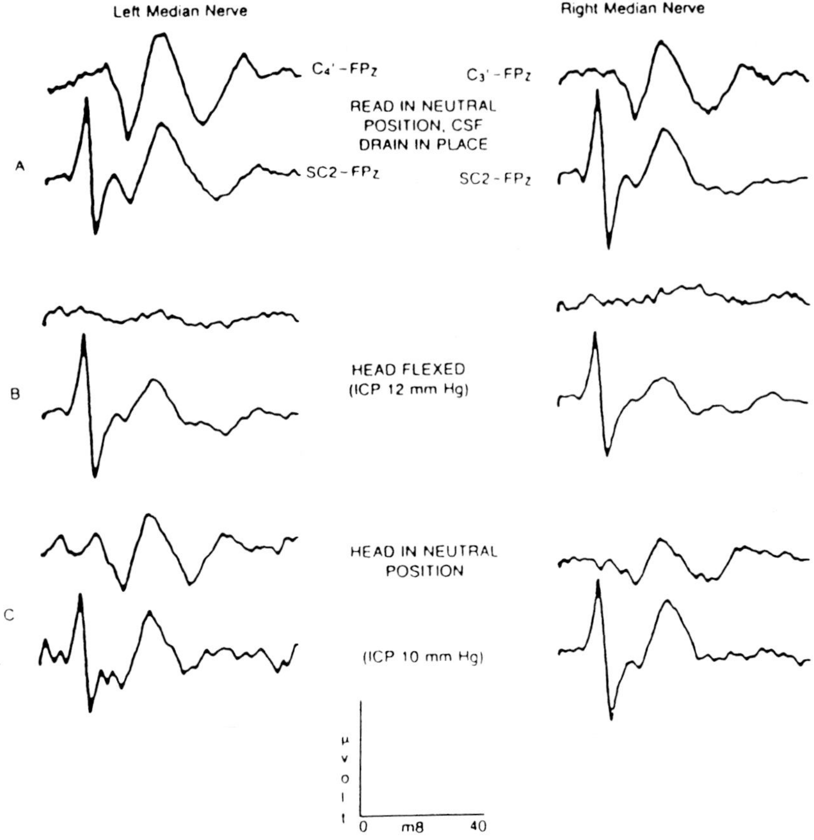

Fig. 14.2 Dramatic change in somatosensory evoked potentials at the scalp, and not at the neck, with head flexion (B), returning to normal as head position is returned to neutral (C). Note that intracranial pressure (ICP) is essentially unchanged. Reproduced with permission from McPherson R W et al 1984.

Jannetta 1983). The brainstem auditory evoked response is generally considered relatively insensitive to anesthetics, and can be monitored effectively during different anesthetic techniques. The visual evoked potential (VEP) is more difficult to monitor intraoperatively because of its likelihood to be lost as a result of much greater sensitivity to anesthetic effects. The VEP is typically stimulated intraoperatively via flashes emitted by light-emitting diodes in eye goggles. Monitoring is at the cortical level, and the potentials are felt to represent transmission via optic pathways. These potentials have not found widespread intraoperative application due to sensitivity to anesthetics and overall difficulty in obtaining satisfactory intraoperative monitoring.

Effects of anesthetic agents

Anesthetic agents may produce alterations of evoked potential waveform latency and amplitude. In general, the sensitivity to waveform changes induced by anesthetic agents in decreasing order of sensitivity is VEP, SSEP, with BAER being the most insensitive. Studies on specific agents show that, with respect to the SSEP, induction doses of thiopental, fentanyl, and etomidate preserved monitoring of SSEP. Thiopental (4 mg/kg^{-1}) and fentanyl (25 $\mu g/kg^{-1}$) produced minor increases in latency and decreases in amplitude of the early cortical components, while 0.4 mg/kg^{-1} of etomidate produced slight increases in latency but dramatic increase in amplitude of the early cortical components (McPherson et al 1986). High dose thiopental has been noted to increase latency and decrease amplitude of the early cortical peaks of the median nerve SSEP, but still preserve ability to monitor, while the BAER showed some increased latency of early peaks with good preservation of monitoring ability (Drummond et al 1985). Etomidate has been shown to have minimal effects on the early peaks of the BAER (Thornton et al 1985). Fentanyl and morphine have been shown, in addition, to have minimal effects on early components of BAER (Samra et al 1984, Samra et al 1985), while producing dose-related latency increases with variable amplitude effects in the SSEP (Pathak et al 1984).

With respect to the BAER, clinically applicable concentrations of the inhaled drugs halothane, enflurane, and isoflurane increased brainstem wave latencies, but preserved wave morphology, thus allowing for continued monitoring ability (Dubois et al 1982, Thornton et al 1983, Thornton et al 1984, Manninen et al 1985). The SSEP demonstrates greater sensitivity to volatile drugs, with significant dose-related alterations in the recorded potentials. For example, increasing dose of isoflurane during isoflurane anesthesia to 2% end-tidal has been shown to produce significant decreases in the amplitude and latency increases of early cortical components (Samra et al 1987), while satisfactory traces could be obtained in all patients at end-tidal concentrations of 0.5% and 1%, with 1.5% being variable. The ability to obtain satisfactory monitoring waveforms after median nerve stimulation has been shown to be greater with halothane than with isoflurane or enflurane (Peterson et al 1986). This study suggested that successful recording could be maintained with 60% N_2O plus 1.0 MAC halothane or 0.5 MAC isoflurane or enflurane. A quantitative difference was found in a study of halothane, enflurane, and isoflurane effects on SSEP generated by posterior tibial nerve stimulation (Pathak et al 1987). These authors found that clinically useful monitoring could be maintained at levels up to 0.75 MAC plus 60% N_2O with all drugs, and at 1.0 MAC plus 60% N_2O with enflurane and isoflurane. It is important, however, to consider the effects of N_2O alone. N_2O has been shown to produce significant decreases in amplitude with minimal latency change in the cortical SSEP (Sebel et al 1984, McPherson et al 1985a, Sloan & Koht 1985). The VEP is also sensitive to the effects of N_2O and isoflurane with latency and amplitude changes (Sebel et al 1984, Chi & Field 1986).

Intraoperative uses of evoked potentials

Monitoring of SEP has been utilized widely with hopes of preventing intraoperative neurologic impairment (Grundy 1982). Typical applications include monitoring of SSEP during spinal surgery (Grundy et al 1982b) and monitoring of BAER during operations in the cerebellopontine angle (Grundy et al 1982a). BAER have been utilized in cerebral posterior circulation vascular surgery as an indicator of brainstem injury (Little et al 1983, Lam et al 1985). SSEP have been monitored during intracranial aneurysm surgery (Grundy et al 1982d, McPherson et al 1983, Carter et al 1984, Symon et al 1984). SSEP monitoring has been compared to EEG during carotid endarterectomy (Moorthy et al 1982, Markand et al 1984, Russ et al 1985, Lam et al 1991, Kearse et al 1992) and to assess potential spinal cord ischemia during aortic operations (Takaki & Okumura 1985, Kaplan et al 1986). VEP have been monitored during operations in the anterior visual pathways (Costa E Silva et al 1985).

Anesthetic management for operations in which evoked potentials are to be monitored should seek to obtain a steady state, so that waveform changes detected are presumed to reflect operative events. In addition, when monitoring SSEP during spinal surgery, consideration must be given to the possibility of performing a 'wake-up test' for intraoperative assessment of motor function (Vauzelle et al 1973). With these factors in mind, thiopental induction with N_2O and opioid infusion for anesthetic maintenance has been suggested for scoliosis surgery (Pathak et al 1983). A technique utilizing volatile agents for maintenance would be appropriate if consideration is given to the fact that higher level of inhalation agents may greatly alter the SSEP waveform. Since the BAER is more resistant to anesthetic effects, a variety of anesthetic agents may be utilized with this technique, but it is still essential to strive for steady-state conditions. Other factors can alter SEP, such as hypotension, hypoxia (Grundy et al 1981), and hypothermia (Stockard et al 1978, Van Rheineck et al 1986), and must be considered if alterations in the SEP waveform occur. Alteration of cortical SEP has also been noted with accumulation of intracranial gas during operations in the sitting position (McPherson et al 1985b, Schubert et al 1986).

Reliability of evoked potentials

As stated previously, evoked potential monitoring seeks to monitor neural pathways at risk and predict and prevent neural dysfunction. Monitoring of BAER in cerebellopontine angle tumor patients has been shown to play a role in hearing preservation (Jannetta et al 1984), but some authors feel that intraoperative BAER are routinely too sensitive, and that changes in operative conditions should be based only on gross changes of the BAER waveform (Friedman et al 1985).

SEP monitoring has found wide application, especially to help preserve function during operations on the spinal cord. In general, reliability has been good, with changes in SSEP predicting postoperative events (Grundy et al 1982c), but concern exists because the SSEP monitors dorsal column function, and not motor function, directly. In fact, postoperative neurologic deficits have occurred despite preserved intraoperative SSEP (Ginsburg et al 1985, Lesser et al 1986). In order to monitor motor function more specifically, evoked potentials obtained via direct motor tract stimulation are being investigated (Levy 1983, Levy 1987).

Intraoperative electromyography

Electromyography (EMG) is a technique widely utilized in the diagnosis of neuromuscular disorders (Buchthal 1985). EMG recording electrodes measure motor unit potentials, which originate from the summated action potentials of the fibers of the motor unit. Adaptation of this monitoring technology, for intraoperative use to monitor and prevent potential nerve injury, is currently being accomplished (Harner et al 1986).

The widest application of intraoperative EMG has been monitoring and preservation of facial nerve function during acoustic neurinoma (vestibular schwannoma) resection (Prass & Luders 1986, Harner et al 1987). The technique of intraoperative EMG for facial nerve preservation involves preoperative placement of indwelling fine wire electrodes into the facial muscles (orbicularis oculi, orbicularis oris, mentalis, frontalis), which is verified by pre-anesthetic recording to verify location, followed by intraoperative recording to determine potential facial nerve damage during tumor resection. Spontaneous muscle action potentials are recorded continuously intraoperatively, and neurotonic discharges that indicate nerve irritation are a signal that surgical maneuvers are affecting the facial nerve. These maneuvers may then be altered to reduce potential nerve damage. In addition, to help localize the facial nerve during the resection, compound muscle action potentials may be recorded from the fine wire electrodes in response to direct electrical stimulation of the facial nerve by the surgeon via a hand-held stimulating electrode. These processes of measuring spontaneous EMG and elicited muscle action potentials are effective in preserving facial nerve function, especially with larger acoustic neurinomas. The use of intraoperative EMG is currently being expanded to provide monitoring of cranial nerve function during surgery in proximity to the brainstem, and for monitoring during spinal surgery.

Anesthetic management of patients who are to undergo intraoperative EMG must be tailored to allow its effective assessment. A major consideration is to avoid further use of muscle relaxants after the initial doses of relaxants necessary for endotracheal intubation. Because of this necessity, anesthesia techniques are chosen that will accomplish immobility as part of the technique. Anesthetic induction is generally accomplished with intravenous administration of thiopental and an intermediate-acting non-depolarizing muscle relaxant, the effects of which will have dissipated prior to the time of intraoperative EMG recording of facial nerve function. No further muscle relaxants are administered. Anesthetic maintenance utilizing a combination of potent inhaled drug and N_2O with small supplemental doses of an intravenous opioid is generally utilized. The patient with an acoustic neurinoma or other cerebellopontine angle tumor can thus provide considerable anesthetic challenge. Anesthetic management must be tailored to allow for effective electrophysiologic monitoring that will involve measurement of brainstem auditory evoked potentials and EMG, and must provide immobility without the use of muscle relaxants at a time when the surgeon is dissecting delicate structures under the operating microscope.

ANESTHETIC MANAGEMENT OF THE TUMOR PATIENT

Supratentorial tumors

Choice of anesthetic agent

The factors in selection of the anesthetic drug are multiple. In neuroanesthesia, the effects of the agent on ICP, cerebral perfusion pressure (CPP), CBF, $CMRO_2$, and promptness of return to consciousness are major considerations. Secondary considerations include drug-related protection from ischemia or edema, blood pressure control, and compatibility with neurophysiologic monitoring techniques.

All of the volatile anesthetics can cause an increase in ICP at deeper levels of anesthesia and normocarbia. These circumstances are rarely used in neoplastic neurosurgery. Moderate hypocarbia with less than 1.0 MAC volatile agent represents the most common application of this anesthetic technique. In cerebrovascular surgery, light volatile anesthesia avoids blood pressure depression, and mild hypocarbia is a reasonable choice to avoid excessive cerebral vasoconstriction.

Halothane produces the greatest reduction in cerebral vascular resistance and the clearest increase in ICP. This can be blunted or even eliminated if hyperventilation of the lungs is established before beginning halothane administration (Adams et al 1972). Isoflurane produces a reduction in cerebral vascular resistance and an elevation of ICP at normocarbia. This response can be blocked by hyperventilation in tumor patients (Adams et al 1981). Other work suggests that patients with a midline shift on CT scan are more likely to show an elevation of ICP during isoflurane anesthesia (Grosslight et al 1985). On balance, human studies suggest that isoflurane is a safe anesthetic drug when used for intracranial tumor surgery (Madsen et al 1987).

Intravenous drugs (e.g. thiopental, fentanyl) are useful in neuroanesthesia because they decrease CBF and $CMRO_2$ together. This allows a reduction in ICP to be accomplished by modification of the vascular compartment without producing cerebral ischemia. Thiopental safely produces a profound linked reduction of CBF and $CMRO_2$ to near half of awake values (Cucchiara & Michenfelder 1973). This is reflected in the dramatic reduction of ICP that can be achieved by utilizing thiopental with this goal in mind. For decades, thiopental has seen waxing and waning of enthusiasm for its use as a constant infusion in combination with N_2O to provide desirable operating conditions for neurosurgical neoplastic cases. The effectiveness of thiopental as a cerebral protective drug should probably be viewed as applicable to the experimental conditions at which that protection is most solidly demonstrated, i.e. cerebral ischemia by vascular occlusion techniques. Cerebral protection by barbiturates in brain tumor patients produced by lowering ICP is a distinctly different, although useful, concept.

In patients with increased ICP propofol has been shown to decrease ICP. This is expected based on its ability to decrease CBF. However, propofol can cause significant decreases in systemic blood pressure. In patients with a tenuous hemodynamic status or severely elevated ICP, this may lead to untoward decreases in CPP (Sebel & Lowdon 1989). Propofol has a unique potential advantage over other available agents for patients with large mass lesions. Volatile anesthetic agents have the potential to increase CBF and ICP, but are compatible with prompt awakening postoperatively. The barbiturates and etomidate, which decrease CBF and ICP, when used as a continuous infusion for a prolonged period will result in delayed awakening postoperatively. Propofol, on the other hand, decreases CBF and ICP. Following termination of prolonged propofol infusions, prompt emergence on completion of the operative procedure is possible. These features may prove to be valuable in certain patients with large intracranial mass lesions.

Fentanyl decreases CBF slightly more than it decreases $CMRO_2$ (Michenfelder & Theye 1971). Theoretically, this imbalance could predispose to cerebral ischemia, but such a consideration does not seem to be clinically important. The usefulness of fentanyl in neurosurgical anesthesia is based on its ability to lower ICP through decreased CBF, and on its control of heart rate and blood pressure during surgical stimulus.

Most craniotomy surgery in the United States today is probably performed following a thiopental induction of anesthesia with intubation of the trachea after a non-depolarizing relaxant, and maintenance with N_2O/isoflurane/fentanyl in various combinations during hypocarbia to $PaCO_2$ levels of 28–33 mmHg.

Choice of muscle relaxants

Muscle relaxant use can probably affect the conduct of a neuroanesthetic as much as the primary agent. Succinylcholine as yet appears unequaled in achieving total rapid paralysis for the rapid sequence intubation of the trachea. There is still controversy regarding succinylcholine-induced increases in ICP (Marsh et al 1980, Minton et al 1985a); however, such increases are probably clinically insignificant except, perhaps, in the most extreme cases of intracranial hypertension. Since complete flaccidity is required to avoid coughing and straining during intubation of the trachea and thus avoid ICP increases, it is reasonable to use a nerve stimulator during induction and intubation in these cases. The shorter acting non-depolarizing relaxants (vecuronium, atracurium) are well suited for intubation paralysis in cases of elevated ICP. They do not increase ICP, and have little or no effect on heart rate and blood pressure (Minton et al 1985b, Unni et al 1986).

Hemiplegia from cerebral ischemia or from cerebral tumor is associated with differences in response to non-depolarizing muscle relaxants on the two sides of the body. The affected extremities are resistant to neuromuscular blockade by non-depolarizing relaxants (Brown & Charlton 1975, Graham 1980). In most operating room arrangements, the face and endotracheal tube are turned toward the anesthetist so that the operative field is uppermost. This places the extremities contralateral to the tumor in a position that allows easy monitoring of neuromuscular transmission. But that arm, for example, is likely to be more resistant to non-depolarizing relaxants than the rest of the body, thus leading us to use a relative overdose of drug. Perhaps this is fortunate, since it ensures that the patient will not move intraoperatively, because we are providing neuromuscular blockade of the most resistant muscles. Succinylcholine is also associated with a special consideration in the hemiplegic patient, that of hyperkalemia (Cooperman et al 1970). The time of sensitivity is not well defined, but cases are reported from 1 week to 6 months following onset of hemiplegia.

Intraoperative fluids

Choice of intraoperative intravenous fluids for tumor patients must take into account the patient's overall fluid and electrolyte status and specific electrolyte imbalances present preoperatively or likely to occur intraoperatively. For most patients, replacement of overnight fluid deficit is not necessary. Angiographic dye used in cerebral studies is osmotically active, however, and substantial intravascular fluid volume can be lost in the urine following such a study. An important factor in fluid administration is the integrity of the blood-brain barrier. For practical purposes, the surgical effort necessary to remove cerebral tumors can always leave the area immediately surrounding the resection with a damaged blood-brain barrier from trauma of resection or retractor ischemia. It is generally felt that limiting fluid administration to what is necessary to maintain hemodynamic stability helps to prevent brain edema; perhaps the converse is more applicable, i.e. large volumes of fluid administered to the injured blood-brain barrier patient contribute to cerebral edema. It is clinically unwise to allow significant intravascular hypervolemia to occur for fear of exacerbation of cerebral edema.

The effect of these fluids on neural tissue that has been injured by trauma or ischemia has been an area of increasing interest. It has long been realized that the use of 5% dextrose in water can result in cerebral edema in the patient with a damaged blood-brain barrier. The mechanism appears to be the passage of sugar and water into the brain tissue, with subsequent metabolism of sugar leaving free water in excess. This phenomenon was actually used in years gone by to increase brain size to fill large intracranial spaces left after removal of subdural hematoma. It is now generally appreciated that isotonic electrolyte solutions provide the most physiologic replacement for neurosurgical patients. Elevated blood glucose has been demonstrated to worsen cerebral ischemic injury in a variety of animal models, including intact primates (Lanier et al 1987). Patients admitted with stroke and elevated blood sugar (>120 mg/dl^{-1}) have increased neurologic damage (Pulsinelli et al 1983). Neurologic deficits are more common and more severe in postcardiac arrest patients with higher blood sugars (Longstreth & Inui 1984). Based on this body of work, it seems reasonable to delete glucose from intravenous fluid administration to patients in whom central neural ischemia is likely to occur. Patients undergoing brain tumor surgery would seem to fall into this category.

The effects of types of fluids with varying osmolarity and osmolality on the injured brain have received some attention. Although it is accepted that hypotonic fluids should not be used in patients with increased intracranial elastance, the choice of isotonic crystalloid versus colloid is somewhat less settled. It is frequently recommended that isotonic crystalloid administration should be limited in neurosurgical patients because of concern that lowering plasma oncotic pressure could result in increases in brain water and ICP. In studies of normal animals, decreases in plasma oncotic pressure by plasmapheresis caused no increase in brain water content, while decreases in plasma osmolality caused significant increases in cortical water content. In animals with cerebral injury, lowering of plasma oncotic pressure by acute hemodilution and isotonic crystalloid infusion caused no increases in brain water or ICP compared with colloid infusions. These results suggest that acute crystalloid infusions to maintain hemodynamic stability and intravascular volume status will not result in increases in ICP.

With the newly appreciated risks of blood transfusion and the shortages of donor blood, more dependence can be placed on colloid products to maintain intravascular volume intraoperatively. Albumin and hetastarch are useful choices. Hetastarch has been anecdotally linked to decreased blood coagulability and to postoperative cerebral hematoma (Symington 1986, Cully et al 1987). It seems reasonable to limit the total volume of hetastarch in the neurosurgical patient to ≤ 20 ml/kg or 1 l, realizing that there are few studies to support or refute such an approach (Layon & Gallagher 1987, Claes et al 1992).

Intraoperative management of 'tight brain'

Intracranial hypertension can result in the extrusion of brain tissue when craniotomy is performed. The first sign of difficulty is usually noted by the neurosurgeon as the craniotomy flap is removed and the dura is bulging and tense. The term 'tight brain' gives no clue as to etiology or course of treatment. Some observations can help assess the severity and tractability of the situation. If the dura is tense and bulging only at the lower portion of the craniectomy, palpation may reveal that the brain tissue is easily displaced upward, and that the superior dura is tense only from being pushed out at the lower level. Surgical exposure may be slightly compromised in this situation, and some maneuvers may improve the situation. If the dura is tense at all edges of the craniectomy and palpation reveals fairly immobile brain beneath, surgical exposure may be severely compromised. Maneuvers may help the situation, but are unlikely to bring the brain profile to the bone edge. A large dural incision will result in brain extrusion with trapping at the edges and little room to achieve exposure. A small dural incision allows the surgeon some control of the brain as he seeks to obtain exposure. Although the usual cause of such extreme tenseness of the dura is not amenable to anesthetic maneuvers, it is important to rule out correctable problems (Table 14.1). The usual cause is intracranial hypertension because of the tumor mass itself. As resection is performed, the dural opening can be enlarged and the offending mass will be removed, eventually leaving a cavity where, previously, there was bulging brain. An ominous cause of such swelling is occult acute bleeding into the tumor. Vital signs give a clue to this. Hypertension may develop without apparent cause, and appears unusually resistant to increasing anesthetic depth. Heart rate may initially rise, but then slows. This response is somewhat masked by the complexity of pharmacologic and surgical interventions superimposed during anesthesia. Timing is also important. If the brain begins to bulge vigorously where it was slack before, intracerebral hemorrhage must be strongly suspected. It is helpful to the surgeon to be informed of the subtle vital sign changes suggesting this etiology, because he/she will need to proceed more rapidly and boldly with decompression. Because of the relationship of cerebral perfusion pressure to ICP and blood pressure, it may be unwise to try to reduce blood pressure before decompression, despite the probability of bleeding.

Table 14.1 Therapeutic maneuvers to improve 'tight brain'

Position, venous return
PCO_2, PO_2
Anesthetic drug
Propofol
Muscle relaxants
Diuretics
Spinal fluid drainage
Steroids
Pneumocephalus

With the use of the operating microscope, the surgeon may adjust the position of the table for best exposure without realizing that the patient is slowly being placed horizontal or head-down. Readjusting the operating room table to allow the head to be slightly elevated can dramatically improve the situation. Venous drainage may be compromised by extreme head positions and go unnoticed until the dura is exposed. Repositioning the alignment of head and chin to body may be necessary.

Because it is a powerful cerebral vasodilator, an increase in $PaCO_2$ may cause a dramatic increase in ICP. Hypoxic cerebral vasodilation may produce the same effect. Reassurance that hypocarbia is achieved and hypoxia is absent can be obtained by arterial blood gas determinations supported by pulse oximetry and capnography.

Despite the overall evidence of safety of volatile anesthetics, it seems prudent to discontinue such drugs and utilize an opioid in the presence of 'tight brain'. There may be no causal connection between volatile drugs and brain size, but changing to an opioid anesthetic eliminates any such possibility. N_2O may increase CBF, but its effect is likely to be less pronounced and easily altered by thiopental or opioids. Acute administration of a sleep dose of thiopental can be expected to reduce ICP. Lack of any visible response of the brain to thiopental suggests a serious situation.

Patients receiving anti-seizure medications may have a shortened response to non-depolarizing muscle relaxants (Messick et al 1982c). Return of abdominal and thoracic muscle tone during light anesthesia can raise central venous pressure and, thus, cerebral venous pressure. Thus, the origin of the anecdote that 'curare relaxes the brain'. Evaluation of the level of neuromuscular blockade is an important subtle step in seeking a cause for 'tight brain'.

Osmotic diuretics have long been shown to be effective at reducing brain size in normal brain tissue by drawing water from the interstitial tissue. In patients with intact autoregulation, mannitol results in no change in CBF and a decrease of ICP by 27% at 25 min. However, in patients with impaired autoregulation, the CBF increases by 5%, and there is less decrease in ICP (18%) at 25 min (Muizelaar et al 1984). Furosemide in fairly large doses (e.g. 80 mg) reduces ICP, but its mechanism of action is not entirely clear (Samson & Beyer 1982).

Drainage of cerebrospinal fluid is a rapid and effective method of reducing intracranial bulk directly. Generally effective methods include subarachnoid needle and catheter techniques. Rarely, pneumocephalus may be present from some previous diagnostic test, and can increase with the use of N_2O.

Monitoring for supratentorial brain tumor surgery

General routine monitoring should be used as for any other case of this magnitude. The use of direct arterial pressure recording is usually appropriate. Specific considerations for additional monitoring and ancillary techniques can aid materially in the management of these patients. Hypocarbia is a part of all neuroanesthetic techniques for tumor resection, and capnography or mass spectrometry is useful for quantitating $PaCO_2$ levels, especially when coupled with blood gas determinations. Meningiomas and metastatic tumors to the brain tend to bleed, suggesting monitoring that provides information on hemodynamic parameters. A lesion invading a major cerebral venous sinus may bleed profusely if venous sinus pressure is high, but may entrain air if venous sinus pressure is subatmospheric. Special monitoring for venous air embolism (VAE) is useful in early detection of air, and a right heart catheter may be lifesaving in a case of massive air embolism through an open cerebral venous sinus. Intracranial pressure monitoring is popular in some centers. Some authors find this particularly useful during induction of and emergence from anesthesia. To be helpful during induction, the ICP monitor must be placed in the awake patient. Induction drugs can then be titrated to produce the desired level of ICP (Bedford & Colley 1986).

Infratentorial tumor surgery

Infratentorial tumors require a change in body and head position to provide surgical access to the posterior fossa. For some lesions, this can be achieved with the patient supine and with the head turned dramatically to the side. For others, the park bench, prone, or sitting position provides the desired surgical exposure.

The sitting position is said to offer some surgical advantages (Table 14.2). Surgeons might weigh these advantages differently, but most would agree that ease of surgical exposure, the amount of blood pooling in the operative field, and the operative position of the surgeon are different among the sitting, lateral, supine, and prone positions. Some anesthesiologists feel that access to the endotracheal tube, the reduction of facial swelling, and the ability to observe facial nerve function are notable advantages of the sitting position in anesthetic management. The two most common procedures performed in the sitting position are cervical laminectomy and posterior fossa exploration. Hazards to the patient having infratentorial surgery

Table 14.2 Practical reasons for selective use of sitting position

Better surgical exposure
Less tissue retraction and damage
Less bleeding
Less cranial nerve damage
More complete resection of the lesion
Ready access to airway, chest extremities
Modern monitoring gives early warning of venous air embolism
Brainstem compromise
Serious problems due to venous air embolism are uncommon

include VAE, hypotension, vital sign changes due to brainstem manipulation, specific cranial nerve stimulation, airway obstruction, and position-related brainstem ischemia. Our management should be directed at the prevention, early detection, and treatment of these problems.

There is much concern about the use of the sitting position, some even suggesting that it is malpractice to use this position for today's surgery. These intimidating statements have some basis in fact, but, in general, do not consider what has become a large body of information about the safety of the sitting position.

Safety

There are several large series of sitting cases that have a remarkably similar and favorable safety record (Standefer et al 1984, Matjasko et al 1985, Young et al 1986, Black et al 1988). The sitting position is being used less, and more posterior fossa procedures are being performed in horizontal positions. The use of the sitting position is becoming a conscious selection, rather than automatic, for any posterior fossa lesion. There is risk and benefit in each position, and these must be weighed in the overall care of the patient.

A recent study puts the problem into perspective, and is consistent with other studies (Black et al 1988). Five hundred and seventy nine posterior fossa craniectomies (333 sitting and 246 horizontal) performed at the Mayo Clinic between 1981 through 1984 were reviewed retrospectively. Intraoperatively, the incidence of hypotension was not different between groups, either from induction of anesthesia to incision or from incision to closure. About 20% of the patients in both groups became hypotensive during each of these periods. All responded to vasopressors and/or fluids. The incidence of VAE in patients monitored with the Doppler was significantly greater in the sitting patients (45%) as compared to the horizontal patients (12%).

An important difference was found in the need for blood transfusion between the two groups, confirming the traditional surgical impression that upright patients 'bleed less'. More than two units of blood were required in 13% of the horizontal patients and in only 3% of the upright patients. Average blood volume transfused was also lower in the sitting patients.

Postoperatively, no differences were found in cardiac or respiratory complications. The perioperative myocardial infarction rate was less than 1% overall, and not different between groups. Respiratory complications were found in 2.5%, and were not different between groups, nor from other studies (Standefer et al 1984).

Thus, the data do not support the general selection of either the sitting or horizontal positions based on outcome. There are certain risks and advantages to each, and selection of position should be made with those in mind.

Table 14.3 Relative contraindications to operative sitting position

Ventriculo-atrial shunt in place and open	
Cerebral ischemia upright awake	
Left atrial pressure < right atrial pressure	
Platypnea-orthodeoxia	
Preoperative demonstration of patent foramen ovale or right-to-left shunt	
? cardiac instability ? age extremes	} chest compression and resuscitation not really better in prone or lateral position

In our opinion, there are some conditions that seem prudent to consider as relative contraindications to the sitting position (Table 14.3), however there are few objective data to support our approach. If a shunt tube is in place from the cerebral ventricular system to the right atrium, air may enter the end of the shunt as CSF drains out and be pulled into the heart. The non-collapsible tubing acts as a non-collapsible vein to allow air to pass unimpeded into the heart. This is not a potential problem with a ventriculo-peritoneal shunt, since the air would have no venous access. We recommend that a patient who has a ventriculo-atrial shunt in place should have the shunt tied off before having an intracranial procedure performed in the sitting position. There are some patients who suffer cerebral ischemia whenever they assume the upright position. Their cardiovascular and cerebral vascular systems may both be implicated in this situation. These patients may present for an extracranial–intracranial bypass procedure for the posterior cerebral circulation. Some surgeons feel the sitting position gives the best exposure for this procedure. We feel that we cannot be sure that we will maintain cerebral circulation in this circumstance, since we must not only put the patient upright, but also give an anesthetic. It seems a reasonable balance of risk:benefit ratio to place such a patient in a horizontal position.

There has been a suggestion that, if the left atrial pressure (as measured by pulmonary artery occlusion pressure [PAOP]) is less than the right atrial pressure in the sitting position, the patient should be operated upon horizontally because of increased risk of paradoxical embolism (Perkins-Pearson et al 1982). This is based on two important assumptions: first, that the left atrial pressure will be greater than the right atrial pressure in the horizontal position; second, that the atrial pressure gradient and its direction is a prognostic indicator of whether VAE will become paradoxical air embolism. Laboratory data indicate that the atrial pressure gradients have little, if any, predictive value during air embolism (Black et al 1989). There are some patients who have a potential right-to-left shunt demonstrated preoperatively. In this unusual cardiovascular illness (platypnea-orthodeoxia) the atrial gradients apparently reverse upon assuming the upright position (Seward et al 1984); the patient is well oxygenated in the supine position, but becomes desaturated in the upright position because of unsaturated blood passing from right to left at the atrial level. There are other patients in whom a patent foramen ovale is demonstrated preoperatively during a cardiac work-up. Still others may have a known right-to-left shunt. It seems that these patients might be at greater risk for paradoxical air embolism should VAE occur, and, therefore, it seems prudent to avoid using the sitting position for them.

Some suggest that patients with cardiac instability or at extremes of age should not be placed in a sitting position, based on a possible need to resuscitate intraoperatively. We feel that it is really no easier to provide chest compression in the prone or lateral position than in the sitting position; they are equally undesirable. The rare occurrence of the need to resuscitate probably does not justify giving up whatever surgical advantage is felt to be gained by using the sitting position. Thus, in our opinion, these last considerations are not really relative contraindications.

Monitoring for infratentorial tumor surgery

In collating the data from many studies, the sitting position seems relatively safe, provided adequate monitoring is used.

Central nervous system. Central nervous system monitoring techniques for patients in the sitting position are directed not only at minimizing the hazards of the position, but also at providing positive information to the surgeon, particularly during posterior fossa exploration. The response of the vital signs to brainstem manipulation and the response of the cranial nerves to stimulation can provide pathophysiologic data that the surgeon can utilize in real time during dissection (Table 14.4).

Blood pressure and pulse rate are monitors of several interrelated systems and factors. Some operations performed in the sitting position tend to be of a type that might result in sudden and extreme changes in heart rate and blood pressure, either because of the surgery or because of VAE. Intra-arterial blood pressure measurements will yield instantaneous information, particularly in regard to cerebral perfusion pressure. This is most easily accomplished when the strain gauge is zeroed to the base of the skull.

The electrocardiogram (ECG) is an effective monitor of brainstem compression. Spontaneous respiration has been advocated as a means of detecting transgression of the respiratory centers during posterior fossa exploration. However, large series indicate that monitoring of the ECG provides adequate warning of brainstem compromise during light anesthesia, while using mechanical ventilation to maintain reduced $PaCO_2$ levels (Michenfelder et al 1969). BAER and SSEP can provide an electrophysiologic monitor for detection of early brainstem compromise. Stimulation of the seventh cranial nerve results in a facial twitch that is visible in the seated patient. Electromyography over the distribution of VII can aid in detecting stimulation of the facial nerve when the face is not accessible to palpation or visual assessment.

Diagnosis of venous air embolism. Monitoring for VAE can be approached from several aspects. Monitors include a precordial Doppler, a right heart catheter, capnograph or mass spectrometer, esophageal stethoscope, transcutaneous O_2, and transesophageal echocardiography (TEE). The most sensitive of these are the TEE and Doppler, followed by expired N_2 (F_EN_2), end-tidal CO_2, transcutaneous O_2, right heart catheter, and, least sensitive, the esophageal stethoscope. None of these monitors is totally reliable. We feel that it is generally necessary to use at least three of these to ensure that VAE can be detected (Fig. 14.3).

The risk of VAE is not eliminated by putting the patient horizontal, but it is reduced. A 12% incidence of Doppler-detected air occurs in supine infratentorial craniectomy cases (Black et al 1988). Once VAE has occurred, about 20% of those patients will have hypotension, regardless of the position of the patient.

The precordial Doppler is advocated as the basic monitoring device for the reduction of hazards due to VAE. It

Table 14.4 Cranial nerve stimulation during posterior fossa surgery

Classic activity description—physical signs	Electronic device
V—motor—jaw jerk	EMG
sensory—hypertension	arterial line
bradycardia	ECG
VII—facial twitch	EMG
X—hypotension	arterial line
bradycardia	ECG
XI—shoulder jerk	EMG
Pons, brainstem compression	BAER, SEP
ectopic cardiac foci	ECG
hyper/hypotension	arterial line
tachy/bradycardia	ECG
gasp, irregular respirations	respirator 'trigger'

EMG, electromyography; ECG, electrocardiogram; BAER, brainstem auditory evoked responses; SEP, sensory evoked potentials.

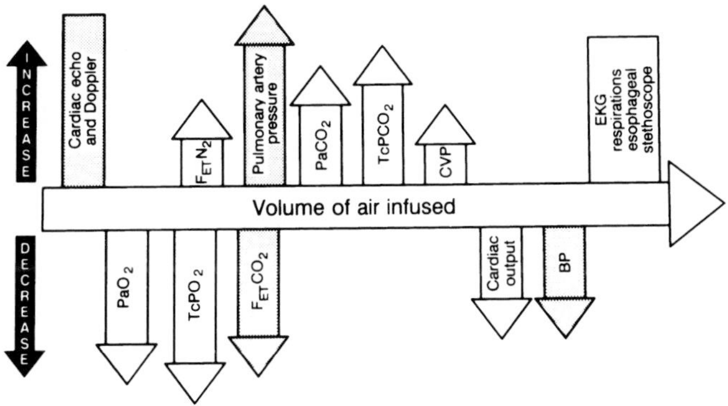

Fig. 14.3 Changes in detection parameters for venous air embolism with increasing air volume. Data are aggregated from human and animal studies under a wide variety of circumstances.

is reasonably priced, relatively easy to use, non-invasive, and very sensitive; its position over the right heart can be verified by rapid injection of saline into the central venous circulation, and its sounds can be heard by both surgeon and anesthesiologist. Its sensitivity has led some to criticize its use as indicating 'insignificant air' before hemodynamic consequences ensue. Protagonists argue that such sensitivity is precisely the early warning needed to identify the occurrence of VAE and stop its entry surgically.

The use of the right heart catheter has evolved and improved such that air can frequently be aspirated when detected on Doppler. But what are the real functions of the right heart catheter? Rapid injection of saline through it can help confirm that the Doppler is properly placed over the right heart. The aspiration of air confirms or establishes the diagnosis of VAE (Michenfelder 1981). The role of the catheter in the treatment of VAE is more anecdotal and less solidly founded. The aspiration of air from the right atrium during VAE is occasionally life-saving, but such occasions must be very rare situations of massive VAE. Whether the routine aspiration of smaller or medium quantities of air from the heart can prevent paradoxical air embolism or cardiopulmonary complications is not known. Right atrial multi-orifice catheters allow a larger amount of air to be aspirated than single-orifice catheters. Proper placement of the right atrial catheter in the high right atrium by ECG control can increase its effectiveness by placing it where the air tends to 'hang up' (Fig. 14.4) (Bunegin et al 1981).

The right heart catheter may be positioned by ECG control, X-ray, or pressure recordings. It is likely that the ECG trace from a multi-orifice catheter comes from the proximal hole, usually 2 cm from the tip (Cucchiara et al 1980). Thus, the tracing sought is a little different with these catheters. The standard concept of a progressively more negative P wave as the catheter is advanced still applies, but the proximal orifice should be placed in the superior vena cava (SVC), allowing the portion of the catheter that has the holes to float at the SVC-high right atrial level (Fig. 14.4). The P wave should be large and negative, with no positive component (Fig. 14.5). This indicates that the proximal orifice is not in the atrium. In practice, one can usually obtain an increasingly negative P wave that finally develops a small positive deflection, and then withdraw slightly to an all negative P wave. Care must be taken when the arm is returned to the side, because the catheter will likely migrate a little more centrally and may need to be withdrawn slightly (Lee et al 1984).

The use of the pulmonary artery catheter for the aspiration of VAE has generally been unsatisfactory, because of the small lumen size and slow speed of blood return; however, other information can be obtained from the pulmonary artery catheter. The entry of air into the pulmonary circulation causes the pulmonary artery (PA) pressure to rise. One can utilize this information to evaluate when

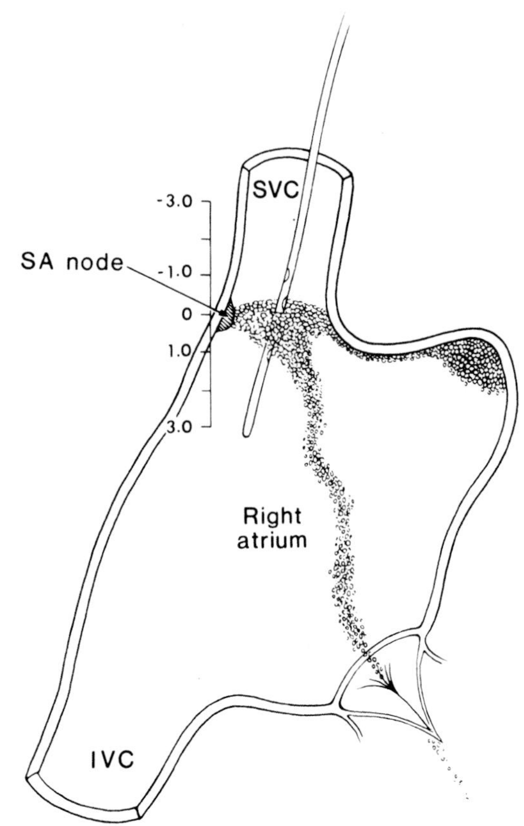

Fig. 14.4 The air tends to localize at the atrial-SVC junction, moving through the tricuspid valve or into upright portions of the atrium. The multi-orifice catheter placement most likely to aspirate air is shown. The electrocardiogram tracing from the catheter in this position is described in Fig. 14.5. Conceptualization of localization of air embolism in the upright heart based on a human cardiac model and human echocardiographic findings.

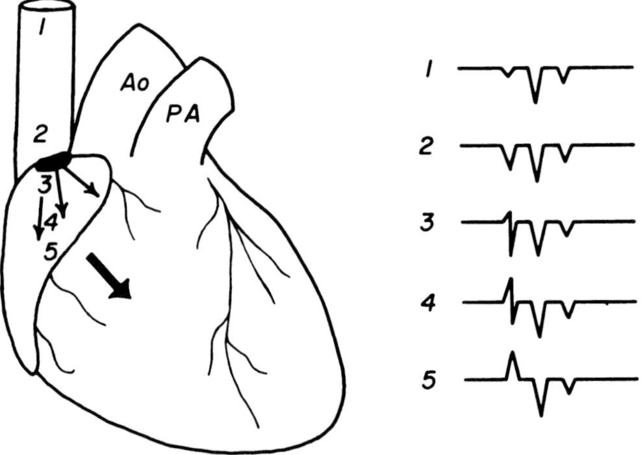

Fig. 14.5 The intracardiac electrocardiogram from each position is shown. With a single orifice catheter, tracing 4 indicates mid-right atrial position. Since the electrocardiogram trace originates from the proximal orifice of a multi-orifice catheter and since placement as shown in Fig. 14.4 is desirable, tracing 2 should be sought. Reproduced with permission from Cucchiara et al 1980.

VAE has cleared the pulmonary circulation. If PA pressure rises during VAE and the Doppler clears, a return of PA pressure to previous levels suggests that the air obstructing the pulmonary circulation has been moved more distally, and probably excreted through the lungs.

Capnography and mass spectrometry demonstrate a decrease in end-tidal CO_2 during VAE with intermediate sensitivity. One can expect to see changes in end-tidal CO_2 after Doppler changes but before hemodynamic changes occur. When enough air is entrained to cause hemodynamic changes, the end-tidal CO_2 will usually drop within a few breaths of the Doppler change. Sensitive mass spectrometry can show increases in F_EN_2 as the VAE is excreted through the lung. Transcutaneous PO_2 is also of intermediate sensitivity, but has more practical and technical problems, making its use in the operating room somewhat less popular (Glenski & Cucchiara 1986).

Transesophageal echocardiography (TEE) is still a research tool, but holds considerable promise in the diagnosis of VAE. It is very sensitive, and allows us to visualize air in the cardiac chambers themselves. This gives us the unique opportunity to identify the occurrence of left heart air (Fig. 14.6) (Cucchiara et al 1984). The only other clinical way to identify paradoxical air embolism during sitting position surgery is for the surgeon to visualize air in the small arteries of the brain or spinal cord. This implies that it is already too late, since the air is already in the vessels to the brain in large enough amounts to be readily seen.

Treatment of venous air embolism. The team approach is critical in achieving a reduction in complications from VAE. The anesthesiologist can make the diagnosis from the devices discussed above. The surgeon often makes the diagnosis at the same time, because (s)he can see that the vein that has been opened is entraining air rather than bleeding back. The role of the anesthesiologist is to support the cardiovascular system so that ischemic injury can be avoided; the role of the surgeon is to stop the influx of air at the surgical site. We can help identify the problem of air in the surgical field by several maneuvers. The surgeon can flood the field with saline to submerge the area of air entry. The application of jugular pressure at the anterior neck for about 15 seconds will frequently raise the venous pressure in the wound enough so that the vessel will back bleed. We would suggest two cautions in applying this pressure. One must attempt to feel the carotid pulsation so that it is not occluded as well. Prolonged occlusion of the jugular veins may raise cerebral venous pressure sufficiently to cause the brain to bulge from the wound. The discontinuation of N_2O will slow the increase in size of the aspirated bubbles and hasten their reabsorption. The use of vasopressors and

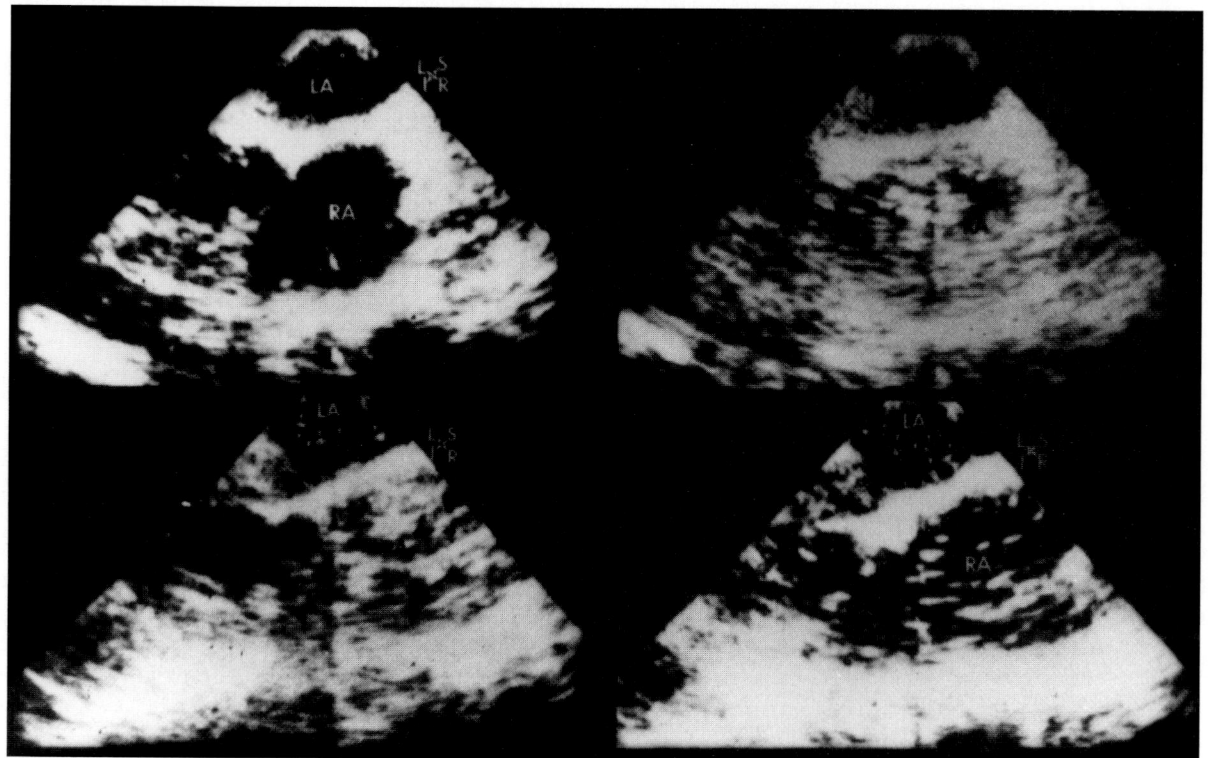

Fig. 14.6 Paradoxical air as noted by transesophageal echocardiography (**top, left**) normal; (**top, right**) air in right atrium; (**bottom, left**) air in left atrium, right atrium nearly opacified; (**bottom, right**) more air in left and right atrium. Reproduced with permission from Cucchiara et al 1984.

volume for pre-load may increase cardiac output and thereby aid in moving the air through the heart to the peripheral pulmonary circulation.

The use of positive end-expiratory pressure (PEEP) in these circumstances is controversial. There is evidence to suggest that, although PEEP may raise the central venous pressure, it may also facilitate the passage of air through a patent foramen ovale. PEEP may raise right atrial pressures to levels which exceed PAOP in seated patients. In examining for patent foramen ovale, cardiologists have shown that a Valsalva maneuver can cause injectate to cross right-to-left at the atrial level on echocardiogram (Lynch et al 1984). The application of PEEP in humans does not eliminate VAE. In dogs, PEEP was less effective in raising cerebral venous pressure than was a neck tourniquet. There are data to suggest that PEEP may not increase paradoxical air embolism, but, when PEEP is released, air tends to move paradoxically (Black et al 1989).

The mechanics of elevation of cerebral venous pressure are not as simple as was previously thought. It appears that cerebral venous flow is carried in both collapsible (jugular veins) and non-collapsible (vertebral venous sinuses) vessels. When venous sinus pressure is highly negative, cerebral venous drainage is carried primarily through non-collapsible vessels that are protected from the neck tourniquet. Neck compression is most effective when venous drainage is through the collapsible channels. That occurs when the venous sinus pressure is only slightly negative or positive. PEEP increased venous sinus pressure when it was very negative only if cardiac output was maintained (Toung et al 1984).

The use of PEEP thus remains controversial, but it is our opinion, based on current literature, that the potential risks of PEEP outweigh its potential benefits.

Anesthetic considerations

There are several viable choices in agent selection for sitting position cases, and each has its advantages and disadvantages. Some of the disadvantages can be minimized by skillful administration. Volatile anesthetics are generally the mainstay for these types of cases at our institution. They provide smooth, easily controlled anesthetic depth; the anesthetic depth can be measured using mass spectrometry; little cardiovascular depression is encountered in the low concentrations required; and a predictable awakening can be accomplished at the end of the case. The supplemental use of N_2O is an area of controversy, particularly in these cases, because of the risk of VAE. When VAE occurs in the presence of N_2O, the bubbles will increase in size as the N_2O diffuses into the bubble faster than the nitrogen can diffuse out. Some have suggested that N_2O should be deleted in sitting cases because of this risk. Many feel that more volatile agents must be used when N_2O is deleted, and it is a little more difficult to end a sitting case without the added analgesia provided by N_2O. These cases can be done with a high dose opioid technique, but, in general, it is difficult to have the patient actively responding at the end of surgery with this technique. The significance of apnea may be confusing, since it may be due to the surgery or to the opioid. Continued intubation of the trachea may be necessary to support ventilation of the lungs. Most use an isoflurane/N_2O/low dose fentanyl technique to circumvent these problems and to allow the versatility required to use or withhold muscle relaxants. The role of propofol in these cases is promising. Most neurosurgeons want to observe the patient awake at the end of the case in the operating room to assess their work and to be sure that a catastrophic event requiring reopening has not occurred. An anesthetic technique that permits this is desirable.

With the advent of SSEP and intraoperative EMG, our use of long-acting muscle relaxants is compromised. Muscle relaxants do not interfere with SSEP monitoring of a cervical laminectomy, for example, but, when cranial nerve motor function (VII, for example) is being tested, we are limited in practice to muscle relaxants for intubation of the trachea and closure only. This poses additional risks, because it is most undesirable to have an open craniotomy patient suddenly strain on the endotracheal tube or move. We have avoided that situation previously by using long-acting non-depolarizing muscle relaxants. As more motor monitoring comes into practice, our use of muscle relaxants will be more limited. This is not only true for sitting cases. These same procedures done in the horizontal position will likely be monitored in the same way. The anesthetic plan must incorporate consideration of these aspects of the procedure. Thus, our overall anesthetic-muscle relaxant technique must be altered to assure, as best we can, that the patient will not move and that the monitoring can be used at critical times.

Emergence from anesthesia

The most serious immediate postoperative complication following posterior fossa craniectomy is apnea. It is very important to be able to define anesthetic-related apnea at the end of the case, since apnea resulting from surgical complications, especially hematoma, may require immediate reoperation. For this reason, it is desirable to return the $PaCO_2$ to near normal and to verify that only the smallest concentration of anesthetic drugs is present, that muscle relaxants are reversed, that temperature is near normal, and that any opioid effects are dissipated. The anesthetic technique should be managed with these goals in mind.

Posterior fossa craniectomy patients are subject to cranial nerve injuries that have implications for the anesthesiologist (Artru et al 1980). Whenever the lower cranial nerves are disturbed, traumatized, or even severed during the procedure, the anesthesiologist should be notified. If cranial nerve V is injured, sensation to the cornea will be impaired, and an eye patch should be used. The most dangerous cranial nerve injuries are to the sensory and motor nerves to the pharynx and larynx. If cranial nerves IX, X, or XI are injured, the patient is at increased risk of aspiration pneumonitis and hypoxia. The pathophysiology seems to involve inability to handle secretions either because the patient is not aware that these are in the pharynx and does not swallow them, or because motor coordination of the pharyngeal muscles is impaired so that swallowing is ineffective. Sometimes the cords are paretic and unable to effectively close the glottis to secretions. The process of aspiration of their own secretions is an insidious one in these patients. We have the clinical impression that they become hypoxic some hours after emerging from anesthesia. If the lower cranial nerves are significantly compromised, the emergence approach we prefer is to leave the patient's trachea intubated at least overnight. We prefer to see the patient swallow on the endotracheal tube before extubation of the trachea to assure ourselves that at least pharyngeal sensation is present. Depending on the anesthetic technique used, this is not always possible, but observation of the event when it occurs can give one a little more confidence in removing the endotracheal tube.

Pneumocephalus occurs regularly in posterior fossa patients, but symptomatic tension pneumocephalus is uncommon. When it occurs, it requires immediate decompression. There is controversy surrounding the use of N_2O and its relationship to the frequency and severity of tension pneumocephalus (Skahen et al 1986, Artru 1987, Domino et al 1992).

Surgery for transsphenoidal tumors

Preoperative assessment of the patient scheduled for transsphenoidal surgery necessitates an evaluation with emphasis on physiologic changes related to endocrine dysfunction (Randall 1982). Glucose tolerance may be disturbed secondary to endocrine dysfunction, and patients should be evaluated for possible hyperglycemia. Adequacy of antidiuretic hormone (ADH) reserve of the posterior pituitary may be determined by measuring urinary concentrating ability following water deprivation (Tindall & McLanahan 1980). Knowledge of baseline function is important, as operative manipulations may alter pituitary function, even if a small adenoma is microscopically removed. This necessitates perioperative provision of glucocorticoids and awareness of the potential postoperative development of diabetes insipidus (Messick et al 1978). In addition to the endocrine evaluation, the radiologic features of the tumor should be reviewed in order to ascertain whether pathology is limited to the sella turcica or involves suprasellar extension.

Special consideration must be given to the patient presenting with Cushing's disease or acromegaly. The patient with Cushing's disease is susceptible to hypertension, hyperglycemia, hyperkalemia, skeletal muscle weakness, and increased intravascular fluid volume (Tasch 1983). The acromegalic may have hypertension, hyperglycemia, and skeletal muscle weakness, as well as skeletal, soft tissue, and connective tissue abnormalities. These may manifest as neuropathies, organomegaly, and alterations in airway anatomy that may make tracheal intubation difficult and may predispose to sleep apnea (Cadieux et al 1982). Airway changes include prognathism, macroglossia, pharyngeal, tonsillar and epiglottic soft tissue hypertrophy, vocal cord fixation, and laryngeal stenosis (Kitahata 1971, Hassan et al 1976). Careful preoperative assessment of the airway in the patient with acromegaly may help to anticipate difficult airway management. This may involve difficulty with obtaining good mask fit and ventilating the patient, visualizing the larynx, and advancing an endotracheal tube (Southwick & Katz 1979). These authors suggest that patients with preoperatively ascertained glottic abnormalities or those with soft tissue abnormalities and glottic abnormalities should be considered for elective tracheostomy preoperatively. Other authors suggest that tracheostomy is rarely necessary in these patients, even with advanced acromegalic changes. Fiberoptic laryngoscopy and intubation of the trachea should be initially considered in acromegalic patients in whom airway management difficulties are anticipated (Ovassapian et al 1981, Messick et al 1982a).

The transsphenoidal approach for microsurgical excision of pituitary adenomas is generally performed under general anesthesia, and principles for management of patients with intracranial lesions should be observed if there is associated suprasellar extension and potential increased intracranial pressure. Patient monitoring routinely includes directly or indirectly measured arterial pressure, ECG, temperature, esophageal auscultation, and urine output. Right atrial/central venous pressure monitoring and precordial Doppler ultrasonic air detection have been suggested by some in order to diagnose and treat potential VAE in operations performed with a 40° head-up tilt (Newfield et al 1978), while others suggest that the monitoring may be omitted if head-up tilt is limited to less than 5–15° (Messick et al 1982b). Induction of general anesthesia can generally be accomplished with intravenous thiopental and a non-depolarizing muscle relaxant to facilitate endotracheal intubation. Succinylcholine may be utilized, especially if a shorter duration of relaxation is desired in cases when difficult airway management is anticipated. The acromegalic airway might be such a case. The transsphenoidal approach to the pituitary usually involves nasal septal and sublabial incisions, thus necessitating oral endotracheal intubation, with the endotracheal tube and esophageal stethoscope secured to the corner of

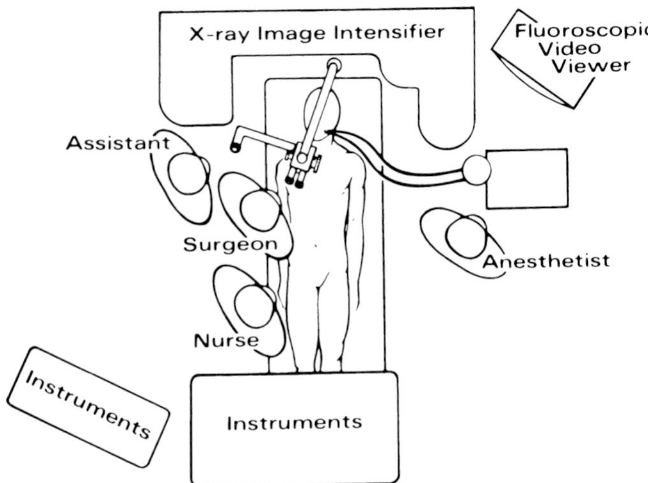

Fig. 14.7 A typical operating room arrangement for transsphenoidal pituitary surgery. Reproduced with permission from Messick J M et al 1982b.

the mouth opposite to the side where the surgeons are operating (Fig. 14.7). The mouth and posterior pharynx may be packed with moist cotton gauze to prevent bleeding into the esophagus and glottic regions and thus prevent postoperative vomiting of blood. Anesthetic maintenance can be achieved either with an opioid-N_2O or inhalation technique. Selection of anesthetic agents must consider the potential hypertensive and arrhythmogenic effects of epinephrine and cocaine used in submucosally injected local anesthetic mixtures by the surgeon (Laws & Kern 1982), with halothane most likely to sensitize toward these effects.

When there is suprasellar extension of the tumor, subarachnoid air may be injected to allow the tumor outline to be visualized on intraoperative fluoroscopy. The elevation of ICP produced by the air may help to deliver the tumor downward into the surgeon's field. Inhaled N_2O will increase the volume of the injected air rapidly. There are several possible approaches to this ancillary technique, none of which has been shown to be clearly superior. One may continue the N_2O and inject smaller volumes of air (e.g. 5 ml), realizing that it will expand as it reaches the cranium. One may discontinue the N_2O and inject subarachnoid air (e.g. 10 ml), or one may draw the gas mixture from the inspired line and inject it. We do not utilize this third option if volatile drugs are in use. The air is injected through a lumbar subarachnoid needle or catheter. As long as CSF can be aspirated from the lumbar drainage system, one can help the surgeon by controlling the degree of downward push on the tumor (related to increased ICP) by removing CSF. Thus, if the air volume proves to be too large as seen from the surgeon's view of the tumor, removal of CSF can optimize the intracranial fluid dynamics. Occasionally, air will be injected but not seen on head fluoroscopy. There may be two reasons for this: (1) the lumbar drain is not subarachnoid (this can be ruled out by withdrawing CSF before and after air injection), and (2) the drain is too caudad, and the air is passing caudad in the subarachnoid space rather than cephalad.

One must bear in mind the potential for operative complications. The sella turcica is bordered laterally by the cavernous sinus, which, in addition to venous structures, contains the intracavernous portion of the internal carotid artery and cranial nerves III, IV, V, and VI. Operative manipulation in the region of the cavernous sinus can thus result in: (1) hemorrhage from the carotid artery or arterial spasm secondary to arterial manipulation, (2) venous hemorrhage and potential entrainment of air into the venous system if head-up tilt is excessive, and (3) cranial nerve weakness secondary to trauma or stretching (Laws & Kern 1982). Visual complications secondary to damage to the optic nerve or chiasm may occur, as well as hypothalamic damage and intracranial hemorrhage. Other complications include postoperative alterations in endocrine function, including the development of diabetes insipidus, which may manifest as a hypotonic polyuria and necessitates frequent reassessment of fluid status. If diabetes insipidus should develop, fluid replacement should include maintenance fluids plus an amount to cover urinary losses. In addition, exogenous vasopressin may need to be administered. This may be accomplished via intranasal administration of DDAVP (desmopressin) once nasal packing is removed (see below).

CRITICAL CARE OF THE PATIENT WHO IS POST-CRANIOTOMY FOR A CEREBRAL TUMOR

How tightly should blood pressure be controlled?

Normal autoregulation of CBF maintains adequate perfusion (CBF = 50 ml/100 g/min) at mean blood pressures ranging from 50–150 torr (Lassen 1974, Lassen & Christensen 1976). Patients who have a history of arterial hypertension shift their cerebral autoregulatory curve to the right, so that a higher pressure is required to maintain adequate perfusion of brain parenchyma (Lassen 1974, Lassen & Christensen 1976). Indeed, the lower limit of autoregulation may be as high as 110–130 torr in hypertensive individuals.

Elevated intracranial pressure impacts on the equation that must be considered when blood pressure control in the post-craniotomy patient is debated (Marsh et al 1977). We normally consider a cerebral perfusion pressure (CPP) (CPP = MAP − ICP)* of ≥ 55 torr to be adequate as long as clinical signs of cerebral dysfunction

*Where MAP is the mean arterial blood pressure:
MAP = diastolic blood pressure + (0.33[systolic − diastolic pressure])
ICP = intracranial pressure

are absent (in an awake patient) or electrophysiologically measured parameters are normal.

In the post-craniotomy patient, in addition to concern about CPP, two other considerations—that of the potentially compromised blood-brain barrier (BBB), and the durability of electrosurgically ablated intracranial blood vessels—enter the discussion. While capillaries in non-neural tissue are permeable to molecules less than about 30 kD in size, the intact BBB has a wide range of permeabilities (Pardridge et al 1986). The relative impermeability of this selectively pervious system protects the brain from external molecules that might upset brain homeostasis, such as lactate from skeletal muscle after severe exertion, and additionally prevents loss of central neurotransmitters (Pardridge et al 1986).

This protective barrier is impaired by certain pathophysiologic events, such as closed head injury, as well as by surgical intervention. Thus, the acutely traumatized brain is at risk of regional blood flow abnormalities that must be taken into account when blood pressure parameters are written for the postoperative period. Areas of local hypoperfusion, related to postoperative regional swelling, can manifest as discrete abnormalities in the neurological examination, or more generally as blunting of the mental status.

During the acute postoperative period concerns of mass effect due to intracranial bleeding are present. Many centers use electrosurgical coagulation of bleeding vessels during the procedure. One aspect of postoperative blood pressure control is aimed at preventing the pressure-related disruption of the electrosurgically coagulated blood vessels. Unfortunately, the literature does not give us any indication as to the pressure limitations of these electrocauterized vessels. As a result of these concerns, we have resolved the issues of blood pressure control, regional perfusion, and cerebral autoregulation in the following manner.

Patients with no history of hypertension

Postoperatively, we maintain the blood pressure in the patient's 'normal range', inasmuch as it is known. This most often results in keeping the systolic blood pressure in the 120–140 torr range. In the first 6–8 h of the acute postoperative period, this control is maintained using continuous intravenous infusion of sodium nitroprusside; we begin at 0.01 μg/kg/min and titrate up to as high as 10 μg/kg/min (although this high-end dose is rarely needed). Thereafter, unless there are specific contraindications such as reactive airways disease or drug allergy, we begin to titrate in another agent, usually the alpha- and beta-blocking drug labetalol, and slowly discontinue the nitroprusside. We initiate the drug at 0.2 mg/kg ideal body weight and double the dose every 5 min until: (1) the blood pressure is adequately controlled (the most common reason for stopping), (2) the pulse rate decreases to 50 beats/min or less (very uncommon), or (3) 1.6 mg/kg has been administered and then repeated twice for a total labetalol dose of 6.2 mg/kg over 30 min (uncommon). After initial control of the blood pressure is obtained, labetalol can usually be administered on an 'as needed' basis every 3–4 h; it can usually be discontinued within a week. Nitroprusside has several problems that make it suboptimal, except for short-term use, in neurosurgical patients. First, the agent increases CBF which, in patients on the steep portion of the cerebral compliance curve, can increase ICP and lower CPP (Orlowski et al 1988, Ziegler 1988). Labetalol, on the other hand, does not appear to cross the BBB, does not affect the ICP, only minimally affects the CPP (Davis R F et al 1981, Gandhi et al 1983) and does not change the intracerebral volume (Davis et al 1981). Further, nitroprusside is metabolized to cyanide which is then rapidly converted to thiocyanate (Van Aken et al 1982). While cyanide toxicity is uncommon when nitroprusside is used at low doses or for a short time at higher doses, thiocyanate, handled by the kidney like chloride, can accumulate in patients with renal failure causing weakness and mental status changes. We thus prefer to use this agent only for the first few hours postoperatively unless no other drug successfully controls blood pressure.

If labetalol is contraindicated or ineffective, we use nifedipine, 10–20 mg sublingually every 4–6 h as needed. In the very rare case in which none of these regimens is effective or all are contraindicated, we switch to the α_2-agonist clonidine and the intravenous form of enalapril, known as enalaprilat. The former agent is placed as a patch of 0.2 mg; approximately 48 h are required before full effect of the drug is noted. The dosage of the patch may be increased weekly if needed; oral clonidine may also be used (Anderson et al 1981, Calhoun & Oparil 1990). Intravenous enalaprilat may be used beginning at 0.625 mg every 6 h; the maximum dose is 20 mg/day, usually given as 5 mg every 6 h. Adverse effects are few, ranging from cough (1.3%), rash (1.3%), taste disturbance (1.4%), angioedema (0.2%), proteinuria (0.7%), and rarely neutropenia; a reversible renal insufficiency due to efferent arteriole dilation with inability to increase renal blood flow may also be seen (Williams 1988).

Blood pressure that is difficult to control may mean the patient has inadequately treated post-craniotomy head pain. Our tendency is to treat this with intravenous morphine sulfate, 0.05 mg/kg ideal body weight. A dose is given every 15 minutes until the pain is brought under control or a total of 0.15 mg/kg has been administered. If the patient becomes somnolent after a dose of morphine, intravenous naloxone, diluted in 0.9% saline to 40 μg/ml, is administered 1 ml every 3–5 minutes until the patient is awake. Obviously, the patient who does not awaken adequately needs to be carefully examined both clinically and radiographically. Intramuscular injection of narcotics borders on the inhumane and, hence, their use is discouraged.

Patients with a history of hypertension

Post-craniotomy patients with a history of arterial hypertension are treated similarly to those without this problem. We do, however, recognize the 'right-shifted' cerebral autoregulatory curve in these patients and, thus, tend to accept a higher systolic blood pressure, in the range of 140–160 torr. If the blood pressure is higher than this, we gain control using the same strategy as mentioned above. As soon as possible, however, we restart the patient on preoperative antihypertensive regimen.

Patients who deteriorate neurologically while blood pressure control is being achieved

Generally, patients who suffer a non-focal deterioration while we are attempting to achieve blood pressure control are more aggressively treated if the blood pressure is still elevated when the deterioration occurs. If, on the other hand, the deterioration occurs while blood pressure is well controlled or lower than desired, we allow it to climb to the highest acceptable value within the 'controlled' range. The rationale behind this is that regional blood flow abnormalities may be responsible: for the earlier formulation, elevation of blood pressure may lead, via Starling forces, to edema formation in areas of the brain that have been surgically traumatized, hence blood pressure control is more rapidly achieved. In the latter formulation, regional edema resulting from surgical trauma may necessitate a higher mean pressure to allow for adequate perfusion. If either of these solutions does not result in rapid correction of the problem, further clinical and radiologic evaluation is required. Focal deteriorations are always aggressively worked-up. We emphasize that these are not definitive answers, simply one way to handle a problem for which inadequate data exist.

Normal perfusion pressure breakthrough syndrome

Even though this is not a problem generally considered of significance in the patient who has undergone a craniotomy for tumor resection, a comment is required. This syndrome is most often seen after resection of an arteriovenous malformation or correction of a high grade carotid stenosis. The mechanism is thought to be paralysis of the vessels that were maximally dilated prior to the operative intervention, resulting in the temporary loss of autoregulation postoperatively. If blood pressure is not aggressively controlled, in the range of 100 torr systolic for the first 2–3 days postoperatively, severe cerebral edema may result (Bernstein et al 1984, Barnett et al 1987). Nitroprusside followed rapidly by labetalol are our agents of choice to obtain control.

Control of intracranial pressure

ICP monitoring and management

With regard to ICP, the most important initial question the clinician must address is which patients will require specific ICP monitoring. After cardiopulmonary resuscitation, head-injured patients with an abnormal computerized axial tomographic (CT) scan are at high risk (53–63%) for elevated ICP and need monitoring (Narayan et al 1982). CT abnormalities include epidural hematoma, subdural hematoma and evidence of diffuse edema. Comatose patients with a normal CT scan of the head are at less risk (13%) for elevated ICP; if they are over the age of 40 years, hypotensive with systolic BP below 90 torr, and show evidence of posturing, the risk of elevated ICP increases (60%) (Narayan et al 1982). Any patient having been paralyzed or heavily sedated as treatment for suspected elevated ICP requires monitoring. Patients who have only mild to moderate head injury, but other traumatic injuries requiring anesthesia for correction may need ICP monitoring during the surgical procedures.

There are both non-invasive and invasive ways to monitor ICP; however, the former methods such as transcranial Doppler (TCD) and visual evoked responses (VER) are not in common clinical use. Nonetheless, both of these may find utility as non-invasive techniques for ICP monitoring in the near future. TCD examines variations in systolic and diastolic peak flows. When ICP increases there is an increase in pulse pressure with higher peak systolic flows and lower diastolic flows. If the ICP becomes higher than diastolic pressure, then diastolic flow velocity disappears. When the ICP exceeds normal arterial flow, then retrograde flow may appear; this tends to be associated with brain death. A major problem of TCD monitoring is its intermittent nature which may result in clinically significant changes being missed. With VER one notes an N_Z waveform at 20 ms associated with a cortical phenomena. Ischemia or increases in ICP alter this waveform latency. ICP is associated with a shift in the latency of N_Z waveform. A confounding factor is papilledema, which can cause artefactual changes (York et al 1984).

The primary methods for direct ICP monitoring are ventriculostomy (the gold standard), subdural bolt, and fiberoptic catheter. Advantages of ventriculostomy are that it is an effective mode for ICP monitoring, and can be easily re-zeroed. Additionally, it carries with it the capacity to drain CSF. A ventriculostomy requires more skill to place properly than the other devices, and is also associated with increased risk of infection, especially if left in place for more than 5–7 days (Kanter & Weiner 1984).

The subdural bolt measures ICP by creating fluid coupling between the CSF and the fluid-filled catheter.

A larger burr hole is required for this technique, and the dura is then opened to expose the CSF. Advantages to this system involve its simplicity and ease of use. Bolts do not require the skill needed for placing a ventriculostomy catheter and, indeed, can be used when edema has collapsed the ventricles. Disadvantages of the system include artefact from tube movement, obstruction by swollen brain, and the need for re-zeroing when head position is changed. Fiberoptic catheters, including the Camino® catheter, are popular, relatively easy to insert, and can be placed in the subdural, intraparenchymal or intraventricular spaces. The disadvantage of this device is that it may slowly drift, and require re-zeroing.

Hyperventilation

Treatment for elevated ICP has traditionally begun with hyperventilation. This represents a relatively easy mode of intervention which can be initiated in the field or the emergency room. Hyperventilation, which decreases $PaCO_2$ to the range of 25–30 torr, causes cerebral vasoconstriction and is a safe and effective initial means for treatment of elevated ICP (Marsh et al 1977). This theory is based on the tenets that elevated ICP is associated with bad outcome, and that hyperventilation can decrease ICP (Marmarou et al 1989). Cerebral lactic acidosis is also associated with poor outcome, and hyperventilation can transiently raise cerebral pH (Cold et al 1975). Muizelaar et al (1991) presented a randomized clinical trial examining hyperventilation versus normoventilation that examined traumatized patients treated in one of three ways: normoventilation, hyperventilation, and hyperventilation with THAM (tris[hydroxymethyl]aminomethane). The results showed that, at three and six months, hyperventilation with THAM had better outcome than controls or hyperventilation alone. The basis suggested for this difference was related to $CMRO_2$ and CBF. When CBF decreases to such an extent that the $CMRO_2$ is not met, the region of the brain involved becomes ischemic. While none of the CBF values from any group was suggestive of ischemia, the hyperventilation group had the highest lactate levels and also had abnormal phosphocreatine/inorganic phosphate ratio, indicative of insufficient oxidative metabolism. Although utilization of hyperventilation and THAM for treatment of elevated ICP has not yet undergone adequate clinical evaluation, standard hyperventilation practices may need re-evaluation as new data are generated.

Sedation/neuromuscular blockade

Patients who have suffered a closed head injury or are post-craniotomy for tumor resection frequently have, at least initially for the latter group, diminished mental status, commonly thrash about in their beds, or 'fight' the ventilator. These actions may raise ICP, especially if the patient is at the steep (or elbow) portion of the intracranial volume-pressure curve. Sedation and/or neuromuscular blockade may be effectively used as adjuncts in the treatment of elevated ICP. Usually, sedation is preferred before neuromuscular blockade, since the former can usually be quickly and completely reversed, and still allows for sequential neurologic examinations. Propofol (Sebel & Lowdon 1989, Albanese et al 1990), beginning at 10 μg/kg/min, is an excellent agent for this purpose as it is a short-acting and powerful sedative. After the redistribution 'sinks' (fat) have been saturated, the drug has a longer effective duration of action as the half-life ($T_{1/2}\beta$) is long. We have found that if the drug dose is progressively titrated *down*, the ability to rapidly arouse the patient for neurologic evaluation is maintained when the agent is discontinued. We use arousability with gentle stimulation as our titration end-point; using the drug in this manner, we have found that an equilibrium is achieved between the triad: drug input-redistribution-metabolism. Additional sedatives are available, including the short-acting benzodiazepine, midazolam. If sedatives are not capable of controlling the patient, then utilization of a neuromuscular blocking agent, in addition to the sedative, may be indicated. While therapy can be initiated with longer-acting agents such as pancuronium, it is our practice to use agents with a shorter $T_{1/2}\beta$, such as vecuronium, mivacurium, or atracurium, titrated to neuromuscular function as measured by twitch or train-of-four response to a supramaximal impulse (Bevan et al 1992, Isenstein et al 1992).

Minimization of stimulation

Along with attempts at sedation, there should be an overall decrease in 'elective' interventions that will be painful or excessively stimulating. This means that suctioning of the endotracheal tube should be minimized if possible. Using intratracheal lidocaine prior to suctioning has been suggested; however, it is our experience that coughing upon instillation obviates its usefulness in this scenario. Thus, we utilize the agent intravenously approximately 90 s prior to stimulation; the dose is 1–2 mg/kg and is usually given as a 4% solution.

Mannitol

Mannitol is also an important therapeutic agent which has substantial effects aside from its ability to decrease cerebral edema. Mannitol's effects on cerebral edema are generally ascribed to its hyperosmolality. One manner by which it functions is to remove brain water from areas of normal brain (Pappius & Dayes 1965); it is also thought to prevent movement of water from the vascular to the intracellular space during membrane pump failure (Fisher

1976, Meyer et al 1987). Mannitol also decreases blood viscosity, decreases microcirculatory vascular resistance, and additionally, it acts as an oxygen free-radical scavenger (Muizelaar et al 1983). Recent work also suggests this agent is helpful in re-establishing perfusion after global ischemia (Shirane & Weinstein 1992). Disadvantages to the use of mannitol are also associated with its hyperosmolality, since with continued use patients may develop rebound cerebral edema, neuronal damage, or renal failure (Stuart et al 1970). Severe dehydration of the brain may result in serious subdural and subarachnoid hemorrhage (Pappius & Dayes 1965). Because of these problems, serum osmolality should not be allowed to rise above 320 mOsm/kg H_2O. The institution of mannitol usually begins with a bolus of 0.25–0.5 g/kg, followed by an infusion of 20% mannitol at 0.06–0.12 g/kg/h. Generally, the infusion is not increased beyond 0.12 g/kg/h, as the risk of a hyperosmolar state and decreased effectiveness of the agent in controlling ICP outweigh the possible benefits. Serum osmolality and sodium are serially checked, respectively, every 8 hours and 4 hours. Utilization of this agent in the presence of widespread disruption of the BBB may result in an aggravation of cerebral edema due to penetration of the agent into the brain (Stuart et al 1970).

Steroids

Interestingly, the utilization of steroids in elevated ICP secondary to severe closed head injury has been shown to result in decreased morbidity and mortality (Marsh et al 1977). The doses used, however, to effect this result were quite high: a 48 mg initial dose of dexamethasone, followed by 8 mg every 2 h on days 1 and 3 post-injury, 4 mg every 2 h on days 2 and 4, and 4 mg every 4 h on days 5 and 8. Using lower doses, a 16 mg initial dose followed by 4 mg every 6 h, resulted in no improvement in outcome compared to patients receiving no drug.

Barbiturates

The last option in the medical armamentarium is barbiturate coma. A great deal of debate has occurred over the usefulness of barbiturate coma in treatment of head injury. The first multi-center randomized trial was concluded in 1988, and suggested that barbiturates were an effective means of controlling ICP in patients refractory to other therapy. The data questionably supported an overall favorable outcome (Eisenberg et al 1988). Patients being placed in barbiturate coma require adequate volume resuscitation, and frequently a pulmonary artery flotation catheter prior to initiation of therapy. These patients may have cardiovascular depression associated with hypotension. Even if volume replacement is adequate, inotropic support with dopamine, dobutamine, or epinephrine will likely be required for hemodynamic instability. The initial loading dose of pentobarbital is 5 mg/kg, followed by 1–2 mg/kg/h as a maintenance infusion. In addition to continued use of an ICP monitor, the drug is titrated to 90% burst suppression on a portable EEG monitor. 90% burst suppression is the most effective means for monitoring barbiturate therapy, while ICP monitoring informs us as to the effectiveness of the treatment. We have also used sodium thiopental for this purpose, although on occasion doses as large as 70 mg/kg, followed by 1–5 mg/kg/h have been required to, respectively, achieve and maintain 90% burst suppression. Usually, within 3–5 days after the event that resulted in elevated ICP, the barbiturate infusion can be tapered, and the patient reassessed for further aggressive ICP control.

Surgical therapy

On rare occasions and in desperate situations, surgical therapies such as unroofing of the cranial vault or temporal lobe resection may be required to save a patient's life. While our experience with this is extremely limited, most often the need for this follows severe closed head injury rather than post-craniotomy for tumor resection.

Evaluation of slow emergence from anesthesia

In the patient who had normal or near-normal mental status prior to operative intervention, a well planned and carried out anesthetic technique frequently allows for the immediate or near-immediate wake-up at the end of the surgical procedure (see above, Anesthetic Management of the Tumor Patient). When, unexpectedly, the patient does not awaken, rapid evaluation, and possibly treatment, is called for. The differential diagnosis (Table 14.5), critically important in the preoperative period when therapeutic intervention is planned, is equally important in the situation we refer to here.

As in any urgent situation in which the diagnosis is not known, the history and physical examination must be rapidly and carefully carried out in a focused manner. The history is obtained from the preintervention and surgical period. Very quickly, the physician will determine if the slow emergence is due to residual anesthetic (either inhaled or intravenous) or neuromuscular blocking agents. Treatment, if appropriate, is provided with naloxone (residual narcotic), flumazenil (residual benzodiazepine), anticholinesterase/anticholinergic combination such as

Table 14.5 Differential diagnosis of failure to awaken

1. Residual anesthetic agent(s)
2. Intracranial bleed
3. Metabolic abnormalities: Na^+, Ca^{+2}, PO_4^{-2}, glucose, hyperosmolality
4. Hypothermia
5. Surgical trauma
6. Hypoxemia

neostigmine and glycopyrrolate (residual neuromuscular blocking agent), or a short period of mechanical ventilation (residual inhaled anesthetic). Residual amounts of several anesthetic agents may result in slow emergence due to additive effects.

Carried out at almost the same time as the review of the anesthetic record is a focused neurologic examination. Any focal finding will result in immediate radiographic evaluation (MRI or CT scanning) followed by intervention, if necessitated by a blood collection that can be surgically removed. Cerebral edema, if noted by MRI or CT, is treated as above (Control of Intracranial Pressure).

If after this initial evaluation no cause is found, a standard battery of studies — including serum Na^+, Ca^{2+}, PO_4^{-2}, osmolarity and glucose — should be done. Even mild to moderate hypothermia, usually defined as between 30 and 35°C, may cause unconsciousness. If no cause can be found, the clinician is left with three possibilities: surgical trauma, unrecognized intraoperative hypoxia, or residual anesthetic agents not reversible by the abovementioned techniques. The neurosurgeon will most often be aware if surgical trauma is a serious contender for the diagnosis. Unrecognized intraoperative hypoxia is (or should be) an event of the past; the availability of relatively inexpensive continuous pulse-oximetry makes the use of this device mandatory in every operating suite. The first two items of this triad will frequently show up as cerebral edema, focal in the former case, diffuse in the latter, on radiographic evaluation. After initial evaluation has shown no focal neurological defects, reversible residual anesthetic, or metabolic abnormalities, watchful waiting will frequently result in emergence. The key to solving this problem is to rapidly rule out the phenomena likely to result in increased patient morbidity or mortality.

Postoperative endotracheal extubation

Decannulation of the trachea after a neurosurgical procedure is generally performed in a manner similar to that followed in other surgical patients. There are, however, some differences. Posterior fossa surgery may result in injury to the brainstem respiratory center or cranial nerves IX, X, and XII or their nuclei. The consequences of this may be a patient who is awake and alert, but is unable to spontaneously breathe or protect the airway for a period of time (usually a few days) postoperatively (Artru et al 1980, Drummond & Todd 1984). Table 14.6 gives the criteria for decannulation.

Of significance, though not widely appreciated, is our preference that imposed work of the breathing apparatus should be zero prior to tracheal decannulation.* Imposed

*This work has been done primarily under the direction of Michael J Banner, PhD, Assistant Professor of Anesthesiology and Physiology, University of Florida College of Medicine.

Table 14.6 Extubation criteria

1. Neurologic status
   a. Awake, alert, cooperative
   b. Intact gag reflex
   c. Able to breathe spontaneously
2. Neuromuscular status
   a. Able to hold head off bed for 5–10 seconds
   b. Negative inspiratory force at least 25 cmH_2O
   c. Forced vital capacity at least 15 ml/kg ideal body weight
   d. Spontaneous tidal volume at least 5 ml/kg ideal body weight
3. Oxygenation status
   a. CPAP $\leq$ 5 cmH_2O
   b. $PaO_2{:}F_iO_2 \geq 300$ torr*
4. Ventilation status
   a. Arterial pH between 7.30 and 7.40
   b. Respiratory rate averages between 10 and 28 breaths/minute
   c. $WOB_{imposed}$ equal to zero

*Such that with an F_iO_2 of 0.3 the PaO_2 would be at least 90 torr.

work of breathing (WOB) is that work performed by the patient while breathing spontaneously through the ventilatory apparatus (endotracheal tube, breathing circuit, ventilator demand-flow system). Total work of breathing (WOB) is that encompassing imposed work and physiologic work and is described by the equation:

$$WOB_{total} = \int P_{es}\, dV$$

where P_{es} is esophageal pressure, used as an inference of intrapleural pressure, and dV is the volume change.

Imposed WOB is described by the equation:

$$WOB_{imposed} = \int P_{ett}\, dV$$

where P_{ett} is the pressure measured at the end of the endotracheal tube. The pressure and volume values are obtained, respectively, from an air-filled 1 mm internal diameter catheter and miniature flow sensor. These data are directed to a portable computerized respiratory monitor (BICORE Monitoring Systems, Inc, Model CP-100, Irvine, CA) from which real-time display of both the pressure-volume loops and the calculations of work are obtained (Banner et al 1993).

Previous work has suggested that imposed WOB may, under certain circumstances‡, be higher than physiologic WOB (= $WOB_{total} - WOB_{imposed}$) (Civetta 1993, Kirton et al 1993). This could result in a patient who appears not to meet the criteria for extubation (Table 14.6) simply due to $WOB_{imposed}$. We generally use the pressure support ventilatory (PSV)§ mode to decrease $WOB_{imposed}$ to zero

‡Such as, for example, breathing through a 7.0 mm internal diameter endotracheal tube, at high peak inspiratory flow rates, on a ventilator with an insensitive demand valve.

§PSV is a pressure limited, flow cycled mode of assisted ventilation in which the patient triggers the ventilator to deliver a preset pressure from which the patient may then obtain the tidal breath. When inspiratory flow drops to (depending on the ventilator in use) about 25% of peak inspiratory flow, the machine cycles off. This mode of assistance is used both as a 'bridge' to wean from mechanical ventilation, and as a means to overcome $WOB_{imposed}$.

prior to extubation of the trachea; we are beginning a formal study to test the hypothesis that patients may be safely extubated at PSV settings corresponding to $WOB_{imposed}$ equal to zero.

Anticonvulsant therapy

Seizures may be a serious problem after tumor resection. Early diagnosis of seizures or new neurologic deficits in the immediate postoperative period may be complicated due to residual anesthetic agent. The seizure may affect the airway or cause the patient to suffer injuries to the extremities resulting from uncontrolled movements during the ictal episode. Seizures themselves may cause structural brain injury thus predisposing the patient to further seizures (Deutschman & Haines 1985). Status epilepticus carries with it serious risk of death, ranging as high as 20%. Seizures may put the postoperative patient at increased risk of cerebral acidosis, cerebral edema or increased ICP (Lee et al 1989).

Patients with a preoperative history of seizures are at greatest risk for ictal activity in the postoperative period (Fukamachi et al 1985). The extent of cortical injury, not necessarily related to cortical resection, is an important determinant of seizure activity, as retraction can be associated with increased risk for postoperative seizures. Extra-axial lesions, such as aneurysms, have a postoperative risk of seizure activity of up to 25% (Kvam et al 1983). Postoperative metabolic derangements, primarily hypoxia, hyper- or hyponatremia, hyperglycemia or acidosis, also increase the risk for seizures. In one study, 80% of patients had a metabolic acidosis immediately prior to seizure and 20% were hyponatremic (Lee et al 1990). Anticonvulsant levels are also of critical importance. North found that inadequate phenytoin levels were a leading cause of postoperative seizures in his examination of postcraniotomy patients (North et al 1983).

Certain tumor types result in an increased risk of associated postoperative seizures. Benign lesions are reported to be associated with a higher relative incidence of seizures, perhaps secondary to longer associated life spans (Deutschman & Haines 1985). Both Lund (1952) and Gamache et al (1982) showed the following seizure frequency: oligodendroglioma 50–81%, astrocytoma 40–66%, ependymoma 33–50%, glioblastoma 30–42%, meningioma 30–40%, metastatic lesions 19–26%. Fukamachi's series showed a predominance of seizures associated with meningiomas, followed by glioblastomas and benign astrocytomas (Fukamachi et al 1985).

Location of the tumor is also a critical factor (Deutschman & Haines 1985). In general, supratentorial tumors are associated with a high degree of seizure activity; Youmans & Cobb (1982) placed the incidence of this association at 50%. This correlated with the statistics quoted by Lund (1952) at 20–80% and with Sach & Furlow (1936) at 35%. While posterior fossa tumors are associated with a decreased incidence of seizure activity, an increased incidence has been noted with medulloblastoma and, to a lesser degree, astrocytomas and meningiomas (Lee et al 1990). Seizures associated with infratentorial masses are rare, and the incidence is further reduced by preoperative shunting procedures (Lee et al 1990). Tumors in close proximity to the motor strip appear to be highly susceptible to epileptic activity (Deutschman & Haines 1985). Correcting Lund's data for orientation to the motor strip results in a particularly high seizure incidence, with ictal activity being seen in 83% of oligodendroglioma/astrocytomas, 71% of meningiomas, and 53% of glioblastomas (Drummond & Todd 1984). Mahaley & Dudka (1981) showed, in a study of tumor patients with preoperative seizures, that frontal, temporal, and parietal lesions all had a seizure incidence of 40%, whereas that for occipital lesions was 14%. Ramamurthi et al (1980) examined 127 patients with meningioma and found that, of the 27/77 patients with preoperative seizures, 35% had frontal or parietal lesions, whereas patients with temporal, occipital, posterior fossa, and miscellaneous locations had a seizure incidence of 20%.

Seizure type may vary with type and location of the neoplasm. The preponderance of data suggest, however, that the qualities of the seizure are the same preoperatively and postoperatively (Ramamurthi et al 1980, Kvam et al 1983, Fukamachi et al 1985, Lee et al 1990). Time to onset of seizure is brief, usually in the immediate postoperative period. Two series (Kvam et al 1983, Lee et al 1990) suggest that most of the seizures that are to occur will do so in the first 24 h postoperatively. This is not, however, uniformly so. North et al (1983) noted that 45% of seizures that were to occur did so within the first week, and 64% within the first month.

Considerable variation of effect of prophylactic anticonvulsants exists. Kvam et al (1983) examined 538 postcraniotomy patients and found 23 of these had postoperative seizures. Preoperative seizures were present in only 5/23, and only 1/23 had therapeutic anticonvulsant levels when examined. These authors suggested an oral loading dose of phenytoin of 10 mg/kg, followed by 5–6 mg/kg in the postoperative period; serial plasma levels of phenytoin should be followed. In a series of 203 patients undergoing craniotomy, randomization to placebo or phenytoin in a double blind manner was performed. All patients with preoperative seizures were excluded and treatment with placebo or study drug was started in the recovery room. 8 of the 101 patients receiving phenytoin had seizures, while 16 patients from the placebo group developed seizures. Only 3 seizure patients from the phenytoin-receiving group had therapeutic phenytoin levels. From these data, the authors suggested that seizure prophylaxis was necessary for 3 months postoperatively. A flaw with the drug regimen in this study, impacting on its ability to prevent postoperative seizures, is the late onset of initiating anticonvulsant prophylaxis (Deutschman & Haines 1985).

While various phenytoin dosing schedules have been suggested by the different investigators (North et al 1983, Deutschman & Haines 1985, Lee et al 1989), our policy is to give an initial dose of 15 mg/kg (about 1 g) over the 20 minutes prior to wound closure. This is followed by 5–6 mg/kg/day postoperatively. Serum levels are followed in conjunction with the clinical pharmacology service.

Syndrome of inappropriate antidiuretic hormone secretion/diabetes insipidus

Derangements of electrolytes involving sodium balance, diabetes insipidus (DI) and the syndrome of inappropriate secretion of antidiuretic hormone (SIADH) are important considerations in patients who have undergone craniotomy for brain tumor resection.

The normal range of serum Na^+ and osmolality are, respectively, 135–145 mEq/l and 282–292 mOsm/kg. The body attempts to maintain this equilibrium through a variety of mechanisms including the hormones ADH, aldosterone, and angiotensin. ADH is produced by the supraoptic/paraventricular nuclei in the hypothalamus. The hormone is transported down long axons to the posterior pituitary. The precursor is then modified to produce three molecules: ADH, neurophysin, and a glycopeptide (Robinson 1988). In this region, baro- and volume-receptors are sensitive to serum Na^+ levels below 135 mEq/l, the serum osmolality, and the volume status. Receptors in the hypothalamus can, in fact, detect a 1% change in osmolality and in this way fine tune ADH secretion (Baylis & Robertson 1980). ADH is normally suppressed when serum osmolality is < 280 mOsm/kg; above this level its secretion increases at a linear rate with osmolality (Ober 1991). Sodium and its associated anions are the most potent solutes capable of stimulating ADH secretion (Robertson 1984).

Receptors for volume status are less sensitive in altering ADH release, as a 5–15% volume change must occur prior to detecting noticeable change in ADH (Robinson 1985, 1988). Once the patient becomes hypovolemic, large amounts of the hormone will be released; a pressor effect may be seen at high levels of ADH. Thirst is also an important but relatively insensitive mechanism for response to osmolar changes. As osmolality increases above 280 mOsm/kg, ADH release is incrementally stimulated; only at about 290–295 mOsm/kg is the thirst mechanism stimulated. Once ADH has been released via these mechanisms, it binds to receptors on renal collecting tubes to increase free water resorption.

The brain is particularly sensitive to changes in serum Na^+ and osmolality, as water freely moves across the BBB along osmotic gradients (Sterns 1991). When the serum sodium is decreased, the relative increase in free water causes the brain to swell. Normally the intracranial contents can increase only by about 10% prior to the precipitation of life-threatening increases in ICP. A 10% decrease in serum Na^+ corresponds roughly to a value of 127 mEq/l; however, patients frequently have a serum Na^+ below this level without life-threatening sequelae (Sterns 1991). The basis for this relates to adaptation by the brain. Acute changes can be responded to within minutes by increasing the bulk flow of water across the brain into the CSF space. Cellular adaptation is much slower, requiring 3–4 h to begin, with maximal effect at 24 h (Sterns 1989, Sterns et al 1989, Berl 1990, Sterns 1990, Sterns & Spital 1990). Initially outward potassium flux increases; later neurons extrude organic solutes. These 'idiogenic osmoles', such as phosphocreatine, myoinositol, glutamate, taurine, and glutamine all decrease their intracellular concentration as part of the adaptation process (Lien et al 1990, Thurston et al 1984, 1989).

Syndrome of inappropriate antidiuretic hormone secretion

Patients post-craniotomy for tumor resection will frequently exhibit decreased urine output; the urine made has decreased free water content and increased osmolality. When volume status is not the reason for the decreased urine output, there may be a relative increase in serum free water; if not noted, acute water intoxication may ensue. Minor symptoms associated with acute water intoxication include headache, nervousness, nausea, emesis, disorientation, and stupor. Serious sequelae can include seizures, coma, and death. These more serious signs are usually associated with an acute drop in serum Na^+ to less than 120–125 mEq/l (Cluitsman & Meinders 1990). Acute hyponatremia is described as that occurring over a time period < 48 h; it may become symptomatic when changes take place at a rate > 12 mEq/l/day. Chronic hyponatremia occurs over a time period > 48 h and is usually asymptomatic until the serum Na^+ is < 115 mEq/l (Cluitsman & Meinders 1990). Potential causes of SIADH include brain tumors, hypothyroidism, glucocorticoid deficiency, and drugs such as vincristine, oxytocin, carbamazepine, clofibrate, chlorpropamide, the non-steroidal anti-inflammatory drugs, and morphine.

Correction of the hyponatremia must be slow or the patient may be left with serious neurologic deficits. The need for slow correction is related to the brain's compensatory mechanisms for edema and hyponatremia. The organic solutes, extruded during the development of the hyponatremia syndrome as a means to prevent cerebral edema, are slow to reaccumulate as the serum Na^+

normalizes (Sterns et al 1989, Thurston et al 1987). Intracellular osmolar normalization must be allowed to occur or the cell will become dehydrated (Sterns et al 1989).

While quite rare, the osmotic demyelination syndrome may occur one to several days after the serum Na^+ has normalized. Initially, patients begin to exhibit behavioral changes, movement disorders, or seizures (Sterns 1989, Sterns 1991). In progressive stages, pseudobulbar palsy, quadriparesis, and coma with pontine demyelination may occur (Sterns et al 1986, Berl 1990, Brunner et al 1990). This is thought to result from inappropriate correction of the hyponatremia. Thus, although there is great controversy (Layon et al 1992), the serum Na^+ should be corrected no faster than 12–24 mEq/l/day (0.5–1 mEq/l/h), particularly if the patient is an alcoholic or has other debilitating diseases.

Treatment begins with volume restriction, initially between 1000 and 1500 ml/day. Fluid restriction decreases intravascular volume with subsequent decreased renal blood flow and glomerular filtration rate, as well as an increased sodium resorption in the proximal tubule; further, increased aldosterone secretion enhances distal tubular sodium resorption. Furosemide is an excellent first-line treatment of SIADH as it impairs the ability of the kidney to concentrate urine and thus increases free water loss. In more extreme cases, 3% NaCl may be used to correct critically low serum Na^+ levels or those that have been refractory to first-line treatment. Although there is some controversy (Layon et al 1992) we generally begin 3% NaCl if the serum Na^+ has acutely dropped to < 125 mEq/l. Conversely, we worry much less about the complications of hyponatremia once the serum Na^+ is ≥ 125 mEq/l. If the patient is having a seizure or is comatose, 3% NaCl can be infused at 1–2 ml/kg/h for 2–3 hours. While this will likely not correct the serum Na^+ to normal, it should take the patient to a value of approximately 125 mEq/l, out of the range of acute danger. In chronic refractory cases, 3% NaCl solution infused initially at rates of 15–25 ml/h are appropriate. In both cases, serial serum Na^+ levels (every 1–2 h until the serum Na^+ is out of the danger range, then every 4 h), hourly urine output and specific gravity, and serum osmolality should be closely followed every 4 hours, particularly over the first 24 hours.

An intriguing syndrome, termed the cerebral salt wasting syndrome, has been described in patients post-subarachnoid hemorrhage (Wijdicks et al 1991). This syndrome has some characteristics similar to those of SIADH. Specifically, serum sodium is low and urine sodium is high. The central difference between these syndromes seems to be that in cerebral salt wasting the patient is hypovolemic and the plasma atrial natriuretic factor is elevated, while in SIADH the patient's volume status is increased and vasopressin levels are relatively increased. Whether this is of significance for patients who have undergone craniotomy for tumor is unclear at this time.

Diabetes insipidus

This syndrome involves an excessive loss of free water as a result of inadequate secretion or action of ADH, with resultant high urine output that can lead to hyperosmolality and elevated serum Na^+. The symptoms usually associated with DI are polydipsia, and production of copious, dilute urine (polyuria). Other general symptoms of DI are impaired mentation, obtundation, weakness, lethargy, coma, seizures, and intracranial bleeding secondary to excessive dehydration. In children, 37% of DI cases are associated with brain tumors, and 10% of such cases occur preoperatively. 25% of adult cases are idiopathic, 17% are associated with intracranial malignancies, and 13% present preoperatively. Interestingly, only 9% of DI cases are associated with hypophysectomy (Moses et al 1976). Central nervous system tumors that may result in DI include craniopharyngioma, pinealomas, meningiomas, dysgerminomas, and pituitary tumors (Vokes & Robertson 1988). Metastatic lesions can also cause DI; in one series these were reported to be the cause of 14% of the total cases (Kimmel & O'Neil 1983). DI may occur as a paraneoplastic syndrome with small cell lung cancer, leukemia, lymphoma and, more rarely, with breast cancer (Kimmel & O'Neill 1983).

Particular care must be paid to the patients who have undergone craniotomy for tumor as they frequently have depressed mental status and may be unable to regulate their volume status with oral fluid intake. Three distinct patterns of DI follow surgery (Verbalis et al 1985). The most common, occurring in at least 50% of patients, consists of acute onset polyuria within 24 hours of surgery, with resolution in 3–5 days; this is the usual pattern associated with post-hypophysectomy patients. The second most common pattern is permanent DI, associated with 33% of trauma and neurosurgery cases in which proximal injury to the pituitary stalk or hypothalamus itself occurs. The third pattern involves a triphasic response. The initial phase is evidenced by abrupt onset of polyuria. This is followed after several days by cessation of diuresis that lasts up to 2 weeks. The second stage is believed secondary to increased release of ADH from injured neurohypophyseal tissue (O'Connor 1952); during the second stage, the patient is at risk for development of hyponatremia and water intoxication. After this, the standard picture of DI returns, reflecting the death of magnocellular neurons by retrograde degeneration (Ober 1991).

Prior to initiation of therapy, an assessment of the free water deficit should be made using the formula:

$$\text{Free } H_2O \text{ deficit} = (Na^+_{actual} - 140)/140 \times (0.6)\ (\text{body weight[kg]})$$

Initially, treatment should begin with isotonic fluid to reverse any hypovolemia that may be present. If persistent elevated urine output continues, with a specific gravity of 1.000–1.005, then hypotonic intravenous fluids (0.45% saline solution, lactated Ringer's solution) should be initiated after a baseline serum Na^+ and osmolality have been obtained. Our practice, in a patient not yet hypovolemic, is to replace urine output greater than 1 ml/kg ideal body weight via intravenous fluids. If the patient has a water deficit requiring correction, it is replaced and then the above noted formula is begun. Our strong bias is to avoid the use of free water (5% dextrose in H_2O = D_5W) if at all possible. DI is almost always diagnosed very rapidly after development, therefore drastic measures such as the utilization of D_5W are only rarely called for. Only with a serum $Na^+ \geq 160$ mEq/l or osmolality ≥ 320 mOsm/kg would we consider rapid correction of the free water deficit. We initially correct about 25% of the calculated deficit rapidly; once the serum Na^+ is approximately 155 mEq/l we correct more gradually.

When possible, patients should be allowed to control themselves with hypotonic oral fluid intake, as the body will tend to maintain proper homeostasis; the altered mental state of the postcraniotomy patient may not allow this option for up to 12–24 h. If drug therapy is required, multiple options exist (Table 14.7). We most frequently use the DDAVP subcutaneously or intravenously, with serial serum Na^+ values to follow progress. This is well tolerated and very effective in treating the DI as onset is < 1 h and duration may be as long as 24 h.

Table 14.7 Drugs for the treatment of diabetes insipidus. Adapted and reproduced with permission from Zaloga 1992

1. Drugs which enhance the effect of intrinsic ADH
   a. Clofibrate 250–500 mg every 6 h
   b. Chlorpropamide 250–750 mg every day
   c. Carbamazepine 400–1000 mg every day
   d. Hydrochlorothiazide 50–100 mg every day
2. ADH analogs
   a. Lysine vasopressin 1–2 sprays in each nostril (5–10 units) every 4–6 h
   b. Vasopressin tannate 2–5 U SC or IM every 24–72 h
   c. Aqueous arginine vasopressin 5–10 U IV, IM, or SC every 4–6 h
   d. DDAVP (desmopressin) 1–2 sprays in each nostril (5–20 μg) every 12–24 h; 2–4 μg IV or SC every 12–24 h

ADH, antidiuretic hormone; SC, subcutaneously; IM, intramuscularly; IV, intravenously.

REFERENCES

Adams R W, Gronert G A, Sundt T M, Michenfelder J D 1972 Halothane, hypocapnia, and cerebrospinal fluid pressure in neurosurgery. Anesthesiology 37: 510–517

Adams R W, Cucchiara R F, Gronert G A, Messick J M, Michenfelder J D 1981 Isoflurane and cerebrospinal fluid pressure in neurosurgical patients. Anesthesiology 54: 97–99

Albanese J, Martin C, Lacarelle B, Saux P, Durand A, Gouin F 1990 Pharmacokinetics of long-term propofol infusion used for sedation in ICU patients. Anesthesiology 73: 214–217

Anderson R J, Hart G R, Crumpler C P, Reed W G, Matthews C A 1981 Oral clonidine loading in hypertensive urgencies. Journal of the American Medical Association 246: 848–850

Artru A A 1983 Relationship between cerebral blood volume and CSF pressure during anesthesia with halothane or enflurane in dogs. Anesthesiology 58: 533–539

Artru A A 1986 Cerebral metabolism and EEG during combination of hypocapnia and isoflurane-induced hypotension in dogs. Anesthesiology 65: 602–608

Artru A A 1987 Breathing nitrous oxide during closure of the dura and cranium is not indicated, letter. Anesthesiology 66: 719

Artru A A, Cucchiara R F, Messick J M 1980 Cardiorespiratory and cranial-nerve sequelae of surgical procedures involving the posterior fossa. Anesthesiology 52: 83–86

Banner M J, Kirby R R, Blanch P B, Layon A J 1993 Decreasing the imposed work of the breathing apparatus to zero using pressure support ventilation. Critical Care Medicine 21: 1333–1338

Barnett G H, Little J R, Ebrahim Z Y, Jones S C, Friel H T 1987 Cerebral circulation during arteriovenous malformation operation. Neurosurgery 20: 836–842

Baylis P H, Robertson G L 1980 Plasma vasopressin response to hypertonic saline infusion to assess posterior pituitary function. Journal of the Royal Society of Medicine 73: 255–260

Bedford R, Colley P 1986 Intracranial tumors. In: Matjasko J, Katz J (eds) Clinical controversies in neuroanesthesia and neurosurgery. Grune & Stratton, Orlando, p 135

Berl T 1990 Treating hyponatremia—damned if we do and damned if we don't. Kidney International 37: 1006–1018

Bernstein M, Fleming J F R, Deck J H N 1984 Cerebral hyperperfusion after carotid endarterectomy—a cause of cerebral hemorrhage. Neurosurgery 15: 50–56

Bevan D R, Donati F, Kopman A F 1992 Reversal of neuromuscular blockade. Anesthesiology 77: 785–805

Black S, Ockert D B, Oliver W C Jr, Cucchiara R 1988 Outcome following posterior fossa craniectomy in patients in the sitting or horizontal positions. Anesthesiology 69: 49–56

Black S, Cuçhiara R F, Nishimura R A, Michenfelder J D 1989 Parameters affecting the occurrence of paradoxical air embolism. Anesthesiology 71: 235–241

Boarini D J, Kassell N F, Coester H C, Butler M, Sokoll M D 1984 Comparison of systemic and cerebrovascular effects of isoflurane and halothane. Neurosurgery 15: 400–409

Brown J C, Charlton J E 1975 Study of sensitivity to curare in certain neurological disorders using a regional technique. Journal of Neurology, Neurosurgery and Psychiatry 38: 34–45

Brunner J E, Redmond J M, Haggar A M, Kruger D F, Elias S B 1990 Central pontine myelinolysis and pontine lesions after rapid correction of hyponatremia—a prospective magnetic resonance imaging study. Annals of Neurology 27: 61–66

Buchthal F 1985 Electromyography in the evaluation of muscle diseases. Neurologic Clinics 3: 573–598

Bunegin L, Albin M, Helsel P E, Hoffman A, Hung T-K 1981 Positioning the right atrial catheter. A model for reappraisal. Anesthesiology 55: 343–348

Cadieux R J, Kales A, Santen R J, Bixler E O, Gordon R 1982 Endoscopic findings in sleep apnea associated with acromegaly. Journal of Clinical Endocrinology and Metabolism 55: 18–22

Calhoun D A, Oparil S 1990 Treatment of hypertensive crisis. New England Journal of Medicine 323: 1177–1183

Carlsson C, Hagerdal M, Kaasik A E, Siesjo B K 1976a The effects of diazepam on cerebral blood flow and oxygen consumption in rats and its synergistic interaction with nitrous oxide. Anesthesiology 45: 319–325

Carlsson C, Hagerdal M, Siesjo B K 1976b The effect of nitrous oxide on oxygen consumption and blood flow in the cerebral cortex of the rat. Acta Anaesthesiologica Scandinavica 20: 91–95

Carlsson C, Keykhah M, Smith D S, Harp J R 1981 Influence of high

dose fentanyl on cerebral blood flow and metabolism. Acta Physiologica Scandinavica 113: 271–272
Carlsson C, Smith D S, Keykhah M M, Englebach I, Harp J R 1982 The effects of high-dose fentanyl on cerebral circulation and metabolism in rats. Anesthesiology 57: 375–380
Carter L P, Raudzens P A, Gaines C, Crowell R M 1984 Somatosensory evoked potentials and cortical blood flow during craniotomy for vascular disease. Neurosurgery 15: 22–28
Chi O Z, Field C 1986 Effects of isoflurane on visual evoked potentials in humans. Anesthesiology 65: 328–330
Civetta J C 1993 Nosocomial respiratory failure or intragenic ventilator dependency. Critical Care Medicine. 21: 171–173
Claes Y, Hemelrijck J V, Gerven M V, Arnout J, Vermylen J 1992 Influence of hydroxyethyl starch on coagulation in patients during the perioperative period. Anesthesia and Analgesia 75: 24–30
Cluitsman F H M, Meinders A E 1990 Management of severe hyponatremia — rapid or slow correction? American Journal of Medicine 88: 161–166
Cold G, Enevoldsen E, Malmros R 1975 Ventricular fluid lactate, pyruvate, bicarbonate, and pH in unconscious brain-injured patients subjected to controlled ventilation. Acta Neurologica Scandinavica 52: 187–195
Cooperman L H, Strobel G E, Kennell E M 1970 Massive hyperkalemia after administration of succinylcholine. Anesthesiology 32: 161–164
Costa E Silva I, Wang A D, Symon L 1985 The application of flash visual evoked potentials during operations on the anterior visual pathways. Neurological Research 7: 11–16
Cucchiara R F, Michenfelder J D 1973 The effect of interruption of the reticular activating system on metabolism in canine cerebral hemispheres before and after thiopental. Anesthesiology 39: 3–12
Cucchiara R F, Theye R A, Michenfelder J D 1974 The effects of isoflurane on canine cerebral metabolism and blood flow. Anesthesiology 40: 571–574
Cucchiara R F, Messick J M, Gronert G A, Michenfelder J D 1980 Time required and success rate of percutaneous right atrial catheterization: description of a technique. Canadian Anaesthetists Society Journal 27: 572–573
Cucchiara R F, Nugent M, Seward J B, Messick J M 1984 Air embolism in upright neurosurgical patients: detection and localization by two-dimensional transesophageal echocardiography. Anesthesiology 60: 353–355
Cully M D, Larson C P Jr, Silverberg G D 1987 Hetastarch coagulopathy in a neurosurgical patient. Anesthesiology 66: 706–707
Dahlgren N, Ingvar M, Yokoyama H, Siesjo B K 1981 Influence of nitrous oxide on local cerebral flow in awake, minimally restrained rats. Journal of Cerebral Blood Flow and Metabolism 1: 211–218
Davis R F, Douglas M E, Heenan T J, Downs J B 1981 Brain tissue pressure during sodium nitroprusside infusion. Critical Care Medicine 9: 17–21
Dawson B, Michenfelder J D, Theye R A 1971 Effects of ketamine on canine cerebral blood flow and metabolism: modification by prior administration of thiopental. Anesthesia and Analgesia 50: 443–447
Deutschman C S, Haines S J 1985 Anticonvulsant prophylaxis in neurologic surgery. Neurosurgery 17: 510–516
Domino K B, Hemstad J R, Lam A M, Laohaprasit V, Maybery T A 1992 Effect of nitrous oxide on intracranial pressure after cranial-dural closure in patients undergoing craniotomy. Anesthesiology 77: 421–425
Drummond J C, Todd M M 1984 Acute sinus arrhythmia during surgery in the fourth ventricle—an indicator of brain stem irritation. Anesthesiology 60: 232–235
Drummond J C, Todd M M, U H S 1985 The effect of high dose sodium thiopental on brainstem auditory and median nerve somatosensory evoked responses in humans. Anesthesiology 63: 249–254
Drummond J C, Todd M M, Scheller M S, Shapiro H M 1986 A comparison of the direct cerebral vasodilating potencies of halothane and isoflurane in the New Zealand white rabbit. Anesthesiology 65: 462–467
Dubois M Y, Sato S, Chassy J, Macnamara T E 1982 Effects of enflurane on brainstem auditory evoked responses in humans. Anesthesia and Analgesia 61: 898–902
Eintrei C, Leszniewski W, Carlsson C 1985 Local application of ^{133}Xenon for measurement of regional cerebral blood flow (rCBF) during halothane, enflurane, and isoflurane anesthesia in humans. Anesthesiology 63: 391–394
Eisenberg H M, Frankowski R F, Contant C F, Marshall L F, Walker M D 1988 High-dose barbiturate control of elevated intracranial pressure in patients with severe head injury. Journal of Neurosurgery 69: 15–23
Fisher E G 1976 Impaired perfusion following cerebrovascular stasis — a review. Archives of Neurology 29: 361–366
Forster A, Juge O, Morel D 1982 Effects of midazolam on cerebral blood flow in human volunteers. Anesthesiology 56: 453–455
Forster A, Juge O, Morel D 1983 Effects of midazolam on cerebral hemodynamics and cerebral vasomotor responsiveness to carbon dioxide. Journal of Cerebral Blood Flow and Metabolism 3: 246–249
Freidman W A, Kaplan B J, Gravenstein D, Rhoton A L Jr 1985 Intraoperative brain-stem auditory evoked potentials during posterior fossa microvascular decompression. Journal of Neurosurgery 62: 552–557
Fukamachi A, Koizumi H, Nukui H 1985 Immediate postoperative seizures — incidence and computed tomographic findings. Surgical Neurology 24: 671–676
Gamache F W, Posner J B, Patterson R H 1982 Metastatic brain tumors. In: Youmans J R (ed) Neurological surgery. W B Saunders, Philadelphia, pp 2872–2898
Gandhi P, Cottrell J E, Scialabba F O, Shwiry B 1983 Deliberate hypotension with labetalol in neurological patients, abstracts. Anesthesiology 59: A360
Ginsburg H H, Shetter A G, Raudzens P A 1985 Postoperative paraplegia with preserved intraoperative somatosensory evoked potentials. Journal of Neurosurgery 63: 296–300
Glenski J A, Cucchiara R F 1986 Transcutaneous O_2 and CO_2 monitoring of neurosurgical patients: detection of an embolism. Anesthesiology 64: 546–550
Graham D 1980 Monitoring neuromuscular block may be unreliable in patients with upper-motor-neuron lesions. Anesthesiology 52: 74–75
Grosslight K, Foster R, Colohan A R, Bedford R F 1985 Isoflurane for neuroanesthesia: risk factors for increases in intracranial pressure. Anesthesiology 63: 533–536
Grundy B L 1982 Monitoring of sensory evoked potentials during neurosurgical operations: methods and applications. Neurosurgery 11: 556–575
Grundy B L 1983 Intraoperative monitoring of sensory-evoked potentials. Anesthesiology 58: 72–87
Grundy B L, Heros R C, Tung A S, Doyle E 1981 Intraoperative hypoxia detected by evoked potential monitoring. Anesthesia and Analgesia 60: 437–439
Grundy B L, Jannetta P J, Procopio P T, Lina A, Boston J R, Doyle E 1982a Intraoperative monitoring of brainstem auditory evoked potentials. Journal of Neurosurgery 57: 674–681
Grundy B L, Nash C L, Brown R H 1982b Deliberate hypotension for spinal fusion: prospective randomized study with evoked potential monitoring. Canadian Anaesthetists Society Journal 29: 452–461
Grundy B L, Nelson P B, Doyle E, Procopio P T 1982c Intraoperative loss of somatosensory-evoked potentials predicts loss of spinal cord function. Anesthesiology 57: 321–322
Grundy B L, Nelson P B, Lina A, Heros R C 1982d Monitoring of cortical somatosensory evoked potentials to determine the safety of sacrificing the anterior cerebral artery. Neurosurgery 11: 64–67
Harner S G, Daube J R, Ebersold M J 1986 Electrophysiologic monitoring of facial nerve during temporal bone surgery. Laryngoscope 96: 65–69
Harner S G, Daube J R, Ebersold M J, Beatty C W 1987 Improved preservation of facial nerve function with use of electrical monitoring during removal of acoustic neuromas. Mayo Clinic Proceedings 62: 92–102
Hassan S Z, Matz G J, Lawrence A M, Collins P A 1976 Laryngeal stenosis in acromegaly: a possible cause of airway difficulties associated with anesthesia. Anesthesia and Analgesia 55: 57–60
Hoffman W E, Miletich D J, Albrecht R F 1986 The effects of midazolam on cerebral blood flow and oxygen consumption and its interaction with nitrous oxide. Anesthesia and Analgesia 65: 729–733

Hougaard K, Hansen A, Brodersen P 1974 The effect of ketamine on regional cerebral blood flow in man. Anesthesiology 41: 562–567

Isenstein D A, Venner D S, Duggan J 1992 Neuromuscular blockade in the intensive care unit. Chest 102: 1258–1266

Jannetta P J, Møller A R, Møller M B 1984 Technique of hearing preservation in small acoustic neuromas. Annals of Surgery 200: 513–523

Jobes D R, Kennell E M, Bush G L, Mull T D, Lecky J H, Behar M G, Wollman H 1977 Cerebral blood flow and metabolism during morphine-nitrous oxide anesthesia in man. Anesthesiology 47: 16–18

Johnston J H, Harper A M 1973 The effect of mannitol on cerebral blood flow. Journal of Neurosurgery 38: 461–471

Kanter R K, Weiner L B 1984 Ventriculostomy-related infections, letter. New England Journal of Medicine 311: 987

Kaplan B J, Friedman W A, Alexander J A, Hampson S R 1986 Somatosensory evoked potential monitoring of spinal cord ischemia during aortic operations. Neurosurgery 19: 82–90

Kassell N F, Hitchon P W, Gerk M K, Sokoll M D, Hill R T 1981 Influence of changes in arterial Pco_2 on cerebral blood flow and metabolism during high-dose barbiturate therapy in dogs. Journal of Neurosurgery 54: 615–619

Kearse L A, Brown E N, McPeck K 1992 Somatosensory evoked potentials sensitivity relative to electroencephalography for carotid ischemia during carotid endarterectomy. Stroke 23: 498–505

Keykhah M M, Smith D S, Carlsson C, Safo Y, Englebach I, Harp J R 1985 Influence of sufentanil on cerebral metabolism and circulation in the rat. Anesthesiology 63: 274–277

Kimmel D W, O'Neill B P 1983 Systemic cancer presenting as diabetes insipidus—clinical and radiologic features of 11 patients with a review of metastatic-induced diabetes insipidus. Cancer 52: 2355–2358

Kirton O, Banner M J, Axelrad A, Drugas G 1993 Detection of unsuspected imposed work of breathing. Case reports. Critical Care Medicine 21: 790–795

Kitahata L M 1971 Airway difficulties associated with anesthesia in acromegaly. British Journal of Anaesthesia 43: 1187–1190

Kvam D A, Loftus C M, Copeland B, Quest D O 1983 Seizures during the immediate postoperative period. Neurosurgery 12: 14–17

Lam A M, Keane J F, Manninen P H 1985 Monitoring of brainstem auditory evoked potentials during basilar artery occlusion in man. British Journal of Anaesthesia 57: 924–928

Lam A M, Manninen P H, Ferguson G G, Nantau W 1991 Monitoring electrophysiologic function during carotid endarterectomy: a comparison of somatosensory evoked potentials and conventional electroencephalogram. Anesthesiology 75: 15–21

Lanier W L, Stangland K J, Scheithauer B W, Milde J H, Michenfelder J D 1987 The effects of dextrose infusion and head position on neurologic outcome after complete cerebral ischemia in primates: examination of a model. Anesthesiology 66: 39–48

Lassen N A 1974 Control of cerebral circulation in health and disease. Circulation Research 34: 749–760

Lassen N A, Christensen M S 1976 Physiology of cerebral blood flow. British Journal of Anaesthesia 48: 719–734

Laws E R, Kern E B 1982 Complications of transsphenoidal surgery. In: Laws E R, Randall R V, Kern E B, Abboud C (eds) Management of pituitary adenomas and related lesions with emphasis on transsphenoidal surgery. Appleton-Century-Crofts, New York, pp 329–346

Layon A J, Gallagher T J 1987 Effects of hetastarch resuscitation on extravascular lung water and cardiopulmonary parameters in a sheep model of hemorrhagic shock. Resuscitation 15: 257–265

Layon A J, Bernards W C, Kirby R R 1992 Fluids and electrolytes in the critically ill. In: Civetta J M, Taylor R W, Kirby R R (eds) Critical care. J B Lippincott, Philadelphia, pp 457–480

Lee D S, Kuhn J, Shaffer M J, Weintraub H D 1984 Migration of tips of central venous catheters in seated patients. Anesthesia and Analgesia 63: 949–952

Lee S T, Lui T N, Chang C N, Cheng W C, Wang D J, Heimbarger R F, Lin C G 1989 Prophylactic anticonvulsants for prevention of immediate and early postcraniotomy seizures. Surgical Neurology 31: 361–364

Lee S T, Lui T N, Chang C N, Cheng W C 1990 Early postoperative seizures after posterior fossa surgery. Journal of Neurosurgery 73: 541–544

Lesser R P, Raudzens P, Luders H et al 1986 Postoperative neurological deficits may occur despite unchanged intraoperative somatosensory evoked potentials. Annals of Neurology 19: 22–25

Levy W J 1983 Spinal evoked potentials from the motor tract. Journal of Neurosurgery 58: 38–44

Levy W J Jr 1987 Clinical experience with motor and cerebellar evoked potential monitoring. Neurosurgery 20: 169–182

Lien Y H, Shapiro J I, Chan L 1990 Effects of hypernatremia on organic brain osmoles. Journal of Clinical Investigation 85: 1427–1435

Little J R, Lesser R P, Lueders H, Furlan A J 1983 Brainstem auditory evoked potentials in posterior circulation surgery. Neurosurgery 12: 496–502

Longstreth W I Jr, Inui T S 1984 High blood glucose level on hospital admission and poor neurological recovery after cardiac arrest. Annals of Neurology 15: 59–63

Lund M 1952 Epilepsy in association with intracranial tumors. Acta Psychiatrica Neurology Scandinavica Suppl 8: 1–149

Lynch J J, Schuchard G H, Gross C M, Wann L S 1984 Prevalence of right-to-left atrial shunting in a healthy population: detection by Valsalva maneuver contrast echocardiography. American Journal of Cardiology 53: 1478–1480

McPherson R W, Niedermeyer E F, Otenasek R J, Hanley D F 1983 Correlation of transient neurological deficit and somatosensory evoked potentials after intracranial aneurysm surgery. Case report. Journal of Neurosurgery 59: 146–149

McPherson R W, Szymanski J, Rogers M 1984 Somatosensory evoked potential changes in position-related brain stem ischemia. Anesthesiology 61: 88

McPherson R W, Mahla M, Johnson R, Traystman R J 1985a Effects of enflurane, isoflurane, and nitrous oxide on somatosensory evoked potentials during fentanyl anesthesia. Anesthesiology 62: 626–633

McPherson R W, Toung T J K, Johnson R M, Rosenbaum A E, Wang H 1985b Intracranial subdural gas: A cause of false-positive change of intraoperative somatosensory evoked potential. Anesthesiology 62: 816–819

McPherson R W, Sell B, Traystman R J 1986 Effects of thiopental, fentanyl and etomidate on upper extremity somatosensory evoked potentials in humans. Anesthesiology 65: 584–589

Madsen J B, Cold G E, Hansen E S, Bardrum B 1987 The effect of isoflurane on cerebral blood flow and metabolism in humans during craniotomy for small supratentorial cerebral tumors. Anesthesiology 66: 332–336

Maekawa T, Sakabe T, Takeshita H 1974 Diazepam blocks cerebral metabolic and circulatory responses to local anesthetic-induced seizures. Anesthesiology 41: 389–391

Mahaley M S, Dudka L 1981 The role of anticonvulsant medications in the management of patients with anaplastic gliomas. Surgical Neurology 16: 399–401

Manninen P H, Lam A M, Nicholas J F 1985 The effects of isoflurane and isoflurane-nitrous oxide anesthesia on brainstem auditory evoked potentials in humans. Anesthesia and Analgesia 64: 43–47

Manohar M, Parks C M 1984 Porcine brain and myocardial perfusion during enflurane anesthesia without and with nitrous oxide. Journal of Cardiovascular Pharmacology 6: 1092–1101

Markand O N, Dilley R S, Moorthy S S, Warren C Jr 1984 Monitoring of somatosensory evoked responses during carotid endarterectomy. Archives of Neurology 41: 375–378

Marmarou A, Anderson R, Ward J D et al 1989 The traumatic coma data bank monitoring of ICP. In: Hoff J T, Bertz A L (eds) Intracranial pressure VII. Springer Verlag, Berlin, pp 549–551

Marsh M L, Marshall L F, Shapiro H M 1977 Neurosurgical intensive care. Anesthesiology 47: 149–163

Marsh M L, Dunlop B J, Shapiro H M, Gagnon R L, Rockoff M A 1980 Succinylcholine—intracranial pressure effects in neurosurgical patients, abstracts. Anesthesia and Analgesia 59: 550–551

Matjasko J, Petrozza P, Cohen M, Steinberg P 1985 Anesthesia and surgery in the seated position: analysis of 554 cases. Neurosurgery 17: 695–702

Matsumiya N, Dohi S 1983 Effects of intravenous or subarachnoid morphine on cerebral and spinal cord hemodynamics and antagonism with naloxone in dogs. Anesthesiology 59: 175–181

Messick J M Jr, Theye R A 1969 Effects of pentobarbital and meperidine on canine cerebral and total oxygen consumption rates. Canadian Anaesthetists Society Journal 16: 321–330

Messick J M Jr, Laws E R Jr, Abboud C F 1978 Anesthesia for transsphenoidal surgery of the hypophyseal region. Anesthesia and Analgesia 57: 206–215

Messick J M, Cucchiara R F, Faust R J 1982a Airway management in patients with acromegaly. Anesthesiology 56: 157

Messick J M, Faust R J, Cucchiara R F 1982b Anesthesia for transsphenoidal microsurgery. In: Laws E R, Randall R V, Kern E B, Abboud C (eds) Management of pituitary adenomas and related lesions with emphasis on transsphenoidal surgery. Appleton-Century-Crofts, New York, pp 253–261

Messick J M, Maass L, Faust R J, Cucchiara R F 1982c Duration of pancuronium neuromuscular blockade in patients taking anticonvulsant mediation. Anesthesia and Analgesia 61: 203–204

Meyer F B, Anderson R E, Sundt T M Jr, Yaksh T L 1987 Treatment of experimental focal cerebral ischemia with mannitol — assessment of intercellular brain pH, cortical blood flow and electroencephalography. Journal of Neurosurgery 66: 109–115

Michenfelder J D 1974 The interdependency of cerebral functional and metabolic effects following massive doses of thiopental in the dog. Anesthesiology 41: 231–236

Michenfelder J D 1981 Central venous catheters in the management of air embolism: whether as well as where. Anesthesiology 55: 339–341

Michenfelder J D, Cucchiara R F 1974 Canine cerebral oxygen consumption during enflurane anesthesia and its modification during induced seizures. Anesthesiology 40: 575–580

Michenfelder J D, Theye R A 1971 Effects of fentanyl, droperidol, and Innovar on canine cerebral metabolism and blood flow. British Journal of Anaesthesia 43: 630–635

Michenfelder J D, Theye R A 1975 In vivo toxic effects of halothane on canine cerebral metabolic pathways. American Journal of Physiology 229: 1050–1055

Michenfelder J D, Gronert G A, Rehder K 1969 Neuroanesthesia. Anesthesiology 30: 65–100

Milde L N, Milde J H, Michenfelder J D 1985 Cerebral functional, metabolic, and hemodynamic effects of etomidate in dogs. Anesthesiology 63: 371–377

Minton M D, Stirt J A, Bedford R F 1985a Increased intracranial pressure from succinylcholine: modification by prior non depolarizing blockade, abstracted. Anesthesiology 63: A391

Minton M D, Stirt J A, Bedford R F, Haworth C 1985b Intracranial pressure after atracurium in neurosurgical patients. Anesthesia and Analgesia 64: 1113–1116

Møller A R, Jannetta P J 1983 Monitoring auditory functions during cranial nerve micro vascular decompression operations by direct recording from the eighth nerve. Journal of Neurosurgery 59: 493–499

Moorthy S S, Markand O N, Dilley R S, McCammon R L, Warren C H Jr 1982 Somatosensory evoked responses during carotid endarterectomy. Anesthesia and Analgesia 61: 879–883

Moses A M, Miller M, Streeten D H P 1976 Pathophysiologic and pharmacologic alterations in the release and action of ADH. Metabolism 25: 697–721

Muizelaar J P, Wei E P, Kontos H A 1983 Mannitol causes compensatory cerebral vasoconstriction and vasodilation in response to blood viscosity changes. Journal of Neurosurgery 59: 822–828

Muizelaar J P, Lutz H A III, Becker D P 1984 Effect of mannitol on ICP and CBF and correlation with pressure autoregulation in severely head-injured patients. Journal of Neurosurgery 61: 700–706

Muizelaar J P, Marmarou A, Ward J D et al 1991 Adverse effects of prolonged hyperventilation in patients with severe head injury—a randomized clinical trial. Journal of Neurosurgery 75: 731–739

Narayan R K, Kishore P R S, Baker D P et al 1982 Intracranial pressure — to monitor or not to monitor? A review of our experience with severe head injury. Journal of Neurosurgery 56: 650–659

Newberg L A, Milde J H, Michenfelder J D 1983 The cerebral metabolic effects of isoflurane at and above concentrations that suppress cortical electrical activity. Anesthesiology 59: 23–28

Newfield P, Albin M S, Chestnut J S, Maroon J 1978 Air embolism during trans-sphenoidal pituitary operations. Neurosurgery 2: 39–42

North J B, Penhall R K, Hanieh A, Frewin D B, Taylor W B 1983 Phenytoin and postoperative epilepsy—a double-blind study. Journal of Neurosurgery 58: 672–677

Ober K P 1991 Diabetes insipidus. Critical Care Clinics 7: 109–125

O'Connor W J 1952 The normal interphase in the polyuria which follows section of the supraoptico-hypophyseal tracts in the dog. Quarterly Journal of Experimental Physiology 37: 1–10

Orlowski J P, Shiesley D, Vidt D G, Barnett G H, Little J R 1988 Labetalol to control blood pressure after cerebrovascular surgery. Critical Care Medicine 16: 765–768

Oshita S, Ishikawa T, Tokutsu Y, Takeshita H 1979 Cerebral circulatory and metabolic stimulation with nitrous oxide in the dog. Acta Anaesthesiologica Scandinavica 23: 177–181

Ovassapian A, Doka J C, Romsa D E 1981 Acromegaly — use of a fiberoptic laryngoscopy to avoid tracheostomy. Anesthesiology 54: 429–430

Pappius H M, Dayes L A 1965 Hypertonic urea — its effects on the distribution of water and electrolytes in normal and edematous brain tissues. Archives of Neurology 13: 395–402

Pardridge W M, Oldendorf W H, Cancilla P, Frank H J L 1986 Blood-brain barrier—interface between internal medicine and the brain. Annals of Internal Medicine 105: 82–95

Pathak K S, Brown R H, Nash C L Jr, Cascorbi H F 1983 Continuous opioid infusion for scoliosis fusion surgery. Anesthesia and Analgesia 62: 841–845

Pathak K S, Brown R H, Cascorbi H F, Nash C L Jr 1984 Effects of fentanyl and morphine on intraoperative somatosensory cortical-evoked potentials. Anesthesia and Analgesia 63: 833–837

Pathak K S, Ammadio M, Kalamchi A, Scoles P V, Shaffer J W, Mackay W 1987 Effects of halothane, enflurane, and isoflurane on somatosensory evoked potentials during nitrous oxide anesthesia. Anesthesiology 66: 753–757

Pelligrino D A, Miletich D J, Hoffman W E, Albrecht R F 1984 Nitrous oxide markedly increases cerebral cortical metabolic rate and blood flow in the goat. Anesthesiology 60: 405–412

Perkins-Pearson N A K, Marshall W K, Bedford R F 1982 Atrial pressures in the seated position: implication of paradoxical air embolism. Anesthesiology 57: 493–497

Peterson D O, Drummond J C, Todd M M 1986 Effects of halothane, enflurane, isoflurane, and nitrous oxide on somatosensory evoked potentials in humans. Anesthesiology 65: 35–40

Phirman J R, Shapiro H M 1977 Modification of nitrous oxide-induced intracranial hypertension by prior induction of anesthesia. Anesthesiology 46: 150–151

Prass R L, Luders H 1986 Acoustic (loudspeaker) facial electromyographic monitoring: part 1. Neurosurgery 19: 392–400

Pulsinelli W A, Levy D E, Sigsbee B, Scherer P, Plum F 1983 Increased damage after ischemic stroke in patients with hyperglycemia with or without established diabetes mellitus. American Journal of Medicine 74: 540–544

Ramamurthi B, Raui R, Ramachandran V 1980 Convulsions with meningiomas—incidence and significance. Surgical Neurology 14: 415–416

Randall R V 1982 Clinical presentation of pituitary adenomas. In: Laws E R, Randall R V, Kern E B, Abboud C (eds) Management of pituitary adenomas and related lesions with emphasis on transsphenoidal surgery. Appleton-Century-Crofts, New York, pp 15–31

Raudzens P A 1982 Intraoperative monitoring of evoked potentials. Annals of the New York Academy of Science 388: 308–326

Renou A M, Vernhiet J, Macrez P, Constant P, Billerey J, Khadaroo M Y, Caille J M 1978 Cerebral blood flow and metabolism during etomidate anesthesia in man. British Journal of Anaesthesia 50: 1047–1051

Robertson G L 1984 Abnormalities of thirst regulation. Kidney International 25: 460–469

Robinson A G 1985 Disorders of antidiuretic hormone secretion. Clinics in Endocrinology and Metabolism 14: 55–88

Robinson A G 1988 Regulation and pathophysiology of posterior pituitary function. In: Collu R, Brown G M, Van Loon G R (eds) Clinical neuroendocrinology. Blackwell Scientific, Boston, pp 65–90

Russ W, Fraedrich G, Hehrlein F W, Hempelmann G 1985 Intraoperative somatosensory evoked potentials as a prognostic factor of neurologic state after carotid endarterectomy. Thoracic and Cardiovascular Surgery 33: 392–396

Sachs E, Furlow F C 1936 The significance of convulsion in the diagnosis of brain tumors. Journal of the Missouri State Medical Association 33: 121–127

Sakabe T, Kuramoto T, Inoue S, Takeshita H 1978 Cerebral effects of nitrous oxide in the dog. Anesthesiology 48: 195–200

Sakabe T, Maekawa T, Fujii S, Ishikawa T, Tateishi A, Takeshita H 1983 Cerebral circulation and metabolism during enflurane anesthesia in humans. Anesthesiology 59: 532–536

Samra S K, Lilly D J, Rush N L, Kirsh M M 1984 Fentanyl anesthesia and human brain stem auditory evoked potentials. Anesthesiology 61: 261–265

Samra S K, Krutak-Krol H, Pohorecki R, Domino E F 1985 Scopolamine, morphine and brain stem auditory evoked potentials in awake monkeys. Anesthesiology 62: 437–441

Samra S K, Vanderzant C W, Domer P A, Sackellarcs C 1987 Differential effects of isoflurane on human median nerve somatosensory evoked potentials. Anesthesiology 66: 29–35

Samson D, Beyer C W Jr 1982 Furosemide in the intraoperative reduction of intracranial pressure in the patient with subarachnoid hemorrhage. Neurosurgery 10: 167–169

Scheller M S, Todd M M, Drummond J C 1986 Isoflurane, halothane, and regional cerebral blood flow at various levels of $PaCO_2$ in rabbits. Anesthesiology 64: 598–604

Schubert A, Zornow M H, Drummond J C, Luerssen T G 1986 Loss of cortical evoked responses due to intracranial gas during posterior fossa craniectomy in the seated position. Anesthesia and Analgesia 65: 203–206

Sebel P S, Lowdon J D 1989 Propofol: a new intravenous anesthetic. Anesthesiology 71: 260–277

Sebel P S, Flynn P J, Ingram D A 1984 Effect of nitrous oxide on visual, auditory and somatosensory evoked potentials. British Journal of Anaesthesia 56: 1403–1407

Seward J B, Hayes D L, Smith H C et al 1984 Platypnea-orthodeoxia: clinical profile, diagnostic workup, management and report of seven cases. Mayo Clinic Proceedings 59: 221–231

Shirane R, Weinstein P K 1992 Effect of mannitol on local cerebral blood flow after temporary complete cerebral ischemia in rats. Journal of Neurosurgery 76: 486–492

Skahen S, Shapiro H M, Drummond J C, Todd M M, Zelman V 1986 Nitrous oxide withdrawal reduces intracranial pressure in the presence of pneumocephalus. Anesthesiology 65: 192–195

Sloan T B, Koht A 1985 Depression of cortical somatosensory evoked potentials by nitrous oxide. British Journal of Anaesthesia 57: 849–852

Southwick J P, Katz J 1979 Unusual airway difficulty in the acromegalic patient—indications for tracheostomy. Anesthesiology 51: 72–73

Standefer M, Bay J W, Trusso D O 1984 The sitting position in neurosurgery: a retrospective analysis of 488 cases. Neurosurgery 14: 649–658

Sterns R H 1989 Neurological deterioration following treatment for hyponatremia. American Journal of Kidney Diseases 13: 434–437

Sterns R H 1990 The management of symptomatic hyponatremia. Seminars in Nephrology 10: 503–514

Sterns R H 1991 The management of hyponatremic emergencies. Critical Care Clinics 7: 127–142

Sterns R H, Spital A 1990 Disorders of water balance. In: Kokko J P, Tannen R L (eds) Fluids and electrolytes, 2nd edn. W B Saunders, Philadelphia, p 139

Sterns R H, Riggs J E, Schochet S S Jr 1986 Osmotic demyelination syndrome following correction of hyponatremia. New England Journal of Medicine 314: 1535–1542

Sterns R H, Thomas D J, Herndon R M 1989 Brain dehydration and neurologic deterioration after rapid correction of hyponatremia. Kidney International 35: 69–75

Stockard J J, Sharbrough F W, Tinker J A 1978 Effects of hypothermia on the human brainstem auditory response. Annals of Neurology 3: 368–370

Stuart F P, Torres E, Fletcher R, Crocker D, Moore F D 1970 Effects of single, repeated and massive mannitol infusion in the dog — structural and functional changes in kidney and brain. Annals of Surgery 172: 190–204

Stullken E H, Milde J H, Michenfelder J D, Tinker J H 1977 The nonlinear responses of cerebral metabolism to low concentrations of halothane, enflurane, isoflurane, and thiopental. Anesthesiology 46: 28–34

Symington B E 1986 Hetastarch and bleeding complications, letter. Annals of Internal Medicine 105: 627–628

Symon L, Wang A D, Costa E Silva I E, Gentili F 1984 Perioperative use of somatosensory evoked responses in aneurysm surgery. Journal of Neurosurgery 60: 269–275

Takaki O, Okumura F 1985 Application and limitation of somatosensory evoked potential monitoring during thoracic aortic aneurysm surgery: a case report. Anesthesiology 63: 700–703

Takeshita H, Okuda Y, Sari A 1972 The effects of ketamine on cerebral circulation and metabolism in man. Anesthesiology 36: 69–75

Tasch M D 1983 Endocrine diseases. In: Stoelting R K, Dierdorf S F (eds) Anesthesia and co-existing disease. Churchill Livingstone, New York, pp 473–515

Theye R A, Michenfelder J D 1968a The effect of halothane on canine cerebral metabolism. Anesthesiology 29: 1113–1118

Theye R A, Michenfelder J D 1968b The effect of nitrous oxide on canine cerebral metabolism. Anesthesiology 29: 1119–1124

Thornton C, Catley D M, Jordon C, Lehane J R, Royston D, Jones J G 1983 Enflurane anaesthesia causes graded changes in the brainstem and early cortical auditory evoked response in man. British Journal of Anaesthesia 55: 479–486

Thornton C, Heneghan C P H, James M F M, Jones J G 1984 Effects of halothane or enflurane with controlled ventilation on auditory evoked potentials. British Journal of Anaesthesia 56: 315–323

Thornton C, Heneghan C P H, Navaratnarajah M, Bateman P E, Jones J G 1985 Effect of etomidate on the auditory evoked response in man. British Journal of Anaesthesia 57: 554–561

Thurston J H, Hauhart R E, Nelson J S 1987 Adaptive decreases in amino acids (taurine in particular), creatine, electrolytes prevent cerebral edema in chronically hyponatremic mice—rapid correction (experimental model of central pontine myelinolysis) causes dehydration and shrinkage of brain. Metabolic Brain Diseases 2: 223–241

Thurston J H, Sherman W R, Hauhart R E, Kloepper R F 1989 Myo-inositol—a newly identified non-nitrogenous osmoregulatory molecule in mammalian brain. Pediatric Research 26: 482–485

Tindall G T, McLanahan C S 1980 Hyperfunctional pituitary tumors: pre- and postoperative management considerations. Clinical Neurosurgery 27: 48–82

Todd M M, Drummond J C 1984 A comparison of the cerebrovascular and metabolic effects of halothane and isoflurane in the cat. Anesthesiology 60: 276–282

Toung T, Ngeow Y K, Long D L, Rogers M C, Traystman R J 1984 Comparison of the effects of positive end-expiratory pressure and jugular venous compression on canine cerebral venous pressure. Anesthesiology 61: 169–172

Unni V K, Gray W J, Young M B 1986 Effects of atracurium on intracranial pressure in man. Anaesthesia 41: 1047–1049

Van Aken H, Puchstein C, Schweppe M-L, Heinecke A 1982 Effect of labetalol on intracranial pressure in dogs with and without intracranial hypertension. Acta Anaesthesiologica Scandinavica 26: 615–619

Van Rheineck Leyssius A T, Kalkman C J, Bovill J G 1986 Influence of moderate hypothermia on posterior tibial nerve somatosensory potentials. Anesthesia and Analgesia 65: 475–480

Vauzelle C, Stagnara P, Jouvinroux P 1973 Functional monitoring of spinal cord activity during spinal surgery. Clinical Orthopaedics and Related Research 93: 173–178

Verbalis J G, Robinson A G, Moses A M 1985 Postoperative and post-traumatic diabetes insipidus. Frontiers of Hormone Research 13: 247–265

Vokes T J, Robertson G L 1988 Disorders of antidiuretic hormone. Endocrinology and Metabolism Clinics of North America 17: 281–299

Wijdicks E F M, Ropper A H, Hunnicutt E J, Richardson G S, Nathanson J A 1991 Atrial natriuretic factor and salt wasting after aneurysmal subarachnoid hemorrhage. Stroke 22: 1519–1524

Williams G H 1988 Converting-enzyme inhibitors in the treatment of hypertension. New England Journal of Medicine 319: 1517–1525

York D, Legan M, Benner S, Watts C 1984 Further studies with a noninvasive method of intracranial pressure estimation. Neurosurgery 14: 456–460

Youmans J R, Cobb C A 1982 Glial and neuronal tumors of the brain in adults. In: Youmans J R (ed) Neurological surgery. W B Saunders, Philadelphia, pp 2759–2835

Young M L, Smith D S, Murtagh F, Vasquez A, Levitt J 1986 Comparison of surgical and anesthetic complications in neurosurgical patients experiencing venous air embolism in the sitting position. Neurosurgery 18: 157–161

Zaloga G P 1992 Hyperosmolar states. In: Givetta J M, Taylor R W, Kirby R R (eds) Critical care. J B Lippincott, Philadelphia, p 455

Ziegler M G 1988 Antihypertensive therapy. In: Chernow B (ed) The pharmacologic approach to the critically ill patient, 2nd edn. Williams & Wilkins, Baltimore, pp 377–378

15. Surgical principles in the management of brain tumors

Robert G. Ojemann

PREOPERATIVE MANAGEMENT

General considerations

The decision to remove a brain tumor is based on an evaluation of the clinical history and findings, the results of the radiographic studies, an evaluation of the benefits and risks of the management options and a detailed discussion with the patient. The surgeon should take a complete history from the patient or, if necessary, from the family to have a clear understanding of the symptoms and how they are affecting the life of the patient. When discussing the operation, it is important to assess the patient's hopes and expectations from the procedure. A clear presentation should be made of the impact of tumor removal on presenting symptoms and the immediate and long-term benefits and risks.

Once the decision has been made to perform surgery, careful planning is required and several management decisions will need to be made. These include an evaluation of the imaging studies and assessment of the overall medical status. Associated hydrocephalus may need to be managed. The operative approach must be carefully considered and decisions made about special equipment needs, the use of intraoperative monitoring and whether a stereotactic biopsy or a stereotactic craniotomy may be needed.

Evaluation of imaging studies

Most brain tumors will be diagnosed by magnetic resonance imaging (MRI) with gadolinium enhancement. The surgeon must decide if this study gives all the information needed to perform the operation. The questions one should consider are:

- Does the type of suspected pathology or the surgical approach being considered require angiography (magnetic resonance or conventional) to evaluate abnormal vascularity, the position of normal blood vessels or the status of the venous sinuses?
- Is computed tomography (CT) needed to evaluate bone anatomy, erosion, calcification or bone pathology?
- Will three-dimensional reconstruction be helpful?
- Would positron emission tomography give useful information?
- If there is abnormal vascular supply to the tumor, should embolization be planned in relation to the operative procedure?
- If the tumor involves the internal carotid artery, should a test occlusion be done?

Medical evaluation and treatment

As part of the initial history the physician must determine if there are any medical problems in the patient's history that require further treatment or evaluation prior to surgery (Allen & Johnston 1990). This assessment should include any adverse response to previous operations, recent medications, and inquiries about bleeding disorders, diabetes, cardiopulmonary problems, allergic reactions, and other types of pathology such as problems in the neck or back that might interfere with positioning. Cardiac and antihypertensive medications are usually continued up to the time of surgery. The patient is advised to avoid aspirin compounds for at least a week prior to operation.

The usual laboratory preoperative evaluation includes blood count, urinalysis, blood sugar, blood urea nitrogen and creatine, electrolytes, coagulation studies (prothrombin time, partial thromboplastin time and platelet count), chest X-ray and electrocardiogram.

The initiation of steroids is another decision that needs attention. If there is significant brain edema, it is this author's practice to prescribe steroids for several days prior to surgery. Even when there is little or no edema but there is going to be significant brain manipulation or retraction, steroids are often begun 48 hours prior to operation unless there is a medical contraindication such as diabetes. Depending on the location of the tumor, a decision will also need to be made about starting anticonvulsant medication.

Management of hydrocephalus

Some patients with brain tumors will have enlarged ventricles on the imaging study. If there are no symptoms or signs of either normal pressure or high-pressure hydrocephalus, nothing needs to be done. If there is a high probability that symptomatic hydrocephalus will be relieved by tumor removal, then the use of perioperative steroids combined in some patients with cerebrospinal fluid drainage at operation is sufficient treatment. In a few patients a ventriculostomy will be left in place for several days and a trial occlusion done to determine if a ventriculo-peritoneal shunt is needed. A ventriculo-peritoneal shunt is done if there is symptomatic hydrocephalus and an adequate decompression of the tumor cannot be accomplished.

In some elderly patients with a symptomatic normal-pressure hydrocephalus syndrome associated with cerebellopontine angle or other skull base tumors, a ventriculo-peritoneal shunt may be the only operation needed. A small group of elderly patients with symptoms from hydrocephalus and with brainstem compression from a large acoustic neurinoma have required a ventriculo-peritoneal shunt and a subtotal removal of the tumor under the same anesthesia, with good results (Ojemann 1993a).

PERIOPERATIVE MANAGEMENT

When the patient arrives in the preoperative area, appropriate intravenous lines are inserted, electrocardiogram leads are placed and a catheter is inserted into the radial artery for continuous monitoring of blood pressure. Intravenous antibiotics are administered. Alternating thigh-high air compression boots are placed on each lower extremity. Careful induction of anesthesia is done to try to avoid episodes of hypotension and hypertension.

After the induction of anesthesia, the eyes are protected with an adhesive patch. A catheter is placed in the bladder. Most patients with a brain tumor are given 10–20 mg of furosemide intravenously shortly after the catheter is inserted. As the surgical area is being prepared, a 20% solution of mannitol is given in a dosage of 1–1.5 g/kg over 20–30 minutes. During the operation, the steroids and antibiotics are continued at 6-hour intervals.

In a situation where adequate cerebrospinal fluid (CSF) drainage may not be possible, particularly when frontal lobe retraction may be required, a lumbar drain is inserted. In some cerebellopontine angle tumors, the cistern is opened and a catheter placed in the area to drain CSF during the operation (Ojemann 1993a).

MONITORING

The anesthesiologist continuously monitors intra-arterial blood pressure, electrocardiogram, oxygen saturation and end-tidal pCO_2. When the semi-sitting position is used or the head is well-elevated, a central venous line and precordial Doppler monitoring are placed.

The surgeon must decide if any special type of intraoperative monitoring will be required. For supratentorial lesions, is cortical electrical stimulation going to be needed to locate the motor cortex? Does the patient need to be awake for language localization? Will electrocorticography be needed in a patient with a seizure disorder?

For infratentorial lesions, plans for cranial nerve monitoring need to be considered. All patients having surgery for cerebellopontine angle tumors should have facial nerve function monitored (Ojemann & Martuza 1990). Monitoring of other cranial nerves is done as indicated.

OPERATIVE MANAGEMENT

Chapters on the general aspects of neurosurgical operative procedures for brain tumors have been included in many publications (see References). Key considerations in removal of a brain tumor include thorough evaluation of the imaging studies, an understanding of the normal and pathologic anatomy, careful positioning of the patient, a well-planned incision and exposure, a familiarity with microsurgical techniques, avoidance of excessive brain retraction, minimal exposure of normal brain tissue, and proper closure. For benign tumors one plans for early interruption of the blood supply, minimal brain retraction whenever possible, internal decompression of the tumor, dissection of the tumor capsule by retraction into the area of decompression, and removal of involved dura and bone if indicated. If the tumor is malignant there should be removal of as much of the tumor as possible while trying to preserve function using stereotactic localization and intraoperative monitoring when indicated.

Microsurgical anatomy

It is essential that the surgeon have a full understanding of the normal anatomy in three dimensions as well as how the tumor is likely to alter the position of the normal anatomic structures. In planning and thinking about the operation the surgeon should not hesitate to consult appropriate surgical or anatomic texts or references. There is nothing wrong with bringing these texts to the operating room if one feels they will be of help, particularly in difficult or rarely performed procedures. Many publications describe the brain anatomy in detail, and the *Stereo Atlas of Operative Microneurosurgery* (Poletti & Ojemann 1985) gives a three-dimensional description of pathological anatomy.

Instrumentation

Instruments needed for brain tumor removal are operating loupes, an operating microscope, a self-retaining retractor system, monopolar and bipolar coagulation, and a full array of microsurgical instruments (Tew & Steiger 1985, Al-Mefty 1989, Rhoton 1990, 1993). It is helpful to have a system to keep the irrigation fluid near body temperature. The many factors that relate to the surgeon's comfort and hand control during the operation have been summarized by Al-Mefty (1989).

Operating loupes are used for the incision, bone removal, dural opening and, depending on the location of the tumor, the initial placement of the self-retaining retractors. In some superficial tumors they are used for the entire operation. Details regarding magnification with the operating microscope in relation to the size and depth of field have been outlined (Tew & Steiger 1985, Rhoton 1990, 1993, Tew & Scodary 1993a). Although this author uses the Greenberg self-retaining retractor system, other satisfactory systems are available (Greenberg 1985). The microsurgical instruments should include bayonet-type bipolar and tumor forceps, straight and curved scissors, needle holders for microsutures, cup forceps, sharp and dull nerve hooks, several types of dissectors and microcurettes (Heifetz 1993, Rhoton 1993). Suction tips of various sizes are necessary, and the suction power should be able to be regulated with a variable control mechanism on the central system. Other essential equipment includes a high-speed air drill, ultrasonic aspirator (Epstein 1985), laser (Cerullo 1985, Boggan & Powers 1990), cautery loops to use with the monopolar coagulation, equipment for ultrasound localization (Dohrmann & Rubin 1985, McGahan et al 1990) and a nerve stimulator.

Heifetz (1993) has outlined principles for the proper use of the bipolar forceps:

1. The current should be set to as low a setting as possible.
2. The coagulation works best if there is a small amount of fluid around the tips.
3. One should wait to start the current flow until the vessel has been grasped.
4. If one blade of an open noninsulated bipolar forceps inadvertently touches tissue while the current is on, the current may try to ground through the tissue with possible damage.
5. When changing from a standard to fine forceps, the current setting should be reduced to lessen the tendency for the forceps to form coagulum and stick to or rupture the blood vessel.
6. The surgeon should slightly open and close the forceps during coagulation.
7. The forceps should be carefully cleaned between each use with a moist sponge.

Position and preparation

Proper positioning of the patient is planned to provide optimal exposure and avoid the need for excessive brain retraction. The position must be comfortable for the surgeon, avoid any abnormal physiologic alteration in the patient, and allow access by the anesthesiologist. In many operations the table is turned so there is a space under the head, allowing the surgeon to sit comfortably with his or her feet under the table. There is usually slight flexion at the knees and hips of the patient. Extra padding is placed as needed to prevent pressure on important structures such as the ulnar and peroneal nerves and bony prominences. If a lateral position is being used, an axillary roll may be needed to prevent compression of the brachial plexus. If the neck is to be flexed or rotated, one must ensure that there is no compromise of venous drainage from the head. In the variations of the supine position, the shoulder on the side of the operation may need to be elevated to avoid excessive rotation of the neck. Illustrations of some of the most important aspects of the different positions and prevention of complications have been presented in chapters in this book and in previous publications (Ojemann 1985, Stewart & Krawchenko 1985, Ojemann et al 1988, Maroon & Abla 1990, Ojemann & Martuza 1990, Ojemann 1991, Kelly & Lyerly 1993, Ojemann 1993a,b,c, Ojemann & Ogilvy 1993, Sekhar & Janecka 1993, Tew & Scodary 1993a,b).

Positioning is facilitated by frequent comparison of the MRI study to external landmarks and the lateral contour of the head. The head is held with the Mayfield-Kees skeletal fixation headrest. It is important to place the three pins so they are as close to perpendicular to the skull as possible. If they are too tangential they may slip or cause a pressure necrosis of the scalp. The Gardner or Sugita headholder may also be used (Heifetz 1993).

The preparation of the surgical site follows standard surgical principles. Hair is clipped well beyond the area to be exposed and the head is shaved after the induction of general anesthesia. Adherent drapes are placed around the margins of the operative field, sealing it from surrounding hair. The scalp is then prepared using appropriate solutions.

Incision

The scalp incision is planned to provide optimal exposure as well as adequate blood supply to the scalp, and is marked with a sterile marking pen. Comparison of external landmarks and measurement to the radiographic images is important. Key external landmarks that can be seen or felt include the midline along the vertex, external ear canal, glabella, occipital protuberance and coronal suture. When determining the incision for midline supratentorial lesions it is often helpful to look at the head from directly lateral and compare the contour of the midline with the midline sagittal MR image. After placing sterile towels around the area, the skin is covered with an adherent steridrape.

After the skin incision is made, bleeding from the scalp is controlled with scalp clips or Dandy clamps placed on the galea. Our routine includes turning the scalp flap with the pericranial tissue and temporalis muscle. A gauze roll is placed under the base of the skin flap to give a rounded contour and prevent a sharp kink that might interfere with the circulation to the flap. When a pericranial graft is needed to replace dura or reinforce an area, it is easily taken from the back of the scalp flap where it has been kept moist with an antibiotic-soaked sponge.

Cranial opening

A free bone flap is this author's preference. To elevate the bone flap, one or more burr holes are used depending on the surgeon's preference. The dura is freed from the overlying bone with a Penfield #3 dissector. The bone flap is then cut with a high speed craniotome. If the dura does not separate easily, which may be the case in some elderly patients, burr holes are made closer together. If the tumor has grown through the dura to extensively involve the bone, a segment of the bone flap may be left attached to the tumor. If there is only slight involvement of the inner table of the skull, the bone flap is separated and the abnormal bone involving the inner table removed with a high speed air drill. Bleeding from the bone is controlled with bone wax. Small drill holes are made at appropriate intervals and fine sutures are placed to tent the dura to the bone edge to control epidural bleeding. These small holes are also used to place stainless steel wires to hold the bone flap. In addition to bipolar coagulation, hemostasis is achieved by using Gelfoam and oxidized regenerated cellulose (Surgicel) (Arand & Sawaya 1990). If one of the air sinuses is entered, special attention is required to prevent infection and the possibility of a cerebrospinal fluid leak. Before opening the dura, the skin margins are covered with antibiotic-soaked sponges and towels are placed around the operative area.

Dural opening

The dura is opened to give adequate visualization, and care is taken to minimize the exposure of normal brain tissue. Normal brain that is exposed or is to be retracted should be protected with a rubber dam covered with a cottonoid. When opening the dura and while doing the initial exposure the venous anatomy needs to be kept in mind. Veins along the anterior third of the sagittal sinus, the middle cerebral vein along the sphenoid wing and the petrosal vein in the cerebellopontine angle can be taken to aid the exposure. Cortical veins along the middle and posterior thirds of the sagittal sinus, the internal cerebral veins, vein of Galen and the vein of Labbe, however, need to be preserved to avoid potential problems with venous infarction.

Surgical approaches

Bifrontal

The patient is placed in the supine position. The elevation and flexion and extension of the head depend on the tumor being treated (Ojemann 1991, 1993c). A coronal incision marked just behind the anterior hairline is made through the galea, taking care to preserve the pericranial tissue (Fig. 15.1). If extra pericranial tissue will be needed to cover the floor of the anterior fossa or be used to patch the convexity dura, the skin along the posterior aspect of the incision is elevated one to two centimeters and the pericranial tissue is incised. The scalp flap and underlying tissue, including the pericranial tissue, are then turned down together. Burr holes are placed just below the end of the anterior temporal line (key hole) and on each side of the sagittal sinus anterior to the skin incision. The bone flap is usually cut in one piece, with the bone cut just above the supraorbital ridge being made from each side as far medially as possible. Because of the irregular bone projecting from the inner table of the skull in this area, it is usually not possible to cut completely across the area. Usually this leaves a centimeter or less of bone in the midline. The outer table of bone is cut with a small burr on the high speed air drill and then the inner table can be broken as the bone is elevated and the free bone flap removed. The frontal sinuses are almost always entered. The mucosa is removed and the sinuses packed with antibiotic-soaked Gelfoam. If the operation is going to be entirely intradural, a small flap of pericranial tissue from the back of the scalp flap is turned down over the sinus

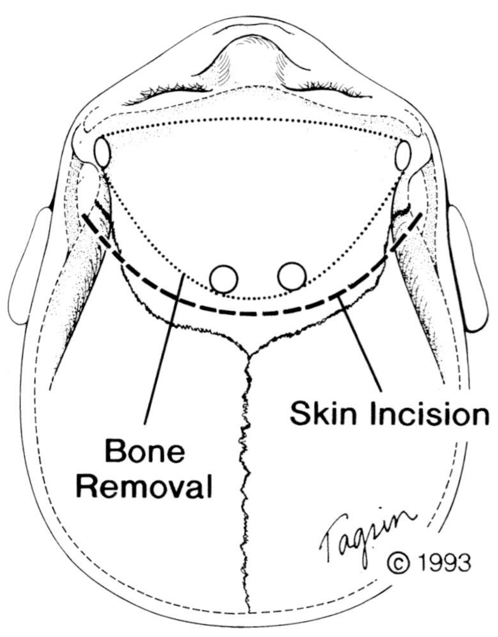

Fig. 15.1 Bifrontal approach.

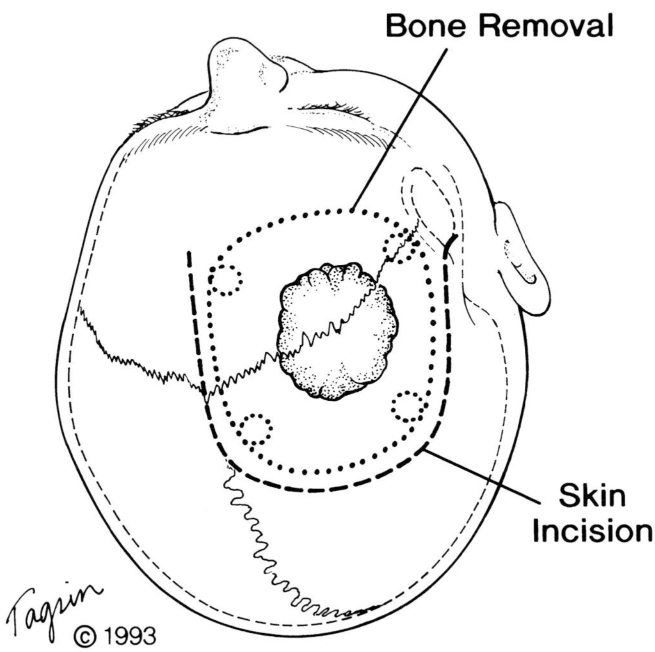

Fig. 15.2 Middle frontal approach.

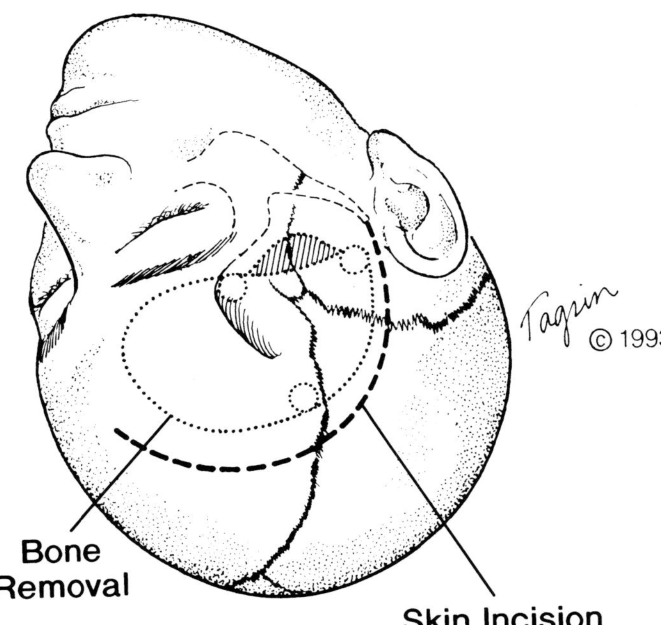

Fig. 15.3 Frontotemporal (pterional) approach.

and sewn to the adjacent dura (Ojemann 1985, 1991, 1993c).

Middle frontal

The patient is in the supine position with the ipsilateral shoulder elevated as needed. The head is elevated so that the convexity over the center of the tumor is at the highest point (Ojemann 1993c, Ojemann & Ogilvy 1993). For tumors in the general region of the coronal suture the skin flap is turned forward (Fig. 15.2). The incision starts at the anterior hairline, extends posteriorly along or parallel to the midline (on the opposite side if necessary) as far as needed, turns inferiorly and then anteriorly to end at about the frontotemporal junction.

Frontotemporal (pterional)

The patient is in the supine position with the ipsilateral shoulder elevated. The degree of head rotation depends on the location of the tumor which is being approached (Ojemann 1985, Ojemann et al 1988, Ojemann 1991, 1993c). The skin incision is made just above the zygomatic process behind the anterior hairline and extends medially to end near the midline at the hairline (Fig. 15.3). If the incision is too far forward the frontal branch of the facial nerve may be injured. The skin, underlying temporalis muscle and pericranial tissue are turned down together, exposing the anterior and lateral inferior frontal and anterior temporal bone. The temporalis muscle may be cut to expose the zygomatic process. A burr hole is placed just below the anterior end of the superior temporal line (key hole). A second burr hole is placed over the anterior temporal lobe and others are used depending on the surgeon's preference. When cutting across the greater wing of the sphenoid bone, resistance may be felt and the cut will need to go superiorly around this area with a craniotome or a burr used to cut through the area. After the bone flap is elevated the lateral portion of the sphenoid wing is removed as is bone over the anterior temporal region.

Frontotemporal (extended temporal)

For tumors in the anterior and medial aspects of the temporal lobe and middle fossa, the pterional exposure may be modified by curving the incision around the top of the ear and extending it medially and anteriorly (Fig. 15.4) (Ojemann et al 1988). The bone removal is similar to that described for the pterional approach but more of the temporal lobe is exposed. This approach allows exposure of the anterior and medial temporal area along the sphenoid wing by providing the ability to retract both the frontal and anterior temporal lobes.

To improve the access to the floor of the middle fossa and sphenoid wing, the skin incision can be carried below the zygoma if it is close to the ear. The zygomatic arch is transected and the temporalis muscle retracted into the space formerly occupied by the zygomatic arch.

Temporal

The patient is placed in a semi-lateral position with the ipsilateral shoulder well elevated. The head is usually

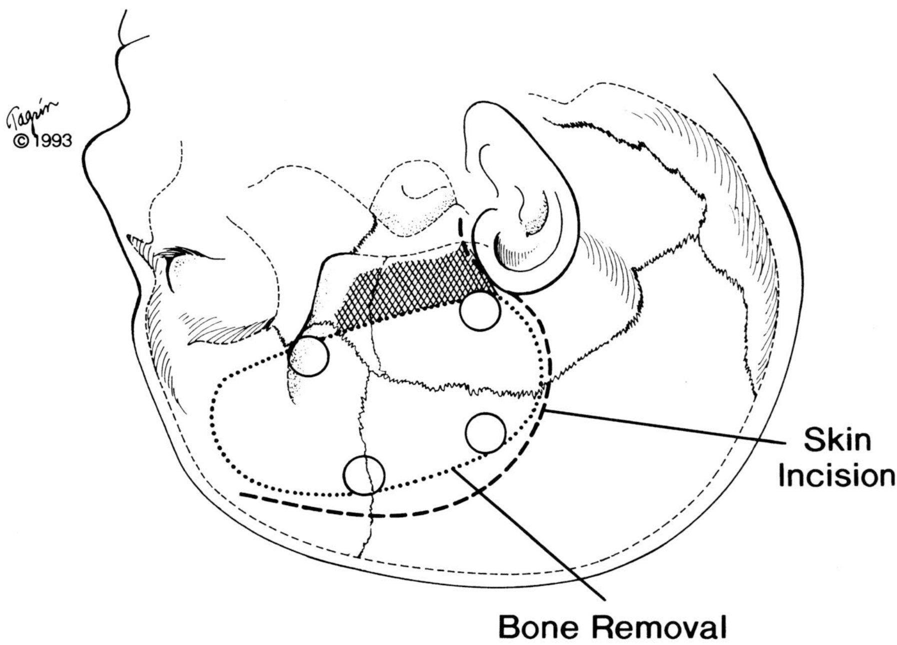

Fig. 15.4 Frontotemporal (extended temporal) approach.

nearly parallel to the floor. The degree of head extension depends on the type of tumor being treated. Tumors in the middle and posterior temporal region can be exposed by a horseshoe-shaped scalp flap based along the floor of the middle fossa (Fig. 15.5). The incision starts just behind the anterior hairline, extends medially to the superior temporal line, goes posteriorly and then inferiorly to end above the mastoid area. If the incision is too far forward or extends below the zygomatic process, the frontal branch of the facial nerve may be injured. After the bone flap is elevated, further bone may be removed to take the exposure to the floor of the middle fossa.

Posterior frontal-parietal (vertex)

The patient is placed in a semi-lateral, semi-sitting position with the head well elevated so that the scalp over the center of the tumor is uppermost (Ojemann et al

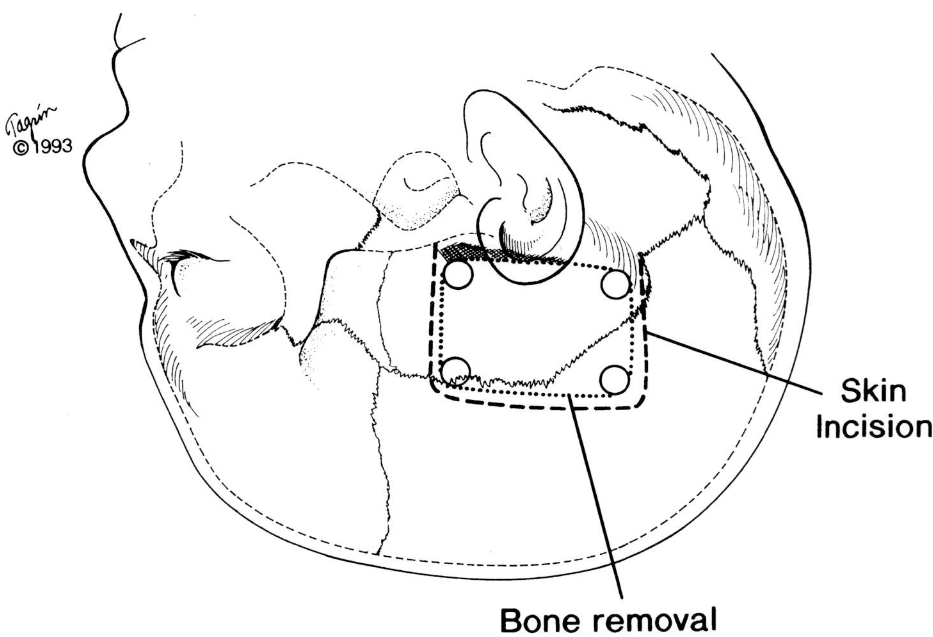

Fig. 15.5 Temporal approach.

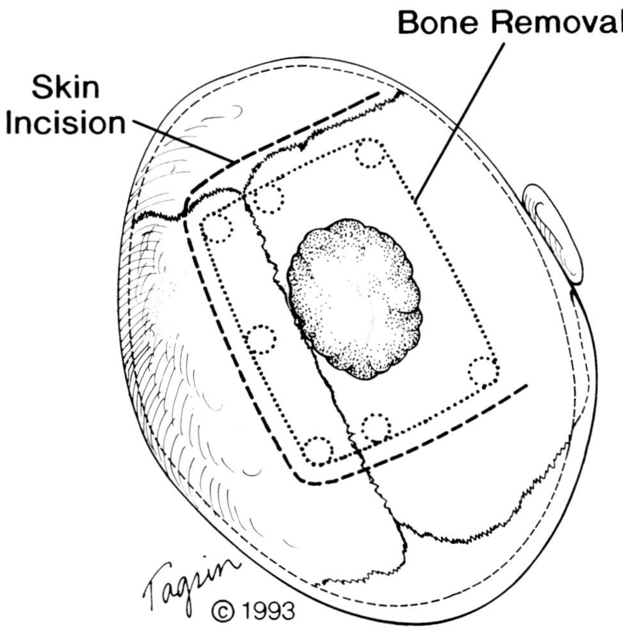

Fig. 15.6 Posterior frontal-parietal (vertex) approach.

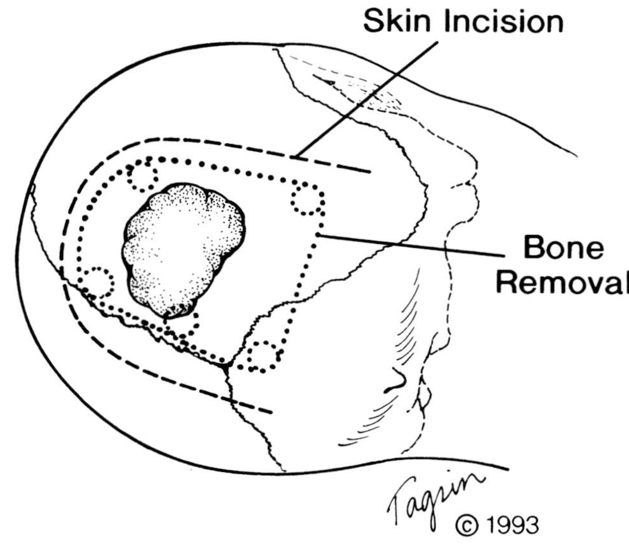

Fig. 15.7 Occipital approach.

1988, Ojemann 1993c, Ojemann & Ogilvy 1993). A horseshoe-shaped incision is made, extending approximately 2 cm across the midline with the anterior and posterior branch of the incision placed to give adequate exposure (Fig. 15.6). Often seven or eight burr holes are used, two on each side of the sagittal sinus, one in the midportion of the contralateral side and two or three across the base. The dural separation and bone cut over the sagittal sinus are done last. As the bone flap is elevated, Gelfoam covered with Surgicel and a cottonoid are placed directly over the sagittal sinus. If the bone is markedly adherent to dura, the bone flap can be elevated in two sections. The first is on the side of the tumor with the medial cut approximately 1 cm from the midline. The second section of bone is then cut and the sagittal sinus exposed under direct vision.

Occipital

The patient is placed in the lateral position using an axillary roll and the head elevated and turned toward the floor to bring the center of the tumor to the highest point (Ojemann 1993c, Ojemann & Ogilvy 1993). The skin incision is horseshoe-shaped, based on the posterior temporal-inferior occipital region, and may be extended across the midline if necessary (Fig. 15.7). The handling of the bone flap is similar to that described in the previous section.

Temporal suboccipital

Modifications of this approach may be used to reach tumors involving the clivus, petrous bone, middle fossa and cerebellopontine angle. The patient is positioned with the ipsilateral shoulder well elevated and the head turned to the opposite side, often nearly parallel to the floor (Ojemann et al 1988). The angle of the exposure can be altered by rotating the table from side to side. The incision starts in front of the ear and curves posteriorly no higher than the superior temporal line. About 2 cm posterior to the mastoid area the incision is carried inferiorly (Fig. 15.8). It can stop just below the level of the mastoid process or can be gently curved onto the neck so that the carotid bifurcation and internal jugular vein can be exposed. A bone flap may be removed above and below the transverse sinus in one or two parts. The same precautions noted with the sagittal sinus are followed. Further bone is removed as needed to expose the sigmoid sinus and the dura anterior to the sinus.

Suboccipital (lateral)

This approach is used for tumors in the cerebellopontine angle and in the lateral cerebellum. The patient is in the supine position with the ipsilateral shoulder slightly elevated and the head turned parallel to the floor (Ojemann & Martuza 1990, Ojemann 1993a). The line of sight may be altered by rotating the table side to side. A vertical incision is made, centered 2 cm medial to the mastoid process (Fig. 15.9). A single burr hole is placed in the bone over the lateral posterior fossa and a bone flap is cut over the lateral two thirds of the cerebellar hemisphere. Further bone is removed as needed to expose the transverse and sigmoid sinuses. Mastoid air cells are usually entered and are occluded with bone wax.

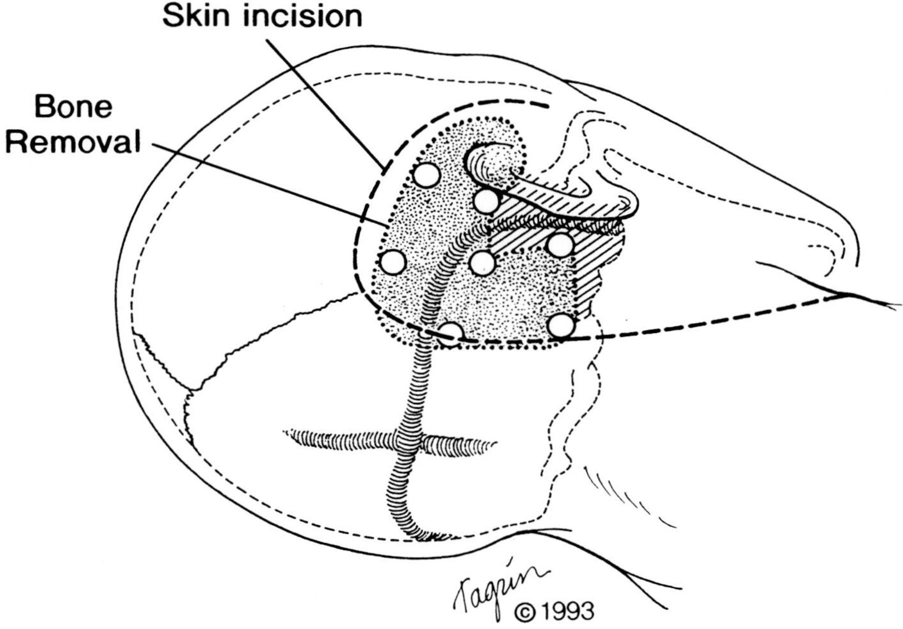

Fig. 15.8 Temporal-suboccipital approach.

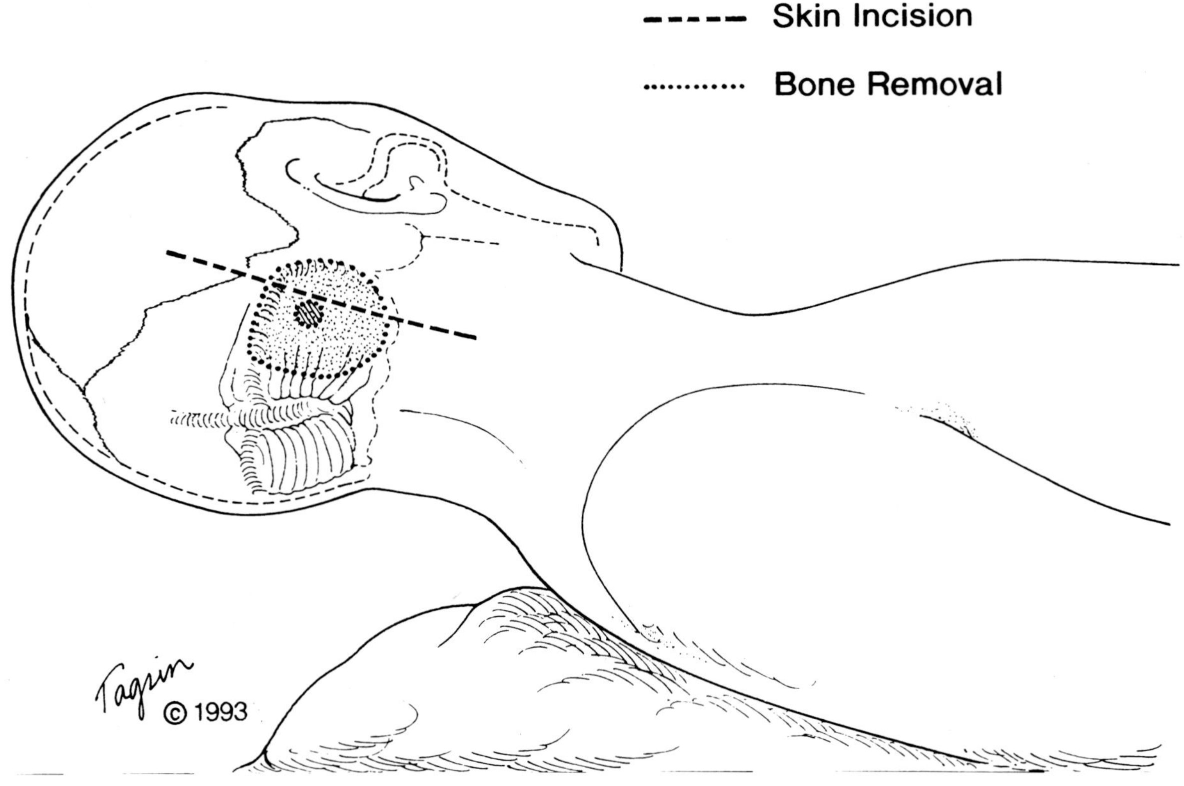

Fig. 15.9 Suboccipital (lateral) approach.

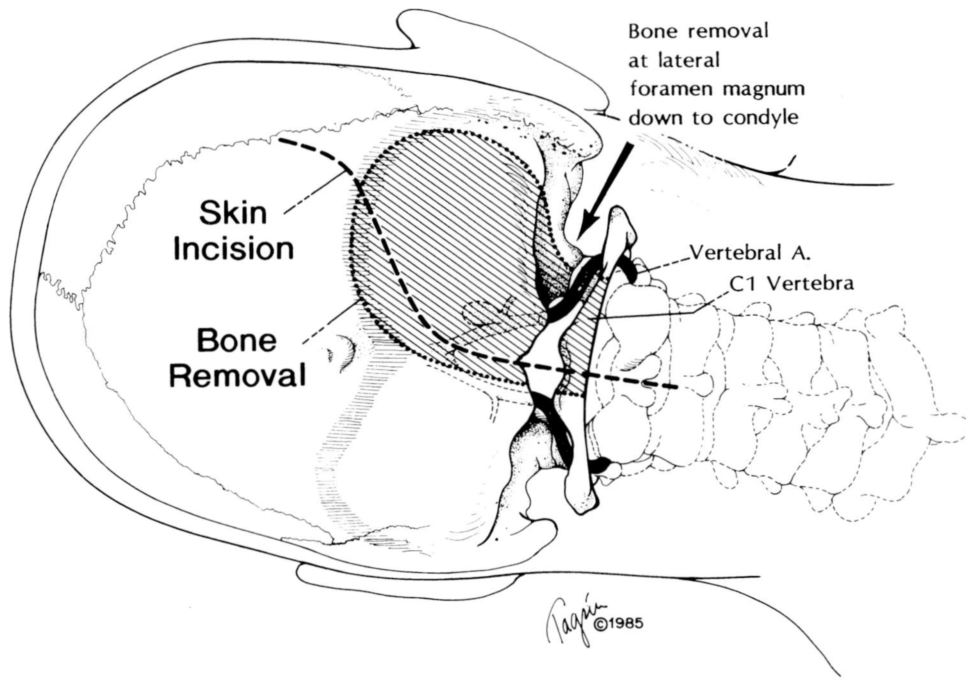

Fig. 15.10 Suboccipital (far lateral) approach.

Suboccipital (far lateral)

The patient is placed in the lateral position with the head slightly elevated and tilted toward the ipsilateral shoulder (Ojemann et al 1988). The skin incision and craniectomy are shown in Figure 15.10. Removal of the rim of the foramen magnum is carried laterally to just behind the occipital condyle. The posterior arch of C1 is removed from the arterial sulcus of the vertebral artery laterally to just beyond the midline medially.

Suboccipital (midline)

I prefer the prone position for most patients but a semi-sitting or lateral oblique position can be used (Tew & Scodary 1993b). A midline incision is made, staying in the plane between the paraspinal-occipital muscles (Fig. 15.11). The muscles are detached to expose the midline bone. A craniectomy is done, removing bone over both medial cerebellar hemispheres including the posterior rim of the foramen magnum. The posterior arch of C1 can be removed if needed. The dura is opened over each cerebellar hemisphere. The incisions are connected across the lower midline and a dural flap rotated superiorly. Bleeding from the occipital sinus is controlled with a running suture. In some patients the dura will also be opened across the foramen magnum and bleeding from the circular sinus may need to be controlled. When a more lateral exposure is needed for a large tumor of the cerebellar hemisphere, the incision is curved laterally (hockey-stick incision — Fig. 15.11).

Other skull base approaches

The surgeon should be familiar with the different approaches that can be used for tumor removal in the skull base (Ojemann 1993b, Sekhar & Janecka 1993). These include craniofacial procedures and approaches to the cavernous sinus. Anterior extradural approaches include transoral, transoral-labimandibular glossotomy, transoral and transpalatal, transsphenoidal, transethmoidal, transmaxillary or combinations of these. Lateral extradural-intradural approaches include translabyrinthine, transcochlear, petrosal and infratemporal.

Tumor removal

The objective of surgical intervention for most benign tumors is usually total removal of the tumor if possible. In some patients involvement with critical structures may prevent a complete excision. The surgeon must remember that the first priority is to try and preserve or improve neurologic function. For patients in whom total removal carries significant risk of morbidity, it may be better judgement to leave some tumor and plan to follow the patient or treat the residual tumor with radiation therapy.

For primary intrinsic brain tumors resection of as much of the tumor tissue as can be reasonably safely excised is planned. In some of these patients with deep tumors or tumors in critical areas, only a stereotactic biopsy may be indicated.

Solitary metastatic tumors are completely removed if they present in an operable location and there is a reason-

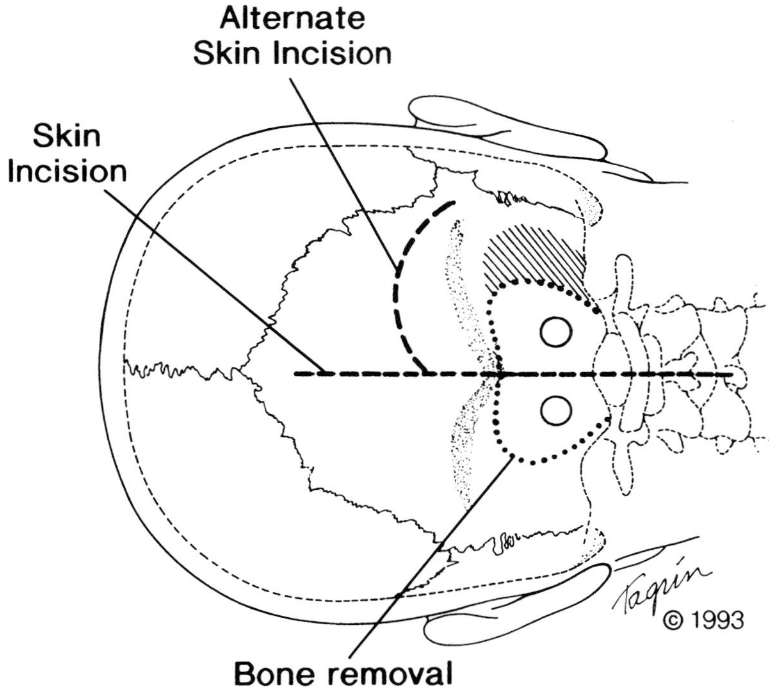

Fig. 15.11 Suboccipital (midline) approach.

able life expectancy. Occasionally, removal of a second metastasis may also be indicated.

The dura is opened to give adequate exposure, being careful not to expose any more brain than necessary. If dura is involved with tumor, such as with a convexity meningioma, it is removed with the tumor. Brain retraction is minimized by position of the patient, the use of furosemide and mannitol, the drainage of cerebrospinal fluid when indicated, and a well-planned exposure. The brain is protected by a rubber sheet covered with a cottonoid when retraction is required.

In many patients with benign tumors, safe removal of the tumor is facilitated by an extensive internal decompression using bipolar coagulation, sharp dissection, cautery loops or the Cavitron. Traction on the tumor capsule away from brain and nerve tissue minimizes the need for retraction of brain tissue and allows separation of vascular and arachnoid attachments. It may be necessary for alternate dissection of the tumor capsule and internal decompression. Cottonoids are also used to protect areas of brain that have been separated from the tumor capsule. Arterial vessels adherent to the capsule of the tumor should be preserved until the surgeon is sure they do not supply important brain tissue. Often, after internal decompression of the tumor, a vessel on the capsule of the tumor can be preserved using microsurgical dissection.

Closure

Careful hemostasis is essential. If not already the case, the patient's blood pressure is often raised to 140 mmHg. If a partial removal of tumor has been done, a single layer of Surgicel is left on the area of the resection as well as on any brain tissue that has been incised.

Usually no attempt is made to pull the retracted, sometimes dried dura together, but a graft of pericranial tissue allows a nice closure to be done. This tissue is also used to replace any defect from dura that was removed with the tumor. The dural closure can be reinforced with a sheet of Gelfoam. Just prior to completion of the dural closure, the subdural space and area of tumor removal are filled with saline (at body temperature) to displace as much air as possible. The bone flap is replaced and held with stainless steel wire inserted through the previously made small drill holes around the craniotomy opening. A wire is also placed across each burr hole and they can be filled with bone dust (collected when the burr holes were made) or acrylic cranioplasty material.

Prior to closing the scalp, the wound is irrigated with an antibiotic solution. The muscle, fascia and galea are closed in separate layers with absorbable sutures.

IMMEDIATE POSTOPERATIVE MANAGEMENT

At the conclusion of the operation, careful attention must be paid to the patient's blood pressure. Continuous monitoring should be done during transfer to the recovery room or intensive care unit and appropriate medications be immediately available to prevent hypertension. The usual precautions regarding an adequate airway are followed.

When a patient does not recover promptly from anesthesia or is not progressing as anticipated from a neurologic standpoint, an immediate CT scan is done to evaluate the presence of hematoma, hydrocephalus, edema, tension pneumocephalus and/or infarction. Subsequent treatment depends on the results of that scan.

Should there be a cerebrospinal fluid leak, a CT scan is done and, if there is no contraindication, a lumbar cerebrospinal fluid drain is placed for 72 hours. Antibiotics, which are usually given for 24 hours after surgery, are continued for as long as the drain is in place.

If the operation involves the pituitary stalk or hypothalamus the patient will need to be carefully observed for diabetes insipidus (see Ch. 14). This is treated with evaluation of electrolytes and osmolarity, fluid replacement and use of vasopressin as needed. After removal of a brain tumor a syndrome of inappropriate antidiuretic secretion hormone may occur. This is generally managed with fluid restriction. If the patient has diabetes, serum glucose is followed and management is done intraoperatively and postoperatively using a sliding scale of insulin.

Depending on the neurologic status and the degree of expected cerebral edema, steroids are gradually tapered over 5–10 days. For supratentorial tumors anticonvulsants are continued. How long they should be continued has not been defined. If there have been no preoperative seizures, this medication is discontinued within 2–3 months. An EEG is then done and the medication continued only if there is an abnormality that suggests a seizure focus. If the patient has had a preoperative seizure disorder, the anticonvulsant will be continued for at least several months and sometimes indefinitely, depending on several factors.

REFERENCES

Allen M B Jr, Johnston K W 1990 Preoperative evaluation: complications, their prevention and treatment. In: Youmans J R (ed) Neurological surgery. W B Saunders, Philadelphia, p 833

Al-Mefty O 1989 1. Ergonomics and cranial-base surgery 2. Power equipment. In: Surgery of the cranial base. Kluwer Academic, Boston, p 3

Arand A G, Sawaya R 1990 Intraoperative use of topical hemostatic agents in neurosurgery. In: Wilkins R H, Rengachary S S (eds) Neurosurgery update I. McGraw-Hill, New York, p 188

Boggan J E, Powers S K 1990 Use of lasers in neurological surgery. In: Youmans J R (ed) Neurological surgery. W B Saunders, Philadelphia, p 992

Cerullo L J 1985 Application of the laser to neurological surgery. In: Wilkins R H, Rengachary S S (eds) Neurosurgery. McGraw-Hill, New York, p 478

Ciric I S, Rosenblatt S 1993 Supratentorial craniotomies. In: Apuzzo M L J (ed) Brain surgery complications avoidance and management. Churchill Livingstone, New York, p 51

Dohrmann G J, Rubin J M 1985 Intraoperative diagnostic ultrasound. In: Wilkins R H, Rengachery S S (eds) Neurosurgery. McGraw-Hill, New York, p 457

Epstein F 1985 Ultrasound dissection. In: Wilkins R H, Rengachary S S (eds) Neurosurgery. McGraw-Hill, New York, p 476

Greenberg I M 1985 Self retaining retractors. In: Wilkins R H, Rengachary S S (eds) Neurosurgery. McGraw-Hill, New York, p 463

Grossman R G 1993 Preoperative and surgical planning for avoiding complications. In: Apuzzo M L J (ed) Brain surgery complications avoidance and management. Churchill Livingstone, New York, p 3

Heifetz M D 1993 Use and misuse of instruments. In: Apuzzo M L J (ed) Brain surgery complications avoidance and management. Churchill Livingstone, New York, p 71

Hoff J T, Clarke H B 1993 Adverse postoperative events. In: Apuzzo M L J (ed) Brain surgery complications avoidance and management. Churchill Livingstone, New York, p 99

Kelly D L Jr, Lyerly M A 1993 Infratentorial procedures — neoplastic disorders — problematical intraoperative events. In: Apuzzo M L J (ed) Brain surgery complications avoidance and management. Churchill Livingstone, New York, p 1671

McGahan J P, Boggan J E, Gooding G A W 1990 Intraoperative use of ultrasound. In: Youmans J R (ed) Neurological surgery. W B Saunders, Philadelphia, p 1033

Maroon J, Abla A 1990 General operative technique. In: Youmans J R (ed) Neurological surgery. W B Saunders, Philadelphia, p 922

Ojemann R G 1985 Meningiomas: Clinical features and surgical management In: Wilkins R H, Rengachary S S (eds) Neurosurgery vol 1. McGraw-Hill, New York, p 312

Ojemann R G 1991 Olfactory groove meningiomas. In: Al-Mefty O (ed) Meningiomas. Raven Press, New York, p 383

Ojemann R G 1993a The surgical management of acoustic neuroma (vestibular schwannoma). Clinical Neurosurgery (In press)

Ojemann R G 1993b Infratentorial procedures — neoplastic disorders — general considerations. In: Apuzzo M L J (ed) Brain surgery complications avoidance and management. Churchill Livingstone, New York, p 1711

Ojemann R G 1993c The surgical management of cranial and spinal meningiomas. Clinical Neurosurgery (In press)

Ojemann R G, Martuza R L 1990 Acoustic neuroma. In: Youmans J R (ed) Neurological surgery. W B Saunders, Philadelphia, p 3316

Ojemann R G, Ogilvy C S 1993 Convexity, parasagittal and parafalcine meningiomas. In: Apuzzo M L J (ed) Brain surgery complications avoidance and management. Churchill Livingstone, New York, p 187

Ojemann R G, Heros R C, Crowell R M 1988 Surgical management of cerebrovascular disease. Williams & Wilkins, Baltimore

Poletti C E, Ojemann R G 1985 Stereo atlas of operative microneurosurgery. C V Mosby, St Louis

Rhoton A L Jr 1990 Micro-operative techniques. In: Youmans J R (ed) Neurological surgery. W B Saunders, Philadelphia, p 941

Rhoton A L Jr 1993 Infratentorial procedures — neoplastic disorders — instrumentation. In: Apuzzo M L J (ed) Brain surgery complications avoidance and management. Churchill Livingstone, New York, p 1647

Sekhar L N, Janecka I P 1993 Surgery of cranial base tumors. Raven Press, New York

Stewart D H Jr, Krawchenko J 1985 Patient positioning. In: Wilkins R H, Rengachary S S (eds) Neurosurgery. McGraw-Hill, New York, p 452

Tew J M Jr, Scodary D J 1993a Supratentorial procedures — basic techniques and surgical positioning. In: Apuzzo M L J (ed) Brain surgery complications avoidance and management. Churchill Livingstone, New York, p 31

Tew J M Jr, Scodary D J 1993b Infratentorial procedures — neoplastic disorders — surgical positioning. In: Apuzzo M L J (ed) Brain surgery complication avoidance and management. Churchill Livingstone, New York, p 1609

Tew J M Jr, Steiger H J 1985 Instrumentation for microneurosurgery. In: Wilkins R H, Rengachary S S (eds) Neurosurgery. McGraw-Hill, New York, p 439

Wilkins R H 1985 Principles of neurosurgical operative technique. In: Wilkins R H, Rengachary S S (eds) Neurosurgery. McGraw-Hill, New York, p 427

16. Stereotaxis in the diagnosis and management of brain tumors

C. H. Rabb M. L. J. Apuzzo

INTRODUCTION

The introduction and subsequent rapid evolution of technology related to computerized imaging has revolutionized the process of neurologic diagnosis. Computerized tomography and magnetic resonance imaging now allow for accurate, non-invasive, structural and functional analysis of intracranial processes previously available only from surgery or autopsy.

These images, though sophisticated, do not replace the need for histologic and microbiological assay in making accurate diagnoses. Given this premise, the application of this technology to stereotactic surgery has provided a rebirth of the field of stereotaxis, a result of improvement in the accuracy of targeting and visualization of critical adjacent structures. The end result is a safer, more accurate method of tissue acquisition as compared to open craniotomy.

The natural evolution of stereotactic methodology has led to the development of various applications of stereotaxis for therapeutic endeavors. In this chapter, we will discuss the role of stereotaxis in the diagnosis and treatment of intracranial neoplasms.

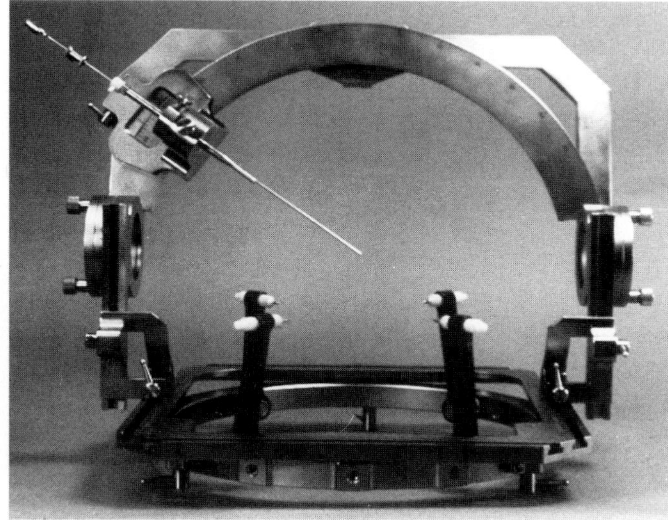

Fig. 16.1 Cosman-Roberts-Wells stereotactic system (Radionics Inc, Burlington, MA). Here the arc is positioned upon the base ring. The latter employs four-point pin fixation to the patient's skull. This arc-radius system allows for multiple entry sites.

STEREOTAXIS IN THE DIAGNOSIS OF BRAIN TUMORS

Methodology

Targeting

Although there are a large number and variety of commercially available stereotactic systems, our experience is derived from the Cosman-Roberts-Wells (CRW) and the Brown-Roberts-Wells apparatus (Radionics Inc, Burlington, MA — Fig. 16.1) (Apuzzo & Sabshin 1983, Heilbrun 1983, Heilbrun et al 1983, Apuzzo et al 1984a, 1987, Couldwell & Apuzzo 1990). Targeting is essentially a result of translation of two-dimensional data from CT or MRI scans into three-dimensional space (Leksell et al 1985, Lunsford et al 1986). This allows subsequent navigation through this stereotactic space in order to access the target. In this chapter, we will focus primarily upon the CT-based system, as this is the most widely used form of image-based stereotaxis.

The first step in the targeting process is application of the base ring, which is accomplished with the aid of local anesthesia and intravenous sedation. We prefer to shave the head prior to base ring application, as this allows visualization of the skull contours, thus optimizing ring placement. For example, the pins are radiopaque, and therefore they must be placed either above or below the target to avoid artefacts. Shaving the head allows proper visualization of external landmarks. The relationship of these landmarks to the target may be determined by inspection of the sagittal views from preoperative MRI scans.

The second step in targeting is imaging. With the

Radionics system, a localizer ring is applied to the base ring. The localizer has a set of nine carbon rods for CT, or a set of rods containing hydrocarbons when using MRI. These rods ultimately serve as fiducial points, once the images are taken.

A lead marker is taped to the patient's head at the anticipated entry site. The entry point is different for each patient, but takes into consideration lesion location, location of potential critical structures, and specific procedural objectives. Although the versatility of the CRW system includes the ability to choose any entry site within the system, it is of benefit to visualize the potential transit of the probe with the use of the lead marker. Once visualized on the CT screen, a wax pencil may be used to mark the position of the lead marker. The subsequent serial scans provide an assessment of the pathway of the stereotactic probe.

Axial images are then obtained, focusing on the target area, as more complete imaging studies are completed prior to the targeting images. The target is then selected using the scanning software's cursor, and Cartesian coordinates are obtained from the scanner. The carbon rods are simultaneously visualized as dots radially arranged around the patient's head (Fig. 16.2). The cursor is then serially advanced to each of these dots, determining the coordinates of these points in space as well. All coordinates are repeated as a check, and the coordinate values are recorded on paper.

The next step is the translational step, during which the data are converted to three-dimensional stereotactic space. These data are entered into the Radionics computer. For the CRW system, the data are analyzed and used to generate the target point in three-dimensional space, with anteroposterior, lateral, and vertical dimensions. These target coordinates are then used to set the target point on the phantom base. The CRW arc itself also has AP, lateral, and vertical parameters, which are set to the same coördinate values as the phantom base. The stereotactic probe is then advanced to the phantom base target to confirm the settings. The stereotactic probe is always set to a depth of 20 cm with the CRW system. Thus, a rehearsal of the procedure is performed.

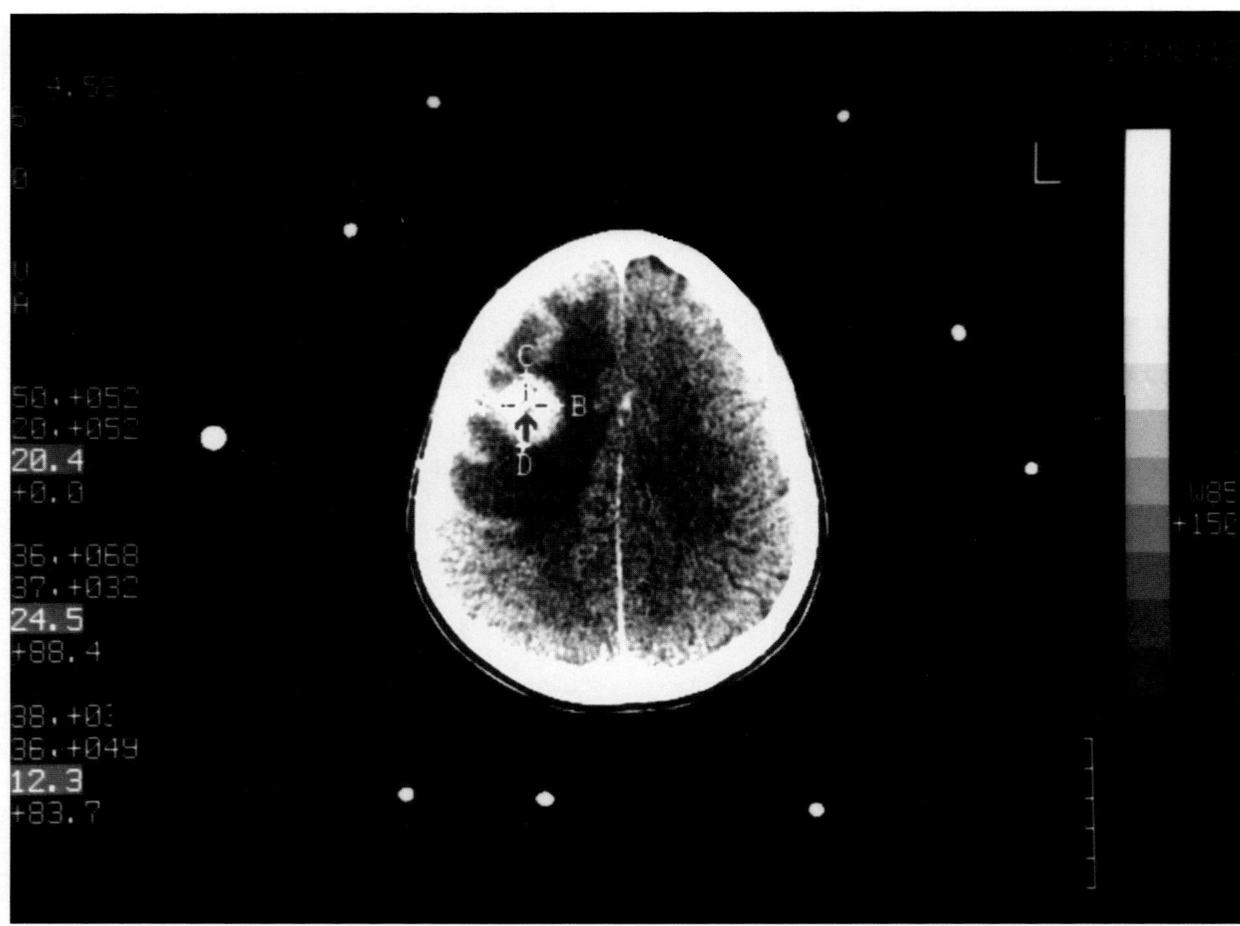

Fig. 16.2 The carbon fiducials are projected on the scanner console as a set of dots radially arranged around the head. These form the references for the computations that result in x, y, and z coordinates of the target.

Tissue acquisition

The target is accessed using the arc. With the CRW system, the base ring is affixed to the Mayfield headrest using an adaptor. After a sterile prep, the scalp is infiltrated with local anesthetic, and a 1.5 cm incision is made over the entry site with a #15 scalpel. The arc is then rotated into place and the probe is advanced into the bushing of the arc to confirm the position of the arc with respect to the entry site. Usually a twist drill hole is made, with the help of a drill guide. Whenever possible, a perpendicular position of the drill on the skull is desired. Once through the inner table, the dura is then penetrated with a sharp probe. If the patient is elderly, preoperative coronal MRI scans will reveal the size of the subarachnoid space. If it is excessively large, a burr hole may be used in lieu of a twist drill so that the underlying dura and cortex may be traversed under direct vision, reducing the risk of intraoperative subdural hematoma.

Biopsy. A number of instruments are available for tissue acquisition (Fig. 16.3). These include the following:

1. a needle core device,
2. a side cutting aspirator,
3. a spiral needle,
4. a side cutting needle, and
5. cup forceps.

The needle core device is a 14 gauge cannula with a stylet for entry, and tissue removal is dependent on aspiration. Tissue removal is dependent on tissue consistency and, in our hands, is unreliable. The aspirator device is similarly dependent on aspiration and, hence, is also unreliable. The spiral needle has also been found to be unsatisfactory for reliable tissue removal. The side cutting needle provides an adequate specimen, but suffers from limitations with accuracy when targeting small lesions in critical locations.

We generally use cupped bronchoscopy forceps. The forceps are advanced through the inner lumen of the stereotactic probe, and are serially opened and closed within the target, withdrawing the desired amount of specimen. These provide reliable tissue sampling in the

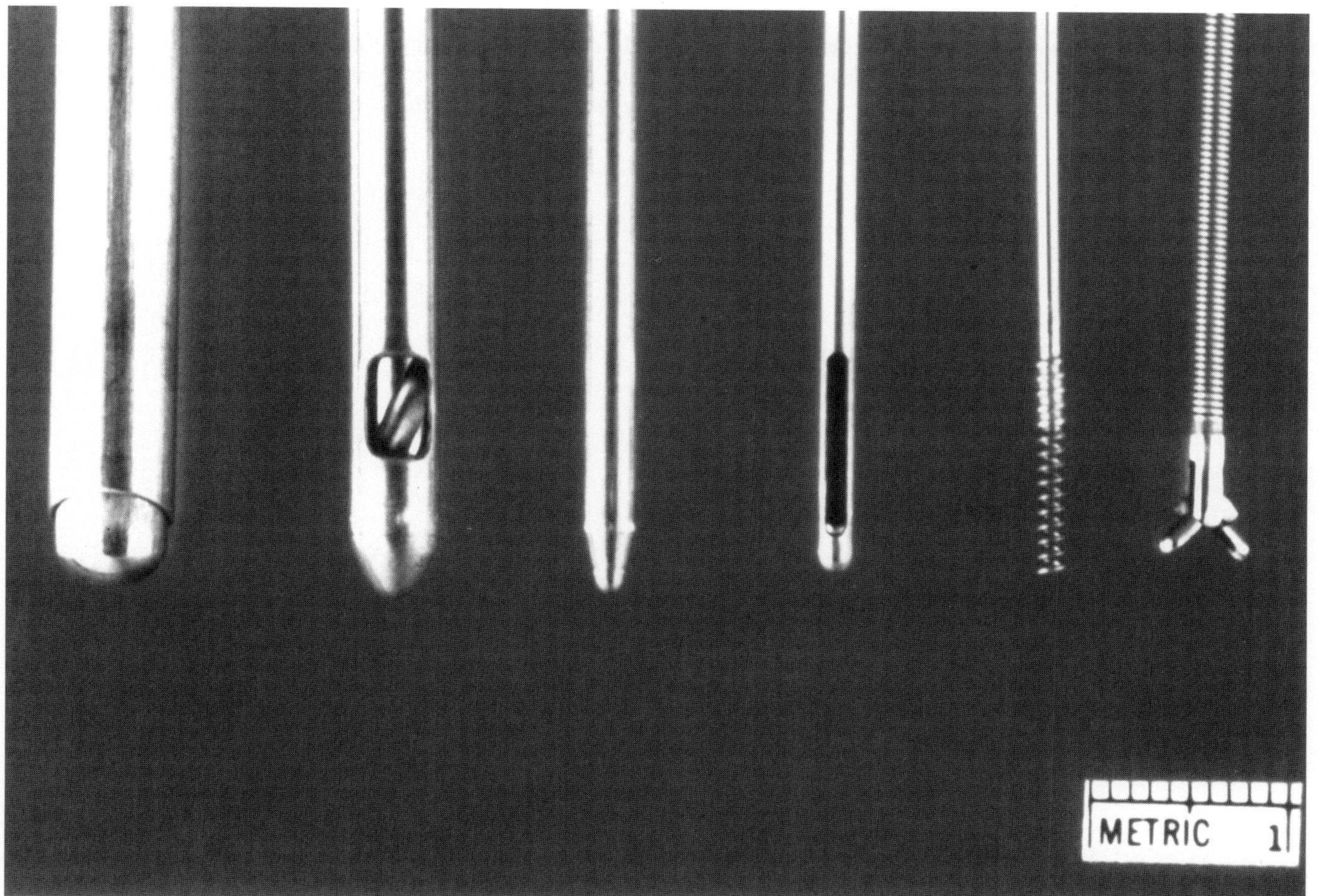

Fig. 16.3 Instrumentation available for tissue sampling. From right to left: flexible cup forceps, spiral needle, side cutting cannula, needle core instrument, Archimedes screw aspirator, and endoscope sheath.

form of 1.5–2 cubic millimeter specimens. The surgeon also gets tactile feedback from the target regarding the consistency of the lesion.

To perform the biopsy, a 14 gauge styleted probe is advanced through the side bushing of the arc to the target. As stated previously, with the CRW system, this is at a depth of 20 cm. The forceps are rotated between each sample, to provide diversity of sampling. To obtain the tissue, the surgeon advances the forceps, while the assistant opens and closes the forceps.

CSF/cyst markers. If the target is cystic in nature, or if the ventricle is traversed while advancing to the target, fluid may be taken for analysis. We have developed a number of cannulae with various gauge lumens and sharp, beveled tips to permit cavity access if the cyst walls appear to be thickened.

Otherwise, the standard 14 gauge probe is used. The probe has a Luer lock at its proximal end; a small syringe may be attached to the probe, and fluid aspirated. This technique may be especially helpful when the differential diagnosis of the lesion includes germ cell tumors, which may secrete hCG or AFP (Dayan et al 1966, Borit 1969, Allen et al 1979, Hasse & Neilsen 1979, Kirschner et al 1981, Arita et al 1983). If the ventricles or cyst are especially large, one must be careful not to withdraw too much fluid, or a subdural hematoma may result from collapse of the cortex away from the inner table.

Endoscopy

A 6.2 mm diameter fiberoptic rigid endoscope with a 20 cm length barrel has been employed for both cerebroscopy and ventriculoscopy (Apuzzo et al 1977). This instrument, produced by Karl Storz Endoscopy (Tuttlingen Germany), provides capabilities of visualization, irrigation, and a port for biopsy forceps (Fig. 16.4). Because of its size, a burr hole is necessary for introduction into the cranial vault. A number of specialized cannulae for cyst wall puncture and aspiration may be utilized (Iizuka 1975). In addition, laser coagulation may be attempted for cauterization.

One of the best applications for endoscopy is colloid cyst aspiration (Powell et al 1983, Apuzzo et al 1984a, Rivas & Lobato 1985). This avoids blind stereotactic puncture, which could potentially damage the fornices. A 13 gauge cannula with a blunt stylet is introduced to the cyst wall; the blunt stylet is subsequently replaced by a sharp one (Fig. 16.5). The latter punctures the cyst wall. The cannula is then advanced into the cyst, the contents of which are aspirated. Kondziolka has recently reported that a low density of the cyst on CT is predictive of treatment success by stereotactic methodologies (Kondziolka & Lunsford 1991). Another application that has been utilized is fenestration of the septum pellucidum for the treatment of unilateral foramen of Munro occlusion (Heilman & Cohen 1991).

Results

Using the methodology described above, 1–2 cubic millimeter tissue samples are submitted to the pathologist. These specimens represent a sample from a much larger tumor mass. This is especially important with respect to glial neoplasms, which often contain heterogeneous cell

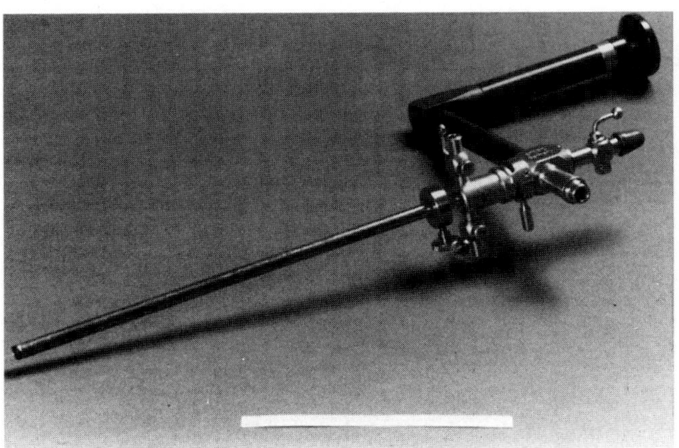

Fig. 16.4 Representative rigid fiberoptic endoscope for ventriculoscopy or cerebroscopy.

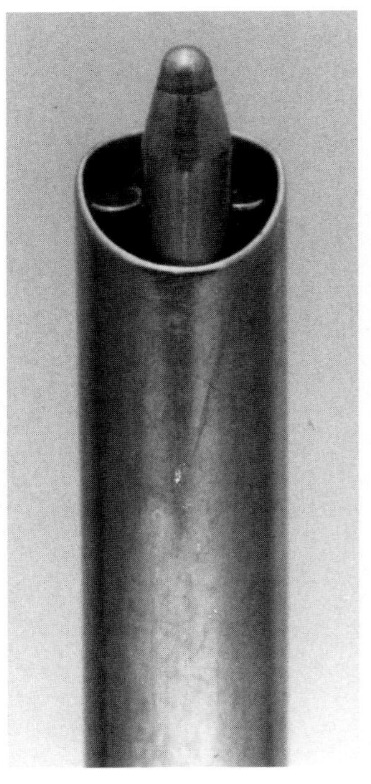

A

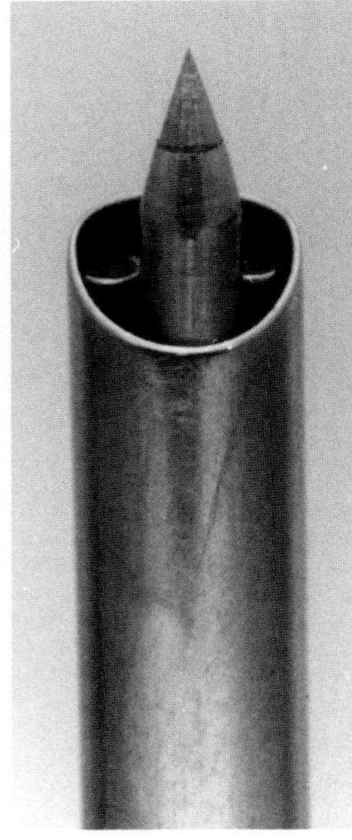

B

Fig. 16.5 Blunt (**A**), and sharp (**B**) probes for use with the fiberoptic endoscope.

populations, and the proper diagnosis affects prognosis. Fortunately, with biopsies obtained stereotactically, the specimen is chosen from a specific portion of the mass as determined by imaging studies. Thus, the clinician must communicate all pertinent clinical and radiographic data to the pathologist in order to maximize the yield from the small specimens and obtain an accurate diagnosis.

The initial step in determining the histopathology of a stereotactically obtained specimen is a smear (Adams et al 1981, Bosch 1980, Eisenhart & Cushing 1930, Russell et al 1937, Morris 1947, Jane & Bertrand 1962, Crain et al 1983, Willems 1983, Linwicz et al 1986). This may be done in nearly all specimens, except when the tissue is especially firm in consistency and will not smear onto the slide. In those cases, one should proceed directly to a frozen section.

To perform a smear, a small piece of tumor is cut with a scalpel blade. Approximately three pieces of the specimen are placed onto a glass slide. A second glass slide is used to crush the specimens, and the smear is then made. The slides are stained with H & E and examined. If the smear is nondiagnostic, a frozen section is performed. If the latter is also nondiagnostic, more specimens are obtained. The remainder of the tissue is stored in formalin and snap frozen for immunoperoxidase staining, such as GFAP, or Ki-67, an antigen indicative of the proliferative potential of tumors.

In our experience, a correct tissue diagnosis can be made in over 95% of cases. Of those nondiagnostic specimens, necrosis was seen in 45%, and inflammatory responses in 41%. Proper target selection may reduce the incidence of failed diagnosis. We usually employ double-dose IV contrast injections prior to imaging, and delay imaging for at least 1 hour after the contrast is given. Sampling from the margin of the mass will reduce the incidence of necrosis within the specimen. Lastly, one may perform tract biopsy, taking multiple biopsies along a tract through the tumor, to decrease the influence of heterogeneous cell populations within a given tumor (Daumas-Duport et al 1982, 1984).

Neuroepithelial tumors

Astrocytic neoplasms. Glial neoplasms constitute the most common type of tumor undergoing stereotactic biopsy. For grading purposes, we use the WHO classification system. The hallmark of glial neoplasms on smear is the presence of abnormal astrocytes which are larger and more angulated than normal astrocytes. These tumors appear to have a fibrillary background on H & E, as opposed to the typical eosinophilic background of normal brain. The presence of endothelial proliferation and the degree of cellularity may also be seen on smears. As we usually sample tumor from the leading edge of the tumor, the necrotic portions of the mass are avoided. This does, however, lead to an underestimation of glioblastomas.

Thus, one may be able to diagnose an astrocytoma (Fig. 16.6) on the basis of the fibrillary background and low cellularity; an anaplastic astrocytoma (Fig. 16.7) may be diagnosed on the basis of pleomorphism, endothelial proliferation, and increased cellularity; glioblastomas (Fig. 16.8) have the hallmark of necrosis (Fulling & Nelson 1984). In addition, with lower tumor grades, the tissue has a firmer consistency; hence, the greater the difficulty in smearing the tissue, the lower the tumor grade.

One difficulty remains, however, for the pathologist: differentiation of tumor from gliosis. The latter tends to have a more heterogeneous cell population that includes fibrillary, protoplasmic, and gemistocytic astrocytes, as well as inflammatory cells (Fig. 16.9). The former tends to have a more uniform degree of hypercellularity. Resolution of this diagnostic dilemma is further aided by the clinical data supplied to the pathologist by the surgeon.

Nonastrocytic glial neoplasms.

Oligodendrogliomas (Fig. 16.10) present as highly cellular when smeared, and have cohesive cells that have uniform round nuclei with a delicate chromatic distribution. The classic ‘fried egg’ appearance only appears, however, on permanent sections as it is a fixation artefact. When this tumor type is suspected, an adequate amount of tissue must be formalin fixed. Central neurocytomas have recently been differentiated from oligodendrogliomas. They occur in the lateral ventricles, and stain positively for synaptophysin.

Ependymomas (Fig. 16.11) are intraventricular tumors that must be differentiated by biopsy from neurocytomas and occasionally meningiomas. These tumors have the classic true and perivascular rosette formation. Unfortunately, these rosettes are seldom seen on smears, and require further preparation.

Choroid plexus papillomas are also seen intraventricularly, and have a classic appearance, with cuboidal epithelium and papillary pattern. Because of the typical clinical and radiographic appearance, these tumors rarely undergo stereotactic biopsy.

Primitive neuroectodermal tumors are tumors that likewise rarely undergo stereotactic biopsy due to their classic presentation in the fourth ventricle. Occasionally these tumors will involve supratentorial structures or pineal region and, if found on stereotactic biopsy, may be aggressively managed. This tumor has a classic basophilic appearance and extreme cellularity. Occasional Homer-Wright rosettes may be seen.

Non-neuroepithelial tumors.

Metastatic tumors may frequently be confused radiographically with glial tumors, and thus may come to stereotactic biopsy. When examining metastatic lesions, two

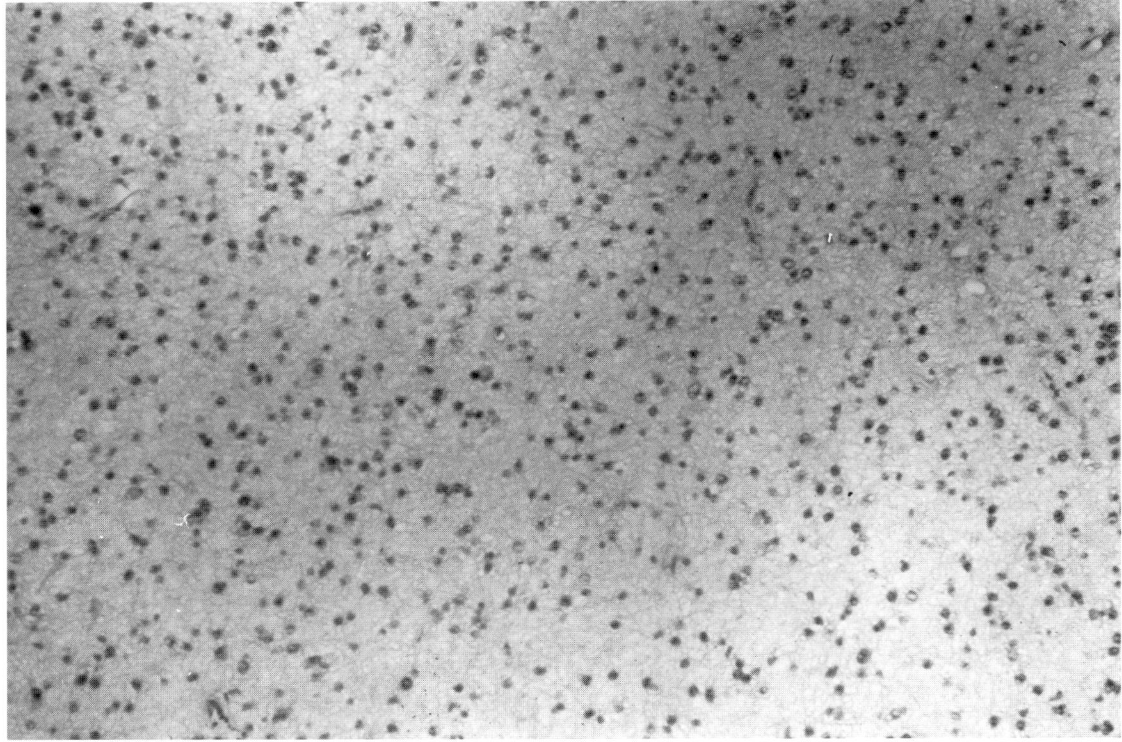

A

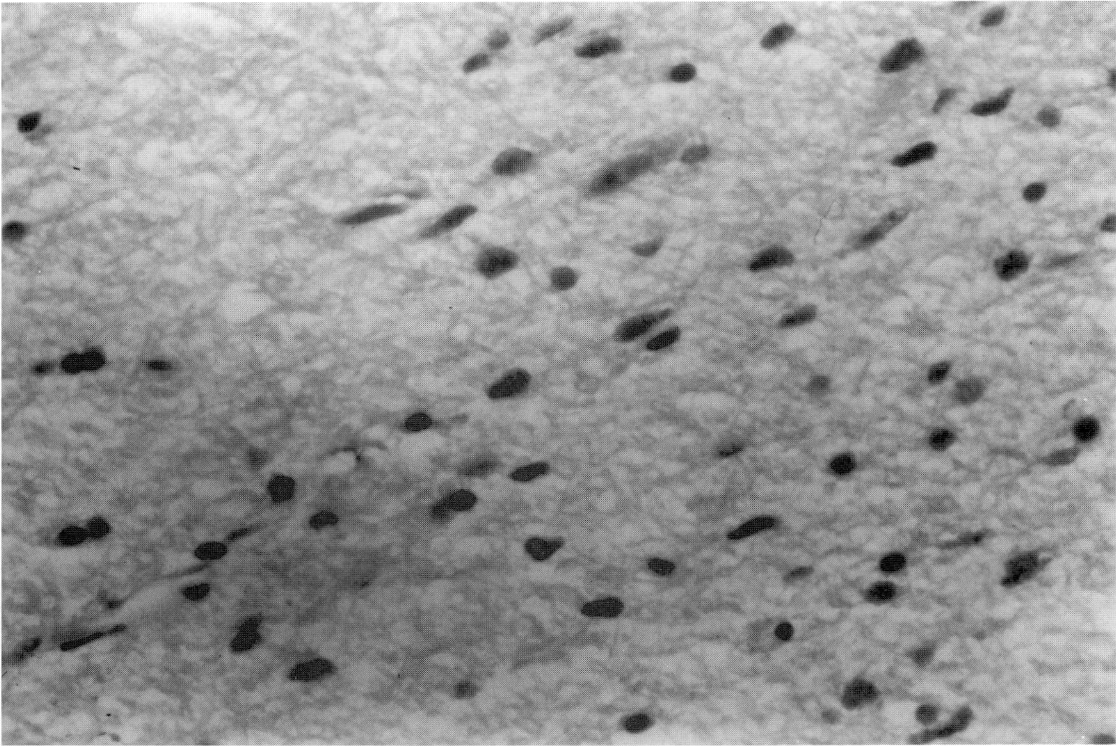

B

Fig. 16.6 Astrocytoma. **A.** Low magnification. The increased cellularity is superimposed upon a prominent fibrillary background. **B.** High magnification. The tumor cells have a variety of nuclear shapes.

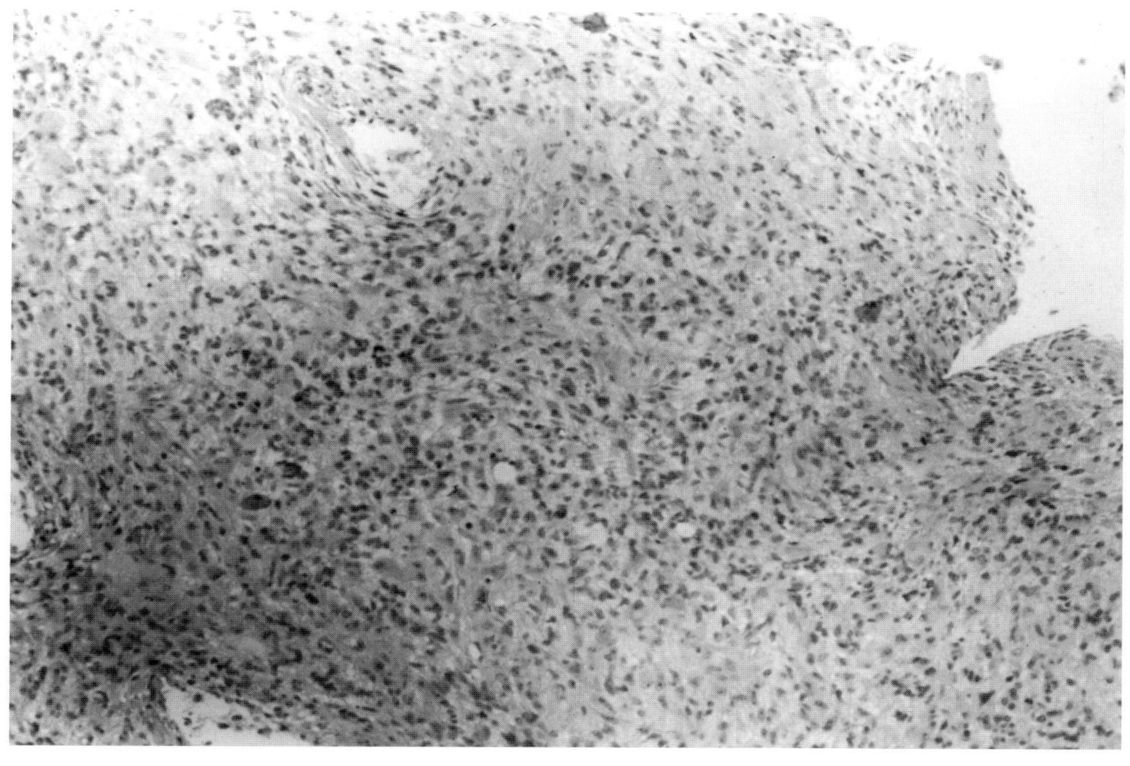

A

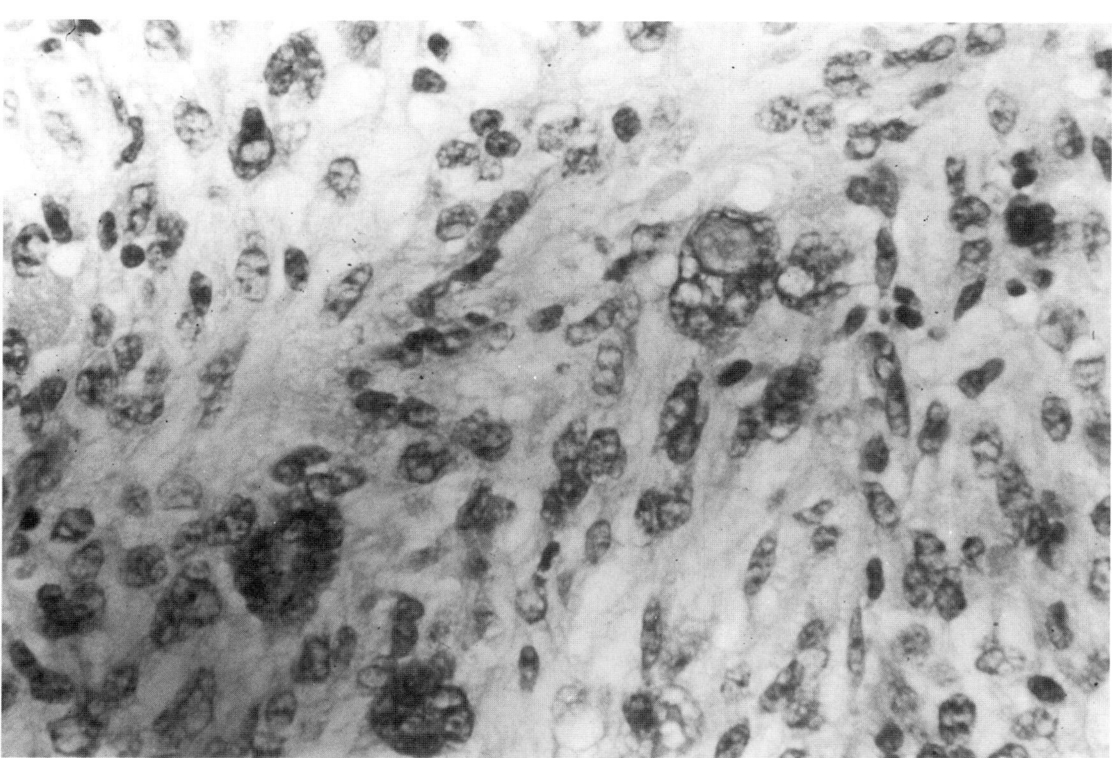

B

Fig. 16.7 Anaplastic astrocytoma. **A.** Low magnification. There is an increase in the cellularity as compared to astrocytoma. **B.** High magnification. Nuclear pleomorphism is more marked, and there are mitotic figures present.

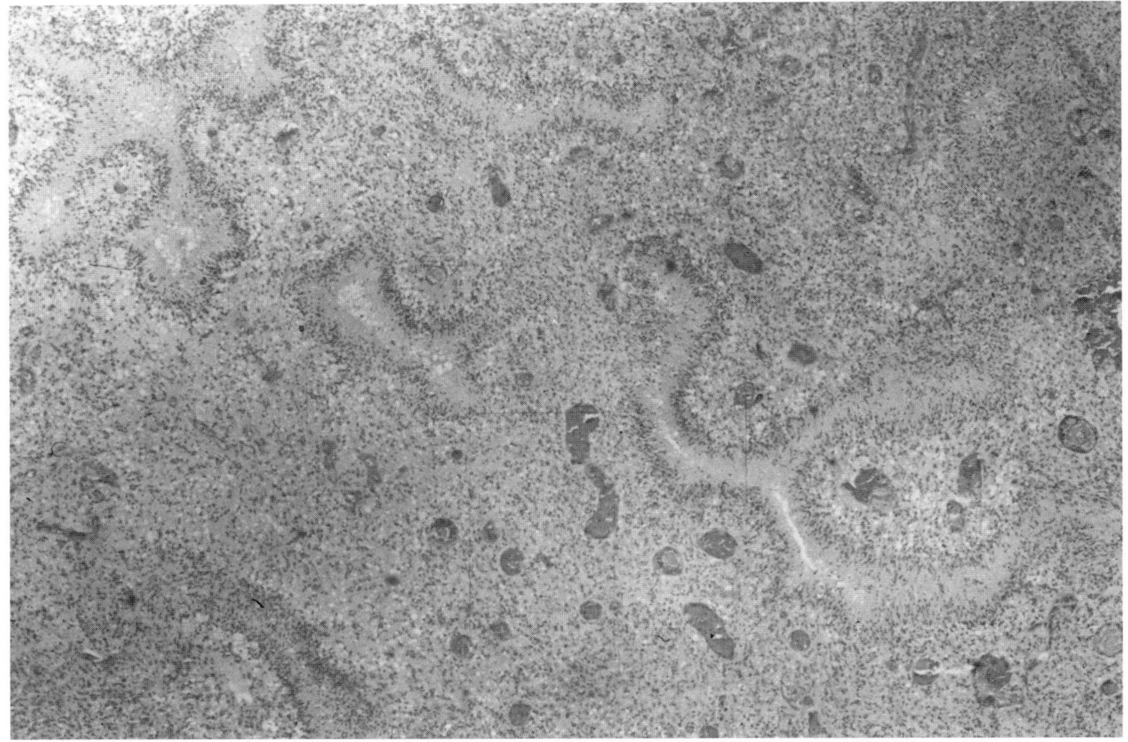

A

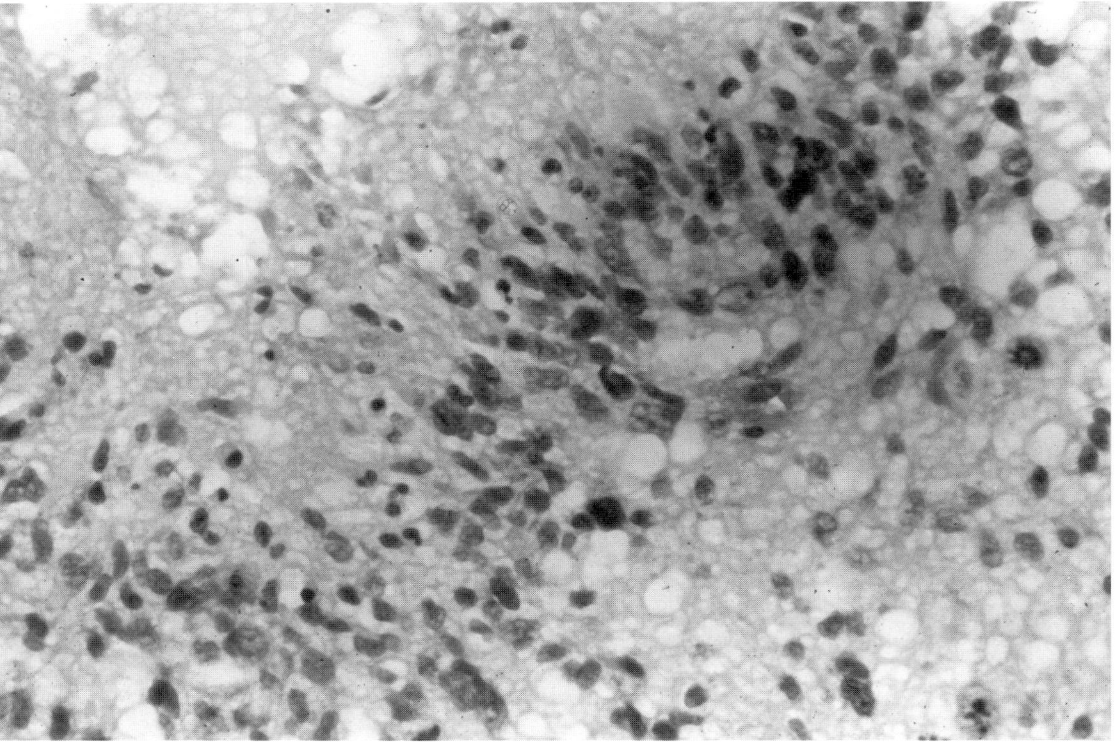

B

Fig. 16.8 Glioblastoma. **A.** Low magnification. The pseudopalisading of cells around areas of necrosis is easily appreciated. **B.** High magnification. Pseudopalisading is again noted.

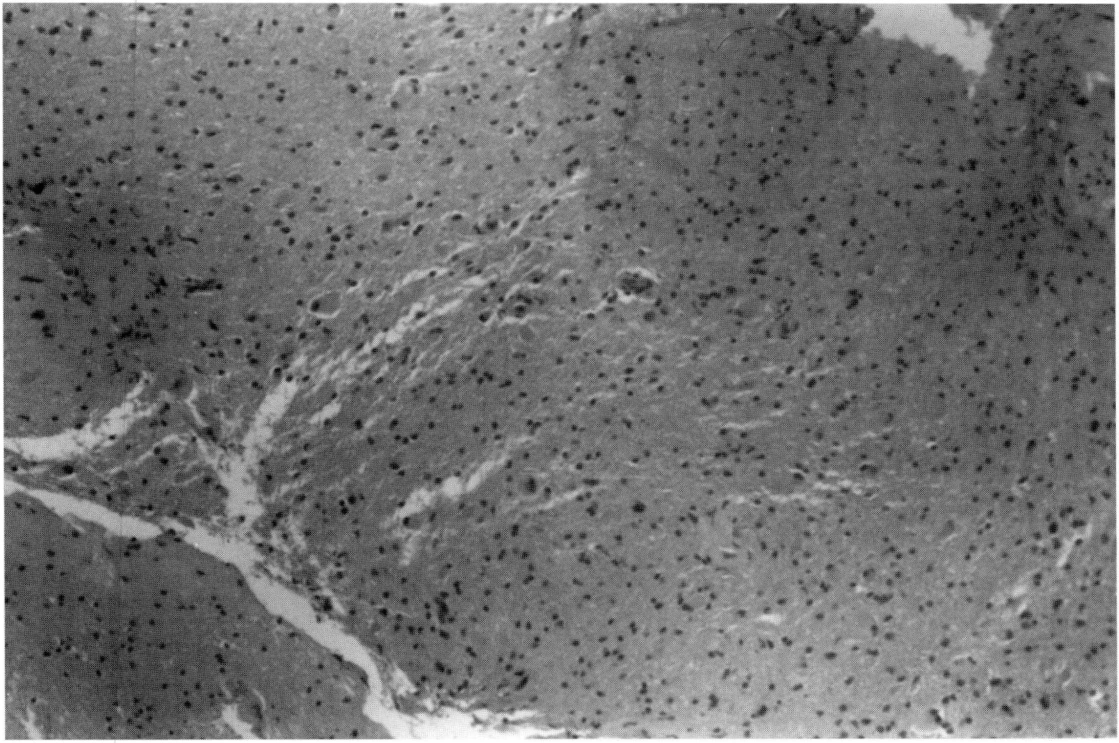

Fig. 16.9 Gliosis. A heterogeneous astrocytic cell population is seen as compared to the cell types of astrocytomas.

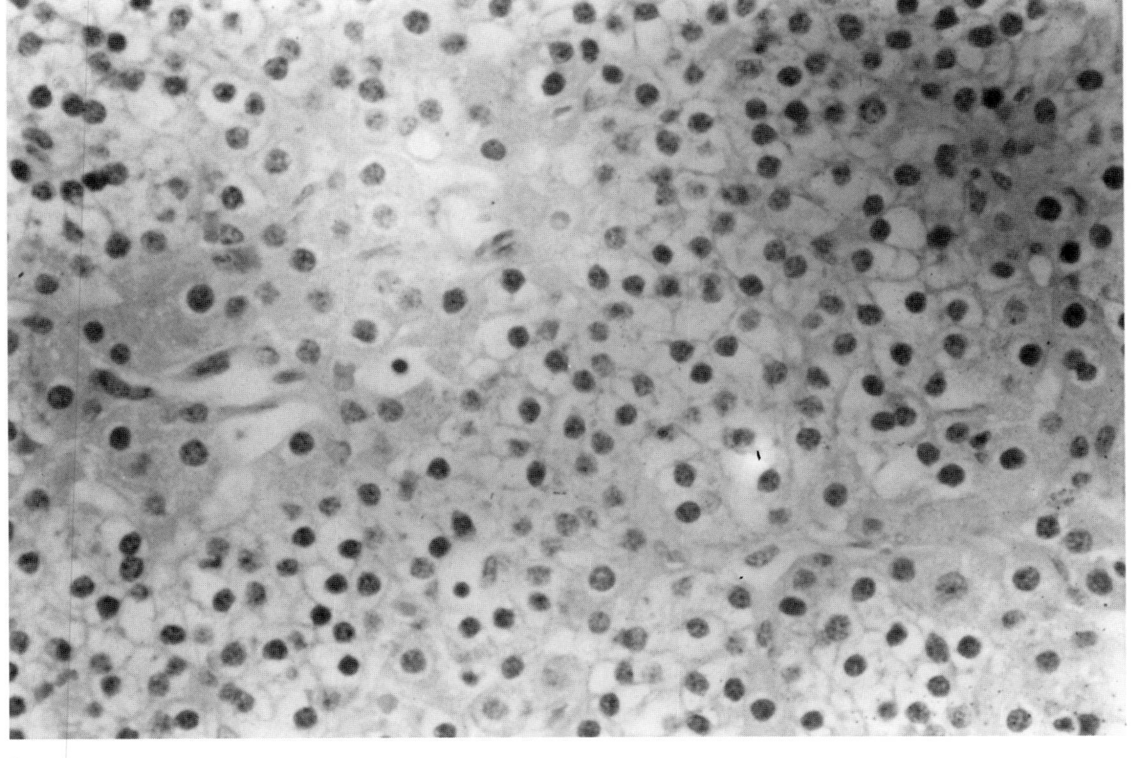

A

Fig. 16.10A

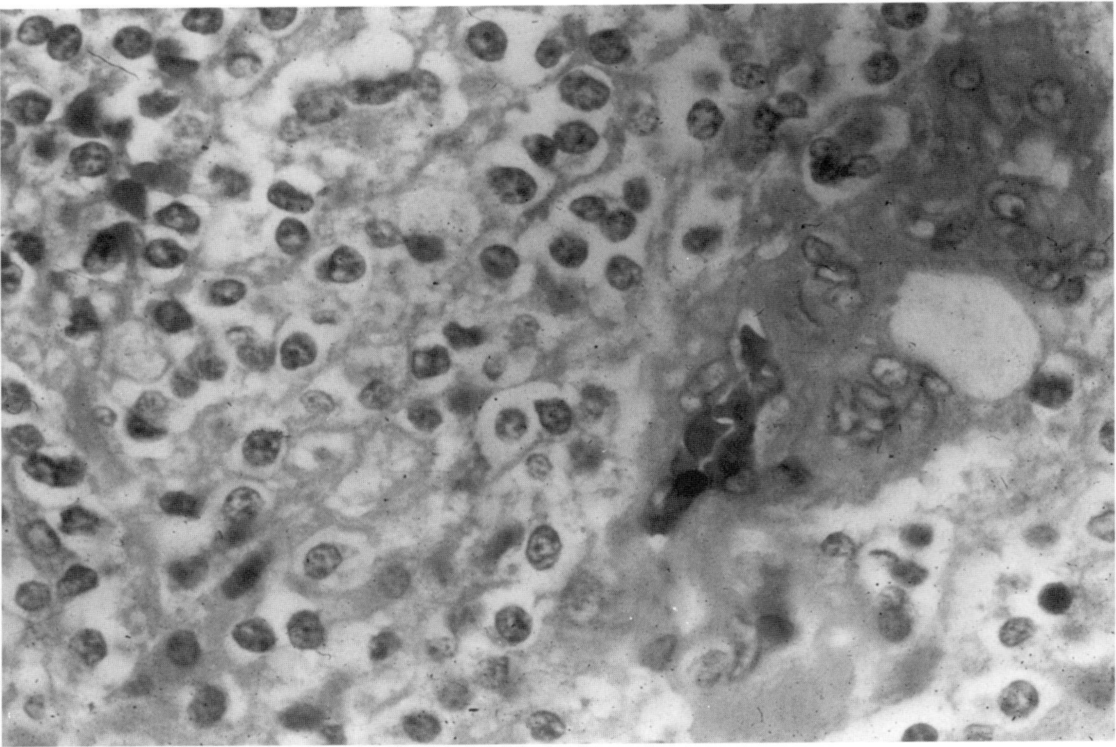

B

Fig. 16.10 Oligodendroglioma. **A.** Low, and **B**, high magnification. The classic 'fried egg' appearance of oligodendroglioma is well represented.

types of smears may be seen. The first is a highly cellular smear composed of cohesive, malignant epithelial cells without a fibrillary background from an area where the neoplasm has replaced normal brain. The second type shows a small number of cohesive cell groups in a background of necrosis or normal brain. Generally, the site of origin is difficult to ascertain, as the specimens are frequently very anaplastic.

Lymphomas are seen with increasing frequency, as the incidence of AIDS rises (Fig. 16.12). These tumors are difficult to classify on smears, and must be examined in detail through immunohistochemistry.

Pineal region tumors are most frequently germ cell in nature. True germinomas typically have a two cell population, one of which is lymphoid in nature. Other germ cell tumors include teratoma, embryonal carcinoma, choriocarcinoma, and yolk sac tumors (Scheithauer 1985). As stated above, CSF markers will aid in the diagnosis. Pineocytomas are primary pineal tumors, composed of uniform round, discohesive cells with scant cytoplasm.

Meningiomas rarely come to stereotactic biopsy, because the diagnosis is usually apparent by clinical and imaging studies. The meningothelial cells are unmistakable, plump cells with central nuclei, clustered together into whorls. Psammoma bodies may also be seen.

STEREOTAXIS IN THE MANAGEMENT OF BRAIN TUMORS

Overview of therapeutic modalities

In addition to diagnostic applications, the principles of stereotactic navigation have been expanded to an increasing role in tumor therapy. These modalities include cyst aspiration, stereotactic craniotomy, interstitial hyperthermia, interstitial chemotherapy, interstitial radiobrachytherapy, interstitial photodynamic therapy, interstitial viral therapy, and stereotactic radiosurgery. In this chapter, we will provide an overview of these forms of applied stereotaxis.

Techniques

Cyst aspiration/drainage

As stated previously, direct aspiration of tumor cysts may be accomplished with the stereotactic apparatus. If the cyst is sizable, we generally implant a subcutaneous catheter-reservoir for repeated aspirations as needed (Fig. 16.13). This may be performed with a 25 gauge needle directly through the skin, obviating the need for additional stereotactic procedures. If the cyst repeatedly

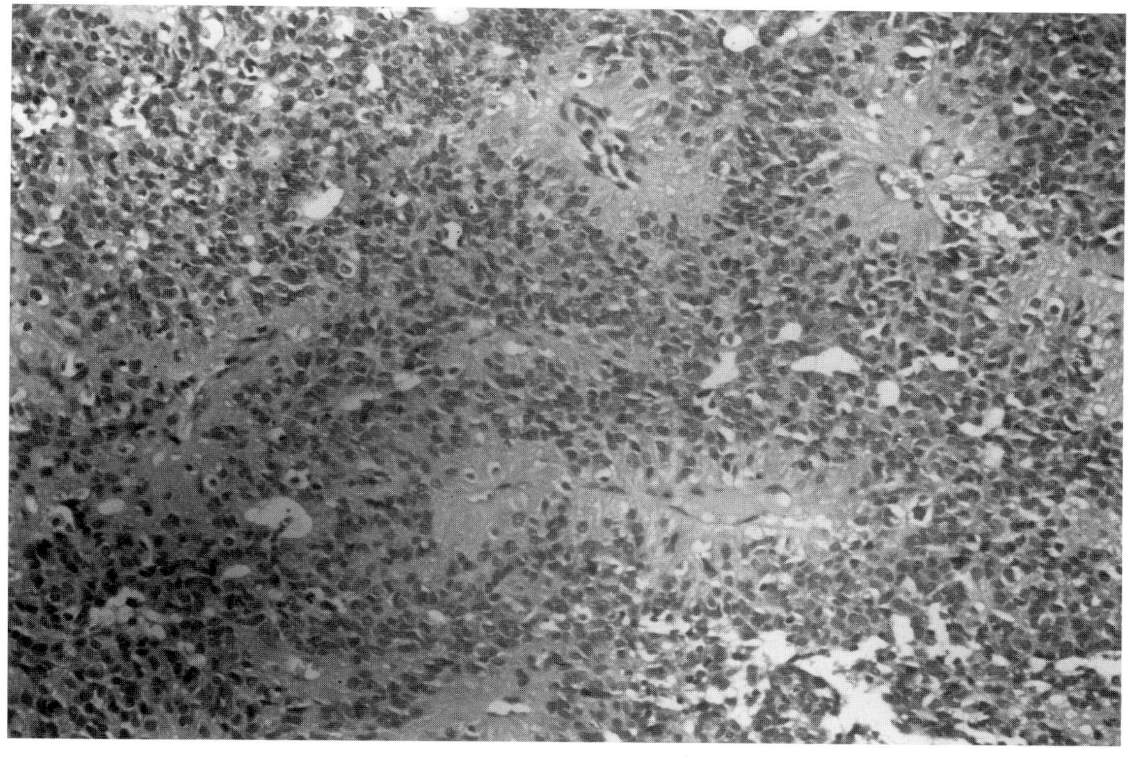

A

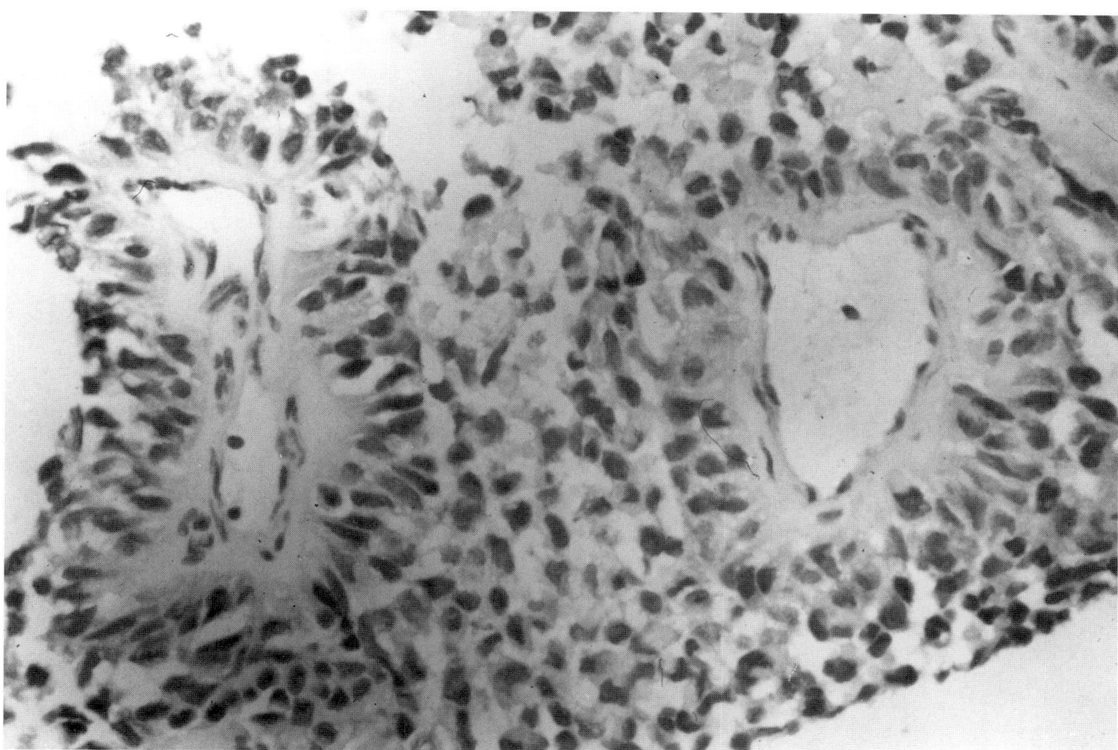

B

Fig. 16.11 Ependymoma. **A.** Low magnification, and **B**, high magnification. Perivascular rosettes are present. True rosettes are also a hallmark of ependymoma.

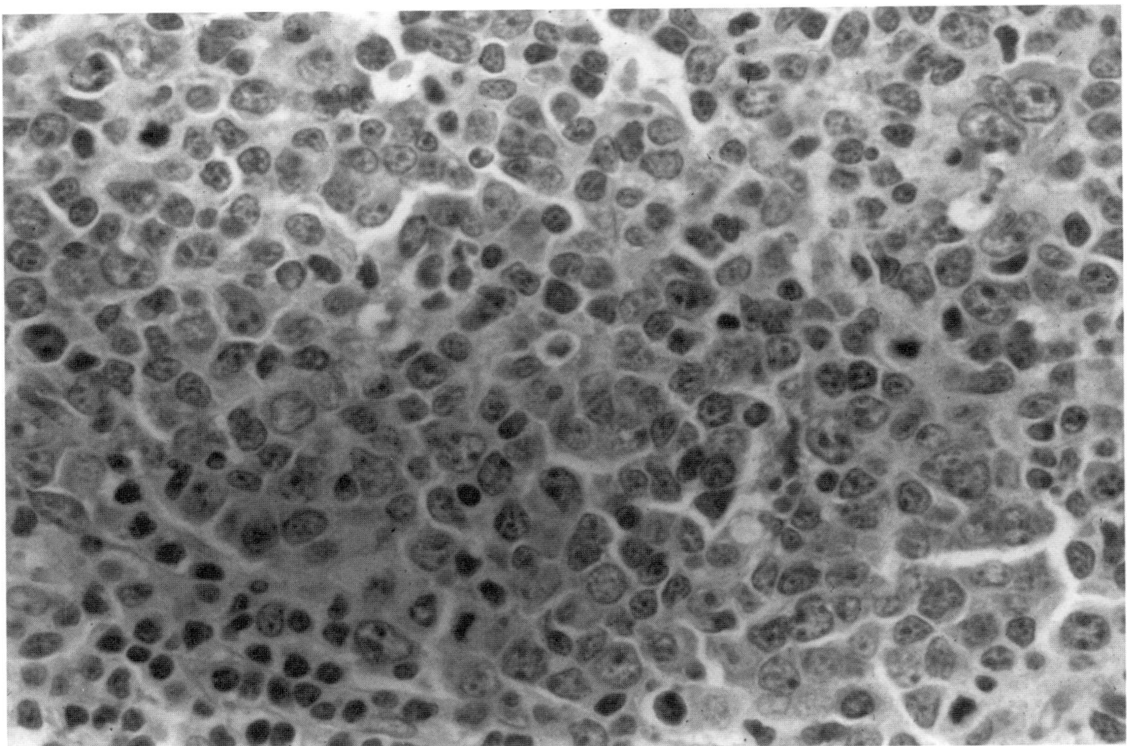

Fig. 16.12 Lymphoma. High cellularity, and the presence of lymphoid cells are characteristics of lymphoma. Most CNS lymphomas are of B-cell origin.

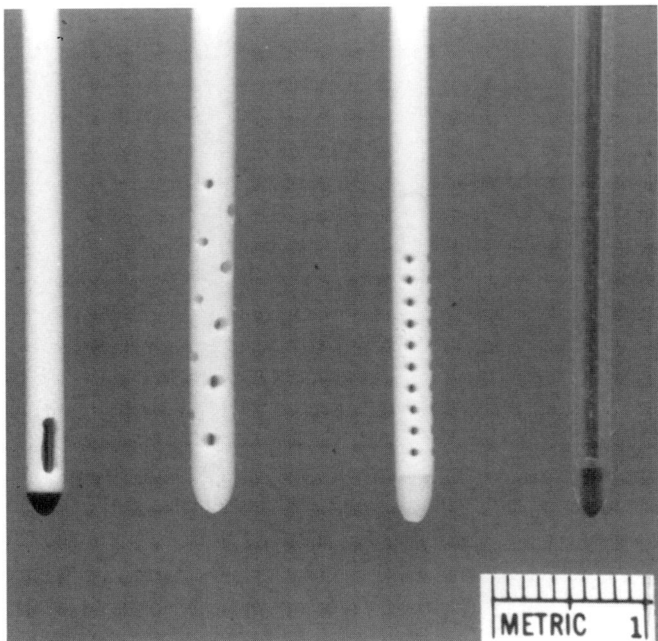

Fig. 16.13 A number of catheters are available for use that are compatible with the stereotactic frame. From left to right: brachytherapy catheter, standard silastic ventriculostomy catheters, and sharp, slotted catheter for cyst drainage procedures. The latter is especially useful for puncture and aspiration of cystic craniopharyngiomas.

reaccumulates after frequent aspirations, we routinely instill ^{32}P colloid, and have found a significant reduction in the need for subsequent aspirations. Communication of the cyst with the ventricular system should be excluded by means of a contrast cystogram, prior to administration of the ^{32}P.

Stereotactic craniotomy

The CRW system is well suited for stereotactically assisted craniotomy (Fig. 16.14). This technique is ideally suited for small lesions located in critical areas of the brain, and has been described recently for localizing small vascular malformations (Sisti et al 1991). Small glial neoplasms or metastases are examples of intra-axial lesions that may be approached in this manner. We have found stereotactic assistance to be superior to ultrasound for locating small lesions.

The lesion is targeted in the usual fashion. Once the craniotomy is performed, the arc may be positioned onto the base ring. The probe may then be positioned to guide the surgeon to the target location. Alternatively, the stereotactic frame may be used to introduce a silastic catheter into place near the lesion. The arc is then removed, and a craniotomy is performed. One then follows the catheter to the lesion.

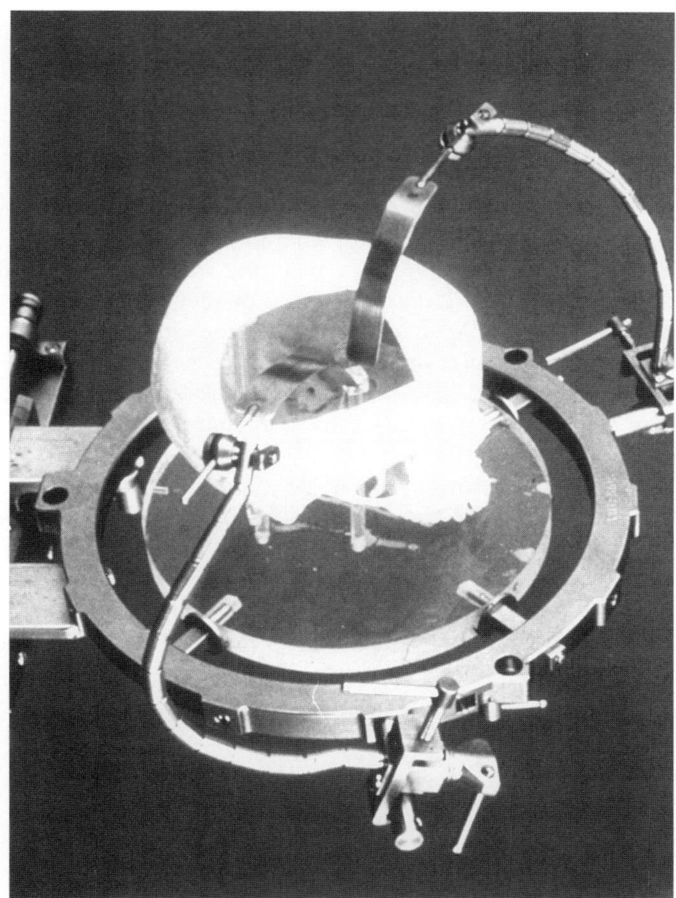

Fig. 16.14 Setup for stereotactically assisted craniotomy. Standard self-retaining retractor systems are compatible with the CRW base ring.

Further extending the principles of stereotaxis, Kelly has developed the concept of volumetric stereotaxis. Using sophisticated computer software, a specially designed cylindrical retractor is advanced to the target. The software then aids the surgeon by directing the microscopic resection until the entire tumor volume as seen on the imaging studies is resected. The resection is accomplished with laser (Kelly et al 1984a,b, 1986, Kelly 1986, 1987).

Intralesional therapy

Chemotherapy. Although extensive laboratory or clinical studies dealing with interstitial chemotherapy are not yet available, a number of reports have implied its potential feasibility and have recommended pursuit of further detailed investigations (Tator 1977, Tator & Wassenar 1977, Tator et al 1977a,b, Kroin & Penn 1982, Bouvier et al 1987). The technical methodology related to imaging-directed stereotaxis no doubt will offer stimulation to those with expertise and interest in this topic.

Hyperthermia. The concept of using elevated temperatures to treat malignancy is not entirely new (Storm 1983, Silberman et al 1986). Within recent years, some investigators have revived interest in the usage of hyperthermia for the treatment of glial neoplasms (Coughlin et al 1983, Brezovich et al 1984, Lyons et al 1984, 1986). The antineoplastic effects of hyperthermia are related to its ability to cause cellular injury, and possibly potentiate the effects of radiation (Dewey & Holahan 1984, Hall & Roisin-Towle 1978). Generally, temperature elevations above 42°C result in death of tumor cell lines. Above this level, the duration of hyperthermia necessary to bring about cell death is reduced (Giovanella 1983). The phenomenon of thermal tolerance is more pronounced in normal cells and, when it occurs, appears to be transient. Some investigators believe that this loss of tolerance is related to the presence of rapid cell division. In the CNS, this assumes a larger role than in other tissues.

As stated above, the mechanism of cellular injury is thought to be related to direct cellular killing, and to possible enhancement of the effects of radiation. The cellular effects are thought to be related to interference with membrane physiology, or possibly damage to chromatin. The role of hyperthermia in radiation therapy relates to interference with DNA repair mechanisms (Emami et al 1984). Some have proposed a role for immune mechanisms in hyperthermia-induced cellular death, but this has not been proven (Hahn 1982).

For neurosurgical procedures employing hyperthermia, the methods for heat delivery are important, as regional, not systemic, heat is desired. This may be accomplished by the use of stereotactically placed needle probes, ferromagnetic seeds, or microwave antennae (Lyons et al 1984). The latter have the theoretical advantage of not heating fat (Atkins 1983). A number of antennae may be implanted in an array within the tumor to provide the appropriate geometry (Salcman & Samaras 1981, Salcman 1984, Winter et al 1985, Roberts et al 1986a).

Several phase I studies have been undertaken for the treatment of glial tumors, most of which employed microwave antenna delivery systems. Few authors reported significant adverse sequelae (Silberman et al 1985).

Photodynamic therapy. Photodynamic therapy relies on the transfer of energy from certain dyes to oxygen, resulting in singlet oxygen, and in turn, free radical induced membrane injury (Dougherty et al 1981, Kaye & Morstyn 1987, Kaye et al 1988). The majority of interest has focused on the study of porphyrins, especially hematoporphyrin derivatives. This compound is preferentially concentrated in neoplastic tissue. As only certain wavelengths of light are absorbed by the hematoporphyrin derivative, the appropriate wavelengths must be delivered to the tumor after administration of the dye. This may be accomplished by stereotactically placed fiberoptic bundles. Phase I trials have been reported, and few side effects were noted (Laws et al 1981). More recently, direct evidence of central tumor necrosis has been demonstrated in human subjects with glial neoplasms, although no response was seen with melanoma (Powers et al 1991).

Radiobrachytherapy. Over the past decade, a great deal of interest has been focused on the use of stereotactically placed interstitial radiation sources for the treatment of malignant glial neoplasms (Mundinger 1966, Backlund 1973a, 1974, Mundinger & Hoefer 1974, Szikla & Peragut 1975, Mundinger 1979, Ostertag et al 1979, Szikla 1979, Szikla et al 1979, Weigel et al 1979, Bernstein & Gutin 1981, Gutin et al 1981, Mundinger 1982, Ostertag 1983, Apuzzo et al 1984b, Gutin et al 1984, Mundinger & Weigel 1984, Ostertag et al 1984, Szikla et al 1984, Backlund 1987, Petrovich et al 1987, Leibel et al 1989). This technique is particularly attractive from a theoretical perspective, as conventional teletherapy has been found to have limitations in effectiveness in the treatment of glial tumors and craniopharyngiomas (Kobayshi et al 1981, Vandenberg et al 1992). With conventional radiotherapy, doses of 50–56 cGy are tolerated reasonably well if the dose is given in fractions of 180 cGy, which reduces the incidence of radiation necrosis. Nevertheless, the vast majority of recurrences in glial tumors occur in the radiated field (Hall 1978, Hochberg & Pruitt 1980). Ideally, one would want a treatment form which effects local tumor kill with minimum radiation to the uninvolved brain. With interstitial implantation, the local dose is increased, and the radiation to the surrounding brain is reduced. Additionally, the radiobiology of the implants is such that a constant dose is given off, resulting in injury to cells, regardless of the cell cycle. Most of the cells in the tumor eventually enter the S phase during the duration of the implantation, increasing the effectiveness of the dose. Further, hypoxic cells become oxygenated during the course of the treatment, thus enhancing the radiation impact.

The most commonly used radiation sources used are ^{192}Ir and ^{125}I. Our experience is primarily derived from the former. Its gamma energy averages 380 KeV and, as such, caution must be exercised by the operating team. Conversely, ^{125}I has an average photon energy of 28 KeV, and is easier to manage (Apuzzo et al 1984b). As the

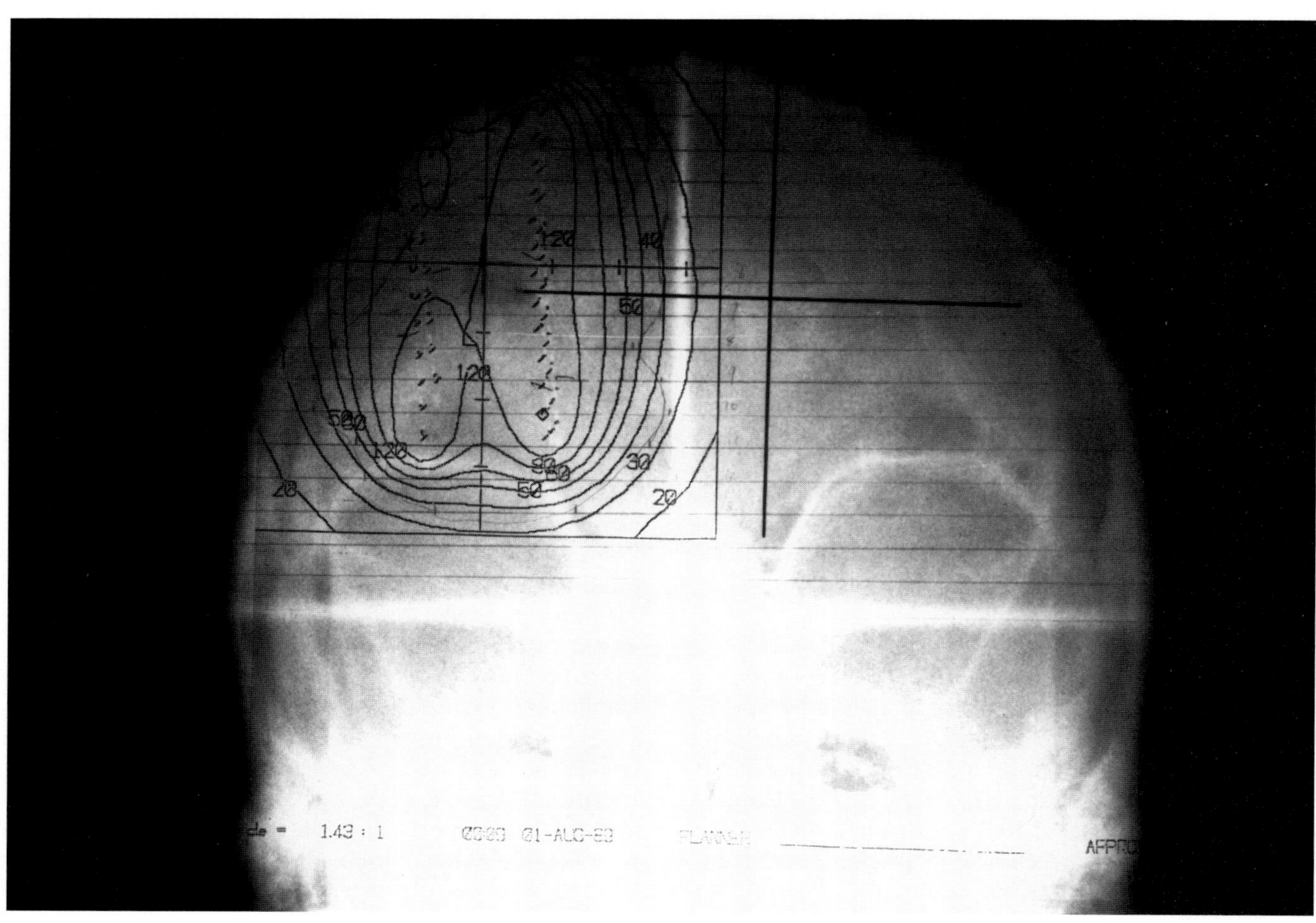

A

Fig. 16.15A (Caption overleaf)

desired dose for brachytherapy is 40–60 cGy/hour, the implants must remain in place for several days.

The extensive and irregular nature of the majority of malignant gliomas dictates the use of multiple catheters which contain these radionuclide sources, spaced at 3 mm intervals to produce a grid effect (Figs 16.15, 16.16). When the target diameter exceeds 5 cm, it is necessary to add additional catheters in the central region to supplement those placed in the periphery in order to avoid cold spots in the central area.

Previously untreated individuals harboring lesions without significant mass effect may be treated primarily following stereotactic biopsy. Regional teletherapy is performed initially, followed approximately two weeks later by a peripheral tumor dose of 45–62 Gy.

Although the frequency with which we employ radio-

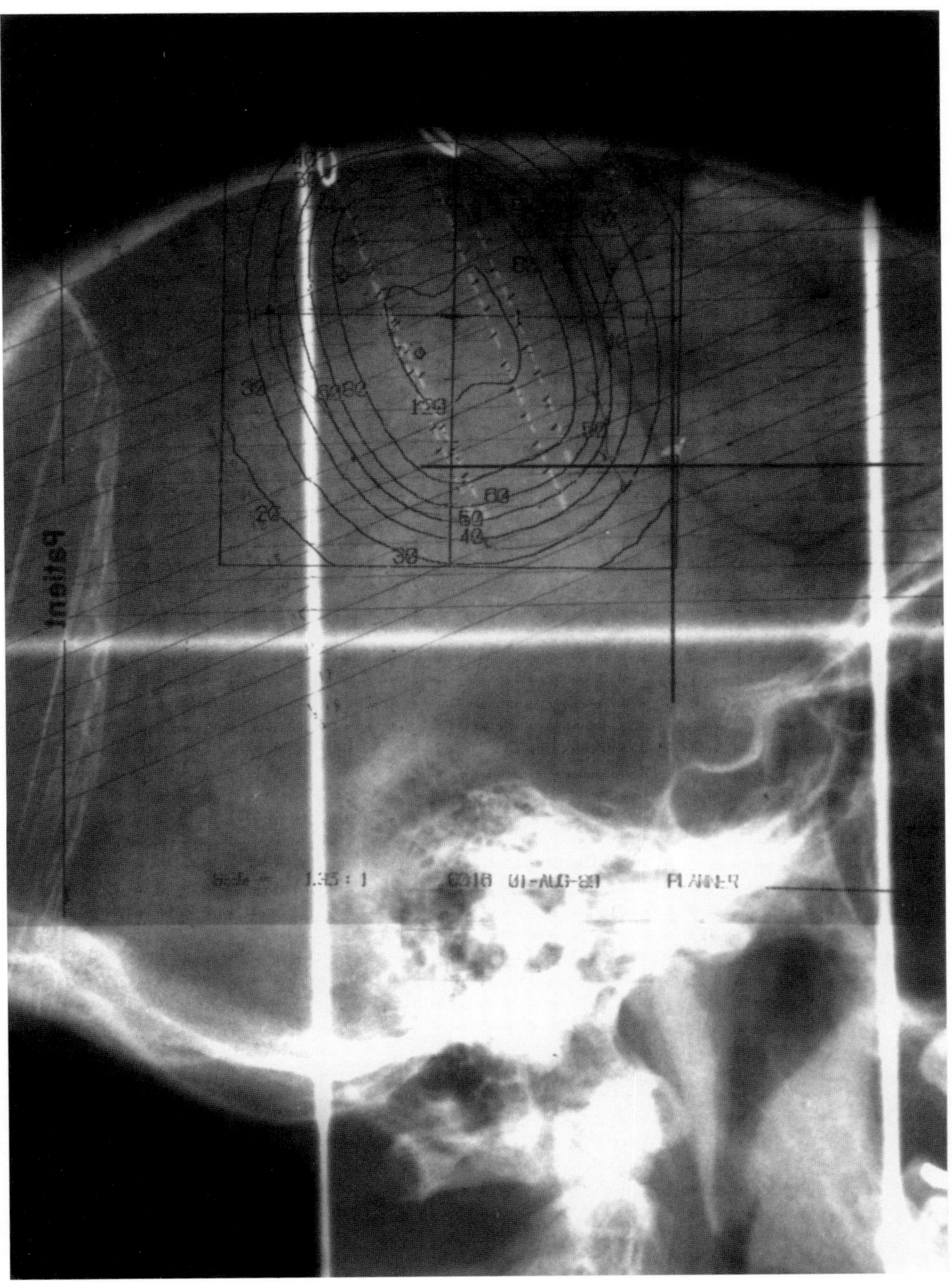

B

Fig. 16.15 **A** and **B.** Example of a brachytherapy dose plan, showing isodose curves for a patient harboring a glioblastoma.

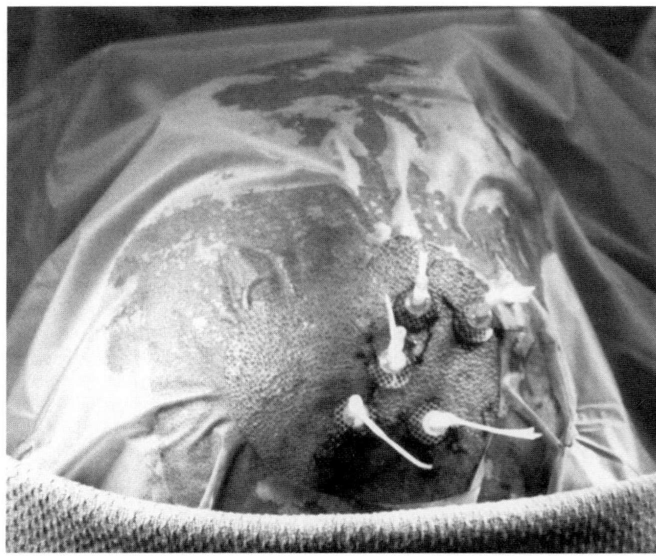

Fig. 16.16 Five-catheter array for instillation of radioisotope for treatment of a glioblastoma.

brachytherapy has diminished in the last 5 years, we will consider for treatment patients who fulfill the following criteria:

a. histology of anaplastic astrocytoma, glioblastoma, recurrent lymphoma, and pineocytoma,
b. age less than 55 years,
c. lesion size of less than 5 cm,
d. peripheral location, and
e. initial Karnofsky performance greater than 70.

One recent large clinical series did indicate a significant improvement in survival in a similarly selected group of patients, and that selection bias played a major role in this observation (Florell et al 1992).

Interstitial viral therapy. The future of intralesional therapy will likely take the form of gene therapy via viral vectors. As this therapy has yet to be fully developed, a novel form of viral therapy has recently been put forward involving herpes viruses (Markert et al 1992). Thymidine kinase-deficient herpes simplex type 1 viruses may be

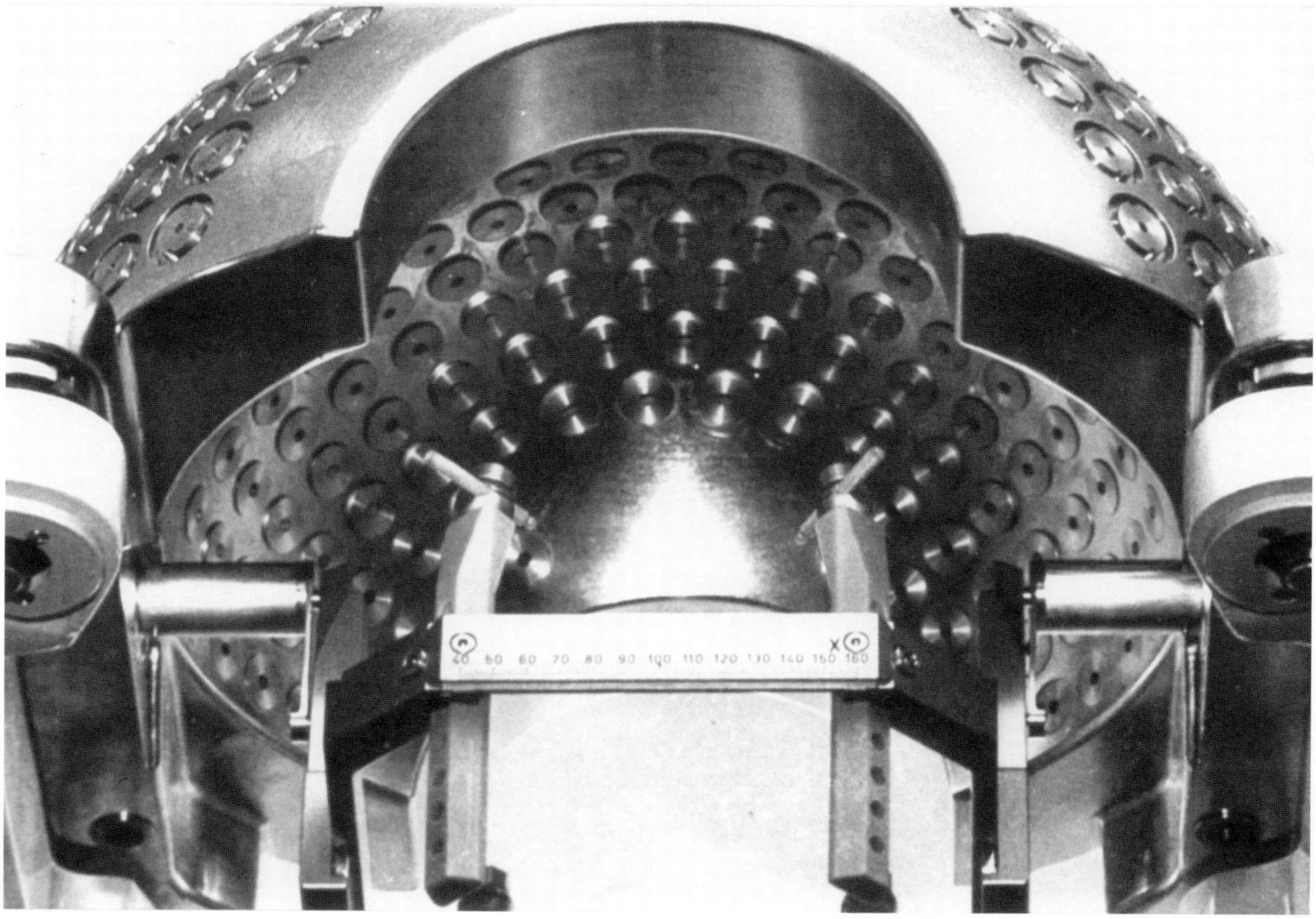

A

Fig. 16.17A (Caption overleaf)

injected into CNS tumors. As these mutants infect only dividing cells, they infect tumor cells preferentially and lyse them. This type of therapy holds great promise, and further studies are anxiously anticipated.

Radiosurgery

Gamma unit. In 1951, Lars Leksell first introduced the term radiation surgery, and in 1968 the first gamma unit was used in Stockholm (Leksell 1951). It employed 179 ^{60}Co sources focused on a specific point in stereotactic space. As a result, the target receives a high dose, with a steep drop-off in the dosage gradient peripherally. The principle involves a single large dose of radiation to effect target necrosis, while sparing the surrounding brain. The primary limitation lay in the volume of tissue that could be treated. In the 1970s, Leksell reported a modification of his radiosurgical method which resulted in an increase in the target volume (Leksell 1971); the current gamma unit design now employs 201 ^{60}Co sources (Leksell & Backlund 1979, Steiner et al 1974, Steiner 1984). The actual treatment involves stereotactic localization using the Leksell system. Once the target is localized in stereotactic space, the patient's head is fixed to the gamma unit, and a collimator helmet is placed over the patient's head (Fig. 16.17). Subsequently, the patient's head and the collimator helmet are advanced into the ^{60}Co sources. The target center is placed at the center of the beams. The treatment is tailored by the use of collimator sizes. In addition, for large lesions, multiple isocenters may be used. Presently, the largest tissue volume that may be treated is 20 cm^3 (Steiner et al 1991).

Particle-beam radiosurgery. The principles of radiosurgery have been expanded to include the usage of protons or helium ions in lieu of photons. This form of radiosurgery actually results in the narrowest isodose curves. This is accomplished by exploiting the Bragg-peak phenomenon (Kjellberg 1979a,b, Kjellberg et al 1983). Unfortunately, particle production requires synchrocyclotrons and, hence, few such facilities are available in the world for this form of radiosurgery.

Linear accelerator (Linac) radiosurgery. As a result of the prohibitive costs associated with the acquisition of the above forms of radiosurgery, alternative methodologies were sought. In the mid 1980s, the linear accelerator was employed as a radiation source for stereotactically directed radiosurgery (Heifetz et al 1984, Hartmann et al 1985, Lutz et al 1988). This form of radiosurgery is based on the concept of stereotactically placing the target in the center of the arc of rotation of the Linac, a widely available source of megavoltage photons. By serially rotating the gantry as well as the patient couch, multiple treatment arcs which overlap at the target may be administered (Luxton et al 1993) (Fig. 16.18).

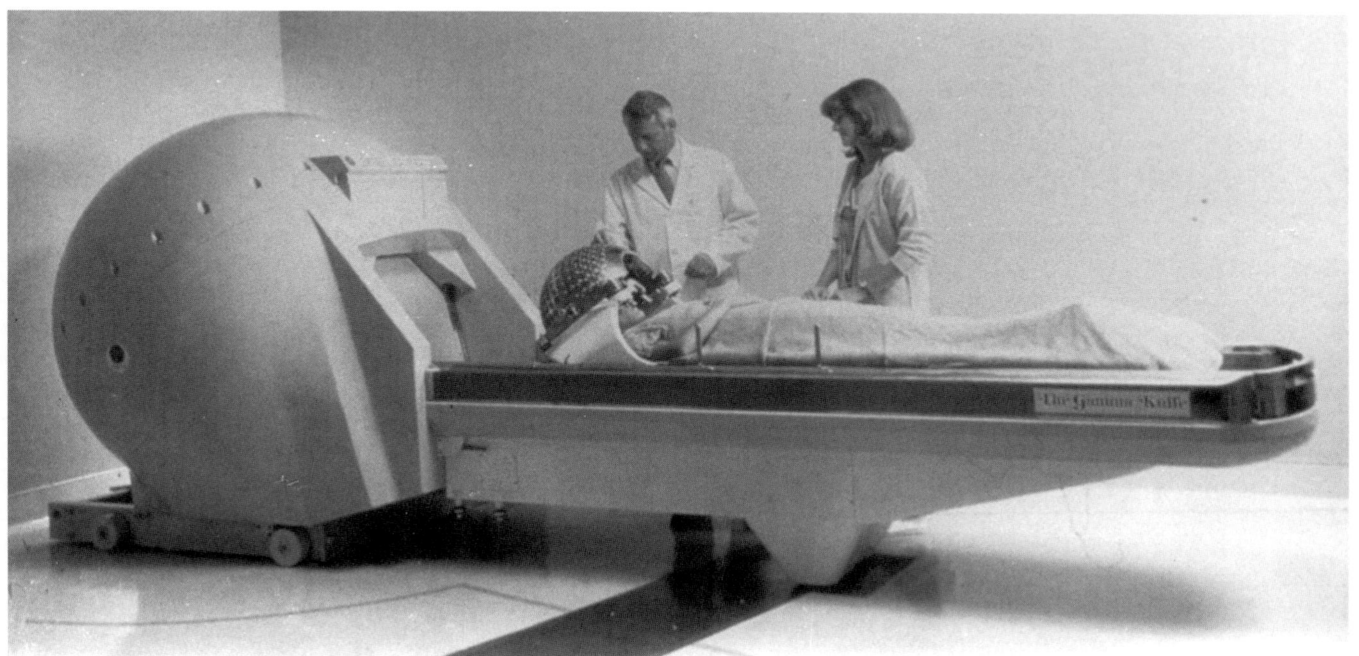

B

Fig. 16.17 **A.** Collimator helmet for the gamma unit. The helmet design allows for adjustment of the collimator size, depending upon lesion diameter. **B.** The patient's head and the collimator helmet are secured to the gamma unit. Together, they are then advanced into the radiation source.

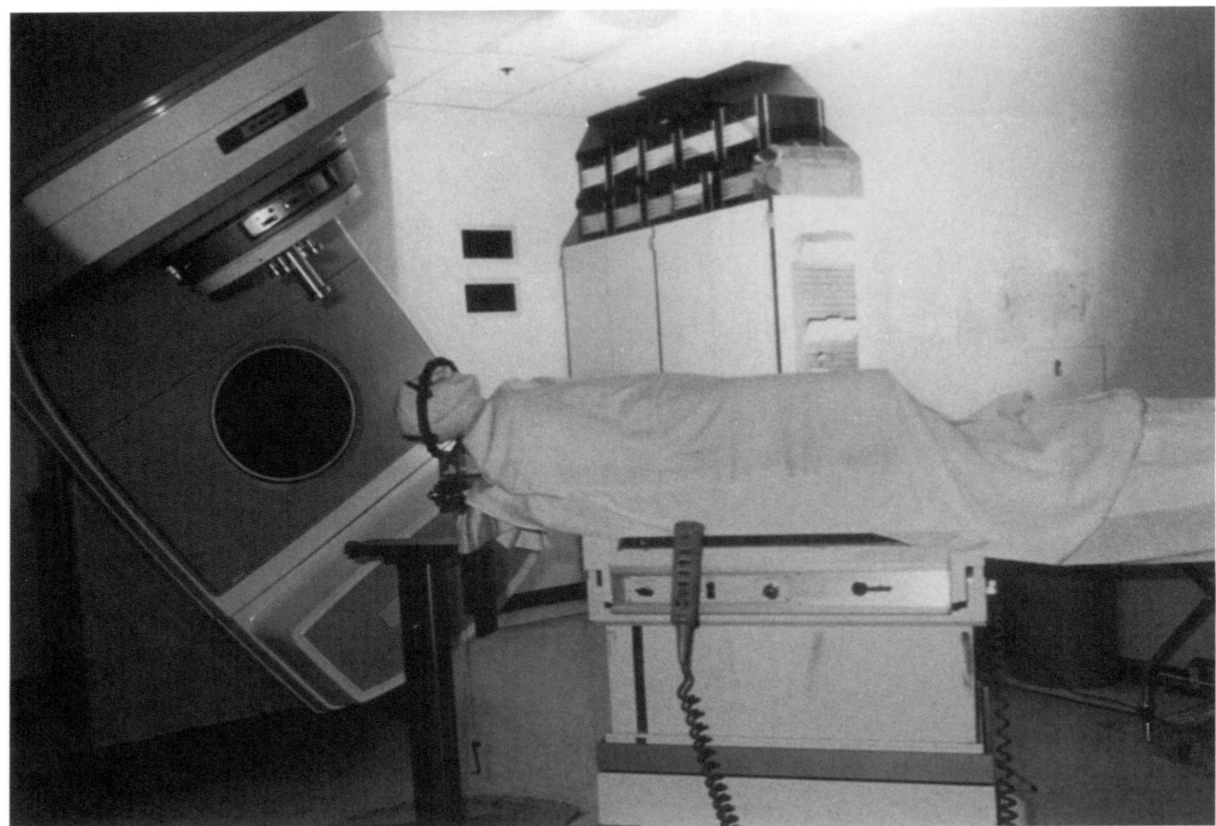

Fig. 16.18 The USC Linac-based radiosurgery system. The floorstand accommodates the base ring, which places the target at the center of the arc of rotation of the Linac. Both the arc and the patient's couch rotate about the axis defined by the target.

The treatment planning is done prior to the treatment session, using MRI scans of the target. The treatment is designed to result in the target receiving a specified dose defined by the 80% isodose line (Figs 16.19, 16.20). This is tailored by changing collimator size and the arcs of rotation of the beam source.

In the near future, fractionated radiosurgery techniques will become widely utilized. This form of radiosurgery combines the tenets of fractionation with standard radiosurgery. The end result will involve frameless methodologies and a probable reduction in the incidence of radionecrosis (Olivier et al 1992).

We presently use the Radionics stereotactic system for target localization using CT imaging. The target is acquired in the same fashion as described previously. Once the target is defined, the stereotactic coordinates are entered into the floorstand in the Linac suite. This places the isocenter in the center of the arc of rotation of the Linac.

To rehearse the treatment, a pointer is placed onto the phantom base ring, and the tip is placed at the target (Fig. 16.21). This pointer is then placed onto the floorstand, the point being the isocenter (Fig. 16.22). Its location is confirmed with the aid of room lasers which intersect at the isocenter. This is further checked by taking X-rays of the pointer at extremes of rotation of the arc, using the beam source. Once the position of the isocenter is confirmed, the treatment is administered.

Results. The technology of radiosurgery has been used to treat arteriovenous malformations and neoplastic disorders, and to effect lesions for functional procedures. In general, the maximum treatment volumes amenable to radiosurgery are those with a diameter 2.5 cm on standard imaging studies. The various neoplasias treated include acoustic neurinomas (vestibular schwannomas), craniopharyngiomas, meningiomas, and metastatic tumors (Lindgren 1958, Backlund 1973b, Barcia-Salorio et al 1984, Colombo et al 1985, Backlund 1987). One recent report analyzed the effectiveness of radiosurgery in growth hormone-secreting pituitary adenomas, but did not show significant benefit (Thoren et al 1991). We have also recently been using radiosurgery to provide a focused boost for gliomas.

With respect to meningiomas, some recent results have been published. Nearly all of these studies have indicated little in the way of tumor size reduction, but nevertheless have demonstrated greater than 90% growth control at 24 months (Kondziolka et al 1991, Steiner et al 1991). Radiosurgery seems ideally suited to treat meningiomas primarily in patients who are prohibitive surgical risks due

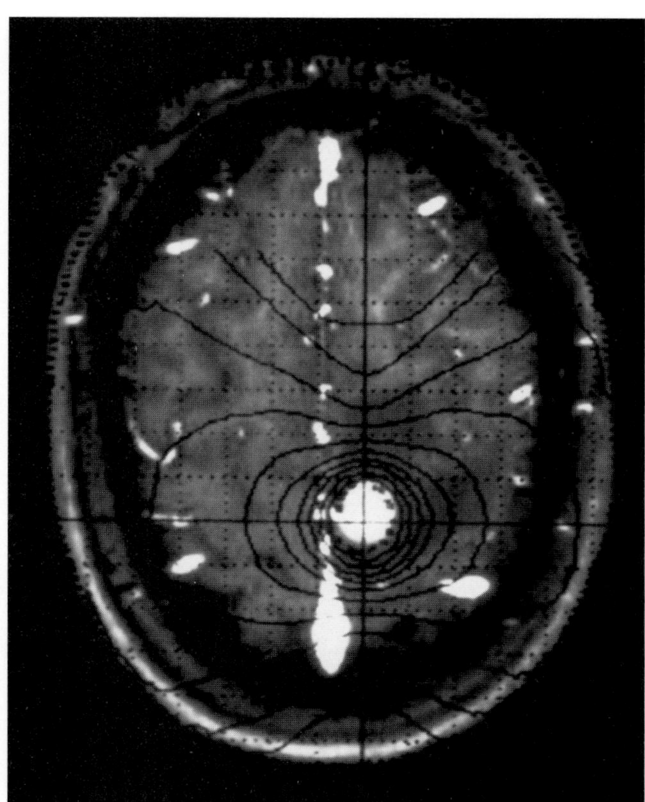

A

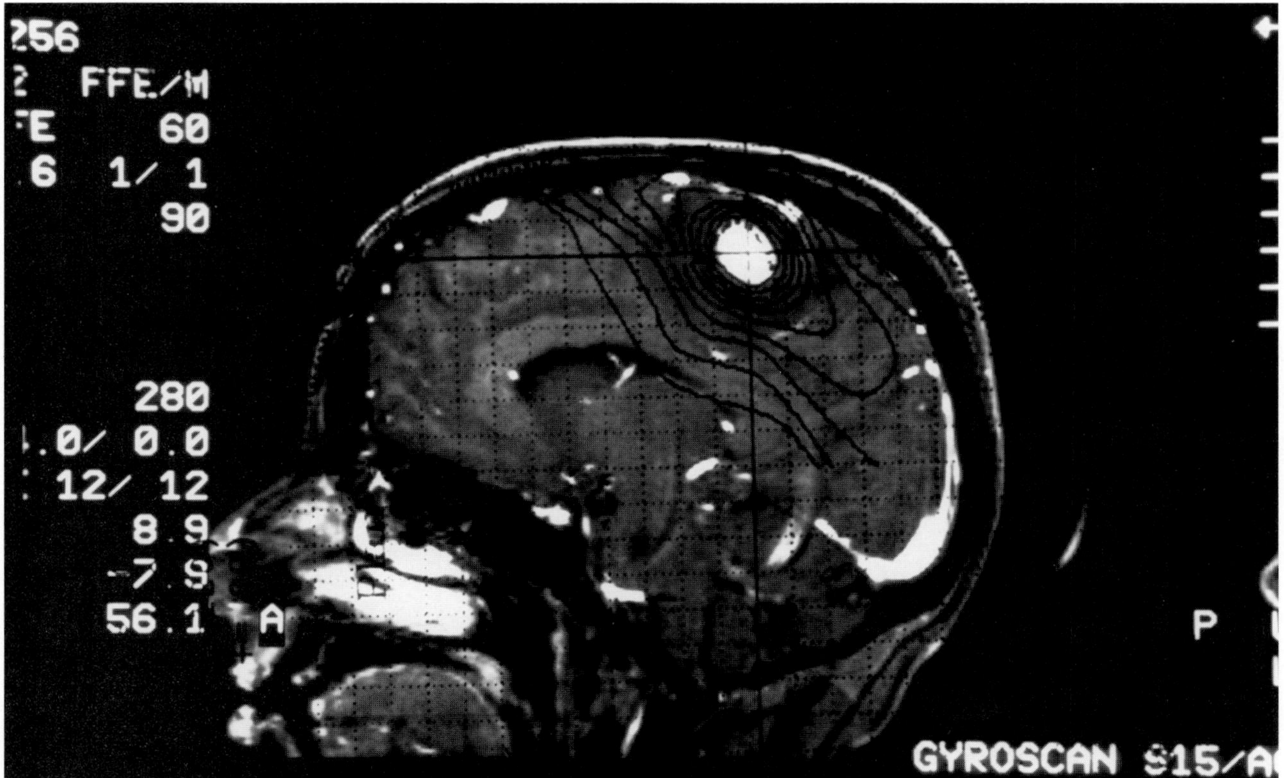

B

Fig. 16.19 Planning session for a metastatic melanoma. Isodose curves are projected in **A** — axial, **B** — sagittal and **C** — coronal planes. **D.** The arcs necessary to deliver the treatment are then calculated.

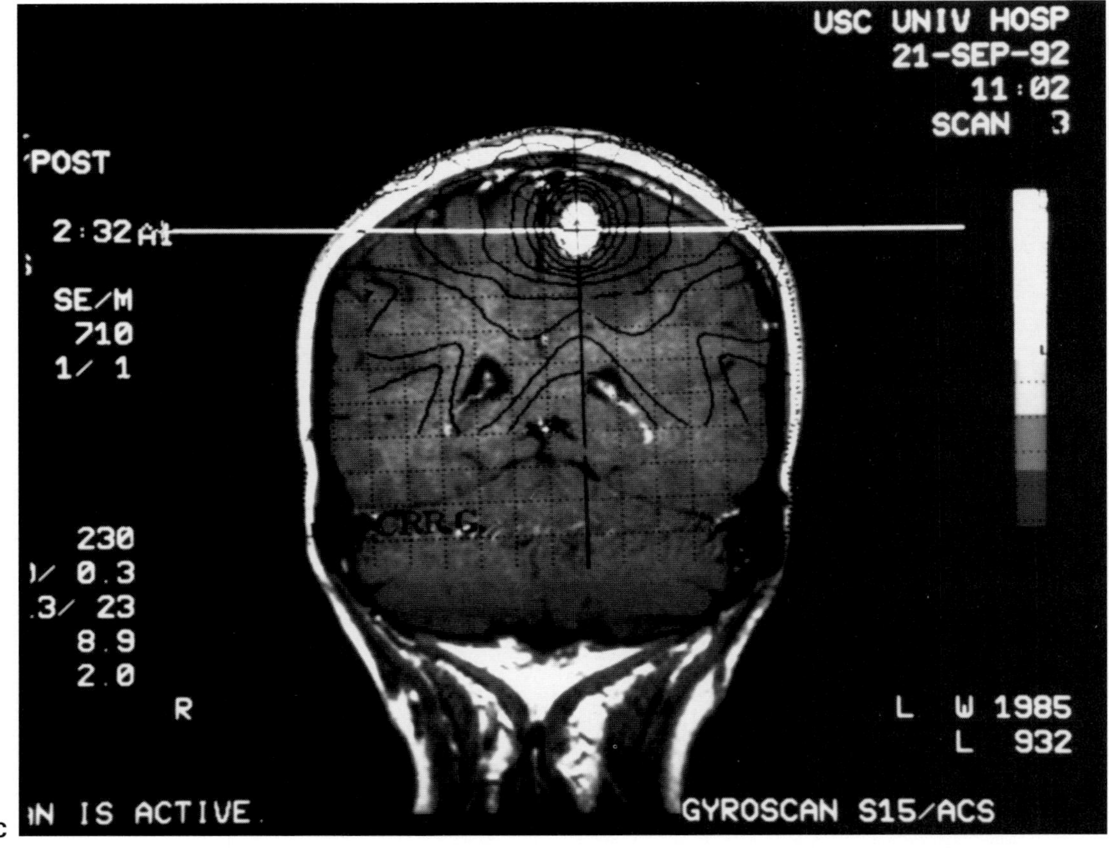

C

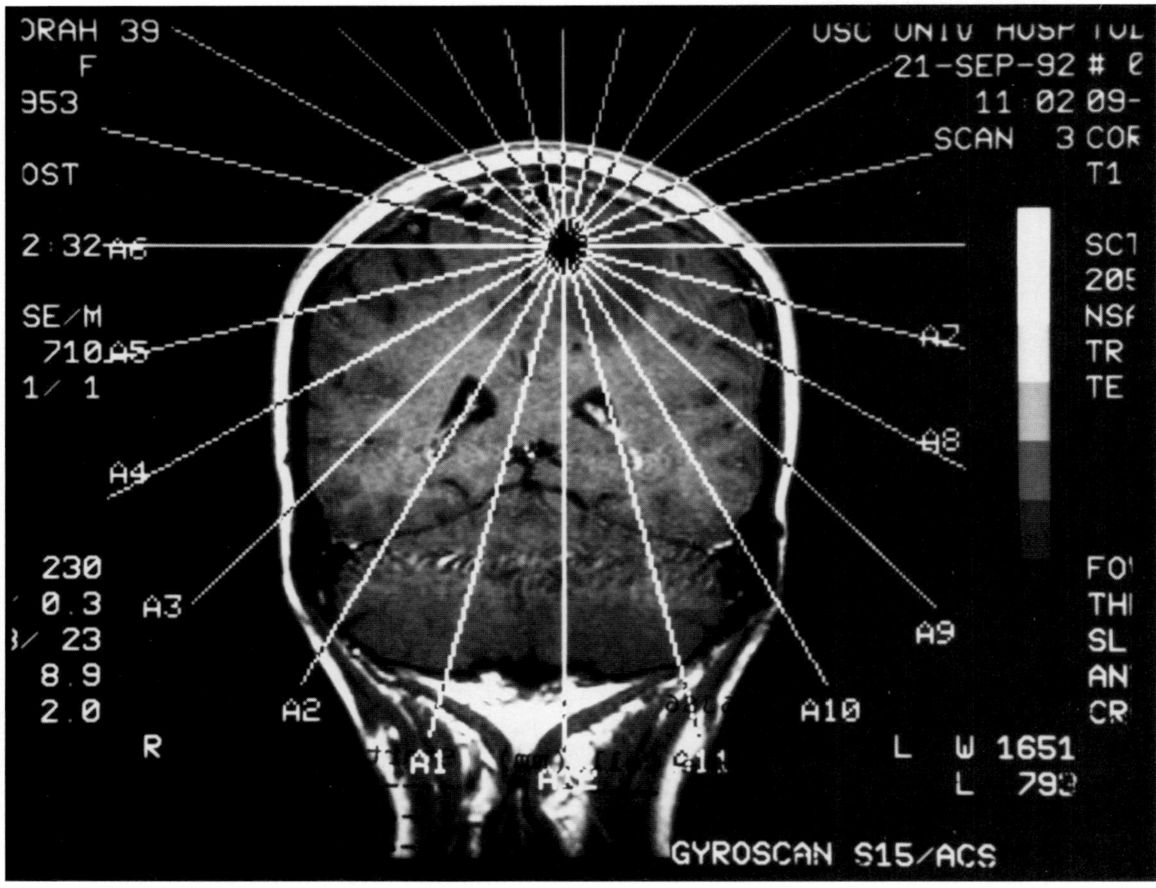

D

Fig. 16.19C & D

Fig. 16.20 A–D. Representative treatment plan for a metastatic renal cell carcinoma.

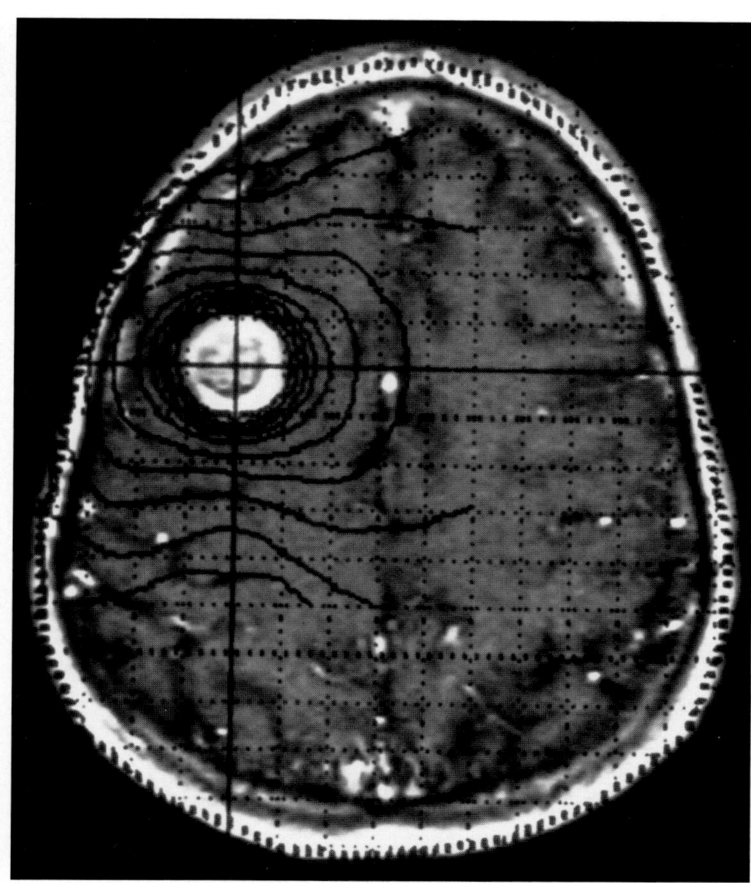

A

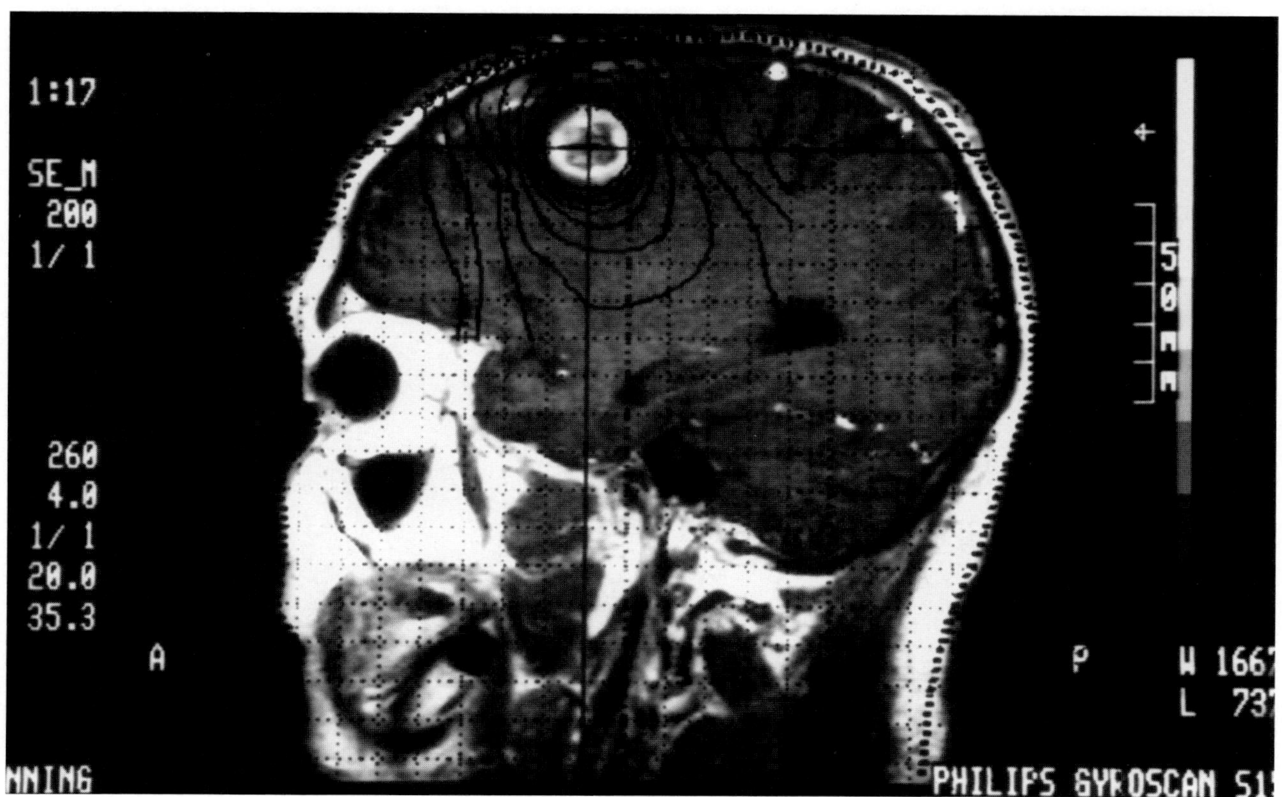

B

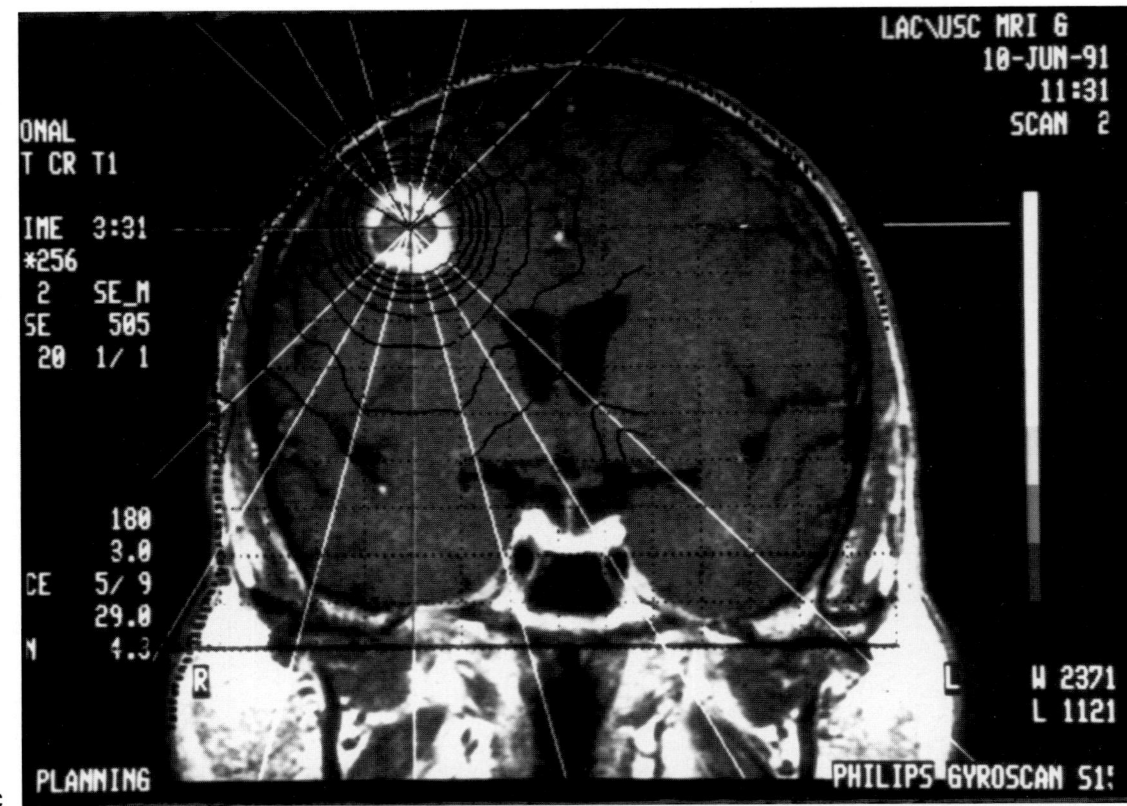

C

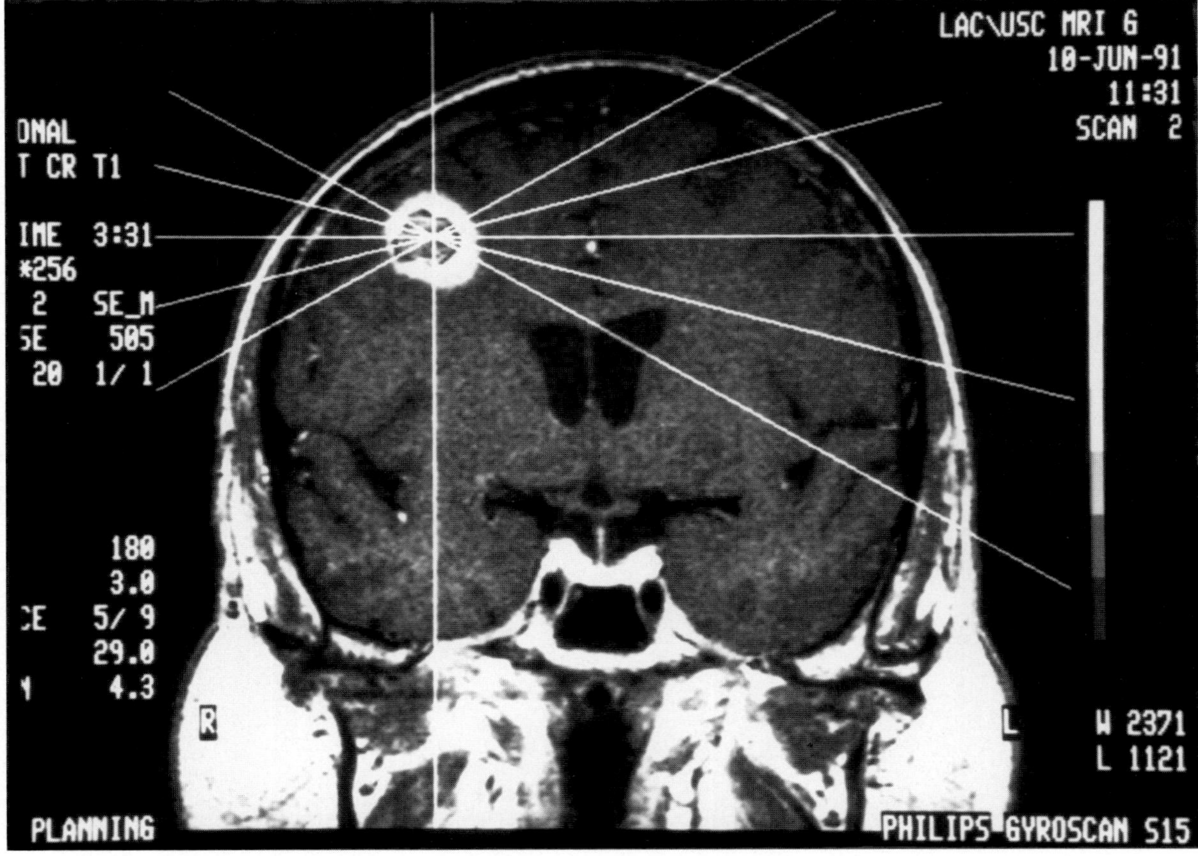

D

Fig. 16.20C & D

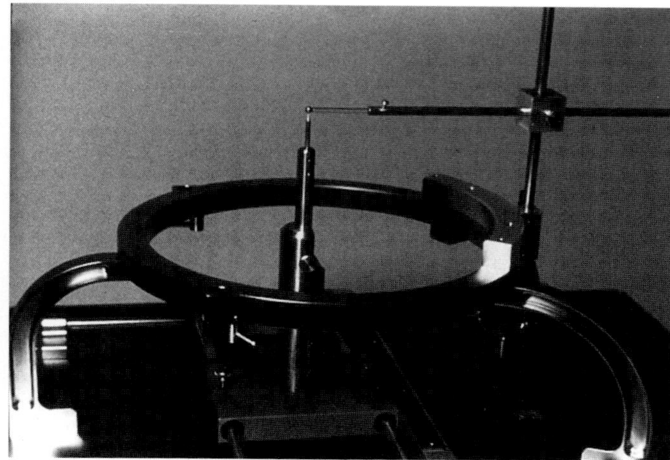

Fig. 16.21 Translational (pointer) device that provides translation of the target's position in stereotactic space to the treatment source. The target is acquired in standard fashion from the computer software, the position is then obtained from the phantom base, and transferred to the floorstand. The position of the pointer thus provides a phantom target to check the target position within the Linac prior to actual treatment.

to tumor location or medical illness, or secondarily for tumor recurrence or residual tumor following craniotomy.

Perhaps even more encouraging, results have recently been published for patients harboring metastatic tumors. In one large series, 80% of patients had either growth stabilization or complete radiographic remission (Adler et al 1992). In our own experience, we have experienced similar results, even in melanoma, a tumor generally thought to be radioresistant (unpublished data). Given the nature of metastatic disease, it is desirable to reduce the number of invasive procedures that patients must incur. As such, we feel that radiosurgery will eventually become the treatment of choice for metastatic tumors involving the CNS.

STEREOTAXIS OF THE FUTURE

Ongoing advances in computer technology are constantly influencing the evolution of stereotaxis. It is inevitable that frameless forms of stereotaxis will soon proliferate (Roberts et al 1986b). These systems will be coupled to advanced graphics systems to allow for real-time interactive imaging capabilities (Watanabe et al 1987). In time, these may eventually consist of three-dimensional holograms. Robotics devices will be integrated to allow the surgeon to interact with the real-time images, giving the robotic assistant instructions via voice-activated input, without having to break the sterile field. Lastly, the use of fiber-optic digitizers may provide for remote surgery using robotics (Kelly 1992).

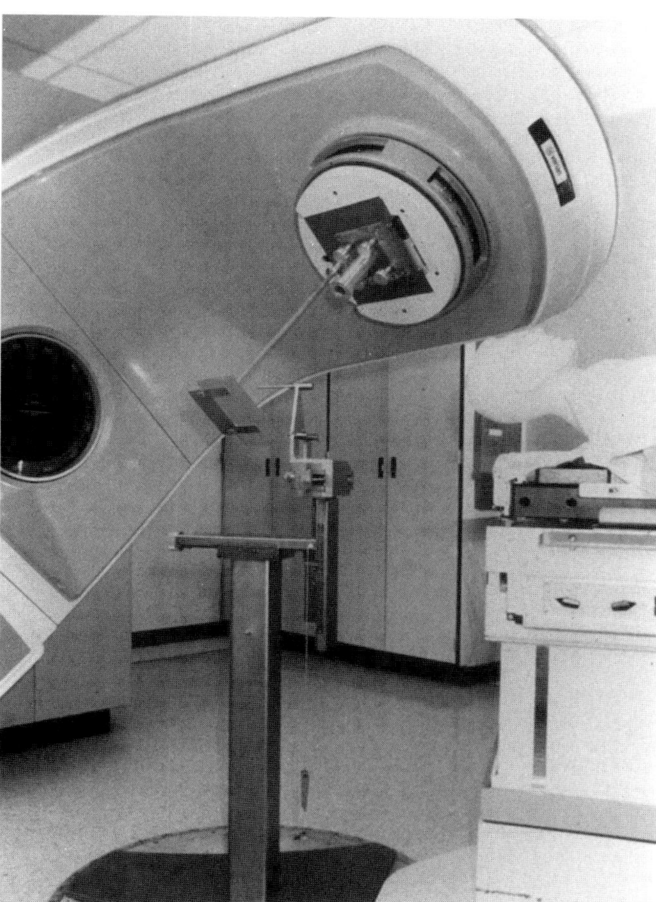

Fig. 16.22 Confirmation of the floorstand position is carried out as a final step prior to proceeding with actual treatment. The Linac is used to take standard X-rays which visualize the position of the pointer tip (target) with reference to the beam source.

CONCLUSIONS

The marriage of contemporary imaging techniques to stereotactic surgical principles has resulted in methodologies that allow for minimally invasive tissue sampling, yet a high diagnostic yield. Application of these principles to therapeutic concepts will continue to expand the goal of modern medicine — safe and effective treatment of disease with minimal intrusion to the patient.

REFERENCES

Adams J H, Graham D, Doyle D 1981 Brain biopsy: The smear technique for neurosurgical procedures. J B Lippincott, Philadelphia, pp 19–23

Adler J R, Cox R S, Kaplan K, Martin D P 1992 Stereotactic radiosurgical treatment of brain metastases. Journal of Neurosurgery 76: 444–449

Allen J C, Nisselbaum J, Epstein F et al 1979 Alpha-fetoprotein and human chorionic gonadotropin determination in cerebrospinal fluid. Journal of Neurosurgery 51: 368–374

Apuzzo M L J, Sabshin J K 1983 Computed tomographic guidance stereotaxis in the management of intracranial mass lesions. Neurosurgery 12: 277–285

Apuzzo M L J, Heifetz M D, Weiss M H, Kurze T 1977 Neurosurgical endoscopy using the side-viewing telescope. Technical note. Journal of Neurosurgery 46: 398–400

Apuzzo M L J, Chandrasoma P T, Zelman V, Giannotta S L, Weiss M H 1984a Computed tomographic guidance stereotaxis in the management of lesions of the third ventricular region. Neurosurgery 15: 502–508

Apuzzo M L J, Jepson J H, Luxton G, Little F M 1984b Ionizing and nonionizing radiation treatment of malignant cerebral gliomas. Specialized approaches. Clin Neurosurg 31: 470–496

Apuzzo M L J, Chandrasoma P T, Cohen D, Zee C S, Zelman V 1987 Computed imaging stereotaxy: Experience and perspective related to 500 procedures applied to brain masses. Neurosurgery 20: 930–937

Arita N, Bitoh S, Ushio Y et al 1983 Primary pineal endodermal sinus tumor with elevated serum and CSF alpha-fetoprotein levels. Journal of Neurosurgery 53: 244–248

Atkins E R 1983 Hyperthermia techniques and instrumentation. In: Storm F K (ed) Hyperthermia in cancer therapy. G K Hall Medical Publishers, Boston, MA, pp 233–256

Backlund E O 1973a Studies on craniopharyngiomas: III. Steteotaxic treatment with intracystic yttrium-90. Acta Chirurgica Scandinavica 139: 344–351

Backlund E O 1973b Studies on craniopharyngiomas. Stereotaxic treatment with radiosurgery. Acta Chirurgica Scandinavica 139: 237–247

Backlund E O 1974 Stereotactic treatment of craniopharyngiomas. Acta Neurochirurgica 21: 177–183

Backlund E O 1987 Role of stereotaxis in the management of midline cerebral lesions. In: Apuzzo M L J (ed) Surgery of the third ventricle. Williams & Wilkins, Baltimore, MD, pp 802–805

Barcia-Salorio J L, Hernandez G, Ciudad J, Bordes V 1984 Stereotactic radiosurgery in acoustic neuromas. Acta Neurochirurgica (Suppl) 33

Bernstein M, Gutin P H 1981 Interstitial irradiation of brain tumors: A review. Neurosurgery 9: 741–750

Borit A 1969 Embryonal carcinoma of the pineal region. Journal of Pathology 97: 165–168

Bosch D A 1980 Indications for stereotactic biopsy in brain tumors. Acta Neurochirurgica (Wein) 54: 167–179

Bouvier G, Penn R D, Kroin J S, Bieque R, Guerard M J 1987 Direct delivery of medication into a brain tumor through multiple chronically implanted catheters. Neurosurgery 20: 286–291

Brezovich I A, Atkinson W J, Lilly M B 1984 Local hyperthermia with interstitial techniques. Cancer Research 44: 4752–4756

Colombo F, Benedetti A, Pozzi F, Avanzp R C, Marchetti C, Chierego G, Zanardo A 1985 External stereotactic irradiation by linear accelerator. Neurosurgery 16: 154–160

Coughlin J C T, Douple E B, Strohbehn J W, Eaton W L, Trembly B S, Wong L T 1983 Interstitial hyperthermia in conjunction with brachytherapy. Radiology 148: 285–288

Couldwell W T, Apuzzo M L J 1990 Initial experience related to the use of the Cosman-Roberts-Wells stereotactic instrument. Technical note. Journal of Neurosurgery 72: 145–148

Crain B J, Bigner S H, Johnston W W 1983 Fine needle aspiration biopsy of deep cerebrum. A comparison of normal and neoplastic morphology. Acta Cytologica (Balt) 26: 772–778

Daumas-Duport C, Monsaingeon V, Szenthe L, Szenthe G 1982 Serial stereotactic biopsies: A double histologic code of gliomas according to malignancy and 3-D configuration, as an aid to therapeutic decision and assessment of results. Applied Neurophysiology 45: 431–437

Daumas-Duport C, Blond S, Vedrenne C L, Szikla G 1984 Radiolesion versus recurrence: Bioptic data in 39 gliomas after interstitial, or combined interstitial and external radiation treatment. Acta Neurochirurgica (Suppl) 33: 291–299

Dayan A D, Marshall A H E, Miller A A et al 1966 Atypical teratomas of the pineal and hypothalamus. Journal of Pathology and Bacteriology 92: 1–28

Dewey W C, Holahan E V 1984 Hyperthermia — basic biology. Progress in Experimental Tumor Research 28: 198–219

Dougherty T J, Thomas R E, Goyle D G, Weishaupt K R 1981 Interstitial photoradiation therapy for primary solid tumors in pet cats and dogs. Cancer Research 41: 401–404

Eisenhart L, Cushing H 1930 Diagnosis of intracranial tumors by supravital technique. American Journal of Pathology 6: 541–552

Emami B, Mittal B M, Sapareto S 1984 Sequencing of the total course of hyperthermia and irradiation. Cancer Research 44: 4731–4732

Florell R C, MacDonald D R, Irish W D, Bernstein M, Leibel S A, Gutin P H, Cairncross J G 1992 Selection bias, survival, and brachytherapy for gliomas. Journal of Neurosurgery 76: 179–183

Fulling K H, Nelson J S 1984 Cerebral astrocytic neoplasms in the adult. Contribution of histologic examination to the assessment of prognosis. Seminars in Diagnostic Pathology 1: 152–163

Giovanella B C 1983 Thermosensitivity of neoplastic cells in vitro. In: Storm F K (ed) Hyperthermia in cancer therapy. G K Hall Medical Publishers, Boston, MA, pp 55–62

Gutin P H, Phillips T L, Hosobuchi Y et al 1981 Permanent and removable implants for the brachytherapy of brain tumors. Int J Radiat Oncol Biol Biophys 7: 1371–1381

Gutin P H, Phillips T L, Wara W M et al 1984 Brachytherapy of recurrent malignant tumors with removable high activity iodine-125 sources. Journal of Neurosurgery 60: 61–68

Hahn G M 1982 Hyperthermia and cancer. Plenum Press, New York

Hall E J 1978 Radiobiology for the radiologists, 2nd edn. Harper & Row, New York

Hall E J, Roizin-Towle L 1978 Biological effects of heat. Cancer Research 44: 4708–4713

Hartmann B, Schlegel W, Sturm V, Bober B, Pastyr O, Lorenz W 1985 Cerebral radiation surgery using moving field irradiation at a linear accelerator facility. Int J Radiat Oncol Phys 11: 1185–1192

Hasse J, Neilsen K 1979 Value of tumor markers in the treatment of endodermal sinus tumors in the pineal region. Neurosurgery 5: 485–488

Heifetz M D, Wexler M, Thompson R 1984 Single-beam radiotherapy knife: A practical theoretical model. Journal of Neurosurgery 60: 814–818

Heilbrun M P 1983 Computed tomography-guided stereotactic systems. Clinical Neurosurgery 31: 564–581

Heilbrun M P, Roberts T S, Apuzzo M L J, Wells T H, Sabshin J K 1983 Preliminary experience with Brown-Roberts-Wells computerized tomography stereotaxic guidance system. Journal of Neurosurgery 59: 217–222

Heilman C B, Cohen A R 1991 Endoscopic ventricular fenestration using a "saline torch." Journal of Neurosurgery 74: 224–229

Hochberg F H, Pruitt A 1980 Assumptions in the radiotherapy of glioblastoma. Neurology 30: 907–911

Iizuka J 1975 Development of a stereotaxic endoscopy of the ventricular system. Confin Neurol 37: 141–149

Jane J A, Bertrand G 1962 A cytological method for the diagnosis of tumors affecting the central nervous system. Journal of Neuropathology and Experimental Neurology 21: 400–409

Kaye A H, Morstyn G 1987 Photoradiation therapy causing selective tumor kill in a rat glioma model. Neurosurgery 20: 408–415

Kaye A H, Morstyn G, Apuzzo M L J 1988 Photoradiation therapy and its potential in the management of neurological tumors. Journal of Neurosurgery 69: 1–14

Kelly P J 1986 Computer assisted stereotaxis: New approaches for the management of intracranial intra-axial tumors. Neurology 36: 535–541

Kelly P J 1987 Computer-assisted stereotaxic laser microsurgery. In: Apuzzo M L J (ed) Surgery of the third ventricle. Williams & Wilkins, Baltimore, MD, pp 811–828

Kelly P J 1992 Prospects for future development in stereotaxy. In: Apuzzo M L J (ed) Neurosurgery of the third millenium. American Association of Neurological Surgeons

Kelly P J, Kall B A, Goerss S 1984a Transposition of volumetric information derived from computed tomography scanning into stereotactic space. Surgical Neurology 21: 465–471

Kelly P J, Kall B A, Goerss S 1984b Computed simulation for the stereotactic placement of interstitial radionuclide sources into computed tomography-defined tumor volumes. Neurosurgery 14: 442–448

Kelly P J, Kall B A, Goerss S, Earnest F IV 1986 Computer-assisted stereotaxic laser resection of intra-axial brain neoplasms. Journal of Neurosurgery 64: 427–439

Kirschner J J, Ginsberg S J, Fitzpatrick A V, Conis R L 1981

Treatment of a primary intracranial germ cell tumor with systemic chemotherapy. Medical Pediatric Oncology 9: 361–365

Kjellberg R N 1979a Isoeffective dose parameters for brain necrosis in relation to proton radiosurgical dosimetry. Stereotactic cerebral irradiation. INSERM Symposium No 12

Kjellberg R N 1979b Stereotactic Bragg-peak proton radiosurgery results. Stereotactic cerebral irradiation. INSERM Symposium No 12

Kjellberg R N, Hanahamura T, Davis K R, Lyons S L, Adams R D 1983 Bragg-peak proton-beam therapy for arteriovenous malformations of the brain. New England Journal of Medicine 309: 269–274

Kobayshi T, Kageyama N, Ohara K 1981 Internal irradiation for cystic craniopharyngioma. Journal of Neurosurgery 55: 896–903

Kondziolka D, Lunsford L D 1991 Stereotactic management of colloid cysts: Factors predicting success. Journal of Neurosurgery 75: 45–51

Kondziolka D, Lunsford L D, Coffey R J, Flickinger J C 1991 Stereotactic radiosurgery of meningiomas. Journal of Neurosurgery 74: 552–559

Kroin J S, Penn R D 1982 Intracerebral chemotherapy: Chronic microinfusion of cis-platinum. Neurosurgery 10: 349–354

Laws E R, Cortese D A, Kinsey J H et al 1981 Photoradiation therapy in the treatment of malignant brain tumors. A phase I (feasability) study. Neurosurgery 9: 672–678

Leibel S A, Gutin P H, Wara W M et al 1989 Survival and quality of life after interstitial implantation of removable high-activity iodine-125 sources for the treatment of patients with recurrent malignant gliomas. Int J Radiat Oncol Biol Phys 17: 1129–1139

Leksell L 1951 The stereotaxic method and radiosurgery of the brain. Acta Chirurgica Scandinavica 102: 316–319

Leksell L 1971 Stereotaxis and radiosurgery: An operative system. Charles C Thomas, Springfield, IL

Leksell L, Backlund E O 1979 Stereotactic gammacapsulotomy. In: Hitchcock E R, Ballantine H T, Meyerson B (eds) Modern concepts in psychiatric surgery. Elsevier, Amsterdam, pp 213–216

Leksell L, Leksell D, Schwebel J 1985 Stereotaxis and nuclear magnetic resonance. Journal of Neurology and Neurosurgical Psychiatry 48: 14–18

Lindgren M 1958 On tolerance of brain tissue and sensitivity of brain tumors to irradiation. Acta Radiol 170: 1–73

Linwicz B H, Henderson K S, Masukawa T, Smith R D 1986 Needle aspiration cytology of intracranial lesions. A review of 84 cases. Acta Cytologica 26: 779–878

Lunsford L D, Martinez A J, Latchaw R E 1986 Stereotaxic surgery with a magnetic resonance and computerized tomographic system. Journal of Neurosurgery 64: 872–878

Lutz W, Winston K R, Meleki N 1988 A system for stereotactic radiosurgery with a linear accelerator. Neurosurgery 22: 454–464

Luxton G, Petrovich Z, Jozef G, Nedzi L A, Apuzzo M L J 1993 Stereotactic radiosurgery: principles and comparison of treatment methods. Neurosurgery 32: 241–259

Lyons E, Britt R H, Strohbehn J W 1984 Localized hyperthermia in the treatment of malignant brain tumors using an interstitial microwave antenna array. IEEE Trans Biomed Engin 31: 53–62

Lyons E, Strohbehn J W, Roberts D W, Wong T Z, Britt R H 1986 Interstitial microwave hyperthermia for the treatment of brain tumors. In: Leopold J, Anghilieri C T, Robert J (eds) Hyperthermia in cancer treatment. CRC Press, Boca Raton, FL, pp 25–45

Markert J M, Coen D M, Malick A, Mineta T, Martuza R L 1992 Expanded spectrum of viral therapy in the treatment of nervous system tumors. Journal of Neurosurgery 77: 590–594

Morris A A 1947 The use of the smear technique in the rapid histologic diagnosis of tumors of the central nervous system: Description of a new staining method. Journal of Neurosurgery 4: 497–504

Mundinger F 1966 The treatment of brain tumors with radioisotopes. Progress in Neurological Surgery 1: 202–257

Mundinger F, Hoefer T 1974 Protracted long-term irradiation of inoperable midbrain tumors by stereotactic Curie-therapy using Iridium-192. Acta Neurochirurgica 21: 93–100

Mundinger F 1979 Rationale and methods of interstitial Ir-192 brachytherapy and Ir-192 and Iodine-125 protracted long-term irradiations. In: Szikla G (ed) Cerebral irradiations. Elsevier, Amsterdam

Mundinger F 1982 Implantation of radioisotopes (Curie-therapy). In: Schaltenbrand G, Walker A E (eds) Stereotaxy of the human brain. Thieme-Stratton, New York

Mundinger F, Weigel K 1984 Long-term results of stereotactic interstitial curietherapy. Acta Neurochirurgica (suppl) 33: 367–371

Olivier A, Sadikot A F, Villemure J G, Pokrupa R, Souham L, Podgorsak E B, Hazel J 1992 Fractionated stereotactic radiotherapy for intracranial neoplasms. Stereotact Funct Neurosurg 59: 193–198

Ostertag C B 1983 Biopsy and interstitial radiation therapy of cerebral gliomas. Italian Journal of Neurological Science (Suppl) 2: 121–128

Ostertag C B, Weigel K, Birg W 1979 CT changes after long-term interstitial iridium-192 irradiation of cerebral gliomas. In: Szikla G (ed) Stereotactic cerebral irradation. Elsevier, Amsterdam

Ostertag C B, Groothuis D, Kleihues P 1984 Effects of tumor and brain: Experimental data on early and late morphologic effects of permanently implanted gamma and beta sources (iridium-192, iodine-125, yttrium-90) in the brain. Acta Neurochirurgica (Suppl) 33: 271–280

Petrovich Z, Apuzzo M L J, Luxton G, Jepson J H, Cohen D 1987 Interstitial radiotherapy of malignant cerebral gliomas. In: Walker M, Kornblith P (eds) Contemporary concepts in neurooncology. Futura Publishers, New York, pp 149–155

Powell M P, Torrens M J, Thomas J L G et al 1983 Isodense colloid cysts of the third ventricle: A diagnostic and therapeutic problem solved by ventriculoscopy. Neurosurgery 13: 234–237

Powers S K, Cush S S, Walstead D L, Kwock L 1991 Stereotactic intratumoral photodynamic therapy for recurrent malignant brain tumors. Neurosurgery 29: 688–696

Rivas J J, Lobato R D 1985 CT-assisted stereotaxic aspiration of colloid cysts of the third ventricle. Journal of Neurosurgery 62: 238–242

Roberts D W, Coughlin C T, Wong T Z, Fratkin J D, Douple E B, Strohbehn J W 1986a Interstitial hyperthermia for malignant glioma. Journal of Neurosurgery 64: 581–587

Roberts D W, Strobehn J W, Hatch J F, Murray W, Kettenberger H 1986b A frameless stereotaxic integration of computerized tomographic imaging and the operating microscope. Journal of Neurosurgery 65: 545–549

Russell D S, Krayenbuhl H, Cairns H 1937 The wet film technique in the histopathological diagnosis of intracranial tumors. A rapid method. Journal of Pathology 45: 501–505

Salcman M 1984 Feasability of microwave hyperthermia for brain tumor therapy. Prog Exp Tumor Res 28: 220–231

Salcman M, Samaras G M 1981 Hyperthermia for brain tumors. Biophysical rationale. Neurosurgery 9: 327–335

Scheithauer B W 1985 Neuropathology of pineal region tumors. Clinical Neurosurgery 32: 351–383

Silberman A W, Rand R W, Storm F K, Drury B, Benz M L, Morton D L 1985 Phase I trial of thermochemotherapy for brain malignancy. Cancer 56: 48–56

Silberman A W, Rand R W, Krag D N, Storm F L, Benz M L, Drury B, Morton D L 1986 Effect of localized magnetic induction hyperthermia on the brain. Cancer 57: 1401–1404

Sisti M B, Solomon R A, Stein B M 1991 Stereotactic craniotomy in the resection of small arteriovenous malformations. Journal of Neurosurgery 75: 40–44

Steiner L 1984 Treatment of arteriovenous malformations by radiosurgery. In: Wilson C B, Stein B M (eds) Intracranial arteriovenous malformations. Williams & Wilkins, Baltimore, MD

Steiner L, Leksell L, Forster D M, Grietz T, Backlund E O 1974 Stereotactic radiosurgery in the intracranial arteriovenous malformations. Acta Neurochirurgica (Suppl) 21: 195–209

Steiner L, Lindquist C, Steiner M 1991 Meningiomas and gamma knife radiosurgery. In: Al-Mefty O (ed) Meningiomas. Raven Press, New York, pp 263–272

Storm F K 1983 Background, principles, and practice. In: Storm F K (ed) Hyperthermia in cancer therapy. G K Hall Medical Publishers, Boston, MA, pp 1–8

Szikla G 1979 Stereotactic cerebral irradiation. Elsevier, North Holland

Szikla G, Peragut J C 1975 Irradiation interstitielle des gliomes. Neurochirurgica (Suppl 2) 21: 187–228

Szikla G, Schlienger M, Betti O et al 1979 Combined interstitial and external irradiation of gliomas. A progress report. In: Szikla G (ed) Stereotactic cerebral irradiation. Elsevier, New York, pp 329–338

Szikla G, Schlienger M, Blind S et al 1984 Interstitial and combined interstitial and external irradiation of supratentorial gliomas. Results in 61 cases treated 1973–1981. Acta Neurochirurgica (Suppl) 33: 355–362

Tator C H 1977 Intraneoplastic injection of CCNU for experimental brain tumor chemotherapy. Surgical Neurology 7: 73–77

Tator C H, Wassenar W 1977 Intraneoplastic injection of methotrexate for experimental brain tumor chemotherapy. Journal of Neurosurgery 46: 175–184

Tator C H, Day A, Ng R, Liberman L 1977a Chemotherapy of an experimental glioma with nitrosoureas. Cancer Research 37: 476–481

Tator C H, Wassenar W, So W S 1977b Therapy of an experimental glioma with systemic or intraneoplastic methotrexate or radiation. Journal of Neurosurgery 46: 175–184

Thoren, Rahn T, Guo W, Werner S 1991 Stereotactic radiosurgery with cobalt-60 gamma unit in the treatment of growth hormone producing pituitary tumors. Neurosurgery 29: 663–668

Vandenberg J H, Blaau G, Breeman W A P, Rahmy A, Wijngaarde R 1992 Intracavitary brachytherapy of cystic craniopharyngioma. Journal of Neurosurgery 77: 545–550

Watanabe E, Watanabe T, Manaka S, Mayanagi Y, Takakura 1987 Three-dimensional digitizer (neuronavigator): new equipment for computed tomography-guided stereotaxic surgery. Surgical Neurology 27: 543–547

Weigel K, Ostertag C B, Mundinger F 1979 Interstitial long-term irradiation of tumors in the pineal region. Stereotactic cerebral irradiation. INSERM, Symposium No 12, pp 283–292

Willems J S 1983 Aspiration biopsy cytology of tumors of the central nervous system and base of the skull. In: Linsk J A, Franzen S (eds) Clinical aspiration cytology. Lippincott, Philadelphia, PA

Winter A, Laing J, Paglione R, Sterzer F 1985 Microwave hyperthermia for brain tumors. Neurosurgery 17: 387–399

17. Radiation therapy and radiosurgery for brain tumors

A. B. M. F. Karim

INTRODUCTION

Many advances have been made regarding the diagnosis and the treatment of brain tumors, particularly in the field of imaging. Tremendous strides in surgical techniques ensure that, at present, virtually no patients are treated empirically without a definite histopathological diagnosis. Unfortunately, a consensus on the criteria of histopathological classification and grading, in spite of many efforts including those from the WHO, has not been reached. Although there are many reports about tumor grading they are not without controversy (Zulch 1979, Smith et al 1983, Daumas–Duport et al 1988, Stam 1991).

Recent developments in radiation oncology for the treatment of brain tumors must be looked at in an arena which deals with developments in neurosurgery, imaging, or pathology. Several attempts are, at present, being undertaken to advance understanding of the biology of brain tumors (Janus et al 1992), particularly those with therapeutic implications. The same is true in the field of radiation neuro-oncology. By collaborating with other neuro-oncologists and incorporating the existing technological excellence within radiation oncology (Schlegel et al 1992), it is hoped that improved treatment results and improved quality of life for the patient are realistic goals in the next century. Some slow but steady trends indicating improvement in the results of treatment are noticeable (Table 17.1). Further improvement may be forthcoming as a result of well-planned prospective studies, specifically randomized clinical trials. Neuro-oncologists must agree that facts and figures from retrospective studies and randomized trials are needed to improve patient care. Not all aspects of radiation therapy and stereotactic 'radiosurgery' will be discussed in this chapter. The attempt here is to cover some important aspects that may not be found in the usually available contemporary literature.

Table 17.1 Improvement trends. Representative percent survival figures after treatment of patients with brain tumors (surgery with postoperative radiotherapy in most situations).

Type of tumor	Average survival %		Years
	1960–1970	1985–1992	
Pilocytic astrocytomas	40–60	80	5
LGG	45	60	5
HGG: grade 3	8	20–30	2
grade 3	<10	15	5
grade 4	0–2	5	2
grade 4	0	0	5
Childhood LGG	70	90	5
Childhood HGG	20	40	3
Ependymoma†	<50	>70	5
Medulloblastomas	40	>50	5
Poor risk group	0	<30	5
Good prognostic group		>65	
Craniopharyngiomas	70	90	10
Pineal blastomas, pineal astrocytomas	<35*	?>50**	5
Germinomas	>70*	90**	5

† Low and high grades of anaplasia have significant prognostic differences.
* Mostly local field.
** Whole brain irradiations.
LGG, low grade glioma
HGG, high grade glioma

CERTAIN GENERAL ASPECTS OF RADIATION THERAPY

Radiation therapy needs modern facilities and a multidisciplinary approach which incorporates the clinical history, operative procedures, histopathology and modern imaging systems. Modern technologies must be individualized for each patient, particularly to deliver adequate dosage to a three-dimensionally (3D) conceived target volume and to avoid unnecessarily high doses to normal tissues. Any tumor may have a spectrum of pathologic elements which can be difficult to differentiate, although many efforts are being undertaken (Janus et al 1992). To counter differing degrees of radiosensitivity, most tumors require a differential dose system (DDS).

The DDS (Karim et al 1991b) means that an inhomogeneous dose distribution to the target volume should be considered, i.e. higher doses to the central core of a tumor and decreasingly less to the surrounding areas. This may be a rather simplistic idea, but is certainly worth trying, particularly when no other data are available describing methods to combat heterogeneity. The DDS also takes

Table 17.2 Percentage of low grade gliomas transformed to a higher grade of malignancy: retrospective studies. From Karim & Kralendonk (1991)

Reference, type of tumor	Astrocytoma (%)	Oligodendroglioma (%)	(%)
Isamat et al (1986)[a]	38		
Müller et al (1977)[a]			
Astrocytoma grade 1 to grade 2	56		
Astrocytoma grade 1 to HGG	31		
Astrocytoma grade 2 to HGG	45		
Afra & Müller (1991)[a]			
Astrocytoma grade 2 to HGG	80		
Oligodendroglioma grade 2 to HGG		52	
Karim et al (unpublished data)[b]			
LGG to HGG			20

HGG = high grade glioma; LGG = low grade glioma.
[a] Most patients not irradiated.
[b] All patients irradiated postoperatively, but with much shorter follow-up.

into account the important question of variable tolerance levels of normal brain tissue and helps to limit late damage. The target volume usually covers not only the tumor area as delineated by the radiological images and as described by the neurosurgeon, but also the possible areas of invasion around the tumor or the routes of possible spread. Even though radiation oncologists enjoy considerable latitude in planning treatment policy compared to that of the surgeon, they must have some intuitive ideas based on objective responses. This latitude is not applicable when a high single dose of radiation is delivered with quality controlled pinpoint accuracy, as practised in the setup for 'radiosurgery' or stereotactic radiotherapy/surgery (STRT/S).

One may assume in a rather uncomplicated way, that 'mis'information or 'mis'interpretation — emanating either from surgery, pathology or images — may be translated into unsuccessful local control or unacceptable morbidity.

Causes of failure

Fortunately, local control for some patients with certain types of brain tumor may mean cure, but in many cases long-term local control is jeopardized because:

- Most tumors are not highly radiosensitive, with the result that recurrence of the same tumor at the same site is rather common in the treatment field. Geographical miss is rather rarely found.
- The vulnerability of normal brain tissue at certain sites means that radiation necrosis may occur, particularly when the threshold dose is surpassed at these sites mediated through one or more column(s) of hot spots in the dose distribution of the target volume.
- The optimum dose to reduce recurrence and to avoid necrosis is difficult to assess.
- Eventually differentiation, i.e. transformation of some tumor cells to higher grades of anaplasia, may occur in an increasing number of patients over a period up to 20 years or even more (Table 17.2).

The occurrence of radionecrosis, recurrence of the tumor at the same site, and dedifferentiation or transformation to a higher grade of malignancy are the principal causes of failure in the treatment of brain tumors. One has to accept that, in spite of progress in many oncological fields, patients with brain tumors are not being cured proportionately. At present, however, in low grade gliomas at least, apparent improvement in overall survival at 5 years by almost 20% has been documented (Karim 1991).

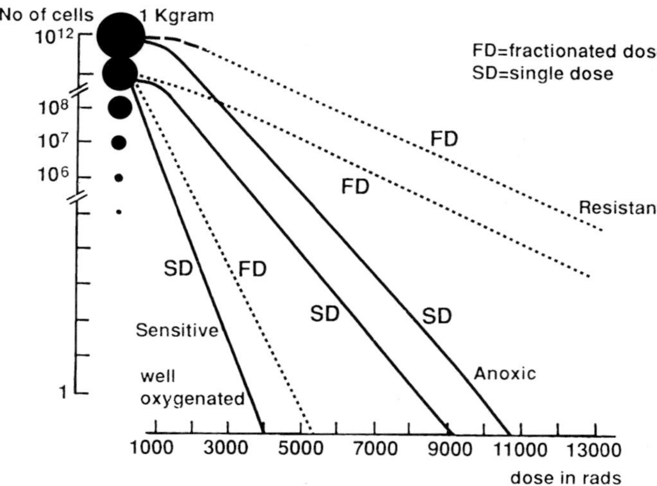

Fig. 17.1 Basic principles of radiobiology for tumor mass, oxygen and fractionation. Greater tumor volume (10^{12} cells = 1 kg) harboring a greater number of anoxic tumor cells requires much higher doses, particularly if fractionation is used. For a smaller number of cells killed, the parallel curves require a lower dose. FD = fractionated dose; SD = single dose. From Karim & Kralendork (1991).

Table 17.3 Prognostic value of amount of tumor removed during surgery in patients treated by postoperative radiotherapy. From Karim & Kralendonk (1991)

Reference, type of study	Survival (years)	Amount of tumor removed			
		<50%	>50%	50–90%	>90%
Sano (1986): LGG (*n* = 2048)	1	72%		76%	92%
	2	60%		65%	85%
	3	52%		57%	78%
Soffietti et al (1989): LGG (*n* = 85)	1	70%		90%	88%
	2	28%		70%	85%
	3	10%		50%	76%
Sano (1986): HGG (glioblastomas) (*n* = 1348)	1	38%		46%	60%
	2	16%		22%	34%
	3	12%		14%	25%
Winger et al (1989): HGG (*n* = 285)	1	15%		40%	64%
	2	5%		15%	35%
	3	5%		10%	21%
Karim et al (1991): HGG (grades 3, 4), (*n* = 88)	1	17%	60%		
	2	11%	25%		
	3	0%	9%		

A pragmatic multidisciplinary approach from a radiobiological point of view

The neurosurgeon in particular does a great service to the patient by removing as much tumor as possible, so that radiation therapy can sterilize a relatively smaller number of tumor cells with an optimum dose (Fig. 17.1), avoiding the risk of radionecrosis. These concepts may not be universally accepted, but the scientific rationale has to be pursued (Guthrie & Laws 1991). Moreover, sufficient clinical data are available at present to show the benefit of aggressive surgical removal of the tumor (Table 17.3, Fig. 17.1).

BASIC FACILITIES, DOSE-TIME AND TECHNICAL ASPECTS OF RADIATION THERAPY

Much technological advancement has already been or is being incorporated in modern radiation therapy, but the motivated radiation oncologist with expertise behind the machines is perhaps most important. Radiation oncologists must be actively supported by a dedicated paramedical staff, e.g. physicists, computer dosimetrists and therapy, simulator and mould-room technicians, among others. The cooperative attitude of all neuro-oncologists in a multidisciplinary team is an essential prerequisite for ensuring better results after treatment for brain tumors.

Linear accelerators are common these days in almost all departments of radiation oncology. These machines with sharper beams offer many treatment possibilities, e.g. multiple fields, moving beams, wedge filters, multileaf and asymmetric collimators, electrons for peripheral small lesions and extra accessories for stereotactic radiotherapy/surgery (STRT/S). Electrons with suitable energy are not usually used but the dose distributions indicate (Karim et al 1991b) that an unnecessarily high dose to normal brain may be avoided if properly planned electron therapy is used (Fig. 17.2). Regrowth of hair may not be as good as with the skin-sparing photons, however, particularly when blocking devices are individually made for sparing the hair roots from a tangenital photon beam.

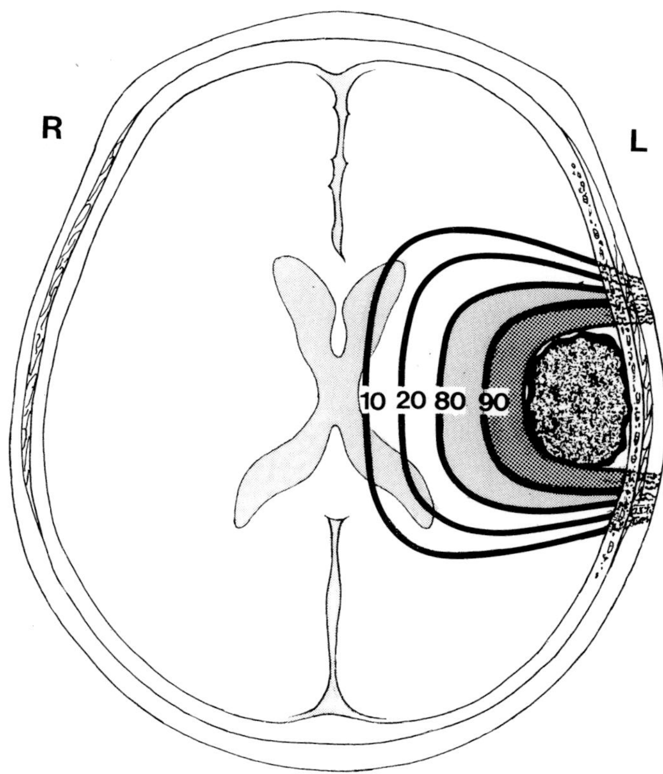

Fig. 17.2 Dose distribution of an electron field for a peripheral tumor.

Essential prerequisites are, of course, knowledge of the anatomical localization of the tumor, its usual pathways of infiltration or spread, the vasculature, the sensitive functional sites in the adjacent normal brain tissue and the different tolerance doses. Much is offered by modern imaging, including 3D techniques, and both CT and

MRI imaging are accepted as complementary (Kaiser & Kralendonk 1991).

Kelly (1992) has recently correlated histologic and CT findings. Integration of all (CT, MRI, angiography) data from images is being accomplished in a planned way in some centers, e.g. Pittsburg, Heidelberg, Boston and others. Positron emission tomography (PET) may provide significant clinical information and is also being incorporated. A CT simulator is ideal but not generally available.

Many departments utilize simulator examination, and the fields are then marked on a CT scan for further modification of field positioning and planning. This method, though time-consuming, may eventually be utilized through a more efficient future CT or MRI simulator. Three-dimensional (3D) viewing and planning based on modern imaging, although important, is not at present universally available. An accurately planned treatment policy should be the norm, incorporating the mould room as an essential facility. Here the patient's head is fixed in an individually made Perspex® shell-mask fixed to a base plate on which the head rests in a comfortable and reproducible way. Accuracy must be high, with less than a 5 mm possibility of displacement of the isocenter, bearing in mind that the daily inaccuracies may negate each other, so that the accuracy may be enhanced; cumulatively enhanced inaccuracy is rare. Localization error is usually defined when the isocenter is displaced more than 5 mm from the original isocenter of the fields and must be avoided. Quality and accuracy may be achieved in many ways, but in any quality control program, one must define these aspects specifically. Calculation of the dose is another important aspect. Many centers follow the ICRU regulation 29 (1978), but even within the framework of these regulations one may sharpen the quality of dose distribution with specificity. It is almost always possible to cover the target volume within 95% isodose distribution, if not higher. It is worthwhile to check the accuracy weekly with a port film, particularly for a complex setup.

On-line portal imaging is an important development and, when routinely available, may be helpful in quality control programs. Expertise from the mould room has routinized accurate fixation, and spared normal tissues by using customized innovative blocking devices. Hair roots are not difficult to spare, and in most situations highly satisfactory regrowth of hair is seen.

Individualization is the key word. Radiation oncologists, physicists and therapy technologists may attain this objective by routine schedules of joint discussions.

In general, complex radiotherapy techniques are not being utilized, although theoretically the need for improvement, particularly to deliver a higher effective tumor dose without surpassing the tolerance dose to the surrounding normal brain tissues, is universally accepted. A few basic assumptions may explain (Karim et al 1991b) this paradox:

- Patients with high grade gliomas or other anaplastic malignant tumors are generally referred for radiation therapy, but for most of these patients the survival benefit is transient. Consequently complex treatment techniques, with higher work load for a department already overburdened with treatment of increasing numbers of cancer patients, are considered futile.
- Low grade gliomas are considered by many as 'benign' tumors and in some institutions are therefore not referred by the surgical team, resulting in a low level of expertise in some radiation oncology centers.
- The guesswork era for localization of the tumor and its extensions has not yet completely ended.

The legacy of inaccuracy with resultant uncertainty creates an unscientific attitude. This leads to simple planning with large opposing fields and, as a result, relatively ineffective doses may be prescribed.

The localization of the tumor, the target volume and the dose determination remain in many situations a difficult proposition (Kaiser & Kralendonk 1991). In the absence of contrast enhancement, it is difficult to be certain of accuracy in encompassing the tumor and its infiltration. Initially one may, in general, be advised to cover a marginal area of 3 cm around a highly malignant tumor and its surrounding edema, while a 2 cm margin may be considered for a low grade glioma. One may consider shrinking the field at 46 Gy and drastically at 54 Gy if a higher dose is contemplated. The usual recommended doses are: 60–64 Gy for highly malignant glioblastomas, 60 Gy for anaplastic grade III tumors and 50–54 Gy for low grade gliomas. Experimentation with different fractionation schemes has not obtained better results (Karim et al 1991b, Fulton et al 1992). Radiosensitive tumors, such as malignant lymphomas or pituitary adenomas, may be adequately treated with lower doses. Elective areas may always receive a lower dose. The maximum doses mentioned here are close to the range of normal brain tissue tolerance.

With meticulous application of DDS using multiple portals, sets of shrinking fields, avoidance of hot spots and individualized blocking devices for all setups, necrosis may be a rare complication. Many have followed these guidelines with 1.8 Gy daily tumor dose for years but, at present, particularly in view of radiobiological considerations (Kogel 1991) and increasing demand on megavoltage space, a daily dose of 2 Gy per fraction (2 Gy/F) is used by some. It should be emphasized that for such a dose (2 Gy/F/day) one must be very careful to avoid hot spots affecting normal brain tissues. Failure to adhere to the above advice may initiate a high incidence of brain necrosis, particularly when the higher total cumulative dose is prescribed. The well-known mathematical models, particularly the usually accepted neuret concept of Sheline (1980), are used as models. Recent critical reviews (Kogel

1991, Rutten 1991) describe details of other models, including the most recently introduced linear-quadratic scheme.

INDICATIONS

Indications or contraindications for treatment of brain lesions are in flux regarding some aspects of lesion treatment in certain situations. These include childhood brain tumors, prophylactic brain irradiation for small cell lung cancer, acute lymphatic leukemia, meningioma and prolactinoma among others. The most universally accepted guidelines are subdivided as follows:

Routinely irradiated in most institutions:

- Anaplastic gliomas grade 3 and 4.
- Medulloblastomas, ependymomas, most pineal tumors (particularly the malignant ones).
- Primary malignant lymphomas of the brain, malignant meningiomas, primitive neuroectodermal tumor (PNET).
- Cerebral metastasis(es).
- Pituitary non-hormone-active adenomas, particularly with supra- or parasellar extensions.
- Pituitary hormone-active tumors resistant to surgical and or medical intervention, e.g. acromegaly, prolactinomas and Cushing's disease.
- Other tumors with threatening symptomatology, e.g. optic gliomas or pituitary adenomas with visual symptoms. Some low grade gliomas with intractable epilepsy.
- Craniopharyngiomas.
- Any deep-seated inoperable tumor or malignancy diagnosed by stereotactic biopsy.

Routinely considered for patients with partially resected or inoperable tumor in many centers:

- Low grade gliomas: in many institutions they are routinely irradiated.
- Pituitary tumors (not amenable to other treatment).
- Craniopharyngiomas.
- Optic gliomas, particularly if vision is threatened.
- Meningiomas. Incompletely resected meningiomas are routinely treated postoperatively in some institutions, but many neurosurgeons refer patients for radiotherapy only after repeated recurrences.
- Childhood brain tumors.
- Sarcomas.

Routinely not considered but should be considered, particularly with recurrence after surgery:

- Meningiomas, particularly the angioblastic types after subtotal removal or after second operation on a recurrence.
- Chordomas. These tumors are now reported to be more amenable to radiotherapy. More effective growth restraint for a prolonged period appears possible after surgery (Fuller & Bloom 1988).

Cerebral metastasis(es)

Multiple metastatic tumors are generally considered for routine whole brain radiation therapy, but for single metastasis surgical removal followed by postoperative radiation therapy is recommended in most centers (Coia 1992, Smalley et al 1992). New data are emerging concerning the effectiveness of stereotactic radiotherapy on single metastasis and also on multiple metastases. Reported controversies (Engenhart et al 1990, Coffey et al 1991, Smalley et al 1992, Coia 1992) are evolving, related to policy of treatment in some centers capable of performing stereotactic single dose or pseudostereotactic fractionated high precision radiation therapy.

It appears justifiable to treat the whole brain to reduce recurrences inside the cranium. Reduction in size and extent of lesions from above 80% to about 20% has been reported (Smalley et al 1992). The important question is (over and above the whole brain irradiation) whether stereotactic or fractionated pseudostereotactic therapy may replace craniotomy to remove a solitary metastatic tumor. This is to be seriously considered when longer life expectancy is presumed in a patient with good performance status and no active disease at the primary site or elsewhere. The morbidity and the hospital stay may thus be limited. The period between the occurrence of the metastasis and the treatment of the primary tumor has, in many situations, been found to have influence on the survival of the patient, but contradictions are also found in the literature (Smalley et al 1992). Randomized trials are being undertaken to resolve some of these issues.

RESULTS

Each of the aforementioned indications should be looked at critically in the light of results of radiotherapy.

Low grade gliomas

It has by no means been proven with randomized studies that patients with low grade gliomas benefit definitively from radiation therapy. The other important unsettled question is that of a dose response. From retrospective studies the presence of a dose–response relationship is strongly indicated. Four randomized trials (Figs 17.3, 17.4) are going on at present and there is hope that the following will be clarified:

- Efficacy of postoperative (or post-biopsy) radiotherapy. There are, at present, two major studies under

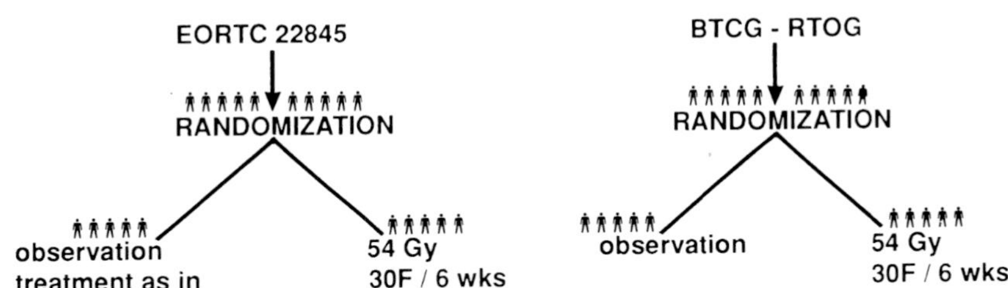

Fig. 17.3 Ongoing trials on efficacy of radiotherapy in low grade gliomas. These are similar studies meant for 'nonbelievers' in radiotherapy. Both use focal irradiation for adult supratentorial low grade gliomas. EORTC = European Organization for Research on Treatment of Cancer; BTCG = Brain Tumor Cooperative Group (USA); RTOG = Radiation Therapy Oncology Group (USA).

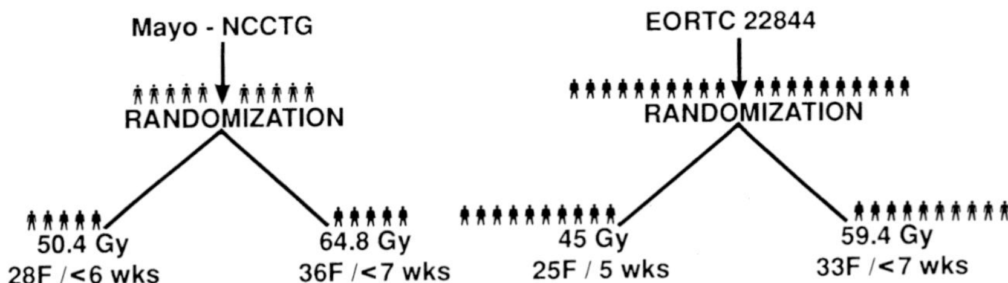

Fig. 17.4 Ongoing trials on dose response for low grade glioma. The American study stratifies biopsied pilocytic astrocytomas separately. Both trials use focal irradiation for adult supratentorial low grade glioma. EORTC = European Organization for Research on Treatment of Cancer; NCCTG = North Central Cancer Treatment Group (USA). From Karim & Kralendonk (1991).

way (EORTC 22845 and BTCG-RTOG). One of them (EORTC) also attempts to determine whether early radiotherapy is more efficient than delayed radiotherapy.

- Controversies surrounding an optimal dose of radiotherapy are being studied in 'dose response' protocols in Europe (EORTC) and USA (Mayo-NCCTG).

The European study is closed for patient accrual but further analysis continues with long-term follow-up of 379 randomized patients. From the emerging preliminary data, it appears at present with the parameters of the EORTC 22844 study that dose response is not in evidence with a large number of patients followed for at least 3 years (total number of patients randomized is 379); this preliminary conclusion may, however, change with time (Fig. 17.5).

The 4-year *overall survival* of 348 patients is a little above, and the disease-free survival is a little below, 60%, however, the overall survival is 70% or above for the:

— small number of patients with grade I tumor
— patients aged between 16 and 30 years
— small T1 (<3 cm, peripherally located) tumors, as defined in this protocol
— patients with higher performance status and/or good neurological status
— oligodendrogliomas as histologic types. Astrocytomas fare worse, and mixed oligo-astrocytomas have fared in between the above two histologic types.

The *disease-free survival* data of these patients do not show significant differences when patients in the different age groups (16–29, 30–39, 40–50, 51–66 years) are analyzed separately. This is in striking contrast to existing data in the literature, where only overall survival has been reported in retrospective studies. It is reported that, while the data on overall survival show highly significant dependency on the parameter of age, corroborating the data available in the literature, the disease-free survival does not. To date, disease-free survival of large numbers of patients has not been analyzed utilizing a prospective study.

The prognostic co-variates and the P-values for the *overall and the disease-free survival* of the patients with

Table 17.4 Preliminary analysis of prognostic factors (co-variates and P-value) with multivariate analysis from EORTC trial 22844

Overall survival	
	P-value
Age	0.00008
Performance and neurologic status (before radiation therapy)	0.0003
'T' (of TGM) parameter as defined in the protocol on preoperative CT scans	0.0013
Histologic type	0.01
Oligodendroglioma and mixed types versus astrocytoma (astrocytoma fares worse)	
The **disease-free survival** (DFS) is dependent on:	
'T' (of TGM) parameter	0.00002
Performance and neurologic status	0.0001
Histologic types (unfavorable for astrocytoma)	0.0004

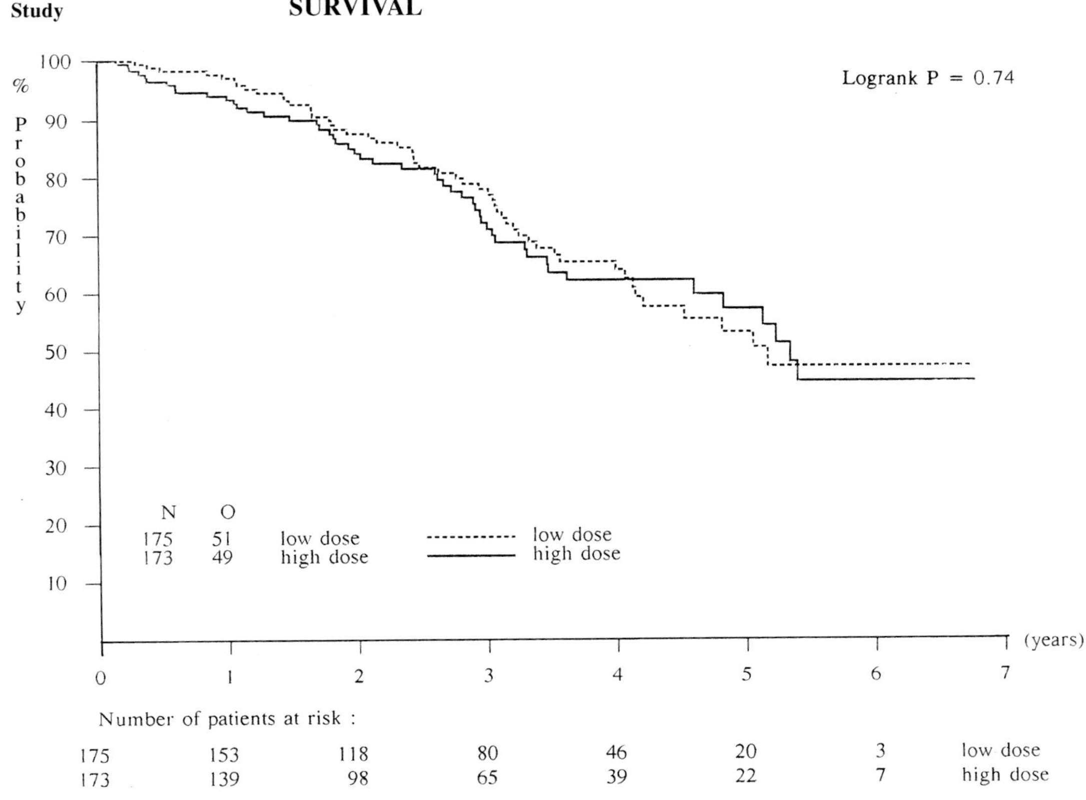

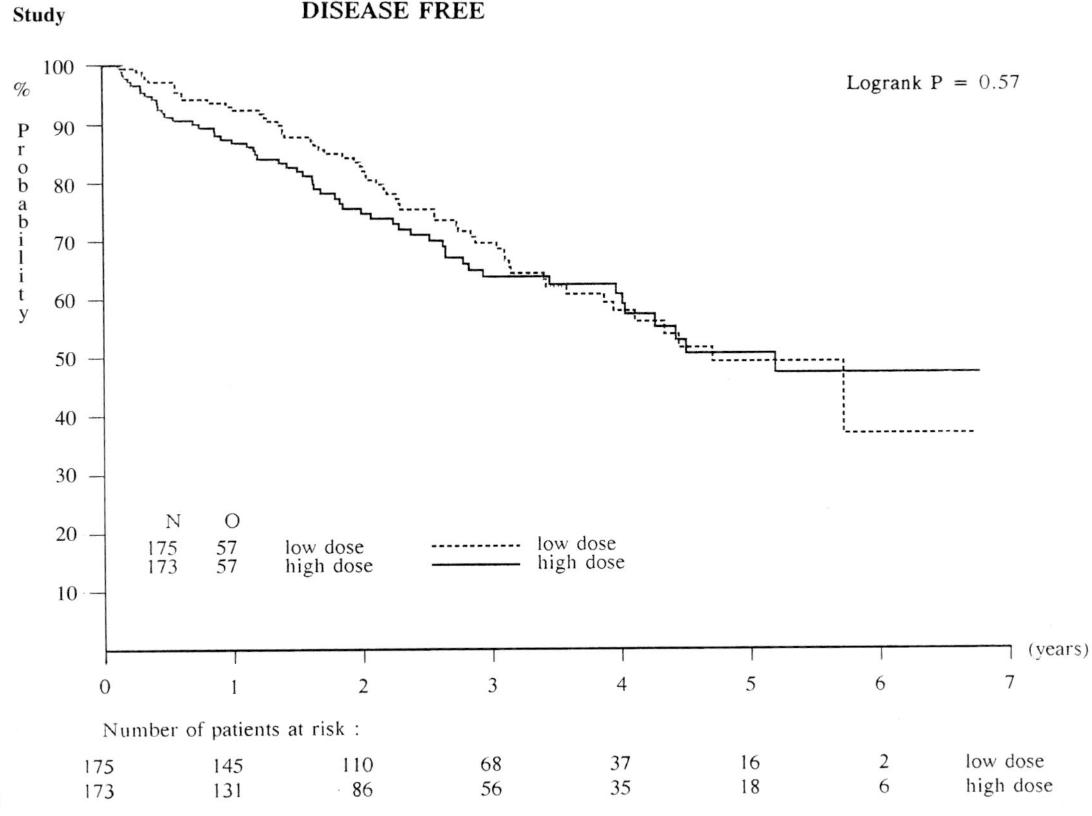

Fig. 17.5 The preliminary survival analysis of 348 evaluable patients with low grade gliomas from the EORTC trial 22844. **A.** The overall survival. **B.** The disease-free survival.

LGG in this trial are shown with multivariate analysis in Table 17.4. From the preliminary results of this prospective study on LGG, the T-staging or the extent of the tumor, as defined in the protocol, seems to be a most important prognostic factor (P-value 0.00002). The question of heterogeneity is perhaps exaggerated and may yield itself to a proper 'T' classification for low grade gliomas.

High grade or malignant gliomas (HGGs)

Recent publications of phase III randomized controlled studies report attempts to improve the results of combined modality treatment: surgery/radiotherapy with or without hypoxic sensitizers or chemo-enhancers or multiple drug chemotherapy. Recently, dose response was not demonstrated in a study using hyperfractionation (Fulton et al 1992). To date no remarkable improvement is evident (from the various trials as reviewed recently by Karim et al 1991a), particularly for patients with grade 4 glioblastoma. Surgery plays the important role of debulking and obtaining a tissue diagnosis. In the Japanese literature, in general, better survival results are reported, particularly when total or near-total removal of the tumor is possible (Sano 1986). A publication reviewing the histopathological parameters of Japanese patients reveals almost no prognostic differences between the Euro-American and Japanese experience (Shibamoto et al 1990).

The prognosis for patients with grade 3 anaplastic gliomas appears to be improving as compared to grade 4 glioblastoma multiforme (Karim et al 1991a).

Strict criteria in histopathological diagnosis, debulking of as much of the tumor as possible, optimum radiotherapy including brachytherapy (Larson et al 1991, Ostertag 1991), in combination with effective selective hypoxic sensitizers or chemotherapeutic enhancers, may result in better survival for patients with grade 3 tumors. It is imperative that the neuro-oncologists study grade 3 gliomas as a separate entity, not mixed with grade 4 glioblastoma multiforme, as has been the case in many recent randomized trials.

Grade 3 tumors may be treated in a randomized controlled study to achieve stepwise improvement, and grade 4 glioblastomas may be treated with more innovative, prospective protocols, e.g. boron neutron capture therapy (BNCT), brachytherapy, multidrug chemotherapy, hyperthermia, etc. Unfortunately, multiple fractionations per day (MFD) have not as yet shown any improvement in survival or local control (Fulton et al 1992). Brachytherapy (Larson et al 1991), particularly after recurrence, and BNCT (Hatanaka 1991) have shown some encouragement. Boosts by stereotactic therapy or incorporation of stereotactic surgery (Guthrie & Adler 1991) may be a promising new field.

A rational approach for management of grade 4 glioblastomas may be to define a group with poor prognostic factors, e.g. massive tumor in an aged patient with low performance and a high grade of neurologic deficit. This group must not, at the present state of our knowledge, be subjected to prolonged periods of futile treatment protocols, particularly when surgical debulking of the tumor is not possible. A short irradiation treatment scheme with comparative effectiveness may be sought, with or without other treatment modalities. On the other hand, patients with better prognostic features (where surgery removes the bulk of the tumor in a younger patient with good performance status and virtually no neurologic deficit) may benefit from innovative efforts to improve survival as well as the quality of life.

Recurrent gliomatous tumors

A treatment strategy for recurrent gliomas has generally not been formulated. It appears useful to consider reoperation and/or reirradiation, at least in some selected patients (Afra & Müller 1991, Larson et al 1991), particularly when the recurrence-free interval after first treatment is more than a year. Most of these patients have been previously irradiated, and tolerance of normal brain tissue must be considered carefully. Our clinical experience suggests, however, that considerable 'regain of therapeutic tolerance' may occur with the passage of time and one may consider 50–55 Gy in about 6–7 weeks, provided meticulously careful planning with DDS is organized. Among such patients irradiated after reoperation, a selected small group have experienced worthwhile survival — 40% at 2 years (Karim, unpublished data). Many tumors dedifferentiate after a period and this phenomenon poses difficulties. Prognosis after recurrence is better if the reoperated tumor has not dedifferentiated into a glioblastoma. Afra & Müller (1991) reported 22.2% survival at 5 years when most tumors, initially grade 2 LGG, changed to grade 3 astrocytomas at the second operation. In this selected series, with a small number of patients, the interval between the first and the second treatment (operation and radiotherapy in most cases) was between 1 and 5 years. Brachytherapy appears to be more effective in HGG, and Larson et al (1991) report 24% and 6% survival at 4 years for patients with anaplastic astrocytoma and glioblastomas, respectively. Recurrent tumors may be prospectively studied with a phase II protocol combining surgery and radiotherapy, with or without chemotherapy. This is a field to be explored carefully in the future with multicentric randomized trials. Larson et al (1991) believe that implantation appears to offer a survival advantage over chemotherapy in the treatment of recurrent malignant gliomas.

Childhood brain tumors

This topic poses different problems, particularly when irradiation is a part of the treatment protocol. Retardation of growth, lower IQ, hormone insufficiency, leukoencephalopathy, etc., are potential dreaded consequences of radiotherapeutic treatment. The long-term quality of life is jeopardized in these children as a result of radiation therapy, particularly when combined with chemotherapy. It is certainly wise to be restrictive if other modalities are available. Unfortunately, children with medulloblastoma, one of the major groups to undergo many clinical trials, still do not exhibit any clearcut evidence of benefit from adjuvant chemotherapy. The current therapy for children with medulloblastoma includes surgical removal followed by craniospinal irradiation with cranial boosts with or without adjuvant chemotherapy. The long-term effects of adjuvant chemotherapy on problems of growth in these children appear to be worse than those treated without adjuvant chemotherapy in a recent study (Olshan et al 1992).

Ependymomas are treated with postoperative radiotherapy. The low grade, less virulent, localized suprasellar tumors may be treated locally with relatively large fields while more virulent or anaplastic tumors require craniospinal irradiation as in medulloblastoma. This policy may not be univerally accepted, as some radiation oncologists tend to treat all ependymomas with craniospinal irradiation. In general, craniospinal radiotherapy plays an important role in the treatment plan of medulloblastomas, ependymomas and PNET tumors.

The technique of craniospinal irradiation is not detailed here and can be found in standard textbooks (Levin et al 1989). One may consider electron therapy with variable energy and half beam techniques to reduce the dose to the vertebral bodies. A small slice of the posterior vertebrae will get almost the same dose as the spinal canal but may not suffer such deleterious effects as with photons. This may be advantageous, particularly in view of problems related to growth and hemopoiesis related to chemotherapy.

Meningiomas

In general, meningiomas are treated by radical surgery. The resectability gives these tumors 'an undeserved reputation' of a benign tumor (Levin et al 1989), particularly because of their well-circumscribed and apparent noninvasive morphology. In many situations, however, total resection is not possible. There is a need for large prospective studies dealing with the natural history of patients with meningiomas (Sankila et al 1992).

Controversies (Taylor et al 1988) surrounding the role of radiotherapy appear to be ever-increasing, with no results from randomized trials currently available. In some of the large neuro-oncological centers data on long-term recurrence have been carefully evaluated to formulate treatment protocols. The recurrence rate of meningioma after complete resection, as reported by the Massachusetts General Hospital, increases with time – 7% at 5, 20% at 10, and 32% at 15 years (Mirimanoff et al 1985). It is well known that the recurrence rate dropped significantly from above 60% to about 25% when the incompletely resected meningiomas were irradiated (Levin et al 1989). The reported median time to recurrence was also significantly different — 125 months with irradiation as against 66 months when radiation therapy was not given. Some of these data are summarized in Table 17.5. The results of stereotactic radiotherapy/surgery appear to be encouraging (Engenhart et al 1990), and long-term follow-up of the patients is eagerly awaited.

Although sparse data are available on the efficacy of radiotherapy for meningiomas at present, clinical indications set the standards for treating patients with incomplete removal of meningiomas postoperatively with adequate dose (about 56 Gy/28F with 2 Gy/F in <6 weeks) and innovative focal field techniques. Fractionated stereotactic radiotherapy boosts may enhance tumor control while morbidity is reduced. Patients with recurrence should be irradiated if possible after reoperation. Inaccessible inoperable meningiomas should be considered for high precision radiotherapy, perhaps with stereotactic methodology.

Cranial base lesions

Pituitary tumors, acromegaly, craniopharyngiomas and rarer tumors e.g. clivus chordomas and glomus jugulare tumors

These tumors are dealt with in detail in other chapters of this book. It appears worthwhile to treat these lesions postoperatively whenever necessary. All hormonally inactive pituitary tumors with suprasellar or parasellar extension, tumors with visual symptoms, and hormonally active tumors resistant to medical intervention may be irradiated. Operated patients with acromegaly with persistent growth hormone levels above 5 and 10 ng/ml in males and females respectively should be considered for irradiation.

We recommend *dose levels* between 44 and 60 Gy in 2Gy/F/d for these tumors. The lower dose is for the pitui-

Table 17.5 Representative recurrence and percent survival rates in the literature for resected meningiomas with or without radiotherapy. Data modified from Simpson (1957), Carella et al (1982), Mirimanoff et al 1985, Taylor et al (1988), Engenhart et al (1990), Glaholm et al (1990).

	1950–1960	1980–1990
Recurrence rates (%) after complete surgical removal		
at 5 years	6	6
at 10 years	20	20
at 15 years		32
*Recurrence rate (%) after incomplete surgical removal**		
surgery alone	70	50
surgery with radiotherapy	3	20
*Survival rate**		
with surgery alone		50
with surgery + radiotherapy		85

* at 10 years

tary adenomas, including acromegaly, and glomus jugulare tumors. Up to 56 Gy maximum is considered for large craniopharyngiomas. Cystic craniopharyngiomas may also be successfully treated by radioactive colloid instillations, particularly when associated with recurring cysts. Both ^{32}P and ^{90}Y have been used. Our 15-year experience follows more than 60 pituitary tumor patients, with minimal follow-up of 3 years, who were treated with shrinking multiple portals (mostly 3–4). The dose range mentioned above has produced no evident eye damage. The tolerance dose of the optic nerve and chiasm is in all probability above this dose level. This was corroborated in one of our studies when a large number of patients with ethmoid cancers were successfully irradiated, delivering with DDS much higher doses to the vicinity (Karim et al 1991b). Clivus chordomas (Fuller & Bloom 1988) or sarcomas should be treated postoperatively with at least 60 Gy over 6 weeks, using a higher dose if feasible. All such radioresistant tumors must be treated with quality controlled multiple shrinking field radiotherapy with blocking devices whenever possible (DDS). Stereotactic radiotherapy/surgery protocols are at present being attempted. These can be recommended as alternatives, preferably with beam shaping (Leavitt et al 1991, Schlegel et al 1992) or as a boost after a reasonable dose has been delivered by conventional therapy techniques.

Pineal region tumors are a group of lesions with heterogeneity in histopathology and also in radiosensitivity. Small localized tumors are usually treated with appropriate time-dose-volume consideration when the exact histopathology and the results of marker studies are known. For example, for germinomas whole brain irradiation with up to 54 Gy in 5–6 weeks with 1.8 Gy/F/day is recommended. The fields may be coned at 45 Gy if feasible to cover the original tumor areas with a rather wide margin. At this stage usually 2 Gy/F/day may be used. After astrocytomas (LGG), pineocytomas, teratomas and other relatively radioresistant tumors are surgically debulked they should be irradiated with local fields only. On the other hand, virulent malignant tumors with seeding capabilities should be treated using combined modality therapy, e.g. craniospinal irradiation up to 36 Gy within about 4 weeks and an additional dose of 20 Gy by focal fields. Chemotherapy should be used when markers (AFP, *B*HCG) are present. Stereotactic biopsies yield diagnostic results in the vast majority of patients, but, if not possible, whole brain irradiation employing a lower dose (e.g. 20–26 Gy in about 3 weeks) may be used as a therapeutic trial. If regression of the tumor occurs, debulking and histopathological diagnosis must be reconsidered before any further treatment decisions are made.

Quality of life after radiation therapy

This important aspect in the evaluation of results of any treatment has elicited attention since Hochberg & Slotnick published their data in 1980. Because of late effects of irradiation developing slowly in normal brain tissue (Sheline 1980, Kogel 1991, Valk & Dillon 1991) it becomes imperative to evaluate the quality of life (QL) of patients with long-term prospective follow-up. This is a difficult task because of multidimensional factors and interactions encompassing physical, emotional, familial, social, intellectual, professional and other levels of day-to-day life.

When treating patients with the most virulent tumors, e.g. glioblastoma, one may justifiably be reluctant to evaluate QL in view of the associated procedures and the short expectancy of life. For others with a reasonably longer life expectancy it is crucial to study QL systematically and prospectively. Of particular importance is the long-term evaluation of the quality of life of younger patients as noted in recent publications (Karim 1991, Mackworth et al 1992, Taphoorn et al 1992); in future more shall be forthcoming. A study on patients with LGG reveals that evaluations are possible and worthwhile. (Table 17.6).

The clinical course during or after radiation therapy

Most patients are clinically improved after surgical removal of a brain tumor, and frequently the improvement continues during radiotherapy. The patients at this stage are usually treated with antiepileptics and corticosteroids although some patients may be tapered off corticosteroids by the second week of radiation therapy. The clinical situation must be carefully followed and an open honest relationship with the patient and his/her family should be

Table 17.6 Preliminary analysis of a prospective study on patients' quality of life after treatment for LGG. From Karim (1991)

	%
Overall quality of life	
Worse	17
Stable	17
Improved	66
Ability to work	
Deteriorated	17*
Stable	17
Improved	66
Occupation of those working	
Full-time housewife	20
Full-time work or student	33
Part-time work	13
Sex life	
Not evaluable	7
Deteriorated	20
Improved	13
Stable (did not worsen)	60

* Not working

established before planning radiation therapy, with at least weekly examinations during radiation therapy. The first planned follow-up at the end of the treatment should be immediate or within a week of completion. The main objective for close follow-up is to monitor carefully the clinical situation. One must look for neurologic deterioration which may be perpetuated by increased intracranial pressure. Treatment-related edema appears to be common although regrowth of the tumor may be a problem when a virulent tumor grows rapidly inside the limited space of the calvarium. Obstruction of the CSF pathways or bleeding may be problems in rare situations. Fluid imbalance, medical causes such as hypertension or infection, excessive epileptogenic activity from a focus in brain may all occasionally cause rapid clinical and neurologic deterioration during or immediately after radiation therapy. Adequate dosages of corticosteroids and or antiepileptics may be considered as the first line of action while searching for causative factors.

RADIATION REACTIONS

While radiation sequelae are touched upon briefly, readers are referred to the literature (Sheline 1980, Kogel 1991, Rutten 1991, Valk & Dillon 1991). Reactions are usually subdivided into three categories: early acute, early delayed, and late.

The classic ***early acute reactions (EAR)*** may occur during the course of radiation therapy but the most severe of these rarely occur when current guidelines are followed, using fraction sizes between 1.5 and 2 Gy. Hyperfractionated radiotherapy (Fulton et al 1992, EORTC trials) with high doses has produced enhanced acute reactions and brain necrosis. The recent trend to use hypofractionated schemes (Tamura et al 1989) with a large dose per fraction must be considered carefully. The multicenter EORTC trial of 59.4 Gy in 6.5 weeks with 1.8 Gy/F/day to part of the brain using DDS has produced moderate to minor acute skin reactions in less than 5% of patients and raised intracranial pressure along with exacerbation of focal symptoms in 1% of the 379 patients. Whole brain treatment with hypofractionated schemes used particularly for palliation, e.g. 30 Gy in 10 F in 2 weeks, with 3 Gy/F and 20 Gy in one week with 4 or 5 Gy/F has produced virtually no acute damage. Rapid palliative effects are usually achieved. It is well known that 15 Gy in 2 F with 7.5 Gy/F or 10 Gy in a single fraction may induce severe early acute reactions, characterized by a sudden deterioration in the clinical situation and severe focal symptoms; such doses are not currently utilized.

Early acute reactions (EAR) are usually treated prophylactically with corticosteroids (up to 16 mg of dexamethasone daily) during the course of radiation therapy. Corticosteroids are usually used initially and tapered off as soon as the clinical situation is improved or stabilized during treatment. In some patients receiving a higher fraction-dose, steroids must not be discontinued until the end of the treatment.

Fatigue commonly occurs during and after radiation therapy, sometimes for prolonged periods. Acute skin reactions can occur during or at the end of the radiotherapy. Dry desquamation with some degree of erythema is often seen and rarely needs extra care. Loss of hair is an important temporary setback, particularly for younger female patients, but satisfactory regrowth of hair is common, particularly with the precautions recommended in this Chapter. Visual sequelae are uncommon in modern radiotherapy but some deafness may be experienced when the temporal lobe receives full dose irradiation; this, however, may improve with the passage of time.

The ***early delayed reaction (EDR)*** may occur several weeks or months after irradiation, in general between 1 and 3 months after completion of therapy. The lethargy and transient somnolence classically noted are analogous to the transient myelopathy syndrome when the spinal cord is irradiated (Jones 1964). Some patients may develop nausea, vomiting, ataxia, dysphagia and nystagmus with a Romberg sign (Rider 1963). This syndrome is usually self-limiting and disappears in about 8 months, but a few patients may experience symptoms for up to 2 years. Other sequelae including local demyelinization, perivascular cellular infiltrates, edema, and endothelial proliferation, among others, have been reported and recently reviewed (Rutten 1991). Histological confirmation is almost impossible because of the self-limiting nature of this pathophysiological phenomenon. The symptoms of EDR should be promptly treated with corticosteroids to counteract fatal herniation of the brain.

Late delayed reactions. The sequelae of radiation may be very insidious in nature, developing after 2–3 years, and they may be focal or diffuse. The incidence is difficult to estimate, but is dose dependent (Jones 1964, Sheline 1980, Marks et al 1985, Kogel 1991, Rutten 1991). Sheline's meticulous study of radiation necrosis detected less than 200 reported patients with unequivocal necrosis. Although focal or diffuse injury may be enhanced by using combined modalities of radiation and chemotherapy, the true incidence is difficult to gauge. Historically a 5% incidence of radiation necrosis has been accepted as a norm, but at present a careful radiation oncologist should encounter this complication only rarely, and must not accept such a norm. Some degree of previously unrecognized injury has been detected with recent developments in neuro-imaging including asymptomatic edema, hypodense 'holes' after postoperative radiotherapy, and diffuse white matter changes on CT or MR scans. Clinical stabilization with some neurological deficit may be noticed. Progression to necrosis is usually observed as a mass lesion producing increased intracranial pressure and focal clinical symptomatology, e.g. epilepsy, motor, sensory, speech disturbances, etc., associated with lethargy. Most patients become symptomatic when necrosis develops. Angiography and PET imaging are able to confirm the diagnosis in most situations. Most necrotic lesions are characterized by vascular changes, edema and a demyelination process. Severe diffuse injury may impair intellectual function causing loss of memory, confusion and dementia, and ultimately may lead to death. In children or young adults the learning process and IQ are compromised. In most cases of severe late effects with clinical manifestations, diffuse white matter changes, gliosis or atrophy of a part of the brain may be seen on the images.

Radiation damage to small vessels is well recognized, and most radiation injuries are mediated through vascular changes. Damage to larger vessels is being reported (Valk & Dillon 1991) with increasing frequency, particularly when young patients have been irradiated and cured. Vascular malformations with vasculopathy (Epstein et al 1992) have been recently described and may be misdiagnosed as tumor recurrences.

Edema and necrosis may be to an extent ameliorated by treatment with corticosteroids but progressive lesions should, whenever possible, be treated by surgical intervention.

COMMENTS ON BRAIN TUMOR STAGING

One of the most important aspects of neuro-oncology (Karim & Kralendonk 1991, Karim et al 1991b) needing urgent attention from all, is the lack of a universally acceptable staging system (Sauwart et al 1989).

The TNM classification (UICC or AJC) has been revised and published (Hermanek & Sobin 1987) quite a few times in the last decades. No system has yet gained universal popularity and innumerable publications appear in the literature, with poorly classified lesions and falsely enhanced notions (Janus et al 1992) on heterogeneity. A proposed staging system incorporating the histological grade (G) and the parameter of the extent of tumor (T) may apply to gliomas. The question of distant metastases (M) is perhaps only to be mentioned for glioblastoma multiforme, medulloblastomas, malignant pineal tumors, high grade ependymomas, PNET, etc. For the low grade gliomas, Karim (as early as 1983) proposed the parameters for 'T' (of TGM) classification for the trials on LGG (EORTC 22844 and 22845) and this has, in a preliminary analysis, proved its value with a large number of patients (379) prospectively studied from 1985 through 1991. The preliminary survival curves of the patients from the EORTC trial 22844 (Fig. 17.6) reveal significant

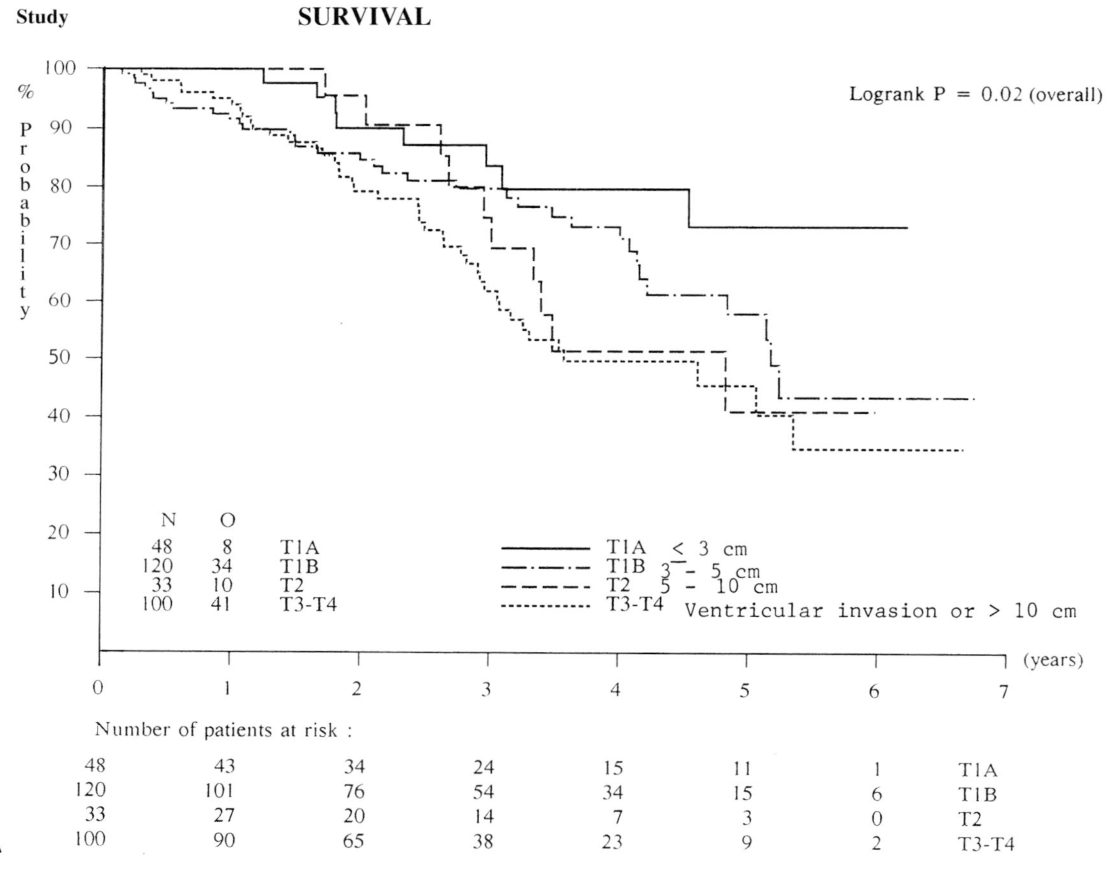

Fig. 17.6A

differences in disease-free survival for the different 'T' groups.

In an attempt to improve on and incorporate these available data one may consider a classification modified from that proposed and used for the EORTC trials so far. The following simple definitions may be proposed:

- T1 tumors may be classified as the smallest tumors, less than 3 cm in maximum diameter.
- T2 tumors may be any tumor between 3 and 5 cm in maximum diameter, not transgressing the midline or lobar boundaries.
- T3 tumors are to be defined when the maximum diameter is beyond 5 cm but less than 10 cm, confined to one side.
- Any tumor beyond 5 cm which crosses the midline or definitely invades the ventricles, or any tumor more than 10 cm in its maximum diameter, should be defined as T4. It is noted that ventricular encroachment or involvement is rare and difficult to define. The subarachnoid space is another such twilight zone.
- For glioblastoma multiforme one may consider only *limited* versus *advanced* tumor, depending on whether the tumor measures less than 3 cm at its maximal diameter.

At present, small cell anaplastic lung cancers with median patient survival of less than one year are classified in this manner, and both these cancers (glioblastomas and small cell lung cancers) have an almost similar mortality potential.

The parameters proposed above may significantly separate the different prognostic subgroups, perhaps to a greater degree than has already been obtained ($P = 0.00002$) in the preliminary results of EORTC trial 22844 by multivariate analysis.

RADIOSURGERY OR STEREOTACTIC RADIOTHERAPY/SURGERY (STRT/S)

The methodology of stereotactic treatment consists of delivering a high dose of radiation in single or multiple fractions to an accurately localized and immobilized small target volume, allowing minimal dose outside that prescribed area. The objective is to reverse the viability or the growth of the lesion through complex radiobiological processes. These radiobiological processes remain ill-defined; attempts have recently been undertaken (Brenner et al 1991, Hall & Brenner 1993) to clarify some aspects.

The well-known innovative Swedish neurosurgeon Lars Leksell (1951) pioneered, improved and developed (1951–1968) his stereotactic system, adding a radio-

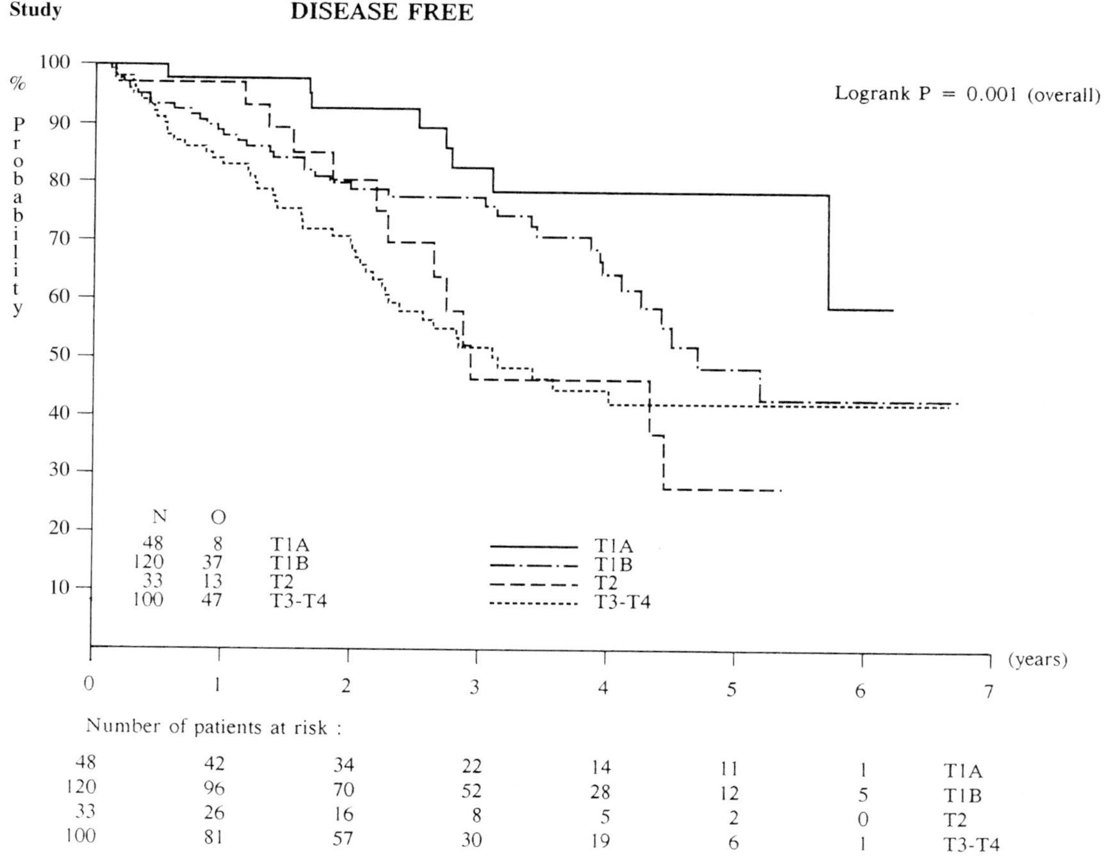

Fig. 17.6 The significant differences of survival of patients with LGG in different 'T' stages. **A.** The overall survival. **B.** The disease-free survival.

therapy apparatus with multiple (more than 200 radioactive ^{60}Co) small sources with all the emanating beams converged and focused on an isocenter. This is popularly known as the Leksell Gamma Knife apparatus. Certain limitations, including the cost of such a dedicated apparatus, have motivated development in another direction. Linear accelerators have been modified and used since the early 1980s. Patients with a stereotactically determined target volume are irradiated with multiple arcs of rotation of the beam. In 1991 there were an estimated (Alexander & Loeffler 1991) 21 Gamma Knives in use while 75 linear accelerators (Linac) were being used for stereotactic treatment all over the world. There is strong belief that there is virtually no difference in the efficacy, accuracy, sharpness and fall-off of the dose distribution between the Gamma Knife and Linac-based STRT/S (Flickinger et al 1990). The former is a dedicated apparatus needing no time-sharing while the latter is in constant use in radiotherapy departments, usually with a heavy work load. A repeat quality check for stringent accuracy is needed before its use for stereotherapy. Linacs need more vigilance, particularly because of the moving beam head and the rotating couch. On the other hand, individualized beam shaping is possible with Linacs (Leavitt et al 1991, Schlegel et al 1992).

A recent development is a dedicated linear accelerator for both STRT/S as well as high quality precision fractionated radiotherapy (Loeffler, personal communication 1992). This dedicated Linac, in use in Boston, has delivered almost 1000 treatment STRT/S sessions in less than 6 months for intracranial lesions; approximately 100 of those were classic single fraction 'radiosurgery'.

As yet there is no consensus on the various terms used, e.g. radiosurgery, radiotherapy, ST radiosurgery, ST radiotherapy, X-knife or photon blade radiotherapy, semi- or pseudo STRT/S, fractionated radiotherapy using stereotactic frames, stereotactic convergent beam radiotherapy, stereotactic single dose radiation therapy. The term radiosurgery was coined by Leksell and as a 'misnomer' has also created controversy (Belli 1990, Heros & Korosue 1990). Apparently it can give the impression that this superspecialty of STRT/S is practised primarily by neurosurgeons, even though the patients treated with STRT/S should be cared for by a team of specialists, including neurosurgeons, neuroradiologists and physicists. In most European countries treatment by radiation is legally permitted only by qualified radiation therapy specialists. These are nothing but teething difficulties in the infancy of STRT/S. The expertise of the demanding superspecialists for a pure high-tech methodology to be combined with highly skilled localization and immobilization procedures, requires constant cooperation among all the neurospecialists with the principal objective of refining and developing the technology for a cure and better quality of life of the patients. It must be emphasized that this new development has given a tremendous impetus to quality controlled radiotherapy and precision stereotactic neurosurgery (Alexander & Loeffler 1991, Guthrie & Adler 1991, Kelly 1992). It is important to realize that there is perhaps no limit for innovations like this, but much hard work needs to be undertaken before the system is perfected and optimally used in day-to-day practice. Systematic studies are needed in the following fields:

- Radiobiology of small fields with high doses: single versus hypofractionated schemes.
- Accuracy of different neurosurgical fixed (Maciunas et al 1992), relocatable and non-invasive frames (Hariz 1990, Delannes et al 1991).
- Selection and indications: brain metastases, angiographically occult vascular malformations, meningiomas, acoustic neurinomas (vestibular schwannomas), etc. Controversies on the latter are being published (Brackmann & Kwartler 1990, Lunsford et al 1990, Thomsen et al 1990). Consensus is needed.
- The limitations and the accuracy of target localization (Serago et al 1992, Spiegelmann et al 1992).
- Cost effectiveness and cost containment (Belli 1990, Steinberg et al 1990).

It is imperative to undertake these studies prospectively and objectively to develop the science of STRT/S with an international consensus.

Indications for treatment

The indications are not yet definitely formulated for all categories of lesions being treated at present. Any deep-seated lesion with all grades of radiosensitivity or radioresistance may be treated by STRT/S. Most frequently inoperable tumors or lesions in a functionally eloquent area are treated by this relatively noninvasive methodology. Commonly treated lesions are: arteriovenous malformations (AVM), cavernomas or angiographically occult vascular malformations (AOVM), residual or recurrent meningiomas, acoustic neurinomas (vestibular schwannomas), pinealomas, pituitary tumors, chordomas, other skull-base lesions, recurrent tumors and solitary or up to 2–3 brain metastases. Small recurrences of malignancies in the head and neck or other regions are being treated. While we have gained experience in such treatments in our center, clinical results of radiosurgery for palliative effects have been reported recently (Kondziolka et al 1991, Kaplan et al 1992). Solitary brain metastasis not associated with any active disease elsewhere may be considered (Coffey et al 1991, Strum et al 1991, Engenhart et al 1992). Boosts by stereotherapy following good regression or stabilization after conventional whole brain irradiation appear to be sound practice. This may be a worthwhile palliative treatment in patients in good general condition with a longer life expectancy. Whole brain radiotherapy is needed to reduce the risk of recurrence from above 60% to about 20% (Coia 1992, Smalley et al 1992). Controversy surrounding this topic has been previously detailed. Multiple brain metastases (2–3) perhaps should not be treated by STRT/S in view of the similar results obtained by simpler radiotherapy procedures and also the important question of cost containment (Belli 1990).

AVMs. These malformations (not tumors) are commonly treated by radiosurgery. The success or obliteration rate depends on the size of the lesions, among other factors, e.g. accuracy and optimum dose. It appears that larger AVMs (> 2.5 cm in diameter) are less curable, and the obliteration rate may drop from 90% to about 60% or less. Hatanaka (1991 and personal communication 1992) has treated selected giant AVMs with boron neutron capture radiation therapy (BNCT) with rewarding results. Initial embolization may be helpful in some selected cases to shrink the abnormal blood vessels, facilitating STRT/S or fractionated high dose radiotherapy (Makoski 1991). Single dose therapy appears effective for AVMs and the threshold dose is probably above 12 Gy. Currently, in most centers, 25 Gy is usually not exceeded for a lesion of about 3 cm diameter. Instances of complications above this level are found in the literature, and the logistic formula as published by Flickinger et al (1990) is a helpful tool used to avoid complications.

Cavernomas (or AOVM) appear to be less amenable to treatment. Controversies are appearing related to the treatment of AOVMs by STRT/S (Kondziolka et al 1990). Results of long-term follow-up with a large number of patients are necessary to guide treatment.

Meningiomas. The prime treatment modality is surgery. These apparently 'benign' tumors (Levin et al 1989) are more radiosensitive than usually thought. In some centers they are routinely irradiated with conventional fractionation schemes if total removal is not possible. STRT/S may be more effective in residual or recurrent meningiomas.

Acoustic neurinomas (vestibular schwannomas). These are usually treated surgically but some neurosurgeons do consider STRT/S in view of the possible morbidity associated with surgery. This view is not without controversy (Brackmann & Kwartler 1990, Lunsford et al 1990). There is morbidity associated with both treatment modalities. The regression pattern after radiotherapy is usually slow and should be monitored carefully. Perhaps one may consider STRT/S as an alternative treatment modality when primary surgery is fraught with unacceptable risks. Patient participation in decision making may help in certain situations.

Gliomas. Small gliomas (HGG or LGG) and other brain tumors may also be boosted with STRT/S, after postoperative conventional radiotherapy. It may be worthwhile to treat a small recurrence by STRT/S after biopsy, particularly if dedifferentiation to glioblastoma is not evidenced.

Radioresistant tumors (e.g. sarcomas, chordomas). Primary surgery may be attempted for these tumors even if only bulk removal is possible. These tumors show, in many situations, relentless progression and should be treated with high dose quality controlled precision radiotherapy. Stereotactic radiotherapy using single or hypofractionated methods is to be considered individually.

The tools

At present, four different types of apparatus are available for STRT/S:

1. The classic dedicated *Gamma Knife* apparatus (Leksell's) with multiple radioactive ^{60}Co sources. This performs STRT/S usually with small field sizes, with collimators from 6–25 mm. There are no moving parts in the apparatus while a patient is being treated. The apparatus is costly.
2. An existing *linear accelerator* (Linac) may be modified for use by ensuring safety and accuracy with new accessories, e.g. frames, head holders, localizers, among others. Multiple collimators, usually from 10–40 mm, with possibilities of single dose treatment or pseudostereotactic fractionated radiotherapy with a number of arcs, with high quality immobilization with invasive or noninvasive frames for fixation may be used. Innovative beam shaping with fixed blocks or moving shadow trays as in conformation therapy is also being developed. This system works on a time-sharing basis.
3. At present *stereotactic linear accelerators* are available, at a commensurate cost, with modifications needed. They meet the demand of daily treatment of patients by conventional as well as stereotactic or pseudostereotactic therapy. This apparatus also works on a time-sharing basis.
4. The most recent development is a *dedicated linear accelerator* designed only for STRT/S. Field sizes up to 10 cm diameter are possible. Loeffler et al 1993, report that about 1000 treatments for intracranial lesions with about 100 classic stereotactic radiosurgical applications have been undertaken by such an apparatus in a period of about 4 months, apparently with high technical satisfaction. This apparatus does not need time-sharing and may become a popular tool, particularly in view of higher accuracy being possible in fractionated radiotherapy. It should be noted that the usual Linacs deliver 8000–9000 treatments each year.

Other important technological accessories for nondedicated existing linear accelerators to be used for STRT/S are a rigid neurosurgical stereoframe or a relocatable frame, and localization frames with markers for angiography, etc. Relocatable frames have been used for fractionated procedures. For charged particle therapy this is essential (Steinberg et al 1990). An analysis of the 'invasive' neurosurgical frames has recently indicated that the accuracy of these frames may be questionable (Maciunas et al 1992).

In some centers pseudostereotactic therapy (i.e. all treatment procedures without the stringent single dose radiosurgery with rigid frames) is being managed with accurate customized masks having some fixation arrangement. It appears that all users find their frames quite satisfactory although the rigid frames fixed to the skull may be considered more accurate.

The major problems

These developments are highly innovative and have a stimulating influence on neurosurgery as well as on conventional and neuroradiotherapy. Stereotactic neurosurgery and neuroradiotherapy with computerized robot arms are developments that may have a great future (Guthrie & Adler 1991).

In this rapidly developing field, time is needed to gather enough data in order to prepare protocols for safe accurate delivery:

- Accuracy currently varies from center to center. The degree of accuracy that is clinically relevant should be examined and incorporated in routine practice of STRT/S or pseudostereotactic radiotherapy.
- Indications must be defined carefully. The benefit accorded to patients must be judged against the work load and the cost effectiveness. We may have the technological expertise to treat cerebral metastases, but the transient survival of the patient may not justify such treatment. Pituitary tumors have been treated with conventional quality radiotherapy with good results for more than 10–15 years. Perhaps it may be difficult to improve upon this record, and increased use of STRT/S may only increase complications.
- Target localization is a problem where integral efforts are needed to incorporate data from modern imaging (CT, MRI, angiography, PET, SPECT, etc.) with 3D viewing.
- Three-dimensional viewing incorporating all imaging data and dosimetry planning is being developed and should be commercially available soon.
- There is an urgent need to define each new term that has been introduced in recent years. Cooperation from all the specialists involved is necessary in order to develop excellent radiotherapeutic protocols.
- The radiobiological aspects are as yet obscure and need to be unfolded systematically and scientifically. The early acute reactions, the early delayed and the late effects of radiobiologically effective proton or heavy particle stereotactic therapy have recently been expertly described by Adams (1991). These effects mimic those of conventional photon radiation but may not be similar to those of STRT/S.
- Quality of life following treatment has not been reported in detail and should be evaluated prospectively with long-term follow-up.
- The issue of fractionation versus single dose treatment is a major one to be settled in the near future, perhaps through multicenter randomized studies. In this era of conventional or superfractionated or hypofractionated radiotherapy, single high dose radiotherapy as in STRT/S is on the other end of the scale and may be considered a contradiction to the time-tested concept of fractionation. Long-term large, comprehensive, prospective evaluations of results and complications are eagerly awaited.

Future studies will determine which methodologies are appropriate for a given clinical situation. One thing is certain, stereotactic radiotherapy/surgery has come to stay.

REFERENCES

Adams R D 1991 The neuropathology of radiosurgery. Stereotact Funct Neurosurg 57: 82–86

Afra D, Müller W 1991 Recurrent low grade gliomas. In: Karim A B M F, Laws E R Jr (eds). Glioma. Springer Verlag, Heidelberg, pp 189–204

Alexander E III, Loeffler J S 1991 Editorial introduction to the Harvard radiosurgery update course in June 1990. Stereotact Funct Neurosurg 57: 5–6

Belli J A 1990 Stereotactic radiation for intracranial arteriovenous malformations. The New England Journal of Medicine 1636 (December 6)

Brackmann D, Kwartler J A 1990 Treatment of acoustic tumors with radiotherapy. Arch Otolaringol Head Neck Surgery 116: 161–162

Brenner D J, Martel M K, Hall E J 1991 Fractionated regimens for stereotactic radiotherapy of recurrent tumors in the brain. International Journal Radiation Oncology Biology Physics 21: 819–824

Carella R J, Ransohoff J, Newall J 1982 Role of radiation therapy in the management of meningioma. Neurosurgery 10: 332–339

Coffey R J, Flickinger J C, Bissonette D J et al 1991 Radiosurgery for solitary brain metastases using Cobalt 60 gamma unit: Methods and results in 24 patients. International Journal of Radiation Oncology, Biology Physics 20: 1287–1295

Coia L R 1992 The role of radiation therapy in the treatment of brain metastases. International Journal Radiation Oncology Biology Physics 23: 229–238

Daumas-Duport C, Scheithauer B, O'Fallon J et al 1988 Grading of astrocytomas. A simple and reproducible method. Cancer 62: 2152–2165

Delannes M, Daly N J, Bonnet J et al 1991 Fractionated radiotherapy of small inoperable lesions of the brain using a non-invasive stereotactic frame. International Journal Radiation Oncology Biology Physics 21: 749–755

Engenhart R, Kimmig B N, Hover K H et al 1990 Stereotactic single high dose radiation therapy of benign intracranial meningiomas. International Journal Radiation Oncology Biology Physics 19: 1021–1026

Engenhart R, Wowra B, Kimmig B et al 1992 Stereotactic convergent beam radiotherapy: Current perspectives based on clinical results (English translation). Strahlentherapie und Onkologie 168: 245–259

Epstein M A, Packer R J, Rorke L B et al 1992 Vascular malformation with radiation vasculopathy after treatment of chiasmatic/hypothalamic glioma. Cancer 70: 887–893

Flickinger J C, Schell M C, Larson D A 1990 Estimation of complications for linear accelerator radiosurgery with the integrated logistic formula. International Journal Radiation Oncology Biology Physics 19: 143–145

Fuller D B, Bloom J G 1988 Radiotherapy for chordoma. International Journal Radiation Oncology Biology Physics 15: 331–339

Fulton D S, Urtasun R C, Scott-Brown I et al 1992 Increasing radiation dose intensity using hyperfractionation in patients with malignant glioma. Journal Neuro-Oncology 14: 63–72

Glaholm J, Bloom H J G, Crow J H 1990 The role of radiotherapy in the management of intracranial meningiomas: the Royal Marsden Hospital experience with 186 patients. International Journal Radiation Oncology Biology Physics 18: 755–761

Guthrie B L, Adler J R 1991 Frameless stereotaxy: computer interactive neurosurgery. Neurological Surgery 2: 1–22

Guthrie B L, Laws E R Jr 1991 Management of supratentorial low grade glioma. In: Karim A B M F, Laws E R (eds) Glioma. Springer Verlag, Heidelberg, pp 75–92

Hall E J, Brenner D J 1993 The radiobiology of radiosurgery: Rationale for different treatment regimes for AVMS and malignancies (Abstr). International conference and course on stereotactic radiotherapy/surgery. May 6–8, Amsterdam p. 21

Hariz M I 1990 A non-invasive adaptation system for computed tomography guided stereotactic neurosurgery. Academic Thesis, University of Umea

Hatanaka H 1991 Boron neutron capture therapy for tumors. In: Karim A B M F, Laws E R Jr (eds) Glioma. Springer Verlag, Heidelberg, pp 233–249

Hermanek P, Sobin L H (eds) 1987 TNM classification of malignant tumors, 4th edn. Springer Verlag, Heidelberg, pp 219–226

Heros R C, Korosue K 1990 Radiation treatment of cerebral arteriovenous malformations. The New England Journal of Medicine 323: 127–129

Hochberg F H, Slotnick B 1980 Neuropsychologic impairment in astrocytoma survivors. Neurology 30: 172–177

ICRU 29 1978 International Commission on Radiation Units and Measurements. Dose specification for reporting external beam therapy with photons and electrons. Report 29. ICRU Publications, Washington DC

Isamat F, Acebes J J, Obarrio L L 1986 Low grade supratentorial astrocytomas. Abstract. International Meeting on Brain Oncology, Rennes, September 1986, VII, p 47

Janus T J, Kysitsis A P, Forman A D et al 1992 Biology and treatment of gliomas. Annals of Oncology 3: 423–433

Jones A 1964 Transient radiation myelopathy. British Journal of Radiology 37: 727–744

Kaplan I D, Adler J R, Hicks W L et al 1992 Radiosurgery for palliation of base skull recurrences from head and neck cancers. Cancer 70: 1980–1984

Kaiser M C, Kralendonk J H 1991 Modern imaging for cerebral gliomas: Breakthroughs and limitations. In: Karim A B M F, Laws E R Jr (eds) Glioma: Principles and practice in neuro-oncology. Springer Verlag, Heidelberg, pp 37–55

Karim A B M F 1991 Cure and quality of life after treatment for glioma. In: Karim A B M F, Laws E R Jr (eds) Glioma. Springer Verlag, Heidelberg, pp 271–282

Karim A B M F, Kralendonk J H 1991 Pitfalls and controversies in the treatment of gliomas. In: Karim A B M F, Laws E R Jr (eds). Glioma. Springer Verlag, Heidelberg, pp 1–16

Karim A B M F, Van der Schueren E, Gonzalez D G et al 1991a Radiotherapy of malignant gliomas. In: Karim A B M F, Laws E R Jr (eds) Glioma. Springer Verlag, Heidelberg, pp 121–124

Karim A B M F, Kralendonk J H, Slotman B J 1991b Advances in neuro-oncology for adult patients with supratentorial gliomas: from the window of radiation oncology. In: Paoletti P et al (eds). Neuro-Oncology Kluwer Academic Publishers, Dordrecht, pp 137–146

Kelly P J 1992 Stereotactic resection and its limitations in glial neoplasms. Stereotact Funct Neurosurg 59: 84–91

Kogel A J 1991 Clinical implications of radiological studies on CNS tolerance. In: Karim A B M F, Laws E R Jr (eds). Glioma. Springer Verlag, Heidelberg, pp 179–188

Kondziolka D, Lunsford L D 1991 Stereotactic radiosurgery for squamous cell carcinoma of the nasopharynx. Laryngoscope 101: 519–522

Kondziolka D, Lunsford L D, Coffey R J et al 1990 Stereotactic radiosurgery of angiographically occult vascular malformations: Indications and preliminary experience. Neurosurgery 27: 892–900

Kondziolka D, Lunsford L D, Coffey R J et al 1991 Gamma Knife radiosurgery. Stereotact Funct Neurosurgery 57: 11–21

Larson D A, Sneed P K, Gutier P H 1991 International brachytherapy for recurrent malignant gliomas. In: Karim A B M F, Laws E R Jr (eds). Glioma. Springer Verlag, Heidelberg, pp 205–215

Leavitt D D, Gibbs F A, Heilbrun M P et al 1991 Dynamic field shaping to optimize stereotactic radiosurgery. International Journal Radiation Oncology Biology Physics 21: 1247–1255

Leksell L 1951 The stereotactic method and radiosurgery of the brain. Acta Chirurgie Scandinavie 102: 316–319

Levin V A, Sheline G I, Gutin P H et al 1989 Neoplasms of the CNS. In: De Vita V T, Hellman S, Rosenberg S A (eds) Principle and practice of oncology. Lippincott, Philadelphia, pp 1557–1611

Loeffler J S, Kooy H M, Alexander E 1993 Stereotactic radiosurgery and radiotherapy using a dedicated linear accelerator. Experience from the Harvard joint center for radiation therapy (abstract). International Conference and Course on Stereotactic Radiotherapy/Surgery, May 6–8, Amsterdam p. 2

Lunsford D D, Kamerer D B, Flickinger J C 1990 Stereotactic radiosurgery for acoustic neuromas. Arch Otolaryngol Head Neck Surgery 116: 907–909

Maciunas R J, Galloway R L, Latimer J et al 1992 An independent application accuracy evaluation of stereotactic frame systems. Stereotact Funct Neurosurg 58: 103–107

Mackworth N, Fobair P, Prados M D 1992 Quality of life self-reports from 200 brain tumor patients: comparisons with Karnofsky performance scores. Journal Neuro-Oncology 14: 243–253

Makoski H B 1991 External stereotactic focal irradiation of arteriovenous malformations by routinely used linear accelerator. In: Sauer R (ed) Medical radiology. Springer Verlag, Heidelberg, pp 95–99

Marks J E, Baglan R J, Prasad S C et al 1981 Cerebral radio necrosis: incidence and risk in relation to dose, time, fractionation and volume. International Journal Radiation Oncology Biology Physics 7: 243–252

Müller W, Afra D, Schröder R 1977 Supratentorial recurrences of gliomas. Morphological studies in relation to time intervals with astrocytomas. Acta Neurochirurgica 37: 75–81

Mirimanoff R O, Dosoretz D E, Linggood R M et al 1985 Meningioma: Analysis of recurrence and progression following neurosurgical resection. Journal of Neurosurgery 62: 18–24

Olshan J S, Gubernick J, Packer R J et al 1992 The effects of adjuvant chemotherapy on growth in children with medulloblastoma. Cancer 70: 2013–2017

Ostertag C B 1991 Stereotactic international radiotherapy in the treatment of gliomas: current status, results and the future. In: Karim A B M F, Laws E R (eds). Glioma. Springer Verlag, Heidelberg, pp 125–137

Rider W D 1963 Radiation damage to the brain — a new syndrome. Journal of the Canadian Association of Radiology 14: 67–69

Rutten E H J M 1991 Radiation injury to the brain. In: Karim A B M F, Laws E R Jr (eds). Glioma. Springer Verlag, Heidelberg, pp 171–178

Sankila R, Kallio M, Jääskeläinen J et al 1992 Long term survival of 1986 patients with intracranial meningioma diagnosed from 1953 to 1984 in Finland. Cancer 15: 1566–1576

Sano K 1986 The future role of neurosurgery in the case of cerebral tumors. Neurosurg Review 9: 13–22

Schlegel W, Pastyr O, Bortfeld T et al 1992 Computer systems and mechanical tools for stereotactically guided conformation therapy with linear accelerators. International Journal Radiation Oncology Biology Physics 24: 781–787

Serago C F, Lewin A A, Houdek P V et al 1992 Radiosurgery target point alignment errors detected with postal film verification.

International Journal Radiation Oncology Biology Physics 24: 777–780
Sheline G E 1980 Irradiation injury of the human brain: a review of clinical experience. In: Gilbert H, Kagan A R (eds) Radiation damage to the nervous system. Raven Press, New York, pp 39–52
Shibamoto J, Jamashita J, Takahashi M et al 1990 Supratentorial malignant glioma: an analysis of radiation therapy in 178 cases. Radiotherapy Oncology 18: 9–17
Simpson D 1957 The recurrence of intracranial meningiomas after surgical treatment. Journal of Neurological Neurosurgery and Psychiatry 20: 22–29
Smalley S R, Laws E R, O'Fallon J R et al 1992 Resection for solitary brain metastasis. Journal of Neurosurgery 77: 531–540
Smith M T, Ludwig C L, Godfrey A D et al 1983 Grading of oligodendrogliomas. Cancer 52: 2107–2114
Soffietti R, Chio A, Giordana M T et al 1989 Prognostic factors in well-differentiated cerebral astrocytomas in the adult. Neurosurgery 24: 686–692
Spiegelmann R, Friedman W A, Bova F J 1992 Limitations of angiographic target localization. Neurosurgery 30: 619–623
Stam F C 1991 The problems of pathological diagnosis. In: Karim A B M F, Laws E R Jr (eds) Glioma. Springer Verlag, Heidelberg, pp 17–36
Steinberg G K, Fabrikant J I, Marks M P et al 1990 Stereotactic heavy-charged-particle bragg-peak radiation for intracranial arteriovenous malformations. New England Journal of Medicine 323: 96–101
Strum V, Kimmig B, Engenhart R et al 1991 Radiosurgical treatment of cerebral metastases. Method, indications and results. Stereotact Funct Neurosurg 57: 7–10
Szuwart U, Bennefeld H, Behr H 1989 Classification of gliomas and medulloblastoma using the new TNM system for cerebral tumors. Neurosurg Review 12: 233–238
Tamura M, Nakamura M, Kunimine H et al 1989 Large dose fraction radiotherapy in the treatment of glioblastoma. Journal of Neuro-Oncology 7: 113–119
Taphoorn M J B, Heimans J J, Snoek F J et al 1992 Assessment of quality of life in patients treated for low grade glioma: a preliminary report. Journal of Neurology, Neurosurgery and Psychiatry 15: 372–376
Taylor B, Marcus R, Freidman W et al 1988 The meningioma controversy: post operative radiation therapy. International Journal Radiation Oncology Biology Physics 15: 299, 304
Thomsen J, Tos M, Borgesen S E 1990 Gamma Knife: hydrocephalus as a complication of stereotactic radiosurgical treatment of an acoustic neuroma. American Journal of Otology 11: 330–333
Valk P E, Dillon W P 1991 Radiation injury of the brain. American Journal of Neurology and Radiology 12: 45–62
Winger M J, MacDonald D R, Cairncross J G 1989 Supratentorial anaplastic gliomas in adults. The prognostic importance of extent of resection and prior low grade glioma. Journal of Neurosurgery 71: 487–493
Zulch K J (ed) 1979 Histological typing of tumors of the central nervous system. International histological classification of tumors, no 21. World Health Organization, Geneva

18. Chemotherapy for brain tumors

Alexandra Flowers Victor A. Levin

The use of cytotoxic drugs is now established in the treatment of brain tumors. Chemotherapy prolongs survival, especially in patients with anaplastic gliomas, medulloblastoma, primitive neuroectodermal tumors (PNET), germ cell tumors and primary central nervous system lymphoma (PNSL). Glioblastoma multiforme tends to be more chemoresistant (Levin 1985).

The choice of the chemotherapeutic agents is determined by multiple factors: sensitivity of the tumor cells to the drugs as demonstrated in vitro and in animal studies, penetrability of the drug into the central nervous system (CNS), the therapeutic index (relationship of efficacy to toxicity) and the pharmacokinetics of the drug (Shapiro 1986, Levin et al 1989).

CLINICAL CONSIDERATIONS

As is also the case with most systemic cancers, chemotherapy of brain tumors is not curative and the goals of treatment are mainly to control the growth of the tumor while maintaining a good performance status and quality of life for the patient (Rodriguez & Levin 1987). Chemotherapy for brain tumors poses special problems, related to the presence of the blood-brain barrier (BBB) and the fact that it is very difficult to obtain an early objective measurement of response to chemotherapy.

The indirect clinical parameters for response are the patient's performance and neurologic status and the most direct measure, the appearance of the tumor on CT or MRI scan. While the performance status can be graded on standardized scales (Karnofsky, Zubrod), the size of the viable tumor cannot be measured accurately on scans due to the infiltrative nature of most of the primary brain tumors and the presence of edema and sometimes blood, and slow dead cell removal. The amount of edema does not correlate with the size of the tumor, as some small but aggressive tumors can cause significant edema and mass effect. On the other hand, even very large low grade tumors may have very little surrounding edema (Shapiro & Byrne 1983). The radiologic picture can also be complicated and confounded by changes due to surgery and prior therapy, especially radiation-induced brain necrosis. For gliomas complete remission with disappearance of the tumor is very unusual; more commonly seen is partial response and stable disease. Complete response can be seen in medulloblastoma, germinoma, occasional pineal region tumors, some PNET and some metastatic lesions. The duration of response and time to progression or recurrence are also dependent on the tumor histology and its sensitivity to chemotherapy. Patient survival is influenced by tumor type and size, performance status, extent of the surgical resection, medical complications related to the tumor itself and to tumor treatment (immunosuppression, radiation necrosis, myelosuppression) (Shapiro & Byrne 1983, Kornblith & Walker 1987).

Age is also an important determinant since children and young adults have a better response to therapy and a significantly better survival than older patients. Age is also important in determining the treatment sequence. For children under the age of six, radiation therapy for brain tumors increases the risk for learning disabilities and personality changes due to radiation necrosis and leukoencephalopathy (Friedman & Oakes 1992). For this age group chemotherapy is the first line of treatment following surgery. In the elderly, even lower grade anaplastic gliomas tend to behave more aggressively than in young adults and are relatively less sensitive to chemotherapy and XRT.

What makes brain tumor chemotherapy more difficult than for other tumor types is the specific tumor environment. The normal brain is a privileged site, protected from noxious agents by skull, meninges and a very effective blood-brain barrier (BBB) (Donelli et al 1992). In the case of brain tumors the skull and meninges limit the expansion of the brain tissue and the edema causes increased intracranial pressure and neurologic problems (Rodriguez & Levin 1987, Donelli et al 1992). The BBB is disrupted within the tumor, but it is not a homogeneous, generalized disruption, and it may be intact in areas of the brain infiltrated with tumor cells. The normal vascular pattern is also changed and there is vascular endothelial cell proliferation and angiogenesis with microvascularization. The new capillaries no longer have the tight junctions seen in normal endothelial cells of the BBB (Levin 1986, Gummerlock & Neuwelt 1987, Donelli et al 1992).

CELLULAR RESISTANCE FACTORS

The sensitivity of brain tumor cells to cytotoxic drugs and drug combinations is first tested in vitro, on tumor cell lines and clones (Bogdahn et al 1987). The in vitro systems are useful for drugs which do not require metabolization to the active ingredients. The problems with tissue cultures are related to the changes occurring in the cell lines through multiple passages and to the selection of clones which no longer resemble the heterogeneous tumor cell populations. The in vitro studies help to define the changes in karyotype and the chromosomal abnormalities that occur with increasing grades of malignancy and to identify some factors for tumor resistance to chemotherapy. The reduced uptake of drugs into tumor cells may be caused by decreased influx, decreased intracellular binding or increased efflux. The reduced influx is determined at the cellular level by defective transmembrane transport systems, as is the case for cells resistant to methotrexate, nitrogen mustard, or melphalan. For cisplatinum, resistant cell lines show both a decreased uptake and increased efflux. In these cell lines there is a decrease in the formation of inter-strand DNA cross-links. Some brain tumors overexpress the multidrug resistance gene (MDR 1) and P-glycoprotein, resulting in resistance to several cytotoxic agents (Evans 1989, Black 1991, Phillips 1991). The overexpression occurs following exposure to cytotoxic agents, and selection of such clones might explain the lack of response of some brain tumors to several different chemotherapy regimens (Shapiro et al 1981, Yung et al 1982, Becker et al 1991, Henson et al 1992, Tishler & Raffel 1992, Tishler et al 1992, Vendrik et al 1992). P-glycoprotein is located in the cell membrane and appears to act as a pump to eliminate the drug from the cell and thus decrease the intracellular levels. This mechanism has been demonstrated for vincristine and doxorubicin. Overexpression of P-glycoprotein has been found in some brain tumors (Henson et al 1992). Another mechanism for multiple drug resistance is related to intracellular levels of glutathione (GSH). Resistance to cisplatin and other alkylating agents has been associated with elevation of GSH levels in tumor cells (Ali-Osman et al 1991, Vendrik et al 1992). Increased efflux of drugs on tumor cells is mediated by glucuronyl-transferase, with formation of drug-glucuronide conjugates which are readily eliminated from the cells (Vendrik et al 1992). Drugs such as calcium-channel blockers (nifedipine, verapamil) and calmodulin interfere with P-glycoprotein and may reverse the multidrug resistance. A proposed mechanism for resistance to purine and pyrimidine analogs (5-fluorouracil, arabinoside cytosine, 6-thioguanine) is a decrease in the activity of phosphorylating enzymes required for nucleotide formation (Vendrik et al 1992). Other resistance mechanisms are gene amplification and increased production of target enzymes for the drug (e.g. dihydrofolate reductase and methotrexate), and increased efficiency of DNA repair enzymes, and salvage pathways.

Most of these resistance mechanisms become operational after exposure to cytotoxic agents, and the design of chemotherapy regimens has to take into account the potential selection of resistant clones. The resistance mechanisms mentioned above are not specific for brain tumor cells; they do apply to many other tumor types.

PHARMACOKINETIC CONSIDERATIONS

The pharmacokinetics of the drug must also be taken into consideration when designing a chemotherapy regimen for treatment of malignant brain tumors. The drugs with the best penetration into the central nervous system (CNS) are small molecules, liposoluble and nonionized. The drugs should also persist in the CNS long enough to ensure exposure of the tumor cells to cytocidal drug concentrations. The half-life of the drug, intracellular binding and capillary-to-cell diffusion are important factors. The drugs' penetration into the tumor is difficult to predict given the heterogeneity of tumors with respect to blood flow, capillary density, and breakdown of the blood-brain barrier (Rall & Zubrod 1962, Levin et al 1980, Levin 1986, Gummerlock & Neuwelt 1987).

For certain types of tumors with potential spread into the cerebrospinal fluid (CSF), such as medulloblastoma, ependymoma, pineal region tumors, and lymphoma, the chemotherapeutic agents used must also have good penetration into the CSF. Again, the half-life of the drug becomes important. Nitrosoureas are generally unstable in water and are cleared very fast from the CSF, and thus are not suitable for treatment of leptomeningeal disease. Unless a continuous infusion of the drug can be established methotrexate, thio-TEPA, and cytosine arabinoside (ara-C) persist longer in the CSF and are used for treatment of leptomeningeal carcinomatosis and lymphomatosis.

CHEMOTHERAPEUTIC AGENTS USED FOR TREATMENT OF MALIGNANT BRAIN TUMORS

Chemotherapy for malignant brain tumors is used as adjuvant or palliative treatment with single agents or drug combinations (Table 18.1). The purpose of drug combinations is to obtain a synergistic or additive effect, to sensitize tumor cells to the action of the most potent drug in the combination and to prevent cellular repair mecha-

Table 18.1 Chemotherapeutic agents used for the treatment of brain tumors

Class and type	Mechanism of action	Drug	Route of adm.	Dose	Tumor
Alkylating agents:					
Nitrosoureas	Cause DNA cross-links and carbamoylation of amino groups	BCNU	IV	200–240 mg/m^2	Malignant gliomas
			IA	160–180 mg/m^{2-}	
		CCNU	PO	100–130 mg/m^{2-}	
		ACNU	IV	100–150 mg/m^2	
			IA	100 mg/m^2	
		MeCNU	PO	130–220 mg/m^2	
		PCNU	IV	60–100 mg/m^2	
	Cause DNA cross-links and inhibit enzymes involved in ribonucleotide reduction pathways	Fotemustine	IV	100 mg/m^2	Malignant gliomas, brain metastases
	Interfere with pyridine nucleotide synthesis	Streptozotocin	IV	500–1500 mg/m^2	Malignant gliomas
Metal salts	Inhibit DNA synthesis through intrastrand cross-links, chelation	Cisplatin	IV	40–120 mg/m^2	Malignant gliomas, PNET, germ cell, medulloblastoma
			IA	90 mg/m^2	
		Carboplatin	IV	300–450 mg/m^{2-}	
			IA	200–400 mg/m^{2-}	
		Iproplatin	IV	300 mg/m^2	
Nitrogen mustard	Produces carbonium ions which react with electron-rich areas in susceptible molecules	Cyclophosphamide	IV	1000–1500 mg/m^2	Medulloblastoma, PNET, germ cell, brain metastases
			PO	60–400 mg/m^2	
		Ifosfamide	IV	1200–3000 mg/m^2	Malignant gliomas, medulloblastoma
		Melphalan	PO	8–10 mg/m^{2-}	
		Nitrogen mustard	IV	6 mg/m^{2-}	
Alkyl sulfone	Interaction with thiol groups	Busulfan	PO	1–4 mg/m^2	Pediatric brain tumors
Ethylimine derivatives	Similar with the nitrogen mustard	Thiotepa	IV	12 mg/m^2	Pediatric brain tumors, meningeal metastases
			IT	2–10 mg/m^2	
Triazine	Formation of diazo compounds	Dacarbazine	IV	150–500 mg/m^2	Malignant meningioma
Benzquinone	Alkylating agent	Pyridinyl-benzquinone (AZQ)	IV	10–15 mg/m^2	Malignant glioma
Antimetabolites					
Folic acid analogs	Inhibit dihydrofolate reductase, blocks thymidilate synthesis	Methotrexate	IV	2000–12000 mg/m^2	Medulloblastoma, PNET, PCNSL
			IT	10–12 mg	
Pyrimidine analogs	Inhibits critical enzymes for nucleic acid synthesis, are incorporated into DNA and RNA	Fluorouracil	IV	1000 mg/m^2	Malignant gliomas, brain metastases
		Cytarabine	IV	100–300 mg/m^2	PCNSL
			IT	100 mg	
Purine analogs	Interfere with normal purine interconversion and thus with RNA and DNA synthesis	Thioguanine	PO	40–100 mg/m^2	Malignant gliomas
		Mercaptopurine	PO	50–100 mg/m^{2-}	
			IV	200–750 mg/m^2	
Natural products					
Vinca alkaloids	Affect microtubular protein, inhibit mitosis	Vincristine	IV	1.4–2 mg/m^2	Malignant gliomas, PNET
Podophyllotoxins	Topoisomerase II inhibitors, cause DNA breakage and arrest of cells in S-phase	Etoposide (VP-16)	IV	50–140 mg/m^2	Malignant gliomas, germ cell, PNET, brain metastases
			PO	50 mg/m^2	
		Teniposide (VM-26)	IV	50–160 mg/m^2	Medulloblastoma
Antibiotics	Cause DNA strand scission	Bleomycin	IV	10–30 units/m^2	Pediatric brain tumors
			IM	10–20 units/m^{2-}	
	Topoisomerase II-dependent DNA cleavage and intercalate with DNA double helix	Doxorubicin	IV	15–75 mg/m^2	Pediatric brain tumors, malignant meningioma
		Idarubicin	IV	10–13 mg/m^{2-}	
Miscellaneous					
Urea analog	Inhibition of enzymatic conversion of ribonucleotides to deoxyribonucleotides	Hydroxyurea	PO	300–1000 mg/m^2	Malignant gliomas
Methylhydrazine derivative	Mechanism not well known, affects DNA, RNA and protein synthesis	Procarbazine	PO	50–150 mg/m^2	Malignant gliomas, PNET, medulloblastoma, PNSL
Halogenated hexitols	Acts as an alkylating agent with effects on DNA, RNA	Dibromodulcitol	PO	100–130 mg/m^2	Malignant gliomas, ependymomas, medulloblastoma, brain metastases
Polyamine inhibitors	Irreversible inhibition of ornithine decarboxylase	Difluoromethyl PO ornithine	PO	2 g/m^2	Malignant glioma

IV = intravenous; PO = oral; IM = intramuscular, IA = intra-arterial; IT = intrathecal
PNET = primitive neuroectodermal tumors; PNSL = primary central nervous system lymphoma

Table 18.2 Chemotherapeutic drug combinations used for the treatment of brain tumors, with emphasis on adult malignant gliomas

Combination	Schedule of administration	Tumor
PCV	**P**rocarbazine 60 mg/m^2/day PO for 14 days, day 8–21, every 6 weeks **CCNU** 110 mg/m^2 PO day 1, every 6 weeks **V**incristine 1.4 mg/m^2 IV days 8 and 29, every 6 weeks	Malignant gliomas
BCNU/CDDP	**BCNU** 80 mg/m^2 IV + **C**isplatin 80 mg/m^2 IV, every 6 weeks or **BCNU** 40 mg/m^2/day IV continuous infusion for 3 days every 4 weeks **C**isplatin 40 mg/m^2/day IV continuous infusion for 3 days every 4 weeks or **BCNU** 100–125 mg/m^2 IA + **C**isplatin 60–120 mg/m^2 IA	Malignant gliomas
BCNU/PV	**BCNU** 200 mg IA on day, 1, every 4 weeks **P**rocarbazine 150 mg PO/day, days 2–9, every 4 weeks **V**incristine 2 mg IV on day 1, every 4 weeks	Malignant gliomas
TPDC-FUHU	6-**T**hioguanine 40 mg/m^2 PO every 6 hours for 12 doses days 1–3, every 6 weeks **P**rocarbazine 50 mg/m^2 PO every 6 hours for 4 doses starting on hour 60, every 6 weeks **D**ibromodulcitol 400 mg/m^2 PO on hour 60, every 6 weeks **CCNU** 110 mg/m^2 PO on hour 72, every 6 weeks 5-**F**luorouracil 1 g/m^2/day IV continuous infusion on days 14–15, every 6 weeks **H**ydroxyurea 1 g/m^2 PO every 4 hours for 3 doses, starting on hour 44 of the fluorouracil infusion, every 6 weeks	Malignant gliomas, brain metastases
'8 drugs in 1 day'	**V**incristine 2 mg, IV, every 4–5 weeks **CCNU** 75 mg/m^2, PO, every 4–5 weeks **P**rocarbazine 75 mg/m^2 PO, every 4–5 weeks **H**ydroxyurea 1500 mg/m^2, PO, every 4–5 weeks **C**isplatin 90 mg/m^2 IV, every 4–5 weeks **C**ytosine arabinoside 300 mg/m^2 IV, every 4–5 weeks **DTIC** 150 mg/m^2 IV, every 4–5 weeks **M**ethylprednisolone 300 mg/m^2 IV every 6 hours for 3 doses, every 4–5 weeks	Malignant gliomas, pediatric brain tumors
CDDP/VP-16	**C**isplatin 100 mg/m^2/day IV for 5 days, every 4 weeks **E**toposide (VP-16) 20 mg/m^2/day IV for 5 days, every 4 weeks	Malignant gliomas, germ cell tumors
BCNU/VM-26	**BCNU** 75 mg/m^2 IV, every 4 weeks **T**eniposide (VM-26) 75 mg/m^2 IV, every week	Malignant gliomas
VP-16/VP	**E**toposide 100 mg/m^2/day IV for 3 days, every 4 weeks **V**incristine 1.4 mg/m^2 IV, every 4 weeks **P**rocarbazine 100 mg/m^2/day PO, for 7 days, every 4 weeks	Malignant gliomas
CBDCA/VP-16	**C**arboplatin (CBDCA) 300 mg/m^2 IV on days 1–3, every 4 weeks **E**toposide 100 mg/m^2 IV on days 1–5, every 4 weeks	Malignant gliomas
CTX/V	**C**yclophosphamide (Cytoxan, CTX) 250–1000 mg/m^2 IV for 2 days, every 3–4 weeks **V**incristine 1.0 mg/m^2 IV, every 3–4 weeks	Malignant gliomas

nisms (Table 18.2) (Wilson et al 1976, Vick et al 1977, Calliauw & Sieben 1986, Day 1986, Shapiro & Shapiro 1986, De Vita 1989, Yung 1990, Hildebrand & Thomas 1991, Mahaley 1991, Shapiro et al 1991, Whittle & Gregor 1991, Horowitz & Poplak 1991). Some drugs are cell-cycle specific, others are cell-cycle nonspecific.

Alkylating agents

Alkylating agents are the most widely used and effective chemotherapeutic agents for the treatment of malignancy. These are cell-cycle nonspecific drugs, however they are most active on rapidly dividing tumor cells, possibly because these cells have less time to repair the DNA damage. Most alkylating agents form positively charged carbonium ions which attack nucleophilic sites on nucleic acids, proteins and amino acids. The alkylation sites on DNA are the 1 and N7 positions on guanine, 1, 3, and 7 positions on adenine; and N3 position on cytosine. The result of these base alkylations can be cross-linking of DNA, single-strand and double-strand breaks and misreading of the DNA code (De Vita 1989).

1. Nitrosoureas are considered to be the most active drugs for CNS tumors, especially for malignant gliomas. The chloroethylnitrosoureas (NU) are highly lipophilic, except for 3 (4-amino-2-methyl-5-pyrimidinyl)methyl-1-(chloroethyl)-1-nitrosourea hydrochloride (ACNU), which is water-soluble, although still lipophilic. Based on their mechanism of action, NU are bifunctional alkylating agents, causing both DNA cross-linking and carbamoylation of amino groups through isocyanate products. The isocyanates deplete glutathione, inhibit DNA repair and interfere with RNA synthesis. Tumor cells resistant to NU have increased levels of glutathione-S-transferase and the repair enzyme guanine-6-methyl transferase. Agents such as misonidazole which deplete intracellular glutathione can restore sensitivity of drug-resistant cells to NU (also to melphalan and cyclophosphamide) (De Vita 1989, Vega et al 1992).

The 1,3-bis(2-chloroethyl)-1 nitrosourea (BCNU) is administered intravenously (IV) or intra-arterially (IA), and 1-(2-chloroethyl)-3-cyclohexyl-1-nitrosourea (CCNU) is given orally. The plasma half-life of both drugs is 15–20 minutes. Laboratory studies showed cross-resistance between BCNU, CCNU, methyl-CCNU, ACNU and PCNU (1-(2-chloroethyl)-2-(2,6-dioxo-3 piperidyl)-1 nitrosourea). The clinical activity is similar for BCNU and CCNU, although some believe that single agent BCNU is slightly superior to CCNU. NU have a synergistic effect with radiation therapy (XRT) and there are clinical studies of BCNU administered IV or IA in conjunction with XRT. The synergistic effect may be due to interference with the cells' repair mechanism as well as synchronization of tumor cells in G_2 phase when there is maximal radiosensitivity (Wilson et al 1972, Walker et al 1980, Levin et al 1984a, Fulton et al 1987). With multiple daily fractions of XRT, practical radiosensitization by BCNU is unattainable.

NU are used for chemotherapy of brain tumors, alone or in drug combinations designed for synergistic effect or to combat resistance to NU and prevent cell repair (Gutin et al 1975, Levin et al 1985, Stewart et al 1987, Shapiro et al 1989, 1992, Watne et al 1992a).

ACNU is another NU, used either IV or IA. Yamashita et al (1991) reported a trial of high dose ACNU with autologous bone marrow transplant (BMT) for treatment of malignant gliomas. The BMT was used to reduce the ACNU-induced myelosuppression.

The dose limiting side effect of NU is myelosuppression, which occurs at 3–5 weeks. Nausea and emesis are the acute side effects, readily controllable with the available antiemetics. Another major side effect which occurs in up to 20% of patients in some studies is pulmonary fibrosis. Renal damage can also occur with high doses of nitrosourea.

Other NU uncommonly used in some brain tumor chemotherapy protocols are streptozotocin and chlorozotocin.

NU are used mainly for the treatment of malignant gliomas (Gutin et al 1975, Levin et al 1985, 1986, Stewart et al 1987, Shapiro et al 1989, Yamashita et al 1991, Levin & Prados 1992, Shapiro et al 1992, Watne et al 1992a) and have shown some activity on metastatic brain tumors (Stewart et al 1987, Levin & Prados 1992).

*2. **Procarbazine*** is a cell-cycle nonspecific alkylating agent, whose mechanism of action is less well defined than that of NU. It inhibits DNA, RNA and protein synthesis. Procarbazine is water-soluble and readily absorbed through the gastrointestinal tract, and it and critical metabolites do cross the BBB. It is also a monoamine oxidase (MAO) inhibitor and can interact with tyramine-containing foods and neuropharmacologically active drugs, causing hypertension and CNS side effects (ataxia, hallucinations). Procarbazine has disulfiram-like activity and when ingested with alcohol can cause gastrointestinal side effects. The dose-limiting side effect is the myelotoxicity (De Vita 1989). Some patients develop allergic reactions (skin rash).

Procarbazine has been used as a single drug for treatment of recurrent malignant gliomas (high dose), and in combination chemotherapy as adjuvant or palliative treatment for malignant gliomas (Levin et al 1986, van Eys et al 1987, Newton et al 1990, Levin & Prados 1992). It is also used in combination chemotherapy for the treatment of poor-risk medulloblastomas and primary CNS lymphoma and for other types of tumors. It is administered orally, but it has also been given IV (van Eys et al 1987).

*3. **Platinum compounds*** are inorganic agents with a planar molecule with a platinum ion which binds to DNA. When administered IV they do not easily cross the BBB, and the levels in the CSF are low except when CNS tumors are present, when the levels in tumor and CSF increase (Riccardi et al 1992).

Cis-platinum (CDDP) is a water-soluble alkylating agent which acts through intrastrand and inter-strand DNA cross-linking. It binds primarily to the guanine base (De Vita 1989).

CDDP is administered IV or IA. The main toxicities are myelosuppression, nephrotoxicity, ototoxicity and peripheral neuropathy. To reduce the risk of renal damage CDDP is administered with high volumes of fluids and sometimes with mannitol to increase renal clearance.

CDDP is active against medulloblastoma, PNET, lymphoma, and germ cell tumors (Patel et al 1992); it is less active against malignant gliomas (Spence et al 1992). CDDP is given in drug combinations (with etoposide, cytoxan, vincristine, and NU) (Madajewics et al 1991, Bobo et al 1992, Yung et al 1992). It is also given IA alone or with BCNU together with XRT (Recht et al 1990, Dropcho 1992).

Carboplatinum is a platinum compound with similar tumor activity as CDDP, but with less renal toxicity and less emesis. It was shown to have moderate activity against pediatric and adult malignant gliomas, similar to CDDP (Poisson et al 1991, Yung et al 1991, Stewart et al 1992a).

*4. **Cyclophosphamide (cytoxan)*** is a chemotherapeutic agent metabolized in the liver to hydroxycyclophosphamide; this is further activated to aldophosphamide, phosphoramide mustard and acrolein. These active compounds account for the alkylating activity of cytoxan (De Vita 1989).

Cytoxan is administered IV in combination chemotherapy regimens for pediatric malignant brain tumors, medulloblastomas, germ cell tumors, and brain metastases.

Ifosfamide is a drug related to cyclophosphamide, with less myelotoxicity. It is used for the treatment of pediatric brain tumors.

Besides myelotoxicity, a common side effect of cyclophosphamide and ifosfamide is hemorrhagic cystitis, which can be prevented by concomitant administration of MESNA.

*5. **Nitrogen mustard*** is the first alkylating agent used for cancer treatment. It has fairly limited use in the therapy of brain tumors. It is used for treatment of medulloblastomas as part of MOPP combination (with vincristine, procarbazine and prednisone) and M-MOPP (with the addition of methotrexate). Myelosuppression is the dose-limiting toxicity. Spirohydantoin mustard is a related compound developed around the phenytoin backbone, with marginal activity for treatment of recurrent malignant gliomas (Prados et al 1979).

*6. **Melphalan (α-methyl-phenylalanine)*** is a phenylalanine derivative with alkylating activity. It crosses the BBB and enters tumor cells through an active amino acid transmembrane transport mechanism. In clinical trials its usefulness against malignant gliomas is minimal, but it showed activity against medulloblastoma (Chamberlain et al 1988). As is the case with the other alkylating agents, its main toxicity is myelosuppression.

*7. **Busulfan*** is an alkylating agent which can be administered orally. It has only limited use in the treatment of malignant brain tumors (Kalifa et al 1992).

*8. **Aziridinyl benzoquinone (AZQ)*** is a water-soluble alkylating agent designed specifically for the treatment of malignant brain tumors due to its ability to cross the BBB in significant amounts. In clinical trials, however, the results have been less encouraging than in animal studies. It has been tested clinically for the treatment of malignant gliomas and ependymomas. Its main toxicity is myelosuppression (Schold et al 1984, Eagan et al 1987).

*9. **Dacarbazine (DTIC)*** (5-(3,3-dimethyl-1-triazeno)-imidazole-4-carboxamide) acts as an alkylating agent and also inhibits purine nucleoside incorporation into the DNA. It is cell-cycle nonspecific. It has limited use for CNS tumors. In combination with adriamycin it is used for the treatment of malignant meningioma. In addition to myelosuppression, a potentially fatal side effect is hepatic veno-occlusive disease and hepatic necrosis (De Vita 1989).

*10. **Dibromodulcitol (mitolactol, DBD)*** is a hexitol biotransformed to mono- and diepoxides. The diepoxide can act as an alkylating agent and produce DNA cross-links. As a single agent, DBD is active against medulloblastoma and ependymomas, but has limited activity against malignant astrocytomas. It can, however, potentiate the activity of nitrosoureas and it is used in combination chemotherapy for primary and metastatic brain tumors (Schuler et al 1992). Its side effects are myelosuppression and, less commonly, nausea and emesis.

Hydroxyurea (HU)

HU is a cell-cycle specific drug, which inhibits ribonucleotide diphosphate reductase, an important enzyme for the synthesis of DNA. This enzyme catalyzes the conversion of ribonucleotides to deoxyribonucleotides. HU crosses the BBB readily. HU is used as a radiosensitizer in conjunction with XRT for the treatment of malignant gliomas. It may also prevent DNA repair of the damage caused by nitrosoureas (Levin et al 1986, Levin & Prados 1992). It is administered orally and is very well tolerated, with only mild side effects such as nausea, loss of appetite, and skin discoloration (Levin 1992).

Plant alkaloids

1. Vinca alkaloids

Vincristine (Oncovin) is a water-soluble alkaloid which acts as a mitotic spindle poison. It causes metaphase arrest by binding to tubulin during S-phase. Although it does not cross the BBB in significant amounts, in combination chemotherapy it has been shown to be active against brain tumors, presumably crossing leaky tumor capillaries and attacking S-phase cells nearby. In combination with CCNU and procarbazine (PCV) it is used for the treatment of malignant gliomas, PNSL and medulloblastoma (Gutin et al 1975, Levin et al 1985, van Eys et al 1988). Vincristine is a bone marrow sparing drug; its main toxicity is peripheral neuropathy.

2. Podophyllotoxins

VM-26 (tenoposide) and VP-16 (etoposide) are highly lipophilic compounds; however, because of their size, they do not readily penetrate into brain and CSF (Kiya et al 1992). They bind to tubulin and inhibit microtubular assembly. Unlike vincristine, the podophyllotoxins arrest cells in G_2 rather than mitosis and cause single-strand and double-strand breaks in DNA. This action is mediated by the formation of a stable complex between the podophyllotoxins, DNA and topoisomerase II (De Vita 1989). VP-16 is used in combination chemotherapy for treatment of pediatric brain tumors, medulloblastoma, germ cell tumors and PNSL (Feun et al 1987, Stewart et al 1987, De Angelis et al 1990). The most important side effect is myelotoxicity, especially leukopenia.

Purine and pyrimidine analogs

*1. **5-Fluorouracil (5FU)*** is a fluorinated pyrimidine analog. It competes with uracil for the enzyme thymidilate synthetase and inhibits thymidine production. By this mechanism 5FU inhibits both DNA and RNA synthesis. After IV administration 5FU crosses the BBB. 5FU as a single agent has no activity against brain tumors. It was shown to have synergistic activity with hydroxyurea and is part of polydrug combinations for treatment of malignant gliomas and metastatic brain tumors (Levin et al 1986, Levin & Prados 1992, Shapiro et al 1992). 5FU also has synergistic activity with carboplatin.

The most significant side-effect is myelosuppression. Rarely an acute cerebellar syndrome may occur.

*2. **Cytosine arabinoside (cytarabine, ara-C)*** is an arabinose nucleoside, recognized enzymatically as an analog of 2′-deoxycytidine and metabolized to ara-CTP. Ara-CTP competes with dCTP and inhibits DNA polymerase. It is also incorporated into DNA leading to a slowing of the elongating chains and defective DNA fragment ligation. Entry of ara-C into tumor cells is a carrier-mediated process. The cytotoxic action of the drug is limited by inactivating enzymes, cytidine deaminase and dCMP deaminase.

Ara-C administered IV crosses the BBB and is used for treatment of PNSL and metastatic lymphoma (DeAngelis et al 1990). It is also administered intrathecally or intraventricularly (through Ommaya-type reservoirs) for treatment of leptomeningeal metastases.

Systemic toxicities include nausea, emesis, and myelotoxicity. An acute pancerebellar syndrome can occur with both IV and intrathecal administration. Other CNS toxicities are encephalopathy and seizures.

*3. **6-Mercaptopurine (6MP) and 6-thioguanine (6TG)*** are purine analogs. Both require activation to monophosphate nucleotides by the enzyme hypoxanthine-guanine phosphoribosyltransferase and inhibit the purine biosynthesis. As triphosphate nucleotides, both are incorporated into DNA. 6TG-induced DNA toxicity is manifested by strand breaks and it also makes DNA more susceptible to alkylation. Both 6TG and 6MP are used in drug combinations for the treatment of malignant gliomas (Levin et al 1986, Levin & Prados 1992). Both are administered orally. The side effects are myelosuppression and immunosuppression.

Methotrexate

Methotrexate is an antifolate antimetabolite. It is a 4-amino-N10 methyl analog of folic acid and it binds tightly to dihydrofolate reductase, thus inhibiting production of tetrahydrofolate (FH4), the active form of the coenzyme. FH4 is necessary for transfer of one-carbon groups for the synthesis of thymidilate and purines. Methotrexate is cell-cycle specific, active only on cells in S-phase.

At conventional doses methotrexate penetrates the CNS very poorly, requiring high doses to produce significant amounts in the brain and CSF.

Methotrexate is used for the treatment of medulloblastoma, PNSL, and PNET. It is not very active against malignant gliomas. It can be administered IV and intrathecally for the treatment of leptomeningeal metastases (Stewart et al 1987).

The toxicities of methotrexate include myelosuppression, immunosuppression, nephrotoxicity and mucositis. When administered with XRT it considerably increases the risk for radiation-induced necrosis and leukoencephalopathy. The CNS toxicity of methotrexate is manifested by encephalopathy. Administration of leucovorin (N5-formyl tetrahydrofolate) reduces the toxic effect of methotrexate on normal cells by competing with methotrexate for binding of dihydrofolate reductase.

Antitumor antibiotics

Commonly used for treatment of systemic malignancies, the antitumor antibiotics have only limited use for the therapy of brain tumors.

*1. **Bleomycin*** is obtained from Streptomyces species; it is a mixture of small molecular weight peptides which binds DNA and produces single-strand and double-strand breaks. It is not cell-cycle specific, however the cells most susceptible are those in premitotic (G_2) and mitotic phase.

Bleomycin is used in some drug combinations for pediatric brain tumors (Stewart et al 1987). Its dose-limiting toxicities are myelosuppression and pulmonary fibrosis.

*2. **Anthracyclines*** are a group of antibiotics also produced from Streptomyces species. Their structure is an anthraquinone nucleus attached to an aminosugar. The mechanism of action of the anthracyclines is complex. Anthracyclines intercalate DNA and block DNA replication and RNA and protein synthesis. DNA intercalation triggers DNA cleavage by topoisomerase II. Another mechanism is formation of semiquinone free radicals which can react with molecular oxygen to form superoxide, hydrogen peroxide and hydroxyl radical.

Although the anthracyclines proved to be very active against systemic cancers, their use for CNS tumors is limited by their poor BBB passage. Adriamycin is used in combination with DTIC for treatment of malignant meningiomas. A new anthracycline, menogaril, has been evaluated, but was found to be of limited activity against malignant gliomas (Stewart et al 1992b).

Myelotoxicity and cardiomyopathy are the dose-limiting toxicities of anthracyclines.

Polyamine inhibitors

The polyamines (putrescine, spermidine, spermine) are implicated in the growth and proliferation of tumor cells (Babuna & Marton 1990, Tsukahara et al 1992). Polyamines also seem to mediate to some degree the radiation-induced brain edema and radiation necrosis, possibly through breakdown of BBB and vascular changes (Gutin et al 1990, Seidenfeld & Prague 1990, Moulinoux et al 1991).

The polyamine inhibitors α-difluoromethyl ornithine

(DFMO, eflornithine) and methyl glyoxal-bisguanylhydrazone (MGBG) have activity against malignant gliomas.

DFMO is an ornithine decarboxylase inhibitor, blocking synthesis of putrescine from ornithine. It does not readily cross the normal BBB; however, because it is not metabolized and does achieve sustained blood levels, diffusion within tumor to adjacent brain does take place. DFMO shows activity against malignant gliomas when administered alone and it potentiates the activity of nitrosoureas (Prados et al 1989, Hunter 1990). Combined administration with MGBG, a competitive inhibitor of S-adenosyl hydrazone, was also shown to be active against malignant gliomas (Levin et al 1987). Experimental intraventricular administration of these drugs on beagle dogs was associated with significant neurotoxicity (Gobbel et al 1991).

In other animal studies DFMO was shown to reduce XRT-induced cerebral edema and necrosis and is presently undergoing clinical trials (Levin et al 1984b).

DFMO can be administered orally or IV, is well tolerated, and its dose-limiting toxicities are myelotoxicity and ototoxicity.

This list of chemotherapeutic agents is not exhaustive, but rather an overview of the cytotoxic drugs used most frequently for treatment of brain tumors.

The response of brain tumors to chemotherapy varies depending on tumor type, the feasibility and extent of surgical resection, prior response to XRT and chemotherapy and the patient's age (De Vita 1983, Shapiro & Byrne 1983, Kornblith & Walker 1987). We will discuss only the chemosensitive primary brain tumors.

CHEMOTHERAPY OF BRAIN TUMORS

Malignant gliomas

Patients with anaplastic astrocytomas (AA) are more likely to benefit from chemotherapy than patients with glioblastoma multiforme (GBM). In the AA group the patients with low to intermediate grade tumors and under the age of 50 have a better response to therapy and longer survival. With all the cytotoxic agents and drug combinations available to date for treatment of malignant gliomas, chemotherapy still benefits mostly the patients in the lower 50th percentile, and especially those below the 25th percentile of surviving patients (Levin 1985).

Nitrosoureas are the most active drugs against malignant gliomas. Nitrosourea-based drug combinations showed increased antitumor efficacy compared with BCNU alone. Significant prolongation of the time to tumor progression (TTP) and survival was demonstrated by Levin et al (1985) for AA patients on the combination procarbazine, CCNU and vincristine (PCV) compared with a group on BCNU (for the 50th percentile 126 weeks and 157 weeks respectively for PCV, and 63 and 82 weeks respectively for BCNU).

Chemotherapy is used as adjuvant following surgery and XRT, or as palliative treatment for patients who failed prior therapy (Walker et al 1980, Levin et al 1985, Shapiro et al 1989, Recht et al 1990, Dropcho et al 1992, Vega et al 1992, Watne et al 1992a,b, Yung et al 1992). There are clinical studies in which chemotherapy is given prior to XRT (Recht et al 1990, Dropcho et al 1992, Watne et al 1992b). The advantage of this approach compared with the conventional post-XRT adjuvant chemotherapy for patients with high grade glioma is yet to be proven. Chemotherapy can be initiated in conjunction with XRT for a dual effect of radiosensitization and drug cytotoxicity. BCNU, cisplatin (IV or IA) and carboplatin are presently used together with XRT in clinical trials.

For recurrent malignant gliomas chemotherapy prolongs survival and also represents the setting for phase I and II clinical trials for new cytotoxic agents. Several drugs and drug combinations such as high dose procarbazine, DFMO, carboplatin, AZQ, PCV and other nitrosourea-based polydrug chemotherapy have shown activity against recurrent malignant gliomas (Gutin et al 1975, Prados et al 1979, Levin et al 1984a, Schold et al 1984, Levin et al 1986, Eagan et al 1987, Fulton et al 1987, Levin et al 1987, Chamberlain et al 1988, Poisson et al 1991, Yung et al 1991, Spence et al 1992, Stewart et al 1992b).

When the duration of radiation therapy is shortened, such as with brachytherapy, radiosurgery or accelerated fractionation schedules, radiosensitization with chemotherapeutic agents becomes more possible as a means to achieve greater tumor cell kill (Phillips et al 1991, Halperin 1992, Fulton et al 1992). To date we lack practical proof of the advantage of this approach, however.

Intracarotid BCNU and cisplatin have been used as adjuvant and palliative chemotherapy, alone or in combination with intravenous chemotherapy and XRT (Stewart et al 1987, Recht et al 1990, Madajewics et al 1991, Bobo et al 1992, Dropcho et al 1992, Shapiro et al 1992, Stewart et al 1992a, Vega et al 1992, Watne et al 1992a). While it has the advantage of improving drug delivery to the tumor, the IA chemotherapy is also associated with increased risk for neurotoxicity and optic nerve damage. A significant increase in survival has not been demonstrated for IA chemotherapy to date.

Brainstem gliomas are treated with the same chemotherapeutic agents as the supratentorial gliomas; no outstanding chemotherapy regimen has been promoted to date.

Anaplastic oligodendroglioma (AO)

Anaplastic oligodendrogliomas appear to be more sensitive to chemotherapy than other types of glioma

(Cairncross et al 1992). Good responses have been reported to the PCV combination. Mixed oligo-astrocytomas also respond better and have a longer time to tumor progression than AA. Pre-XRT chemotherapy with PCV for malignant oligodendroglioma induced complete or partial response in 11 of 14 patients in a study by Glass et al (1992) and it may also improve the outcome after XRT.

Still, even with good response to chemotherapy, AO do recur and the search continues for new treatment alternatives.

Anaplastic ependymoma (AE)

The treatment of anaplastic ependymoma is complicated by the propensity of these tumors to spread into the CSF. There are no chemotherapy regimens designed specifically for the treatment of AE. The same drugs used for the treatment of malignant gliomas are used for AE following craniospinal radiation therapy, either with single drugs (BCNU, DBD) or drug combinations.

Medulloblastoma

Chemotherapy is used for treatment of poor-risk medulloblastoma and for recurrent medulloblastoma. For children with medulloblastoma, chemotherapy with MOPP or M-MOPP or vincristine and cisplatin proved very effective. For older children and adults with poor-risk medulloblastoma, good responses are obtained with craniospinal XRT followed by chemotherapy with drug combinations (M-MOPP, cytoxan with VP-16 and cisplatin) or single drugs. Chemotherapy can also start before XRT or concomitantly. Unfortunately, in spite of demonstrated chemosensitivity, medulloblastomas tend to recur once the chemotherapy is discontinued. Aggressive chemotherapy with bone marrow transplantation is undergoing clinical trials (Lundberg et al 1992).

Germ cell tumors

When occurring as primary intracranial tumors, germ cell tumors are frequently found in the pineal region. The diagnosis is established at surgery and by detecting high levels of chorionic gonadotrophins or α-fetoprotein in the CSF. Germ cell tumors are chemosensitive and good responses have been obtained with combination chemotherapy with cisplatin, VP-16 and bleomycin or cytoxan, and also with actinomycin D, methotrexate, and vinblastine (Levin 1985, Mahaley 1991, Patel et al 1992). Greater use of chemotherapy before and instead of XRT is currently receiving attention in most centres worldwide.

Primary central nervous system lymphoma (PNSL)

The incidence of PNSL, both non-AIDS and AIDS-related is increasing. Treatment with XRT and chemotherapy is only palliative. Like the systemic lymphoma, PNSL is chemosensitive. Combination chemotherapy with ara-C, cytoxan, adriamycin, methotrexate, 6-MP, vincristine, and prednisone is effective and used in clinical studies prior to and in conjunction with whole brain XRT. For patients with leptomeningeal spread intraventricular ara-C or methotrexate is also administered (Hochberg & Miller 1988, DeAngelis et al 1990, Chamberlain & Levin 1992). There is no doubt, however, that the addition of chemotherapy has increased survival over XRT alone.

FUTURE DIRECTIONS

Chemotherapy has contributed to prolonged survival of patients with malignant brain tumors, but has not increased the cure rate. To improve response to chemotherapy the design of future drugs and drug combinations must be aimed at overcoming tumor cell resistance, improving drug delivery to the tumor and improving the therapeutic index (Grossman et al 1987, Takada et al 1991, Boiardi et al 1992).

Increased drug delivery to the tumor can be achieved by maintaining blood levels (continuous infusion), intra-arterial administration, manipulation of the blood-brain barrier and direct intratumoral administration. Intra-arterial administration of chemotherapy increases drug delivery to the tumor but is associated with increased risk for neurotoxicity.

Manipulation of the BBB — temporary osmotic BBB disruption with mannitol — followed by chemotherapy is well tolerated, however it has not shown a survival advantage over the more conventional chemotherapy (Gummerlock et al 1992, Jamshidi et al 1992).

Intratumoral administration of chemotherapeutic agents is a new modality to improve drug delivery to the tumor and surrounding brain tissue while at the same time minimizing the systemic toxicity. In animal studies intratumoral injection of AZQ showed a much better response than intravenous administration, while cis-platinum had dose-limiting acute neurotoxicity (Tomita 1991, Ogasawara et al 1992). Grossman et al (1992) obtained a sustained high local concentration of BCNU delivered by surgically implanted biodegradable polymers. Early edema and necrosis at injection site were noted, which resolved with time. The problem with this approach, as with systemic administration, is the uneven drug distribution within the tumor and adjacent brain tissue.

High dose chemotherapy with bone marrow transplantation rescue is also undergoing investigation; however this approach is still limited due to severe toxicity and immunosuppression (Yamashita et al 1991, Kalifa et al 1992). Colony stimulating factors such as granulocyte colony stimulating factors (G-CSF) and granulocyte-macrophage colony stimulating factor (GM-CSF) as well as cytokines — interleukin 1 (IL-1) and IL-6 — can help prevent or reduce myelosuppression and thus support the patients receiving high dose chemotherapy. The recombinant human IL-1 has hematopoietic regulative effects, induces the production of hematopoietic growth factors and activates primitive hematopoietic progenitor cells, preventing both leukopenia and thrombocytopenia (Tanaka et al 1992).

As we gain a better understanding of the molecular biology of brain tumors, with the multitude of genetic alterations and growth factors and their influence on response to chemotherapy, new therapeutic approaches may emerge, which may hold the promise for cure.

REFERENCES

Ali-Osman F, Sriram R, Raikar A 1991 Inhibition of repair of DNA-interstrand cross-links in human malignant astrocytoma cells: Mediation by glutathione depletion. (meeting abstr). Proceedings of the Annual Meeting of the American Association for Cancer Research 32: A2579

Babuna O, Marton L J 1990 Polyamine accumulation and vasogenic edema in the genesis of late delayed radiation injury in the central nervous system (CNS). Acta Neurochir Suppl 51: 372–374

Becker I, Becker K F, Meyermann R, Holt V 1991 The multidrug resistance gene MDR1 is expressed in human glial tumors. Acta Neuropathol 82: 516–519

Black P McL 1991 Brain tumors. New England Journal of Medicine 324: 1471–1476

Bobo H, Kapp J P, Vance R 1992 Effect of intra-arterial cisplatin and 1,3-bis(2 chloroethyl)-1-nitrosourea (BCNU) dosage on radiographic response and regional toxicity in malignant glioma patients: proposal of a new method of intra-arterial dosage calculation. Journal of Neuro-oncology 13: 291–299

Boiardi C, Silvani A, Milanesi I et al 1992 Efficacy of "8-drugs-in-one-day" combination in treatment of recurrent GBM patients. Journal of Neuro-oncology 12: 153–158

Bogdahn U, Weber H, Zapf J et al 1987 Therapy of malignant brain tumors: Comparison of the in vitro activities of vidarabine monophosphate, BCNU and 5-fluorouracil. Acta Neurologica Scandinavica 75: 28–36

Cairncross J G, MacDonald D R, Ramsay D A 1992 Aggressive oligodendroglioma: a chemosensitive tumor. Neurosurgery 31: 78–82

Calliauw L, Sieben G 1986 The future of chemotherapy in malignant brain tumors. Neurosurgical Review 9: 27–30

Chamberlain M C, Levin V A 1992 Primary central nervous system lymphoma: a role for adjuvant chemotherapy. Journal of Neuro-oncology 14: 271–275

Chamberlain M C, Prados M D, Silver P, Levin V A 1988 A phase II trial of oral melphalan in recurrent primary brain tumors. American Journal of Clinical Oncology 11: 52–54

Day R S 1986 Treatment sequencing, asymmetry and uncertainty: protocol strategies for combination chemotherapy. Cancer Research 46: 3876–3885

DeAngelis L M, Yahalom J, Heinemann M H et al 1990 Primary CNS lymphoma. Combined treatment with chemotherapy and radiotherapy. Neurology 40: 80–86

De Vita V T Jr 1983 The relationship between tumor mass and resistance to chemotherapy. Implication for surgical adjuvant treatment of cancer. Cancer 51: 1209

De Vita V T Jr 1989 Principles of chemotherapy. In: De Vita Jr V T, Hellman S, Rosenberg S A (eds) Cancer. Principles and practice of oncology. J B Lippincott, pp 276–301

Donelli M G, Zucchetti M, D'Incalci M 1992 Do anticancer agents reach the tumor target in the human brain? Cancer Chemother Pharmacol 30: 251–260

Dropcho E, Rosenfeld S S, Morawetz R B et al 1992 Preradiation intracarotid cisplatin treatment of newly diagnosed anaplastic gliomas. Journal of Clinical Oncology 10: 425–458

Eagan R T, Dinapoli R P, Cascino T L et al 1987 Comprehensive phase II evaluation of Aziridinyl-benzoquinone (AZQ, diaziquone) in recurrent human primary brain tumors. Journal of Neuro-oncology 5: 309–314

Evans C A 1989 Mechanisms of resistance to alkylating agents in brain tumor cells. Abstr Int "B" 50: 1307

Feun L G, Lee Y Y, Yung W K et al 1987 Intracarotid VP-16 in malignant brain tumors. Journal of Neuro-oncology 4: 397–401

Friedman H S, Oakes W J 1992 New treatment options in the management of childhood brain tumors. Oncology 6: 27–36

Fulton D S, Urtasun R C, McKinnon S, Tanasichuk H 1987 Misonidazole and CCNU chemotherapy for recurrent primary brain tumors. Journal of Neuro-oncology 4: 383–388

Fulton D S, Urtasun R C, Scott-Brown I et al 1992 Increasing radiation dose intensity using hyperfractionation in patients with malignant gliomas. Final report of a prospective phase I–II dose response study. Journal of Neuro-oncology 14: 63–72

Glass J, Hochberg F H, Grubeer M L et al 1992 The treatment of oligodendroglioma and mixed oligodendroglioma-astrocytomas with PCV chemotherapy. Journal of Neurosurgery 76: 741–745

Gobbel G T, Marton L J, Seilhan T M, Fike J R 1991 Modification of radiation-induced brain injury by alpha-difluoromethyl ornithine. Radiation Research 128: 306–315

Grossman S, Sheidler V, Weissman D et al 1987 Continuous infusion (CI) therapy for primary brain tumors: a new approach with a high response rate (meeting abstr). Proceedings of the Annual Meeting of the American Society Clin Oncol 6: A279

Grossman S A, Reinhard C, Colvin M D et al 1992 The intracerebral distribution of BCNU delivered by surgically implanted biodegradable polymers. Journal of Neurosurgery 76: 640–647

Gummerlock M K, Neuwelt E A 1987 Principles of chemotherapy in brain neoplasms. In: Jellinger K (ed) Therapy of malignant brain tumors. Springer Verlag, New York, pp 277–348

Gummerlock M K, Belshe B D, Masden R, Watts C 1992 Osmotic blood-brain barrier disruption and chemotherapy in the treatment of high grade malignant glioma: patient series and literature review. Journal of Neuro-oncology 12: 33–46

Gutin P H, Wilson C B, Kumar A R V et al 1975 Phase II study of procarbazine, CCNU, vincristine combination chemotherapy in the treatment of malignant brain tumors. Cancer 35: 1389

Gutin P H, McDermott M W, Ross G, Chan P H 1990 Polyamine accumulation and vasogenic edema in the genesis of late delayed radiation injury of the central nervous system. Acta Neurochir Suppl 51: 372–374

Halperin E C 1992 Multiple-fraction-per day external beam radiotherapy for adults with supratentorial malignant gliomas. Journal of Neuro-oncology 14: 255–262

Henson J W, Cordon-Cardo C, Posner J B 1992 P-glycoprotein expression in brain tumors. Journal of Neuro-oncology 14: 37–43

Hildebrand J, Thomas D G T 1991 Report of a workshop sponsored by the European Organization for Research and Treatment of Cancer (EORTC) on the treatment of primary malignant brain tumors. Journal of Neurology, Neurosurgery and Psychiatry 54: 182–183

Hochberg F H, Miller D C 1988 Primary central nervous system lymphoma. Journal of Neurosurgery 68: 835–853

Horowitz M E, Poplak D G 1991 Development of chemotherapy treatment for brain tumors. Neurol Clin 9: 363–373

Hunter L J 1990 Effect of alpha-difluoromethyl ornithine on 1,3-bis-(2 chloroethyl)-1-nitrosourea and cis-diamino-dichloroplatinum (II) cytotoxicity, DNA interstrand cross-linking and growth in human brain tumor cell lines in vitro. Cancer Research 50: 2768–2772

Jamshidi J, Yoshimine T, Ushio Y, Hayaskawa T 1992 Effects of glucocorticoid and chemotherapy on the peritumoral edema and astrocytic reaction in experimental brain tumors. Journal of Neuro-oncology 12: 197–204

Kalifa C, Hartmann O, Demecocq F et al 1992 High-dose busulfan and thiotepa with autologous bone marrow transplantation in childhood malignant brain tumors: a phase II study. Bone Marrow Transplantation 9: 227–233

Kiya K, Uozumi T, Ogasawa H et al 1992 Penetration of etoposide into human malignant brain tumors after intravenous and oral administration. Cancer Chemotherapy and Pharmacology 29: 339–342

Kornblith P L, Walker M 1987 Chemotherapy for malignant intracranial tumors. Cancer Treatment Research 36: 185–203

Levin V A 1985 Chemotherapy of primary brain tumors. In: Vick N A, Bigner D D (eds) Neuro-Oncology. Neurologic Clinics of North America, 3rd edn. P B Saunders, p 855

Levin V A 1986 Pharmacokinetics and central nervous system chemotherapy. In: Hellman K, Carter S K (eds) Fundamentals of cancer chemotherapy. McGraw-Hill, pp 28–40

Levin V A 1992 The place of hydroxyurea in the treatment of primary brain tumors. Seminars in Oncology 19 (suppl 9): 34–39

Levin V A, Prados M D 1992 Treatment of recurrent gliomas and metastatic brain tumors with a polydrug protocol designed to combat nitrosourea resistance. Journal of Clinical Oncology 10: 766–771

Levin V A, Patlak C S, Landahl H D 1980 Heuristic modeling of drug delivery to malignant brain tumors. J Pharmacokinet Biopharm 8: 251

Levin V A, Resser K, McGrath L et al 1984a PCNU treatment for recurrent malignant glioma. Cancer Treatment Rep 68: 969

Levin V A, Byrd D, Campbell J et al 1984b CNS toxicity and CSF pharmacokinetics of intraventricular DFMO and MGBG in beagle dogs. Cancer Chemotherapy and Pharmacology 13: 200–205

Levin V A, Wara W M, Davis R L et al 1985 Phase III comparison of chemotherapy with BCNU and the combination procarbazine, CCNU and vincristine administered after radiation therapy with hydroxyurea to patients with malignant gliomas. Journal of Neurosurgery 63: 218

Levin V A, Phuphanich S, Liu H C et al 1986 Phase II study of combined lomustine, 5-fluorouracil, hydroxyurea and 6-mercaptopurine (BFHM) for the treatment of malignant glioma. Cancer Treat Rep 70: 1271–1274

Levin V A, Chamberlain M C, Prados M D et al 1987 Phase I–II study of eflornithine and mitozoguazine combined in the treatment of recurrent primary brain tumors. Cancer Treat Rep 71: 459–464

Levin V A, Sheline G E, Gutin P H 1989 Neoplasms of the central nervous system. In: De Vita V T Jr, Hellman S, Rosenberg S A (eds) Cancer. Principles and practice of oncology. J B Lippincott, pp 1557–1611

Lundberg J H, Weissman D E, Beatty P A, Ash R C 1992 Treatment of recurrent metastatic medulloblastoma with intensive chemotherapy and allogeneic bone marrow transplantation. Journal of Neuro-Oncology 13: 151–155

Madajewics S, Chowhan N, Iliya A et al 1991 Intracarotid chemotherapy with etoposide and cisplatin for malignant brain tumors. Cancer 67: 2844–2849

Mahaley M S 1991 Neuro-Oncology index and review (adult primary brain tumors). Radiotherapy, chemotherapy, immunotherapy, photodynamic therapy. Journal of Neuro-Oncology 11: 85–142

Moulinoux J P, Daarcwel F, Quemener V et al 1991 Inhibition of the growth of U251 human glioblastoma in nude mice by polyamine deprivation. Anticancer Research 11: 175–179

Newton H B, Junck L, Bromberg J et al 1990 Procarbazine chemotherapy in the treatment of recurrent malignant astrocytomas after radiation and nitrosourea failure. Neurology 40: 1743–1746

Ogasawara H, Kiya K, Kurisu K et al 1992 Effect of intracarotid infusion of etoposide with angiotensin II-induced hypertension on the blood-brain barrier and the brain tissue. Journal of Neuro-Oncology 13: 111–117

Patel S R, Buckner J C, Smithson W A et al 1992 Cisplatin-based chemotherapy in primary central nervous system germ cell tumors. Journal of Neuro-Oncology 12: 47–52

Phillips P C 1991 Antineoplastic drug resistance in brain tumors. Neurol Clin 9: 383–404

Phillips T L, Levin V A, Ahn D K et al 1991 Evaluation of bromodeoxyuridine in glioblastoma multiforme: A Northern California Cancer Center phase II study. Int J Radiat Oncol Biol Phys 21: 709–714

Poisson M, Pereon Y, Chiras J, Delattre J Y 1991 Treatment of recurrent malignant supratentorial gliomas with carboplatin (CBDCA). Journal of Neuro-Oncology 10: 130–144

Prados M D, Rodriguez C, Seager M et al 1979 Phase II study of spirohydantoin mustard for the treatment of recurrent malignant gliomas. Journal of Neurosurgery 51: 526

Prados M, Rodriguez L, Chamberlain M et al 1989 Treatment with 1,3-bis(2 chloroethyl)-1-nitrosourea and alphadi-fluoromethyl ornithine. Neurosurgery 24: 806–809

Rall D P, Zubrod C G 1962 Mechanism of drug absorption and excretion. Passage of drugs in and out of the central nervous system. Annual Review of Pharmacology 2: 109–128

Recht L, Fram R J, Strauss G et al 1990 Preirradiation chemotherapy of supratentorial malignant primary brain tumors with intracarotid cis-platinum (CDDP) and I.V. BCNU. A phase II trial. American Journal of Clinical Oncology 13: 125–131

Riccardi R, Riccardi A, Di Rocco C et al 1992 Cerebrospinal fluid pharmacokinetics of carboplatin in children with brain tumors. Cancer Chemother Pharmacol 30: 21–24

Rodriguez L A, Levin V A 1987 Does chemotherapy benefit patients with a central nervous system glioma? Oncology 1: 29–36

Schold S C, Friedman H S, Bjornsson T D et al 1984 Treatment of patients with recurrent primary brain tumor with AZQ. Neurology 34: 615

Schuler D, Somlo P, Koos R et al 1992 Treatment of malignant posterior brain tumors in children: the chemotherapy of relapsed medulloblastoma with a dibromodulcitol containing regimen and pharmacokinetic studies of dibromodulcitol in children. Medical Pediatric Oncology 20: 312–314

Seidenfeld J, Prague W S 1990 Comparison between sensitive and resistant tumor cell lines regarding effect of polyamine depletion on chloroethylnitrosourea efficacy. Cancer Research 50: 521–526

Shapiro W R 1986 Therapy of adult malignant brain tumors. What have the clinical trials taught us? Seminars in Oncology 13: 38

Shapiro W R, Byrne T N 1983 Chemotherapy of brain tumors. Basic concepts. In: Walker M D (ed) Oncology of the nervous system. Martinus Nijhoff, pp 65–100

Shapiro W R, Shapiro J R 1986 Principles of brain tumor chemotherapy (Review). Seminars in Oncology 13: 56–69

Shapiro W R, Yung W A, Basler G A et al 1981 heterogenous response to chemotherapy of human gliomas grown in nude mice and as clones in vitro. Cancer Treat Resp 65 (Suppl 2): 55–59

Shapiro W R, Green S B, Burger P L 1989 Randomized trial of three chemotherapy regimens and two radiotherapy regimens in postoperative treatment of malignant glioma. Brain Tumor Cooperative Group Trial 8001. Journal of Neurosurgery 7: 1–9

Shapiro W R, Green S B, Burger P C et al 1991 Recent results in the chemotherapy of brain tumors — BTCG studies. Developments in Oncology 66: 147–152

Shapiro W R, Green S B, Burger P C et al 1992 A randomized comparison of intra-arterial versus intravenous BCNU, with or without intravenous 5-fluorouracil, for newly diagnosed patients with malignant glioma. Journal of Neurosurgery 76: 772–781

Spence A M, Berger M S W, Livingston R B et al 1992 Phase II evaluation of high-dose intravenous cisplatin for treatment of adult malignant gliomas recurrent after chloro-ethylnitrosourea failure. Journal of Neuro-oncology 12: 187–191

Stewart D J, Grahovac Z, Hugenholtz H et al 1987 Combined intra-arterial and systemic chemotherapy for intracerebral tumors. Neurosurgery 21: 207–214

Stewart D J, Belanger J M, Grahovac Z, et al 1992a Phase I study of intracarotid administration of carboplatin. Neurosurgery 30: 512–516

Stewart D J, Hugenholtz H, Da Silva V F et al 1992b Phase II study of weekly intravenous menogaril in the treatment of recurrent astrocytomas in adults. Journal of Neuro-Oncology 13: 183–188

Takada Y, Greig N H, Vistica D et al 1991 Affinity of antineoplastic amino-acid transporter of the blood-brain barrier. Cancer Chemotherapy and Pharmacology 29: 89–94

Tanaka S, Taguchi S, Watanabe K et al 1992 Preventive effects of interleukin 1b for ACNU induced myelosuppression in malignant brain tumors: the experimental and preliminary clinical studies. Journal of Neuro-oncology 14: 159–168

Tishler D M, Raffel C 1992 Development of multidrug resistance in a primitive neuroectodermal cell line. Journal of Neurosurgery 76: 502–506

Tishler D M, Weinberg K I, Sender L S et al 1992 Multidrug resistance gene expression in pediatric primitive neuroectodermal tumors of the central nervous system. Journal of Neurosurgery 76: 507–512

Tomita T 1991 Interstitial chemotherapy for brain tumors. Review. Journal of Neuro-oncology 10: 37–47

Tsukahara T, Tamura M, Yamazaki H et al 1992 The additive effect of alpha-difluoromethyl ornithine (DFMO) and radiation therapy in a rat glioma model. Journal of Cancer Research and Clinical Oncology 118: 171–175

van Eys J, Cangir A, Pack R, Baram T 1987 Phase I trial of procarbazine as a 5-day continuous infusion in children with central nervous system tumors. Cancer Treat Rep 71: 973–974

van Eys J, Baram T Z, Cangir A et al 1988 Salvage chemotherapy for recurrent primary brain tumors in children. Journal of Pediatrics 113: 601–606

Vega F, Davila L, Chatellier G et al 1992 Treatment of malignant gliomas with surgery, intraarterial chemotherapy with ACNU and radiation therapy. Journal of Neuro-oncology 13: 131–135

Vendrik C P J, Bergers J J, De Jong W H, Steernberg P A 1992 Resistance to cytostatic drugs at the cellular level. Cancer Chemother Pharmacol 29: 413–429

Vick N A, Khandekar J D, Bigner D D 1977 Chemotherapy of brain tumors: The blood-brain barrier is not a factor. Archives of Neurology 34: 523–526

Walker M D, Green S B, Byar D P 1980 Randomized comparison of radiotherapy and nitrosoureas for the treatment of malignant glioma after surgery. New England Journal of Medicine 303: 1323–1329

Watne K, Hannisdal E, Nome O et al 1992a Combined intra-arterial chemotherapy followed by radiation in astrocytomas. Journal of Neuro-oncology 14: 73–80

Watne K, Nome O, Hager B, Hirschberg H 1992b Preradiation chemotherapy in glioma patients with poor prognostic factors. Journal of Neuro-oncology 13: 261–264

Whittle I R, Gregor A 1991 The treatment of primary malignant brain tumors. Journal of Neurology, Neurosurgery and Psychiatry 54: 101–103

Wilson C B, Gutin P H, Boldrey E B et al 1972 Phase II study of 1-(2 chloroethyl)-3-cyclohexyl-nitrosourea (CCNU) in the treatment of brain tumors. Cancer Chemother Rep 56: 421

Wilson C B, Gutin P H, Boldrey E B et al 1976 Single agent chemotherapy of brain tumors. Archives of Neurology 33: 739

Yamashita J, Shoin K, Soma M 1991 High dose ACNU chemotherapy with autologous bone marrow transplantation for human malignant brain tumors. Developments in Oncology 66: 897–899

Yung W K 1990 Chemotherapy for malignant brain tumors. Current Opinions in Oncology 2: 673–678

Yung W K A, Shapiro J R, Shapiro W R 1982 Heterogenous chemosensitivities of subpopulations of human glioma cells in culture. Cancer Research 42: 992–998

Yung W K A, Janus T J, Maor M, Feun L G 1992 Adjuvant chemotherapy with carmustine and cisplatin for patients with malignant gliomas. Journal of Neuro-oncology 112: 131–135

Yung W K A, Mechtler L, Gleason M J 1991 Intravenous carboplatin for recurrent malignant gliomas: a phase II study. Journal of Neuro-oncology 9: 860–864

19. Brain tumor therapy protocols and combined modality therapy

Michael Prados Susan Chang

INTRODUCTION

The incidence of tumors of the central nervous system is increasing, especially in the elderly population. In the United States, about 1–2% of the population are affected and this is associated with tremendous morbidity and mortality, as evident from the 11 000 deaths of the 15 000 patients diagnosed in 1989 (Walker et al 1985, Silverberg & Lubara 1989).

One of the strategies to improve upon the outcome of patients treated is to emphasize the multidisciplinary approach to their management. In terms of direct patient care, a number of subspecialists are involved including neurosurgeons, medical and radiation oncologists, pediatric oncologists, neurologists, and neuro-oncologists. Neuroradiologists and pathologists also play an important role in the management of these patients. More and more emphasis is being placed on the role of laboratory research and work of basic scientists in helping to understand the genesis and behavior of brain tumors, so that relevant treatment strategies can be designed and developed. Scientists in the fields of immunology, molecular biology, genetics, radiobiology, biochemistry, research pharmacology and organic chemistry are part of the multidisciplinary team. With the development of novel diagnostic techniques in the fields of molecular genetics and gene therapy, a correlation between tissue diagnosis and treatment outcome may be possible, hence the importance of tissue banks so that these specimens may be available for future study.

TREATMENT

In general, surgery serves to make a diagnosis, alleviate symptoms and to remove as much tumor as is safely possible with the intention of prolonging life. Since most brain tumors tend to be infiltrative, it is often impossible to remove all microscopic disease. This is the basis for the multimodality therapy of most tumors of the central nervous system.

Radiotherapy is one of the more effective treatment modalities in the treatment of brain tumors. In addition to conventional dose fractionation, there are studies investigating the role of hyperfractionated schedules, accelerated hyperfractionation, brachytherapy with and without hyperthermia, stereotactic radiosurgery and high linear energy transfer irradiation in the treatment of these patients.

A modification of radiation therapy is the use of a chemical agent to enhance the effect of radiation. These include hypoxic cell sensitizers, halogenated pyrimidines, and platinum analogs.

Initial treatment of malignant gliomas (glioblastoma and anaplastic astrocytoma)

Historical perspective

Because of the dismal survival results of patients with malignant gliomas treated with surgery alone, a combined modality approach has been applied to the treatment of these patients. Irradiation is an effective adjuvant to surgery and in prospective studies has afforded better survival over either surgery alone or surgery and chemotherapy.

The initial studies of irradiation and chemotherapy adjuvant to surgery were conducted by the BTSG in 1969 (Walker et al 1978). Patients who had undergone surgery were randomized to four groups: (1) supportive care only; (2) carmustine 80 mg/m^2 given on three successive days every 6 weeks for a year; (3) whole-brain irradiation to a total of 50–60 Gy; (4) whole brain irradiation to a total of 50–60 Gy and carmustine 80 mg/m^2 given on three successive days every 6 weeks for a year. Patients with glioblastoma constituted 90% of the treated groups. The median survival of the groups were 14, 19, 36 and 35 weeks respectively. Surgery and radiation offered a significantly improved survival time over surgery alone or with chemotherapy. The addition of carmustine to radiation did not affect the median survival significantly.

Further studies looking at the role of adjuvant nitrosourea chemotherapy followed. A study undertaken by the

BTSG randomized patients with malignant gliomas who had undergone surgery to 4 groups: (1) semustine; (2) radiation; (3) semustine and radiation; (4) carmustine and radiation (Walker et al 1980). This study confirmed the benefit of radiotherapy with the median survival of the groups being 31, 37, 43 and 49 weeks respectively. The survival rates with carmustine and radiation were not significantly longer than radiation alone or with radiation and semustine. To enhance the survival advantage with postoperative irradiation, higher doses of radiation were investigated. The BTSG retrospectively analyzed data on patients treated in randomized studies with median doses of 50, 55 and 60 Gy and found a dose-effect relationship with median survivals of 28, 36 and 42 weeks respectively (Walker et al 1979).

In a randomized study by the RTOG and the ECOG groups (Chang et al 1983), patients with biopsy-proven supratentorial malignant gliomas were treated with: (1) whole brain radiation therapy to a dose of 60 Gy as the control radiation; (2) control radiation plus a boost of 10 Gy to the tumor bed; (3) control radiation plus carmustine; (4) control radiation plus semustine and imidazolecarboxamide (DTIC). The median survivals were 9.9, 8.4, 10 and 9.8 months respectively. There was no advantage to adding a boost of radiation to the tumor bed. Only in the patients 40–60 years of age was an advantage seen to adding chemotherapy to radiation. The semustine and DTIC combination was more toxic than the carmustine treatment.

Chemotherapeutic agents may be used before, during or after radiotherapy. Most treatment strategies use chemotherapy after radiotherapy; a major exception is in the pediatric population, in which the modality of radiation therapy is reserved until the patient is as old as possible, preferably older than 3 years, so that the long-term effects of radiation are spared. The most common drug group used for brain tumors is the nitrosoureas. These agents are lipid-soluble and can cross the blood-brain barrier. Many other chemotherapeutic agents have been used in the treatment of brain tumors, but tumor cell resistance and limitations in drug delivery are the major barriers in the efficacy of these agents. Some experimental strategies in the delivery of chemotherapeutic agents include intra-arterial, intratumoral and interstitial administration, and the use of monoclonal antibodies as carriers. High dose chemotherapy with autologous bone marrow transplantation is another strategy to try to improve on the efficacy of chemotherapy. Agents that overcome multidrug resistance are also being investigated.

As more is being learned about the relationship of defects in immune surveillance and the development of malignancies, strategies involving modulation of the immune system are being tested in the treatment of brain tumors.

Intense laboratory research in the various fields of cell biology and genetics that add insight into the complex process of oncogenesis has resulted in the development of exciting approaches in gene therapy for the treatment of brain tumors. An example of one novel approach is the introduction of an exogenous gene into proliferating tumors. This gene encodes a susceptibility factor that would then make the tumor sensitive to a chemotherapeutic agent that ideally does not have toxic effects on normal tissues. Experiments incorporating the exogenous gene that encodes the herpes simplex enzyme thymidine kinase into patients with brain tumors, with the subsequent administration of the antiviral agent ganciclovir, are currently being undertaken. Brain tumors are ideal in the investigation of this strategy, since the surrounding tissue is nonproliferating and as a result does not incorporate the exogenous gene and would theoretically be immune to the effect of the chemotherapeutic agent.

The role of combination chemotherapy as an adjunct to radiation therapy (60 Gy with hydroxyurea as a sensitizer) in patients with malignant glioma was studied by the Northern California Oncology Group. (Levin et al 1990a). This randomized trial compared the effects of adjuvant carmustine versus the combination PCV regimen (procarbazine, lomustine and vincristine). Patients with anaplastic gliomas treated with PCV had a survival advantage with a median survival of 152 weeks compared to 82 weeks for those treated with carmustine alone. There was no difference in the two groups of patients with glioblastoma multiforme.

Attempts at modifications in the administration of radiation therapy to improve upon the results of standard fractionation have included the use of hyperfractionation. This involves dividing the daily dose in multiple fractions and is believed to enhance the radiation effect since the tumor cells are less resistant to frequent radiation fractions than normal brain cells. This technique would also allow for minimization of radiation injury to normal brain. Urtasun and colleagues (1989) treated patients with malignant gliomas three times daily to a total dose of 61.41, 71.20 or 80.00 Gy, and when there was a recurrence, the patients received lomustine chemotherapy. Median survivals were 45.8, 37.2 and 60.5 weeks, no better than historical controls. Accelerated hyperfractionation involving the use of higher doses per fraction is being investigated.

Another modification to improve the efficacy of radiation is the use of radiation sensitizers. The halogenated pyrimidine bromodeoxyuridine (BUdR) incorporates into the DNA of dividing cells and enhances the effect of radiation. Greenberg and colleagues (1988) studied 18 patients treated with intra-arterial BUdR and found a small survival advantage compared to historical controls. Preliminary data from the NCOG (Levin et al 1990b) suggest a survival advantage with the halogenated pyrimidine bromodeoxyuridine given intravenously in patients with anaplastic gliomas but not in those with glioblastoma multiforme. This is currently being investigated in a phase III trial.

Other forms of radiation therapy have also been studied in the treatment of malignant gliomas. The RTOG conducted a randomized dose-finding study of neutrons given as a boost to conventional whole brain photon beam radiation to a dose of 45 Gy (Laramore et al 1988). There was no difference in the overall survival among six different neutron dose levels, but for patients with less aggressive histology (anaplastic astrocytomas versus glioblastoma multiforme) there was a suggestion that patients on the higher dose levels had poorer survival.

Interstitial brachytherapy using iodine-125 radioactive sources implanted within a tumor has been used in the treatment of recurrent malignant gliomas with some impressive results. Gutin and colleagues treated 45 patients with recurrent glioblastoma and 50 patients with recurrent anaplastic astrocytoma with median survivals of 54 weeks and 87 weeks respectively. The evaluation of this technique at the time of initial diagnosis is being studied. A summary of the current phase I, II and III trials in patients with newly diagnosed malignant gliomas is presented in Tables 19.1–19.3.

Treatment of recurrent malignant gliomas

Once it is determined that a tumor has progressed, further treatment may include surgical resection, re-irradiation (for example using brachytherapy or radiosurgery), chemotherapy, immunotherapy, gene therapy and palliative care. Most of the current protocols for the treatment of recurrent gliomas are trials aimed at identifying new

Table 19.1 Current protocols for the initial treatment of malignant gliomas (Phase III trials)

Institution	Tumor type	Objective
NCI-T91-00560 NCOG-6G90-3	Anaplastic astrocytoma	Radiotherapy vs radiotherapy/BUdR, followed by PCV
NCI-T91-00470 NCOG-6G90-1	Glioblastoma multiforme	Accelerated hyperfractionation +/– DFMO vs single fraction radiation +/– DFMO
MDA-Dm-92035 NCI-T92-0114C	Malignant glioma	DFMO + PCV vs PCV, following radiotherapy
EU-90007 MRC-BR05	Grade 3/4 astrocytoma	PCV vs no chemotherapy, following radiotherapy
RTOG-9006	Malignant astrocytoma and glioblastoma multiforme	Single fraction radiation +BCNU vs hyperfractionation
BTCG-8901	Malignant glioma	Radiation + BCNU vs radiation +BCNU + intra-arterial cisplatin vs radiation + piroxantrone
MAYO-887252 NCCTG-887252	High grade glioma	Radiation + BCNU vs radiation + BCNU + interferon-α
BTCG-8701	Malignant glioma	Brachytherapy with ^{125}I implants vs no therapy, following radiation

Table 19.2 Current protocols for the initial treatment of malignant gliomas (Phase II trials)

Institution	Tumor type	Objective
NCI-V91-0036 NCOG-6G90–2	Glioblastoma multiforme	Radiation + HU followed by brachytherapy +/– hyperthermia
E-2392 EST-PC-390	High grade glioma	Radiation + VCR/VR-16/PCB
NCI-V91-01154 SUNY-HSC-2166	High grade malignant glioma	MOP prior to radiation
NCI-T88-0130D NCOG-6G872	Glioblastoma multiforme	Radiation with Neon beam
JHOC-8813 NCI-V88-0408	High grade glioma	3 cycles of BCNU + cisplatin followed by radiation
NOR-NRH-BN	Inoperable brain tumors	Intra-arterial BCNU + VCR/PCB followed by radiation
MICH-T87-0015 NCI-T87-00150	Malignant glioma	Radiosensitization with intra-arterial BUdR/5FU plus cranial radiotherapy
NCI-T91-00170 NYMC-T91-0017	Grade III/IV astrocytoma	High dose diaziquone plus autologous bone marrow transplantation

Table 19.3 Current protocols for the initial treatment of malignant gliomas (Phase I trials)

Institution	Tumor type	Objective
CCUM-9242 NCI-T92-0056D	Malignant glioma	Intra-arterial BUdR/BCNU infusion
MDA-ID-92005 NCI-T92-0053D	Malignant glioma	BUdR + accelerated fractionation radiation followed by PCV
CAN-OTT-9001 NCI-V91-0078	Grade III/IV astrocytoma	Preoperative radiation and surgery
NCI-T90-0023D UCCRC-5853	Anaplastic astrocytoma and glioblastoma multiforme	5-FU, hydroxyurea and escalating doses of IUdR

agents, or combinations of agents that have activity and may be used in phase III trials.

There are a number of phase II trials using new drugs such as edatrexate, temozolomide, tretinoin, cystemustine, amonafide, acivicin, merbarone and didemnin B. Combination chemotherapy trials include 5FU and high dose leucovorin; continuous infusion carboplatin and 5FU with oral procarbazine; and thiotepa, etoposide and carboplatin with autologous bone marrow transplantation.

The EORTC (26881) has a phase III trial looking at patients with recurrent malignant gliomas randomized to BCNU vs BCNU/VCR/nimodipine. The group at UCSF also has a phase III trial of BCNU vs BCNU/fluosol/oxygen for patients with recurrent astrocytomas.

The NCI has an immunotherapy trial (NCI-T89-023711) using intracavitary IL-2 and LAK cells for recurrent primary brain tumors as well as monoclonal antibody OKT3 with low dose cytoxan for recurrent advanced malignancies (NCI-V90-0206).

The current radiation protocols for the treatment of recurrent malignant gliomas include three brachytherapy trials and one radiosurgery trial. The group in Pittsburgh (WPH-1) has a phase I/II study evaluating interstitial brachytherapy while the BTRC has a phase I trial (9101) using BUDR or IUDR with ^{125}I seed implants. The group in Michigan (M1184) is investigating intra-arterial BUdR with ^{125}I seed implants.

The RTOG (9005) is evaluating small field stereotactic external beam radiation in a phase I study of recurrent primary brain tumors.

An exciting therapeutic approach is being investigated by the NIH. Accrual has begun into the gene therapy trial using stereotactically placed murine cells engineered to produce a retroviral vector which carries the gene for herpes simplex thymidine kinase. Patients are then treated with ganciclovir. This trial is open for patients with recurrent anaplastic astrocytoma or glioblastoma.

Ependymoma

Historical perspective

Ependymomas are classified as either differentiated (low grade) or anaplastic (malignant) tumors. There are, however, conflicting data concerning the prognostic implications of anaplasia in these tumors (Ernestus et al 1989). Since there are no formal prospective studies of ependymoma, treatment recommendations remain controversial.

The goal of surgery in the treatment of ependymoma is gross total removal. This is often limited by the location in the posterior fossa or spinal cord involving the cauda equina. Historically, trials have documented the radiosensitivity of ependymomas. In a series by Ernestus and colleagues (1989), for example, median disease-free survival for patients with grade II supratentorial ependymoma treated with radiation was 185 months versus 38 months if no radiation was administered. For patients who underwent only a partial resection, median survival without recurrence was 9 months if only surgery was performed versus 108 months in those who received postoperative radiation therapy.

What is still unclear from the historical reviews is the perimeter of the radiation field and whether the craniospinal axis should be treated adjuvantly. The primary site of recurrence of low grade ependymoma is usually within the local radiation field (Garrett & Simpson 1983, Wallner et al 1986) and as such whole brain radiation or craniospinal irradiation for supratentorial ependymoma is not indicated, if initial staging investigations with MR imaging of the spine and CSF cytology are negative. The risk of spinal subarachnoid metastasis is greatest with infratentorial anaplastic ependymomas and many groups (Salazar et al 1983) suggest irradiation of the entire craniospinal axis for anaplastic ependymomas.

Ependymomas are sensitive to several agents, including the nitrosoureas, platinum compounds, procarbazine and dibromodulcitol (Friedman & Oakes 1987). Most of these agents are used at the time of recurrence. The role of adjuvant chemotherapy after radiation therapy has not been established in the treatment of ependymomas. A recent retrospective review of the UCSF experience suggests that a multimodality approach at initial diagnosis has helped to achieve significantly longer survival in patients with anaplastic ependymoma than previously reported in the literature.

Medulloblastoma

Medulloblastoma (MB) and primitive neuroectodermal tumors (PNET) are a group of diverse tumors that most commonly occur within the pediatric age group (Parks et al 1983). The primitive nature of the tumor on histological preparations accounts for the name, with several components possible, representing different cell lineages (Packer et al 1984). Thus a tumor may have neuronal, glial or ependymal elements, as well as undifferentiated cells. A true cell of origin has not been defined. These lesions have the unique property of dissemination within the neuroaxis, and treatment has included the primary tumor, as well as uninvolved areas of the brain and spinal cord (Allen & Epstein 1982). The use of craniospinal radiotherapy has consistently produced the longest disease-free survival, and in some cases, this survival is enhanced with the use of adjuvant chemotherapy (Bloom et al 1990). A series of multi-institutional trials have documented aspects of disease which are known to increase the risk of relapse, and currently patients have been treated according to this risk status (Evans et al 1900, Tait et al 1990, Krischer et al 1991, Packer et al 1991). Patients with good risk features have minimal residual disease remaining following surgical resection, and no evidence of distant disease as measured by staging of the spine and brain, as well as sampling of the CSF to evaluate the presence of malignant tumor cells. Known poor risk factors include the presence of malignant cells within the spinal fluid (M-1), disease in the brain (M-2) or spine (M-3), or extraneural metastasis (M-4). Factors that are less clear include the presence of microscopic invasion of the brainstem, and the extent of postoperative residual disease (Parks et al 1983, Packer et al 1984). Currently, the Children's Cancer Group (CCG) and the Pediatric Oncology Group (POG) define poor risk residual disease as postoperative tumor greater than 1.5 cm, measured by MRI or contrast CT. Tumors that arise within the brainstem, spinal cord, and pineal regions are also considered poor risk features, and tumors that occur in infants less than 2 or 3 years of age often will relapse irrespective of staging. Recommended staging procedures include postoperative MRI within 48–72 hours of surgery, spinal MRI with and without contrast either preoperative (if MB/PNET is clinically suspected) or postoperatively, and CSF cytology from the lumbar CSF no sooner than 2 weeks postoperatively. Extraneural metastasis is most often to bone or bone marrow, and in patients with significant tumor burdens, it may be appropriate to obtain a bone scan and bone marrow biopsy. These risk factors were based upon a staging system described by Chang, a 'TNM' system that now does not appear to be predictive for relapse when the T stage has been evaluated. In the Chang system, the T or 'Tumor' stage was subdivided by extent of disease defined by the neurosurgeon, and was graded from 1–4 based upon extent of tumor and location. A further subdivision of the T stage has recently been used, T-3a and T-3b, but again, recent data would seem to suggest that this staging system is not predictive. Thus, the current favored approach to T staging is to measure the postoperative tumor size with contrast images. This latter approach has not yet been validated by a prospective trial, and also awaits confirmation. It is likely that biological markers will add significantly to our understanding of risk, and techniques of molecular genetics have advanced to a stage where hopefully a biological staging system will soon become available.

Treatment consists of a multidisciplinary approach that includes the neurosurgeon, neuropathologist, neuroradiologist, radiation oncologist and pediatric neurologist and oncologist. Surgical resection is done with the goal of maximal tumor debulking and the re-establishment of CSF flow if obstructed. Since the residual tumor burden influences both survival and treatment decision, it is crucial that neurosurgical planning is for maximal resection whenever possible. Current multi-institutional trials strongly request that tissue be processed for routine pathological analysis, as well as biological testing, often requiring the storage of tissue in tissue banks or sending of samples to reference laboratories for unique testing. Neuroradiological assessment of the extent of postoperative tumor volume is a requisite for tumor staging and thus early radiological staging is encouraged to minimize the impact of normal postoperative changes that may over- or underestimate the remaining tumor. Postoperative MRI of the brain and spine must also be carefully analyzed to exclude otherwise reversible findings such as the presence of blood or inflammatory changes. Spinal CSF analysis is recommended to be done prior to treatment, or longer than 2 weeks postoperatively. False positive findings of tumor cells shed as a consequence of the surgical procedure are more commonly found when the sampling is done immediately or 1–2 weeks following surgery. Once the risk status is accurately evaluated, treatment decisions become more precise. Entering a patient into one of a number of clinical research trials is also strongly encouraged, to increase our knowledge of the effects of treatment and to study the biology of this tumor. It is because of controlled clinical research trials that this disease is now potentially curable.

Good risk patients are treated with craniospinal radiation. The primary tumor volume is usually treated to a dose of 54 Gy, using single fractions delivered 5 days a week. The uninvolved brain and spine are treated to a dose of 36 Gy. Patients with poor risk factors are treated with adjuvant chemotherapy, usually with drugs such as the nitrosoureas and vincristine. A series of clinical research studies have been conducted over the last several years investigating the use of chemotherapy (Evans et al 1990, Tait et al 1990, Krischer et al 1991, Packer et al 1991). In general, it appears that a subset of patients with poor risk factors benefit from combined modality therapy. Patients with good risk factors have yet to be shown to have any benefit with additional therapy other than craniospinal radiation. It is possible, however, that the best drug or drug combination has not been tested and that even good risk patients will have prolonged disease-free survival using adjuvant chemotherapy. The major pediatric oncology research groups, the Children's Cancer Group (CCG), the Pediatric Oncology Group (POG), and the International Society of Pediatric Oncology (SIOP) have all demonstrated an increase in progression-free survival in patients with poor risk factors when adjuvant chemotherapy was given, with no benefit for good risk patients. These trials have been controlled, randomized trials, testing this hypothesis. Clinical research studies continue in this disease. Patients with good risk factors have been studied with the goal of lowering the radiation dose to the brain and spine, in an attempt to try and reduce the late effects of radiation, such as neuroendocrine abnormalities, neurocognitive decline, and abnormalities of bone growth, especially of the spine (Tomita & McLone 1986, Halberg et al 1991). One recently conducted trial tested the dose of 24 Gy to the craniospinal axis compared with a more standard dose of 36 Gy in patients with good risk features. Unfortunately, a statistically increased incidence of exoprimary relapse in the spine was observed in the lower dose arms and thus the study was closed early. Other attempts are continuing, with the same goal of reducing the dose. One strategy is to reduce the dose of radiation, but to add adjuvant chemotherapy, hoping that the addition of chemotherapy will additionally protect the brain and spine 'at risk'. This strategy will soon be tested in a controlled randomized trial conducted by the CCG and the POG. Patients with good risk features have a 70–80% chance of survival at 5 years using radiation therapy alone.

For patients with poor risk features, current modalities of therapy are still inadequate. Disease-free survival is often only 30–40% at 5 years despite radiotherapy and chemotherapy. Current strategies being tested include the use of more intensive chemotherapy, and different radiation schemes. One new approach will be to deliver intensive chemotherapy prior to hyperfractionated radiotherapy (Allen et al 1991). A new trial at the CCG, for instance, will treat patients with alternating cycles of cisplatin, cytoxan, etoposide, and vincristine with carboplatin, ifosfamide, and etoposide for 4–5 cycles, followed by radiation delivered twice a day to a total dose of 72 Gy to the primary site and 40 Gy to the brain and spine.

Children under the age of 3 are treated with chemotherapy rather than with radiotherapy, in order to spare the serious sequelae of neurotoxicity using radiotherapy in this young age group. Many of the chemotherapy regimens being tested for recurrent disease or for intensive adjuvant or neoadjuvant treatment come from experiences in the treatment of infants. It is clear that salvage is possible with chemotherapy alone, and in some cases prolonged disease-free survival is possible without the use of radiotherapy. This is especially true for infants with tumors that are completely resected, with no other evidence of neuroaxis spread, who are treated with multiagent chemotherapy. Infants and young children with large residual tumor burdens often fail all attempts at treatment.

It is strongly encouraged that clinicians enter children with MB/PNET into clinical research studies. It is through this mechanism of clinical research that all children will benefit, hopefully with an expectation of cure.

Current investigative protocols for medulloblastoma and primitive neuroectodermal tumors

POG. 9233
POG. 9234
Phase III randomized trial of standard vs dose-intense chemotherapy with cytoxan/vincristine and cisplatin/etoposide, with or without radiotherapy in children under 3 years of age with a CNS malignancy

POG. 9031
Phase III comparison of pre- vs post-irradiation chemotherapy with cisplatin/etoposide in children with advanced medulloblastoma

NCI-T92-0146
Phase II evaluation of topotecan in recurrent or progressive pediatric central nervous system tumors, including medulloblastoma

CCG-0921
Phase II study of idarubicin in children with recurrent malignant brain tumors, including medulloblastoma

POG-9237
Phase II study of idarubicin with G-CSF support in children with recurrent and progressive brain tumors

CCG-0902
Phase II study of fazarabine in children with recurrent solid tumors, including medulloblastoma

CCG-0894
Phase II randomized study of ICE (ifosfamide, carboplatin, etoposide) with high vs low dose G-CSF in children with recurrent malignant tumors, including medulloblastoma

CCG-9892
Phase II pilot study of reduced neuroaxis radiotherapy and adjuvant chemotherapy with CCNU/cisplatin/vincristine in children between 18 and 120 months of age with medulloblastoma or PNET of the posterior fossa

MDA-P-88006
Phase II study of MMOPP (methotrexate plus nitrogen mustard, vincristine, procarbazine, prednisone) as primary therapy for infants and young children with PNET

Proposed new trials for medulloblastoma

CCG-9014
POG-9231
Intergroup randomized phase III trial for newly diagnosed good risk medulloblastoma. Patients will be treated either with craniospinal radiation to standard doses (36 Gy to brain and spine, 54 Gy to posterior fossa), or reduced radiation to brain and spine (2340 rads, 54 Gy to posterior fossa) with adjuvant chemotherapy using cisplatin, cyclophosphamide and vincristine.

CCG-9012
Pre-irradiation chemotherapy followed by hyperfractionated radiotherapy in patients with newly diagnosed poor risk medulloblastoma and cortical or spinal PNET. Chemotherapy will use alternating cycles of cisplatin, etoposide, cyclophosphamide, vincristine (Regimen A) with carboplatin, ifosfamide, and etoposide. Radiation will begin following the 5th cycle of chemotherapy using twice a day treatment of 100 cGy to a dose of 72 Gy to primary site, and 40 Gy to the craniospinal axis.

REFERENCES

Allen J C, Epstein F 1982 Medulloblastoma and other primary malignant neuroectodermal tumors of the CNS — the effects of patients' age and extent of disease on prognosis. Journal of Neurosurgery 57: 446–451

Allen J, Nirenberg A, Donahue B 1991 A Phase I/II pilot study employing hyperfractionated radiotherapy and adjuvant chemotherapy for high-risk primitive neuroectodermal tumors. Annals of Neurology 30: 457–458

Bloom H J G, Glees J, Bell J 1990 The treatment and long term prognosis of children with intracranial tumors: A study of 610 cases, 1950–1981. Int J Radiat Oncol Biol Phys 18: 723–745

Chang C H, Horton J, Schoenfeld D et al 1983 Comparison of postoperative radiotherapy and combined postoperative radiotherapy and chemotherapy in the multidisciplinary management of malignant gliomas. Cancer 52: 997–1007

Ernestus R-I, Wilcke O, Schroder R 1989 Intracranial ependymomas: prognostic aspects. Neurosurgical Review 12: 157–163

Evans A E, Jenkins R D T, Sposto R et al 1990 The treatment of medulloblastoma: the results of a prospective randomized trial of radiation therapy with and without chloroethylcyclohexyl nitrosourea, vincristine and prednisone. Journal of Neurosurgery 72: 572–582

Friedman H S, Oakes W J 1987 The chemotherapy of posterior fossa tumors in childhood. Journal of Neuro-oncology 5: 217

Garrett P G, Simpson W J K 1983 Ependymoma: Results of radiation therapy. Int J Radiation Oncology Biol Phys 9: 1121–1124

Greenberg H S, Chandler W F, Diaz R F et al 1988 Intra-arterial bromodeoxyuridine radiosensitization and radiation in treatment of malignant astrocytomas. Journal of Neurosurgery 69: 500–506

Halberg F E, Wara W M, Fippin L F et al 1991 Low-dose craniospinal radiation therapy for medulloblastoma. Int J Radiat Oncol Biol Phys 20: 651–654

Krischer J P, Ragab A H, Kun L et al 1991 Nitrogen mustard, vincristine, procarbazine, and prednisone as adjuvant chemotherapy in the treatment of medulloblastoma — a Pediatric Oncology Group Study. Journal of Neurosurgery 74: 905–909

Laramore G E, Diener-West M, Griffin T W et al 1988 Randomized neutron dose searching study for malignant gliomas of the brain: results of an RTOG study. Int J Radiation Oncology Biol Phys 14: 1093–1102

Levin V A, Silver P, Hannigan J et al 1990a Superiority of post-radiotherapy adjuvant chemotherapy with CCNU, Procarbazine and vincristine (PCV) over BCNU for anaplastic gliomas: NCOG 6G61 final report. Int J Radiation Oncology Biol Phys 18: 321–324

Levin V A, Wara W M, Gutin P H et al 1990b Initial analysis of NCOG 6G 82–1: Bromodeoxyuridine (BUdR) during irradiation followed by CCNU, procarbazine and vincristine (PCV) chemotherapy for malignant gliomas. Proc Am Soc Clin Oncol (abstract) 9: 91

Packer R, Sutton L, Rorke L et al 1984 Prognostic importance of cellular differentiation in medulloblastoma of childhood. Journal of Neurosurgery 61: 296–301

Packer R J, Sutton L N, Goldwein J W et al 1991 Improved survival with the use of adjuvant chemotherapy in the treatment of medulloblastoma. Journal of Neurosurgery 74: 433–440

Parks T, Hoffman J, Hendrich E et al 1983 Medulloblastoma, clinical presentation and management: experience at the Hospital for Sick Children, Toronto, 1950–1980. Journal of Neurosurgery 58: 543–552

Salazar O, Castro-Vita H, VanHoutta P et al 1983 Improved survival in cases of intracranial ependymoma after radiation therapy. Late report and recommendations. Journal of Neurosurgery 59: 652

Silverberg E, Lubara J A 1989 Cancer Statistics CA 39: 3

Tait D M, Thornton-Jones H, Bloom H J G et al 1990 Adjuvant chemotherapy for medulloblastoma: The first multi-center control trial of the International Society of Paediatric Oncology (SIOP 1). European Journal of Cancer 26 (4): 464–469

Tomita T, McLone D G 1986 Medulloblastoma in childhood: results of radical resection and low-dose neuroaxis radiation therapy. Journal of Neurosurgery 64: 238–242

Urtasun R, Fulton D, Huyser-Wierenga D et al 1989 Dose intensity in radiotherapy: "Is more better" for patients with malignant glioma? Proc Am Soc Clin Oncol (abstract) 8: 84

Walker M D, Alexander E Jr, Hunt W E et al 1978 Evaluation of BCNU and/or radiotherapy in the treatment of anaplastic gliomas. Journal of Neurosurgery 49: 333–343

Walker M D, Strike T A, Sheline G E 1979 An analysis of dose-effect relationship in the radiotherapy of malignant gliomas. Int J Radiation Oncology Biol Phys 5: 1725–1731

Walker M D, Green S B, Byar D P et al 1980 Randomized comparisons of radiotherapy and nitrosoureas for the treatment of malignant glioma after surgery. New England Journal of Medicine 303: 1323–1329

Walker A E, Robins M, Weinfeld F D 1985 Epidemiology of brain tumors: the national survey of intracranial neoplasms. Neurology 35: 219

Wallner K E, Wara W M, Sheline G E, Davis R L 1986 Intracranial ependymomas: results of treatment with partial or whole brain irradiation without spinal irradiation. Int J Radiation Oncology Biol Phys 12: 1937–1941

20. Experimental therapy for brain tumors

Michael Salcman

INTRODUCTION

The development and application of innovative treatments for brain tumors has entered an exciting new era, one in which the evolution of therapeutic strategies is based on an improved understanding of the biology of the tumor rather than empirical trial and error. The neurobiology of brain tumors is a much wider subject than oncogenesis and the molecular properties of neoplastic cells, it also subsumes important information about the interactive relationship of the tumor to its target organ and its host, since the physiology of the brain and the biologic milieu of the patient often represent critical limitations in regard to the safety and efficacy of therapy (Salcman 1991a). As a general rule, therapeutic agents must be delivered in doses sufficient to produce cell-killing or some other desired effect in the tumor without concomitant production of toxicity in the surrounding brain. Apart from such problems with delivery and safety, inherent resistance of the tumor to any given agent remains the primary reason for therapeutic failure, an obstacle not easily comprehended or likely to be overcome without some understanding of the relevant molecular biology. At the present time, less than 5% of all brain tumor patients are involved in investigative protocols (Lee et al 1991); clinicians must accept the responsibility for promoting the advancement of brain tumor therapy through increased entry of their patients into prospective trials.

GENETIC IMPLICATIONS FOR THERAPY

The neoplastic phenotype probably represents the result of multiple genetic alterations, the ultimate effect of which is uncontrolled cellular proliferation. In normal cells and tissues, control of proliferation and growth is achieved through the balanced activity of growth-promoting proto-oncogenes and the braking effect of growth-constraining suppressor genes (Weinberg 1991). Inferences about the importance of genetic events in the development of brain tumors were first made with the initial demonstration of visible chromosomal abnormalities by karyotype analysis and chromosomal banding techniques (Mark 1970, Solomon et al 1991). Monosomy 22 was first detected in a benign meningioma and large scale alterations were subsequently demonstrated in a variety of other neuroectodermal lesions (Solomon et al 1991). In more recent years, sophisticated techniques, such as restriction fragment length polymorphism (RFLP) analysis, have been used to detect deletions and alterations of ever smaller amounts of genetic material, usually containing tumor suppressor genes, at specific sites on individual chromosomes. Although more than 1500 cloned genes have been reported, thus far, fewer than 20% have been incorporated into genetic maps; it is expected, therefore, that genetic analysis will yield further discoveries in the future (NIH/CEPH Collaborative Mapping Group 1992).

The overexpression of dominant oncogenes in brain tumors has been demonstrated by molecular probes that detect reduplication, amplification or rearrangement of the gene itself and by electrochemical and isotopic techniques that measure an increase in the amount of mRNA or protein product (usually a growth factor or growth factor receptor) associated with the gene (McDonald & Dohrmann 1988). In the current view, development of the neoplastic phenotype requires more than a single genetic event, and a sequence of such events is probably responsible for progressive anaplasia and dedifferentiation. Such a sequence has been demonstrated for colon carcinoma and is thought to occur during the evolution of a glioblastoma from a pre-existing astrocytoma (James et al 1988, Vogelstein et al 1988). Since genetic loss and chromosomal rearrangement are more likely in mitotically and metabolically active tissue, the length of time that a cellular population is at risk for such genetic events at a specific stage in the development of the nervous system may explain the relative frequency and age-related incidence of most neuroectodermal tumors (Rubinstein 1991). Rubinstein has termed this period of risk 'the window of neoplastic vulnerability'; in the case of astrocytic populations, for example, the window extends into the postnatal period and involves large numbers of cells — hence the potential role of environmental exposure to carcinogens in the development of astrocytic tumors during adult life as well as in utero (Selikoff & Hammond 1982).

For astrocytic tumors, the frequency with which chromosomal abnormalities are detected increases with the degree of anaplasia (Bigner et al 1988). Abnormalities observed in glioblastoma include an extra copy of chromosome 7 (50–80%), loss of chromosome 10 (30–60%), deletion or translocation of 9p (about 30%), and a variety of cytogenetic changes in chromosomes 22, 1p, 6q, 7q, 11q, 13q, and 19p (Bigner et al 1984, 1990). Thus, the highly variable morphology and biological behavior of some brain tumors may be a consequence of the karyotypic heterogeneity of cell populations within the tumor (Bigner et al 1981, Shapiro et al 1981). The double minute chromosomes observed in some examples of glioblastoma may contain amplified or extra copies of the erb-B gene for the epidermal growth factor receptor (EGFr).

In addition to observable chromosomal abnormalities, RFLP analysis indicates loss of heterozygosity on chromosome 10 in the majority of glioblastomas but in no tumors of lower grade (James et al 1988, Fults et al 1989). In contrast, almost equal numbers of anaplastic astrocytomas and glioblastomas (about 40%) demonstrate loss of heterozygosity on 17p (El-Azouzi et al 1989, Fults et al 1989, James et al 1989, Fults et al 1990). Hence, the progressive development of a glioblastoma from an anaplastic astrocytoma may involve the loss of tumor suppressor genes on chromosome 10 subsequent to the loss or alteration of the p53 gene on 17p (Fig. 20.1). Studies by James and others confirm the suspicion that glioblastoma is clonal in origin and may represent the common phenotypic terminus for all glial tumors (James et al 1988, 1989, Kim & Harsh 1993). Development of progressive anaplasia coincident with the occurrence of sequential genetic

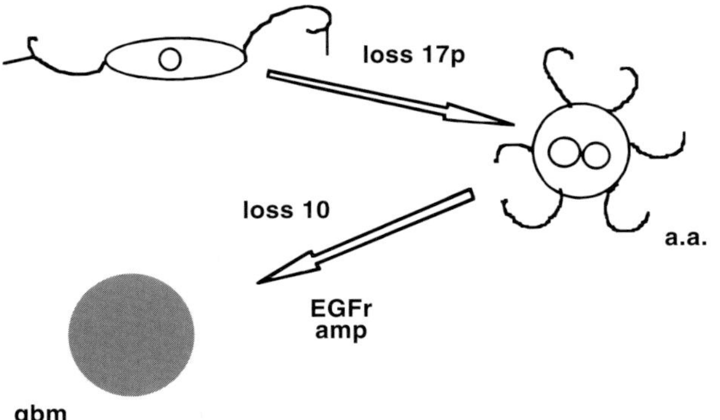

Fig. 20.1 Genetic model of progressive anaplasia in astrocytoma. Loss of heterozygosity on chromosome 17p is a key step in the development of anaplastic astrocytoma cells (a.a.) from phenotypically normal astrocytes. Further genetic loss on chromosome 10 either prior to or concomitant with amplification of the gene for the epidermal growth factor receptor protein (EGFr) contributes towards the evolution of an a.a. into a glioblastoma multiforme (gbm).

events is consistent with the results of repeat biopsies performed at the time of tumor recurrence (Muller et al 1977).

Loss of wild-type p53 suppressor activity is the most common cancer-related genetic event and has been implicated in the oncogenesis of a wide variety of tumors. Conversely, mutant p53 activity favors cell growth and acts in a dominant fashion with respect to the wild-type allele (Weinberg 1991). Frequency of the p53 mutation appears to correlate with the grade of the tumor and is more often present at time of recurrence (Sidransky et al 1992). Mutant p53 alleles can be passed through the germline where they can serve as inherited determinants of a generalized predisposition to cancer formation, as seen in the Li-Fraumani syndrome and in some families with glioblastoma (Salcman & Solomon 1984, Malkin et al 1990, 1992, Toguchida et al 1992). Cellular heat shock protein (Hsc 70) is often bound up with mixtures of mutant and wild-type p53 molecules, thus depriving the nucleus of the active p53 complexes that are required for negative growth regulation (Weinberg 1991). Therefore, aspects of the p53 regulatory system share the properties of both oncogenes and tumor suppressor genes.

Loss of tumor suppressor genes may be involved in the genesis of benign central nervous system tumors (Martuza 1991). Type 1 neurofibromatosis or von Recklinghausen's disease (NF-1) is associated with loss of heterozygosity for a gene on 17q thought to be involved in the down-regulation of the p21 ras oncogene. The gene for familial breast cancer has also been localized to chromosome 17 (NIH-CEPH Collaborative Mapping Group 1992). Loss of heterozygosity on chromosome 22q has been associated with type 2 neurofibromatosis, meningioma, and acoustic schwannoma (Seizinger et al 1986). Therapeutic strategies based on the loss of suppressor genes during oncogenesis and anaplasia might include gene replacement or the use of differentiating agents to re-establish normal growth control and a less anaplastic phenotype.

Overexpression of oncogenes may be important to both the initiation and maintenance of the malignant phenotype. The epidermal growth factor receptor (EGFr) gene has been mapped to chromosome 7 and, as we have already seen, extra copies of this chromosome as well as double minutes are frequently observed in glioblastoma (Bigner et al 1984). Moreover, amplification and rearrangement of the EGFr gene have been shown to correlate with increased amounts of its mRNA and receptor protein, the quantities of which generally increase with the degree of anaplasia in astrocytomas (Libermann et al 1985). EGFr is a polygamous receptor capable of binding a number of growth factors to its external domain, including EGF and transforming growth factor alpha (TGF-α), while its cytoplasmic domain consists of a tyrosine kinase that can stimulate DNA synthesis through a second messenger system (Aaronson 1991). Amplification of the

EGFr oncogene is seen in 40–50% of glioblastomas and increased levels of its mRNA have been detected in lower grade astrocytomas (Ekstrand et al 1991). Monoclonal antibodies have been used to stain for EGFr in the vascular stroma of benign tumors such as meningiomas, and anti-EGFr therapy has been used to inhibit meningioma growth in vitro (Adams et al 1990). Since amplification of other oncogenes, such as N-myc, has been shown to correlate inversely with the length of survival of patients with neuroblastoma (Seeger et al 1985), the reported association of EGFr overexpression with anaplastic change in astrocytoma probably has real prognostic implications. Whether amplification of the erb-B oncogene is a primary event in the development of glioblastoma is open to question since loss of chromosome 10 and a possible tumor suppressor gene appears to precede EGFr overexpression (von Deimling et al 1992).

Another growth factor strongly implicated in the clinical behavior of astrocytomas is the beta chain of platelet-derived growth factor (PDGF) produced by the c-sis proto-oncogene located on chromosome 22. In embryonic tissue, PDGF delays differentiation and promotes proliferation of glial precursor cells. The gene for the PDGF-β chain has a strong homology to the simian sarcoma virus (v-sis) oncogene. In tissue culture, a combination of PDGF and EGF can sustain astrocytic growth in the absence of fetal calf serum and at nearly the same level as a full complement of other nutrient factors (Pollack et al 1990a, b). Many tumor cell lines coexpress both EGFr and PDGF (Harsh et al 1989). Increased PDGF expression without c-sis gene amplification or rearrangement has been demonstrated in glioma cell lines and glioblastoma (Press et al 1989, Harsh et al 1990); this is unlike the situation with overexpression of the EGFr gene. The mRNA for the PDGF α-chain has been detected in neuroectodermal tumors of virtually every type but mRNA for the β-chain is usually seen only in high grade astrocytomas (Mapstone 1991). Some tumors overexpress both a PDGF-like mitogen and the PDGF receptor (Harsh et al 1990, Maxwell et al 1990) and are therefore capable of autonomous growth through the mechanism of autocrine stimulation (Fig. 20.2). The development of sarcomatous elements in a glioblastoma may represent an example of paracrine stimulation in which the production of growth factors by neoplastic astrocytes induces uncontrolled growth and anaplasia in capillary endothelial cells.

Normal tissues and tumor cells possess receptor proteins for many other growth factors and hormones. It is likely that the induction and maintenance of the malignant phenotype is a multifactorial process (Mapstone et al 1991). Transforming growth factor β (TGF) has been detected in normal cells as well as in many glial cell lines without any direct relation to the degree of malignancy (Mapstone 1991, Mapstone et al 1991). Detection of increased levels of high molecular weight TGF-α in the urine of brain tumor patients has been proposed as a therapeutic and diagnostic marker for cancer (Kanno et al 1988). TGF-α competes with EGF for binding on the EGF receptor but appears to have its own receptor as well, at least on sensory neurons (Chalazonitis et al 1992). Some mitogenic polypeptides also behave as neurotrophic factors required for neural maintenance and repair. TGF-α mRNA levels have been found to be 15–170 times higher than those of EGF in the normal adult and developing mouse brain (Lazar & Blum 1992). Hence, anti-TGF-α therapy is unlikely to be selective for neoplastic tissue in the brain.

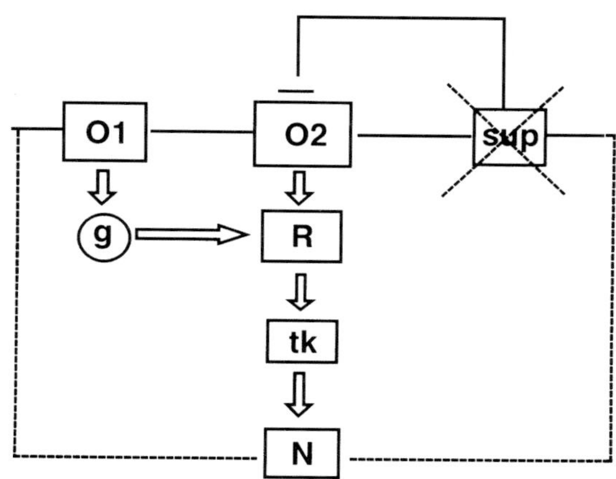

Fig. 20.2 Diagram of therapeutic targets based on model of growth control in normal and neoplastic cells. Dominant oncogenes (O1 and O2) code for growth factors (g) and growth factor receptors (R). Overexpression of both oncogenes in the same cell results in autocrine growth as does autonomous activity in the second messenger system or signal pathway that leads to the nucleus (N) and produces cell division. Thymidine kinase (tk) and protein kinase C are frequent components of the signal pathway. Loss of suppressor gene activity (sup) can also result in overexpression of oncogenes and autonomous activity in the signal pathway.

Flow cytometry and immunoblot analysis has been used to demonstrate overexpression of the c-myc oncoprotein, a mediator of cellular proliferation, in glioblastomas but not in benign brain tissue (Engelhard et al 1989). Correlation between the degree of malignancy and the amount of myc expression has been demonstrated but n-myc expression appears to be restricted to tumors of neuronal lineage (Fujimoto et al 1988, U et al 1989). As opposed to amplification of the N-myc proto-oncogene, increased expression of the TRK gene for the high-affinity receptor complex that binds the neurotrophic nerve growth factor (NGF) is associated with a good outcome in neuroblastoma (Nakagawara et al 1993). PDGF can stimulate rapid and transient expression of both myc and fos as well as their protein products in quiescent cells. In some cell systems, overexpression of c-myc abrogates the requirement for PDGF growth stimulation.

Fifty-fold amplification of a novel gene (gli) mapped to chromosome 12 has been reported in glioblastoma (Kinzler et al 1987); such a finding may represent yet another example of tumor heterogeneity. The neu gene is an erb-B homologue that does not code for EGFr and maps to chromosome 17 (Schechter et al 1985). Cytokine gene expression for interleukins and basic fibroblast growth factor (bFGF) has also been reported in some cell lines (Lichtor et al 1990). The gene for bFGF has been mapped to chromosome 4, and bFGF may be identical with tumor angiogenesis factor in gliomas (Westphal & Herrmann 1989). The distribution of basic fibroblast growth factor in the brain is largely restricted to astrocytes where it may play a role in the differentiation of these cells (Woodward et al 1992). Finally, benign tumors may demonstrate a spectrum of genetic expression and growth factor sensitivity distinct from that observed in malignant tumors. For example, insulin binding has been found to be higher in meningiomas than in glioblastomas although both types of tumor demonstrate elevated insulin-like growth factor (IGF)-I binding (somatomedin C) and undergo insulin-induced growth stimulation (Glick et al 1989). The relative importance of IGF-related peptides to other growth factors and hormones is unknown.

Therapeutic strategies based on the activity of dominant oncogenes in benign and malignant brain tumors can be directed at three or four potential targets (Fig. 20.2): (1) the gene itself; (2) the intracellular signal pathway (e.g. the tyrosine kinase or protein kinase C systems); (3) the gene product, either a growth factor (e.g. PDGF or bFGF) or its associated receptor (e.g. EGFr), especially if the gene or gene product are structurally dissimilar from their analogs in the surrounding brain (Westphal & Herrmann 1989).

THE PROBLEM OF HETEROGENEITY

Once tumor growth has been initiated, progressive anaplasia is accompanied by an accumulation of chromosomal abnormalities, transpositions, mutations and genetic loss, in addition to further elaboration of growth factors, the general result of which is an increase in cellular diversity and tumor heterogeneity (Bigner 1981). A natural consequence of such heterogeneity is the development of subpopulations of cells with highly variable metabolic, kinetic and antigenic properties, such that the tumor mass can be conceived of as a collection of cell compartments likely to differ in their susceptibility to different treatment modalities (Salcman et al 1982). Gross cytoarchitectonic differences across the tumor mass in regard to blood supply, oxygenation, necrosis and the status of the blood-brain barrier are likely to add further variability to any therapeutic response since the efficacy of many agents is dependent on the local environment and the proportion of non-cycling cells. Even in glioblastoma, the ^{3}H-thymidine labeling index or growth fraction represents less than 10% of the viable cells in the tumor mass (Hoshino 1984, 1991). Hence, there are advantages to be gained from non-cell cycle specific therapies. Furthermore sequential treatment with individual agents risks the development of resistant cell lines and recurrence of the entire tumor mass from any cell compartment inherently resistant to the agent currently in use. A possible strategy for addressing tumor heterogeneity is the use of a true multimodality treatment plan in which each cell compartment within the tumor is simultaneously targeted by the modality to which it is most susceptible (Table 20.1). Combinations of surgery and chemotherapy (Tel et al 1980, Brem et al 1991), chemotherapy and radiation (Gutin et al 1984), radiation and hyperthermia (Roberts et al 1985, Cohen et al 1990, Salcman 1991a, Sneed et al 1991), or radiation and immunotherapy (Colapinto et al 1990) are but a few examples of this approach. As a strategy to combat tumor heterogeneity, multimodality therapy may also uncover useful treatment interactions that result in the potentiation of individual agents (Salcman & Ebert 1991).

Table 20.1 Biological problem: tumor heterogeneity. Solution: multimodality therapy.

I. Main tumor mass:	Local agents:
A. Non-dividing, hypoxic cells	Surgery
	Hyperthermia
	Radiosensitizers: fluosol; BUdR
B. Vascularized, dividing cells	Chemotherapy: temozolomide; polyamine depletion; verapamil
	Radiation
	Photochemotherapy
II. Cells in periphery:	Blood-borne agents:
	Monoclonal antibodies
	Cytokines: TNF-α; IL-2
	Differentiators: neurotrophins; phorbol esters
	Recombinant toxins: ricin; diphtheria; pseudomonas exotoxin
	Viral vectors
	Transduced cells

REGIONAL THERAPY: SURGERY AND RADIATION

Surgery and radiation are prototypical examples of therapeutic modalities, the benefits and risks of which are sharply restricted to the treatment volume defined by imaging. Local therapy may result in a cure if relatively few tumor cells extend beyond the treatment volume, but only if a sufficient dose of the treating agent is delivered to the tumor and only if the surrounding brain is spared the toxic effects of the treatment (Sheline et al 1980, Salcman 1993). Patients with metastatic carcinoma to the brain who die of systemic disease without autopsy evidence of residual tumor at the site of surgery are examples of local cure; conversely, most patients with glioblastoma die of local tumor recurrence and are examples of the failure of this strategy (Salcman 1980). We know from serial stereotactic biopsies that a large number of tumor cells extend out into the surrounding brain and that the enhanced MR or CT scan, commonly used to define surgical and brachytherapy margins, seriously underestimate the extent of the tumor (Kelly et al 1987, Burger et al 1988, Schiffer 1991). Further, the intimate relationship of neoplastic cells to the surrounding neuropil and vascular supply makes it unlikely that the treatment volume for surgery or radiation can be safely extended outside the enhancing rim. Nevertheless, the length of survival for patients with most types of tumor correlates with the post-excision residual tumor volume and the total dose of radiation (Walker et al 1979, Salcman 1990). In addition, reoperation and interstitial brachytherapy are currently the two most successful rescue therapies in patients with recurrent astrocytoma (Salcman et al 1982, 1986, Leibel et al 1989, Loeffler et al 1990, Gutin et al 1991, Salcman 1993; see also Ch. 26). Therefore, local tumor control must be important, especially since the majority of treatment failures in patients with glioblastoma occur within 2–3 cm of the enhancing rim used in treatment planning (Hochberg & Pruitt 1980, Liang et al 1991). Nevertheless, our experience with surgery and image-guided radiation often fails to produce a cure and tells us that tumor cells in the surrounding brain are probably underdosed by conventional therapy. In addition, further enhancement of the therapeutic effect in this region is unlikely to be achieved without significant risk.

These theoretical limitations probably apply to virtually any image-based, sharply localized treatment modality so that the survival advantages (if any) provided by combined brachytherapy and interstitial hyperthermia, stereotactic radiosurgery, intraoperative afterloading, californium implants for interstitial neutron capture therapy, interstitial phototherapy and interstitial chemotherapy are likely to be modest. This does not mean that we should stop investigating these modalities since low-level exposure of the surrounding brain to some agents may provide useful potentiation of radiopharmaceuticals, monoclonal antibodies, conventional chemotherapy and immunobiologicals directed at the surround. It does mean that sharply localized therapy based solely on the delivery of some type of energy to an image-defined target is unlikely to produce a cure for an infiltrating tumor unless the lesion is small and situated in a non-critical area of the brain.

Various methods of increasing the radiosensitivity of tumor cells have been studied, including hyperbaric oxygen, hyperthermia, electron affinic drugs, halogenated pyrimidines, hyperfractionation and alternative energy sources. In addition to tissue hypoxia, the inherent radioresistance of brain tumors may depend on genetic mechanisms for producing DNA repair in sublethally damaged cells (Gerweck et al 1977, Kayama et al 1991, Zhang et al 1993a). For example, protein kinase C (PKC) phosphorylates a plasma membrane protein that plays an important role in multidrug resistance and may also contribute to radioresistance (Zhang et al 1993b). Hyperbaric oxygen and electron affinic agents have failed to prolong survival in clinical trials (Coleman et al 1992). Laboratory studies indicate, however, that hyperthermia and alkylating agents such as BCNU or a combination of thymidine and hyperthermia can produce greater radiosensitization than either modality used alone (Cohen et al 1990, Salcman & Ebert 1991). Furthermore, administration of staurosporine, a potent PKC inhibitor, prior to radiation can attenuate the repair of damaged DNA in C6 cells (Zhang et al 1993b). It remains to be seen, however, if radiosensitization in the surround can be produced safely without increasing neuronal and vascular toxicity from external radiotherapy. Intra-arterial administration of bromodeoxyuridine (BUdR) two weeks before and during focal external beam radiotherapy has been carried out without undue toxicity and has led to a median survival of 20 months in 23 patients with malignant glioma (Hegarty et al 1990). Iododeoxyuridine (IUdR) also has been proposed as a radiation sensitizer, especially for interstitial brachytherapy (Goodman et al 1990a). Although hyperbaric chambers have failed to produce prolonged survival, presumably in an attempt to overcome the radioresistance produced by tissue hypoxia, non-toxic oxygen carriers such as the perflorochemical emulsion fluosol have been shown to have some therapeutic benefit in early clinical trials (Evans et al 1990).

Hyperthermia represents a powerful method by which the cell-killing of both radiation and chemotherapy can be potentiated (Salcman & Samaras 1981, 1983, Salcman 1991b, Salcman & Ebert 1991). Unfortunately, safe and efficacious delivery of hyperthermia into the brain remains a technical challenge. The production of a nearly homogeneous temperature field may require greater knowledge of the thermal properties of the brain than we possess or the use of a large number of catheters and mechanically injurious seeds (Salcman et al 1989, Kobayashi et al 1991). Nevertheless, new catheters and technologies are under development and several clinical trials combining hyperthermia with radiation or other modalities have demonstrated safety and feasibility (Roberts et al 1985, Ferraro et al 1989, Salcman 1991b, Sneed et al 1991, Stea et al 1991). Optical fibers and lasers used in photochemotherapy (see below) can be used to deliver hyperthermia as well.

The rationale for the use of hyperfractionation or heavy particles such as neutrons, pions or protons is discussed in Chapter 26; to date, there is no evidence to indicate that survival in glioblastoma can be prolonged by such methods (Griffin et al 1983, Goodman et al 1990b, Greiner et al 1990, Kolker et al 1990). Proton beam therapy has been of demonstrable benefit, however, in the management of low grade malignancies and skull base tumors such as anaplastic meningioma and chondrosarcoma (Austin-Seymour et al 1990). Interstitial brachytherapy with permanent implants has also been used in the treatment of such lesions (Kumar et al 1991, Salcman et al 1992). Stereotactic radiosurgery represents a possible alternative to implant therapy for some types of tumor and is of proven benefit in the treatment of slower growing benign lesions such as acoustic schwannoma, meningioma and pituitary adenoma. Experience with this modality in the treatment of malignant brain tumors is quite preliminary in nature and enthusiasm should be tempered by our knowledge of the biological considerations discussed previously (Kimmel et al 1987, Kondziolka & Lunsford 1993). The radiobiology of radiosurgery is currently under study in the rat C6 glioma, a relatively circumscribed tumor with occasional distant spread (Kondziolka et al 1992). Variations in the maximum treatment dose, from 30–100 Gy, did not produce observed differences in tumor response. Nevertheless, a median survival of 16 months has been achieved in patients with small glioblastomas treated with adjuvant stereotactic radiosurgery, and even better results have been observed in lower grade neoplasms (Kondziolka & Lunsford 1993).

Radiolabeled monoclonal antibodies (see below) and boron neutron capture therapy represent at least two methods by which radiation can be selectively delivered to individual cells throughout the tumor. Boron neutron capture therapy or BNCT is based on a nuclear reaction in which the bombardment of ^{10}B with low energy or thermal neutrons results in the release of stripped down helium nuclei (α-particles) and ^{7}Li nuclei (Barth et al 1990). These particles have path lengths of approximately 1 cell diameter (10–14 μm), theoretically limiting the radiation effect to those tumor cells that have taken up sufficient ^{10}B and simultaneously sparing normal cells in their immediate vicinity. Early clinical trials probably failed because of the rapid attenuation of thermal neutrons in tissue, thus limiting the effective depth of penetration to 3 or 4 cm, and the non-selective uptake of freely diffusable, low molecular weight boron compounds. Later trials incorporated sulfhydryl-containing boron hydride anions with greater tumor uptake and no apparent toxicity (Hatanaka 1975). Enhanced survival in F98 brain tumor-bearing rats and in vitro experiments suggest that even better results may be achieved if tumor concentrations of ^{10}B can be increased (Clendenon et al 1990). Based on the experience with drug localization in photodynamic therapy, boron-containing porphyrins and phthalocyanines are under study. Preliminary experiments utilizing boron compounds conjugated to monoclonal antibodies have not been successful. Implanted isotopic sources of neutrons such as californium-252 are an attractive alternative to expensive nuclear reactors and may overcome limitations based on beam penetration (Beach et al 1990).

Heretofore, the use of photodynamic therapy also has been limited by problems related to the tissue penetration of light at the wavelengths required for activation of drugs selectively taken up by tumor tissue (Powers et al 1991). Stereotactic techniques utilizing optical fibers and new drugs may overcome some of these limitations but recent data indicate that the uptake of photosensitizers may be non-uniform in individual patients (Origitano et al 1993).

LESSONS LEARNED FROM CHEMOTHERAPY

Single agent chemotherapy in the up-front treatment of malignant gliomas has been singularly unsuccessful in prolonging survival, even though almost 40% of patients with favorable prognostic factors respond to BCNU or procarbazine (PBZ) at time of recurrence (see Ch. 26). The modest results obtained with the use of chemotherapy for intracranial tumors are similar to those observed in the treatment of solid cancers in other organ systems such as the lung and gastrointestinal tract. The fundamental resistance of glioblastoma to chemotherapy is highlighted by the fact that no combination of chemical agents has been demonstrated to be superior to monotherapy with BCNU (Walker et al 1980, Grossman 1991, Kramer & Packer 1992). The combination of PBZ, CCNU and vincristine (PCV) has, however, shown modest efficacy in the treatment of lower grade tumors such as oligodendroglioma, anaplastic astrocytoma and optic nerve glioma (Levin et al 1990, Cairncross et al 1992). Median survival in patients with malignant astrocytoma treated with BCNU after surgery and radiation was 82 weeks in comparison to 157 weeks after adjuvant treatment with PCV (Levin et al 1990); unfortunately, there was no difference in survival between the two treatment arms in patients with glioblastoma. A few new drugs are now entering clinical trials, the most promising of which may be temozolomide, an imidazotetrazine derivative, an oral agent without significant drug toxicity (Newlands et al 1992).

Attempts at improving the therapeutic response to chemotherapy by increasing drug delivery have largely failed; the complications observed with the intra-arterial administration of various nitrosoureas and platinum compounds are not justified by the modest benefits (Mahaley et al 1986, Fauchon et al 1990). For example, a recent trial of intra-arterial HECNU in combination with surgery and radiation produced a median survival of 10.5 months in glioblastoma patients and a 10% incidence of monocular blindness and leukoencephalopathy (Fauchon et al 1990). Similarly, transient disruption of the blood-brain barrier would appear to have little or no place in the treatment of primary brain tumors (Neuwelt et al 1983, Salcman & Broadwell 1991). Of real interest is the recent demonstration that leukotrienes can selectively alter tumor capillary permeability without disrupting normal endothelial function in the surrounding brain (Black et al 1990).

Nevertheless, the leaky capillaries present in the majority of malignant brain tumors do not block efficient drug entry and most small lipophilic agents are delivered in satisfactory concentrations. The inherent drug resistance of the tumor, the real risk of brain toxicity (Kaplan & Wiernik 1982), and the cellular diversity and structural complexity of the neoplasm remain the chief obstacles to effective chemotherapy.

Some tumors and tumor cell lines appear to be especially resistant to chemotherapy, even when the drug is delivered in adequate doses and in proper relation to the cell cycle. Some of this resistance is age-dependent and much of it is due to increased drug metabolism and repair of sublethal damage through activation of the multidrug resistance gene (MDR) and the elaboration of protective proteins (Rosenblum et al 1982, Matsumoto et al 1990, Berger & Ali-Osman 1991). One experimental approach to this problem is the use of chemosensitizing agents. Verapamil, a calcium channel blocker, alters the intracellular accumulation of drugs and may affect the activity of DNA repair enzymes (Bowles et al 1990). One might also be able to develop antibodies to the MDR gene or alter its expression through the concomitant administration of differentiating agents such as retinoic acid, butyric acid, cyclic AMP or hyperthermia (Ebert & Salcman 1993). Depletion of polyamines by such inhibitors as DFMO (α-difluoromethylornithine) and MGBG (methylglyoxal bis guanylhydrazone) has been shown to potentiate the activity of BCNU against the 9L intracerebral rat tumor but this combination has failed to produce prolonged survival in glioblastoma patients (Prados et al 1989).

Because even glioblastomas have a low labeling index, continuous exposure of the entire cell mass to effective levels of chemotherapeutic agents is not possible without significant systemic toxicity, hence the current interest in interstitial chemotherapy (Brem et al 1991, Tomita 1991). The recent development of non-toxic drug-impregnated polymers provides the first opportunity for the controlled release of drugs directly into the tumor on a long-term basis. Release of BCNU from the polyanhydride continues for up to three weeks. Twenty one patients entered into a Phase II study demonstrated a median survival of 48 weeks from the time of reoperation (Brem et al 1991). Conceptually, diffusion of drug directly into the tumor may produce conditions similar to those obtained during in vitro drug sensitivity testing. In such circumstances, a clinical response to a chemotherapeutic agent is correctly predicted in only 50–70% of cases despite uniformly high drug levels and no difficulties with tumor access (Kimmel et al 1987). Inherent drug resistance and tumor heterogeneity in vivo are likely to pose major problems for interstitial chemotherapy. Individualization of therapy based on in vitro drug testing remains a hope rather than a reality in most clinics (Rosenblum et al 1983).

BIOLOGIC RESPONSE MODIFIERS AND IMMUNOTHERAPY

That immunotherapy has failed to improve the survival of patients with malignant brain tumors is not surprising given its modest record in the treatment of solid tumors outside the nervous system (Young et al 1991, Herberman 1992). The most extensively examined strategies have included the use of various cytokines, vaccination against tumors, the use of monoclonal antibodies to tumor-associated antigens and adoptive cellular therapy. Unfortunately, most immunological agents suffer from either low activity or low potency. The latter problem is further complicated in the nervous system by lack of a tumor-specific antigen, thus negating the exquisite selectivity of most immunological techniques and the potential for systemic delivery. Most tumor-associated antigens (TAAs) are differentiation antigens that may be expressed in small amounts on normal cells at some stage in development but not at maturity (Herberman 1992). Furthermore, glial tumors are capable of shedding or internalizing surface proteins and can produce blocking factors (including overexpressed growth factors) against antibodies and activated lymphocytes. There is also evidence to suggest that expression of surface proteins by astrocytoma cells is age dependent (Hunt & Sherbet 1989). An additional problem is posed by the immunologically impaired status of many patients with malignant gliomas (Young et al 1991). Finally, insufficient attention has been paid to the mechanisms by which surgery may alter tumor burden, vascular access and immunocompetence to the benefit of immunotherapy (Brooks & Roszman 1980).

Among potential antigen targets, marker proteins used in the immunostaining of tumors, such as glial fibrillary acidic protein (GFAP), the fibroblast intermediate filament, vimentin, and S-100 protein are all expressed in normal cells as well as in astrocytomas and oligodendrogliomas (Tabuchi et al 1982, Yung et al 1985, Lee et al 1991, Molenaar & Trojanowski 1991). In gliosarcomas, vimentin staining is restricted to the sarcomatous portion of the tumor; factor VIII staining of the endothelium supports the theory that these are the cells of origin for the mesenchymal elements of the tumor (Schiffer et al 1984). Fibronectin, the major non-collagenous component of the extracellular matrix, is confined to the vasculature in astrocytoma tissue but can be expressed by GFAP-positive glioma cells in vitro (Davenport & McKeever 1987). The concentration of fibronectin in the vicinity of the tumor is such that it can serve as an antigenic target for radiolabeled monoclonal antibodies, especially since fibronectin, collagen and laminin are absent in the extracellular matrix of normal brain parenchyma (McComb & Bigner 1985). Unfortunately, elevated levels of fibronectin can be detected in the plasma of brain tumor patients as well as in patients with a wide variety of other conditions and this is likely to limit the potential for systemic delivery of antifibronectin immunologicals (Sawaya et al 1985), hence, the continued importance of developing antibodies to glioma-mesenchymal extracellular matrix antigens that are distinct from fibronectin and laminin (McComb & Bigner 1985).

Some of the activity and potency problems of humoral-based immunotherapy can be overcome by conjugating monoclonal antibodies to radioactive isotopes or to plant and bacterial toxins (Zovickian et al 1987, Zovickian & Youle 1988, Johnson et al 1989). The transferrin receptor (TR), a transmembrane glycoprotein that mediates cellular uptake of iron, is overexpressed in glioblastoma and other tumors; it may represent a suitable tumor Ag in that its concentration in non-proliferating neural tissue, save the capillary endothelium, is virtually nil. Furthermore, antibodies raised to TR are likely to enter tumor cells by receptor-mediated endocytosis. A ricin-labeled monoclonal Ab to TR has produced significant in vitro cytotoxicity against both glioblastoma and medulloblastoma cell lines (Recht et al 1990). These results have been replicated after intrathecal delivery in an animal model of leptomeningeal neoplasia (Zovickian & Youle 1988). A genetically engineered diphtheria toxin can maintain the tumor-killing efficiency of the complete plant toxin (ricin) without demonstrating non-specific binding to normal cells (Johnson et al 1989). Unfortunately, the modified antibody-toxin conjugate is still too large for transvascular delivery. However, recombinant toxins can be linked to growth factors or single chain antigen-binding proteins that are smaller than complete antibodies (Pastan & Fitzgerald 1991). When the cDNA for TGF-α is recombinantly bound to pseudomonas exotoxin, the resulting chimera selectively binds to and kills cells that express the epidermal growth factor receptor (EGFr). Additionally, it may be possible to use liposomes to act as delivery modules for polarized and high molecular weight substances. Not only can liposomes cross blood vessels but antibodies coupled to them may provide for even more selective delivery of cytotoxic agents. For example, this technique has been used to increase the in vitro cytotoxicity of encapsulated methotrexate against glioma cells by 100-fold in comparison to free drug (Kito et al 1989).

In experimental animals, F(ab′)2 fragments of monoclonal antibody [Mel-14F(ab′)2] have been used to deliver iodine-131 to human intracerebral xenografts in athymic mice; survival was prolonged and uptake increased by the concomitant use of hyperthermia at 42°C (Colapinto et al 1990, Cope et al 1990). Selective uptake of indium-111 or ^{90}Y-labeled monoclonal antibody has been demonstrated in other animal studies and similar agents have been used for imaging and treatment in glioma patients (Bergh et al 1990, Williams et al 1990). Thus far, the most encouraging application of this technology has been its use in the intrathecal treatment of disseminated leptomeningeal glioblastoma and medulloblastoma (Lashford et al 1988). Four of five patients in a pilot study achieved an objective response with excellent clinical tolerance to ^{131}I-labeled antibodies. Of course, many of the problems involved in the treatment of an intracranial tumor, such as large cellular volumes, uncertain vascular access and low antibody potency and specificity, are not issues of moment in the subarachnoid space. Recently, hybridoma technology has been used to produce a panel of five human antiglioma monoclonal antibodies (IgM) that recognize cell surface glycolipids (Dan et al 1992). These reagents have been shown to cross-react with relatively few nongliomatous tumor cell lines and fail to react with normal human astrocytes.

Thus far, neither biologic response modifiers nor cellular-based therapy has demonstrated any greater promise as single-agent treatments than antibody-based immunotherapy. Intratumoral injection of interleukin-2-activated lymphocytes and interferon-β has failed to improve survival of glioblastoma patients and only a modest response in a few patients has been observed with systemic interferon (Fetell et al 1990, Lillehei et al 1991). Intracarotid administration of tumor necrosis factor-α (TNF) represents a new and more aggressive example of the use of biologic response modifiers in the treatment of malignant gliomas (Yoshida et al 1992). Such agents may find a role in the devascularization of benign tumors such as meningioma. TNF is a cytokine of macrophage origin capable of inducing hemorrhagic necrosis in vivo and tumor cell death in vitro. Unfortunately, the 20% response rate observed in glioma patients is similar to the results obtained in systemic tumors of other types (Yoshida et al 1992). In conclusion, immunotherapy is unlikely to succeed as single modality treatment; however, it would appear to have great potential as a carrier and targeting technology in combination with other agents.

MOLECULAR TARGETS AND DIFFERENTIATION THERAPY

As illustrated diagramatically in Figure 20.2, the growth control system of a cell consists of a number of dominant growth-promoting genes (O1 and O2) responsible for the production of growth factors (g) and growth factor receptor proteins (R). When a single cell is capable of producing both a growth factor and the appropriate receptor, we speak of autocrine stimulation. In some tumors, the receptor proteins are structurally altered so that they do not require the presence of a growth factor in order to be active. Most receptors of oncogenic importance contain a cytoplasmic domain that functions as a tyrosine kinase (tk), the activation of which results in the phosphorylation of proteins important in either cytoplasmic transcription or in the signaling of other genes within the nucleus (N). In this fashion, the activation of a receptor at the surface of the cell can alter the regulation of other oncogenes more directly associated with DNA replication (e.g. myc) and cell division. In a normal cell, this chain of events is under negative feedback control and is usually braked by the activity of recessive genes known as tumor suppressors (sup), the loss of which is associated with progressive degrees of anaplasia. This simple schema can serve as the basis for a number of potential therapeutic strategies (see Tables 20.2, 20.3), including inhibition or neutralization of a dominant oncogene (O1 and O2), destruction or blockage of its growth factor (g) and associated receptor protein (R), down-regulation and inhibition of the intracellular signal pathway (tk), and replacement of the activity or product of a lost suppressor gene (sup).

In fact, almost as soon as overexpression of the EGFr gene (v-erb-B) was detected in human gliomas, clinical trials based on this information were initiated (Epenetos et al 1985). As demonstrated by CT, regression of a grade 4 tumor was produced by the intra-arterial infusion of an anti-EGFr antibody labeled with iodine-131 (45 mCi) that cross-reacted with blood type A antigen. The antibody was developed against a human epidermoid carcinoma line that expressed high concentrations of EGFr. More recently, a Phase II clinical trial has been carried out in 25 patients exposed intravenously or intra-arterially to iodine-125 (25 mCi) labeled to a more specific anti-EGFr antibody (Brady et al 1992). The antibody causes down-regulation of the receptor without stimulation of tyrosine kinase activity, and the high energy transfer (HET) of iodine-125 produces less sublethal damage repair that is susceptible to the influence of hypoxia and the cell cycle. The average total dose of iodine-125 in the trial was 151 mCi. The first infusion was carried out 3–4 weeks after the completion of conventional external beam radiation to an average total dose of 61 Gy (6100 rads). The projected median survival obtained in 10 patients with anaplastic astrocytoma and 15 patients with GBM was 15.6 months (Brady et al 1992). A randomized multicenter study is currently under way to better define the clinical response to this novel form of adjuvant therapy. Not all malignant astrocytomas, however, overexpress the EGFr gene or its receptor protein and not all cells in a given tumor stain with anti-EGFr antibody. As a result, glioma cell lines demonstrate a variable response to epidermal growth factor stimulation in serum-free media (Pollack et al 1990b).

Table 20.2 Biological problem: dominant oncogene expression. Solution: blocking agents.

Monoclonal antibody vs
- Gene
- Growth factor
- GF receptor
- Transduction pathway

Chemical block vs
- Gene
- Growth factor:
  - antisense oligonucleotide vs IGF-I trapidil vs PDGF
- GF receptor:
  - recombinant toxin: TGF-α pseudomonas
  - suramin
- Transduction pathway:
  - PKC inhibitors:
    - staurosporine
    - tamoxifen
    - polymyxin B
    - phorbol esters
  - Tyrosine kinase:
    - erbstatin
    - tyrphostin

Table 20.3 Biological problem: loss of suppressor gene activity. Solution: replace activity or differentiation.

Replace activity:
- Gene therapy:
  - Gene insertion
  - Viral vector
  - Cellular vector

Reverse process:
- Differentiating agents:
  - Retinoids
  - cAMP
  - Butyroids
  - Hyperthermia?

Drugs can be designed to block phosphorylation of tyrosine residues and thus interfere with mitogenic signal transduction; erbstatin, a tyrosine analog, and tyrphostins are prototypes of such agents (Aaronson 1991). Tamoxifen, a nonsteroidal antiestrogen, may act through inhibition of protein kinase C. In a Phase II study, tamoxifen has shown some efficacy in glioma patients who have already failed other therapy without evidence for toxicity or side effects (Vertosick et al 1992). Modulators of the protein kinase C system have been shown to inhibit the in vitro growth of established glioma cell lines (Couldwell et al 1990). Tamoxifen administered orally in very high doses (80–100 mg, b.i.d.) has produced radiographic tumor reduction in 3 of 11 patients who had already failed other treatments (Couldwell et al 1993). Staurosporine is an even more potent inhibitor of PKC and should enter clinical trial shortly.

Attempts to inhibit the activity of platelet-derived growth factor (PDGF) represent an example of an anti-growth factor strategy. In serum-free media, glioma cell lines exposed to the combination of PDGF and EGF grow almost as well as they do in response to fetal calf serum, and many glioma cell lines exhibit PDGF receptor activity, increased PDGF mRNA or produce a PDGF mitogen (Harsh et al 1990, Pollack et al 1990b, Mapstone 1991). Use of an anti-PDGF antibody in vitro strongly inhibits DNA synthesis and cell proliferation without eliminating the effect of fetal calf serum on DNA synthesis (Pollack et al 1990a). In these studies, trapidil (1–100 μg/ml), a PDGF-blocking agent, and polymyxin B (10 to

50 μg/ml), a protein kinase C inhibitor, were all very effective in blocking baseline and serum-stimulated DNA synthesis and cell proliferation in vitro (Pollack et al 1990a). Trapidil competes for receptor binding with PDGF and should work if the cell line produces a PDGF-like mitogen (Kuratsu & Ushio 1990).

Some of the mitogenic effects of PDGF may result from protein kinase C-mediated phosphorylation of appropriate substrates. Phorbol esters, such as 4-β-phorbol-12,13-dibutyrate (PDB) and phorbol-12-myristate-13-acetate (PMA), can activate the PKC second messenger system and inhibit the in vitro growth of human glioma cell lines (Couldwell et al 1990). This may occur through down-regulation of already high intrinsic PKC activity and produces an increase in the degree of glial fibrillary acidic protein (GFAP) staining, a possible marker of increased cellular differentiation (Couldwell et al 1990). In response to the administration of phorbol esters and cyclic AMP in vitro, primitive cells can be induced to differentiate toward a more mature astrocytic morphology, at which time their growth rate slows and eventually ceases (Ebert & Salcman 1993). The effects of such agents are, however, not necessarily beneficial in all respects. Although PMA was shown to promote differentiation and slowed growth in the SNB19 glioblastoma cell line, it also decreased susceptibility of the cells to lymphokine-activated killer cell activity (Maleci et al 1990). Neurotrophins such as nerve growth factor (NGF) also might be used to induce differentiation toward a more benign phenotype in NGF-dependent tumors, or their withdrawal might be used to induce cell death (Nakagawara et al 1993).

Despite such difficulties, chemical differentiation may represent a therapeutic strategy by which downstream signal transduction of growth factor-GF receptor stimulation can be inhibited and reversal of the malignant phenotype achieved. Several in vitro studies have now demonstrated the feasibility of combination therapy utilizing conventional alkylating agents and either chemical differentiation or anti-PDGF agents (Kuratsu & Ushio 1990, Ebert & Salcman 1993). In comparison to 1 μg/ml of ACNU alone, trapidil at 100 μg/ml decreased the growth rate of U251MG cells from 63% to 31% (Kuratsu & Ushio 1990). Suramin has attracted attention for its use in clinical trials precisely because it inhibits the binding of a number of growth factors (PDGF, EGF and tumor growth factor-β) to their receptors (Stein et al 1989). In the human U87MG glioma cell line and in a model canine glioma cell line, the combination of cyclic AMP and sodium butyrate, a phorbol ester, has been shown to increase the degree of cell killing produced by BCNU, cis-platinum, and hyperthermia (Fig. 20.3; Tables 20.4, 20.5; Ebert & Salcman 1993).

Because of their inherently low toxicity, the retinoids, a class of differentiation agents distinct from phorbol esters and cyclic AMP, have received widespread clinical interest. Vitamin A (retinol) and its derivatives, such as tretinoin (all-trans-retinoic acid) and isotretinoin (13-cis-retinoic acid), induce in vitro differentiation in a variety of

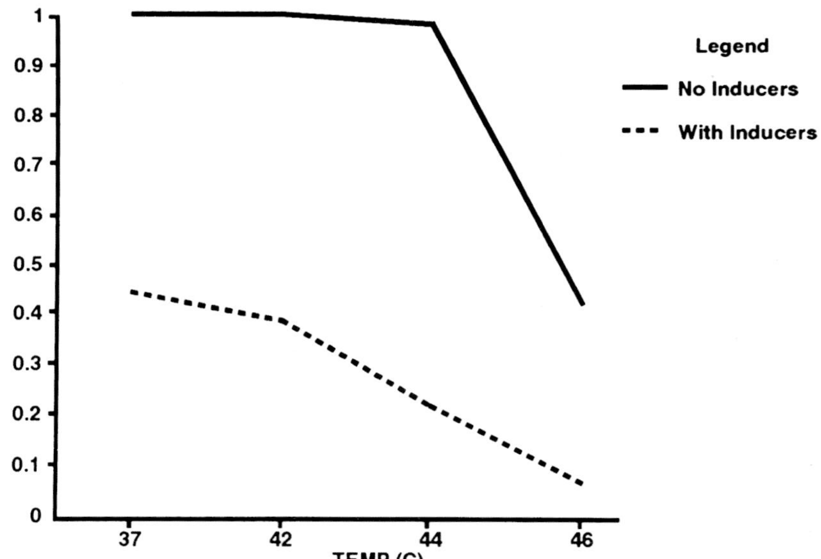

Fig. 20.3 Effect of chemical inducers on thermal sensitivity. Administration of cyclic AMP and sodium butyrate to either canine glioma cells or the human U87MG glioblastoma cell line results in heightened sensitivity to 30 minutes of hyperthermia at temperatures of 42–46°C as demonstrated by the decreased surviving fraction by colony formation assay. Based on data from Ebert & Salcman (1993).

Table 20.4 Sequential BCNU-differentiation therapy in CBT and U87MG

Treatment	Day	Surviving fraction *CBT*	*U-87MG*
Control	—	1.00 +/– 0.07	1.00 +/– 0.02
BCNU	0	0.42 +/– 0.10	0.77 +/– 0.06
BCNU	3	0.17 +/– 0.03	0.48 +/– 0.05
cAMP/butyrate	0–3	0.57 +/– 0.06	0.53 +/– 0.04
BCNU + cAMP/butyrate	0		
	0–3	0.05 +/– 0.01	0.27 +/– 0.01
BCNU + cAMP/butyrate	3		
	0–3	0.06 +/– 0.01	0.31 +/– 0.03

Table 20.5 Sequential cisplatin-differentiation therapy in U87MG

Treatment	Day	Surviving fraction
Control	—	1.00 +/– 0.02
Cisplatin	0	0.76 +/– 0.05
Cisplatin	3	0.69 +/– 0.06
cAMP/butyrate	0–3	0.68 +/– 0.05
Cisplatin + cAMP/butyrate	0	
	0–3	0.19 +/– 0.01
Cisplatin + cAMP/butyrate	3	
	0–3	0.31 +/– 0.01

tumor cells and have produced clinical responses in many patients with acute promyelocytic leukemia. For example, isotretinoin has been shown to be more effective than β-carotene in the prevention of oral carcinogenesis from leukoplakia, a premalignant lesion (Lippman et al 1993). The retinoic acid receptor-α (RAR-α) on chromosome 17 appears to regulate the transcription of many genes and may also control cellular differentiation as a result of interactions with nuclear proto-oncogenes (Cheson 1992). In vitro and in vivo retinoid resistance can be reversed with cytochrome p450 inhibitors such as ketoconazole.

GENE THERAPY

Manipulation of the genetic machinery of the cell represents the most exciting as well as the most controversial new approach in cancer therapy, and may take a number of forms (Table 20.6). Potential types of gene therapy include the random insertion of a normal copy of the gene into the target tissue or cell; gene modification or correction of the defective gene in situ; and gene surgery or substitution, whereby the defective gene is excised and physically replaced with its normal counterpart (Larrick & Burck 1991). In addition, a gene can be activated or shut down through modification of its in situ control elements or through the use of combined strategies. Retroviruses, adenoviruses and genetically altered cells, such as lymphocytes and fibroblasts, can be used as vectors to carry gene therapy into the tumor and are far more efficient at gene transfer than chemical or physical techniques. The transient persistence of transferred genes represents the most serious limitation of in vivo techniques, and problems involved in the transplantation of transduced cells have thus far limited the application of ex vivo gene therapies (Mulligan 1993). Innumerable technical and ethical considerations are likely to restrict gene therapy to somatic rather than germline cellular targets for the foreseeable future.

Table 20.6 Potential forms of gene therapy

1. Somatic vs germline therapy
2. Random gene insertion or addition
3. Targeted approaches:
   - Gene modification (in situ)
   - Gene substitution or replacement
   - Gene activation (modify control in situ)
4. Combined approaches after ex-vivo insertion:
   - Herpes simplex mutant (tk–)
   - Fibroblast with HSV tk+
   - Cytosine deaminase + cells
   - Antisense oligonucleotide + cells
   - TNF-α + cells
   - GM-CSF + cells

Clinical gene transfer in an approved protocol, insertion of a marker gene for assistance in the correction of an enzyme deficiency, first took place on May 22, 1989; in the subsequent period of less than three years, more than 30 other clinical trials entered various stages of development (Anderson 1992, Rosenberg 1992). The earliest examples of gene therapy in cancer involved the use of genetically altered tumor-infiltrating lymphocytes (TIL) as vectors to carry tumor necrosis factor (TNF) into malignant melanoma and the addition of cytokine genes (for TNF or interleukin-2, IL-2) to the patient's own tumor cells so as to evoke a more pronounced systemic T-cell-mediated antitumor immunity (Rosenberg 1992). Thus far, side effects from retroviral-mediated gene transfer in patients and other primates have not been observed and no example of malignancy due to a replication-defective retroviral vector has been found. As already intimated, gene therapy is unlikely to have major impact on the general treatment of human diseases until efficient vectors are engineered that 'target specific cell types, insert their genetic information into a safe site in the genome, and (are) regulated by normal physiologic signals' (Anderson 1992).

Herpes virus vectors may provide a unique strategy for persistence of foreign DNA in the central nervous system. For example, the genetically engineered herpes simplex virus (HSV-1) mutant dlsptk completely lacks thymidine kinase (tk) activity and, as a result, cannot replicate in non-dividing cells such as neurons and normal glia (Martuza et al 1991). Hence, such a virus might preferentially divide in and prove cytopathic to neoplastic cells in the brain. In cell culture, dlsptk has been shown to efficiently kill a number of human glioma cell lines, and intraneoplastic injection of the virus in nude mice bearing intracerebral U87 gliomas successfully prolonged survival (Martuza et al 1991). Since the mutant virus is as sensitive to vidarabine and foscarnet as wild-type virus, these drugs could be used to protect normal replicating tissues from unintended viral exposure. Recently, this approach has successfully been applied in vitro and in the nude mouse to a variety of human brain tumors including medulloblastoma, malignant meningioma and neurofibrosarcoma (Markert et al 1992). However, even replication-incompetent herpes virus can kill cells through the elaboration of toxic viral gene products (Mulligan 1993).

Rather than using direct viral transfer of genes, transduced cells can be used to carry genetic material into the nervous system. For example, the HSV-1 thymidine kinase gene was inserted into murine fibroblasts by retroviral-mediated gene transfer and the transduced cells were stereotactically injected into rats bearing intracerebral gliomas (Culver et al 1992). Continuous production of retroviral vector particles in the immediate environment of the tumor makes the particles available to transduce other cells whenever they enter DNA synthesis. Subsequent treatment with ganciclovir (GCV) preferentially kills tumor containing the tk gene without affecting normal brain cells that are tk–. In 11 of 14 GCV-treated rats with 9L tumors previously injected with HS-tk retroviral vector-producing murine fibroblasts, there was complete macroscopic and microscopic regression of the tumor (Culver et al 1992). A clinical trial utilizing this methodology has received NIH approval. A related strategy is the injection of cells modified to express cytosine deaminase, a bacterial enzyme capable of converting the ordinarily nontoxic drug 5′-fluorocytosine to the cytotoxic compound 5-fluorouracil (5FU), thus killing the gene-modified cells.

Cells altered by gene insertion can also be used as vectors for therapeutic strategies directed at growth factors and growth factor receptors. In rats with established C6 gliomas, the subsequent injection of tumor cells transfected with the gene for antisense insulin-like growth factor I (IGF-I) produced regression of the tumors (Trojan et al 1993). Antisense oligonucleotides block the transcription and activity of naturally occurring peptide sequences produced by normal mRNA. In the C6 model, antisense IGF-I not only prevented growth factor activity but also increased the immunogenicity of the tumor and heightened the degree of CD8+ lymphocyte invasion (Trojan et al 1993). In this example, tumor immunogenicity was increased by blocking a naturally occurring cytokine that may normally act to help the tumor escape immune surveillance. In another study, the in vitro glioma cytotoxicity of lymphokine-activated killer cells (LAK cells) was increased three-fold by using liposomes to transfect them with the gene for tumor necrosis factor α (TNF-α) (Tashiro et al 1993). This methodology involves the simultaneous application of three novel technologies.

The selective chemosensitivity and enhanced immunogenicity produced by some gene insertion strategies are truly elegant examples of the concept of combined modality therapy. In the treatment of enzyme deficiency disorders, it is the goal of gene insertion to provide the patient with replacement therapy at the molecular level; this may also prove to be a highly effective strategy in the treatment of some cancers. The tumor suppressor p53 is a nuclear phosphoprotein with characteristics of a transcription factor; as previously discussed, loss of the wild-type p53 gene and/or possession of a p53 mutant is associated with many different types of cancer as well as with a general proclivity for tumor development as expressed in the cancer family syndrome. Loss of wild-type p53 function might transcriptionally activate those genes normally repressed by p53, and this pattern of wild-type p53 repression and mutant p53 activation has been observed in regard to the multidrug resistance gene (MDR) and the heat shock protein (hsp70) promoter gene (Agoff et al 1993). Regulation of the cell cycle at the late G1/early S phase by p53 may depend on protein–protein interactions while the effect of p53 on transcription may involve direct contact of p53 with a specific DNA sequence (Kern et al 1992). The heat shock proteins, including members of the hsp70 and hsp60 families, are important components of the non-specific stress response of mammalian cells and function to prevent denaturation or act to renature damaged proteins by protecting or promoting protein folding (Martin et al 1992). For example, in bacteria, yeast, and mammalian cells, a slight elevation in temperature results in a two- to three-fold increase in the amount of mitochondrial hsp. It is conceivable, therefore, that the use of gene insertion to increase the amount of wild-type p53 activity might simultaneously inhibit cell growth, reverse the neoplastic phenotype, and promote increased sensitivity to both hyperthermia and chemotherapy. Germline therapy with the p53 gene or its protein product might reduce the susceptibility of individuals in cancer family pedigrees to develop tumors. Early success has been reported with the use of a retrovirus to insert wild-type retinoblastoma (RB) genes into osteosarcoma and prostate cancer cells that lack them; the tumor cells not only grow more slowly in vitro but lose their tumorigenicity in nude mice (Weinberg 1991). Nevertheless, the technical and social difficulties involved in the successful implementation of somatic gene therapy remain formidable and should not be underestimated in the near term.

CONCLUSIONS

Successful treatment of malignant brain tumors is likely to depend on a multimodality approach in which at least three important biological problems are specifically addressed: (1) cellular diversity and heterogeneity, (2) oncogene overactivity, and (3) suppressor gene loss. In theory, control of the central mass of the tumor can be achieved by some combination of local and regional agents such as surgery, radiation and hyperthermia, when used together rather than sequentially. Scattered nests of tumor cells in the surrounding brain, however, are unlikely to be controlled by this method without insupportable neurotoxicity. Successful treatment of the surround is likely to depend on agents that specifically recognize molecular biologic differences between tumor cells and normal neurons or glia. This may be achieved either through the use of agents that block oncogene expression or through reversal of the malignant phenotype. The latter may require the induction of cellular differentiation or the insertion of lost genetic material (Table 20.6).

REFERENCES

Aaronson S A 1991 Growth factors and cancer. Science 254: 1146–1153

Adams E F, Schrell U M H, Fahlbusch R et al 1990 Hormonal dependency of cerebral meningiomas. Part 2: In vitro effect of steroids, bromocriptine, and epidermal growth factor on growth of meningiomas. Journal of Neurosurgery 73: 750–755

Agoff S N, Hou J, Linzer D I H et al 1993 Regulation of the human hsp70 promoter by p53. Science 259: 84–87

Anderson W F 1992 Human gene therapy. Science 256: 808–813

Austin-Seymour M, Munzenrider J, Linggood R et al 1990 Fractionated proton radiation therapy of cranial and intracranial tumors. American Journal of Clinical Oncology 13: 327–330

Barth R F, Soloway A H, Fairchild R G 1990 Boron neutron capture therapy of cancer. Cancer Research 50: 1061–1070

Beach J L, Schroy C B, Ashtari M et al 1990 Boron neutron capture enhancement of 252Cf brachytherapy. International Journal of Radiation Oncology and Biological Physics 18: 1421–1427

Berger M S, Ali-Osman F 1991 Mutagenesis and DNA repair mechanisms. In: Salcman M (ed) Neurobiology of brain tumors. Williams & Wilkins, Baltimore, pp 63–72

Bergh J, Nilsson S, Liljedahl C et al 1990 In vivo imaging and treatment of human brain tumors utilizing the radiolabeled monoclonal antibody MUC 2–63. Anticancer Research 10: 655–660

Bernstein M, Ginsberg H, Glen J 1992 Brachytherapy: brain injury in the rat with the 21-aminosteroid V74398F. Neurosurgery 31: 923–929

Bigner D D 1981 Biology of gliomas: potential clinical implications of glioma cellular heterogeneity. Neurosurgery 9: 320–326

Bigner D D, Bigner S H, Ponten J et al 1981 Heterogeneity of genotypic and phenotypic characteristics of fifteen permanent cell lines derived from human gliomas. Journal of Neuropathology and Experimental Neurology 40: 201–229

Bigner S H, Mark J, Mahaley M S et al 1984 Patterns of the early, gross chromosomal changes in malignant human gliomas. Hereditas 101: 103–113

Bigner S H, Mark J, Burger P et al 1988 Specific chromosomal abnormalities in malignant human gliomas. Cancer Research 48: 405–411

Bigner S H, Mark J, Bigner D D 1990 Cytogenetics of human brain tumors. Cancer Genetics and Cytogenetics 47: 141–154

Black K L, King W A, Ikezaki K 1990 Selective opening of the blood-brain barrier by intracarotid infusion of leukotriene C4. Journal of Neurosurgery 72: 912–916

Bowles A P, Pantazis C G, Wansley W 1990 Use of verapamil to enhance the antiproliferative activity of BCNU in human glioma cells: an in vitro and in vivo study. Journal of Neurosurgery 73: 248–253

Brady L W, Miyamoto C, Woo D V et al 1992 Malignant astrocytomas treated with iodine-125 labeled monoclonal antibody against epidermal growth factor receptor: a phase II trial. International Journal of Radiation Oncology and Biological Physics 22: 225–230

Brem H, Mahaley S, Vick N et al 1991 Interstitial chemotherapy with drug polymer implants for the treatment of recurrent gliomas. Journal of Neurosurgery 74: 441–446

Brooks W H, Roszman T L 1980 Cellular immune responsiveness of patients with primary intracranial tumors. In: Thomas D G T, Graham D I (eds) Brain tumors: scientific basis, clinical investigation, and current therapy. Butterworth, London, pp 121–132

Burger P C, Heinz E R, Shibata T et al 1988 Topographic anatomy and CT correlations in the untreated glioblastoma multiforme. Journal of Neurosurgery 68: 698–704

Cairncross J G, Macdonald D R, Ramsay D A 1992 Aggressive oligodendroglioma: a chemosensitive tumor. Neurosurgery 31: 78–82

Chalazonitis A, Kessler J A, Twardzik D R et al 1992 Transforming growth factor alpha, but not epidermal growth factor, promotes the survival of sensory neurons in vitro. Journal of Neuroscience 12: 583–594

Cheson B D 1992 The maturation of differentiation therapy. Editorial. New England Journal of Medicine 327: 422–423

Clendenon N R, Barth R F, Gordon W A et al 1990 Boron neutron capture therapy of a rat glioma. Neurosurgery 26: 47–55

Coffey R J, Lunsford D, Flinkinger J C 1991 The role of radiosurgery in the treatment of malignant brain tumors. Neurosurgery Clinics of North America 3(1): 231–244

Cohen J D, Robins H I, Javid M J 1990 Radiosensitization of C6 glioma by thymidine and 41.8°C hyperthermia. Journal of Neurosurgery 72: 732–785

Colapinto E V, Zalusky M R, Archer G E et al 1990 Radioimmunotherapy of intracerebral human glioma xenografts with 131I labeled F(ab′)2 fragments of monoclonal antibody Mel-14. Cancer Research 50: 1822–1827

Coleman C N, Noll L, Riese N et al 1992 Final report of the phase I trial of continuous infusion etanidazole (SR 2508): A radiation therapy oncology group study. International Journal of Radiation Oncology and Biological Physics 22: 577–580

Cope D A, Dewhirst W, Friedman H S et al 1990 Enhanced delivery of a monoclonal antibody F(ab′)2 fragment to subcutaneous human glioma xenografts using local hyperthermia. Cancer Research 50: 1803–1809

Couldwell W T, Antel J P, Apuzzo M L J et al 1990 Inhibition of growth of established human glioma cell lines by modulators of the protein kinase-C system. Journal of Neurosurgery 73: 594–600

Couldwell W T, Weiss M H, DeGiorgio C M et al 1993 Clinical and radiographic response in a minority of patients with recurrent malignant gliomas treated with high-dose tamoxifen. Neurosurgery 32: 485–490

Culver K W, Ram Z, Wallbridge S et al 1992 In vivo gene transfer with retroviral vector-producer cells for treatment of experimental brain tumors. Science 256: 1550–1552

Dan M D, Schlachta C M, Guy J et al 1992 Human antiglioma monoclonal antibodies from patients with astrocytic tumors. Journal of Neurosurgery 76: 660–669

Davenport R D, McKeever P E 1987 DNA content and marker expression in human glioma explants. Acta Neuropathol (Berlin) 74: 362–365

Ebert P S, Salcman M 1993 Differentiation of human and canine brain tumor cells enhances therapeutic sensitivity to hyperthermia and chemotherapy in vitro. Neurosurgery (submitted)

Ekstrand A J, James C D, Cavenee W et al 1991 Genes for epidermal growth factor receptor, transforming growth factor alpha, and epidermal growth factor and their expression in human gliomas in vivo. Cancer Research 51: 2164–2172

El-Azouzi M, Chung R Y, Farmer G E et al 1989 Loss of distinct regions on the short arm of chromosome 17 associated with tumorigenesis of human astrocytomas. Proceedings of the National Academy of Sciences of the USA 86: 7186–7190

Engelhard H H, Bulter A B, Bauer K D 1989 Quantification of the c-myc oncoprotein in human glioblastoma cells and tumor tissue. Journal of Neurosurgery 71: 224–232

Epenetos A A, Courtenay-Luck N, Pickering D et al 1985 Antibody guided irradiation of brain glioma by arterial infusion of radioactive monoclonal antibody against epidermal growth factor receptor and blood group A antigen. British Medical Journal 290: 1463–1466

Evans R G, Kimler B F, Morantz R A et al 1990 A phase I/II study of the use of fluosol as an adjuvant to radiation therapy in the treatment of primary high-grade brain tumors. International Journal of Radiation Oncology and Biological Physics 19: 415–420

Fauchon F, Davila L, Chatellier G et al 1990 Treatment of malignant gliomas with surgery, intra-arterial infusion of 1-(2-hydroxyethyl) chloroethylnitrosourea, and radiation therapy: a phase II study. Neurosurgery 27: 231–234

Ferraro F T, Salcman M, Broadwell R D et al 1989 Alumina ceramic as a biomaterial for use in afterloading radiation catheters for hyperthermia. Neurosurgery 25: 209–213

Fetell M R, Housepian E M, Oster M W et al 1990 Intratumor administration of beta-interferon in recurrent malignant gliomas: a phase I clinical and laboratory study. Cancer 65: 78–83

Fujimoto M, Weaker F J, Herbert D C et al 1988 Expression of three viral oncogenes (v-sis, v-myc, v-fos) in primary human brain tumors of neuroectodermal origin. Neurology 38: 289–293

Fults D, Tippets R, Thomas G et al 1989 Loss of heterozygosity for loci on chromosome 17p in human malignant astrocytoma. Cancer Research 49: 6572–6577

Fults D, Pedrone C, Thomas G et al 1990 Allelotype of human malignant astrocytoma. Cancer Research 50: 5784–5780

Gerweck L E, Kornblith P L, Burlett P et al 1977 Radiation sensitivity of cultured human glioblastoma cells. Radiology 125: 231–241

Glick R P, Gettleman R, Patel K et al 1989 Insulin and insulin-like growth factor I in brain tumors: binding and in vitro effects. Neurosurgery 24: 791–797

Goodman J H, Gahbauer R A, Kanellitsas C et al 1990a Theoretical basis and clinical methodology for stereotactic interstitial brain tumor irradiation using iododeoxy-uridine as a radiation sensitizer and 145 Sm as a brachytherapy source. Stereotact Funct Neurosurgery 54 & 55: 531–534

Goodman G B, Skarsgard L D, Thompson G B et al 1990b Pion therapy at TRIUMF: treatment results for astrocytoma grade 3, 4: a pilot study. Radiother Oncol 17: 21–28

Greiner R, Blattmann H, Thum P et al 1990 Anaplastic astrocytoma and glioblastoma: pion irradiation with the dynamic conformation technique at the Swiss Institute for Nuclear Research (SIN). Radiother Oncol 17: 37–46

Griffin T W, Davis R, Larramore G et al 1983 Fast neutron radiation therapy for glioblastoma multiforme: Results of an RTOG study. American Journal of Clinical Oncology (CCT) 6: 661–667

Grossman S A 1991 Chemotherapy of brain tumors. In: Salcman M (ed) Neurobiology of brain tumors. Williams & Wilkins, Baltimore, pp 321–340

Gutin P H, Bernstein M, Sano Y et al 1984 Combination therapy with 1,3-bis (2-chloroethyl)-1-nitrosourea and low dose rate radiation in the 9L rat brain tumor and spheroid models: implications for brain tumor brachytherapy. Neurosurgery 15: 781–786

Gutin P H, Prados M D, Phillips T L et al 1991 External irradiation followed by an interstitial high-activity iodine-125 implant "boost" in the initial treatment of malignant gliomas: NCOG study 6G-82-2. International Journal of Radiation Oncology and Biological Physics 21: 601–606

Harsh G R IV, Rosenblum M L, Williams L T 1989 Oncogene-related growth factors and growth factor receptors in human malignant glioma-derived cell lines. Journal of Neuro-Oncology 7: 47–56

Harsh G R, Keating M T, Escobedo J A et al 1990 Platelet derived growth factor (PDGF) autocrine components in human tumor cell lines. Journal of Neuro-Oncology 8: 1–12

Hatanaka H 1975 A revised boron-neutron capture theory for malignant brain tumors. II. Interim clinical results with the patients excluding previous treatments. Journal of Neurology 209: 81–94

Hegarty T J, Thornton A F, Diaz R F et al 1990 Intra-arterial bromodeoxyuridine radiosensitization of malignant gliomas. International Journal of Radiation Oncology and Biological Physics 19: 421–428

Herberman R B 1992 Tumor immunology. Journal of the American Medical Association 268: 2935–2939

Hermansson M, Nister M, Betsholtz C et al 1988 Endothelial cell hyperplasia in human glioblastoma: coexpression of mRNA for platelet-derived growth factor (PDGF) B chain and PDGF receptor suggests autocrine growth stimulation. Proceedings of the National Academy of Sciences of the USA 85: 7748–7752

Hochberg F H, Pruitt A 1980 Assumptions in the radiotherapy of glioblastoma. Neurology 30: 907–911

Hoshino T 1984 A commentary on the biology and growth kinetics of low grade and high grade gliomas. Journal of Neurosurgery 61: 895–900

Hoshino T 1991 Cell kinetics of brain tumors. In: Salcman M (ed) Neurobiology of brain tumors. Williams & Wilkins, Baltimore, pp 145–159

Hunt G, Sherbet G V 1989 Age-related cell surface proteins of human astrocytoma cells in culture. Anticancer Research 9: 157–160

James C D, Carlbom E, Dumanski J P et al 1988 Clonal genomic alterations in glioma malignancy stages. Cancer Research 48: 5546–5551

James C D, Carlbom E, Nordenskjold et al 1989 Mitotic recombination of chromosome 17 in astrocytomas. Proceedings of the National Academy of Sciences of the USA 86: 2858–2862

Johnson V G, Wrobel C, Wilson D et al 1989 Improved tumor-specific immunotoxins in the treatment of CNS and leptomeningeal neoplasia. Journal of Neurosurgery 70: 240–248

Kanno H, Kawabara T, Yasumitsu H et al 1988 Transforming growth factors in urine from patients with primary brain tumors. Journal of Neurosurgery 68: 775–780

Kaplan R S, Wiernik P H 1982 Neurotoxicity of antineoplastic drugs. Seminars in Oncology 9: 103–130

Kayama T, Yoshimoto T, Fujimoto S et al 1991 Intratumoral oxygen pressure in malignant brain tumor. Journal of Neurosurgery 74: 55–59

Kelly P J, Daumas-Duport C, Kispert D B et al 1987 Imaging-based stereotaxic serial biopsies in untreated intracranial glial neoplasms. Journal of Neurosurgery 66: 865–874

Kern S E, Pietenpol J A, Thiagalingam S et al 1992 Oncogenic forms of p53 inhibit p53-regulated gene expression. Science 256: 827–830

Kim D H, Harsh G R 1993 Advances in brain tumor biology: the genetics of astrocytoma. In: Salcman M (ed) Current techniques in neurosurgery. Current Science, Philadelphia, pp 1.1–1.8

Kimmel D W, Shapiro J R, Shapiro W R 1987 In vitro drug sensitivity testing in human gliomas. Journal of Neurosurgery 66: 161–171

Kinzler K W, Bigner S H, Bigner D D et al 1987 Identification of an amplified, highly expressed gene in a human glioma. Science 236: 70–73

Kito A, Yoshida J, Kageyama N et al 1989 Liposomes coupled with monoclonal antibodies against glioma-associated antigen for targeting chemotherapy of glioma. Journal of Neurosurgery 71: 382–387

Kobayashi T, Kida Y, Tanaka T et al 1991 Interstitial hyperthermia of malignant brain tumors by implant heating system: clinical experience. Journal of Neuro-Oncology 10: 153–163

Kolker J D, Halpern H J, Krishnasamy S et al 1990 "Instant-mix" whole brain photon with neutron boost radiotherapy for malignant gliomas. International Journal of Radiat Biol Phys 19: 409–414

Kondziolka D, Lunsford L D 1993 Stereotactic radiosurgery for brain tumors. In: Salcman M (ed) Current techniques in neurosurgery. Current Science, Philadelphia, pp 5.1–5.11

Kondziolka D, Lunsford L D, Claassen D et al 1992 Radiobiology of radiosurgery: Part II. The rat C6 glioma model. Neurosurgery 31: 280–288

Kramer E D, Packer R J 1992 Chemotherapy of malignant brain tumors in children. Clinical Neuropharmacology 15: 163–185

Kumar P P, Patil A A, Leibrock L G et al 1991 Brachytherapy: a viable alternative in the management of basal meningiomas. Neurosurgery 29: 676–680

Kuratsu J-I, Ushio Y 1990 Antiproliferative effect of trapidil, a platelet-derived growth factor antagonist, on a glioma cell line in vitro. Journal of Neurosurgery 73: 436–440

Larrick J W, Burck K L 1991 Gene therapy. Application of molecular biology. Elsevier, New York, p 276
Lashford L S, Davies A G, Richardson R B et al 1988 A pilot study of 131I monoclonal antibodies in the therapy of leptomeningeal tumors. Cancer 61: 857–868
Lazar L M, Blum M 1992 Regional distribution and developmental expression of epidermal growth factor and transforming growth factor-alpha mRNA in mouse brain by a quantitative nuclease protection assay. Journal of Neuroscience 12: 1688–1697
Lee Y, Wikstrand C J, Humphrey P A et al 1991 In vitro growth of brain tumors. In: Salcman M (ed) Neurobiology of brain tumors. Williams & Wilkins, Baltimore, pp 163–183
Leibel S A, Gutin P H, Wara W M et al 1989 Survival and quality of life after interstitial implantation of removable high-activity iodine-125 sources for the treatment of patients with recurrent malignant gliomas. International Journal of Radiation Oncology and Biological Physics 17: 1129–1139
Levin V A, Silver P, Hannigan J et al 1990 Superiority of post-radiotherapy adjuvant chemotherapy with CCNU, procarbazine, and vincristine (PCV) over BCNU for anaplastic gliomas: NCOG 6G61 final report. International Journal of Radiation Oncology and Biological Physics 18: 321–324
Liang B C, Thornton A F, Sandler H M et al 1991 Malignant astrocytomas: focal tumor recurrence after focal external beam radiation therapy. Journal of Neurosurgery 75: 559–563
Libermann T A, Nusbaum H R, Razon N et al 1985 Amplification, enhanced expression and possible rearrangement of EGF receptor gene in primary human brain tumors of glial origin. Nature 313: 144–147
Lichtor T, Dohrmann G J, Gurney M E 1990 Cytokine gene expression by human gliomas. Neurosurgery 26: 788–793
Lillehei K O, Mitchell D H, Johnson S D et al 1991 Long-term follow-up of patients with recurrent malignant gliomas treated with adjuvant adoptive immunotherapy. Neurosurgery 28: 16–23
Lippman S M, Batsakis J G, Toth B B 1993 Comparison of low-dose isoretinoin with beta carotene to prevent oral carcinogenesis. New England Journal of Medicine 328: 15–20
Loeffler J S, Alexander E III, Wen P Y et al 1990 Results of stereotactic brachytherapy used in the initial management of patients with glioblastoma. Journal of the National Cancer Institute 82: 1918–1921
McComb R D, Bigner D D 1985 Immunolocalization of monoclonal antibody-defined extracellular matrix antigens in human brain tumors. Journal of Neuro-Oncology 3: 181–186
McDonald J D, Dohrmann G J 1988 Molecular biology of brain tumors. Neurosurgery 23: 537–544
Mahaley M S, Whaley R A, Blue M et al 1986 Central neurotoxicity following intracarotid BCNU chemotherapy for malignant gliomas. Journal of Neuro-Oncology 3: 297–314
Mahaley M S, Mettlin C, Natarajan R et al 1989 National survey of patterns of care for brain-tumor patients. Journal of Neurosurgery 71: 826–836
Maleci A, Alterman R L, Sundstrom et al 1990 Effect of phorbol esters on the susceptibility of a glioma cell line to lymphokine-activated killer cell activity. Journal of Neurosurgery 73: 91–97
Malkin D, Li F P, Strong L C et al 1990 Germline p53 mutation in a familial syndrome of breast cancer, sarcomas, and other neoplasms. Science 250: 1233–1250
Malkin D, Jolly K W, Barbier N et al 1992 Germline mutations of the p53 tumor-suppressor gene in children and young adults with second malignant neoplasms. New England Journal of Medicine 326: 1309–1315
Mapstone T B 1991 Expression of platelet-derived growth factor and transforming growth factor and their correlation with cellular morphology in glial tumors. Journal of Neurosurgery 75: 447–451
Mapstone T B, McMichael M, Goldthwait D 1991 Expression of platelet-derived growth factors, transforming growth factors, and the ros gene in a variety of primary human brain tumors. Neurosurgery 28: 216–222
Mark J 1970 Chromosomal patterns in human meningiomas. European Journal of Cancer 6: 489–498
Markert J M, Coen D M, Malick A et al 1992 Expanded spectrum of viral therapy in the treatment of nervous system tumors. Journal of Neurosurgery 77: 590–594
Martin J, Horwich A L, Hartl F U 1992 Prevention of protein denaturation under heat stress by the chaperonin Hsp60. Science 258: 995–998
Martuza R L 1991 Neurofibromatosis as a model for tumor formation in the human nervous system. In: Salcman M (ed) Neurobiology of brain tumors. Williams & Wilkins, Baltimore, pp 53–62
Martuza R L, Malick A, Markert J M et al 1991 Experimental therapy of human glioma by means of a genetically engineered virus mutant. Science 252: 854–855
Matsumoto T, Tani E, Kaba K et al 1990 Amplification and expression of a multidrug resistance gene in human glioma cell lines. Journal of Neurosurgery 72: 96–100
Maxwell M, Naber S P, Wolfe H J et al 1990 Coexpression of platelet derived growth factor (PDGF) and PDGF-receptor genes by primary human astrocytomas may contribute to their development and maintenance. Journal of Clinical Investigation 86: 131–140
Molenaar W M, Trojanowski J Q 1991 Biological markers of glial and primitive tumors. In: Salcman M (ed) Neurobiology of brain tumors. Williams & Wilkins, Baltimore, pp 185–210
Muller W, Afra D, Schroder R 1977 Supratentorial recurrences of gliomas: morphological studies in relation to time intervals with astrocytomas. Acta Neurochirurgica 37: 75–91
Mulligan R C 1993 The basic science of gene therapy. Science 260: 926–931
Nakagawara A, Arima-Nakagawara M, Scavarda N J et al 1993 Association between high levels of expression of the TRK gene and favorable outcome in human neuroblastoma. New England Journal of Medicine 328: 847–854
Neuwelt E A, Frenkel E P, Diehl J et al 1983 Reversible osmotic blood-brain barrier disruption in humans: implications for the chemotherapy of malignant brain tumors. Neurosurgery 12: 662–671
Newlands E S, Backledge G R P, Slack J A et al 1992 Phase I trial of temozolomide (CCRG 81045: M&B 39831: NSC 362856). British Journal of Cancer 65: 287–291
NIH/CEPH Collaborative Mapping Group 1992 A comprehensive genetic linkage map of the human genome. Science 258: 67–86
Origitano T C, Karesh S M, Hennkin R E et al 1993 Photodynamic therapy for intracranial neoplasms: investigations of photosensitizer uptake and distribution using indium-111 photofrin-II single photon emission computed tomography scans in humans with intracranial neoplasms. Neurosurgery 32: 357–364
Pastan I, Fitzgerald D 1991 Recombinant toxins for cancer treatment. Science 254: 1173–1177
Pollack I F, Randall M S, Kristofik M P et al 1990a Response of malignant glioma cell lines to activation and inhibition of protein kinase C-mediated pathways. Journal of Neurosurgery 73: 98–105
Pollack I F, Randall M S, Kristofik M P et al 1990b Response of malignant glioma cell lines to epidermal growth factor and platelet-derived growth factor in a serum-free medium. Journal of Neurosurgery 73: 106–112
Powers S K, Cush S S, Walstad D L et al 1991 Stereotactic intratumoral photodynamic therapy for recurrent malignant brain tumors. Neurosurgery 29: 688–696
Prados M, Rodriguez L, Chamberlain M et al 1989 Treatment of recurrent gliomas with 1,3-bis(2-chloroethyl)-1-nitrosourea and alpha-difluoromethylornithine. Neurosurgery 24: 806–809
Press R D, Misra A, Samols D et al 1989 Major structural alterations of the c-sis gene are not observed in a series of tumors of the human central nervous system. Journal of Neuro-Oncology 7: 345–356
Recht L, Torres C O, Smith T W et al 1990 Transferrin receptor in normal and neoplastic tissue: implications for brain-tumor immunotherapy. Journal of Neurosurgery 72: 941–945
Roberts D W, Coughlin C T, Wong T Z et al 1985 Interstitial hyperthermia and iridium brachytherapy in treatment of malignant glioma: a phase I clinical trial. Journal of Neurosurgery 64: 581–587
Rosenberg S A 1992 Gene therapy for cancer. Journal of the American Medical Association 268: 2416–2419
Rosenblum M L, Dougherty D V, Barger G R et al 1982 Age-related chemosensitivity of stem cells from human malignant brain tumors. Lancet 1: 885–887

Rosenblum M L, Gerosa M A, Wilson C B et al 1983 Stem cell studies of human malignant brain tumors. Part I: development of the stem cell assay and its potential. Journal of Neurosurgery 58: 170–176

Rubinstein L J 1991 Glioma cytogeny and differentiation viewed through the window of neoplastic vulnerability. In: Salcman M (ed) Neurobiology of brain tumors. Williams & Wilkins, Baltimore, pp 35–52

Salcman M 1980 Survival in glioblastoma: Historical perspective. Neurosurgery 7: 435–439

Salcman M 1990 Epidemiology and factors affecting survival. In: Apuzzo M L J (ed) Malignant cerebral glioma. American Association of Neurological Surgeons, Park Ridge, Illinois, pp 95–109

Salcman M (ed) 1991a Neurobiology of brain tumors. Vol 4, Concepts in neurosurgery. Williams & Wilkins, Baltimore, p 386

Salcman M 1991b Hyperthermia. In: Salcman M (ed) Neurobiology of brain tumors. Williams & Wilkins, Baltimore, pp 359–373

Salcman M 1993 Recent advances and future directions in interstitial brachytherapy. In: Salcman M (ed) Current techniques in neurosurgery. Current Science, Philadelphia, pp 4.1–4.14

Salcman M, Broadwell R D 1991 The blood-brain barrier. In: Neurobiology of brain tumors, Salcman M (ed). Vol 4, Concepts in Neurosurgery. Williams & Wilkins, Baltimore, pp 229–249

Salcman M, Ebert P S 1991 In vitro response of human glioblastoma and canine glioma cells to hyperthermia, radiation, and chemotherapy. Neurosurgery 29: 526–531

Salcman M, Samaras G M 1981 Hyperthermia for brain tumors: biophysical rationale. Neurosurgery 9: 327–335

Salcman M, Samaras G M 1983 Interstitial microwave hyperthermia for brain tumors. Results of a phase 1 clinical trial. Journal of Neuro-Oncology 1: 225–236

Salcman M, Solomon L 1984 Occurrence of glioblastoma multiforme in three generations of a cancer family. Neurosurgery 14: 557–561

Salcman M, Kaplan R S, Ducker T B et al 1982 The effect of age and reoperation on survival in the combined modality treatment of malignant astrocytoma. Neurosurgery 10: 454–463

Salcman M, Sewchand W, Amin P P et al 1986 Technique and preliminary results of interstitial irradiation for primary brain tumors. Journal of Neuro-Oncology 4: 141–149

Salcman M, Corradino G, Moriyama E et al 1989 Cerebral blood flow and the thermal properties of the brain: a preliminary analysis. Journal of Neurosurgery 70: 592–598

Salcman M, Scholtz H, Krist D et al 1992 Extraskeletal myxoid chondrosarcoma of the falx. Neurosurgery 31: 344–348

Sawaya R, Cummins C J, Smith B H et al 1985 Plasma fibronectin in patients with brain tumors. Neurosurgery 16: 161–165

Schechter A L, Hung M-C, Weinberg R A et al 1985 The neu gene: an erbB-homologous gene distinct from and unlinked to the gene encoding the EGF receptor. Science 229: 976–978

Schiffer D 1991 Patterns of tumor growth. In: Salcman M (ed) Neurobiology of brain tumors. Williams & Wilkins, Baltimore, pp 229–249

Schiffer D, Giordana M T, Mauro A et al 1984 GFAP, F VIII/RAg, laminin, and fibronectin in gliosarcomas: an immunohistochemical study. Acta Neuropathologica (Berlin) 63: 108–116

Schoenberg B S 1991 Epidemiology of primary intracranial neoplasms: disease distribution and risk factors. In: Salcman M (ed) Neurobiology of brain tumors. Williams & Wilkins, Baltimore, pp 3–18

Seeger R C, Brodeur G M, Sather H et al 1985 Association of multiple copies of N-myc oncogene with rapid progression of neuroblastomas. New England Journal of Medicine 313: 1111–1116

Seizinger B R, Martuza R L, Gusella J F 1986 Loss of genes on chromosome 22 in tumorigenesis of human acoustic neuroma. Nature 322: 644–647

Selikoff I J, Hammond E C 1982 Brain tumors in the chemical industry. Annals of the New York Academy of Science 381: 1–364

Shapiro J R, Yung W-K, Shapiro W R 1981 Isolation, karyotype, and clonal growth of heterogeneous subpopulations of human malignant gliomas. Cancer Research 41: 2349–2359

Sheline G E, Wara W M, Smith V 1980 Therapeutic irradiation and brain injury. International Journal of Radiation Oncology and Biological Physics 6: 1215–1228

Sidransky D, Mikklesen T, Schwechheimer K et al 1992 Clonal expansion of p53 mutant cells is associated with brain tumour progression. Nature 355: 846–847

Sneed P K, Stauffer P R, Gutin P H et al 1991 Interstitial irradiation and hyperthermia for the treatment of recurrent malignant brain tumors. Neurosurgery 28: 206–215

Solomon E, Borrow J, Goddard A D 1991 Chromosome aberrations and cancer. Science 254: 1153–1160

Stea B, Cetas T C, Cassady J R et al 1991 Interstitial thermoradiotherapy of brain tumors: preliminary results of a phase I clinical trial. International Journal of Radiation Oncology and Biological Physics 19: 1463–1471

Stein C A, LaRocca R V, Thomas R et al 1989 Suramin: an anticancer drug with a unique mechanism of action. Journal of Clinical Oncology 7: 499–508

Tabuchi K, Moriya Y, Furuta T et al 1982 S-100 protein in human glial tumours. Qualitative and quantitative studies. Acta Neurochirurgica 65: 239–251

Tashiro T, Yoshida J, Mizuno M et al 1993 Reinforced cytotoxicity of lymphokine-activated killer cells toward glioma cells by transfection with the tumor necrosis factor-alpha gene. Journal of Neurosurgery 78: 252–256

Tel E, Hoshino T, Barker M et al 1980 Effect of surgery on BCNU chemotherapy in a rat brain tumor model. Journal of Neurosurgery 52: 529–532

Toguchida J, Yamaguchi T, Dayton S H et al 1992 Prevalence and spectrum of germline mutations of the p53 gene among patients with sarcoma. New England Journal of Medicine 326: 1301–1308

Tomita T 1991 Interstitial chemotherapy for brain tumors: review. Journal of Neuro-Oncology 10: 57–74

Trojan J, Johnson T R, Rudin S D et al 1993 Treatment and prevention of rat glioblastoma by immunogenic C6 cells expressing antisense insulin-like growth factor I RNA. Science 259: 94–97

U H S, Kelley P Y, Hatton J D et al 1989 Proto-oncogene abnormalities and their relationship to tumorigenicity in some human glioblastomas. Journal of Neurosurgery 71: 83–90

Vertosick F T, Selker R G, Pollack I F et al 1992 The treatment of intracranial malignant gliomas using orally administered tamoxifen therapy: preliminary results in a series of "failed" patients. Neurosurgery 30: 897–902

Vogelstein B, Fearon E, Hamilton S et al 1988 Genetic alterations during colorectal-tumor development. New England Journal of Medicine 319: 525–532

von Deimling A, Louis D N, von Ammon K et al 1992 Association of epidermal growth factor receptor gene amplification with loss of chromosome 10 in human glioblastoma multiforme. Journal of Neurosurgery 77: 295–301

Walker M D, Strike T A, Sheline G E 1979 An analysis of dose-effect relationship in the radiotherapy of malignant gliomas. International Journal of Radiation Oncology and Biological Physics 5: 1725–1731

Walker M D, Green S B, Byar D P et al 1980 Randomized comparisons of radiotherapy and nitrosoureas for the treatment of malignant glioma after surgery. New England Journal of Medicine 303: 1323–1329

Weinberg R A 1991 Tumor suppressor genes. Science 254: 1138–1146

Westphal M, Herrmann H-D 1989 Growth factor biology and oncogene activation in human gliomas and their implications for specific therapeutic concepts. Neurosurgery 25: 681–694

Williams J A, Wessels B W, Edwards J A et al 1990 Targeting and therapy of human glioma xenografts in vivo utilizing radiolabeled antibodies. Cancer Research 50: 974s-979s

Woodward W R, Nishi R, Meshul C K et al 1992 Nuclear and cytoplasmic localization of basic fibroblast growth factor in astrocytes and CA2 hippocampal neurons. Journal of Neuroscience 12: 142–152

Yoshida J, Wakabayashi T, Mizuno M et al 1992 Clinical effect of intra-arterial tumor necrosis factor-alpha for malignant glioma. Journal of Neurosurgery 77: 78–83

Young H F, Merchant R E, Apuzzo M L J 1991 Immunocompetence of patients with malignant glioma. In: Salcman M (ed) Neurobiology of brain tumors. Williams & Wilkins, Baltimore, pp 211–227

Yung W-K A, Luna M, Borit A 1985 Vimentin and glial fibrillary acidic protein in human brain tumors. Journal of Neuro-Oncology 3: 35–38

Zhang W, Hara A, Sakai N et al 1993a Radiosensitization and inhibition of deoxyribonucleic acid repair in rat glioma cells by long-term treatment with 12-O-tetradecanoylphorbol 13-acetate. Neurosurgery 32: 432–437

Zhang W, Yamada H, Sakai N et al 1993b Sensitization of C6 glioma cells to radiation by staurosporine, a potent protein kinase C inhibitor. Journal of Neuro-Oncology 15: 1–7

Zovickian J, Youle R J 1988 Efficacy of intrathecal immunotoxin therapy in an animal model of leptomeningeal neoplasia. Journal of Neurosurgery 68: 767–774

Zovickian J, Johnson V G, Youle R J 1987 Potent and specific killing of human malignant brain tumor cells by an anti-transferrin receptor antibody-ricin immunotoxin. Journal of Neurosurgery 66: 850–861

21. Experimental models of brain tumors

Norbert Roosen Mark L. Rosenblum

INTRODUCTION

Effective treatment of brain tumors depends upon the detailed knowledge physicians have of these neoplasms, i.e. their biology, genetics, neuropathology, pathophysiology, and clinical peculiarities. Scientific advances in these areas are imperative to improve upon the still dismal prognosis of most brain tumors. This progress depends on rigorous scientific testing of hypotheses concerning the etiology, the pathogenesis, and the different treatment modalities of brain tumors. Therefore, although it is highly desirable that as many patients as possible participate in clinical studies addressing these questions, many aspects cannot be investigated adequately in the clinical setting and a variety of laboratory models of brain tumors should be available for study.

We provide an overview of several different experimental models that have been used for brain tumor research. We have attempted to survey the field as exhaustively as possible, but a truly comprehensive review of the literature on experimental brain tumor models surpasses the scope of this chapter.

We refer the interested reader to several available excellent reviews on neuro-oncology and brain tumor models published during the past decades. An early, very detailed and comprehensive review published in German by Jänisch & Schreiber in 1969 has been translated and updated in English by Bigner & Swenberg (1977). The use of brain tumor models for experimental chemotherapy in neuro-oncology has been detailed by Barker (1976), and transplantable brain tumors have been specifically addressed by Wilson & Bates (1972). Rubinstein (1977) made correlations between various animal brain tumor models and human neuropathology. Chemical and viral induction of brain tumors has been reviewed by Swenberg (1977), Crafts & Wilson (1977) outlined available animal models of brain tumor, and more recently animal brain tumor models have been reviewed by Schold & Bigner (1983). The study of brain tumor invasion using in vivo and in vitro model systems has been described by Laerum et al (1984). Invasion has been addressed in depth in a monograph by Mareel et al (1991). The use of spheroids in cancer research has been exhaustively summarized by Bjerkvig (1992) in a book which also includes numerous details about their usefulness for neuro-oncology.

First we will address in vitro models for the study of brain tumors and then in vivo models. We will describe these models and highlight their useful features as well as their limitations. It is not the intent of this chapter, however, to discuss the applications of different brain tumor models in detail. Indeed, almost any of these models can be used for a variety of purposes, ranging from the study of basic cell biology to therapeutic applications such as chemosensitivity testing.

IN VITRO MODELS

Cell and tissue culture

The most simple and basic brain tumor model involves the culture of cells in vitro. Early investigators attempted to culture different surgically resected brain tumors as well as tumors that had been induced in animal models. Human tumors have been explanted in vitro and researchers have developed continuously growing cell lines from these tumors. Some cell lines have enjoyed wide use in scientific research, such as a few of the originally derived cell lines by J. Pontén and B. Westermark at the University of Uppsala in Sweden (e.g. U87MG, U105MG, U118MG, U138MG, U178MG, U251MG, U343MG, U373MG, U410MG, U1231MG — Pontén & MacIntyre 1968, Westermark et al 1968, Pontén 1975, Westermark 1973, Pontén & Westermark 1978). Manoury (1977) described the establishment of glial cell lines, as did Manuelidis (1969) and Manuelidis & Manuelidis (1979). Glial fibrillary acidic protein (GFAP) positive cell lines have been described by Manoury et al (1979), Pontén & MacIntyre (1968), Pontén (1975), Black et al (1982), and Studer et al (1985). Other tumors such as neurofibromas (Pleasure et al 1986), meningiomas, and medulloblastomas (McAllister et al 1977, Friedman et al 1983, 1985, Jacobsen et al 1985) have also been developed into cell lines. Neurofibroma cells usually show two predominant cell types: elongated, bipolar or multipolar Schwann-like cells; and flat, pleomorphic fibroblast-like cells (Pleasure et al 1986). Meningioma cells are easily cultured and have a uniform aspect in cell culture despite their variable histological features (Kepes 1982). Different cell populations, such as flat fusiform cells, spindle cells, and flat polygonal cells, can be identified in all these cultures, but the overall aspect does not differ significantly from one tumor culture to another (Bland & Russell 1938). It has not been easy to establish medulloblastoma cell lines. Only a few are available. These medulloblastoma cell lines tend to grow in suspension culture (e.g. D283Med, D384Med, D425Med, D458Med, and D341Med — Friedman et al 1985, 1988, He et al 1989, Bigner et al 1990, He 1990). The Duke lines, as well as the ONS medulloblastoma lines reported by Tamura et al (1989), exhibit a neuronal phenotype. Overall they are negative for glioma-associated antigens such as GFAP and positive for synaptophysin and neurofilament proteins (Friedman et al 1991). The Daoy cell line grows as an adherent monolayer culture (Jacobson et al 1985, He et al 1989). Daoy is positive for glioma-associated antigens, epidermal growth factor receptor, tenascin, and synaptophysin as well (Friedman et al 1991).

These efforts have led to the development of many established tumor cell lines of human and non-human origin. Established cell lines are well characterized with regard to their growth properties, medium requirements, immunocytochemical characteristics, biochemical features, karyotypes, etc. Because established cell lines are so well defined as compared to primary explant cultures, they are often used in experimental studies, and consistent and reproducible results are far more easily obtained with them than with primary explants or early passages from surgically obtained specimens. A series of established human glioma and medulloblastoma cell lines has been characterized and described by Bigner et al (1981) and Studer et al (1985) as well as He et al (1989) and Friedman et al (1991), respectively.

Some basic difficulties exist in cell line characterization. For example, a problem in establishing tumor cell lines is overgrowth by non-neoplastic cells such as fibroblasts, endothelial cells, macrophages, and leptomeningeal cells (Raedler & Raedler 1984, Rutka et al 1986). Also, cells tend to change their characteristics during prolonged culture time. Westphal et al (1990) studied the changes in antigenic properties as revealed by immunocytochemistry during the course of tumor biopsy culturing. Although GFAP staining was positive in most of the early cultures of glioblastomas and low and high grade astrocytomas, the frequency of positively staining cells was much reduced after only 6 weeks in culture. On the other hand, these authors reported one example of a culture in which initially only 1% of cells stained for GFAP, but which finally developed into a 99% positive cell line. Loss of GFAP positivity is usually accompanied by an increase in fibronectin positivity. However, coexpression of fibronectin and GFAP has been shown occasionally (Rutka et al 1987). The differences in findings as reported by Westphal et al (1990) and other investigators such as Kennedy et al (1987) have been attributed to different culture conditions, e.g. the cell cultures reported by Westphal et al (1990) have all been originated on a substrate coated with an extracellular matrix (Westphal et al 1987). A further difficulty is that cell lines may become contaminated by other cell lines carried in the same laboratory (Nelson-Rees & Flandermeyer 1976, Harris et al 1981). The human rhabdomyosarcoma line TE-671 is an example of this phenomenon: initially derived in 1969 (McAllister et al 1969), another cell line has been reported to be of medulloblastoma origin (McAllister et al 1977) but turned out to be the original rhabdomyosarcoma line (Stratton et al 1989a,b). HeLa cells have been known to contaminate several in vitro cell lines (Gartler 1968, Culliton 1974, Nelson-Rees et al 1981). Modern techniques such as DNA finger printing are extremely helpful to identify differences and similarities in various cell populations (Jeffreys et al 1985a,b, Thacker et al 1988, Van Helden et al 1988, Gilbert et al 1990, Honma et al 1992). Finally, as in any type of cell culture, it is important to monitor for mycoplasma infection (Hayflick 1965) because this might invalidate any results obtained.

Evaluation of proliferation and clonogenic capacity

Overall growth potential of cell lines can be evaluated with growth curves and crystal violet and MTT assays. Growth curves are a basic technique for evaluation of in vitro cultured cells and the methodology has been described well in every handbook on cell culture (e.g. Kruse & Patterson 1973, Freshney 1987). A crystal violet assay is performed in tissue culture wells. The cells are stained and the total staining intensity is measured quantitatively by optical absorbance. An image analysis system can be used advantageously. This procedure gives an estimate of the total number of cells in the culture wells. The assay has been used by Frappaz et al (1988) to evaluate the effects of various concentrations of epidermal growth factor on the growth of primary and metastatic central nervous system tumors. The MTT assay is based upon the reduction of tetrazolium compounds by actively metabolizing cells; the assay was initially developed by Mossman (1983) and is now widely used because it is a miniaturized and easily performed assay, e.g. very useful for drug testing. The reduction of MTT by actively metabolizing cells results in the formation of insoluble formazan crystals. These can be redissolved in DMSO or mineral oil. The optical density of the resulting purplish stain can be measured by a computerized microplate absorption reader. The absorption value correlates with the number of living cells in each well. XTT, also a tetrazolium compound, has been used in a similar type of assay (Scudiero et al 1988). A similar method has been described by Skehan et al (1990). These authors selected the dye sulforhodamine B to stain the cells in microwells which can be read by a microplate reader in a similar way as the MTT plates.

Chemosensitivity testing has always been an important field of research in oncology and brain tumor research, and many of the aforementioned techniques have been used for that purpose. These studies are addressed in another chapter of this book. Newly developed drugs must be tested for their cytotoxic efficacy against brain tumor cell lines, and clinicians are interested in obtaining a drug sensitivity profile for the tumor of a particular patient. In vitro cell culture models have been used to perform such chemosensitivity assays. Murray et al (1954) studied chemosensitivity of glioblastoma cells using a double coverslip lying-drop culture. Other investigators followed in publishing their results with in vitro chemosensitivity assaying of brain tumors (Walker & Wright 1961, Easty & Wylie 1963, Gazso & Afra 1969). Colony-forming efficiency assays as developed by Rosenblum et al (1978) have proven useful. More recently, because of its convenience, the MTT or XTT assay has been adopted by many researchers for purposes of chemosensitivity assaying (Carmichael et al 1987, Scudiero et al 1988). The MTT assay's usefulness and limitations for the study of short-term cultures have been worked out by Nikkhah et al (1992a,b). These authors evaluated biopsy specimens from 150 patients (mostly astrocytomas and glioblastomas but other tumors as well, such as oligodendroglioma, ependymoma, and medulloblastoma) for chemosensitivity against carmustine (BCNU), vincristine (ACNU), DIAC, DAG, mitomycin C, and mitoxantrone. MTT assays were performed on cells of passage 1 or passage 2. In 45 cases they did simultaneous colony-forming efficiency assays. Overall, a 10–20% higher resistance against cytotoxic drugs was found with the MTT assay than with the colony-forming efficiency assay. The correlation between histopathological diagnosis and chemosensitivity generally was not good, paralleling clinical findings. A prospective clinical trial to assess the predictive value of the MTT chemosensitivity assay was suggested and is now being performed by the British Medical Research Council's group on brain tumor therapy.

Human tumor stem cell assays that have been developed measure the presence and growth potential of clonogenic tumor cells. These assays commonly use agar layers to inhibit tumor cell migration and to facilitate colony formation. Courtenay & Mills (1978) described the in vitro study of tumor stem cells that originated from human tumors which have been subcultured in immunosuppressed mice. This was a modification of a previous reported technique for mouse tumor stem cells (Courtenay 1976). Hamburger & Salmon (1977) reported an improved human tumor stem cell assay that did not require subculturing of tumor specimens in mice.

Another commonly used assay for the evaluation of growth, more specifically clonogenic growth, of brain tumors is the colony-forming efficiency assay developed by Rosenblum et al (1975a, 1978). This assay has been used advantageously for in vitro evaluation of in vivo chemotherapy (Rosenblum et al 1975a,b, 1981).

Three-dimensional culture models

A different field of research is the development of in vitro culture methods by which the cells can grow in a three-dimensional fashion. This can be realized in different ways: by having cells grow in gels and form three-dimensional colonies, because cell migration is markedly reduced by the gel-containing growth medium; by culturing cells in suspension allowing them to aggregate and form spheroids; and by providing a three-dimensional matrix support for cell growth such as sponges, gelfoam, cellulose polyacetate, etc. Colony formation in gels was first observed by Sanders & Burford (1964) and MacPherson & Montagnier (1964) in hamster kidney cells. This method has been used in radiation research (Nias & Fox 1968), for isolation of single cells (MacPherson 1973), and for cell spheroid culture (Folkman et al 1974, Carlsson 1977). The three-dimensional growth pattern in these cultures results in a tissue-like cell arrangement which in all likelihood is more physiological. Significant, sometimes even surprisingly large differences in chemosensitivity have been described between cells grown in monolayer and those grown in three-dimensional culture (Jung et al 1991). A further three-dimensional culture model uses sponge-gel-supporting matrix (Hoffman 1991). Overall, the properties of three-dimensionally cultured tumor cells seem to equal the properties of in vivo growing tumors better than do monolayer cells (Hoffman 1993). Studies have shown that glioblastoma can be maintained in three-dimensional culture using gelfoam matrix culture (Rubinstein et al 1973, Rubinstein & Herman 1975, Keohane et al 1990).

Although three-dimensional tumor growth in vitro has been used for different purposes, one of the most fruitful areas of scientific study is the problem of tumor cell invasion.

Tumor spheroids have been described by Bradford et al (1990a) and Steinsvåg & Laerum (1985), and many human and experimental brain tumors can be easily cultured as spheroids (Deen et al 1980, Dertinger & Hülser 1981, Darling et al 1983). Although a wide variety of tumor cell lines form spheroids, not all do: of 27 human tumor cell lines examined by Carlsson et al (1983), only 16 formed spheroids, of which 15 also grew as spheroids. Normal tissue did not grow as spheroids, although 7 of 8 tissues examined formed spheroids. Normal lymphoid tissue, however, was successful in spheroid forming and growing as spheroids. The 9L rat brain tumor has been cultured in spheroids to assess its response to radiation and BCNU (Deen et al 1980). Interestingly, the 9L spheroids were more resistant to radiation and to BCNU than were the 9L single cell suspensions. This is in concordance with observations in other cell types grown in three-dimensional culture conditions (Hoffman 1993).

Glioma spheroids have been co-cultured with spheroids obtained from non-tumoral tissues such as fetal rat brain or chicken heart. In these systems spheroids from tumors and from normal tissues come into contact and stick together, and invasion of the normal tissue spheroid by the neoplastic cells can be observed (Fig. 21.1). This model, as well as others, has been used for invasion studies (Mareel 1983).

A wide variety of host cells have been used to study brain tumor cells in confrontation type of assays: e.g. chick embryo heart (de Ridder & Laerum 1981), chick chorioallantoic membrane (Dexter et al 1983), developing chick wing bud (Tickle et al 1978), and fetal rat brain aggregates (Steinsvåg et al 1985). These aggregates of fetal rat brain are particularly interesting because they develop into organoid structures consisting of immature brain tissue (Garber & Moscona 1972, Seeds & Haffke 1978, Bjerkvig 1986). The confrontation model developed by Steinsvåg et al (1985) has been studied in comparison with in vitro invasion using the same neurogenic tumor cell lines BT4Cn and BT5C (Laerum et al 1977).

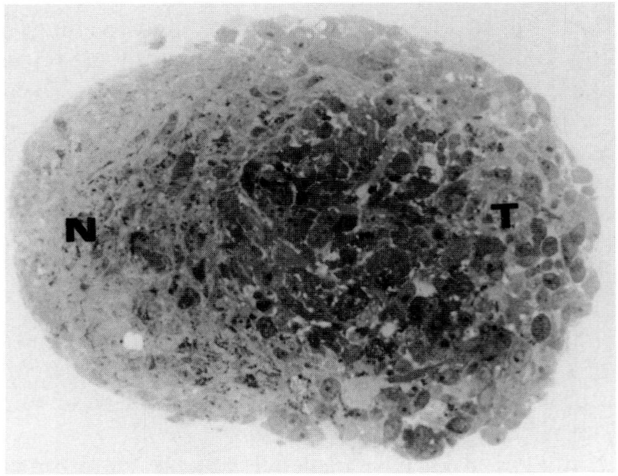

Fig. 21.1 This toluidine blue stained Epon section shows a spheroid grown from BT4CN cells that has been confronted with a fetal rat brain aggregate. The spheroid confrontation assay allows the evaluation of growth and invasion of the tumor cells (T) into the fetal rat brain aggregate (N) in a three-dimensional and almost organotypic way. Microphotograph courtesy of Dr T Mikkelsen and Dr R Bjerkvig.

The authors found a striking similarity between the in vivo and in vitro findings (Bjerkvig et al 1986). Indeed, both cell lines showed the same pattern of invasion in vitro as was found in vivo in syngeneic BD IX rats (Bjerkvig et al 1986). This observation is in the same line as the finding of close similarity in chemosensitivity between in vivo growing tumor cells and three-dimensionally growing tumor cells (Hoffman 1993).

Clinical correlation of in vitro invasiveness with clinical invasiveness has been reported to be excellent in the embryonic chick heart confrontation assay (de Ridder & Calliauw 1992). These authors found that the replacement of heart tissue by tumor-derived cells was observed only in confrontation assays using cells derived from malignant tumors with invasive and metastatic characteristics in vivo. They described three different morphologic patterns of interaction between non-neoplastic and neoplastic cells. Type I showed progressive engulfment of tumor-derived tissue by heart tissue. In type II both tissues remained present. Type III demonstrated progressive replacement of heart tissue by tumor-derived cells. Interestingly, a considerable proportion of metastatic tumors (6 of 21) and glioblastomas (9 of 18) revealed a type I result, i.e. non-invasive, and even non-survival of the tumor-derived cells in the confrontation assay. The cells seemed to die by an apoptotic process. The remaining metastatic and glioblastomatous tumors tested in the assay all belonged to type III. None of these tumors belonged to type II in the assay. All meningiomas in their series were convexity meningiomas and macroscopically radically resected. Of the 34 meningiomas, 4 exhibited a type III confrontation assay; histologically, these tumors were either malignant (2 cases) or non-malignant (2 cases). These 4 patients had an unfavorable clinical course, with early death in the case of the 2 malignant meningiomas and early recurrence in the case of one of the two other tumors. All other 30 meningiomas had type I or II confrontation assays.

Unfortunately, cells from freshly dissociated tumor specimens do not survive in these confrontation assays (Backlund & Bjerkvig 1989, de Ridder & Calliauw 1990), and even a considerable number of monolayer flaps used in these assays do not survive (de Ridder & Calliauw 1992). The reasons for this phenomenon are unclear. The requirement for initial subculturing of tissue in vitro makes the technique somewhat less attractive.

Wang & Nicolson (1983) evaluated a subpopulation of murine B16 melanoma cells, specifically selected for rapid brain colonization and invasion, in an in vitro assay using neonatal mouse cerebrum or cerebellum tissue cultured on cellulose polyacetate substrate. These authors favored cellulose polyacetate as a culture substrate because it allowed the neurogenic cells such as glia and neurons to anchor, but did not promote tumor cell spreading and migration. They found that most of the B16 melanoma cells extended pseudopodia and filopodia during their invasion of the brain tissue, which took place quite rapidly. Indeed, within 4 hours invading cells were found deep within the brain tissue. Although some cells retained their spherical shape with a surface covered with numerous microvilli, these cells also were found to invade.

Steinsvåg (1985) described the interactions between malignant rat glioma cells from the BT5C line (Laerum & Rajewsky 1975) and fetal rat brain aggregates, a model developed to mimic more closely clinical invasion of gliomas (Steinsvåg & Laerum 1985). The tumor cells at the border area developed numerous lamellopodia that were present only on the side directed toward the normal brain tissue. Tumor cells covered the surface of the normal brain aggregate and also produced cytoplasmic extensions into the normal tissue aggregate with subsequent invasion. This model is interesting and useful because it uses differentiated brain tissue as a target for invasion by neoplastic glial cells. In vivo the preferred routes of invasion, as seen in a C6 glioma model in rat brain, are on basal lamina and following nerve fiber bundles, intersecting as well as parallel (Bernstein et al 1990).

In vitro models of invasion using basement membrane-like coatings on filters have been developed for the study of invasion and the screening of anti-invasive agents (Hendrix et al 1987, Welch et al 1989). In our laboratory at the University of California, San Francisco, an invasion model for brain tumor cell lines using a single cell suspension has been developed (Amar 1993 personal communication). This model is based upon the cells' ability to penetrate a Matrigel-coated filter with small pore size. Quantification can be performed and correlated with in vivo invasiveness.

IN VIVO MODELS

In vivo brain tumor models can be classified into several categories. Some animals spontaneously develop brain tumors. Different animal models have been described in which the tumors were induced by various carcinogenic agents, most commonly chemical compounds or viruses, more seldom radiation. A major effort toward standardization of brain tumor growth has been done by establishing transplantable brain tumor models. These are either syngeneic or heterogeneic, as well as orthotopic or heterotopic. Most animal tumor models use small rodents such as mice and rats as the host organism. These animals have the advantage of being small, easily available in larger numbers, and manageable with regard to experimental procedures as well as caging and housing. Studies with larger animals, such as rabbits, cats, dogs, even primates, have been reported. The obvious advantage of these larger animal models is the larger brain, which allows for a longer clinical course due to more room for tumor growth. Disadvantages are that the experimental procedures quickly become more elaborate, the number of animals to be used or available is limited, and caging and housing pose a larger financial and personnel burden.

Overall, the main advantage of using animal models as opposed to purely in vitro work is that in vivo studies of chemosensitivity and anticancer drug pharmacology can take advantage of the growth of glioma cells as a tumor within a living organism.

Spontaneous brain tumors in animals

Spontaneous brain tumors in animals are considered rare, but probably are much more frequent than generally presumed (Zülch 1986). McGrath (1962) found 2.83% brain tumors in a series of 6175 dogs. Luginbühl et al (1968) described a large series of animal brain tumors (330 cases). Most tumors occurred in dogs. Meningiomas were found most often in cats.

Spontaneous murine astrocytomas have been described and used to develop cell lines for s.c. or i.c. tumor models, such as the 497-P(1) line from a VM spontaneous murine astrocytoma (Bradford et al 1989, 1990a,b).

A variety of neoplasms have been described in fish (Dawe & Harschbarger 1975), in which peripheral nerve tumors seem to occur relatively frequently (Mawdesly-Thomas 1975). The bicolor damselfish (*Pomacentrus partitus*) of the Florida, Bahamas, and Caribbean sea reefs has been proposed as a suitable model for the study of neurofibromatosis because it is often afflicted with a condition named damselfish neurofibromatosis (Schmale et al 1986). These fish develop numerous pigmented and non-pigmented cutaneous lesions, also involving the fins. On microscopic examination these lesions are identical to neurofibromas. Prevalence rates among this species have been reported between 0.3% and 24% of adults (Schmale 1985).

However, due to their relative rarity and unpredictability, spontaneously occurring brain tumors in animals are not a convenient tumor model for neuro-oncologic research.

Brain tumor induction in animals

Brain tumors have been induced in mice, rats, and other experimental animals with carcinogenic compounds such as aromatic hydrocarbons, N-nitrosoureas, triazenes, etc. The first experimentally induced brain tumors in laboratory animals were reported by Weil (1938), who used white rats and the chemical compound styril-430, an antitrypanosomiasis chemotherapeutic agent. He induced several brain tumors, including meningiomas. 20-methylcholanthrene, 3,4-benzpyrene, and 1,2,5,6-dibenzanthracene are other chemical compounds that have been used for the purpose of chemically inducing experimental brain tumors (Seligman et al 1939, Sweet & Bailey 1941, Zimmerman & Arnold 1941, Arnold & Zimmerman 1943). A mouse ependymoblastoma induced by i.c. application of methylcholanthrene (Zimmerman & Arnold 1941) has been used as an i.c. model to study methotrexate therapy that has been either systemically or intraneoplastically administered (Tator & Wassenaar 1977, Tator et al 1977). Benda et al (1971) developed several glial tumor cell lines in CD Fisher rats that have been injected regularly with N-nitrosomethylurea. One of these tumors (tumor #9) was later carried in culture at the Brain Tumor Research Center of the University of California, San Francisco, under the designation 9L (Fig. 21.2), and developed into one of the most frequently used in vitro and in vivo models (Barker et al 1973). Vazquez-Lopez (1945) first reported feeding of a carcinogen-induced experimental brain tumor. He and others (Hoch-Ligeti & Russell 1951, Oyasu et al 1970) used 2-acetylaminofluorene. The specific type of tumor induced by chemicals cannot be predicted, although some chemicals are more prone to induce particular tumor types, e.g. MNUs are effective inducers of PNS tumors when given intravenously to rats (Denlingger et al 1973). Transplacental induction of brain tumors has been studied in rats (Nir et al 1989, Shibata et al 1989) and in non-human primates (Rice et al 1989). The offspring of these carcinogen-treated animals exhibit a wide variety of brain tumors. Depending upon the exact conditions of the experiment, the tumor incidence can reach as high as 100%, and the induction of certain tumors can be preferentially stimulated. Methylnitrosourea has been used to induce Schwann cell tumors in rats. Jay et al (1986) used this model to study the effects of tamoxifen and estradiol on the tumor development. A high percentage of animals (93% surviving 150 or more days) developed benign and malignant Schwann cell tumors, and daily administration of estradiol and tamoxifen significantly decreased the number of tumors developing. Susceptibility of rats to trigeminal schwannoma induction by neonatal administration of N-ethyl-N-nitrosourea was studied by Naito et al (1985). Males were found to be more susceptible than females.

Radiation is far less effective in inducing brain tumors than carcinogenic compounds or viruses. Mostly mesenchymal tumors were induced, but gliomatous neoplasms have been reported too (McDonald 1970).

Viruses reportedly are able to induce brain tumors, including RNA oncornaviruses such as avian sarcoma virus (ASV), simian sarcoma virus (SSV), and murine sarcoma virus (MSV); DNA papovaviruses such as bovine papilloma virus (BPV), polyomavirus, simian vacuolating virus (SV-40), human papovavirus, and SV-40-human adenovirus 7 hybrids; and DNA adenoviruses such as human adenovirus, simian adenovirus, simian virus 20 (SV-20), and avian adenovirus. Rous sarcoma virus has been reported to induce glial and meningial tumors in dogs (Rabotti et al 1966, Bucciarelli et al 1967, Haguenau et al 1972), as well as in other animals such as the guinea pig (Ahlstrom et al 1974). Meningiomas have been induced with BPV in calves (Lancaster et al 1967), in cats (Gordon & Olson 1968), and in hamsters (Robl et al 1972). Examples of well-known tumors induced by

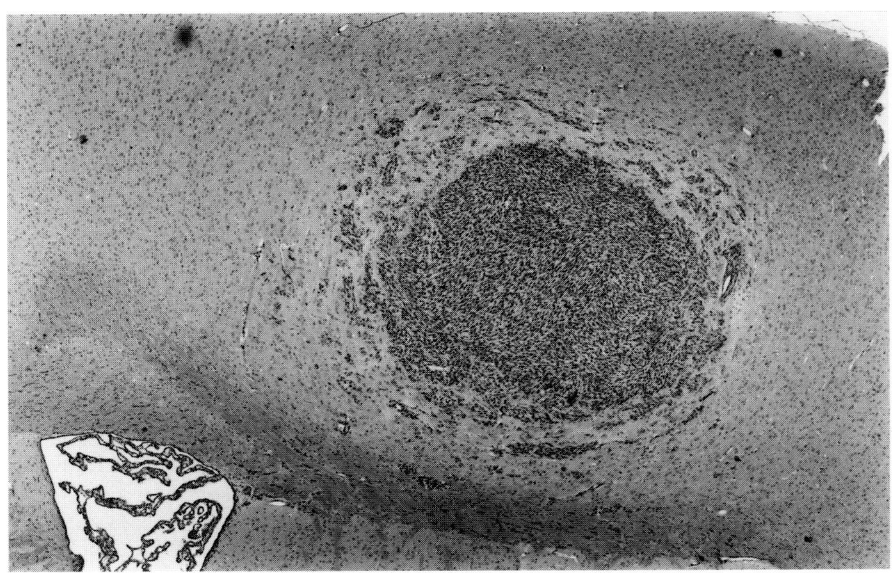

Fig. 21.2 Syngeneic 9L gliosarcoma cells have been used extensively to grow intracerebral brain tumors in F344 rats. In addition to its predominantly spherical growth pattern, a rim of invasively proliferating cells at the tumor periphery can be seen. H&E.

chemical or viral carcinogenesis include 9L, C6, RG2, RT2 (ASV induced), SR-B10.A (Rous sarcoma virus induced — Sakamoto et al 1989), etc. More recently molecular biology techniques have been applied to the study of viral oncogenesis. Entire viral genomes or part of these have been introduced into fertilized mouse eggs and transgenic animals have been developed (Feigenbaum et al 1993). Olfactory neuroblastomas developed in mice that carried the entire early (E1) region of human adenovirus type 12 under control of mouse mammary tumor virus long terminal repeat, and a large number of mature retrovirus particles were present in these tumors (Koike et al 1990). Clinical observations have associated the human DNA virus, JCV, which causes progressive multifocal leukencephalopathy, with an increased incidence of gliomas (Castaigne et al 1974, Sima et al 1983). Interestingly, transgenic mice containing the entire early region of JCV express a marked neurotropism and develop tumors of the adrenal medulla that resemble adrenal medulla neuroblastoma, and tumors of the myenteric plexus, arising from the ganglion cells (Small et al 1986a,b, Feigenbaum et al 1992). The tissue specificity of JCV, i.e. its neurotropism, seems to be determined by its enhancer/promotor region, because the incorporation of a different enhancer/promotor region such as from SV-40, a highly related virus, resulted in tumors of epithelial cells in the choroid plexus, the thyroid, and kidneys (Feigenbaum et al 1992). These JCV transgenic mice did not develop brain tumors, but direct inoculation of JCV has caused the development of brain tumors in hamsters and owl monkeys, albeit after a long latency (Padgett et al 1977, Nagashima et al 1984, Major et al 1987). Transgenic mice expressing the *Tax* protein of human T-cell leukemia virus type I have been found to develop neurofibromas of nerve sheets that are strikingly similar to the neurofibromas seen in von Recklinghausen disease (Nerenberg et al 1987, Hinrichs et al 1987). Tumors of the peripheral as well as cranial nerves have been found. Among the cranial nerves, the trigeminal nerve was often affected, a finding which parallels clinical experience in neurofibromatosis patients. The high incidence of spontaneously occurring, nonfamilial neurofibromatosis in the population (about 50% of patients not having a family history) has been used as evidence for an infectious etiology of the disease, and the results of the cited transgenic mice studies indeed support such a hypothesis. The main difference between the JCV-induced tumors and the HTLV-I-related tumors is that the expression of the JCV T antigen is restricted to neural cells by the viral transcriptional regulatory element, whereas the HTLV-I *Tax* protein, although being expressed in all tissues, does not cause tumors in non-nerve sheath cells, probably because of an as yet unknown host factor (Feigenbaum et al 1993). Transgenic mice expressing SV-40 large T-antigen under control of a complete SV-40 enhancer and the SV-40 promotor showed the development of neuroectodermal tumors originating in the pineal gland (Theuring et al 1990).

Brain tumors implanted into small rodent animals

Brain tumors can be implanted into the brain of animals in different ways, such as freehand injection of cell suspensions or alternatively stereotactic injections or implantation into aspiration pockets in the brain cortex. They can also be implanted into the subarachnoid space. Furthermore, implantation into extracerebral sites is an option: the subcutaneous tissue has been used frequently, as has the subrenal capsule tissue. In some tumor model systems the tumor cells to be implanted originate from in vitro cultures, whereas in other systems the tumors are serially passed from animal to animal. The optimal technique for needle injection of cell suspensions has been addressed in several papers. The use of a skull screw and bone wax to reduce the amount of reflux has been described (Barker et al 1973). Other authors use an agar-containing cell suspension (Kobayashi et al 1980). The parameters of cell injection such as volume and velocity of injection have been studied by Plunkett et al (1988, 1989), who found optimal results with a relatively slow (i.e. ± 5 μl/min) injection of up to 10 μl of cell suspension.

Davaki & Lantos (1980) compared the pathology of brain tumors of murine origin transplanted into syngeneic rats, according to the passage level of the in vitro cultures in which the A15A5 cell line was maintained. Earlier passages showed less malignant tumors intracranially, whereas older passages led to a more malignant phenotype with major variability in cellular size, shape, extracellular space, hemorrhage into the tumor, vascularity, and invasion of peritumoral tissues. These same authors (Davaki & Lantos 1981) described the ultrastructure of a rat brain tumor model in which A15A5 tumor cells have been implanted into syngeneic BD IX rats.

The 9L rat gliosarcoma was used to develop an intracerebral tumor model by Barker et al (1979). (The 9L subline was one reconstituted in the early 1970s from a culture sent to the University of California San Francisco from the Brain Tumor Research Center of the National Cancer Institute.) The model has been well defined and characterized and has since been extensively used in neurooncologic research (Fig. 21.2). Henderson et al (1981) used it to evaluate radiation therapy in rats carrying the 9L tumor i.c. Barker et al (1979) investigated combined BCNU and radiation therapy with the 9L intracerebral tumor model, whereas Kimler et al (1992) studied various chemotherapy agents such as BCNU, bleomycin, AZQ, CDDP, and acivicin, and applied these agents s.c., i.p., or i.c.

Other implantation models include a syngeneic intracerebral model in rats with implantation of BT4An into rat brain (Mella et al 1990) and metastatic tumors such as Walker 256 tumors implanted into rats (King et al 1991).

The murine C6 glioma has been derived from an MNU-induced rat glioma (Benda et al 1971) and has been used frequently in experimental neuro-oncology. It was derived from the cloned cells of an MNU-induced rat glioma (Bissell et al 1974, Benda et al 1968). C6 murine glioma has been implanted i.c. by Mineura et al (1992), who have studied the effect of intracarotid chemotherapy with nimustine on the proliferation characteristics of the glioma.

Glioma cell invasion and migration have been studied using the C6 glioma in rat brain (Bernstein et al 1990). Elaborating on these studies with C6, human malignant glioma xenografts have been introduced into the brain of Sprague-Dawley rats and the migration of these tumor cells followed (Bernstein et al 1989). Grafted astrocytoma cells were found on the glia limitans, in the Virchow-Robin spaces, migrating along the blood vessels and between sub- and ependymal layers in the ventricles. The presence of basal lamina and of parallel nerve bundles was a common feature in these migration routes. In a further study, these authors implanted human brain tumors (low and high grade astrocytomas) in non-immunosuppressed Sprague-Dawley rats to study brain invasion by these tumors (Bernstein et al 1993). These authors were able to follow the invasive migration of human tumor cells into rat brain by staining these cells for the human specific $p185^{c\text{-}neu.}$ An alternative method of tracking human cells within a population of non-human cells takes advantage of genomic *alu* sequences, highly specific for human DNA (Jelinek & Schmid 1982, Lee et al 1990, DeArmond 1993 personal communication).

Vogel & Berry (1975) transplanted human meningiomas into the chorioallantoic membrane of the chick embryo.

Metastatic tumors have been used as intracerebral models. In the study of brain metastasis an important distinction needs to be made between models that use carcinomas or sarcomas for i.c. inoculation and models in which the tumor cells are administered through the arterial circulation. The latter models are probably more relevant for the study of metastasis and invasion of non-cerebral tumor cells through the blood-brain barrier and into nervous tissue.

The use of carcinoma cells for i.c. inoculation has been reported by many authors. Norrell & Wilson (1965) reported the use of a methylcholanthrene-induced rat mammary carcinoma to study experimental intra-arterial chemotherapy in the rat.

Some publications have addressed the methodology of administering the neoplastic cells through the circulation. McCutcheon et al (1990) used intracardiac injection of KHT sarcoma cells to develop brain metastases in mice. Lymphomas have been studied by Keyaki et al (1988) in mouse brain. K-1735 melanoma cells were injected into the carotid arteries of mice by Schackert & Fidler (1988), who were successful in establishing brain metastases of these tumor cells. The number of animal models of brain metastasis is relatively limited. Melanoma has been used by Brunson et al (1978), Raz & Hart (1980), and Kawaguchi et al (1985). Ballinger & Schimpff (1979) used other models. Conley (1979, 1982a,b, 1984) used KHT fibrosarcoma cells. Ushio et al (1977) and Hasegawa et al (1983) introduced Walker 256 carcinoma cells selectively into the intracranial internal carotid artery of rats.

Intracerebellar growth of RG2 (a well-established rat glioma transplacentally induced by N-nitrosourea — Ko et al 1980) after subdural implantation of multicellular tumor spheroids has been reported as a model for invasion of normal brain tissue (Krajewski et al 1986). This experimental model is of interest because it does not involve an implantation procedure that disrupts nervous tissue.

Subrenal capsule assays have been used in experimental neuro-oncology, as by Weiszäcker et al (1983). Experimental neurinomas and also human meningiomas have been studied with this type of assay (Krajewski et al 1984, Medhkour et al 1989). Acoustic neurinomas (vestibular schwannomas), neurofibromas, and schwannomas, however, appear to grow better in the sciatic nerve than in a subrenal capsule assay in nude mice (Lee et al 1990, 1992).

The host can be of importance in determining the features of a transplanted brain tumor. San-Galli et al (1989) reported that implantation of C6 glioma cells into Wistar rats resulted in tumors that were histologically much closer to spontaneous glioblastomas than C6 tumors implanted into other rat strains.

Xenografting human brain tumors into animals

Human brain tumors can be introduced into other species. Sometimes animals are not prepared specifically and therefore implanted tumors will not grow well or even not take at all due to the immunocompetence of the host. Nevertheless, human malignant astrocytomas have been xenotransplanted into the brains of non-immunosuppressed or immunodeficient Sprague-Dawley rats with an acceptable take rate of 2 in 3 (Strömblad et al 1982), probably taking advantage of the brain's immunoprivileged site. In any case, this might be sufficient for short-term studies. Another example is a xenografted human oligodendroglioma-derived line that was used in rat experiments with i.p. and intracisternal methotrexate application (Wilson et al 1967). Antithymocyte serum was used in neonatal F344 rats to make them immunosuppressed, and subsequently the human glioma cell line D54MG was implanted intracerebrally (Vriesendorp et al 1987).

In order to achieve a better take rate and especially to obtain long-term tumor growth, however, it is necessary to decrease the host's immunocompetence. Several methods are available to achieve this purpose. Antithymocyte serum was used in neonatal F344 rats to make them immunosuppressed, and subsequently the human glioma cell line D54MG was implanted intracerebrally (Vriesendorp et al 1987). Nowadays, the athymic nude mouse xenograft model is the most commonly used (Fig. 21.3). Because of the nude mouse's immunodeficiency, xenografts have a high take rate. On the other hand, these mice are still sufficiently immunocompetent not to make their handling in the laboratory and animal care facilities too cumbersome and difficult, as compared to other mice strains that have more severe and/or combined immunodeficiencies. Tumor take rate after s.c. implantation has been reported to be even higher when the cells are admixed with Matrigel, a complex mixture of basement membrane components rich in laminin (Sweeney et al 1991). Gliomas usually are implanted subcutaneously in nude mice, as reported by many authors (Shapiro et al 1979, Horten et al 1981, Bamberg et al 1988). The subcutaneous xenograft is an easily accessible and evaluable tumor model because of its subcutaneous localization. Tumor growth is conveniently measurable and tumors can be grown relatively large, ensuring a generous supply of tissues for study. For example, medulloblastoma has been implanted subcutaneously in athymic mice and this model has been used for blood flow and blood-to-tissue transport studies with quantitative autoradiography (Warnke et al 1987). The rhabdomyosarcoma cell line TE671 (McAllister et al 1977) has been introduced subcutaneously into nude mice for chemotherapy studies (Houchens et al 1983). Although cited as a medulloblastoma-derived cell line in some publications, the TE671 line has been shown to be of rhabdomyosarcomatous origin (Stratton et al 1989a,b).

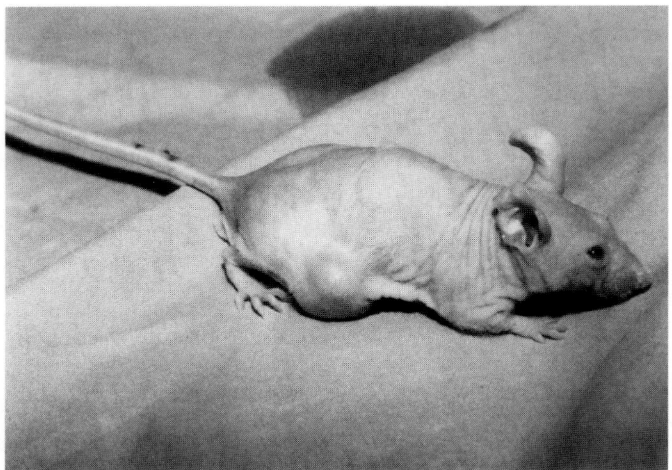

Fig. 21.3 The immunodeficient athymic 'nude' mouse is a convenient host animal for several brain tumor cell lines. This mouse carries a subcutaneous xenograft of the tumorigenic glioblastoma line U251MG. The tumor is seen as a conspicuous nodule in the flank of the depicted animal just in front of the right hindleg.

In some reports other sites, such as intracerebral, have been used (Shapiro et al 1979, Horten et al 1981). Intracerebrally implanted astrocytomas grew in three different patterns (Basler & Shapiro 1982). Some tumors grew diffusely infiltrating the hemispheres, some grew as discrete nodules, and a few grew as discrete nodules with some diffuse borders towards the surrounding brain. A predominantly infiltrating type of growth has been reported by Horten et al (1981).

An intrathecal model has been developed by Abernathey et al (1988). These authors injected glioma line U87MG into the lumbar subarachnoid space by lumbar puncture and were able to obtain a spinal syndrome in all mice inoculated with tumor.

Human acoustic neurinomas (vestibular schwannomas), neurofibromas, and schwannomas have been transplanted into nude mice by Lee et al (1992). They compared the subrenal capsule assay with implantation into the sciatic nerve and found these tumors grew more readily in the sciatic nerve of the experimental animals, better retaining their original histologic characteristics. Appenzeller et al (1986) made mice immuno-incompetent and transplanted Schwann cells from normal sural nerve, neurofibroma, and malignant schwannoma from neurofibromatosis patients into the sciatic nerves of these mice. They showed that sural nerve Schwann cells of a patient with neurofibromatosis myelinated the mouse axons regularly, whereas neurofibroma and malignant schwannoma Schwann cells could not do this. Meningiomas have been implanted with a high take rate, either as solid tissue fragments or as cell suspensions, into kidneys of nude mice for use in a subrenal capsule assay (Medhkour et al 1989).

Except for gliomas, other tumors such as carcinomas and metastases or even craniopharyngiomas have been implanted into nude mice (Bullard & Bigner 1979, Bamberg et al 1988, Stranahan et al 1992).

Effects from chemotherapy as well as from other therapeutic modalities can be easily monitored in tumors carried as a xenograft by nude mice. The D54MG cell line has been implanted intracerebrally in nude athymic mice and its sensitivity against procarbazine, BCNU, AZQ, and CDDP determined (Schold et al 1983). Other cell lines have also been used for testing BCNU in s.c. xenografts in nude mice (Bullard et al 1981).

Four different medulloblastoma cell lines have been used in extensive phenotypic characterization studies in vitro as well as in vivo using i.c. xenografts in nude athymic rats (He et al 1989).

Nude rats (Fig. 21.4) have only infrequently been used for intracerebral tumor models as mentioned in a few reports. Magnetic resonance imaging (MRI) of sodium ions

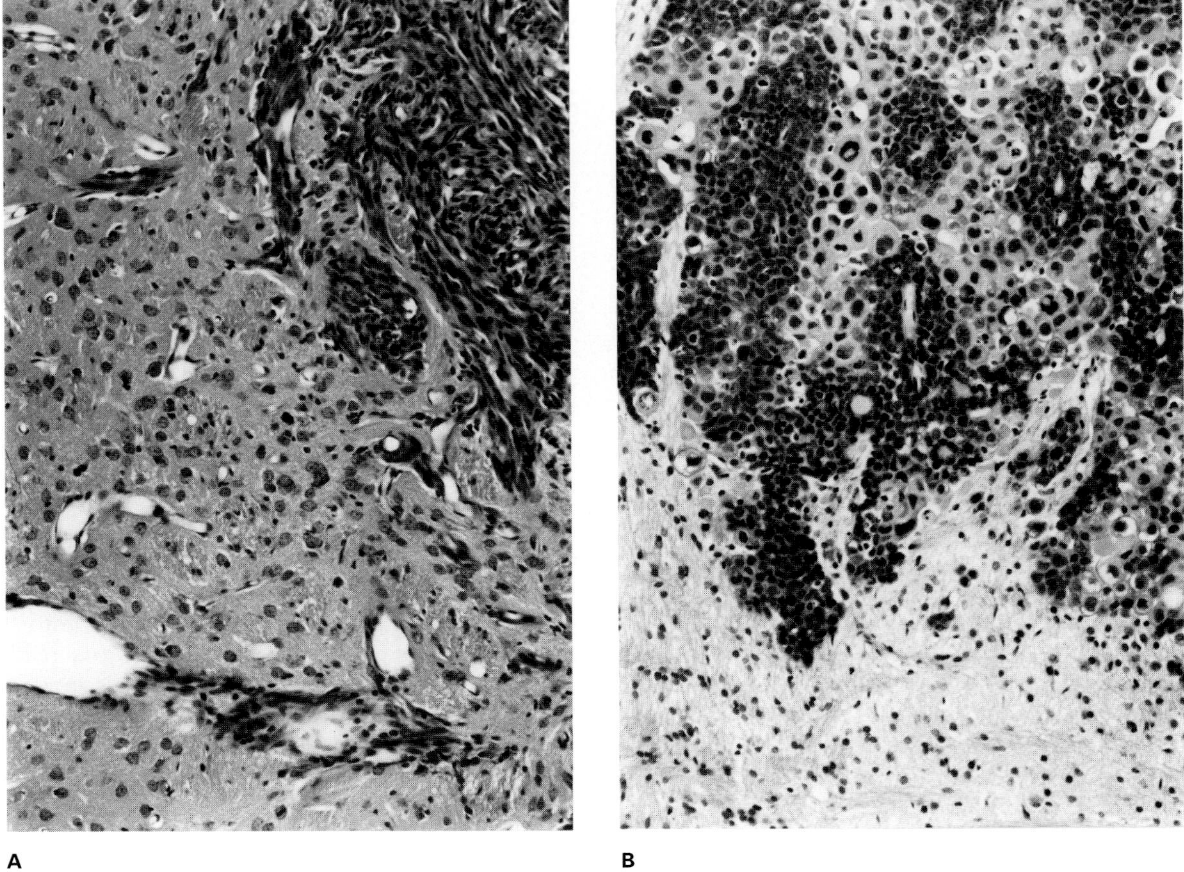

Fig. 21.4 Intracerebral xenografts offer a distinct advantage for experimental studies as compared to other implantation sites. Intracerebral xenografts in immunodeficient athymic 'nude' rats show different growth patterns, as exemplified by 251MG **A** and SF767 **B**. U251MG exhibits an irregular border with cellular infiltration into peritumoral brain whereas SF767 remains well circumscribed and reveals almost no cell invasion. H&E.

has been described in such a model (Griffey et al 1990). Wrobel et al (1990) grew the human small cell lung carcinoma N417D intracerebrally in the nude rat. They used the model to evaluate intravenous diphtheria toxin as a therapeutic modality. Control animals had a median survival of 15 days, whereas animals treated with 1.0 μg/animal had extended median survival times of 26.5 days ($p < 0.0002$). This showed adequate permeability of the blood-tumor barrier for large-size molecules such as diphtheria toxin and possibly also immunotoxins. Neuwelt et al (1985) have described the permeability characteristics of this particular brain tumor model.

Rhabdomyosarcoma also has been grown intracerebrally in nude rats and used for blood flow and blood-to-tissue transport measurements (Warnke et al 1987).

Bernsen et al (1992) have reported the development of a human brain tumor model in the nude rat. Astrocytoma grade III and IV were passaged subcutaneously 4 times in nude mice prior to inoculation into the brains of nude rats. Tumor growth was demonstrated in 16 of 21 nude rats by histologic methods. Nuclear magnetic resonance (NMR) studies of these animals were done with a 6.3 T magnet using a spin-echo T_2-weighted imaging sequence for growth monitoring and image-guided ^1H NMR spectroscopy for the assessment of regional differences in choline-containing compounds, phosphocreatine, N-acetyl-aspartate, and lactate. Histologically, tumors usually grew as spherical masses. Brain adjacent to tumor demonstrated a variable amount of infiltration and invasion. Edema was also present. Tumor growth was variable and became detectable by NMR imaging after a few weeks up to several months. Increases in the signals of lactate and choline-containing compounds were seen over time accompanying continuous growth of the tumors, as well as decreases in phosphocreatine and N-acetyl-aspartate signals. These results are comparable to the experimental findings in C6 rat gliomas implanted in rat brain (Remy et al 1989) and to clinical findings in ^1H NMR spectroscopy of human astrocytomas in situ (Bruhn et al 1989, Segebarth et al 1990, Gill et al 1990).

Schuster et al (1993) reported encouraging results of intra-arterial chemotherapy with 4-hydroperoxycyclophosphamide in the treatment of the human-derived D54MG glioma cell line, xenografted into the brain of nude rats.

A particular problem with nude rats is that they are less efficient in the acceptance of xenografts than are nude mice. As in nude mice, the best take rate is obtained in younger animals (Colston et al 1981, Maruo et al 1982). The same authors also reported a much higher spontaneous regression of initially growing tumors in nude rats than in nude mice (Colston et al 1981, Maruo et al 1982).

Experimental cerebrospinal fluid pathway gliomatosis has been established in a rat model by Rewers et al (1990). The 9L gliosarcoma has been used for this purpose. The model was reproducible in the development of neurologic symptoms. Most animals developed hydrocephalus after the injection of 9L cells into the lateral ventricle. The survival time was highly dependent upon the number of cells injected: 5×10^5 cells resulting in 18 days, 5×10^4 in 24 days, and 5×10^3 cells in 29 days survival. Yoshida et al (1986) used C6 and 9L glioma cells to develop experimental meningeal gliomatosis in rats. Injection of at least 10^6 cells resulted in reliable tumor growth. Fuchs et al (1990) used two different cell lines to develop an experimental model of neoplastic meningitis in the nude rat. They used the human rhabdomyosarcoma line TE671 (McAllister et al 1969, 1977, Stratton et al 1989a,b) and the human glioma line D54MG (Giard et al 1973).

Schabet et al (1987, 1989) developed a meningeal melanomatosis model in nude rats with the B16 mouse melanoma cells. This model was used by Martos et al (1992) to evaluate tumor growth and progression with MRI, using also the paramagnetic contrast agent gadolinium-DTPA. It was also used to investigate the efficacy of ACNU for therapy of this condition (Schabet et al 1992).

Molecular genetics and transgenic animal models

Examples of molecular biological manipulations used in neuro-oncologic research have been mentioned in the subsection on viral induction of brain tumors in animals. Additional examples will be given here. The techniques are used to elucidate neuro-oncogenesis or to design novel and promising therapies.

Rat C6 gliomas (Benda et al 1968), normally expressing high amounts of insulin-like growth factor I (IGF-I), have been stably transfected with an antisense IGF-I cDNA (Trojan et al 1992). This resulted in abrogation of their tumorigenicity in syngeneic rats. Also s.c. injection of transfected C6 cells prevented formation of s.c. as well as i.c. tumors by subsequent injection of non-transfected C6 cells (Trojan et al 1993). Furthermore, antisense IGF-I cDNA transfected cells caused regression of existing C6 tumors if injected at a distant site of these tumors (Trojan et al 1993).

Subcutaneous and intracranial U87MG glioblastoma cells were used in a nude mouse model by Martuza (1991) to evaluate a new antiglioma therapy using genetically engineered strains of the neurotropic virus herpes simplex-1. The thymidine kinase-deficient mutant strains cannot replicate in non-dividing cells (i.e. in normal brain), whereas they can replicate in dividing cells (i.e. tumor cells), thereby causing lysis of glioma cells (Martuza et al 1991, Markert et al 1993). Initial studies showed an amazing activity against the glioma cells, although a considerable incidence of herpes encephalitis was also found (Martuza et al 1991, Markert et al 1993). Newly developed herpes simplex-1 strains, however, seem to obviate this problem (Markert et al 1993). Interestingly, some of the mutant attenuated herpes simplex-1 strains used in these studies still show an acceptable sensitivity for the commonly used antiherpetic drugs acyclovir and ganciclovir (Markert et al 1993). This may allow treatment of encephalitic side effects should this brain tumor treatment concept be introduced into clinical trial.

Transgenic mice have been developed that have inheritable retinoblastomas bilaterally and multifocally in their eyes (O'Brien et al 1990, Marcus et al 1991). These animals developed retinoblastomas in 100% of cases and also central nervous system tumors in 15–27% of cases. These cerebral tumors have been characterized as primitive neuroectodermal tumors of the midbrain. They arose from the subependymal cells of the cerebral aqueduct.

Large animal models of brain tumors

Bayens-Simmonds et al (1988, 1989) reported on the establishment of 9L tumors in cat brains. No immunosuppression was required and an 88% take rate was obtained. The F98 rat glioma clone was xenotransplanted into the internal capsule of cats by Wechsler et al (1989) and Hossmann et al (1989) who studied the neuropathology as well as edema formation and protein and water content of edematous regions in the cat brains by MRI. In another publication from the same research group, biochemical studies were reported (Linn et al 1989). Kabuto et al (1990) used cats to grow the rat glioma C6 intracerebrally. The cats were not immunosuppressed and survived on average 3 weeks after implantation of 5×10^5 cells. A large animal human brain tumor xenograft model was developed in immunosuppressed cats by Krushelnycky et al (1991). These authors used the cell line D54MG, derived from a human glioblastoma multiforme, and the TE671 human rhabdomyosarcoma cell line. Reproducible results after stereotactic implantation were obtained after pretreating the cats with 120 mg/day of cyclosporine A orally for at least 10 days prior to implantation of 10×10^6 tumor cells. This animal model could be used very well for MRI studies. The tumors were reasonably well circumscribed anaplastic gliomas with some invasion of surrounding normal brain tissue. Although some perivascular lymphocytic cuffing was seen, there was only negligible intratumoral lymphocyte infiltration.

A canine intracerebral gliosarcoma model has been used by Whelan et al (1988) to study gadolinium-enhanced MRI methodology in brain tumors and to compare this to computed tomography and the histologic features of the tumors.

A rabbit brain tumor model was used (Weissman & Grossman 1988, Zagzag et al 1989) to study the development of angiogenesis and the evaluation of brain edema. These authors used the VX2 carcinoma as a tumor model.

Non-human primates also have been used to develop a brain tumor model. Ausman et al (1977) reported on the implantation of choriocarcinoma into the brain of rhesus monkeys, as first described by Lewis et al (1968). Dexamethasone effects on tumor-induced brain edema and dexamethasone's distribution within the brain of monkeys have also been investigated with this model (Yamada et al 1979).

Overall, large animal models have the advantage of being better suitable for imaging studies and therapeutic studies than mice and rats; however, they are much more expensive and labor-intensive than small animal brain tumor models.

Experimental tumor models in humans

Although now inconceivable, in the early days of neuro-oncological research brain tumors have been transplanted as autotransplantation in man for the purpose of studying the growth and therapeutic responses of the implants (Bloom et al 1960, Battista et al 1961, Grace et al 1961, Mitts & Walker 1964).

Battista et al (1961) reported follow-up on a patient included in Bloom et al's report (1960). These authors made a saline tumor suspension of an anaplastic astrocytoma that had recurred within 4 months after a previous operation, and injected this solution subcutaneously into six different areas of the patient's anterior thighs. 34 days after implantation they noted the first evidence of subcutaneous tumor growth. These implants were biopsied several times and demonstrated actively growing anaplastic astrocytoma similar to the original tumor. Radiation therapy was given to one of the implants, and repeated biopsies allowed the authors to describe the radiation-induced changes in the tumor tissue.

Grace et al (1961) reported 6 patients in whom they autotransplanted gliomas. The subcutaneous transplants survived in only 2 of the cases, and these tumors were described as 'typical' glioblastoma. Interestingly, 2 of the 4 patients in whom the transplants did not survive showed a positive delayed hypersensitivity reaction against intradermal challenge with normal brain or tumor substance. On the other hand, the 2 patients in whom the transplants grew did not demonstrate similar immunologic phenomena.

Mitts & Walker (1964) described 5 patients with glioblastomas in whom they performed autologous subcutaneous tumor implants. In addition, for control purposes, they implanted 'normal' brain in some of these patients. The tumor implants survived only in 2 patients; the 'normal' brain implants did not survive in any of the patients. The intracerebral tumors in these cases had been described microscopically as glioblastoma with a major sarcomatous component. In the implant the sarcomatous component was very conspicuous and dominated the histologic picture. Malignant glial cells did grow but were not as active as the reticulin fiber-producing sarcomatous cells.

CONCLUSIONS

A variety of tumor models are available in neuro-oncology. This ensures that the appropriate research model can be chosen by individual investigators to answer the research question(s) as accurately as possible. The applications of these various brain tumor models encompass the whole field of neuro-oncology ranging from basic cell biology, biochemistry and physiology to clinically oriented disciplines such as pharmacology and preclinical therapeutics. Accordingly, some of the reviewed models will be described in other chapters of this book, where their discussion will be much more focused on their practical application.

Despite the many models available, additional brain tumor models need to be developed because so many questions in neuro-oncology remain unanswered. We anticipate an increasingly important role for molecular biologic and molecular genetic research systems to elucidate more basic enigmas of brain tumor genesis and to develop better and more efficient therapies. Another area that will show much activity in the near future is the establishment of more clinically relevant brain tumor models using human cell lines and primary cultures in immunodeficient animals, specifically mice and rats. Such models will prove to be invaluable for preclinical research.

REFERENCES

Abernathey C D, Kooistra K L, Wilcox G L, Laws E R Jr 1988 New xenograft model for assessing experimental therapy of central nervous system tumors: human glioblastomas in the intrathecal compartment of the nude mouse. Neurosurgery 22: 877–881

Ahlstrom C G, Olin T, Smitterberg B 1974 Intracranial tumors induced in guinea pigs with Rous sarcoma virus. Acta Pathologica et Microbiologica Scandinavica [C] 82: 326–336

Appenzeller O, Kornfeld M, Atkinson R, Snyder R D 1986

Neurofibromatosis xenografts. Contribution to pathogenesis. Journal of Neurological Sciences 74: 69–77

Arnold H, Zimmerman H M 1943 Experimental brain tumors. III. Tumors produced with dibenzathracene. Cancer Research 3: 682–665

Ausman J I, Levin V A, Brown W E, Rall D P, Fenstermacher J D 1977 Brain tumor chemotherapy. Pharmacological principles derived from a monkey brain-tumor model. Journal of Neurosurgery 46: 155–164

Backlund E, Bjerkvig R 1989 Stereotactic biopsies as a model for studying the interaction between gliomas and normal brain tissue in vitro. Journal of Neurosurgical Science 33: 31–33

Ballinger W E, Schimpff R D 1979 An experimental model for cerebral metastasis: preliminary light and ultrastructural studies. Journal of Neuropathology and Experimental Neurology 38: 19–34

Bamberg M, Budach V, Stuschke M, Gerhard L, Streffer C 1988 Heterotransplantation of a human glioma and brain metastases in the athymic nude mouse — a preclinical model for radiation oncology. 1. Basic principles and methodology. Strahlenklinik und Onkologie 164: 235–243

Barker M 1976 Experimental chemotherapy models. In: Fewer D, Wilson C B, Levin V A (eds) Brain tumor chemotherapy. Charles C Thomas, Springfield, IL, pp 75–95

Barker M, Hoshino T, Gurcay O, Wilson C B, Nielsen S L, Downie R, Eliason J 1973 Development of an animal brain tumor model and its response to therapy with 1,3-bis(2-chloroethyl)-1-nitrosourea. Cancer Research 33: 976–986

Barker M, Deen D F, Baker D G 1979 BCNU and X-ray therapy of intracerebral 9L rat tumors. International Journal of Radiation Oncology Biology Physics 5: 1581–1583

Basler G A, Shapiro W R 1982 Brain tumor research with nude mice. The Nude Mouse in Experimental and Clinical Research 2: 475–490

Battista A F, Bloom W, Loffman M, Feigin I 1961 Autotransplantation of anaplastic astrocytoma into the subcutaneous tissue of man. Neurology 11: 977–981

Bayens-Simmonds J, Boisvert D P, Castro M E, Johnson E S 1988 A feline model for experimental studies of peritumor brain edema. Journal of Neuro-Oncology 6: 371–378

Bayens-Simmonds J, Boisvert D P, Baker G B 1989 Regional monoamine and metabolite levels in a feline brain tumor model. Molecular and Chemical Neuropathology 10: 63–75

Benda P, Lightbody J, Sato G, Levine L, Sweet W 1968 Differentiated rat glial cell strain in tissue culture. Science 161: 370–371

Benda P, Someda K, Messer J, Sweet W H 1971 Morphological and immunochemical studies of rat glial tumors and clonal strains propagated in culture. Journal of Neurosurgery 34: 310–323

Bernsen H J J A, Heerschap A, van der Kogel A J et al 1992 Image-guided 1H NMR spectroscopical and histological characterization of a human brain tumor model in the nude rat; a new approach to monitor changes in tumor metabolism. Journal of Neuro-Oncology 13: 119–130

Bernstein J J, Goldberg W J, Laws E R Jr 1989 Human malignant astrocytoma xenografts migrate in rat brain: a model for central nervous system cancer research. Journal of Neuroscience Research 22: 134–143

Bernstein J J, Goldberg W J, Laws E R Jr, Conger D, Morreale V, Wood L R 1990 C6 glioma cell invasion and migration of rat brain after neural homografting: ultrastructure. Neurosurgery 26: 622–628

Bernstein J J, Anagnostopoulos A V, Hattwick E A, Laws E R Jr 1993 Human-specific c-*neu* proto-oncogene protein overexpression in human malignant astrocytomas before and after xenografting. Journal of Neurosurgery 78: 240–251

Bigner D D, Swenberg J A (eds) 1977 Jänisch and Schreiber's experimental tumors of the central nervous system. The Upjohn Company, Kalamazoo, MI, p 160

Bigner D D, Bigner S H, Pontén J et al 1981 Heterogeneity of morphologic and other phenotypic characteristics of fifteen permanent cell lines derived from human gliomas. Journal of Neuropathology and Experimental Neurology 40: 201–229

Bigner S H, Friedman H S, Vogelstein B, Oakes W J, Bigner D D 1990 Amplification of the c-*myc* gene in human medulloblastoma cell lines and xenografts. Cancer Research 50: 2347–2350

Bissell M G, Rubinstein L J, Bignami A, Herman M M 1974 Characterization of the rat C-6 glioma maintained in organ culture systems. Production of glial fibrillary acidic protein in the absence of gliofibrillogenesis. Brain Research 82: 77

Bjerkvig R 1986 Reaggregation of fetal rat brain cells in a stationary culture system. II. Ultrastructural characterization. In Vitro 22: 192–200

Bjerkvig R 1992 Spheroid culture in cancer research. C R C Press, Boca Raton, FL, p 334

Bjerkvig R, Laerum O D, Mella O 1986 Glioma cell interactions with fetal rat brain aggregates in vitro and with brain tissue in vivo. Cancer Research 46: 4071–4079

Black P McL, Kornblith P L, Davison P F et al 1982 Immunological, biochemical, ultrastructural, and electrophysiological characteristics of a human glioblastoma-derived cell culture line. Journal of Neurosurgery 56: 62–72

Bland J O W, Russell D 1938 Histological types of meningiomata and a comparison of their behavior in tissue culture with that of certain normal human tissues. Journal of Pathology and Bacteriology 50: 53–59

Bloom W, Carstairs K, Crompton M, McKissock W 1960 Autologous glioma transplantation. Lancet ii: 77–78

Bradford R, Darling J L, Thomas D G 1989 The development of an animal model of glioma for use in experimental neuro-oncology. British Journal of Neurosurgery 3: 197–210

Bradford R, Darling J L, Sier N, Thomas D G 1990a The VM model of glioma: preparation of multicellular tumour spheroids (MTS) and their response to chemotherapy. Journal of Neuro-Oncology 9: 105–114

Bradford R, Darling J L, Thomas D G 1990b The chemotherapeutic response of a murine (VM) model of human glioma. British Journal of Cancer 61: 46–50

Bruhn H, Frahm J, Gryngell M L, Merboldt K D, Sauter R, Hamburger C 1989 Noninvasive differentiation of tumors with the use of localized ^{1}H spectroscopy in vivo. Initial experiments in patients with brain tumors. Radiology 172: 541–548

Brunson K W, Beattie G, Nicolson G L 1978 Selection and altered properties of brain-colonising metastatic melanoma. Nature 272: 543–545

Bucciarelli E, Rabiotti G F, Dalton A J 1967 Ultrastructure of meningeal tumors induced in dogs with Rous sarcoma virus. Journal of the National Cancer Institute 38: 359–381

Bullard D E, Bigner D D 1979 Heterotransplantation of human craniopharyngiomas in athymic nude mice. Neurosurgery 4: 308–314

Bullard D E, Schold S C Jr, Bigner S H, Bigner D D 1981 Growth and chemotherapeutic response in athymic mice of tumors arising from human glioma-derived cell lines. Journal of Neuropathology and Experimental Neurology 40: 410–427

Carlsson J 1977 A proliferation gradient in three-dimensional colonies of cultured human glioma cells. International Journal of Cancer 20: 129–136

Carlsson J, Nilsson K, Westermark B et al 1983 Formation and growth of multicellular spheroids of human origin. International Journal of Cancer 31: 523–533

Carmichael J, DeGraff W G, Gazdar A F, Minna J D, Mitchell J B 1987 Evaluation of tetrazolium-based semiautomated colorimetric assay: assessment of chemosensitivity testing. Cancer Research 47: 936–942

Castaigne P, Rondot P, Escourolle R, Ribadeau Dumas J L, Cathala F, Hauw J J 1974 Leucoencéphalopathie multifocale progressive et 'gliomes' multiples. Revue Neurologique (Paris) 130: 379–392

Colston M J, Fieldsteel A H, Dawson P J 1981 Growth and regression of human tumor cell lines in congenitally athymic (rnu/rnu) rats. Journal of the National Cancer Institute 66: 843–848

Conley F K 1979 Development of a metastatic brain tumor model in mice. Cancer Research 39: 1001–1007

Conley F K 1982a Murine models of metastatic neoplasia to the central nervous system. Cancer Metastasis Reviews 1: 203–213

Conley F K 1982b Effect of immunomodulation on the fate of tumor cells in the central nervous system and systemic organs of mice. Distribution of [125I]-5-iodo-2′-deoxyuridine-labeled KHT cells after left intracardial injection. Journal of the National Cancer Institute 69: 465–473

Conley F K 1984 Metastatic brain tumor model in mice that mimics the neoplastic cascade in humans. Neurosurgery 14: 187–192
Courtenay V D 1976 A soft agar colony assay for Lewis lung tumour and B16 melanoma taken directly from the mouse. British Journal of Cancer 34: 39
Courtenay V D, Mills J 1978 An in vitro colony assay for human tumours grown in immune-suppressed mice and treated in vivo with cytotoxic agents. British Journal of Cancer 37: 261–268
Crafts D, Wilson C B 1977 Animals models of brain tumors. National Cancer Institute Monograph 46: 11–17
Culliton B J 1974 HeLa cells: contaminating culture around the world. Science 184: 1058–1059
Darling J L, Oktar N, Thomas D G T 1983 Multicellular tumour spheroid derived from human brain tumours. Cell Biology International Report 7: 23–30
Davaki P, Lantos P L 1980 Morphological analysis of malignancy: A comparative study of transplanted brain tumours. British Journal of Experimental Pathology 61: 655–660
Davaki P, Lantos P L 1981 The development of brain tumours produced in rats by the intracerebral injection of neoplastic glial cells: a fine ultrastructural study. Neuropathology and Applied Neurobiology 7: 49–61
Dawe C J, Harshbarger J C 1975 Neoplasms in feral fishes: their significance to cancer research. In: Ribelin W E, Migaki G (eds) The pathology of fishes. University of Wisconsin Press, Madison, WI, pp 871–894
Deen D F, Hoshino T, Williams M E, Muraoka I, Knebel K D, Barker M 1980 Development of a 9L rat brain tumor cell multicellular spheroid system and its response to 1,3-bis(2-chloroethyl)-1-nitrosourea and radiation. Journal of the National Cancer Institute 64: 1373–1382
Denlingger R H, Koestner A, Swenberg J A 1973 An experimental model for selective production of neoplasms of the peripheral nervous system. Acta Neuropathologica 23: 219–228
de Ridder L, Calliauw L 1990 Invasion of human brain tumors in vitro: relationship to clinical evolution. Journal of Neurosurgery 72: 589–593
de Ridder L, Calliauw L 1992 Invasiveness of primary and secondary brain tumors in vitro correlated with clinical results. Neurosurgery 31: 1043–1048
de Ridder L, Laerum O D 1981 Invasion of rat neurogenic cell lines in embryonic chick heart fragments in vitro. Journal of the National Cancer Institute 66: 723–728
Dertinger H, Hülser D 1981 Increased radioresistance of cells in cultured multicell spheroids. Radiation Environmental Biophysics 19: 101–107
Dexter D L, Lee E S, DeFusco D J, Libbey N P, Spermulli E N, Calabresi P 1983 Selection of metastatic variants using chicken chorioallantoic membrane and nude mice. Cancer Research 43: 1733–1740
Easty D M, Wylie J A 1963 Screening of 12 gliomata against chemotherapeutic agents in vitro. British Medical Journal 5345: 1589
Feigenbaum L, Hinrichs S H, Jay G 1992 JCV and SV40 enhancers and transforming proteins: role in determining tissue specificity and pathogenicity in transgenic mice. Journal of Virology 66: 1176–1182
Feigenbaum L, Ueda H, Jay G 1993 Viral etiology of neurological malignancies in transgenic mice: olfactory neuroblastoma, adrenal and myenteric plexus tumors, and nonfamilial von Recklinghausen neurofibromatosis. In: Levine A J, Schmidek H H (eds) Molecular genetics of nervous system tumors. Wiley Liss, New York, NY, pp 153–161
Folkman J, Hochberg M, Knighton D 1974 Self-regulation of growth in three dimensions: the role of surface area limitation. In: Clarkson B, Baserga R (eds) Control of proliferation in animal cells. Cold Spring Harbor Laboratory Press, Cold Spring Harbor, pp 833–860
Frappaz D, Singletary S E, Spitzer G, Yung A 1988 Enhancement of growth of primary metastatic fresh human tumors of the nervous system by epidermal growth factor in serum-free short term culture. Neurosurgery 23: 355–359
Freshney R I 1987 Culture of animal cells. A manual of basic technique, 2nd edn. Alan R Liss, New York, NY, p 397
Friedman H S, Bigner S H, McComb R D et al 1983 A model for human medulloblastoma: growth, morphology, and chromosomal analysis in vitro and in athymic mice. Journal of Neuropathology and Experimental Neurology 42: 485–503
Friedman H S, Burger P C, Bigner S H, Trojanowski J Q, Wikstrand C J, Halperin E C, Bigner D D 1985 Establishment and characterization of the human medulloblastoma cell line and transplantable xenograft D283 Med. Journal of Neuropathology and Experimental Neurology 44: 592–605
Friedman H S, Burger P C, Bigner S H et al 1988 Phenotypic and genotypic analysis of a human medulloblastoma cell line and transplantable xenograft (D341Med) demonstrating amplification of c-myc. American Journal of Pathology 130: 472–484
Friedman H S, Oakes W J, Bigner S H, Wikstrand C J, Bigner D D 1991 Medulloblastoma: tumor biological and clinical perspectives. Journal of Neuro-Oncology 11: 1–15
Fuchs H E, Archer G E, Colvin O M et al 1990 Activity of intrathecal 4-hydroperoxycyclophosphamide in a nude rat model of human neoplastic meningitis. Cancer Research 50: 1954–1959
Garber B B, Moscona A A 1972 Reconstruction of brain tissue from cell suspensions. II. Specific enhancement of aggregation of embryonic cerebral cells by supernatant from homologous cell cultures. Developmental Biology 27: 235–243
Gartler S M 1968 Apparent HeLa contamination of human heteroploid cell lines: Nature 217: 750–751
Gazso L R, Afra D 1969 Study on the effect of actinomycins in tissue cultures from human brain tumors. Acta Neurochirurgica (Wien) 21: 139
Giard D J, Aaronson S A, Todaro G J, Arnstein P, Kersey J H, Dosile H, Parks W P 1973 In vitro cultivation of human tumors: establishment of cell lines derived from a series of solid tumors. Journal of the National Cancer Institute 51: 1417–1423
Gilbert D A, Reid Y A, Gail M H, Pee D, White C, Hay R J, O'Brien S J 1990 Application of DNA fingerprints for cell-line individualization. American Journal of Human Genetics 47: 499–514
Gill S S, Thomas D G T, Van Bruggen N et al 1990 Proton MR Spectroscopy of intracranial tumors: in vivo and in vitro studies. Journal of Computer Assisted Tomography 14: 497–504
Gordon D E, Olson C 1968 Meningiomas and fibroblastic neoplasia in calves induced with the bovine papilloma virus. Cancer Research 28: 2423–2431
Grace J, Perese D, Metzgar R, Sasabe T, Holdrige B 1961 Tumor autograft responses in patients with glioblastoma multiforme. Journal of Neurosurgery 18: 159–167
Griffey R H, Griffey B V, Mortwiyoff N A 1990 Triple-quantum-wherence-filtered imaging of sodium ions in vivo at 4.7 tesla. Magnetic Resonance in Medicine 13: 305–313
Haguenau F, Rabiotti G F, Lyon G, Moraillon A 1972 Tumeurs cérébrales expérimentales d'étiologie virale chez le chien. Leur similitude histologique avec les tumeurs humaines démontrée par un épendymome. Revue Neurologique (Paris) 126: 347–370
Hamburger A W, Salmon S E 1977 Primary bioassay of human tumor stem cells. Science 197: 461–463
Harris N L, Gang D L, Quay S C, Poppema S, Zamecnik P C, Nelson-Rees W A, O'Brien S J 1981 Contamination of Hodgkin's disease cell culture. Nature 289: 228–230
Hasegawa H, Ushio Y, Hayakawa T, Yamada K, Mogami H 1983 Changes of the blood-brain barrier in experimental metastatic brain tumors. Journal of Neurosurgery 59: 304–310
Hayflick L 1965 Tissue cultures and mycoplasmas. Texas Report in Biology and Medicine 23: 285–303
He X, Skapek S X, Wikstrand C J et al 1989 Phenotypic analysis of four human medulloblastoma cell lines and transplantable xenografts. Journal of Neuropathology and Experimental Neurology 1989: 48–68
He X 1990 Phenotypic analysis of human medulloblastoma and distribution of the gangliosides GD3 and GD2 in human neuroectodermal tumors. Duke University, PhD Thesis, p 197
Henderson S D, Kimler B F, Morantz R A 1981 Radiation therapy of 9L rat brain tumors. International Journal of Radiation Oncology, Biology, Physics 7: 497–502
Hendrix M J C, Seftor E A, Seftor R E B, Fidler I J 1987 A simple quantitative assay for studying the invasive potential of high and low human metastatic variants. Cancer Letters 38: 137–147

Hinrichs S H, Nerenberg M, Reynolds R K, Khoury S, Jay G 1987 A transgenic mouse model for human neurofibromatosis. Science 237: 1340–1343

Hoch-Ligeti C, Russell D S 1951 Primary tumors of the brain and meninges in rats fed 2-acetylaminofluorene. Acta Unionis Internationalis Contra Cancrum 7: 126–129

Hoffman R M 1991 In vitro sensitivity assays in cancer: a review, analysis and prognosis. Journal of Clinical Laboratory Analysis 5: 133–143

Hoffman R M 1993 To do tissue culture in two or three dimensions? That is the question. Stem Cells 11: 105–111

Honma M, Kataoka E, Ohnishi K, Ohno T, Takeuchi M, Nomura N, Mizusawa H 1992 A new DNA profiling system for cell line identification for use in cell banks in Japan. In Vitro Cellular and Developmental Biology 28A: 24–28

Horten B C, Basler G A, Shapiro W R 1981 Xenograft of human malignant glial tumors into brains of nude mice. A histopathological study. Journal of Neuropathology and Experimental Neurology 40: 493–511

Hossmann K A, Szymas J, Seo K, Assheuer J, Krajewski S 1989 Experimental transplantation gliomas in the adult cat brain. 2. Pathophysiology and magnetic resonance imaging. Acta Neurochirurgica 98: 189–200

Houchens D P, Ovejera A A, Riblet S M, Slagel D E 1983 Human brain tumor xenografts in nude mice as a chemotherapy model. European Journal of Cancer and Clinical Oncology 19: 799–805

Jacobsen P F, Jenkyn D J, Papadimitriou J M 1985 Establishment of a human medulloblastoma cell line and its heterotransplantation into nude mice. Journal of Neuropathology and Experimental Neurology 44: 472–485

Jänisch W, Schreiber D 1969 Experimentelle Geschwülste des Zentralnervensystems. VEB Gustav Fischer, Jena, GDR

Jay J R, MacLaughlin D T, Badger T M, Miller D C, Martuza R L 1986 Hormonal modulation of Schwann cell tumors. 1. The effects of estradiol and tamoxifen on methylnitrosourea-induced rat schwann cell tumors. Annals of the New York Academy of Sciences 486: 371–382

Jeffreys A J, Wilson V, Thein S L 1985a Hypervariable minisatellite regions in human DNA. Nature 314: 67–73

Jeffreys A J, Wilson V, Thein S L 1985b Individual specific 'fingerprints' of human DNA. Nature 316: 76–79

Jelinek W R, Schmid C W 1982 Repetitive sequences in eukaryotic DNA and their expression. Annual Review of Biochemistry 51: 813–844

Jung H W, Berens M E, Krouwer H G J, Rosenblum M L 1991 A three-dimensional micro-organ culture system optimized for in vitro growth of human malignant brain tumors. Neurosurgery 29: 390–398

Kabuto M, Hayashi M, Nakagawa T et al 1990 Experimental brain tumor in adult mongrel cat. Brain & Nerve 42: 339–343

Kawaguchi I, Kawaguchi M, Dulski K M, Nicolson G L 1985 Cellular behavior of metastatic B16 melanoma in experimental blood-borne implantation and cerebral invasion. Invasion and Metastasis 5: 16–30

Kennedy P G E, Watkins B A, Thomas D G T, Noble M D 1987 Antigenic expression by cells derived from human gliomas does not correlate with morphologic classification. Neuropathology and Applied Neurobiology 13: 327–347

Keohane M E, Hall S W, VandenBerg S R, Gonias S L 1990 Secretion of alpha2-macroglobulin, alpha2-antiplasmin, and plasminogen activator inhibitor-1 by glioblastoma multiforme in primary organ culture. Journal of Neurosurgery 73: 234–241

Kepes J J 1982 Meningiomas. Biology, pathology, and differential diagnosis. Masson Publishing, New York, NY, p 206

Keyaki A, Handa H, Yamashita J, Kuribayashi K, Masuda T 1988 Immunological response in the mouse brain: II. Experimental immunotherapy model against transplanted mouse lymphoma in the brain. Archiv für Japanische Chirurgie 57: 202–214

Kimler B F, Liu C, Evans R G, Morantz R A 1992 Intracerebral chemotherapy in the 9L rat brain tumor model. Journal of Neuro-Oncology 14: 191–200

King W A, Black K L, Ikezaki K, Conklin S, Becker D P 1991 Tumor-associated neurological dysfunction prevented by lazaroids in rats. Journal of Neurosurgery 74: 112–115

Ko L, Koestner A, Wechsler W 1980 Morphological characterization of nitrosourea-induced glioma cell lines and clones. Acta Neuropathologica 51: 23–31

Kobayashi N, Allen N, Clendenon N R, Ko L W 1980 An improved rat brain-tumor model. Journal of Neurosurgery 53: 808–815

Koike K, Jay G, Hartley J W, Schrenzel M D, Higgins R J, Himrichs S J 1990 Activation of retrovirus in transgenic mice: association with development of olfactory neuroblastoma. Journal of Virology 64: 3988–3991

Krajewski S, Tauber H, Wechsler W 1984 Syngeneic and allogeneic transplantations of RN6-neurinoma spheroids into subrenal capsule of adult rats. Strahlentherapie 160: 54–55

Krajewski S, Kiwit J C W, Wechsler W 1986 RG2 glioma growth in rat cerebellum after subdural implantation. Journal of Neurosurgery 65: 222–229

Kruse P F Jr, Patterson M K Jr 1973 Tissue culture. Methods and applications. Academic Press, New York, NY, p 868

Krushelnycky B W, Farr-Jones M A, Mielke B, McKean J D, Weir B K, Petruk K C 1991 Development of a large-animal human brain tumor xenograft model in immunosuppressed cats. Cancer Research 51: 2430–2437

Laerum O D, Rajewsky M F 1975 Neoplastic transformation of fetal rat brain cells in culture after exposure to ethylnitrosourea in vivo. Journal of the National Cancer Institute 55: 1177–1187

Laerum O D, Rajewsky M F, Schachner M, Stavrou D, Haglid K H, Haugen Å 1977 Phenotypic properties of neoplastic cell lines developed from fetal rat brain cells in culture after exposure to ethylnitrosourea in vivo. Zeitschrift für Krebsforschung 89: 273–295

Laerum O D, Bjerkvig R, Steinsvåg S K, de Ridder L 1984 Invasiveness of primary brain tumors. Cancer Metastasis Reviews 3: 223–236

Lancaster W D, Olson C, Meinke W 1967 Quantitation of bovine papilloma viral DNA in viral-induced tumors. Journal of Virology 17: 824–831

Lee J K, Kim T S, Chiocca E A, Medhkour A, Martuza R L 1990 Growth of human schwannomas in the subrenal capsule of the nude mouse. Neurosurgery 26: 598–605

Lee J K, Sobel R A, Chiocca E A, Kim T S, Martuza R L 1992 Growth of human acoustic neuromas, neurofibromas and schwannomas in the subrenal capsule and sciatic nerve of the nude mouse. Journal of Neuro-Oncology 14: 101–114

Lewis J L Jr, Brown W E Jr, Hertz R, Davis R C, Johnson R H 1968 Heterotransplantation of human choriocarcinoma in monkeys. Cancer Research 28: 2032–2038

Linn F, Seo K, Kossmann K A 1989 Experimental transplantation gliomas in the adult cat brain. 3. Regional biochemistry. Acta Neurochirurgica 99: 85–93

Luginbühl H, Fankhauser R, McGrath J T 1968 Spontaneous neoplasms of the nervous system in animals. Progress in Neurological Surgery 2: 85–86

McAllister R M, Melnyk J, Finklestein J Z, Adams E C, Gardner M B 1969 Cultivation in vitro of cells derived from a human rhabdomyosarcoma. Cancer 24: 520–526

McAllister R M, Isaacs H, Rongey R, Peer M, Au W, Soulap S W, Gardner M B 1977 Establishment of a human medulloblastoma cell line. International Journal of Cancer 20: 206–212

McCutcheon I E, Baranco R A, Katz D A, Saris S C 1990 Adoptive immunotherapy of intracerebral metastases in mice. Journal of Neurosurgery 72: 102–109

McDonald L W 1970 Interaction of chemical carcinogens, radiation and viruses in the production of glial tumors of the central nervous system: Preliminary report of induction of glioma by ionizing radiation. Proceedings of VIth International Congress of Neuropathology. Masson, Paris, pp 564–565

McGrath J T 1962 Intracranial pathology of the dog. Acta Neuropathologica [suppl] 1: 3–4

MacPherson I 1973 Soft agar techniques. In: Kruse P F, Patterson M K (eds) Tissue culture methods and applications. Academic Press, London, pp 276–280

MacPherson I, Montagnier L 1964 Agar suspension culture for the selective assay of cells transformed by polyoma virus. Virology 23: 291–294

Major E O, Vacante D A, Traub R G, London W T, Sever J L 1987 Owl monkey astrocytoma cells in culture spontaneously produce infectious JC virus which demonstrates altered biological properties. Journal of Virology 61: 1435–1441

Manoury R 1977 Establishment and characterization of five human cell lines derived from a series of fifty primary intracranial tumors. Acta Neuropathologica 39: 33–41

Manoury R, Daumas-Duport C, Fontaime C, Vedrenne C 1979 Ultrastructural localization of glial fibrillary acidic protein (GFAP) in human glioma culture by immunoperoxidase method. Brain Research 170: 392–398

Manuelidis E E 1969 Experiments with tissue culture and heterologous transplantation of tumors. Annals of the New York Academy of Sciences 159: 409–431

Manuelidis L, Manuelidis E E 1979 Surface growth characteristics of defined normal and neoplastic neuroectodermal cells in vitro. Progress in Neuropathology 4: 235–266

Marcus D M, Carpenter J L, O'Brien J M et al 1991 Primitive neuroectodermal tumor of the midbrain in a murine model of retinoblastoma. Investigative Ophthalmology and Visual Science 32: 293–301

Mareel M M 1983 Invasion in vitro. Methods of analysis. Cancer Metastasis Reviews 2: 201–218

Mareel M M, De Baetselier P, Van Roy F M 1991 Mechanisms of invasion and metastasis. CRC Press, Boca Raton, FL, p 565

Markert J M, Malick A, Coen D M, Martuza R L 1993 Reduction and elimination of encephalitis in an experimental glioma therapy model with attenuated herpes simplex mutants that retain susceptibility to acyclovir. Neurosurgery 32: 597–603

Martos J, Petersen D, Klose U et al 1992 MR imaging of experimental meningeal melanomatosis in nude rats. Journal of Neuro-Oncology 14: 207–211

Martuza R L, Malick A, Markert J M, Ruffner K L, Coen D M 1991 Experimental therapy of human glioma by means of a genetically engineered virus mutant. Science 252: 854–856

Maruo K, Ueyama Y, Kuwahara Y, Hioki K, Saito M, Nomura T, Tamaoki N 1982 Human tumour xenografts in athymic rats and their age dependence. British Journal of Cancer 45: 786–789

Mawdesly-Thomas L E 1975 Neoplasia in fish. In: Ribelin W E, Migaki G (eds) The pathology of fishes. University of Wisconsin Press, Madison, Wisconsin, pp 871–894

Medhkour A, Van Roey M, Sobel R A, Fingert H J, Lee J, Martuza R L 1989 Implantation of human meningiomas into the subrenal capsule of the nude mouse. A model for studies of tumor growth. Journal of Neurosurgery 71: 545–550

Mella O, Bjerkvig R, Schem B C, Dahl O, Laerum O D 1990 A cerebral glioma model for experimental therapy and in vivo invasion studies in syngeneic BDIX rats. Journal of Neuro-Oncology 9: 93–104

Mineura K, Watanabe K, Izumi I, Kowada M 1992 Modulation of BUdR labeling index in rat brain tumors following intracarotid ACNU administration. Journal of Neuro-Oncology 14: 201–205

Mitts M G, Walker A E 1964 Autotransplantation of gliomas. Journal of Neuropathology and Experimental Neurology 23: 324–333

Mossman M 1983 Rapid colorimetric assay for cellular growth and survival: application to proliferation and cytotoxicity assays. Journal of Immunological Methods 65: 55–63

Murray M R, Petersen E R, Hirschberg E, Pool J L 1954 Metabolic and chemotherapeutic investigation of human glioblastoma in vitro. Annals of the New York Academy of Sciences 58: 1147–1171

Nagashima K, Yasui K, Kimura J et al 1984 Induction of brain tumors by a newly isolated JC virus (Tokyo-1 strain). American Journal of Pathology 116: 455–463

Naito M, Ito A, Ayoama H 1985 Genetics of susceptibility of rats to trigeminal schwannomas induced by neonatal administration of N-ethyl-N-nitrosourea. Journal of the National Cancer Institute 74: 241–245

Nelson-Rees W A, Flandermeyer R R 1976 Inter- and intraspecies contamination of human breast tumor cell lines HBC and BeCa5 and other cell culture. Science 195: 1343–1344

Nelson-Rees W A, Daniels D W, Flandermeyer R R 1981 Cross-contamination of cell culture. Science 212: 446–452

Nerenberg M, Hinrichs S H, Reynolds R K, Khoury G, Jay G 1987 The *tat* gene human T-lymphotropic virus type 1 induces mesenchymal tumors in transgenic mice. Science 237: 1324–1329

Neuwelt E A, Frenkel E P, D'Agostino A N et al 1985 Growth of human lung tumor in the brain of the nude rat as a model to evaluate antitumor agent delivery across the blood-brain barrier. Cancer Research 45: 2827–2833

Nias A H W, Fox M 1968 Minimum clone size for estimating normal reproductive capacity of cultured cells. British Journal of Radiology 41: 468–474

Nikkhah G, Tonn J C, Hoffman O, Kraemer H P, Darling J L, Schachenmayr W, Schönmayr R 1992a The MTT assay for chemosensitivity testing of human tumors of the central nervous system. Part II: Evaluation of patient- and drug-specific variables. Journal of Neuro-Oncology 13: 13–24

Nikkhah G, Tonn J C, Hoffman O, Kraemer H P, Darling J L, Schönmayr R, Schachenmayr W 1992b The MTT assay for chemosensitivity testing of human tumors of the central nervous system. Part I: Evaluation of test specific variables. Journal of Neuro-Oncology 13: 1–11

Nir I, Levanon D, Iosilevsky G 1989 Permeability of experimental gliomas: uptake of 99mTc-glucoheptonate and alteration in blood-brain barrier as determined by cytochemistry and electron microscopy. Neurosurgery 25: 523–531

Norrell H A Jr, Wilson C B 1965 Chemotherapy of experimental brain tumors by arterial infusion. Surgical Forum 16: 429–431

O'Brien J M, Marcus D M, Bernards R, Carpenter J L, Windle J J, Mellon P, Albert D M 1990 A transgenic mouse model for trilateral retinoblastoma. Archives of Ophthalmology 108: 1145–1151

Oyasu R, Battifora H A, Clasen R A, McDonald J H, Hass G M 1970 Induction of cerebral gliomas in rats with dietary lead subacetate and 2-acetylaminofluorene. Cancer Research 30: 1248–1261

Padgett B L, Walker D L, ZuRhein G M, Varakis J N 1977 Differential neurooncogenicity of strains of JC virus, a human polyoma virus, in newborn Syrian hamsters. Cancer Research 37: 718–720

Pleasure D, Kreider B, Sobue G, Ross A H, Koprowski H, Sonnefeld K H, Rubenstein A E 1986 Schwann-like cells cultured from human dermal neurofibromas. Immunohistological identification and response to Schwann cell mitogens. Annals of the New York Academy of Sciences 486: 227–240

Plunkett R J, Weber R J, Oldfield E H 1988 Stereotaxic implantation of dispersed cell suspensions into brain. A systematic appraisal of cell placement and survival. Journal of Neurosurgery 69: 228–233

Plunkett R J, Saris S C, Bankiewicz K S, Ikejiri B, Weber R J 1989 Implantation of dispersed cells into primate brain. Journal of Neurosurgery 70: 441–445

Pontén J 1975 Neoplastic human glia cells in culture. In: Fogh J (ed) Human tumor cells in vitro. Plenum, New York, NY, pp 175–206

Pontén J, MacIntyre E 1968 Long term culture of normal and neoplastic human glia. Acta Pathologica et Microbiologica Scandinavica 74: 465–486

Pontén J, Westermark B 1978 Properties of human malignant glioma cells in vitro. Medical Biology 56: 184–193

Rabotti G F, Grove A S, Sellers R L, Anderson W R 1966 Induction of multiple brain tumors (gliomata and leptomeningeal sarcomata) in dogs. Nature 209: 884–886

Raedler E, Raedler A 1984 Local proliferation of macrophages in central nervous system tissue cultures. Journal of Neuropathology and Experimental Neurology 43: 531–540

Raz A, Hart I R 1980 Murine melanoma: a model for intracranial metastasis. British Journal of Cancer 42: 331–341

Remy C, von Kienlin M, François A, Benabid A L, Decorps M 1989 In vivo 1H spectroscopy of an intracerebral glioma in the rat. Magnetic Resonance in Medicine 9: 395–401

Rewers A B, Redgate E S, Deutsch M, Fisher E R, Boggs S S 1990 A new rat brain tumor model: glioma disseminated via the cerebral spinal fluid pathways. Journal of Neuro-Oncology 8: 213–219

Rice J M, Rehm S, Donovan P J, Perantoni A O 1989 Comparative transplacental carcinogenesis by directly acting and metabolism-dependent alkylating agents in rodents and nonhuman primates. IARC Scientific Publications, Lyon 96: 17–34

Robl M G, Gordon D E, Lee K P, Olson C 1972 Intracranial fibroblastic neoplasms in the hamster from bovine papilloma virus. Cancer Research 32: 2221–2223

Rosenblum M L, Knebel K D, Wheeler K T et al 1975a Development of an in vitro colony formation assay for the evaluation of in vivo chemotherapy of a rat brain tumor. In Vitro 11: 264–273
Rosenblum M L, Wheeler K T, Wilson C B et al 1975b In vitro evaluation of in vivo brain tumor chemotherapy with 1,3-bis(2-chloroethyl)-1-nitrosourea. Cancer Research 35: 1387–1391
Rosenblum M L, Vasquez D A, Hoshino T, Wilson C B 1978 Development of a clonogenic cell assay for human brain tumors. Cancer 41: 2305–2314
Rosenblum M L, Dougherty D V, Reese C, Wilson C B 1981 Potentials and possible pitfalls of human stem cell analysis. Cancer Chemotherapy and Pharmacology 6: 227–235
Rubinstein L J 1977 Correlation of animal brain tumor models with human neuro-oncology. National Cancer Institute Monographs 46: 43–49
Rubinstein L J, Herman M M 1975 Studies on the differentiation of human and experimental gliomas in organ culture systems. Recent Results in Cancer Research 51: 35–51
Rubinstein L J, Herman M M, Foley V L 1973 In vitro characteristics of human glioblastomas maintained in organ culture systems. Light microscopy observations. American Journal of Pathology 71: 61–70
Rutka J T, Kleppe-Hoifodt H, Emma D A et al 1986 Characterization of normal human brain cultures. Evidence for the outgrowth of leptomeningeal cells. Laboratory Investigation 55: 71–85
Rutka J T, Giblin J R, Dougherty D V et al 1987 Establishment and characterization of five cell lines derived from human malignant gliomas. Acta Neuropathologica 75: 92–103
Sakamoto K, Hoshino H, Kiuchi Y, Nakano G, Nagamachi Y 1989 Potential usefulness of a cultured glioma cell line induced by Rous sarcoma virus in B10. A mouse as an immunotherapy model. Japanese Journal of Experimental Medicine 59: 173–180
Sanders F K, Burford B O 1964 Ascites tumours from BHK-21 cells transformed in vitro by polyoma virus. Nature 201: 786–789
San-Galli F, Vrignaud P, Robert J, Coindre J M, Cohadon F 1989 Assessment of the experimental model of transplanted C6 glioblastoma in Wistar rats. Journal of Neuro-Oncology 7: 299–304
Schabet M, Wiethölter H, Meier D 1987 Experimental meningeal neoplasia in nude rats. Neurology 37(suppl 1): 311
Schabet M, Wiethölter H, Meier D, Birchmeier W 1989 Experimental meningeal melanomatosis. Strahlentherapie und Onkologie 165: 491–492
Schabet M, Ohneseit P, Buchholz R, Santo-Höltje L, Schmidberger H 1992 Intrathecal ACNU treatment of B16 melanoma leptomeningeal metastasis in a new athymic rat model. Journal of Neuro-Oncology 14: 169–175
Schackert G, Fidler I J 1988 Development of in vivo models for studies of brain metastasis. International Journal of Cancer 41: 589–594
Schmale M C 1985 Histopathology, distribution, and development of a neoplastic disease in the bicolor damselfish (*Pomacentrus partitus*) from Florida reefs. Ph D dissertation. University of Miami, Miami, FL
Schmale M C, Hensley G T, Udey L R 1986 Neurofibromatosis in the binocular damselfish (*Pomacentrus partitus*) as a model of von Recklinghausen neurofibromatosis. Annals of the New York Academy of Sciences 486: 386–402
Schold S C, Bigner D D 1983 A review of animal brain tumor models that have been used for therapeutic studies. In: Walker M D (ed) Oncology of the nervous system. Martinus Nijhoff, Boston, MA, pp 31–63
Schold S C Jr, Rawlings C E III, Bigner S H, Bigner D D 1983 Intracerebral growth of a human glioma tumor line in athymic mice and treatment with procarbazine, 1,3-bis(2-chloroethyl)-1-nitrosourea, aziridinylbenzoquinone, and cis-platinum. Neurosurgery 12: 672–677
Schuster J M, Friedman H S, Archer G E, Fuchs H E, McLendon R E, Colvin O M, Bigner D D 1993 Intraarterial therapy of human glioma xenografts in athymic rats using 4-hydroperoxycyclophosphamide. Cancer Research 53: 2338–2343
Scudiero D A, Shoemaker R H, Paul K D et al 1988 Evaluation of a soluble tetrazolium/formazan assay for cell growth and drug sensitivity in culture using human and other tumor lines. Cancer Research 48: 4827–4833
Seeds N W, Haffke S C 1978 Cell junctions and ultrastructural development of reaggregated mouse brain cell cultures. Developmental Neuroscience 1: 69–79
Segebarth C, Baleriaux D F, Luyten P R, den Hollander J A 1990 Detection of metabolic heterogeneity of human intracranial tumors in vivo by ^{1}H NMR spectroscopic imaging. Magnetic Resonance in Medicine 13: 62–76
Seligman A M, Shear M J, Alexander L 1939 Studies in carcinogenesis. VIII. Experimental production of brain tumors in mice with methylcholanthrene. American Journal of Cancer 37: 364–399
Shapiro W R, Basler G A, Chernik N L, Posner J B 1979 Human brain tumor transplantation into nude mice. Journal of the National Cancer Institute 62: 447–453
Shibata S, Jinnouchi T, Mori K 1989 Ultrastructural study of capillary permeability of liposome-encapsulated cisplatin in an experimental rat brain tumor model. Neurologia Medico-Chirurgica 29: 696–700
Sima A A F, Finkelstein S D, McLachlan D R 1983 Multiple malignant astrocytomas in a patient with spontaneous progressive multifocal leukoencephalopathy. Annals of Neurology 14: 183–188
Skehan P, Storeng R, Scudiero D et al 1990 New colorimetric cytotoxicity assay for anti-cancer-drug screening. Journal of the National Cancer Institute 82: 1107–1112
Small J A, Khoury G, Jay G, Howley P M, Scangos G A 1986a Early regions of JC virus and BK virus induce distinct and tissue-specific tumors in transgenic mice. Proceedings of the National Academy of Sciences of the USA 83: 8288–8292
Small J A, Scangos G A, Cork L, Jay G, Khoury G 1986b The early region of human papovavirus JC induces dysmyelination in transgenic mice. Cell 46: 13–18
Steinsvåg S K 1985 Interaction between glioma cells and normal brain tissue in organ culture studied by scanning electron microscopy. Invasion Metastasis 5: 255–269
Steinsvåg S K, Laerum O D 1985 Invasion of glioma cells into brain tissue in organ culture. Journal of the National Cancer Institute 74: 24–32
Steinsvåg S K, Laerum O D, Bjerkvig R 1985 Interaction between rat glioma cells and normal rat brain tissue in organ culture. Journal of the National Cancer Institute 74: 1095–1104
Stranahan P L, Howard R B, Pfenninger O, Cowen M E, Johnston M R, Pettijohn D E 1992 Mucin gel formed by tumorigenic squamous lung carcinoma cells has $Le^{(a)-X}$ oligosaccharides and excludes antibodies from underlying cells. Cancer Research 52: 2923–2930
Stratton M R, Darling J L, Pilkington G J, Lantos P L, Reeves B R, Cooper C S 1989a Characterization of the human cell line TE-671. Carcinogenesis 10: 899–905
Stratton M R, Reeves B R, Cooper C S 1989b Misidentified cell. Nature 337: 311–312
Strömblad L G, Brun A, Salford L G, Steveni U 1982 A model for xenotransplantation of human malignant astrocytomas into the brain of normal adult rats. Acta Neurochirurgica 65: 217–226
Studer A, de Tribolet N, Diserens A C, Gaide A C, Matthieu J M, Carrel S, Stavrou D 1985 Characterization of four human malignant glioma cell lines. Acta Neuropathologica 66: 208–217
Sweeney T M, Kibbey M C, Zain M, Fridman R, Kleinman H K 1991 Basement membrane and the SIKVAV laminin-derived peptide promote tumor growth and metastases. Cancer and Metastasis Reviews 10: 245–254
Sweet W H, Bailey P 1941 Experimental production of intracranial tumors in the white rat. Archives of Neurology and Psychiatry 45: 1047–1049
Swenberg J A 1977 Chemical- and virus-induced brain tumors. National Cancer Institute Monographs 46: 3–10
Tamura K, Shimizu K, Yamada M et al 1989 Expression of major histocompatibility complex on human medulloblastoma cells with neuronal differentiation. Cancer Research 49: 5380–5384
Tator C H, Wassenaar W 1977 Intraneoplastic injection of methotrexate for experimental brain-tumor chemotherapy. Journal of Neurosurgery 46: 165–174
Tator C H, Wassenaar W, Day A, So W S 1977 Therapy of an experimental glioma with systemic or intraneoplastic methotrexate or radiation. Journal of Neurosurgery 46: 175–184

Thacker J, Webb M B T, Debenham P G 1988 Fingerprinting cell lines: use of human hypervariable DNA probes to characterize mammalian cell cultures. Somatic and Cell Molecular Genetics 14: 519–525

Theuring F, Gotz W, Balling R, Korf H W, Schulze F, Herken R, Gruss P 1990 Tumorigenesis and eye abnormalities in transgenic mice expressing MSV-SV40 large T-antigen. Oncogene 5: 225–232

Tickle C, Crawley A, Goodman M 1978 Cell movement and the mechanism of invasiveness: a survey of the behaviour of some normal and malignant cells implanted into the developing chick wing bud. Journal of Cellular Science 31: 293–322

Trojan J, Blossey B K, Johnson T R, Rudin S D, Tykocinski M, Ilan J, Ilan J 1992 Loss of tumorigenicity of rat glioblastoma directed by episome-based antisense cDNA transcription of insulin-like growth factor I. Proceedings of the National Academy of Sciences of the United States of America 89: 4874–4878

Trojan J, Johnson T R, Rudin S D, Ilan J, Tykocinski M L, Ilan J 1993 Treatment and prevention of rat glioblastoma by immunogenic C6 cells expressing antisense insulin-like growth factor I RNA. Science 259: 94–97

Ushio Y, Chernik N L, Shapiro W R, Posner J B 1977 Metastatic tumor of the brain: development of an experimental model. Annals of Neurology 2: 20–29

Van Helden P D, Wiid I J F, Albrecht C F et al 1988 Cross-contamination of human esophageal squamous carcinoma cell lines detected by DNA fingerprint analysis. Cancer Research 48: 5660–5662

Vasquez-Lopez E 1945 Glioma in a rat fed with 2-acetyl-amino-fluorene. Nature 156: 296–297

Vogel H B, Berry R G 1975 Chorioallantoic membrane heterotransplantation of human brain tumors. International Journal of Cancer 15: 401–408

Vriesendorp F J, Peagram C, Bigner D D, Groothuis D R 1987 Concurrent measurements of blood flow and transcapillary transport in xenotransplanted human gliomas in immunosuppressed rats. Journal of the National Cancer Institute 79: 123–130

Walker D G, Wright J C 1961 The effect of vincaleukoblastine on primary cultures of human neoplasms. A preliminary report. Cancer Chemotherapy Reports 14: 139

Wang T Y, Nicolson G L 1983 Metastatic tumor cell invasion of brain organ tissue cultured on cellulose polyacetate strips. Clinical and Experimental Metastasis 1: 327–339

Warnke P C, Friedman H S, Bigner D D, Groothuis D R 1987 Simultaneous measurements of blood flow and blood-to-tissue transport in xenotransplanted medulloblastomas. Cancer Research 47: 1687–1690

Wechsler W, Szymas J, Bilzer T, Hossmann K A 1989 Experimental transplantation gliomas in the adult cat brain. 1. Experimental model and neuropathology. Acta Neurochirurgica 98: 77–89

Weil A 1938 Experimental production of tumors in the brains of white rats. Archives of Pathology 26: 777–790

Weissman D E, Grossman S A 1988 A model for quantitation of peritumoral brain edema. Journal of Neuroscience Methods 23: 207–210

Weiszäcker M, Nagamune A, Rathmer K, Wechsler W 1983 Brain tumor growth and response to chemotherapy in the subrenal capsule assay. Journal of Cancer Research and Clinical Oncology 106: 229–233

Welch D R, Lobl T J, Seftor E A et al 1989 Use of the membrane invasion culture system (MICS) as a screen for anti-invasive agents. International Journal of Cancer 43: 449–457

Westermark B 1973 The deficient density-dependent growth control of human malignant glioma cells and virus-transformed glia-like cells in culture. International Journal of Cancer 12: 438–451

Westermark B, Pontén J, Hugosson R 1968 Determinants for the establishment of permanent tissue culture lines from human gliomas. Acta Pathologica et Microbiologica Scandinavica 74: 465–486

Westphal M, Hänsel M, Brunken M, König A, Köppen J A, Herrmann H D 1987 Initiation of primary cell cultures from human intracranial tumors on extracellular matrix from bovine corneal endothelial cells. Experimental Cell Biology 55: 152–163

Westphal M, Nausch H, Herrmann H D 1990 Antigenic staining patterns of human glioma cultures: primary cultures, long-term cultures and cell lines. Journal of Neurocytology 19: 466–477

Whelan H T, Clanton J A, Wilson R E, Tulipan N B 1988 Comparison of CT and MRI brain tumor imaging using a canine glioma model. Pediatric Neurology 4: 279–283

Wilson C B, Bates E A 1972 Transplantable brain tumors. In: Kirsch W M, Paoletti G, Paoletti P (eds) The experimental biology of brain tumors. Charles C Thomas, Springfield, Illinois, pp 19–56

Wilson C B, Norrell H Jr, Barker M 1967 Intrathecal injection of methotrexate (NSC-740) in transplanted brain tumors. Cancer Chemotherapy Reports 51: 1–6

Wrobel C J, Wright D C, Dedrick R L, Youle R J 1990 Diphtheria toxin effects on brain-tumor xenografts. Implications for protein-based brain-tumor chemotherapy. Journal of Neurosurgery 72: 946–950

Yamada K, Bremer A M, West C R 1979 Effects of dexamethasone on tumor-induced brain edema and its distribution in the brain of monkeys. Journal of Neurosurgery 50: 361–367

Yoshida T, Shimizu K, Ushio Y, Hayakawa T, Arita N, Mogami H 1986 Development of experimental meningeal gliomatosis models in rats. Journal of Neurosurgery 65: 503–507

Zagzag D, Goldenberg M, Brem S 1989 Angiogenesis and blood-brain barrier breakdown modulate CT contrast enhancement: an experimental study in a rabbit brain-tumor model. American Journal of Radiology 153: 141–146

Zimmermann H M, Arnold H 1941 Experimental brain tumors. I. Tumors produced with methylcholanthrene. Cancer Research 1: 919–938

Zimmerman H M, Arnold H 1943 Experimental brain tumors. II. Tumors produced with benzpyrene. American Journal of Pathology 19: 939–956

Zülch K J 1986 Brain tumors. Their biology and pathology, 3rd edn. Springer, Berlin, Germany, p 704

22. Management of brain tumors in the pediatric patient

John A. Duncan III   Harold J. Hoffman

INTRODUCTION

This chapter discusses general principles in the management of pediatric brain tumors. Specific operative techniques and neuroanesthetic procedures have been developed over the past 30 years at The Hospital for Sick Children in Toronto, and advances have been made in other areas of special consideration. The guidelines and suggestions presented in this chapter reflect this evolution and summarize our current understanding and treatment of brain tumors in children.

PREOPERATIVE CEREBROSPINAL FLUID (CSF) DIVERSION

Modern radiologic techniques such as computed tomography (CT) and magnetic resonance imaging (MRI) provide superb anatomic and pathologic detail. As the availability of these facilities becomes increasingly widespread, children with brain tumors are being diagnosed earlier and therefore do not become as critically ill as in the past. The use of these imaging techniques has eliminated more invasive diagnostic tests, such as ventriculography, pneumoencephalography and cerebral angiography, in the investigation of intracranial neoplastic disease. Surgical intervention can now take place earlier, and as a result, the need for temporary preoperative CSF diversion has virtually disappeared. In patients with hydrocephalus secondary to tumor, a preoperative ventriculo-peritoneal (VP) shunt is not only unnecessary but may be dangerous. Instead of undergoing CSF diversion, the patient is placed on dexamethasone, 0.5 mg/kg per day, and prepared for surgery. Preoperative diuresis with frusemide or mannitol is unnecessary; the condition of most children will stabilize or improve before surgery after receiving steroids.

The complications of preoperative CSF diversion include shunt malfunction, infection, rapid decompression with subdural hematoma formation, upward herniation with brainstem compression, intratumoral hemorrhage, and tumor metastasis to the peritoneal cavity with subsequent widespread dissemination (Hoffman et al 1976, Epstein & Murali 1978, Vaquero et al 1981, Waga et al 1981, Hoffman 1988).

At the time of surgery, the combination of hyperventilation and mannitol (1.5 g/kg) will consistently produce a 'slack' brain, negating the need for ventricular drainage. Occasionally, a hemispheric tumor cyst will need to be aspirated with a brain needle, adequately decompressing the contents of the posterior fossa, prior to opening the dura. In children with tumors in the fourth ventricle, we prefer to cannulate the aqueduct of Sylvius with a Lapras catheter in cases where normal CSF circulation will not be re-established by surgery (Fig. 22.1). In such patients, the aqueduct of Sylvius is dilated and can be easily catheterized under direct vision after tumor removal.

NEUROANESTHESIA

Success in pediatric neurosurgery depends on expert neuroanesthesia (Kleinman & Bissonette 1992). In most cases, routine use of preoperative sedation should be avoided. Sedatives and narcotics should not be given to unmonitored pediatric patients because they may precipitate respiratory depression with consequent hypercarbia or loss of airway integrity. Upon arrival in the operating room, all infants and children are preoxygenated with 100% oxygen by mask. Often neurosurgical patients will have increased intracranial pressure (ICP), which predisposes the child to gastric content regurgitation and subsequent aspiration. Therefore, anesthesia is induced in a rapid sequence, using intravenous thiopental (4–6 mg/kg) and atropine (0.02 mg/kg), followed by succinylcholine (2 mg/kg) or a fast-acting, non-depolarizing muscle relaxant to facilitate tracheal intubation. The anticholinergic effects of atropine help to prevent the deleterious vagal responses that often occur after succinylcholine administration and laryngoscopy. Intravenous lidocaine (1.0–1.5 mg/kg) suppresses coughing and straining with airway manipulation, preventing a precipitous rise in ICP during intubation. In children operated upon in the prone

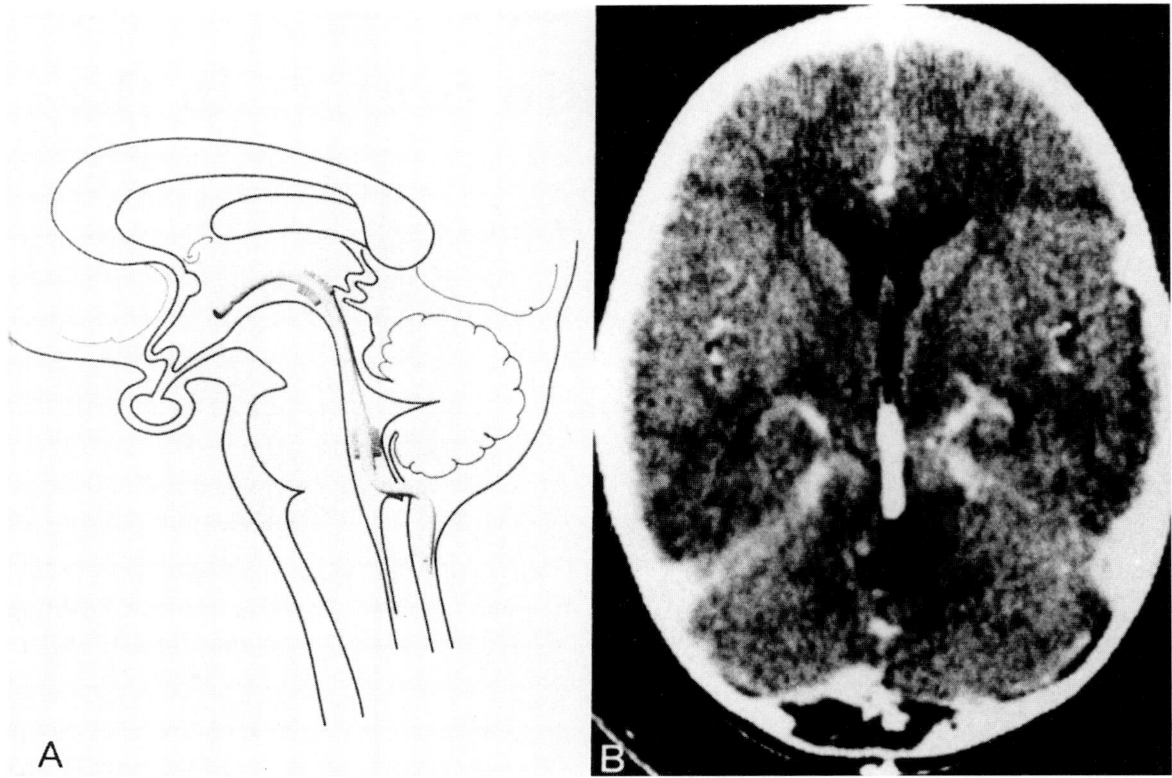

Fig. 22.1 **A.** Correct anatomical position of Lapras catheter. **B.** Axial computed tomography scan with catheter in third ventricle and aqueduct of Sylvius.

position, placement of a nasal endotracheal tube avoids kinking and airway obstruction when the neck is flexed. Anesthesia is maintained by the combination of a volatile anesthetic such as isoflurane, a long-acting, non-depolarizing muscle relaxant (pancuronium, 0.15 mg/kg), and a narcotic (fentanyl, 1–5 μg/kg). Unlike other inhalation anesthetics, isoflurane does not significantly increase cerebral blood flow (Leon & Bissonette 1991) and helps control ICP. The association of intermittent positive-pressure ventilation with hyperventilation ($PaCO_2$ 25–30 mmHg), and the administration of mannitol (1.0–1.5 g/kg) with frusemide (0.4–0.6 mg/kg) during induction, provide excellent brain relaxation.

Careful intraoperative monitoring is mandatory. Oximetry and electrocardiography leads are fixed to the patient. An esophageal stethoscope is placed to monitor heart rate, heart sounds and ventilation. A Foley catheter to monitor urine output and a rectal temperature probe are inserted. An arterial line is placed in all patients to monitor blood pressure and obtain arterial blood gas samples. A precordial Doppler is placed during all procedures in which the possibility of air embolism exists. End-tidal CO_2 is also measured to detect air embolism. Air in the pulmonary vessels interferes with gaseous exchange and causes retention of arterial CO_2, leading to a rapid fall in end-tidal CO_2 (Matjasko et al 1985). In the older child, a central venous pressure line is inserted and used to help manage air embolism, once detected. A large-bore intravenous catheter placed percutaneously into the long saphenous or other large vein is used for fluid administration during and after surgery.

In cases requiring electrocortical mapping, neuroleptic analgesia with the patient awake and cooperative is used in children 4 years and older (Nebbin & Bissonette 1993). This allows localization of the sensory and motor cortex, mapping of speech areas, and identification of epileptogenic foci using intraoperative electrocorticography. The child is first premedicated with atropine (0.02 mg/kg), then neuroleptic analgesia is induced with intravenous fentanyl (0.002 mg/kg) and droperidol (0.1 mg/kg). The scalp is infiltrated with local anesthetic (0.25% marcaine and epinephrine 1/200 000) (Hartley et al 1991). Anesthesia or analgesia is maintained with both droperidol and fentanyl. To ensure an alert, cooperative patient, droperidol is restricted after the first hour and should not exceed a total dose of 0.25 mg/kg. Fentanyl is given to maintain a respiratory rate between 9 and 15 respirations/min. Supplemental nitrous oxide can be given by mask, but must be stopped in advance of intraoperative electrocorticography. At The Hospital for Sick Children (HSC) in Toronto, such anesthesia is used for children 4 years of age and older for procedures lasting up to 6 hours without serious ill effect (Creighton 1982). Nausea, vomiting, depressed respiration, and altered level of consciousness can all occur, but are easily managed by experienced pediatric neuroanesthesiologists.

PATIENT POSITIONING

Patient positioning is dependent on tumor location. For over 30 years, the prone position has been used exclusively at HSC for children with posterior fossa tumors (Fig. 22.2). This position is easily maintained and the operative table can be tilted to improve venous drainage. The microscope can be used in a greater variety of approaches than is possible with the patient in a sitting position, thus significantly reducing the tiring effect on the surgeon's arms, neck and shoulders. In addition, the risk of air embolism, systemic hypotension, and frontal pneumocephalus is dramatically reduced. The risk in the sitting position has been reported to vary between 2 and 45% (Hurter & Sebel 1979, Cucchiara & Bowers 1982), whereas in the prone position, experience at HSC over the past 25 years shows no clear evidence of air embolism resulting in permanent neurologic injury in children after surgery.

At HSC, the heads of patients less than 1 year old are placed on a well-padded horseshoe headholder. The level of the head is always slightly above the heart and the face is well-padded in the prone position. In patients between 1 and 5 years old, the Sugita 4- to 6-pin fixation headholder, with infant pins, is used. Fixation with six pins is used in children 1–3 years old who have a relatively thin skull, with all six pins tightened to light finger tension. In children between 6 and 12 years, either the Sugita or Mayfield headholder with infant pins is used. The heads of patients 12 and older are held with adult pins. Care must be taken to avoid overtightening the pins, as this could cause inadvertent skull fracture, epidural hematoma, dural laceration, and/or brain injury.

OPERATIVE TECHNIQUES

When a craniotomy is performed, patient size and blood volume should be calculated and the expected blood loss anticipated. The normal blood volume of infants and children is 8.5% and 7.0% of body weight, respectively. After the skin is prepared, marked and incised, scalp bleeding

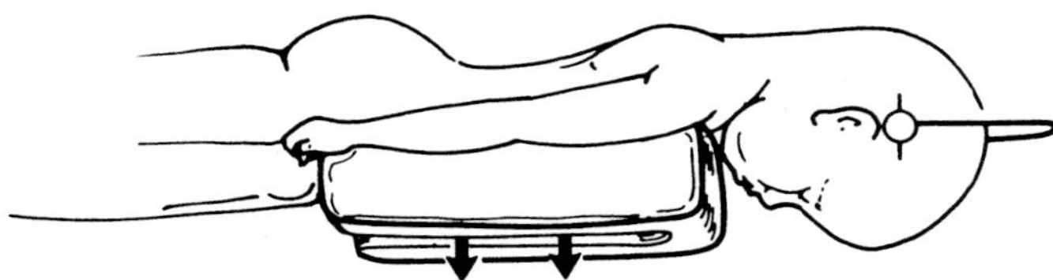

Fig. 22.2 Prone position with patient on padded U-shaped bolster used at The Hospital for Sick Children.

must be meticulously controlled. Excessive blood loss from the scalp is not acceptable and only increases the need for later transfusion. Before the incision is made, the scalp is infiltrated with local anesthetic and adrenalin (1/100 000), which helps to reduce blood loss. Raney clips placed on the skin edge provide for hemostasis. After the scalp is reflected, skull thickness must be estimated before the placement of burr holes. Care must be taken to avoid plunging through thin bone. The dura adjacent to open sutures may be exposed without a perforator. The bone edge is identified and a small portion is cut or rongeured away. In an infant or young child, opening the dura before adequate brain relaxation may be catastrophic. Because of the relative lack of myelination in a very young brain, brain easily herniates through a dural opening when ICP is elevated. An effective method of decompression before opening the dura is to cannulate the ipsilateral lateral ventricle with a fine brain needle connected to an open gravity drain. After the ventricle is decompressed, the needle is removed. The dura is then tacked to the free bone edge, obliterating the potential epidural space and promoting hemostasis. The dura is opened under direct vision. It is flapped or hinged parallel to a venous sinus or the skull base. Care must be taken to expose only as much brain as necessary. After a watertight dural closure, the bone flap is secured with sutures. At HSC, we often use an osteoplastic flap, which promotes bone growth and wound healing and helps prevent infection. Burr holes need not be covered, since in almost all children they will completely fill in within 6–12 months. Packed red blood cells or whole blood must be available in the operating room throughout the entire craniotomy; a transfusion should be given when the surgeon and/or anesthesiologist determines it necessary.

When a posterior fossa craniectomy is performed, the head is flexed in the headholder to open up the space between the foramen magnum and the arch of C1. Excessive flexion should be avoided, especially if the tumor or cerebellar tonsils have descended beneath the foramen magnum. A midline skin incision is made from just above the inion to the midcervical region. Care must be taken to visualize the median raphe. Placing a self-retaining retractor too quickly may distort the anatomy and take the surgeon down a paramedian course through muscle, producing brisk bleeding. Once the spinous processes are identified, the retractor is placed and the paravertebral muscles are reflected from the upper cervical lamina. A horizontal incision is made in the paraspinal muscles in the midoccipital region to help in the eventual closing of the musculature (Fig. 22.3). The muscle is then taken off the occipital bone and any bleeding occipital emissary veins are coagulated and the orifices filled with wax. Sharp dissection is used to cut the periosteum over the arch of C1 on either side of the midline. The periosteum is stripped off the arch of C1, using an index finger covered

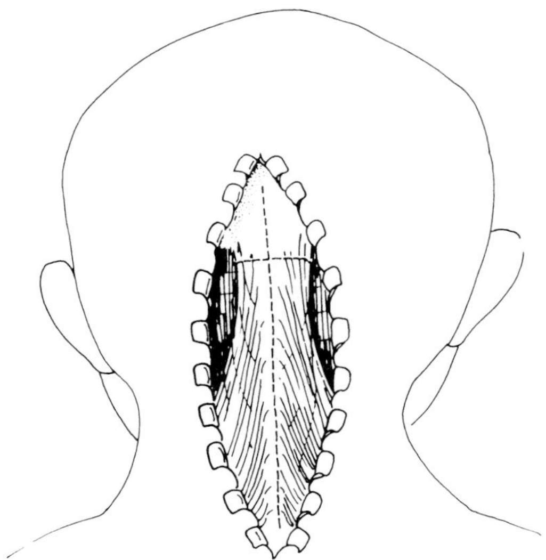

Fig. 22.3 Horizontal and vertical incisions made in suboccipital paraspinal muscles during opening.

with gauze, thus avoiding injury to the vertebral arteries (Fig. 22.4). With a power craniotome, a burr hole is placed on either side of the midline below the inion. The occipital bone is rongeured between the burr holes across the midline and then downward on either side towards the foramen magnum. The bone is then grasped with the rongeur and taken off the underlying dura, leaving the remaining attachment of the atlanto–occipital membrane intact. This membrane, which extends from the lip of the foramen magnum to the arch of C1, is sharply divided at its attachment to the arch of C1, and the occipital bone is removed in one piece (Fig. 22.5). The arch of C1 is then removed (Hoffman 1988).

It is important to remember that the posterior arch of C1 can be bifid in a small child. A deep, initial midline incision with the scalpel or cautery may pass through dura, possibly injuring the spinal cord. For this reason, when approaching C1 in the midline, the surgeon must take great care in reflecting adherent soft tissues (Rutka et al 1993).

In children under the age of 3 years, especially infants, the occipital sinus is often a plexus of veins at the foramen magnum. Therefore, placement of the dural opening is extremely important so as to minimize blood loss. If one 'V's the dural incision below the foramen magnum, one should avoid brisk bleeding. Any bleeding from the cut dural edge should be coagulated promptly. Occasionally there may be a midline falx cerebelli; by opening the dura in the midline below the foramen magnum, the surgeon avoids the difficulty of cutting across the falx (Hoffman 1988). The dura is then hinged upward by a ligature placed around the occipital sinus at its inferior extent. The dural incision is now extended into a Y-shape by dividing the dura over the cervical region (Fig. 22.6).

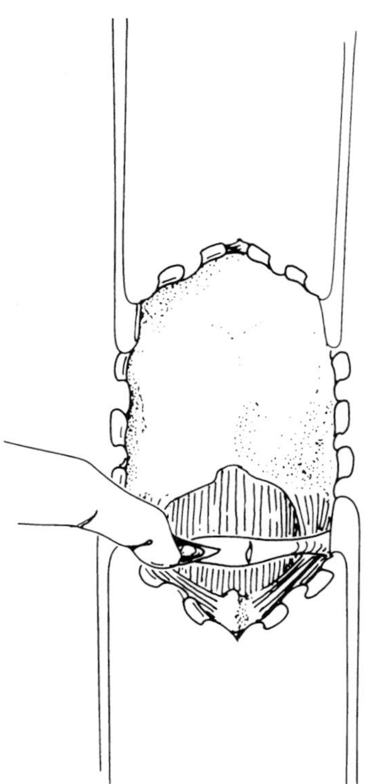

Fig. 22.4 Periosteum stripped from C1 using a gauze-covered index finger.

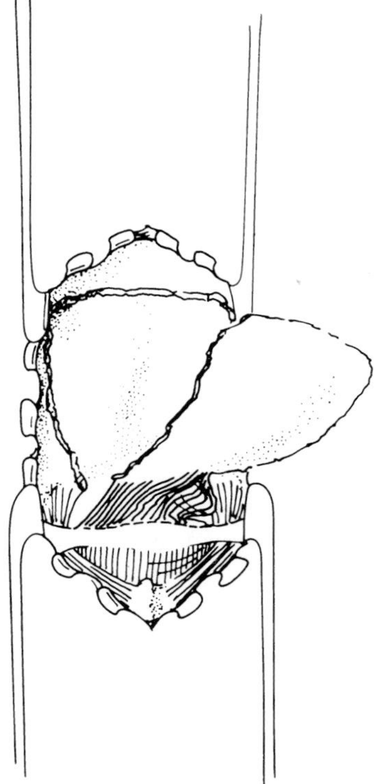

Fig. 22.5 Removal of occipital bone and division of atlanto-occipital membrane.

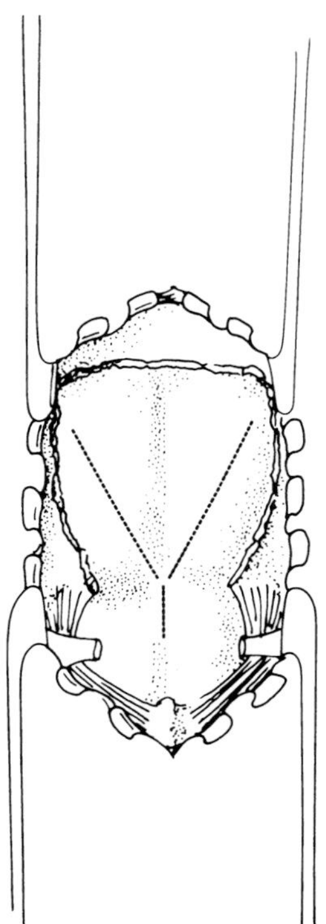

Fig. 22.6 Dural incision in suboccipital region.

The cisterna magna arachnoid is then opened, allowing a view of the cerebellar tonsils, the upper cervical cord, and tumor. Early in the operation on a fourth ventricular tumor, the floor of the fourth ventricle should be identified and protected by a cotton patty (Hoffman 1988).

In the case of a hemispheric posterior fossa tumor such as a cerebellar astrocytoma, care must be taken to avoid contaminating the CSF space with cyst fluid or blood. These fluids may be irritating and cause a chemical meningitis. In young children, this meningitis increases the likelihood of hydrocephalus requiring a VP shunt (Lunardi et al 1989) or of a pseudomeningocele. Therefore, whenever technically possible, we advise against opening into the cisterna magna in children with such tumors. Instead, a horizontal incision is made in the involved hemisphere, providing direct access to the tumor.

POSTOPERATIVE CARE

All children receive a contrast-enhanced CT or MRI scan within 24 hours after surgery. These early scans document the extent of tumor resection, provide a baseline for tumor progression and/or development of hydrocephalus, detect silent postoperative hematomas, but do not yet show surgical enhancement artefact.

The incidence of postoperative hydrocephalus following posterior fossa craniectomy depends on tumor type and age of the child. In general, 25% of all children will require a VP shunt. This incidence is higher in the younger child, and is more common in children under 3 years of age. In addition, tectal brainstem and dorsally exophytic fourth ventricular tumors, in contrast to cerebellar astrocytomas, almost always require a VP shunt or placement of a Lapras catheter, respectively. If a Lapras catheter is placed into the aqueduct of Sylvius, a postoperative lumbar puncture is performed the following day to improve CSF flow.

Cervical pseudomeningoceles develop in approximately 10–15% of children following tumor removal. They may or may not be associated with developing hydrocephalus and can be avoided by not opening the cisterna magna in patients with cerebellar hemispheric astrocytoma. They can become problematic when the incision is threatened but may be ameliorated by serial lumbar punctures. Persistent, large, tense pseudomeningoceles often reflect communicating hydrocephalus (extraventricular) and require a VP shunt. Alternatively, a cyst-peritoneal or lumboperitoneal shunt may be needed, preventing CSF leakage through the wound (Rutka et al 1993). However, if present, CSF leaks and subsequent meningitis must be treated with appropriate antibiotics and temporary CSF diversion before definitive shunting.

RADIATION THERAPY

Today, we are acutely aware of the detrimental effects of radiation therapy on the developing brain. Some of the well-known complications of radiation therapy include endocrinopathy (usually manifest initially as growth hormone deficiency), cognitive intellectual deficits, behavioral disturbance, visual loss, vascular injury, and secondary malignancy (Duffner et al 1985, Packer et al 1989, Rappaport & Brauner 1989, Rutka et al 1993). We therefore strongly advocate a policy of delayed radiotherapy for malignant tumors in children under the age of 3 years. These tumors are best managed with surgery and chemotherapy. Re-resection and delayed radiation after age 3 seem most appropriate in cases of tumor progression. Numerous cases of malignant transformation several years after radiotherapy have been identified in children with cerebellar astrocytoma, optic nerve glioma, and craniopharyngioma (Bernell et al 1972, Scott & Ballantine 1973, Kleinman et al 1978, Ushio et al 1987, Wisoff & Llena 1989, Schwartz & Ghatak 1990). We believe that radiation therapy can play a role in the induction of a malignant tumor; therefore, its use and effectiveness with benign pediatric tumors must be carefully considered.

Many childhood tumors are benign gliomas. Examples include optic nerve gliomas, focal brainstem tumors, and thalamic gliomas. Surgical decompression, accurate histologic diagnosis, and subsequent observation with frequent CT or MR scans are recommended. Radiation therapy should be avoided in these benign glial tumors, even if partially resected. Often the tumors will remain quiescent for long periods after partial resection; in fact, many will involute and some will disappear. If tumor progression does occur or if neurologic function becomes compromised, chemotherapy with or without surgical re-exploration should be initiated. The decision to reoperate on any benign tumor should be based on its size and location, time interval to recurrence, need for repeat tissue diagnosis, condition of the patient, operative risk, and the benefit of additional decompression.

CHEMOTHERAPY

Since the efficacy of chemotherapy for many pediatric tumors is still largely unknown, several multicenter trials designed to test its effectiveness are currently under way. In the meantime, the following recent observations are being used as a guide to treatment at our institution. First, preoperative chemotherapy may play an important role in both choroid plexus carcinomas and craniopharyngiomas by increasing the possibility of total surgical removal. For choroid plexus carcinomas, chemotherapy with ifosphamide, carboplatinum and VP-16 shrinks and devitalizes a vascular and highly invasive tumor (Weitzman et al 1988) (Fig. 22.7). In craniopharyngiomas, injection of intracystic bleomycin (Takahashi et al 1985) one month before surgery thickens the capsular wall (Fig. 22.8). Both techniques aid the surgeon by facilitating total removal of these difficult tumors. Second, postoperative chemotherapy significantly prolongs the survival of infants and young children with malignant supratentorial hemispheric tumors (Sanford et al 1992). These children now show a 55–90% progression-free survival rate after surgery and chemotherapy. Third, in children with medulloblastoma, chemotherapy plus surgery and radiotherapy has resulted in a 5-year survival rate of over 70% for high risk patients (Packer et al 1991).

It is now apparent that malignant tumors in children are often biologically different from their histologic counterparts in adults, and frequently respond favorably to aggressive chemotherapeutic treatments. In addition, the acute hematologic, gastrointestinal, renal and neurologic side effects of chemotherapy, although possibly severe, are usually readily managed, well tolerated, and often reversible in children. The judicious use of chemotherapy avoids the devastating long-term effects of radiation therapy.

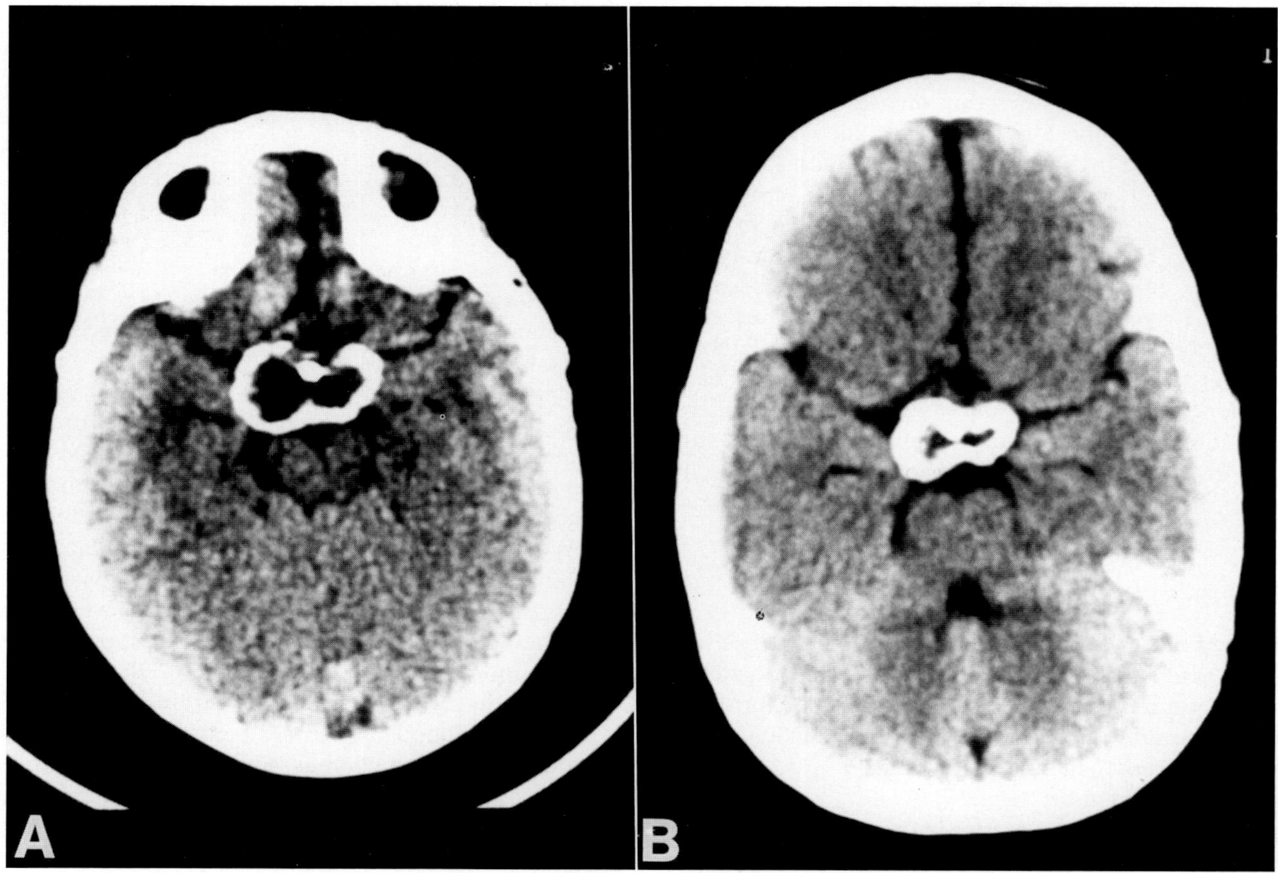

Fig. 22.7 Axial computed tomography scan of cystic craniopharyngioma. **A.** Before treatment with bleomycin. **B.** After 1 month of intracystic injection of bleomycin, showing thickening of cyst wall and collapse of cyst.

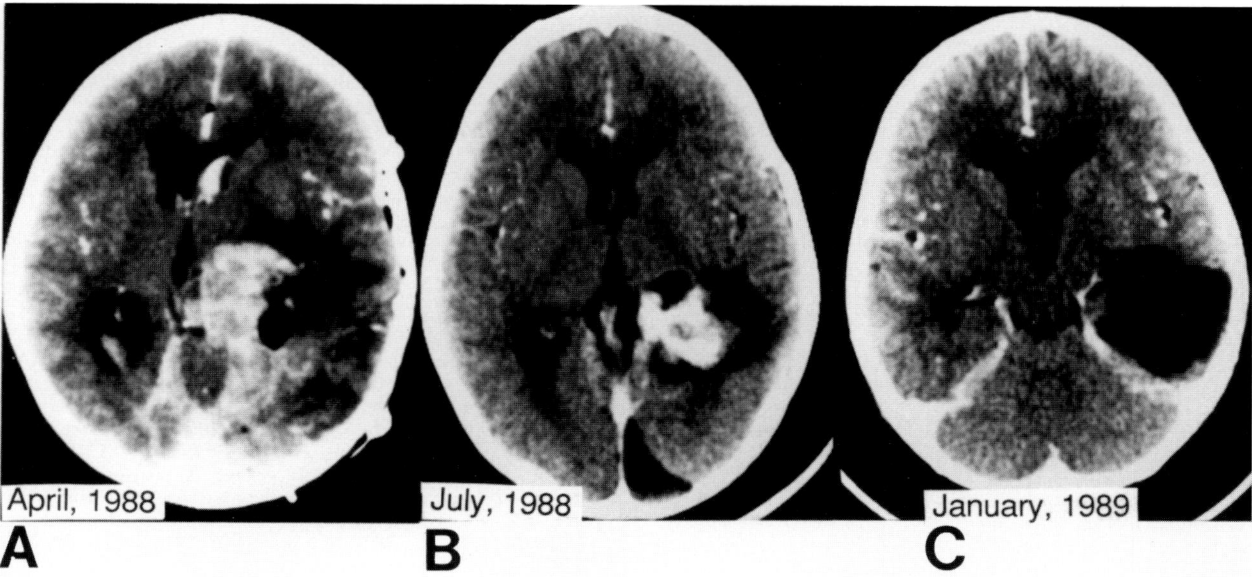

Fig. 22.8 Enhanced axial computed tomography scan of left choroid plexus carcinoma. **A.** Before chemotherapy. **B.** After three courses of chemotherapy, showing shrinkage of tumor. **C.** After complete resection.

Clearly, as current investigations continue to add to our knowledge, new and effective chemotherapeutic regimens will be developed to treat an even broader range of pediatric tumors.

STEREOTAXY

The role of stereotaxy in treating pediatric tumors is expanding quickly. With surgical advances, such as the frameless stereotactic techniques, and the increased efficacy of chemotherapy, the use of simple stereotactic biopsy followed by radiation therapy is no longer the only available treatment for many axial tumors. Today, brainstem gliomas, pineal region tumors, intraventricular tumors, and suprasellar lesions can be safely surgically removed. Sampling error resulting from inadequate tumor volume is avoided. New techniques, such as use of the intraoperative arm, allow for safe and complete or near complete surgical resection. The ISG viewing wand (ISG Technologies, Mississauga, Ont) has been found to be particularly useful. Over the past 15 months, this device has been used at HSC to locate subcortical lesions, guide the operative approach through areas adjacent to eloquent brain, estimate the extent of intraoperative tumor resection, and define regional anatomy before catastrophic surgical injury occurs to major blood vessels and cranial nerves. Because many pediatric tumors involve deep midline structures, we have found when operating on them that intraoperative shift of critical anatomy is minimal and subsequent localization reasonably accurate. Without doubt, continued progress with intraoperative stereotaxy will contribute to the safe and complete removal of benign lesions.

NEUROENDOSCOPY

Another area of special interest and future promise is neuroendoscopy, which permits small ventricular tumors or cysts to be biopsied or removed with a minimally invasive procedure. Although neuroendoscopy is still at an early stage in its development and application to the treatment of brain tumors, it is not unreasonable to predict its use in the management of numerous benign intraventricular tumors, such as colloid cysts, giant cell subependymomas, exophytic thalamic gliomas, and pineal region tumors. Concomitant ventriculostomy for the treatment of hydrocephalus resulting from obstruction at the foramen of Monro or aqueduct of Sylvius has already become an accepted practice in patients with these intraventricular lesions.

CONSULTANT SERVICES

Most important to the ultimate success of the treatment of pediatric brain tumors is the expertise offered by various consultant services. An expert pediatric neuropathologist is an absolute necessity to ensure the accurate tissue diagnoses needed to guide the course of treatment. Highly qualified pediatric neuro-oncologists and radiation therapists must be involved in all patient care decisions. Such specialists should participate in and help supervise multicenter trials. Consultants in endocrinology, intensive care medicine and pediatrics must also be involved early in the postoperative course. Management of fluids and electrolyte disturbance is often best handled by such experts rather than by the surgical team alone. In such a coordinated team approach, led by the surgeon, lies the most promising road to success in the management of children with brain tumors.

REFERENCES

Bernell W R, Kepes J J, Seitz E P 1972 Late malignant recurrence of childhood cerebellar astrocytoma. Journal of Neurosurgery 37: 470–474

Creighton R E 1982 Paediatric neuroanaesthesia. In: Steward D J (ed) Some aspects of paediatric anesthesia. Elsevier/North Holland, Amsterdam, the Netherlands, pp 199–210

Cucchiara R F, Bowers B 1982 Air embolism in children undergoing suboccipital craniotomy. Anesthesiology 57: 338–339

Duffner P K, Cohen M E, Thomas P R M, Lansky S B 1985 The long-term effects of cranial irradiation on the central nervous system. Cancer 56: 1841–1846

Epstein F, Murali R 1978 Pediatric posterior fossa tumors: hazards of the "preoperative" shunt. Neurosurgery 3: 348–350

Hartley E J, Bissonnette B, St Louis P, Rybczynski J, McLeod M E 1991 Scalp infiltration with bupivacaine in pediatric brain surgery. Anesthesia Analgesia 73: 29–32

Hoffman H J 1988 Tumors of the fourth ventricle: technical considerations in tumor surgery. Clinical Neurosurgery 34: 523–545

Hoffman H J, Hendrick E B, Humphreys R P 1976 Metastasis via ventriculoperitoneal shunt in patients with medulloblastoma. Journal of Neurosurgery 44: 562–566

Hurter D, Sebel P S 1979 Detection of venous air embolism. A clinical report using end-tidal carbon dioxide monitoring during neurosurgery. Anaesthesia 34: 578–582

Kleinman G M, Schoene W C, Walshe T M III, Richardson E P Jr 1978 Malignant transformation in benign cerebellar astrocytoma. Case report. Journal of Neurosurgery 49: 111–118

Kleinman S E, Bissonnette B 1992 Management of successful pediatric neuroanesthesia. Anesthetic Clinics of North America 10: 537–561

Leon J E, Bissonnette B 1991 Cerebrovascular responses to carbon dioxide in children anaesthetized with halothane and isoflurane. Canadian Journal of Anaesthesia 38: 817–826

Lunardi P, Missori P, Fraioli B 1989 Chemical meningitis: unusual presentation of a cerebellar astrocytoma: case report and review of the literature. Neurosurgery 25: 264–270

Matjasko J, Petrozza P, Mackenzie C F 1985 Sensitivity of end-tidal nitrogen in venous air embolism detection in dogs. Anesthesiology 63: 418–423

Nebbin S N, Bissonnette B 1993 Neurolept anesthesia: nearly gone but not forgotten. Canadian Journal of Anaesthesia (in press)

Packer R J, Sutton L N, Atkins T E et al 1989 A prospective study of cognitive function in children receiving whole-brain radiotherapy and chemotherapy: 2-year results. Journal of Neurosurgery 70: 707–713

Packer R J, Sutton L N, Goldwein J W et al 1991 Improved survival with the use of adjuvant chemotherapy in the treatment of medulloblastoma. Journal of Neurosurgery 74: 433–440

Rappaport R, Brauner R 1989 Growth and endocrine disorders secondary to cranial irradiation. Pediatric Research 25: 561–567

Rutka J T, Hoffman H J, Duncan J A III 1993 Astrocytomas of the fourth ventricle. In: Cohen A (ed). Surgical disorders of the IVth ventricle. Blackwell Scientific Cambridge, Mass, (in press)

Sanford R A, Duffner P, Krischen J et al 1992 Effect of gross total resection on malignant brain tumors of infancy. Presented at the annual meeting of the American Association of Neurosurgeons, San Francisco, CA, April 14,1992. Scientific Program, p 126 (abstract 736)

Schwartz A M, Ghatak N R 1990 Malignant transformation of benign cerebellar astrocytoma. Cancer 65: 333–336

Scott R M, Ballantine H T Jr 1973 Cerebellar astrocytoma: malignant recurrence after prolonged postoperative survival. Case report. Journal of Neurosurgery 39: 777–779

Takahashi H, Nakazawa S, Shimura T 1985 Evaluation of postoperative intratumoral injection of bleomycin for craniopharyngioma in children. Journal of Neurosurgery 62: 120–127

Ushio Y, Arita N, Yoshimine T, Ikeda T, Mogami H 1987 Malignant recurrence of childhood cerebellar astrocytoma: case report. Neurosurgery 21: 251–255

Vaquero J, Cabezudo J M, De Sola R G, Nombela L 1981 Intratumoral hemorrhage in posterior fossa tumors after ventricular drainage. Journal of Neurosurgery 54: 406–408

Waga S, Shimizu T, Shimosaka S, Tochio H 1981 Intratumoral hemorrhage after a ventriculoperitoneal shunting procedure. Neurosurgery 9: 249–252

Weitzman S, Greenberg M L, Becker L E, Hoffman H J 1988 Choroid plexus carcinoma — response to neoadjuvant combination chemotherapy. Pediatric Neuroscience 14: 165 abstract

Wisoff H S, Llena J F 1989 Glioblastoma multiforme of the cerebellum five decades after irradiation of a cerebellar tumor. Journal of Neuro-Oncology 7: 339–344

23. Management of recurrent gliomas and meningiomas

Griffith R. Harsh IV

INTRODUCTION

Renewed growth of a mass at the site of a previously treated brain tumor raises the issues of indications for and choices of treatment. Important considerations include the following: (1) is the mass a recurrence of the original tumor; (2) why did the tumor regrow; (3) what threat to the patient's neurologic function and survival does this regrowth pose; and (4) what additional therapy is appropriate?

I. CONFIRMATION OF RECURRENCE

When recurrent growth of a tumor is suspected clinically or radiographically, the full set of imaging studies should be reviewed with careful notice of change of imaging signals and documentation of lesion size. The original pathology specimen should be reviewed.

A. Differential diagnosis

An enlarging lesion at the site of a previously treated tumor likely represents renewed growth of an incompletely eradicated initial tumor rather than the development of a new pathologic entity. Exceptions are infrequent:

- A distinctly new tumor may arise at the site of an eradicated tumor. This is more likely if there is a genetic predisposition to tumor development shared by cells in the area; e.g. multiple neurofibromas can develop along the same nerve root in a patient with neurofibromatosis or multiple gliomas in a patient with tuberous sclerosis.
- A tumor of related histology may supplant the original tumor; e.g. the astrocytic component may replace the oligodendrocytic component as the predominant subtype of a mixed glioma, or a gliosarcoma may arise from a previously treated glioblastoma.
- The initial therapy may induce a secondary tumor of a different type; e.g. a parasellar sarcoma after irradiation for a pituitary adenoma, or a glioblastoma in the radiation field of a meningioma.
- A metastatic tumor may grow in the original tumor; e.g. a breast metastasis within a pituitary adenoma.
- Non-neoplastic lesions may mimic tumor growth; e.g. an abscess at the site of resection of a tumor, or radiation necrosis following focal high dose irradiation.

These alternative diagnoses must be excluded before prognosis is addressed and therapy is chosen. Neurodiagnostic imaging usually permits accurate prediction of the diagnosis. Usually, recurrent tumors have imaging features similar to those of the original lesion. A recurrent meningioma usually is dural-based and homogeneously enhances, whereas a recurrent malignant glioma will likely have central low intensity, rim enhancement, and hypodense surround on CT scans. In some cases, however, attention to subtle differences may be required: a dural tail may differentiate a radiation-induced meningioma from a recurrent pituitary adenoma; a more spherical, sharply demarcated shape may suggest abscess rather than recurrent malignant glioma.

Two scenarios often pose particular diagnostic difficulty. In each case, alternative diagnoses are often impossible to distinguish by imaging criteria alone.

B. Malignant progression

The first situation is the renewed growth of a low grade tumor. When low grade gliomas regrow after therapy, approximately half remain non-anaplastic, but the other 50% have progressed to a more malignant form (Wilson 1975, Muller et al 1977, Laws et al 1984, Kaye 1992, McCormack et al 1992). Molecular analyses have delineated genetic correlates of this progression (Von Diemling et al 1993). Enlarging low grade tumors will likely resemble the original tumor on imaging studies. When progression in grade has occurred, the new tumor may also resemble the old one, especially if the original tumor enhanced with contrast. Enhancement is highly predictive of recurrence; low grade enhancing tumors are 6.8 times as likely to recur as non-enhancing ones (McCormack et al 1992). Most commonly, new malignant growth in a previously non-enhancing glioma enhances and is thus readily identified. In one study, only 30% (16/42) of low grade tumors enhanced initially, but 92% (22/24) enhanced at recurrence (McCormack et al 1992). Occasionally, however, an enlarging malignant focus may not enhance. It might, however, be apparent as a region of hypermetabolism on a 2-deoxyglucose PET study or an area of increased cerebral blood volume on a functional MRI scan (DiChiro et al 1985, Alavi et al 1988, Le Bihan et al 1993). Usually, however, histologic analysis after biopsy or resection is warranted to verify malignant transformation.

Malignant change in meningiomas occurs less frequently than in low grade gliomas. Features such as mitosis, nuclear pleomorphism including large nucleoli, hypervascularity, hemosiderin, necrosis, and alterations in the architectural pattern, such as separation of meningotheliomatous and fibroblastic areas and invasion of cortex, muscle, and bone predict rapid growth, early clinical deterioration after treatment of recurrence and brief survival (de la Monte et al 1986). Hypermetabolism and increased cerebral blood volume might also be discernible in tumors with atypical histologic features and aggressive clinical behavior (DiChiro et al 1987). Radiographic features such as multinodularity, central hypodensity, extensive edema, and limited demarcation from cortex and surrounding dura suggest the presence of atypical histology, but many neuropathologists reserve the term malignant meningioma for those with extracranial metastases (New et al 1982). Since most recurrent meningiomas retain their original histologic features at recurrence and meningiomas of benign histology account for the majority of meningiomas that metastasize, the development of atypical histologic features in a meningioma cannot be accurately predicted without tissue examination.

C. Radiation effects

The second scenario which causes diagnostic difficulty is renewed enlargement of a tumor mass following radiation. Often, CT and MRI imaging inadequately distinguish recurrent tumor from radiation-induced necrosis. Radiation can cause tumor enlargement by an early reaction, which is likely edema occurring during or shortly after irradiation, by an early delayed reaction that involves edema and demyelination arising a few weeks to a few months after radiation, and by a late delayed reaction that occurs 6–24 months after radiation and reflects radiation-induced necrosis (Leibel & Sheline 1987). Only large, very malignant tumors grow sufficiently fast to show significant enlargement during, or within three months of completing, a course of radiation. In most cases, tumor enlargement from early or early delayed effects represents edema, is transient, and responds to a short course of corticosteroids. In contrast, radiation-induced necrosis appears at about the time malignant tumors might be expected to recur. It is thus more likely to be mistaken for recurrent tumor growth.

The risk of radiation necrosis increases with the volume treated, dose delivered, and fraction size (Marks et al 1981). Regional teletherapy to a dose of 60 Gy is the current standard radiation treatment for most gliomas (Walker et al 1978). It has a low risk of inducing radiation necrosis. Radiation-induced changes following regional teletherapy are relatively diffuse. The CT and MRI enhancement is patchy and irregularly marginated. The low-density, T1 hypointense, T2 hyperintense regions of edema correspond to the area irradiated. Often, delayed late radiation change after regional teletherapy is distinguishable from the more focal appearance of recurrent tumor.

In contrast, radiation necrosis following focal radiation treatments such as brachytherapy and radiosurgery is more difficult to distinguish from recurrent tumor. These methods deliver high doses of radiation to relatively small volumes over a short time period (Loeffler et al 1990, Scharfen et al 1992). A common protocol for brachytherapy is a 60 Gy boost (to 60 Gy of regional external beam radiotherapy) to a 0–5 cm tumor delivered over approximately one week. The radiosurgery equivalent is a 10–20 Gy boost to a 0–3 cm diameter tumor delivered in less than one hour (Li et al 1992). Necrosis occurs in almost all cases. Radiographically, radiation-induced necrosis is a ring contrast-enhancing mass similar to a malignant tumor. It has a CT hypodense, T1 hypointense, T2 hyperintense center, an enhancing annular region, and a hypodense, T1 hypointense, T2 hyperintense surround. The surround corresponds to edema that strikingly conforms to the patterns of white matter tract radiations. The similarity of this appearance to that of recurrent tumors and the time course of its occurrence presents great difficulty in distinguishing recurrent tumor from radiation-induced necrosis. A variety of functional neurodiagnostic imaging techniques are currently being studied for their ability to distinguish between these two possibilities. These include PET scans, thallium studies, and cerebral blood volume mapping. Regions of high activity are thought to distinguish recurrent tumor from relatively metabolically inactive and hypovascular radiation necrosis (DiChiro et al 1985, Alavi et al 1988, Valk et al 1988, Le Bihan et al 1993).

In many cases, the data from these studies are inconclusive and the diagnosis is revealed either by the clinical course or by analysis of a pathology specimen. When an enlarging mass that is either recurrent tumor, radiation necrosis, or both becomes symptomatic, corticosteroid therapy is required (Edwards & Wilson 1980). About half the patients receiving brachytherapy and radiosurgery develop symptoms that either prove refractory to corticosteroids or require debilitating long-term steroid use (Loeffler et al 1990a,b, Alexander & Loeffler 1992, Scharfen et al 1992). Surgery for resection of an enlarging, symptomatic mass is needed in 20% to 40% of cases following brachytherapy or radiosurgery of a malignant glioma, and approximately 10% of cases of radiosurgery for metastatic tumors (Loeffler et al 1990a,b Alexander & Loeffler 1992, Scharfen et al 1992). At reoperation for presumed radiation necrosis following focal radiation treatment of a malignant glioma, necrosis was found in 5% of cases, tumor alone in 2%, and a mixture of radiation necrosis and tumor in 66% (Scharfen et al 1992). In almost all cases, the tumor that is seen is of reduced viability (Daumas-Duport et al 1984, Rosenblum et al 1985).

II. CAUSES OF RECURRENCE

Renewed growth of a brain tumor following surgery and possibly radiation and chemotherapy indicates failure of these therapies to reduce the tumor mass to a size (approximately 10^5 cells) (Salcman 1982a, Shapiro 1982) permitting eradication by the patient's immune system (Fig. 23.1) (Harsh & Wilson 1990). Failure arises from a number of factors that limit the efficacy of each modality.

A. Recurrence after surgery

Surgery may fail because of anatomical considerations, pathologic features, or errors in judgement or technique. The involvement of critical structures may limit the initial resection. Tumor investment of the carotid artery or ocular motor nerves by a parasellar meningioma or proximity of a glioma to eloquent cortex often warrant incomplete removal. Tumor recurrence, despite removal of all macroscopically evident tumor, can occur if there is microscopic infiltration of adjacent structures. Even low grade cerebral gliomas are usually infiltrative, and microscopic foci of neoplastic cells are frequently found about the margins of the resected dural base of a meningioma (Borovich & Doron 1986). Malignant meningiomas and anaplastic astrocytomas characteristically are widely invasive. Finally, errors in judgement, such as preoperatively underestimating the amount of tumor that can be safely removed or intraoperatively failing to remove tumor that was targeted, result in leaving potentially resectable tumor as a nidus of regrowth.

B. Recurrence after radiation

Radiation therapy may fail because of inadequate targeting, underutilization of tolerable dose, or radiation resistance of the tumor cells. The correlations between imaging abnormality and tumor extent are incomplete. Pathologic studies have shown that individual tumor cells can be found throughout and even beyond CT hypodense and MRI T2 hyperintense areas of malignant glioma (Kelly et al 1987, Burger et al 1988). The choice of field size for irradiation of such a lesion is difficult and relies as much on the trade-off between target volume and tolerable dose

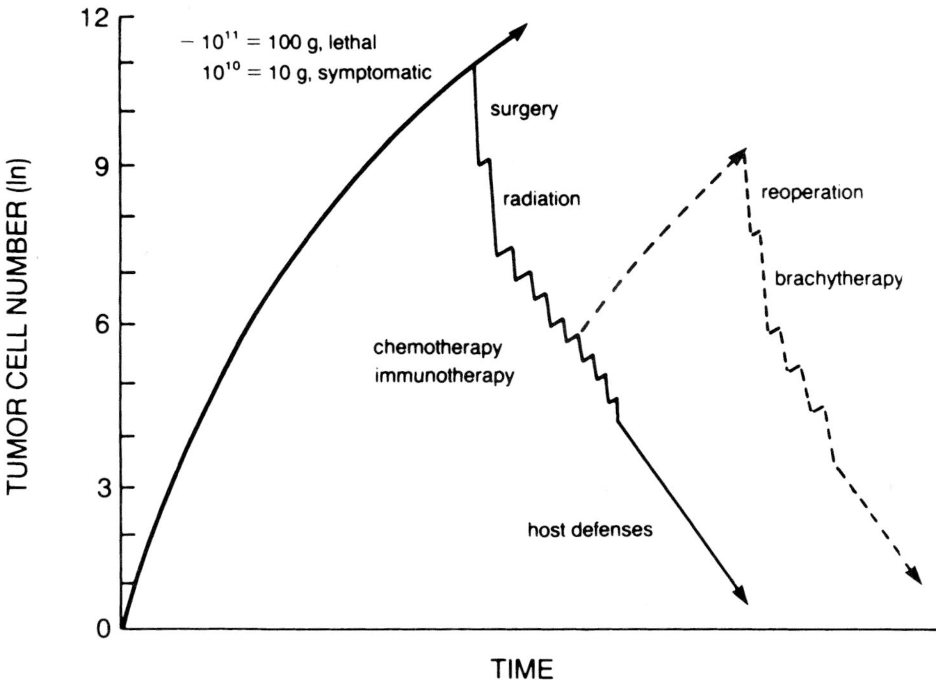

Fig. 23.1 Multimodality therapy of malignant gliomas. Combined use of various therapeutic methods, including reoperation, attempts reduction of tumor cell number.

as on the accurate delineation of tumor boundaries. Similarly, the portion of the dural tail of a meningioma that contains tumor cells and the extent of brain invasion from the contrast-enhancing margin of a metastasis are incompletely known; failure to include an adequate annulus of tissue about the tumor to accommodate imaging uncertainty and technical error may leave tumor cells incompletely irradiated (Borovich et al 1986). Even if the maximal dose tolerated by infiltrative surrounding brain is delivered, tumor cells may remain viable. Hypoxic, nonproliferating cells are particularly radioresistant; with time or change in the physiologic conditions following therapy, re-entry of cells into the cell cycle permits the proliferation that results in clinically apparent tumor recurrence (Hoshino 1984).

C. Recurrence after chemotherapy

Chemotherapy fails as a result of inadequate drug delivery, toxicity, or cell resistance. The blood-brain barrier is deficient in the contrast-enhancing region of the tumor, but surrounding brain usually has an intact blood-brain barrier; lipid-insoluble drugs thus have limited access to tumor cells infiltrating peripheral regions. The margin between drug efficacy and neurotoxicity, bone marrow suppression, pulmonary injury, and intestinal side effects is often narrow. Noncycling cells are resistant to cell cycle-specific drugs, and potentially vulnerable cells often rapidly develop biochemical means of resistance to chemotherapeutic agents (Hoshino 1984, Kornblith & Walker 1988).

Even if these therapies significantly reduce the tumor burden, the patient's immune response may be rendered ineffective by chemotherapy and by the tumor's secretion of factors antagonistic to immune cytokines (Kikuchi & Neuwelt 1983). Each of these limitations of each component of multimodality therapy may contribute to failure to prevent tumor regrowth. At the time of tumor recurrence, consideration of these reasons for failure is essential to assessment of prognosis and to the choice of subsequent therapy.

III. PROGNOSTIC IMPLICATIONS OF RESIDUAL AND RECURRENT TUMOR

In the management of a recurrent brain tumor, consideration of the prognostic implications of regrowth is essential. The presence of residual tumor and the occurrence of tumor regrowth likely have different prognostic implications.

A. Residual tumor

Radiologic demonstration of residual tumor after initial treatment may be consistent with preoperative goals and expectations; the prognosis would be that originally formulated. If, however, residual tumor is identified unexpectedly, the prognosis may need to be altered. The prognostic import of residual tumor is best seen in the relationship between extent of resection and likelihood of tumor recurrence.

1. Residual meningiomas

For meningiomas, the extent of resection dramatically affects patient outcome. The incidence of symptomatic recurrence varies with the amount of tumor remaining after the initial operation: 44% following partial removal; 29% following removal of tumor down to its dural base; 19% after removal of tumor and coagulation of its dural base; and 9% following removal of all tumor and infiltrated dura and bone (Simpson 1957). That resection of the dural base of an otherwise completely removed tumor reduces the recurrence rate by half (10% vs 20%) has been confirmed by subsequent reports (Yamashita et al 1980, Chan & Thompson 1984). In a more recent study, total removal produced a much higher chance of freedom from recurrence than did partial removal (93%, 80%, and 68% vs 63%, 45%, and 9% after 5, 10, and 15 years respectively) (Mirimanoff et al 1985). The probabilities of a second operation were 6%, 15%, and 20% at intervals of 5, 10, and 15 years after a total resection but 25%, 44%, and 84% at the same intervals following partial resection.

Tumor location is a critical determinant of resectability and, thus, of recurrence frequency. Reported 5–10-year recurrence rates are approximately 5% for intraventricular meningiomas, 20% for parasagittal, falcine, cerebral convexity, parabasal convexity (lateral sphenoid wing and olfactory groove) and cerebellar convexity tumors, and 50% for basal (medial sphenoid, cavernous, orbital, clival, petrous, and tentorial) meningiomas (Phillipon & Cornu 1991). In one series, 96% of convexity meningiomas were totally removed and only 3% had recurred at 5 years, but for sphenoid ridge meningiomas, the total resection rate was 28% and the 5-year recurrence rate was 34% (Mirimanoff et al 1985). High rates of incomplete removal likely reflect tumor investment of cranial nerves, the brainstem, the internal carotid, vertebral, or basilar arteries, or invasion of dural sinuses. Widespread invasion of bone, particularly if lytic rather than hyperostotic changes are seen, and infiltration of cortex are also prognostic of frequent and early recurrence. In one series, 40% (12/30) of tumors causing skull lysis recurred, but only 13% (4/31) of hyperostosing tumors recurred — despite the observation that hyperostotic bone almost invariably contains tumor cells (Olmsted & McGee 1977). Similarly, invasion of cortex is ominous; it was noted in 22% of multiply recurrent tumors, 9% of singly recurrent tumors, and only 1% of non-recurrent tumors (Boker et al 1985).

Other atypical pathologic features correlating with a tendency to recur are necrosis and frequent mitoses. Necrosis occurred in 26% of tumors that eventually recurred but in only 6% of nonrecurring tumors. The comparable incidences for high mitotic frequency were 20% and 8%, respectively (Boker et al 1985, de la Monte et al 1986). High proliferation indices — BUdR labeling index greater than 1% and flow cytometric index greater than 19% — separate tumors prone to recurrence from nonrecurring ones and correlate with tumor doubling rates of several months rather than years and with time to tumor recurrence of 1–3 years rather than 5–10 years (Jaaskelainen et al 1985, Cho et al 1986, Crone et al 1988). Almost all meningiomas with multiple atypical characteristics recur, regardless of the extent of their resection (de la Monte et al 1986, Jaaskelainen 1986, Jaaskelainen et al 1986).

Young age correlates with the likelihood of recurrence of meningiomas because of the longer time at risk and more aggressive tumor behavior. In one series, tumors that eventually recurred initially presented at a mean age of 43 years, as opposed to 53 years for nonrecurrent tumors. This relationship holds for the risk of recurrence after reoperation as well; tumors with multiple recurrences initially presented at 36.4 years vs. 46.7 years for singly recurrent tumors (Phillipon & Cornu 1991). These prognostic indicators should influence the decisions regarding the management of both residual and recurrent meningiomas.

When residual tumor is identified by postoperative imaging, the management options include reoperation, irradiation, and observation. Unless a readily correctible technical or medical consideration limited the initial resection, early reoperation will not be warranted. Radiation of residual meningiomas is relatively safe and effective; in one study, radiation following surgery reduced the rate of recurrence of incompletely resected meningiomas from 60% to 32% and increased the interval to recurrence from 66 to 125 months (Carella et al 1982, Barbaro et al 1987, Goldsmith et al 1992). Nevertheless, the ability to detect small changes in tumor size radiographically, their relatively slow growth, and the infrequency of malignant transformation argue for delaying reoperation or irradiation of residual tumor mass until renewed growth is documented. Follow-up of such cases must be regular (usually annual neurologic and radiographic examinations) and sustained, as the cumulative risk of recurrence continues to increase after 5 and 10 years (Mirimanoff et al 1985). Atypical and malignant meningiomas, with their high likelihood of rapid regrowth, however, warrant adjuvant radiation, even if gross total resection is achieved.

2. Residual gliomas

Cytoreductive surgery is a fundamental part of the treatment of most systemic malignancies (Devita 1983). In most cases, there is a strong relationship between the extent of resection and outcome. For gliomas, the relationship between extent of resection or, more significantly, size of residual tumor, and outcome measures, such as interval to tumor progression and survival, is less clear.

Correlation of survival with extent of resection for low grade gliomas has been suggested by retrospective uncontrolled reviews and comparisons with historical controls (Ammirati et al 1987a, Vertosick et al 1991, McCormack et al 1992). One study of 461 adult patients with low grade cerebral gliomas found that gross total surgical removal correlated with length of survival (Laws et al 1984). Another reported a median survival of 7.4 years following maximal surgical resection. The median survival of a subgroup of hemispheric tumors compared favorably (10 years vs 8 years) with that of a comparable series treated with biopsy and radiation alone (Vertosick et al 1991, McCormack et al 1992).

For high grade gliomas, the correlations between the extent of resection at the initial operation and both the time to tumor recurrence and the duration of patient survival are disputed (Coffey et al 1988). Historical reports and reviews of large series have noted the association of survival and extent of resection for both astrocytomas and oligodendrogliomas (Jelsma & Bucy 1969, Walker et al 1978, Chang et al 1983, Nelson et al 1985, Shaw et al 1992). Extensive reviews of the literature, however, have failed to locate randomized, controlled clinical trials comparing survival after biopsy with that after radical resection of malignant gliomas (Nazzaro & Neuwelt 1990, Quigley & Maroon 1991). Nevertheless, the benefit of surgical cytoreduction has been strongly suggested:

1. Reviews of multicentered trials have shown that the more complete the resection, the longer the patient lived (Shapiro 1982, Wood et al 1988).
2. In another study of 243 patients, multivariate regression analysis identified extent of resection as an important prognostic factor ($p < 0.0001$) for survival (Vecht et al 1990).
3. Single center studies have confirmed this relationship: in one study containing 21 glioblastomas and 10 anaplastic astrocytomas, median survival after gross total resection was 90 weeks versus only 43 weeks following subtotal resection, and the 2-year survival rates were 19% and 0%, respectively, even though the two groups were well matched for other prognostically significant variables (Ammirati 1987b, Ciric et al 1989); in another, patients with gross total resection of malignant glioma lived longer (76 versus 19 weeks) than those who underwent only a biopsy, even after correction for tumor accessibility and all other prognostically significant variables (Winger et al 1989).

4. In two larger series, patients with resected cortical and subcortical grade IV gliomas lived longer (50.6 vs 33.0 weeks — Devaux et al 1993; and 39.5 vs 32.0 weeks — Kreth et al 1993) after surgery and radiation than those who underwent biopsy and radiation.

5. Small postoperative tumor volume has been shown to correlate with time to tumor progression after surgery (Levin et al 1980) and longer patient survival (Androeu et 1983).

Although less than ideal, the data which exist for gliomas and experience with tumors outside the central nervous system suggest the benefit of cytoreduction when a near-total removal (1–2 log reduction of tumor cell number) of a glial tumor can be achieved. Thus, failure to identify and remove readily accessible tumor mass at an initial operation might warrant reoperation before regrowth occurs.

B. Recurrent tumor

Regrowth of tumors after an initial response (diminution or stability) to surgery and radiation therapy is ominous. This is particularly true if the growth is more rapid or more infiltrative than that of the original tumor. Such growth often manifests changes in the basic biology of the tumor that make it less responsive to subsequent therapy. A short interval between initial treatment and recurrence of symptoms often indicates rapid regrowth and a poor prognosis. Factors to be considered in estimating prognosis include the biology of the tumor (its pathology, growth rate, and invasiveness), its resectability, its prior response to radiation and chemotherapy, and the age and performance status of the patient. Estimates of the recurrent tumor's size, growth rate, invasiveness, and location must be made in assessing its potential for causing both neurologic deficit and death. Reappearance of a slowly growing, well-demarcated frontal convexity meningioma in a middle-aged patient of good neurologic condition after a 10-year interval of postsurgical quiescence clearly carries a much different prognosis than diffuse diencephalic spread of a glioblastoma multiforme in an elderly patient with a poor performance status three months after treatment with surgery, radiation, and chemotherapy.

IV. THERAPY OF RECURRENT TUMORS

The choice of therapy of a recurrent tumor is based upon a comparison of the natural history of the regrowing tumor with the risk/benefit calculus of potential therapies.

A. Therapy of recurrent meningiomas

Meningiomas that recur may warrant reoperation and/or radiation. Recurrent meningiomas can cause neurologic deficit and threaten survival by direct compression of eloquent tissue or by increasing intracranial pressure. An enlarging tumor, even if asymptomatic, should be treated unless anatomical considerations, severe medical problems, or limited life expectancy preclude it. The decision to reoperate must weigh the natural history of the recurrent tumor, its likelihood of causing neurologic injury or death within the patient's expected lifetime, the technical feasibility of achieving a radical resection, and the patient's medical condition.

The pattern of recurrence will influence the choice of therapy. Recurrence is almost always local, although multifocal recurrence and spread of tumor in different directions from the original site can occur. Multifocal recurrence was found in 16% (7/45) of cases in one series of recurrent meningiomas; multifocality of recurrence was associated with younger age, atypical and malignant histologies, and a tendency to recur multiple times (Phillipon & Cornu 1991). These types of meningiomas require more extensive surgical exposure and mandate radiation after reoperation.

Recurrent tumors may recapitulate the pattern of growth of the original tumor or they may behave differently. In the former case, the surgical considerations will be similar to those of the original operation. In the latter, a different surgical approach may be needed: (1) a convexity meningioma that was intradural initially may regrow extradurally, extend through a trephination, and erode the scalp — excision may necessitate a larger scalp flap which requires tissue transfer for closure and piecemeal removal of a bone flap anchored to the dura by a dumbbell extension of the tumor through the trephination (Fig. 23.2); (2) a falx meningioma may regrow contralaterally requiring a bilateral exposure; (3) a parasagittal meningioma may completely occlude a previously patent superior sagittal sinus such that excision of the sinus and complete removal of the tumor is possible; and, (4) a globoid clinoidal meningioma may recur as an en plaque tumor extending through the optic canal or invading the cavernous sinus such that a more extensive resection of the skull base is necessary.

If surgery is not feasible, or if tumor remains after reoperation, radiation should be given, particularly if the meningioma's histology is atypical or malignant. The probability of another recurrence after reoperation alone is 42% at 5 years and 56% after 10 years; and the mean recurrence-free interval is shorter following each successive surgery: 6 years, 3 years and 10 months, 3 years, and 1 year and 7 months after the first, second, third, and fourth operations, respectively (Mirimanoff et al 1985, Phillipon & Cornu 1991). If the tumor is small (less than 10 cm^3 in volume), the histology is typical, and MRI with gadolinium enhancement shows the tumor to be discrete, then radiosurgery is an excellent alternative to fractionated teletherapy. Stereotactic radiosurgery of cavernous sinus meningiomas remaining after radical surgery has provided a 100% control rate at a median follow-up of 2 years

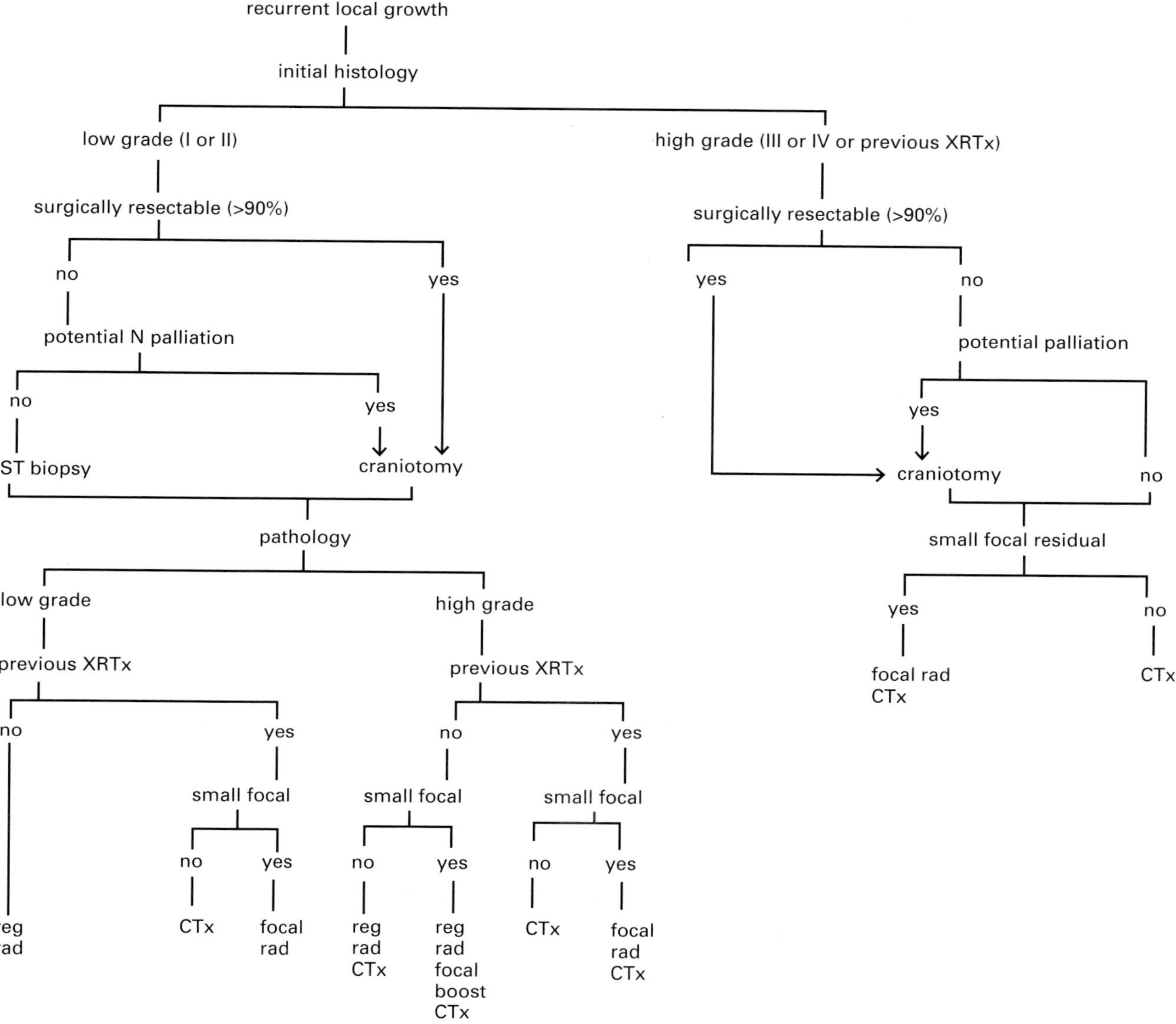

Fig. 23.2 Management of a recurrent glioma. Decisions in the management of a recurrent tumor should consider grade, resectability and prior therapy.

(range 6–54 months); 19/34 (56%) tumors regressed; 24% of patients had neurologic improvement; 70% were unchanged, and 2 patients (6%) developed permanent new neurologic deficits (Duma et al 1993). If the tumor is large, appears more malignant, and grows diffusely, fractionated teletherapy, which permits treatment of a larger volume, is appropriate (Carella et al 1982, Barbaro et al 1987, Goldsmith et al 1992). In a subset of one series treated with treatment planning based on CT or MR imaging, an actuarial progression-free survival rate of 98% at 5 years was achieved (Goldsmith et al 1992). Tumor remaining after reoperation should also be irradiated. Anti-steroid receptor chemotherapy (e.g. RU486) may be beneficial (Tilzer et al 1982). Other, more standard forms of chemotherapy are of little value for recurrent meningiomas, even those with a malignant histology. Following retreatment of a meningioma, just as with the original tumor, rigorous, long-term follow-up is necessary.

B. Therapy of recurrent gliomas

Gliomas that recur warrant aggressive multimodality therapy if the patient is in acceptable neurologic and general medical condition and therapeutic options offer a realistic chance for significant palliation of neurologic status or extension of survival (Salcman et al 1982a).

1. *Patterns of recurrence of gliomas*

When gliomas recur, most do so locally. More than

80% of recurrent glioblastoma multiforme arise within 2 cm of the original margin of contrast-enhancing tumor (Hochberg & Pruitt 1980, Wallner et al 1989a). This tendency to recur locally is a function of tumor cell distribution. There is a gradient of tumor cell density in which tumor cell number decreases rapidly at increasing distances from the contrast-enhancing rim of solid tumor. Thus, although there are individual tumor cells spread through the brain at great distances from the primary site, there are so many more cells locally that odds favor local reaccumulation of tumor mass (Burger et al 1983, Kelly et al 1987). Factors contributing to the likelihood of local recurrence include: (1) the relative predominance of tumor cell mass in the region; (2) the statistical likelihood that a local cell will be the cell that first develops a competitive proliferative advantage; (3) the possibility that the physiologic milieu (hypervascularity, disrupted tissue architecture, and paracrine growth factor stimuli) at the site is particularly conducive to regrowth.

As tumor cell proliferation resumes at the initial tumor site, cells again spread rapidly and diffusely. Tumor cell proliferation resumes at distant sites as a result of the influx of these new, mitotically active cells or the renewed growth of cells that spread before the initial treatment (Fig. 23.3) (Choucair et al 1986). Consequently, treatments targeting local recurrence alone will, at best, be briefly palliative. Treatment of tumor recurrences thus usually involves a combination of modalities aimed at both local and distant disease.

2. *Multimodality therapy of recurrent malignant glioma*

An enlarging lesion that was originally a low grade glioma should undergo biopsy (stereotactically or, if resection is anatomically feasible, by open craniotomy) to confirm histology (Fig. 23.4). If the tumor remains low grade and a majority of the lesion can be resected without inflicting significant neurologic deficit, it should be removed; if previously irradiated to less than maximal tolerable dose, the tumor bed and surrounding area should receive fractionated teletherapy. If the tumor is inaccessible to surgery, radiation alone should be prescribed. If a previously irradiated low grade tumor recurs as a low grade glioma, it should be resected, if possible. If it is inaccessible, stereotactically delivered focal radiation should be given (Ostertag 1983).

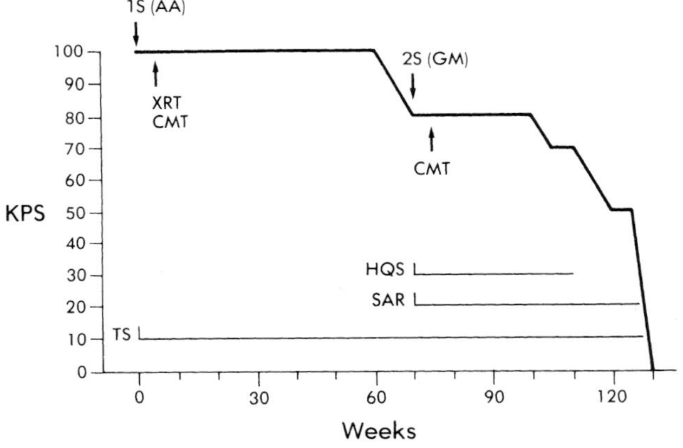

Fig. 23.3 Quality of life considerations in the management of patients with malignant gliomas. Maintenance of high performance status is a critical feature of outcome. The Karnofsky score (KPS) as a function of time indicates the quality of the survival time that follows each intervention. 1S = initial surgery; XRT = radiation therapy; CMT = chemotherapy; 2S = reoperation; TS = total survival; HQS = high quality survival (K =/>70); SAR = survival after reoperation; AA = anaplastic astrocytoma; GM = glioblastoma multiforme.

If the low grade tumor recurs as a high grade tumor or if a high grade tumor recurs, reoperation should be attempted if the patient has a Karnofsky score of at least 70 and removal of all or almost all of the contrast-enhancing tumor is potentially attainable, or if the tumor mass is causing neurologic symptoms that might be palliated by its reduction. If previously unirradiated, the tumor bed and its annular margin should receive regional teletherapy; a stereotactically delivered focal boost of interstitial brachytherapy or radiosurgery should be given to any contrast-enhancing residual, particularly if the recurrent tumor is a glioblastoma (Loeffler et al 1990b, Alexander & Loeffler 1992, Scharfen et al 1992).

Brachytherapy has proven valuable in treating glioblastomas, both initially and at the time of recurrence. The median survival following brachytherapy was 49 weeks for recurrent glioblastomas but only 52 weeks for anaplastic astrocytomas (Scharfen et al 1992). Patients receiving brachytherapy were highly selected; only about 20% of recurrent tumors met the criteria of size and focality. Almost 10% of patients suffered severe acute toxicity and approximately 40% required reoperation for medically refractory neurologic deterioration and intracranial mass effect. Although tumor was identified in 95% of the specimens harvested at reoperation, reoperation was associated with a longer survival after brachytherapy (90 versus 37 weeks for those not undergoing reoperation). The authors suggested that this morbidity was justified by the prolongation of survival achieved in patients with glioblastomas but not by that for those with anaplastic astrocytomas (Scharfen et al 1992). Stereotactic radiosurgery is a less invasive way of inducing tumor necrosis. Reported median survival following radiosurgery of recurrent glioblastomas is 40 weeks and for recurrent anaplastic astrocytomas it is at least 16 months. Here, too, patients were highly selected and significant radiation injury was frequent (21% of cases) (Alexander & Loeffler 1992).

Chemotherapy of recurrent astrocytomas is often valuable. Low grade tumors will generally not have been treated by chemotherapy at the time of initial presentation unless a predominant oligodendrocytic component warranted PCV (procarbazine, CCNU, vincristine) chemotherapy (Glass et al 1992). Adjuvant chemotherapy of

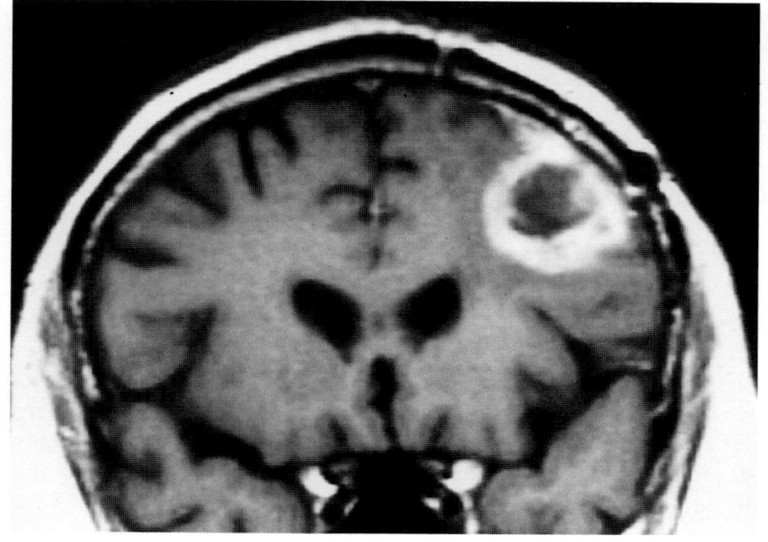

A

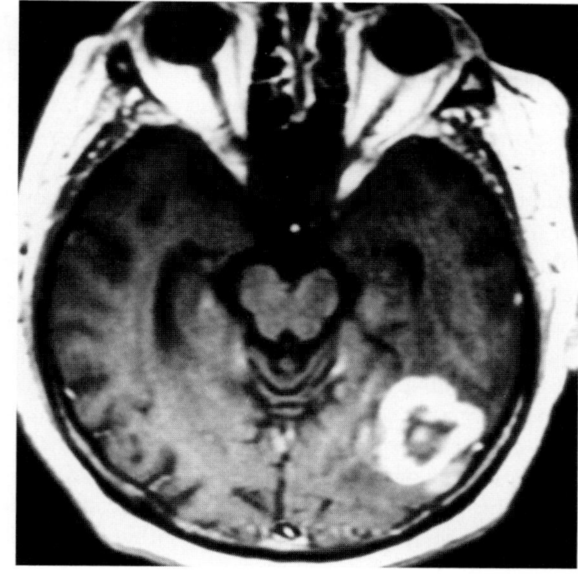

C

B

Fig. 23.4 Recurrent malignant glioma. **A.** A 34-year-old man developed local recurrence of a left frontal glioblastoma multiforme 6 months following treatment with surgery and radiation therapy. **B.** This was treated by reoperation and chemotherapy. **C.** Four months later, he developed a left occipital tumor that also was resected. He received additional chemotherapy and survived for 5 months following the second reoperation.

malignant gliomas, in combination with radiation and surgery, increases the percentage of patients surviving at 1 year by 10% (a relative increase of 23.4%) and at 2 years of 8.6% (a 52.4% relative increase) (Fine et al 1993, Shapiro et al 1989). For grade IV tumors, BCNU and PCV provide similar results, but the PCV combination is superior for grade III tumors (Fine et al 1993, Levin et al 1990, Prados et al 1992). At the time of renewed growth of a high grade tumor, if the tumor has not previously been exposed to a nitrosourea, BCNU or the PCV combination should be tried (Deutsch et al 1989). If nitrosourea therapy is unsuccessful, non-nitrosourea alternatives such as carboplatin, cisplatin, or tamoxifen might be appropriate. The response rates (partial response or stable disease) to such chemotherapy at the time of recurrence range from 20–50%. In a recent study using intravenous carboplatin, a response occurred in 48% of patients (57% of patients with recurrent anaplastic astrocytomas and 40% of patients with glioblastoma multiforme); responders had a median time to tumor progression of 26 weeks compared to a median of 11 weeks for the entire group (Yung et al 1991).

3. *Rationale for reoperation*

Early reoperation, within months of the initial procedure, might be indicated for complications such as intracerebral, subdural, or epidural hematoma, wound dehiscence and infection, or hydrocephalus and CSF leakage. Occasionally, failure to identify and remove readily accessible tumor mass might warrant reoperation. In the Royal Melbourne Hospital experience, 5 of 200 patients underwent early reoperation (Kaye 1992).

More frequently, true tumor recurrence after an interval of response to the initial therapy is the reason for considering reoperation. Reoperation is justified if it produces sustained improvement of neurologic condition and quality of life and/or significant enhancement of response rates to adjuvant therapy. Palliation of neurologic symptoms by surgery results from reduction of the local mass effect produced by the tumor and tumor-induced edema. Multiple studies have shown that surgical cytoreduction can both improve neurologic deficits and promote maintenance of high performance status. One review of 82 patients examined 5 categories of neurologic function in each patient. 191 neurologic deficits were noted preoperatively. Postoperatively, 151 deficits were improved or stable and 40 were worse (Shapiro et al 1989). Another study showed that patients undergoing gross total resection of their malignant gliomas were likely to have improved neurologic benefit (97% of 36 patients had either improved or stable neurologic examinations), improved functional status (mean Karnofsky score improvement of 6.8%) and extended maintenance of good functional status (185 weeks) (Ammirati et al 1987b, Ciric et al 1989). A third confirmed that extent of surgery was correlated with better immediate postoperative performance, lower 1-month mortality rate, and longer survival — 43% of patients with malignant gliomas improved, 50% remained unchanged, and 7% suffered deterioration in their neurologic condition following resection of at least 75% of their tumor, as opposed to 28% improved, 51% unchanged, and 21% worse after a more limited resection (Vecht et al 1990).

Similar results can be achieved by reoperation. In one series 45% of the patients had an improved Karnofsky score following reoperation (Ammirati et al 1987a). In another reoperation series, when gross tumor resection was achieved, 82% (32/39) of patients had improvement or stability in their Karnofsky score (Wallner et al 1989b).

The doubling rate of malignant gliomas is so high, however, that the benefit from reoperation will be very brief unless there are adjuvant therapies able to induce remission of tumor growth. Surgical resection is especially beneficial when reduction of tumor burden improves the response rate to such therapies. Studies from UCSF, Memorial Sloan-Kettering and the University of Washington at Seattle have shown that reoperation followed by chemotherapy leads to stabilization of performance score for significant intervals (Ammirati et al 1987a, Harsh et al 1987, Berger et al 1992). At UCSF, 44% of patients with glioblastomas maintained a performance level of at least 70 (a level consistent with self care and judged to be survival of high quality — Karnofsky et al 1951) for at least 6 months after reoperation; 18% maintained this level for at least a year; and 3 patients did so for longer than 3 years. Most (52% of 31) patients with anaplastic astrocytomas maintained this performance level for at

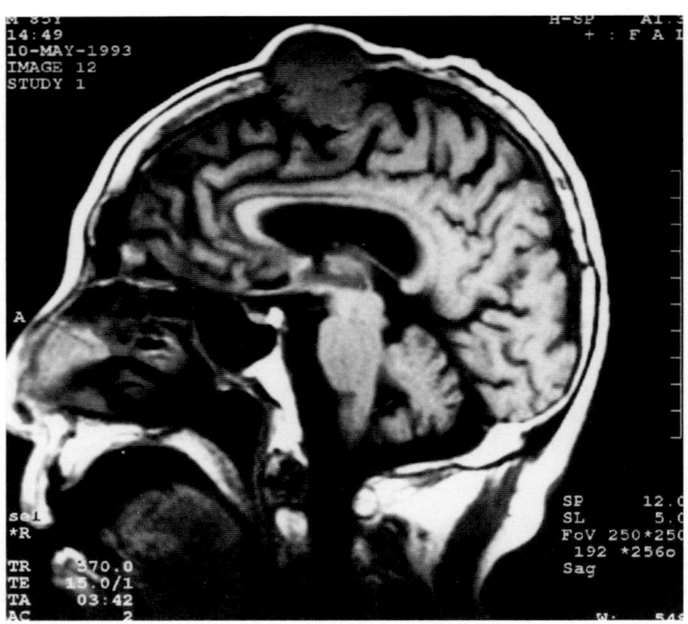

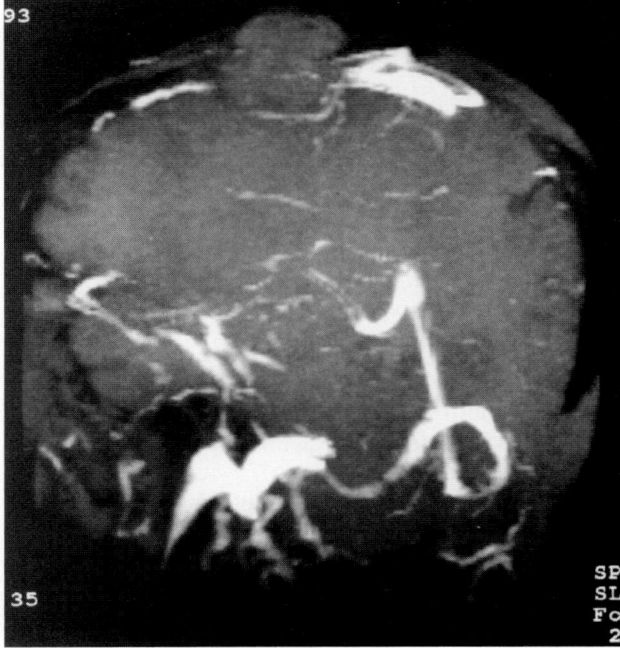

Fig. 23.5 Recurrent meningioma. **A.** A 78-year-old man developed a convexity skull mass at the site of a falx meningioma that had been resected previously. Extension of the recurrent tumor through the skull and falx was apparent. **B.** The superior sagittal sinus was occluded by tumor such that it could be sacrificed and the tumor totally removed.

least 12 months after reoperation; 13% had more than 4 years of high quality survival. Approximately 90% of the survival after reoperation for anaplastic meningioma was of high quality (Harsh et al 1987) (Fig. 23.5). In the Memorial Sloan-Kettering group, the median duration of maintenance of independent status (Karnofsky score of at least 80) was 34 weeks. In the Seattle series, patients with a Karnofsky score of at least 70 maintained this high level of function for an average of 37 weeks after reoperation for glioblastoma and for 70 weeks after reoperation for anaplastic astrocytoma (Berger et al 1992).

Aggressive surgical cytoreduction at the time of recurrence increases the duration as well as the quality of patient survival (Salcman 1985). Support for reoperation is found in comparisons of the outcomes in cases in which different degrees of tumor removal were accomplished and in comparisons of the survival of patients following reoperation with that of historical controls not receiving reoperation. Patients in whom gross total resection of a glioblastoma is achieved survive longer (45.6 versus 25.6 weeks) than do those receiving near-total or subtotal resections; for anaplastic astrocytomas, the effect of extent of resection is similar (87.5 versus 55.7 weeks) (Berger et al 1992). In the Sloan-Kettering series that grouped glioblastomas and anaplastic astrocytomas together, a similar difference was found (51.2 versus 23.3 weeks) (Ammirati et al 1987a). In the UCSF series, survival of patients undergoing reoperation and chemotherapy for either anaplastic astrocytoma or glioblastoma was longer than that of patients receiving chemotherapy alone at the time of tumor recurrence (Harsh et al 1987).

The benefit of reoperative surgery is also suggested by experience with brachytherapy. Patients undergoing reoperation for tumor recurrence and/or radiation necrosis following brachytherapy for glioblastomas, either initially or at first recurrence, survived longer than those not receiving reoperation, with median total survival of 120 versus 62 weeks for patients with primarily treated tumors and 90 versus 37 weeks for patients treated with brachytherapy at the time of first recurrence (Scharfen et al 1992).

Reoperation as a part of the multimodality treatment of recurrent gliomas is further supported by study of long-term survivors of glioblastoma multiforme. A review of the UCSF experience identified 22/449 (5%) patients with glioblastomas who survived at least 5 years after diagnosis. 16 of 22 had tumor recurrence that was treated; 9 underwent between one and three reoperations. For 8 of the 16 patients with treated recurrence, survival after treatment of recurrence (median of 4.5 years) was longer than the remission produced by the initial treatment (Chandler et al 1993).

4. *Selection of patients for reoperation*

Case selection is critical to outcome. The patient's profile of prognostic factors, his/her predicted tolerance of the procedure, and the feasibility of extensive tumor resection without undue risk of new neurologic morbidity must all be considered. Multiple characteristics have been identified as predictive of a good response to reoperation (Table 23.1). Foremost among these are tumor histology, patient

Table 23.1 Reoperation for recurrent gliomas

Author	# pts	Path	SAR	HOS	Morb	Mort	↓K	Cx	Px Relations	Weeks
Young et al 1981	24	GM	14		52%	17%	25%	25%	$K \geq 60 \rightarrow$ SAR	22 v 9
									II > 12m → SAR	16.5 v 8.5
Salcman 1982	40	MG	37			0%		8%	Age < 40 → SAR	57 v 36
Ammirati et al 1987	55	64% GM	36	34	16%	64%	45%	18%	K > 70 → SAR	48.5 v 19
									Grade → SAR	61 v 29
									Ext. resect. → SAR	51.2 v 23.3
Harsh et al 1987	49	GM	36		5.7%		0%		Age → SAR	
									$K \geq 70 \rightarrow$ HQS	
Harsh et al 1987	21	AA	88	83	5.7%		0%		Age → HQS	
									Grade → SAR	
Berger et al 1992	56	GM							$K \geq 70 \rightarrow$ SAR	70.7 v 36.5
									$K \geq 70 \rightarrow$ SOE	36.6 v 8.4
									$Age \leq 60 \rightarrow$ SOE	35.1 v 9.4
									II > 12m → SAR	150 v 48
Berger et al 1992	14	AA							II > 12m → SOE	99.5 v 22.4
Kaye 1992	50	GM				16%	0%	52%	Age → SAR	
									Grade → SAR	
									II → SAR	
									Age → HQS	
									Grade → HQS	
									II → HQS	
Scharfen 1992	18	GM	52				40%			
	27	AA	153							

Key: Path = pathology; GM = glioblastoma multiforme; AA = anaplastic astrocytoma; SAR = survival after reoperation; HQS = high quality survival (K=/≥ 70); Morb = morbidity; Mort = mortality; ↓K = decreased performance score; Cx = complications; II = interoperative interval; Ext resect = extent of resection.

age, performance status, interoperative interval, and extent of resection.

The prognostic significance of tumor grade is evident in most series. Median survival after reoperation was 88 weeks for patients with anaplastic astrocytomas but only 36 weeks for those with glioblastomas at UCSF, and 61 weeks and 29 weeks, respectively, at Sloan-Kettering (Ammirati et al 1987a, Harsh et al 1987).

The effect of age may overwhelm that of tumor grade. In one series, survival after reoperation was 57 weeks for those younger than 40 years but only 36 weeks for older patients (Salcman et al 1982a,b). Other authors found an association between youth and total survival after diagnosis and between youth and quality of survival after reoperation, but not duration of survival after reoperation (Ammirati et al 1987a, Harsh et al 1987).

Preoperative performance score significantly affected outcome. At Kentucky, survival after reoperation was 22 weeks for patients with performance scores of at least 70 but only 9 weeks for more disabled patients (Young et al 1981). In the Seattle series, for glioblastomas, survival after reoperation was almost twice as long (71 versus 36 weeks) for patients with Karnofsky scores of at least 70 (Berger et al 1992).

The prognostic importance of the interval between initial treatment and recurrence is disputed (Wilson 1975). The Kentucky series found survival to be twice as long if the interval between operations exceeded 6 months. In Seattle, a three-fold difference (150 versus 48 weeks for glioblastoma, and 164 versus 52 weeks for anaplastic astrocytomas) was noted when the time to progression exceeded 3 years (Berger et al 1992). Others, however, have found either no relation, or an inverse relation between the interoperative interval and survival after reoperation (Salcman et al 1982b, Ammirati et al 1987a, Harsh et al 1987).

A more complete resection of recurrent tumor portends longer survival. At Sloan-Kettering, gross total resection afforded a median survival of 51.2 weeks versus 23.3 weeks for a more limited resection (Ammirati et al 1987a, Wallner et al 1989b). Others have noted a strong trend in the correlation between a more complete removal of tumor and survival duration (Berger et al 1992). The ability to remove sufficient tumor mass to reduce intracranial pressure and palliate neurologic symptoms depends on the location of the tumor and its physical characteristics. Removal is facilitated by a more superficial location in noneloquent areas; a discrete pseudoencapsulated mass is more easily removed than a less well-marginated diffuse one; drainage of a cystic component will often provide immediate reduction of mass, as well as an avenue for further resection of tumor.

During the interval between initial surgery and tumor recurrence, the patient will usually undergo therapy that might affect his/her tolerance of surgery. The decision to reoperate must consider overall physical condition, tissue viability, blood coagulability, hematologic reserve, and immune function following surgery, radiation, corticosteroids, and chemotherapy. High risk of multisystem failure, failure to thrive, intracranial hemorrhage, anemia, wound infection, pneumonia, and neurologic damage may exist. This risk should be assessed for each patient by obtaining preoperative chemical, hematologic, and radiographic studies.

In choosing patients for reoperation, consideration of the individual patient's profile of these prognostically significant factors permits a reasonable estimate of the likelihood of his benefiting from the procedure.

5. *Preparation for reoperation*

Preoperatively the patient is likely to be receiving corticosteroids; these should be continued. At the time of induction of anesthesia, the patient is fitted with elastic stockings and thigh-high intermittent-compression airboots. He/she is given additional steroids, prophylactic antibiotics, an anticonvulsant, and osmotic and loop diuretics and is hyperventilated. In positioning the patient, the likelihood of elevated intracranial pressure makes attention to elevation of the head above the level of the heart particularly important.

6. *Reoperative exposure*

In planning the needed exposure, the location of the tumor can be specified by its relationship to the margins of the craniotomy plate on CT scan, to the cortical pattern of gyri and sulci on the MRI scan, or by intraoperative stereotactic localization techniques. The procedure should be planned in advance to ensure adequate skin opening, craniotomy, and durotomy to expose the recurrent mass. All may need enlarging due to the increased extent of the tumor or a desire to perform corticography for mapping of motor and/or speech function.

The previous skin incision is usually used. The skin opening can be increased by additional incisions. They should be external to the previous flap, avoid its base and other vascular pedicles, and intersect the previous incision at right angles. The margins of the prior craniotomy flap should be defined. Generally, this is best accomplished with a curet, beginning at the prior trephination. Only rarely does the prior flap need to be recut. Dissection in the epidural plane can be begun with a curet followed by a #3 and then a #2 Penfield dissector. The craniotomy plate is further elevated as the dura is stripped from its inner surface with a periosteal elevator. Epidural adhesions fixing dura to the craniotomy margin should be preserved as prophylaxis against postoperative extension of an epidural fluid collection unless the craniotomy needs to be enlarged. In this case, these adhesions are dissected with a curet and trimmed. After the dura is stripped from the undersurface of the cranial plate, an additional segment of bone can be removed with a craniotome.

The durotomy may need to be enlarged, but often it can be limited to part of the dural exposure. It should be planned to minimize traverse of cortical adhesions. For instance, in re-exposing a temporal lesion, the durotomy can be placed over the cyst remaining from the prior resection. Flapping the dura superiorly then allows adhesions to be put on traction such that they may be dissected from cortex, coagulated, and sharply divided. Extending a durotomy along an old incision line should be avoided. The old incision line should be traversed perpendicularly and as infrequently as possible in that it is often the site of the densest adhesions. Microdissection of larger vessels from dural attachments may be necessary.

Once the dura is opened and retracted, the exposed cortex is inspected for the surface presentation of the tumor, apparent as abnormal color, consistency, and vascularity.

Localization of the subcortical extent of the tumor is then undertaken. Again, the preoperative imaging studies and stereotactic techniques are of value (Kelly 1989). Transcortical ultrasonography is often helpful, although this technique tends to overestimate the volume of recurrent tumor (Le Roux et al 1989). Tumor may also be found by locating a cystic resection cavity or encephalomalacic brain left after the previous operation. In that almost all tumors recur within 2 cm of the original tumor's margin, exposure of the initial tumor's surgical bed will usually reveal at least part of the recurrent mass.

Electrocorticographic mapping of motor, sensory, and speech areas may reduce the chance of inflicting neurologic deficit and may encourage a more extensive resection by revealing the relationship of the site of cortical traverse and of the subsequent subcortical dissection to eloquent brain (Berger et al 1990). This technique is often more difficult at the time of reoperation because of cortical disruption by the tumor and prior surgery. An intraoperative photograph from cortical mapping at the time of the initial craniotomy may suffice.

Generally, the appearance of the tumor itself is the best guide to its extent. Tumor-infiltrated cortex is likely to have increased vascular markings, a pink to gray color, and a firm consistency. Its central core may vary from yellow cystic fluid of low viscosity to high viscosity, soupy, white necrosis that resembles pus, to a yellow-gray, granular, honeycomb-like material. Generally, the center is relatively avascular although it may be traversed by thrombosed blood vessels.

Some advocate incision into the tumor mass and internal debulking with an ultrasonic aspirator or laser as an initial step. However, this often induces significant hemorrhage. Enucleation by circumferential dissection in the pseudoplane about the rim of solid tumor is usually more satisfactory. Arteries supplying the tumor and veins draining it can be coagulated and divided as they enter the tumor mass, much as the vascular supply of an arteriovenous malformation is handled. Particularly in areas of noneloquent brain, the softened, necrotic, highly edematous white matter around the tumor provides an excellent plane of dissection. The use of bipolar cautery forceps and suction together accomplishes this dissection while reducing local mass. Beyond the encephalomalacic brain lies more normal brain that, although edematous and possibly injured by prior retraction and radiation therapy, is often functional and should be preserved.

Often, the tumor can be removed as a single specimen without the need for significant retraction of surrounding brain. In general, gentle, temporary displacement of a cottonoid paddy lying on the margin of resection provides sufficient exposure of the dissection plane that fixed self-retaining retractors are unnecessary. Retraction of the tumor mass is preferable to retraction of surrounding brain. Often, identification of the appropriate plane for the circumferential dissection is facilitated by this retraction on the tumor; coherence of the tumor mass helps delineate the plane between solid tumor and tumor-infiltrated brain.

Once the tumor mass has been removed, the margins of resection should be inspected to verify completeness of the excision. The margins should be free of tumor that is more firm, glassy, opaque, and hypervascular. Biopsies of the surrounding edematous brain should be sent for frozen-section analysis to verify absence of tumor. If solid tumor or tumor infiltrating into non-eloquent areas remains, it should be removed. In some cases, extension of tumor into eloquent areas or diencephalic structures will preclude resection of the entire mass. In such cases, the tumor should be divided. This often entails coagulation of numerous strands of small, thin-walled blood vessels. This is particularly true if the extension is in the direction of the vascular supply, e.g. medial extension of a temporal lobe tumor toward the posterior aspect of the Sylvian fissure. Particular care should be taken to coagulate and sharply divide these vessels. Tearing them without prior coagulation will leave a loose end which will retract and continue to bleed. Such loose ends should be directly coagulated rather than tamponaded with hemostatic packing, which may encourage deeper dissection of a hematoma.

After the resection has been completed, hemostasis should be confirmed by filling the tumor cavity with saline and, during a Valsalva maneuver, observing for wisps of continuing hemorrhage. This should be performed with the patient's blood pressure at least as high as his/her normal pressure. The cavity is then aspirated, lined with a single layer of Surgicel, and filled again with irrigation fluid. Hyperventilation is then reversed to permit expansion of the brain during closure.

Watertight dural closure is essential. Often, this can be attained by primary suturing, given the decompression from the operation. If the dura is incompetent, it may be supplemented by a pericranial graft. Peripheral and central dural tacking sutures are placed. The bone fragments are wired together, and then the craniotomy plate is fixed with either stainless steel wire or non-absorbable monofilament suture. The wound is irrigated multiple times with antibiotic solution and then closed in layers with 2–0 absorbable suture in muscle, fascia, and galea. The galeal sutures should be inverted and the knots should be cut short to avoid erosion superficially. They should be placed in sufficient proximity that tension-free closure of the skin is possible. Simple running 4-0 nylon skin sutures provide adequate skin closure except at sites of attenuation where horizontal mattress sutures may be less likely to compromise blood supply.

Postoperatively, the patient should be closely monitored for at least 72 hours for signs of increased intracranial pressure from hematoma or edema. Fluid restriction, dehydration, and corticosteroids should be continued throughout this period. The patient should be mobilized as soon as possible, and a gadolinium-enhanced MRI scan should be obtained as soon as he/she is able to tolerate it.

REFERENCES

Alavi J B, Alavi A, Chawluk J et al 1988 Positron emission tomography in patients with gliomas. A predictor of prognosis. Cancer 62: 1074–1078

Alexander E A, Loeffler J S 1992 Radiosurgery using a modified linear accelerator. Neurosurgical Clinics of North America 3: 174–176

Ammirati M, Galicich J H, Arbit B 1987a Reoperation in the treatment of recurrent intracranial malignant gliomas. Neurosurgery 21: 607–614

Ammirati M, Vick N, Liao Y, Ciric I, Mikhael M 1987b Effect of the extent of surgical resection on survival and quality of life in patients with supratentorial glioblastomas and anaplastic astrocytomas. Neurosurgery 21: 201–206

Androeu J, George A E, Wise A et al 1983 CT prognostic criteria of survival after malignant glioma surgery. AJNR 4: 488–490

Barbaro N M, Gutin P H, Wilson C B, Sheline G E, Boldrey E B, Wara W M 1987 Radiation therapy in the treatment of partially resected meningiomas. Neurosurgery 20: 525–528

Berger M S, Ojemann G A, Lettich E 1990 Neurophysiological monitoring during astrocytoma surgery. Neurosurgical Clinics of North America 1: 65–80

Berger M S, Tucker A, Spence A, Winn H R 1992 Reoperation for glioma. Clinical Neurosurgery 39: 172–186

Boker D K, Meurer H, Gullotta F 1985 Recurrent intracranial meningiomas. Evaluation of some factors predisposing for tumor recurrence. Journal of Neurosurgical Science 29: 11–17

Borovich B, Doron Y 1986 Recurrence of intracranial meningiomas: the role played by regional multicentricity. Journal of Neurosurgery 64: 58–63

Borovich B, Doron Y, Braun J et al 1986 Recurrence of intracranial meningiomas: the role played by regional multicentricity. Part 2: clinical and radiological aspects. Journal of Neurosurgery 65: 168–171

Burger P C, Dubois P J, Schold S C Jr et al 1983 Computerized tomography and pathologic studies of the untreated, quiescent, and recurrent glioblastoma multiforme. Journal of Neurosurgery 58: 159–169

Burger P C, Heinz E R, Shibata T et al 1988 Topographic anatomy and CT correlations in the untreated glioblastoma multiforme. Journal of Neurosurgery 68: 698–704

Carella R J, Ransohoff J, Newall J 1982 Role of radiation therapy in the management of meningioma. Neurosurgery 10: 332–339

Chan R C, Thompson G B 1984 Morbidity, mortality and quality of life following surgery for intracranial meningiomas: a retrospective study in 257 cases. Journal of Neurosurgery 60: 52–60

Chang C H, Horton J, Schoenfeld O et al 1983 Comparison of postoperative radiotherapy and combined postoperative radiotherapy and chemotherapy in the multidisciplinary management of malignant gliomas. Cancer 52: 997–1007

Chandler K L, Prados M D, Malec M, Wilson C B 1993 Long-term survival in patients with glioblastoma multiforme. Neurosurgery 32: 716–720

Cho K G, Hoshino T, Nagashima T, Murovic J A, Wilson C B 1986 Prediction of tumor doubling time in recurrent meningiomas: cell kinetics studies with bromodeoxyuridine labelling. Journal of Neurosurgery 65: 790–794

Choucair A K, Levin V A, Gutin P H, Davis R L, Silver P, Edwards S M B, Wilson C B 1986 Development of multiple lesions during radiation therapy and chemotherapy in patients with gliomas. Journal of Neurosurgery 65: 654–658

Ciric I, Ammirati M, Vick N et al 1989 Supratentorial gliomas: surgical considerations and immediate postoperative results. Gross total resection versus partial resection. Neurosurgery 21: 21–26

Coffey R J, Lunsford L D, Taylor F H 1988 Survival after stereotactic biopsy of malignant gliomas. Neurosurgery 22: 465–473

Crone K R, Challa V R, Kute T E, Moody D M, Kelly D L Jr 1988 Relationship between flow cytometric features and clinical behaviour of meningiomas. Neurosurgery 23: 720–724

Daumas-Duport C, Blond S, Vedrenee C, Szikla G 1984 Radiolesion versus recurrence: bioptic data in 30 gliomas after interstitial implant or combined interstitial and external radiation treatment. Acta Neurochirurgica 33 (suppl): 291–299

de la Monte S, Flickinger J, Linggood R M 1986 Histopathologic features predicting recurrence of meningiomas following subtotal resection. American Journal of Surgical Pathology 10: 836–843

Deutsch M, Green S B, Strike T A et al 1989 Results of a randomized trial comparing BCNU plus radiotherapy, streptozotocin plus radiotherapy, BCNU plus hyperfractionated radiotherapy and BCNU following misonidazole plus radiotherapy in the postoperative treatment of malignant glioma. International Journal of Radiation Oncology Biology Physics 16: 1389–1396

Devaux B C, O'Fallon J R, Kelly P J 1993 Resection, biopsy, and survival in malignant gliomas. A retrospective study of clinical parameters, therapy, and outcome. Journal of Neurosurgery 78: 767–775

Devita V T 1983 The relationship between tumor mass and resistance to chemotherapy. Cancer 51: 1209–1220

DiChiro G, Brooks R, Bairamian D et al 1985 Diagnostic and prognostic value of positron emission tomography using [18F]-fluorodeoxyglucose in brain tumors. In: Reivich M, Alavi A (eds) Positron emission tomography. Alan R Liss, New York, NY, pp 291–309

DiChiro G, Hatazawa J, Katz D A et al 1987 Glucose utilization by intracranial meningiomas as an index of tumor aggressivity and probability of recurrence: an ET study. Radiology 164: 521–526

Duma C M, Lunsford L D, Kondziolka D, Harsh G R, Flickinger J 1993 Stereotactic radiosurgery of cavernous sinus meningiomas as an addition or alternative to microsurgery. Neurosurgery 32: 699–705

Edwards M S, Wilson C B. Treatment of radiation necrosis. In: Gilbert H A, Kagan A R (eds) Radiation damage to the nervous system. A delayed therapeutic hazard. Raven Press, New York, pp 120–143

Fine H A, Dear K B G, Loeffler J S, Black P McL, Canellos G P 1971 Meta-analysis of radiation therapy with and without adjuvant chemotherapy for malignant gliomas in adults. Cancer 71: 2585–2587

Glass J, Hochberg F H, Gruber M L, Louis D N, Smith D, Rattner B 1992 The treatment of oligodendrogliomas and mixed oligodendroglioma-astrocytomas with PCV chemotherapy. Journal of Neurosurgery 76: 741–745

Goldsmith B, Wara W, Wilson C B, Larson D 1992 Postoperative external beam irradiation for subtotally resected meningiomas. International Journal Radiation Oncology Biology Physics 24 (suppl 1): 126–127

Harsh G R, Wilson C B 1990 Neuroepithelial tumors in adults. In: Youmans J R (ed) Neurological surgery, ch 107 W B Saunders, Philadelphia pp 3040–3136

Harsh G R, Levin V A, Gutin P H et al 1987 Reoperation for recurrent glioblastoma and anaplastic astrocytoma. Neurosurgery 21: 615–621

Hochberg F H, Pruitt A 1980 Assumptions in the radiotherapy of glioblastoma. Neurology 30: 407–911

Hoshino T A 1984 A commentary on the biology and growth kinetics of low-grade and high-grade gliomas. Journal of Neurosurgery 61: 895–900

Jaaskelainen J 1986 Seemingly complete removal of histologically benign intracranial meningioma: late recurrence rate and factors predicting recurrence in 657 patients. Surgical Neurology 26: 461–469

Jaaskelainen J, Haltia M, Laasonen E, Wahlstrom T, Valtonen S 1985 The growth rate of intracranial meningiomas and its relation to histology: an analysis of 43 patients. Surgical Neurology 24: 165–172

Jaaskelainen H et al 1986 Atypical and anaplastic meningiomas: radiology, surgery, radiotherapy, and outcome. Surgical Neurology 25: 233–242

Jelsma R, Bucy P C 1969 Glioblastoma multiforme. Its treatment and some factors effecting survival. Archives of Neurology 20: 161–171

Karnofsky D, Burchenal J H, Armistead G C Jr et al 1951 Triethylene melamine in the treatment of neoplastic disease. AMA Arch Intern Med 87: 477–516

Kaye A H 1992 Malignant brain tumors. In: Rothenberg R E (ed) Reoperative surgery. McGraw-Hill, New York, pp 51–76

Kelly P J 1989 Stereotactic biopsy and resection in thalamic astrocytomas. Neurosurgery 25: 185–195

Kelly P J, Daumas-Duport C, Scheithauer B et al 1987 Stereotactic histologic correlation of computed tomography and magnetic resonance imaging defined abnormalities in patients with glial neoplasms. Mayo Clinic Proceedings 62: 450–459

Kikuchi K, Neuwelt E A 1983 Presence of immunosuppressive factors in brain tumor cyst fluid. Journal of Neurosurgery 59: 790–799

Kornblith P L, Walker M 1988 Chemotherapy of gliomas. Journal of Neurosurgery 68: 1–17

Kreth F W, Warnke P C, Scheremet R, Osterstag C B 1993 Surgical resection and radiation therapy in the treatment of glioblastoma multiforme. Journal of Neurosurgery 78: 762–766

Laws E R, Taylor W F, Clifton M B, Okazaki H 1984 Neurosurgical management of low-grade astrocytoma of the cerebral hemispheres. Journal of Neurosurgery 61: 665–673

Le Bihan D, Douek M, Argyropoulou M et al 1993 Diffusion and profusion magnetic resonance imaging in brain tumors. Top Magnetic Resonance Imaging 5: 25–31

Leibel S A, Sheline G E 1987 Radiation therapy for neoplasms of the brain. Journal of Neurosurgery 66: 1–22

LeRoux P D, Berger M S, Ojemann G A et al 1989 Correlation of intraoperative ultrasound tumor volumes and margins with preoperative computerized tomography scans. Journal of Neurosurgery 71: 691–698

Levin V A, Hoffman W F, Heilbron D C et al 1980 Prognostic significance of the pretreatment CT scan on time to progression for patients with malignant gliomas. Journal of Neurosurgery 52: 642–647

Levin V A, Silver P, Hannigan J et al 1990 Superiority of post radiotherapy adjuvant chemotherapy with CCNU, procarbazine, and vicristine (PCV) over BCNU for anaplastic gliomas NCOG 6G 61 final report. International Journal of Radiation Oncology Biology Physics 18: 321–324

Li A, Shea W M, Wyn C J, Fine H A, Black P A 1992 Radiosurgery as part of the initial management of patients with malignant glioma. Journal of Clinical Oncology 10: 1379–1385

Loeffler J S, Alexander III E, Wen P Y et al 1990a Results of stereotactic brachytherapy used in the initial management of patients with glioblastoma. JNCI 82: 1918–1921

Loeffler J S, Alexander III E, Hochberg F H et al 1990b Clinical patterns of failure following stereotactic interstitial irradiation for malignant gliomas. International Journal Radiation Oncology Biology Physics 19: 1455–1462

Marks J E, Boylan R J, Prossal S C et al 1981 Cerebral radionecrosis; incidence and risk in relation to dose, time, fractionation, and volume. International Journal Radiation Oncology Biology Physics 7: 243–252

McCormack B M, Miller D C, Budzilovich G N, Voostrees G J, Ransohoff J 1992 Treatment and survival of low grade astrocytoma in adults. 1977–1988. Neurosurgery 31: 636–642

Mirimanoff R O, Dosoretz D E, Linggood R M, Ojemann R G, Martuza R L 1985 Meningioma: analysis of recurrence and progression following neurosurgical resection. Journal of Neurosurgery 62: 18–24

Muller W, Aftra D, Schroder R 1977 Supratentorial recurrences of gliomas: Morphological studies in relation to time intervals with astrocytomas. Acta Neurochirurgica (Wien) 37: 75–91

Nazzaro J, Neuwelt E 1990 The role of surgery in the management of supratentorial intermediate and high-grade astrocytomas in adults. Journal of Neurosurgery 73: 331–344

Nelson D F, Nelson J S, Davis D R, Chang C H, Griffin T W, Pajak T F 1985 Survival and prognosis of patients with astrocytoma with atypical or anaplastic features. Journal of Neuro-Oncology 3: 99–103

New P F J, Hesselink J R, O'Carroll C P, Kleinman G M 1982 Malignant meningiomas: CT and histologic criteria, including a new CT sign. AJNR 3: 267–276

Olmsted W W, McGee T P 1977 Prognosis in meningiomas through evaluation of skull bone patterns. Radiology 123: 375–377

Osterstag C B 1983 Biopsy and interstitial radiation therapy of cerebral gliomas. Italian Journal of Neurological Science 2 (suppl): 121–128

Phillipon J, Cornu P 1991 The recurrence of meningiomas. In: Al-Mefty O (ed) Meningiomas, ch 7. Raven Press, New York, pp 87–105

Prados M B, Gutin P H, Phillips T L et al 1992 Highly anaplastic astrocytoma: a review of 357 patients treated between 1977 and 1989. International Journal Radiation Oncology Biology Physics 23: 3–8

Quigley M R, Maroon J C 1991 The relationship between survival and the extent of the resection in patients with supratentorial malignant gliomas. Neurosurgery 29: 385–389

Rosenblum M L, Chiu-Liu H, Davis R L, Gutin P H 1985 Radiation necrosis versus tumor recurrence following interstitial brachytherapy: Utility of tissue culture studies. Proceedings of the American Association of Neurological Surgeons p 264

Salcman M. Resection and reoperation in neuro-oncology. Neurology Clinics 3: 831–841

Salcman M, Kaplan R S, Samaras G M et al 1982a Aggressive multimodality therapy based on a multicompartmental model of glioblastoma. Surgery 92: 250–259

Salcman M, Kaplan R S, Durken T B et al 1982b Effect of age and reoperation on survival in the combined modality treatment of malignant astrocytomas. Neurosurgery 10: 454–463

Scharfen C D, Sneed P K, Wara W M et al 1992 high activity iodine-125 interstitial implant for gliomas. International Journal Radiation Oncology Biology Physics 24: 583–591

Shapiro W R 1982 Treatment of neuroectodermal brain tumors. Annals of Neurology 12: 231–237

Shapiro W R, Green S B, Burger P C et al 1989 Randomized trial of three chemotherapeutic regimens in postoperative treatment of malignant glioma. Journal of Neurosurgery 71: 1–9

Shaw E G, Scheithauer B W, O'Fallon J R, Tazellar H D, David D H 1992 Oligodendrogliomas: the Mayo experience. Journal of Neurosurgery 76: 428–434

Simpson D 1957 The recurrence of intracranial meningiomas after surgical treatment. Journal of Neurology, Neurosurgery and Psychiatry 20: 22–39

Tilzer L L, Plapp F V, Evans J P et al 1982 Steroid receptor proteins in human meningiomas. Cancer 49: 633–636

Valk P E, Budinger T F, Levin V A, Silver P, Gutin P, Doyle W K 1988 PET of malignant cerebral tumors after interstitial brachytherapy. Demonstration of metabolic activity and correlation with clinical outcome. Journal of Neurosurgery 69: 830–838

Vecht C J, Avezaat C J, van Patten W L, Eijkenboom W M, Stefanko S Z 1990 The influence of the extent of surgery on the neurologic function and survival in malignant glioma. A retrooperation analysis in 243 patients. Journal of Neurology, Neurosurgery and Psychiatry 53: 466–471

Vertosick F T, Selker R G, Arena V C 1991 Survival of patients with well differentiated astrocytomas diagnosed in the era of computed tomography. Neurosurgery 28: 496–501

Von Diemling A, Louis D M, Von Ammon K, Schoenfeld D, Wiestler O D, Seranger B R 1993 Subsets of glioblastoma multiforme defined by molecular genetic analysis. Brain Pathology 3: 19–26

Walker M D, Alexander E, Hunt W E et al 1978 Evaluation of BCNU and/or radiotherapy in the treatment of anaplastic gliomas. Journal of Neurosurgery 49: 333–343

Wallner K E, Galicich J H, Krol G, et al 1989a Patterns of failure following treatment for glioblastoma multiforme and anaplastic astrocytoma. International Journal Radiation Oncology Biology Physics 16: 1405–1409

Wallner K E, Galicich J H, Malkin M G 1989b Inability of computed tomography appearance of recurrent malignant astrocytoma to predict survival following reoperation. Journal of Clinical Oncology 7: 1492–1496

Wilson C B 1980 Reoperation for primary tumors. Seminars in Oncology 2: 19–20

Winger M J, Macdonald D R, Cairncross J G 1989 Supratentorial anaplastic gliomas in adults. The prognostic importance of extent of resection and prior low grade glioma. Journal of Neurosurgery 71: 487–493

Wood J R, Green S B, Shapiro W R 1988 The prognostic importance of tumor size in malignant gliomas: a computed tomographic scan study by the Brain Tumor Cooperative Group. Journal of Clinical Oncology 6: 338–343

Yamashita J, Handa H, Iwaki K, Abe M 1980 Recurrence of intracranial meningiomas with special reference to radiotherapy. Surgical Neurology 14: 33–40

Young B, Oldfield E H, Markesberry W R et al 1981 Reoperation for glioblastoma. Journal of Neurosurgery 55: 917–921

Yung W K A, Mechtler L, Gleason M J 1991 Intravenous carboplatin for recurrent malignant glioma: a phase II study. Journal of Clinical Oncology 9: 860–864

Specific brain tumors

PART I

Gliomas

24. Low grade astrocytomas

Robert A. Morantz

The tumors that we shall be concerned with in this chapter are those that arise from the supporting cells of the central nervous system. These tumors have been called astrocytomas in the recent three-tier World Health Organization classification. They correspond to the grade I and grade II astrocytomas of the Kernohan classification, or what have been called 'low grade' astrocytomas in the past. Under the more recent classification schema proposed by Daumas-Duport et al (1988) these tumors would be called grade II. This group includes tumors that previously were classified descriptively by such terms as *fibrillary* or *protoplasmic*.

Some types of astrocytomas would appear to have a well-defined prognosis that is unique unto themselves and therefore will not be included in this chapter. Specifically, the 'gemistocytic' astrocytoma seems to have a high incidence of conversion into more malignant forms and thus a worse prognosis than other low grade astrocytomas (Krouwer et al 1991); conversely, the 'pilocytic' astrocytoma appears to have an excellent prognosis no matter how radical the surgical resection or type of postoperative adjuvant therapy (Clark et al 1985, Palma & Guidetti 1985). Both the ganglioglioma and the pleomorphic xanthoastrocytoma share certain favorable prognostic features with the low grade astrocytoma; in each case, however, their unique features make it best that these tumors be considered as separate entities (Kepes et al 1979, Silver et al 1991). Finally, this chapter specifically excludes tumors with a pathologic diagnosis of malignant glioma, anaplastic astrocytoma, or astrocytoma grade III. While certain of the conclusions of this chapter might also apply to low grade oligodendroglioma and mixed oligodendroglioma-astrocytoma, there is little agreement as to how such lesions should be graded and few studies in the literature as to their optimal treatment. Thus, this chapter will focus on the low grade astrocytomas rather than the low grade gliomas.

INCIDENCE AND PREVALENCE

Low grade astrocytomas constitute approximately 15% of brain tumors in adults and approximately 25% of brain tumors in children (Guthrie & Laws 1990). Since studies conducted in different parts of the world have indicated that the average annual incidence rate per 100 000 population of gliomas is approximately 5.4 (Radhakrishnan et al 1994), we can calculate that the incidence rate of low grade astrocytomas in adults is approximately 0.9 per 100 000 population. The general incidence of brain tumors in children (from birth to 12 years) is approximately 2.4 per 100 000 per year (Radhakrishnan et al 1994). Consequently, the incidence of low grade astrocytoma in this population is quite similar to adults — i.e. approximately 0.8 per 100 000 per year.

AGE AND SEX DISTRIBUTION

The median age of patients with low grade astrocytomas is considerably lower than that of patients with more malignant gliomas, and is approximately 35 years. Most studies have shown that males constitute between 55 and 65% of these patients (Guthrie & Laws 1990).

FAMILY HISTORY AND GENETIC FACTORS

There has been no indication in the literature that low grade astrocytomas are either more or less prevalent among different racial or national groups. In a similar manner, with the exception of those families whose members are suffering from one of the phakomatoses, it has not been documented that genetic factors play a role in the development of these tumors. In the case of families with neurofibromatosis, those with type 1 have an increased incidence of optic pathway gliomas. In addition, nearly 15% of gliomas associated with the NF-1 syndrome are located in the brainstem, cerebral cortex or the cerebellum. In general, the low grade gliomas found in patients with neurofibromatosis behave in a more malignant fashion than those found in the general population (Warnick 1994). Patients with tuberous sclerosis will have subependymal giant cell astrocytoma occurring in approximately 5% of affected individuals. These tumors usually occur during the teenage years, and typically occur in the region of the foramen of Monro.

SITES OF PREDILECTION

Low grade astrocytomas arise predominantly within the convexity of the brain, roughly in proportion to the relative mass of the different lobes. The frontal lobe is the most common location, followed by the temporal lobe (Zülch 1986).

CLINICAL PRESENTATION

As with other intrinsic brain tumors, low grade astrocytomas may produce signs and symptoms by several mechanisms:

1. By direct infiltration into and destruction of the neurons within a given area of the brain,
2. By local pressure upon neighboring structures,
3. By producing a generalized increase in intracranial pressure.

Headache, lethargy, and personality change are the most common symptoms produced by the third mechanism, while papilledema is the most common sign. The nature of the focal neurologic deficit produced by local infiltration of tumor cells will of course depend on the location of the lesion. By far the most common presenting symptom is an epileptic seizure, which in the present era has been reported to occur in more than one half of all low grade astrocytoma patients. Focal symptoms (and especially epileptic seizures) may occur for many years prior to the diagnosis of low grade astrocytoma being made.

IMAGING DIAGNOSIS

In past years, the neuroradiologic procedures used to diagnose a low grade astrocytoma included isotope brain scanning and cerebral angiography. The isotope brain scan might or might not demonstrate the lesion; the angiogram would usually demonstrate a mass lesion without evidence of abnormal vascularity. At the present time such diagnostic procedures are of historical interest only.

In recent years the diagnostic procedures of choice have become CT and/or MR imaging. Since it is not uncommon to find low grade astrocytomas which are detected only on MR imaging (after normal CT scans), most believe that MR imaging is the most sensitive test available today to diagnose these lesions. At surgery, the use of intraoperative ultrasonography has been reported to be extremely helpful in outlining the extent of the lesion (LeRoux et al 1992).

Whether or not enhancement of the lesion on CT scan is correlated with a poorer prognosis in patients with low grade astrocytomas is controversial. An early paper reported that contrast enhancement had no prognostic value in patients with these tumors (Silverman & Marks 1981). A more recent larger series, however, concluded that those patients whose tumors enhanced on CT scanning had a poorer prognosis than those whose lesions did not enhance after the administration of an intravenous contrast agent (Piepmeier 1987). This poorer prognosis was evident even when adjustment was made for the age of the patient, which is the strongest of all prognosticators. This later finding has recently been strongly supported by a retrospective study, which found that contrast enhancement on the CT scan was associated with almost seven times the risk of tumor recurrence relative to those tumors not showing such enhancement (McCormack et al 1992).

CT scanning in a typical case reveals a non-enhancing lesion whose density is lower than that of the surrounding brain (Fig. 24.1). A mass effect upon surrounding ventricular structures is common. When enhancement does occur, it is generally faint and homogeneous.

On MR images, the lesion typically presents as a low intensity area on the T1 images, whereas there is almost always an increase in signal intensity corresponding with an increase in relaxation time on T2-weighted images (Figs 24.2, 24.3). The area of increased signal is usually homogeneous and well circumscribed, with no evidence of hemorrhage or necrosis (Drayer et al 1987). In many cases, on MR scans it is difficult to differentiate the tumor itself from surrounding areas of edema. Although the data are still not definitive, it does *not* appear that the use of an MRI contrast agent such as gadolinium appreciably improves the ability to detect small lesions. There also would appear to be a role for PET scanning in the diagnosis and treatment of these patients. A low grade astrocytoma will be hypometabolic and therefore 'cold' on PET scanning. If, however, dedifferentiation to a more malignant state occurs within a low grade astrocytoma, this area will be hypermetabolic and consequently will appear as a 'hot spot' on PET scanning. This information may be extremely valuable in determining a site for stereotactic biopsy and/or determining whether the patient should be treated with postoperative radiation therapy (Worthington et al 1987, Francavilla et al 1989).

Other than the neuroradiologic tests outlined above, there are as yet no specific blood or CSF tests which are diagnostic of a low grade astrocytoma.

GROSS MORPHOLOGIC FEATURES

The gross morphology of these tumors varies somewhat depending on whether they are of the protoplasmic or fibrillary types. In general, the protoplasmic astrocytoma

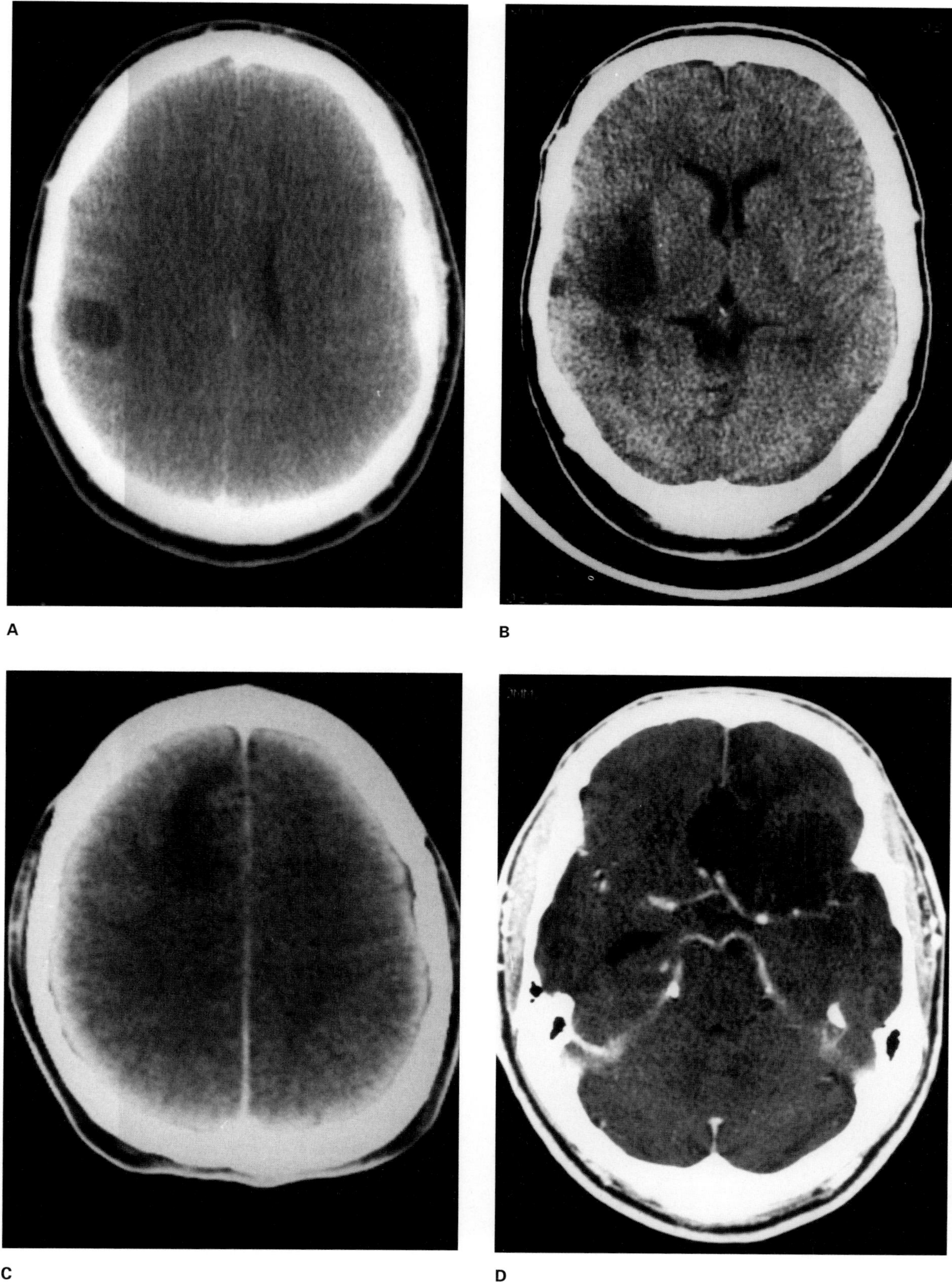

Fig. 24.1 Typical CT scans (contrast-enhanced) of 4 patients **A–D** with pathologically proven low grade astrocytomas.

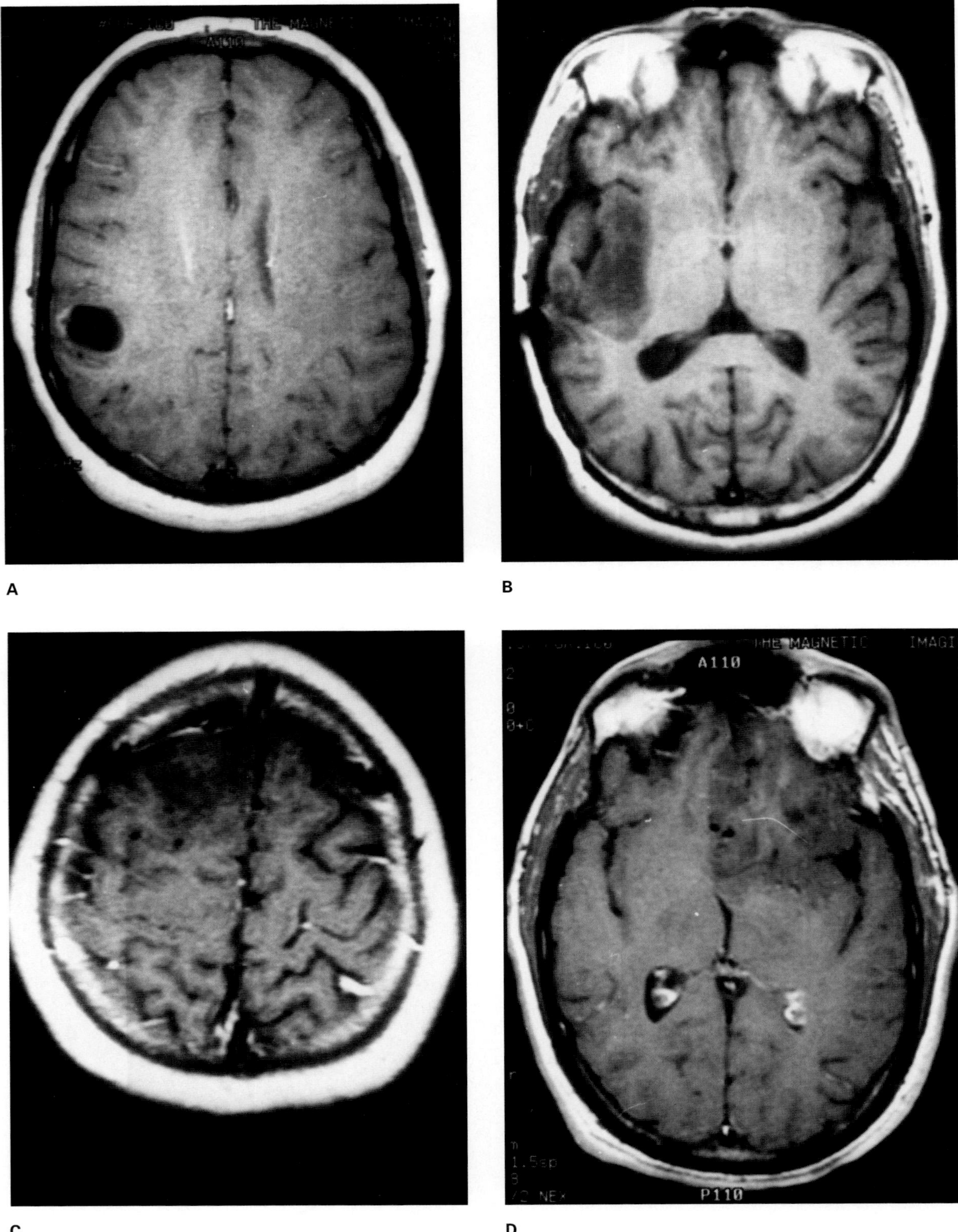

Fig. 24.2 MRI scans (T1 images) of same 4 patients as in Fig. 24.1 **A–D** with pathologically proven low grade astrocytomas.

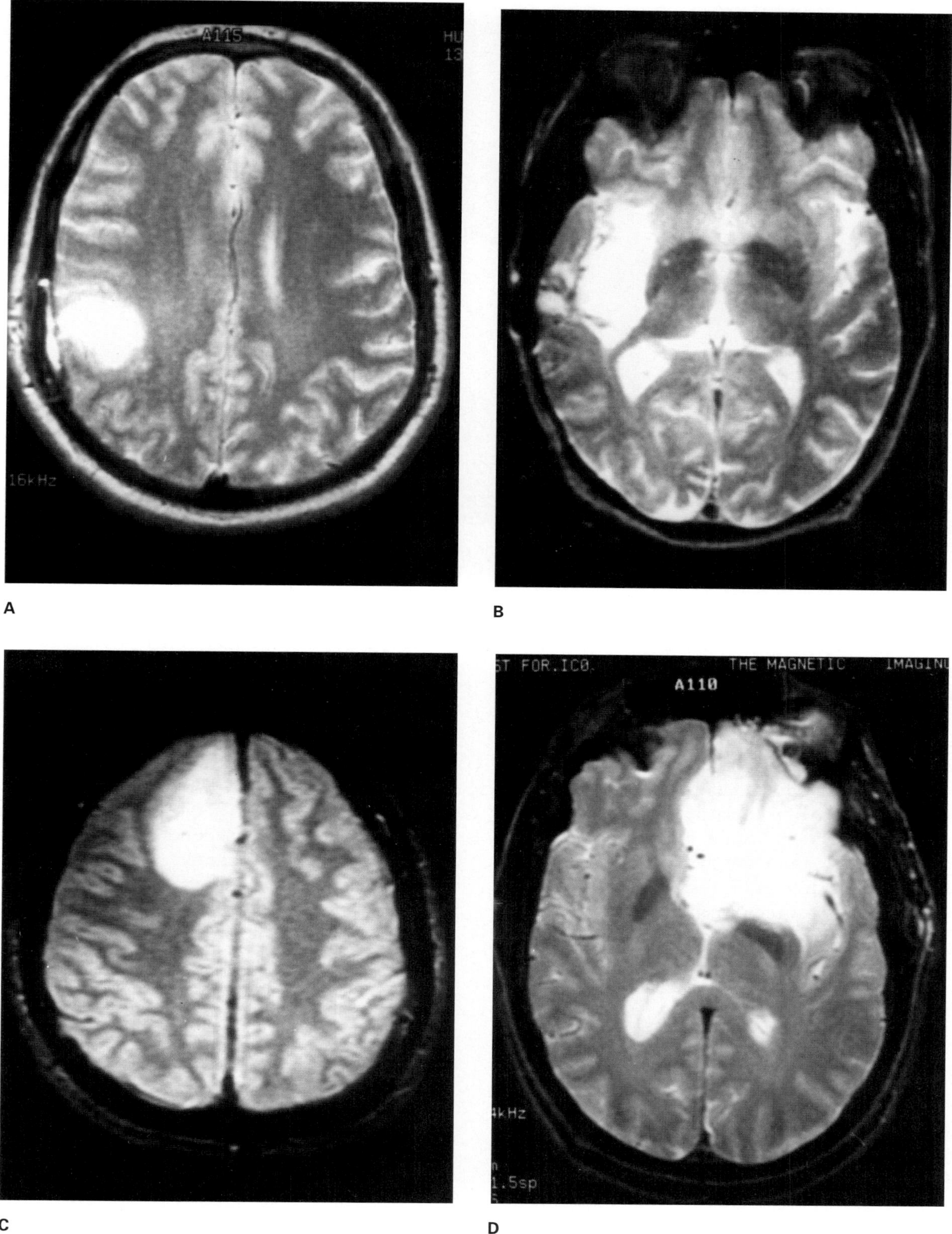

Fig. 24.3 MRI scans (T2 images) of same 4 patients as in Figs 24.1, 24.2 **A–D** with pathologically proven low grade astrocytomas.

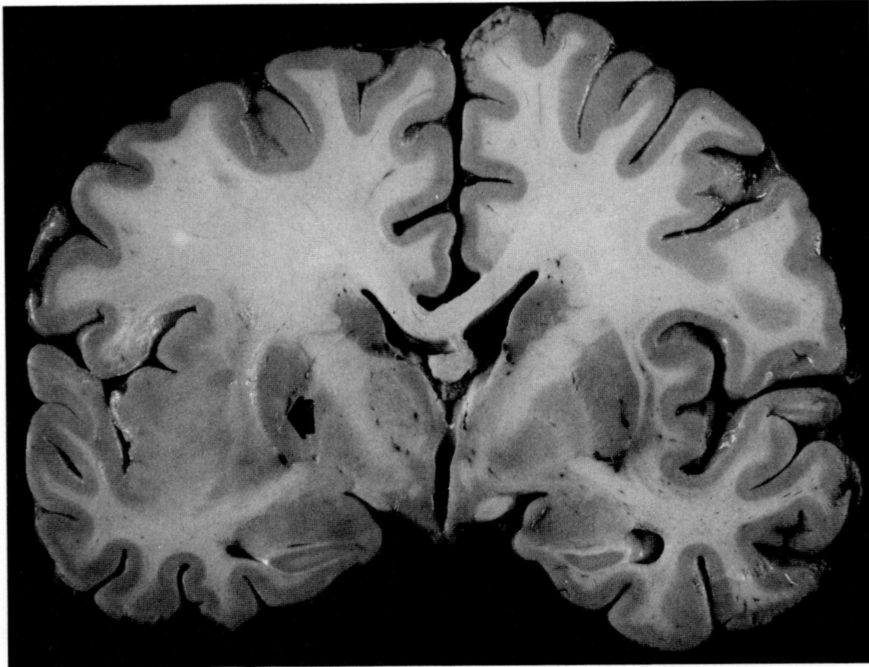

Fig. 24.4 Gross photograph of a protoplasmic astrocytoma showing expansion of the cortex. Note the edema in the white matter of the ipsilateral hemisphere.

of the cerebrum will appear grossly as a superficial soft-gray expansion of the cortex, although more careful examination of the cut surface will usually reveal involvement of the subjacent white matter (Fig. 24.4). The borders of the tumor are poorly defined and cyst formation is common, especially with deeply seated lesions. The tissue itself is soft, homogeneous, and rather gelatinous in texture. The fibrillary astrocytoma will usually be tougher and more firm than the protoplasmic variety; it may feel quite rubbery to the touch. Since the appearance of the cut surface is whiter than that of the protoplasmic variety, it is more difficult to distinguish tumor from surrounding white matter. Because of tumor cell infiltration, the adjacent cortex will appear paler than surrounding tissue, with the demarkation of the gray matter from the subjacent white matter being obliterated (Russell & Rubinstein 1989).

HISTOPATHOLOGIC FEATURES

The histopathologic features once again vary somewhat, depending on the specific tumor type. The protoplasmic astrocytoma is composed of evenly distributed tumor cells within an eosinophilic matrix. These cells are usually arranged in a fine cobweb network. On higher power examination, the individual tumor cells are seen to be rather plump astrocytes, whose cytoplasm may be unusually swollen. These cells have fewer and shorter cellular processes than normal astrocytes. Microcystic degenerative changes are seen characteristically, especially in the deeper parts of the tumor. The intrinsic blood vessels are usually relatively scanty (Fig. 24.5).

In the fibrillary astrocytoma, both fine and coarse neuroglial fibrils occupy the matrix and in some cases can achieve a considerable length. The cells' bodies are dispersed unevenly throughout this matrix. In some cases of fibrillary astrocytoma, the tumor cells are small, and usually contain fine fibrils. Mitoses are, in general, difficult to find, and the nuclei do not show much variability. When the cortex is infiltrated it is common to find a subpial zone in which the cell bodies are more densely collected than in the brain parenchyma. The superficial leptomeninges may be invaded by the tumor, and the sylvian fissure may be bridged by neoplastic cells over a considerable portion of its length. Cerebrospinal dissemination is decidedly rare.

The infiltrated brain tissues are usually well preserved; in the cortex the pre-existing neurons are separated by the tumor cells whereas in the white matter demyelinated nerve fibers are forced apart. The blood vessels are also forced apart by the infiltrating tumor cells, but they almost never demonstrate endothelial hyperplasia. Degenerative changes with the formation of microcysts are frequent, and calcification may occasionally occur.

On electron microscopy, one will usually note the presence of bundles of intermediate filaments which range in size from 7–11 nanometers in diameter. These occur in the perikaryon as well as the cell processes. Microtubules

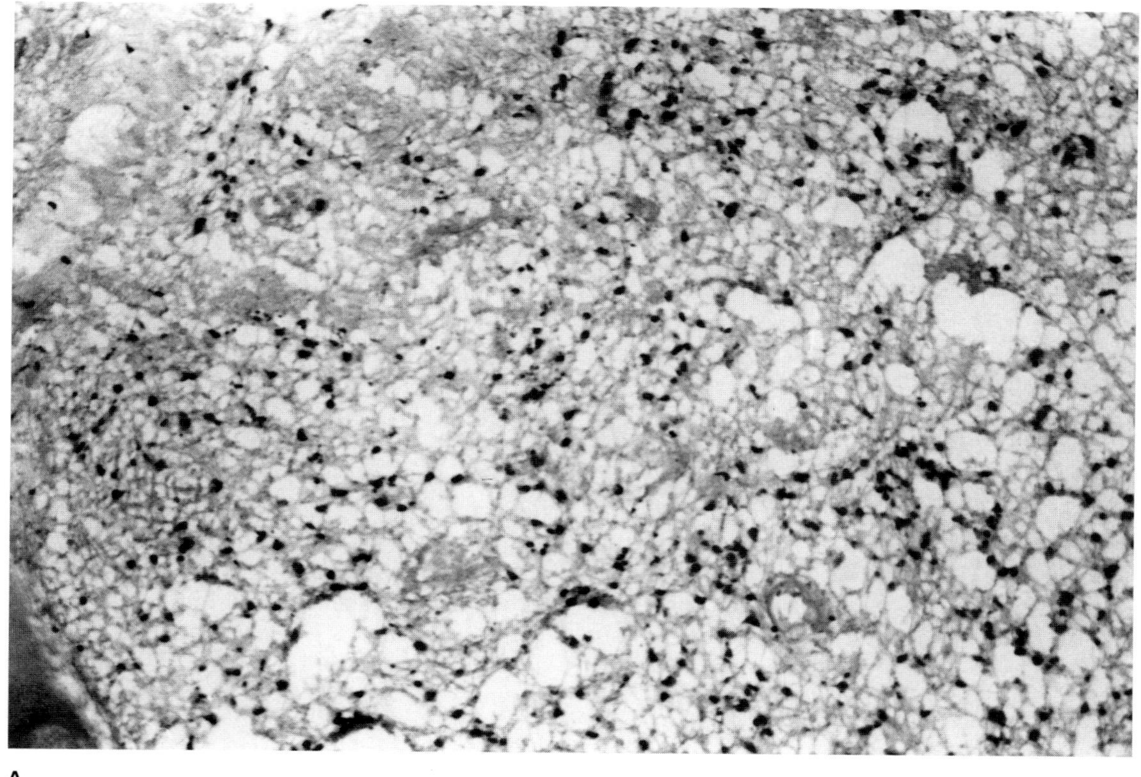

A

B

Fig. 24.5 Low power (**A**) and high power (**B**) microscopic view of a typical low grade astrocytoma.

may be found in some of the cell processes. Scanning electron microscopy will demonstrate the network that is formed by the radiating and interlacing cell processes.

In the case of the protoplasmic variant of low grade astrocytoma, immunohistochemical evaluation reveals that staining for GFA protein is usually negative, probably due to the relative lack of filaments in the tumor cells. On the other hand, in the case of the fibrillary astrocytoma, stains for GFA protein are uniformly positive. These tumors have also been demonstrated to be immunopositive for glutamine synthetase, the aldolase C isoenzyme, the S-100 protein, and vimentin (Russell & Rubinstein 1989).

INCIDENCE OF MALIGNANCY

The incidence of more 'malignant' areas within a low grade astrocytoma is an extremely important issue. In order to analyze it further, we must first briefly discuss the question of sampling and dedifferentiation. Scherer was one of the first to emphasize that great care must be taken to examine all areas of a low grade astrocytoma before deciding that anaplastic foci are not present (Scherer 1940). In his classic study, he made careful sections of the cerebral hemispheres of 18 patients with astrocytomas and found foci of anaplasia in 13. In a similar manner, Russell & Rubinstein examined 55 autopsy specimens of patients who had been diagnosed clinically as having an astrocytoma. In more than 50% of these cases, areas of anaplastic change were found. Looked at from another perspective, these same authors analyzed a series of 129 autopsied cases of glioblastoma multiforme and concluded that approximately 28% could be considered to have arisen from pre-existing astrocytoma (Russell & Rubinstein 1989).

The frequency of dedifferentiation, or change to a more malignant form, has been studied by several authors. Müller & associates examined 72 patients whose pathologic diagnosis at the time of initial operation was astrocytoma. At the time of recurrence, 14% of the tumors were unchanged pathologically, whereas 55% were now classified as anaplastic astrocytoma, and 30% were now classified as glioblastoma multiforme. The time between the initial pathologic diagnosis and the second operation averaged 31 months. The authors concluded that in approximately two thirds of all astrocytomas (i.e. including both the low grade and anaplastic astrocytomas) one can expect dedifferentiation to a more malignant state to occur (Müller et al 1977).

In 79 patients with recurrent tumor growth documented at either subsequent surgery or autopsy, Laws et al found that a change to astrocytoma grade III or IV had occurred in approximately 50% of the cases (Laws et al 1984). A more recent series from Italy reported that 79% of their astrocytoma patients who had recurrent tumor were found to have anaplastic areas at either reoperation or autopsy (Soffretti et al 1989). Another recent study of 25 patients found that none of the 8 deaths was due to the progressive growth of the low grade astrocytoma, but rather 7 of the 8 deaths occurred in patients whose tumors had dedifferentiated into an anaplastic astrocytoma or a glioblastoma (Vertosick et al 1991). McCormack et al also found that dedifferentiation occurred in 6 of 7 patients with recurrent tumor (McCormack et al 1992).

The literature is not unanimous, however, in reporting that such a high incidence of dedifferentiation will occur in these tumors, since Piepmeier found that malignant transformation was seen in only 13% of his patients at the time of second operation or autopsy (Piepmeier 1987). This number is almost certainly an understatement, however, because the patient population reviewed in his study had a median follow-up of only 5 years, and such malignant dedifferentiation would undoubtedly occur in more patients if the follow-up time were increased.

Although this is still a subject of some debate and no definite answer can be given, it is probably fair to suggest that the presence of anaplastic areas at the time of a second resection or biopsy in a patient with a previously diagnosed low grade astrocytoma is not necessarily due to an initial sampling error. Rather, in up to one half of cases, dedifferentiation of a low grade astrocytoma to a more malignant form occurs.

Recent basic research may offer insight as to the molecular-genetic basis of the process of dedifferentiation. In the case of colonic cancer, the progression from the more benign polyp to the overt cancer is reflected in an increasing number of genetic abnormalities within the genome of the tumor cell. Several studies would seem to indicate that a similar process may be occurring in the progression (or dedifferentiation) of an astrocytoma through the stage of anaplastic astrocytoma and ultimately to glioblastoma multiforme. One recent study found mutations in the p53 tumor suppressor gene in 0% of low grade astrocytomas, 36% of anaplastic astrocytomas and 28% of glioblastomas, while abnormalities on chromosome 10 were found in 0% of low grade astrocytomas, 23% of anaplastic astrocytomas and 61% of glioblastomas (Fults et al 1992). Another investigation reported that, in patients who were shown to have undergone dedifferentiation at a second operation, the percentage of cells showing a mutation at the p53 gene had increased markedly, perhaps due to a selective growth advantage of these mutated cells (Sidransky et al 1992).

A reasonable hypothesis of the events underlying dedifferentiation, then, would be that a glial cell experiences a small number of 'genetic hits' to change it into a low grade astrocytoma. If these same cells then experience further alteration in their genetic make-up (e.g. by mutation on a tumor suppressor gene such as p53) they will then undergo dedifferentiation to a more malignant phenotype.

Even in those low grade astrocytomas which do not

undergo dedifferentiation, the prognosis may be poor if the lesion is deep-seated. McCormack reported that the outlook for patients with such lesions is far worse than that for those with hemispheric tumors — i.e. such patients had a median survival of only 2 years. Furthermore, they may experience progressive decline and death as a result of the spread of their low grade tumor rather than necessarily as a consequence of dedifferentiation to a higher grade of malignancy (McCormack et al 1992).

SURGICAL MANAGEMENT

The overall management plan for the patient diagnosed as having a low grade astrocytoma is controversial. It is a general rule of surgical oncology that surgery should be carried out as early in the course of malignancy as possible. However, it has never been proved that earlier treatment of a low grade astrocytoma produces an increase in life span as measured from the time of diagnosis. Furthermore, because more and more patients are having their tumors detected while they are neurologically intact, and because operative intervention in some locations will carry a significant risk of postoperative morbidity, some have made the case that surgery should be delayed in lesions that do not show a change in appearance on sequential radiologic studies.

One retrospective study compared the outcome of a group of 26 patients who had radiologic evidence strongly suggestive of a low grade astrocytoma and who were initially not operated upon to a similar group of 20 patients who were subjected to immediate surgical intervention (Recht et al 1992). These authors found no significant difference in the incidence of dedifferentiation or survival time between the two groups and thus could not demonstrate that deferring surgery led to a worse outcome for patients with low grade astrocytomas.

Nevertheless, we are still faced with the problem that, even at the present time, it is impossible to determine pathology conclusively by radiologic procedures, as is proven by the fact that one study found that CT scan enhancement was absent in over 30% of patients with highly anaplastic astrocytoma and even in 4% of patients with glioblastoma multiforme (Chamberlain et al 1988). Since the adjuvant treatment recommended in the latter two instances would likely be different than in the case of the low grade astrocytoma, the desire to forego surgery is almost always outweighed by the necessity of obtaining a precise pathologic diagnosis.

If we are committed to surgical management then we must ask ourselves questions as to the type of surgical procedure to be carried out. Most, but certainly not all of the retrospective studies that have been published have indicated that patients who underwent a 'gross total' removal of their lesion experienced a longer survival than those who did not. We must be quite careful in evaluating such data, however, since it is quite likely that patients in these two groups were not comparable — i.e. in those patients whose tumors were widely infiltrating into vital areas, surgical judgement was at variance with an attempt at 'gross total' removal. Given the general oncologic principle, however, that one should try to obtain the maximum reduction of tumor burden possible and the known propensity of residual cells to undergo malignant dedifferentiation, it would appear prudent to attempt a 'gross total' removal in those lesions where this can be done without producing a postoperative neurologic deficit.

If a standard craniotomy is to be carried out, then certain technical aspects should be considered. In many instances the Cavitron ultrasonic aspirator (CUSA) will be helpful. As in the case of surgery for other intrinsic brain tumors, the tumor should be entered as close to the center as possible and then progressively removed towards the periphery (Guthrie & Laws 1990). In many instances it is quite difficult to be certain of the interface between tumor tissue and edematous surrounding brain. Studies by Kelly and others have shown that in low grade astrocytomas there may be no such clear interface (Kelly et al 1987). Consequently, the surgeon should err on the conservative side when potentially important areas of brain are nearby. Other technical adjuncts that may be helpful include the use of an ultrasound device for tumor localization and cortical electrophysiologic monitoring to outline contiguous eloquent areas of the brain.

Since in many instances it is quite difficult for the surgeon to determine the precise location of a low grade tumor at surgery, these tumors in many cases are ideal for a 'stereotactic craniotomy'. In this instance, the quite clear delineation of the tumor as seen on the CT or MRI scan can be used to allow one to pass a catheter stereotactically into the center of the lesion. At the time of craniotomy, the surgeon then follows this catheter to the tumor and thus is certain that he is removing the abnormal area that has been seen on the radiologic study.

In the present era many patients have MRI or CT scans which show quite small lesions with no evidence of mass effect. In such an instance, CT or MRI guided stereotactic biopsy is an excellent means of obtaining a definitive tissue diagnosis without subjecting the patient to the risks and inconvenience of a standard craniotomy. In many cases such patients may be discharged from the hospital the following day. Within the last several years, stereotactic biopsy has proven itself to be an extremely accurate, low risk technique which is therefore ideal for the definitive diagnosis of many low grade astrocytomas. It is presently the procedure of choice over the previously utilized open biopsy technique in most cases.

RADIATION THERAPY

Perhaps the most controversial area in the treatment of

low grade astrocytomas is the question of whether postoperative radiation therapy should be used as an adjunctive form of treatment (Morantz 1987). The answer to this question should be relatively easy to come by. Ideally, such an answer would be forthcoming from what is probably our most powerful tool for scientifically answering clinical questions such as this one — the randomized, controlled, prospective clinical trial. In this case one would have to carry out a multigroup, long-term (perhaps as long as 10-year) study in which two large groups of patients (containing individuals who are balanced with respect to important variables such as age, tumor location, histologic classification, etc.) were treated identically in every respect (i.e. extent of operation, use of steroids, etc.) except that one group received an exactly specified course of radiation therapy and the other group did not. Whether there was a statistically significant difference in the length and/or quality of survival between these two groups could then be determined. Such a study has never been completed, although at the present time several such cooperative endeavors are in progress both in the United States and in Europe. Unfortunately the results of these studies will not be available for many years to come.

Because no single neurosurgeon's experience is adequate to answer properly how patients with a low grade astrocytoma should be optimally treated postoperatively, and the results of the present cooperative trials will not be available for many years, we are faced with the question of how to manage this group of patients at present. The imperfect present-day solution would seem to be a review of the major studies that have been published to date to determine whether they can furnish any guidance.

What is immediately apparent in carrying out such a review, however, is that the reports previously published on this topic have not satisfied even the minimal criteria that could be set forth for a study that could properly answer this question (Table 24.1). More specifically, the previous studies have been *retrospective* analyses in which the irradiated and non-irradiated groups of patients have not been similar in important characteristics (e.g. age, Karnofsky rating, etc.). The pathologic classification of the lesions has been different (e.g. varying numbers of grade I and grade II tumors). The location and size of the tumors have been different, and the extent of operation has not been uniform (e.g. biopsy versus complete resection). Finally, the parameters of the treatment being tested (i.e. radiation therapy) have not been standardized with respect to total dose, duration of therapy, field size, etc. With these objections clearly in mind let us review the previous literature such as it is, in an attempt to discover whether there is any trend that can provide us with at least some general guidelines (Table 24.2).

Table 24.1 Difficulties with previous studies of the role of radiation therapy in the treatment of astrocytoma

No uniformity of patient selection
No uniformity in the varying neurologic status of the patients (e.g. Karnofsky scale)
No uniform system of pathologic classification
No uniformity of radiation therapy dosage and field size
No uniformity in the extent of surgical removal of the tumor (i.e. gross total removal vs biopsy)
No uniformity in the location of the lesion (i.e. cerebrum vs cerebellum vs brainstem)
No simultaneous control group of patients who were not treated with radiation therapy

One of the earliest reports reviewed 176 cases that were treated at the Montreal Neurologic Institute between 1940 and 1949 (Levy & Elvidge 1956). These authors found what has been confirmed subsequently by many others — that the 'gemistocytic' type of astrocytoma has a poorer prognosis than that of other variants and that patients with cerebellar astrocytomas did better than those with cerebral lesions, even in the face of incomplete resection. Several years later another study was carried out at the same institution over a much longer period and compared the survival of 81 low grade astrocytoma patients who had received radiation therapy with a group of 71 patients who had not (Bouchard & Peirce 1960). They found that, although the 3-year survival rate was virtually identical (i.e. 62 versus 59%), the 5-year survival statistics showed an increased longevity in those who had received radiation therapy (i.e. 49 versus 38%). From this data, they concluded that ionizing radiation should be used as an adjunctive form of therapy in the treatment of such patients.

In 1961 a review was published which looked at 194 cases of cerebral astrocytoma seen at the Baylor University College of Medicine (Gol 1961). Two thirds of the postoperative patients were given radiation therapy. Gol found that, irrespective of whether biopsy or resection was the surgical procedure used, the addition of radiation therapy caused an increase in survival (biopsy, 10 versus 2 months; resection 32 versus 23 months). In addition, this study was the first indicating that patients whose tumor was resected rather than just biopsied did better, irrespective of what other therapy was utilized.

In 1966, the first of four major studies utilizing the clinical material of the Mayo Clinic was published (Uihlein et al 1966). This report reviewed 83 patients with astrocytoma treated between 1955 and 1959. Thirty three of their patients underwent operation alone and 50 were treated with operation followed by radiation therapy. They found that 65% of those treated with operation alone were alive at 5 years and only 54% of those treated by operation and radiation therapy were alive at 5 years. If anything, this indicated a decreased survival after the addition of radiation therapy. When they separated the irradiated cases into those that had received 35 Gy or more and those who had received a lower dosage, however, the 5-year survival rates were 63 and 42%. From this

Table 24.2 Treatment of cerebral astrocytoma

Author(s)	Years of study	Type of astrocytoma	No. of cases	Radiation dose	Survival (%) 3-yr Surgery	3-yr Surgery & radiation	5-yr Surgery	5-yr Surgery & radiation	10-yr Surgery	10-yr Surgery & radiation
Levy & Elvidge (1956)	1940–1949	Astrocytomas grade I & II	176	?	52	62	26	36	—	—
Bouchard & Peirce (1960)	1939–1959	Astrocytomas	152	5000–6000 Gy	59	61.7	38	49	—	—
Gol (1961)	?	Astrocytomas grade I & II	194	?		*Median survival:*	Biopsy alone: 2 mo Biopsy + RT: 10 mo		Resection alone: 23 mo Resection + RT: 32 mo	
Uihlein et al (1966)	1955–1959	Astrocytomas grade I & II	83	2000–6000 Gy	63.6	64	65	54	—	—
Stage & Stein (1974)	1956–1970	Cerebral astrocytomas grade II	45	3500–6500 Gy	—	—	20	42	—	—
Marsa et al (1975)	1957–1973	Astrocytomas	40	4900–6650 Gy	—	62	—	~41	—	~22
Leibel et al (1975)	1942–1967	Astrocytomas grade I & II	147	3500–5000 Gy	27	59	19	46	11	35
Weir & Grace (1976)	1960–1970	Astrocytomas grade I & II	107	?		*Average survival:*	Surgery: 28 mo Surgery + RT: 35 mo			
Fazekas (1977)	1958–1974	Astrocytomas grade I & II	68	850–1400 rads	—	—	32	54	32	26
Scanlon & Taylor (1979)	1960–1969	Astrocytomas grade I & II	134	1400 rads	—	—	—	64	—	—
Bloom (1980)	1952–1970	Astrocytomas grade I & II	120 (adults)	?	—	—	Grade I: 33 Grade II: 21			Grade I: 16 Grade II: 6
Laws et al (1984)	1915–1975	Astrocytomas low grade	461	4000–7900 rads	—	—	~35	~50	~10	~15
Garcia et al (1985)	1950–1979	Astrocytomas grade I, II, III	86 (adults)	3500–6100 rads	35	61	22	40	9	9
Piepmeier (1987)	1975–1985	Astrocytomas low grade	60	5000–6000 rads	*Mean survival:* Biopsy alone: 6.67 yr STR alone: 9.58 yr TR alone: 5.10 yr Biopsy + RT: 6.01 yr TR + RT: 6.34 yr TR + RT: 7.65 yr					
Medbery et al (1988)	1960–1986	Astrocytomas grade I & II	60	3200–6480 rads		STR: TR:	25 100	43 67	— —	32 —
Soffietti et al (1989)	1950–1982	Astrocytomas 'well differentiated'	85	?	58	>4000 rads = 73 <4000 rads = 40	30	>4000 rads = 9 <4000 rads = 25	7	>4000 rads = 9 <4000 rads = 0
Shaw et al (1989)	1960–1982	Astrocytomas grades I & II Pilocytic astrocytomas and oligoastrocytomas	167	600–6500 rads	—	—	32	>5300 rads = 68 <5300 rads = 47	11	>5300 rads = 39 <5300 rads = 21
Whitton & Bloom (1990)	1960–1985	Astrocytomas grade I & II	60	5000–5500 rads		62		36		28
North et al (1990)	1975–1984	Astrocytomas grade I & II	77 (25 children)	5000–5500 rads				55		43
Vertosick et al (1991)	1978–1988	Astrocytomas grade I & II	25	5400–6000 rads	(all pts: median = 8.2 yrs)		all pts. 65		all pts. 36	
McCormack et al (1992)	1977–1988	Astrocytomas grade I & II	53	2400–6800 rads	(all pts. median = 7.5 yrs			64		48

analysis it was concluded that there is a 'suggestion' that irradiation may be helpful in the treatment of the low grade astrocytoma.

A 1974 study reviewed the University of California, Los Angeles, experience with supratentorial brain tumors and found 6 patients with grade I lesions and 45 patients with grade II lesions (Stage & Stein 1974). An analysis of their survival curves indicated a 40% 5-year survival for those treated with resection and radiation therapy compared to a 20% 5-year survival for those treated with operation alone.

In 1975, a study reviewed the survival rate for all patients treated with radiation therapy at Stanford University between 1957 and 1973 (Marsa et al 1975). They found a 5-year survival rate of approximately 41% and a 10-year survival rate of approximately 22%. In addition, they confirmed that dedifferentiation to a higher grade of malignancy seemed to occur in a substantial proportion of patients in whom the surgical diagnosis was compared to that which was found at subsequent autopsy.

A 1975 study reviewed the experience at the University of California, San Francisco, in the treatment of astrocytoma (Leibel et al 1975). They found 147 patients who were treated at this institution between 1942 and 1967. If the patients who had complete resection of their lesion were excluded from the analysis, there was a clear-cut increased survival in the group undergoing radiation therapy (i.e. 5-year survival of 46 versus 19%; 10-year survival of 35 versus 11%). Based on their analysis, patients with complete removal of their tumor did well even if they did not receive radiation therapy, and patients with cerebellar lesions also did well irrespective of whether radiation therapy was given. Finally, they indicated that the quality of life was acceptable in long-term survivors and that there were no instances of radiation damage in those who experienced long-term survival.

A Canadian study published in 1976 reviewed 107 patients with a grade I or grade II supratentorial astrocytoma treated in the Province of Alberta between 1960 and 1970 (Weir & Grace 1976). They analyzed the patients with respect to prognostic factors that might be related to survival and found that young age, lower grade at operation (i.e. grade I > grade II), and the addition of radiation therapy were correlated with an increased survival. The following year a study was published which reviewed 68 patients with grade I or grade II lesions treated at the Geisinger Clinic between 1958 and 1974 (Fazekas 1977). He concluded that completely excised lesions and those in the cerebellum did well whether or not radiation was given. For those with incomplete resection, radiation increased the 5-year survival from 32 to 54%, although by 10 years this difference was thought not to be significant (i.e. 26 versus 32%).

In 1979, the second report from the Mayo Clinic was published which reviewed 134 cases of low grade glioma treated between 1960 and 1969 (Scanlon & Taylor 1979). Specifically eliminated were patients with complete resection of the lesion because they were not referred for radiation therapy. After analyzing their data, they concluded that young age and location in the cerebellum were important positive prognostic factors. In contrast to previous findings, they were able to show no advantage of subtotal resection over biopsy. In addition, they found that patients receiving less than 1400 rads did just as well as those receiving a larger dose and that there was a worsening of survival when whole brain rather than localized radiation therapy was given.

In a European study published in 1982, Bloom reviewed the experience at the Royal Marsden Hospital in treating brain tumors with radiation therapy. His treatment group consisted of 120 patients with grade I or grade II lesions. Although survival data are given only for those treated with operation and radiation therapy (grade I, 5-year survival of 33%; 10-year survival, 16%; grade II, 5-year survival, 21%; 10-year survival, 6%), he concluded that 'delay of recurrence and greater survival can be expected following postoperative radiation therapy than after surgery alone'.

In 1984, Laws et al again used the patient population at the Mayo Clinic to review 461 astrocytoma patients treated between 1915 and 1971 (Laws et al 1984). These cases were selected from a much larger group of patients and represented only those with supratentorial tumors who survived at least 30 days postoperatively and for whom follow-up data were available. Multiple prognostic factors were analyzed for possible correlation with an increase in survival. The authors found that the age of the patient was the most important variable and surpassed all others in its positive correlation with long-term survival. This important finding has been confirmed by almost all subsequent studies. In addition, they interpreted the data as supporting radical operation, and a beneficial effect of radiation therapy only in those patients with poor prognostic factors (e.g. older age). Their data have been reinterpreted by Sheline as showing a survival advantage for the irradiated group if one considers only those receiving > 4000 cGy as having been adequately irradiated (Sheline 1986).

In the following year a study was published which reported a retrospective analysis of 86 patients treated at Washington University between 1950 and 1979 (Garcia et al 1985). Although the number of patients with well-differentiated astrocytomas was small, they found that those with the juvenile pilocytic type did well regardless of treatment and did not require radiation therapy, a conclusion that has been confirmed in several other studies (Clark et al 1985, Palma & Guidetti 1985).

In 1987, Piepmeier reviewed the records of 60 patients with low grade astrocytomas seen at the Yale-New Haven Hospital between 1975 and 1985 (Piepmeier 1987). In this retrospective review there was no significant difference found in survival between those patients who received radiation therapy in addition to surgery and those who did not. What is important in this study is that all patients who were irradiated received between 50 and 60 Gy delivered over 5–6 weeks to fields that were constructed using CT scanning to include the tumor plus a wide margin of surrounding brain. One caveat expressed by the author, however, was that since the patient population reviewed was treated over the last decade, the mean follow-up time was slightly less than 5 years and thus this may have been insufficient time to allow a potential effect of radiation to become evident. It should also be noted, however, that most previous studies which did indicate a beneficial effect of radiation therapy did so mainly at 5 years, with such beneficial effect if anything decreasing at 10 years or longer.

A 1988 study reviewed 60 patients with low grade

astrocytomas who were treated at the Bethesda Naval Hospital between 1960 and 1986 (Medbery et al 1988). The series compared 50 patients who received postoperative radiation therapy and 10 patients who did not. Although the numbers were small, there appeared to be a survival advantage at 5 years for those with incompletely resected lesions who received radiation therapy.

In 1989 the fourth study from the Mayo Clinic was published. This paper reported on 167 patients, of whom 139 (83%) received surgery plus radiation therapy with a mean tumor dose of 50 Gy. The 5-year survival rate for those receiving high dose (> 53 Gy) radiation therapy was 68% whereas the survival rate was 47% for those who received low dose irradiation (< 53 Gy) and 32% for those who had surgery but were not irradiated (Shaw et al 1989). The comparable 10-year survival rates were 39%, 21% and 11% respectively. In contrast to these data for the grade I and II astrocytomas indicating a beneficial effect of radiation therapy, they found that postoperative irradiation was not associated with improved survival in the patient with pilocytic astrocytomas.

A paper from France in 1989 reported on 22 pediatric patients (≤ 15 years old) who were operated on for grade I or II astrocytomas (Hirsch et al 1989). None of these patients was initially given radiation therapy. Since only 3 recurrences (8%) were seen in the entire group of 42 patients (which included 8 patients with oligodendroglioma and 12 patients with oligoastrocytoma), the authors concluded that postoperative radiation therapy should *not* be given to pediatric patients with low grade cerebral gliomas.

In 1990 North et al reported on a series of 77 patients from the Johns Hopkins Medical Center who were treated with a uniform radiation dose of 50–55 Gy over a period of 5½–6 weeks (North et al 1990). More importantly, in this study quality of life was determined at one and two years postoperatively and at last follow-up 2–12 years after surgery. They observed that mental retardation was observed in 50% of the children who had received radiation therapy. Overall, however, 80% of short-term survivors and 67% of long-term survivors were intellectually and physically intact and without major neurologic deficit.

In that same year another study reviewed 88 patients with cerebral low grade gliomas who were treated with postoperative radiotherapy at the Royal Marsden Hospital between 1960 and 1985 (Whitton & Bloom 1990). Treatments were given 5 times a week to a total dose of 50–55 Gy. They were able to confirm that age was a very important prognostic factor, but indicated that it was still unclear whether or not postoperative radiotherapy was effective.

A 1991 study from the University of Pittsburgh analyzed treatment results in 25 patients with well-differentiated cerebral astrocytomas (Vertosick et al 1991). The median survival for their entire group of patients was 8.2 years, which is the longest that has thus far been reported. They attributed this long-term survival to earlier diagnosis in the CT/MRI scan era rather than to the specific efficacy of any modern form of adjuvant therapy. Approximately 70% of their patients received postoperative radiation therapy, whereas 30% did not. In this series, the use of radiotherapy did not have a significant impact upon the time to differentiation or the time to death, although they cautioned that the number of patients in each group was small.

Most recently, there was a report of a retrospective series of 53 patients with supratentorial astrocytomas who were treated at the NYU Medical Center (McCormack et al 1992). Since fully 98% of their patients received postoperative radiation therapy, it could not be determined whether or not such patients lived longer than those who did not receive such adjuvant therapy.

There have been several recent reports on the use of alternative forms of radiation therapy in the treatment of low grade astrocytomas. Three authors have reported on the use of interstitial radiation therapy with implanted ^{125}I seeds. The first paper detailed a series of 45 patients, and concluded that its use should be limited to patients less than 40 years of age whose tumors were not in the optic chiasm, hypothalamus, or lower brainstem (Frank et al 1987). In 1990, there was a report on the use of interstitial radiation in 13 children which indicated that tumor shrinkage was seen on CT scan in all children by 6 months postimplantation (Voges et al 1990). In 1991, there was a report on the use of interstitial radiation in 89 patients harboring nonresectable low grade brainstem astrocytomas (Mundinger et al 1991). Since these tumors differ from cerebral tumors in many respects, one cannot extrapolate from these data as to the possible effectiveness of this technique in the treatment of *cerebral* low grade tumors. The paper does, however, indicate that interstitial radiation therapy when carried out with ^{125}I via an implanted catheter is a safe and feasible technique.

There has also been one report on the use of stereotactic radiosurgery in the treatment of low grade astrocytomas. This paper reported on 14 patients with nonoperable low grade astrocytomas who were treated with unconventionally fractionated stereotactic radiosurgery (Pozza et al 1989). A total of 16–50 Gy was administered in either one or two fractions 8 days apart. They indicated that 12 of 14 patients demonstrated a partial or complete response as demonstrated by CT scanning.

Finally, there has even been a recent case report on the use of *re-irradiation* in a patient with a low grade astrocytoma who had been irradiated 8 years previously (Selbergeld et al 1992). In this single instance, there was no evidence of clinical or radiologic brain injury at the time of 3-year follow-up.

As indicated in the literature review above, the majority of the major English-language studies have found that radiation therapy has been effective when added to surgery in the treatment of cerebral astrocytoma (Table 24.2). One must, however, be extremely cautious in interpreting these retrospective data. As I have indicated previously, it is mandatory to take into account the various prognostic factors that may be present in different degrees in the two groups of patients that are being compared. Age, functional status for the patient, extent of surgical removal and pathologic grade (i.e. grade I or II) are at least some of the important variables that must be known. In almost none of the studies reviewed is this information available. Consequently, any conclusions reached must be considered only tentative until the proper studies are carried out.

Future advances in technology may allow a subgroup of patients with low grade astrocytomas to be selected who would most benefit from receiving postoperative radiation therapy. Currently, procedures have been developed that can measure the proliferative potential of low grade astrocytomas using immunohistochemical techniques such as in vivo labeling with ^{3}H-thymidine (Hoshino 1984), in vivo (Hoshino et al 1988) or in vitro (Nishizak et al 1988) labeling with 5-bromodeoxyuridine (BUdR) or labeling with the monoclonal antibody Ki-67 (Zuber et al 1988). A more simple technique may involve the measurement of nucleolar organizer regions (Hara et al 1990). Preliminary data appear to reveal a correlation between a poor prognosis and an increase in proliferative potential. Furthermore, a study of 12 patients with low grade astrocytomas who underwent PET scanning with ^{18}F-fluorodeoxyglucose (FDG) indicated that malignant change may be associated with a focal area of hypermetabolism that develops within an area that in general is hypometabolic (Francavilla et al 1989). If this is confirmed in other studies, then perhaps only those patients whose tumors have a labeling index above a certain level or who have a hypermetabolic area on PET scanning should receive radiation therapy.

The issue of whether radiation therapy should be utilized in these patients is not one that can be taken lightly. In patients with anaplastic astrocytoma or glioblastoma multiforme, it is quite probable that the relatively short survival time prevents the long-term deleterious effects of radiation therapy from becoming evident. This would not be the case in this group of patients, who have a 5-year survival rate of approximately 50–60% and a 10-year survival rate of perhaps 40%.

There have been many studies of the complications that may be produced by cerebral radiation therapy. One such study reported on patients in whom malignant gliomas developed after radiation therapy that had been previously administered for other conditions (Shapiro et al 1989). At least 7 such cases have been documented; patients who experienced this complication tended to be young (as is the case in most patients with low grade astrocytomas who are given radiation therapy). A recent review from the Mount Sinai Hospital in New York City found 7 cases of radiation-induced meningiomas (Harrison et al 1991). The overwhelming majority of these patients had received low dose radiation therapy (8 Gy) to the scalp for tinea capitis. The second largest group, however, were patients who received high dose radiation for primary brain tumors.

Although the reported incidence of radiation necrosis varies widely, white matter changes are being seen more and more frequently on MRI scans of patients who have previously undergone radiation therapy. A recent study indicates the presence of radiation necrosis in 9% of a series of 76 patients treated with whole brain radiation for various intrinsic brain tumors (Hohwieler et al 1986). In this regard, it is of interest that a review of 371 irradiated brain tumor patients found the incidence of radiation necrosis to be 1.5% at 55 Gy and 4% at 60 Gy, with a substantial increase after higher doses (Marks & Wong 1985). Since it is generally accepted that the risks of untoward sequelae from radiation therapy are greater after whole brain therapy than after more localized treatment, it would seem most prudent to carry out only localized radiation if one decides to use this adjuvant form of therapy.

CHEMOTHERAPY

Let us now look at the question of whether or not chemotherapy is useful as a postoperative adjuvant therapy in the treatment of these patients. Over the years there have been several anecdotal reports on the use of various chemotherapeutic agents in small numbers of patients with low grade astrocytomas (Eagan et al 1982, Djerassi et al 1985). Invariably one has been unable to draw conclusions with respect to efficacy from such case reports. There has been one recent analysis which compared 75 patients who were treated with radiation plus intra-arterial BCNU as well as vincristine and procarbazine to 57 patients treated with radiation alone (Watne et al 1992). This study appeared to show a longer survival in those treated with this aggressive chemotherapy regimen.

There has, however, been a prospective randomized study which came to the opposite conclusion. This study, which was conducted by the Southwest Oncology Group, demonstrated that the addition of CCNU to radiation therapy did *not* result in an increase in survival (Eyre et al 1993). At the present time, therefore, it appears that there is no proven beneficial effect of chemotherapy in the treatment of patients with low grade astrocytomas.

Currently, there are no studies which document a beneficial effect as a result of experimental methods of treatment such as immunotherapy, radiosensitizers, hyperthermia, etc. in the treatment of these tumors.

PATTERNS OF FAILURE

The failure of the previously described treatment modalities is almost always due to local recurrence. This can be the result either of the continued growth of the low grade neoplasm (which can result in the death of the patient if the tumor is located in the deeper part of the brain) or of the dedifferentiation of a low grade tumor into a more malignant glioma.

MANAGEMENT OF RECURRENT DISEASE

The treatment of such a recurrence depends on establishing the tumor grade. This implies that repeat biopsy will be necessary in most cases. If the tumor remains low grade, then the patient may be followed by periodic CT/MRI scans and/or PET scans. Observation may also be warranted if the patient's clinical status is stable. If such a tumor is enlarging and causing significant mass effect or CSF obstruction, then repeat resection alone should be considered. On the other hand, if the neuroradiologic studies, clinical course and/or biopsy indicate that malignant transformation has occurred, a more aggressive treatment regimen consisting of repeat surgical resection, interstitial radiation therapy and/or chemotherapy may now be considered. Since the time period between the initial radiation which may have been given and the recurrence may be quite long, re-irradiation may also be considered. As indicated, a good result after re-irradiation has recently been described in a single patient whose tumor recurred 8½ years after the initial radiation (Selbergeld et al 1992).

MANAGEMENT OUTCOME

What length of survival, then, can we expect in patients harboring a low grade astrocytoma? A review of the several series that have been carried out prior to 1990 would indicate a 5-year survival rate of approximately 40–50% and a 10-year survival of approximately 20–30%. The two most recent series however (which included patients who were diagnosed solely within the CT scan era) indicate a current median survival for the entire group of patients of approximately 7½ years, with a 5-year survival of approximately 65% and a 10-year survival of approximately 40% (Vertosick et al 1991, McCormack et al 1992).

REFERENCES

Bloom H J G 1982 Intracranial tumors: response and resistance to therapeutic endeavors, 1970–1980. International Journal Radiation Oncology Biology Physics 8: 1083–1113

Bouchard J, Peirce B C 1960 Radiation therapy in the management of neoplasms of the central nervous system with a special note in regard to children: twenty years' experience 1939–1958. American Journal of Radiology 84: 610–628

Chamberlain M C, Murovic J A, Levin V A 1988 Absence of contrast enhancement on CT brain scans of patients with supratentorial malignant gliomas. Neurology 38: 1371–1374

Clark G B, Henry J M, McKeever P E 1985 Cerebral pilocytic astrocytoma. Cancer 56: 1128–1133

Daumas-Duport C, Scheithauer B, O'Fallon J et al 1988 Grading of astrocytomas. Cancer 62: 2152–2165

Djerassi I, Kim J S, Rigger A 1985 Response of astrocytomas to high-dose methotrexate with citrovorum factor rescue. Cancer 55: 2741–2747

Drayer B P, Johnson P C, Bird C R 1987 Magnetic resonance imaging and glioma. Barrow Neurological Institute Quarterly 3: 44–55

Eagan R T, Dinapoli R P, Herman R C et al 1982 Combination carmustine (BCNU) and dihydrogalactilol in the treatment of primary brain tumors recurring after irradiation. Cancer Treatment Reports 66: 1647–1649

Eyre H J, Eltringham J R, Crowley J, Morantz R A 1993 A randomized trial of radiotherapy versus radiotherapy plus CCNU for incompletely resected low-grade gliomas: Southwest Oncology Group study. Journal of Neurosurgery 78: 909–914

Fazekas J T 1977 Treatment of grades I and II brain astrocytomas: the role of radiotherapy. International Journal Radiation Oncology Biology Physics 2: 661–666

Francavilla T L, Miletich R S, DiChiro G et al 1989 Positron emission tomography in the detection of malignant degeneration of low-grade gliomas. Neurosurgery 26: 1–5

Frank F, Fabrizi A P, Garst G et al 1987 Late considerations in the treatment of low-grade malignant cerebral tumors with Iodine-125 brachytherapy. Applied Neurophysiology 50: 302–309

Fults D, Brockmeyer D, Tullous M W et al 1992 P53 mutation and loss of heterozygosity on chromosome 17 and 10 during human astrocytoma progression. Cancer Research 52: 674–679

Garcia D M, Fulling K H, Marks J E 1985 The value of radiation therapy in addition to surgery for astrocytomas of the adult cerebrum. Cancer 55: 919–927

Gol A 1961 The relatively benign astrocytomas of the cerebrum: a clinical study of 194 verified cases. Journal of Neurosurgery 18: 501–506

Guthrie B L, Laws E R 1990 Supratentorial low-grade gliomas. Neurosurgery Clinics of North America 1: 37–48

Hara A, Hirayoma H, Sakai N 1990 Correlation between nucleolar organizer region staining and Ki-67 immunostaining in human gliomas. Surgical Neurology 33: 320–324

Harrison M J, Wolfe D E, Lau T S 1991 Radiation induced meningiomas: experience at the Mount Sinai Hospital and review of the literature. Journal of Neurosurgery 75: 564–574

Hirsch J F, Sainte Rose C, Pierre-Kahn A et al 1989 Benign astrocytic and oligodendrocytic tumors of the cerebral hemispheres in children. Journal of Neurosurgery 70: 568–572

Hohwieler M L, Lo T C, Silverman M L, Friedberg S R 1986 Brain necrosis after radiotherapy for primary intracerebral tumor. Neurosurgery 18: 67–74

Hoshino T 1984 A commentary on the biology and growth kinetics of low-grade and high-grade gliomas. Journal of Neurosurgery 61: 895–900

Hoshino T, Rodriguez L A, Cho K G et al 1988 Prognostic implications of the proliferative potential of low-grade astrocytomas. Journal of Neurosurgery 69: 839–842

Kelly P J, Daumas-Duport C, Scheithauer B W et al 1987 Stereotactic histologic correlations of computed tomography and magnetic resonance imaging-defined abnormalities in patients with glial neoplasm. Mayo Clinic Procedings 62: 450–459

Kepes J J, Rubinstein L J, Eng L V 1979 Pleomorphic xanthoastrocytoma: a distinctive meningocerebral glioma of young subjects with relatively favorable prognosis; a study of 12 cases. Cancer 44: 1839–1852

Krouwer H G, Davis R L, Silver P et al 1991 Gemistocytic astrocytomas: a reappraisal. Journal of Neurosurgery 74: 399–406

Laws E R Jr, Taylor W F, Clifton M B et al 1984 Neurosurgical management of low-grade astrocytomas of the cerebral hemispheres. Journal of Neurosurgery 61: 665–673

Leibel S A, Sheline G E, Wara W M et al 1975 The role of radiation therapy in the treatment of astrocytomas. Cancer 35: 1551–1557

LeRoux P D, Berger M S, Wang K et al 1992 Low-grade gliomas: comparison of intraoperative ultrasound characteristics with preoperative imaging studies. Journal of Neurological Oncology 13: 189–198

Levy L F, Elvidge A R 1956 Astrocytoma of the brain and spinal cord: a review of 176 cases, 1940–1949. Journal of Neurosurgery 13: 413–443

McCormack B M, Miller D C, Budzilovich G N 1992 Treatment and survival of low-grade astrocytoma in adults — 1977–1988. Neurosurgery 31: 636–642

Marks J E, Wong I 1985 The risk of cerebral radionecrosis in relation to dose, time and fractionation: a follow-up study. Progress in Experimental Tumor Research 29: 210–218

Marsa G W, Goffinet D R, Rubinstein L J et al 1975 Megavoltage irradiation in the treatment of gliomas of the brain and spinal cord. Cancer 36: 1681–1689

Medbery C A, Straus K L, Steinberg S M, Cotelingam J D, Fisher W S 1988 Low-grade astrocytomas: treatment results and prognostic variables. International Journal Radiation Oncology Biology Physics 15: 837–841

Morantz R A 1987 Radiation therapy in the treatment of cerebral astrocytomas. Neurosurgery 20: 975–982

Müller W, Afra D, Schröder R 1977 Supratentorial recurrences of gliomas: morphological studies in relation to time intervals with astrocytomas. Acta Neurochirurgica (Wien) 37: 75–91

Mundinger F, Braus D F, Krauss J K et al 1991 Long-term outcome of 89 low-grade brain-stem gliomas after interstitial radiation therapy. Journal of Neurosurgery 75: 740–746

Nishizak T, Orita T, Saiki M, Furutani Y, Aoki H 1988 Cell kinetic studies of human brain tumors by in-vitro labeling using anti-BUDR monoclonal antibody. Journal of Neurosurgery 69: 371–374

North C A, North R B, Epstein J A et al 1990 Low-grade cerebral astrocytomas: survival and quality of life after radiation therapy. Cancer 66: 6–14

Palma L, Guidetti B 1985 Cystic pilocytic astrocytomas of the cerebral hemispheres; surgical experience with 51 cases and long-term results. Journal of Neurosurgery 62: 811–815

Piepmeier J M 1987 Observations on the current treatment of low-grade astrocytic tumors of the cerebral hemispheres. Journal of Neurosurgery 67: 177–181

Pozza F, Colombo F, Chierego G et al 1989 Low-grade astrocytomas: treatment with unconventionally fractionated external beam stereotactic radiation therapy. Radiology 171: 565–569

Radhakrishnan K, Bohnen N I, Kurland L T 1993 Epidemiology of brain tumors. In: Morantz R A, Walsh J (eds) Brain tumors: a comprehensive text. Marcel Dekker, New York

Recht L D, Lew R, Smith T W 1992 Suspected low-grade glioma: is deferring treatment safe? Annals of Neurology 31: 431–436

Russell D S, Rubinstein L J 1989 Pathology of tumors of the nervous system, 5th edn. Williams & Wilkins, Baltimore, pp 126–225

Scanlon P W, Taylor W F 1979 Radiotherapy of intracranial astrocytomas: analysis of 417 cases treated from 1960 through 1969. Neurosurgery 5: 301–308

Scherer J H 1940 Cerebral astrocytomas and their derivatives. American Journal of Cancer 40: 159–198

Schiffer D, Giordana M T, Sofietti R et al 1984 Effects of radiotherapy on the astrocytomatous areas of malignant gliomas. Journal of Neuro-Oncology 2: 167–175

Selbergeld D L, Griffin B K, Ojemann G 1992 Reirradiation for recurrent cerebral astrocytoma. Journal of Neuro-Oncology 12: 145–151

Shapiro S, Mealey J Jr, Sartorius C 1989 Radiation-induced intracranial malignant gliomas. Journal of Neurosurgery 71: 77–82

Shaw E G, Daumas-Duport C, Scheithauer B W et al 1989 Radiation therapy in the management of low-grade supratentorial astrocytomas. Journal of Neurosurgery 70: 853–861

Sheline G E 1986 The role of radiation therapy in the treatment of low-grade gliomas. Clinical Neurosurgery 33: 563–574

Sidransky D, Mikkelsen T, Schwechheimer K et al 1992 Clonal expansion of p53 mutant cells is associated with brain tumor progression. Nature 355: 846–847

Silver J M, Rawlings C E, Rossitch E et al 1991 Ganglioglioma: a clinical study with long-term follow-up. Surgical Neurology 35: 261–266

Silverman C, Marks J E 1981 Prognostic significance of contrast enhancement in low-grade astrocytomas of the adult cerebrum. Radiology 139: 211–213

Soffietti R, Chio A, Giordana M T et al 1989 Prognostic factors in well-differentiated cerebral astrocytomas in the adult. Neurosurgery 24: 686–692

Stage W S, Stein J J 1974 Treatment of malignant astrocytomas. American Journal of Radiology 120: 7–18

Uihlein A, Colby M Y Jr, Layton D D et al 1966 Comparison of surgery and surgery plus irradiation in the treatment of supratentorial gliomas. Acta Radiologica 5: 67–78

Vertosick F T, Selker R G, Arena V C 1991 Survival of patients with well-differentiated astrocytomas diagnosed in the era of computed tomography. Neurosurgery 28: 496–501

Voges J, Sturm V, Berthold F et al 1990 Interstitial irradiation of cerebral gliomas in childhood by permanently implanted 125-iodine: Preliminary results. Klin Padiatr 202: 270–274

Warnick R E 1993 Tumors associated with the phakomatoses. In Morantz R A, Walsh J (eds) Brain tumors: a comprehensive text. Marcel Dekker, New York

Watne K, Hannisdal E, Nome O 1992 Combined intra-arterial chemotherapy followed by radiation in astrocytomas. Journal of Neuro-Oncology 14: 73–80

Weir B, Grace M 1976 The relative significance of factors affecting post-operative survival in astrocytomas, grades I and II. Canadian Journal of Neurological Science 3: 47–50

Whitton A C, Bloom H J G 1990 Low-grade glioma of the cerebral hemispheres in adults: a retrospective study of 88 cases. International Journal Radiation Oncology Biology Physics 18: 783–786

Worthington C, Tyler J F, Villemare J G 1987 Stereotactic biopsy and positron emission tomography correlation of cerebral gliomas. Surgical Neurology 27: 87–92

Zuber P, Hamou M, de Tribolet N 1988 Identification of proliferating cells in human gliomas using the monoclonal antibody Ki-67. Neurosurgery 22: 364–368

Zülch K J 1986 Brain tumors: their biology and pathology, 3rd edn. Springer-Verlag, Berlin, pp 210–213

25. Glioblastoma and malignant astrocytoma

Michael Salcman

INTRODUCTION

Anaplastic astrocytoma and glioblastoma multiforme are the most frequent primary brain tumors in the adult age group and represent a major cause of morbidity and mortality in neurologic practice. Overall, brain tumors are the third or fourth most frequent cause of cancer-related deaths in middle-aged males and the second commonest cause of cancer deaths in children. In the pediatric population, the incidence of malignant astrocytoma among hemispheric lesions is surprisingly high (Schoenberg et al 1976). Although primary malignant brain tumors constitute only about 2% of all cancers, they are associated with severe disability and a high risk of death. Patients with malignant astrocytoma are often struck in the most productive period of their lives; frequent deterioration of mental faculties and a high case:fatality ratio contribute to the unique personal and social impact of these tumors. Unfortunately, the public health implications of anaplastic astrocytoma and glioblastoma multiforme are not fully appreciated. Advances in the treatment of other brain tumors should not blind us to the enormity of the challenges we still face in the successful management of malignant gliomas (Salcman 1985a, 1991b).

INCIDENCE AND PREVALENCE

The distribution of primary brain tumors in the general population is strongly age specific, so that the probability of histologic malignancy in an astrocytoma is only 0.34 between the years of 30 and 34 and is 0.85 after the age of 60 (Trouillas et al 1975). The incidence per 100 000 population of glioblastoma and astrocytoma rises from 0.2 and 0.5 in the under-14 age group to 4.5 and 1.7 respectively after the age of 45 (Cohen & Modan 1968). This age-related shift in histology is accompanied by an age-associated shift in tumor site so that, under the age of 25 years, 67% of astrocytomas are located in the posterior fossa but in patients older than 25, 90% of tumors are supratentorial in location. In Israel, the incidence of glioblastoma as a percentage of the total number of gliomas and medulloblastomas increases from 11% in the under-14 age group to 23, 35, 50 and 58% in the 15–29, 30–44, 45–59 and over-60 age groups, respectively (Cohen & Modan 1968). The relative frequency of glioblastoma and anaplastic astrocytoma among all primary brain tumors ranges from more than a fifth to nearly one half of all cases (Table 25.1). In the United States, a national survey of patterns of care for patients with brain tumors revealed that 27.7% of the cases were glioblastomas and 26.6% were astrocytomas (Mahaley et al 1989). In children less than 14 years of age, glioblastoma represents 20% of all primary brain tumors, but it accounts for more than half of histologically confirmed cases in adults (Schoenberg et al 1976).

When examining the incidence and prevalence of a particular tumor in a given population, the age and sex distribution of the survey must be taken into account (Schoenberg 1991). Such factors help to explain the difference in magnitude between the overall incidence and prevalence of a tumor in a given population and the peak

Table 25.1 The incidence of glioblastoma and anaplastic astrocytoma among all primary brain tumors

Series	Area	Tumor	Percent
Barker et al (1976)	England	G3 & G4	47.9
Trouillas et al (1975)	Lyon	GBM	41.3
Schoenberg et al (1976)	Conn.	GBM	20.3
Annegers et al (1981)	Rochester	Glioma	34.9
Ohaegbula et al (1980)	Nigeria	Glioma	20.8
Mahaley et al (1989)	USA	GBM	27.7
		AA	2.8
		Astro	26.6
Salcman (1985)	Baltimore	GBM	42.8
Walker et al (1985)	USA	GBM	20.0
		Astro	34.8
Cohen & Modan (1968)	Israel	GBM	20.2
		Astro	
Mao et al (1991)	Canada	GBM	37.0
		Astro	21.0

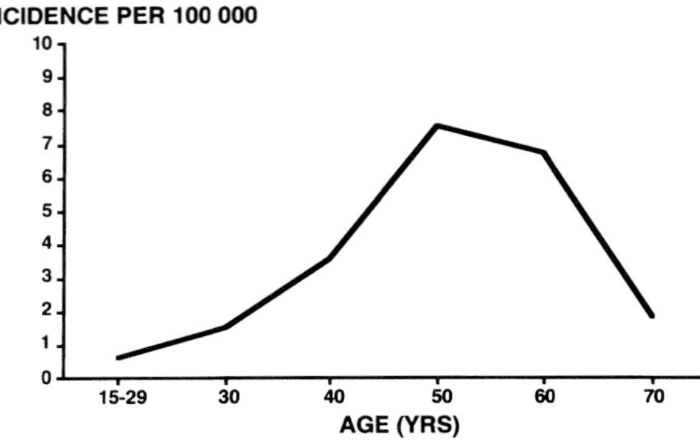

Fig. 25.1 Incidence of glioblastoma as a function of age. The incidence of glioblastoma per 100 000 population as a function of age, based on data from the United Kingdom prior to 1980. A broad peak exists between the ages of 45 and 60. Recent data indicate that the age-related incidence continues its steady rise into the seventh and eighth decades.

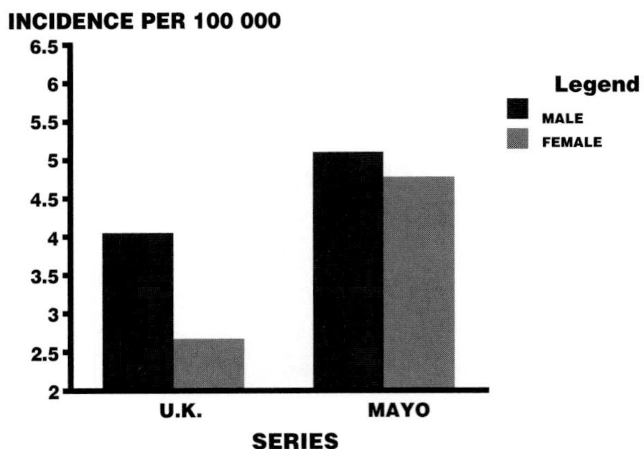

Fig. 25.2 Incidence of malignant astrocytoma as a function of sex. The incidence of glioblastoma per 100 000 in adult men and women presented as a series of bar graphs; a slight preponderance of males is seen in most series. U.K. = United Kingdom data; Mayo = Rochester, Minn. data

incidence or prevalence (Fig. 25.1). In England, for example, the peak incidence of glioblastoma multiforme is 7.53 per 100 000 population and occurs in the 50–59-year age group (Barker et al 1976). In Sweden, the overall incidence from 1958–1975 was 4.2 per 100 000 (Salford et al 1988). In the United States, glioblastoma multiforme occurs at the greatest mean age of all brain tumors (60.2 years); patients with astrocytoma and anaplastic astrocytoma have mean ages a full decade younger ($p < 0.01$) (Mahaley et al 1989). In some surgical series, nearly half of operated tumors in patients older than 65 have been glioblastomas (Tomita & Raimondi 1981). In Canada, the age-specific death rate between 1965 and 1967 peaked in the 55–60-year age group but has recently been shown to increase continuously to 75–79 years of age in the 1985–1987 period (Mao et al 1991).

From 1973–1974, there were 17 030 new cases of primary brain tumor diagnosed per year in the United States for an age-corrected incidence of 8.2 per 100 000, and more than half of these tumors were gliomas (Walker et al 1985). Twenty % of the pathologically confirmed cases were glioblastoma. Since then, some investigators have claimed that the incidence of malignant brain tumors has increased in developed countries as a part of a general increase in cancer frequency and death (Davis et al 1990). This increase has been most striking in the older age groups. In the United States and Canada, there has been at least a two-fold increase in the number of glioblastomas seen in patients over 75 years of age (Greig et al 1990, Mao et al 1991). From 1969–1985, the incidence of brain cancer in elderly Canadian men and women increased 89% and 139% respectively (Mao et al 1991). For example, the incidence of glioblastoma in this group was 5 per 100 000 in 1971 and increased to more than 8 per 100 000 by 1985. Some have claimed that the increase is due to a higher detection rate, brought about through the application of improved technology. For example, prior to the advent of MR and CT, perhaps 6% of brain tumors were misclassified as strokes. Nevertheless, even a 20% improvement in detection rate provided by modern imaging has been shown inadequate to explain the absolute increase observed in the incidence of malignant brain tumors, especially in the elderly (Desmeules et al 1992).

Considerable evidence indicates that glioblastomas and anaplastic astrocytomas are slightly more common in men than in women (Fig. 25.2; Table 25.2) and are more frequently observed in whites than in blacks (Trouillas et al 1975, Ohaegbula et al 1980). The male:female sex ratio for glioblastoma is about 1.6 and for astrocytoma about 1.5 (Trouillas et al 1975). For all types of brain cancer, the male:female incidence ratio is about 1.37 (Mao et al 1991). The relative infrequency of malignant gliomas in blacks is supported by comparisons of the racial incidence of these tumors in the United States and in Africa as well as by an examination of the incidence in Israeli immigrants by continent of origin (Cohen & Modan 1968). In seven published series, gliomas in Africans represented only 36.8% of treated primary brain tumors as opposed to

Table 25.2 Incidence of glioblastoma and anaplastic astrocytoma by sex

Series	Area	Tumor	M:F Ratio
Barker et al (1976)	England	G3 & G4	1.5:1
Trouillas et al (1975)	Lyon	GBM	1.66:1
		Astro	1.48:1
Annegers et al (1981)	Rochester	Glioma	1.06:1
Mahaley et al (1989)	USA	GBM	1.23:1
		AA	1.25:1
Walker et al (1985)	USA	GBM	1.11:1
		Astro	1.17:1
Cohen & Modan (1968)	Israel	Malig.	1.4:1
Mao et al (1991)	Canada	Malig.	1.4:1
Salcman (1993)	Baltimore	G3&G4	1.4:1

about 50% of such tumors in the West (Ohaegbula et al 1980). Once racial differences and the state of economic development are taken into account, the incidence of glioblastoma and malignant astrocytoma generally does not vary from nation to nation around the world (Cheng 1982). However, the rate of increase in brain cancer death rates for Japan is far greater than that of other developed countries, perhaps because the absolute levels are somewhat lower (Davis et al 1990).

FAMILY HISTORY, GENETICS AND ONCOGENESIS

Glioblastoma multiforme and anaplastic astrocytoma usually occur as sporadic tumors without evidence of any familial tendency or identification of environmental risk factors. However, an increased incidence of malignant gliomas has been observed in the context of the cancer family syndrome, usually in association with breast carcinoma, soft tissue sarcomas and leukemia (Lynch et al 1973, Li & Fraumeni 1982). In some family pedigrees, the tendency to develop either an anaplastic astrocytoma or an extraneural malignancy appears to be a dominantly inherited trait (Lynch et al 1973, Li & Fraumeni 1982, Salcman & Solomon 1984). Mutation of the p53 gene on chromosome 17 may occur as a dominant allelotype and has been detected in some cancer family members. The pedigree of such a family is presented in Figure 25.3; the middle son in each of three successive generations developed a glioblastoma, and the overall risk of cancer in the paternal line was approximately 50% (Salcman & Solomon 1984). In this example, malignant astrocytoma presumably occurs because of the inheritance of a general predisposition to the development of tumors. Coexistence of astrocytoma and colonic carcinoma (Turcot syndrome) has also been reported (Todd et al 1981) and occasional astrocytomas occur in patients with such classic heredofamilial disorders as tuberous sclerosis and neurofibromatosis. Patients with these diseases are at risk of developing brain tumors of many different histologies (Schoenberg 1977). The recent demonstration of the genetic defect in neurofibromatosis is an important clue to the molecular etiology of astrocytic tumors (Seizinger et al 1986).

At the present time, several authors have put forward the theory that the development of a glioblastoma from a low grade astrocytoma represents a stepwise process in which progressive loss of tumor suppressor genes on chromosomes 17 and 10 is associated with the development of anaplasia and that the activation of dominant oncogenes results in further promotion of growth and heterogeneity through the elaboration of growth factors (James et al 1988, 1989; see also Ch. 20). This theory is attractive in a number of respects. Stepwise loss of tumor suppressor genes has been demonstrated in the development of colon carcinoma, a tumor frequently associated with astrocytoma in cancer family pedigrees. Overexpression of onco-

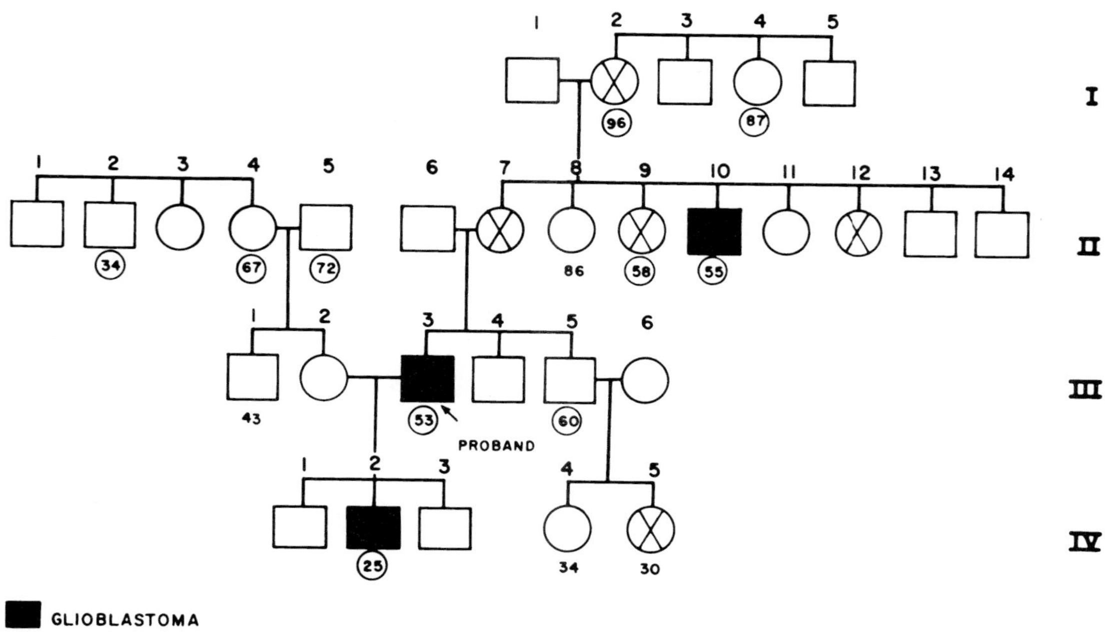

Fig. 25.3 Occurrence of glioblastoma in the cancer family syndrome. The pedigree demonstrates that family members on the paternal side have a 50% chance of developing a glioblastoma (filled squares), a breast carcinoma (crossed circles) or other solid malignancy. In some families, the tendency to develop tumors is associated with inheritance of a dominant but mutant gene for the p53 protein. Reproduced with permission from Salcman & Solomon (1984).

genes has been shown to correlate inversely with length of survival in patients with tumors derived from the neural crest (Seeger et al 1985). Chromosomal abnormalities on chromosomes 10 and 17 are frequently observed in glioma patients, and the p53 tumor suppressor gene, important in the genesis of the cancer family syndrome, as well as the NF-1 gene, have been mapped to chromosome 17. Loss of genetic material on chromosome 10 has predicted biological malignancy in oligodendroglioma as well as in astrocytoma (Wu et al 1992). PDGFr and EGFr activation are the most powerful in vitro stimulants to glioma growth, even in the absence of fetal calf serum (Pollack et al 1990). The degree of anaplasia in astrocytomas has been correlated with the level of EGFr protein and amplification of the EGFr gene (Libermann et al 1985). Astrocytomas are capable of autocrine stimulation and growth when they coexpress mRNA for both PDGF and its receptor (Hermansson et al 1988, Maxwell et al 1990). Growth factors like PDGF and TGF have angiogenic properties and may be responsible for sarcomatous transformation in glioblastoma. Stepwise anaplasia of astrocytomas has been frequently observed by serial biopsy at time of recurrence (Muller et al 1977). Furthermore, a theory based on multiple genetic events is consistent with Rubinstein's concept of a window of neoplastic vulnerability during which genetic and environmental factors have their greatest impact in utero and postnatally (Rubinstein 1991). Finally, the loci of genetic abnormalities observed in sporadic glioblastoma and anaplastic astrocytoma are frequently the same as those seen in neurofibromatosis. Nevertheless, glioblastoma and malignant astrocytoma almost never occur as inheritable diseases except when they form part of the spectrum of tumors observed in the cancer family syndrome. Attempts to identify environmental risk factors have been generally unsuccessful although clusters of brain tumor cases have been reported in association with petrochemical plants and childhood radiation (Selikoff & Hammond 1982, Schoenberg 1991).

SITES OF PREDILECTION

Glioblastoma multiforme and anaplastic astrocytoma are usually centered in the deep white matter of the cerebral hemispheres (Fig. 25.4). Although the majority of tumors are described as occurring in different lobes of the brain, many of the frontal and occipital lesions border on the parietal lobe and straddle more than one functional area. This topographic tendency increases the difficulty of surgical removal and often brings the tumor into proximity of the thalamus or basal ganglia. Of course, glioblastoma and anaplastic astrocytoma occur in a wide variety of other locations. For example, nearly half of gliomas of the brainstem and spinal cord, frequently assumed to be low grade without histologic confirmation, are discovered to

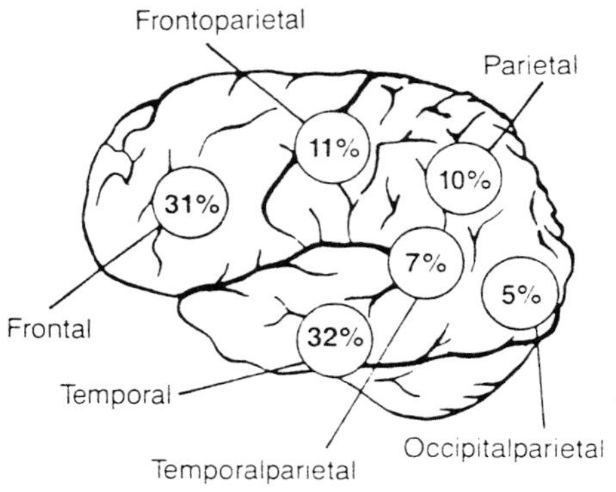

Fig. 25.4 Topographic distribution of glioblastoma in the brain. The topographic distribution of 901 cases of glioblastoma and malignant astrocytoma as reported in the literature. Although the frontal and temporal lobes are the most frequently involved single areas, the number of lesions bordering the central parietal region from all possible directions is equally large. Reproduced with permission from Salcman (1988).

be malignant. On the other hand, fewer than 50 glioblastomas of the cerebellum have been described in the literature, some of which represent late degeneration of previously diagnosed solid astrocytomas in this location. Nevertheless, de novo glioblastoma of the cerebellum has been observed on a number of occasions in both adults and children (Fig. 25.5). Finally, since 10% of glioblastomas present on the surface of the brain with an epicenter

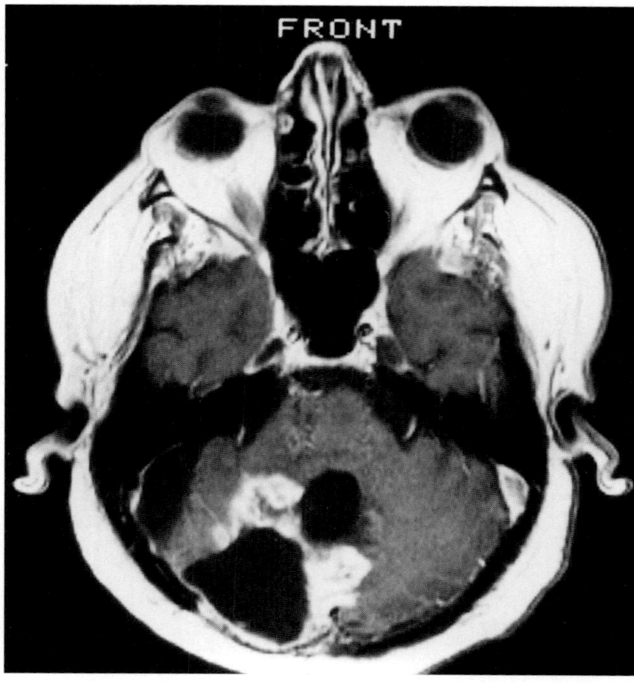

Fig. 25.5 Primary glioblastoma of the cerebellum. A rare case of glioblastoma in the posterior fossa of a 46-year-old male demonstrates some of the classic radiographic features of the disease, including dense enhancement with gadolinium in a ring-shaped pattern. Less than 50 such cases have been described in the literature. The patient died 27 months after diagnosis.

located at the gray-white junction, radiographic demonstration of a malignant tumor in this location should not be assumed to represent a metastatic lesion without definitive histologic verification.

CLINICAL PRESENTATION

The signs and symptoms produced by any intracranial lesion are a function of location rather than histology. Since glioblastoma and anaplastic astrocytoma may occur anywhere within the intracranial cavity, the likelihood of any given mode of presentation is entirely dependent on the topographic distribution of the tumor (Fig. 25.4). Signs and symptoms due to raised intracranial pressure are general in nature and may include headache, drowsiness, stiff neck, and involvement of the 3rd and 6th cranial nerves. These findings are usually produced through volumetric enlargement of the tumor and its zone of peritumoral edema beyond the compensatory mechanisms of the brain (Salcman 1990d). Since malignant astrocytomas rarely involve the ventricular pathway, nonspecific signs and symptoms are rarely due to hydrocephalus. On occasion, a thalamic tumor may produce blockage of the third ventricle through coaptation of the opposite ventricular wall. In addition, up to 5% of tumors in the pineal region and vicinity of the cerebral aqueduct are glioblastomas and anaplastic astrocytomas (Stein & Bruce 1992). Drowsiness and stiff neck are ominous signs produced by transtentorial and tonsillar herniation respectively. Since the introduction of CT and MR scanning, early diagnosis has been facilitated and presentation of brain tumor patients in a state of depressed consciousness has become a distinct rarity.

Site-specific findings depend entirely on the location of the tumor and are due to a combination of irritative (i.e. epileptic) and destructive mechanisms. Seizures are more likely to occur when the tumor arises in an epileptogenic area of the brain such as the frontoparietal region or the temporal lobe; the site of origin then determines the type of seizure phenomena observed. Similarly, weakness and sensory neglect are hallmarks of tumors arising in the frontoparietal and thalamic regions, while difficulties with memory, judgement and personality betoken tumor and swelling in one or both frontal lobes. Elderly patients who present with an organic mental syndrome have an exceedingly poor prognosis because their tumors usually involve the corpus callosum. Visual field defects are relatively infrequent complaints in patients with malignant astrocytoma because very few of the tumors arise in the occipital lobe and patients are generally unaware of the slow onset of a cortically-based hemianopsia. The classic triad of headache, seizures and hemiparesis is seen in less than half of patients; the relative frequency of signs and symptoms in malignant gliomas are summarized in Tables 25.3 and 25.4.

Table 25.3 Symptoms at assessment in glioma patients

Symptom	All gliomas*	GBM†	Oligo#
Headache	71.4	76.8	23.1
Seizures	53.9	29.2	86.5
Grand mal	20.4		
Focal	22.8	—	36.5
Psychomotor	8.6	—	28.8
Minor absence	2.1	—	17.3
Mental change	52.2	43.8	38.5
Hemiparesis	43.3	42.8	19.2
Vomiting	31.5	30.7	
Dysphasia	27.0	29.0	3.8
Impaired l.o.c.	24.8	27.7	
Hemianesthesia	13.6	14.1	5.8
Hemianopsia	8.1	1.0	

*McKeran & Thomas (1980); N = 653
†Compiled from Roth & Elvidge (1960); Frankel & German (1958); Jelsma & Bucy (1967); N = 870
#Chin et al (1980); N = 52
l.o.c. = level of consciousness

Table 25.4 Physical signs at assessment in glioma patients

Sign	Astro Gr.1*	Astro Gr.2/3†	GBM#	Oligo
Hemiparesis	45.8	58.6	66.9	58.3
Cranial nerve@	64.6	45.5	63.5	41.7
Papilledema	56.3	47.2	58.2	50.0
Mental change~	39.6	50.4	38.3	52.8
Hemianesthesia$	20.5	32.5	37.9	27.8
Depressed sensorium			37.3	
Hemianopsia	18.8	32.2	31.7	33.3
Dysphasia	22.9	24.3	29.2	25.0

* McKeran & Thomas (1980); includes some cerebellar tumors; N = 48
† McKeran & Thomas (1980); N = 341
# Compiled from Roth & Elvidge (1960); Jelsma & Bucy (1967); McKeran & Thomas (1980); N = 826
@ Includes facial palsy
~ Includes confusion and disorientation
$ Includes parietal lobe syndromes, sensory loss, astereognosis

The tempo with which signs and symptoms develop is extremely important in the diagnosis of intracranial diseases. The acute presentation of a glioblastoma may be preceded by a several-year history of seizures during which imaging studies have remained negative or inconclusive; in some cases involving younger patients, an imaging study may never have been obtained. There is some evidence to indicate that a prolonged history of seizures is associated with a better prognosis since it may correlate with the gradual development of a malignant tumor in a more benign pre-existing focus of low grade tumor or astrocytosis (McKeran & Thomas 1980, Medical Research Council Brain Tumour Working Party 1990). A seizure history longer than 18 months or a duration of other symptoms for more than 6 months have been looked upon as favorable prognostic criteria (Roth & Elvidge 1960, Walker et al 1980). More typically, the presentation of adult patients with glioblastoma involves several months of gradual neurologic deterioration in

Table 25.5 Incidence of hemorrhage by tumor type. Modified from Salcman (1992)

Tumor	No. cases	No. bleeding	% Bleeding
Astrocytoma	472	12	2.5
Oligodendroglioma	72	6	8.3
Ependymoma	105	7	6.6
Glioblastoma	399	25	6.3
Medulloblastoma	145	2	1.4
Metastatic CA	104	3	2.9

contradistinction to the much briefer clinical course of metastatic tumor and the rapid evolution of signs and symptoms over hours to days in patients with cerebrovascular disorders. Only 20% of patients have a history shorter than 1 month and only 10% have had symptoms for longer than a year (Roth & Elvidge 1960). Subtle personality and memory changes may occur in almost half of patients with malignant astrocytoma and are often denied by both patient and family until further reflection has occurred in the postoperative period. Glioblastomas are among the most frequent tumors to undergo hemorrhagic change, and their clinical presentation may mimic a stroke in evolution. The sudden onset of a hemiplegia or depressed level of consciousness in a brain tumor suspect should raise the possibility of intratumoral bleeding. Approximately 3% of patients admitted with the diagnosis of 'stroke' are subsequently discovered to have a tumor, and about 3% of all tumors present with hemorrhage or in a stroke-like fashion (Salcman 1992). The clinical management of patients who suffer acute deterioration from a brain tumor is extremely difficult and the prognosis for such patients is very bleak. The data on incidence of hemorrhage by tumor type are summarized in Table 25.5.

IMAGING DIAGNOSIS

Any patient suspected of harboring a brain tumor should immediately undergo CT or MR imaging. The study should always be carried out in both a plain and enhanced manner so that the pattern of contrast enhancement can be properly evaluated and evidence for bleeding, calcification and edema delineated prior to administration of radiographic contrast or gadolinium. Although the diagnosis of a grade 3 or grade 4 astrocytoma is seriously in doubt in the absence of contrast enhancement, it can never be excluded since examples of malignant astrocytoma with almost negative scans have been published (Fig. 25.6A). On the other hand, dense contrast enhancement in either a uniform or ring-shaped pattern almost always excludes the presence of a low grade tumor. A single ring-shaped lesion in the hemispheric white matter of an adult with an appropriate history should be assumed to be a malignant astrocytoma until proven otherwise (Fig. 25.6). Typically, neoplastic ring-shaped lesions have walls of non-uniform thickness with one or more areas projecting inward into a region of central lucency. Conversely, the pattern of enhancement seen with a mature brain abscess usually consists of a thin rim of uniform thickness without any mushrooming or protrusions. Although a glioblastoma may produce a uniform pattern of enhancement, virtually no grade 3 or intermediate grade astrocytoma produces a ring-shaped lesion on CT or MR. The area of peritumoral edema around a malignant astrocytoma or glioblastoma is usually of the same diameter as the tumor itself, while the low density area around a metastatic tumor may be considerably larger than the lesion. Metastatic tumors are usually located at the gray-white junction and may be multiple in number. The epicenter of a glioblastoma is usually in the deep white matter, and fewer than 3% of tumors appear to be multicentric. The intensity of enhancement has little to do with the degree of tumor vascularity but is almost entirely due to breakdown of the blood-brain barrier (Salcman & Broadwell 1991). In almost all cases, the zone of safe resection and the target volume used for brachytherapy is contained within the zone of enhancement.

Both MR and CT imaging can be used to locate the tumor with respect to the motor strip and other important anatomical boundaries (Salcman 1985b, Berger et al 1990). Today, preoperative angiography is rarely useful for this purpose. If needed, the localizing information provided by the pattern of superficial venous drainage can now be obtained from magnetic resonance angiography or MRA. Positron emission tomography (PET) can be used to differentiate radiation necrosis from recurrent tumor but is not useful in the initial diagnosis of high grade gliomas because image quality and resolution on PET are inferior to both CT and MRI. Plain film radiography and air contrast studies are now of historical interest only. Myelography and combined myelography and CT scanning are sometimes useful in detecting drop metastases in patients complaining of radicular or myelopathic symptoms. However, MRI is often superior in such circumstances (Fig. 25.11).

LABORATORY DIAGNOSIS

There are no reliable blood tests presently available to establish the diagnosis of a malignant astrocytoma although elevated levels of human chorionic gonadotropin (HCG), carcinoembryonic antigen (CEA) and α-fetoprotein (AFP) would point to other malignant processes of a primitive, congenital or metastatic nature. Levels of tumor markers are almost always higher in the CSF than in peripheral blood but it is usually impractical or dangerous to obtain CSF in tumor suspects. On rare occasions, metastatic glioblastomas can present with a clinical picture similar to that of meningeal carcinomatosis; elevation

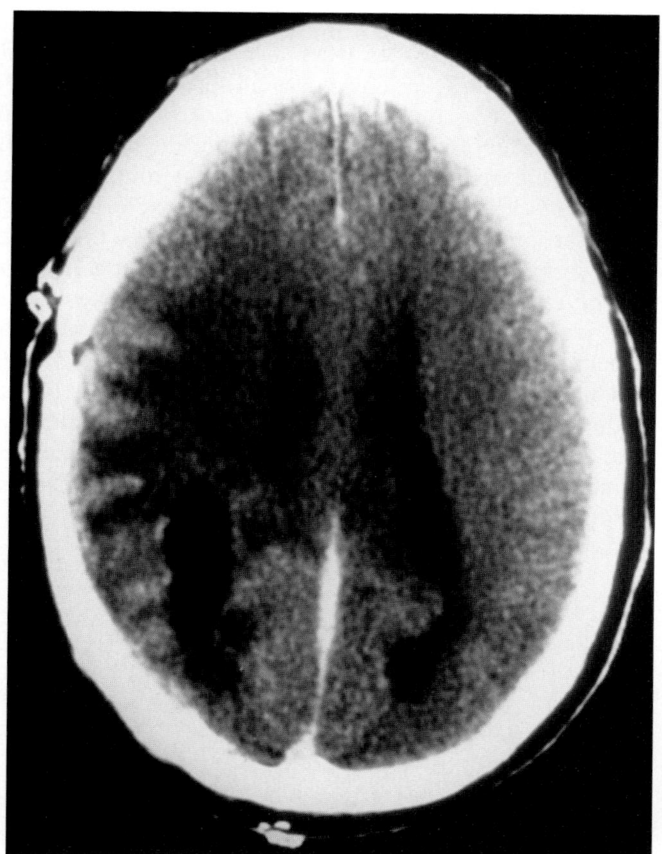

A

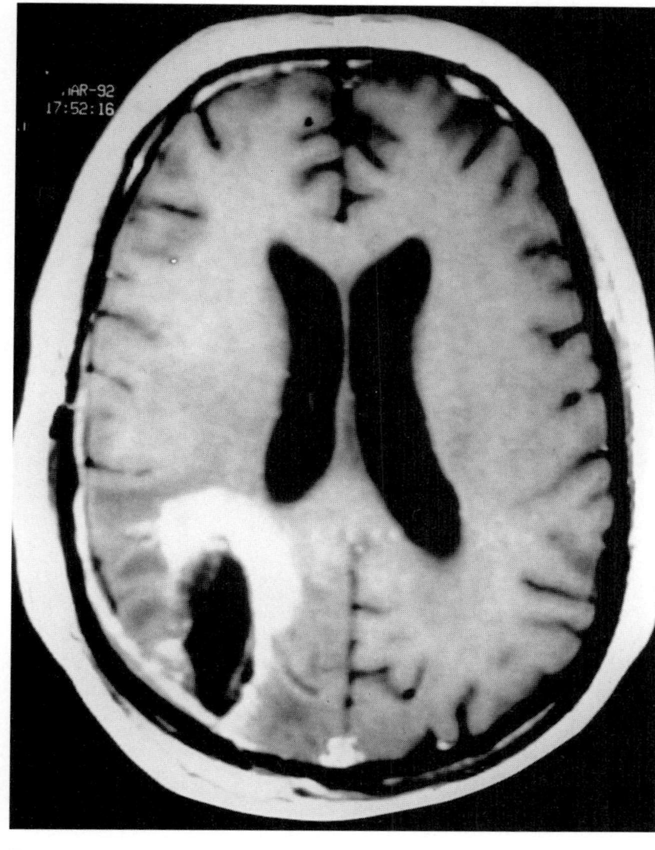

B

Fig. 25.6 Radiographic appearance of hemispheric glioblastoma. This case of a recurrent tumor in an adult is unusual in that the CT scan (**A**) demonstrated so little enhancement in comparison to an MRI scan (**B**) obtained only 5 days later. The area of low density change on the CT is approximately equal in diameter to the size of the enhancing tumor on MRI. On the latter, small pockets of enhancement can be seen outside the main mass.

of CSF β-glucuronidase is seen in the latter process but not with GBM. Levels of CSF polyamines have been used by some investigators to monitor the impact of therapy on neuroectodermal tumors, especially medulloblastoma, and as a screen for recurrence, but are probably not superior to regular scanning and neurologic examination in astrocytoma patients. Since no tumor-specific antigen has been identified for astrocytoma, it has not been possible to devise a definitive blood or CSF assay. The recent demonstration of transforming growth factors in the urine of some patients with primary brain tumors raises the future possibility of clinical testing based on molecular biology (Kanno et al 1988).

In addition to chemical markers, the CSF can be examined for the presence of malignant cells and elevated protein. The latter is a nonspecific finding and the cells can be difficult to identify without appropriate immunostaining for GFAP, S-100 protein or epithelial antigens. Without direct invasion of the CSF pathways, intrinsic tumors of the brain rarely produce an elevated cell count in CSF or recoverable material for cytology. In the absence of an unusual clinical presentation (i.e. meningeal seeding), these tests are superfluous and potentially dangerous or misleading.

GROSS MORPHOLOGY

Malignant astrocytoma and glioblastoma multiforme represent two of the more dramatic lesions encountered in the operating theater or during autopsy. The multiform histology of the tumor (see below) is reflected in the multiple colors, textures and consistencies of the gross specimen (Fig. 25.7). In the first textbook devoted to the subject of brain tumors (1888), Bramwell described the glioma as follows:

> [the] tendency to infiltrate the nervous structures is
> the most characteristic feature of the gliomatous tumour. The
> tumour tissue is never limited by a capsule, and it
> is impossible to say, without microscopical examination, where
> the tumour tissue ceases and the normal brain

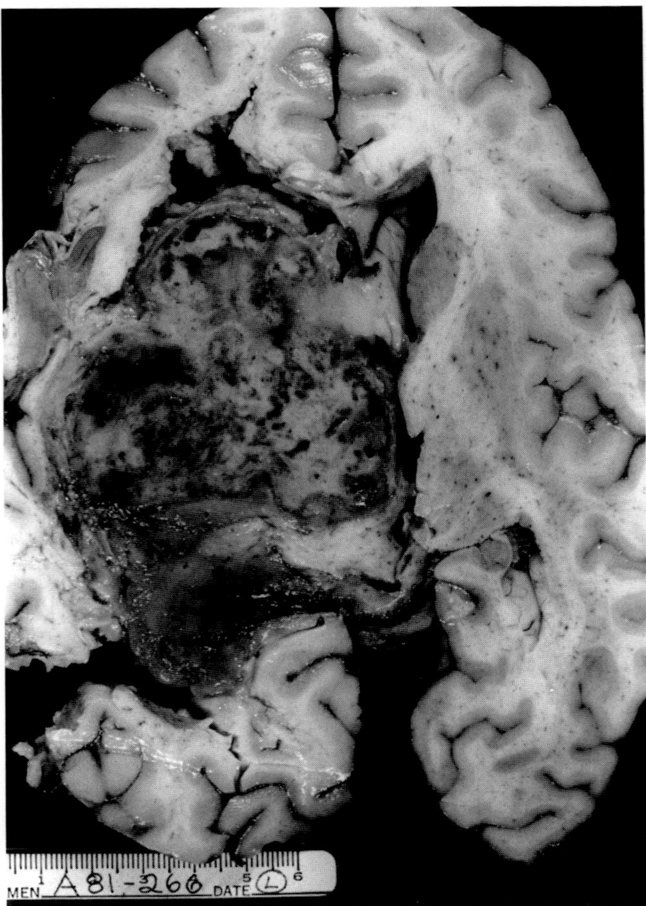

Fig. 25.7 Gross appearance of glioblastoma at autopsy. This photograph was taken of a fresh specimen sectioned in the plane of an axial CT or MRI slice. The variegated shades and texture of the tumor is readily apparent, as is the mass effect on midline structures.

tissue begins. The affected part of the brain often appears to be swollen, and is usually of a delicate pink, or purplish pink colour. In other cases the normal colour of the affected part is retained; in others again, nodules of firm, old, yellow and caseous-looking, or recent, black blood clot are scattered throughout the affected tissue. The corpus callosum or basal ganglia may, in consequence of this gliomatous infiltration, be swollen to twice or three times their usual size. Bramwell (1888).

The tumor is usually solid with small zones of central liquefaction or necrosis and may contain microcysts rather than the gross cystic spaces of benign cerebellar tumors. Although some tumors appear to be grossly demarcated from the surrounding brain in the manner of metastatic carcinoma, most are diffusely infiltrating with interdigitating fingers of tumor and normal tissue. The tumor is often gray-brown in color but can be meat-red like a meningioma and may contain areas of purple and greenish change due to hypervascularity and hemorrhage. Although no true capsule exists, glioblastoma only rarely invades non-neural tissues such as dura, bone or skin. Indeed, dura is a very effective barrier to the spread of the tumor. On occasion, milky effusions can be seen in the subarachnoid spaces when a malignant astrocytoma reaches the surface. The surrounding white matter is shiny and edematous; edema fluid can be seen to pour from its surfaces beneath the operating microscope. The tumor itself can be smooth and shiny or rough and dull with a cobblestone or ligneous feel to the exploring finger. Calcification is almost never present unless the tumor arises in a pre-existing lesion. Gray-yellow cheesy material can be evacuated from the necrotic center, especially in recurrent tumors after radiation and chemotherapy. Subarachnoid spread of the tumor may result in the encasement of nerves but the epineurium serves as a barrier to direct invasion. The cranial nerves usually do not contain tumor unless a malignant astrocytoma originates in an area such as the hypothalamus and directly extends into the chiasm.

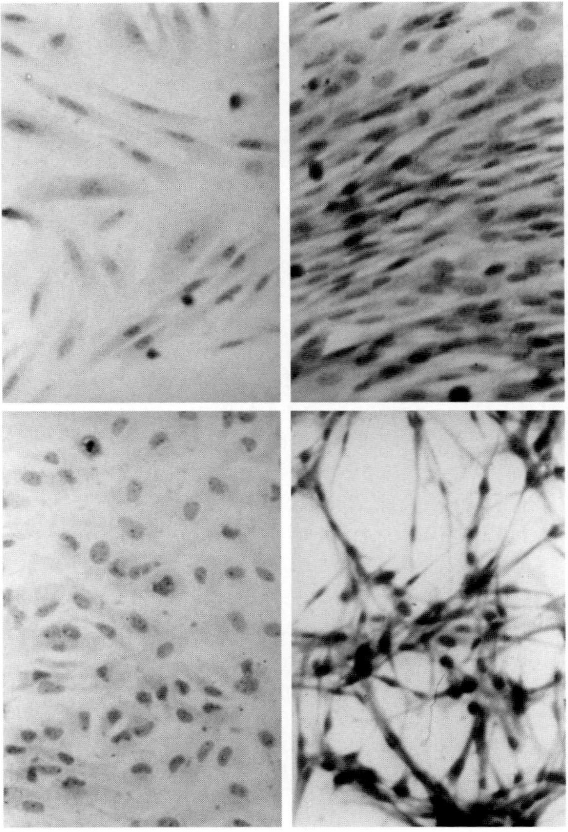

Fig. 25.8 Microphotograph of glioblastoma cell lines. Glioblastoma multiforme may contain within it cells of a variety of shapes and sizes, some resembling mature astrocytes, others that are small and dark like lymphocytes, and still others that are spindle-shaped like fibroblasts. Each cell type may be seen in different tumors from separate patients or in combinations in a single tumor in an individual patient. Courtesy of Darrell Bigner, Duke University.

HISTOPATHOLOGIC FEATURES

Glioblastoma multiforme was named for the extreme variability of cell morphology and tissue architecture observed with the light microscope after routine staining with standard techniques such as hematoxylin and eosin (H&E). In the Kernohan grading system, glioblastoma multiforme is equivalent to a grade 4 astrocytoma. Tissue culture studies have confirmed an extreme degree of cell diversity by isolating distinctly different cell types from different tumors and from different areas in single tumors (Bigner 1981) (Fig. 25.8). The majority of cells have small dark nuclei ('blue tumors') with scant pink cytoplasm and multiple fibrillary processes containing sucker feet like mature astrocytes. The cells can be bipolar or multipolar, and the nuclei vary in shape and size. Small dark cells resembling lymphocytes are also frequently present and multinucleated giant cells are occasionally seen. Mitotic figures are always present and secondary structures such as pseudopalisading may be observed (Fig. 25.9). Endothelial hyperplasia and intercellular areas of necrosis are two of the principal hallmarks of progressive anaplasia in astrocytoma. A diagnosis of glioblastoma should not be made in the absence of microscopic areas of necrosis and vascular change. Anaplastic astrocytomas or Kernohan grade 3 tumors have increased cell density, frequent mitotic figures and atypical nuclear or cytoplasmic morphology, but lack evidence of intercellular necrosis. Some of the histologic features in astrocytic tumors, such as cell density, nuclear variability, endothelial hyperplasia and necrosis, correlate with the length of survival and are of predictive value (Cohadon et al 1985, Nelson et al 1985).

Special stains are unnecessary to make the diagnosis of glioblastoma except when the tumor is so undifferentiated that no characteristic features can be discerned. Unfortunately, such tumors are also likely to be negative for immunostaining against GFAP and S-100 protein. Glial fibrillary acidic protein (GFAP) is the classic intermediate filament contained within the cytoplasm of astrocytes and astrocytic tumors but it can be absent in highly undifferentiated tumors. Carcinomas and lymphomas are almost always positive for epithelial antigen and other characteristic proteins, while GBM is always negative except for extremely rare examples of collision tumors or

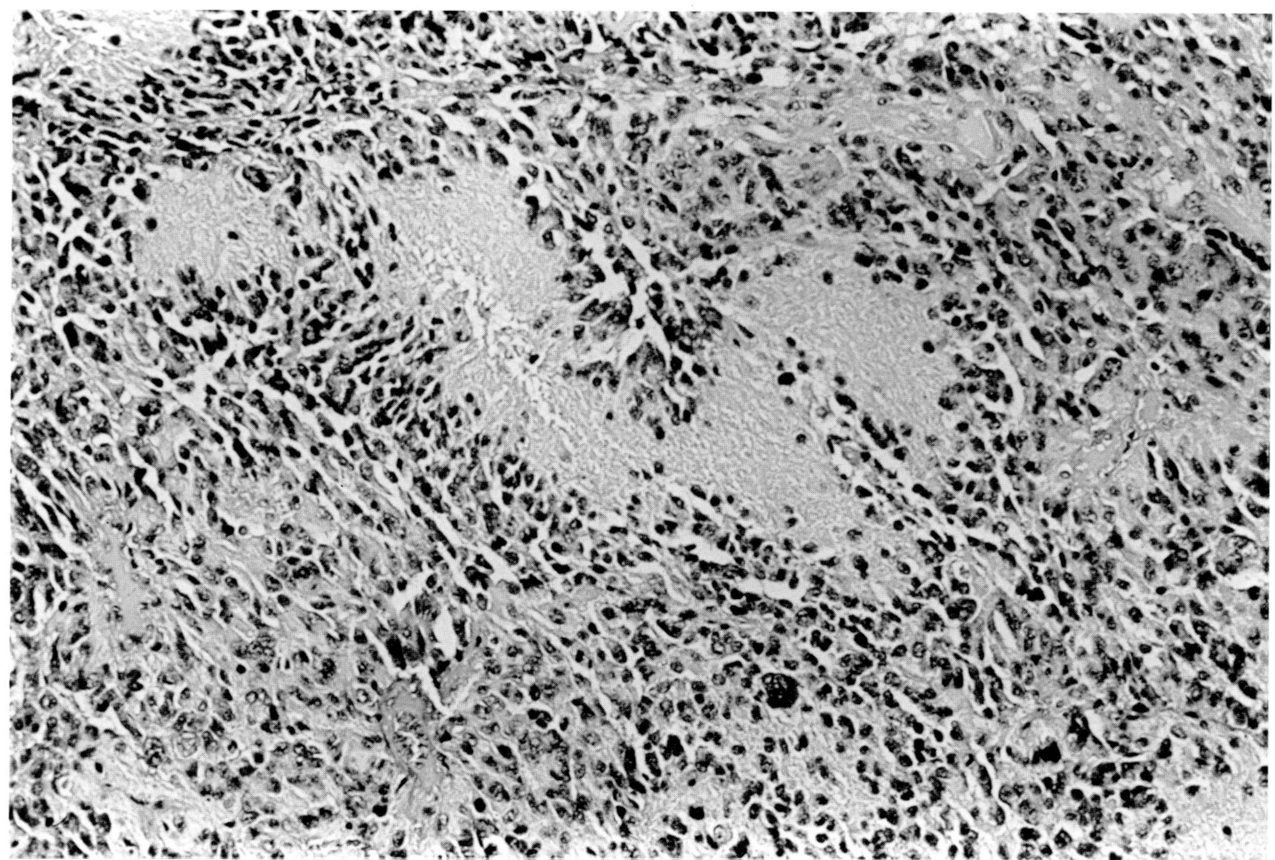

Fig. 25.9 Microphotograph of glioblastoma multiforme. The presence of necrosis is pathognomonic of glioblastoma and serves to separate its histologic appearance from that of anaplastic astrocytoma. Both tumors demonstrate hypercellularity, cellular pleomorphism, atypical nuclei and numerous mitotic figures. Classic pseudopalisading of cell nuclei (as seen here) occurs when tumor cells are arranged in picket-fence formation around a central area of necrosis.

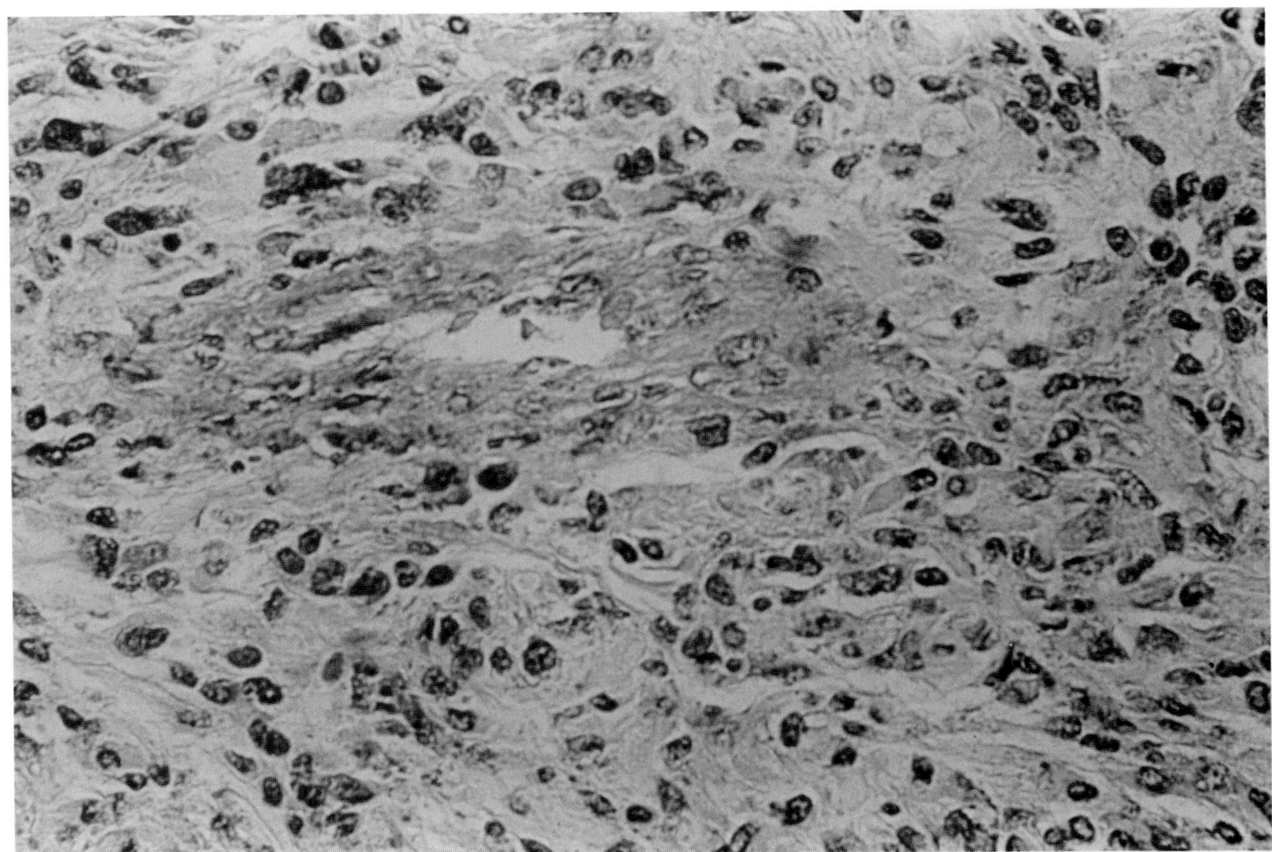

Fig. 25.10 Histopathology of gliosarcoma. Gliosarcoma represents a variant of glioblastoma in which neoplastic transformation of mesenchymal tissue, primarily cells from the capillary endothelium, results in areas of fibrosarcoma and glioblastoma coexisting within single microscopic fields. The plump hyperplastic capillary seen in the center of this figure is frequently observed in malignant astrocytomas of high grade.

metaplasia of a portion of GBM into carcinoma, often the subject of a case report. Gliosarcoma is a more frequent diagnostic problem (Fig. 25.10); reticulin stains and collagen stains often prove useful in delineating areas of fibrosarcomatous change. The sarcomatous portion of the tumor probably arises from mesenchymal cells in the walls of hyperplastic vessels. Some of the growth factors involved in the development and progression of astrocytomas are also powerful inducers of angiogenesis. It is much less likely for an astrocytoma to develop within a pre-existing sarcoma but plausible examples of this sequence also have been demonstrated.

Some of the newest staining techniques provide information in regard to growth rate and tumor kinetics. Silver stains can pick up nucleolar organizer regions (NORs) on both formalin-fixed and paraffin-embedded sections. The NORs represent loops of ribosomal DNA that are present in the nucleoli; these loops contain ribosomal RNA genes that are transcribed by RNA polymerase I (Hara et al 1990). It has been shown that visualization of the argyrophilia depends on active transcription of the genes (Plate et al 1990). Furthermore, the mean number of NORs has been shown to correlate with the histologic grade of astrocytic tumors and with the labeling index (LI) as estimated by immunostaining for the Ki-67 antigen. The latter is a nuclear protein associated with cell proliferation, present throughout all phases of the cell cycle except the G_O phase. Recently, both the AgNOR technique and Ki-67 immunostaining have been successfully applied to smear preparations and frozen sections (Hara et al 1990, Plate et al 1990), thus offering the potential for obtaining kinetic information from stereotactic biopsies. Heretofore, the gold standard for estimating the growth fraction (GF) of intracranial tumors has involved the preoperative injection of bromodeoxyuridine (BUdR), a thymidine analog, and the use of a monoclonal antibody against BUdR on the specimens (Hoshino 1991). Labeling indices defined by Ki-67 are generally somewhat higher than those obtained with BUdR because the latter technique is restricted to S-phase cells. In vitro determination of the LI by anti-BUdR staining has been shown to correlate with patient prognosis and does not involve a preoperative injection; survival and recurrence-free survival for patients with either gliomas or meningiomas was prolonged with

LIs <4% and LIs <1% respectively (Nishizaki et al 1990). Presumably, rapid determination of such data with either Ki-67 or the AgNOR technique would provide similarly useful information.

DEFINITION OF MALIGNANCY

The evolution of neuro-oncology as a special field of study is partially based on the difficulties one encounters in applying the usual criteria of malignancy to most tumors of the central nervous system. The location of a tumor is often more important in determining patient survival than any single combination of histologic features, and the most malignant primary tumors of the neuraxis usually kill by local recurrence without evidence of metastatic spread or cachexia, clinical features commonly associated with systemic cancers. Absent also, is the usual tight correlation between histology, malignancy and metastatic spread. Tumors of the central nervous system are usually defined as malignant by the somewhat circular observation that they almost invariably kill the patient. By any such criteria, anaplastic astrocytoma and glioblastoma multiforme are truly malignant tumors although their clinical behaviour is sufficiently unique that they should not be considered 'cancers' in the commonly accepted sense.

It is also difficult to know when a malignant astrocytoma has been 'cured', another word best avoided in the presence of patients and families beset with this condition. Although measurable 5-year survival rates are now reported, it is not uncommon to have patients whose tumors recur and who die several years after they have been taken off all therapy, the CT or MRI scan remaining negative until shortly before the final recurrence and death. Until quite recently, the 3-year survival rate for glioblastoma was 3% and the 5-year survival rate was zero, a situation quite without parallel to solid malignancies in the lung, pancreas and esophagus (Salcman 1980). Now that a few well-documented patients have lived 10 years or more after histologic diagnosis, often with significant disabilities secondary to the intensity of their treatment, one may still wonder whether 'cure' has been achieved even in these exceptional cases.

As indicated in a previous section, anaplastic astrocytoma and glioblastoma form a histologic continuum with lower grade glial tumors, differing from these more 'benign' lesions by their cell density and pleomorphism. In addition, a malignant astrocytoma may demonstrate endothelial hyperplasia, and glioblastoma is hallmarked by the presence of focal necrosis. Unlike their lower grade brethren, the malignant astrocytomas always recur, sometimes on a regional basis at the original site and often in a more widespread pattern. Since 10% of the tumors reach the cortical surface, spread in the subarachnoid space and into the Virchow-Robin spaces occurs. Subependymal spread is a truly ominous mode of recurrence in young patients after intensive therapy and usually heralds short survival after its radiographic demonstration. The most common pattern of spread is along the path of the deep white matter tracts, especially the corpus callosum (Schiffer 1991). In this manner, astrocytic tumors cross from one hemisphere to the other ('butterfly glioma') in either the rostrum or the splenium. Tumors thought to be multicentric by radiographic criteria are usually discovered to have travelled from one pole to the other of an ipsilateral hemisphere by means of the deep white matter when carefully examined by serial sections. These patterns of spread have been beautifully demonstrated in classic texts of histopathology and have been replicated with experimental tumors in animals (Schiffer 1991). Isolated malignant cells often extend several centimeters beyond the enhancing rim of the tumor and sometimes are found in far distant sites (Burger 1983, Kelly et al 1987). The degree to which a glioblastoma can be considered a localized or regional disease is thereby called into question.

Nevertheless, a number of investigators have demonstrated that the majority of recurrences occur within a 2 cm border of the original lesion (Hochberg & Pruitt 1980), and this fact has been used to support the aggressive application of interstitial brachytherapy, hyperthermia and reoperation in the treatment of these lesions. After conventional radiation, more than 90% of gliomas have been shown to recur at the site of the original tumor (Choucair et al 1986). Such data have resulted in the adoption of smaller treatment fields for use during postoperative external beam radiation therapy. In a series of 42 patients, when focal brain irradiation was restricted to an area within 3 cm of the tumor margin, all recurrences were within 2 cm of the original lesion (Liang et al 1991). Four of the patients also experienced a second recurrent area, 2 of which were outside the 2 cm margin. Whether it is the strictly local recurrence of the tumor that results in the death of the patient remains a moot point in my judgement. If only a few cells invade the hypothalamus or use the U-fibers from the frontal to the temporal lobes to cross the Sylvian fissure, the patient may become functionally doomed despite the fact that the MRI or CT scan indicates a pattern of recurrence that is predominantly local. In truth, there are both regional and more widespread features to the dissemination of glial tumors, and therapeutic plans need to be designed with both aspects in mind.

Metastatic spread of malignant astrocytomas is decidedly unusual and occurs in less than 5% of cases. In 600 cases of supratentorial glioblastoma seen over a 10-year period, only 11 patients (i.e. 2%) with brainstem or spinal cord metastases were identified (Vertosick & Selker 1990). The mean time interval between diagnosis of intracranial disease and diagnosis of metastases was 14.1 months in this series; this finding supports the notion that clinical metastases occur relatively late in the course of glioblastoma and that most patients do not live long enough to develop this complication. The usual route for metastatic spread is by way of the cerebrospinal fluid; patients late in their clinical course may complain of foot drop and pain caused by drop metastases (Fig. 25.11). The clinical incidence of spinal involvement is so low that it does not seem to justify the use of prophylactic craniospinal irradiation as employed in the treatment of medulloblastoma. However, the incidence of meningeal gliomatosis at autopsy can be as high as 21% (Cerame et al 1985). Spread to the viscera is even more uncommon but glioblastoma may go to the lungs, pleura, lymph nodes, bone marrow and liver. Extraneural metastasis has been reported in 0.4–0.5% of patients with neuroectodermal tumors (Smith et al 1969, Schuster et al 1976). Only 2% of such cases appear to occur in the absence of a defense-altering procedure such as craniotomy or shunting; and gliosarcoma is somewhat more likely to exhibit extraneural spread than glioblastoma (Cerame et al 1985). Local dissemination to the subcutaneous tissues of the scalp, face and neck usually occurs only after multiple operations and failure to close the dura. The latter represents a remarkably effective barrier to the local or regional spread of tumors of all types and must be preserved at all costs during the course of surgery. During radiation and chemotherapy, 5% of patients with glioblastoma and 8.6% of patients with anaplastic gliomas develop multiple lesions. In a series of 72 patients with spread of this type, only 15 developed lesions in the spinal cord (1.5%), only one extraneural deposit was documented (0.1%) and more than 90% of the gliomas recurred at the original site (Choucair et al 1986). A summary of the incidence of multiple lesions from various series is given in Table 25.6.

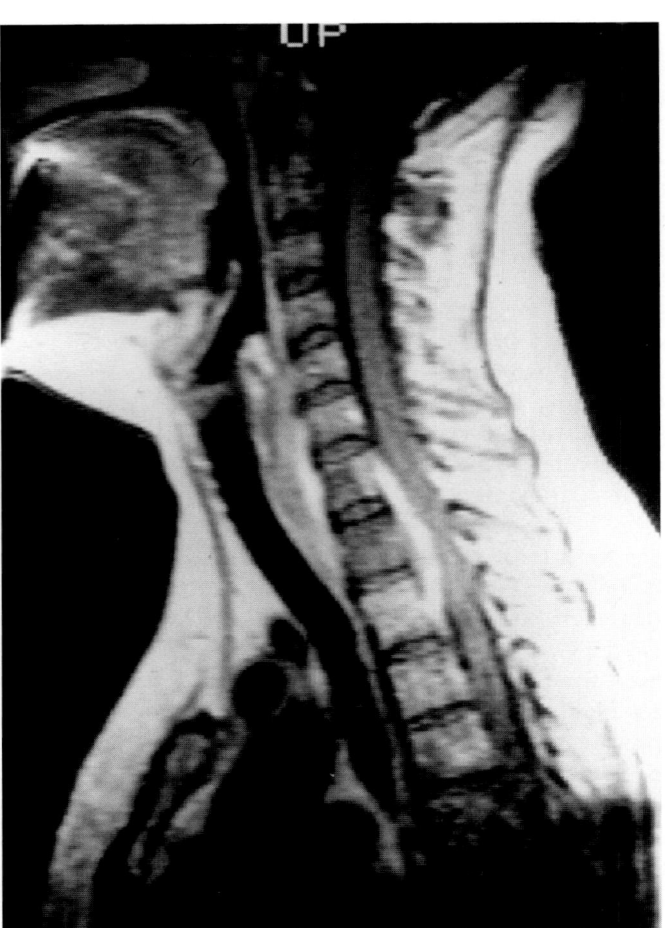

Fig. 25.11 Radiographic appearance of metastatic glioblastoma. Metastatic dissemination of glioblastoma usually occurs within the CSF pathways and can be demonstrated by myelography at spinal levels or by MRI. In this example, an enhancing lesion is present ventral to the spinal cord at C7 through T2.

GENERAL MANAGEMENT PLAN

The diagnosis of brain tumor must be entertained in any adult who presents with personality change, headache, seizures or hemiparesis. The initial diagnostic study should be an enhanced CT or MRI scan and, if a single lesion is detected, with or without a ring-shaped pattern of enhancement, then a diagnosis of malignant astrocytoma or glioblastoma should be assumed until proven otherwise. Except under very unusual circumstances, no patient with an intracranial mass should be subjected to therapy without a definitive histologic diagnosis. The radiographic appearance of malignant astrocytoma can be mimicked by a number of other tumors and non-neoplastic processes including metastatic carcinoma, primary lymphoma, atypical meningioma, bacterial abscess and infarction. Since patients known to have systemic cancer are more likely to develop a second primary than the population at large, a solitary lesion should not be assumed to be metastatic in nature. An image-guided stereotactic biopsy can be carried out under local anesthesia without complication in almost any patient, irrespective of age and general frailty. In general, however, tissue should be obtained at

Table 25.6 The incidence of multiple lesions in malignant glioma. Modified from Choucair et al (1986)

Authors & year	No. cases	Incidence
Courville (1936)		7.8%
Scherer (1940)	120	10%
Manzini & Serra (1952)		7.3%
Moertel et al (1961)	135	4.9%
Batzdorf & Malamud (1963)	209	16.3%
Rubinstein (1976)		10.5%
Hochberg & Pruitt (1980)	127	4%
Choucair et al (1986)	1047	7%
Liang et al (1991)	42	4.7%

craniotomy when a reasonable attempt can be made to perform a radical excision of the lesion.

In most patients with malignant astrocytoma, a craniotomy should be carried out with the goal of removing as much tumor as possible while, at the same time, preserving the structural and functional integrity of the surrounding brain. All adult patients with grade 3 or grade 4 astrocytomas should then be given a course of external radiation to a region rather than to the entire brain. Enhanced CT scans or MRI scans should be obtained in the postoperative period and at one month following the conclusion of radiotherapy to check on the extent of the resection and the radiosensitivity of the tumor. The wide field radiation should be supplemented by either a coned-down external boost to the tumor site or by an interstitial radiation implant. Patients younger than 40 years of age with grade 3 tumors are then followed with regular neurologic evaluations and enhanced scans every 3 months until radiographic recurrence or progression is detected. Young patients with grade 4 lesions may benefit from nitrosourea chemotherapy after the conclusion of radiation if residual tumor is still visible on their post-RT scan. Older patients with glioblastoma are unlikely to respond to conventional chemotherapy and should be entered into therapeutic trials if interstitial brachytherapy up-front fails or if they are not appropriate candidates for this modality at the time of recurrence or progression. Patients should undergo neurologic evaluation and scanning just prior to each course of chemotherapy, and if progression is documented, there is usually no justification for giving another course of the same agent. Reoperation should be considered whenever a major change in the therapeutic plan is entertained or when resection is likely to improve the functional status of the patient (Salcman et al 1982).

Conventional management of patients with malignant astrocytoma, as outlined above, is generally unsatisfactory because a linear or sequential treatment plan cannot deal effectively with the extreme cellular heterogeneity and therapeutic resistance of the tumor. Most solid tumors contain a diversity of cells that differ in their morphology, kinetics, metabolism, vascular access, oxygenation, genetics and antigenic expression (Salcman 1991b). These cell compartments within the tumor may also be assumed to differ in regard to their therapeutic sensitivity to different treatment modalities. In the future, the initial management of patients with glioblastoma is likely to be based on the near-simultaneous application of surgery, radiation and chemotherapy to the central tumor mass in a way that potentiates their individual effects and minimizes cumulative toxicity. More remotely, one can expect that recent advances in molecular biology will result in the use of gene-based therapy, as well as immunological and differentiation agents, for treatment of the cells scattered throughout the surrounding neuropil where the toxic side effects of conventional agents at effective doses are unacceptable (see also Ch. 20).

SURGICAL MANAGEMENT

The surgical management of patients with malignant astrocytoma has evolved tremendously since the original report in 1884 by Bennett & Godlee on the first successful removal of a glial tumor (Bennett & Godlee 1884). Critics and advocates of extensive resection have debated the merits and available data for more than fifty years, frequently without noticing that the framework of their discussion has been in continuous flux. Technological advances in surgery and changes in the availability and efficacy of adjuvant therapy must, of necessity, alter the feasibility and purpose of procedures carried out in a variety of circumstances throughout the patient's clinical course. As previously stated, the general goal should be to remove as much tumor as possible with as little structural or functional disturbance to the brain as necessary. Unlike the lymphomas and leukemias, malignant astrocytoma is a solid and heterogeneous tumor, the optimal treatment of which is likely to resemble that of other solid malignancies such as lung or colon carcinoma. It is generally agreed that survival with systemic cancers is closely linked to the surgical stage of the disease and that when the extent of the surgical resection is not properly considered, the results of randomized trials of radiation and chemotherapy are likely to indicate false benefits where none exist (Gastrointestinal Tumor Study Group 1984). Moreover, this general oncologic principle has been shown to apply to a variety of neuroectodermal tumors along a full spectrum of benign and malignant histologies, including meningioma, medulloblastoma, cerebellar astrocytoma, and gemistocytic astrocytoma (Adegbite et al 1983, Park et al 1983, Hoshino 1984, Laws et al 1984, Mirimanoff et al 1985, Salcman 1990c, Krouwer et al 1991). A randomized trial has recently demonstrated the superiority of results obtained when surgery precedes radiation in the treatment of solitary metastatic carcinoma in the brain (Patchell et al 1990). For a variety of practical and ethical reasons, it is unlikely that a randomized trial on the use of craniotomy in malignant astrocytoma will ever be mounted. However, retrospective data are available on more than 600 patients in the literature who received surgery as their only therapy and whose operations can be classified as a simple biopsy, limited excision or radical removal (Salcman 1985b); as can be seen, the data demonstrate a general association between the length of survival and the extent of resection (Fig. 25.12). Furthermore, when the randomized patients of the Brain Tumor Study Group were stratified according to the amount of residual tumor visible on the postoperative CT scan, a clear association with survival was demonstrated

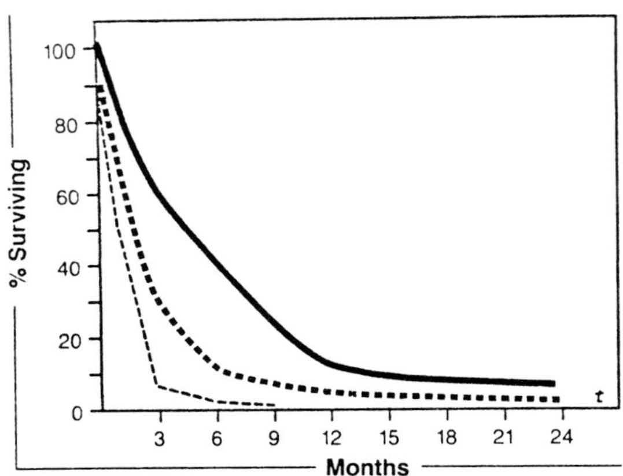

Fig. 25.12 Relation of survival to extent of resection. A retrospective analysis of 603 glioblastoma patients reported in the literature who were treated only with surgery. Prolonged survival appears to be associated with more extensive surgery (solid line, 172 cases). In the absence of radiation and chemotherapy, patients undergoing partial resections (heavy broken line, 301 cases) and simple biopsy (light broken line, 130 cases) did not fare as well. Reprinted with permission from Salcman (1985b).

($p < 0.001$) despite lack of a similar correlation between length of survival and preoperative tumor size (Wood et al 1988). Surgery also has been identified as one of the four most important prognostic variables in a series of randomized trials on postoperative radiation and radiosensitizers (Medical Research Council Brain Tumour Working Party 1990). A number of other prospective and retrospective studies have shown that the extent of surgery is a strong predictor of survival, especially if postoperative scans rather than the surgeon's impression are used to gauge the amount of tumor removed (Andreou et al 1983, Hirakawa et al 1984, Ammirati et al 1987b, Ciric et al 1987).

Extensive resection offers the patient a variety of practical and theoretical advantages over simple biopsy (Table 25.7). Mechanical cytoreduction is the most rapid and effective means known of removing large numbers of cells potentially resistant to radiation or chemotherapy. Surgery is safest in the center of the tumor mass where the cells are metabolically and kinetically quiescent; these cells also have poor vascular access and low oxygen tensions. Furthermore, their removal may alter the cell kinetics of the remaining tumor through a decrease in population pressure, thus inducing the entry of non-cycling cells into active division and increasing their susceptibility to chemotherapy and radiation (Hoshino 1984). Potentiation of nitrosourea chemotherapy by surgery has been demonstrated in the laboratory, as has its beneficial effect on immunotherapy (Brooks & Roszman 1980, Tel et al 1980). The latter may occur through a reduction in tumor burden and mechanical disturbance of the blood-brain barrier (Salcman & Broadwell 1991). It has also been shown that resection almost always maintains or improves the functionality of the patient and produces beneficial metabolic effects even in regions of the brain remote from the operative site (Shapiro 1982, Beaney et al 1985). It is not surprising, therefore, that the quality of survival in glioblastoma patients improves when the postoperative scan has been surgically 'cleared' of all enhancing tumor (Ammirati et al 1987b).

Table 25.7 Rationale for extensive resection in glioma patients

Mechanical cytoreduction can:
provide rapid 2-log cell kill
remove resistant cells
prolong survival
Surgical decompression can:
decrease intracranial hypertension
improve neurologic function
Resection may potentiate or facilitate:
radiation therapy
chemotherapy
immunotherapy
brachytherapy and hyperthermia
Extensive tissue sampling

An even stronger case may exist for the use of reoperation as rescue therapy in patients with recurrent tumors (Young et al 1981, Salcman et al 1982, Ammirati et al 1987a, Harsh et al 1987, Salcman et al 1993a). Three separate clinical series have now documented a median additional survival of 37 weeks from the time of the second operation until either an additional procedure or death (Salcman et al 1982, Ammirati et al 1987a, Harsh et al 1987). Not only is the functional status of the patient maintained or improved but the sharply decreased tumor burden provides optimal conditions for the next treatment (e.g. interstitial brachytherapy, hyperthermia or chemotherapy) to succeed (Fig. 25.13). Reoperation should always be used in the context of other therapies since surgery alone adds only 3 months to the survival of the patient and has no effect on the many tumor cells situated outside the operative field defined by the enhanced scan.

The technical details of glioma excision at initial presentation and at recurrence have been extensively discussed on a number of occasions (Salcman 1985b, Pia 1986, Salcman et al 1986a, Salcman 1990a, Rostomily et al 1991, Salcman 1993) and will not be exhaustively treated in this chapter. Nevertheless, a number of key points should be mentioned. Preoperative planning is just as critical to the success of these procedures as the precision and gentleness with which the operation is carried out. Careful measurements of the tumor along the three major axes should be made and the tumor volume related to the important anatomical structures on every side of it. An approach should be chosen that minimizes the length of the cortical incision as well as the length of the transcortical tunnel through which the operation must be carried out. In general, this means taking the most direct approach possible to the tumor, even in the vicinity of the parietal cortex. Short incisions and deep transcortical

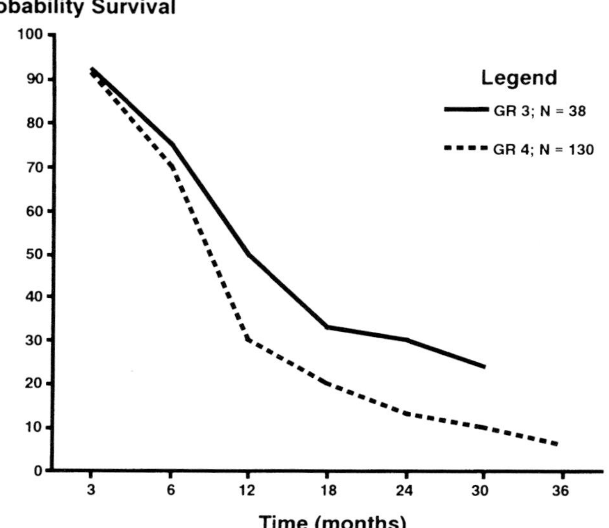

Fig. 25.13 Survival after repeat craniotomy for glioblastoma. These Kaplan-Meier survival curves represent 168 adult patients with malignant astrocytoma and a minimum 3-year follow-up who underwent reoperation. The median additional survival time from the second craniotomy to the next operation or until death was about 9 months in both groups of patients. Salcman et al (1993, unpublished data).

Table 25.8 Morbidity and mortality of craniotomy for glioma

Series & year	Tumor	No. cases	Mortality	Morbidity
Cushing (1932)	Glioma	1173	17.2	
Davis et al (1949)	GBM	187	41.1	
Grant (1956)	Astro	279	20.0	
	GBM	350	38.0	
	Oligo	48	19.0	
Frankel & German (1958)	GBM	183	18.5	
Roth & Elvidge (1960)	GBM	399	21.5	
Ley et al (1962)	Astro	37	16.2	
	GBM	207	31.4	
	Oligo	40	30.0	
Hitchcock & Sato (1964)	GBM	222	19.0	
Jelsma & Bucy (1967)#	GBM	122	27.9	
	GBM	35	2.9	
Leibel et al (1975)	Astro	147	17.0	
Salcman et al (1982)	GBM	74	0.7	
Ammirati et al (1987b)	GBM/AA	31	0.0	16.0 t
Ciric et al (1987)	Glioma	42	0.0	7.0
Fadul et al (1988)	Glioma	104	3.3	19.7
Hollerhage et al (1991)	GBM	118	3.4*	17.0
Salcman et al (1993)@	GBM	509	2.7	8.0
	GBM	220	3.5	8.0

Notes: 1-month mortality rates except as noted (* = 1 week)
#, First series 1948–1961; second is 1962–1964
@, First series is all cases; second is reoperations only; morbidity rates are neurologic except as noted (t = total)
GBM = glioblastoma; Astro = astrocytoma; Oligo = oligodendroglioma; Glioma = all glial tumors

exposures require magnification and illumination; the microscope and self-retaining retractors should be employed whenever possible (Salcman 1985b). Microsurgical techniques can be used to approach the tumor through a sulcus or fissure, thus avoiding a transcortical tunnel altogether (Pia 1986, Salcman 1993). Stereotactically guided craniotomies are more precise than intraoperative ultrasound in locating small tumors in critical anatomical regions, and intraoperative electrophysiologic mapping is more precise in defining eloquent tissue than preoperative estimates based on the MRI scan or superficial landmarks (Rubin & Dohrmann 1983, Moore et al 1989, Berger et al 1990, Salcman 1990a, 1993). The resection should be continued until the dimensions of the resection cavity in every direction match those of the preoperative measurements and edematous white matter is seen glistening on every wall of the tumor bed (Salcman 1985b, 1990a, 1993). These criteria usually bring the surgeon to the outer margin of the enhancing rim of the tumor where a few extra millimeters of tissue can be safely excised with the use of a two-point suction cautery or the carbon dioxide laser (Salcman et al 1986a). The resection should then be halted so as to avoid entering the surrounding brain and the attendant risk of a postoperative deficit. Gentleness in treatment of the superficial tissues is quite important because of the high incidence of wound infections in reoperated patients previously exposed to radiation and chemotherapy (Tenney et al 1985).

The morbidity and mortality of both primary and repeat craniotomies for glioblastoma have steadily dropped since the advent of modern anesthesia, corticosteroids, the operating microscope and CT and MR imaging (Table 25.8). A recent review of our experience with 509 operations carried out in 289 adult patients with malignant astrocytoma indicated a neurologic morbidity rate of 8% and a 2.7% 30-day operative mortality; similar figures were obtained in the subgroup of patients undergoing reoperation (Salcman et al 1993a). Other contemporary series have produced similar results (Ammirati et al 1987b, Ciric et al 1987, Fadul et al 1988). Early morbidity is decreased by the use of microsurgical techniques (Hollerhage et al 1991) and is increased in older patients with deep tumors (Fadul et al 1988). In general, the neurologic condition and performance status of patients with malignant glioma is either improved or stabilized by surgery (Table 25.9).

Under some circumstances, it is neither safe nor advisable to carry out an extensive resection of a malignant astrocytoma (Table 25.10) and an image-guided stereotactic biopsy should be offered to the patient instead.

Table 25.9 Rate of neurologic stability or improvement by type of operation

Series	No.	Incomplete	Complete
Ciric et al (1987)	42	60%	96%
Fadul et al (1988)	138	61–70%	80%
Hollerhage et al (1991)	118	50–91%*	74–77%

*Partial resections with and without lobectomy

Table 25.10 Relative indications for stereotactic surgery

Tumor:	Is centrally located Is poorly defined by CT or MR Is smaller than 2 cm Is primarily cystic Has changed character
Patient:	Is too ill for craniotomy Is neurologically intact
Therapy:	Deliver brachytherapy Interstitial hyperthermia Interstitial phototherapy Stereotactic radiosurgery Requires repeat tissue sampling

Table 25.11 Stereotactic series 1983–1990

Procedure	No.
Biopsy	171
Astrocytoma Gr I & II	24
Astrocytoma Gr III & IV	56
Oligodendroglioma-astro	6
Oligodendroglioma	5
Metastatic carcinoma	9
Lymphoma	5
Other tumors	3
Infections	17
Vascular	8
Gliosis & misc.	27
No diagnosis	11
Tumor cyst drainage	6
Depth electrodes and marking	9
Radiation and hyperthermia implants	55
	241

Stereotactic procedures are extremely safe and can usually be performed with less than a 3% morbidity, a 1% mortality and less than a 3% incidence of hemorrhage (Ostertag et al 1980, Apuzzo et al 1987, Salcman et al 1989, Salcman 1990a). In more than 90% of cases, a correct histopathologic diagnosis is obtained and there is little or no justification at present for exposing any patient to radiation without obtaining a tissue sample first (Taratuto et al 1991). The most important complication of stereotactic procedures is intracerebral hemorrhage. This is seen on less than 3% of all postoperative CT scans and is clinically significant in less than 1% of all patients (Salcman 1990a). When intraoperative bleeding occurs at the mouth of the biopsy cannula, gentle irrigation should be performed across the mouth and not forced down into the cannula. Similarly, resist the temptation to replace the stylet into the catheter since this will only serve to trap the blood within the brain and convert minor bleeding into a major intraparenchymal mass. The Backlund biopsy needle (a spiral instrument resembling a spring) or a side cutting biopsy catheter (Nashold type) usually provide enough tissue for diagnosis and are much less dangerous than grasping or biting forceps. Even in a neuro-oncology service with a strong emphasis on extensive use of open resection, about 20% of all operations carried out for tumor were stereotactic procedures (Salcman 1990; Table 25.11). Stereotactic surgery is especially appropriate for poorly defined or non-enhancing lesions in deep or critical locations in patients who are neurologically intact (see Table 25.10). Even when the majority of targets are located in the brainstem, basal ganglia and thalamus, the morbidity and mortality of stereotactic biopsy is surprisingly low (Ostertag et al 1980). In some patients, a stereotactic biopsy and external radiation can produce results comparable to those achieved by more extensive procedures (Coffey et al 1988).

As previously indicated, image-guided stereotaxy can be used to direct the placement of bone flaps and cortical incisions for open craniotomy (Moore et al 1989, Salcman 1990a). In addition, stereotactic techniques and computer-activated stepping motors have been used to drive carbon dioxide lasers during volumetric resection of intra-axial lesions (Kelly et al 1986, Kelly 1988). Unfortunately, such procedures carried out in the basal ganglia and thalamus failed to prolong the survival of patients with glioblastoma beyond an average of 37 weeks (Kelly et al 1986). A number of robot arms are currently under investigation as intraoperative aids for the excision of small lesions (Watanabe et al 1991) and represent first steps in the development of frameless stereotaxy.

RADIATION THERAPY

As demonstrated by numerous retrospective studies and controlled clinical trials, radiation remains the single most effective treatment for malignant astrocytoma (Andersen 1978, Walker et al 1978, Salcman 1980, Walker et al 1980). The major cellular effect of ionizing radiation consists of damage produced in the DNA helix by electrons and free radicals (Bernstein & Gutin 1981). The free radicals are created through the interaction of X-ray and gamma-ray photons with water or by fast electrons ejected from their orbitals in biological molecules. The ultimate effect of radiation on DNA is to produce single- or double-strand breaks, some of which can be prevented or repaired through the restorative action of endogenous sulfhydryl compounds. Since permanent damage depends on the production of peroxide and the presence of oxygen, sulfhydryl radioprotection is more effective in competing for the available oxygen when oxygen tensions are low. Recent studies have confirmed the presence of significantly lower oxygen tensions in malignant brain tumors ($p < 0.005$) than in surrounding cortex (Kayama et al 1991); this finding is one of the reasons for the relative radioresistance of these neoplasms. The sensitivity of virtually all biologic systems to ionizing radiation is decreased perhaps as much as three-fold in the absence of oxygen (Kinsella & Bloomer 1981). In addition, in vitro testing has demonstrated that some astrocytoma cell lines are inherently more radioresistant than cells from other types of tumors (Gerweck et al 1977). Nevertheless, survival of patients with malignant astrocytoma and glioblastoma from 12 months after diagnosis or into the second year is almost entirely due to the use of radiation (Salcman 1980). Patient survival also correlates with the total dose of radiation used until 70 Gy is reached (Walker et al 1979); at that point, further increases are circumscribed by the toxic effects of radiation on the surrounding brain and its vasculature. In addition to total dose, the incidence of radiation necrosis is a function of the number of fractions employed and the elapsed time of treatment (Sheline et al 1980).

In an analysis of 1561 patients drawn from the literature, each of whom at least had an attempt at a radical excision of their malignant astrocytoma, the median survival of patients undergoing surgery alone was 4 months in comparison to 9.25 months for those receiving radiation as well as excision (Salcman 1980). In a small but early randomized trial, the survival benefit of radiation at 6 months was significant at $p < 0.005$ if early deaths before two months were excluded from both treatment arms (Andersen 1978). There were no 1-year survivors in the non-irradiated group. The value of postoperative radiation was conclusively established by the multicenter randomized trial of the Brain Tumor Study Group during its evaluation of BCNU chemotherapy (Walker et al 1978). The median survival of adequately treated patients receiving surgery alone was 17 weeks in comparison to 37.5 weeks for those undergoing surgery plus radiation ($p < 0.001$); the addition of chemotherapy did not appear to provide prolonged survival. In the randomized trials of the Radiation Therapy Oncology Group (RTOG), increasing the dose of radiation to 7000 rads given over 8–9 weeks did not further increase the length of survival (Chang et al 1983). Clinical experience has taught us that growth of the tumor during the course of radiation is an extremely poor prognostic sign and this effect has recently been quantitated. In a series of 510 patients, the size of the tumor on the post-irradiation scan was related to survival at the $p < 0.00001$ level (Wood et al 1988). Patients whose tumors remained unchanged in size or actually became smaller on comparison of the pre- and post-irradiation scans had much better survival than those patients whose tumors grew during treatment ($p < 0.0001$). Since the mechanism of action and the means of repair for some chemotherapeutic agents is similar to that of ionizing radiation, growth of the tumor during radiotherapy often predicts therapeutic resistance to the nitrosoureas and other alkylating agents.

Not all patients who worsen during the course of radiation do so because of tumor growth. Evaluation of patients in the first 18 weeks after radiation by neurologic examination, CT scanning and glucocorticoid requirements, has revealed that up to 28% show some subsequent improvement (Hoffman et al 1979). This time course is consistent with the subacute effects of radiation on the brain, some of which are reversed by remyelination, repair of the blood-brain barrier and a decrease in interstitial edema (Sheline et al 1980). For this reason, it is important to maintain all patients on adequate doses of glucocorticoids during the course of radiation therapy and especially when the lesion and the radiation field are centered on the diencephalon or brainstem. Prolonged survival of some glioma patients has further emphasized the necessity to decrease the toxicity of treatment so that quality of survival can be maximized, hence the current practice of restricting radiation to a region around the enhancing margin of the tumor rather than using holohemispheric or whole brain fields. At the present time, there is no evidence to indicate that whole brain irradiation confers any additional survival in comparison to regional treatment with suitably generous margins.

Many of the experimental approaches in radiation therapy have been designed to augment the oxygen effect since the radiosensitivity of biologic systems is decreased as much as three-fold in the absence of oxygen (Kinsella & Bloomer 1981). In superfractionation radiation therapy, multiple low dose fractions of radiation are administered each day on the theory that the higher total dose achieved over a shorter time span results in increased tumor reoxygenation, a decreased oxygen enhancement ratio, and decreased tumor repopulation from cells able to repair sublethal injury. Repair of sublethal damage in hypoxic or neoplastic tissue is slower than in normal tissue and should be incomplete from one fraction to the next. In addition, the normal surrounding tissue is relatively protected from radionecrosis by the increased number of fractions, each at a relatively smaller dose. A randomized trial of conventional radiation to 6000 rads over 5 weeks versus superfractionation at 3 doses a day to 5000 rads over 4 weeks did not produce a significant difference in survival (Shin et al 1983). In another randomized study, there was no difference in the 5-year survival rate between patients receiving conventional whole brain irradiation at 200 cGy per day to a total of 4000 cGy prior to a focal boost of 1000 cGy, and a group of patients undergoing 3 fractions a day (76 cGy per fraction) to a total dose of 4760 cGy prior to the focal boost (Ludgate et al 1988). Attempts at using hyperbaric chambers to overcome tissue hypoxia have not been successful (Chang 1977). Certain electron-affinic drugs, such as metronidazole and misonidazole, are capable of sensitizing hypoxic cells to ionizing radiation in all phases of the cell cycle and like oxygen can interfere with molecular repair mechanisms (Gutin et al 1980, Bloom 1982). Unlike oxygen, however, their uptake and metabolism by cells is much slower and they should penetrate more deeply into oxygen-depleted tissue (Gutin et al 1980). Unfortunately, a randomized trial has demonstrated that the survival curves of patients receiving either radiation alone, radiation plus misonidazole or radiation plus metronidazole were identical (Urtasun et al 1982). The dose-limiting factor in the use of these agents has been the incidence of central and peripheral neurotoxicity at higher doses.

Heavy particle beams consisting of neutrons, pi-mesons and heavy ions produce cell-killing by mechanisms that are less dependent on oxygen or the phase of the cell cycle than the less dense ionization produced by conventional photons (Bloom 1982). At small daily fractions, particles are more cytotoxic than photons because cells repair more photon damage than particle damage. However, early clinical trials failed to take into account the relative biologic effectiveness of neutrons on normal brain tissue, and survival did not improve despite apparent sterilization of tumor at autopsy (Laramore et al 1978, Shaw et al 1978). To mitigate the production of degenerative changes in the brain, protocols were designed in which whole brain irradiation was carried out by photons and only the coned-down boost was carried out by neutrons. In a prospective RTOG study, 166 patients with malignant astrocytoma were randomized to receive either a 1500 rad photon boost or the equivalent neutron boost after 5000 rads of conventional whole brain irradiation; there were no statistical differences in the survival curves of the two groups, but autopsy examination continued to reveal the qualitative superiority of neutron sterilization (Griffin et al 1983). It is hoped that further modifications of dose-time relationships and neutron-photon mixes will result in improved survival and tissue tolerance. Alternative means for achieving these aims depend on absolute restriction of the neutron effect to the tumor mass alone. Californium-252 is a fast neutron-emitting isotope that can be afterloaded into interstitial radiation catheters previously placed into residual tumor or into the tumor resection cavity. In the most extensive clinical trial thus far, 56 patients were implanted within two weeks of surgical resection and the catheters were removed after 300 neutron rads had been delivered (Patchell et al 1988). Following removal of the isotope sources, patients received conventional external beam photon irradiation (6000–7000 rads over 5–7 weeks) until a total photon-equivalent dose to the tumor site of 8100–9000 rads was achieved; the median survival time was 10 months, and survival rates at 18 and 24 months were 28% and 19% respectively. These results are not significantly different from those of conventional therapy. On the other hand, it is possible that interstitial californium may provide the solution to the technical problems that have heretofore frustrated the application of boron-neutron capture therapy in the treatment of malignant brain tumors (Hatanaka 1975, Beach et al 1990).

Interstitial brachytherapy has received a great deal of interest because it represents a method by which high doses of radiation can be delivered to the target with relative sparing of the surrounding brain. Continuous low dose irradiation at 40–100 rads per hour over the course of several days allows tumor tissue to reoxygenate and permits more cells to enter active division during the course of therapy. The usual total dose is in the range of 5000–7500 rads (cGY) delivered to the edge of the enhancing tumor or to some point 5–15 mm beyond it. The technique can be used up-front to deliver a focal boost after 4500 rads of regional external radiation in newly diagnosed patients or it can be employed as rescue therapy at the time of recurrence. In a series of 95 patients with malignant astrocytoma implanted with ^{125}I, a median survival of 81 weeks was achieved in grade 3 tumors and a median survival of 54 weeks was observed in grade 4 tumors from the time of recurrence (Leibel et al 1989). In our own experience, 37 patients with malignant astrocytoma implanted with ^{192}Ir achieved a median survival of 34 weeks (Salcman et al 1986b, 1993b). It is safe to say, therefore, that interstitial brachytherapy represents the single most effective rescue therapy presently available for patients with recurrent lesions (Fig. 25.14). Unfortunately, only 20–30% of patients are eligible to receive implantation because of limitations on the size and disposition of the tumor as well as the general condition of the patient (Loeffler et al 1990b). Candidates for brachytherapy must have a relatively good performance status in order to assist with their care in the ICU. The tumor must be unifocal, less than 5 cm in greatest diameter, and susceptible to implantation by relatively few catheters, none of which requires a trajectory through or in the vicin-

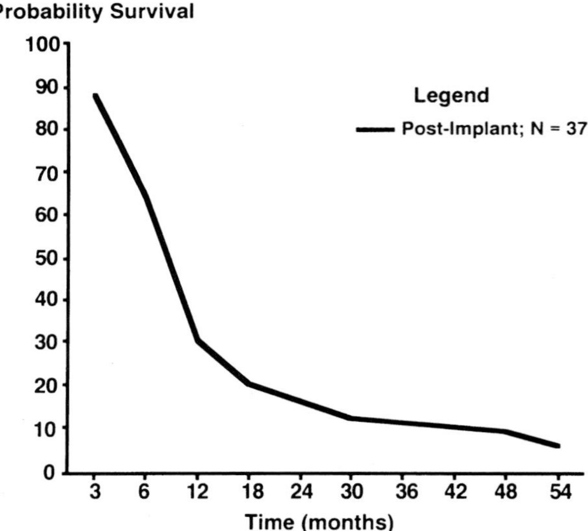

Fig. 25.14 Survival after brachytherapy for recurrent glioblastoma. The Kaplan-Meier survival curve is based on 37 adult patients with malignant astrocytoma who underwent interstitial brachytherapy with ^{192}Ir at recurrence; only 3 patients received concomitant hyperthermia. The median additional survival until the next craniotomy or death was about 9 months. Salcman et al (1993, unpublished data).

ity of a major vessel or other important structure. Thus, candidates for brachytherapy are also the patients most likely to do well after any number of other rescue strategies and are usually younger and healthier than glioblastoma patients in general. Hence, the precise value of brachytherapy needs to be established in a randomized clinical trial (Loeffler et al 1990a, Florell et al 1992). For these reasons among others, the role of brachytherapy in the up-front treatment of malignant gliomas has not as yet been established. Preliminary data indicate a good response among grade 3 patients but no overall improvement in survival for glioblastoma patients (Loeffler et al 1990b, Gutin et al 1991). Stereotactic radiosurgery may prove to be a viable alternative to the use of radiation implants (Coffey et al 1991).

A number of centers are currently investigating methods of further increasing the efficacy of interstitial radiation by combining it with chemotherapy or interstitial hyperthermia (Roberts et al 1985, Salcman 1991a, Sneed et al 1991). Hyperthermia has a direct cell-killing effect on poorly oxygenated, poorly vascularized, non-cycling tissues of the kind that are inherently resistant to radiation (Salcman & Samaras 1981). In vitro studies in both animal and human glioma cell lines have shown that the combination of radiation and hyperthermia is more effective than any other type of combined modality therapy and that addition of BCNU or platinum adds only a modest further increase in cell-killing (Salcman & Ebert 1991). Most clinical trials have employed microwave antennas operating at 2450 or 915 MHz to deliver heat for one hour at 45°C before and after 3–5 days of interstitial brachytherapy (Salcman & Samaras 1983, Roberts et al 1985, Salcman 1991a, Sneed et al 1991). The antennas are usually loaded into the same afterloading catheters used to deliver the radiation, and complications have been few. The data are too preliminary to comment on patient survival. Other centers in Japan and the United States have been investigating the use of implanted Curie-point ferromagnetic seeds to deliver heat through the activation of an external electrical field (Kobayashi et al 1991).

In general, stereotactically guided brachytherapy, with or without concomitant hyperthermia, is well tolerated. From 20–40% of patients implanted with ^{125}I develop radionecrosis to a degree requiring reoperation; it is interesting to note that this group of recurrent patients demonstrates the best response to therapy and the longest survival (Gutin et al 1987). Whether this excellent response is due to the fact that the patient has been taken to the edge of toxicity or whether the patient is responding to the combination of radiation and surgery is unknown. In the dog brain and in tumor model, the area of necrosis surrounding permanently implanted iodine-125 seeds is very sharply delineated (Ostertag et al 1984). The majority of patients with glioblastoma eventually fail brachytherapy, with recurrences at the edge of the treatment field and sometimes more distantly (Loeffler et al 1990a). In a very real sense, the great advantage of brachytherapy is also its greatest limitation: a therapeutic effect that is sharply limited to the treatment field as defined by CT or MR imaging, but one that cannot take into account the many scattered tumor cells just outside the treatment volume.

CHEMOTHERAPY

In the early 1970s, great expectations were raised that chemotherapy would provide the answer to the problem of the malignant glioma but were subsequently unfulfilled. Medical oncologists, buoyed by their recent successes in the treatment of lymphomas and leukemias, ignored the special biological properties of intracranial tumors in the hope that blood-borne agents might effectively treat complex and cellularly diverse lesions within the intracranial cavity. The extreme structural heterogeneity of malignant astrocytoma is only one aspect of its inherent drug resistance. Some tumor cells have the capacity to elaborate DNA repair enzymes and other factors through activation of a multidrug resistance (MDR) gene that confers protection from several agents after exposure to but a single drug (Matsumoto et al 1990). Although some of the problems involved with drug resistance and tumor access might be overcome through extreme elevations in dose, this tactic risks the occurrence of neurotoxicity, yet another important limitation on successful chemotherapy in the nervous system (Kaplan & Wiernik 1982, Salcman & Broadwell 1991).

The introduction of the nitrosoureas remains the earliest and most significant contribution of chemotherapy to the treatment of malignant glioma. In 1970, two groups of investigators simultaneously reported Phase II data indicating the activity of BCNU in patients with recurrent tumors (Walker & Hurwitz 1970, Wilson et al 1970). The 40% response rate achieved with the use of BCNU alone has never been surpassed by any other agent or combination of agents. CCNU and procarbazine are approximately as active and can be given orally but are probably not quite as effective as BCNU when given up-front in an adjuvant mode. Unfortunately, the adjuvant use of BCNU in combination with radiation or shortly after the completion of radiation adds only a modest survival benefit to the patient (Walker et al 1978, 1980). In an extensive analysis of the literature, the median survival of patients with grade 4 tumors after excisional surgery, radiation and chemotherapy was only 10 months, in comparison to the 9.25-month survival obtained after surgery and radiation alone (Salcman 1980). In a prospective randomized trial there was no statistically significant difference between the survival curves with and without BCNU (Walker et al 1980). However, careful attention to the published data indicates that the only measurable long-term (i.e. 24-month) survival rate was in the BCNU arm, in comparison to almost no long-term survivors without BCNU (Walker et al 1980). In a recent analysis of 58 patients alive more than 36 months after tissue diagnosis, almost all had received prolonged nitrosourea chemotherapy, and this helped to differentiate them from short-term survivors at a modest level of significance ($p < 0.02$) (Salcman et al 1993b).

It has been our experience that a clinical or radiographic response to BCNU is much more likely to occur in patients less than 40 years of age and that growth of the tumor during radiotherapy is an almost certain predictor of BCNU failure. Tumor cells from young patients less than 50 years of age exposed in vitro to BCNU appear to be inherently more sensitive than cells grown from older patients (Rosenblum et al 1982). This remarkable finding needs to be replicated and the work extended to other possible factors that might explain the overwhelming importance of age as a prognostic factor in the survival of patients with glioblastoma. In at least one randomized trial, the addition of BCNU (but not methyl-CCNU and DTIC) to surgery and radiation produced increased survival among patients in the 40–60-year age group (Chang et al 1983). Since BCNU acts as an alkylating agent in its attack on nucleic acids, it is understandable that radioresistance might be useful in predicting drug resistance. In vitro techniques for testing the chemosensitivity of tumor cells from patients have proved more valuable in predicting drug resistance than in predicting drug sensitivity (Kornblith et al 1981, Bogdahn 1983, Rosenblum et al 1983).

BCNU is a lipophilic, non-polar, low molecular weight substance that rapidly crosses cell membranes during its first or second pass in the cerebral circulation. Its clinical effectiveness probably has been limited more by the inherent drug resistance of the tumor and the sensitivity of the surrounding brain than by any problem with drug delivery or tumor access. Attempts to improve the response rate through the use of massive systemic doses and autologous bone marrow rescue, or by intracarotid infusion and osmotic opening of the blood-brain barrier have largely failed (Hochberg et al 1981, Neuwelt et al 1983) and have caused considerable toxicity (Mahaley et al 1986). Although intratumoral delivery of nitrosoureas is likely to decrease neurotoxicity, it remains to be seen whether this technique can overcome the inherent resistance of the tumor (Brem et al 1991). Surgery has been shown to potentiate the efficacy of BCNU in animal tumor models (Tel et al 1980), and reoperation is frequently employed prior to the implantation of drug-containing wafers. Recent in vitro data on human glioma cells indicate that there may be real advantages to the simultaneous use of radiation, hyperthermia and chemotherapy (Salcman & Ebert 1991).

For the time being, BCNU should continue to be considered the first drug of choice in the adjuvant treatment of young patients with tumors that have either stayed the same size or have been reduced in size during the course of radiation. The usual starting dose is 80–100 mg/m^2 given intravenously over 1–3 days. In patients with scans that are free of enhancing tumor at the conclusion of radiation, BCNU may be held in reserve and used at recurrence, usually after reoperation. Treatment is repeated every 8–10 weeks after reversal of the thrombocytopenia and low white count that is usually observed by week 4 or 5. An enhanced scan should always be repeated just prior to the next dose and if it shows deterioration (even after just one course), BCNU should be stopped and another agent considered. In addition to bone marrow suppression, cumulative doses of BCNU above 1.2–1.5 g/m^2 expose the patient to the risk of pulmonary toxicity (Aronin et al 1980, Selker et al 1980, O'Driscoll et al 1990). Since this complication of nitrosourea therapy is frequently fatal, it is unfortunately necessary to stop BCNU in most drug-responding patients after 12–18 months even if careful pulmonary testing is carried out on a routine basis. Other complications of BCNU include renal toxicity, neurotoxicity and secondary tumors (Boice et al 1983). Persistent thrombocytopenia or low blood cell counts require downscaling of the dose; BCNU is probably not effective at doses less than 60 mg/m^2 and sometimes has to be stopped because of myelosuppression.

In older patients, alternatives to BCNU need to be considered since there is little evidence to indicate that its adjuvant use is of benefit and relatively few older patients with recurrent tumors respond. After initial surgery and radiation have failed, patients older than 50 years of age with recurrent tumors should be offered reoperation and interstitial brachytherapy, if the lesion is appropriately sized and situated, or reoperation and an experimental drug if the latter is available and the tumor cannot be implanted. In many older patients, physical and social limitations make the use of an oral agent such as procarbazine or CCNU the preferable choice when other alternatives have been considered and rejected. The usual dose of procarbazine is 150 mg/m^2 every 28 days. Some patients with anaplastic astrocytoma (but not glioblastoma) do better with the combination of procarbazine, CCNU and vincristine (PCV) than they do with BCNU alone (Levin et al 1990). A few patients who fail nitrosourea chemotherapy respond to one of the platinum compounds, although this agent is generally more useful in pediatric tumors (Khan et al 1982, Kramer & Packer 1992). Attempts at increasing the efficacy of platinum through intracarotid infusion and blood-brain barrier manipulation have produced tremendous neurotoxicity without comparable improvement in the length of survival. Despite the ability of pharmacologists to custom-design drugs such as spirohydantoin mustard and AZQ that rapidly cross lipid membranes, tumor resistance and neurotoxicity have remained major limiting factors in the development of successful chemotherapy for malignant astrocytoma (Egorin et al 1984, Grossman 1991).

OTHER ADJUNCTIVE THERAPY

Surgery, radiation and nitrosourea chemotherapy are the only established treatments for glioblastoma and anaplastic astrocytoma. Hyperthermia is reaching clinical application in some clinics as an adjunctive modality to interstitial brachytherapy. At the present time, all other types of treatment should be considered experimental and of unproven efficacy. Various forms of immunotherapy have been evaluated in clinical trials and none has succeeded in lengthening survival (Young et al 1991). Attempts to infuse mixtures of activated lymphocytes and biological response modifiers such as interleukin have failed, as have methods for boosting the native immunocompetence of glioma patients. Without a tumor-specific antigen, it has not been possible to develop a monoclonal antibody that is specific for glioblastoma but antibodies have been raised against growth factors and related gene products such as the EGF receptor; the latter technique is currently undergoing clinical trial with radiolabeled antibody (Brady et al 1992). The use of gene therapy or differentiating agents is far in the future although laboratory studies have demonstrated feasibility (see also Ch. 20). Photoactivated chemotherapy has been piloted in patients with recurrent tumors, usually at open craniotomy but most recently via stereotactic techniques (Powers et al 1991). A number of new chemotherapeutic agents are also on the horizon, the most promising of which may be tamoxifen because of its ability to moderate drug resistance (Vertosick et al 1992).

MANAGEMENT OF ASSOCIATED PHENOMENA

Patients with glioblastoma and malignant astrocytoma frequently develop raised intracranial pressure at some time in their clinical course. Unlike the volumetric competition with brain usually observed with extra-axial lesions, an elevated ICP may develop gradually or not at all if normal parenchyma is slowly replaced by an infiltrating tumor. Peritumoral edema increases the effective diameter of the tumor and may precipitate decompensation of the normal intracranial pressure–volume relationship (Salcman 1990d). Corticosteroids remain the most effective agents available for the chronic management of edema and borderline ICP. Unfortunately, some patients are quite sensitive to the side effects of chronic steroid administration and may suffer from altered body image, obesity, psychosis and stress fractures. The general rule is to use the lowest possible dose that remains effective in alleviating headache and drowsiness. Attempts at tapering the patient from steroids may temporarily worsen a hemiparesis or precipitate a neurologic crisis. Sometimes the inability to taper a patient is a strong indication that reoperation and a switch in therapy are necessary. A typical postoperative corticosteroid dose is 4–10 mg of dexamethasone given intravenously or by mouth every 6 hours. The immediate postoperative taper is carried out over 7–10 days until the patient is left on some low dose (0.5–1 mg twice a day) for use during the course of radiotherapy. After several weeks of steroid treatment, the final stages of tapering should be carried out very gradually so as to avoid symptomatic hypoadrenalism. Patients on chronic steroids are more susceptible to infection and may have difficulty healing reoperated incisions. Steroids can also uncover subclinical diabetes mellitus and patients may require active therapy for hyperglycemia. During the final stages of the illness, steroids may be the only means available for keeping the patient alert and functioning within his or her family; the dose can safely be increased until a level of 40–80 mg of dexamethasone a day is reached. Steroids can also be withdrawn as needed in preterminal patients with a depressed level of consciousness.

Acute elevations of ICP are sometimes precipitated by impaired respiration and CO_2 retention or by sudden hemorrhage into the tumor. These situations are best handled in the usual way with hyperventilation, intravenous mannitol (0.5–1.0 gram per kg body weight) and expeditious removal of the tumor, the blood clot or the swollen brain. Mannitol should not be given as a 'push' but dripped in over 20–30 minutes in the dose indicated and then maintained on an hourly basis of 10–20 grams until resolution of the crisis. Unless hydrocephalus is a significant contributor to the problem, CSF drainage should not be employed since it may be difficult to tap the shifted ventricle without further damaging the brain or causing hemorrhage in the tumor. Sometimes drainage of the ventricle contralateral to the tumor further accentuates the degree of shift and precipitates central herniation. Fortunately, relatively few patients with malignant astrocytoma ever suffer from hydrocephalus unless a thalamic tumor causes coaptation of the ventricular walls or widespread intraventricular seeding has occurred from metastatic glioblastoma. In such situations, the practical benefits of ventriculo-peritoneal shunting probably outweigh the theoretical risk of spreading the tumor into the peritoneal cavity. Paraneoplastic syndromes do not occur with malignant gliomas, and the occurrence of myelopathy, neuropathy or pituitary disturbance should always be considered either a complication of therapy or secondary to direct spread of tumor.

PATTERNS OF FAILURE

As indicated in preceding sections, glioblastoma and anaplastic astrocytoma tend to recur locally until the patient succumbs from microscopic invasion or compression of vital centers in the brain. More than 90% of malignant gliomas recur within 2 cm of their original site of presentation after treatment with either regional or interstitial radiation (Hochberg & Pruitt 1980, Choucair et al 1986, Liang et al 1991). Some patients (5–10%) may develop enhancing lesions at some distance from the original tumor, either in the ipsilateral hemisphere or on the opposite side. This is not surprising if one recalls the widespread distribution of scattered malignant cells detected at autopsy and during methodical stereotactic biopsy studies (Burger 1983, Kelly et al 1987). The cells tend to traffic along white matter tracts such as long association pathways and the corpus callosum (Burger 1990, Schiffer 1991). No more than 2% of patients demonstrate clinical seeding within the CSF or outside the central nervous system (Choucair et al 1986). Direct extension of the tumor into the soft tissues of the scalp and face is unusual without preceding craniotomy and incompetence of the dura. Seeding into the CSF usually produces a lumbosacral syndrome of pain and weakness in the lower extremities. This syndrome can be documented by myelography and CT scanning and sometimes can be treated with focal radiation or intrathecal administration of radiolabeled monoclonal antibodies against astrocytoma-related antigens. The incidence of spinal cord involvement at recurrence is about 1.5%, and the incidence of extraneural metastasis is 0.1–0.5% (Choucair et al 1986).

MANAGEMENT OF RECURRENT DISEASE

At the present time, the two most successful management techniques for recurrent astrocytoma are reoperation and interstitial brachytherapy. Several major series all indicate an additional median survival time of 36–37 weeks in patients with malignant astrocytoma and glioblastoma who undergo reoperation in the context of further therapy (Table 25.12). In a recent review of our experience with 220 reoperations in 168 patients, the neurologic morbidity was 8% and the 30-day operative mortality was 3%. Patients with grade 3 tumors did better than those with glioblastoma and, unlike the latter, their response to reoperation was not age dependent. Among our long-term (> 36-month) survivors, representing 20% of 289 patients with a 3-year follow-up, multiple operations were significantly associated with survival ($p < 0.001$) (Salcman et al

Table 25.12 Results of reoperation in malignant astrocytoma

Series/year	No. cases	Median survival (wks)				
		All	*G3*	*G4*	*Morb.*	*Mort.*
Young et al (1981)	24	14				
Salcman et al (1982)	40	37				0.0%
Ammirati et al (1987)	55	36	61	29	18%	1.4%
Harsh et al (1987)	70		88	36	5.7%	4.3%
Salcman (1993)	168	39	52	35	8%	3.5%

1993a,b). In patients with recurrent glioblastoma, interstitial brachytherapy also provides a median additional survival time of about 9 months (Gutin et al 1987, Salcman et al 1993a) (Fig. 25.14). Once again, patients with malignant astrocytoma or grade 3 tumors do considerably better than patients with glioblastoma and sometimes achieve an additional 2 years of survival (Gutin et al 1987). Unfortunately, only 20–30% of patients with recurrent tumors are suitable candidates for brachytherapy based on such criteria as the size and location of the tumor and the condition of the patient. A much wider group of patients can be offered reoperation prior to some form of additional therapy.

Patients less than 40 years of age who have not been previously exposed to chemotherapy should be treated with BCNU after reoperation. Since many young patients have already received this drug, their treatment options are limited to more experimental agents if they are not candidates for brachytherapy. Such patients should be entered into therapeutic trials of Phase I or Phase II investigational drugs, biological response modifiers, monoclonal antibodies to growth factors and receptors, stereotactic radiosurgery and vector-mediated gene therapy (see Ch. 20). Patients older than 40 years of age are less likely to respond to any type of rescue therapy other than reoperation and brachytherapy. BCNU is often withheld from older patients at the time of initial presentation and may be used at recurrence after reoperation. Procarbazine is well-tolerated in older patients and is given orally for 2 weeks alternating with a rest period of similar length. It can be used in patients who have already received BCNU or in older patients who have never received chemotherapy. The biological effectiveness of some drugs can be increased by coadministration with other agents such as tamoxifen or 5FU (Levin et al 1978, Vertosick et al 1992). Tamoxifen may act to partially reverse multidrug resistance. The combination of cyclophosphamide and vincristine has proved useful in some recurrent tumors (Longee et al 1990). Older patients with good performance scores should also be encouraged to enter clinical trials of investigational agents since the likelihood of their responding to conventional drugs at time of recurrence is relatively remote.

For those few patients with metastatic disease, only palliative therapy is available. Intrathecal methotrexate and monoclonal antibodies to neural crest antigens can be injected into the CSF in the hope of treating subarachnoid seeding. More discrete areas of tumor in the spine or in extraneural sites such as bone can be treated with focal radiation. Soft tissue metastases sometimes respond in dramatic fashion to systemic chemotherapy with BCNU and 5FU even when the intracranial tumor has demonstrated relative resistance.

Intracranial patterns of spread that preclude the use of reoperation or brachytherapy are usually associated with a poor prognosis. Spread of the tumor through the corpus callosum and into the opposite frontal lobe or through the posterior forceps from one hemisphere into the other, intraventricular tumor in the thalamus and basal ganglia, as well as subependymal spread within the CSF are all ominous findings on the enhanced MR or CT scan. In such circumstances, only modest expectations from conventional agents should be conveyed to the patient and the family. If entry into a clinical trial is out of the question, then careful consideration should be given to the intensity and location of care-giving during the remaining months of the patient's life. Some patients can be managed for a considerable period of time with high doses of corticosteroids (40 mg/day of dexamethasone or its equivalent) until systemic intolerance to the drug or mental status changes supervene. The goal should always be to maximize the amount of time that the patient can pleasurably interact with the family and to minimize the amount of time spent in an essentially unresponsive state. Such a condition is not only undignified for the patient but also represents a tremendous emotional and financial burden for the family.

RESULTS OF THERAPY

Malignant astrocytoma and glioblastoma multiforme remain among the most difficult tumors to treat in the field of oncology. Until quite recently, the length of survival for patients with glioblastoma was distinctly inferior to the results observed in patients with carcinomas of the lung, esophagus and pancreas. The median survival of glioblastoma patients after conventional surgery and radiation is 37 weeks (Walker et al 1978, Salcman 1980) and is much worse for patients older than 60 years of age (Table 25.13). Prior to 1980, only 10% of patients were alive 18–24 months after diagnosis and virtually no patients were alive 5 years after conventional therapy (Salcman 1980). These figures were obtained from a retrospective analysis of more than 1500 patients in the pre-1980 literature in whom an attempt had been made at radical resection. This survival curve can be compared to one obtained from a similar analysis carried out on more than 1500 cases drawn from the post-1980 literature (Fig. 25.15). These patients all received surgery and conventional radiation in the modern era, and the majority of them were also exposed to investigational agents such as chemotherapy and brachytherapy. Note that the number of long-term survivors at 24–36 months has increased without any significant change in the shape of the survival curve (Salcman 1990b). The upper curve in Figure 25.15 is based on a consecutive unselected series of patients exposed to aggressive multimodality therapy by an interdisciplinary team on our neuro-oncology service in Baltimore. Although measurable 3- and 5-year survival rates are evident, there is still no significant change in the overall shape of the survival curve. Unlike recent survival curves constructed for patients with medulloblastoma and meningioma, there is no shoulder and no tail-like plateau to indicate probability of cure.

In our series of 289 patients with more than 36 months of available follow-up, 58 patients or 20% lived more than 3 years after tissue diagnosis (Salcman et al 1993b). An examination of these long-term survivors indicates a number of prognostic factors common to all astrocytoma

Table 25.13 Therapeutic results of selected major series

Series/year	Treatment	Median S	2-yr	5-yr
Walker et al (1978)	S	17 wks	0	0
	S + BCNU	25	0	—
	S + RT	37.5	1	—
	S + RT + BCNU	40.5	5	—
Walker et al (1980)	S + MeCCNU	24	7.5	—
	S + RT	36	9.7	—
	S + RT + BCNU	51	15.2	—
	S + RT + MeCCNU	42	12.2	—
Green et al (1983)	S + RT + medrol	40		
	S + RT + PBZ	47		
	S + RT + BCNU	50		
Salcman et al (1993)	S + RT	20 m vs 7 m*		
	S + RT + BCNU	26 m vs 11 m		
	S + RT + chemo	24 m vs 16 m		
	S + RT + implant	29 m vs 14 m		

*Medians in months for patients <40 and >40 years of age

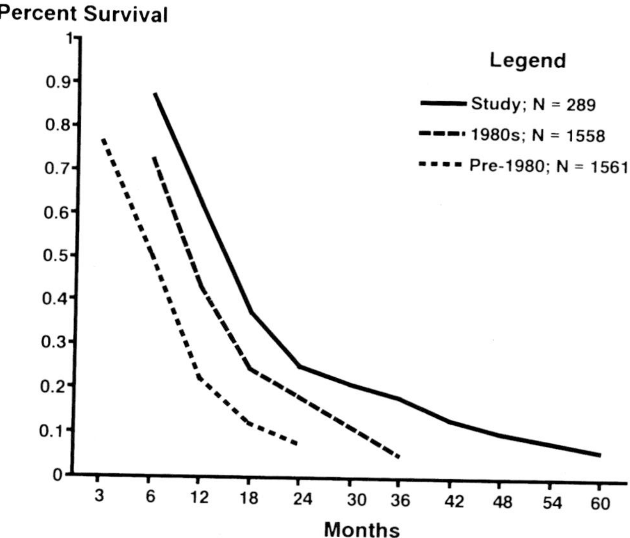

Fig. 25.15 Historical survival curves for patients with glioblastoma multiforme. The bottom curve is a retrospective analysis of 1561 cases of malignant astrocytoma and glioblastoma drawn from the pre-1980 literature; in each patient a radical excision was either achieved or attempted prior to further therapy (see Salcman 1980). The middle curve represents a retrospective analysis of 1558 further cases published from 1980 to 1990 (see Salcman 1990b). The uppermost curve is based on 289 patients with malignant astrocytoma treated in our neuro-oncology service from 1978 to 1988 (Salcman et al, 1993, unpublished data). These curves represent the accumulated experience with more than 3000 cases and may be taken to represent the natural treated history of the disease. Most published survival curves should fall between the upper and lower curves of this figure.

Table 25.14 Prognostic variables for survival in glioblastoma. Modified from Salcman (1990b)

Variable	Significance
Patient:	
Age	$p < 0.0002$ to 0.00001
Sex	NS
Performance preop	$p < 0.001$ to 0.00001
Performance postop	$p < 0.005$
Blood type	NS to $p = 0.05$
Tumor:	
Kernohan grade	NS to $p < 0.00001$
Neovascularity	$p < 0.001$
Necrosis	$p < 0.001$
Lymphocyte infiltration	NS to $p < 0.01$
Therapy:	
Extent of resection	$p < 0.001$ to 0.0001
Post-RT volume	$p < 0.0001$ to 0.00001

patients who do well (Table 25.14). As already noted in this article and demonstrated in the literature, age is the single most important variable in the prognosis of the patient (Salcman 1980, Walker et al 1980). Older patients may be less immunocompetent and their tumors may be inherently more resistant to chemotherapy and other agents. Next to age, the presence of necrosis and the histologic grade of the tumor are the most important prognostic variables (Fig. 25.16, 25.17). In some studies, the performance grade of the patient has also been highly significant (Walker et al 1978, 1980). Positive treatment factors include extensive resection and an adequate dose

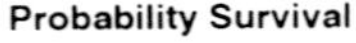

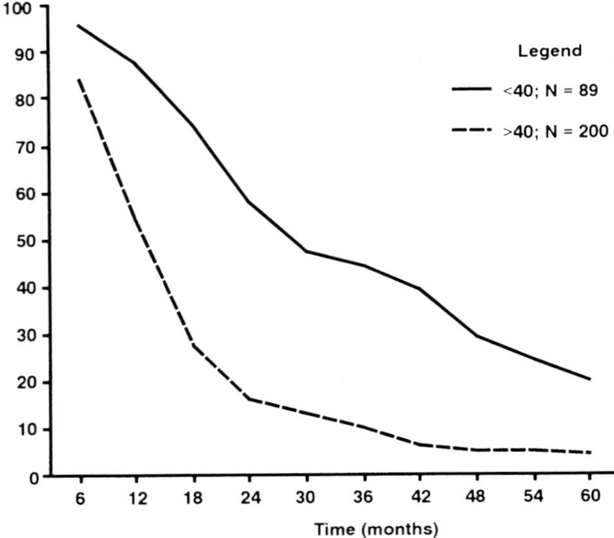

Fig. 25.16 The influence of age on survival in patients with glioblastoma and anaplastic astrocytoma. In 289 patients with a minimum follow-up of 36 months, the length of survival was related to age less than or greater than 40 years at $p < 0.001$. Salcman et al (1993).

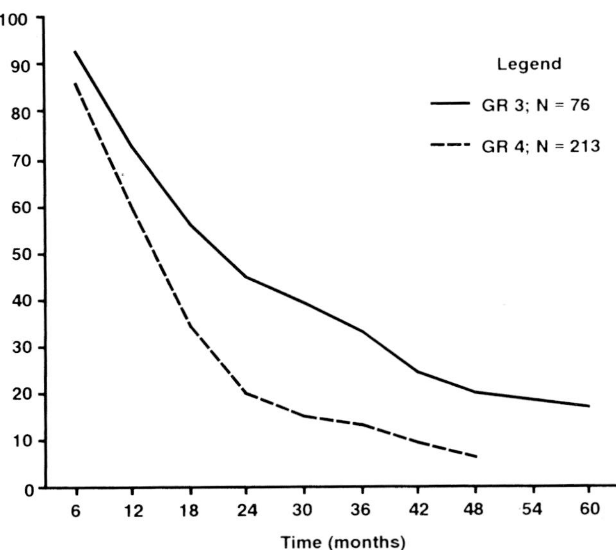

Fig. 25.17 The influence of histology on survival in patients with glioblastoma and anaplastic astrocytoma. In 289 patients with a minimum follow-up of 36 months, the length of survival was related to classification of the tumor as a grade 3 or grade 4 astrocytoma at $p < 0.001$. Salcman et al (1993).

of radiation at or above 6000 cGy (rads). In our series, there was more frequent use of reoperation and more intensive treatment with nitrosourea chemotherapy in long-term survivors than in patients who lived less than 3 years. Conflicting data in the literature on the importance of uncommon histologic features such as lymphocyte invasion and patient characteristics such as blood type have not been supported in recent studies (Salcman 1990b).

Unfortunately, many of the tumor and patient characteristics generally considered favorable are those used to select patients for more aggressive treatments such as interstitial radiation and hyperthermia (Loeffler et al 1990a, Florell et al 1992). Even in radiation and chemotherapy trials, study patients are frequently not representative of all tumor patients; in general, they tend to be younger, have a better performance status and live longer than unselected patients (Winger et al 1989). Given these limitations on the available data, it is advisable to view reported statistics as the outer bounds of what can be achieved under the most favorable circumstances. For example, the 20% 3-year survival rate and 5% incidence of 5-year survivors demonstrated in Figure 25.18 were achieved through aggressive application of multimodality therapy and reoperation by an experienced interdisciplinary team working on a referral population (Salcman et al 1993b). However, even without extraordinary measures, and for no apparent reason, an occasional patient with favorable prognostic variables will tend to do well. A Scandinavian survey of 1147 patients with grade 3 and 4 astrocytomas treated in a variety of clinics revealed 6 pa-

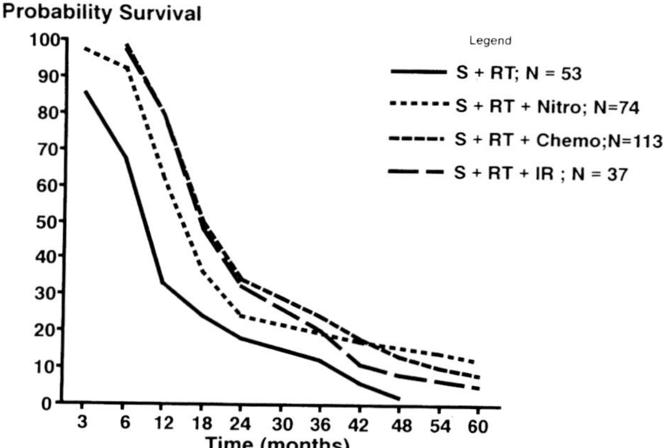

Fig. 25.18 The influence of therapy on survival in patients with glioblastoma and anaplastic astrocytoma. In 289 patients with a minimum follow-up of 36 months, survival in patients less than 40 years of age was unrelated to the type of therapy received beyond surgery and radiation (S + RT; N = 53). Patients were prospectively assigned in a non-random fashion to different experimental protocols. The majority received a nitrosourea in addition to surgery and radiation (S + RT + Nitro; N = 74) while others received experimental chemotherapy or biologic response modifiers in addition to or in place of nitrosoureas (S + RT + Chemo; N = 113). Finally, some patients underwent interstitial brachytherapy at the time of recurrence, usually without concomitant hyperthermia (S + RT + IR; N = 37).

tients in good condition at 12–28 years after surgery for a 10-year survival rate of 0.5%; all of the patients were 38 years of age or less at the time of their first procedure (Salford et al 1988). In the majority of clinical situations, however, it is best to assume that only 10–20% of patients will live 18–24 months after diagnosis of a glioblastoma, and that less than 5% will live 3 years or longer. In children with high grade gliomas, the 5-year survival rate may be as high as 25%, and 10% may live longer than 10 years (Kramer & Packer 1992). The histologic and biologic spectrum of tumors with the same name varies greatly with age at diagnosis, a concern voiced in some of the very first survival studies (Busch & Christensen 1947).

As the number of long-term survivors begins slowly to increase, the quality of survival becomes an issue of equal importance. An early study reviewing the postoperative and postradiation course in 260 patients with gliomas of all types indicated that 12.6% returned to work or full time domestic duty, 53.4% remained at home, where almost half had a major neurologic deficit, and 18.4% were confined to chronic sick beds until time of death (Betty 1964). Almost equal numbers of patients with left and right sided lesions returned to work. Even in the 1950s, reported percentages of glioblastoma patients returning to full or part time work varied between 8.5 and 45% (Frankel & German 1958, Betty 1964). The quality of survival in more than 300 patients with glioblastoma, based on neurologic disability, was good or unchanged in almost 40% and fair (walking and looking after themselves) in another 26% (Roth & Elvidge 1960). Only 19% had severe deficits like hemiplegia and dysphasia but another 14.1% were very severely disabled and in need of terminal nursing care. In a more contemporary series of 74 patients with glioblastoma, all were capable of self-care in the postoperative period and 40% were capable of at least partial employment during chemotherapy (Hochberg et al 1979). Satisfactory levels of function were stable for more than 70% of the average postoperative course of 8 months. The same investigators performed neuropsychologic evaluations on 13 patients who survived more than one year but failed to return to premorbid educational or vocational levels (Hochberg & Slotnick 1980). In the absence of tumor regrowth, these survivors demonstrated diffuse deficits in problem solving and coping with novel situations, deficits that were ascribed to therapy. More recently, in a series of 9 long-term survivors drawn from a total patient population of 160, 30% became demented and 2 others suffered from impaired short-term memory or other neurologic deficits such as gait apraxia (Imperato et al 1990). One 23-year-old patient with glioblastoma died of recurrent tumor 10 years after diagnosis. Based on their experience with malignant astrocytoma, these authors suggested restraint in the application of radiation and chemotherapy to patients with lower grade tumors. However, as indicated above, the long-term functional results in patients with high grade lesions are not always so grim. There is evidence to suggest that function is maintained until shortly before the preterminal period and that once deterioration in ambulation or mental status is observed the end is usually no more than 2–4 months distant. Hence, it is very worthwhile to prolong the survival of patients with malignant astrocytoma since most of the additional time is 'good' time and functional decompensation usually occurs late in the clinical course. The deleterious effects of present forms of therapy cannot be denied, however, and research into more effective means for moderating neurotoxicity may prove almost as important as discovering new methods for further prolonging the survival of our patients.

REFERENCES

Adegbite A B, Khan M I, Paine K W E et al 1983 The recurrence of intracranial meningioma after surgical treatment. Journal of Neurosurgery 58: 51–56

Ammirati M, Galicich J H, Arbit E et al 1987a Reoperation in the treatment of recurrent intracranial malignant gliomas. Neurosurgery 21: 601–614

Ammirati M, Vick N, Liao Y et al 1987b Effect of the extent of surgical resection on survival and quality of life in patients with supratentorial glioblastomas and anaplastic astrocytomas. Neurosurgery 21: 201–206

Andersen A P 1978 Postoperative irradiation of glioblastomas. Results in a randomized series. Acta Radiologica Oncology 17: 475–484

Andreou J, George A E, Wise A et al 1983 CT prognostic criteria of survival after malignant glioma surgery. American Journal of Neuroradiology 4: 488–490
Annegers J F, Schoenberg B S, Okazaki H et al 1981 Epidemiologic study of primary intracranial neoplasms. Archives of Neurology 38: 217–219
Apuzzo M L J, Chandrasoma P T, Cohen D et al 1987 Computed imaging stereotaxy: Experience and perspective related to 500 procedures applied to brain masses. Neurosurgery 20: 930–937
Aronin P A, Mahaley M S, Rudnick S A et al 1980 Prediction of BCNU pulmonary toxicity in patients with malignant gliomas: an assessment of risk factors. New England Journal of Medicine 303: 183–188
Barker D J P, Weller R O, Garfield J S 1976 Epidemiology of primary tumors of the brain and spinal cord: a regional survey in southern England. Journal of Neurology, Neurosurgery and Psychiatry 39: 290–296
Beach J L, Schroy C B, Ashtari et al 1990 Boron neutron capture enhancement of 252Cf brachytherapy. International Journal of Radiation Oncology Biology Physics 18: 1421–1427
Beaney R P, Brooks D J, Leenders K L et al 1985 Blood flow and oxygen utilization in the contralateral cerebral cortex of patients with untreated intracranial tumors as studied by positron emission tomography, with observations on the effect of decompressive surgery. Journal of Neurology, Neurosurgery and Psychiatry 48: 310–319
Bennett H, Godlee R J 1884 Excision of a tumor from the brain. Lancet 2: 1090–1091
Berger M S, Cohen W A, Ojemann G A 1990 Correlation of motor cortex brain mapping data with magnetic resonance imaging. Journal of Neurosurgery 72: 383–3877
Bernstein M, Gutin P H 1981 Interstitial irradiation of brain tumors: a review. Neurosurgery 9: 741–750
Bernstein M, Laperriet N A, Leung P et al 1990 Interstitial brachytherapy for malignant brain tumors: preliminary results. Neurosurgery 26: 371–380
Betty M J 1964 Quality of survival in treated patients with supratentorial gliomata. Journal of Neurology, Neurosurgery and Psychiatry 27: 556–561
Bigner D D 1981 Biology of gliomas: potential clinical implications of glioma cellular heterogeneity. Neurosurgery 9: 320–326
Bloom H J G 1982 Intracranial tumors: Response and resistance to therapeutic endeavors, 1970–1980. International Journal of Radiation Oncology Biology Physics 8: 1083–1113
Bogdahn U 1983 Chemosensitivity of malignant human brain tumors. Preliminary results. Journal of Neuro-Oncology 1: 149–166
Boice J D, Greene M H, Killen J Y et al 1983 Leukemia and preleukemia after adjuvant treatment of gastrointestinal cancer with semustine (methyl-CCNU). New England Journal of Medicine 309: 1079–1084
Brady L W, Miyamoto C, Woo D et al 1992 Malignant astrocytomas treated with iodine-125 labeled monoclonal antibody against epidermal growth factor receptor: a phase II trial. International Journal of Radiation Oncology Biology Physics 22: 225–230
Bramwell B 1888 Intracranial tumours. Pentland, Edinburgh, p 222
Brem H, Mahaley S, Vick N et al 1991 Interstitial chemotherapy with drug polymer implants for the treatment of recurrent gliomas. Journal of Neurosurgery 74: 441–446
Brooks W H, Roszman T L 1980 Cellular immune responsiveness of patients with primary intracranial tumors. In: Thomas D G T, Graham D I (eds) Brain tumors: Scientific basis, clinical investigation, and current therapy. Butterworth, London, pp 121–132
Burger P C 1983 Pathologic anatomy and CT correlations in the glioblastoma multiforme. Applied Neurophysiology 46: 180–187
Burger P C 1990 Classification, grading, and patterns of spread of malignant gliomas. In: Apuzzo M L J (ed) Malignant cerebral glioma. American Association of Neurological Surgeons, Park Ridge, pp 3–17
Busch E, Christensen E 1947 The three types of glioblastoma. Journal of Neurosurgery 4: 200–220
Cerame M A, Guthikonda M, Kohli C M 1985 Extraneural metastases in gliosarcoma. A case report and review of the literature. Neurosurgery 17: 413–418
Chang C H 1977 Hyperbaric oxygen and radiation therapy in the management of glioblastoma. National Cancer Institute Monograph 46: 163–169
Chang C H, Horton J, Schoenfeld D et al 1983 Comparison of postoperative radiotherapy and combined postoperative radiotherapy and chemotherapy in the multidisciplinary management of malignant gliomas. A Joint Radiation Therapy Oncology Group and Eastern Cooperative Oncology Group Study. Cancer 52: 997–1007
Cheng M K 1982 Brain tumor in the People's Republic of China: a statistical review. Neurosurgery 10: 16–21
Choucair A K, Levin V A, Gutin P H et al 1986 Development of multiple lesions during radiation therapy and chemotherapy in patients with gliomas. Journal of Neurosurgery 65: 654–658
Ciric I, Ammirati M, Vick N et al 1987 Supratentorial gliomas: Surgical considerations and immediate postoperative results. Gross total resection versus partial resection. Neurosurgery 21: 21–26
Coffey R J, Lunsford L D, Taylor F H 1988 Survival after stereotactic biopsy of malignant gliomas. Neurosurgery 22: 465–473
Coffey R J, Lunsford D, Flinkinger J C 1991 The role of radiosurgery in the treatment of malignant brain tumors. Neurosurgery Clinics of North America 3(1): 231–244
Cohadon F, Aouad N, Rougier A et al 1985 Histologic and non-histologic factors correlated with survival time in supratentorial astrocytic tumors. Journal of Neuro-Oncology 3: 105–111
Cohen A, Modan B 1968 Some epidemiologic aspects of neoplastic diseases in Israeli immigrant population. III. Brain tumors. Cancer 22: 1323–1328
Davis D L, Hoel D, Fox J et al 1990 International trends in cancer mortality in France, West Germany, Italy, Japan, England and Wales, and the USA. Lancet 336: 474–481
Desmeules M, Mikkelsen T, Mao Y 1992 Increasing incidence of primary malignant brain tumors: influence of diagnostic methods. Journal of the National Cancer Institute 84: 442–445
Egorin M J, Bellis E H, Salcman M et al 1984 The pharmacology of diaziquone given by intravenous or intracarotid infusion to normal and intracranial tumor bearing puppies. Journal of Neurosurgery 60: 1005–1013
El-Azouzi M, Chung R Y, Farmer G E et al 1989 Loss of distinct regions on the short arm of chromosome 17 associated with tumorigenesis of human astrocytomas. Proceedings of the National Academy of Sciences of the USA 86: 7186–7190
Fadul C, Wood J, Thaler H et al 1988 Morbidity and mortality of craniotomy for excision of supratentorial gliomas. Neurology 38: 1374–1379
Florell R C, MacDonald D R, Irish W D et al 1992 Selection bias, survival and brachytherapy for glioma. Journal of Neurosurgery 76: 179–183
Frankel S A, German W J 1958 Glioblastoma multiforme: Review of 219 cases with regard to natural history, pathology, diagnostic methods and treatment. Journal of Neurosurgery 15: 489–503
Gastrointestinal Tumor Study Group 1984 Adjuvant therapy of colon cancer: Results of a prospectively randomized trial. New England Journal of Medicine 310: 737–743
Gerweck L E, Kornblith P L, Burlett P et al 1977 Radiation sensitivity of cultured human glioblastoma cells. Radiology 125: 231–241
Green S B, Byar D P, Walker M D et al 1983 Comparisons of carmustine, procarbazine, and high-dose methylprednisolone as additions to surgery and radiotherapy for the treatment of malignant glioma. Cancer Treatment Report 67: 121–132
Greig N H, Ries L G, Yancik R et al 1990 Increasing annual incidence of primary malignant brain tumors in the elderly. Journal of the National Cancer Institute 82: 1621–1624
Griffin T W, Davis R, Larramore G et al 1983 Fast neutron radiation therapy for glioblastoma multiforme: Results of an RTOG study. American Journal of Clinical Oncology (CCT) 6: 661–667
Grossman S A 1991 Chemotherapy of brain tumors. In: Salcman M (ed) Neurobiology of brain tumors. Williams & Wilkins, Baltimore, pp 321–340
Gutin P H, Wara W M, Phillips T L et al 1980 Hypoxic cell radiosensitizers in the treatment of malignant brain tumors. Neurosurgery 6: 567–576
Gutin P H, Leibel S A, Wara W M et al 1987 Recurrent malignant

gliomas: Survival following interstitial brachytherapy with high-activity iodine-125 sources. Journal of Neurosurgery 67: 864–973

Gutin P H, Prados M D, Phillips T L et al 1991 External irradiation followed by an interstitial high-activity iodine-125 implant "boost" in the initial treatment of malignant gliomas: NCOG study 6G-82-2. International Journal of Radiation Oncology Biology Physics 21: 601–606

Hara A, Hirayama H, Sakai N et al 1990 Correlation between nucleolar organizer region staining and Ki-67 immunostaining in human gliomas. Surgical Neurology 33: 320–324

Harsh G R IV, Levin V A, Gutin P H et al 1987 Reoperation for recurrent glioblastoma and anaplastic astrocytoma. Neurosurgery 21: 615–621

Hatanaka H 1975 A revised boron-neutron capture theory for malignant brain tumors. II. Interim clinical results with the patients excluding previous treatments. Journal of Neurology 209: 81–94

Hermansson M, Nister M, Betsholtz C et al 1988 Endothelial cell hyperplasia in human glioblastoma: coexpression of mRNA for platelet-derived growth factor (PDGF) B chain and PDGF receptor suggests autocrine growth stimulation. Proceedings of the National Academy of Sciences of the USA 85: 7748–7752

Hirakawa K, Suzuki K, Ueda S et al 1984 Multivariate analysis of factors affecting postoperative survival in malignant astrocytoma. Journal of Neuro-Oncology 2: 331–340

Hitchcock E, Sato F 1964 Treatment of malignant gliomata. Journal of Neurosurgery 21: 497–505

Hochberg F H, Pruitt A 1980 Assumptions in the radiotherapy of glioblastoma. Neurology 30: 907–911

Hochberg F H, Slotnick B 1980 Neuropsychologic impairment in astrocytoma survivors. Neurology 30: 172–177

Hochberg F H, Linggood R, Wolfson L et al 1979 Quality and duration of survival in glioblastoma multiforme. Combined surgical, radiation, and lomustine therapy. Journal of the American Medical Association 241: 1016–1018

Hochberg F H, Parker L M, Takvorian T et al 1981 High-dose BCNU with autologous bone marrow rescue for recurrent glioblastoma multiforme. Journal of Neurosurgery 54: 455–460

Hoffman W F, Levin V A, Wilson C B 1979 Evaluation of malignant glioma patients during the postirradiation period. Journal of Neurosurgery 50: 624–628

Hollerhage H-G, Zumkeller M, Becker M et al 1991 Influence of type and extent of surgery on early results and survival time in glioblastoma multiforme. Acta Neurochirurgica (Wien) 113: 31–37

Hoshino T 1984 A commentary on the biology and growth kinetics of low grade and high grade gliomas. Journal of Neurosurgery 61: 895–900

Hoshino T 1991 Cell kinetics of brain tumors. In: Salcman M (ed) Neurobiology of brain tumors. Williams & Wilkins, Baltimore, pp 145–159

Imperato J P, Paleologos N A, Vick N A 1990 Effects of treatment on long-term survivors with malignant astrocytomas. Annals of Neurology 28: 818–822

James C D, Carlbom E, Dumanski J P et al 1988 Clonal genomic alterations in glioma malignancy stages. Cancer Research 48: 5546–5551

James C D, Carlbom E, Nordenskjold et al 1989 Mitotic recombination of chromosome 17 in astrocytomas. Proceedings of the National Academy of Sciences of the USA 86: 2858–2862

Jelsma R, Bucy P C 1967 The treatment of glioblastoma multiforme of the brain. Journal of Neurosurgery 27: 388–400

Kanno H, Kawabara T, Yasumitsu H et al 1988 Transforming growth factors in urine from patients with primary brain tumors. Journal of Neurosurgery 68: 775–780

Kaplan R S, Weirnik P H 1982 Neurotoxicity of antineoplastic drugs. Seminars in Oncology 9: 103–130

Kayama T, Yoshimoto T, Fujimoto S et al 1991 Intratumoral oxygen pressure in malignant brain tumor. Journal of Neurosurgery 74: 55–59

Kelly P J 1988 Volumetric stereotactic surgical resection of intra-axial brain mass lesions. Mayo Clinic Proceedings 63: 1186–1198

Kelly P J, Kall B A, Goerss S et al 1986 Computer-assisted stereotaxic laser resection of intra-axial brain neoplasms. Journal of Neurosurgery 64: 427–439

Kelly P J, Daumas-Duport C, Kispert D B et al 1987 Imaging-based stereotaxic serial biopsies in untreated intracranial glial neoplasms. Journal of Neurosurgery 66: 865–874

Khan A B, D'Souza B J, Wharam M D et al 1982 Cisplatin therapy in recurrent childhood brain tumors. Cancer Treatment Report 66: 2013–2020

Kinsella T J, Bloomer W D 1981 New therapeutic strategies in radiation therapy. Journal of the American Medical Association 245: 1669–1674

Kobayashi T, Kida Y, Tanaka T et al 1991 Interstitial hyperthermia of malignant brain tumors by implant heating system: clinical experience. Journal of Neuro-Oncology 10: 153–163

Kornblith P L, Smith B H, Leonard L A 1981 Response of cultured human brain tumors to nitrosoureas: Correlation with clinical data. Cancer 47: 255–265

Kramer E D, Packer R J 1992 Chemotherapy of malignant brain tumors in children. Clinical Neuropharmacology 15: 163–185

Krouwer H G J, Davis R L, Silver P et al 1991 Gemistocytic astrocytomas: a reappraisal. Journal of Neurosurgery 74: 399–406

Laramore G E, Griffin T W, Gerdes A J et al 1978 Fast neutron and mixed (neutron/photon) beam teletherapy for grades III and IV astrocytomas. Cancer 42: 96–103

Laws E R, Taylor W F, Clifton M B et al 1984 Neurosurgical management of low grade astrocytoma of the cerebral hemispheres. Journal of Neurosurgery 61: 665–673

Leibel S A, Gutin P H, Wara W M et al 1989 Survival and quality of life after interstitial implantation of removable high-activity iodine-125 sources for the treatment of patients with recurrent malignant gliomas. International Journal of Radiation Oncology Biology Physics 17: 1129–1139

Levin V A, Hoffman W F, Pischer T L et al 1978 BCNU-5-fluorouracil combination therapy for recurrent malignant brain tumors. Cancer Treatment Report 62: 2071–2076

Levin V A, Silver P, Hannigan J et al 1990 Superiority of post-radiotherapy adjuvant chemotherapy with CCNU, procarbazine, and vincristine (PCV) over BCNU for anaplastic gliomas: NCOG 6G61 final report. International Journal of Radiation Oncology Biology Physics 18: 321–324

Li F P, Fraumeni J F 1982 Prospective study of a family cancer syndrome. Journal of the American Medical Association 247: 2692–2694

Liang B C, Thornton A F, Sandler H M et al 1991 Malignant astrocytomas: focal tumor recurrence after focal external beam radiation therapy. Journal of Neurosurgery 75: 559–563

Libermann T A, Nusbaum H R, Razon N et al 1985 Amplification, enhanced expression and possible rearrangement of EGF receptor gene in primary human brain tumors of glial origin. Nature 313: 144–147

Loeffler J S, Alexander E III, Hochberg F H et al 1990a Clinical patterns of failure following stereotactic interstitial irradiation for malignant gliomas. International Journal of Radiation Oncology Biology Physics 19: 1455–1462

Loeffler J S, Alexander E III, Wen P Y et al 1990b Results of stereotactic brachytherapy used in the initial management of patients with glioblastoma. Journal of the National Cancer Institute 82: 1918–1921

Longee D C, Friedman H S, Albright R E et al 1990 Treatment of patients with recurrent gliomas with cyclophosphamide and vincristine. Journal of Neurosurgery 72: 583–588

Ludgate C M, Douglas B G, Dixon P F et al 1988 Superfractionated radiotherapy in grade III, IV intracranial gliomas. International Journal of Radiation Oncology Biology Physics 15: 1091–1095

Lynch H T, Krush A J, Harlan W L et al 1973 Association of soft tissue sarcoma, leukemia, and brain tumors in families affected with breast cancer. Am. Surg. 39: 199–206

McKeran R O, Thomas D G T 1980 The clinical study of gliomas. In: Thomas D G T, Graham D I (eds) Brain tumors: scientific basis, clinical investigation, and current therapy. Butterworth, London, pp 194–230

Mahaley M S, Whaley R A, Blue M et al 1986 Central neurotoxicity following intracarotid BCNU chemotherapy for malignant gliomas. Journal of Neuro-Oncology 3: 297–314

Mahaley M S, Mettlin C, Natarajan et al 1989 National survey of

patterns of care for brain-tumor patients. Journal of Neurosurgery 71: 826–836
Mao Y, Desmeules M R, Semenciw R et al 1991 Increasing brain cancer rates in Canada. Canadian Medical Association Journal 145: 1583–1591
Matsumoto T, Tani E, Kaba K et al 1990 Amplification and expression of a multidrug resistance gene in human glioma cell lines. Journal of Neurosurgery 72: 96–100
Maxwell M, Naber S P, Wolfe H J et al 1990 Coexpression of platelet derived growth factor (PDGF) and PDGF-receptor genes by primary human astrocytomas may contribute to their development and maintenance. Journal of Clinical Investigation 86: 131–40
Medical Research Council Brain Tumor Working Party 1990 Prognostic factors for high-grade malignant glioma: development of a prognostic index. Journal of Neuro-Oncology 9: 47–55
Mirimanoff R O, Dosoretz D E, Linggood R M et al 1985 Meningioma: Analysis of recurrence and progression following neurosurgical resection. Journal of Neurosurgery 62: 18–24
Moore M R, Black P McL, Ellenbogen R et al 1989 Stereotactic craniotomy: methods and results using the Brown-Roberts-Wells stereotactic frame. Neurosurgery 25: 572–578
Muller W, Afra D, Schroder R 1977 Supratentorial recurrences of gliomas: morphological studies in relation to time intervals with astrocytomas. Acta Neurochirurgica 37: 75–91
Nelson D F, Nelson J S, Davis D R et al 1985 Survival and prognosis of patients with astrocytoma with atypical or anaplastic features. Journal of Neuro-Oncology 3: 99–103
Neuwelt E A, Frenkel E P, Diehl J et al 1983 Reversible osmotic blood-brain barrier disruption in humans: implications for the chemotherapy of malignant brain tumors. Neurosurgery 12: 662–671
Nishizaki T, Orita T, Kajiwara K et al 1990 Correlation of in vitro bromodeoxyuridine labeling index and DNA aneuploidy with survival or recurrence in brain tumor patients. Journal of Neurosurgery 73: 396–400
O'Driscoll B R, Hasleton P S, Taylor P M et al 1990 Active lung fibrosis up to 17 years after chemotherapy with carmustine (BCNU) in childhood. New England Journal of Medicine 323: 378–382
Ohaegbula S C, Saddeqi N, Ikerionwu S 1980 Intracranial tumors in Enugu, Nigeria. Cancer 46: 2322–2324
Ostertag C B, Mennel H D, Kiessling M 1980 Stereotactic biopsy of brain tumors. Surgical Neurology 14: 275–283
Ostertag C B, Groothuis D, Kleihues P 1984 Experimental data on early and late morphologic effects of permanently implanted gamma and beta sources (iridium-192, iodine-125 and yttrium-90) in the brain. Acta Neurochirurgica (suppl) 33: 271–280
Park T S, Hoffman H J, Hendrick E B et al 1983 Medulloblastoma: Clinical presentation and management: Experience at the Hospital for Sick Children, Toronto, 1950–1980. Journal of Neurosurgery 58: 543–552
Patchell R A, Maruyama Y, Tibbs P A et al 1988 Neutron interstitial brachytherapy for malignant gliomas: a pilot study. Journal of Neurosurgery 68: 67–72
Patchell R A, Tibbs P A, Walsh J W et al 1990 A randomized trial of surgery in the treatment of single metastases to the brain. New England Journal of Medicine 322: 494–499
Pia H W 1986 Microsurgery of gliomas. Acta Neurochirurgica 80: 1–11
Plate K H, Ruschoff J, Behnke J et al 1990 Proliferative potential of human brain tumours as assessed by nucleolar organizer regions (AgNORs) and Ki-67-immunoreactivity. Acta Neurochirurgica 104: 103–109
Pollack I F, Randall M S, Kristofik M P et al 1990 Response of malignant glioma cell lines to epidermal growth factor and platelet-derived growth factor in a serum-free medium. Journal of Neurosurgery 73: 106–112
Powers S K, Cush S S, Walstad D L et al 1991 Stereotactic intratumoral photodynamic therapy for recurrent malignant brain tumors. Neurosurgery 29: 688–696
Roberts D W, Coughlin C T, Wong T Z et al 1985 Interstitial hyperthermia and iridium brachytherapy in treatment of malignant glioma: a phase I clinical trial. Journal of Neurosurgery 64: 581–587
Rosenblum M L, Dougherty D V, Barger G R et al 1982 Age-related chemosensitivity of stem cells from human malignant brain tumors. Lancet 1: 885–887
Rosenblum M L, Gerosa M A, Wilson C B et al 1983 Stem cell studies of human malignant brain tumors. Part I: development of the stem cell assay and its potential. Journal of Neurosurgery 58: 170–176
Rostomily R C, Berger M S, Ojemann G A et al 1991 Postoperative deficits and functional recovery following removal of tumors involving the dominant hemisphere supplementary motor area. Journal of Neurosurgery 75: 62–68
Roth J G, Elvidge A R 1960 Glioblastoma multiforme: a clinical survey. Journal of Neurosurgery 17: 736–750
Rubin J M, Dohrmann G 1983 Intraoperative neurosurgical ultrasound in the localization and characterization of intracranial masses. Radiology 148: 519–524
Rubinstein L J 1991 Glioma cytogeny and differentiation viewed through the window of neoplastic vulnerability. In: Salcman M (ed) Neurobiology of brain tumors. Williams & Wilkins, Baltimore, pp 35–52
Salcman M 1980 Survival in glioblastoma: Historical perspective. Neurosurgery 7: 435–439
Salcman M 1985a The morbidity and mortality of brain tumors: A perspective on recent advances in therapy. Neurol Clin 3: 1–29
Salcman M 1985b Supratentorial gliomas: Clinical features and surgical therapy. In: Wilkins R H, Rengachary S S (eds) Neurosurgery. McGraw-Hill, New York, pp 550–579
Salcman M 1985c Resection and reoperation in neuro-oncology. Rationale and approach. Neurol Clin 3: 831–842
Salcman M 1988 The role of surgical resection in the treatment of malignant brain tumors: Who benefits? Oncology 2: 47–59
Salcman M 1990a Malignant glioma management. Neurosurgery Clinics of North America 1: 49–63
Salcman M 1990b Epidemiology and factors affecting survival. In: Apuzzo M L J (ed) Malignant cerebral glioma. American Association of Neurological Surgeons, Park Ridge, Illionois, pp 95–109
Salcman M 1990c Radical surgery for low-grade glioma. Clinical Neurosurgery 36: 353–366
Salcman M 1990d The unconscious patient. In: Salcman M (ed) Neurologic emergencies, recognition and management, 2nd edn. Raven Press, New York, pp 17–38
Salcman M 1991a Hyperthermia. In: Salcman M (ed) Neurobiology of brain tumors. Williams & Wilkins, Baltimore, pp 359–373
Salcman M (ed) 1991b The neurobiology of brain tumors. Vol 4. Concepts in neurosurgery. Williams & Wilkins, Baltimore, p 386
Salcman M 1992 Intracranial hemorrhage caused by brain tumor. In: Kaufman H H (ed) Intracerebral hematomas. Raven Press, New York, pp 95–106
Salcman M 1993 Intrinsic cerebral glioma. In: Apuzzo M L J (ed) Brain surgery, complication avoidance and management. Churchill Livingstone, New York, pp 379–390
Salcman M, Broadwell R D 1991 The blood-brain barrier. In: Salcman M (ed) Neurobiology of brain tumors. Vol 4. Concepts in neurosurgery. Williams & Wilkins, Baltimore, pp 229–249
Salcman M, Ebert P S 1991 In vitro response of human glioblastoma and canine glioma cells to hyperthermia, radiation, and chemotherapy. Neurosurgery 29: 526–531
Salcman M, Samaras G M 1981 Hyperthermia for brain tumors: biophysical rationale. Neurosurgery 9: 327–335
Salcman M, Samaras G M 1983 Interstitial microwave hyperthermia for brain tumors. Results of a phase 1 clinical trial. Journal of Neuro-Oncology 1: 225–236
Salcman M, Solomon L 1984 Occurrence of glioblastoma multiforme in three generations of a cancer family. Neurosurgery 14: 557–561
Salcman M, Kaplan R S, Ducker T B et al 1982 Effect of age and reoperation on survival in the combined modality treatment of malignant astrocytoma. Neurosurgery 10: 454–463
Salcman M, Robinson W, Montgomery E 1986a Laser microsurgery: A review of 105 intracranial tumors. Journal of Neuro-oncology 3: 363–371
Salcman M, Sewchand W, Amin P P et al 1986b Technique and preliminary results of interstitial irradiation for primary brain tumors. Journal of Neuro-Oncology 4: 141–149
Salcman M, Bellis E H, Sewchand W et al 1989 Technical aids for the flexible use of the Leksell stereotactic system. Neurological Research 11: 89–96

Salcman M, Scholtz H, Kaplan R S 1993a The role of reoperation in the multimodality treatment of malignant astrocytoma. (in preparation)

Salcman M, Scholtz H, Kaplan R S et al 1993b Long term survival in patients with malignant astrocytoma. (in preparation)

Salford L G, Brun A, Nirfalk S 1988 Ten-year survival among patients with supratentorial astrocytomas grade III and IV. Journal of Neurosurgery 69: 506–509

Schiffer D 1991 Patterns of tumor growth. In: Salcman M (ed) Neurobiology of brain tumors. Williams & Wilkins, Baltimore, pp 229–249

Schoenberg B S 1977 Multiple primary neoplasms and the nervous system. Cancer 40: 1961–1967

Schoenberg B S 1991 Epidemiology of primary intracranial neoplasms: disease distribution and risk factors. In: Salcman M (ed) Neurobiology of brain tumors. Williams & Wilkins, Baltimore, pp 3–18

Schoenberg B S, Schoenberg D C, Christine B W et al 1976 The epidemiology of primary intracranial neoplasms of childhood: a population study. Mayo Clinic Proceedings 51: 51–56

Schuster H, Jellinger K, Gund A et al 1976 Extracranial metastases of anaplastic cerebral gliomas. Acta Neurochirurgica 35: 247–259

Seeger R C, Brodeur G M, Sather H et al 1985 Association of multiple copies of N-myc oncogene with rapid progression of neuroblastomas. New England Journal of Medicine 313: 1111–1116

Seizinger B R, Martuza R L, Gusella J F 1986 Loss of genes on chromosome 22 in tumorigenesis of human acoustic neuroma. Nature 322: 644–647

Selikoff I J, Hammond E C 1982 Brain tumors in the chemical industry. Annals of the New York Academy of Science 381: 1–364

Selker R G, Jacobs S A, Moore P B et al 1980 1,3-Bis(2-chloroethyl)-1-nitrosourea (BCNU)-induced pulmonary fibrosis. Neurosurgery 7: 560–565

Shapiro W R 1982 Treatment of neuroectodermal brain tumors. Annals of Neurology 12: 231–237

Shaw C-M, Sumi S M, Alvord E C et al 1978 Fast-neutron irradiation of glioblastoma multiforme. Neuropathological analysis. Journal of Neurosurgery 49: 1–12

Sheline G E, Wara W M, Smith V 1980 Therapeutic irradiation and brain injury. International Journal of Radiation Oncology Biology Physics 6: 1215–1228

Shin K H, Muller P J, Geggie P H S 1983 Superfractionation radiation therapy in the treatment of malignant astrocytoma. Cancer 52: 2040–2043

Smith D R, Hardman J M, Earle K M 1969 Metastasizing neuroectodermal tumors of the central nervous system. Journal of Neurosurgery 31: 50–58

Sneed P K, Stauffer P R, Gutin P H et al 1991 Interstitial irradiation and hyperthermia for the treatment of recurrent malignant brain tumors. Neurosurgery 28: 206–215

Stein B M, Bruce J N 1992 Surgical management of pineal region tumors. Clinical Neurosurgery 39: 509–532

Taratuto A, Sevlever G, Piccardo P 1991 Clues and pitfalls in stereotactic biopsy of the central nervous system. Archives of Pathology and Laboratory Medicine 115: 596–602

Tel E, Hoshino T, Barker M et al 1980 Effect of surgery on BCNU chemotherapy in a rat brain tumor model. Journal of Neurosurgery 52: 529–532

Tenney J H, Vlahov D, Salcman M et al 1985 Wide variation in risk of wound infection following clean neurosurgery: Implications for perioperative antibiotic prophylaxis. Journal of Neurosurgery 62: 243–247

Todd D W, Christoferson L A, Leech R W et al 1981 A family affected with intestinal polyposis and gliomas. Annals of Neurology 10: 390–392

Tomita T, Raimondi A J 1981 Brain tumors in the elderly. Journal of the American Medical Association 246: 53–55

Trouillas P, Menaud G, De The G et al 1975 Etude epidemiologique des tumeurs primitives du neuraxe dans la region Rhone-Alphes. Rev Neurol 131: 691–708

Urtasun R, Feldstein M L, Partington J et al 1982 Radiation and nitroimidazoles in supratentorial high grade gliomas: A second clinical trial. British Journal of Cancer 46: 101–108

Vertosick F T, Selker R G 1990 Brain stem and spinal metastases of supratentorial glioblastoma multiforme. A clinical series. Neurosurgery 27: 516–522

Vertosick F T, Selker R G, Pollack I F et al 1992 The treatment of intracranial malignant gliomas using orally administered tamoxifen therapy: preliminary results in a series of "failed" patients. Neurosurgery 30: 897–903

Walker A E, Robins M, Weinfeld F D 1985 Epidemiology of brain tumors: the national survey of intracranial neoplasms. Neurology 35: 219–226

Walker M D, Hurwitz B S 1970 BCNU (1,3-bis(2-chloroethyl)-1-nitrosourea, NSC-409962) in the treatment of malignant brain tumor. A preliminary report. Cancer Chemotherapy Report 54: 263–271

Walker M D, Alexander E, Hunt W E et al 1978 Evaluation of BCNU and/or radiotherapy in the treatment of anaplastic gliomas: A cooperative clinical trial. Journal of Neurosurgery 49: 333–343

Walker M D, Strike T A, Sheline G E 1979 An analysis of dose-effect relationship in the radiotherapy of malignant gliomas. International Journal of Radiation Oncology Biology Physics 5: 1725–1731

Walker M D, Green S B, Byar D P et al 1980 Randomized comparisons of radiotherapy and nitrosoureas for the treatment of malignant glioma after surgery. New England Journal of Medicine 303: 1323–1329

Watanabe E, Mayanagi Y, Kosugi Y et al 1991 Open surgery assisted by the neuronavigator, a stereotactic, articulated, sensitive arm. Neurosurgery 28: 792–800

Wilson C B, Boldrey E B, Enot K J 1970 1,3-bis(2-chloroethyl)-1-nitrosourea (NSC-409962) in the treatment of brain tumors. Cancer Chemotherapy Report 54: 273–281

Winger M J, Macdonald D R, Schold S C et al 1989 Selection bias in clinical trials of anaplastic glioma. Annals of Neurology 26: 531–534

Wood J R, Greene S B, Shapiro W R 1988 The prognostic importance of tumor size in malignant gliomas: A computed tomographic scan study by the Brain Tumor Cooperative Group. Journal of Clinical Oncology 6: 338–343

Wu J K, Folkerth R D, Ye Z et al 1992 Aggressive oligodendroglioma predicted by chromosome 10 restriction fragment length polymorphism analysis. Case study. Journal of Neuro-Oncology 15: 29–35

Young B, Oldfield E H, Markesbery W R et al 1981 Reoperation for glioblastoma. Journal of Neurosurgery 55: 917–921

Young H F, Merchant R E, Apuzzo M L J 1991 Immunocompetence of patients with malignant glioma. In: Salcman M (ed) Neurobiology of brain tumors. Williams & Wilkins, Baltimore, pp 211–227

26. Oligodendroglioma

William T. Couldwell   David R. Hinton

HISTORICAL BACKGROUND

The first description of an oligodendroglioma was published in an historic classification of the glioma group by Bailey & Cushing in 1926. Subsequently, Bailey & Bucy reported their classic description of 13 cases of oligodendrogliomas in 1929, a milestone work which first correlated the tumor's histologic description and clinical behavior. This was a remarkably insightful publication, which laid a foundation of knowledge of the behavior of this tumor which changed remarkably little in the subsequent half century. This may in part be attributable to the relatively uncommon occurrence of these lesions, resulting in the reporting of small retrospective series, lack of universality of histologic grading and variability of treatment protocols for patients harboring these tumors. Recently published series, however, have dramatically increased our insight into the response of these tumors to therapy.

INCIDENCE AND PREVALENCE OF OLIGODENDROGLIOMA

Oligodendrogliomas are not common intracranial neoplasms; they represent approximately 4–7% of all primary intracranial gliomas (Rubinstein 1972, Mørk et al 1985), with occasional series reporting a higher incidence (10–15% — Burger et al 1991, 18.8% — Zülch 1986). They represent the third most common gliomas following glioblastoma and astrocytoma. They are reported to be equally distributed between sexes (Rubinstein 1972), though some report a higher incidence in males (3:2–2:1 males: females — Russell and Rubinstein 1977, Mørk et al 1985). In a similar age prevalence with the much more common astrocytomas, they most frequently occur in the fourth and fifth decades of life. There is a biphasic age distribution to the tumors, with two peak incidences at 6–12 years and 26–46 years. Although the smaller peak of incidence of oligodendrogliomas occurs in childhood, the overall incidence in this age group makes presentation uncommon (Wilkinson et al 1987); clinical series in childhood, however, have been reported (Hirsch et al 1989).

SITES OF PREDILECTION

Oligodendrogliomas occur most frequently within the cerebral hemispheres, often in a frontal location (Fig. 26.1). These lesions predominate in the white matter of the cerebral hemispheres in rough proportion to the mass of each lobe (frontal:parietal:temporal:occipital; 3:2:2:1 — Earnest et al 1950, Roberts & German 1966, Chin et al 1980, Burger & Vogel 1982). Often they involve the

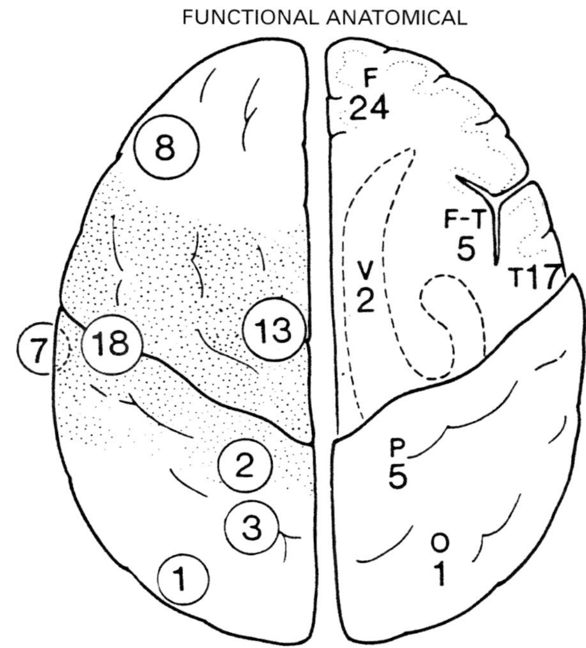

Fig. 26.1 Tumor distribution in a series of 54 cases of oligodendroglioma; anatomical (right) and functional (left) views. Most tumors are concentrated in the functionally important frontotemporal region (motor-sensory-speech) in contrast to frontal predilection, anatomically. From Chin et al (1980), with permission.

frontotemporal-perisylvian region, with extension up to the paracentral regions, producing neurologic compromise.

Although they may occur in any supratentorial location, a primary infratentorial tumor is distinctly uncommon (Wilkinson et al 1987). A report of 4 oligodendrogliomas of the posterior fossa in childhood (Packer et al 1985) suggested that these tumors may behave aggressively in this location and may require presymptomatic craniospinal radiation. Oligodendrogliomas of the spinal cord are rare (Fortuna et al 1980), with very rare case reports describing 'holocord' localization (Pagni et al 1991).

These tumors are infiltrative; however, in contrast to astrocytomas, there is often an abrupt interface between the tumor and the adjacent white matter. Oligodendrogliomas characteristically infiltrate into the cortex and may extend into the leptomeninges; on occasion they may adhere to dura and mimic the appearance of a meningioma. Very rarely, the tumor cells may widely infiltrate through the white matter, deep grey matter and brainstem resulting in *gliomatosis cerebri* (Balko et al 1992). In lesions that are adjacent to the ventricular system or the subarachnoid spaces, seeding of cerebrospinal fluid pathways may occur (Blumenfeld & Gardner 1945, Burger 1990). In this regard, intraventricular oligodendrogliomas have been infrequently reported (Garza-Mercado et al, 1987, most recently by Tekkok et al 1992). Intraventricular oligodendrogliomas must be differentiated from the histologically similar-appearing central neurocytoma (Kim et al 1992). The neurocytoma typically occurs in young adults and has a good prognosis; it may present with intraventricular hemorrhage. Neurocytomas are discrete, often calcified tumors which usually protrude into the ventricular system. They are distinguished by their immunohistochemical expression of neuronal markers (neuron-specific enolase, synaptophysin) and by the presence of dense-core vesicles on ultrastructural examination (Kubota et al 1991, von Deimling et al 1991). Oligodendrogliomas, like other gliomas, have rarely been noted to metastasize (James & Pagel 1951), though multiple intracranial lesions have been reported (Ogasawara et al 1990).

CLINICAL PRESENTATION

Classically it has been reported that most patients harboring oligodendrogliomas present with a long preceding history of epilepsy and a tumor with radiologic evidence of calcification (Wilkinson et al 1987). Typically, middle-aged individuals present with a several-year history of seizures (Shaw et al 1992). Though various types of seizures may occur, generalized convulsions occur at a significantly higher rate (Chin et al 1980). Often these seizures develop gradually in the early stages of the illness, which prompted Bailey & Cushing to describe in their 1926 treatise: 'when people of middle life begin in this way to have epileptiform attacks of obscure etiology, the possible existence of one of these slow-growing lesions must always be borne in mind'. Epilepsy may, for many years, be the only manifestation of intracerebral tumors which behave in a relatively benign manner (Smith et al 1991). In this regard, epilepsy has been shown clinically to be a favorable prognostic factor for oligodendrogliomas (Walker et al 1978). Such observations have supported the consensus that epilepsy as a first symptom appears to be one of the most important ways of identifying primary brain tumors with good quality survival.

Clinical studies, however, have indicated that up to one half of patients with oligodendrogliomas do not present with seizures. The remainder of patients present with a variety of symptoms, usually including focal neurologic deficit and headache. In cases of intraventricular tumors, the most common presenting symptom is increased intracranial pressure, with headache, usually associated with visual disturbances and papilledema. Tumors with these alternate presentations are more likely to exhibit a more aggressive clinical course.

Rarely, oligodendroglioma has been reported to occur following external beam radiotherapy for another primary tumor (Huang et al 1987).

RADIOGRAPHIC EVALUATION

Radiographic evaluation of a patient suspected of harboring an intracranial mass lesion should be initiated with a computed tomographic (CT) or magnetic resonance (MR) scan. As mentioned above, in the case of oligodendroglioma, these lesions are usually supratentorial and as many as 60% of them calcify, often in clumps (Lee & Van Tassel 1989, Segall et al 1990). In consideration of this large percentage with associated calcification, the use of CT with superior visualization of calcium may be valuable. Thus CT and MR imaging are suitable complementary methods to characterize the tumor and evaluate its extension (Margain et al 1991). Both of these modalities should be obtained with and without contrast enhancement (intravenous gadolinium-DTPA contrast for MR; iodinated contrast for CT). The tumor is often seen as a large, calcified, poorly-enhancing peripheral frontal lesion (Fig. 26.2). Higher grade lesions, and those with mixed components (astroglial-oligodendroglial) in which the astrocytic component is anaplastic will more often enhance, and be associated with hemorrhagic and necrotic areas.

PATHOLOGIC FEATURES OF OLIGODENDROGLIOMAS

Gross morphological features

Oligodendrogliomas are usually solid, relatively well-

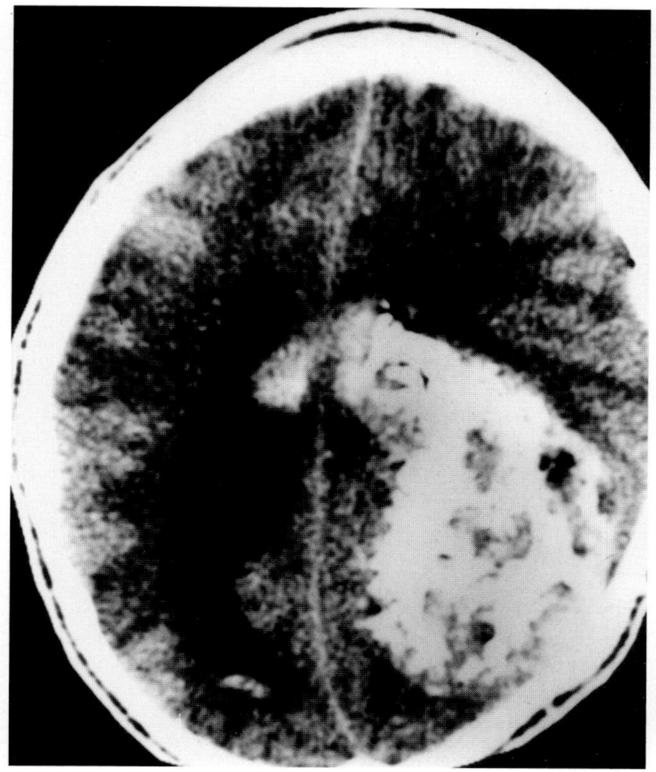

A

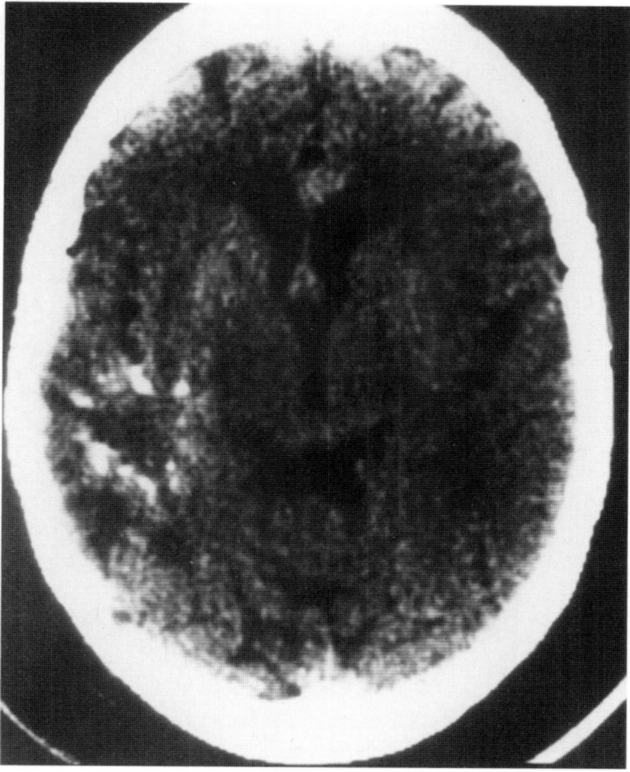

B

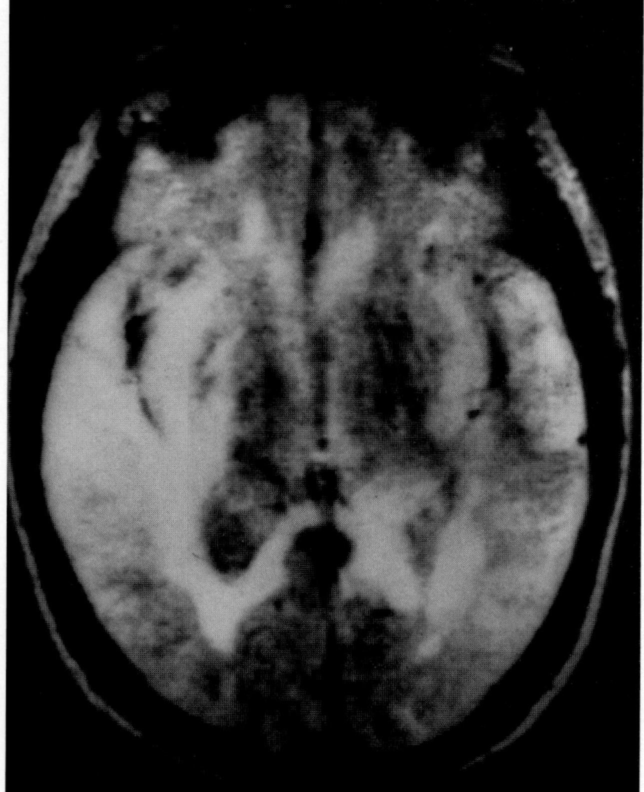

C

Fig. 26.2 A. CT without contrast enhancement demonstrating a large left parietal calcified tumor which subsequently was demonstrated to be oligodendroglioma on histologic analysis. Because of the presence of calcification in the majority of these lesions, CT may offer complementary information to MRI. This is illustrated in the right posterior temporal lesion seen on CT examination **B**, which is more evident than on the T2-weighted MRI of the same patient **C**.

defined, soft gray-pink tumors (Fig. 26.3). Those tumors with mucinous change may be gelatinous. Larger tumors may show areas of necrosis and cyst formation. Calcification is frequent and may impart a gritty texture to the tumor. The tumor may be associated with or present with spontaneous intracerebral hemorrhage, a complication that may be related to the structure of the neoplastic capillary bed.

Microscopic features

Well-differentiated oligodendrogliomas are composed of cells with uniform, round to oval nuclei and fine chromatin pattern with small nucleoli (Fig. 26.4). The cytoplasm shows minimal process formation so that a fibrillary background appearance is lacking. Perinuclear haloes are characteristic of oligodendrogliomas and are a result of autolysis due to delay in fixation (Fig. 26.4); haloes are

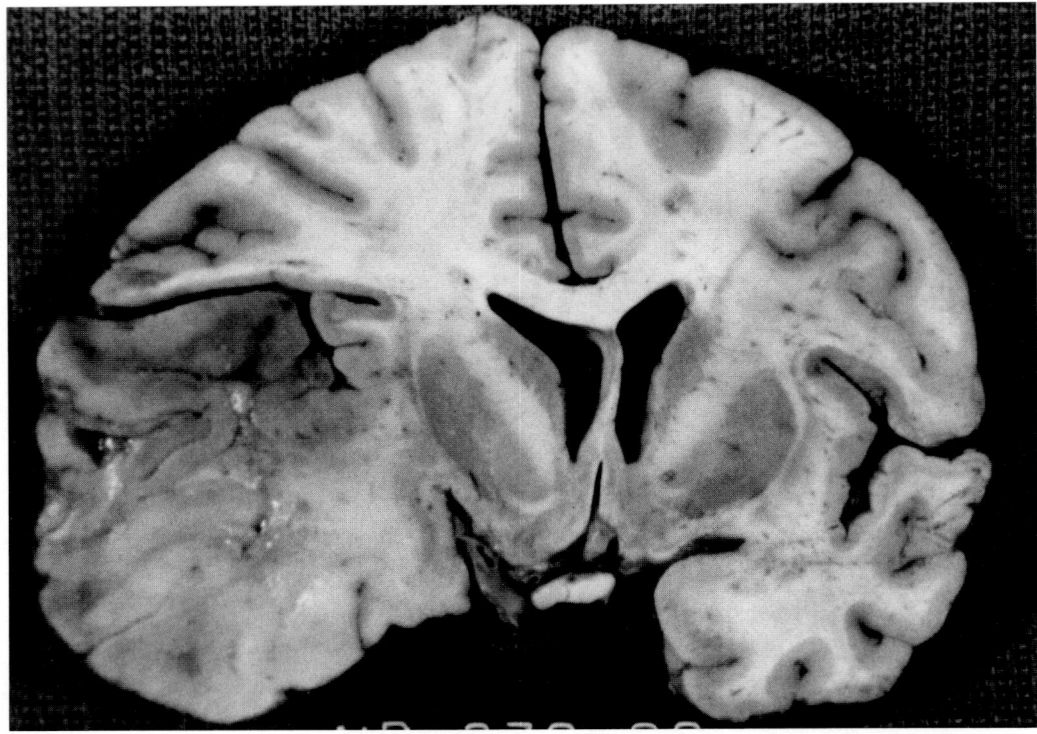

Fig. 26.3 Pathologic specimen of an oligodendroglioma. Note the large right temporal calcified lesion on this autopsy specimen. Photograph provided by Dr Bernadette Curry.

therefore absent in frozen sections. The tumor cells are present in sheets and lobular groups between a prominent vascular network composed of distinctive short curvilinear capillaries. Infiltration of the tumor into cerebral cortex results in perineuronal satellitosis, and perivascular and subpial tumor cell aggregates. Calcification is very frequent in these tumors and may be found as calcospherites in the tumor or adjacent brain, or as mineralization of tumor vessels. The grading of oligodendrogliomas is described in detail in a later section. As the tumors become more anaplastic they typically become more cellular, with increased nuclear pleomorphism, developing vascular proliferation and areas of focal tumor necrosis. While low grade oligodendrogliomas lack astrocytic features,

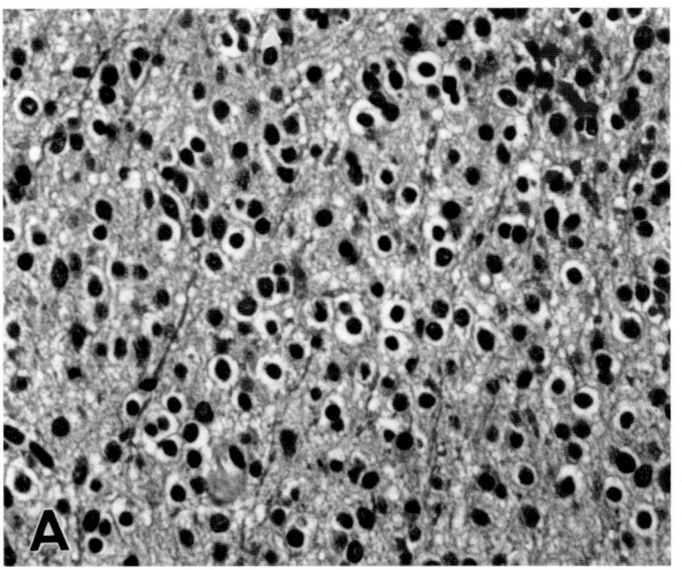

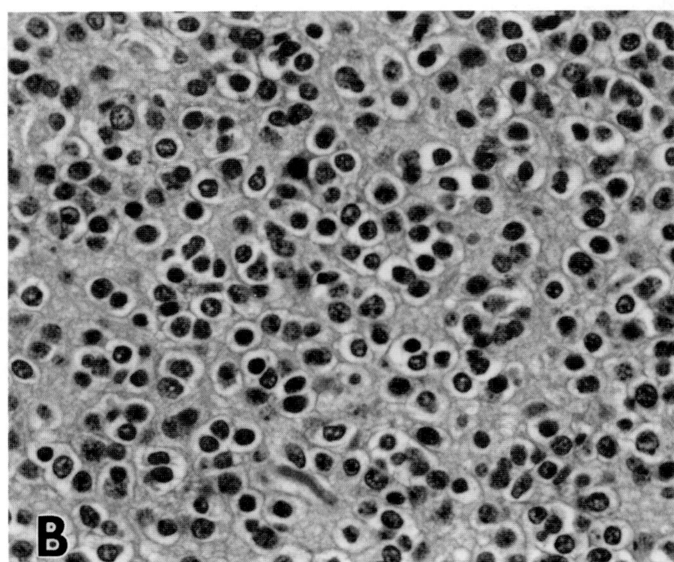

Fig. 26.4 A & B

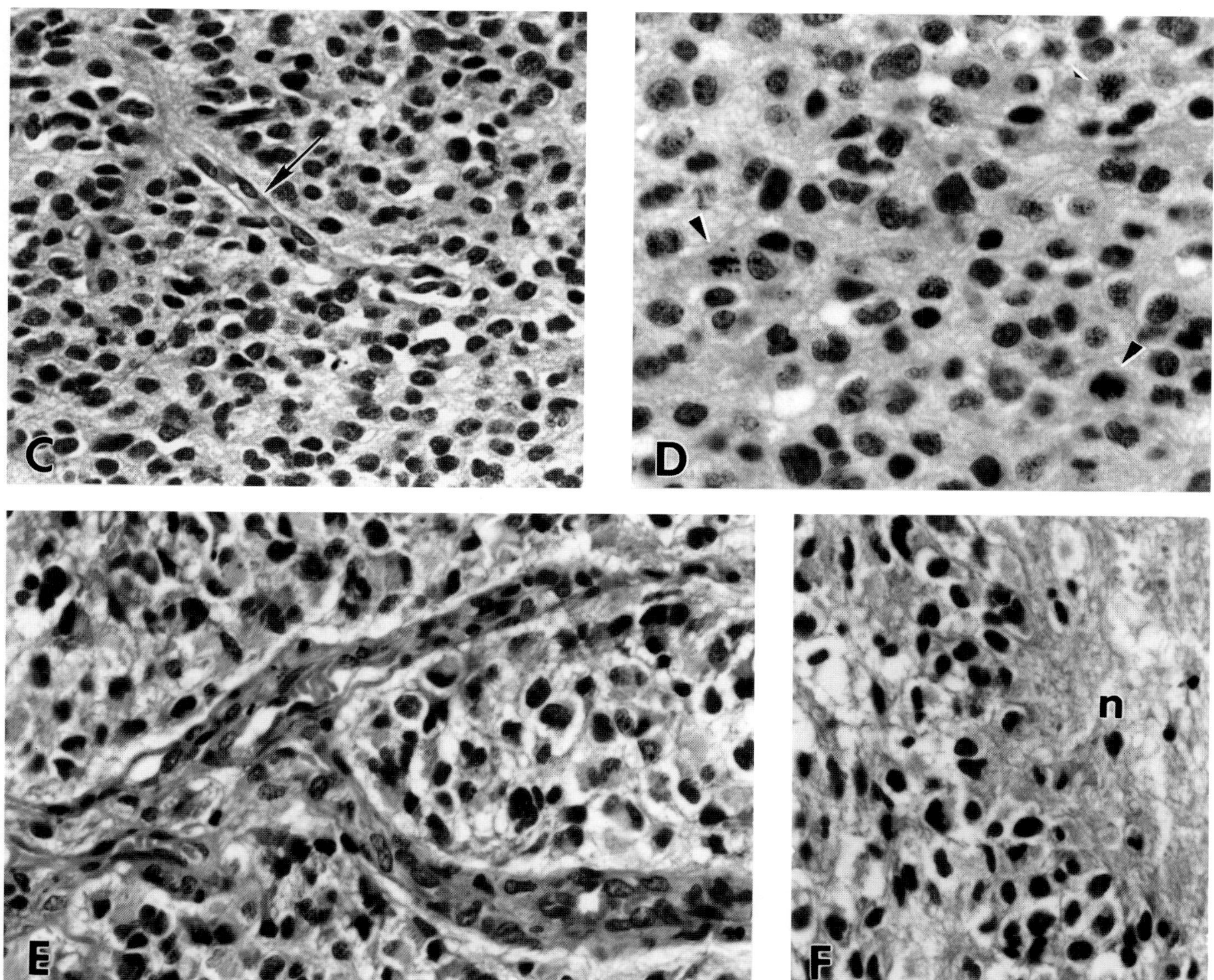

Fig. 26.4 Microscopic features of oligodendroglioma. Typical histologic features of oligodendrogliomas using Kernohan/Smith tumor grades. Grade 1/A **A.** Round-to-oval uniform appearing nuclei with preservation of neuropil (H&E × 300). Grade 2/B **B.** Tumor is moderately hypercellular with less preservation of neuropil. Nuclei show mild-to-moderate pleomorphism and perinuclear haloes are well developed (H&E × 325). Grade 3/B **C.** Tumor is moderately hypercellular. Nuclei show more prominent pleomorphism and atypia. There is little persistent neuropil, perinuclear haloes are less apparent, but typical thin-walled arcuate vessels are seen (H&E × 325). **D.** Grade 3 neoplasms characteristically show mitotic activity (arrowheads) (H&E ×500). Grade 4/C **E.** There is increased cellularity with more prominent pleomorphism and no apparent residual neuropil. Microgemistocytes, with eccentric eosinophilic cytoplasm, are present. Blood vessel walls show branching and increased numbers of endothelial cell nuclei (H&E × 350). Grade 4/D **F.** Necrosis is present in grade 4 tumors (H&E × 350). Reprinted with permission from Coons et al (1994).

histologically malignant oligodendroglial tumors tend to develop certain astrocytic features. These tumors have a propensity to include large entrapped reactive astrocytes as well as small tumor cells with eccentric non-fibrillar glassy cytoplasm strongly positive for glial fibrillary acidic protein (minigemistocytes).

Ultrastructural features

Oligodendroglial tumor cells show variable amounts of cytoplasm which is often rich in organelles including numerous microtubules, free ribosomes, and mitochondria. There may be an associated prominent Golgi apparatus. While occasional intermediate filaments may be present, large compact bundles of glial filaments as seen in astrocytomas are absent except in the included reactive gemistocytes or transitional gliofibrillary astrocytes (minigemistocytes). Ultrastructural studies have confirmed that the perinuclear halo found in formalin-fixed/paraffin-embedded material is secondary to autolysis.

Immunohistochemistry

Normal oligodendroglial cells can be identified by several specific marker proteins including myelin basic protein (MBP), myelin-associated glycoprotein (MAG), galactocerebrosidase and carbonic anhydrase C; however, none of these proteins is consistently expressed in neoplastic oligodendrocytes (Schwechheimer et al 1992). Some oligodendrogliomas show focal or patchy staining for S-100 or neuron-specific enolase (NSE), but this is generally not sensitive or specific enough to be of use. A high percentage of oligodendrogliomas are immunoreactive for the cell surface antigen Leu 7 (Nakagawa et al 1986). All oligodendrogliomas studied by de la Monte (1981) showed immunoreactivity for A2B5, a marker of progenitors of oligodendroglial cells and type 2 astrocytes; however, the specificity of this marker has not yet been confirmed. While most well-differentiated neoplastic oligodendrocytes are negative for glial fibrillary acidic protein (GFAP), occasional entrapped reactive astrocytes and large gemistocytes may be found in oligodendrogliomas. A recent report by Kros et al (1990) indicated that tumors containing large classic gemistocytes were associated with a worse prognosis. Scattered neoplastic cells with morphologic characteristics of oligodendroglial cells may also be GFAP positive and are then termed gliofibrillary oligodendrocytes. Tumors may also contain small gemistocytic tumor cells (minigemistocytes) which may represent transitional or intermediate forms between oligodendroglial and astrocytic phenotype.

Cytogenetic and molecular studies

Relatively few oligodendrogliomas have been studied by cytogenetic and molecular methods. Most oligodendrogliomas (90%) have karyotypically normal stemlines although secondary lines have shown loss of the Y chromosome; rare tumors have demonstrated abnormalities involving chromosomes 7 (+7), 22 (−22), 1(p) and 9(p) (Rey et al 1987, Bigner 1990, Jenkins et al 1989, Griffin et al 1992). A large DNA flow cytometric study of 85 oligodendrogliomas found that there was no association between ploidy status and survival (Kros et al 1992). Molecular studies have not revealed specific allelic deletions (on chromosomes 9, 10, or 17 — James et al 1988), and have only rarely shown abnormalities in proto-oncogene expression (a single mixed glioma with EGFR amplification — Fuller & Bigner 1992) or p53 mutations (2/17 oligodendrogliomas showing missense p53 mutations — Ohgaki et al 1991).

Differential diagnosis

Oligodendrogliomas must be differentiated pathologically from a host of lesions that may imitate their appearance or complicate their identification. The availability of only small stereotactic biopsies may make this differentiation more difficult. The distinction between a well-differentiated fibrillary astrocytoma and oligodendroglioma may be difficult on intraoperative frozen section because of the lack of 'fried egg' appearance in these preparations. While true mixed gliomas show distinct areas of oligodendroglioma along with areas of astrocytoma, other gliomas may show cells which imitate oligodendroglioma. Oligodendroglial appearing areas may be found in juvenile pilocytic astrocytomas and cellular ependymomas (clear cell ependymoma). Vascular malformations may show areas of oligodendroglial proliferation which may imitate an oligodendroglioma. The dysembryonic neuroepithelial tumor is a distinct childhood tumor which frequently contains foci similar in appearance to oligodendroglioma. As described previously, intraventricular oligodendrogliomas must be differentiated from the similar appearing central neurocytomas (neuronal tumors with an excellent prognosis). Infiltration of an oligodendroglioma through the leptomeninges with attachment to the dura may result in confusion with a meningioma. Poorly differentiated oligodendrogliomas may be confused with other anaplastic gliomas or possibly with metastatic carcinoma. Finally, oligodendrogliomas may present with intracerebral hemorrhage; fragments of tumor may only be found after careful examination of evacuated blood clot (Hinton et al 1984).

Histological grading

Grading of oligodendrogliomas has not yet been standardized internationally (Table 26.1). The three-tiered system as suggested by Ringertz (1950) is used by many neuropathologists. The well-differentiated oligodendroglioma is characterized by its lack of nuclear pleomorphism, minimal mitotic activity, and absence of vascular proliferation and necrosis. Anaplastic oligodendrogliomas are more cellular with significant nuclear pleomorphism, elevated mitotic rate, vascular proliferation and often necrosis. The presence of tumor necrosis alone does not upgrade the tumor to glioblastoma multiforme. Typical glioblastoma multiforme is only rarely found as a progressive change in oligodendroglioma but is the most malignant form of this tumor. Another grading system from the Armed Forces Institute of Pathology (AFIP) (Smith et al 1983) uses a four-tiered system based on the presence of five features: cellularity, cellular atypia, mitotic index, endothelial proliferation, and necrosis. The St. Anne/Mayo system was devised for use in the assessment of diffuse fibrillary astrocytomas but has recently been applied in the analysis of oligodendrogliomas (Shaw et al 1992). This approach is based on the presence or absence of four specific features (nuclear abnormalities, mitoses, endothelial proliferation, necrosis) and is very reproducible. This system of classification has been incorporated into the new

Table 26.1 A comparison of grading systems currently used in the pathologic description of oligodendrogliomas. Note that overlap exists between categories in the 3- and 4-tiered systems, thus definition of the system used is essential.

3-TIERED SYSTEM		4-TIERED SYSTEMS			
GRADE	RINGERTZ		AFIP (Smith et al 1983)	KERNOHAN	ST. ANNE-MAYO
1 Well-diff.	Nuclear pleomorphism — minimal Mitotic activity — minimal Vascular proliferation — absent Necrosis — absent	1 (A)	Absent or low degree of following features: • endothelial proliferation • necrosis • ↑ nuclear:cytoplasmic (n/e) ratio • ↑ cell density • pleomorphism	Anaplasia — absent Cellularity — mild Endothelial prolif. — minimal Transition to brain — broad Mitoses — absent	None of the following criteria: • nuclear abnormalities • mitosis • endothelial prolif. • necrosis
2 Anaplastic or malignant	Cellularity — increased Nuclear pleomorphism — significant Mitotic rate — elevated Vascular proliferation — present Necrosis — often present	2 (B)	Presence of pleomorphism and/or ↑ cell density and ↑ n/c ratio	Anaplasia — focal Cellularity — mild Mitoses — absent Endothelial proliferation — minimal Transition to brain — less broad	One of above criteria
		3(C)	Presence of: • pleomorphism • endothelial proliferation • ↑ cell density • ↑ n:c ratio	Anaplasia — ½ of cells Cellularity — increased Mitoses — present Endothelial prolif. — more frequent Necrosis — frequent Transition to brain — narrow	Two of above criteria
3 GBM	Cellularity — high Nuclear pleomorphism — high Mitotic rate — high Vascular proliferation — present Necrosis — present with pseudopalisading	4(D)	All 5 features present at high level	Anaplasia — extensive Cellularity — marked Mitoses — numerous Necrosis — extensive Transition to brain — may be sharp	Three or four of above criteria

World Health Organization (WHO) classification of brain tumors (Kleihues et al 1993). Note that there is overlap in the criteria for these grading systems, such that precise definition of the system utilized is essential (Table 26.1).

While earlier studies suggested that grading had little value, more recent literature indicates significant prognostic value for tumor grade. Early reports described the clinical course of patients with oligodendroglioma to be unpredictable, with a poor correlation between histologic evidence of malignancy and survival (Roberts & German 1966, Russell & Rubinstein 1977, Chin et al 1980, Reedy et al 1983). However, recent reports advocate that general management strategies should be predicated upon the histologic grade (Ludwig et al 1986). Weir & Elvidge (1968) first noted that there was a slight tendency for patients with marked nuclear pleomorphism to survive for shorter periods than those whose tumors were marked by a uniform 'honeycomb' appearance. Subsequently Smith et al (1983) found in their retrospective study that neoplasms of higher grade had a significantly decreased survival. While this study found that pleomorphism was the most significant variable, subsequent studies have shown that increased cell density, necrosis (Mørk et al 1986, Bullard et al 1987, Burger et al 1987), vascular proliferation and mitoses (Mørk et al 1986, Burger et al 1987) were negative prognostic indicators. The Scandinavian study reported by Mørk et al (1985) found that microcystic change was a good prognostic indicator. Other authors have reported similar conclusions, with histologic grade being the single most important prognostic variable in both univariate and multivariate analyses (Ludwig et al 1986, Sun et al 1988). Most recently, Shaw et al (1992) reviewed the Mayo Clinic experience of 81 oligodendrogliomas. They classified tumors according to two different four-tiered systems, the Kernohan and the St. Anne-Mayo, which utilize similar criteria to the above classification (Table 26.1). In their analysis of 13 possible prognosticating factors, tumor grade was most strongly associated with survival.

Assessment of growth fraction in oligodendroglial tumors by means of the proliferation-associated antigen Ki-67 may be useful in assigning tumor grade, particularly in small biopsies or tumors of intermediate histology. There is a good correlation reported between tumor grade and Ki-67 index (Shibata et al 1988, Deckert et al 1989). For Shibata's and Deckert's series, oligodendroglial tumors were found to have a Ki-67 index of 2.2% and 4.2% respectively, while atypical or recurrent oligodendrogliomas had a Ki-67 index of 5.3% and 14.4% respectively.

GENERAL MANAGEMENT PLAN

There is still significant controversy in the literature as to the optimal management of a patient harboring an oligodendroglioma. The reason for this is multifactorial, but in part includes the conflicting data regarding the role of tumor grading in prognostication, the benefit of surgical resection, and the efficacy of radiation therapy for low grade tumors.

Collectively, it would seem most rational to tailor the individual patient's therapy to the location of the tumor, histologic grade, clinical presentation, and general medical condition (including Karnofsky performance score). Treatment options for these relatively slow-growing lesions include observation following biopsy, or surgical resection with or without postoperative radiation and/or chemotherapy.

For oligodendrogliomas of low grade, the decision is most difficult. Perhaps it is safest to concede initially that we currently do not know how best to manage intrinsic supratentorial tumors with a relatively long natural history. The dilemma is whether or not these patients should be subjected to the risks of treatment (surgery or radiation) as soon as the diagnosis is made (Cairncross & Laperriere 1989). The situation is even more difficult when the lesion is low density, non-enhancing (on CT or MRI) and the patient is neurologically intact. It is our current practice to obtain tissue (by stereotactic biopsy or by excisional biopsy in selected cases) in *all* cases of suspected oligodendroglioma to verify histologic diagnosis. Subsequent treatment options (surgical resection, radiotherapy, chemotherapy) with associated risks are then discussed with the patient. It must be emphasized that all risks must be considered when planning subsequent management strategies.

As oligodendroglial tumors commonly present with epilepsy, the role of surgical resection in seizure management deserves comment. Epilepsy due to intracerebral tumors may be refractory to drugs, with significant remission of seizures being rare (Smith et al 1991). Efficacy of surgical resection in decreasing seizure frequency has been clearly demonstrated by some authors (Page et al 1969, Lee et al 1989), while other authors have reported variable results (30–50% response to surgery as reported by Smith et al 1991).

SURGICAL MANAGEMENT

The role of surgical resection of low grade tumors is somewhat controversial. While some studies report efficacy of surgical resection in patients with low grade astrocytomas (Laws et al 1984, Soffietti et al 1990), other authors are less enthusiastic, suggesting that such results may be the result of selection bias (i.e. tumors in more accessible locations, in younger individuals or those with higher Karnofsky scores, with fewer underlying medical problems — Sandeman et al 1990, Winger et al 1989b, Smith et al 1991). Furthermore, it is unknown if results of studies of predominantly low grade astrocytomas will extrapolate to the management of oligodendrogliomas.

Several series have emphasized the importance of extent of resection on survival in patients with oligodendrogliomas (Horrax & Wu 1951, Roberts & German 1966, Reedy et al 1983). In a recent published study reviewing the Mayo Clinic experience (Shaw et al 1992), patients who underwent gross total resection had improved survival times in comparison with patients who underwent only subtotal resections. However, the patients who underwent gross total removal were often younger with lower grade tumors, factors which favor improved survival. In a series of 82 patients, these authors reported median survival time of 12.6 years, and 5- and 10-year survival rates of 74% and 59% in patients who had undergone gross total surgical resection, in comparison to 4.9 years, 48% and 26% respectively for those patients who underwent a subtotal resection. In the series of Mørk et al (1985), similar results were seen, with a median survival of 3.8 years compared with 2.7 years in patients with subtotal resection. Similar results have been noted in other recent series: Lindegaard et al (1987), in a review of 170 cases of oligodendroglioma, reported a favorable median survival time of 7 years, and 5- and 10-year survival rates of 54% and 38% respectively if gross surgical removal was achieved. Whitton & Bloom (1990) reported 84% 5-year survival in patients with total or subtotal resection in comparison to 41% in patients in whom only a biopsy or partial resection had been performed. A limited number of other studies, however, have failed to demonstrate statistical significance of the extent of resection on survival (Sun et al 1988). In a review of 424 cases, performed by the Brain Tumor Registry of Japan (Committee of Brain Tumor Registry in Japan 1987), a significant difference in survival was noted between the biopsy group and the subtotally or totally resected group, but no significant difference was noted between the 50–75% resected group and the total removal group.

In summary, review of the contemporary literature suggests that the survival of patients with pure oligodendroglioma is improved when surgical cytoreductive therapy has been performed. In consideration of this, we would advocate aggressive surgical resection in patients harboring lesions in accessible locations, which are deemed resectable with minimal morbidity and which pose little risk for an increase in neurologic deficit. In lesions adjacent to eloquent cortical regions, (speech, motor or sensory cortex) the use of intraoperative electrophysiologic mapping techniques may be helpful to maximize resection of the tumor. Performing the resection under local anesthesia may facilitate localization of speech and enable resection of tumors in patients with lesions of the dominant hemisphere in which resection would seemingly otherwise pose a prohibitive risk of postoperative aphasia.

RADIATION THERAPY

The role of radiotherapy in the management of low grade gliomas has not been definitively established (Cairncross & Laperierre 1989, Shaw 1990). The sensitivity of these tumors to radiotherapy is difficult to assess, due largely to the limited number of patients reported (Lindegaard et al 1987). This, together with the lack of uniformity of pathologic grades of tumors treated, differences in treatment doses, and lack of randomization have made interpretation of the efficacy of radiotherapy in these tumors difficult.

Sheline et al (1964) originally compared rates of survival between radiated and non-radiated patients with oligodendrogliomas, and concluded that these tumors were radiosensitive. Chin et al (1980) also reported efficacy of postoperative radiotherapy in 24 patients (of a series of 54) receiving from 53–70 Gy. Subsequently, Lindegaard et al (1987), in their review of 170 patients, reported that in those patients with partially resected lesions, median survival was increased from 26–37 months (statistically significant) with postoperative radiation therapy. However, they noted no benefit from radiation therapy in patients who underwent 'total' removal (these authors admit that 'total removal' must be used with caution in reference to cerebral gliomas). Indeed, they state that radiotherapy in such patients may be detrimental, in that these particular patients had better survival times without irradiation. Moreover, though they noted a significant increase in the median survival time, radiotherapy did not influence the cure rate in oligodendroglioma patients with subtotal resections. In addition, they noted that radiation doses between 40 and 50 Gy were as effective as doses between 50 and 60 Gy, and therefore suggested that the lower dose be utilized to decrease the risk of radiation necrosis, for which the risk increases proportionately with the dose delivered. Two recently published series reported the 5-year survival of oligodendroglioma to be 54–57%, which is approximately double that for anaplastic astrocytomas treated with radiation therapy alone (Wallner et al 1988, Shaw et al 1992). Conversely, there exist several reports of no increase in significant survival with postoperative radiation therapy (Müller et al 1977, Áfra et al 1978, Dohrmann et al 1978, Reedy et al 1983). The interpretation of these studies is confounded by other strong prognostic factors being associated with both survival and receiving radiotherapy (Lindegaard et al 1987).

The confusing issue of the efficacy of postoperative radiotherapy will undoubtedly require a proper prospective, randomized study for resolution (Leibel & Sheline 1987). At the present time, considering the questionable efficacy reported in the literature, the risks of such therapy must be carefully considered before a decision is made (Marks et al 1981).

Taken together, for the adult patient we would concur with the management strategy as proposed by Morantz (1988), in which radiation should be considered in that group of patients whose oligodendroglioma on pathologic examination exhibits poor prognostic features (i.e. pleomorphism, necrosis, endothelial proliferation, and high cell density and nuclear:cytoplasmic ratio, as suggested by Ludwig et al 1986) and is subtotally resected.

In children, the necessity of radiation therapy for benign oligodendrogliomas has not been demonstrated. Moreover, its efficacy has been questioned in consideration of the added risks of radiation to the developing nervous system (Dohrmann et al 1978, Reedy et al 1983, Hirsch et al 1989). In children with complete surgical resection, the incidence of recurrence is low (Hirsch et al 1989) and the risk of exposing the childhood brain to the deleterious effects of radiation hardly seems justified.

The increasing use of stereotactic radiosurgery at multiple neurosurgical centers offers another alternative to standard external beam radiation therapy (RT) for lesions located in deep or eloquent areas. Stereotactic radiosurgery was conceived to be more analogous to conventional surgery than conventional radiotherapy, and refers to single-fraction, high dose irradiation of a limited target volume of tissue. This may be delivered by charged-particle heavy ion beam, e.g. proton-beam (the Leksell cobalt-60 Gamma Knife, and the conventional linear accelerator (LINAC) generators recently reviewed by Luxton et al 1993). Radiobiological considerations of normal tissue tolerance are thought to limit effective radiosurgery to targets no larger than 3–4 cm. Intuitively, if the benign oligodendroglioma is localized, this type of therapy may be a rational alternative to surgical resection. Though few data are as yet available in the literature, clinical trials are currently being undertaken to evaluate the efficacy of such techniques.

CHEMOTHERAPY

The prognosis for most patients with recurrent malignant glioma following surgical resection and radiotherapy is poor. Because of their rarity, oligodendrogliomas have routinely been grouped with other glioma tumors in various clinical chemotherapy studies, with little distinction being made concerning their response to chemotherapy and survival (Kyritsis et al 1993). For this reason, chemotherapeutic protocols and data regarding the sensitivity of these tumors have been limited to a few oncology centers.

Recent reports have indicated that chemosensitivity of malignant oligodendrogliomas may be distinct from that of other glial tumors (Cairncross & Macdonald 1988, 1991, Macdonald et al 1990, Glass et al 1992). Cairncross & Macdonald (1988) have observed that oligodendrogliomas that had regrown after one or more resections and RT invariably responded to chemotherapy. Histologic analysis of these tumors indicated that they were anaplastic and behaved in a clinically aggressive manner. In the 10 consecutively treated anaplastic recurrent tumors, the majority of the patients received procarbazine, CCNU and vincristine (PCV; Table 26.2), with one each receiving BCNU and diazoquone (AZQ). The median duration of response in these previously irradiated patients was 15 months. Patients with recurrent anaplastic tumors responded to the chemotherapy, but were not cured. Treatment of such patients with 'salvage' chemotherapy is much less optimistic; while some patients may have achieved partial responses, they occurred with different chemotherapeutic agents (PCV, melphalan) and tended to be of short duration (Cairncross et al 1992).

Encouraged by the success of chemotherapy for recurrent tumors following RT, the same group has treated newly-diagnosed aggressive tumors (defined as those tumors displaying radiologic and histologic features of aggressiveness, such as increasing symptoms, growth, and contrast enhancement on imaging studies) with chemotherapy before administering local RT (Macdonald et al 1990). The rationale for administering chemotherapy prior to RT is to circumvent the theoretical concern that RT-induced vascular injury impairs drug delivery, and thus to afford an opportunity to assess the response to chemotherapy alone (Cairncross et al 1992). In the limited number of patients (5) given PCV chemotherapy, 4 have responded, the majority completely. From this limited experience, the authors have advocated early aggressive therapy for such tumors (see below).

In support of the above results from the London (Ontario) Regional Cancer Center, the combination of PCV given for 2–5 42-day cycles has demonstrated a 79% response (greater than 50% tumor reduction) in a small series of 14 patients (Glass et al 1992). Carboplatin has been advocated for use in recurrent anaplastic gliomas (including oligodendrogliomas) following failure on nitrosourea therapy (Poisson et al 1991).

In partial contrast to the above results is the study recently reported by Kyritsis et al (1993), who compared treatment outcome in a series of 17 patients with anaplastic oligodendroglioma and 17 patients with anaplastic mixed oligodendroglioma-astrocytoma. They concluded that aggressive initial treatment of anaplastic oligodendroglioma offered minimal advantage over conventional radiotherapy alone, but was advantageous for recurrent anaplastic oligodendroglioma and mixed tumors: of recurrent anaplastic oligodendrogliomas, 75% of the tumors responded or exhibited stable disease, resulting in long response duration and long survival (15–132+ months). The surprising fact with this study was that the initial anaplastic oligodendroglioma patients who were treated aggressively did worse than any other group, which was difficult to rationalize.

At this time, it is unknown whether PCV, which has been the most frequently reported combinational chemotherapeutic protocol utilized with successful results in these tumors, is superior to other cytotoxic drugs with demonstrated activity against oligodendroglioma (BCNU, AZQ, or melphalan (Cairncross & Macdonald 1988, Schold et al 1989, Brown et al 1990). However, Levin et al (1990) have reported that patients with moderately aggressive anaplastic gliomas (other than GBM) lived longer after treatment with PCV than after treatment with BCNU. PCV, melphalan, and thiotepa may be equally effective (Cairncross et al 1992).

Collectively, however, these results suggest a unique chemotherapeutic sensitivity for tumors with an oligodendroglial component (Glass et al 1992). The postulate that these tumors share a common progenitor lineage (A2B5+ — de la Monte 1989) may offer a rationale for this sensitivity.

Of interest is a report of a complete response of a recurrent malignant oligodendroglioma to high dose thiotepa with autologous bone marrow rescue (Saarinen et al 1990), suggesting that these tumors may be amenable to the use of this agent, which exhibits good CNS penetration and may require only one course of treatment.

Based upon the above review of the current salient literature, adjuvant chemotherapy should be considered in those cases with residual or recurrent anaplastic oligodendroglioma, or in those tumors which behave clinically and radiographically in an aggressive manner. Most clinically and radiologically aggressive oligodendrogliomas are anaplastic, and anaplastic oligodendrogliomas behave aggressively, as do some non-anaplastic tumors (Macdonald et al 1990); in these patients a trial of chemotherapy is justified. In patients with stable non-enhancing lesions on

Table 26.2 One current protocol for PCV[a] chemotherapy, as administered by Cairncross et al at the London Regional Cancer Centre. From Cairncross et al (1992), with permission.

Drug	Dosage and schedule	Frequency
CCNU (lomustine)	Day 1: 110 mg/m^2, by mouth	
Vincristine[b]	Day 8: 1.4 mg/m^2, intravenously	
Procarbazine	Days 8–21: 60 mg/m^2/day, by mouth	Every 8 weeks
Vincristine[b]	Day 29 1.4 mg/m^2, intravenously	

[a]PCV = procarbazine, CCNU (lomustine), and vincristine
[b]Maximum dose, 2 mg

serial radiographic studies (i.e. indolent), that histologically show no evidence of aggressive features, then a course of observation would be warranted.

MANAGEMENT OUTCOME

Patients with anaplastic oligodendrogliomas live longer than those with glioblastoma, anaplastic astrocytoma, or anaplastic mixed glioma (Winger et al 1989a). Such longer survival may reflect a better natural history, and may be amplified by a better response to treatment. In London, Ontario, the median survival of patients with anaplastic oligodendrogliomas is 278 weeks, and these patients represent 30% of those with anaplastic gliomas who survive 5 years (Winger et al 1989a). Patients with anaplastic mixed gliomas (astrocytoma-oligodendroglioma) had comparable survival times to those with anaplastic astrocytomas (57 vs 63 weeks). Other groups have supported the opinion that patients with oligodendrogliomas appear to have a better prognosis than those with tumors of pure astrocytic lineage (Kyritsis & Levin 1992). While comparing favorably with the prognosis for patients with anaplastic astrocytoma or glioblastoma multiforme, the overall outlook for patients with oligodendroglioma is only fair, with 5-year survival ranging from 24% (Wilkinson et al 1987) to up to 60% (Chin et al 1980). In general, over 50% of patients undergoing surgical treatment for oligodendroglioma fail to survive longer than 5 years postoperatively (Mørk et al 1985, Ludwig et al 1986, Lindegaard et al 1987, Wilkinson et al 1987).

Table 26.3 summarizes postoperative survival in selected series of patients with oligodendroglioma.

There are several factors which may have some prognostic importance in these tumors:

1. As mentioned above, the most important of these factors may relate to histologic grade. Recent series have reported the significance of histologic grading in outcome (Smith et al 1983, Wilkinson et al 1987). Mørk et al (1985) have reported that patients with calcified and grossly well-demarcated tumors had a significantly longer postoperative survival; however, Sun et al (1988) found no such relation.

2. In a similar fashion to astrocytoma, age at the time of diagnosis has been shown to be a predominant and statistically significant factor in prognosis (Wilkinson et al 1987). It has long been known that the prognosis of benign supratentorial gliomas is different in children and adults (Gol 1962, Heiskanen 1977); it is unclear if the negative impact of greater age at the time of diagnosis is a result of the inability of an older person to survive the disability of the tumor or a true biological difference in tumor behavior.

3. The improved prognosis of a patient with a history of a prior low grade tumor had been alluded to some five decades ago (Sherer 1940). Recent published data indicate that this may be a significant prognostic variable, suggesting that there may be molecular genetic differences in those tumors that represent progression of a low grade tumor versus a de novo anaplastic lesion.

4. Some authors report the negative prognostic implications of presentation with a focal neurologic deficit.

While a younger age at diagnosis, longer duration of symptoms, and history of a low grade glioma in anaplastic oligodendroglioma patients may in part account for an increased survival when compared to astrocytomas, the sensitivity of these tumors to chemotherapy when recurrent (Cairncross & Macdonald 1988) also favorably influences prognosis.

Table 26.3 Postoperative survival in selected series of patients with cerebral oligodendroglioma*. Reproduced from Lindegaard et al (1987), with permission.

Authors & year	No. of cases	Treatment	Cumulative proportion surviving				
			1 yr	3 yrs	5 yrs	8 yrs	10 yrs
Earnest et al 1950	107	S			(0.23)		
Richmond 1959	22	SR			(0.53)		
Sheline et al 1964	13	S			(0.31)		(0.25)
	13	SR			(0.85)		(0.55)
Reedy et al 1983	21	S	0.85	0.74	0.54		
	27	SR	0.81	0.68	0.51		
Lindegaard et al 1987	62‡	S	0.65	0.35	0.27	0.14	0.12
	108§	SR	0.89	0.53	0.36	0.17	0.08

*S = surgery only: SR = surgery + postoperative radiotherapy. Numbers in parentheses denote the survival rate.
‡Median postoperative survival = 26.5 months
§Median postoperative survival = 38 months

REFERENCES

Áfra D, Müller W, Benoist G, Schröder R 1978 Supratentorial recurrences of gliomas: results of reoperations on astrocytomas and oligodendrogliomas. Acta Neurochirurgica (Wien) 43: 217–227

Bailey P, Bucy P C 1929 Oligodendrogliomas of the brain. Journal of Pathology and Bacteriology 32: 735–751

Bailey P, Cushing H 1926 Clinical correlation. In: A classification of the tumors of the glioma group on a histogenetic basis with a correlated study of prognosis. J B Lippincott, Philadelphia, pp 105–165

Balko M G, Blisard K S, Samaha F J 1992 Oligodendroglial gliomatosis cerebri. Human Pathology 23: 706–707

Bigner S H 1990 Cytogenetics of human brain tumors. Cancer Genetics Cytogenetics 47: 141–154

Blumenfeld C M, Gardner W J 1945 Disseminated oligodendroglioma. Archives of Neurology and Psychiatry 54: 274–279

Brown M, Cairncross J G, Vick N A, Macdonald D R, Freidman H S, Dropcho E J, Schold S C Jr 1990 Differential response of recurrent oligodendroglioma versus astrocytoma to intravenous melphalan. Neurology 40 (suppl 1): 397–398 (abstr)

Bullard D E, Rawlings C E, Phillips B, McLendon R E, Schold S C, Bullard D E 1987 Oligodendroglioma. An analysis of the value of radiation therapy. Cancer 60: 2179–2188

Burger P C 1900 Classification, grading and patterns of spread of malignant gliomas. In: Apuzzo M L J (ed) Malignant cerebral glioma. AANS Publications Committee, Park Ridge, IL, pp 3–17

Burger P C, Vogel F 1982 Oligodendroglioma. In: Surgical pathology of the nervous system and its coverings, 2nd edn. John Wiley and Sons, New York

Burger P C, Rawlings C E, Cox E B et al 1987 Clinicopathological correlations in the oligodendroglioma. Cancer 59: 1345–1352

Burger P C, Scheithauer B W, Vogel F 1991 Oligodendroglioma. In: Surgical pathology of the nervous system and its coverings, 3rd edn. John Wiley and Sons, New York, pp 306–327

Cairncross J G, Laperriere N J 1989 Low-grade glioma. To treat or not to treat? Archives of Neurology 46: 1238–1239

Cairncross J G, Macdonald D R 1988 Successful chemotherapy for recurrent malignant oligodendroglioma. Annals of Neurology 23: 360–364

Cairncross J G, Macdonald D R 1991 Chemotherapy for oligodendroglioma. Archives of Neurology 48: 225–227

Cairncross J G, Macdonald D R, Ramsay D A 1992 Aggressive oligodendroglioma: a chemosensitive tumor. Neurosurgery 31: 78–82

Chin H W, Hazel J J, Kim T H, Webster J H 1980 Oligodendrogliomas I. A clinical study of cerebral oligodendrogliomas. Cancer 45: 1458–1466

Committee of Brain Tumor Registry in Japan 1987 Brain Tumor Registry in Japan, vol 6.

Deckert M, Reifenberger G, Wechsler W 1989 Determination of the proliferative potential of human brain tumors using the monoclonal antibody Ki-67. Cancer Research and Clinical Oncology 115: 179–188

de la Monte S M 1990 Immunohistochemical diagnosis of nervous system neoplasms. Clinics in Laboratory Medicine 10: 151–178

de la Monte S M 1989 Uniform lineage of oligodendrogliomas. American Journal of Pathology 135: 529–540

Dohrmann G J, Farwell J R, Flannery J T 1979 Oligodendrogliomas in children. Surgical Neurology 10: 21–25

Earnest F III, Kernohan J W, Craig W M 1950 Oligodendrogliomas. A review of two hundred cases. Archives of Neurology and Psychiatry 63: 964–976

Fortuna A, Celli P, Palma L 1980 Oligodendroglioma of the spinal cord. Acta Neurochirurgica (Wien) 52: 305–329

Fuller G N, Bigner S H 1992 Amplified cellular oncogenes in neoplasms of the human central nervous system. Mutation Research 276: 299–306

Garza-Mercado R, Campa H, Grajeda J 1987 Primary oligodendroglioma of the septum pellucidum. Neurosurgery 21: 78–80

Glass J G, Hochberg F H, Gruber M L, Louis D N, Smith D, Rattner B 1992 The treatment of oligodendrogliomas and mixed oligodendrogliomas-astrocytomas with PCV chemotherapy. Journal of Neurosurgery 76: 741–745

Gol A 1962 Cerebral astrocytomas in childhood. A clinical study. Journal of Neurosurgery 19: 577–582

Griffin C A, Long P P, Carson B S, Brem H 1992 Chromosome abnormalities in low-grade central nervous system tumors. Cancer Genetics Cytogenetics 60: 67–73

Heiskanen O 1977 Intracranial tumors of children. Child's Brain 3: 69–78

Hinton D R, Dolan E, Sima A A F 1984 The value of histopathologic examination of surgically removed blood clot in determining the etiology of spontaneous intracerebral hemorrhage. Stroke 15: 517–520

Hirsch J F, Sainte Rose C, Pierre-Khan A, Pfister A, Hoppe-Hirsch E 1989 Benign astrocytic and oligodendrocytic tumors of the cerebral hemispheres in children. Journal of Neurosurgery 70: 568–572

Horrax G, Wu W Q 1951 Postoperative survival of patients with intracranial oligodendroglioma with special reference to radical tumor removal: a study of 26 patients. Journal of Neurosurgery 8: 473–479

Huang C I, Chiou W H, Ho D M 1987 Oligodendroglioma occurring after radiation therapy for pituitary adenoma. Journal of Neurology, Neurosurgery and Psychiatry 50: 1619–1624

James C D, Carlbom E, Dumanski J P, Hansen M, Nordenskjold M, Collins V P, Cavenee W 1988 Clonal genomic alterations in glioma malignancy stages. Cancer Research 48: 5546–5551

James T G I, Pagel W 1951 Oligodendroglioma with extracranial metastases. British Journal of Surgery 39: 56–65

Jenkins R B, Kimmel D W, Moertel C A, Schultz C G, Scheithauer B W, Kelly P J, DeWald G W 1989 A cytogenetic study of 53 human gliomas. Cancer Genetics Cytogenetics 39: 253–279

Kim D G, Chi J G, Park S H et al 1992 Intraventricular neurocytoma: clinicopathological analysis of seven cases. Journal of Neurosurgery 76: 759–765

Kleihves P, Burger P C Scheithauer B W 1993 The new WHO classification of brain tumors. Brain Pathology 3: 255–268

Kros J M, Troost D, van Eden C G, van der Werf A J M, Uylings H B M 1988 Oligodendroglioma. A comparison of two grading systems. Cancer 61: 2251–2259

Kros J M, van Eden C G, Stefanko S Z, Waayer-van Batenburg M, van der Kwast T H 1990 Prognostic implications of glial fibrillary acidic protein containing cell types in oligodendrogliomas. Cancer 66: 1204–1212

Kros J M, van Eden C G, Vissers C J, Mulder A H, van der Kwast T H 1992 Prognostic relevance of DNA flow cytometry in oligodendroglioma. Cancer 69: 1791–1798

Kubota T, Hayashi M, Kawano H et al 1991 Central neurocytoma: immunohistochemical and ultrastructural study. Acta Neuropathologica 81: 418–427

Kyritsis A P, Levin V A 1992 Chemotherapeutic approaches to the treatment of malignant gliomas. Advances in Oncology 8: 9–13

Kyritsis A P, Yung W K, Bruner J, Gleason M J, Levin V A 1993 The treatment of anaplastic oligodendrogliomas and mixed gliomas. Neurosurgery 32: 365–371

Laws E R, Taylor W F, Clifton M B, Okazaki H 1984 Neurosurgical management of low grade astrocytoma of the cerebral hemispheres. Journal of Neurosurgery 61: 665–673

Lee T K Y, Nakasu Y, Jeffree M A et al 1989 Indolent glioma: a cause of epilepsy. Archives of Diseases of Childhood 64: 1666–1671

Lee Y Y, Van Tassel P 1989 Intracranial oligodendrogliomas: imaging findings in 35 untreated cases. AJNR 10: 119–127

Leibel S A, Sheline G E 1987 Radiation therapy for neoplasms of the brain. Journal of Neurosurgery 66: 1–22

Levin V A, Silver P, Hannigan J, Wara W M, Gutin P H, Davis R L, Wilson C B 1990 Superiority of post-radiotherapy adjuvant chemotherapy with CCNU, procarbazine, and vincristine (PCV) over BCNU for anaplastic gliomas: NCOG 6G61 final report. International Journal of Radiation Oncology Biology Physics 18: 321–324

Lindegaard K F, Mørk S J, Eide G E et al 1987 Statistical analysis of clinicopathological features, radiotherapy, and survival in 170 cases of oligodendroglioma. Journal of Neurosurgery 67: 224–230

Ludwig C L, Smith M T, Godfrey A D, Armbrustmacher V W 1986 A clinicopathological study of 323 patients with oligodendrogliomas. Annals of Neurology 19: 15–21

Luxton G, Petrovich Z, Jozsef G, Nedzi L A, Apuzzo M L J 1993 Stereotactic radiosurgery: principles and comparison of treatment methods. Neurosurgery 32: 241–259

Macdonald D R, Gaspar L E, Cairncross J G 1990 Successful chemotherapy for newly diagnosed aggressive oligodendroglioma. Annals of Neurology 27: 573–574

Margain D, Peretti-Viton P, Perez-Castillo A M, Martini P, Salamon G 1991 Oligodendrogliomas. Journal de Neuroradiologie 18: 153–160

Marks J E, Baglan R J, Prassad S C, Blank W F 1981 Cerebral necrosis: incidence and risk in relation to dose, time, fractionation and volume. International Journal of Radiation Oncology Biology Physics 7: 243–252

Morantz R A 1988 Editorial comment. Neurosurgery 22: 890–891

Mørk S J, Lindegaard K F, Halvorsen T B et al 1985 Oligodendroglioma: incidence and biological behavior in a defined population. Journal of Neurosurgery 63: 881–889

Mørk S J, Halvorsen T B, Lindegaard K F, Eide G E 1986 Oligodendroglioma: histological evaluation and prognosis. Journal of Neuropathology and Experimental Neurology 45: 65–78

Müller W, Áfra D, Schröder R 1977 Supratentorial recurrences of gliomas: morphological studies in relation to time intervals with oligodendrogliomas. Acta Neurochirurgica (Wien) 39: 15–25

Nakagawa Y, Perentes E, Rubinstein L J 1986 Immunohistochemical characterization of oligodendrogliomas: an analysis of multiple markers. Acta Neuropathologica 1986: 15–22

Ohgaki H, Eibl R H, Wiestler O D, Yasargil M G, Newcomb E W, Kleihues P 1991 p53 mutations in nonastrocytic human brain tumors. Cancer Research 51: 6202–6205

Ogasawara H, Kiya K, Uozumi T, Sugiyama K, Kawamoto K, Ohta M 1990 Multiple oligodendroglioma. Case report. Neurologia Medica-Chirugica 30: 127–131

Packer R J, Sutton L N, Rorke L B, Zimmerman R A, Littman P, Bruce D A, Schut L 1985 Oligodendroglioma of the posterior fossa in childhood. Cancer 56: 195–199

Page L K, Lombroso C T, Matson D D 1969 Childhood epilepsy with late detection of cerebral glioma. Journal of Neurosurgery 31: 253–261

Pagni C A, Canavero S, Gaidolfi E 1991 Intramedullary "holocord" oligodendroglioma: case report. Acta Neurochirurgica 113: 96–99

Poisson M, Pereon Y, Chiras J, Delattre J Y 1991 Treatment of recurrent malignant supratentorial gliomas with carboplatin (CBDCA). Journal of Neuro-Oncology 10: 139–144

Reedy D P, Bay J W, Hahn J F 1983 Role of irradiation therapy in the treatment of cerebral oligodendroglioma: and analysis of 57 cases and a literature review. Neurosurgery 13: 499–503

Rey J A, Bello M J, de Campos J M, Kusak M E, Moreno S 1987 Chromosome composition of a series of 22 human low-grade gliomas. Cancer Genetics Cytogenetics 29: 223–237

Ringertz N 1950 Grading of gliomas. APMIS 27: 51–64

Roberts M, German W J 1966 A long term study of patients with oligodendrogliomas. Follow-up of 50 cases including Dr. Harvey Cushing's series. Journal of Neurosurgery 24: 697–700

Rubinstein L J 1972 Oligodendrogliomas. In: Tumors of the central nervous system. Armed Forces Institute of Pathology, Washington DC, pp 85–104

Russell D S, Rubinstein L J 1977 Oligodendroglioma. In: Pathology of tumors of the central nervous system. Edward Arnold, London

Russell D S, Rubinstein L J 1989 Oligodendroglioma. In: Pathology of tumors of the central nervous system, 5th edn. Edward Arnold, London, pp 172–187

Saarinen U M, Pihko H, Mäkipernaa A 1990 High-dose thiotepa with autologous bone marrow rescue in recurrent malignant oligodendroglioma: a case report. Journal of Neuro-Oncology 9: 57–61

Sandeman D R, Sandeman A P, Buston P et al 1990 The management of patients with an intrinsic brain tumor. British Journal of Neurosurgery 4: 299–312

Schold S C, Cairncross J G, Bullard D E 1985 Chemotherapy of primary brain tumors. In: Wilkins R H, Rengachary SS (eds) Neurosurgery. McGraw-Hill, New York, pp 1143–1153

Schwechheimer K, Gass P, Berlet H H 1992 Expression of oligodendroglia and Schwann cell markers in human nervous system tumors. Acta Neuropathologica 83: 283–291

Segall H D, Destian S, Nelson M D, Zee C-S, Ahmadi J 1990 CT and MR imaging in malignant gliomas. In: Apuzzo M L J (ed) Malignant cerebral glioma. AANS Publications Committee, Park Ridge, IL, pp 63–77

Shaw E G 1990 Low-grade gliomas. To treat or not to treat? A radiation oncologist's viewpoint. Archives of Neurology 47: 1138–1139

Shaw E G, Scheithauer B W, O-Fallon J R, Tazelaar H D, Davis D H 1992 Oligodendrogliomas: the Mayo Clinic experience. Journal of Neurosurgery 76: 428–434

Sheline G E, Boldrey E, Karlsberg P, Phillips T L 1964 Therapeutic considerations in tumors affecting the central nervous system: Oligodendrogliomas. Radiology 82: 84–89

Sherer H J 1940 Cerebral astrocytomas and their derivatives. American Journal of Cancer 40: 159–198

Shibata T, Burger P C, Kleihaus P 1988 Ki-67 immunoperoxidase stain as a marker for the histologic grading of nervous system tumors. Acta Neurochirurgica Suppl 43: 103–106

Smith D F, Hutton J L, Sandemann D, Foy P M, Shaw M D, Williams I R, Chadwick D W 1991 The prognosis of primary intracerebral tumors presenting with epilepsy: the outcome of medical and surgical management. Journal of Neurology, Neurosurgery and Psychiatry 54: 915–920

Smith M T, Ludwig C L, Godfrey A D, Armbrustmacher V W 1983 Grading of oligodendrogliomas. Cancer 52: 2107–2114

Soffietti 1990 Histologic and clinical factors of prognostic significance in astrocytic gliomas. Journal of Neurological Science 34: 231–234

Sun Z M, Gnka S, Shitara N, Akanuma A, Takakura K 1988 Factors possibly influencing the prognosis of oligodendroglioma. Neurosurgery 22: 886–891

Tekkok I H, Ayberk G, Saglam S, Onol B 1992 Primary intraventricular oligodendroglioma. Neurochirurgia 35: 63–66

von Deimling A, Kleihaus P, Saremaslani P, Yasargil M G, Spoerri O, Sudhof T C, Wiestler O D 1991 Histogenesis and differentiation potential of central neurocytomas. Laboratory Investigation 64: 585–591

Walker M D, Alexander E, Hunt W E et al 1978 Evaluation of BCNU and/or radiotherapy in treatment of anaplastic gliomas. Journal of Neurosurgery 49: 323–343

Wallner K E, Gonzales M, Sheline G E 1988 Treatment of oligodendrogliomas with or without postoperative irradiation. Journal of Neurosurgery 68: 684–688

Weir B, Elvidge A R 1968 Oligodendrogliomas: an analysis of 63 cases. Journal of Neurosurgery 29: 500–505

Whitton A C, Bloom H J G 1990 Low grade glioma of the cerebral hemispheres in adults: a retrospective analysis of 88 cases. International Journal of Radiation Oncology Biology Physics 18: 783–786

Winger M J, Macdonald D R, Cairncross J G 1989a Supratentorial anaplastic gliomas in adults. The prognostic importance of extent of resection and prior low-grade glioma. Journal of Neurosurgery 71: 487–493

Winger M J, Macdonald M D, Schold S C, Cairncross J G 1989b Selection bias in clinical trials of anaplastic glioma. Annals of Neurology 26: 531–534

Wilkinson I M S, Anderson J R, Holmes A E 1987 Oligodendroglioma: an analysis of 42 cases. Journal of Neurology, Neurosurgery and Psychiatry 50: 304–312

Zülch K J 1986 Brain tumors. Their biology and pathology, 3rd edn., Springer Verlag, Berlin, p 241

27. Intracranial ependymomas

John A. Duncan III   Harold J. Hoffman

Ependymomas are tumors derived from ependymal cells, found lining the cerebral ventricles and central canal of the spinal cord (Dohrmann et al 1976). Intracranial ependymomas are infrequent tumors that account for 1.9–7.8% of all neoplasms of the CNS (Svien et al 1953, Barone & Elvidge 1970, Russell & Rubinstein 1977), and at least half present in the first two decades of life. Tumors of the posterior fossa predominate in young children, while supratentorial tumors are more common in older children, adolescents, and adults (Oi & Raimondi 1982). Intradural spinal cord tumors are of two types: intramedullary ependymomas or myxopapillary ependymomas of the filum terminale. For the purpose of this discussion, only intracranial ependymomas will be considered.

DEMOGRAPHICS

In childhood, ependymomas are the third most common intracranial neoplasm (Wallner et al 1986), accounting for 6–12% of all intracranial tumors (Matson 1969, Koos & Miller 1971, Liu et al 1976, Coulon & Till 1977, Russell & Rubinstein 1977, Dohrmann 1985, Duffner & Cohen 1985, Becker & Halliday 1987, Liebel & Sheline 1987) and up to 30% of all those in children under the age of 3 years (Choux 1983). Two thirds of these neoplasms are infratentorial (Mabon et al 1949, Ringertz & Reymond 1949, Svien et al 1953, Kricheff et al 1963, Fokes & Earle 1969, Matson 1969, Barone & Elvidge 1970, Koos & Miller 1971, Dohrmann et al 1976, Liu et al 1976, Coulon & Till 1977, Bloom 1982, Jenkins 1982, Pierre-Khan et al 1983, Salazar et al 1983, Dohrmann 1985, Gilles et al 1987), and 50% of the affected children present before the age of 3 years (Matson 1969, Dohrmann et al 1976, Coulon & Till 1977, Salazar et al 1983).

At The Hospital for Sick Children (HSC) in Toronto, 67 patients with intracranial ependymomas were treated between 1950 and 1983. The age at presentation ranged from 7 weeks to 16 years, with a mean of 3.7 years. Ependymomas have no sex predilection; of the 67 patients reported, 38 were boys and 29 girls (a ratio of 1.3:1) (Hendrick & Raffel 1989). In the most recent series, reported by Nazar et al (1990), 35 patients with infratentorial ependymoma were treated between 1970 and 1987. The mean age at diagnosis was 70.5 months, without sex predilection (18 males, 17 females) (Fig. 27.1).

SIGNS AND SYMPTOMS

In posterior fossa ependymomas, the most common presenting symptoms are nausea and vomiting followed by headache. These symptoms are related to hydrocephalus, caused by obstruction of the fourth ventricle. Other symptoms, including ataxia, visual disturbances, dizziness, neck pain, and hemiparesis, are related to compression of posterior fossa structures (Hendrick & Raffel 1989). Children less than 2 years of age present with vomiting, irritability, and lethargy, reflecting the presence of their open sutures (which provide room for hydrocephalus) and their neurologic immaturity (Shuman et al 1975).

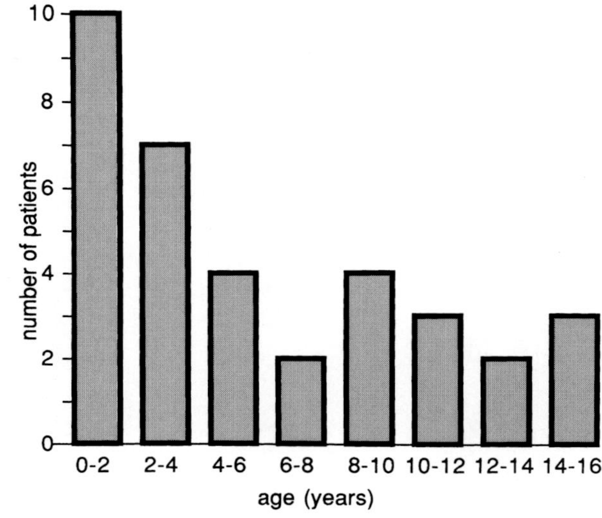

Fig. 27.1 Age distribution in 35 children treated at The Hospital for Sick Children, 1970–1987.

Table 27.1 Symptoms of children at The Hospital for Sick Children, Toronto, with intracranial ependymomas.

Symptom	Series 1950–1983 All children (n = 67)	Series 1970–1987 < 2 yrs (n = 10)	> 2 yrs (n = 25)
Nausea and vomiting	61%	80%	80%
Headache	52%	0	68%
Ataxia	33%	30%	28%
Irritability	8%	60%	0
Weight loss	13%	20%	16%

In the two previous HSC series, nausea and vomiting were present in the majority of patients, followed by headache, ataxia, and weight loss (Hendrick & Raffel 1989, Nazar et al 1990) (Table 27.1). The duration of symptoms was approximately 3 months on average and ranged from 4–450 days.

The most common presenting signs in children are papilledema, ataxia, nystagmus, gaze palsy, lower cranial nerve palsy, and increased head circumference in children less than 2 years old. Again, these are related to increased intracranial pressure (papilledema, sixth-nerve palsy, increased head circumference) or the tumor mass compressing or infiltrating adjacent cerebellum or brainstem. In the earlier HSC series, papilledema was present in 39 patients (58%), ataxia in 30 (45%), nystagmus in 24 (36%), gaze palsy in 18 (27%), and lower cranial nerve palsy in 7 (11%) (Hendrick & Raffel 1989). Focal cerebellar, brainstem, or lower cranial nerve signs have been shown to correlate well with tumor invasion of these structures.

As with any tumor in young children, many presenting signs and symptoms are nonspecific (irritability, fever, lethargy, weight loss, developmental delay) and require a high index of suspicion.

Supratentorial ependymomas are more common in older children and adults. These are usually accompanied by signs and symptoms of mass effect or focal neurologic deficit, including headache, nausea, vomiting, seizure, lethargy, behavioral change, intellectual impairment, papilledema, hemiparesis, apraxia, or visual field loss. Approximately one half of the supratentorial tumors arise from the wall of the ventricle; the remainder arise in areas remote from the ventricular wall from presumed fetal ependymal cell rests in adjacent white matter. Supratentorial ependymomas often result in ventricular compression and midline shift.

HISTOLOGY

Histologically, ependymomas are characterized by three features: true ependymal rosettes, perivascular pseudorosettes, and blepharoplasts. Blepharoplasts are the basal bodies of cilia and are contained in cells arranged around a lumen. Anaplastic (malignant) ependymomas contain

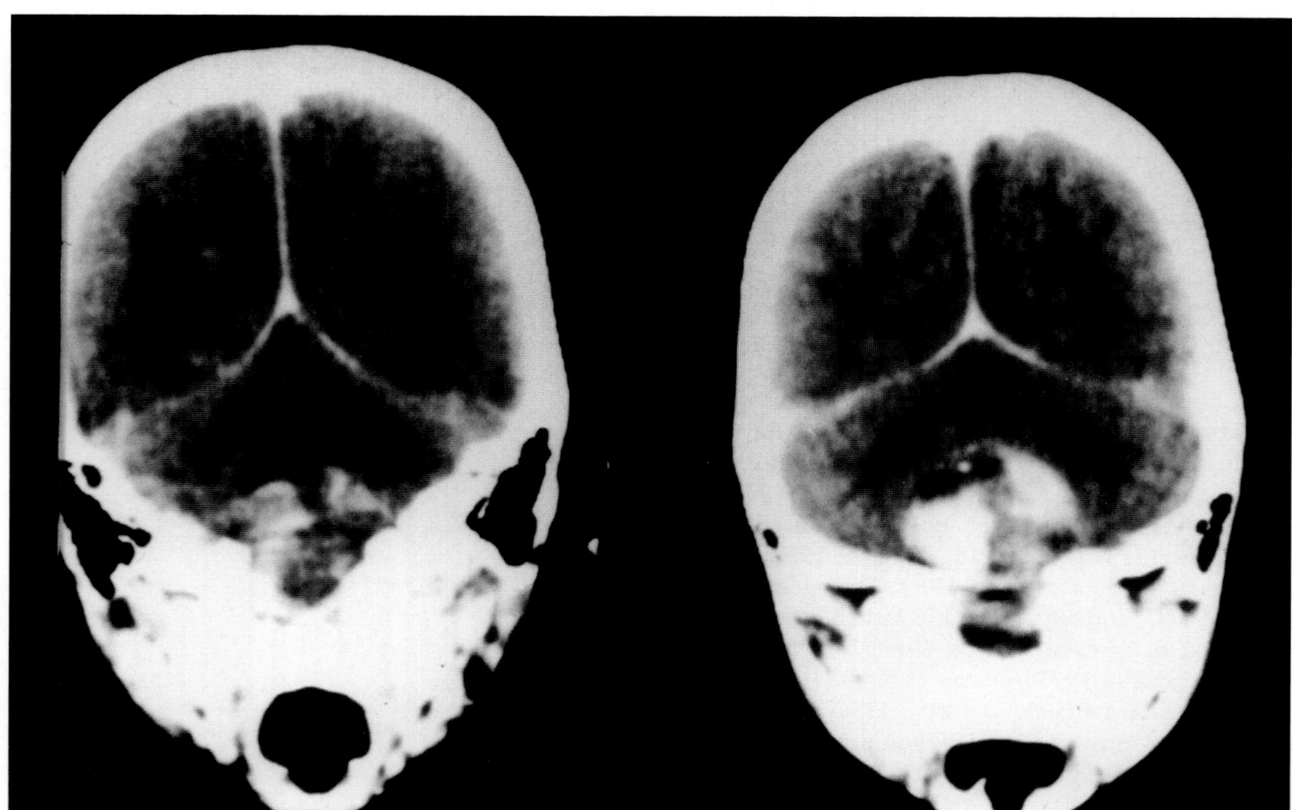

Fig. 27.2 Coronal computed tomography with contrast, showing extension of tumor through foramen magnum.

all of the above structures, in addition to nuclear hyperchromatism, cytoplasmic and nuclear pleomorphism, disorganized cytoarchitecture, mitosis, necrosis, and other features of anaplasia.

Many histologic classification schemes have been proposed for ependymomas (Kernohan & Fletcher-Kernohan 1937, Kernohan & Sayre 1952, Rubinstein 1972, Russell & Rubinstein 1977). Although each uses different nomenclature and criteria, the underlying common denominator is that of either low or high grade with regard to malignant histologic features. Supratentorial tumors are reported to be more mitotically active than infratentorial tumors (Zülch 1986). Yet the degree of malignancy varies highly according to intracranial tumor location, and may in fact be more a function of patient age. High grade, anaplastic tumors tend to be more common in the posterior fossa of young children (< 5) and in the cerebral hemispheres of adults.

NEUROIMAGING

On computed tomography (CT) scans, intracranial ependymomas may be of high density, isodense with brain, or of mixed density on precontrast scan. They usually show some enhancement after IV contrast infusion. Calcification occurs in 50% of all tumors. Supratentorial tumors are often cystic, whereas infratentorial tumors are usually solid with downward extension through the vallecula and below the foramen magnum (Fig. 27.2). Hydrocephalus, with obstruction at the level of the fourth ventricle, is very common (Svien et al 1953, Zee et al 1983).

Nuclear magnetic resonance imaging (MRI) better defines anatomical detail in the transaxial, coronal, and sagittal planes. Beam-hardening artefacts, common in the posterior fossa with CT, are not present, and the level of extension is well defined.

Multiplanar MRI evaluation of both the brain and spinal cord is critical for optimal surgical planning and adjuvant radiotherapy. Multiple MRI parameters should be examined (T1, proton density, and T2), as the relationship of tumor to normal brain structures is better determined on T2 and proton density images. The degree of tumor extension into the cerebrospinal fluid (CSF) spaces around the brainstem and spinal cord is better delineated on T1 or proton density images (Fig. 27.3). Enhancement with gadolinium is necessary for optimal spinal cord imaging and thus accurate clinical staging of CNS disease (Spoto et al 1990, Healey et al 1991).

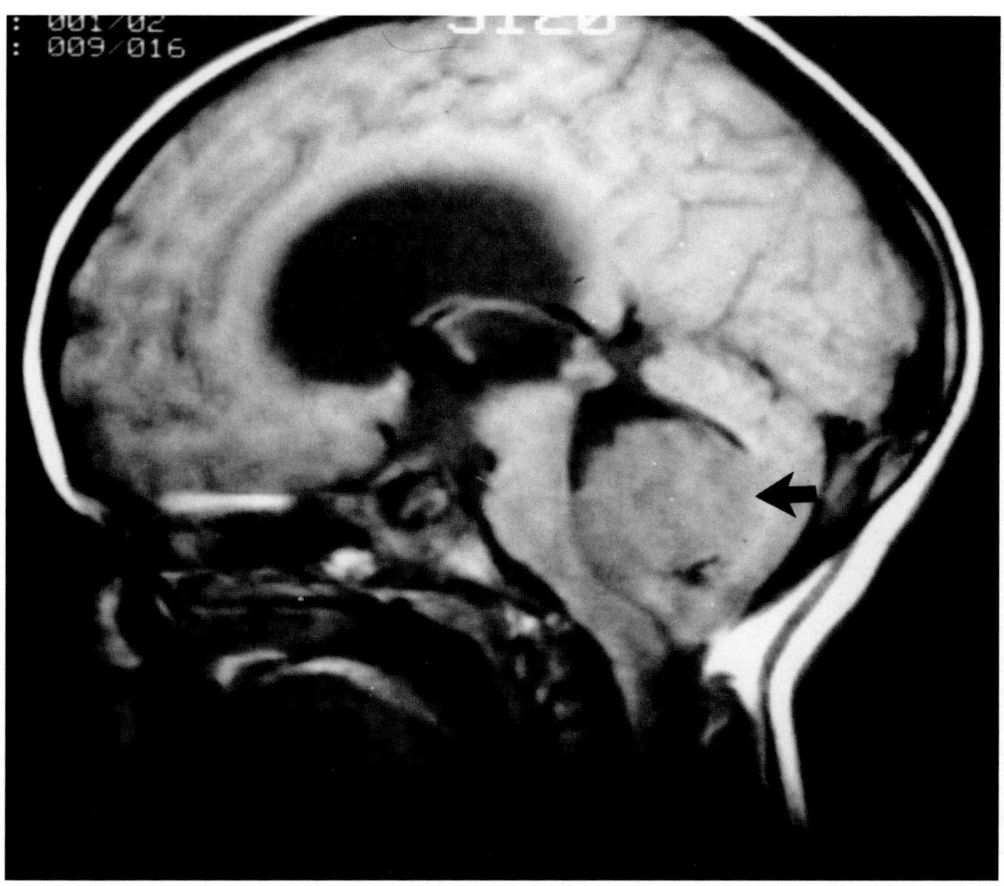

Fig. 27.3 Sagittal magnetic resonance imaging, showing tumor in fourth ventricle (arrow) with hydrocephalus and brainstem displacement.

Angiography is no longer necessary as an investigative tool for a patient with an ependymoma.

DIFFERENTIAL DIAGNOSIS

The differential diagnosis of mass lesions in or near the fourth ventricle in children includes medulloblastoma, astrocytoma, ependymoma, choroid plexus papilloma, brainstem glioma, dermoid cyst, and meningioma. Other than routine preoperative laboratory examinations, no specific tests are needed or helpful in narrowing the differential diagnosis. Cytologic evaluation of CSF needs to be performed only for staging purposes and may be omitted if the perioperative spinal MRI finding is definitive and the operative tissue diagnosis is well established.

Preoperative neuroimaging may help to narrow the differential diagnosis but is not diagnostic. Medulloblastoma is commonly hyperdense on noncontrast CT and enhances more uniformly after IV contrast infusion. In addition, this lesion tends to extend upward to the incisura, in contrast to the downward projection of ependymomas. Juvenile pilocytic astrocytomas are cystic, partially solid tumors, arising off midline in the cerebellar hemisphere, and are hypodense on precontrast CT scans. Enhancement of the solid component and cyst wall is variable. Other tumors, such as the choroid plexus papilloma and meningioma, enhance strongly and homogeneously. Both are intraventricular tumors, often filling the fourth ventricle. Brainstem gliomas and dermoid/epidermoid tumors are best localized and differentiated with MRI.

SURGICAL THERAPY

At present, surgery remains the most effective mode of treatment. It has three goals: establishment of tissue diagnosis, total removal of tumor, and re-establishment of normal CSF flow. Historically, operative mortality is reported to range from 17–50% (Ringertz & Reymond 1949, Phillips et al 1964, Dohrmann et al 1976), but more recent studies suggest it is now less than 8% for resection of posterior fossa tumors (Nazar et al 1990, Sutton et al 1990, Lyons & Kelly 1991). At highly specialized centers, such as HSC, mortality is less than 1% (Tomita et al 1988). Perioperative morbidity, however, continues to remain high (10–30%), with most deficits related to brainstem injury.

Preoperative shunting is not necessary and can be dangerous. Adequate decompression of the posterior fossa can be achieved with preoperative steroids, osmotic diuresis, and hyperventilation. Only rarely is CSF diversion required, and if needed is best performed intraoperatively via an occipital or frontal burr hole. Upward herniation, intratumoral hemorrhage, and postoperative subdural hematoma are avoided if shunting is not performed (Barone & Elvidge 1970, Tomita et al 1988, Hendrick & Raffel 1989). The possibility of upward herniation or hemorrhage within the ependymoma is real and can be fatal. Even if the patient's neurologic condition is initially stable or improves after shunting, the tumor within the fourth ventricle can subsequently shift upward by decompression of the supratentorial hydrocephalus, leading to hemorrhage and/or brainstem compression (Tomita et al 1988).

Operative approach

The patient is placed prone with the neck flexed. A Sugita four-pin fixation head holder is used in patients 2 years of age and older. A midline incision is made, extending from just above the inion to the spinous process of C3–4. Paraspinal musculature is reflected from the occiput and C1. A suboccipital craniectomy that includes the foramen magnum inferiorly is then performed. The transverse sinus should be defined superiorly. The posterior arch of C1 is then removed, as well as additional cervical lamina, depending on the inferior extent of tumor as shown on radiographs. The dura is opened with a standard Y-shaped incision. The foramen of Magendie is defined and the tumor exposed. The tumor is soft and gelatinous, not encapsulated, reddish grey in color, and typically found in the midline. It can also be found in the lateral recesses with extension out of the foramen of Luschka. The vermis is split inferiorly to give wide access to the tumor in the fourth ventricle. The tumor is removed by bipolar electrocautery and the ultrasonic aspirator; care is taken not to injure structures in the floor of the fourth ventricle. Most tumors are easily removed from the walls and roof of the fourth ventricle (Hendrick & Raffel 1989). 'Plastic' ependymomas (Courville & Broussalian 1961) are a distinct type of tumor and will often mold themselves to available spaces in the posterior fossa, without being adherent (Fig. 27.4). They often present bilaterally in the cerebellopontine angle and are easy to remove.

Ependymomas found unilaterally in the cerebellopontine or cerebellomedullary cistern, however, often pose difficult surgical problems, as the regional arteries and cranial nerves are compressed or engulfed by the tumor, and the brainstem may be compressed or invaded (Tomita et al 1988). It may be possible to remove these tumors with minimal damage to cranial nerves and arteries with magnification and meticulous dissection. The cerebellopontine angle is approached extra-axially, requiring additional lateral bone removal from the midline suboccipital craniectomy. The vertebral artery and its branches must be identified and preserved. Patients may show transient dysfunction of respective cranial nerves, but as a rule enjoy complete or nearly complete recovery over several months if the continuity of these nerves is preserved (Tomita et al 1988).

The major difficulty is encountered at the end of tumor removal when the site of invasion is determined. This can

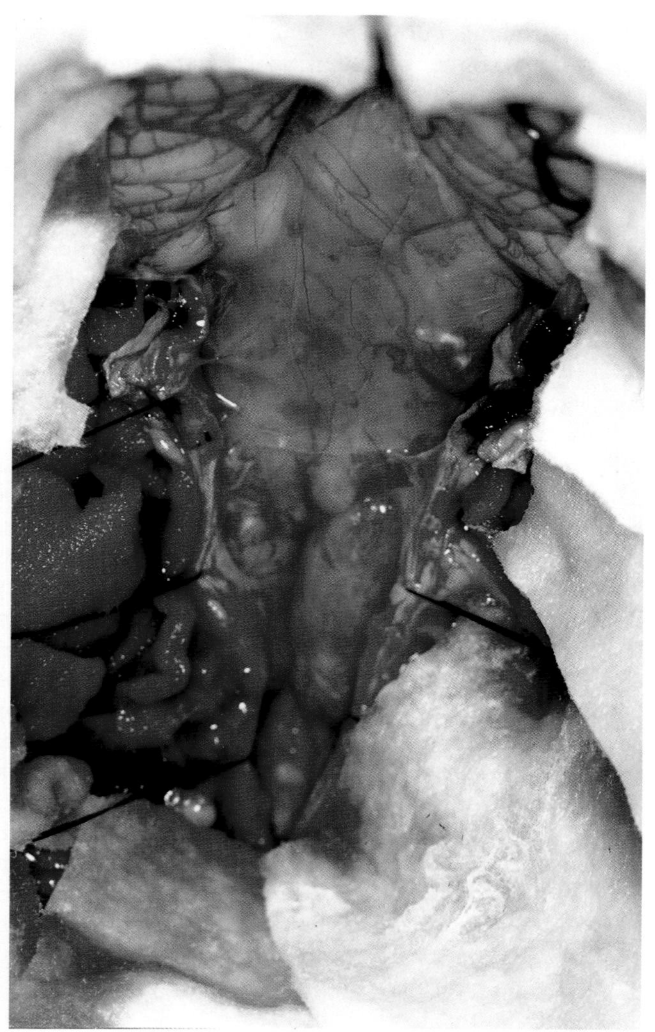

Fig. 27.4 Intraoperative photograph of desmoplastic ependymoma at the foramen magnum.

be the floor of the fourth ventricle, where the tumor remains adherent. In order to avoid significant morbidity, the surgeon must frequently leave behind a small amount of tumor extending into the floor. Some surgeons advocate use of the CO_2 laser for near-total removal of infiltrative tumor, but this practice increases the risk of brainstem injury (Tomita et al 1988). Tumor extension up the aqueduct of Sylvius can often be removed completely. A watertight dural closure is achieved and the wound closed in layers. A dural graft is usually necessary; cadaveric, lyophilized dura is frequently used (Hendrick & Raffel 1989).

SURVIVAL

Today, the 5-year survival rate for patients (children and adults) with intracranial ependymoma is approximately 50% (Phillips et al 1964, Dohrmann et al 1976, Oi & Raimondi 1982, Pierre-Khan et al 1983, Nazar et al 1990, Healey et al 1991, Lyons & Kelly 1991). Healey et al (1991), recently reported actuarial survival rates for their entire cohort of 61% for 5 years and 46% for 10 years. This broad range, however, disregards patient age and tumor location. When grouped according to these factors, the 5-year survival rate in children with posterior fossa tumors ranges from 14–45%, with increased survival reported in the most recent series with similar population profiles (Dohrmann et al 1976, Coulon & Till 1977, Tomita et al 1988, Nazar et al 1990, Sutton et al 1990). Studies of children with either supratentorial or infratentorial tumors show an increase in the 5-year survival rate ranging from 26% to 51%, reflecting longer survival in children with supratentorial ependymomas (Bloom 1982, Pierre-Khan et al 1983, Cohen & Duffner 1985, Tomita et al 1988, Sutton et al 1990).

Determinants of outcome

Age

Patient age strongly correlates with outcome. In a report by Lyons & Kelly (1991), 5-year survival rates for adults and children with posterior fossa tumors were 76% and 14% respectively. This observation has been made in numerous studies (Garrett & Simpson 1983, Ilgren et al 1984, West et al 1985), irrespective of tumor location, and may be an important prognostic factor. The prognosis is reported to be significantly worse in children 5 years of age and younger, and dismal when children are less than 24 months old (Pierre-Khan et al 1983, Goldwein et al 1988, Lefkowitz et al 1988, Nazar et al 1990, Healey et al 1991, Lyons & Kelly 1991). Healey et al (1991) reported an overall actuarial survival of 0% at 12 years of age in infants 24 months and younger at the time of diagnosis, in contrast to 62% in older children.

In other combined series, older patients fared worse than young children (Chin et al 1982, Salazar et al 1983, Lejeune et al 1987). This discrepancy is partially explained by inconsistency in defining the age of children and the increased incidence of malignant supratentorial ependymoma in adults. Our experience at HCS, however, strongly supports the conclusion that the younger the child, the worse the prognosis (Fig. 27.5).

Location

Numerous studies demonstrate a worse prognosis associated with tumors of the fourth ventricle than with supratentorial tumors (Dohrmann et al 1976, Oi & Raimondi 1982, Pierre-Khan et al 1983). In children less than 5 years of age, almost all tumors arise in the midline of the posterior fossa and, in our experience, carry the worst prognosis.

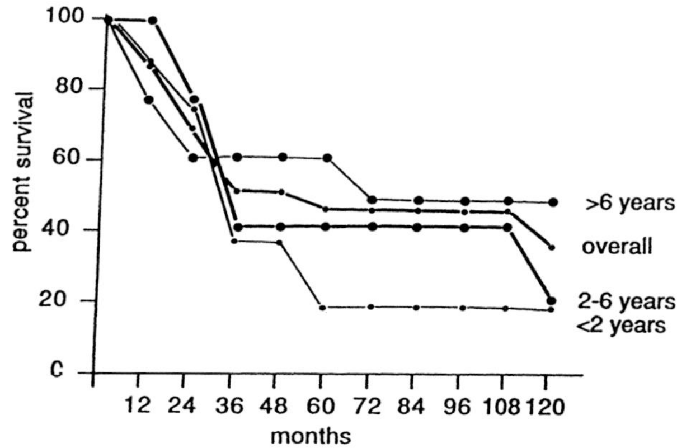

Fig. 27.5 Age-related survival, The Hospital for Sick Children, 1970–1987.

A 1993 report by Ikezaki et al that considered only tumors in the posterior fossa correlates microanatomical location with degree of resection and postoperative survival. In this series, tumors were classified into three types — mid-floor, lateral, and roof — based on their primary location relative to the fourth ventricle. Total removal was never achieved in lateral tumors, and 5-year survival was markedly reduced compared with the other two groups (Ikezaki et al 1993). This study emphasizes the difficulty in achieving a gross total resection in this location, doubtless because of the tumor's proximity to cranial nerves and blood vessels, and tumor invasion of the brainstem. It is hoped that this method of classification may prove prognostically useful and aid in the management of children with a posterior fossa ependymoma.

Tumor grade

The relationship of histopathologic findings to survival is not clear. In some series, the median survival rate in patients with a malignant ependymoma is less than in those with benign ependymoma (Kernohan & Sayre 1952, Rubinstein 1970, Renaudin et al 1979), whereas in others it is unaltered (Fokes & Earle 1969, Barone & Elvidge 1970, Dohrmann et al 1976). The reason for this discrepancy, although unknown, is probably related to variations in tumor biology for histologically similar neoplasms, to inconsistency and lack of uniformity in histologic diagnosis, or possibly to wide intratumoral histologic variability resulting in incorrect tissue diagnosis.

Today, most institutions use the two-tiered World Health Organization (WHO) classification of ependymomas (Table 27.2). Ependymoblastomas are not included in this scheme and are classified as primitive neuroectodermal tumors (PNET) with ependymal differentiation (Rorke 1983, Rorke et al 1985). These malignant tumors differ significantly from ependymomas in both biologic activity and response to irradiation or various chemotherapeutic agents, and will not be considered further.

On the basis of the WHO classification system for ependymomas, many authors believe that tumor histology (grade) is a useful prognostic indicator — a view with which we agree (Dohrmann et al 1976, Kim & Fayos 1977, Bloom 1982, Chin et al 1982, Garrett & Simpson 1983, Salazar 1983, Marsh & Laws 1987, Shaw et al 1987, Nazar et al 1990). Other series do not support this view; in these, tumor grade has had either no or poor correlation with outcome (Kricheff et al 1963, Fokes & Earle 1969, Barone & Elvidge 1970, Shapiro 1975, Mørk & Loken 1977, Oi & Raimondi 1982, Ilgren et al 1984, Rorke 1987, Rawlings et al 1988, Ross & Rubinstein 1989). Because of these conflicting reports and the known diversity of histologic features both between tumors and within different areas of the same specimen, Nazar et al (1990) developed a three-tiered system for infratentorial ependymomas based on mitotic activity, cellularity, and necrosis (categories I–III, Table 27.3). In the most recent HSC series reported (Nazar et al 1990), these three categories had a significant association with survival rate, especially the mitotic index. Five-year survival rates of 70.5%, 49.5%, and 12.1% were observed for categories I, II and III, respectively, and more important, the difference in outcome was significant between categories I and III (Fig. 27.6). Not surprisingly, category I tumors showed

Table 27.2 World Health Organization Classification (Zurich, 1990)

	True rosettes	Pseudorosettes	Blepharoplasts	Dense cellularity	Necrosis	Mitosis
Benign	+	+	+	–	–	+/–
Anaplastic	+	+	+	+	+	++

Table 27.3 Histologic categorization of ependymoma. Source: Nazar et al (1990)

Feature	Category I	Category II	Category III					
Mitotic index	low	low	mod	mod	mod	high	high	high
Dense cellularity	–	+	+	–	+	–	+	+
Necrosis	–	+	–	+	+	+	–	+

mod = moderate

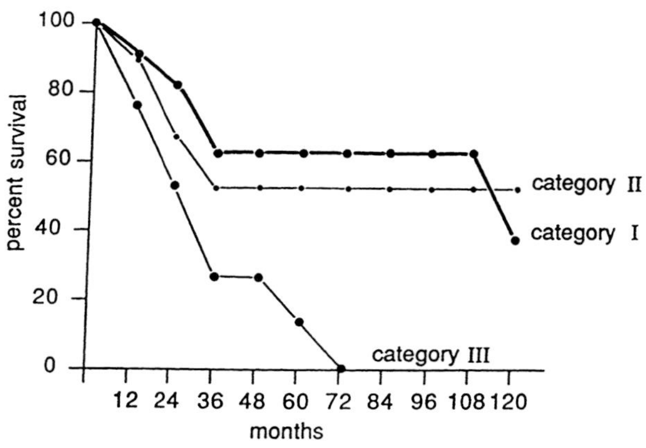

Fig. 27.6 Survival related to histology, categories I–III, The Hospital for Sick Children, 1970–1980 (see Table 28.2).

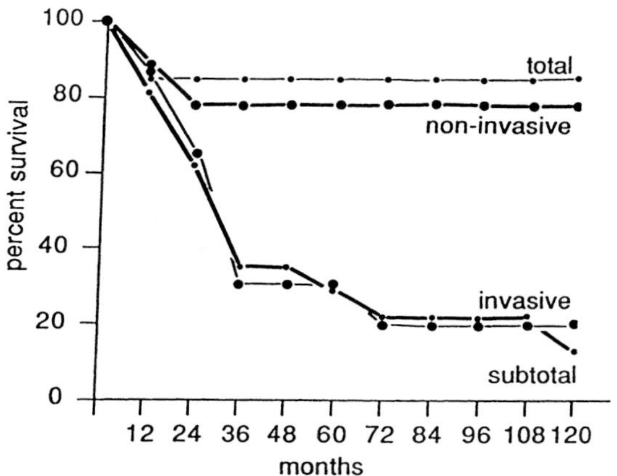

Fig. 27.7 Survival related to tumor removal (total vs subtotal) and degree of invasion, The Hospital for Sick Children, 1970–1987. Differences were significant at 60 months ($p < 0.05$).

the lowest incidence of patients presenting with focal cerebellar, brainstem, or cranial nerve signs (25%), the lowest incidence of invasion (22.2%), and the highest rate for gross total resection (71%) among all noninvasive tumors.

Tumor resection

Numerous recent studies have shown a high correlation between gross total removal of tumor and improved survival, and thus the extent of tumor resection has become the major determinant of outcome (Oi & Raimondi 1982, Hendrick & Raffel 1989, Nazar et al 1990, Papadopoulos et al 1990, Sutton et al 1990, Healey et al 1991). This relationship has been shown in studies of infratentorial as well as intracranial tumors from both infra- and supratentorial locations. In 1991, Healey et al reported a 75% 5-year freedom from progressive disease (FPD) in patients with no residual postoperative tumor, in contrast to a 5-year FPD of 0% in those with residual disease. In their study, residual disease was based on immediate postoperative neuroimaging (CT or MRI) and, not surprisingly, correlated poorly with surgical assessment of the extent of tumor resection (< 70%).

The effect of resection in patients with supratentorial tumors is not as clear. Some recent reports show no or little effect on survival, whereas others suggest a trend toward better survival in those who have undergone more extensive resection (Sutton et al 1990, Lyons & Kelly 1991). Interestingly, in these studies, those heavily weighted with children show correlation with survival, whereas those composed predominantly of adults do not. Once again, tumor grade, degree of invasion, and location probably determine the extent of surgical resection.

The more radical the resection, the greater the likelihood of postoperative neurologic deficit. The favorable outcomes seen with more aggressive resections may not be due solely to the resection itself but may reflect tumor biology (i.e. grade, invasiveness, etc.) that makes radical resection possible or even probable (Fig. 27.7). Nonetheless, an attempt at aggressive surgical resection seems appropriate, even though it may result in postoperative morbidity in some patients (Sutton et al 1990).

RATE OF RECURRENCE AND PATTERN OF FAILURE

Although the majority of ependymomas are histologically 'benign' in appearance, the outlook remains poor because of the high rate of recurrence. The median time to recurrence after total resection is considered to be 22–24 months; recurrences are infrequent after 36 months and few, if any, have been seen past 62 months (Hendrick & Raffel 1989, Nazar et al 1990). Tumors recur in virtually all patients with subtotal resection within 12–14 months, regardless of adjuvant treatment. Unfortunately, gross total resection is possible in fewer than 25% of cases as a result of the infiltrative, invasive nature of this tumor; the prognosis is therefore generally poor.

Goldwein et al (1990) recently reported a 2-year actuarial survival rate of 29% and a progression-free survival of 23% in children with recurrent ependymoma. Overall survival was much higher for patients with histologically benign lesions at relapse (53% vs 9%) and for those treated at first relapse compared with those treated subsequently (39% vs 7%). Other factors, including interval to relapse (< 1 year), extent of surgery, patient age (< 4 years), or tumor location (supratentorial vs infratentorial) had no impact on survival.

Ependymomas recur almost invariably at the primary site, with CSF metastasis ranging from 0–64% in different historical series (Svien et al 1953, Kricheff et al 1963, Sagerman et al 1965, Barone & Elvidge 1970, Shuman et al 1975, Dohrmann et al 1976, Liu et al 1976, Coulon & Till 1977, Kim & Fayos 1977, Mørk & Loken 1977, Bouchard 1980, Bloom 1982, Chin et al 1982, Marks &

Adler 1982, Pierre-Khan et al 1983, Salazar et al 1983, Wallner et al 1986, Marsh & Laws 1987, Nazar et al 1990). Yet, although CNS dissemination is possible, isolated distant metastases are rare. Even though autopsy series can show spinal cord seeding in approximately 30% of patients (Salazar 1983, Nazar et al 1990), average overall seeding from recent combined series of infratentorial and supratentorial tumors was 10–13% (Nazar et al 1990). More important, symptomatic spinal cord metastases occur in only 4–6% (Nazar et al 1990, Lyons & Kelly 1991) of patients with infratentorial tumors.

Although a higher incidence has been noted for infratentorial ependymomas of poorly differentiated tumors of the fourth ventricle (Kim & Fayos 1977, Oi & Raimondi 1982, Pierre-Khan et al 1983), metastases are *almost always* found in association with tumor recurrence at the primary site. This finding suggests that local recurrence is responsible for tumor seeding and that isolated, distant metastasis is rare, thus underlining the importance of local control.

ADJUVANT THERAPY

Radiation

Historically, 5-year survival rates for intracranial ependymomas treated by surgery alone ranged from 17–27% (Cushing 1932, Ringertz & Reymond 1949, Fokes & Earle 1969, Gilles et al 1987). These rates were substantially improved by the addition of postoperative irradiation, which has resulted in a 5-year survival rate of 40–87% in patients receiving doses of 45 Gy or higher (Sheline 1975, Dohrmann et al 1976, Bloom 1982, Salazar et al 1983, Liebel & Sheline 1987). Although not proven, a dose-response relationship probably exists. In a review of the literature, Liebel & Sheline reported in 1987 that doses less than 45 Gy resulted in a 5-year survival rate of approximately 50% (range 36–70%) for intracranial tumors. The rate increased to 46–87% in patients who received doses greater than or equal to 45 Gy.

Today the benefit of postoperative irradiation is well accepted, even though the radiosensitivity of ependymomas is highly variable, contrary to earlier optimistic reports (Sheline 1975). It should be stressed that tumor histology does not correlate with response to irradiation and that both low and high grade tumors are equally likely to recur quickly.

The main controversy today centers on the field size of irradiation. It has not been well established whether whole brain irradiation (WBI) or craniospinal irradiation (CSI) significantly improves outcome compared with involved field irradiation (IFI) (Sagerman et al 1965, Salazar et al 1975, Bloom 1982, Marks & Adler 1982, Garrett & Simpson 1983, Salazar et al 1983, Wara 1985, Wallner et al 1986, Liebel & Sheline 1987, Marsh & Laws 1987, Shaw et al 1987, Kun et al 1988, Hendrick & Raffel 1989). It has also been suggested that craniospinal irradiation may not prevent spread of tumor through the CSF (Oi & Raimondi 1982). Earlier reports that relatively high rates of CSF seeding necessitate CSI seem unjustified, considering that failure invariably occurs at the primary site and that isolated spinal cord metastases are rare. Efforts should be directed toward achieving local control and developing new protocols.

Chemotherapy

The failure of surgery and irradiation to achieve long-term survival has led to the use of various chemotherapeutic drugs in the treatment of both primary and recurrent disease. In recurrent ependymomas, several centers have reported some benefit from treatment with cisplatin and VP-16 (Goldwein et al 1990), but as yet no conclusive evidence supports the use of any agent to treat either newly diagnosed or recurrent tumors (Khan et al 1982, Walker & Allen 1983, Sexauer et al 1985, Gaynon et al 1987, Bertolone et al 1989, Goldwein et al 1990, Sutton et al 1990, Tamura et al 1990).

Of special interest are several reports of histologic change after irradiation and chemotherapy. In the recent report by Goldwein et al (1990), the histology of recurrent tumor differed from that at initial diagnosis in 12 of 33 specimens examined. Differentiation along more benign ependymal lines was seen in a significant number of patients. This phenomenon has been observed at several centers in patients with prolonged survival, but evidence of its occurrence remains anecdotal. It was illustrated in a patient treated recently at HSC. An 8.5-year-old white male had presented at 20 months of age with a rapidly progressive left sixth-nerve palsy, unsteadiness of gait, irritability, vomiting, and weight loss. CT and MRI scans showed a large posterior fossa mass, filling the fourth ventricle and extending into the left cerebellopontine angle (Fig. 27.8). This mass enhanced with contrast, showed no calcification, and was associated with minimal to moderate hydrocephalus.

In March 1986, the patient underwent a suboccipital craniectomy and subtotal resection of tumor. Clinical staging showed no spread of disease. The child underwent adjuvant therapy consisting of 50 Gy of IFI (25 fractions) and seven cycles of '8 in 1' chemotherapy (Geyer et al 1988) after completion of radiotherapy. This regimen includes cisplatinum. Over the next 2 years, he improved clinically, with resolution of the hemiparesis and ataxia and increased function of the left facial nerve. Histologic diagnosis showed an anaplastic ependymoma with areas of increased cellularity, mitosis, and focal areas of necrosis.

The patient did well until December 1989, when he developed recurrent tumor in the left foramen of Luschka. He was reoperated on and a gross total resection was achieved. Histologic examination of the entire surgical specimen revealed only benign ependymoma (Fig. 27.9).

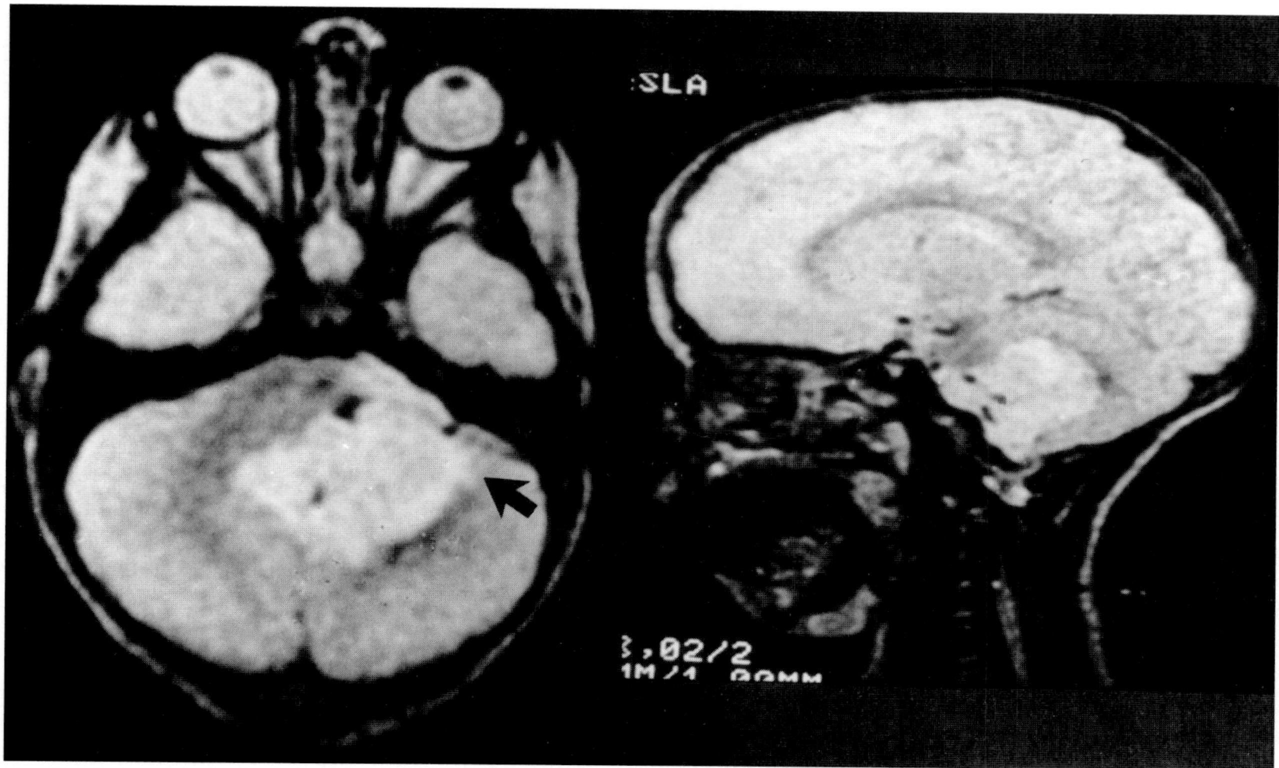

Fig. 27.8 Magnetic resonance imaging (axial, sagittal), showing midline tumor with extension into left cerebellopontine angle (arrow).

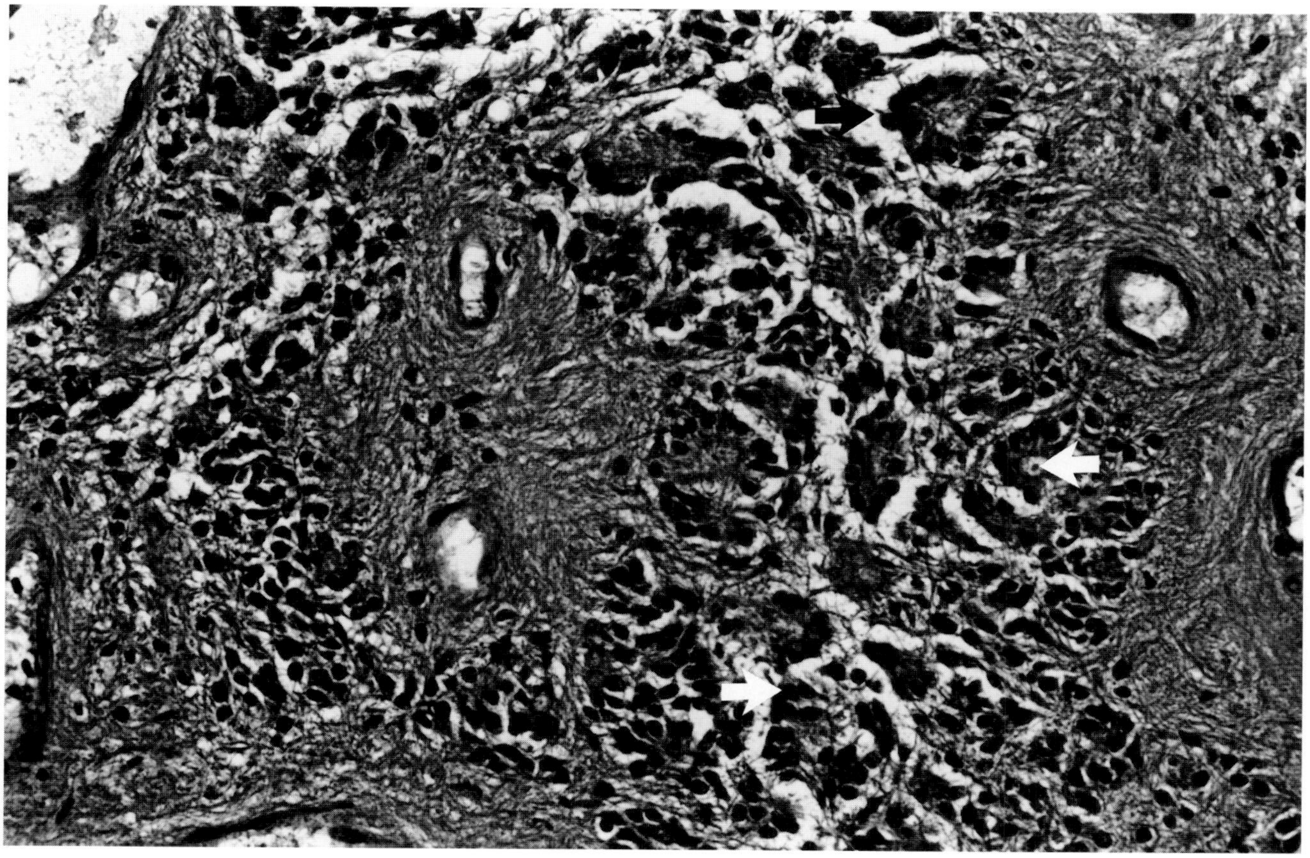

Fig. 27.9 Benign ependymoma with true rosettes (arrows). Hematoxylin and eosin, × 300.

The child required one additional surgical resection for a small local recurrence of a tumor that was histologically identical to the previous specimen. Today he is essentially asymptomatic; his left facial palsy has improved and he suffers only moderate left sensorineural hearing loss.

Thus, surgery, conventional radiation, and chemotherapeutic regimens that include cisplatinum or carboplatinum and VP-16 may significantly alter the histology and biologic behavior of aggressive tumors (i.e. category III), resulting in local control in high risk patients.

OVERALL MANAGEMENT PLAN

In 1990, on the basis of results obtained at HSC, Nazar et al (1990) proposed the treatment protocol referred to earlier for children with infratentorial ependymoma in which patients are grouped into categories I–III, based on tumor histology. All cases are appropriately staged with spinal MRI and/or CSF cytology, and those with spinal seeding receive CSI after surgery. Surgery is attempted in all primary cases with the intent of achieving a gross total resection. Tumor invasiveness, histologic findings, and degree of tumor removal determine whether patients receive surgery alone, surgery with radiation, or a combination of surgery, radiation, and chemotherapy (Fig. 27.10). In children less than 3 years of age, a schedule of chemotherapy followed by delayed radiotherapy is employed for all invasive or subtotally resected tumors.

Today, for all patients with intracranial ependymoma, we continue to advocate the use of this protocol with minor modifications. Because of the growing number of permanent cures reported (Ringertz & Reymond 1949, Koos & Miller 1971, Dohrmann et al 1976, Mørk & Loken 1977, Oi & Raimondi 1982, Nazar et al 1990) following total removal of histologically benign, noninvasive tumors (category I and plastic ependymomas), we strongly recommend surgery *alone* followed by frequent, scheduled, high-quality neuroimaging. Unfortunately, the percentage of patients in this situation is small — probably fewer than 20–25% of all patients initially treated.

Most patients will require adjuvant treatment with radiation, chemotherapy, or both. Because tumor recurrence is almost always at the primary site, great emphasis should be placed on achieving local control. Since no evidence to date clearly supports one type of radiotherapy, IFI (50–55 Gy) with broad margins (> 2 cm) seems most appropriate for infratentorial tumors. An argument can still be made for WBI, especially in more diffuse supratentorial and anaplastic tumors; however, IFI significantly reduces the overall radiation exposure and late deleterious effects on cognitive function and growth seen with the use of WBI in children.

The addition of chemotherapy, specifically the choice of drug, remains controversial. Regimens including VP-16, cis- or carboplatinum seem partially efficacious in recurrent cases, although there is no evidence to support an improved outcome in the treatment of either primary or recurrent disease. Because of anecdotal reports, such as the case we describe, however, aggressive protocols employing these agents in initial postoperative treatment regimens *must* be pursued and are strongly advocated here.

Treatments achieving local control must be aggressively sought. Second-look operations for unexpected residual disease on postoperative imaging are encouraged in patients with noninvasive, benign histologic findings. New treatments such as radiosurgery, use of radiosensitizers, and immunotherapy hold promise for the future. Well-designed, multicenter trials are needed to test new treatment methods, improve local tumor control, and achieve a better outcome for patients with intracranial ependymoma.

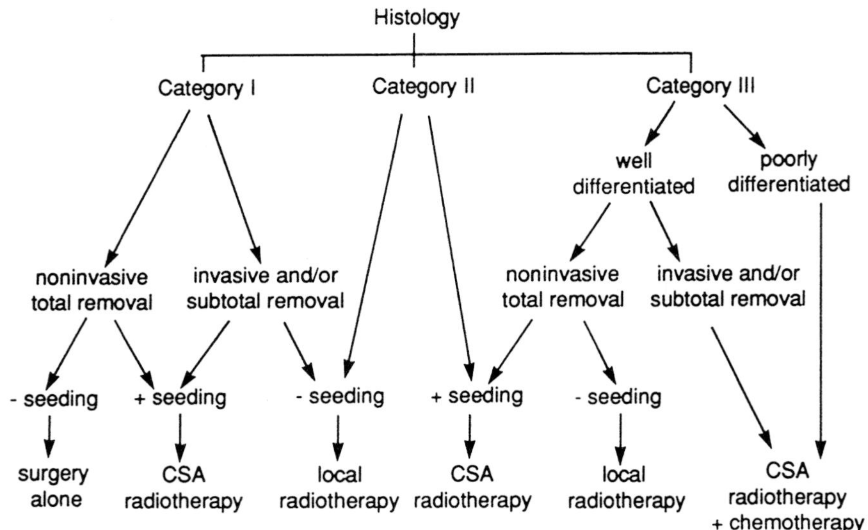

Fig. 27.10 Treatment protocol in patients 3 years and older at The Hospital for Sick Children.

REFERENCES

Barone B M, Elvidge A R 1970 Ependymomas. A clinical study. Journal of Neurosurgery 33: 428–438

Becker L E, Halliday W C 1987 Central nervous system tumors of childhood. Perspectives in Pediatric Pathology 10: 86–134

Bertolone S J, Baum E S, Krivit W et al 1989 A phase II study of cisplatin therapy in recurrent childhood brain tumors. A report from the Children's Cancer Study Group. Journal of Neuro-Oncology 7: 5–11

Bloom H J G 1982 Intracranial tumors: response and resistance to therapeutic endeavors, 1970–1980. International Journal of Radiation Oncology Biology Physics 8: 1083–1113

Bouchard J 1980 Central nervous system. In: Fletcher G (ed) Textbook of radiology, 3rd edn. Lea & Febiger, Philadelphia, pp 444–498

Chin H W, Maruyama Y, Markesbery W et al 1982 Intracranial ependymoma: results of radiotherapy at the University of Kentucky. Cancer 49: 2276–2280

Choux M 1983 Ependymomas of the posterior fossa in children. In: Amador L V (ed) Brain tumors in the young. Charles C Thomas, Springfield, Ill; pp 526–545

Cohen M E, Duffner P K 1985 Current therapy in childhood brain tumors. Neurology Clinics 3: 147–164

Coulon R A, Till K 1977 Intracranial ependymomas in children. Child's Brain 3: 154–168

Courville C B, Broussalian S L 1961 Plastic ependymoma of the lateral recess. Report of eight verified cases. Journal of Neurosurgery 18: 792–798

Cushing H 1932 Intracranial tumors. Notes upon a series of two thousand verified cases with surgical-mortality percentages pertaining thereto. Charles C Thomas, Springfield, Ill, p 56

Dohrmann G J 1985 Ependymomas. In: Wilkins R H, Rengachary S S (eds) Neurosurgery, vol 1. McGraw-Hill, New York; pp 767–771

Dohrmann G J, Farwell J R, Flannery J T 1976 Ependymomas and ependymoblastomas in children. Journal of Neurosurgery 45: 273

Duffner P K, Cohen M E 1985 Treatment of brain tumors in babies and very young children. Pediatric Neuroscience 12: 304–310

Fokes E C Jr, Earle K M 1969 Ependymomas: Clinical and pathological aspects. Journal of Neurosurgery 30: 585–594

Garrett P G, Simpson W J 1983 Ependymomas: results of radiation treatment. International Journal of Radiation Oncology Biology Physics 9: 1121–1124

Gaynon P S, Ettinger L J, Moel D et al 1987 Pediatric phase I trial of carboplatin: a CCSG report. Cancer Treatment Report 71: 1039–1042

Geyer J R, Pendergast T W, Millstein J N et al 1988 Eight drugs in one day for children with brain tumors. Journal of Clinical Oncology 6: 996–1000

Gilles F H, Leviton A, Hedley-White E T et al 1987 Childhood brain tumor update. Human Pathology 14: 834–845

Goldwein J W, Leahy J M, Packer R J 1988 Intracranial ependymomas in children. Pediatric Neuroscience 14: 153 [abstract]

Goldwein J W, Glauser T A, Packer R J et al 1990 Recurrent intracranial ependymomas in children. Cancer 66: 557

Healey E A, Barnes P D, Kupsky W J et al 1991 The prognostic significance of postoperative residual tumor in ependymoma. Neurosurgery 28: 666–672

Hendrick E B, Raffel C 1989 Tumors of the fourth ventricle: ependymomas, choroid plexus papillomas and dermoid cysts. In: Pediatric Neurosurgery. W B Saunders, Philadelphia, pp 366–371

Ikezaki K, Matsushima T, Inoue T et al 1993 Correlation of microanatomical localization with postoperative survival in posterior fossa ependymomas. Neurosurgery 32: 38–44

Ilgren E B, Stiller C A, Hughes J T et al 1984 Ependymomas: A clinical and pathologic study: Part I. Biologic features. Clinical Neuropathology 3: 113–121

Jenkins R D T 1982 Childhood ependymoma — radiation treatment results. In: Chang C H, Housepian E M (eds) Tumors of the central nervous system: Modern radiotherapy in multidisciplinary management. Masson, Paris, pp 128–132

Kernohan J W, Fletcher-Kernohan E M 1937 Ependymomas. A study of 109 cases. Res Publ Assoc Res Nerv Ment Dis 16: 182

Kernohan J W, Sayre G P 1952 Tumors of the central nervous system, fasc 35. Atlas of tumor pathology, Sect X, fasc 35. Armed Forces Institute of Pathology, Washington, DC, p 129

Khan A B, D'Souza B J, Wharam M D et al 1982 Cis-platinum therapy in recurrent childhood brain tumors. Cancer Treatment Report 66: 2013

Kim Y H, Fayos J V 1977 Intracranial ependymomas. Radiology 124: 805–808

Koos W T, Miller M H 1971 Intracranial tumors of infants and children. CV Mosby, St Louis, pp 331–334

Kricheff I I, Becker M, Schneck S A et al 1963 Intracranial ependymomas: factors influencing prognosis. Journal of Neurosurgery 21: 7–14

Kun L E, Kovnar E H, Sanford R A 1988 Ependymomas in children. Pediatric Neuroscience 14: 57–63

Lefkowitz I, Evans A, Sposto R et al 1988 Adjuvant chemotherapy of posterior fossa ependymoma: Craniospinal radiation with or without CCNU, vincristine and prednisone. Pediatric Neuroscience 14: 149 [abstract]

Lejeune J P, Dhellemmes P, Dupard T et al 1987 Les ependymomas intracraniens. Neurochirurgie 33: 118–123

Liebel S A, Sheline G E 1987 Radiation therapy of neoplasms of the brain. Journal of Neurosurgery 66: 1–22

Liu H M, Boggs J, Kidd J 1976 Ependymomas in childhood. I. Histological survey and clinicopathological correlation. Child's Brain 2: 92–110

Lyons M K, Kelly P J 1991 Posterior fossa ependymomas: report of 30 cases and review of the literature. Neurosurgery 28: 659–665

Mabon F R, Svien H J, Kernohan J W et al 1949 Ependymomas. Proceedings of the Staff Meetings of the Mayo Clinic 24: 65–71

Marks J E, Adler S J 1982 A comparative study of ependymomas by site of orgin. International Journal of Radiation Oncology Biology Physics 8: 37–43

Marsh W R Jr, Laws E R Jr 1987 Intracranial ependymomas. Progress in Experimental Tumor Research 30: 175–180

Matson D D 1969 Tumors of the posterior fossa. In: Matson D D (ed) Neurosurgery of infancy and childhood, 2nd edn. Charles C Thomas, Springfield, Ill, pp 410–479

Mørk S J, Loken A C 1977 Ependymoma. A follow-up study of 101 cases. Cancer 40: 907–915

Nazar G B, Hoffman H J, Becker L E et al 1990 Infratentorial ependymomas in childhood: prognostic factors and treatment. Journal of Neurosurgery 72: 408–417

Oi S, Raimondi A J 1982 Ependymoma in children. Pediatric neurosurgery. Surgery of the developing nervous system. Grune & Stratton, New York, pp 419–428

Papadopoulos D P, Giri S, Evans R G 1990 Prognostic factors and management of intracranial ependymomas. Anticancer Research 10: 689–692

Phillips T L, Sheline G E, Boldrey E 1964 Therapeutic considerations in tumors affecting the central nervous system: ependymomas. Radiology 83: 98–105

Pierre-Khan A, Hirsch J F, Roux F X et al 1983 Intracranial ependymomas in childhood. Survival and functional results of 47 cases. Child's Brain 10: 145

Rawlings C E III, Giangaspero F, Burger P C et al 1988 Ependymomas: a clinicopathologic study. Surgical Neurology 29: 271–281

Renaudin J W, DiTullio M V, Brown W J 1979 Seeding of intracranial ependymomas in children. Child's Brain 5: 408

Ringertz N, Reymond A 1949 Ependymomas and choroid plexus papillomas. Journal of Neuropathology and Experimental Neurology 8: 355–380

Rorke L B 1983 The cerebellar medulloblastoma and its relationship to primitive neuroectodermal tumors. Journal of Neuropathology and Experimental Neurology 42: 1–15

Rorke L B 1987 Relationship of morphology of ependymomas in children to prognosis. Progress in Experimental Tumor Research 30: 170–174

Rorke L B, Gilles F H, Davis R L et al 1985 Revision of the World Health Organization classification of brain tumors for childhood brain tumors. Cancer 56: 1869–1886

Ross G W, Rubinstein L J 1989 Lack of histopathological correlation of malignant ependymomas with postoperative survival. Journal of Neurosurgery 70: 31–36
Rubinstein L J 1970 The definition of ependymoblastoma. Archives of Pathology 90: 35
Rubinstein L J 1972 Tumors of the central nervous system. Atlas of tumor pathology, series II, fasc 6. Armed Forces Institute of Pathology, Washington, DC, pp 104–126
Russell D S, Rubinstein L J 1977 Pathology of tumors of the nervous system, 4th edn. Arnold Press, London; pp 203–226
Sagerman R H, Bagshaw M A, Hanberry J 1965 Considerations in the treatment of ependymoma. Radiology 84: 401–408
Salazar O M 1983 A better understanding of CNS seeding and a brighter outlook of postoperatively irradiated patients with ependymomas. International Journal of Radiation Oncology Biology Physics 9: 1231–1234
Salazar O M, Rubin P, Bassano D et al 1975 Improved survival in cases of intracranial ependymomas by irradiation: dose selection and field extension. Cancer 35: 1563–1573
Salazar O M, Castro-Vita H, Van Houtie P et al 1983 Improved survival in cases of ependymoma after radiation therapy: late report and recommendations. Journal of Neurosurgery 59: 652–659
Sexauer C L, Khan A, Burger P C et al 1985 Cisplatin in recurrent pediatric brain tumors. A POG Phase II study. Cancer 56(7): 1497–1501
Shapiro W R 1975 Chemotherapy of primary malignant brain tumors in children. Cancer 35: 965–972
Shaw E G, Evans R G, Scheithauer B W et al 1987 Postoperative radiotherapy of intracraial ependymoma in pediatric and adult patients. International Journal of Radiation Oncology Biology Physics 13: 1457–1462
Sheline G E 1975 Radiation therapy of tumors of the central nervous system in childhood. Cancer 35: 957
Shuman R M, Alvord E C Jr, Leech R W 1975 The biology of childhood ependymomas. Archives of Neurology 32: 731–739
Spoto G P, Press G A, Hesselink J R, Solomon M 1990 Intracranial ependymomas: MR manifestations. AJNR 11: 83–91
Sutton L N, Goldwein G, Perilongo B et al 1990 Prognostic factors in childhood ependymomas. Pediatric Neurosurgery 16: 57–65
Svien H J, Mabon R F, Kernohan J W et al 1953 Ependymoma of the brain: pathologic aspects. Neurology 3: 1–15
Tamura M, Ono N, Kurihara H et al 1990 Adjunctive treatment for recurrent childhood ependymoma of the IV ventricle: chemotherapy with CDDP and MCNU. Child's Nervous System 6: 186
Tomita T, McLone D G, Lakshmi D et al 1988 Benign ependymomas of the posterior fossa in childhood. Pediatric Neuroscience 14: 277–285
Walker R W, Allen J C 1983 Treatment of recurrent primary intracranial childhood tumors with cis-diaminedichloroplatinum. Annals of Neurology 14: 371
Wallner K E, Wara W M, Sheline G E et al 1986 Intracranial ependymomas: results of treatment with partial or whole brain irradiation without spinal irradiation. International Journal of Radiation Oncology Biology Physics 12: 1937–1941
Wara W M 1985 Radiation therapy for brain tumors. Cancer 55: 2291–2295
West C R, Bruce D A, Duffner P K 1985 Ependymomas: factors in clinical and diagnostic staging. Cancer 56: 1812–1816
Zee C S, Segall H D, Ahmadi J et al 1983 Computed tomography of posterior fossa ependymomas in childhood. Surgical Neurology 20: 221
Zülch K J 1986 Brain tumors: their biology and pathology, 3rd edn. Springer-Verlag, New York, pp 258–276

28. Choroid plexus papilloma

R. Michael Scott   John Knightly

INCIDENCE AND PREVALENCE

Choroid plexus tumors (CPT) are rare lesions of the central nervous system (CNS). After first being described by Guerard (1883), CPTs were found in the literature usually as case reports until the midpart of this century when larger series of cases were reported (see Table 28.1). Davis & Cushing (1925) and Zülch (1986) each found a CPT incidence of 0.6% in their series of 964 and 9000 patients respectively. Norlen (1949) and Bohm & Strang (1961) reported an incidence of 0.4%. In Matsuda's (1991) description of the Japanese tumor registry, CPTs were found in 0.5% of patients. Thus, over several large series, an incidence rate between 0.4 and 0.6% is reported.

Although the rate of CPT found in the general population is low, different rates can be found in the pediatric population. Several of these series are presented in Table 28.1. Matson & Crofton (1960) were the first to report this age difference, with a 3.9% incidence in patients with CNS tumors less than 12 years old at Boston Children's Hospital. Rovit et al (1970) found a similar rate of 4.0% in his series of patients. Ellenbogen et al (1989), describing one of the largest groups of CPTs, including Matson's original series, reported an incidence of 2.9%. The Toronto series of Yates et al (1979), Felix et al (1987), and Humphreys et al (1987) reported incidence rates between 1.8% and 2.2%. The Finnish survey of Heiskanen (1977) revealed a CPT incidence of 1.5%, the British series of Hawkins (1980) reported a 2.3% incidence, and the Taiwanese study of Ho et al (1991), 2.3%. All these series contained patients less than 16 years of age. In Pascual-Castroviejo et al's (1983) series of patients less than 8 years old, a 6.4% incidence was found, with all patients having CPT being less than 2 years old. Jooma et al (1984) and Haddad et al (1991) found even higher rates of 12.5% and 13.6% in series of patients under the age of one. These series indicate an incidence rate of between 1.5% and 3.9% in the general pediatric population of CNS tumors, with a higher incidence in children less than 2 years old.

Table 28.1 Incidence and sex predilection for CPTs in published series: pediatric centers. Data obtained from selected series which included specific case numbers and data.

Author	Year	Center	Incidence	Sex (M:F)
Matson & Crofton	1961	Boston, US	3.9	8:8
Thompson et al	1973	Toronto, Canada	2.3	10:4
Hawkins	1980	London, UK	2.3	13:4
Pascual-Castroviejo et al	1983	Madrid, Spain	6.4	8:6
Humphreys et al	1987	Toronto, Canada	1.8	15:8
Ellenbogen et al	1989	Boston, US	2.9	24:16
Knierim	1990	Loma Linda, US	?	5:2
Lena et al	1990	Marseille, France	?	13:11
Spallone et al	1990	Rome, Italy	3.0	6:9
Ho et al	1991	Taipei, ROC	2.3	6:2
		General population		
Davis & Cushing	1925	Boston, US	0.6	4:2
Bohm & Strang	1961	Stockholm, Sweden	0.4	10:15
Zülch	1986	Köln, Germany	0.6	'equal'
Boyd & Steinbok	1987	Vancouver, Canada	?	6:5
Palazzi et al	1989	Verona, Italy	?	3:5
Paulus & Jänisch	1990	Germany	?	29:23

While most CPTs consist of choroid plexus papilloma (CPP), significant numbers of these lesions are the more aggressive choroid plexus carcinoma (CPC). Most large series of CPTs have variable rates of CPC, ranging from 10–35% (Matson & Crofton 1960, Raimondi & Gutierrez 1975, Ellenbogen et al 1989, Johnson 1989, Knierim 1990). Similar rates are found outside of the US in Italy (12.5%, Palazzi et al 1989), England (17.6%, Hawkins 1980) and Canada (18.2%, Boyd & Steinbok 1987; 26.7%, Felix et al 1987; 26%, Humphreys et al 1987). In Taipei, Ho et al (1991) found 25% of CPTs to be CPC, while in Japan, only 8.1% were CPCs (Matsuda et al 1991).

AGE DISTRIBUTION

As noted above, CPTs can be found at any age, but they appear to be more common in childhood. Figure 28.1 represents the age distribution of patients with CPTs in several large pediatric series in which the ages of individual patients were reported. Most patients presented in the first two years of life. In Ellenbogen et al's (1989) series of 40 patients, the range in ages was 6 days to 16 years (median 10 months). Of these cases, 65% occurred before age 2, with an additional 25% between 2 and 12 years. Lena et al (1990) had similar results, with 58% of patients less than 2 years old and 76% under age 5. All of Pascual-Castroviejo et al's (1983) 14 patients presented before age 2, with 78.6% presenting before age 1. Spallone et al (1990) had older children with CPTs in their pediatric series, with 33% of patients between ages 9 and 15.

There are several studies that report cases in the general population and they are represented graphically in Figure 28.2. This again shows the increased incidence of this disease in children. Boyd & Steinbok's (1987) series of both adults and children had 73% of patients less than 18 months (mean 12 months), with 3 adults ranging from 21–58 years. McGirr et al (1988), reporting on the experience of the Mayo Clinic, found a mean age of 29.7 years. The distribution of ages was: 4% less than 1 year, 15% between 1 and 10 years, 8% between 10 and 16 years, and 73% adults. Bohm & Strang (1961) had an almost identical distribution, with a mean age of 27.3 years (range of 7 months to 60 years), and 4% less than 1 year, 16% between 1 and 10 years, 4% between 10 and 16 years, and 76% adults. Based on these series, there do not appear to be any additional age groups with increased incidence rates during adulthood.

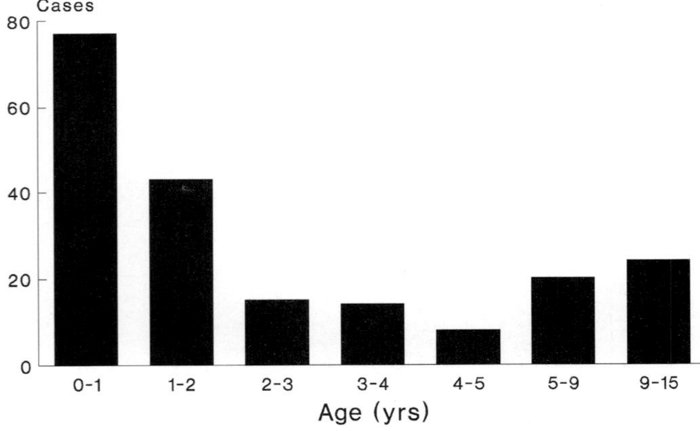

Fig. 28.1 Histogram of the age distribution in CPTs from several pediatric centers in which the report gives specific ages for patients. The majority of cases are found in the first two years of life, with the highest incidence in patients less than age 1. Data obtained from Matson & Crofton 1960, Thompson et al 1973, Hawkins 1980, Pascual-Castroviejo et al 1983, Knierim 1990, Spallone et al 1990, Ho et al 1991.

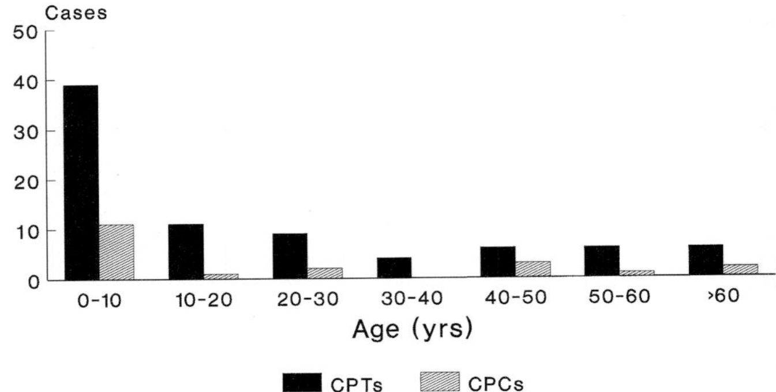

Fig. 28.2 Histogram of the age distribution of CPTs in the general population from series reporting specific age data. Again, the higher incidence for both CPP and CPC is seen in younger patients. Data obtained from Bohm & Strang 1961, Coffin et al 1986, Boyd & Steinbok 1987, Palazzi et al 1989, Paulus & Jänisch 1990.

SEX DISTRIBUTION

The sex ratio of CPTs is presented in Table 28.1. While some older series of patients with CPTs indicated a female predominance (Bohm & Strang 1961), most recent series indicate either an equal incidence (Matson & Crofton 1960, Thompson et al 1973, Pascual-Castroviejo et al 1983) or a higher incidence in males (Hawkins 1980, Felix et al 1987, Ellenbogen et al 1989, Johnson 1989). A similar finding is found in the CPC data, with either an equal predilection (Boyd & Steinbok 1987, Ellenbogen et al 1989) or slightly higher in males (Allen et al 1992, Packer et al 1992).

RACIAL, NATIONAL, GEOGRAPHICAL CONSIDERATIONS

There are no racial, ethnic, or geographic factors which can be implicated in either the incidence or etiology of choroid plexus tumors.

FAMILY HISTORY AND GENETIC FACTORS

While no clear familial or genetic factors have been implicated in the development of CPTs, the fact that many of these tumors are found in childhood and neonates indicates that many of these lesions are congenital (Ellenbogen et al 1989). Bergsagel et al (1992) have suggested an etiologic role for the polyomavirus SV-40. The SV-40 virus has been shown to induce CPP in transgenic mice (Chen & Van Dyke 1991). Probes for this virus reacted to 50% of the CPP tumors tested. Though 80% of the population up to the age of 20 is seropositive for this ubiquitous virus, these tumors are rare (Bergsagel et al 1992). The virus can be spread to the brain only during the limited period in utero when the blood-brain barrier is permeable and a seronegative mother is infected for the first time.

Another reason the probes may have reacted to the tumors is the presence of the appropriate DNA sequences in the germline of the tumor (Bergsagel et al 1992). There are several reports of CPP associated with Li-Fraumeni syndrome and Aicardi's syndrome (Robinow et al 1984, Garber et al 1990, Yuasa et al 1993). There have also been reports of CPP associated with von-Hippel Lindau (VHL) disease (Blamires et al 1992). Of interest in this case was the loss of an allele on chromosome 3 in the CPP tissue, similar to the deletion found in other tumors associated with VHL disease. Though no firm genetic predisposition has been proven, there have been several case reports of CPTs in siblings, with Zwetsloot et al (1991) proposing an autosomal recessive mode of inheritance.

SITES OF PREDILECTION

As seen in Table 28.2 and Figure 28.3, CPTs present in age-dependent locations. In McGirr et al's (1988) series, all lesions in patients less than 16 years old were localized to the lateral ventricles. Similarly, all CPTs in adults were in the posterior fossa. Bohm & Strang (1961) found no

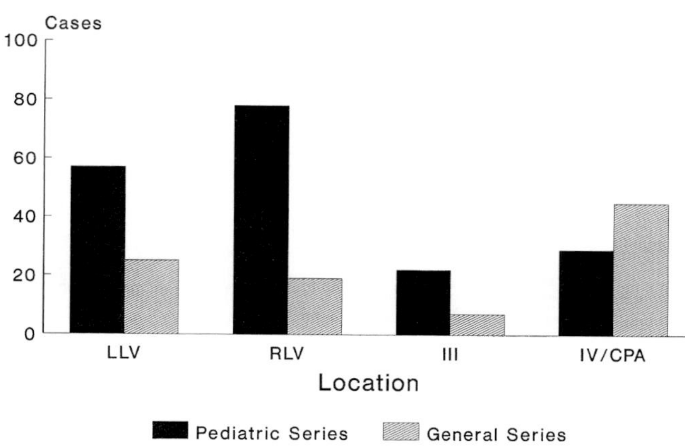

Fig. 28.3 Histogram representing the reported anatomic locations of CPTs in both the pediatric and general population. Note the increased incidence of lateral ventricle occurrence in younger patients, with a posterior fossa predominance in the general population with older patients. Data obtained from Table 29.2.

children with posterior fossa tumors, but a few adults had tumors in the lateral ventricle. Similar results have been found in other reports (Thompson et al 1973, Carpenter et al 1982, Russell & Rubinstein 1989).

When examining the pediatric literature (Table 28.2, Fig. 28.3.), there appears to be a predilection of CPTs for the lateral ventricles and, in particular, the atrium of the ventricles. Ellenbogen et al (1989) found 75% of CPTs to be in the lateral ventricles, with Felix et al (1987) describing 79% occurrence in this location. While some have suggested a majority of lateral ventricle CPTs localizing to the left (van Wagenen 1930, Russell & Rubinstein 1989), other large series have found an equal distribution (Matson & Crofton 1960, Dohrmann & Collias 1975, Felix et al 1987, Ellenbogen et al 1989, Johnson 1989). It has been noted by some that CPP is the most common

Table 28.2 Location of CPTs in published series: pediatric centers. Data obtained from reports including exact numbers of lesions at each anatomic site. Ellenbogen et al (1989) and Knierim (1990) each have 1 case of bilateral CPP.

Author	Year	LLV	RLV	III	IV/CPA
Thompson et al	1973	14	26	2	4
Hawkins	1980	4	9	0	4
Pascual-Castroviejo et al	1983	4	6	2	3
Humphreys et al	1987	7	10	4	4
Ellenbogen et al	1989	15	16	4	6
Knierim	1990	5	3	1	0
Lena et al	1990	6	5	7	6
Ho et al	1991	2	3	2	2
Totals		57 (31%)	78 (42%)	22 (12%)	29 (15%)
General population					
Bohm & Strang	1961	5	3	2	15
Boyd & Steinbok	1987	3	1	3	4
Palazzi et al	1989	1	0	1	6
Paulus & Jänisch	1990	16	15	1	20
Totals		25 (26%)	19 (20%)	7 (7%)	45 (47%)

hemispheric tumor in the first year of life (Jooma et al 1984, Johnson 1989). While this seems to be the overall tendency, other series have found fourth ventricle CPTs in children to be from 15–25% of cases (Matson & Crofton 1960, Hawkins 1980, Boyd & Steinbok 1987, Ellenbogen et al 1989).

In adults, most lesions are found in the posterior fossa (Table 28.2, Fig. 28.3). All of McGirr et al's (1988) adult cases of CPP were infratentorial, with 79% of the lesions in the fourth ventricle and the remainder in the cerebellopontine angle (CPA). Bohm & Strang (1961) reported 79% of adult cases localized to the fourth ventricle, 16% in the lateral ventricle, and 5% in the third ventricle.

While there have been numerous reported cases of CPTs in the CPA, this is an unusual location for these lesions, and their point of origin is unclear. Some believe these to be fourth ventricular lesions with extension into the CPA (Bohm & Strang 1961). Others indicate that these lesions arise from tufts of choroid plexus present at the exit of the foramen of Luschka (Hammock et al 1976, Piquet & de Tribolet 1984, van Swieten et al 1987). CPTs present in the CPA are usually more common in adults, with few cases found in the pediatric literature (Hammock et al 1976, Piquet & de Tribolet 1984). These lesions can also be found in the cerebellomedullary cistern by the foramen of Magendie (van Swieten et al 1987).

The least common location for CPTs is the third ventricle (Schijman et al 1990). As of 1983, there were only 20 reported cases in the literature (Gradin et al 1984). In most series, CPTs in the third ventricle make up between 2% and 10% of cases (Matson & Crofton 1960, Bohm & Strang 1961, Rovit et al 1970, Ellenbogen et al 1989, Knierim 1990, Paulus & Jänisch 1990). While some series found no patients with CPTs in the area (Hawkins 1980, McGirr et al 1988), Boyd & Steinbok (1987) found 3 out of 11 patients with CPTs localized to the third ventricle. The low incidence in the third ventricle for CPTs appears to be true for both children and adults.

An interesting phenomenon associated with CPTs is villous hypertrophy. Originally described by Davis in 1924, villous hypertrophy is the occurrence of bilateral CPP of the lateral ventricles. These lesions can produce significant hydrocephalus from overproduction of CSF (Welch et al 1983). These are very rare lesions which were not encountered in several large series, and only as isolated cases in others, and may not represent true tumors.

PRESENTING FEATURES

Patients with CPTs usually present with symptoms referable to increased intracranial pressure (ICP). In children, these symptoms are manifested as nausea/vomiting, headache, irritability/malaise, visual disturbances/strabismus, and ataxia. Seizures can also be a presenting symptom in up to 18% of patients (Ellenbogen et al 1989). Rarely CPTs can present as meningismus secondary to subarachnoid hemorrhage in either children or adults. Other presenting symptoms have been head tilt, titubation, exophthalmos, and failure to thrive (Boyd & Steinbok 1987, McGirr et al 1988, Ellenbogen et al 1989, Johnson 1989).

In the adult population, headaches are the most commonly encountered symptom (McGirr et al 1988). There are frequently symptoms associated with cranial nerve dysfunction, especially in those patients with tumors localized to the posterior fossa. Other symptoms include visual changes, syncope, nystagmus, vertigo, ataxia, hemiparesis, nausea and vomiting, tinnitus, and excessive fatigue (Bohm & Strang 1961, Boyd & Steinbok 1987, McGirr et al 1988).

The physical signs commonly found at presentation are also related to increased ICP. In children less than 2 years of age, craniomegaly secondary to hydrocephalus is the most common physical finding in most series. After this age, in both children and adults, ataxia, papilledema, and extraocular motility dysfunction (including sunsetting of eyes) are the usual presenting signs. Failure to thrive and developmental delay can also be seen as well as stupor and coma (Lena et al 1990). Cranial nerve involvement can include II through X in varying combinations. Other physical features of CPTs include hemiparesis, sensory and reflex changes, cerebellar dysfunction, and nystagmus.

In both children and adults, the effects of increased ICP and hydrocephalus cause many of the general signs and symptoms seen with CPTs. The hydrocephalus associated with CPTs is unique among all CNS tumors as it is caused not only by obstruction of flow, but also by CSF overproduction from the tumor tissue itself (Knierim 1990). This phenomenon is described in greater detail later in the chapter. More focal symptoms and deficits are due to the location of the tumor, especially those arising in the posterior fossa. In regard to duration of symptoms prior to diagnosis, there appears to be no difference between CPC and CPP, though some have argued that CPC will present earlier than CPP (Johnson 1989).

IMAGING DIAGNOSIS

Prior to the advent of computerized tomography (CT) and magnetic resonance imaging (MRI), pneumoencephalography and ventriculography were standard diagnostic tests in the evaluation of CPTs. These procedures are mentioned for historical purposes only, as they play no current role in the management of these patients.

Plain films

While CT has supplanted plain roentgenograms of the

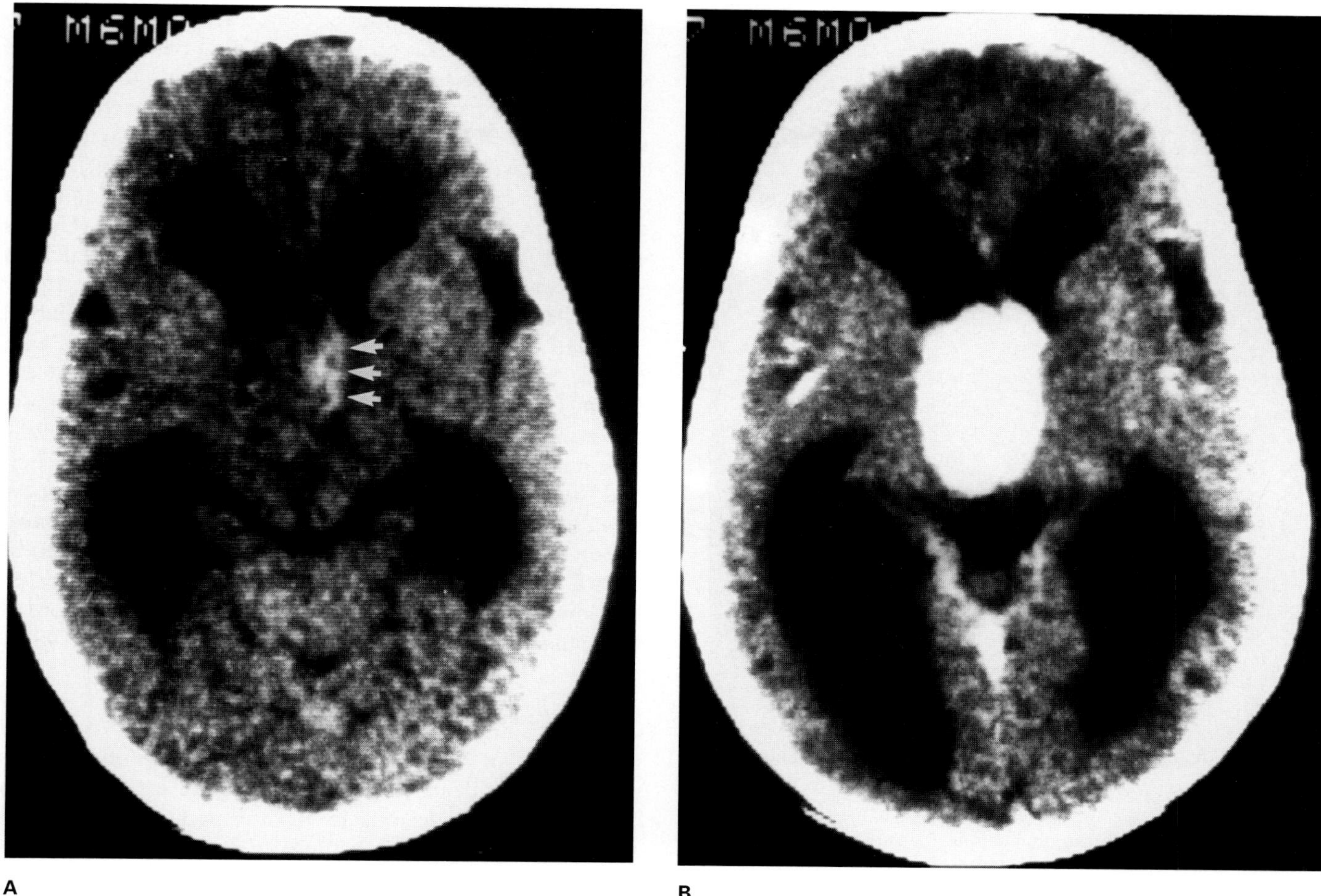

Fig. 28.4 This 6 month-old patient with a third ventricular choroid plexus papilloma presented with signs and symptoms of increased intracranial pressure and rapidly enlarging head. **A.** CT scan, non-enhanced. The mass occludes both foramina of Monro and its attenuation characteristics are similar to the surrounding brain. There is a band of calcification along its left border (arrows). **B.** With intravenous contrast administration, the mass has a bright, homogeneous enhancement which clarifies its borders and suggests a papillary character.

head as the initial study in patients with evidence of increased ICP, these studies are nevertheless occasionally obtained. Depending on the age of the patient, calcification or other features may be found — split sutures, cranial lacunae in infants, sella changes in older patients. The clinical significance of calcification is unclear. Various studies have shown an incidence of calcification of CPTs from 0–20% on plain films (Matson & Crofton 1960, Rovit et al 1970, Hawkins 1980, Pascual-Castroviejo et al 1983). While calcification in the region of any of the ventricles or CPA may indicate CPT in the presence of other signs of elevated ICP (Rovit et al 1970), other studies are of course required to define the radiographic diagnosis.

Computerized tomography

In patients with CPTs, CT scanning is frequently the initial diagnostic test obtained. The CT characteristics of both CPP and CPC are well characterized (Pascual-Castroviejo et al 1983, Coates et al 1989). In CPP, these lesions can attain a large size before presenting clinically. The majority of cases will show varying degrees of hydrocephalus. Depending upon the location of the tumor, this may be seen as communicating or non-communicating hydrocephalus. On non-enhanced studies (see Fig. 28.4A), the tumor appears as a smooth or lobulated mass, homogeneous in texture, which is isodense to slightly hyperdense in relation to surrounding brain parenchyma. This increase in attenuation is due to the highly vascular nature of these tumors, and their location adjacent to hypodense CSF (Coates et al 1989). There is usually no evidence of local invasion. With intravenous contrast, there is marked, homogeneous enhancement (Figs 28.4B, 28.5). In cases of villous hypertrophy, there is bilateral enlargement of all the choroid plexus in the lateral ventricle (Johnson 1989). There are some differences between CPP and CPC on CT. A CPC will appear as an inhomogeneous mass on both contrast and non-contrast CT scans, but

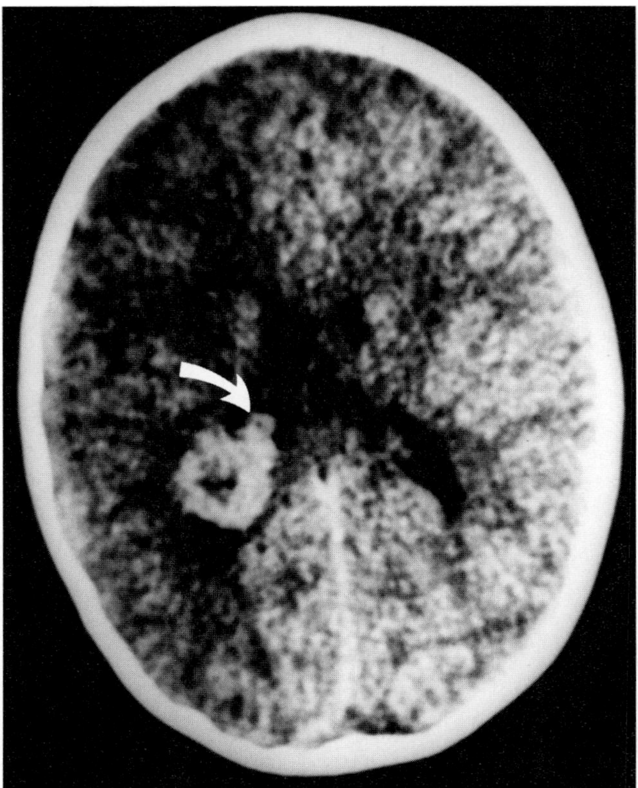

Fig. 28.5 This 3-year-old patient presented with headaches due to a lateral ventricular choroid plexus papilloma. The CT scan following intravenous contrast administration demonstrates a lobular mass with central low attenuation and slight anterior extension along the attachment of the choroid plexus (curved arrow). The lateral ventricle is widened and the occipital horn enlarged.

may densely contrast enhance (Fig. 28.7A). CPCs are iso- to hyperdense in relation to surrounding parenchyma and will show evidence of local brain invasion. In addition, some authors have suggested there is less severe hydrocephalus in CPC patients compared to those with CPP (Pascual-Castroviejo et al 1983, Coates et al 1989).

An additional finding with CT imaging of CPTs is the presence of calcification in up to 24–80% of cases (Coates et al 1989). The normal choroid plexus is not calcified in childhood. It is frequently calcified in adults, especially in the lateral ventricle. A calcified tumor in childhood localized to the ventricular system and associated with hydrocephalus should suggest the presence of a CPT (Coates et al 1989). Similarly, calcified tumors in the third and fourth ventricles, as well as the CPA, in adults may indicate a CPT. The differential diagnosis of a calcified ventricular tumor includes ependymoma, astrocytoma, oligodendroglioma, meningioma, teratoma, pineal region tumors, and craniopharyngioma (Coates et al 1989). The CPP has a stippled, punctate pattern of calcification on CT, with the calcium in a CPC having more of a globular appearance (Coates et al 1989, Johnson 1989).

Magnetic resonance imaging

The advent of MRI has further eased the ability to diagnose CPP, utilizing differences in signal intensity. With T2 weighting, the lesions are of intermediate or increased signal intensity (T2 lengthening) (Coates et al 1989). Also seen are areas of signal void. When curvilinear in appear-

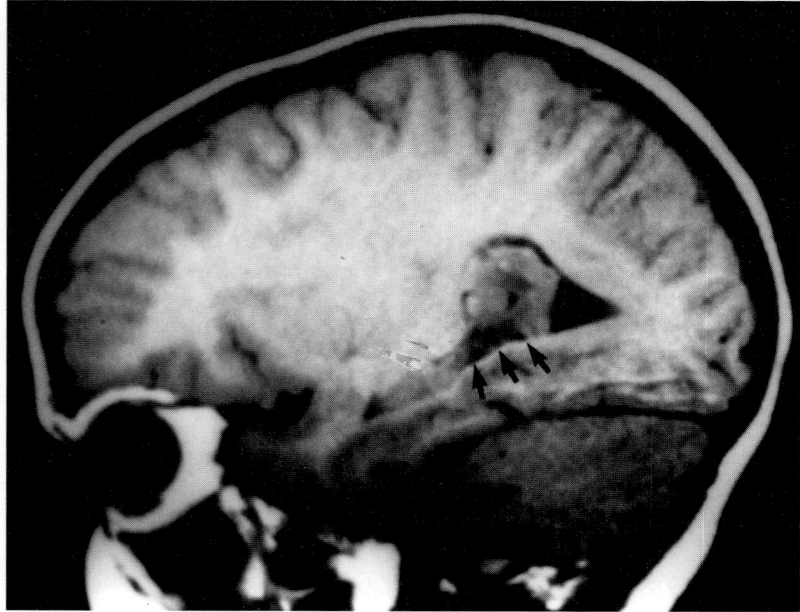

A

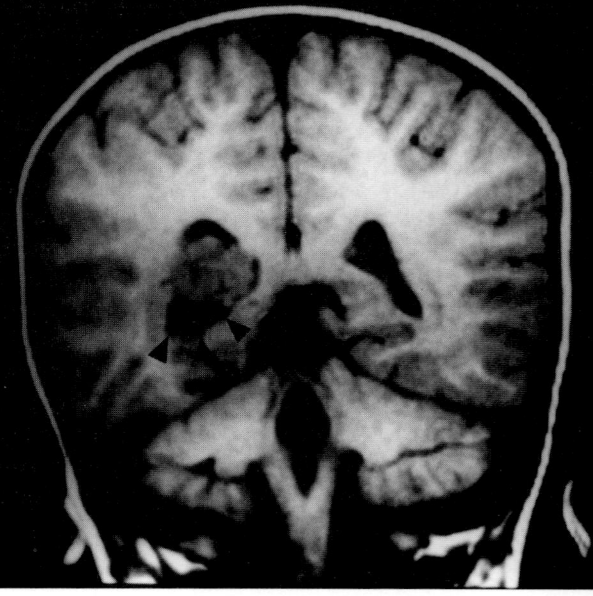

B

Fig. 28.6 MRI scan, same patient as Fig. 29.5. **A.** Parasagittal image, T1-weighted, demonstrating continuity with temporal horn choroid plexus, dilated occipital horn, and mixed signal intensities within the lesion. Inferiorly located signal voids suggest the location of hypertrophied feeding choroidal vessels (arrows). **B.** Coronal image, T1-weighted, demonstrating the mass within the enlarged ventricular system and flow voids below the mass (arrowheads) suggesting hypertrophied feeding choroidal vessels.

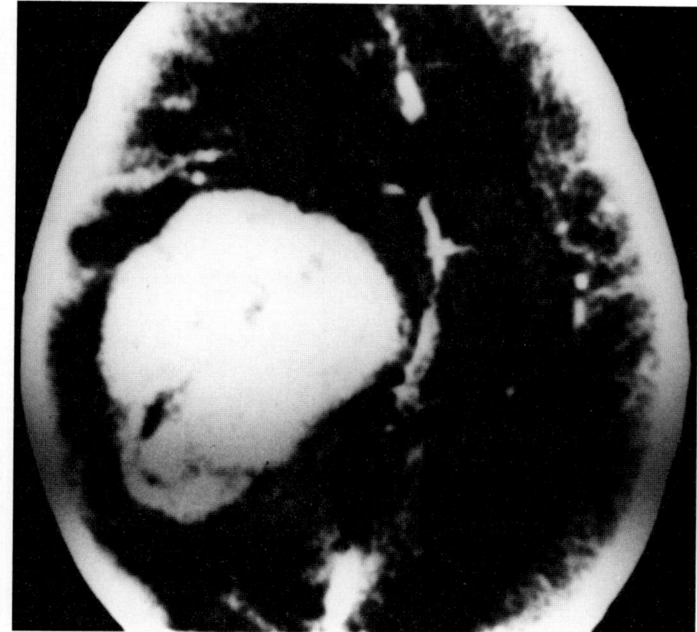

A

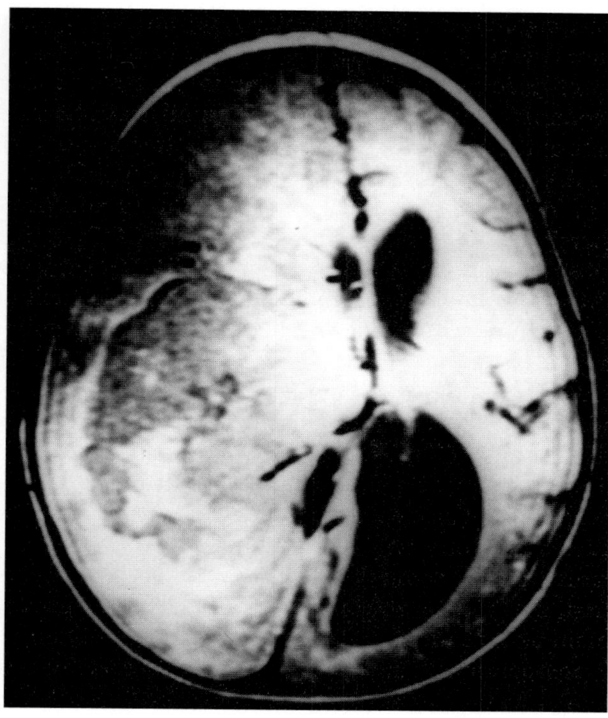

B

Fig. 28.7 1-year-old child with choroid plexus carcinoma, right lateral ventricle. **A.** CT scan following enhancement with intravenous contrast reveals large, densely enhancing mass lesion with midline shift; the scan suggests some intratumoral necrosis. **B.** MRI, axial view, T1-weighted, confirms variegated appearance and intraventricular location of neoplasm. **C.** The parasagittal MRI, T1-weighted, demonstrates trapped and dilated temporal horn (arrows) which could be tapped at surgery to relieve mass effect.

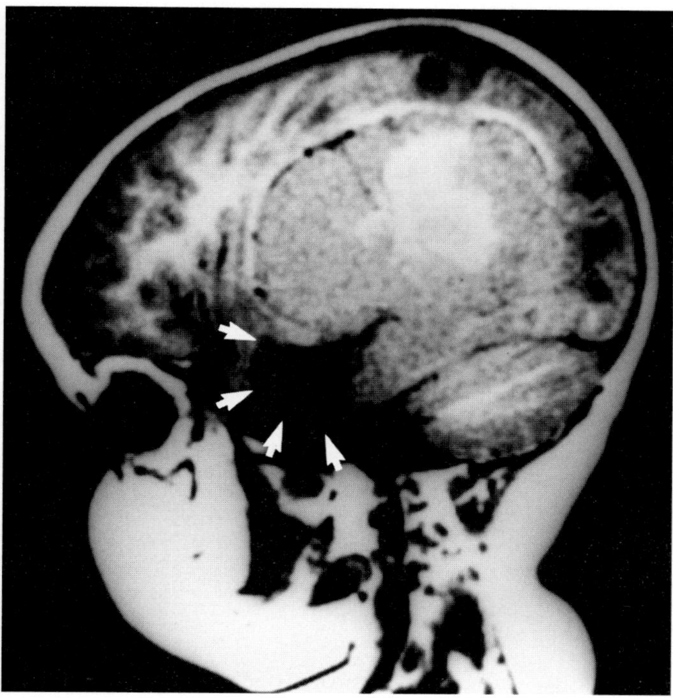

C

ance, these most likely represent intratumoral blood vessels (Coates et al 1989). When the areas of decreased signal intensity are more inhomogeneous or diffuse, calcification and old hemorrhage should be considered. These findings can be more clearly differentiated with CT. The MRI study can also be used to localize blood vessels feeding or draining the tumor (Figs 28.6A, B). This information may, in some cases, obviate the need for cerebral angiography. Additional benefits of MRI over CT are superior anatomical localization of the tumor in relation to surrounding normal structures and delineation of tumor extension into adjacent brain or through intraventricular foramen. The dynamics of CSF circulation can also be evaluated with MRI (Coates et al 1989).

The MRI findings in CPC are similar to those found with CT (Figs 28.7B, C). These tumors are again of intermediate signal intensity, but are inhomogeneous in character in T1, T2 and proton-density weighted sequences (Coates et al 1989). Areas of low signal intensity on T1 weighting, and high signal intensity on T2 weighting in the center of the tumor have been found histologically to be consistent with necrosis (Coates et al 1989). These tumors invade local parenchyma and induce significant peritumoral edema with increased signal intensity in the surrounding white matter on T2 sequences. Other nonspecific changes readily seen on MRI include mass effect resulting from the tumor and/or edema, and periventricular transependymal edema (increased signal on T2 and proton-weighted images) secondary to the hydrostatic pressure effects of hydrocephalus (Coates et al 1989).

Use of gadolinium diethylenetriaminepentaacetic acid as a contrast agent with MRI elicits similar effects as a contrast-enhanced CT scan, but with better anatomical detail. A contrast MRI is also superior to CT with contrast in delineating residual or recurrent tumor postoperatively, as well as detecting seeding by CPTs within the subarachnoid space (Coates et al 1989). Recent work with MRI has shown its usefulness for volumetric analysis of serial studies to better evaluate changes in tumor volume after different therapeutic interventions (Filipek et al 1991).

Both CT and MRI can be extremely useful in detecting and diagnosing CPTs. Though MRI gives better anatomic detail and some information about the surrounding vasculature, the acquisition time for these studies must be considered. As Johnson (1989) points out, these patients can present in extremis and, especially in the case of children, may not be able to tolerate the sedation needed to obtain an adequate study. The decision to obtain an MRI preoperatively must be made on a case-by-case basis.

Cerebral angiography

Although CT and MRI have replaced cerebral angiography as the imaging procedure of choice in CPT management, it remains an important diagnostic test. A detailed description of the angiographic appearance of CPTs is found in Raimondi & Gutierrez (1975). Their angiographic criteria for the diagnosis of CPTs of the lateral ventricle include:

1. Asymmetrical hydrocephalus with shift away from the side of the larger ventricle.
2. The 'double tumor' sign: a vascular deformity of the parietal, occipital, and posterior temporal arteries from the mass in the trigone, and another area of expansion in the temporal or occipital region from trapping of the temporal or occipital horn.
3. A granular stain from tumor blush which, while not enabling distinction of CPP from CPC, can be used to identify projections of tumor away from the main mass.
4. Hypertrophy of the feeding vessels, usually the anterior choroidal artery, posterior lateral perforating branches, or the lateral posterior choroidal artery. These vessels can become quite tortuous. In larger tumors, more than one of these may enlarge. The medial posterior choroidal artery may hypertrophy when the tumor involves the third ventricle or the quadrigeminal cistern.
5. Inferior and medial displacement of the vein of Rosenthal by the combination of hydrocephalus, trapping of the temporal horn, and the bulk of the tumor itself.
6. Anterior and inferior displacement of the thalamus as well as a shift medially.
7. In some cases, an arteriovenous malformation or venous aneurysm can be seen on the surface of the tumor.

While the classic finding of a tortuous, hypertrophied anterior choroidal artery leading to a tumor blush in the region of the trigone is suggestive of a CPT, other lesions must also be considered. Meningiomas of the ventricle can have a similar angiographic appearance, though they are rare in the pediatric population (Johnson 1989). The information is useful to supplement findings found on CT or MRI.

Raimondi & Gutierrez (1975) also described the angiographic findings found with CPTs involving the fourth ventricle and CPA. Nonspecific criteria include a pattern of noncommunicating hydrocephalus involving the third and lateral ventricles, with evidence of a mass involving the fourth ventricle or adjacent cisterns. More specific for a CPT is the presence of a tumor blush, and hypertrophy with tortuosity of the precentral branches of the superior cerebellar artery or the medullary and vermian branches of the posterior inferior cerebellar artery (Raimondi & Gutierrez 1975). With tumors involving the CPA, there is typically hypertrophy and tortuosity of the anterior inferior cerebellar artery (AICA) (van Swieten et al 1987). While all these findings together may be suggestive of a CPT, other tumors such as medulloblastoma, ependymoma, and hemangioblastoma cannot be excluded (Johnson 1989).

The venous drainage of CPTs is through the quadrigeminal, Galenic, or subependymal venous systems. Choroid tumors involving the fourth ventricle are usually drained via the precentral veins (Johnson 1989).

The primary indication for cerebral angiography is to obtain more definitive localization of the vascular structures feeding and draining the CPT than can be found with CT or MRI. Certainly, for large, complex tumors with extensions out of the primary ventricle, cerebral angiography might be utilized to help plan the operative approach. With smaller and more localized lesions, angiography is rarely indicated. MRI angiographic techniques will probably prove to be of value in the evaluation of certain patients with CPTs.

Ultrasonography

Ultrasound (US) can also be used to diagnose CPTs in infants. In many instances of infants presenting with hydrocephalus, US is the initial diagnostic test. In cases of CPT, an echogenic mass is found within a dilated ventricle (Chow et al 1986, Ivan et al 1986). Though intraventricular hemorrhage can produce a similar finding, newer generation scanners with Doppler flow scanning can show the increased vascularity within the lesion. While CT and MRI give much better anatomic resolution, US offers an inexpensive, bedside alternative for diagnosis and postoperative follow-up in patients who may be too

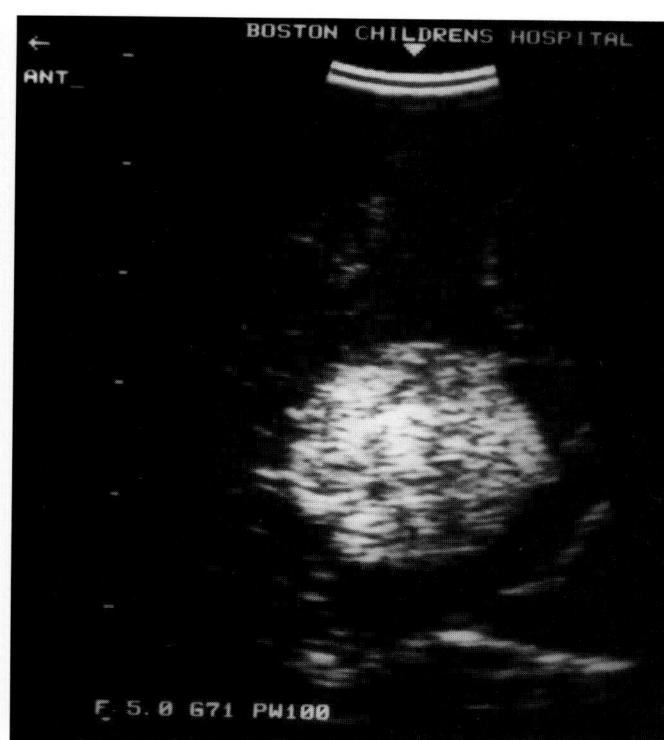

A

critically ill for the use of CT or MRI, and is an important aid in intraoperative localization (see Figs 28.8A, B).

LABORATORY DIAGNOSIS

The diagnosis of a CPT is made predominantly on the basis of radiographic evaluation. There are currently no tests or screening techniques for use with blood or serum. Although some findings on analysis of the CSF may suggest the presence of a choroid plexus tumor, such as xanthochromic fluid or a high protein content, the risks of obtaining CSF in this patient population and the non-specificity of the test results are contraindications for routine assessment of the CSF by lumbar puncture.

Recently Qualman and colleagues (1992) have suggested using CSF nephelometry for following patients with CPTs. In their nephelometry technique, serial post-operative CSF samples are obtained and α_1-antitrypsin (A1AT) is quantitatively measured. The levels of A1AT have been found to be increased over those of controls in a patient with CPC, with a decrease noted after treatment, followed by another increase when the tumor recurred. These authors suggest that A1AT levels can be used for tumor surveillance after treatment (Qualman et al 1992).

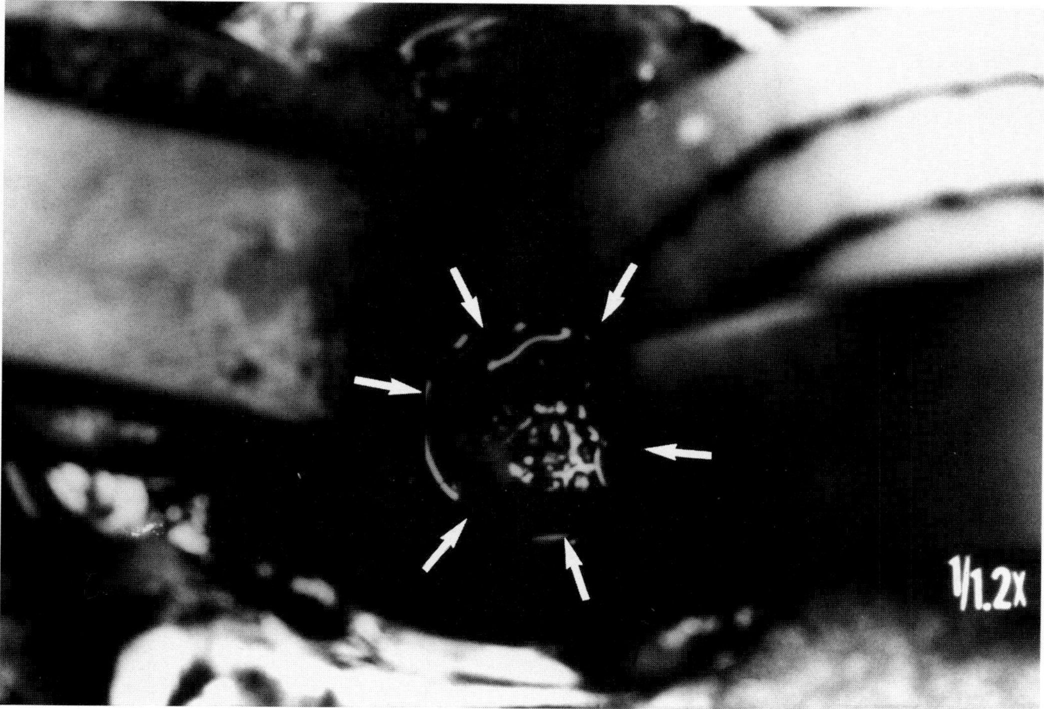

B

Fig. 28.8 **A.** Intraoperative ultrasound, same patient as Fig. 28.5. This diagnostic modality is an important surgical aid in intraoperative localization of choroid plexus tumors because of lesion echogenicity and proximity to the echolucent ventricular system, and permits precise targeting of the tumor from the brain surface. **B.** Intraoperative view, same patient. The tumor (arrows) has been exposed through a small corticectomy, and its mulberry-like appearance is demonstrated.

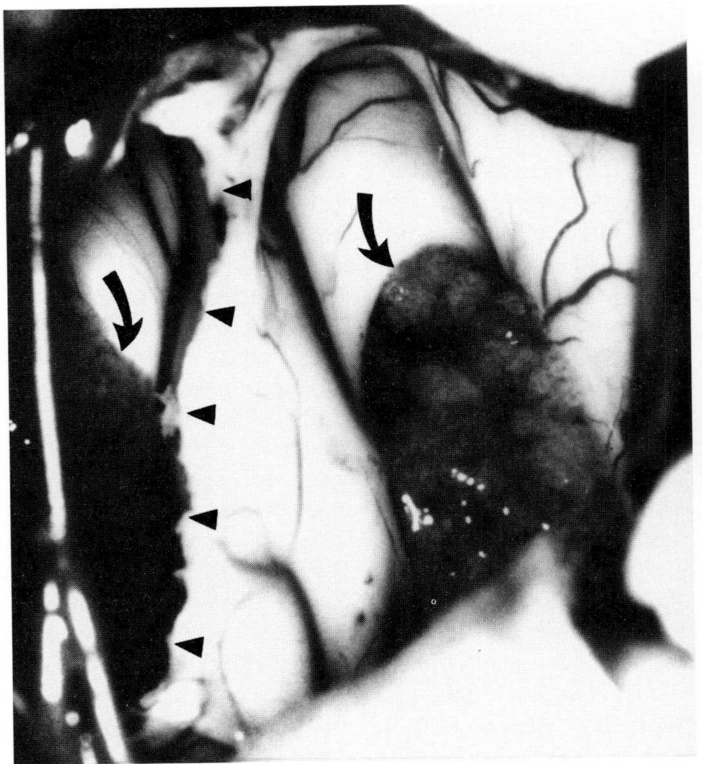

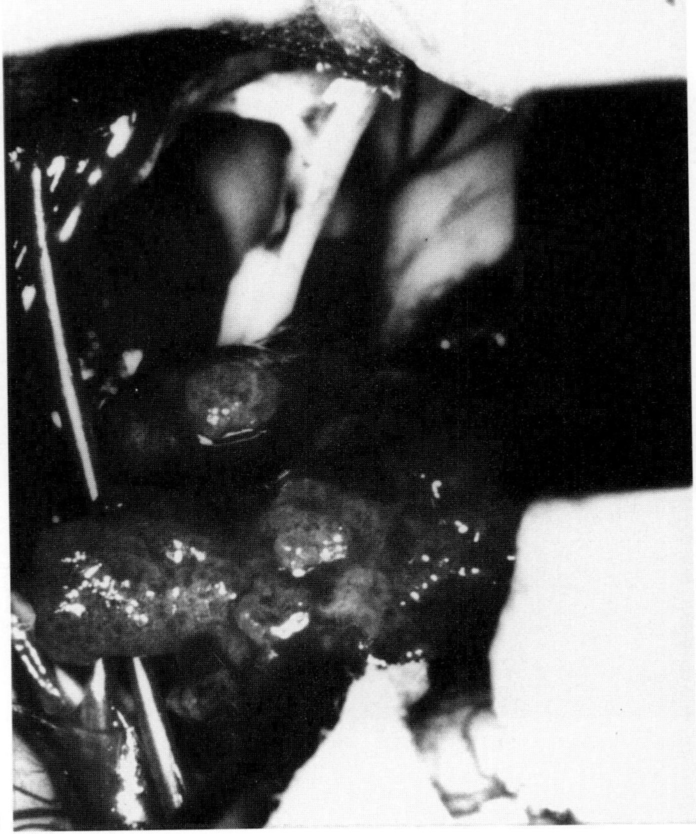

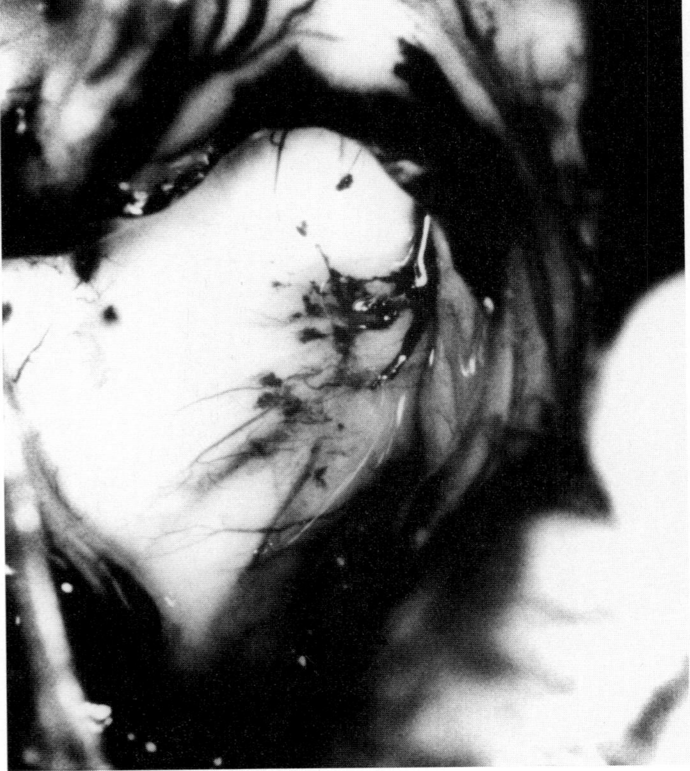

Fig. 28.9 Intraoperative photographs, same patient as in Fig. 28.4. The choroid plexus papilloma of the third ventricle has been approached through the corpus callosum. **A.** Initial exposure, with fronds of tumors (curved black arrows) presenting at both foramina of Monro. The septum pellucidum (arrowheads) has been widely fenestrated to gain access to the left lateral ventricle. **B.** Tumor is being extracted from the right foramen of Monro; the papillary nature of the tumor is apparent as it is draped, during removal, over the pericallosal branch of the right anterior cerebral artery. **C.** The tumor has been removed, and the clean white walls of the third ventricle can be visualized.

GROSS MORPHOLOGIC FEATURES

The macroscopic appearance of CPP is that of a lobulated, well-demarcated mass within the ventricular system. The average size of these tumors at presentation was 4 cm in Ellenbogen et al's (1989) series, with over 30% being larger than 6 cm. As depicted in Figure 28.9, the tumors are pink to reddish-grey or purple in color with an irregular, frondlike, papillary surface resembling a cauliflower (McGirr et al 1988). There is usually local expansion of the involved ventricle. Those tumors arising from the lateral ventricle usually are found in the plexus at the confluence of the inferior and posterior horns (Russell & Rubinstein 1989). As the tumor expands, it may extend through the foramen of Monro and into the third ventricle, or through the choroidal fissure and into the quadrigeminal cistern and even the contralateral lateral ventricle (Raimondi 1987, 1989). In cases of CPP, there is a clear distinction between the tumor and normal brain.

In the fourth ventricle, extension can occur through the foramen of Luschka and into the CPA or through the foramen of Magendie and into the cisterna magna. There is local compression of the cerebellum and brainstem. Those CPPs arising primarily in the CPA (from tufts of choroid plexus in the lateral recesses of the fourth ventricle) will produce compression and local distortion similar to other CPA masses (Rubinstein 1972).

The texture of a CPP has been described as both firm and soft, but invariably will be vascular with a friable surface. There may be areas of focal hemorrhage which can be old or new (Rubinstein 1972). Calcification can be appreciated in approximately 20% of specimens, and can lead to difficulties performing frozen sections. Russell & Rubinstein (1989) describe a case with calcification so dense as to appear bonelike.

HISTOPATHOLOGIC FEATURES

Choroid plexus epithelium is derived from neuroectodermal tissue that has been induced to change by infolding of mesoderm into the primitive ventricular system. Its structure and function are similar to those of surface epithelium (Russell & Rubinstein 1989). These similarities are also found in their respective neoplasms, with CPP and CPC closely resembling papillomas and carcinomas of surface epithelium.

Light microscopy

In CPP, the histologic appearance is similar to that of normal choroid plexus. The tumor has an arborizing pattern of papillae (see Fig. 28.9B) covered by a single layer of pseudostratified cuboidal or columnar epithelium (McGirr et al 1988). The nuclei are oval in shape and basally located. The papillae have a stroma of vascularized collagen. The connective tissue stroma, which separates CPP from papillary ependymoma, will have fibrillary neuroglia (Russell & Rubinstein 1989). The cells are fairly uniform and regular in pattern and shape. Cytologic anaplasia, multinucleation and giant cell formation are not seen and mitotic figures are rare (Rubinstein 1972). Lamellar microcalcification, present in most cases, was mild in extent in 50% of cases, moderate in 8%, and severe in 12% (McGirr et al 1988). Cilia were present in some infantile cases, indicating that the tumor developed in fetal life when cilia are transiently present in the epithelium of normal choroid plexus (Russell & Rubinstein 1989).

Special stains

For most cases, no special stains are needed to make the diagnosis of CPP other than hematoxylin and eosin. With PAS stains, occasional cells may contain PAS-positive material, a finding also seen in normal choroid plexus. Rubinstein (1972) describes a variant of CPP — a cystic tumor with a more acinar arrangement which stains intensely with PAS. These tumors are exceedingly rare, do arise from the choroid plexus in areas similar to CPP, and have been termed 'papillary and acinar mucus-secreting adenomas' (Rubinstein 1972).

Cytology

Cytologic evaluation of CSF in patients with CPTs is not always diagnostic or of high yield. When present, CPP cells are seen singularly or in clusters (> 10 per slide) with regular, round to oval nuclei (Buchino & Mason 1992). The nuclei have a uniform chromatin pattern, and there is abundant cytoplasm. This is similar to the features seen in papillary ependymoma. However, in CPTs there is no nuclear molding, in contrast to papillary ependymomas, which will also have a multilayered arrangement not seen in CPTs. Primitive neuroectodermal tumors are also to be considered in the differential diagnosis of cell clusters seen in the CSF, but usually are more hyperchromatic with evidence of molding (Buchino & Mason 1992). The cytologic findings of CPC include variability in nuclear size and shape; a high nuclear: cytoplasmic ratio; scant, pale, granular cytoplasm; and single or multiple micronucleoli (Kim et al 1985).

Immunohistochemistry

In recent years, several different immunohistochemical probes have been examined for use as markers of CPTs. These tests can aid not only in differentiating CPTs from other primary tumors and metastatic disease, but also in differentiating between CPP and CPC.

The most sensitive immunohistochemical marker for CPTs has been transthyretin (TTR, prealbumin), a protein synthesized in the brain exclusively by the CP. Production of TTR is found early on in the embryonic development of the choroid plexus and it is one of the major biosynthetic products of CP (Herbert et al 1990). After initial inconsistent findings by various authors, Herbert et al (1990) changed the methodology of the assay which improved the consistency of the findings. Several studies have now found TTR expressed in all CPTs (Matsushima et al 1988, Herbert et al 1990, Ho et al 1991). There is no clear difference in the pattern between CPP and CPC. The only other CNS tumors to show reactivity to TTR were a myxopapillary ependymoma of the filum terminale and a metastatic papillary thyroid carcinoma, both of which are histologically different from CPTs and had a much weaker staining pattern (Herbert et al 1990).

Another marker that may be specific for CPTs versus other primary brain tumors is laminin. As CPTs are an epithelial-based tumor, they have a basement membrane with a laminin subcomponent. Furness et al (1990) found immunoreactivity to laminin in all the CPTs (both CPP and CPC) they examined, but none in the ependymomas studied. In addition, there was a difference between CPP and CPC. The CPP had a continuous linear pattern consistent with other benign epithelial tumors, while the CPC showed a less intense, fragmented staining pattern.

Glial fibrillary acidic protein (GFAP) has also been associated with CPTs to varying degrees by many authors (Felix et al 1987, Russell & Rubinstein 1989, Furness et al 1990, Paulus & Jänisch 1990, Ho et al 1991, Cruz-Sanchez et al 1992, Gianella-Borradori et al 1992). Mature CP is normally negative for GFAP (Miettinen et al 1986) and the finding of GFAP within CPTs is considered to be indicative of ependymal differentiation owing to the neuroepithelial origin of CP (Russell & Rubinstein 1989). The presence of GFAP reactivity can be due to local glial differentiation, phagocytosis of the antigen by tumor cells, or origination of the tumor from transitional cells between CP and normal ependyma. Though the specificity of GFAP staining will not differentiate CPTs from other primary CNS lesions (specifically papillary ependymoma), it will exclude metastatic disease from the diagnosis (Ho et al 1991). Another nonspecific protein, S-100, has also been found to be expressed in CPTs (Felix et al 1987, Paulus and Jänisch 1990). Felix at al (1987) found a high association of S-100 in CPP, but to a lesser degree in CPC.

Cytokeratins and vimentin are another group of intermediate filament proteins that are produced by normal CP and by CPTs (Coffin et al 1986, Miettinen et al 1986). Several authors (Miettinen et al 1986, Mannoji & Becker 1988, Furness et al 1990) have found that cytokeratins are seen in CPTs but not in intracranial ependymomas. It is interesting to note that Furness and co-workers (1990) did find expression of cytokeratins in myxopapillary ependymomas of the cauda equina, though at lesser levels than found in CPTs.

Carcinoembryonic antigen (CEA) has been implicated in the past as a marker of CPC and as an indicator of poor prognosis. Several authors (Coffin et al 1986, Felix et al 1987, Matsushima et al 1988) found CEA consistently in CPC, with little or no reactivity found in CPP. However, this has not been confirmed by other studies (Furness et al 1990, Paulus & Jänisch 1990, Ho et al 1991). Paulus & Jänisch (1990) believe CEA activity is more consistent with a metastatic carcinoma to the CP, and not a CPC.

Electron microscopy

The electron microscopic features of CPTs are similar to those found in normal CP, with some minor variations. The typical findings include tumor cells resting on a continuous basement membrane (Felix et al 1987, Russell & Rubinstein 1989). The apical surface of the cells contain microvilli and junctional complexes, these tight junctions forming a blood-cerebrospinal fluid barrier (Russell & Rubinstein 1989). Within the cells are bundles of intermediate filaments (Felix et al 1987, Russell & Rubinstein 1989) and, in the infantile and childhood cases, large aggregates of glycogen granules (Russell & Rubinstein 1989). Cilia have been observed on the surface of the tumor cells and may be diagnostically important as they are not routinely found in normal choroid plexus except early in development (Russell & Rubinstein 1989). In addition, some cilia have an abnormal microtubular arrangement of 8+1 or 5+0 as opposed to the normal 9+0 (Felix et al 1987).

It should be noted that these findings are consistent with epithelium involved in fluid transport (Carter et al 1972). This provides some evidence for CSF overproduction by CPTs.

Molecular markers

Most known markers for CPTs use immunohistochemical analysis of monoclonal antibodies to different antigens in the cells, as discussed above. Gianella-Borradori et al (1992) have described an immunophenotypic pattern of CPTs which includes positive findings of cytokeratin, GFAP, two neuroectodermal markers — PI-153/3 and UJ 223.8, and a neural and leukocyte marker — Thy-1. Use of these markers, as well as additional markers for laminin and TTR, can help define the diagnosis of CPT when a question exists on morphologic criteria.

DEFINITION AND INCIDENCE OF 'MALIGNANCY'

Choroid plexus carcinoma, as mentioned earlier, is a rare tumor accounting for up to 20–30% of CPTs (Johnson 1989, Allen et al 1992). The majority of these cases occur in children. Most cases are localized to the lateral ventricles. The tumor is seen with equal frequency in males and females throughout all age ranges (Matsuda et al 1991). When CPC occurs in adults, the average age has been found to be 39 (Dohrmann & Collias 1975), with no predilection found between the posterior fossa and lateral ventricles (Matsuda et al 1991). In adults, the diagnosis of CPC must be carefully made. Not only are they rare in this age group, but confusion with a metastatic adenocarcinoma can easily occur (Lewis 1967, Dohrmann & Collias 1975, Russell & Rubinstein 1989). Metastatic adenocarcinoma is highly unlikely in children. Patients with CPC will usually present with symptoms of increased ICP similar to patients with CPP (Ellenbogen et al 1989). Packer et al (1992) found in addition an increase in focal neurologic deficits as presenting symptoms in patients with CPC.

The histologic criteria for CPC have been promoted by Lewis (1967) and Russell & Rubinstein (1989). These include: (1) transition from normal to abnormal choroid plexus; (2) nuclear atypia; and (3) invasion into adjacent neural tissue. Transition between normal CP and CPC can help confirm the lesion as originating in the CP. With this transition occurs a loss of the normal papillary architecture that is seen with both normal CP and CPP (Ellenbogen et al 1989, Russell & Rubinstein 1989). Cellular immaturity is found ultrastructurally (Anguilar et al 1983). There is also neoplastic invasion of the connective tissue stroma of the papillary structure (Johnson 1989).

The nuclear atypia seen with CPC includes nuclear pleomorphism (some with giant cells), cellular anaplasia, variations in chromatin content, glandular and acinar structures, solid sheets of anaplastic cells, and necrosis (Lewis 1967, Johnson 1989, Russell & Rubinstein 1989). Mitotic figures are commonly found in CPC, and their presence in what is thought to be a CPP should raise the suspicion of malignant change (Russell & Rubinstein 1989). Large areas of necrosis are not usually seen in CPC and may indicate a metastatic papillary adenocarcinoma (Lewis 1967).

Invasion of normal neural tissue is present in CPC with the infiltrating cells assuming a diffuse and ill-defined pattern (Russell & Rubinstein 1989). Focal infiltration occurring in what otherwise appears to be a CPP does not necessarily denote malignancy. If the infiltration is accompanied by mitotic activity and cellular irregularity, then suspicion should be raised for development of malignant change and tumor recurrence (Russell & Rubinstein 1989). Infiltration without other evidence of atypia has the same benign course as CPP (Ellenbogen et al 1989, Russell & Rubinstein 1989).

The electron microscopic findings of CPC include two layers of tumor cells with a basement membrane separating the tumor cells from the fibrovascular stroma (Felix et al 1987). Desmosomes, bundles of intermediate filaments, and microvilli are found, as they are in CPP; however, cilia are not appreciated (Felix et al 1987). These findings do not help in differentiating a CPP from a CPC, but can distinguish CPC from other lesions such as an ependymoma (Matsuda et al 1991).

Metastatic spread via seeding is a common finding in CPTs, with an overall incidence of 10–20% (Johnson 1989), but it is not pathognomonic of CPC as CPP can also show seeding (Lewis 1967, Russell & Rubinstein 1989). Seeding by CPP is an uncommon occurrence, but one with a benign course. The 'shed' cells retain the benign morphologic characteristics of the parent tumor (Lewis 1967). In CPC, metastatic seeding is found in 44% of cases (Ausman et al 1984) throughout the leptomeninges and walls of the ventricular system (Russell & Rubinstein 1989). Cases of extraneural metastasis are extremely rare, but have been reported in the lung (St Clair et al 1991).

The outcome of patients with CPC is largely dependent on the ability to excise the tumor. In most older series, the prognosis was poor. Recent series (Ellenbogen et al 1989, Packer et al 1992) have shown more encouraging results. Packer et al (1992), combining their patients with others in the literature, found 11 of 14 children having prolonged disease-free interval after total surgical excision, while only 2 of 20 patients with partial excisions were reported to be alive and free of progressive disease. Ellenbogen et al (1989) report a 50% 5-year survival rate with most deaths occurring before 1960. Local recurrence, when it occurs, should be treated with aggressive surgical excision despite the histologic findings (Ellenbogen et al 1989).

There are no good predictors of the activity of CPC based on tumor markers. Furness et al (1990) consider that the behavior of the lesion is best predicted by morphologic criteria and how the histologic appearance of the tumor differs from normal choroid plexus.

GENERAL MANAGEMENT PLAN

The mainstay of treatment of CPTs is early diagnosis and surgical excision. With the advent of CT and MRI, diagnosis of an intraventricular mass in a patient with evidence of increased ICP can be made early in the evaluation. After obtaining the appropriate imaging studies, and stabilizing the patient clinically, surgery can then be performed with the goal of gross total resection (GTR). Postoperatively, some patients may require a shunting procedure. If the lesion is a CPP and has been removed in toto, no additional treatment is needed other than radiographic surveillance for recurrence. In cases where there is residual or recurrent disease, some form of adjunctive therapy may be considered. However, surgical resection is the only proven form of therapy for this benign lesion. If the diagnosis is CPC, imaging of the neuraxis must be done to rule out seeding. Adjunctive therapy for this lesion is age-dependent, with chemotherapy becoming the preferred treatment both pre- and postoperatively. A diagnosis of CPC with subtotal removal will make some form of adjunctive treatment necessary.

SURGICAL MANAGEMENT

The primary treatment modality for CPTs is gross total resection of the lesion. After establishing the diagnosis of an intraventricular mass with hydrocephalus and raised ICP, the first decision involves the need for preoperative shunting or CSF diversion (i.e. ventriculostomy with external ventricular draining). This decision must be based on the clinical condition of the patient, and the radiographic findings on CT or MRI. All patients should be started on corticosteroids as soon as the diagnosis is made in an attempt to decrease any cerebral edema that may be present, and possibly to decrease CSF production. Many patients have rapid clinical improvement with the administration of steroids, obviating the need for early ventricular draining. Johnson (1989) uses obliteration of the basal cisterns as an absolute indication for ventriculostomy, with failure of the patient to improve clinically 4 hours after starting steroids as another indication for ventriculostomy. Some authors recommend shunting preoperatively to allow for resolution of the hydrocephalus, clinical improvement of the patient, and cortical mantle thickening which may lessen the chance of hemispheric collapse postoperatively (Raimondi & Gutierrez 1975, Lena et al 1990). One problem with preoperative ventriculo-peritoneal shunts is the development of ascites in some patients because of the high rate of CSF production by some of these tumors (Knierim 1990, Schijman et al 1990). The ability to make a radiographic diagnosis early in the management of a patient may make close clinical observation an option prior to any surgical intervention. These decisions are made on a case-by-case basis.

Another preoperative concern in CPTs is the possibility of blood loss, the most common operative complication in most series (Bohm & Strang 1961, Hawkins 1980, Ellenbogen et al 1989). Ensuring adequate hydration, and availability of blood products is imperative. This is especially true in the very young children who make up the majority of patients and may present with significant fluid deficit from losses secondary to vomiting and anorexia due to increased ICP. All patients should also be started on anticonvulsants preoperatively (Shillito & Matson 1982).

The surgical approach is determined by careful analysis of the radiographic studies. If the lesion is large, or if there is any doubt as to its vascular supply, then arteriography should be used to supplement other imaging modalities. In many cases, high resolution CT and MRI may give all the information necessary for planning a safe operative approach.

A thorough discussion of operative techniques employed for CPT resection can be found in Shillito & Matson (1982) and Raimondi (1987, 1989). These authors and others (Matson & Crofton 1960, Hawkins 1980, Ellenbogen et al 1989) recommend 'en bloc' excision of the tumor whenever possible after first gaining control of the vascular supply. They do not recommend piecemeal resection of the tumor because of the danger of blood loss. Advances in operative technology — including the operative microscope, bipolar electrocautery, and safe retractor systems — have made surgical excision of these lesions safer. Raimondi (1989) advocates the use of bipolar electrocautery to shrink the tumor and allow better visibility of the vascular pedicle before removal. Some authors recommend the tandem use of ultrasonic aspiration and bipolar electrocautery to debulk the tumor and maintain hemostasis, allowing the vasculature to be exposed in this fashion (Ivan et al 1986, Johnson 1989). For some large tumors, it may be advisable to remove the lesion in a staged fashion, especially in children where ongoing fluid loss may pose difficulties (Ellenbogen et al 1989).

For tumors in the region of the trigone, most authors prefer an approach in the region posterior to the angular gyrus (Shillito & Matson 1982, Johnson 1989, Raimondi 1987, 1989). This provides access to the tumor and its vascular pedicle, which is usually on the inferomedial surface (Shillito & Matson 1982, Raimondi 1989). Tumors extending into the foramen of Monro may require an additional cerebrotomy in the frontal region (Raimondi 1987). Prior to the dural incision, a ventricular needle may be inserted into the dilated temporal horn to relax the brain if it is under tension (Shillito & Matson 1982). After localizing the tumor within the ventricle, cotton pledgets should be used to isolate the tumor, preventing blood from escaping into the ventricular system. After the tumor is removed, the ventricles should be re-expanded with normal saline prior to closure to remove air and decrease the subdural space (Johnson 1989). The tumor bed should be inspected for 10 minutes prior to closure to ensure no bleeding persists (Raimondi 1989).

In cases where there is extension of the tumor through the choroidal fissure and into the quadrigeminal cistern, two approaches must be made. Raimondi (1987, 1989) recommends going transcortically as described above (bilaterally if needed) and then parasagittally to expose the quadrigeminal cistern. Here the arterial supply is from the medial and lateral posterior choroidal arteries, which must be secured. Care must also be taken not to damage the major veins which are tributaries of and in close proximity to the galenic system.

When a CPT arises in, or extends into the third ventricle, there are several different possible approaches. Some authors prefer a transcallosal approach (Raimondi & Gutierrez 1975, Fortuna 1979, Ellenbogen et al 1989, Knierim 1991). This approach obviates the need for a cortical incision (Fig. 29.7). The transfrontal, transventricular approach to CPTs in the third ventricle has also been recommended by other authors (Gradin et al 1983, Raimondi 1989, Schijman et al 1990).

Posterior fossa CPTs are approached through a suboccipital craniotomy (Ellenbogen et al 1989) or craniectomy (Raimondi & Gutierrez 1975). For lesions localized mainly in the fourth ventricle, the vermis, tonsils and upper cervical cord are first exposed. The tonsils can then be retracted laterally to expose the base of the vermis and the vermian and medullary branches of PICA which feed the tumor. These can then be occluded and divided so the vascular supply to the tumor is controlled prior to manipulation of the tumor mass (Raimondi 1987). The surgeon should also be aware of possible feeding branches from AICA in the lateral recess, where a bleeding vessel may retract if not adequately controlled (Raimondi 1987). Care must be taken when removing the tumor to limit manipulation of the tumor which may have adhesions with the floor of the fourth ventricle resulting in torsion on the brainstem. In addition, venous drainage may involve the superior medullary velum and precentral veins which can be torn by removal of the tumor prior to their visualization and control (Raimondi & Gutierrez 1975).

Tumors localized to the CPA can be removed via a lateral suboccipital approach with attention given to branches of PICA or AICA which are the predominant arterial supply (Piguet & de Tribolet 1984, van Swieten et al 1987). Another potential arterial feeder is the tentorial branch from the meningohypophyseal trunk (artery of Bernasconi) (van Swieten et al 1987).

Regardless of the location, the main goal is total resection of the lesion. This is true for both CPP and CPC. Even if there is gross infiltration of normal brain, a total resection should be attempted if possible (Boyd & Steinbok 1987, McGirr et al 1988, Ellenbogen et al 1989, Johnson 1989, Knierim 1991). In cases where there is localized recurrence of tumor, regardless of histologic type, the treatment plan should first consider additional surgical resection if the patient's clinical condition permits (Ellenbogen et al 1989). If the lesion is considered to be surgically inaccessible, additional adjunctive therapies must be considered.

INDICATIONS FOR AND RESULTS OF RADIATION THERAPY/RADIOSURGERY

The use of radiation therapy (RTx) in the management of CPTs is controversial. As noted above, the primary treatment of these lesions is GTR. However, in cases where only a subtotal resection can be safely performed, or surgery is contraindicated, consideration may be given to the use of adjunctive RTx. Regardless of the histologic diagnosis, most authors agree that RTx is contraindicated in children less than 3 years of age (Johnson 1989, Knierim 1990, Allen et al 1992).

The difficulty in determining the best RTx protocol for the treatment of CPTs is their overall rarity, with no large series of patients treated in a consistent pattern. Problems in evaluating these series include inconsistencies in reporting exact doses, fraction schedules, and the type of fields used. For patients with CPP and GTR, there is no indication for additional treatment with RTx (McGirr et al 1988, Ellenbogen et al 1989, Johnson 1989, Knierim 1991, Packer et al 1992). In cases of residual CPP, there has been no clear indication that RTx has any effect. While some authors report good results with RTx (Palazzi et al 1989, Packer et al 1992), others found no clear benefit (Matson & Crofton 1960, Bohm & Strang 1961, McGirr et al 1989). McGirr et al (1989) found a 50% recurrence rate in patients with subtotal resections treated with RTx, and had two patients with subtotal resection remain disease-free with no RTx. They recommended against using routine RTx in CPP patients with subtotal resections.

In cases of CPC with GTR and no evidence of seeding, most authors recommend the use of RTx (Matson and Crofton 1960, Bohm and Strang 1961, Carpenter et al 1982, Ausman et al 1984, Johnson 1989, Palazzi et al 1989). In cases of residual CPC (Fig. 28.10), some authors use standard RTx (Knierim 1991, Allen et al 1992). Others use full craniospinal radiation in CPC cases because of the risk of disseminated disease (Ausman et al 1984, Palazzi et al 1989, Packer et al 1992).

In cases of recurrent CPTs, surgery is again the recommended initial treatment, with RTx also playing a role. Several series suggest RTx in cases of recurrent disease (McGirr et al 1988). Packer et al (1992), however, found no response in patients treated with RTx at relapse.

Preoperative RTx has been suggested in the hope of decreasing tumor vasculature (Hawkins 1980). This has been done only in isolated cases and no data have been presented to suggest this as standard practice. No series using stereotactic radiosurgical procedures or the Gamma Knife have been published, but they may play a role in managing recurrent or residual CPCs that are surgically inaccessible.

INDICATIONS FOR AND RESULTS OF CHEMOTHERAPY

In the past, adjunctive treatment of CPT consisted primarily of RTx. Recently, several reports have appeared on the possible usefulness of chemotherapy (CTx) for those patients not treated adequately with surgery. This is especially true in patients less than 3 years of age, in whom RTx is a relative contraindication. The difficulty in deciding on the proper use of CTx is emphasized by reviewing the pertinent literature. Very few large series are available in which CTx was used, and none in which a prospective protocol was followed. Most reports consist of limited number of patients with varying combinations of CTx agents. Another difficulty in examining these series is the grouping together of patients undergoing GTR (theoretically a cure by itself) and subtotal resections and then receiving CTx, making comparison of outcomes difficult. The main problem with the CTx literature, as with the RTx literature, stems from the relative rarity of CPTs.

The clearest indications for CTx are in the management of young children with residual CPC after an adequate attempt at surgical resection, or in the presence of metastatic spread (Johnson 1989, Duffner et al 1989, Allen et al 1992, Packer et al 1992). Duffner et al (1989) used the Infant Pediatric Oncology Group (POG) protocol alone (cyclophosphamide, vincristine, cisplatin, and

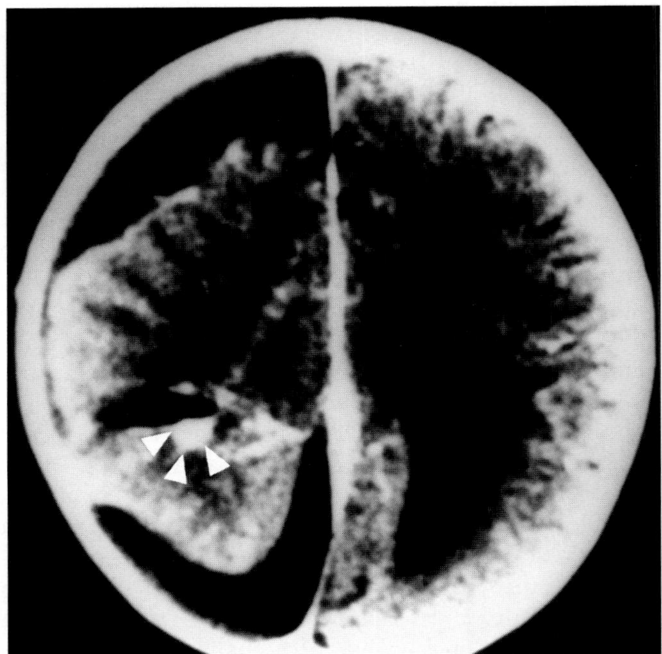

A

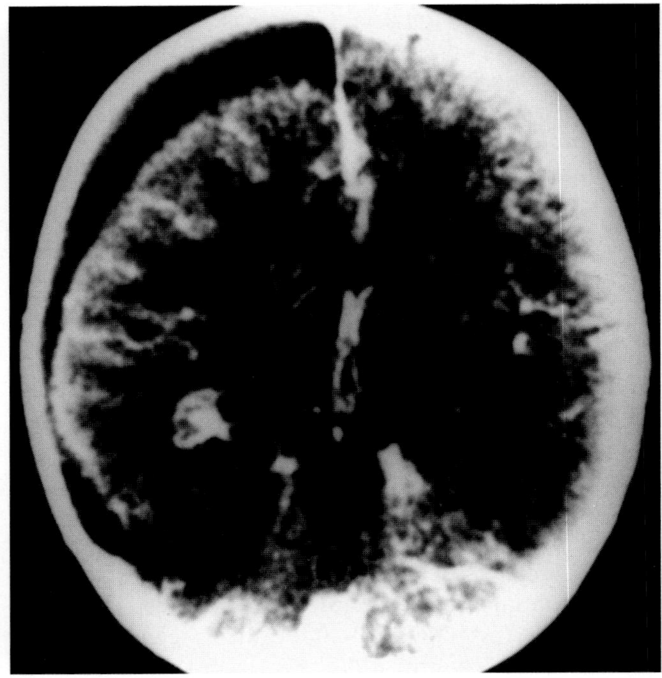

B

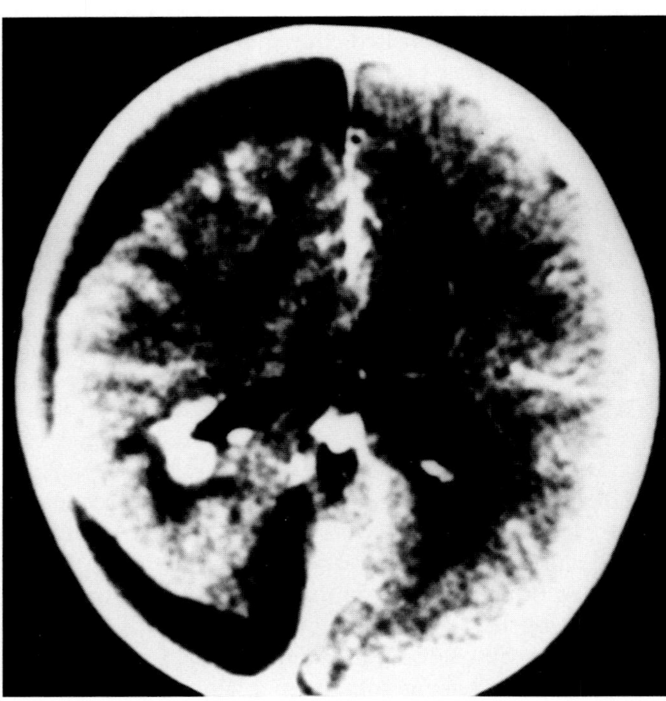

C

Fig. 28.10 Same patient as Fig. 28.7; postoperative enhanced CT scans. **A.** 1 month postoperative scan, demonstrating subdural fluid collection, a common finding after removal of large choroid plexus tumors. A small focus of enhancement suggests residual neoplasm (arrowheads). **B, C.** Repeat scans, 2 and 3 months postoperative, demonstrating enlargement of the contrast-enhancing area. The patient was reoperated upon to excise the residual tumor confirmed by pathological examination, with no subsequent recurrence.

etoposide) on 5 patients with CPC, 3 with residual tumor after surgery, with a good response in 3 patients, including the 2 patients with GTR. Allen et al (1992) used a similar protocol in 3 cases (cisplatin and etoposide) with 1 patient having a sustained remission (this patient also underwent a second surgical procedure which was reported to be a GTR). Packer et al (1992) used several combinations of cisplatin and etoposide (and thiotepa in 1 patient) as a salvage attempt in 4 of 6 patients with relapse after partial resection and RTx, with only 1 response. Gianella-Borradori et al (1992) administered the 8-drugs-in-1-day protocol to 2 patients with residual disease, with no evidence of progression and follow-up over 4 years. Boyd & Steinbok (1987) used the same protocol with no success in 1 patient.

St Clair et al (1991) have advocated the use of CTx as an interim measure to increase the possibility of GTR. Using etoposide (VP-16), ifosfamide and carboplatinum, they showed a decrease in tumor size and vascularity after treatment. These patients initially had partial resections or biopsies and after CTX were able to have GTR with less intraoperative blood loss. The use of preoperative CTx should be considered with large lesions in small children to decrease operative risks and help ensure GTR which carries the best prognosis.

The current recommendations for CTx are in the management of patients under 36 months of age who have residual or recurrent CPC after surgical resection. Depending upon the clinical presentation of the patient, preoperative CTx should be considered as a prelude to an attempt at GTR (St Clair et al 1991). If a response is seen, further treatment can consist of maintenance CTx (Allen et al [1992] recommend carboplatin, cyclophosphamide and vincristine), or an additional attempt at surgical resection. The use of RTx should be used as a last resort, given the potential for damage to the developing brain. The role CTx should play in the management of adults with recurrent or residual CPTs has not been thoroughly explored, but could be used depending on the patient's clinical status. If future studies confirm the benefits of CTx, it may become the primary adjunctive therapy in the management of CPTs (Duffner et al 1989, St Clair et al 1991, Allen et al 1992).

OTHER ADJUNCTIVE THERAPY

Given the scarcity of CPTs, and the success rates obtained with GTR, most adjunctive therapy has centered on the use of RTx and CTx. The clinical effects of other treatment modalities such as adoptive immunotherapy, hyperthermia, photoradiation, etc. remain unknown.

MANAGEMENT OF ASSOCIATED PHENOMENA

An important clinical phenomenon seen with CPTs is the large degree of hydrocephalus associated with these lesions which usually brings the patient to clinical attention. The hydrocephalus produced by choroid plexus tumors is interesting because it is apparently produced not only by blockage of CSF pathways within the brain or over its surface, but also by overproduction of CSF, a unique feature of these neoplasms. There are numerous reports of patients with choroid plexus tumors whose hydrocephalus is refractory to shunting or who develop ascites after shunting (Eisenberg et al 1974, Milhorat et al 1976, Knierim 1990). Eisenberg et al (1974) measured CSF production at greater than four times the normal rate in a child with a CPP of the left ventricle. Milhorat et al (1976) found a similar rate which decreased to normal range after the complete removal of the tumor. Matson & Crofton (1960) believed that complete resection of a CPP was curative for hydrocephalus and that shunting was not indicated in the routine postoperative management of these patients. While some series have patients whose hydrocephalus resolves after GTR, the experience of other authors is that patients will need shunting after surgery (Raimondi & Gutierrez 1975, Lena et al 1990). Subarachnoid blood, from tumor hemorrhage or surgery, desquamation of necrotic tumor, proteinaceous CSF, basal meningitis, inflammatory ependymitis and metastatic tumor cells can lead to communicating hydrocephalus in spite of GTR (Raimondi & Gutierrez 1975, Ellenbogen et al 1989, Russell & Rubinstein 1989). Most authors currently recommend no shunting at the time of the initial surgery and close CT follow-up of the patients (Hawkins 1980, Boyd & Steinbok 1987, Ellenbogen et al 1989, Johnson 1989). Any patient with persistent or increasing hydrocephalus should then be treated with the appropriate shunting technique. Shillito & Matson (1982) caution that intraventricular clot with obstruction of the foramen of Monro may also be a cause of postoperative hydrocephalus.

Subdural effusions are another problem frequently encountered in the postoperative management of CPTs, especially when transcortical incisions are used (Fig. 28.8). This problem develops when the thinned cortical mantle produced by ventriculomegaly collapses after decompression of the ventricle. Another explanation may be persistent hydrocephalus with fluid flowing out of the cortical incision into the subdural space created at surgery. These subdural effusions can have a significant effect on neurologic recovery (Pascual-Castroviejo et al 1983). Several techniques can be used in the management of this problem. Before dural closure, the ventricle should be re-expanded with saline (Boyd & Steinbok 1987, Johnson 1989). Boyd & Steinbok (1987) recommend attempting pial closure, especially in patients with thinned cortical mantles, to prevent the development of ventriculo-subdural fistulas. Johnson (1989) recommends a subdural drain postoperatively set to the level of the bed. Shillito & Matson (1982) recommend against drains to prevent spinal fluid fistulas from developing. If hydrocephalus exists in conjunction with the effusion, a ventriculo-peritoneal shunt (VPS) may be useful on the ipsilateral side. Routine use of VPS, however, may lead to subdural formation by overdraining the ventricles (Pascual-Castroviejo et al 1983). In some patients, a combination of ventricular and subdural shunting may be needed. Regardless of the techniques used, it is the authors' experience that such collections are an almost invariable sequel of surgery for CPTs associated with hydrocephalus in children.

PATTERNS OF FAILURE

There is a difference between CPP and CPC in the presentation of persistent disease. For CPP undergoing GTR, treatment failure will usually manifest as local tumor recurrence. In most recent studies, this problem is rare. McGirr et al (1988) treated 14 patients with GTR, with 12 patients surviving and only 1 recurrence in this group occurring 11 years after surgery with the patient doing well after a second procedure with GTR. Ellenbogen et al (1989) reported no recurrences in their patients with GTR with an average follow-up period of 4.5 years. Knierim (1990) also reported no recurrences, but had a shorter follow-up period. Other series have similar experiences (Hawkins 1980, Boyd & Steinbok 1987). These same series also report a higher rate of recurrence, or continued growth in patients with subtotal resections. Raimondi (1989) warns of the possibility of subependymal spread of tumor or spread into adjacent cisterns. With CT and MRI, this phenomenon should be appreciated before surgery, but it can also be a factor in tumor recurrence at sites adjacent to the original lesion. As noted above, CSF examination can sometimes find abnormal cells consistent with CPP, but this appears not to be of clinical significance.

In cases of CPC, local recurrence and subependymal spread are more common, as well as metastatic spread throughout the subarachnoid space. For patients undergoing GTR, Ellenbogen et al (1989) found tumor recurrence at the primary site in 3 out of 9 patients. Packer et al (1992) reported that 1 in 5 of their patients had a recurrence after GTR, and that patient had positive cytology on postoperative staging. Patients with partial resections and evidence of seeding had poor clinical outcomes. Boyd & Steinbok (1987) and Hawkins (1980) had 5 patients with CPC, all dying within 5 months except 1 who was alive after RTx but with follow-up less than 2 years. All of Ellenbogen et al's (1989) CPC patients with subtotal resections died within 7 months, all having residual tumor at autopsy. Packer et al (1992) found 2 patients with disseminated disease at diagnosis; both patients died within 5 months with evidence of both local and metastatic recurrence. These authors also found 5 of 6 patients with subtotal resections developing recurrences a median of 3 months after treatment (1 patient had a late recurrence 52 months after treatment including RTx). Of Allen et al's (1992) 3 patients, 2 developed recurrences after partial resections, one dying 11 months and the other 57 months after diagnosis; both patients were treated with adjunctive CTx.

MANAGEMENT OF RECURRENT DISEASE

The definitive treatment for recurrent disease is another attempt at surgical resection. This is true for both CPP and CPC (Ellenbogen et al 1989). In most patients with residual CPP, conservative management is the prudent course of action until the patient can tolerate further surgery or tumor growth resumes. The role of CTx in residual CPP has not been well studied.

After GTR in recurrent CPC, some authors would advocate some form of adjunctive therapy regardless of the extent of resection. The clinical condition and age of the patient should determine the treatment course. Adjunctive therapy is mainly indicated in CPC not amenable to complete surgical excision, or with evidence of seeding or distant disease. If the recurrence is limited to the local site and staging is clear, CTx should be used in infants and possibly all patients in the hope of controlling the disease or as an interim measure before further surgery. This protocol is controversial, since some would advocate craniospinal RTx with boosts to the primary site. In cases where there is evidence of metastatic disease on staging, there is clear evidence that adjunctive treatment should be given, as the outcome without additional therapy is bleak. Most studies have used craniospinal RTx in the management of widespread disease, but further studies may indicate that CTx is a better option, and it is certainly the treatment of choice in patients less than 36 months of age.

Several series attempted combination treatment with RTx and CTx. Maria et al (1985) reported salvaging a patient with a recurrent CPC after two subtotal resections and RTx, using a combination of cisplatin, bleomycin, and vinblastine. Kim et al (1985) successfully treated a patient with metastatic disease using a combination of RTx, intrathecal methotrexate and systemic BCNU and 5-fluorouracil. Ellenbogen et al (1989) treated 3 patients with recurrent CPC using vincristine and cisplatin with mixed results, the only patient having a good response also receiving RTx.

MANAGEMENT OUTCOME

The survival rates are different for CPP and CPC and have significantly improved in the era of modern neurosurgery. Bohm & Strang (1961), in their series from 1926 to 1958, had a surgical mortality of 40%, higher (62.5%) in patients with lesions in the lateral ventricles (6 out of 8 patients here being children). Patients with tumors in the fourth ventricle, all adults, had an average survival of 13.4 years. Matson & Crofton (1960) reported a 27% overall perioperative mortality rate with the surviving patients doing well, follow-up ranging up to 7 years. Hawkins (1980) had an operative mortality of 24%. Long-term results were good in 35% and fair ('moderately handicapped') in 24% (46% and 31% if only the surviving patients are accounted for). Boyd & Steinbok (1987) had 2 of 11 patients die within 2 months of surgery (both had CPC). The remaining 9 patients were followed for a mean of 5.5 years (range 5 months to 9 years) with only one tumor-related death; there were no deaths in patients with GTR. McGirr et al (1988) reported a perioperative mortality rate of 15%, all deaths occurring before 1950. The average follow-up for the remaining patients was 10.8 years, ranging from 6 months to 40 years. All patients with GTR survived. In surviving patients with subtotal resection, 2 out of 10 received no RTx and are clinically well 6 and 8 years after surgery. The remaining 8 patients received RTx: 4 are doing well at follow-up (time frame not reported); the other 4 died, with tumor recurrence within the radiation ports in 3 of these patients (unknown in the other case). Ellenbogen et al (1989) had an 88% survival rate in patients with CPP, the last death occurring in 1961. The overall 5-year survival rate was 84%, 100% if only the patients treated after 1961 are counted. The median follow-up period was 4.5 years (ranging from 9 months to 30 years). Knierim (1990) reported a 0% operative mortality and no deaths in their patients with

CPP, all with GTR (mean follow-up 40 months, range 11.5–74 months). These results show an increase in safety (lower surgical mortality) and better outcome (increased survival) with the advent of newer surgical techniques.

While the results for patients with CPC have not been as good as with CPP, the trends noted above are also seen with CPC. In the early studies, CPC carried a grave prognosis with only rare patients having sustained survival. Recent studies have shown some encouragement. Ellenbogen et al (1989) reported a 5-year survival rate of 50%. Nine patients underwent GTR: 4 had no recurrence (median follow-up 9.8 years); 1 patient received RTx and subsequently developed a meningioma within the radiation field 18 years after surgery, but no recurrence of the CPC; 3 patients had recurrences and were treated with combinations of surgery, CTx and RTx, with 1 death; and a patient initially biopsied and treated with CTx and then GTR had no recurrence at 3 years. All patients with subtotal resections died. Packer et al (1992) had similar results with 45% (5/11 patients) being in remission a median of 48 months after diagnosis, and 55% (6/11) having relapse at a median of 6 months. Of the 5 patients in remission, 4 had GTR; the other patient with GTR had a recurrence at 5 months and was receiving CTx at the time of the report. Of the 6 patients with subtotal resections, only 1 survived (RTx given, 44+ months of remission). Allen et al (1992) treated 3 patients initially with subtotal resection and CTX; the only patient having a complete response (46+ months) had an additional GTR procedure, the other 2 died of recurrences 5 and 57 months after diagnosis.

It is clear from the above statistics that GTR is the goal in the management of CPP and CPC. If total resection is obtained, patient survival is far better than if subtotal resection is performed. However, new regimens of CTx, combined in some cases with RTx, may offer substantial palliative therapy to patients with residual and recurrent disease. Advances in neurosurgery and modern neurosurgical techniques have considerably improved the outlook for patients with CPTs.

REFERENCES

Allen J, Wisoff J, Helson L, Pearce J, Arenson E 1992 Choroid plexus carcinoma — responses to chemotherapy alone in newly diagnosed young children. Journal of Neuro-Oncology 12: 69–74

Anguilar D, Martin J M, Aneiros J, Arjona V, Lara J L, Nogales F 1983 The fine structure of choroid plexus carcinoma. Histopathology 7: 939–946

Ausman J I, Shrontz C, Chason J, Knighton R S, Pak H, Patel S 1984 Aggressive choroid plexus papilloma. Surgical Neurology 22: 472–476

Bergsagel D J, Finegold M J, Butel J S, Kupsky W H, Garcea R L 1992 DNA sequences similar to those of simian virus 40 in ependymomas and choroid plexus tumors of childhood. The New England Journal of Medicine 326: 988–993

Blamires T L, Friedmann I, Moffat D A 1992 Von Hippel-Lindau disease associated with an invasive choroid plexus tumor presenting as a middle ear mass. The Journal of Laryngology and Otology 106: 429–435

Bohm E, Strang R 1961 Choroid plexus papillomas. Journal of Neurosurgery 18: 493–500

Boyd M C, Steinbok M B 1987 Choroid plexus tumors: problems in diagnosis and management. Journal of Neurosurgery 66: 800–805

Buchino J J, Mason K G 1992 Choroid plexus papilloma. Report of a case with cytologic differential diagnosis. Acta Cytologica 36: 95–97

Carpenter D B, Michelsen W J, Hays A P 1982 Carcinoma of the choroid plexus. Case report. Journal of Neurosurgery 56: 722–727

Carter L P, Beggs J, Waggener J D 1972 Ultrastructure of three choroid plexus papillomas. Cancer 30: 1130–1136

Chen J, Van Dyke T 1991 Uniform cell-autonomous tumorigenesis of the choroid plexus by papovavirus large T antigens. Molecular and Cellular Biology 11 (12): 5968–5976

Chow P P, Horgan J G, Burns P N, Weltin G, Taylor K J W 1986 Choroid plexus papilloma: detection by real-time and doppler sonography. American Journal of Neuroradiology 7: 168–170

Coates T L, Hinshaw D B Jr, Peckman N et al 1989 Pediatric choroid plexus neoplasms: MR, CT, and pathologic correlation. Radiology 173: 81–88

Coffin C M, Wick M R, Braun J T, Dehner L P 1986 Choroid plexus neoplasms. Clinicopathologic and immunohistochemical studies. American Journal of Surgical Pathology 10: 394–404

Cruz-Sanchez F F, Garcia-Bachs M, Rossi M L et al 1992 Epithelial differentiation in gliomas, meningiomas and choroid plexus papillomas. Virchows Archiv B Cell Pathology 62: 25–34

Davis L E 1924 A physiopathological study of the choroid plexus with the report of a case of villous hypertrophy. Medical Research 44: 521–534

Davis L E, Cushing H 1925 Papilloma of the choroid plexus: with the report of six cases. Archives of Neurology and Psychiatry 13: 681–710

Dohrmann G J, Collias J C 1975 Choroid plexus carcinoma. Journal of Neurosurgery 43: 225–232

Duffner P K, Cohen M E, Horowitz M et al 1989 The treatment of choroid plexus carcinoma in infancy with chemotherapy. Annals of Neurology 26: 460

Eisenberg H E, McComb J G, Lorenzo A V 1974 Cerebrospinal fluid overproduction and hydrocephalus associated with choroid plexus papilloma. Journal of Neurosurgery 40: 381–385

Ellenbogen R G, Winston K R, Kupsky W J 1989 Tumors of the choroid plexus in children. Neurosurgery 25: 327–335

Felix I, Phudhichareonrat S, Halliday W C, Becker L E 1987 Choroid plexus tumors in children: immunohistochemical and scanning-electron-microscopic features. Pediatric Neuroscience 13: 263–269

Filipek P A, Kennedy D N, Caviness V S Jr 1991 Volumetric analyses of central nervous system neoplasm based on MRI. Pediatric Neurology 7: 347–351

Furness P N, Lowe J, Tarrant G S 1990 Subepithelial basement membrane deposition and intermediate filament expression in choroid plexus neoplasms and ependymomas. Histopathology 16: 251–255

Garber J E, Burke E M, Lavally B L et al 1990 Choroid plexus tumors in the breast cancer-sarcoma syndrome. Cancer 66: 2658–2660

Gianella-Borradori A, Zeltzer P M, Bodey B, Nelson M, Britton H, Marlin A 1992 Choroid plexus tumors in childhood: response to chemotherapy, and immunophenotypic profile using a panel of monoclonal antibodies. Cancer 69: 809–816

Gradin W C, Taylon C, Fruin A H 1983 Choroid plexus papilloma of the third ventricle: case report and review of the literature. Neurosurgery 12: 217–220

Guerard M 1832 Tumeur fongeuse dans le ventricle droit du cerveau chez une petite fille de trois ans. Bulletin of the Society of Anatomy of Paris 8: 211–214

Haddad S F, Menezes A H, Bell W E, Godersky J C, Afifi A K, Bale J F 1991 Brain tumors occurring before 1 year of age: a retrospective review of 22 cases in an 11-year period (1977–1987). Neurosurgery 29: 8–13

Hammock M K, Milhorat T H, Breckbill D L 1976 Primary choroid plexus papilloma of the cerebellopontine angle presenting as a brain stem tumor in a child. Child's Brain 2: 132–142
Hawkins J C III 1980 Treatment of choroid plexus papillomas in children: a brief analysis of twenty years' experience. Neurosurgery 6: 380–384
Heiskanen O 1977 Intracranial tumors of children. Child's Brain 3: 69–78
Herbert J, Cavallaro T, Dwork A J 1990 A marker for primary choroid plexus neoplasms. American Journal of Pathology 136: 1317–1325
Ho D M, Wong T T, Liu H C 1991 Choroid plexus tumors in childhood. Histopathologic study and clinico-pathological correlation. Child's Nervous System 7: 437–441
Humphreys R P, Nemoto S, Hendrick E B, Hoffman H J 1987 Childhood choroid plexus tumors. Concepts in Pediatric Neurosurgery 7: 1–18
Ivan L P, Martin D J, Mallya K B, Schneider E 1986 Choroid plexus papilloma in a 4-month-old child: a case report. Journal of Child Neurology 1: 53–55
Johnson D L 1989 Management of choroid plexus tumors in children: Pediatric Neuroscience 15: 195–206
Jooma R, Hayward R D, Grant D N 1984 Intracranial neoplasms during the first year of life: analysis of one hundred consecutive cases. Neurosurgery 14: 31–41
Kim K, Greenblatt S H, Robinson M G 1985 Choroid plexus carcinoma. Report of a case with cytopathologic differential diagnosis. Acta Cytologica 29: 846–849
Knierim D S 1990 Choroid plexus tumors in infants. Pediatric Neurosurgery 16: 276–280
Lena G, Genitori L, Molina J, Legatte J R S, Choux M 1990 Choroid plexus tumours in children. Review of 24 cases. Acta Neurochirurgica (Wien) 106: 68–72
Lewis P 1967 Carcinoma of the choroid plexus. Brain 90: 177–186
McGirr S J, Ebersold M J, Scheithauer B W, Quast L M, Shaw E G 1988 Choroid plexus papillomas: long-term follow-up results in a surgically treated series. Journal of Neurosurgery 69: 843–849
Mannoji H, Becker L E 1988 Ependymal and choroid plexus tumors. Cytokeratin and GFAP expression. Cancer 61: 1377–1385
Maria B L, Graham M L, Strauss L C, Wharam M D 1985 Response of a recurrent choroid plexus tumor to combination chemotherapy. Journal of Neuro-Oncology 3: 259–262
Matson D D, Crofton F D L 1960 Papilloma of the choroid plexus in childhood. Journal of Neurosurgery 17: 1002–1027
Matsuda M, Uzura S, Nakasu S, Handa J 1991 Primary carcinoma of the choroid plexus in the lateral ventricle. Surgical Neurology 36: 294–299
Matsushima T, Inoue T, Takeshita I, Fukui M, Iwaki T, Kitamoto T 1988 Choroid plexus papillomas: an immunohistochemical study with particular reference to the coexpression of prealbumin. Neurosurgery 23: 384–389
Miettinen M, Clark R, Virtanen I 1986 Intermediate filament proteins in choroid plexus and ependyma and their tumors. American Journal of Pathology 123: 231–240
Milhorat T H, Hammock M K, Davis D A, Fenstermacher J D 1976 Choroid plexus papilloma. Proof of cerebrospinal overproduction. Child's Brain 2: 273–289
Norlen G 1949 Papillomas of the choroid plexus: with report of a successfully removed tumor of the left lateral ventricle in a 7 months old child. Acta Chirurgica Scandinavia 98: 279–297
Packer R J, Perilongo G, Johnson D et al 1992 Choroid plexus carcinoma of childhood. Cancer 69: 580–585
Palazzi M, Di Marco A, Campostrini F, Grandinetti A, Bontempini L 1989 The role of radiotherapy in the management of choroid plexus neoplasms. Tumori 75: 463–469
Pascual-Castroviejo I, Villarejo F, Perez-Higueras A, Morales C, Pascual-Pascual S I 1983 Childhood choroid plexus neoplasms. A study of 14 cases less than 2 years old. European Journal of Pediatrics 140: 51–56
Paulus W, Jänisch W 1990 Clinicopathologic correlations in epithelial choroid plexus neoplasms: a study of 52 cases. Acta Neuropathologica (Berl) 80: 635–641
Piguet V, de Tribolet N 1984 Choroid plexus papilloma of the cerebellopontine angle presenting as a subarachnoid hemorrhage: case report. Neurosurgery 15: 114–116
Qualman S J, Shannon B T, Boesel C P, Jacobs D, Jinkens C, Hayes J 1992 Ploidy analysis and cerebrospinal fluid nephelometry as measures of clinical outcome in childhood choroid plexus neoplasia. Pathology Annual 27 (Pt 1): 305–320
Raimondi A J 1987 Pediatric neurosurgery. Theoretical principles art of surgical techniques. Springer-Verlag, New York
Raimondi A J 1989 Intraventricular tumors. In: McLaurin R L, Schut L, Venes J L, Epstein F (eds) Pediatric neurosurgery. Surgery of the developing nervous system, 2nd edn. W B Saunders, Philadelphia, p 383
Raimondi A J, Gutierrez F A 1975 Diagnosis and surgical treatment of choroid plexus papillomas. Child's Brain 1: 81–115
Robinow M, Johnson G F, Minella P A 1984 Aicardi syndrome, papilloma of the choroid plexus, cleft lip, and cleft of the posterior palate. Journal of Pediatrics 104: 404–405
Rovit R L, Schechter M M, Chodroff P 1970 Choroid plexus papilloma. Observations on radiographic diagnosis. American Journal of Roentgenology 110: 608–617
Rubinstein L J 1972 Tumors of the central nervous system, 2nd edn. Armed Forces Institute of Pathology, Bethesda
Russell D S, Rubinstein L J 1989 Pathology of tumours of the nervous system, 5th edn. Williams & Wilkins, Baltimore
Schijman E, Monges J, Raimondi A J, Tomita T 1990 Choroid plexus papillomas of the III ventricle in childhood. Their diagnosis and surgical management. Child's Nervous System 6: 331–334
Shillito J Jr, Matson D D 1982 An atlas of pediatric neurosurgical operations. W B Saunders, Philadelphia
Spallone A, Pastore F S, Giuffre R, Guidetti B 1990 Choroid plexus papillomas in infancy and childhood. Child's Nervous System 6: 71–74
St Clair S K, Humphreys R P, Pillay P K, Hoffman H J, Blaser S I, Becker L E 1991 Current management of choroid plexus carcinoma in children. Pediatric Neurosurgery 17: 225–233
Thompson J R, Harwood-Nash D C, Fitz C R 1973 The neuroradiology of childhood choroid plexus neoplasms. American Journal of Roentgenology 118: 116–133
Van Swieten J C, Thomeer R T W M, Vielvoye G J, Bots G T A M 1987 Choroid plexus papilloma in the posterior fossa. Surgical Neurology 28: 129–134
Van Wagenen W P 1930 Papillomas of the choroid plexus. Report of two cases, one with removal of tumor and one with "seeding" of the tumor in the ventricular system. Archives of Surgery 20: 199–231
Welch K, Strand R, Bresnan M, Cavazzuti V 1983 Congenital hydrocephalus due to villous hypertrophy of the telencephalic choroid plexuses. Case report. Journal of Neurosurgery 59: 172–175
Yates A J, Becker L E, Sachs L A 1979 Brain tumors in childhood. Child's Brain 5: 31–39
Yuasa H, Tokito S, Tokunaga M 1993 Primary carcinoma of the choroid plexus in Li-Fraumeni syndrome: case report. Neurosurgery 32: 131–133
Zülch K J 1986 Brain tumors: their biology and pathology, 3rd edn. Springer-Verlag, Berlin
Zwetsloot C P, Kros J M, Paz G 1991 Familial occurrence of tumours of the choroid plexus. Journal of Medical Genetics 28: 492–494

29. Uncommon glial tumors

Thomas C. Chen Ignacio Gonzalez-Gomez J Gordon McComb

INTRODUCTION

This chapter's focus is a constellation of neoplastic lesions entitled 'uncommon glial tumors'. Unlike the tumors covered elsewhere, most of these tumors are rarely encountered. Some tumors (dysembryoblastic neuroepithelial and desmoplastic infantile ganglioglioma) have only recently been recognized as independent tumors under the World Health Organization classification (VandenBerg et al 1987a, Daumas-Duport et al 1988). Some of the tumors are associated with medical problems such as precocious puberty in patients with hypothalamic hamartomas (Albright & Lee 1993), and tumors of the kidneys, heart, and lungs in patients with subependymal giant cell astrocytomas (Donegani et al 1972). In some of these tumors, the histopathologic characteristics do not reflect biologic behavior. The appearance of subependymal giant cell astrocytomas is consistent with a malignant astrocytoma, although its growth potential is limited and surgical resection curative (Nagib et al 1984). Pleomorphic xanthoastrocytoma generally has a good prognosis despite the appearance of cellular atypia and pleomorphic cells (Kepes et al 1979).

The nine tumors discussed in this chapter are classified depending upon whether the predominant cell type is of astrocytic, neuronal, or ganglionic origin (Table 29.1).

Table 29.1 Uncommon glial tumors

I. Tumors of predominantly astrocytic origin
- astroblastoma
- gliomatosis cerebri
- pleomorphic xanthoastrocytoma
- subependymal giant cell astrocytoma

II. Tumors of neuronal/glial origin
- desmoplastic infantile ganglioglioma
- dysembryoblastic neuroepithelial tumor
- ganglioglioma
- spongioblastoma
- central neurocytoma

III. Tumors of predominantly ganglionic origin
- gangliocytoma
- hypothalamic hamartomas

ASTROBLASTOMA

Demographics

Astroblastoma is a rare glial tumor first described by Bailey & Bucy in 1930. Since then, it has received little formal attention in the literature. It is estimated that astroblastomas make up 0.45–2.8% of all gliomas (Husain & Leetsma 1986). The peak age incidence is in the first three decades (Russell & Rubinstein 1989); however, the age distribution ranges from 3 years old to 67 years old (Hoag et al 1986, Husain & Leetsma 1986). There is no sex, familial or racial predilection (Bailey & Bucy 1930, Bonnin & Rubinstein 1989). Astroblastomas are commonly supratentorial tumors, located cortically or subcortically (Bailey & Bucy 1930). Cerebellar locations have been reported (Steinberg et al 1985).

Diagnosis

Patients usually present with signs and symptoms of cortical dysfunction, i.e. hemiparesis, personality change, or seizures (Bailey & Bucy 1930, Bonnin & Rubinstein 1989). Imaging diagnosis has been limited. Angiography usually shows a vascular tumor. Computed tomography (CT) appearances range from a poorly-defined hypodense tumor with irregular enhancement to a well-defined tumor with intense enhancement (Hoag et al 1986, Husain & Leetsma 1986). There have been no documented magnetic resonance (MR) studies showing the signal intensities of this tumor. Skull X-rays are of limited value in the diagnostic evaluation of this tumor and of others in this chapter. By utilizing the scout film and bone windows of the CT scan, better information may be obtained. Skull X-rays will not be subsequently mentioned.

Pathology

The cell of origin of astroblastomas is controversial. Bailey & Bucy believed that they are derived from astroblasts (embryonal unipolar cells with 'sucker' feet attached to

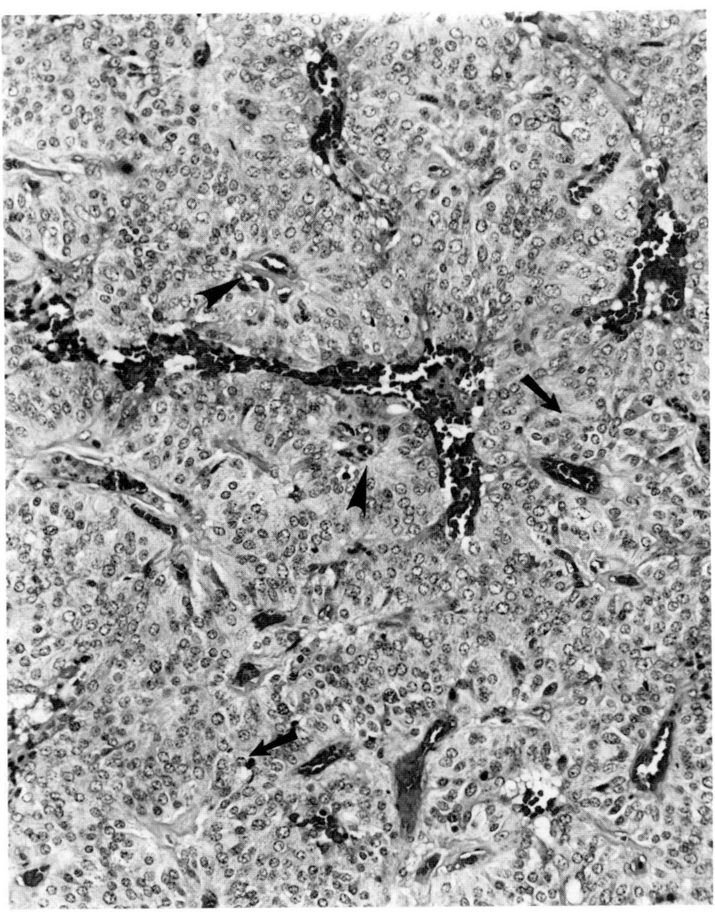

Fig. 29.1 **A.** Astroblastoma showing the characteristic astroblastic pseudorosettes (arrowheads). The cellular population is fairly uniform with occasional mitosis and no endothelial proliferation. The cellularity between pseudorosettes is scanty (arrows). H&E ×80. **B.** Astroblastoma with perivascular pseudorosettes formed of a centrally located blood vessel surrounded by large cells with the nucleus distant from the vascular core and their cytoplasm extending radially toward the vascular wall (arrowhead). The nucleus is slightly convoluted with coarse granular chromatin and one or more inconspicuous nucleoli. H&E ×160.

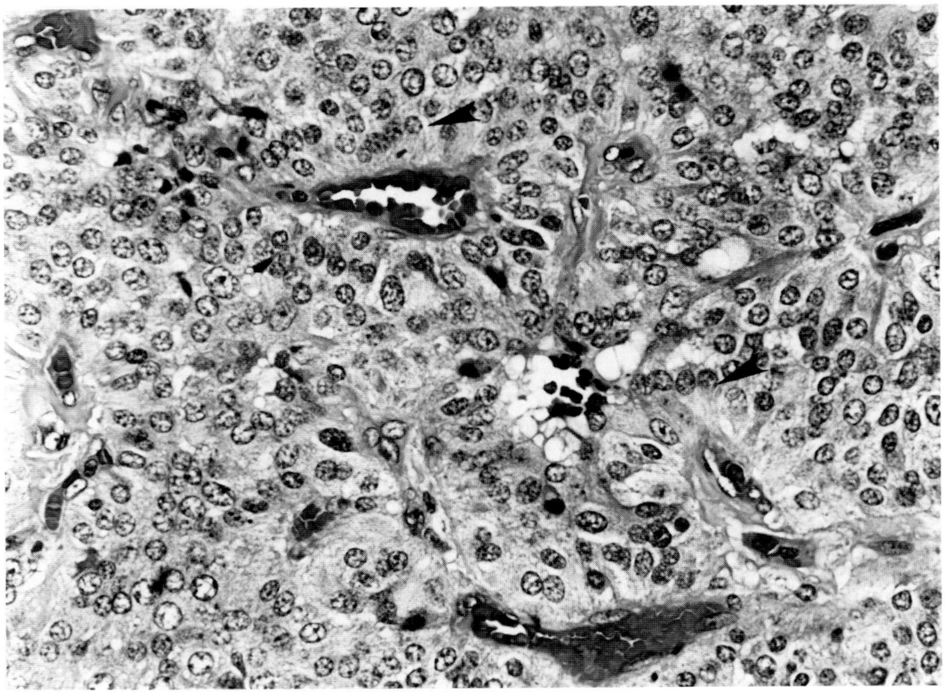

A

B

vessels), which are the precursors of adult astroglia (Bailey & Bucy 1930). Others have proposed the theory that astroblastomas arise by 'dedifferentiation' from mature astroglial cells by an unknown process (Russell & Rubinstein 1989). Rubinstein has further proposed that astroblastomas arise from the tanycyte, a glial precursor cell which is normally found scattered along the ependymal lining of the embryonal and neonatal mammalian brain (Rubinstein & Herman 1989).

Grossly, astroblastomas are not well encapsulated, appear grayish-pink in color, and range from soft to extremely firm in consistency. Central areas of necrosis, or hemorrhage into cystic cavities may be seen. The size ranges from a few millimeters to greater than 8 cm in size (Bailey & Bucy 1930). Microscopically astroblastomas have a characteristic appearance. Prominent elongated tumor cells with footplates form pseudorosettes around blood vessels. Slight or moderate nuclear pleomorphism with limited mitotic activity is present (Fig. 29.1) (Burger et al 1991).

Astroblastomas grown in cell culture demonstrate outgrowths of flattened, angulated cells with epithelial features of early developing normal astrocytes (Russell & Rubinstein 1989).

Immunohistochemistry demonstrates occasional positivity for glial fibrillary acidic protein (GFAP), and extensive positivity for vimentin, neuron-specific enolase, S-100, and epithelial membrane antigen (Cabello et al 1991). Astroblastomas are anti-Leu 7 positive, a natural killer cell antibody positive for cells of neuroepithelial origin, but not for cells of oligodendroglial or embryonal origin (Perentes & Rubinstein 1986). Ultrastructural studies with electron microscopy demonstrate blood vessels with fenestrated endothelial cells, surrounded by a lamellated basal lamina compactly invested by neoplastic cells. Coated vesicles and abundant intermediate filaments are present in tumoral cell cytoplasm (Kubota et al 1985, Cabello et al 1991). Bonnin and Rubinstein have characterized two types of pathologies, low grade and high grade astroblastomas. Low grade tumors are characterized by a uniform perivascular arrangement of pseudorosettes, low to moderate number of mitotic figures, little cellular atypia, minimal or no vascular endothelial proliferation, and prominent sclerosis of the vascular walls. High grade tumors have evidence of cytological atypia, compact cellularity, perivascular cells in multiple layers with high mitotic rates, and hypertrophy of vascular endothelium. Necrosis is seen in up to 70% of the tumors, irrespective of tumor grade, but does not appear to have prognostic significance (Bonnin & Rubinstein 1989).

Differential diagnosis

The differential diagnosis of astroblastomas includes those malignant gliomas which may form pseudorosettes. Gemistocytic astrocytomas may show pseudorosettes, but are strongly fibrillated. Ependymomas form pseudorosettes but have a more compact structure between perivascular pseudorosettes, and are strongly fibrillated. Some metastatic tumors such as carcinoma, melanoma, and sarcoma also form pseudorosettes (Rubinstein 1972).

Treatment

Surgical resection is the mainstay of treatment. Astroblastomas are often fairly circumscribed, located in the superficial cortex, and not difficult to remove. Radiation therapy was given to one patient with a suprasellar mass after a biopsy, with good control of tumor growth (Bonnin & Rubinstein 1989). Chemotherapy was administered to five patients in the same series with no real change in the prognosis (Bonnin & Rubinstein 1989). One patient received bleomycin without radiation, and was doing well 3.5 years postoperatively (Kubota et al 1985).

Clinical outcome

Due to the small number of these tumors and variance within this small group, the clinical outcome of astroblastomas is hard to predict. The prognosis appears to be intermediate between that of astrocytoma and glioblastoma. Most of the patients in Bailey and Bucy's original series died within one year secondary to postoperative fatality or increased tumor size (Bailey & Bucy 1930). Bonnin's series attempted to correlate the prognosis between low grade and high grade astroblastomas. In 5 of 8 patients followed with low grade tumors, survival ranged from 3–20 years post-treatment. However, one tumor converted to a fatal glioblastoma multiforme. On the other hand, in 3 of 4 patients followed with high grade astroblastomas, the survival ranged from 1.5–2.5 years post-treatment. One patient had a long-term survival. The authors concluded that it was difficult to predict prognosis as some tumors converted to more malignant tumor types (Bonnin & Rubinstein 1989, Russell & Rubinstein 1989).

GLIOMATOSIS CEREBRI

Demographics

Gliomatosis cerebri was initially described by Nevin as a clinically distinct entity in 1938 and is recognized by the World Health Organization as a specific diagnostic entity among neuroepithelial tumors (Nevin 1938, Zülch 1979). Nevin considered that the histopathological appearances were consistent with a diffuse glial process rather than spread from one or more foci (Nevin 1938). Since his initial report, just over 60 cases have been reported in the literature (Bebin & Tytus 1956, Sarhaddi et al 1973, Cough & Weiss 1974, Nahser 1974, Kawano et al 1978,

Miller et al 1981, Simonati et al 1981, Artigas et al 1985, Balakrishnan et al 1985, Spagnoli et al 1987, Dickson et al 1988, Rippe et al 1990, Wilson et al 1990, Gottesman et al 1991, Hara et al 1991, Kandler et al 1991, Ross et al 1991, Yanaka et al 1992). The age span ranges from 9 years to a patient in the sixth decade, with most patients presenting between the third and fourth decades (Sarhaddi et al 1973). There does not appear to be a racial, familial, or sexual predilection. Gliomatosis cerebri presents as a diffuse involvement of the cerebral hemisphere, usually without brainstem or cerebellar involvement.

Diagnosis

The presenting history is often insidious, with a progressive history of personality changes, headaches, and eventual impaired mental status. Increased intracranial pressure is usually present secondary to diffuse tumor infiltration (Cough & Weiss 1974). One patient presented with hydrocephalus and dementia possibly secondary to massive enlargement of the white matter commissural tracts (corpus callosum, anterior commissure, and fornices) that may have been directly responsible for obstruction of cerebrospinal fluid (CSF) pathways (Dickson et al 1988). The duration of symptoms may be several months to many years (Couch & Weiss 1974). Moreover, previous imaging studies with cerebral angiography and pneumoencephalography were usually nondiagnostic. CT scanning shows diffuse low density and white matter hypertrophy, with minimal contrast enhancement (Nahser et al 1981, Kandler et al 1991, Yanaka et al 1992). EEG findings are those of diffuse slow waves only. CSF analysis is also unremarkable except for a slightly increased protein, however, cytological analysis may yield enough abnormal cells to suggest a diagnosis (Miller et al 1981). As a result, many of these patients are diagnosed with gliomatosis cerebri only at autopsy (Balakrishnan et al 1985). MR scanning is currently the diagnostic imaging technique of choice, providing a clear picture of the diffuse enlargement of the involved structures. On T1-weighted images, the lesions appear isointense or hypointense relative to gray matter, with diffuse enlargement of the cerebral hemispheres (Fig. 29.2). There is minimal contrast enhancement with gadolinium (Gd-DTPA), however, focal areas of enhancement may be present secondary to tumor deposits eliciting localized edema and blood-brain barrier

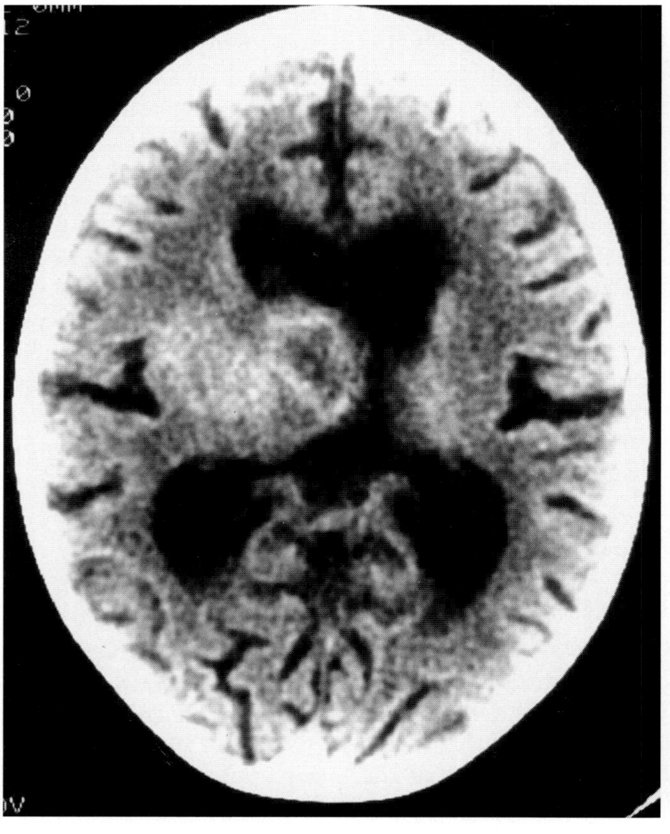

A

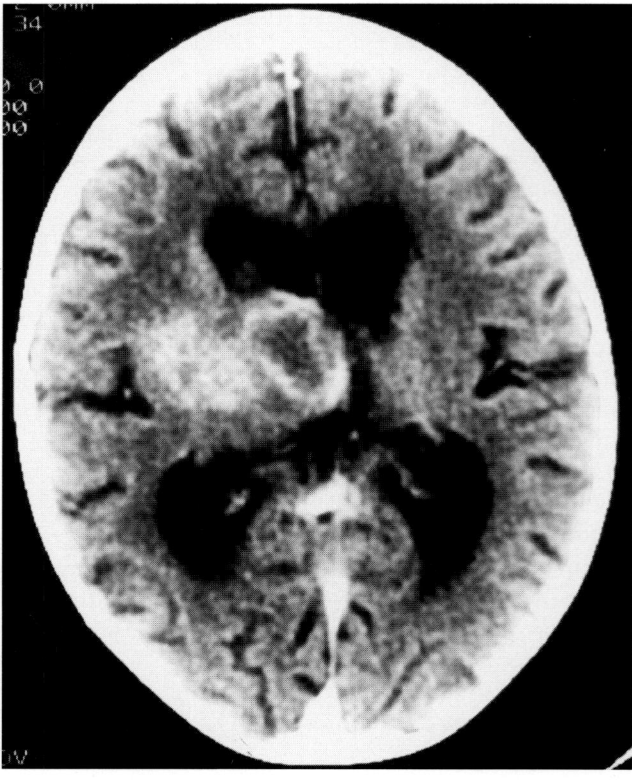

B

Fig. 29.2 Gliomatosis cerebri. This 5-year-old boy presented with headaches, vomiting, and a left hemiparesis. MR scan with and without contrast demonstrates a diffuse right thalamic tumor, isointense to gray matter, with poor enhancement **A, B.** The patient underwent a stereotactic biopsy for diagnosis and followed by chemotherapy and radiation. He expired 6 months after his initial diagnosis.

permeability changes. These enhancement patterns may simulate leptomeningeal tumor dissemination (Rippe et al 1990). T2-weighted images provide the clearest representation. The involved white matter has diffuse, enlarged, hyperintense lesions (Spagnoli et al 1987, Ross et al 1991, Yanaka et al 1992). Positron emission tomography (PET) scans using ^{11}C-L-methionine show isotope accumulation in the diffusely infiltrative tumorous area with greater accuracy than CT or MR, when confirmed at autopsy (Mineura et al 1991).

Pathology

Grossly, the brain involved with gliomatosis cerebri is characterized by diffuse enlargement. The gyri may be slightly enlarged; however, the normal architecture is maintained. On light microscopy, diffuse infiltration by glioma cells along anatomic pathways throughout the central nervous system, sparing of cortical structures, and extensive white matter demyelination, with no areas of necrosis or hemorrhage, is seen (Fig. 29.3) (Sarhaddi et al 1973, Simonati et al 1981). Rubinstein maintains that gliomatosis cerebri is really a diffuse cerebral astrocytoma and does not represent a distinct neoplastic process (Russell & Rubinstein 1989). The unusual presentation, diagnostic difficulties, and distinct pathological process arising from one or more foci of frank neoplasia, however, led many pathologists to consider it a distinct neuroepithelial tumor (Cough & Weiss 1974). Ultrastructure studies showed that four main types of tumor cells are present: anaplastic astrocytes poor in organelles with a variable number of glial microfilaments; atypical oligodendrocytes with scanty cytoplasm in which microtubules are present; intermediate forms with abundant cytoplasm containing organelles, microtubules and microfilaments; and small cells with round nuclei and a very scanty rim of cytoplasm (Cervos-Navarro et al 1987). In keeping with ultrastructural studies, gliomatosis cerebri with predominantly neoplastic oligodendroglia infiltration has been reported (Balko et al 1992). Conversion of gliomatosis cerebri to glioblastoma multiforme has been reported (Romero et al 1988). A one-step silver colloid method for nucleolar organizer region-associated protein (AgNOR) has been used in gliomatosis cerebri to estimate its proliferative potential. AgNOR stain is similar to that of low grade gliomas, suggesting invasive characteristics, but with a proliferative potential lower than high grade gliomas (Hara et al 1991).

Differential diagnosis

The differential diagnosis for gliomatosis cerebri is that of a low grade glioma or oligodendroglioma. Although it would have been difficult in the past to distinguish gliomatosis cerebri from these forms of glioma without an autopsy, current MR imaging should be able to show an accurate representation (Spagnoli et al 1987, Yanaka et al 1992). It should be noted that some patients may not have imaging documentation until later in their course (Wilson et al 1990, Gottesman et al 1991). In that case, presentation with increased intracranial pressure without focal radiologic abnormalities may be interpreted initially as pseudotumor cerebri (Gottesman et al 1991).

Treatment

Because of the diffuse infiltrative nature of this tumor, it is impossible to attempt a surgical resection. Instead, biopsy for a diagnosis followed by radiation is currently the treatment of choice (Schober et al 1991). If hydrocephalus develops, a ventriculo-peritoneal shunt for control of intracranial pressure (ICP) may be temporarily helpful (Dickson et al 1988). Radiation therapy has been shown to be beneficial in some cases, however, the data are still anecdotal (Wilson et al 1990, Gottesman et al 1991). No specific benefit from any chemotherapy regimen has been reported.

Clinical outcome

The outcome is dismal. Although survival periods up to 4 years have been reported from onset of symptoms, most patients die within months (Nevin 1938). No effective treatment has been reported.

PLEOMORPHIC XANTHOASTROCYTOMA

Demographics

Pleomorphic xanthoastrocytoma (PXA) is a rare glioma initially reported in 1979 by Kepes et al in 12 patients (Kepes et al 1979). Since then, more than 50 cases have been reported (Kuhajda et al 1981, Saikai et al 1981, Jones et al 1983, Maleki et al 1983, Strom & Skullerud 1983, Weldon-Linne et al 1983, Goldring et al 1985, Gomez et al 1985, Palma et al 1985, Grant & Gallagher 1986, Iwaki et al 1987, Mackenzie 1987, Gaskill et al 1988, Stuart et al 1988, Kepes et al 1989, Whittle et al 1989, Guo & Zhang 1990, Ng et al 1990b, Sarkar et al 1990, Sugita et al 1990, Allegranza et al 1991, Hosokawa et al 1991, Kros et al 1991, Loiseau et al 1991, Sawyer et al 1991, Furuta et al 1992, Lindboe et al 1992, Sawyer et al 1992, Yoshino & Lucio 1992, Zorzi et al 1992). The patients are generally young, usually in their late teens to early 30s; the youngest patient was 3 years of age, and the oldest 62 (Strom & Skullerud 1983, Mackenzie 1987). There does not appear to be a sexual, racial, or familial predisposition. PXA has been reported throughout the brain, but more commonly on the surface of the temporal and parietal lobes (Russell & Rubinstein 1989).

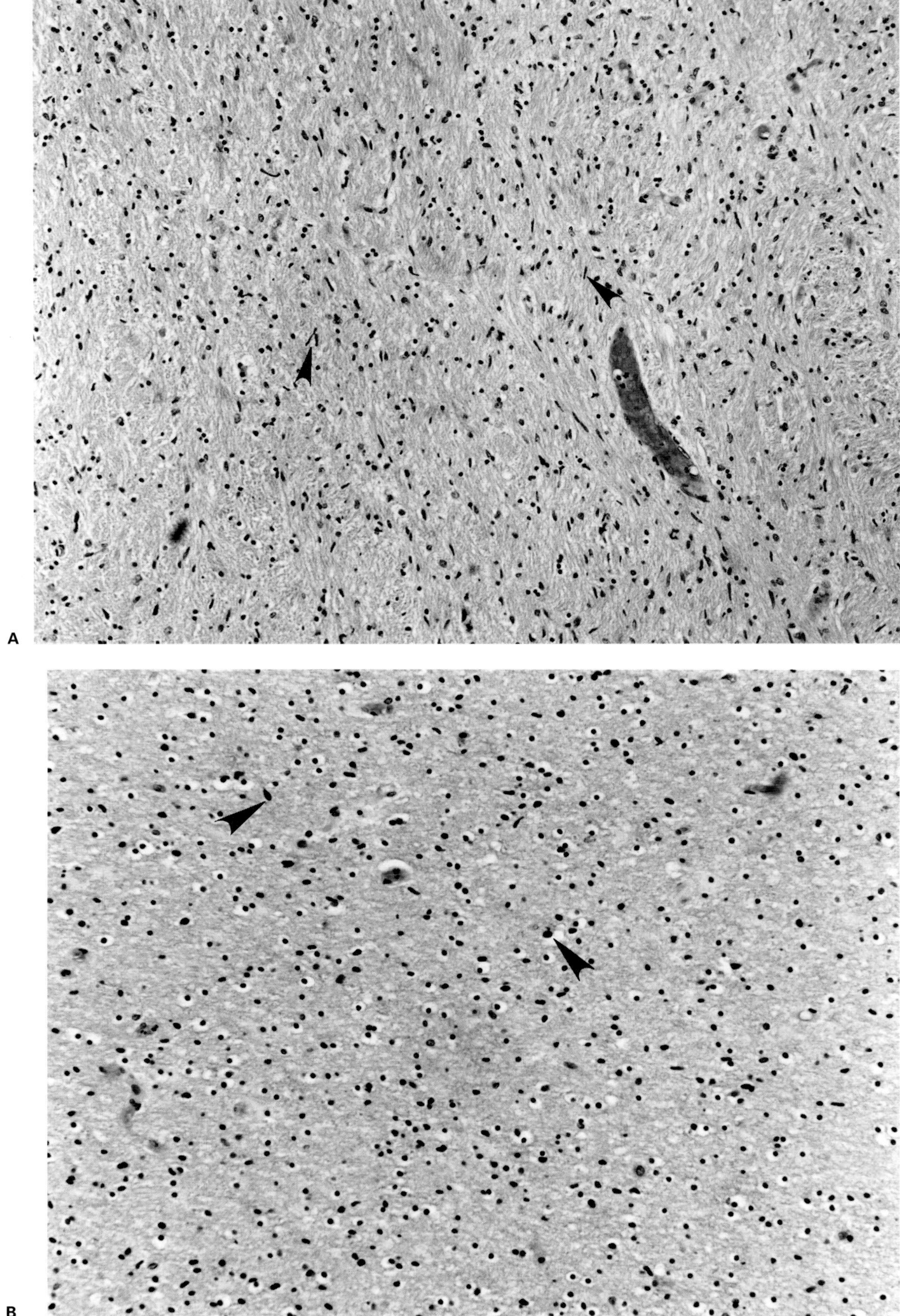

Fig. 29.3A & B

Fig. 29.3 A. Gliomatosis cerebri with focal areas showing increased cell density with numerous neoplastic astrocytes infiltrating the intersecting bundles at the centrum semiovale (arrowheads). H&E ×100. **B.** Gliomatosis cerebri showing scattered neoplastic cells between normal glial elements of the hemispheric white matter that are characterized by their increased nuclear size, pleomorphism, and hyperchromatism (arrowheads). H&E ×160.

Diagnosis

A history of chronic seizures and headaches is the usual presentation (Kepes et al 1979, Goldring et al 1985, Russell & Rubinstein 1989). Occasionally, increased intracranial pressure with papilledema may be present. Focal neurologic deficits are uncommon (Maleki et al 1983, Iwaki et al 1987).

CT scans often demonstrate a cystic tumor with nodular enhancement, usually on the surface of the temporal or parietal lobes (Weldon-Linne et al 1983, Blom 1988, Kros et al 1991), however, PXA has also been reported in the thalamus and cerebellum (Kros et al 1991, Lindboe et al 1992). Recently, Yoshino & Lucio (1992) reported two cases of PXA using MR imaging. No increased signal on T1-weighted image was observed in the tumor prior to contrast administration, but on post-Gd-DTPA, the nodular portion of the tumor was markedly enhanced. Increased signal intensity on proton-density and T2-weighted images was seen in both the cystic and solid components of the tumor (Yoshino & Lucio 1992). Cerebral angiography demonstrates an avascular to moderately vascular tumor, with derivation of blood supply from meningeal feeders (Maleki et al 1983, Yoshino & Lucio 1992).

Pathology

The tumor is often located superficially in the temporal or parietal cortex, involving the leptomeninges, but not the dura mater. A mural nodule of yellowish or reddish tissue, encapsulated by a proteinaceous cyst, is often found (Russell & Rubinstein 1989).

The cell of origin of PXA has been the subject of much debate. Kepes initially established the glial nature of xanthoastrocytomas on the basis of their positive GFAP staining, and proposed the subpial astrocyte, which is known to be partially covered by basal lamina, as this neoplasm's cell of origin (Kepes 1979). Paulus disputed the astrocytic origin of this tumor, pointing out that not all tumors classified as xanthoastrocytomas were GFAP positive. Moreover, a spectrum of immunostains for mesenchymal tumors, such as α_1-antichymotrypsin, tartrate-resistant acid phosphatase, common leukocyte antigen, and OKM-1, were positive in xanthoastrocytomas (Paulus & Peiffer 1988).

Histologically, PXA shows cellular atypia and nuclear pleomorphism. The cells are often xanthomatous in appearance. Giant cells are present, along with a variable number of lymphocytes and plasma cells (Zorzi et al 1992). Few if any mitoses are present, and there is no evidence of intratumoral necrosis or endothelial proliferation (Fig. 29.4) (Kepes et al 1979, Loiseau et al 1991). Electron microscopy (EM) demonstrates epithelial properties such as intercellular junctions, interdigitations between apposing tumor cells, and a well-defined basal lamina surrounding the tumor nests (Iwaki et al 1987). On the basis of the EM characteristics, Sugita has proposed two PXA subtypes: an 'epithelial' form and an 'angiomatous variant'. The angiomatous variant is very vascular with surrounding desmoplastic reaction secondary to protein leakage from vessels (Sugita et al 1990).

Immunohistochemistry is helpful in characterizing these tumors. Most PXA are GFAP positive; however, some tumors with PXA characteristics have been reported to be GFAP negative. Reticulin stains show a rich reticulin network (Kepes et al 1979). Ki-67, a marker for actively proliferating cells, has been tested for on one tumor, which was < 1% positive (Sugita et al 1990).

Cytogenetics performed on one PXA revealed a karyotype of 48 X,Y, with trisomies for chromosomes 3, 5, 7, 15 and monosomy for chromosome 22 (Sawyer et al 1992). Telomeric association, evolving to ring chromosomes, has been reported in a recurrent pleomorphic xanthoastrocytoma (Sawyer et al 1992). Despite the degree of pleomorphism present in the tumor, cytofluorometric analysis of one PXA revealed that the main mode of the tumor was diploid with polyploid classes (no aneuploidy) (Hosokawa et al 1991).

There have been two reported cases of mixed ganglioglioma-PXA. In one case, the two tumors were clearly separated. In Lindboe et al's case, however, abnormal ganglion cells were clearly within the PXA component (Furuta et al 1992, Lindboe et al 1992).

Differential diagnosis

Imaging differential diagnoses for a peripheral enhancing lesion in a child or young adult include: (1) glioblastoma, (2) ganglioglioma, (3) gangliosarcoma, (4) astrocytoma, (5) meningioma, (6) meningosarcoma, (7) oligodendroglioma, (8) juvenile pilocytic astrocytoma, (9) solitary metastasis (Yoshino & Lucio 1992). From the histopathological standpoint, three tumors must be distinguished from PXA. Juvenile pilocytic astrocytoma is a common tumor of astrocytic origin which can be readily distinguished from PXA by the numerous hairlike fibrils that abound in the cytoplasm and the processes of the neoplastic cells present in the pilocytic astrocytoma (Gomez et al 1985, Russell & Rubinstein 1989). Fibrous xanthomas have gross features of a meningioma, but the histological characteristics of a fibrous histiocytoma. All cells

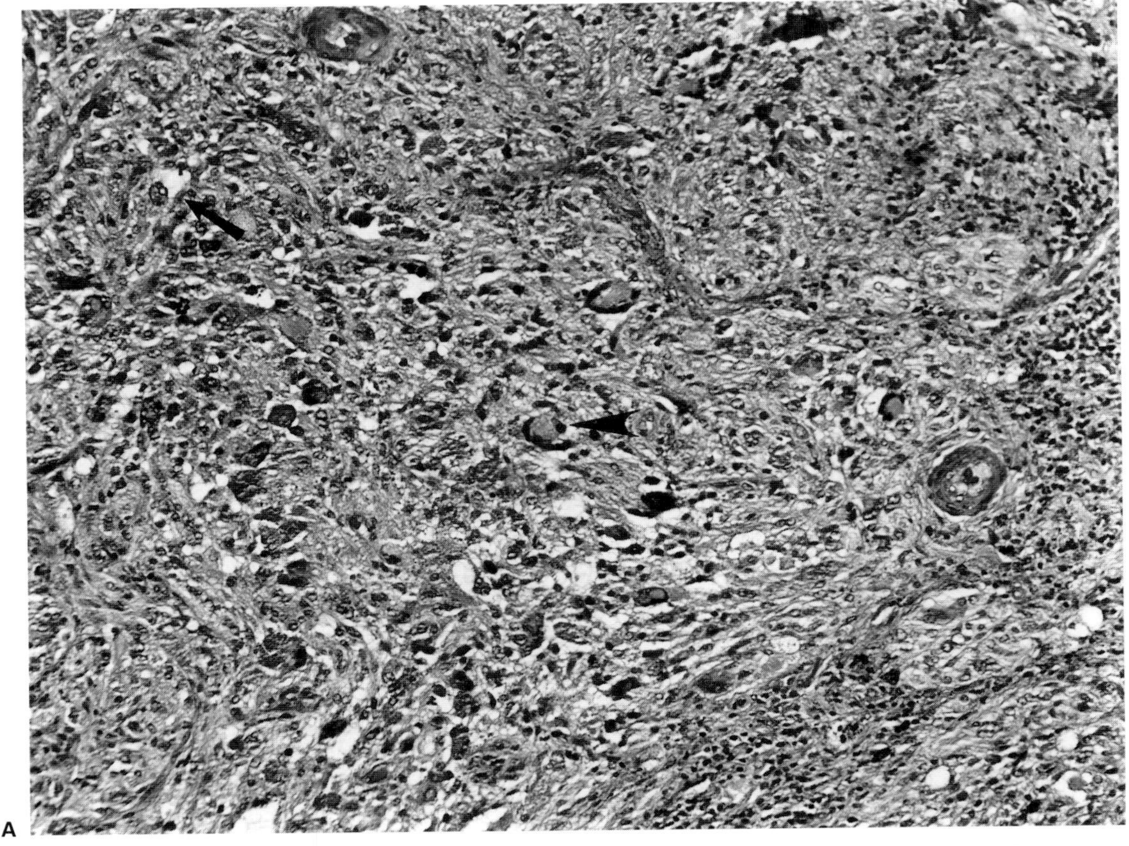

A

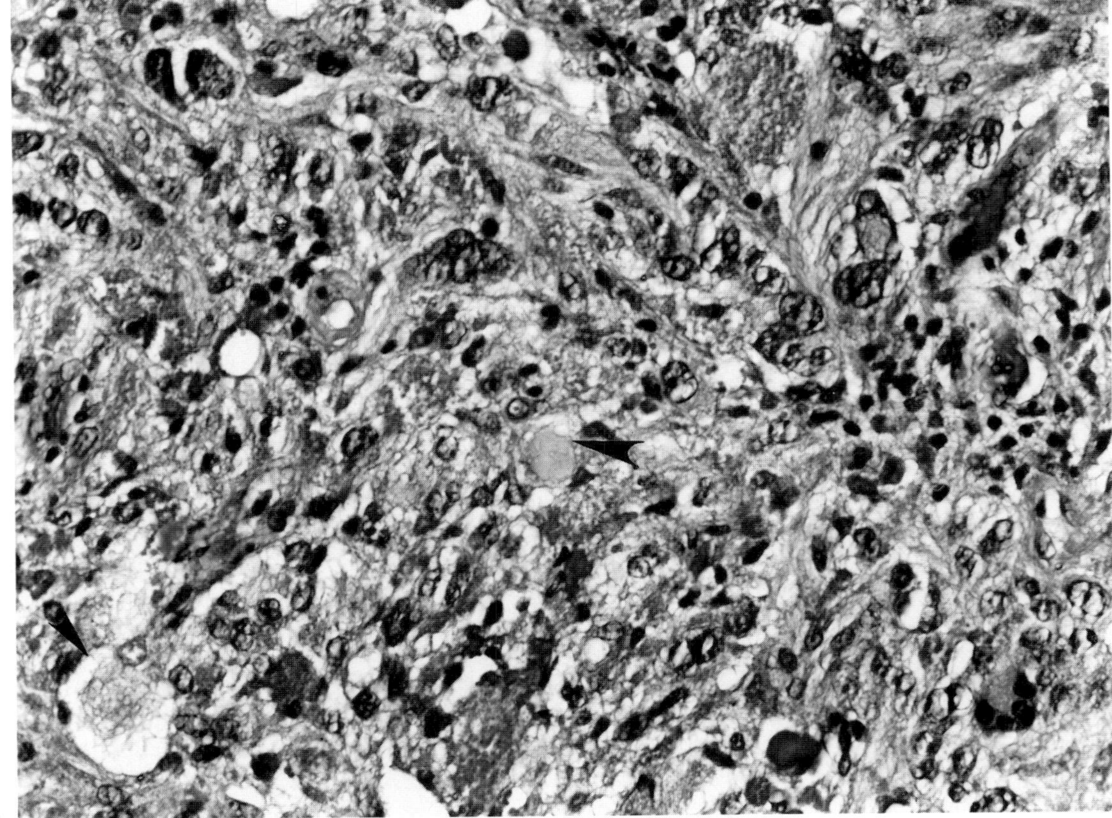

B

Fig. 29.4A & B

Fig. 29.4 **A.** Pleomorphic xanthoastrocytoma composed of pleomorphic cells (arrow) of variable size and shape with one or more nuclei. These cells are forming clusters or bundles (arrowhead). H&E ×100. **B.** Pleomorphic xanthoastrocytoma showing the proliferating tumor cells containing a large convoluted nucleus and prominent nucleolus, some of which are binucleated or multinucleated. The cytoplasm is abundant and in some cells vacuolated by numerous lipid droplets (arrowheads). Mitotic figures, necrosis, and vascular proliferation are remarkably absent. H&E ×200.

are GFAP negative (Kepes 1979). PXA must be differentiated from a malignant astrocytoma with xanthomatous changes, as the pleomorphic appearance and bizarre multinucleated giant cells resemble glioblastoma (Grant & Gallagher 1986, Sarkar et al 1990). However, superficial location with leptomeningeal involvement, relative paucity of mitoses, and the absence of intratumoral necrosis point towards the diagnosis of PXA.

Treatment

Surgical excision is the initial mode of treatment. Most tumors are superficially located, and gross total resection is usually possible. Seizures and increased intracranial pressure are often successfully treated with tumor removal. Whole brain radiation, using doses ranging from 30–60 Gy, has been used in cases where gross total resection was not achieved. There have not been enough patients with long-term follow-up to determine whether postoperative radiation actually improves the prognosis. Chemotherapy is not usually given. Sugita reported the use of ACNU (1-(4-amino-2-methylpyrimidine-5-yl)-methyl-3-(2-chloroethyl)-3-nitrosurea) in one asymptomatic patient with a 2 year follow-up (Sugita et al 1990).

Clinical outcome

The overall outcome is generally good. Seizures, if initially present, are well-controlled with surgery (Kepes et al 1979, Goldring et al 1985). Despite the cellular pleomorphism, long-term survival is the general rule, even in patients who have not received any form of adjunctive therapy or have not had a gross total resection. Asymptomatic survival rates of more than 10–20 years are common (Kepes et al 1979, Palma et al 1985, Paulus & Peiffer 1988). The number one prognostic factor in patient survival or future tumor recurrence is the completeness of tumor removal. Local recurrence may occur. Some patients, however, despite a prolonged period of asymptomatic survival, may undergo rapid deterioration (Weldon-Linne et al 1983). Kepes reported 3 cases of pleomorphic xanthoastrocytoma with malignant degeneration to small cell glioblastoma multiforme (GBM) over a period of 6 years, 15 years, and 6 months. The degeneration of these cells into GBM has been cited as further proof of the astrocytic origin of these tumors (Kepes et al 1989).

SUBEPENDYMAL GIANT CELL ASTROCYTOMA

Demographics

Tuberous sclerosis is an autosomal dominant phakomatosis characterized by the classic triad of mental retardation, seizures, and adenoma sebaceum first described by Vogt in 1908 (Vogt 1908). The incidence of tuberous sclerosis has been estimated to range from 1/100 000 to 1/50 000 (Nagib et al 1984). In one large series of 345 tuberous sclerosis patients, 6.1% of the patients had subependymal giant cell astrocytoma (SGCA) (Shepherd et al 1991). The age range for initial presentation and discovery of SGCA ranges from neonatal (Painter et al 1984, Rikonen & Simell 1990, Tien et al 1990, Hahn et al 1991) to 50 years old (Burger et al 1991). Most patients have clinical manifestations before age 20 (Burger et al 1991). There is no sex or racial predilection. SGCAs arise from subependymal nodules located in the walls of the lateral ventricle adjacent to the foramen of Monro (Nagib et al 1984).

Diagnosis

The initial diagnosis of tuberous sclerosis is based on a multitude of signs and symptoms including dermatological manifestations (adenoma sebaceum, shagreen patches, areas of altered pigmentation, depigmented nevi, subungual fibromas), retinal tumors, seizures, and mental retardation (Fig. 29.5). Other systemic manifestations include tumors of the kidneys, heart, and lung. Lesions of the spleen, pancreas, and genitalia are less common (Donegani et al 1972, Nagib et al 1984). Patients' usual presentation with SGCA in earlier series was with the presence of increased intracranial pressure when the tumor resulted in obstruction at the foramen of Monro (Kapp et al 1967). Current imaging allows for diagnosis of SGCA before the development of increased intracranial pressure. In neonates, cranial ultrasound can be used initially to establish the presence of the tumor, followed by a CT scan for better anatomical detail (Hahn et al 1991). CT scans are useful in following the course of tubers. Fujiwara followed a 7-month-old child with CT scans until he was 10 years of age, demonstrating sequential growth of subependymal nodules to a SGCA which was subsequently resected (Fujiwara et al 1989). Calcifications can be seen on CT scans both within the SGCA and in tubers adjacent to the ventricular systems. Unlike gliomas, which often have a variable degree of contrast enhancement, SGCAs have fairly uniform enhancement (Nagib et al 1984, Jelinek et al 1990, Martin et al 1990). The various intracranial manifestations of tuberous sclerosis — including multiple subependymal nodules, tubers

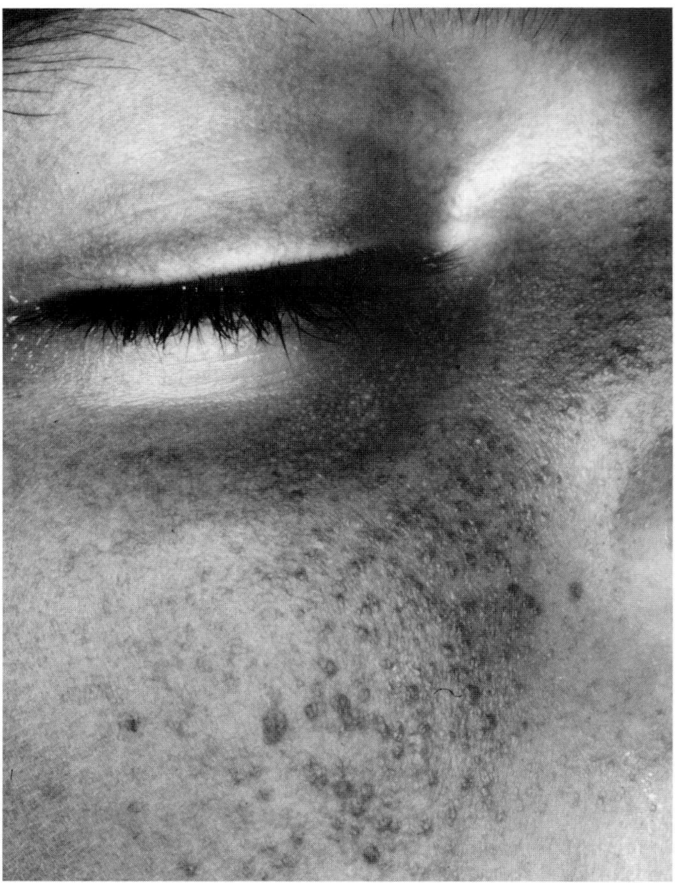

Fig. 29.5 Adenoma sebaceum in a child with tuberous sclerosis.

(seen as areas of high signal intensity on T2-weighted images), disruption of cortical architecture, and dilated ventricles — are well seen on MR imaging (McMurdo et al 1987, Braffman et al 1992). The current imaging diagnosis of choice for SGCA is MR scanning with and without gadolinium, with coronal sections through the region of the foramen of Monro. SGCAs are isointense to gray matter on T1-weighted images. They are hyperintense to gray matter on T2-weighted images with signal voids secondary to calcification and enhance markedly with contrast (Fig. 29.6) (Martin et al 1990).

Pathology

Grossly, SGCAs are fairly well circumscribed, gray to pinkish red in color, and occasionally hemorrhagic because of increased vascularity (Rubinstein 1972). Giant cells, which are also found in cortical tubers, are characteristically seen, with regular nuclei on light microscopy (Trombley & Mirra 1981). The cytoplasm is abundant and eosinophilic (Nardelli et al 1986, Burger et al 1991). Evidence of necrosis and focal areas of mitosis may be present; however, no correlation exists with a worse prognosis in these patients (Fig. 29.7) (Chow et al 1983). On electron microscopy, giant cells appear as large cells with abundant cytoplasm and numerous astrocytic filaments (Boesel et al 1979). Cytomorphology of SGCA shows spindle and epithelioid shaped tumor cells with dense eosinophilic cytoplasm, eccentric nuclei, prominent nu-

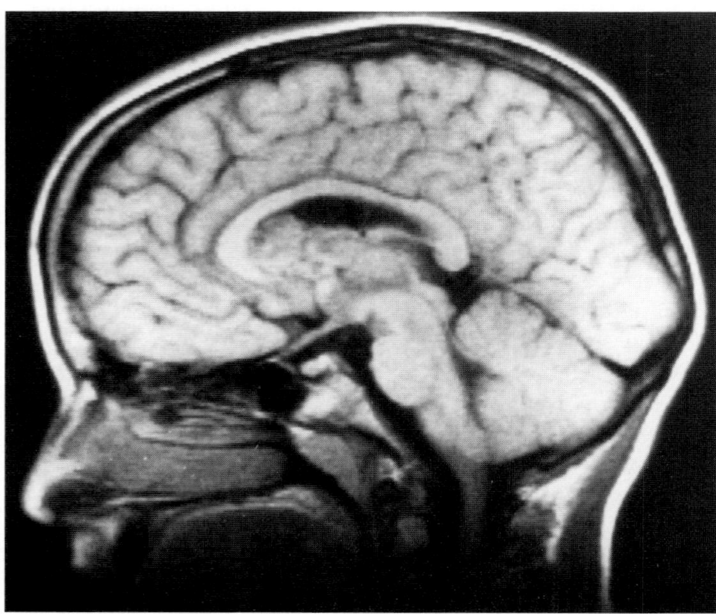

A

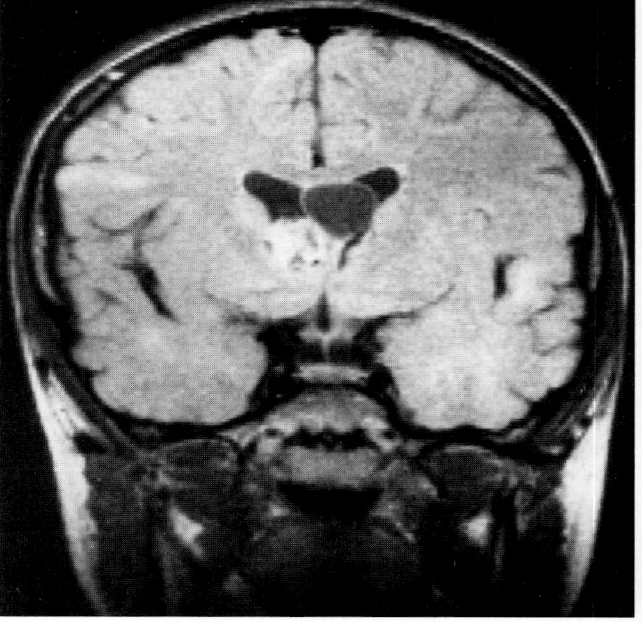

B

Fig. 29.6 Subependymal giant cell astrocytoma. This 9-year-old boy presented with recurrent headaches. **A.** MR scan (T1-weighted) shows a tumor isointense to gray matter in the lateral ventricle. **B.** The tumor enhances evenly with contrast, and a cystic component is seen in the coronal section. The patient underwent a gross total resection without further recurrence.

cleoli, and nuclear cytoplasmic inclusions (Altermatt & Scheithauer 1991). In order to determine whether SGCAs are astrocytic or neuronal in origin, Nakamura et al performed glial fibrillary and S-100 stains. They found that half of the tumors were GFAP positive, and 6 out of 7 of the tumors were S-100 positive, suggesting that SGCAs may originate from germinal matrix cells that have not differentiated into astrocytic or neuronal tumors (Nakamura & Becker 1983). Bonnin et al (1984) showed that in patients with tuberous sclerosis, most of the tumors were GFAP negative. If the tumors were GFAP positive, they were not associated with tuberous sclerosis. This paper points out that the potential for astrocytic or neuronal differentiation may be incompletely expressed if tuberous sclerosis is present (Bonnin et al 1984). Rarely is there an association between malignant glial tumors and patients with tuberous sclerosis (Padmalatha et al 1980). Staining for αB crystallin is positive in subependymal giant cells and in astrocytic tumors among neuroectodermal neoplasms. αB crystallin is negative in ependymal/choroid plexus tumors, suggesting that αB crystallin is selectively secreted by astrocytic tumors (Iwaki et al 1991). Flow cytometry showed that almost all of the tumors were diploid. No correlation was found between histological features such as atypia, mitoses, endothelial proliferations, or necrosis with flow cytometric characteristics (Shepherd et al 1991).

Differential diagnosis

The differential diagnosis for tumors of the lateral ventricle in addition to SGCA includes ependymoma, subependymoma, primary cerebral neuroblastoma, astrocytoma, oligodendroglioma, meningioma, neurocytoma, and choroid plexus papilloma (Nishio et al 1990). Other tumors commonly described in the tuberous sclerosis complex include cerebral hemangiomas, spongioblastomas, neurinomas, and ependymomas (Shepherd et al 1991). In one series of 47 pathologically proven lateral ventricular neoplasms, Jelinek found that the clinical characteristics most consistent with SGCA include presentation in the first three decades of life, location at the foramen of Monro, and tumor enhancement with contrast on CT scan (Jelinek et al 1990). Histologically, the differential diagnosis of a giant cell astrocytoma includes gemistocytic astrocytoma and giant cell glioblastoma. Giant cells may look like the giant cells of GBM or like gemistocytic cells (Boesel et al 1979). Gemistocytic astrocytomas are usually nondiscrete infiltrating lesions in the white matter of older individuals. Histologically, they are intensely GFAP positive, with exceptionally large component cells characterized by an eosinophilic cytoplasm (Russell & Rubinstein 1989). Giant cell glioblastomas are not found in the subependymal location, and occur in the older population. Histologically, giant cell glioblastomas are anaplastic tumors with vascular proliferation, necrosis, or pseudopalisading as in GBM (Burger et al 1991).

Treatment

The treatment of choice is surgical resection, with gross total removal if possible. Subtotal resection is often adequate as these tumors are slow growing and may have limited growth potential in any remaining tumor, similar to that of a pilocytic astrocytoma (Kapp et al 1967, Nagib et al 1984). Follow-up imaging should be obtained at regular intervals, however, to rule out tumor regrowth or hydrocephalus. Patients with unresolved hydrocephalus despite tumor removal need to be shunted. Neonates suspected of having tuberous sclerosis should have a cardiac evaluation as part of the diagnostic work-up prior to surgical removal of an intraventricular tumor. Painter et al (1984) reported their experience with two neonates who underwent attempted surgical resection but died secondary to refractory intraoperative cardiac arrhythmias. Both were found at autopsy to have multiple cardiac rhabdomyomas (Painter et al 1984). Radiotherapy has been employed in the past, however, there is no evidence documenting any difference in survival (Boesel et al 1979). No chemotherapy trials have been conducted.

In summary, the treatment of SGCA is surgical, both for the original tumor and recurrences that might occur, with radiation and chemotherapy playing no role.

Clinical outcome

The clinical outcome for the SGCA alone is generally favorable and patients have been stable at 15-year follow-ups despite subtotal resections (Kapp et al 1967, Nagib et al 1984). The prognosis has no bearing on the tumor having focal areas of active mitoses or necrosis (Chow et al 1983). The severity of seizure disorders and degree of mental retardation have no relationship to the status of an SGCA (Webb et al 1991). Adequate treatment of the hydrocephalus present in some of these patients also reflects on outcome.

DESMOPLASTIC INFANTILE GANGLIOGLIOMA

Demographics

Desmoplastic infantile gangliogliomas (desmoplastic supratentorial neuroepithelial tumors) are rare glial tumors of infancy first described by VandenBerg et al in 1987 (VandenBerg et al 1987a). The tumors were initially described by Taratuto et al as superficial cerebral astrocytomas with dural attachment (Taratuto et al 1984). Currently, 26 cases have been reported in the literature (Paulus et al 1992). Patient ages range from 2 months to 4 years old. There is no sex, familial, or racial predilection.

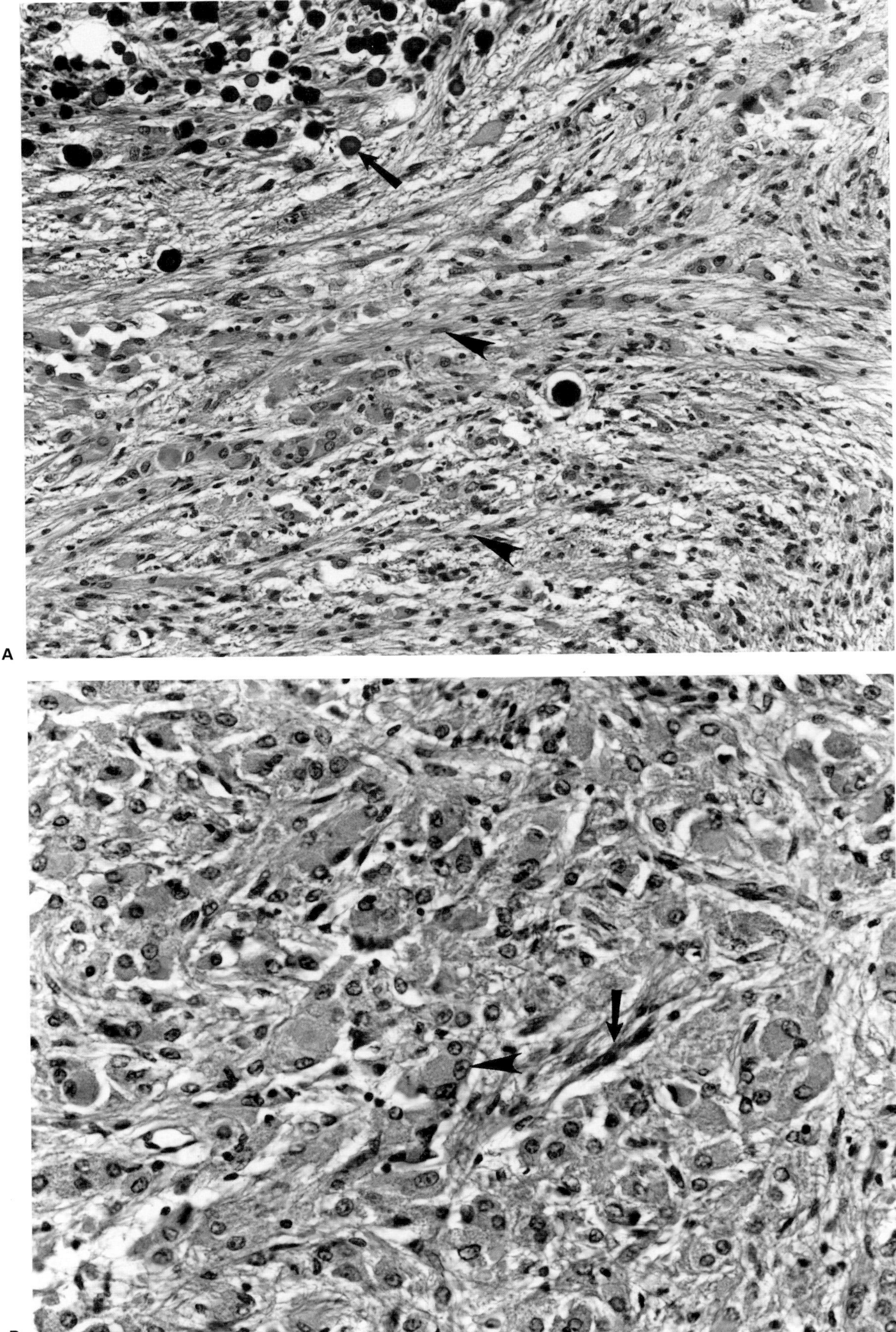

Fig. 29.7A & B

Fig. 29.7 **A.** Subependymal giant cell astrocytoma containing a mixed cell population of large cells, bundles of fibrillary astrocytes (arrowheads) and calcifications (arrow). H&E ×100. **B.** Subependymal giant cell astrocytoma exhibiting the typical clusters of large gemistocytic cells (arrowhead) and fibrillary astrocytes (arrow) arranged in a compact pattern of growth. H&E ×200.

Diagnosis

Most patients present with new-onset seizures. As these tumors often occur in infants, very large tumors may present with progressive increase in head circumference only. The neurological exam is usually nonfocal, and signs and symptoms of increased intracranial pressure may be the only findings. CT scan shows a large cystic tumor with an enhancing solid component (Taratuto et al 1983, Ng et al 1990a). T1-weighted images on MR show the cystic component of the tumor as hypointense to gray matter, with an isointense solid component (Fig. 29.8). T2-weighted images demonstrate T2 prolongation in the cyst with variable signal intensity of the tumor. The tumor usually abuts on the meningeal surface, with an intense contrast enhancement pattern (Martin et al 1991).

Pathology

Grossly, desmoplastic infantile gangliogliomas are large superficially located lesions, firmly attached to the dura, with prominent uni- or multiloculated cysts. The tumors are firm and avascular, with a dense desmoplastic component, superficially resembling a moderately cellular fibroma. No connections with the ventricular system are present. Microscopically, desmoplastic infantile gangliogliomas show evidence of glial and ganglionic differentiation accompanied by an extreme desmoplastic reaction. The fibroblastic elements are often admixed with variable numbers of pleomorphic neuroepithelial cells. The tumors are composed of fibroblast-like spindle-shaped cells with elongated nuclei. No necrosis or endothelial proliferation is seen (Fig. 29.9) (VandenBerg et al 1987a, Paulus et al 1992). Electron microscopy studies demonstrate elongated cells with abundant cytoplasm, lobulated nuclei, and prominent nucleoli, partly invested by a pericytoplasmic basal lamina. Tumor cells of both neuronal and glial origin were readily demonstrable by immunohistochemistry in that the cells were either GFAP or neurofilament positive, but not both. The cell of origin for these tumors is presumed to be superficial undifferentiated bipotential neuroepithelial cells which can give rise to both neuronal and glial tumor cells (Vandenberg et al 1987b). In one report, Schwann cell differentiation in addition to neuronal and glial differentiation was present (Ng et al 1990a).

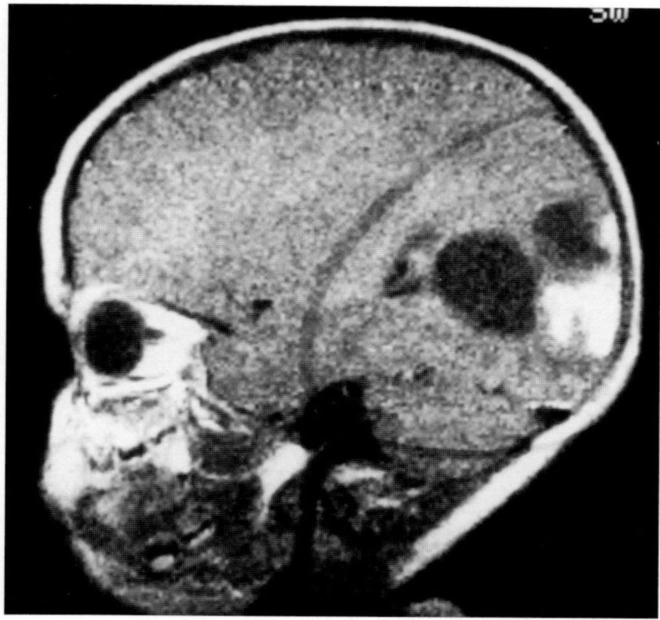

Fig. 29.8 Desmoplastic infantile ganglioglioma. This 1-year-old girl presented with a 3-week history of seizures. MR scan (T1-weighted image) shows a left occipital tumor with a hypointense cystic component and an evenly enhancing solid portion. Minimal mass effect is present. The patient underwent a gross total resection of her tumor with no further recurrence.

Differential diagnosis

The differential diagnosis of a large superficially located tumor in infants includes primitive neuroectodermal tumor (PNET), supratentorial ependymoma, and astrocytoma. Pathologically, desmoplastic infantile gangliogliomas must be distinguished from PXAs, gangliogliomas, and astrocytomas. PXA shares characteristics, including an astrocytic cell population, prominent leptomeningeal involvement with desmoplasia, presence of basal lamina covering part of the cytoplasmic membrane of the tumor cells, and a favorable prognosis. However, PXAs occur in an older age group, are predominantly located in the temporal lobe, and do not have neuronal differentiation (Kepes et al 1979). The name desmoplastic infantile ganglioglioma suggests a kinship to the gangliogliomas. Differences include presentation in infancy, more frequent inclusion of immature neuroepithelial cells, characteristic dense desmoplasia, and lack of a predominant localization in the temporal lobe. Unlike astrocytomas, the presence of a large component of primitive cells, abundant mitoses, and necrosis does not necessarily imply a worse prognosis (VandenBerg et al 1987a).

Treatment

The treatment of choice is gross total resection. The tumors are not well vascularized, often have a large cystic component, and are superficially located. Long-term survival is possible even if subtotal resection is performed. Although a good number of the patients reported received

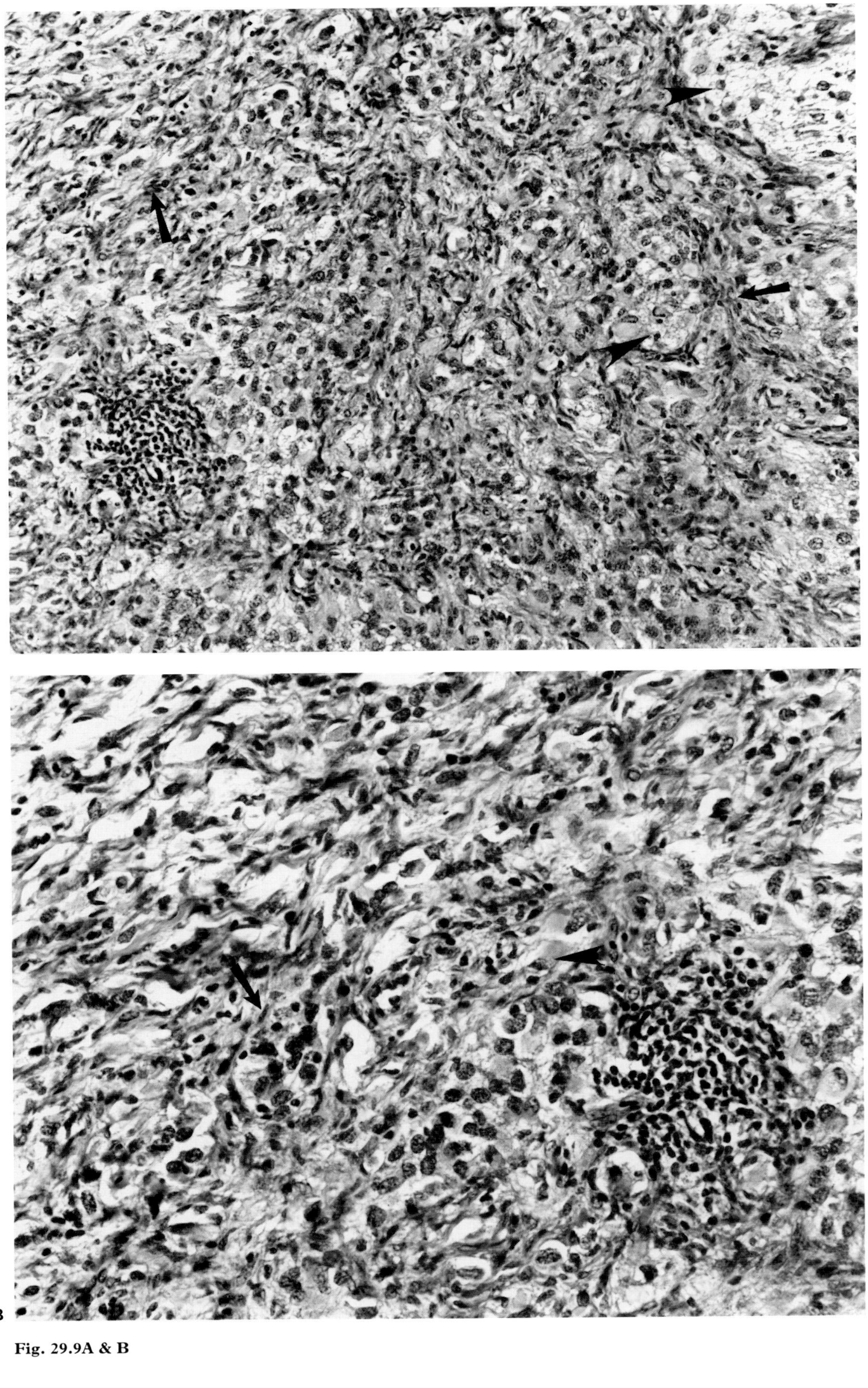

A

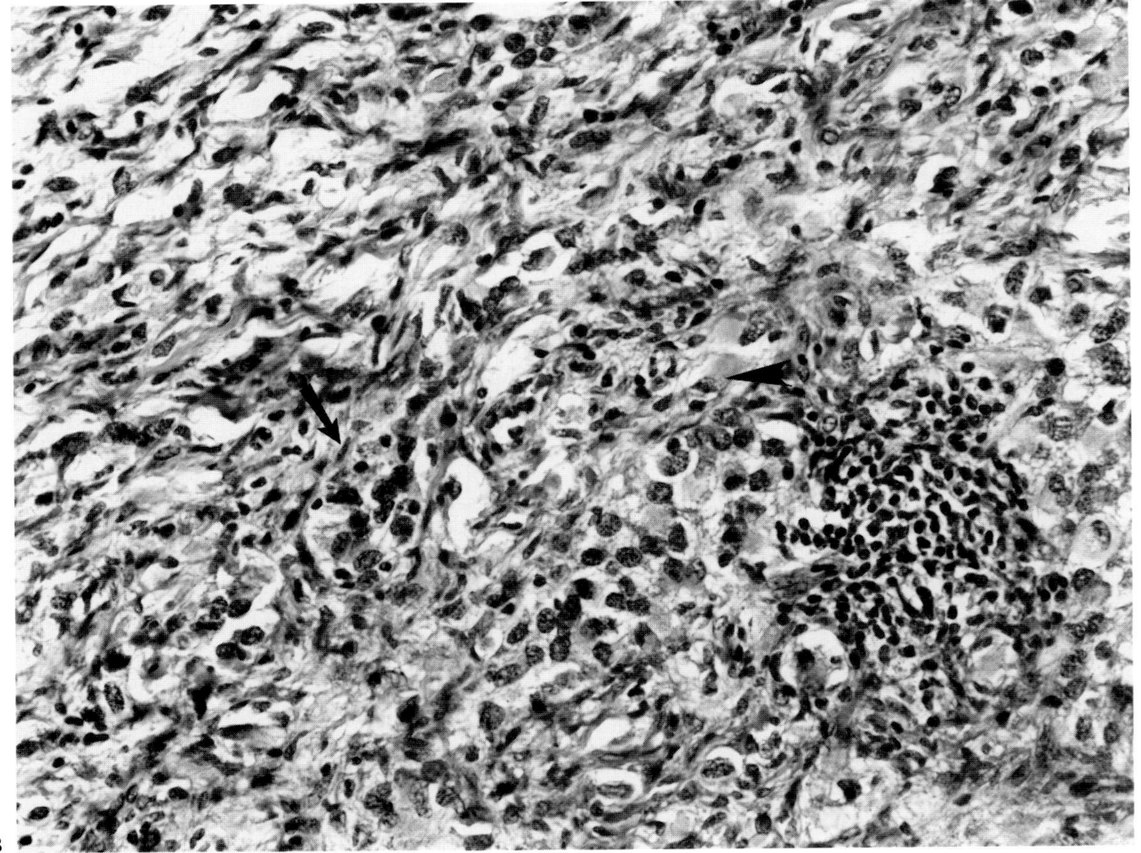

B

Fig. 29.9A & B

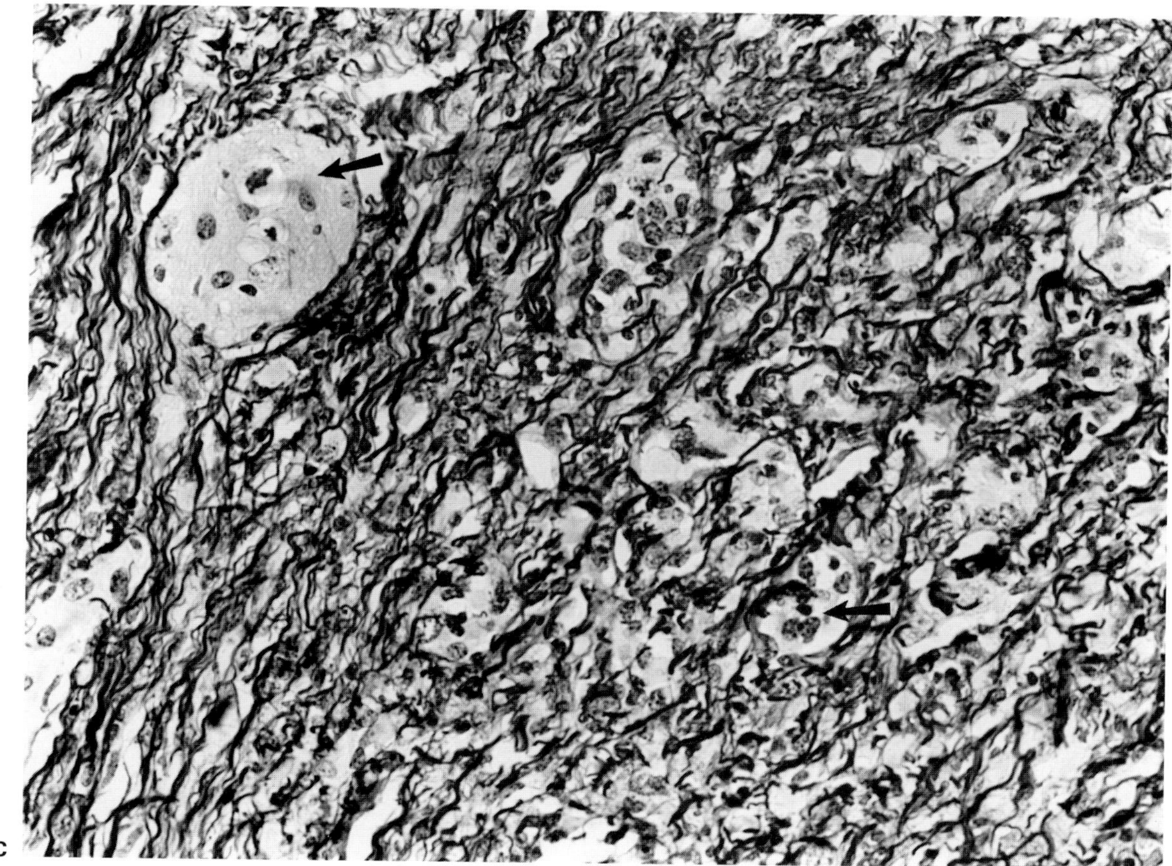

Fig. 29.9 **A.** Desmoplastic infantile ganglioglioma showing a mixture of glial and neuronal elements which are found scattered and forming clusters (arrowheads) surrounded by fibrous septa (arrows). H&E ×100. **B.** Desmoplastic infantile ganglioglioma with a composite cellular element. Most of the elongated cells are fibroblasts (arrow), intermingled with fibrillary and gemistocytic astrocytes (arrowhead). A small lymphocytic aggregate and scattered neurons are present. H&E ×200. **C.** Desmoplastic infantile ganglioglioma showing extensive accumulation of reticulin fibers (darkly stained) separating neuroglial islands (arrows). Reticulin fiber stain ×100.

radiation therapy, the data available have not shown any difference in survival. There was also no difference in survival following chemotherapy (VandenBerg et al 1987a). Adjuvant therapy is therefore not indicated. Recurrent tumor is treated with repeat surgical excision.

Clinical outcome

The clinical outcome after surgery is good. In VandenBerg et al's series, 8 of 9 patients with complete or near-total surgical resection of their tumors have survived 1.5–14 years following surgery (VandenBerg et al 1987a).

DYSEMBRYOPLASTIC NEUROEPITHELIAL TUMOR

Demographics

Dysembryoplastic neuroepithelial tumors (DNTs) were initially described by Daumas-Duport et al in 1988. Since then, a total of 72 cases have been reported in the literature (Daumas-Duport et al 1988, Koeller & Dillon 1992, Kirkpatrick et al 1993). The age range is from 1 year old to 19 years old, with a mean of 9 years. The sex distribution is M:F = 1.5:1. There does not seem to be a racial or genetic predisposition.

Diagnosis

The most common presentation is seizures, followed by headaches. Most of the patients have a nonfocal neurological exam. CT scan shows a supratentorial hypodense 'pseudocystic' lesion, especially in the temporal lobe (Daumas-Duport et al 1988). On MR scanning, the lesion is hypointense to gray matter on T1-weighted images, and hyperintense to gray matter on T2-weighted images, with variable contrast enhancement. Proton-density images demonstrate slightly higher signal intensity in the lesion than in cerebrospinal fluid (Koeller & Dillon 1992). A variable degree of calcification may be demonstrated by either MR or CT scans (Daumas-Duport et al 1992, Koeller & Dillon 1992).

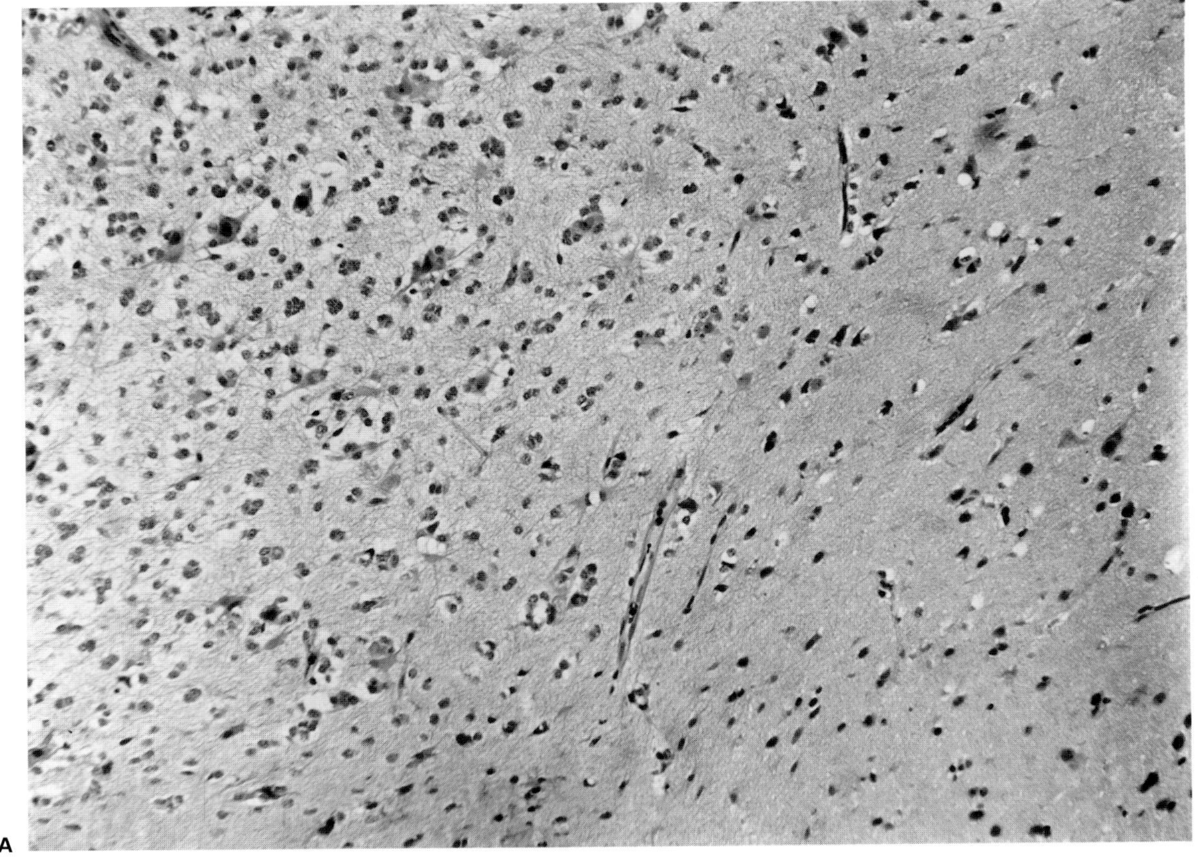
A

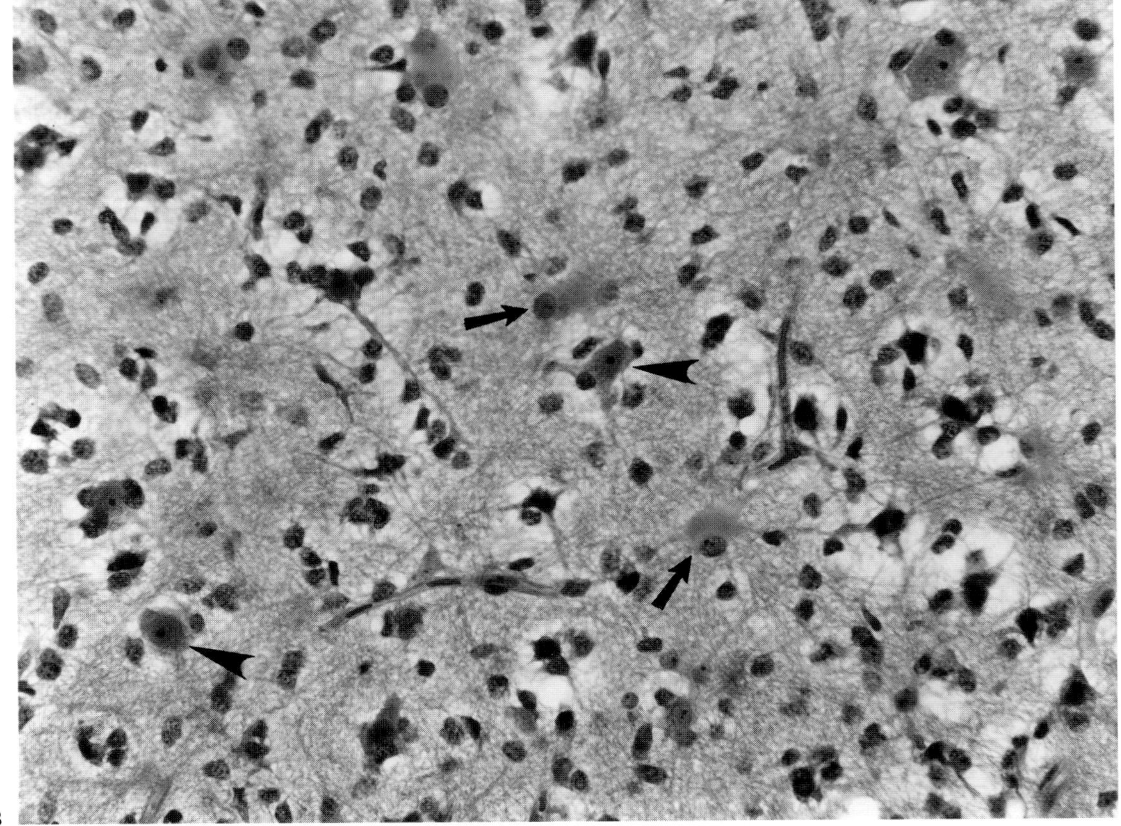
B

Fig. 29.10A & B

Fig. 29.10 **A.** Dysembryoplastic neuroepithelial tumor showing the characteristic nodular pattern of growth involving the cortex. Rarification of the neuropil and a prominent vascular meshwork are present. H&E ×100. **B.** Dysembryoplastic neuroepithelial tumor with a mixed population of glial and neuronal elements. The neurons have normal morphology (arrowhead) and the glial component is composed of astrocytes and oligodendrocytes exhibiting mild nuclear pleomorphism. Several hypertrophic (gemistocytic) astrocytes are seen in this field (arrows). H&E ×200.

Pathology

Most of the tumors are located in the temporal lobe, followed by the frontal, occipital, and parietal lobes. The tumor is macroscopically visible on the surface, well demarcated in some, and poorly demarcated in others. There is no uniform tumor consistency. Microscopically, dysembryoplastic neuroepithelial tumors are characterized by a 'specific glioneuronal element', a nodular component, and associated cortical dysplasia (Fig. 29.10). The 'specific glioneuronal element' is composed of both neurons and glial cells, which may range from compact to alveolar in structure, depending upon the degree of extracellular mucoid substance accumulation. While the 'specific glioneuronal element' is similar from one case to another, the nodular component varies. It is made up of neurons, astrocytes, and oligodendrocytes, often with evidence of cellular atypia. Foci of cortical dysplasia are also present. Daumas-Duport et al (1988) suggest that DNT results from disorganized embryogenesis, i.e. dysembryoplastic, and the site of origin is most likely from the subpial granular layer. The presence of foci of cortical dysplasia strongly suggests that DNTs arise during the formation of the cortex (Daumas-Duport et al 1988).

Differential diagnosis

The differential diagnoses of DNT include ganglioglioma, mixed oligoastrocytoma, and hamartoma. Histologically, gangliogliomas do not exhibit a multinodular architecture. Unlike DNT, they are not intracortical, but are randomly situated. Bizarre neurons or giant ganglion-like cells are present in gangliogliomas, but not in DNT. The abundant connective tissue stroma and perivascular lymphocytic infiltrates that characterize the ganglion cell-rich part of ganglioglioma are not present in DNT. Lastly, the oligodendroglial component found in DNT is usually not prominent in gangliogliomas (Haddad et al 1992). Oligoastrocytomas may include nodular foci which should not be misinterpreted as DNT. Conversely, cortical infiltration by oligoastrocytoma should not be confused with the characteristic neuroglial component of DNT (Russell & Rubinstein 1989). Hamartomas are characterized only by the presence of neuronal elements, without evidence of astrocytic and oligodendroglial components or cortical dysplasia (Albright & Lee 1993).

Treatment

The treatment is surgical excision. DNTs have a good prognosis whether total or subtotal resection is performed. In one series of 39 cases, 17 patients underwent subtotal resections with no clinical or radiological evidence of recurrence on long-term follow-up (Daumas-Duport et al 1988). Kirkpatrick et al found that the pathology in a group of seizure patients was predominantly DNT (27/31 patients). Patients with gross total resections did not have evidence of recurrence, and there was good seizure control despite subtotal resection in a majority of the patients (Kirkpatrick et al 1993). Radiotherapy itself does not appear to confer any obvious benefit. There was no difference in survival or recurrence in 13 subjects who had undergone postoperative radiotherapy compared with 26 subjects who had not had postoperative radiotherapy (Daumas-Duport et al 1988). No data on chemotherapy are available. Therefore, the treatment for the original tumor, as well as any recurrence, is surgical.

Clinical outcome

Although newly recognized as a distinct pathological entity, diagnosis of DNT is important as it has a benign prognosis. Recognition of DNT will spare young patients the deleterious effects of radio- or chemotherapy. Moreover, DNT is an important etiology of temporal lobe epilepsy, and subsequent removal will result in long-term control of seizures.

GANGLIOGLIOMA

Demographics

Gangliogliomas were first named by Courville in 1930 to describe a set of neoplasms with both astrocytic and neuronal components (Courville 1930). Gangliogliomas make up 0.4–7.6% of all brain tumors, and 1% of all intramedullary spinal cord tumors (Kalyan-Raman & Olivero 1987, Miller et al 1990). Most of the patients are less than 30 years old; however, the age span ranges from 2 months to 70 years (Benitez et al 1990, Castillo et al 1990). There does not appear to be a sex, familial, or racial preference. There are no other associations with this tumor, although one patient had both neurofibromatosis type 1 (NF-1) and a ganglioglioma (Parizel et al 1991). Although gangliogliomas were initially thought by Courville to be located predominantly in the floor of the third ventricle, subsequent series have shown that the majority of gangliogliomas are located in the cerebral hemispheres, especially in the frontal and temporal lobes (Courville 1930). In the younger age population, Haddad notes an increased incidence of midline tumors (Haddad et al 1992). Less common locations in the optic nerve, chiasm, and tract (Bergin et al 1988, Chilton et al 1990,

Sugiyama et al 1992), brainstem (Garcia et al 1984, Davidson et al 1992), cerebellum (Mizuno et al 1987) and spinal cord (Johannson et al 1981) have been reported. Although metastasis is rare, leptomeningeal and subarachnoid spread have been reported (Tien et al 1992, Wacker et al 1992).

Diagnosis

The overwhelming presenting history of patients with gangliogliomas is a progressive seizure disorder. Seizures may be present from months to several years before the diagnosis is established (Demierre et al 1986, Chamberlain & Press 1990, Diepholder et al 1991). Presenting signs and symptoms vary depending on patient age, tumor location, and the aggressiveness of the tumor (Fletcher et al 1988). In very young patients, increasing head circumference would usually indicate increased intracranial pressure (Demierre et al 1986, Hunt & Johnson 1989, Diepholder et al 1991). Patients with intraorbital gangliogliomas may present with proptosis and visual loss (Bergin et al 1988, Chilton et al 1990), while those with brainstem gangliogliomas may exhibit hemiparesis and cranial nerve deficits (Fig. 29.11) (Garcia et al 1984, Nelson et al 1987, Davidson et al 1992). One patient's initial symptoms were hearing loss and ataxia from a left cerebellar mass (Dhillon 1987). The findings are usually longstanding due to the nonaggressive nature of gangliogliomas in most cases. One patient with a ganglioglioma in the superior part of the medulla had a 46-year history of neurological dysfunction before she finally died from pneumonia (Davidson et al 1992).

Cerebral angiography does not yield additional information apart from confirming that these tumors are not vascular (Silver et al 1991). CT scan usually demonstrates a hypodense or isodense lesion with poor contrast enhancement (Rommel & Hamer 1983). Castillo found that gangliogliomas may be divided into solid and cystic components on the basis of their CT characteristics. Cystic tumors were located, with decreasing frequency, in the cerebellum, temporal, frontal, and parietal lobes. Solid tumors were usually in the temporal lobe. Better contrast enhancement was found with the solid tumors (Fig. 29.12) (Castillo et al 1990). Calcification is seen in approximately 1 in 3 of the tumors (Dorne et al 1986). Anaplastic tumors may show a heterogeneous appearance on CT, with excellent contrast enhancement (Hall et al 1986). MR imaging is useful in distinguishing the cystic tumor component (Fig. 29.11) (Furuta et al 1992, Haddad et al 1992). The majority of tumors are hypointense relative to gray matter on T1-weighted images, and hyperintense relative to gray matter on T2-weighted

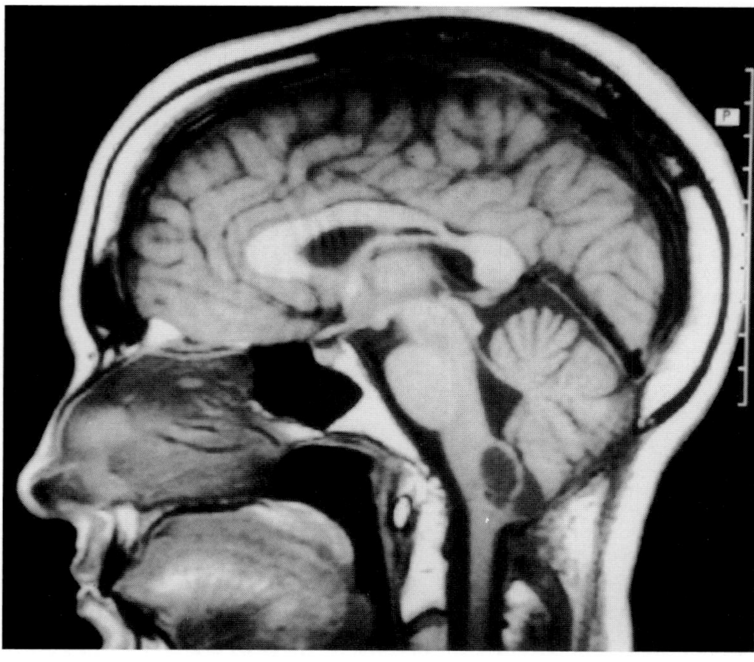

A

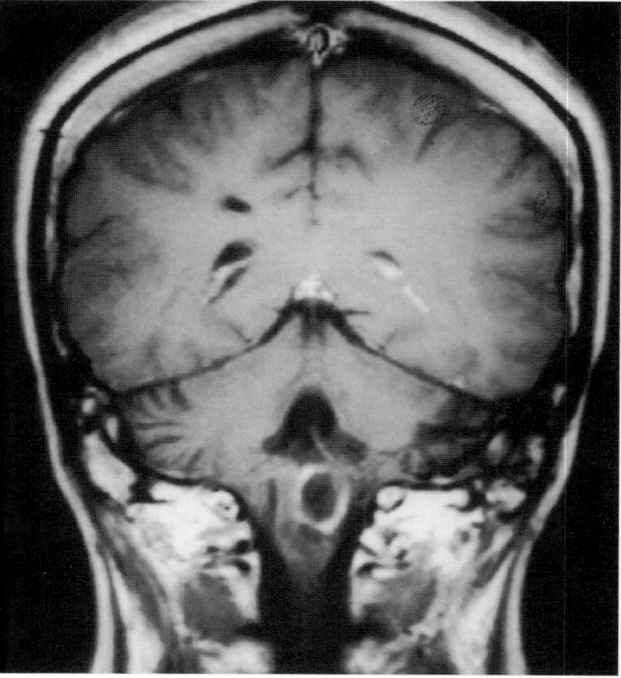

B

Fig. 29.11 Ganglioglioma. This 18-year-old woman presented with a one-year history of nausea, vomiting, and weight loss. Neurological examination revealed multiple left lower cranial nerve (IX, X, XII) dysfunction and a left sensory deficit. MR scan (T1-weighted image) reveals a cystic tumor, hypointense to gray matter, in the medulla (**A**) with mild enhancement (**B**). The patient underwent a subtotal resection of her tumor, radiation, and ventriculo-peritoneal shunt placement. It is now 13 years since her original surgery and she is neurologically stable.

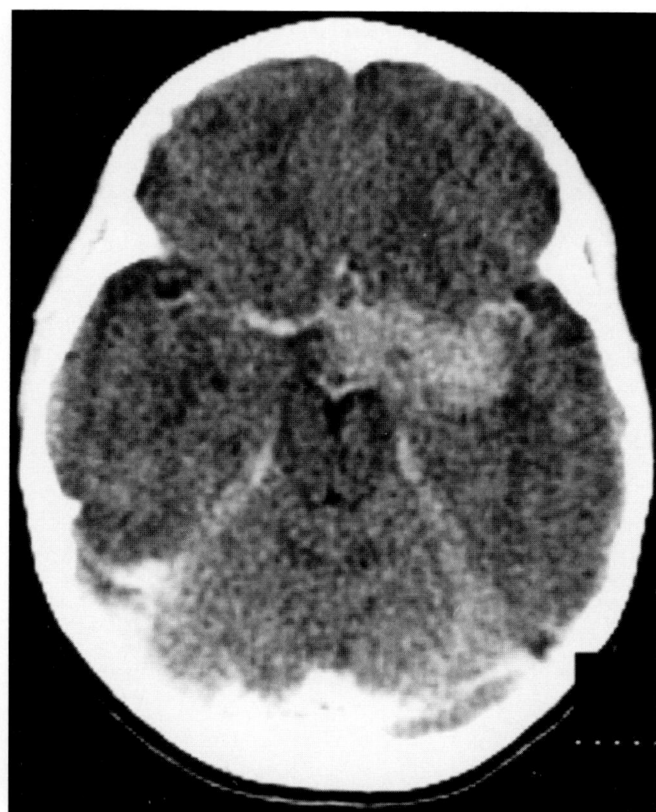

Fig. 29.12 Ganglioglioma. This 10-year-old boy presented with uncinate fits and a mild right hemiparesis. CT scan with contrast reveals an enhancing tumor extending from the left sylvian fissure to the suprasellar cistern with engulfment of the left middle cerebral artery. The patient underwent a partial resection of his tumor with no adjunctive therapy. Tumor recurrence led to a repeat resection and stereotactic radiosurgery. The patient subsequently underwent chemotherapy and a repeat resection elsewhere with further neurological deficits. He is currently 9 years from his original diagnosis with progressive disease.

images (Benitez et al 1990, Tampieri et al 1991). MR was able to demonstrate leptomeningeal and subarachnoid spread along the middle cerebral artery and right sylvian fissure in a patient with leptomeningeal metastasis (Tien et al 1992).

Pathology

Grossly, gangliogliomas are firm, grayish tumors which may have cystic components (Henry et al 1978). On light microscopy, both neuronal and astrocytic components are readily apparent. Mild to moderate cellularity, minimal pleomorphism, and rare mitotic figures are present (Fig. 29.13). Anaplastic degeneration, should it occur, is usually detected in the glial component of the tumor (Allegranza 1990). Occasionally, other tumors including pleomorphic xanthoastrocytoma (Furuta et al 1992), osteomas (Hori et al 1988), and melanotic cells (Hunt & Johnson 1989) may be interspersed within the ganglioglioma. On electron microscopy, three main cell types may be seen: (1) ganglion cells with dense core vesicles, (2) glial cells with processes filled with filament, and (3) probable mesenchymal cells adjacent to abundant collagen fibrils (Rubinstein & Herman 1972). Features of neuronal degeneration have been found in gangliogliomas including neurofilament aggregates, and Hirano, Lafora, and zebra bodies (Takahashi et al 1987). Neoplastic ganglion cells show intense immunoreactivity for synaptophysin, a 38 kilodalton glycoprotein located in synaptic vesicle membranes that outlines the borders of cell bodies (Miller D C et al 1990, Diepholder et al 1991). Kawai has demonstrated the presence of tyrosine hydroxylase (a rate-limiting enzyme in the catecholamine synthesizing pathway), and numerous dense core vesicles in the neuronal component of gangliogliomas, suggesting that the origin of these cells may have been from ectopic neural crest tissues (Kawai et al 1987, Diepholder et al 1991, Issidorides & Arvanitis 1993). Other neuroendocrine markers including serotonin, somatostatin, met-enkephalin, leu-enkephalin, and substance P have been variably demonstrated in the dense core granules (Takahashi et al 1989). Flow cytometry of a ganglioglioma demonstrated aneuploidy in both necrotic regions of the tumor and sections with atypical findings (Bowles et al 1988). Fujimoto has looked at mRNA expression of various oncogenes including v-sis, v-myc and v-fos, and found increased v-sis and v-fos expression for gangliogliomas and other benign tumors (Fujimoto et al 1988). Mapstone found increased mRNA expression for PFGF-β and the ras gene for malignant tumors, but not in benign tumors, including a single case of ganglioglioma (Mapstone et al 1991). Wacker has demonstrated loss of chromosome 17p in a child with a malignant ganglioglioma (Wacker et al 1992).

Differential diagnosis

Differential diagnosis of gangliogliomas includes gangliocytomas, low grade gliomas, dysembryoplastic neuroepithelial tumors, and oligodendrogliomas. Gangliocytomas usually occur in the cerebellum (Lhermitte-Duclos disease), and are characterized by alteration of the normal cerebellar architecture, resulting in hypertrophied neuronal cells in the granule cell layer. No glial component is present (Reznik & Schoenen 1983). Low grade gliomas may be differentiated from gangliogliomas as they do not have neuronal components (Russell & Rubinstein 1989). Dysembryoplastic neuroepithelial tumors, which also commonly occur in the temporal lobe, have a characteristic glioneuronal element, nodular component, and association with cortical dysplasia (Daumas-Duport et al 1988). Lastly, oligodendrogliomas may be differentiated from gangliogliomas since they do not have neuronal elements, and are derived from oligodendrocytes (Russell & Rubinstein 1989).

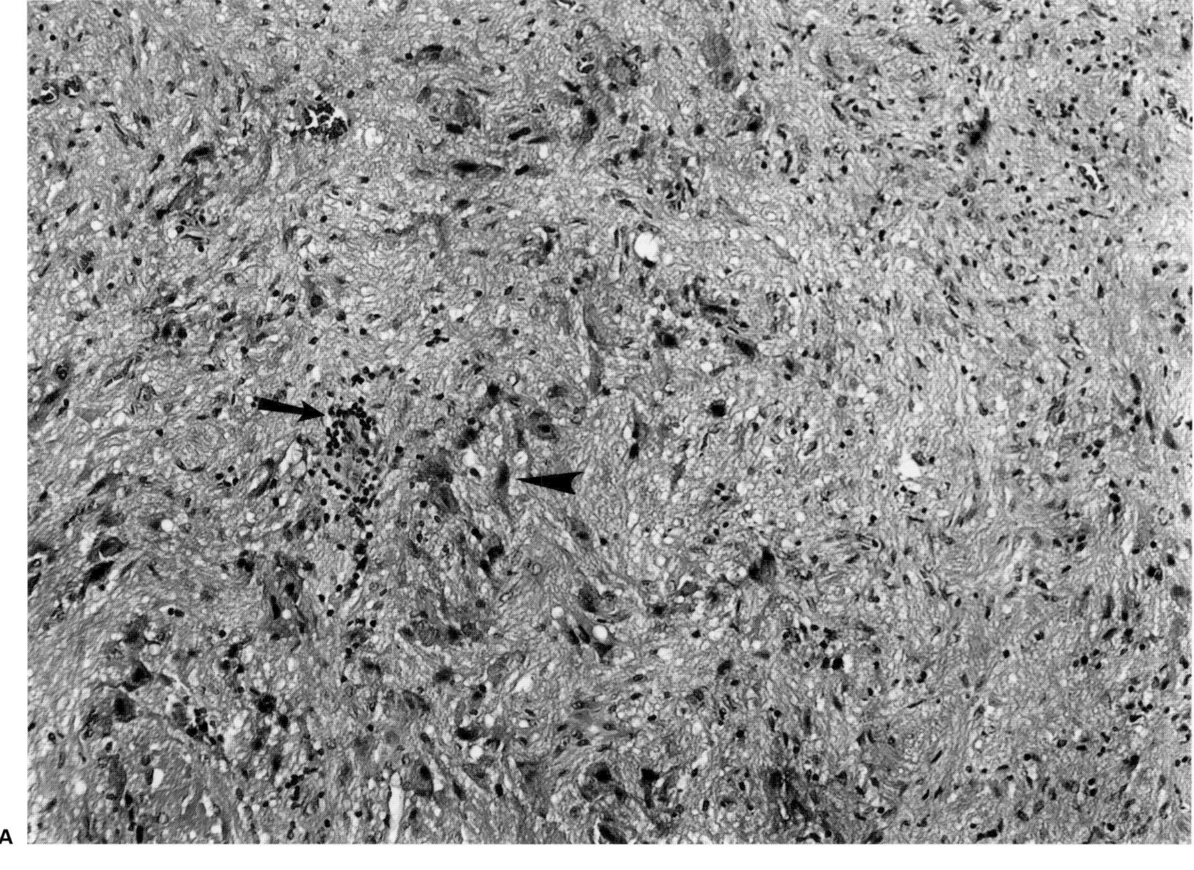

A

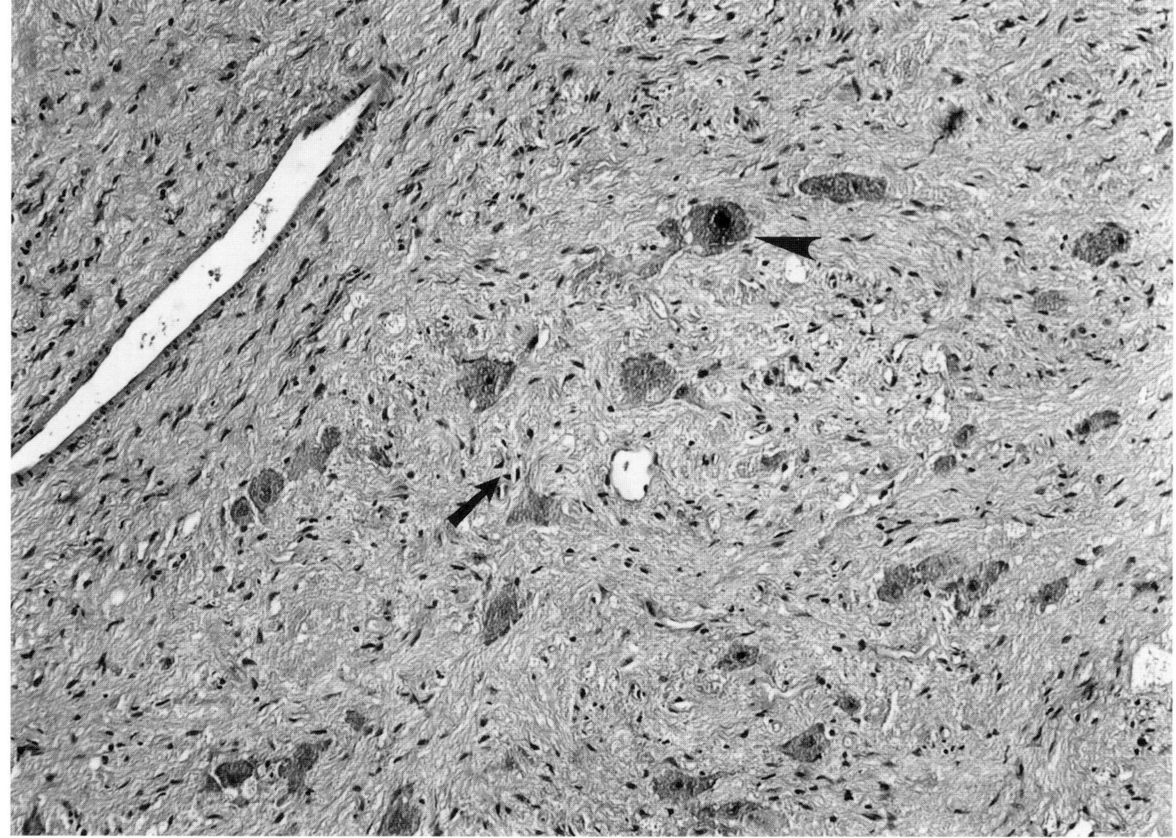

B

Fig. 29.13A & B

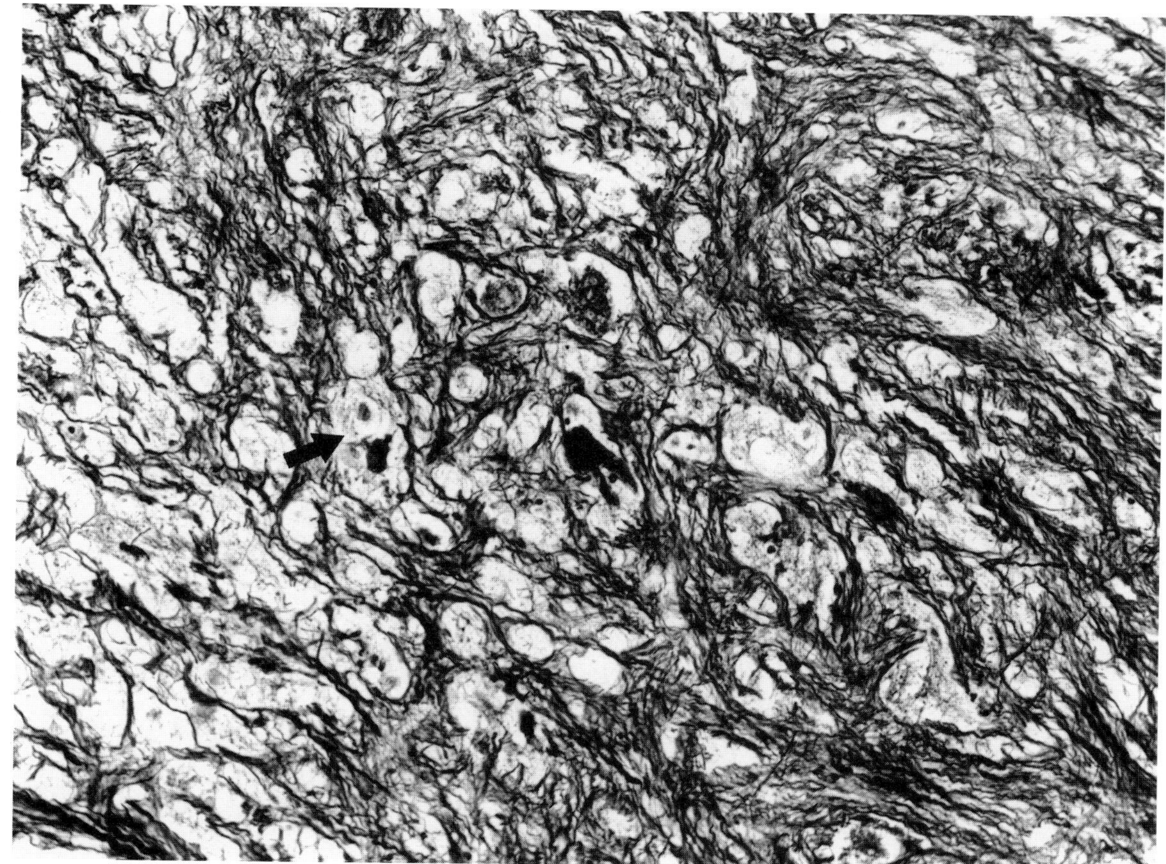

C

Fig. 29.13 **A.** Ganglioglioma showing the characteristic mixed composition of neuronal (arrowhead), glial, mesenchymal elements and focal lymphocytic aggregates (arrow). H&E ×100. **B.** Ganglioglioma showing clusters of haphazardly arranged neurons which exhibit marked variation in size and shape (arrowhead). The glial component contains astrocytic and few oligodendroglial elements with no atypia (arrow). H&E ×200. **C.** Ganglioglioma showing neuroglial islands and individual neurons (arrow) surrounded by dense bands of connective tissue rich in darkly stained reticulin fibers. Reticulin fiber stain ×100.

Treatment

In accessible tumors, the treatment for gangliogliomas is surgical. Gross total removal is the best chance for a cure (Sutton et al 1991, Haddad et al 1992). An attempt at gross total resection is still the goal even if the ganglioglioma is anaplastic. Hall has reported long-term survival in a 6-month-old girl with an anaplastic ganglioglioma after a gross total resection (Hall et al 1986). Subtotal resection of exophytic components of ganglioglomas located in the brainstem and optic tracts may be the only option (Garcia et al 1984, Chilton et al 1990). Only partial excisions are usually possible with midline tumors, and carry a greater chance of recurrence (Haddad et al 1992). The result of radiotherapy for gangliogliomas is inconclusive. Radiotherapy (40–60 Gy) is most commonly given to patients with tumors for whom only a subtotal resection could be achieved and who have recurrence, or to patients with anaplastic components to their tumors (Cox et al 1982, Silver et al 1991). Patients with complete resections and benign histologies should not be given radiotherapy. Consideration of the patient's age should be taken into account as intracranial radiation in younger children will result in substantial deterioration of intellectual and endocrine development (Ellenberg et al 1987). Only a few patients have received chemotherapy, and there does not appear to be a substantial benefit (Silver et al 1991).

Clinical outcome

Long-term survival is excellent if a gross total resection is achieved. Seizure control is much improved in patients with gross total tumor resection (Sutton et al 1983, 1987, Otsubo et al 1990, Silver et al 1991, Haddad et al 1992). Leptomeningeal spread of a tumor with a malignant component has been reported, but is rare (Tien et al 1992, Wacker et al 1992).

POLAR SPONGIOBLASTOMA

Demographics

Polar spongioblastomas, first described by Russell & Cairns

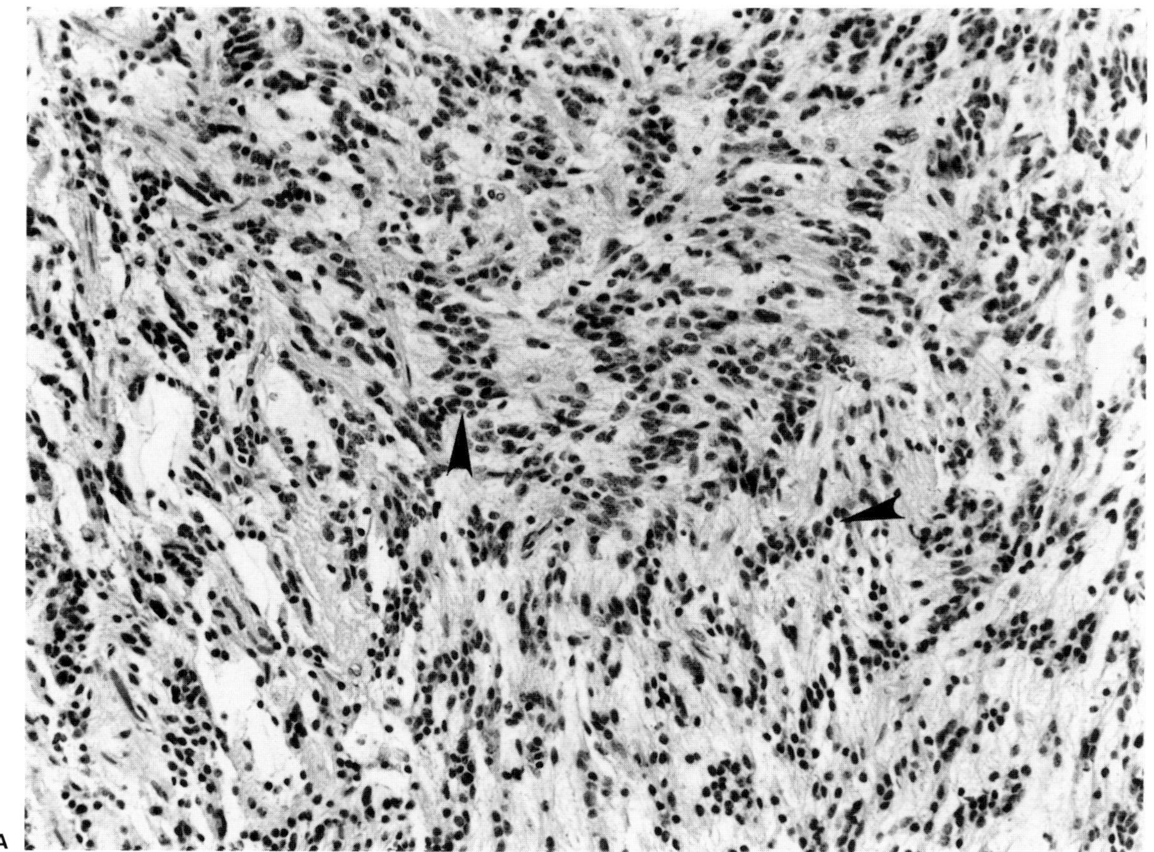

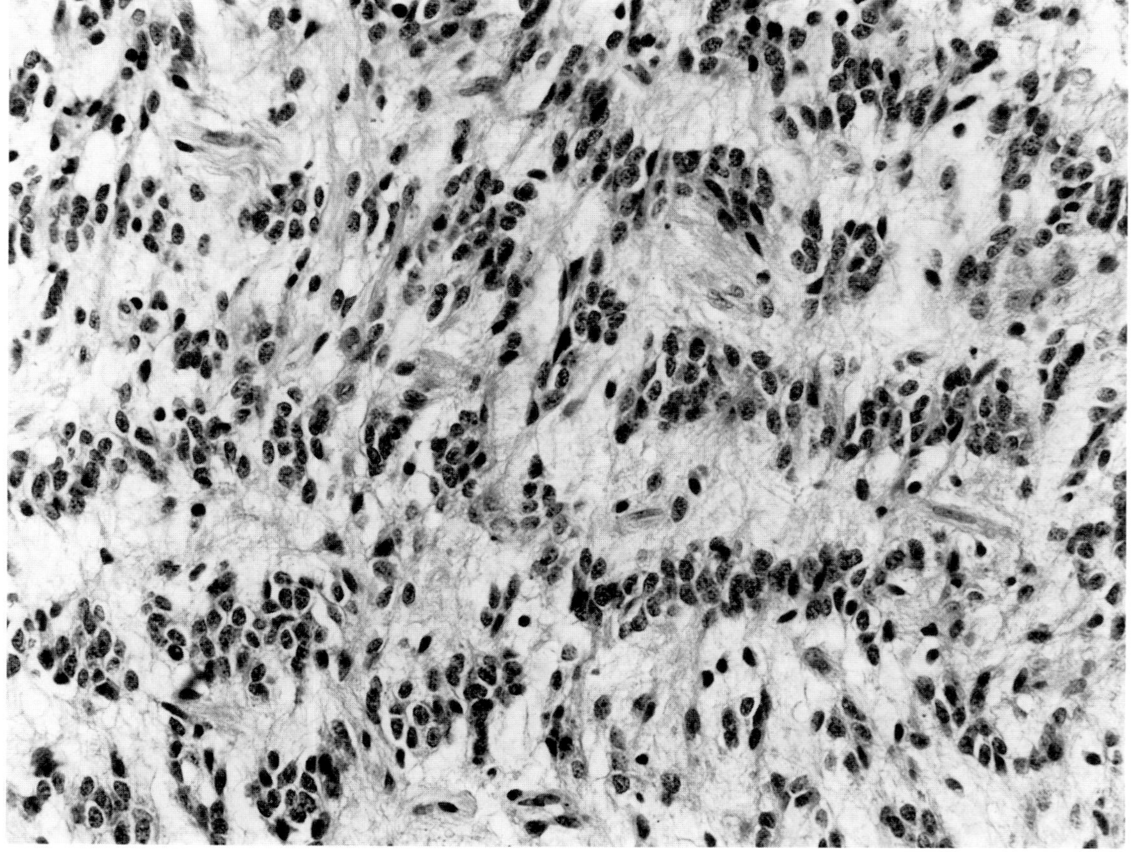

Fig. 29.14A & B

Fig. 29.14 **A.** Polar spongioblastoma showing characteristic uniform histologic pattern of growth with parallel arrangement of tumor cells and nuclear palisades (arrowheads). H&E ×160. **B.** Polar spongioblastoma with compact rhythmic bands of neoplastic cells in a loose fibrillary background. The tumor cell nuclei are oval with finely granular chromatin and no pleomorphism. H&E ×200.

in 1947, are rare neoplasms involving midline structures (Russell & Cairns 1947). Since then, 12 cases have been reported. The hypothalamus, lateral walls of the third ventricle, fourth ventricle, and optic chiasm are the most commonly involved. It has been reported in the spinal cord and frontal lobe as well. The age range is from 6 months to 46 years, with a median age of 8.5 years (Jansen et al 1990). No sexual, familial, or racial predilection can be estimated because of the rarity of the tumor.

Diagnosis

The presenting signs and symptoms, depending on the location of the tumor, range from the diencephalic syndrome to seizures (de Chadarevian et al 1984, Jansen et al 1990). Information as to the radiological diagnosis is limited. A CT scan in one patient showed a hypodense lesion in the frontal lobe with evidence of calcification (Jansen et al 1990). No MR data are available.

Pathology

Grossly, the tumor is grayish-white in color, firm, and usually well demarcated. If subarachnoid metastasis has occurred, thick sheets of soft grey tissue may be present (Rubinstein 1972). Light microscopy shows tumor cells arranged in characteristic parallel fashion, like a step-ladder, forming compact bands secondary to palisading of the nuclei. The cells are thin, unipolar or bipolar in shape, with dark oval nuclei. Neuroglial fibrils, if present, are more prominent in regions of astrocytic differentiation (Fig. 29.14) (Rubinstein 1972).

Although the polar spongioblastoma has been thought to be cytogenetically related to the embryonal radial glial cell and was considered, therefore, as a primitive glial tumor in the WHO classification of 1979, it has been set aside as a neuroepithelial tumor of uncertain origin in the new WHO classification (Zülch 1979, Kleihues et al 1993). Ultrastructural studies and immunohistochemistry suggest a neuroendocrine nature. Electron microscopy demonstrates three zones of differentiation: (1) a densely cellular zone corresponding to the palisades seen by light microscopy, (2) a fibrillary zone composed of elongated cytoplasmic processes, intervening between the palisades and the vascular walls, and (3) a perivascular zone with corresponding vessels. This three-tiered arrangement has led de Chadarevian et al to propose that the organization is similar to that of the hypothalamic neuroendocrine system, with a perivascular cellular arrangement, intracytoplasmic microtubules, and membrane-bound dense core granules (de Chadarevian et al 1984). Jansen et al have also noted prominent endoplasmic reticulum and microtubules in the tumor cytoplasm, suggesting a neuronal origin. Immunohistochemistry demonstrates that some of the tumor cells are neuron-specific enolase positive. Most of the tumor cells are GFAP negative except in portions of the tumor with more prominent astrocytic differentiation (Jansen et al 1990). Bignami et al have shown that glial hyaluronate binding protein (GHA) is negative in neuroepithelial tumors such as astrocytomas, oligodendrogliomas, medulloblastomas, and ependymomas. Spongioblastomas are GHA positive, however, suggesting that they are derived from a more primitive glial precursor, as immature glial cells forming the periventricular germinal layer are GHA positive in 22-week-old human embryos (Bignami et al 1989).

Differential diagnosis

Differential diagnosis of spongioblastomas includes any neuroepithelial tumor which may contain palisades of tumor: ependymomas, oligodendrogliomas, pilocytic astrocytomas, cerebellar astrocytomas, medulloblastomas, and cerebral neuroblastomas. Schiffer et al believe that polar spongioblastomas should not be considered a tumor entity. They feel that even in cases where nuclear palisading represents the predominant histological characteristic, evidence can be found that it is only an architectural feature of another neuroepithelial tumor (Schiffer et al 1993).

Treatment

The treatment of choice is surgical resection. The first cases reported by Russell & Cairns presented with subarachnoid spread and survived only about a year (Russell & Cairns 1947). Recently long-term survival in patients with frontal or parietal lobe tumors who had undergone a gross total resection has been documented (Bignami et al 1989, Jansen et al 1990). Steinberg reported a patient with a subtotally resected fourth ventricular spongioblastoma who had undergone radiotherapy without recurrence on a 15-year follow-up (Steinberg et al 1985). The effect of radiotherapy is mixed. Although anecdotal reports suggest that it may be helpful, the survival of some patients has not improved (Jansen et al 1990). No data on chemotherapy are available.

Clinical outcome

Clinical outcome in this small group of patients appears to be varied. Long-term survival, even after subtotal resection followed by radiation, may be achieved (Jansen et al 1990).

GANGLIOCYTOMA

Demographics

Lhermitte-Duclos disease, or dysplastic gangliocytoma of the cerebellum, is a rare tumor first reported in 1920 by Lhermitte & Duclos, with more than 60 cases reported in the literature since then (Lhermitte & Duclos 1920, Sabin et al 1988). Although this tumor has been reported in the hypothalamus and spinal cord, the majority arise from the cerebellum (Bevan et al 1989, Azzarelli et al 1991). The age of presentation ranges from birth to the sixth decade; but most commonly the tumor is initially seen in the third and fourth decades of life. There is no sexual or racial predilection (Roessman & Wongmongkolrit 1984, Faillot et al 1990). There is no hereditary basis for Lhermitte-Duclos disease, but a case of mother and son has been reported (Ambler et al 1969).

Diagnosis

Most patients present with signs and symptoms of cerebellar dysfunction (ataxia, dysdiadochokinesia, nystagmus), or increased intracranial pressure secondary to hydrocephalus. Lhermitte-Duclos disease may be associated with other CNS malformations including hydromyelia, brain heterotopia, and megalencephaly (Reznik & Schoenen 1983). It has been found in association with Cowden disease, an autosomal dominant multiple hamartomatous condition of the skin and mucous membranes, with frequent involvement of the thyroid, breast, colon, and adnexa (Padberg et al 1991).

CT scanning shows a hypodense lesion in the cerebellum with minimal contrast enhancement (Fig. 29.15) (di Lorenzo et al 1984, Smith et al 1989). Areas of calcification may be present. MR scanning shows the tumor to be hypointense to gray matter on T1-weighted images, and hyperintense to gray matter on T2-weighted images. As with CT, there is minimal enhancement of the tumor on MR. The lamellar appearance of the tumor may be appreciated on T2-weighted images, corresponding to the pathological finding of thickened cerebellar folia. As would be expected from CT and MR, the tumor on angiography is an avascular mass (Roski et al 1981, Sabin et al 1988, Faillot et al 1990). MR may also be useful in determining the presence of residual tumor (Marano et al 1988, Reeder et al 1988, Smith et al 1989, Ashley et al 1990, Faillot et al 1990).

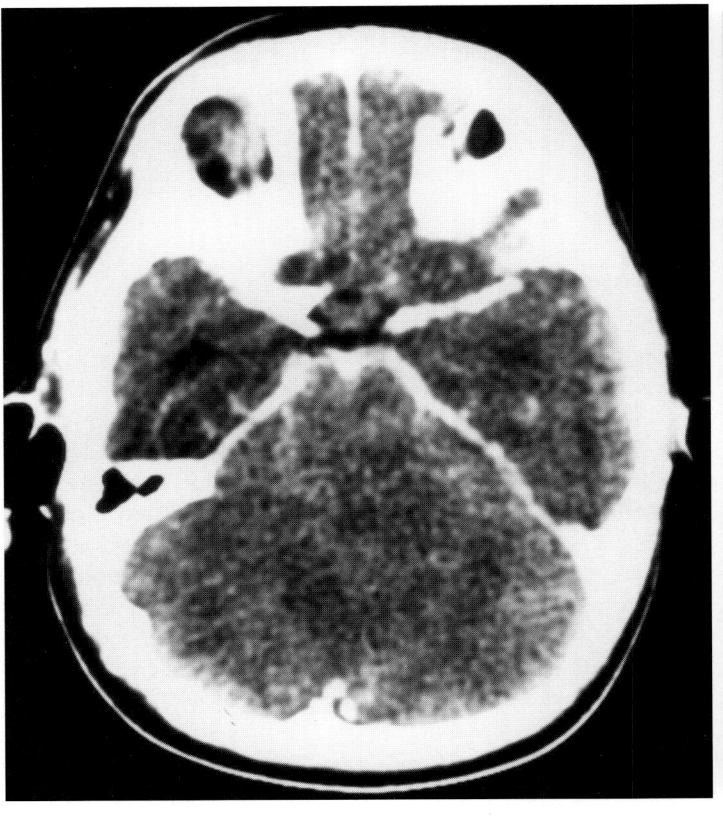

A

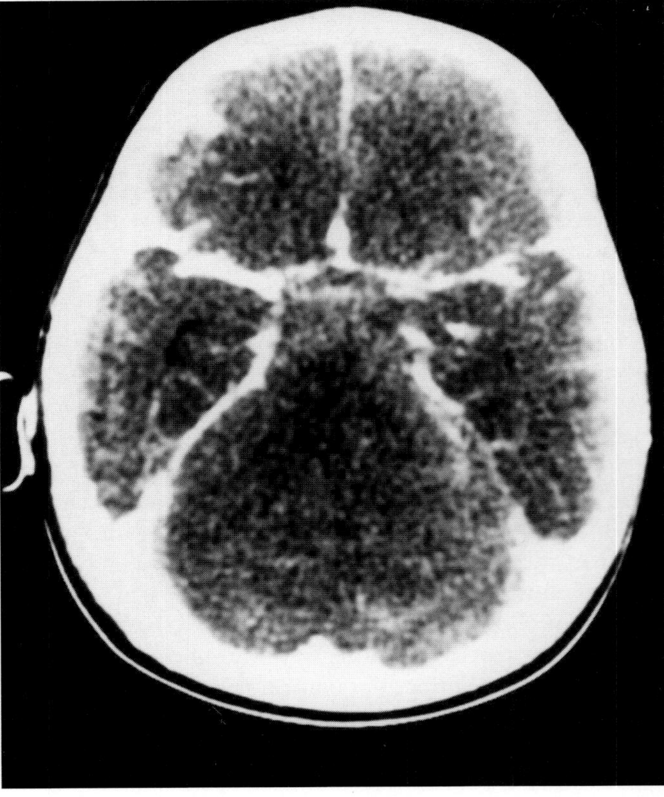

B

Fig. 29.15 Gangliocytoma (Lhermitte-Duclos). This 7-year-old boy with a history of developmental delay expired from acute hydrocephalus. CT scan revealed a non-enhancing hypodense lesion occupying most of the cerebellum with obstruction of the basilar cisterns **A, B**. The diagnosis of gangliocytoma was obtained post mortem.

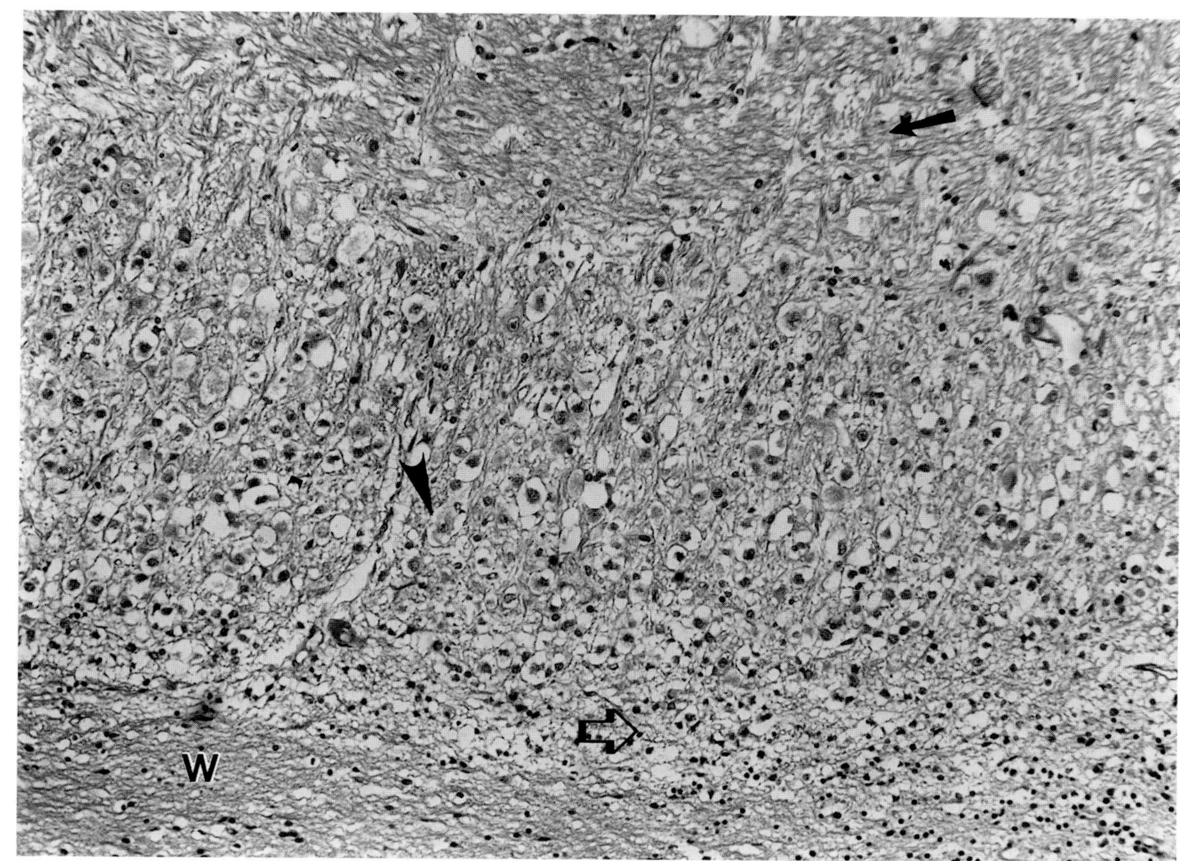

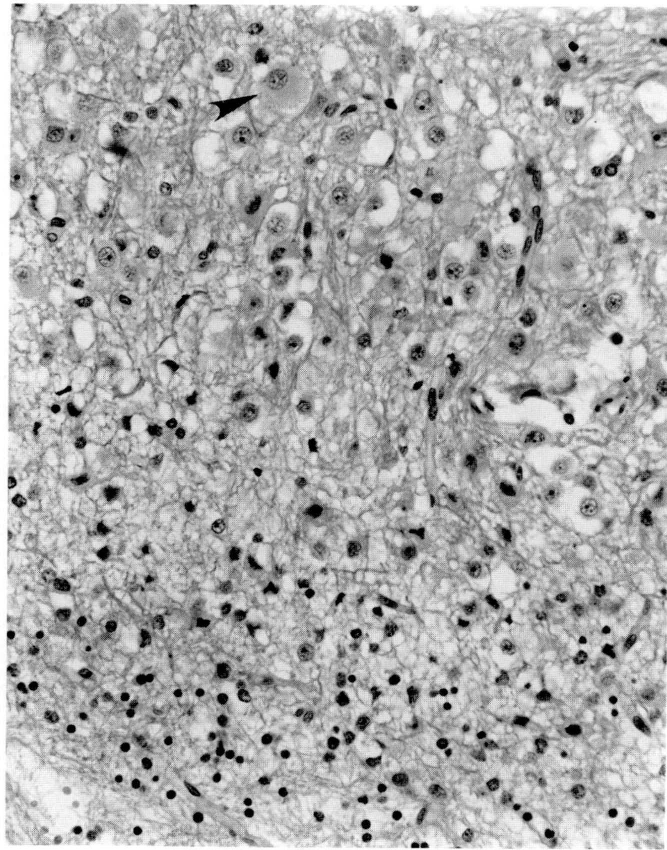

Fig. 29.16 **A.** Gangliocytoma showing proliferation of neuronal cells (arrowhead) that are replacing the internal granular cell layer (white arrow); their arborizations form a thick plexus in the molecular layer (arrow). The subcortical white matter is thin (W), H&E ×100. **B.** Gangliocytoma showing diffuse hypertrophy of the cerebellar folia with proliferating small neurons, some of which are as large as Purkinje cells (arrowhead). H&E ×150.

Pathology

Grossly, cerebellar gangliocytomas present as widened cerebellar folia (Sabin et al 1988). It is often difficult to establish a plane between the gangliocytoma and normal cerebellum. Microscopically, the normal cerebellar architecture is altered, with the three layers of the cerebellar cortex (molecular, Purkinje, and granular) disrupted. Instead, there is thickening of the molecular layer, widening of the granule cell layer, disappearance of the Purkinje cell layer, and a decrease in the arbor vitae of the cerebellum. Pleomorphic ganglion cells without invasive characteristics replace the granule cell layer. Neovascular proliferation may be present in areas with the highest neuronal concentration. Excessive numbers of large myelinated axons exist within the molecular layer (Fig. 29.16) (Roski et al 1981, Reznik & Schoenen 1983, di Lorenzo et al 1984, Reeder et al 1988, Sabin et al 1988, Smith et al 1989, Padberg et al 1991). One patient with an intramedullary spinal cord gangliocytoma experienced a hypertensive episode during surgery. The immunohistochemistry of this patient's tumor with anti-tyrosine hydroxylase antibody for mature ganglion cells demonstrated dense core vesicles, suggesting that the transient hypertension was secondary to catecholamine release (Azzarelli et al 1991).

Differential diagnosis

The differential diagnosis of gangliocytomas includes low grade gliomas versus hamartomas. Definitive diagnosis is made by demonstration of disruption of cerebellar architecture with proliferation of ganglion cells in the granule cell layer.

Treatment

The treatment of choice is surgical resection. However, total resection is almost never obtained because of the difficulty in obtaining a plane between normal cerebellum and the gangliocytoma. Subtotal resection, however, may be sufficient for diminishing the mass effect, and repeat debulking may be necessary (Marano et al 1988). Adjunctive radiotherapy and chemotherapy may be employed; however, their efficacy is unknown.

Clinical outcome

The overall outcome in gangliocytomas of the cerebellum is good. Although all the reports emphasize subtotal resections only, follow-up of the patients usually shows them to be doing well up to 4 years after surgery (Roski et al 1981, Reznik & Schoenen 1983, Marano et al 1988).

HYPOTHALAMIC HAMARTOMA

Demographics

The first case of hypothalamic hamartoma was reported in 1934 (Le Marquand & Russell 1934). Since then, over 90 cases have been reported in the world literature, of which 56 cases have been reported since 1980 (Albright & Lee 1993). The vast majority of the tumors are found in the ventral aspect of the hypothalamus, ranging in position from the tuber cinereum to the mamillary body, and are either sessile or pedunculated in appearance (Yamada & Sano 1992). Although most children present with precocious puberty before the age of 3, patients as old as 8 years old have been reported (Zuniga et al 1983, Starceski et al 1990). In one survey of hypothalamic hamartomas, 84% of the children presented with sexual precocity before age 3 (Hibi & Fujiwara 1987). There does not appear to be a sexual, familial, or racial predilection. Hypothalamic hamartomas may be associated with midline deformities including callosal agenesis, optic malformations, and hemispheric dysgenesis (Boyko et al 1991, Yamada et al 1992).

Diagnosis

Most of the patients present with isosexual precocious puberty. Males have voice deepening, muscular development, acne, pubic hair, and enlarged testes and penis. In females, breast development, menses, pubic hair, and excessive muscularity are noted (Albright & Lee 1993). The children are large for their age, and bone age is advanced by at least 3 years (Markin et al 1987). Commonly, the parents will note behavioral changes, complaining of an 'adolescent personality' in their children (Albright & Lee 1993). Neurological findings are often present. Gelastic seizures or laughing fits occur in up to 21% of the patients. Mental retardation is not uncommon (Judge et al 1977). Boyko believes that pedunculated lesions present with precocious puberty, and sessile lesions present with seizures (Boyko et al 1991). Other findings include headaches, visual disturbances, or evidence of autonomic dysfunction (hyperphagia, hyperactivity, or somnolence) (Yamada et al 1992).

Precocious puberty may be confirmed by elevated LH, FSH, estradiol, or testosterone levels (Hibi & Fujiwara 1987). Suppression of LH and FSH occurs by GnRH continuous stimulation. Prolactin levels may also be elevated, but GH and TSH levels are usually normal (Culler et al 1985). The hypothalamic-pituitary axis is usually immature. In one male patient with precocious puberty, the hypothalamic-pituitary axis was found to be unresponsive to clomiphene. A stimulatory response to this drug is found only in the middle to late stages of sexual maturation. The absent stimulatory response suggests a lack of maturation of the usual central nervous system events associated with normal puberty. Negative feedback was intact, but was partially resistant to steroid suppression (Judge et al 1977).

MR is the imaging diagnosis of choice. T1-weighted images show good resolution of the hamartoma from the surrounding brain. No enhancement of the tumor is found with gadolinium (Fig. 29.17). T2-weighted images show the hamartoma to be isointense or hyperintense relative to gray matter. T2-weighted images may be harder to interpret, however, because of the difficulty in distinguishing tumor from the surrounding CSF in the suprasellar cisterns (Beningfield et al 1988, Albright & Lee 1993). Although there are no large series of hamartomas examined with MR scans, there does not appear to be any difference in MR signal characteristics and histopathology (Boyko et al 1991). CT scanning has been used in the past. The tumors appear isodense to gray matter on CT, and do not enhance with contrast (Hahn et al 1987, Markin et al 1987). Cerebral angiography does not yield a tumor blush (Hahn et al 1987).

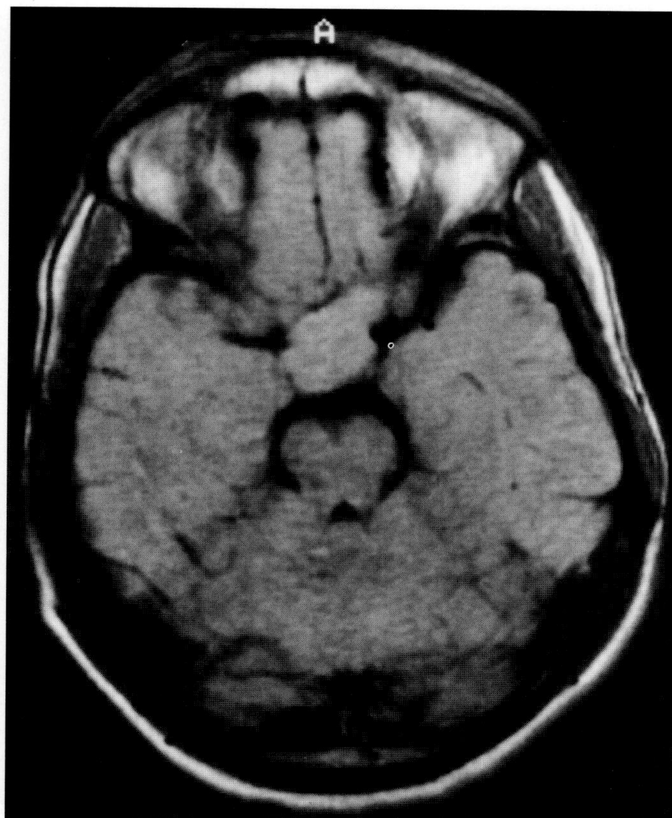

Fig. 29.17 MR scan (T1-weighted image) showing the sessile form of hypothalamic hamartoma, isointense to gray matter.

Pathology

The majority of hamartomas are pedunculated into the interpeduncular cistern, on a stalk containing myelinated fibers (Yamada et al 1992). Other hamartomas are sessile, with a wide attachment to the ventral surface of the hypothalamus or embodied in the hypothalamus itself (Yamada et al 1992). Hamartomas are usually firm, and vary in size from 0.5–4.0 cm in diameter. In asymptomatic patients, they are usually less than 1.5 cm in diameter (Albright & Lee 1993). Microscopically, hypothalamic hamartomas are primarily composed of mature neurons interspersed with glial cells. There is moderate glial cellularity over a fibrillar background, without neoplastic differentiation (Fig. 29.18) (Alvarez-Garijo et al 1983, Yamada et al 1992). Independent neuroendocrine units with neurons containing neurosecretory granules, blood vessels with fenestrated endothelium, and double basement membranes may be present (Judge et al 1977). Dense core granules may be seen on electron microscopy (Judge et al 1977). These pathological findings suggest two possible mechanisms for precocious puberty: (1) mechanical compression of inhibitory pathways from the hypothalamus and posterior pituitary, and (2) direct neurosecretory function in the hamartomas. In both instances, there is an oversecretion of GnRH, leading to inappropriate production of LH and FSH in the anterior pituitary (Judge et al 1977, Boyko et al 1991).

Differential diagnosis

The differential diagnosis of a child presenting with precocious puberty includes hypothalamic astrocytoma, optic nerve/chiasm glioma, germinoma, craniopharyngioma, and a suprasellar cyst (Markin et al 1987). These lesions can usually be distinguished on MR scanning. Pathologically, hamartomas need to be differentiated from low grade gliomas, gangliogliomas, and gangliocytomas. Low grade gliomas have evidence of astrocytic neoplastic differentiation, without the presence of neuronal elements. Gangliogliomas will show glial neoplastic differentiation, but also have ganglionic components. Gangliocytomas are usually located in the cerebellum (Lhermitte-Duclos disease), however, they have been reported in the hypothalamus (Reznik & Schoenen 1983, Bevan et al 1989). They are distinguished by the presence of pleomorphic ganglionic cells.

Treatment

Treatment of hypothalamic hamartomas may be based on medical therapy or surgical excision. Nonsurgical treatment of hamartomas is now possible with long-acting GnRH analogs. Since pulsatile GnRH release is necessary to initiate puberty, continuous GnRH stimulation will inhibit gonadotropin secretion (Conn & Crowley 1991). The disadvantages with GnRH therapy are severalfold: (1) GnRH therapy is expensive (approximately $3600/year), (2) it may not reverse the muscularity, increased appetite, and 'adolescent' personality often found in these patients, and (3) it may need to be used for many years depending on the age of the child (Albright & Lee 1993). It should be noted, however, that GnRH has been administered up to 13 years without significant sequelae. In an older patient who may be close to starting puberty, no treatment may be appropriate. Starceski et al reported an 8 years 7 months old boy who was not given any treatment, and was able to obtain an acceptable adult height. Moreover, it should be pointed out that, even without any form of medical treatment in the younger patients, the undesirable side effects are limited to accelerated growth with tall stature for age, premature sexual childhood development and adult stature shorter than would have been ordinarily obtained (Starceski et al 1990).

The ideal surgical candidate is a young patient, who otherwise would need to be on long-term GnRH analog therapy, with precocious puberty but normal pubertal endocrine makeup, in whom a cessation of premature pubertal development is desired. A pedunculated tumor would be ideal for surgical removal (Starceski et al 1990).

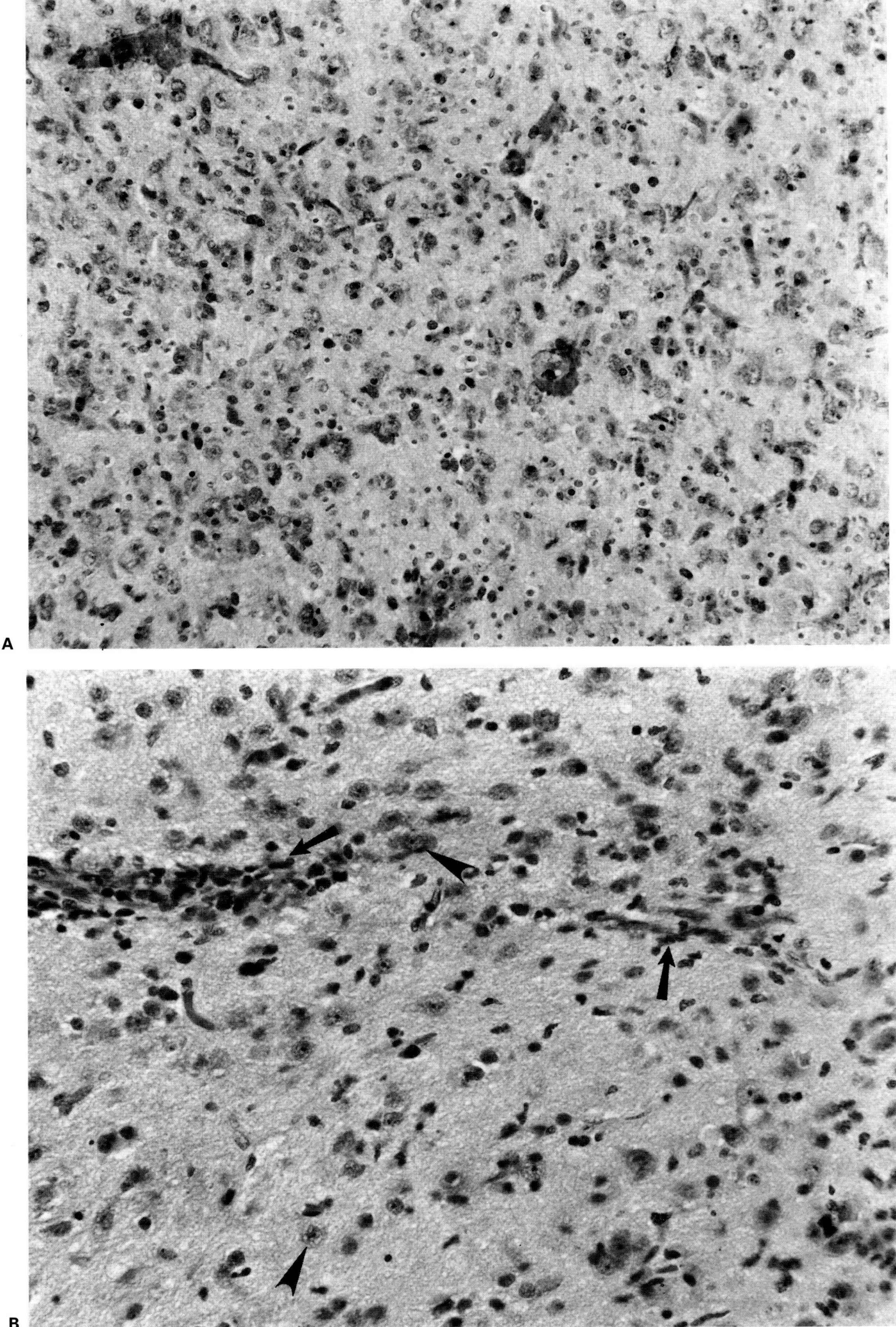

Fig. 29.18A & B

Fig. 29.18 **A.** Hypothalamic hamartoma with a high and irregularly distributed neuronal density. Clustering of neurons forming a definitive nuclear conglomerate is not present. H & E × 100. **B.** Hypothalamic hamartoma composed predominantly of normal appearing neurons varying in size and shape (arrowheads); the glial component in this case is small and mostly located around blood vessels (arrows). H&E ×200.

Albright & Lee have reported good results in the removal of both pedunculated and sessile tumors. A subtemporal approach allows the best visualization of the normal anatomy (Judge et al 1977, Price et al 1984, Markin et al 1987, Albright & Lee 1993). As the posterior surface of the hamartoma is often adherent to the anterior brainstem with adhesions to the basilar artery, an approach that allows visualization of the basilar artery is needed (Albright & Lee 1993). Theoretically, a pedunculated lesion transected at the stalk without removal of the hamartoma should cure the endocrine disturbances, however, removal of the hamartoma allows surgical confirmation of the diagnosis. Sessile lesions are harder to remove, and often a total removal is not possible when they extend into the hypothalamus. In that case, a subtotal removal so that the tumor is flush with the ventral surface of the hypothalamus is the treatment of choice (Albright & Lee 1993).

The most likely surgical morbidity from an attempt at removal is transient oculomotor paresis secondary to oculomotor nerve manipulation (Albright & Lee 1993). Surgical therapy, on the other hand, has not always been successful (Hibi & Fujiwara 1987, Albright & Lee 1993). In one series, 7 of 13 male patients underwent radiation after surgery, with no difference in survival (Hibi & Fujiwara 1987). The use of antineoplastic agents is not warranted.

Clinical outcome

The clinical outcome is generally good. Few patients die from hypothalamic hamartomas even if the lesion is incompletely removed. A cure of the endocrinopathy by surgical intervention is most likely if the lesion is pedunculated, however, partial removal may be sufficient to restore a normal endocrine axis (Albright & Lee 1993). Once a chemical cure is achieved, return to basal endocrine status may be obtained. Previous adolescent bodily changes (i.e. pubic hair, enlarged testes, breast development) will return to normal (Albright & Lee 1993). Operative intervention is only indicated in selected cases where GnRH suppression or no treatment are not viable options.

REFERENCES

Albright A L, Lee P A 1993 Neurosurgical treatment of hypothalamic hamartomas causing precocious puberty. Journal of Neurosurgery 78: 77–82

Allegranza A, Pileri S, Frank G, Ferracini R 1990 Cerebral ganglioglioma with anaplastic oligodendroglial component. Histopathology 17: 439–441

Allegranza A, Ferraresi S, Bruzzone M, Giombini S 1991 Cerebromeningeal pleomorphic xanthoastrocytoma. Report on four cases: clinical, radiological, and pathological features. Neurosurgical Review 14: 43–49

Altermatt J H, Scheithauer B W 1991 Cytomorphology of subependymal giant cell astrocytoma. Acta Cytologica 36: 171–175

Alvarez-Garijo J A, Albiach V J, Vila M M et al 1983 Precocious puberty and hypothalamic hamartoma with total recovery after surgical treatment. Journal of Neurosurgery 58: 583–585

Ambler M, Pogacar S, Sidman R 1969 Lhermitte-Duclos disease (granule cell hypertrophy of the cerebellum): pathological analysis of the first family cases. Journal of Neuropathology and Experimental Neurology 28: 622–647

Artigas J, Cervos-Navarro J, Iglesisas J R et al 1985 Gliomatosis cerebri: clinical and histological findings. Clinical Neuropathology 4: 135–148

Ashley D G, Zee C S, Chandrasoma P T, Segall H D 1990 Lhermitte-Duclos disease: CT and MR findings. Journal of Computer Assisted Tomography 14 (6): 984–987

Azzarelli B, Luerssen T G, Wolfe T M 1991 Intramedullary secretory gangliocytoma. Acta Neuropathologica 82: 402–407

Bailey P, Bucy P C 1930 Astroblastomas of the brain. Acta Psychiatrica Scandinavia 5: 439–461

Balakrishnan V, Hornabrook R W, Alexander W S 1985 Gliomatosis cerebri: report of a case. Pathology 17: 123–126

Balko M G, Blisard K S, Samaha F J 1992 Oligodendroglial gliomatosis cerebri. Human Pathology 23: 706–707

Bebin J, Tytus J S 1956 Gliomatosis cerebri. Report of a case. Neurology 6: 815–822

Beningfield S J, Bonnici F, Cremin B J 1988 Magnetic resonance imaging of hypothalamic hamartomas. British Journal of Radiology 61: 1177–1180

Benitez W I, Glasier C M, Husain M, Angtuaco E J C, Chadduck W M 1990 MR findings in childhood gangliogliomas. Journal of Computer Assisted Tomography 14: 711–716

Bergin D J, Johnson T E, Spencer W H, McCord C D 1988 Ganglioglioma of the optic nerve. American Journal of Ophthalmology 105: 146–149

Bevan J S, Asa S L, Rossi M L, Esiri M M, Adams C B T, Burke C W 1989 Intrasellar gangliocytoma containing gastrin and growth hormone-releasing hormone associated with a growth hormone-secreting pituitary adenoma. Clinical Endocrinology 30: 213–224

Bignami A, Adelman L S, Perides G, Dahl D 1989 Glial hyaluronate-binding protein in polar spongioblastoma. Journal of Neuropathology and Experimental Neurology 48: 187–196

Blom R J 1988 Pleomorphic xanthoastrocytoma: CT appearance. Journal of Computer Assisted Tomography 12: 351–352

Boesel C P, Paulson G W, Kosnik E, Earle K M 1979 Brain hamartomas and tumors associated with tuberous sclerosis. Neurosurgery 4: 410–417

Bonnin J M, Rubinstein L J 1989 Astroblastomas: a pathological study of 23 tumors, with a postoperative follow-up in 13 patients. Neurosurgery 25: 6–13

Bonnin J M, Rubinstein L J, Papasozomenos S Ch, Marangos P J 1984 Subependymal giant cell astrocytoma. Significance and possible cytogenetic implications of an immunohistochemical study. Acta Neuropathologica (Berlin) 62: 185–193

Bowles A P, Pantazis C G, Allen M B, Martinez J, Allsbrook W C 1988 Ganglioglioma, a malignant tumor? Correlation with flow dexoyribonucleic acid cytometric analysis. Neurosurgery 23: 376–381

Boyko O B, Curnes J T, Oakes W J, Burger P C 1991 Hamartomas of the tuber cinereum: CT, MR, and pathologic findings. American Journal of Neuroradiology 12: 309–314

Braffman B H, Bilaniuk L T, Naidich T P et al 1992 MR imaging of tuberous sclerosis: pathogenesis of this phakamatosis, use of gadopentetate dimeglumine, and literature review. Radiology 183: 227–238
Burger P C, Scheithauer B W, Vogel F S 1991 Primary neoplasms. In: Surgical pathology of the nervous system and its coverings, 3rd edn. Churchill Livingstone, Edinburgh
Cabello A, Madero S, Castresana A, Diaz-Lobato R 1991 Astroblastoma: electron microscopy and immunohistochemical findings: case report. Surgical Neurology 35: 116–121
Castillo M, Davis P C, Takei Y, Hoffman J C 1990 Intracranial ganglioglioma: MR, CT, and clinical findings in 18 patients. American Journal of Radiology 154: 607–612
Cervos-Navarro J, Artigas J, Aruffo C, Iglesias J 1987 The fine structure of gliomatosis cerebri. Virchows Archiv 411: 93–98
Chamberlain M C, Press G A 1990 Temporal lobe ganglioglioma in refractory epilepsy: CT and MR in three cases. Journal of Neuro-Oncology 9: 81–87
Chilton J, Caughron M R, Kepes J J 1990 Gangliogliomas of the optic chiasm: case report and review of the literature. Neurosurgery 26: 1042–1045
Chow C W, Klug G L, Lewis E A 1983 Subependymal giant-cell astrocytoma in children: an unusual discrepancy between histological and clinical features. Journal of Neurosurgery 68: 880–883
Conn P M, Crowley W F Jr 1991 Gonadotropin-releasing hormone and its analogues. New England Journal of Medicine 324: 93–103
Couch J R, Weiss S A 1974 Gliomatosis cerebri: report of four cases and review of the literature. Neurology 24: 504–511
Courville C B 1930 Ganglioglioma. Tumor of the central nervous system: review of the literature and report of two cases. Archives of Neurology and Psychiatry 24: 439–491
Cox J D, Zimmerman H M, Haughton V M 1982 Microcystic ganglioglioma treated by partial removal and radiation therapy. Cancer 50: 473–477
Culler F L, James H E, Simon M L, Jones K L 1985 Identification of gonadotropin-releasing hormone in neurons of a hypothalamic hamartoma in a boy with precocious puberty. Neurosurgery 17: 408–412
Daumas-Duport C, Scheithauer B W, Chodkiewicz J P, Laws E R, Vedrenne C 1988 Dysembryoplastic neuroepithelial tumor: a surgically curable tumor of young patients with intractable partial seizures. Neurosurgery 23: 545–556
Davidson L A, Graham D I, Carey F A 1992 Chronic neurological dysfunction attributable to a ganglioglioma. Histopathology 21: 275–278
de Chaderevian J P, Guyda H J, Hollenberg R D 1984 Hypothalamic polar spongioblastoma associated with the diencephalic syndrome. Virchows Archiv 402: 465–474
Demierre B, Stichnoth F A, Hori A, Spoerri O 1986 Intracerebral ganglioglioma. Journal of Neurosurgery 65: 117–182
Dhillon R S 1987 Posterior fossa ganglioglioma — an unusual cause of hearing loss. Journal of Laryngology and Otology 101: 714–717
Dickson D W, Horoupian D S, Thal L J, Lantos G 1988 Gliomatosis cerebri presenting with hydrocephalus and dementia. AJNR 9: 200–202
Diepholder H M, Schwecheimer K, Mohadjer M, Knoth R, Volk B 1991 A clinicopathologic and immunomorphologic study of 13 cases of ganglioglioma. Cancer 68: 2192–2201
Di Lorenzo N, Lunardi P, Fortuna A 1984 Granulomolecular hypertrophy of the cerebellum (Lhermitte-Duclos disease). Journal of Neurosurgery 60: 644–646
Donegani R, Grattarola F R, Wildi E 1972 Tuberous sclerosis: Bourneville disease. In: Jinkin P J, Bruyn G W (eds) Handbook of clinical neurology: the phakamatoses. Elsevier, New York, NY; pp 340–389
Dorne H L, O'Gorman A M, Melanson D 1986 Computed tomography of intracranial gangliogliomas. American Journal of Neuroradiology 7: 281–285
Ellenberg L, McComb J G, Siegel S E, Stone S 1987 Factors affecting intellectual outcome in pediatric brain tumor patients. Neurosurgery 21: 638–644
Faillot T, Sichez J P, Brault J L et al 1990 Lhermitte-Duclos disease (dysplastic gangliocytoma of the cerebellum). Acta Neurochirurgica 105: 44–49
Fletcher W A, Hoyt W F, Narahara M H 1988 Congenital quadrantanopia with occipital lobe ganglioglioma. Neurology 38: 1892–1894
Fujimoto M, Weaker F J, Herbert D C, Sharp Z D, Sheridan P J, Story J L 1988 Expression of three viral oncogenes (v-sis, v-myc, v-fos) in primary human brain tumors of neuroectodermal tumors. Neurology 38: 289–293
Fujiwara S, Takaki T, Hikita T, Nishio S 1989 Subependymal giant-cell astrocytoma associated with tuberous sclerosis. Do subependymal nodules grow? Child's Nervous System 5: 43–44
Furuta A, Takahasi H, Ikuta F, Onda K, Takeda N, Tanaka R 1992 Temporal lobe tumor demonstrating ganglioglioma and pleomorphic xanthoastrocytoma components. Case report. Journal of Neurosurgery 77: 143–147
Garcia C A, McGarry P A, Collada M 1984 Ganglioglioma of the brain stem. Journal of Neurosurgery 60: 431–434
Gaskill S J, Marlin A E, Saldivar V 1988 Glioblastoma multiforme masquerading as a pleomorphic xanthoastrocytoma. Child's Nervous System 4: 237–240
Goldring S, Rich K M, Picker S 1985 Experience with gliomas in patients presenting with a chronic seizure disorder. Clinical Neurosurgery 33: 15–42
Gomez J G, Garcia J H, Colon L E 1985 A variant of cerebral glioma called pleomorphic xanthoastrocytoma: case report. Neurosurgery 16: 703–706
Gottesman M, Laufer H, Patel M 1991 Gliomatosis cerebri: a case report. Clinical Neuropathology 10: 303–305
Grant J W, Gallagher P J 1986 Pleomorphic xanthoastrocytoma: immunohistochemical methods for differentiation from fibrous histiocytomas with similar morphology. American Journal of Surgical Pathology 10(5): 335–341
Guo L X, Zhang R L 1990 Pleomorphic xanthoastrocytoma: a case report. Chung-Hua Chung Liu Tsa Chih (Chinese Journal of Oncology) 12: 477–478
Haddad S F, Moore S A, Menezes A H, Vangilder J C 1992 Ganglioglioma: 13 years of experience. Neurosurgery 31: 171–178
Hahn F J, Leibrock L G, Huseman C A, Makos M M 1988 The MR appearance of hypothalamic hamartoma. Neuroradiology 30: 65–68
Hahn J S, Bejar R, Gladson C L 1991 Neonatal subependymal giant cell astrocytoma associated with tuberous sclerosis: MRI, CT, and ultrasound correlation. Neurology 41: 124–128
Hall W A, Yunis E J, Albright A L 1986 Anaplastic ganglioglioma in an infant: case report and review of the literature. Neurosurgery 19: 1016–1020
Hara A, Sakai N, Yamada H, Tanaka T, Mori H 1991 Assessment of proliferative potential in gliomatosis cerebri. Journal of Neurology 238: 80–82
Henry J M, Heffner R R, Earle K M 1978 Gangliogliomas of CNS: a clinico-pathological study of 50 cases. Journal of Neuropathology and Experimental Neurology 37: 626 (abstract)
Hibi I, Fujiwara K 1987 Precocious puberty of cerebral origin: a cooperative study in Japan. Progress in Experimental Tumor Research 30: 224–238
Hoag G, Sima A A F, Rozdilsky B 1986 Astroblastoma revisited: a report of three cases. Acta Neuropathologica 70: 10–16
Hori A, Weiss R, Schaake T 1988 Ganglioglioma containing osseous tissue and neurofibrillary tangles. Archives of Pathology and Laboratory Medicine 112: 653–655
Hosokawa Y, Tsuchihashi Y, Okabe H et al 1991 Pleomorphic xanthoastrocytoma: ultrastructural, immunohistochemical, and DNA cytofluorometric study of a case. Cancer 68: 853–859
Hunt S J, Johnson P C 1989 Melanotic ganglioglioma of the pineal region. Acta Neuropathologica 79: 222–225
Husain A N, Leestma J E 1986 Cerebral astroblastoma: immunohistochemical and ultrastructural features. Case report. Journal of Neurosurgery 64: 657–661
Issidorides M R, Arvanitis D 1993 Histochemical marker of human catecholamine neurons in ganglion cells and processes of a temporal lobe ganglioglioma. Surgical Neurology 39: 66–71
Iwaki I, Fukui M, Kondo A, Matshushima T, Takeshita I 1987 Epithelial properties of pleomorphic xanthoastrocytomas determined

in ultrastructural and immunohistochemical studies. Acta Neuropathologica 74: 142–150

Iwaki T, Iwaki A, Miyazono M, Goldman J E 1991 Preferential expression of αB-crystallin in astrocytic elements of neuroectodermal tumors. Cancer 68: 2230–2240

Jansen G H, Troost D, Dingemans K P 1990 Polar spongioblastoma: an immunohistochemical and electron microscopical study. Acta Neuropathologica 81: 228–232

Jelinek J, Smirniotopoulos J G, Parisi J E, Kanzer M 1990 Lateral ventricular neoplasms of the brain: differential diagnosis based on clinical, CT, and MR findings. American Journal of Neuroradiology 11: 567–574

Johannson J H, Rekate H L, Roessmann U 1981 Gangliogliomas: pathological and clinical correlation. Journal of Neurosurgery 54: 58–63

Jones M C, Drut R, Raglia G 1983 Pleomorphic xanthoastrocytoma. A report of 2 cases. Pediatric Pathology 1: 459–467

Judge D M, Kulin H E, Page R, Santen R et al 1977 Hypothalamic hamartoma: a source of luteinizing-hormone-releasing factor in precocious puberty. New England Journal of Medicine 296: 7–10

Kalyan-Raman U P, Olivero W C 1987 Ganglioglioma: a correlative clinicopathological and radiological study of ten surgically treated cases with follow-up. Neurosurgery 20: 428–433

Kandler R H, Smith C M L, Broome J C, Davies-Jones M B 1991 Gliomatosis cerebri: a clinical, radiological and pathological report of four cases. British Journal of Neurosurgery 5: 187–193

Kapp J P, Paulson G W, Odom G L 1967 Brain tumors with tuberous sclerosis. Journal of Neurosurgery 26: 191–202

Kawai K, Takahashi H, Ikuta F, Tanimura K, Honda Y, Yamazaki H 1987 The occurrence of catecholamine neurons in a parietal lobe ganglioglioma. Cancer 60: 1532–1536

Kawano N, Miyasaka Y, Yada K et al 1978 Diffuse cerebrospinal gliomatosis. Journal of Neurosurgery 49: 303–307

Kepes J J 1979 "Xanthomatous" lesions of the central nervous system. Definition, classification and some recent observations. Progress in Neuropathology 4: 179–213

Kepes J J, Rubinstein L J, Eng L F 1979 Pleomorphic xanthoastrocytoma: a distinctive meningocerebral glioma of young subjects with relatively favorable prognosis: a study of 12 cases. Cancer 44: 1839–1852

Kepes J J, Rubinstein L J, Ansbacher L, Schreiber D J 1989 Histopathological features of recurrent pleomorphic xanthoastrocytomas: further corroboration of the glial nature of this neoplasm. A study of 3 cases. Acta Neuropathologica 78: 585–593

Kirkpatrick P J, Honavar M, Janota I, Polkey C E 1993 Control of temporal lobe epilepsy following *en bloc* resection of low-grade tumors. Journal of Neurosurgery 78: 19–25

Kleihues P, Burger P C, Scheithauer B W 1993 Histological typing of tumours of the central nervous system, 2nd edn. Springer-Verlag, Berlin, (in press)

Koeller K K, Dillon W P 1992 Dysembryoplastic neuroepithelial tumors: MR appearance. American Journal of Neuroradiology 13: 1319–1325

Kros J M, Vecht C J, Stefanko S Z 1991 The pleomorphic xanthoastrocytoma and its differential diagnosis: a study of five cases. Human Pathology 22: 1128–1135

Kubota T, Hirano A, Sato K, Yamamoto S 1985 The fine structure of astroblastoma. Cancer 55: 745–750

Kuhajda F P, Mendelson G, Taxy J B, Long D M 1981 Pleomorphic xanthoastrocytoma: report of a case with light and electron microscopy. Ultrastructural Pathology 2: 25–32

Le Marquand H S, Russell D S 1934 A case of pubertas praecox (macrogenitosomia praecox) in a boy associated with a tumor in the floor of the third ventricle. Berkeley Hospital Report 3: 31–61

Lhermitte J, Duclos P 1920 Sur un ganglioneurome diffus du cortex du cervelet. Bulletin of Association of French Cancer 9: 99–107

Lindboe C F, Cappelen J, Kepes J J 1992 Pleomorphic xanthoastrocytoma as a component of a cerebellar ganglioglioma: case report. Neurosurgery 31: 353–355

Loiseau H, Rivel J, Vital C, Rougier A, Cohadon F 1991 Pleomorphic xanthoastrocytoma: Apropos of 3 new cases. Review of the literature. Neuro-chirurgie 37: 338–347

Mackenzie J M 1987 Pleomorphic xanthoastrocytoma in a 62-year old male. Neuropathology and Applied Neurobiology 13: 481–487

McMurdo S K, Moore S G, Brant-Zawadzki M et al 1987 MR imaging of intracranial tuberous sclerosis. American Journal of Neuroradiology 8: 77–82

Maleki M, Robitaille Y, Bertrand G 1983 Atypical xanthoastrocytoma presenting as a meningioma. Surgical Neurology 20: 235–238

Mapstone T, McMichael M, Goldthwait D 1991 Expression of platelet-derived growth factors, transforming growth factors, and the ros gene in a variety of primary human brain tumors. Neurosurgery 28: 216–222

Marano S R, Johnson P C, Spetzler R F 1988 Recurrent Lhermitte-Duclos disease in a child. Journal of Neurosurgery 69: 599–603

Markin R S, Leibrock L G, Huseman C A, McComb R D 1987 Hypothalamic hamartoma: a report of 2 cases. Pediatric Neurosciences 13: 19–26

Martin D S, Levy B, Awwad E E, Pittman T 1991 Desmoplastic infantile ganglioglioma: CT and MR features. American Journal of Neuroradiology 12: 1195–1197

Martin N, Debussche C, DeBroucker T, Mompoint D, Marsault C, Nahum H 1990 Gadolinium-DTPA enhanced MR imaging in tuberous sclerosis. Neuroradiology 31: 492–497

Miller D C, Koslow M, Budzilovich G N, Burstein D E 1990 Synaptophysin: a sensitive and specific marker for ganglion cells in central nervous system neoplasms. Human Pathology 21: 271–276

Miller G, Towfighi J, Page R B 1990 Spinal cord ganglioglioma presenting as hydrocephalus. Journal of Neuro-Oncology 9: 147–152

Miller R R, Lin F, Mallonee M M 1981 Cytologic diagnosis of gliomatosis cerebri. Acta Cytologica 25: 37–39

Mineura K, Sasajima T, Kowada M, Uesaka Y, Shishido F 1991 Innovative approach in the diagnosis of gliomatosis cerebri using carbon-11-L-methionine positron emission tomography. Journal of Nuclear Medicine 32: 726–728

Mizuno J, Nishio S, Barrow D, Davis P C, Tindall G T 1987 Ganglioglioma of the cerebellum: case report. Neurosurgery 21: 584–588

Nagib M G, Haines S J, Erickson D L, Mastri A R 1984 Tuberous sclerosis: a review for the neurosurgeon. Neurosurgery 14: 93–98

Nahser H C, Gerhard L, Reinhardt V, Nau H E, Bamberg M 1981 Diffuse and multicentric brain tumors: correlation of histological, clinical, and CT appearance. Acta Neuropathologica (Berlin) (suppl VII): 101–104

Nakamura Y, Becker L E 1983 Subependymal giant-cell tumor: astrocytic or neuronal? Acta Neuropathologica 60: 271–277

Nardelli E, Benedictis G De, La Stilla G, Nicolardi G 1986 Tuberous sclerosis — a neuropathological and immunohistochemical (PAP) study. Clinical Neuropathology 5: 261–266

Nelson J, Frost J L, Schochet S S 1987 Sudden, unexpected death in a 5 year old boy with an unusual primary intracranial neoplasm. American Journal of Forensic Medicine and Pathology 8: 148–152

Nevin S 1938 Gliomatosis cerebri. Brain 61: 170–191

Ng T H K, Fung C F, Ma L T 1990a The pathological spectrum of desmoplastic infantile gangliogliomas. Histopathology 16: 235–241

Ng T H K, Fung C F, Ma L T 1990b Test and teach: Number 64. Diagnosis: pleomorphic xanthoastrocytoma. Pathology 22: 201–202, 243–244

Nishio S, Fujiwara S, Tashima T, Takeshita I, Fujii K, Fukui M 1990 Tumors of the lateral ventricular wall, especially the septum pellucidum: clinical presentation and variations in pathological features. Neurosurgery 27: 224–230

Otsubo H, Hoffman H J, Humphreys R P et al 1990 Evaluation, surgical approach and outcome of seizure patients with gangliogliomas. Pediatric Neurosurgery 16: 208–212

Padberg G W, Schot J D L, Vielvoye G J, Bots G T A M, de Beer F C 1991 Lhermitte-Duclos Disease and Cowden Disease: a single phakamatoses. Annals of Neurology 29: 517–523

Padmalatha C, Harruff R C, Ganick D, Hafez G R 1980 Glioblastoma multiforme with tuberous sclerosis: report of a case. Archives of Pathology and Laboratory Medicine 104: 649–650

Painter M J, Pang D, Ahdab-Barmada M, Bergman I 1984 Conatal brain tumors in patients with tuberous sclerosis. Neurosurgery 14: 570–573

Palma L, Maleci A, di Lorenzo N, Lauro G M 1985 Pleomorphic xanthoastrocytoma with 18-year survival: case report. Journal of Neurosurgery 63: 808–810
Parizel P M, Martin J J, Van Vyve M, van den Hauwe L, De Schepper A M 1991 Cerebral ganglioglioma and neurofibromatosis type I: case report and review of the literature. Neuroradiology 33: 357–359
Paulus W, Peiffer J 1988 Does the pleomorphic xanthoastrocytoma exist? Problems in the application of immunological techniques to the classification of brain tumors. Acta Neuropathologica 76: 245–252
Paulus W, Schlote W, Perentes E, Jacobi G, Warmuth-Metz M, Roggendorf W 1992 Desmoplastic supratentorial neuroepithelial tumours of infancy. Histopathology 21: 43–49
Perentes E, Rubinstein L J 1986 Immunohistochemical recognition of human neuroepithelial tumors by anti-Leu 7 (HNK-1) monoclonal antibody. Acta Neuropathologica 69: 227–233
Price R A, Lee P A, Albright A L, Ronnekleiv O K et al 1984 Treatment of sexual precocity by removal of a luteinizing hormone-releasing hormone secreting hamartoma. Journal of American Medical Association 251: 2247–2249
Reeder R F, Saunders R L, Roberts D W, Fratkin J D, Cromwell L D 1988 Magnetic resonance imaging in the diagnosis and treatment of Lhermitte-Duclos disease (dysplastic gangliocytoma of the cerebellum). Neurosurgery 23: 240–245
Reznik M, Schoenen J 1983 Lhermitte-Duclos disease. Acta Neuropathologica 59: 88–94
Rikonen R, Simell O 1990 Tuberous sclerosis and infantile spasms. Developmental Medicine and Child Neurology 32: 203–209
Rippe D J, Boyko O B, Fuller G N, Friedman H S, Oakes W J, Schold S C 1990 Gadopentetate-dimeglumine-enhanced MR imaging of gliomatosis cerebri: appearance mimicking leptomeningeal tumor dissemination. American Journal of Neuroradiology 11: 800–801
Roessman U, Wongmongkolrit T 1984 Dysplastic gangliocytoma of the cerebellum in a newborn. Case report. Journal of Neurosurgery 60: 845–847
Romero F J, Ortega A, Titus F, Ibarra B, Navarro C, Rovira M 1988 Gliomatosis cerebri with formation of a glioblastoma multiform: study and follow-up by magnetic resonance and computed tomography. Journal of Computed Tomography 12: 253–257
Rommel T, Hamer J 1983 Development of ganglioglioma in computed tomography. Neuroradiology 24: 237–239
Roski R A, Roessmann U, Spetzler R F, Kaufman B, Nulsen F E 1981 Clinical and pathological study of dysplastic gangliocytoma. Journal of Neurosurgery 55: 318–321
Ross I B, Robitaille Y, Villemure J G, Tampieri D 1991 Diagnosis and management of gliomatosis cerebri: recent trends. Surgical Neurology 36: 431–440
Rubinstein L J 1972 Tumors of the central nervous system. Air Force Institute of Pathology, Bethesda
Rubinstein L J, Herman M M 1972 A light and electron-microscopic study of a temporal-lobe ganglioglioma. Journal of Neurological Sciences 16: 27–48
Rubinstein L J, Herman M M 1989 The astroblastoma and its possible cytogenic relationship to the tanycyte: an electron microscopic, immunohistochemical, tissue- and organ-culture study. Acta Neuropathologica 78: 472–483
Russell D S, Cairns H 1947 Polar spongioblastomas. Archives of Histology (B. Aires) 3: 423–441
Russell D S, Rubinstein L J 1989 Pathology of tumours of the nervous system, 5th edn. Edward Arnold, London
Sabin H I, Kidov H G W, Kendall B E, Symon L 1988 Lhermitte-Duclos Disease (dysplastic gangliocytoma): a case report with CT and MRI. Acta Neurochirurgica 93: 149–153
Saikai H, Kawano N, Okada K, Tanabe T, Yada K, Yagishita S 1981 A case of pleomorphic xanthoastrocytoma. No Shinkei Geka. Neurological Surgery 9: 1519–1524
Sarhaddi S, Bravo E, Cyrus A E 1973 Gliomatosis cerebri: a case report and review of the literature. Southern Medical Journal 66: 883–888
Sarkar C, Roy S, Bhatia S 1990 Xanthomatous change in tumours of glial origin. Indian Journal of Medical Research 92: 324–331
Sawyer J R, Roloson G J, Chadduck W M, Boop F A 1991 Cytogenetic findings in a pleomorphic xanthoastrocytoma. Cancer Genetics and Cytogenetics 55: 225–230
Sawyer J R, Thomas E L, Roloson G J, Chadduck W M, Boop F A 1992 Telomeric associations evolving to ring chromosomes in a recurrent pleomorphic xanthoastrocytoma. Cancer Genetics and Cytogenetics 60: 152–157
Schiffer D, Cravioto H, Giordana M T, Migheli A, Pezzulo T, Vigliani M C 1993 Is polar spongioblastoma a tumor entity? Journal of Neurosurgery 78: 587–591
Schober R, Mai J K, Wechsler W 1991 Gliomatosis cerebri: bioptical approach and neuropathological verification. Acta Neurochirurgica 113: 131–137
Shepherd C W, Scheithauer B W, Gomez M R, Altermatt H J, Katzmann J A 1991 Subependymal giant cell astrocytoma: a clinical, pathological, and flow cytometric study. Neurosurgery 28: 864–868
Silver J M, Rawlings C E, Rossitch E, Zeidman S M, Friedman A H 1991 Ganglioglioma: a clinical study with long-term follow-up. Surgical Neurology 35: 261–266
Simonati A, Vio M, Iannucci A M, Toso V, Morello F, Rizzuto N 1981 Gliomatosis cerebri diffusa: a case report. Acta Neuropathologica 54: 311–314
Smith R R, Gross R I, Goldberg H I, Hackney D B, Bilaniuk L T, Zimmerman R A 1989 MR imaging of Lhermitte-Duclos disease: a case report. American Journal of Neuroradiology 10: 187–189
Spagnoli M V, Grossman R I, Packer R J et al 1987 Magnetic resonance imaging determination of gliomatosis cerebri. Neuroradiology 29: 15–18
Starceski P J, Lee P A, Albright A L, Migeon C J 1990 Hypothalamic hamartomas and sexual precocity. Evaluation of treatment options. American Journal of Diseases of Childhood 144: 225–228
Steinberg G K, Shuer L M, Conley F K, Hanbery J W 1985 Evolution and outcome in malignant astroglial neoplasms of the cerebellum. Journal of Neurosurgery 62: 9–17
Strom E H, Skullerud K 1983 Pleomorphic xanthoastrocytoma: report of 5 cases. Clinical Neuropathology 2: 188–191
Stuart G, Appleton D B, Cooke R 1988 Pleomorphic xanthoastrocytoma: report of two cases. Neurosurgery 22: 422–427
Sugita Y, Kepes J J, Shigemori M et al 1990 Pleomorphic xanthoastrocytoma with desmoplastic reaction: angiomatous variant. Report of two cases. Clinical Neuropathology 9: 271–278
Sugiyama K, Goishi J, Sogabe T, Uozumi T, Hotta T, Kiya K 1992 Ganglioglioma of the optic pathway: a case report. Surgical Neurology 37: 22–25
Sutton L N, Packer R J, Rorke L B, Bruce D A, Schut L 1983 Cerebral gangliogliomas during childhood. Neurosurgery 13: 124–128
Sutton L N, Packer R J, Zimmerman R A, Bruce D A, Schut L 1987 Cerebral gangliogliomas of childhood. Progress in Experimental Tumor Research 30: 239–246
Sutton L N, Packer R J, Schut L 1991 Gangliogliomas. In: Wilkins R H, Rengachary S (eds) Neurosurgery update I: Diagnosis, operative techniques, and neuro-oncology, vol I. McGraw-Hill, New York, pp 461–463
Takahashi H, Ikuta F, Tsuchida T, Tanaka R 1987 Ultrastructural alterations of neuronal cells in a brain stem ganglioma. Acta Neuropathologica 74: 307–312
Takahashi H, Wakabayashi K, Kawai K et al 1989 Neuroendocrine markers in central nervous system neuronal tumors (gangliocytoma and ganglioglioma). Acta Neuropathologica 77: 237–243
Tampieri D, Moumdjian R, Melanson D, Ethier R 1991 Intracerebral gangliogliomas in patients with partial complex seizures: CT and MR imaging findings. American Journal of Neuroradiology 12: 749–755
Taratuto A L, Monges J, Lylyk P, Leiguarda R 1984 Superficial cerebral astrocytoma attached to dura. Report of six cases in infants. Cancer 54: 2505–2512
Tien R D, Hesselink J R, Duberg A 1990 Rare subependymal giant-cell astrocytoma in a neonate with tuberous sclerosis. American Journal of Neuroradiology 11: 1251–1252
Tien R D, Tuori S L, Pulkingham N, Burger P C 1992 Ganglioglioma with leptomeningeal and subarachnoid spread: results of CT, MR, and PET imaging. American Journal of Radiology 159: 391–393

Trombley I K, Mirra S S 1981 Ultrastructure of tuberous sclerosis: cortical tuber and subependymal tumor. Annals of Neurology 9: 174–181

VandenBerg S R, May E E, Rubinstein L J et al 1987a Desmoplastic supratentorial neuroepithelial tumors of infancy with divergent differentiation potential ("desmoplastic infantile gangliogliomas"). Journal of Neurosurgery 66: 58–71

VandenBerg S R, Herman M M, Rubinstein L J 1987b Embryonal central neuroepithelial tumors: current concepts and future challenges. Cancer and Metastasis Reviews 5: 343–364

Vogt H 1908 Zur pathologie und pathologishen Anatomie der verschiedenen idiotie-formen: Tuberose sklerose. Monatsschrift Psychiatry Neurology 24: 106–150

Wacker M R, Cogen P H, Etzell J E, Daneshvar L, Davis R L, Prados M D 1992 Diffuse leptomeningeal involvement by a ganglioglioma in a child. Journal of Neurosurgery 77: 302–306

Webb D W, Thomson J L G, Osborne J P 1991 Cranial magnetic resonance imaging in patients with tuberous sclerosis and normal intellect. Archives of Diseases of Childhood 66: 1375–1377

Weldon-Linne C M, Victor T A, Groothius D R, Vick N A 1983 Pleomorphic xanthoastrocytoma: ultrastructural and immunohistochemical study of a case with a rapidly fatal outcome following surgery. Cancer 52: 2055–2063

Whittle I R, Gordon A, Misra B K, Shaw J F, Steers A J W 1989 Pleomorphic xanthoastrocytoma: report of four cases. Journal of Neurosurgery 70: 463–468

Wilson W B, Kosmorsky G S, deMasters B K et al 1990 Diffusely infiltrating brainstem gliomas: a report of the diagnostic difficulties in 2 cases. Neurology 40: 1237–1241

Yamada S, Sano T 1992 Neuropathology of the hypothalamus. In: Barrow D L, Selman W (eds) Neuroendocrinology. Williams & Wilkins, Baltimore, pp 259–288

Yanaka K, Kamezaki T, Kobayashi E, Matsueda K, Yoshii Y, Nose T 1992 MR imaging of diffuse glioma. American Journal of Neuroradiology 13: 349–351

Yoshino M R, Lucio R 1992 Pleomorphic xanthoastrocytoma. American Journal of Neuroradiology 13: 1330–1332

Zorzi F, Facchetti F, Baronchelli C, Cani E 1992 Pleomorphic xanthoastrocytoma: an immunohistochemical study of three cases. Histopathology 20: 267–269

Zülch K J 1979 Histological typing of tumours of the central nervous system. In: International histological classification of tumors, no. 21. World Health Organization, Geneva, Switzerland, pp 19–20

Zuniga O F, Tanner S M, Wild W O, Mosier H D 1983 Hamartoma of CNS associated with precocious puberty. American Journal of Diseases of Childhood 137: 127–133

PART II

Neuronal and neuronal precursor tumors

30. Medulloblastoma and primitive neuroectodermal tumors

Mitchel S. Berger Lorenzo Magrassi Russ Geyer

EPIDEMIOLOGY

Medulloblastoma, also referred to as an infratentorial primitive neuroectodermal tumor (iPNET), accounts for approximately 7–8% of all intracranial tumors, and nearly 30% of childhood central nervous system (CNS) neoplasms (Russell & Rubinstein 1989). In this chapter, the two terms will be used interchangeably and designated as medulloblastoma (iPNET). When actual population-based studies are considered, these figures are somewhat diminished. The Norwegian Cancer Registry reported that medulloblastomas represented 3.1% of all primary brain tumors in all age groups between 1955 and 1984 (Helseth & Mørk 1989). In a population-based study from the Swedish Cancer Registry, medulloblastomas (iPNET) represented 21% of all primary brain tumors in the pediatric age group (Lannering et al 1990). Similar figures were provided by British Tumor Registries between 1971 and 1985 (Stiller & Bunch 1992), and from the United States, using data from the Surveillance, Epidemiology and End Results (SEER) program (Duffner et al 1986). In the United States alone, approximately 350 new cases of medulloblastoma are identified each year (Friedman et al 1991). Medulloblastoma (iPNET) represented 5.6% of all intracranial and intraspinal tumors treated at the Seoul National University Hospital and Children's Hospital from 1980–1987 (Chi & Khang 1989). If the analysis is limited to the pediatric population, the incidence rises to 25.6% of all CNS tumors. Similar numbers were also reported from smaller population territories such as Barbados, West Indies, between 1978 and 1988 (Lashley et al 1991).

Males are traditionally more affected than female children. In the Swedish Cancer Registry study, the overall male to female ratio for primary brain tumors was 1.01:1, however, for medulloblastoma (iPNET), the ratio was 1.8:1 (Lannering et al 1990). A population-based study conducted in the United States confirmed that sex and age were statistically significant factors in the incidence rates of this lesion (Roberts et al 1991). That study also reported a male to female ratio of 1:6 and a median age at diagnosis of 9 years. Overall, about half of medulloblastoma (iPNET) occurs in the first 10 years of life (Russell & Rubinstein 1989); however, sporadic cases of this tumor type occurring as late as the eighth decade are well documented (Kepes et al 1987). The average age at presentation of clinical signs and symptoms in adult patients is 34.1 years. The incidence of medulloblastoma (iPNET) in adults, e.g. 20 years of age and greater, as documented in the Connecticut Tumor Registry, was 0.058/100 000 population per year (Farwell & Flannery 1987). Data from the Third National Cancer Survey and the SEER program has demonstrated that the incidence rates for Caucasians were slightly higher than for blacks (Bunin 1987). In this same study, the male to female ratio for medulloblastoma (iPNET) differed between Caucasians (1.7:1) and blacks (1:1).

FAMILY HISTORY AND GENETIC FACTORS

Medulloblastoma (iPNET) is a sporadically occurring tumor in both children and adults. An extensive literature search identified 14 familial cases (Tijssen 1986, Hung et al 1990). 4 of these tumors involved monozygotic twins, while the remaining 10 lesions were identified in siblings.

Genetic analysis of medulloblastoma (iPNET) has demonstrated a frequent loss of genetic material consistently from the short arm of chromosome 17 (Bigner et al 1988, James et al 1990, Raffel et al 1990), where the region commonly lost spanned 17p13.3 to 17pter (Thomas & Raffel 1991, Biegel et al 1992). These data have suggested, perhaps, a new tumor-associated locus on 17p, distinct from and removed from the p53 gene. Alterations in this supposed new locus may be involved in initiating or in the progression of at least a subset of medulloblastoma (iPNET) (Thomas & Raffel 1991, Biegel et al 1992). The loss of genetic material from chromosome 17p, when cytogenetically evident, appears to impact negatively in terms of prognosis for patients with these tumors (Cogen 1991), and thus is of prognostic importance.

Medulloblastoma (iPNET) may accompany other clinical features of certain hereditary syndromes. Nevoid basal cell carcinoma (Gorlin syndrome) is an autosomal dominant disorder that predisposes an individual to have basal cell skin cancer, ovarian fibromas and widespread developmental defects (Gorlin 1987). The genetic basis for this syndrome has recently been mapped to a locus in close proximity of 9q31 (Farndon et al 1992, Gailani et al 1992, Reis et al 1992). A British study, based on cases diagnosed between 1954 and 1989 involving an area under the auspices of the Northwest Regional Health Authority, demonstrated that 1–2% of all patients with medulloblastoma (iPNET) have Gorlin syndrome. This is in contrast to 3–5% of patients affected by this hereditary disease who develop the infratentorial malignancy (Evans et al 1991). Medulloblastoma (iPNET) has also been associated with the blue rubber bleb nevus syndrome (Rice & Fischer 1962), an autosomal dominant disease characterized by hemangiomas of the trunk and upper arms, and less commonly involving internal organs (27). When this tumor is found in patients with familial polyposis, Turcot's syndrome should be suspected (Jarvis et al 1988). Medulloblastoma (iPNET) has been diagnosed in a 3-year-old child who came from a family affected by the Li-Fraumeni syndrome. In this setting, there is a germline mutation in the p53 gene leading to the substitution of glutamic acid for the wild-type arginine at position 248 (Santibanez-Koref et al 1991); however, mutations in the p53 gene have been identified in only 10% of medulloblastoma (iPNET) not associated with the Li-Fraumeni syndrome (Ohgaki et al 1991, Cogen et al 1992).

Amplification of the c-myc oncogene and an increased level of c-myc expression have been demonstrated in some medulloblastoma (iPNET) tumor samples. N-myc expression, however, is usually not elevated (MacGregor & Ziff 1990, Raffel et al 1990). The incidence of N-ras activation, e.g. mutations at codons 12, 13 and 61, has been reported to be greater in medulloblastoma (iPNET) than in other CNS tumors evaluated thus far (Olascon et al 1991).

CLINICAL AND LABORATORY FINDINGS

No specific presenting sign or symptom is pathognomonic of medulloblastoma (iPNET) when compared to other lesions originating in the cerebellum (Choux & Lena 1982, Edwards & Hudgins 1989). Unilateral cerebellar findings associated with astrocytomas and intense neck pain and stiffness, seen more often with ependymomas, are not overwhelming features of medulloblastoma (iPNET). Early symptoms identified in children with this lesion are usually demonstrated by changes in behavior, e.g. irritability, lethargy, decreased social interactions, and loss of appetite. These symptoms are usually followed by intermittent vomiting and headache, the former being worse when the patient awakens in the morning, and associated with steady improvement throughout the day. Intracranial hypertension due mainly to obstructive hydrocephalus secondary to occlusion of the cerebral aqueduct or fourth ventricle by the mass, is a very common finding. This may be associated with a sixth cranial nerve palsy resulting from pressure and trapping of the nerve as it enters the posterior cavernous sinus under the petroclival ligament and traverses through Dorello's canal.

Nausea as a distinct symptom from vomiting is unusual unless the tumor infiltrates the floor of the fourth ventricle. When that occurs, it is often associated with some form of gaze palsy. Head tilt and mild neck stiffness resulting in an abnormal head posture, are also relatively common and result from meningeal irritation at the level of the foramen magnum. Midline cerebellar findings, e.g. wide-based stance, ataxic gait and nystagmus, or lateral tumor involvement resulting in unilateral dysdiadochokinesia, hypotonia, dysmetria and intention tremor are typical in patients with this common infratentorial tumor. A lateral cerebellar syndrome is more frequently seen with the desmoplastic variant of medulloblastoma (iPNET) that often arises unilaterally in the cerebellar hemisphere.

No specific biochemical test has been identified to help make the diagnosis of medulloblastoma (iPNET); however, several markers have been documented in the cerebrospinal fluid (CSF) in these children (Koskiniemi 1988). Human glioma-associated antigen has been quantified in the CSF of medulloblastoma (iPNET) patients using radioimmune assays with the G-22 monoclonal antibody (Yoshida et al 1990). The level of detection of this antigen has been found to be greater than in those patients affected by other non-PNET-type tumors of the posterior fossa (Yoshida et al 1990), and may serve as a useful marker of tumor progression or recurrence. Demosterol and putrescine levels are elevated in the CSF of medulloblastoma (iPNET) patients and may correspond to their clinical status of disease progression (Koskiniemi 1988). Increased CSF levels of putrescine and spermidine, compared with their immediate postoperative values, may be an early predictor of tumor relapse (Marton et al 1979, 1981).

CSF cytological assessment is not always a reliable method to differentiate medulloblastoma (iPNET) cells from disseminated tumor cells of other posterior fossa tumors. Certainly, CSF cytology may be negative in the presence of bulky disease on preoperative imaging studies. Little experience is available on preoperative CSF analysis because of the accompanying risks of cerebellar tonsillar herniation resulting from a lumbar puncture. Likewise, cytology is difficult to assess, as normal cells may appear microscopically abnormal after sloughing off into the CSF following intrathecal chemotherapy and craniospinal radiation.

DIAGNOSTIC IMAGING STUDIES

Current diagnostic imaging methods of choice for medulloblastoma (iPNET) are contrast-enhanced magnetic resonance (MR) and computed tomography (CT) scans (Kingsley & Kendall 1979), although the former modality is preferred (Heafner et al 1985). Both methods will readily identify changes in the ventricular system and the point of CSF obstruction caused by the tumor. MR imaging is superior to CT scans due to the multiplanar views obtained of the mass, i.e. axial, coronal, sagittal, and detection of secondary tumor deposits in the subarachnoid spaces or in the intrathecal compartment. Some investigators still consider the density of the lesion on non-contrast-enhanced CT scans to be the most reliable means of distinguishing this tumor, which is often hyperdense, from the cerebellar astrocytoma (hypo- or isodense) (Barkovich 1992).

Myelography with CT scans has been the most precise method in the past for evaluating spinal metastases from any posterior fossa mass (Deutsch & Reigel 1980, Dorwart et al 1981). Because of the invasive nature of this imaging modality and the increased sensitivity of spinal MR studies augmented with contrast enhancement, however, the latter technique is now preferred for the initial staging evaluation and subsequent follow-up studies (Dickman et al 1989, Barkovich 1992).

As a result of its typical midline position, CT often depicts medulloblastoma (iPNET) as a hyperdense mass with either uniform or heterogeneous contrast enhancement (Zimmerman et al 1978, Kingsley & Kendall 1979). Rarely is more than one mass present in the cerebellum at the initial presentation (Shen & Yang 1988, Spagnoli et al 1990). Lack of contrast enhancement and other atypical features, e.g. hemorrhage, cysts, eccentric location, can be identified in up to 47% of all patients (Zee et al 1982). Cysts of large dimensions are quite unusual (Mahapatra et al 1989).

The appearance of medulloblastoma (iPNET) on MR imaging studies may be variable and nonspecific (Barkovich 1992, Meyers et al 1992). T1-weighted images usually demonstrate a hypointense mass that alters the morphology of the fourth ventricle (Meyers et al 1992). Since calcification is atypical, the signal void that this mineral produces is not a common feature, thus indicating that any evidence of a signal dropout in the mass represents a flow void from a vascular structure. T2-weighted sequences often reveal a hyperintense lesion

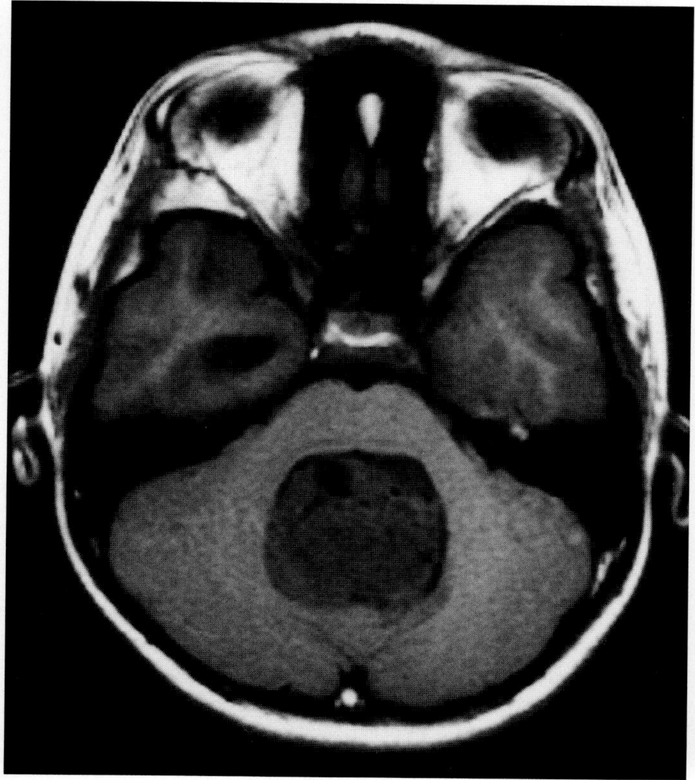
A

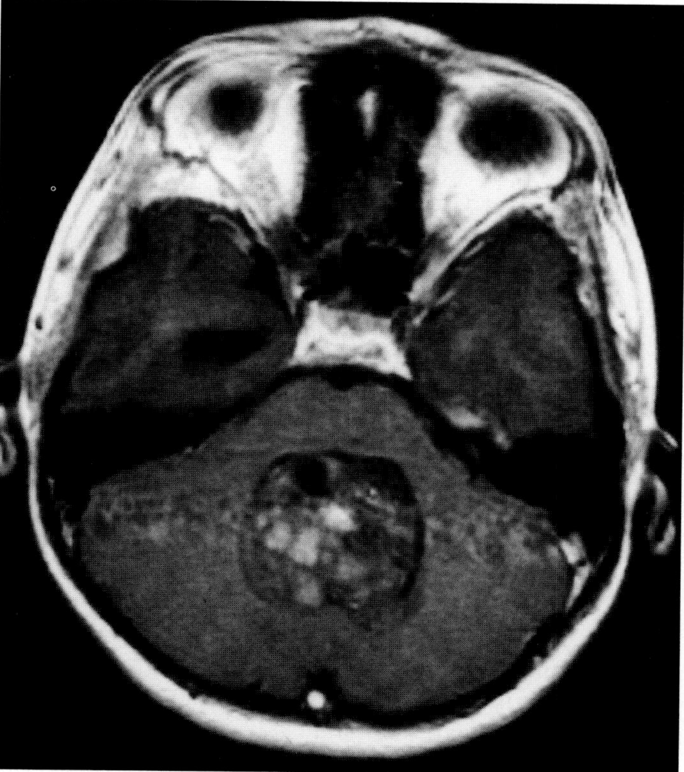
B

Fig. 30.1 T1-weighted axial MR images of a fourth ventricular medulloblastoma (iPNET) without (**A**) and with (**B**) intravenous gadolinium (DPTA). The tumor is primarily attached to the roof of the fourth ventricle, and demonstrates a heterogeneous contrast enhancement pattern typical of this tumor type.

with occasional foci of hypo- or isotense signals. Hypointense medulloblastoma (iPNET) as seen with long TR/TE sequences has also been described (Barkovich 1992), and according to some investigators, this is strongly suggestive of a medulloblastoma since it is very seldom identified with other posterior fossa tumors (Berkovich & Edwards 1990). Because of the peritumoral edema which is often present, administration of paramagnetic contrast agents, e.g. gadolinium DTPA, will readily identify the tumor margins (Waluch & Dyck 1990), despite an often-seen heterogeneous enhancement pattern (Meyers et al 1992) (Figs 30.1A,B). At the time of tumor recurrence, gadolinium enhancement may be minimal or may be present around the tumor bed as a result of radiation-induced changes in the blood-brain barrier (Rollins et al 1990). Similarly, metastatic lesions often demonstrate sparse enhancement following intravenous contrast administration (Meyers et al 1992). It should also be noted that when a child with medulloblastoma (iPNET) presents with bone pain, a metastatic lesion must be ruled out, using a standard skeletal survey looking for osteolytic or osteosclerotic foci (Vieco et al 1989).

Contrary to children, adults often have laterally situated tumors involving the cerebellar hemispheres with poorly defined margins or small degenerative cysts (Bourgouin et al 1990). Medulloblastoma (iPNET) in adults, although unusual, is more common than posterior fossa astrocytic gliomas and less frequent than metastases in middle and older age groups, respectively.

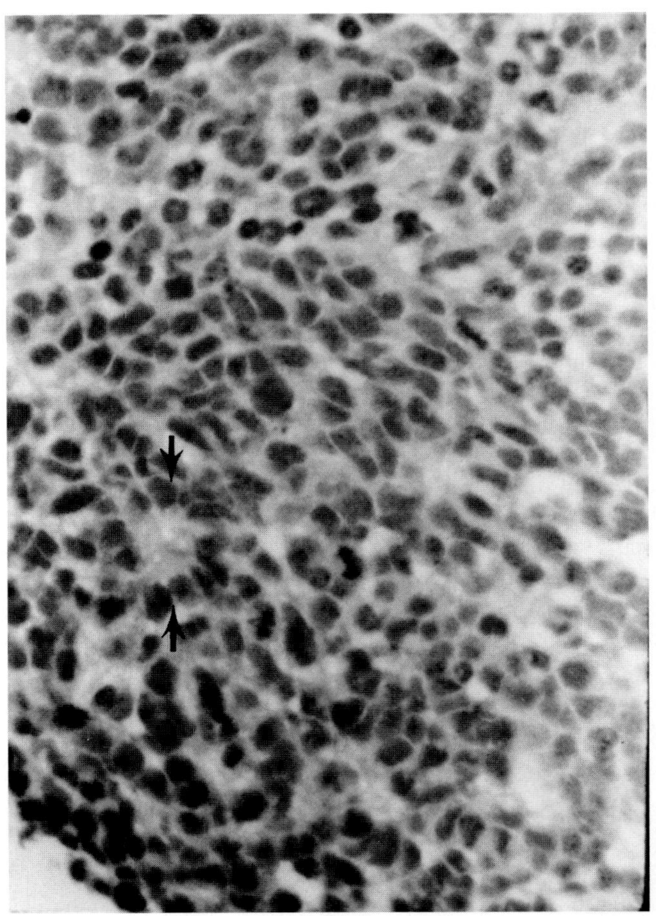

Fig. 30.2 Microscopic (×310) appearance of a medulloblastoma (iPNET) reveals typical features of small, round hyperchromatic nuclei with numerous mitoses and a Homer Wright rosette (arrows).

PATHOLOGY

Grossly, the medulloblastoma (iPNET) appears as a pinkish-gray mass with tiny vessels insinuated within the tumor capsule. Although highly unusual, this tumor may grow en plaque along the surface of the cerebellum without an associated parenchymal mass (Ferrara et al 1989). Intratumoral calcifications and cysts are unusual (Mahapatra et al 1989), as is the grossly evident necrosis typical of glioblastoma multiforme.

Histologically, the medulloblastoma (iPNET) is composed of small, poorly differentiated cells with minimal cytoplasm (Fig. 30.2). Occasionally, Homer Wright rosettes, i.e. pseudorosettes, may be identified. Microscopically, cellular differentiation with astrocytic, neuronal and ependymal features has resulted in the concept of designating medulloblastomas (iPNET) as primitive neuroectodermal tumors with and without differentiation (Burger et al 1991). It is debatable whether or not glial differentiation, as determined immunohistochemically with glial fibrillary acid protein (GFAP), is predictive of patient outcome (Szymas et al 1987, Taomoto et al 1987, Goldberg-Stern et al 1991). It may be that GFAP-positive cells are indicative of reactive astrocytes trapped within a medulloblastoma and not intrinsic to the tumor (Coffin et al 1983). Recent evidence from our laboratory indicates, however, that GFAP-negative medulloblastoma cells are capable of expressing this intermediate filament protein when exposed to glial maturation factor (Keles et al 1993). Thus, the question of histogenesis may be partially answered, assuming that undifferentiated cells have the capability to express GFAP under certain circumstances, which strongly suggests astrocytic lineage in some of these tumors.

Some medulloblastomas (iPNET) have, in addition to the typical cytological features, an abundant network of reticulin fibers. This is quite typical when the lesions originate in the cerebellar hemisphere close to the pia-arachnoid surface; and these lesions are designated as desmoplastic medulloblastomas (iPNET) (Burger et al 1991) (Fig. 30.3). The cells may display a nodular morphology with linear patterns. In one series, over 90% of the desmoplastic medulloblastomas (iPNET) demonstrated a diploid DNA content (Giangaspero et al 1991). It has also been proposed recently that the desmoplastic

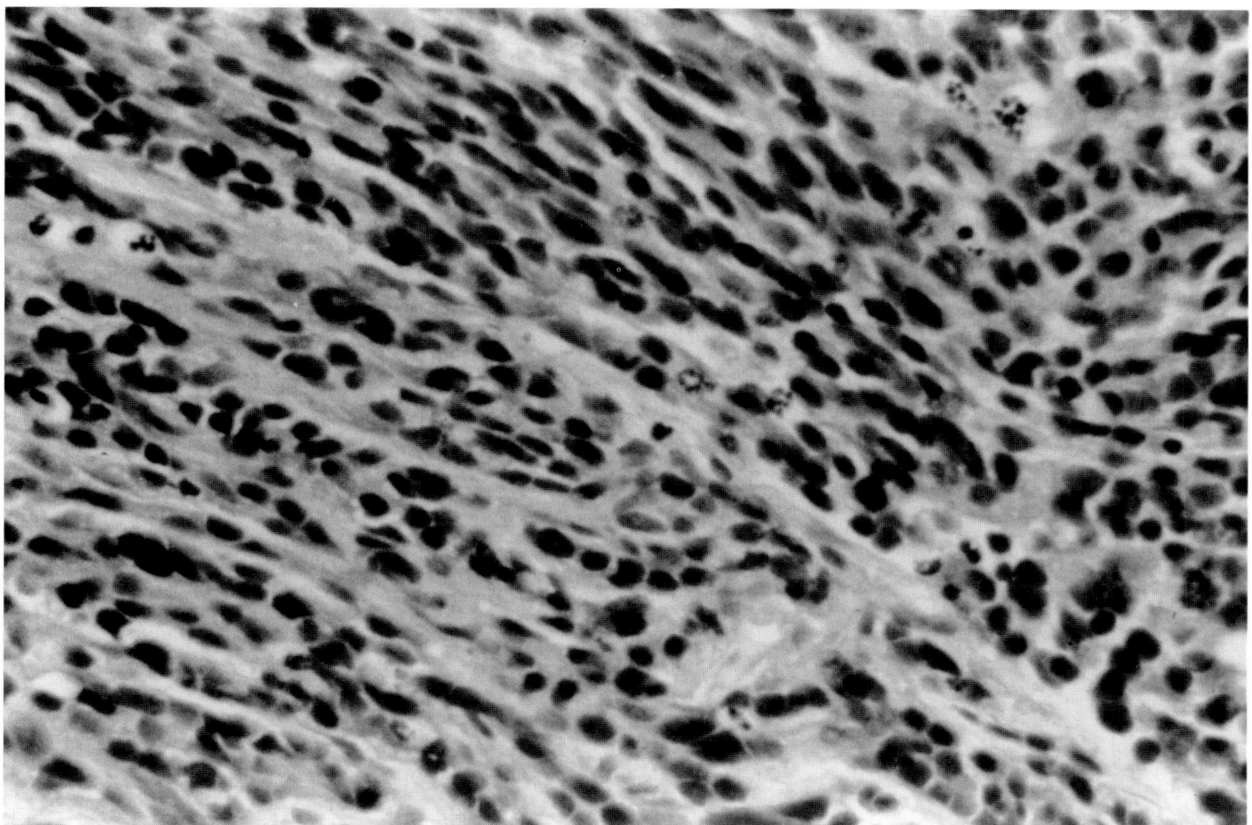

Fig. 30.3 In addition to the typical histologic features of this medulloblastoma (iPNET), desmoplastic elements, composed of connective tissue stroma, may be present, especially in laterally based tumors (× 258).

variant and the cerebellar neuroblastoma are possibly the same tumor phenotype (Burger et al 1991).

Three additional histologic variants of medulloblastoma (iPNET) previously described are medullomyoblastoma, melanotic and large cell medulloblastomas. In the former tumor type, striated and, occasionally, smooth muscle cells are present. In addition, neuronal and glial cell differentiation may coexist in the same lesion (Schiffer et al 1992). When the medullomyoblastoma contains differentiated cells along ectodermal, mesodermal and endodermal lines, it must be reclassified as a teratoma. Melanin-containing cells may be found between the typical small undifferentiated medulloblastoma (iPNET) cells (Dolman 1988). So-called melanotic medulloblastomas are quite unusual (Maire et al 1992). More recently, neuropathologists have described a tumor variant characterized by cells with large vesicular nuclei and prominent nucleoli. These cells exhibit strong immunoreactivity for synaptophysin. This large cell medulloblastoma (iPNET) appears to be linked with a more aggressive clinical course (Giangaspero et al 1992).

Attempts at correlating histopathological features with prognosis have often been unsuccessful. The majority of these studies are retrospective and encompass various treatment protocols which make correlation of outcome with histology difficult. Nonetheless, these parameters — including cell kinetic and DNA content data — will be reviewed in this context.

Increased vascularity and endothelial hyperplasia, traditionally known to predict a bad clinical outcome for malignant gliomas, have also been linked to a poor prognosis in terms of tumor progression and recurrence by some investigators (Taomoto et al 1987, Maire et al 1992), but not by others (Caputy et al 1987). The presence of necrosis seems to be an important indicator of early relapse (Caputy et al 1987) and a diminished 5-year survival rate (Packer et al 1984, Maire et al 1992). A high mitotic index is variable in terms of predicting a shorter relapse-free survival (Caputy et al 1987, Taomoto et al 1987, Schiffer et al 1989, Maire et al 1992).

As previously stated, cellular differentiation may influence prognosis (Schoefield 1992); however, uncertainties regarding its significance are related to the sensitivity and specificity of the antigens evaluated in documenting differentiation. Small variations in routinely used tissue fixation protocols may influence the qualitative results.

Paraffin-embedded tumors have also yielded inconsistent immunostaining. Also, as alluded to before, normal reactive astrocytes and neurons may be trapped within the tumor, ultimately influencing the interpretation of the immunohistochemistry (Schiffer et al 1989).

Although the large cell medulloblastoma (iPNET) is associated with a more aggressive clinical behavior, the medullomyoblastoma appears to have a similar outcome to the classic type of medulloblastoma (Schiffer et al 1992). The desmoplastic variant, however, behaves less aggressively (Chatty & Earle 1971, Caputy et al 1987, Vieco et al 1991), or similarly to the classic histologic phenotype (Park et al 1983, Schiffer et al 1989).

Proliferative parameters and DNA ploidy have also been analyzed in an attempt to predict clinical outcome. In a retrospective flow cytometry study using paraffin-embedded specimens from brain tumor patients who received bromodeoxyuridine (BUdR) at the time of surgery, 66.7% of the medulloblastoma (iPNET) specimens demonstrated an aneuploid DNA content (Cho et al 1988), which did not specifically correlate with the percentage of S-phase cells labeled with BUdR. This labeling index determined by BUdR or tritiated thymidine administration has demonstrated a relatively high value, compared with other neuroectodermal tumors, of 11.7% ± 1.3%. The labeling index also appears to correlate with patient age — i.e. higher in younger children — but not with survival. As expected, low levels of statin, a nuclear protein specifically expressed in quiescent (noncycling, G_O) cells, complements the high number of BUdR-positive cells (Tsanaclis et al 1991). The duration of cells in the S-phase, estimated with a double labeling method, was 6.1–11.3 hours (mean, 8.0 ± 0.8 h), and the calculated doubling time was 25–82 hours (Ito et al 1992). Since the initial report by Tomita et al (1988) demonstrating that an aneuploid DNA content yields a better prognosis than diploid medulloblastomas (iPNET), other investigators have confirmed the results, especially when a gross total resection is achieved (Schofield et al 1992). These data, however, have been recently questioned by others (Zebrini et al 1993). Until this issue is resolved for medulloblastomas, tissue specimens should always be sent for DNA content analysis. Interestingly enough, one report has demonstrated that desmoplastic tumors are almost always near diploid, which is inconsistent with a better prognosis for this particular phenotype.

SURGICAL MANAGEMENT

The goals of surgery are to alleviate the symptoms of obstructive hydrocephalus and achieve a radical tumor resection. Because most children present to a physician with mild to moderately severe signs and symptoms of intracranial hypertension due to ventriculomegaly, the clinical condition is usually stable enough to be managed conservatively with steroid administration for several days. Infrequently, it is necessary to place an external ventricular drain (EVD) preoperatively due to lethargy or severe headaches. The EVD should drain only 3–5 ml/h so as to avoid rapid supratentorial decompression, which has been associated with upward cerebellar herniation and coma (Epstein & Murali 1978, McLaurin 1983). In our experience (Berger & Culley 1993), children with medulloblastoma (iPNET) will ultimately require a permanent CSF diversion procedure 40% of the time; this rate is influenced by a number of factors, including young age, use of cadaveric dura during the dural closure, midline tumor location, smaller extent of tumor resection, and the formation of a pseudomeningocele secondary to aseptic meningitis. This rate is less than the nearly 60% requirement for a permanent shunt reported at some time during the perioperative period in a recent Childrens Cancer Group (CCG) analysis (Albright 1989). Therefore, with the likelihood that a shunt may only be necessary in half of patients with medulloblastomas (iPNET), it is contraindicated to place a preoperative permanent CSF diversion device.

Previous concerns regarding an increased risk of systemic metastases promoted via a CSF shunt placed in the abdomen or atrium (Tarbell et al 1991) have not been substantiated in the modern era (Lefkowitz et al 1988). Thus, in-line filters are not routinely recommended as part of the shunt procedure.

Most pediatric neurosurgeons prefer the prone position or a variation of this, i.e. Concorde (Kobayashi et al 1983). It is interesting to note that in the CCG study analyzing the current neurosurgical management of medulloblastomas (iPNET), over 75% of sitting position craniotomies were performed by general, i.e. nonpediatric, neurosurgeons, despite the higher incidence of serious complications while the patient is upright (Martin 1987). Prior to the skin incision during the operation, and postoperatively, as long as the EVD is in place, intravenous antibiotics, e.g. vancomycin (10 mg/kg) and gentamicin (2 mg/kg), are administered. Depending upon the patient's size, 2–4 mg of dexamethasone are given every 6 hours and tapered off completely at 7–10 days following the operation.

A midline incision and craniectomy are performed unless the lesion is primarily located within the cerebellar hemisphere. It is unnecessary to remove the lamina of C1 for any posterior fossa medulloblastoma (iPNET) to achieve a complete resection. Although it is safe in terms of stability, performing laminectomies of C2 and below may lead to an unstable cervical spine and a swan neck deformity in children and adolescents (Steinbok et al 1989). The dura is opened in a Y-shaped fashion and secured superiorly to the occipital periosteum to avoid epidural bleeding from the torcula. In very young children, large dural venous lakes and a circular sinus at the foramen magnum may make the dural opening quite difficult. Weck clips are often helpful to occlude venous bleeding and are compatible with postoperative magnetic resonance imaging studies (Raimondi 1987).

Once the dura is opened, the surgeon must inspect the cerebellar surface for signs of subarachnoid tumor dissemination, i.e. sugar-coating (Schut 1985). The tumor may not be obvious at first unless it is bulging out from the fourth ventricle and into the cisterna magna. The cerebellar tonsils are retracted laterally and the inferior vermis is exposed and kept intact unless grossly infiltrated with tumor. In our experience, postoperative mutism and pharyngeal dysfunction are seen only when inferior vermian structures are violated. Fortunately, this is a transient phenomenon and is typically described in the pediatric population (Rekate et al 1985, Dietze & Mickle 1990, Ferrante et al 1990), although it has rarely been documented in adults (Salvati et al 1991). The mutism is usually evident a few hours after the operation and may last for 16–20 weeks. Following that, dysarthria is evident before a return to normal, fluent speech.

The tumor is quite vascular and easily aspirated with suction or the ultrasonic aspirator. Gross total removal of all tumor is usually the rule, although several caveats are critical for the surgeon to appreciate, namely, that the tumor may invade the brainstem and hide in the foramina of Luschka. The use of small dental mirrors will identify tumor in these lateral fourth ventricular recesses. If the inferior vermis is intact and tumor extends above into the superior aspect of the ventricle, right-angled curettes are used to extract the tumor without having to damage or split the inferior vermis. A 90% or greater tumor removal was achieved in over 80% of operations performed in the previously cited CCG study (Albright 1989). In addition, there was a significant difference favoring radical and complete resections when the surgery was performed by a pediatric specialist as opposed to a general neurosurgeon.

Following tumor removal, which should always include unblocking the aqueduct within the fourth ventricle to re-establish CSF flow, the dura is reapproximated and closed in an attempted watertight fashion using periosteum from the occipital region. If an EVD is in place at the end of surgery, it should be elevated each day and subsequently removed some time during the first postoperative week. If the patient develops headaches and lethargy with evidence of enlarged ventricles on a CT scan during this process, a permanent shunt will almost always be necessary. Likewise, a large pseudomeningocele is cosmetically unacceptable and should be treated with a CSF diversion procedure. A postoperative CT scan, with and without intravenous contrast administration, should be performed within 2–3 days of surgery to minimize the spurious enhancement at the resection margins secondary to surgical trauma (Jeffries et al 1981, Cairncross et al 1985, Wakai et al 1990).

In addition to the postoperative mutism previously described, additional complications include a transient inability to elevate the eyelids (Gaskill & Marlin 1991), tension pneumocephalus, especially over the frontal lobes following the sitting position in a patient with large ventricles (Lunsford et al 1979, Ramet al 1992), and early postoperative seizures (Lee et al 1990). The latter morbidity is uncommon and usually a result of electrolyte abnormalities (Lee et al 1990).

It remains questionable whether the extent of resection favorably affects survival, primarily because all studies to date either rely on the surgeon's subjective impression or the qualitative appearance of the resection cavity seen on postoperative imaging studies. Notwithstanding, several reports fail to find a significant advantage in terms of event-free survival between patients who underwent total or near-total removal versus a less aggressive resection (Evans et al 1990, Garton et al 1990, Geyer et al 1991). Contrary to this, a tumor resection of 90% or better has been correlated with a longer survival period (Raimondi & Tomita 1979, Noms et al 1981, Tomita et al 1988). This advantage reached statistical significance in an International Society of Pediatric Oncologists (SIOP) study reported over a decade ago (Gerosa et al 1981).

Overall, there is no disagreement regarding the aggressive tumor removal approach that neurosurgeons should pursue for medulloblastomas (iPNET). If a subtotal resection is performed initially, and residual disease is present on follow-up imaging studies at one year postoperatively, relapse is the rule despite adjuvant therapy (Bourne et al 1992). Therefore, second-look surgery to rule out residual tumor, which should include an attempt at a complete resection, is currently recommended when diagnostic imaging studies show persistent disease.

RADIOTHERAPY

An extremely poor progress was reported for medulloblastoma (iPNET) through the early 1950s, despite the use of involved field radiotherapy (Bloom et al 1969). In 1953, Patterson first reported results of irradiation of the entire neuraxis, with 7 of 13 children alive 3 years after treatment. Bloom et al (1969) reported the largest series to date, in which 71 children received 4500–5000 cGy to the spine. With this approach, the 5- and 10-year survival rates were 40% and 30%, respectively. Poor prognostic indicators were noted to be brainstem invasion and a less than complete tumor excision. Failure was most often seen as recurrence of the original primary tumor.

Subsequent single-institution studies have reported improved results in the megavoltage radiotherapy era, with 5- and 10-year actuarial survival rates of 46–68%, and 42–46%, respectively (Bellani et al 1956, Hirsch et al 1979, Berry et al 1981, Jenkin et al 1990, Hughes et al 1992). An important dose-response relationship is apparent in these studies, as local tumor control in the posterior fossa is clearly dose dependent. Patients receiving greater than 5000–5400 cGy to this region have less than a 25% local failure rate compared with a greater than 50% local failure rate in those patients receiving less than this dose.

The dose of radiation required to prevent recurrences outside the primary tumor site is less clear because routine evaluation of the neuraxis was not commonplace until the early 1980s in many centers. Patients presumed on clinical grounds to be free of metastasis at diagnosis may, in fact, have had disseminated disease. A range of doses from approximately 2400–4000 cGy delivered to the cranium and spine have been reported, while doses from 3000–3600 cGy have become the convention. With this latter dose range, most series report an incidence of recurrence in the lower dose 'prophylactic' irradiation field of approximately 15%.

Several institutions have investigated the use of lower doses of craniospinal irradiation, i.e. less than 3000 cGy, both with and without adjuvant chemotherapy, and reported survival rates no different from those obtained with higher doses (Brand et al 1987, Levin et al 1988, Hughes et al 1992). In these studies, survival was independent of the spinal and whole brain radiation dose, and failure occurred initially in the posterior fossa in the majority of patients.

In the light of these promising single institution reports, two multi-institution trials were opened in the 1980s to investigate the hypothesis that a lower dose of craniospinal irradiation would result in equivalent tumor control rates, and decreased late sequelae as opposed to the conventional dose of irradiation. The two cooperative pediatric groups in the United States randomized patients to receive either 2400 or 3600 cGy to the neuraxis with a boost to 5400 cGy to the posterior fossa in both treatment arms. The trial was limited to average risk patients (minimal postoperative residual tumor, no metastasis at diagnosis and no brainstem involvement), and did not include adjuvant chemotherapy. The trial, however, was terminated early because of an excessive number of failures in the low dose treatment arm, both in and outside of the primary site (Deutsch et al 1991). A similar trial was conducted by the SIOP in Europe, and although preradiation chemotherapy was administered, reduction of craniospinal dose resulted in a poorer tumor control (Gnekow et al 1991). Thus, it appears, even in good risk patients, that a total craniospinal dose of 2400 cGy is associated with a higher failure rate than the conventional neuraxis dose.

In addition to the dose of irradiation used, the technique of irradiation is critical to outcome in medulloblastoma (iPNET), e.g. recurrence in the region of the cribriform plate has been associated with excessively large eyeblocks. Several recent reports of multi-institutional trials have demonstrated evidence of failure related to radiotherapeutic techniques (Carrie et al 1992, Rottinger et al 1992). In one study, upon central review, 10 of 22 failures were determined to be due to improper field size or technique (Carrie et al 1992).

Attempts to minimize late sequelae of craniospinal irradiation, in addition to lowering the total dose, have included the use of electron beam radiation to the spinal canal, and the use of intrathecal radioactive gold. However, late complications have been reported with both modalities (Gaspar et al 1991).

Failure at the primary site continues to be the predominant barrier to cure in patients with medulloblastoma (iPNET). New approaches to improve local control include the use of hyperfractionated radiotherapy to higher total doses of radiation, which is under investigation in several centers. This technique is based on the hypothesis that for normal brain tissue, fraction size reduction can result in tissue sparing, and, theoretically, neoplastic tissue has less capacity for repair following irradiation. It remains to be determined whether increasing the posterior fossa dose (to approximately 600 cGy) with conventional fractions might result in increased tumor control without unacceptable toxicity.

In summary, adjuvant radiotherapy alone, with posterior fossa doses of at least 5000 cGy and neuraxis doses of at least 3000 cGy result in a 50–70% 5-year event-free survival (EFS), and in some subsets of patients with favorable features, i.e. no metastatic disease, complete resection may result in even higher tumor control rates. It is not clear, however, that further gains in survival are possible with improvement in current radiotherapeutic techniques. It does appear that lower than standard doses of craniospinal irradiation, at least without chemotherapy, are less effective and potentially dangerous.

CHEMOTHERAPY

The rationale for exploring the use of chemotherapy in patients with medulloblastoma (iPNET) has been developed for patients with recurrent tumor. For newly diagnosed patients, its use in an adjuvant fashion in combination with radiotherapy is an attempt to decrease the frequency of tumor recurrence and to allow for reduction of the total dose of irradiation. Over the last 20 years, the use of chemotherapy in patients with medulloblastoma (iPNET) has resulted in promising suggestions of efficacy, but clear proof of its value, except in selected subsets of patients, remains elusive.

A number of chemotherapeutic agents have been demonstrated to have activity in recurrent medulloblastoma (iPNET), namely cyclophosphamide, cisplatin and carboplatin, which in small series have shown at least 25% objective response rates (Abrahamsen et al 1992, Allen & Helson 1981, Friedman et al 1986, Bertolone et al 1989, Gaynon et al 1990). In addition, several multi-regimen combinations, such as CCNU, vincristine and cisplatin

(Lefkowitz et al 1990) and '8 drugs in 1 day' (vincristine, CCNU, cisplatin, hydroxyurea, prednisone, cyclophosphamide, Ara-C and procarbazine) have shown significant activity (Pendergrass et al 1987). In general, an objective response to therapy is defined as at least a 50% reduction in the cross-sectional area of tumor as seen on MRI or CT scans.

In addition to assessment of chemotherapeutic activity in patients with recurrent tumors who are often heavily pretreated, 'neo-adjuvant', i.e. preradiation treatment, in newly diagnosed patients with residual disease, has provided the setting in which to evaluate chemotherapy response for medulloblastoma (iPNET). In fact, this setting may be more relevant to the assessment of the potential value as adjuvant therapy in newly diagnosed patients. Such a strategy has recently demonstrated the significant activity of the combination of vincristine, cisplatin and cyclophosphamide (48% response) (Mosijczuk et al 1991), and of cisplatin and etoposide (80% response) (Kovnar et al 1990). In addition to allowing for the assessment of chemotherapeutic agents, administration of chemotherapy prior to irradiation has several potential advantages: (1) intensive chemotherapy is likely to be better tolerated prior to marrow suppressive craniospinal irradiation, and agents such as cisplatin may have less ototoxicity when administered in this fashion; and (2) reducing tumor burden prior to irradiation might result in improved tumor control. Conversely, delaying the use of a proven modality of treatment, i.e. radiotherapy, may result in disease progression at an early stage. Intervals from 1–3 months of preradiation chemotherapy appear to be safe. Disease recurrence in infants treated only with chemotherapy, however, occurs at a median of approximately 6 months (Geyer et al 1993).

The relative rarity of medulloblastoma (iPNET) necessitates randomized multi-institutional trials. Four such trials have been reported and another recently concluded in which adjuvant chemotherapy, in addition to craniospinal irradiation, was evaluated. In the late 1970s and early 1980s, the Childrens Cancer Group (CCG) in the United States and SIOP conducted randomized trials comparing craniospinal irradiation plus chemotherapy (CCNU, vincristine) with irradiation alone. These studies began before computerized tomography was readily available, and all patients were not completely staged with myelograms. Overall, the 5-year EFS was not different between the two treatment arms in either study. In the CCG study, the 5-year EFS was 60% for patients treated with chemotherapy and irradiation and 50% for patients treated with irradiation alone (Evans et al 1990). Comparable results were also obtained in the SIOP study (55% versus 45%, respectively) (Tait et al 1990). In both studies, however, chemotherapy was of benefit in subsets of patients with poor-risk features, i.e. those with large tumors, tumors invading the brainstem, partially resected tumors and disseminated tumors at diagnosis. A subsequent SIOP trial using preirradiation chemotherapy with vincristine, procarbazine and methotrexate did not clarify the role of chemotherapy for either high risk or average risk patients (Gnekow et al 1991). The CCG has just concluded a study for poor risk medulloblastoma (iPNET) patients comparing CCNU, prednisone and vincristine to '8 drugs in 1 day'.

In a randomized trial conducted by the Pediatric Oncology Group (POG), adjuvant postirradiation chemotherapy consisting of nitrogen mustard, vincristine, procarbazine and prednisone was compared to the treatment of patients with irradiation alone. There was a statistically significant increase in 5-year survival rate for the chemotherapeutic group, but the study did not show a statistically significant advantage for irradiation plus MOPP in EFS (Krishner 1991).

In a single-treatment arm, single-institution study, investigators at the Children's Hospital of Philadelphia using adjuvant chemotherapy (cisplatin, CCNU, vincristine) and standard dose craniospinal irradiation in the treatment of poor risk patients with medulloblastoma (iPNET) have reported the best results to date. Actuarial 5-year EFS is greater than 80% among 51 patients. This compares to a group of patients with standard risk disease (10 patients) treated concurrently with identical radiotherapy, but without chemotherapy in whom the disease-free survival (DFS) is 52%.

Use of chemotherapy in very young children with medulloblastoma (iPNET), in an attempt to delay or avoid radiotherapy, has been recently investigated. Using MOPP, infants with medulloblastoma (iPNET) at the MD Anderson Cancer Center had a 50% 5-year EFS (Ater et al 1988). The Pediatric Oncology Group (POG) recently concluded a trial for children less than 3 years of age with malignant brain tumors, and the 2-year EFS was approximately 40% for patients with medulloblastoma (iPNET). Radiotherapy was administered to these patients after the completion of chemotherapy (1–2 years). Most patients who progressed did so very early in treatment, and the role of radiotherapy in contributing to long-term EFS is uncertain. A similar study utilizing '8 drugs in 1 day' chemotherapy was recently concluded by the CCG. Those children with medulloblastoma (iPNET) had approximately a 25% 2-year EFS. Unlike the POG study, few of these patients received irradiation at any given time (Geyer 1992). Both groups have recently opened new trials, in which intensified chemotherapy is utilized in an attempt to decrease the rate of early disease progression.

As previously discussed, reduction of radiation dose delivered to the neuraxis in an attempt to decrease the long-term deficits associated with craniospinal irradiation, has resulted in an excessive rate of progression compared to standard radiation in two randomized multi-institutional trials. Several trials are currently investigating the hypothesis that the use of effective adjuvant chemotherapy will 'make up the difference'. The CCG is currently piloting the combination of low dose (2500 cGy) craniospinal irradiation and standard posterior fossa dose (5400 cGy) with adjuvant chemotherapy (CCNU, cisplatin and vincristine). A trial including both the CCG and the POG, randomizing standard radiotherapy (3600 cGy craniospinal) versus reduced dose craniospinal irradiation and adjuvant chemotherapy (vincristine, cyclophosphamide, cisplatin) is currently being discussed for patients with average risk medulloblastoma. Such trials, in addition to standard outcome measures in terms of EFS, must also be rigorously designed to assess late effects, particularly endocrine and psychological function.

Although chemotherapy is clearly of benefit to those patients with high risk medulloblastoma, particularly those with large invasive tumors and metastatic disease at diagnosis, this group of patients continues to have a poor overall survival. New strategies for their treatment include the use of high dose chemotherapy prior to the use of aggressive radiotherapy, perhaps delivered by hyperfractionation. The use of very high dose chemotherapy followed by reinfusion of previously harvested autologous bone marrow may have a role in intensifying therapy prior to irradiation in these high risk patients. New chemotherapeutic agents and combinations of established agents are very much needed. The use of in vitro medulloblastoma cell lines, and, in particular, the use of these cell lines in nude mice, is a rational approach for developing new therapeutic strategies. A nude mouse model of disseminated leptomeningeal medulloblastoma has recently been used to demonstrate the value of a cyclophosphamide derivative when administered intrathecally (Schuster et al 1991), and this agent is now under evaluation in Phase I/II clinical trials.

PATTERNS OF FAILURE

Systemic metastases occur in 5–15% of the patients with medulloblastoma, involving the bone marrow, lymph nodes and liver in decreasing order (Anzil 1970, Amador 1983). In patients treated only with surgery and radiotherapy, a 5-year cumulative incidence of up to 18% for bone metastases and posterior fossa relapses has been reported. Typically, there is usually a much higher failure rate in the posterior fossa (79%) compared to any site outside the CNS (21%) for medulloblastoma (Brust et al 1968). Supratentorial relapse is also not uncommon, and may be present in 44–47% of all medulloblastoma recurrences (Brust et al 1968, Brutschin & Culver 1973). Direct spread of the tumor to adjacent cervical tissues via an open dura is uncommon but may explain why the lymphatic system becomes involved (Campbell et al 1984). Although prediction of the greatest period of risk for medulloblastoma recurrence is still not clearly defined (Berger & Ewidge 1963), most of the tumors relapse at a period equal to the age at diagnosis plus 9 months, i.e. Collins' law (Brander & Turner 1975, Gerosa et al 1981).

LATE EFFECTS OF TREATMENT

With the development of effective therapy resulting in long-term survival in the majority of children with medulloblastoma, the consequences of treatment on the physical and neuropsychological growth of these children have become increasingly apparent.

A recent analysis of 22 studies of the neuropsychological status of children with primary brain tumors attempted to identify those factors that placed children at greatest risk of psychological impairment. The adverse effects of radiation therapy increased with treatment volume, as nonirradiated children had the highest performance, and those who received whole brain irradiation the lowest. Younger children exhibited a lower IQ overall than that of older children. Among children who had received cranial irradiation, those who were younger than 4 years old had significantly lower IQs than those who were older (mean 73.4 versus 87.0; $p < 0.05$) (Mulhern et al 1992).

In a prospective study, intelligence testing was performed in 43 children with brain tumors (Ellensburg et al 1987) within one month of diagnosis, 3 months after diagnosis and at sequential 6-month follow-up periods. Whole brain irradiation was closely associated with a decrease in cognitive function, especially in younger children. Of 9 patients under the age of 7 years who received whole brain irradiation, 8 had an IQ loss. All 7 children who were given whole brain irradiation before 5 years of age had below average IQs at follow-up, with declines of up to 47 points. This study showed no consistent deficits in children receiving local irradiation or in those given chemotherapy.

Packer et al (1989) prospectively studied children with medulloblastoma who received 2400 cGy whole brain irradiation if they were 18–36 months of age at diagnosis, and 3600 cGy if older. Children less than 18 months of age were not studied. Children less than 7 years of age at diagnosis had a mean fall in full scale IQ of 25 points at 2 years following treatment. The 3 youngest children, all of whom received 2400 cGy, had a fall of 34–37 points in full scale IQ with retesting after 2 years following treatment. Children with cerebellar astrocytomas who were not irradiated did not show a significant decline over time in any measure of intelligence.

Thus, there is strong evidence that whole brain irradiation can result in intellectual deficits, particularly in the very young child. The relationship between total dose of irradiation and degree of intellectual impairment is less clear. As discussed above, the most severe deficits in one study were observed in children who received 2400 cGy whole brain irradiation; however, these were also the youngest children at the time of treatment. An analysis of IQ in children receiving whole brain irradiation for acute lymphoblastic leukemia (ALL) or primary brain tumors was recently reported. Using a regression model to correct for initial IQ and age at treatment, patients who received 3600 cGy of whole brain irradiation were estimated to score 8.2 points less on IQ testing than those who received 2400 cGy, and 12.3 points less than those receiving 1800 cGy.

The role of chemotherapy in the development of intellectual deficits is less clear than that of irradiation. There is evidence that the addition of chemotherapy, particularly methotrexate, to whole brain irradiation has contributed to intellectual decline, both in patients with acute lymphoblastic leukemia and in those with brain tumors (Bleyer & Griffin 1980). There is little evidence that systemic chemotherapy alone is responsible for IQ loss. Children receiving systemic chemotherapy only appear to have less neuropsychological morbidity than those receiving irradiation in one recently published study (Moore et al 1992).

The adverse effect of radiotherapy on growth and development has been well documented. Irradiation in the pituitary and hypothalamus results in decreased growth hormone responses to provocative stimulation and growth retardation in the majority of patients with medulloblastoma using standard radiation (Kanev et al 1991). There is evidence that children less than 10 years of age at the time of radiotherapy are more vulnerable to these effects (Oberfield et al 1986). Spinal irradiation can result in impaired spinal growth, the severity of which is directly related to the age at which the radiation therapy is administered, as well as to the total dose delivered. The addition of adjuvant chemotherapy to craniospinal irradiation may result in more severe growth retardation (Olshan et al 1992).

Acknowledgements

This work was supported by NIH Grant KO8 NS01253–01, American Cancer Society Professor of Clinical Oncology #071 (M. S. Berger), NIH-NINCDS T32 NS07289, and American Cancer Society's Arthur Campbell Fellowship Training Grant (M. S. Berger); also by NIH Clinical Investigator Award KO8 CA-01451–02 (J. R. Geyer).

REFERENCES

Abrahamsen T, Lange B, Packer R et al 1992 High-dose cyclophosphamide with granulocyte/macrophage colony-stimulating factor (GM-CSF) in malignant brain tumors in children. SIOP XXIV Meeting: 381 (proceedings)

Albright A L 1989 Current neurosurgical treatment of medulloblastoma in children: A report from the Children's Cancer Group. Pediatric Neuroscience 15: 276–282

Allen J C, Helson L 1981 High-dose cyclophosphamide chemotherapy for recurrent CNS tumors. Journal of Neurosurgery 55: 749–756

Amador L V 1983 Brain tumors in the young. Charles C Thomas, Springfield, Ill, pp 3–22

Anzil A P 1970 Glioblastoma multiforme with extracranial metastases in the absence of previous chemotherapy. Case report. Journal of Neurosurgery 33: 88–94

Ater J L, Woo S Y, vanEys J 1988 Update on MOPP chemotherapy as primary therapy for infant brain tumors (abstract). Pediatric Neuroscience 14: 153

Barkovich A J, Edwards M 1990 Brain tumors of childhood In: Barkovich A J (ed) Pediatric neuroimaging. Raven Press, New York, p 149

Barkovich A J 1992 Neuroimaging of pediatric brain tumors. In: Berger M S (ed) Pediatric Neuro-Oncology. Neurosurg Clin 3: 739–769

Bellani F F, Gasparini M, Lombardi F et al 1984 Medulloblastoma: Results of a sequential combined treatment. Cancer 54: 1956–1961

Berger E C, Elvidge A R 1963 Medulloblastomas and cerebellar sarcomas. A clinical survey. Journal of Neurosurgery 20: 139–144

Berger M S, Culley D J 1993 Requirements for ventriculoperitoneal shunts following posterior fossa tumor surgery: a retrospective analysis. Neurosurgery (accepted for publication)

Berry M P, Jenkin R D, Keen C W et al 1981 Radiation treatment of medulloblastoma: A 21-year review. Journal of Neurosurgery 55: 43–51

Bertolone S J, Baum E S, Krivit W et al 1989 A Phase II study of cisplatin therapy in recurrent childhood brain tumors: A report from the Children's Cancer Study Group. Journal of Neurology and Oncology 7: 5–11

Biegel J A, Burk C D, Barr F G, Emanuel B S 1992 Evidence for a 17p tumor related locus distinct from p53 in pediatric primitive neuroectodermal tumors. Cancer Research 52: 3391–3395

Bigner S H, Mark J, Friedma H S, Biegel J A, Bigner D D 1988 Structural chromosomal abnormalities in human medulloblastoma. Cancer Genetics and Cytogenetics 30: 91–101

Bleyer W, Griffin W 1980 White matter necrosis, mineralizing microangiopathy in intellectual abilities in survivors of childhood leukemia. In: Gilbert H, Kagen R (eds) Radiation damage to the central nervous system. Raven Press, New York, pp 155–173

Bloom H J, Wallace E N, Henk J M 1969 The treatment and prognosis of medulloblastoma in children: A study of 82 verified cases. AJR 105: 43–62

Bourgouin P M, Tampieri D, Grahovac S Z, L'eger C, Del Carpio R, Melancon D 1992 CT and MR imaging findings in adults with cerebellar medulloblastoma: comparison with findings in children. American Journal of Roentgenology 159: 609–612

Bourne J P, Geyer J R, Berger M S, Griffin B, Milstein J 1992 The prognostic significance of postoperative residual contrast enhancement on CT scan in pediatric medulloblastoma patients. Journal of Neuro-Oncology 14: 263–270

Brand W N, Schneider P A, Tokars R P 1987 Long-term results for a pilot study of low dose cranial-spinal irradiation for cerebellar medulloblastoma. International Journal of Radiation Oncology Biology Physics 13: 1641–1645

Brander W L, Turner D R 1975 Extracranial metastases from a glioma in the absence of surgical intervention. Journal of Neurology Neurosurgery and Psychiatry 38: 1133–1135

Brust J C M, Moiel R H, Rosenberg R N 1968 Glial tumor metastases through a ventriculopleural shunt. Resultant massive pleural effusion. Archives of Neurology 18: 649–653

Brutschin P, Culver G J 1973 Extracranial metastases from medulloblastomas. Radiology 107: 359–362

Bunin G 1987 Racial patterns of childhood brain cancer by histologic type. Journal of the National Cancer Institute 78: 875–880

Burger P, Scheithauer B W, Vogel F S 1991 Surgical pathology of the nervous system and its coverings, 3rd edn. Churchill Livingstone, New York, NY, pp 339–350

Cairncross J G, Pexman J H W, Rathbone M P 1985 Postoperative contrast enhancement in patients with brain tumor. Annals of Neurology 17: 570–572

Campbell A N, Chan H S L, Becker L E et al 1984 Extracranial metastases in childhood primary intracranial tumors: a report of 21 cases and review of the literature. Cancer 53: 974–981

Caputy A J, McCullogh D C, Manz H J, Patterson K, Hammock M K 1987 A review of the factors influencing the prognosis of medulloblastoma. The importance of cell differentiation. Journal of Neurosurgery 66: 80–87

Carrie C, Alapetite C, Mere P et al 1992 Quality control of radiotherapeutic treatment of medulloblastoma in a multicentric study: the contribution of radiotherapy technique to tumor relapse. Radiotherapy and Oncology 24: 77–81

Chatty E M, Earle K M 1971 Medulloblastoma. A report of 201 cases with emphasis on the relationship of histologic variants to survival. Cancer 28: 977–983

Chi J G, Khang S K 1989 Central nervous system tumors among Koreans — a statistical study on 697 cases. Journal of Korean Medical Science 4: 77–90

Cho K G, Nagashima T, Barnwell S, Hoshino T 1988 Flow cytometric determination of modal DNA population in relation to proliferative potential of human intracranial neoplasms. Journal of Neurosurgery 69: 588–592

Choux M, Lena G 1982 Le medulloblastome. Neurochirurgie 28(suppl): 1–229

Coffin C M, Mukai K, Dehner P 1983 Glial differentiation in medulloblastomas. American Journal of Surgical Pathology 7: 555–565

Cogen P H 1991 Prognostic significance of molecular genetic markers in childhood brain tumors. Pediatric Neurosurgery 17: 245–250

Cogen P H, Daneshvar L, Metzger A K, Duyk G, Edwards M S, Sheffield V C 1992 Involvement of multiple chromosome 17p loci in medulloblastoma tumorigenesis. American Journal of Human Genetics 50: 584–589

Deutsch M, Reigel D H 1980 The value of myelography in the management of childhood medulloblastoma. Cancer 45: 2194–2197

Deutsch M, Thomas P, Boyett J et al 1991 Low stage medulloblastoma: A Children's Cancer Study Group (CCSG) and Pediatric Oncology Group (POG) randomized study of standard versus reduced neuroaxis irradiation. Proceedings of ASCO 10: 124

Dickman C, Rekate H, Bird C et al 1989 Unenhanced and gadolinium-DTPA-enhanced MR imaging in postoperative evaluation of pediatric brain tumors. Journal of Neurosurgery 71: 49–53

Dietze D D Jr, Mickle J P 1990 Cerebellar mutism after posterior fossa surgery. Pediatric Neurosurgery 16: 25–31

Dolman C L 1988 Melanotic medulloblastoma. A case report with immunohistochemical and ultrastructural examination. Acta Neuropathologica 76: 528–531

Dorwart R H, Wara W M, Normal D et al 1981 Complete myelographic evaluation of spinal metastases from medulloblastoma. Radiology 139: 403–408

Duffner P K, Cohen M E, Myers M H et al 1986 Survival of children with brain tumors: SEER program 1973–1980. Neurology 36: 597–601

Edwards M S B, Hudgins R J 1989 Medulloblastomas and primitive neuroectodermal tumors of the posterior fossa. In: McLaurin R L, Venes J L, Schut L, Epstein F (eds). Pediatric neurosurgery, 2nd edn. W B Saunders, Philadelphia, pp 347–356

Ellensburg L, McComb J G, Siegel S E et al 1987 Factors affecting intellectual outcome in pediatric brain tumor patients. Neurosurgery 21: 638–644

Epstein F, Murali R 1978 Pediatric posterior fossa tumors: hazards of the "preoperative" shunt. Neurosurgery 3: 348–350

Evans A E, Jenkin R D, Sposto R et al 1990 The treatment of medulloblastoma. Results of a prospective randomized trial of radiation therapy with and without CCNU, vincristine and prednisone. Journal of Neurosurgery 72: 572–582

Evans D G, Farndon P A, Burnell L D, Gattamaneni H R, Birch J M 1991 The incidence of Gorlin syndrome in 173 consecutive cases of medulloblastoma. British Journal of Cancer 64: 959–961

Farndon P A, DelMastro R G, Evans D G R, Kilpatric M W 1992 Location of the gene for Gorlin syndrome. Lancet 339: 581–582

Farwell J R, Flannery J T 1987 Adult occurrence of medulloblastoma. Acta Neurochirurgica (Wien) 86: 1–5

Ferrante L, Mastronardi L, Acqui M, Fortuna A 1990 Mutism after posterior fossa surgery in children. Report of 3 cases [published erratum appears in Journal of Neurosurgery 1991; 74: 314]. Journal of Neurosurgery 72: 959–963

Ferrara M, Bizzozzero L, Fiumara E, D'Angelo V, Corona C, Colombo N 1989 Primary leptomeningeal dissemination of medulloblastoma. Report of an unusual case. Journal of Neurosurgical Science 33: 219–223

Friedman H S, Mahaley M S, Schold S C et al 1986 Efficacy of vincristine and cyclophosphamide in the therapy of recurrent medulloblastoma. Neurosurgery 18: 335–340

Friedman H S, Oakes W J, Bigner S H, Wikstrand C J, Bigner D D 1991 Medulloblastoma: tumor biological and clinical perspectives. Journal of Neuro-Oncology 11: 1–15

Gailani M R, Bale S J, Leffell D J et al 1992 Developmental defects in Gorlin syndrome related to a putative tumor suppressor gene on Chromosome 9. Cell 69: 111–117

Garton G R, Schomberg P J, Scheithauer B W et al 1990 Medulloblastoma — prognostic factors and outcome of treatment: review of the Mayo Clinic experience. Mayo Clinic Proceedings 65: 1077–1086

Gaskill S J, Marlin A E 1991 Transient eye closure after posterior fossa tumor surgery in children. Pediatric Neurosurgery 17: 196–198

Gaspar L E, Dawson D J, Tilley G S et al 1991 Medulloblastoma: long-term follow-up of patients treated with electron irradiation of the spinal field. Radiology 180: 867–870

Gaynon P S, Ettinger L J, Baum E S et al 1990 Carboplatin in childhood brain tumors — A Children's Cancer Study Group Phase II trial. Cancer 66: 2465–2469

Gerosa M A, DiStefano E, Olivi A et al 1981 Multidisciplinary treatment of medulloblastoma: a 5-year experience with the SIOP trial. Child's Brain 8: 107–118

Geyer R, Zeltzer P, Finlay J et al 1992 Chemotherapy for infants with malignant brain tumors: report of the Children's Cancer Study group trials CCG-921 and CCG-945. Proceedings of ASCO, 11 March, 1258

Geyer R, Levy M, Berger M S, Milstein J, Griffin B, Bleyer W A 1991 Infants with medulloblastoma: a single institution review of survival. Neurosurgery 29: 707–710

Geyer R, Berger M S, Allen J, Finlay J, Jakacki R, Jennings M et al 1993 Intensive chemotherapy pilot for infants with malignant brain tumors. Proceedings of ASCO, 12 March

Giangaspero F, Chieco P, Ceccarelli C et al 1991 "Desmoplastic" versus "classic" medulloblastoma: comparison of DNA content, histopathology and differentiation. Virchows Arch A Pathol Anat Histopathol 418: 207–214

Giangaspero F, Rigobello L, Badiali M et al 1992 Large-cell medulloblastomas. A distinct variant with highly aggressive behavior. American Journal of Surgical Pathology 16: 687–693

Gnekow A, Bailey C, Michaelis J et al 1991 SIOP/GPO medulloblastoma trial II — Med 84: Annual status report. SIOP XXIII Meeting: 435 (proceedings)

Goldberg-Stern H, Gadothin N, Stern S, Cohen I J, Zaizov R, Sandbank U 1991 The prognostic significance of glial fibrillary acidic protein staining in medulloblastoma. Cancer 68: 568–573

Gorlin R J 1987 Nevoid basal-cell carcinoma syndrome. Medicine (Baltimore) 66: 98–113

Heafner M D, Schut L, Packer R J et al 1985 Discrepancy between CT and MRI in a case of medulloblastoma. Neurosurgery 17: 487–489

Helseth A, Mørk S J 1989 Neoplasms of the central nervous system in Norway. III Epidemiological characteristics of intracranial gliomas according to histology. APMIS 97: 547–555

Hirsch J F, Renier D, Czernichow P et al 1979 Medulloblastoma in childhood: survival and functional results. Acta Neurochirurgica (Wien) 48: 1–15

Hughes E N, Shillito J, Sallan S E et al 1992 Medulloblastoma at the Joint Center for Radiation Therapy between 1968 and 1984: The influence of radiation dose on the patterns of failure and survival. Cancer 61: 1992–1998

Hung K L, Wu C M, Huang J S, How S W 1990 Familial medulloblastoma in siblings: report in one family and review of the literature. Surgical Neurology 33: 341–346. (Familial medulloblastoma in siblings: report in one family and review of the literature (letter) [corrected and republished letter originally printed in Surgical Neurology 1991 July; 36(1): 70]; Surgical Neurology 1991 Sept., 36(3): 234

Ito S, Hoshino T, Prados M D, Edwards M S 1992 Cell kinetics of medulloblastomas. Cancer 70: 671–678

James C D, He J, Carlbom E, Mikkelsen T, Ridderheim P A, Cavenee W K, Collins V P 1990 Loss of genetic information in central nervous system tumors common to children and young adults. Genes Chromosome Cancer 2: 94–102

Jarvis L, Bathurst N, Mohan D, Beckly D 1988 Turcot's syndrome: a review. Diseases of the Colon and Rectum 31: 907–914

Jeffries B F, Kishore P R S, Singh K S 1981 Contrast enhancement in the postoperative brain. Radiology 139: 409–413

Jenkin D, Goddard K, Armstrong D et al 1990 Posterior fossa medulloblastoma in childhood: Treatment results and a proposal for a new staging system. International Journal of Radiation Oncology Biology Physics 19: 265–274

Kanev P M, Berger M S, Lefebvre J F, Mauseth R S 1991 Growth hormone deficiency following radiation therapy of primary brain tumors in children. Journal of Neurosurgery 74: 743–748

Keles G E, Berger M S, Lim R, Silber J 1993 Antiproliferative effect and induction of GFAP expression in human medulloblastoma cells by Glia Maturation Factor-B. Oncology Research 4: 431–437

Kepes J J, Morantz R A, Dorzab W E 1987 Cerebellar medulloblastoma in a 73 year old woman. Neurosurgery 21: 81–83

Kingsley D F E, Kendall E 1979 The CT scanner in posterior fossa tumors of childhood. British Journal of Radiology 52: 769–776

Kobayashi S, Sugita K, Tanaka Y et al 1983 Infratentorial approach to the pineal region in the prone position: Concorde position. Journal of Neurosurgery 58: 141–143

Koskiniemi M 1988 Malignancy markers in the cerebrospinal fluid. European Journal of Pediatrics 148: 3–8

Kovnar E, Kellie S, Horowitz M et al 1990 Preirradiation cisplatin and etoposide in the treatment of high-risk medulloblastoma and other malignant embryonal tumors of the Central Nervous System. A Phase II study. Journal of Clinical Oncology 8: 330–336

Krischer J P, Ragab A H, Kun L et al 1991 Nitrogen mustard, vincristine, procarbazine and prednisone as adjuvant chemotherapy in the treatment of medulloblastoma. Journal of Neurosurgery 74: 905–909

Lannering B, Marky I, Nordborg C 1990 Brain tumors in childhood and adolescence in west Sweden 1970–1984. Epidemiology and survival. Cancer 66: 604–609

Lashley P M, Clarke H, Archer E Y 1991 Primary pediatric brain tumors in Barbados: 10-year analysis (1978–1988). Journal of Tropical Pediatrics 37: 64–66

Lee S T, Lui T N, Chang C N, Cheng W C 1990 Early postoperative seizures after posterior fossa surgery. Journal of Neurosurgery 73: 541–544

Lefkowitz I B, Packer R J, Ryan S G et al 1988 Late recurrence of primitive neuroectodermal tumor/medulloblastoma. Cancer 62: 826–830

Lefkowitz I, Packer R, Siegel K et al 1990 Results of treatment of children with recurrent medulloblastoma/primitive neuroectodermal tumors with lomustine, cisplatin and vincristine. Cancer 65: 412–417

Levin V A, Rodriguez L A, Edwards M W et al 1988 Treatment of medulloblastoma with procarbazine, hydroxyurea and reduced radiation doses to whole brain and spine. Journal of Neurosurgery 68: 383–387

Lunsford L D, Maroon J C, Sheptak P E, Albin M S 1979 Subdural tension pneumocephalus: report of two cases. Journal of Neurosurgery 50: 525–527

MacGregor D N, Ziff E B 1990 Elevated c-myc expression in childhood medulloblastomas. Pediatric Research 28: 63–68

McKusick V A 1992 Mendelian inheritance in man: catalogs of autosomal dominant, autosomal recessive, and X-linked phenotypes, Johns Hopkins University Press, Baltimore

McLaurin R L 1983 Disadvantages of the preoperative shunt in posterior fossa tumors. Clinical Neurosurgery 30: 286–292

Mahapatra A K, Paul H K, Sarkar C 1989 Cystic medulloblastoma. Neuroradiology 31: 369–370

Maire J P, Gu'erin J, Rivel J, San-Galli F, Bernard C, Dautheribes M, Caudry M 1992 Le medulloblastome de l'enfant incidence prognostique de l'hyperplasie vasculaire de la necrose de coagulation et de l'etat clinique post-operatoire sur la survie. Neurochirurgie 38: 80–8

Martin J T 1987 Positioning in anesthesia and surgery, 2nd edn. W B Saunders, Philadelphia, pp 79–106

Marton L J, Edwards M S, Levin V A 1979 Predictive value of cerebrospinal fluid polyamines in medulloblastoma. Cancer Res 39: 993–997

Marton L J, Edwards M S, Levin V A et al 1981 CSF polyamines: a new and important means of monitoring patients with medulloblastoma. Cancer 47: 757–760

Meyers S P, Kemp S S, Tarr R W 1992 MR imaging features of medulloblastomas. American Journal of Roentgenology 158: 859–865

Moore B, Ater J, Copeland D 1992 Improved neuropsychological outcome in children with brain tumors diagnosed during infancy and treated without cranial irradiation. Journal of Child Neurology 7: 281–290

Mosijczuk A, Burger P, Freeman A et al 1991 Pre-radiation chemotherapy in advanced medulloblastoma: POG pilot 8695 study. SIOP XIII Meeting: 434 (proceedings)

Mulhern R K, Hancock J, Fairclough D et al 1992 Neuropsychological status of children treated for brain tumors. A critical review and integrative analysis. Medical and Pediatric Oncology 20: 181–191

Norris D G, Bruce D A, Byrd R L et al 1981 Improved relapse-free survival in medulloblastoma utilizing modern techniques. Neurosurgery 9: 661–664

Oberfield S, Allen J, Pollack J et al 1986 Long term endocrine sequelae after treatment of medulloblastoma: prospective studies on growth and thyroid function. Journal of Pediatrics 108: 219–223

Ohgaki H, Eibl R H, Wiestler O D, Yasargil M G, Newcomb E W, Kleihues P 1991 p53 mutations in non astrocytic human brain tumors. Cancer Research 51: 6202–6205

Olascon A, Lania A, Badiali M et al 1991 Analysis of N-ras gene mutations in medulloblastomas by polymerase chain reaction and oligonucleotide probes in formalin-fixed paraffin-embedded tissues. Medical Pediatric Oncology 19: 240–245

Olshan J, Gubernick J, Packer R et al 1992 The effects of adjuvant chemotherapy on growth in children with medulloblastoma. Cancer 70: 2013–2017

Packer R J, Sutton L N, Rorke L B et al 1984 Prognostic importance of cellular differentiation in medulloblastoma of childhood. Journal of Neurosurgery 61: 291–301

Packer R J, Sutton L N, Atkins T E et al 1989 A prospective study of cognitive function in children receiving whole brain radiotherapy and chemotherapy: 2-year results. Journal of Neurosurgery 70: 707–713

Park T S, Hoffman H J, Hendrick E B 1983 Medulloblastoma: clinical presentation and management. Experience at the Hospital for Sick Children. Journal of Neurosurgery 58: 543–552

Pendergrass T W, Milstein J M, Geyer J R et al 1987 Eight drugs in one day chemotherapy for brain tumors: experience in 107 children and rationale for preradiation chemotherapy. Journal of Clinical Oncology 5: 1221–1281

Raffel C, Gilles F E, Weinberg K I 1990 Reduction to homozygosity and gene amplification in central nervous system primitive neuroectodermal tumors of childhood. Cancer Research 50: 587–591

Raimondi A J Pediatric neurosurgery. Theoretical principles, art of surgical techniques, 2nd edn. New York, Springer

Raimondi A J, Tomita T 1979 Advantages of "total resection" of medulloblastoma and disadvantages of full head postoperative radiation therapy. Child's Brain 5: 550–555

Ram Z, Knoller N, Findler G, Sahar A 1992 Delayed intraventricular tension pneumocephalus complicating posterior fossa surgery for cerebellar medulloblastoma. Child's Nervous System 8: 351–353

Reis A, Kuster W, Linss G et al 1992 Localisation of gene for the nevoid basal-cell carcinoma syndrome. Lancet 339: 617

Rekate H L, Grubb R L, Aram D M 1985 Muteness of cerebellar origin. Archives of Neurology 42: 697–698

Rice J S, Fischer D S 1962 Blue rubber bleb nevus syndrome. Archives of Dermatology 86: 503–511

Roberts R O, Lynch C F, Jones M P, Hart M N 1991 Medulloblastoma: a population-based study of 532 cases. Journal of Neuropathology and Experimental Neurology 50: 134–144

Rollins N, Mendelsohn D, Mulne A, Barton R, Diehl J, Reyes N, Sklar F 1990 Recurrent medulloblastoma: frequency of tumor enhancement on Gd-DTPA MR imaging. American Journal of Neuroradiology 11: 583–587

Rottinger E, Bailey C, Bamberg M et al 1992 Medulloblastoma: Influence of quality of radiotherapy on prognosis. SIOP XXIV Meeting: 387 (proceedings)

Russell D S, Rubinstein L J 1989 Pathology of tumors of the nervous system, 5th edn. Edward Arnold, London

Salvati M, Missori P, Lunardi P, Orlando E R 1991 Transient cerebellar mutism after posterior cranial fossa surgery in an adult. Case report and review of the literature. Clinical Neurology and Neurosurgery 93: 313–316

Santibanez-Koref M F, Birch J M et al 1991 p53 germline mutations in Li-Fraumeni syndrome. Lancet 338: 1490–1491

Schiffer D, Giordana M T, Vigliani M C 1989 Brain tumors of childhood: nosological and diagnostic problems. Child's Nervous System 5: 220–229

Schiffer D, Giordana M T, Pezzotta S, Pezzulo T, Vigliani M C 1992 Medullomyoblastoma: report of two cases. Child's Nervous System 8: 268–272

Schoefield D E 1992 Diagnostic histopathology, cytogenetics and molecular markers of pediatric brain tumors. Neurosurgical Clinics of North America 3: 723–738

Schofield D E, Yunis E J, Geyer J R, Albright A L, Berger M S, Taylor S R 1992 DNA content and other prognostic features in childhood medulloblastoma. Proposal of a scoring system. Cancer 69: 1307–1314

Schuster J, Friedman H, Bigner D 1991 Therapeutic analysis of in vitro and in vivo brain tumor models. Neurology Clinics 9: 375–382

Schut L, Bruce D A, Sutton L N 1985 Medulloblastoma. In: Wilkins R H, Rengachary J J (eds) Neurosurgety I. McGraw-Hill, New York, pp. 758–761

Shen W C, Yang C F 1988 Multifocal cerebellar medulloblastoma: CT findings. Journal of Computer Assisted Tomography 12: 894

Spagnoli D, Tomei G, Masini B, DeSantis A, Grimoldi N, Lucarini C, Gaini S M 1990 A case of multifocal cerebellar medulloblastoma in an adult patient. Journal of Neurosurgical Science 34: 323–325

Steinbok P, Boyd M, Cochrane D 1989 Cervical spine deformity following craniotomy and upper cervical laminectomy for posterior fossa tumors in children. Child's Nervous System 5: 25–28

Stiller C A, Bunch K J 1992 Brain and spinal tumours in children aged under two years: incidence and survival in Britain, 1971–85. British Journal of Cancer (suppl) Aug. 18: S50–53

Szymas J, Biczysko W, Gabryel P, Morkowski S 1987 Medulloblastoma: histological evaluation and prognosis. Child's Nervous System 3: 74–80

Tait D M, Thornton J H, Bloom H et al 1990 Adjuvant chemotherapy for medulloblastoma: The first multi-centre control trial of the International Society of Paediatric Oncology (SIOPI). European Journal of Cancer 26: 464–469

Taomoto K, Tomita T, Raimondi A J, Leetsma J E 1987 Medulloblastoma in childhood: histological factors influencing patient's outcome. Child's Nervous System 3: 345–360

Tarbell N J, Loeffler J S, Silver B et al 1991 The change in patterns of relapse in medulloblastoma. Cancer 68: 1600–1604

Thomas G A, Raffel C 1991 Loss of heterozygosity on 6q, 16q and 17p in human central nervous system primitive neuroectodermal tumors. Cancer Research 51: 639–643

Tijssen C C 1986 Genetic factors and family studies in medulloblastoma. In: Zeltzer P M, Pochedly C (eds). Praeger, New York

Tomita T, Yasue M, Engelhard H H, McLone D G, Gonzalez-Crussi F, Bauer K D 1988 Flow cytometric DNA analysis of medulloblastoma. Prognostic implication of aneuploidy. Cancer 61: 744–749

Tsanaclis A M, Brem S S, Gately S, Schipper H M, Wang E 1991 Statin immunolocalization in human brain tumors. Detection of noncycling cells using a novel marker of cell quiescence. Cancer 68(4): 786–792

Vieco P T, Azooz E M, Hoeffel J C 1989 Metastases to bone in medulloblastoma. A report of 5 cases. Skeletal Radiology 18: 445–449

Vieco P T, Azooz E M, Hoeffel J C et al 1991 Medulloblastoma: freedom from relapse longer than 8 years — a therapeutic cure? Journal of Neurosurgery 75: 575–582

Wakai S, Andoh Y, Ochiai C 1990 Postoperative contrast enhancement in brain tumors and intracerebral hematomas; CT study. Journal of Computer Assisted Tomography 14: 267–271

Waluch V, Dyck P 1990 Magnetic resonance imaging of posterior fossa masses. In: Wilkins R H, Rengachary S S (eds) Neurosurgery update I. McGraw-Hill, New York, pp 30–46

Yoshida J, Yamamoto R, Wakabayashi T, Nagata M, Seo H 1990 Radioimmunoassay of glioma-associated antigen in cerebrospinal fluid and its usefulness for the diagnosis and monitoring of human glioma [see Comments]. CM Comment in Journal of Neuro-Oncology 1991, Aug. 11 81. SOJ Neuro-Oncology, 1990 Feb. 8: 23–31

Zebrini C, Gelber R D, Weinberg D et al 1993 Prognostic factors in medulloblastoma, including DNA ploidy. Journal of Clinical Oncology 11: 616–622

Zee C S, Segall H D, Miller C et al 1982 Less common CT features of medulloblastoma. Radiology 144: 97–102

Zimmerman R A, Bilawick C T, Pahlajani H 1978 Spectrum of medulloblastoma demonstrated by computer tomography. Radiology 126: 137–141

PART III

Nerve sheath tumors

31. Acoustic neurinoma (vestibular schwannoma)

Robert Macfarlane   T. T. King

INCIDENCE AND PREVALENCE OF TUMOR

Epidemiology

Acoustic neurinomas (vestibular schwannomas) account for approximately 6–8% of all primary intracranial tumors, and are responsible for about 78% of lesions which develop within the cerebellopontine angle (Cushing 1932, Revilla 1947). However, the percentage differs considerably in more recent series, due probably to variations in the referral base. Tumors are bilateral in around 4–5% of cases.

With one exception, there have been no large studies to determine the incidence of acoustic neurinoma in a well-defined geographic population. Tos et al (1992a) have estimated an annual detection rate of 9.4 tumors per year per million inhabitants of Denmark. This is much lower than estimates based upon anatomic studies of autopsy material. Hardy & Crowe (1936) found 6 minute and asymptomatic schwannomas in a study of 250 temporal bones, an incidence of 2.4%. In a similar study, Leonard & Talbot (1970) suggested an incidence of around 1.7%. However, postmortem studies may have overestimated the true incidence of this condition. The fact that audiometry was available in the cadavers studied, and that the specimens were not consecutive, suggests that the material may have been biased to temporal bones with pre-existing hearing disorders. In a more recent and unselected postmortem study of 298 temporal bones, Karjalainen et al (1984) found no occult neurinomas. In a clinical series of 9176 patients investigated for otoneurological disorders, only 0.76% were found to harbor a cerebellopontine angle tumor, some of which were acoustic neurinomas (Guyot et al 1992).

Whatever the true incidence of the condition, the disparity between clinical and pathological studies does suggest that a substantial number of lesions remain asymptomatic or undiagnosed, and that occult neurinomas may follow a benign course (Brackmann & Kwartler 1990a). An increase in the number of tumors treated in the last decade is more likely to represent better awareness of the condition and earlier diagnosis, than to suggest a true increase in the prevalence of the disease (Glasscock 1987, Tos et al 1992a).

Growth rate

The natural history of acoustic neurinomas is variable, and is reflected in marked differences in the duration of symptoms at the time of presentation. Usually such tumors are slow-growing. In some series, around 40% of tumors treated conservatively did not enlarge at all, or even regressed over the period of observation (Luetje et al 1988, Valvassori & Guzman 1989, Thomsen & Tos 1990). On average, lesion diameter will increase at a rate of less than 2 mm per year in around 78% of patients (Nedzelski et al 1992). In other instances the rate of growth is more rapid, at between 2.5 and 4 mm per year (Wazen et al 1985, Laasonen & Troupp 1986). The rate of expansion may however be considerably slower in the elderly, where a mean enlargement of 1.4 mm per year has been reported (Sterkers et al 1992). This is in contrast to a study by Valvassori & Guzman (1989), who concluded that there is no correlation between the rate of tumor growth and patient age. Yet there does exist an inverse relationship between age and tumor size at presentation. Large tumors are significantly more common in the younger age groups (Thomsen et al 1992).

It is believed that the future behavior of a tumor can be predicted radiologically within a relatively short period of observation. A pattern of slow or absent growth over a period of 18 months to 3 years makes it unlikely that subsequent enlargement will be significant (Nedzelski et al 1992). Valvassori & Guzman (1989) reached a similar conclusion in a study of 35 patients managed expectantly. Any further growth was evident usually within the first year. On the other hand, Norén & Greitz (1992) studied 98 tumors in 93 patients over a period of 12–183 months and observed that 66% of tumors increased in size over 1–2 years, that 86% enlarged when observed for 3–4 years, but that 100% had expanded if follow-up was continued for more than 4 years.

Flow cytometric studies have confirmed a variable mitotic rate in acoustic neurinomas, and have shown that this correlates clinically with the speed of tumor growth (Wennerberg & Mercke 1989). DNA cytofluorometric analysis has been used also to establish the proportion of cells in the 'S' phase of the cell cycle, but this is not linked to tumor size, nor to the duration of symptoms at the time of presentation (Rasmussen et al 1984). These data are supported by the results of clinical studies, which have shown no statistical correlation between tumor size at diagnosis and the rate of subsequent growth (Nedzelski et al 1992). Large tumors do not necessarily grow faster than smaller ones. Factors other than mitotic activity which govern the rate of expansion of these lesions include hemorrhage, cystic degeneration, and peritumoral edema. Any of these may, on occasion, result in precipitate enlargement of the tumor (Nager 1969, Lee & Wang 1989).

A hormone related closely to bovine pituitary growth factor may play a role in Schwann cell proliferation in acoustic neurinoma (Brockes et al 1986). Other hormone receptors have also been identified in a varying proportion of tumors. Amongst them are estrogen and progesterone receptors, although neither of these is thought to govern growth behavior, despite a female preponderance of tumors (Markwalder et al 1986, Whittle et al 1987). Estrogen binding receptors are present in 45% of male and 48% of female neurinomas (Martuza et al 1981). There are, however, reports of an increase in size and vascularity of tumors in women, particularly during pregnancy (Allen et al 1974). Recent evidence suggests that a variety of tumors may secrete their own ('autocrine') growth factors, which bind to specific receptors on the cell membrane and stimulate it to traverse the cell cycle more quickly (for review see Rutka et al 1990).

The growth rate of bilateral tumors is also very variable, but is on average considerably faster than for unilateral lesions (Kasantikul et al 1980a). However it is uncertain whether this reflects a different biology for these neoplasms, or the fact that they occur in a younger patient population — a subgroup which are known already to exhibit a more rapid rate of growth (Graham & Sataloff 1984).

AGE DISTRIBUTION

Acoustic neurinomas occur most frequently in middle age. In a series of 500 cases reported by the House group, approximately 50% of patients were in either their fifth or sixth decades, and only 15% of tumors developed in people under the age of 30 (Fig. 31.1). Acoustic neurinomas which develop in patients suffering from neurofibromatosis tend to present earlier, with a peak incidence around the third decade (Revilla 1947, Eldridge 1981, Evans et al 1992a). It is very rare for acoustic neurinomas to develop in children, except those who have neurofibromatosis type 2 (Allcutt et al 1991). The youngest recorded patient was 12 months of age (Fabiani et al 1975). Presentation often occurs late in children because unilateral deafness may be overlooked (Allcutt et al 1991). An association between acoustic neurinoma, salivary gland tumors, and childhood cranial irradiation has been reported (Shore-Freedman et al 1983).

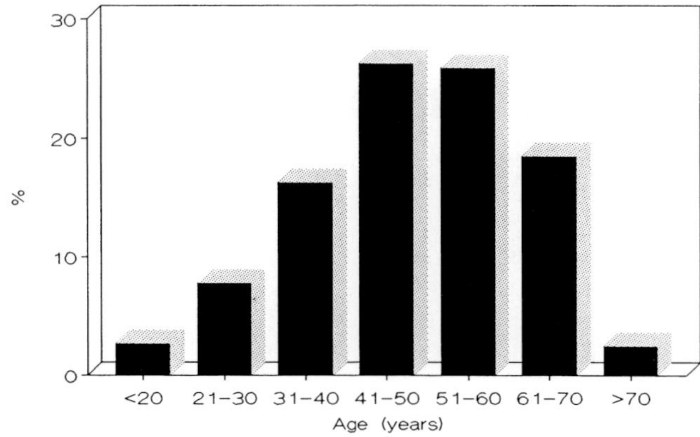

Fig. 31.1 Age distribution of a cumulative series of 1113 cases of acoustic neurinoma.

SEX DISTRIBUTION

Cumulative results from large series in the literature show a consistent preponderance of tumors in women who are affected in around 57%, and men in 43% of cases (Fig. 31.2). This however is not true of tumors in childhood, where an equal sex distribution is seen (Hernanz-Schulman et al 1986). A difference in the age distribution of tumors between the sexes was noted by Borck & Zulch (1951). Men had an earlier peak prevalence (36–42 years) than women (42–56 years), although this finding has not been confirmed by later work.

RACIAL, NATIONAL, AND GEOGRAPHIC CONSIDERATIONS

There have to date been no large multinational studies to determine demographic factors relating to acoustic

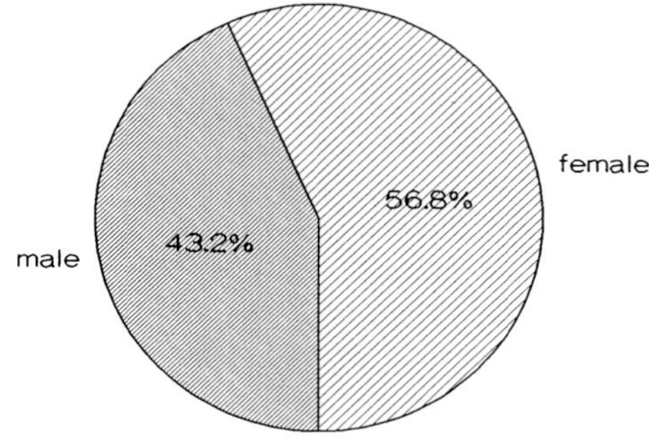

Fig. 31.2 Distribution of tumors by sex.

neurinoma. However, the proportion which these tumors contribute to the total number of primary intracranial neoplasms varies considerably in different populations. Unfortunately this does not provide a complete profile of the condition because it depends also on the prevalence of other primary tumors. The incidence of acoustic neurinoma appears to be greatest in the Far East, where they account for 10.6% of primary intracranial neoplasms in India (Dastur et al 1968) and 10.2% of those which occur in China (Huang et al 1982). In the Middle East, a 9% incidence is found in Egypt (Sorour et al 1973). Rates of 4.9% and 4% are reported in England (Barker et al 1976) and the USA respectively (Kurland et al 1982). The lowest incidence is found in African negroes, with figures of 2.6% recorded in Kenya (Ruberti & Poppi 1971), 0.9% in Nigeria (Adeloye 1979), and 0.5% in what was formerly Rhodesia. The latter can be contrasted with a 3.7% incidence in the white population of the same country (Levy & Auchterlonie 1975). Misdiagnosis may, however, play some part in the low incidence rates reported in Africans. With the use of immunohistochemical markers Simpson et al (1990) established that some acoustic neurinomas had been misdiagnosed as meningiomas, and they concluded that the true incidence in black South Africans was 3.7%. In our experience acoustic neurinomas are very uncommon in negroes, and few if any such families have ever been documented to develop bilateral forms of the disease. Although we are not aware of any studies on social factors, the condition appears to be more common in middle than lower social classes. This may be because the latter are less likely to seek medical attention for relatively minor symptoms.

GENETIC FACTORS

Acoustic neurinomas occur in both sporadic and hereditary forms. Unilateral sporadic tumors account for 96% of cases, and the presence of such a lesion does not predispose the patient to develop other neoplasms, nor is there genetic transmission to their offspring. Hereditary acoustic neurinomas result from NF-2 (bilateral acoustic neurinomas; central neurofibromatosis) or, doubtfully, from NF-1 (von Recklinghausen's disease; peripheral neurofibromatosis). Both are autosomal dominant conditions with a high degree of penetrance. Bilateral acoustic neurinoma was, until recently, regarded as a central form of von Recklinghausen's disease. However, in 1980, Kanter et al concluded that the two conditions were distinct, and this has been confirmed subsequently by chromosomal studies. NF-1 is much more common than NF-2, and has an incidence of 1/4000 population (Korf 1990). It is characterized by widespread neuromas occurring both intra- and extracranially. With the use of recombinant DNA studies the genetic defect in NF-1 has been localized to chromosome 17 (Barker et al 1987). However, unilateral acoustic neurinomas are seen in only 2–4% of patients with NF-1 (Holt 1978), and bilateral tumors are exceptionally rare (Rubinstein 1986). A recent study demonstrated no increase in the incidence of acoustic neurinoma in NF-1, and reports of bilateral tumors may in fact represent misdiagnosis of what should correctly be defined as NF-2 (Huson et al 1988). Given the heterogeneity of neurofibromatosis (for review see Riccardi & Eichner 1986), some variations in classification are inevitable.

NF-2 occurs in about 1/33–50 000 individuals (Evans et al 1992a). The spontaneous mutation rate is around 50%. Bilateral acoustic neurinomas are pathognomonic of this condition, but are not fully penetrant. Other cranial and spinal tumors may also develop. The mean age at onset of symptoms is 22 years, and at diagnosis 28 years (Evans et al 1992a). Café-au-lait patches are found in 41% of patients, and presenile lens opacity or subcapsular cataract in 38% (Evans et al 1992b). As well as bilateral acoustic neurinomas, the definition of NF-2 also encompasses individuals who have a first-degree relative suffering from the condition and who have either a unilateral acoustic neurinoma or two of the following: a neurofibroma or schwannoma, meningioma, glioma, or juvenile posterior subcapsular lenticular opacity. The natural history of NF-2 is variable, and males may sometimes have a milder form of the disease than that which is seen in females. The age at onset of symptoms is significantly younger in maternally than paternally affected cases (18.2 vs 24.5 years; Evans et al 1992a). Both the acoustic neurinomas do not always develop simultaneously, although this is usual. A span of a few months or several years may at times separate them.

Using the technique of linkage analysis, the gene responsible for the control of Schwann cell growth has been localized to the long arm of chromosome 22 (Martuza & Eldridge 1988). Chromosome 22, although one of the smallest, is genetically very active, and spontaneous mutations are thought to be common. Genes on this chromosome are believed to be responsible for a number of inherited and acquired tumors (Kaplan et al 1987). Regulation of Schwann cell growth is under the control of a suppressor gene, the NF-2 gene. This nomenclature is both unfortunate and rather confusing, in that a defect in the NF-2 gene is thought to be responsible for both sporadic and bilateral (NF-2) forms of the tumor (Seizinger et al 1986). Using polymorphic DNA markers to search for loss of particular chromosome regions, Seizinger and co-workers were able to identify that 44% of 16 sporadic acoustic neurinomas showed loss of constitutional heterozygosity on chromosome 22. The difference between sporadic and hereditary forms of the disease is that the defect in bilateral acoustic neurinoma is present in the germ cell line. The patient inherits only one copy of the tumor suppressor gene, and undergoes spontaneous mutation of the other antioncogene in a somatic cell. In sporadic forms, homozygous mutation of both NF-2 genes has to occur in one specific Schwann cell precursor. A subset of NF-2 patients (called NF-2 deletional) inherit a defect in the NF-2 genes, not only of Schwann cells, but in all cells. In addition to bilateral acoustic neurinoma, these patients are prone also to develop multiple meningiomas (Lanser 1992).

The gene responsible for NF-2 has been localized to chromosome 22 (Seizinger et al 1986, Rouleau et al 1987), determined in part from showing loss of heterozygosity for portions of the long arm of that chromosome in vestibular schwannomas that occur sporadically, separate from NF-2, or in such tumors occurring as part of NF-2. The gene for NF-2 was specifically identified and its characterization begun in early 1993 (Bianchi et al 1994). A recent report from Harvard has added further information (Trofatter et al 1993). The product of this gene is a novel protein related to other cytoskeletal proteins that link the cell membrane to the cytoskeleton. Until such time that the gene can be reproducibly screened for, Evans et al (1992b) have described a protocol for the screening of subjects at risk of NF-2. (The references for Seizinger, Rouleau and Bianchi are in Chapter 34, the reference for Trofatter is in Chapter 35.)

Acoustic neurinoma has been described also as a component of Carney's complex — a syndrome comprising myxomas, spotty pigmentation, and endocrine overactivity (Carney et al 1985, 1986, Mansell et al 1991). This syndrome is usually sporadic, although autosomal dominant inheritance has been reported (Carney et al 1986).

SITES OF PREDILECTION

Acoustic neurinomas are thought to arise at the point where glial (central) nerve sheaths are replaced by those of Schwann (peripheral) cells and fibroblasts. This transition (the Obersteiner-Redlich zone) is located usually within the internal auditory canal. The variability of this demarcation, however, means that some tumors arise laterally within the internal auditory meatus, whilst others lie entirely within the cerebellopontine angle (Neely & Hough 1986). Although it was at one time believed that tumors arose primarily from the superior vestibular nerve, evidence now suggests an almost equal incidence of superior and inferior vestibular nerve lesions (Clemis et al 1986). Only rarely is the cochlear division involved (Bebin 1979). Clemis et al (1986) concluded that 50–60% of tumors arose from the superior vestibular nerve, 40–50% from the inferior vestibular nerve, and that less than 10% were derived from the cochlear nerve. The reason why this neoplasm should arise so frequently from the vestibular nerve is unknown, but it does contain an excess of the embryonic precursors of Schwann cells (Bebin 1979). Neurinomas can arise from other nerves within the temporal bone, and at times it may be impossible to determine their nerve of origin (Best 1968).

PRESENTING FEATURES

Unilateral sensorineural hearing loss, tinnitus, and dysequilibrium are the most common presenting symptoms, although only about 10% of patients with such features will be found on investigation to harbor an acoustic neurinoma (Valvassori & Potter 1982). The mode of presentation is dependent on tumor size, and whether or not early symptoms are overlooked. In the past four decades there has been a steady increase in the proportion of small tumors detected and, therefore, a shift in the pattern of symptoms away from those due to mass effect (Symon et al 1989). The most common symptoms of acoustic neurinoma are unilateral sensorineural hearing loss (96%), unsteadiness (77%), tinnitus (71%), mastoid pain or otalgia (28%), headache (29%), facial numbness (7%) and diplopia (7%) (Hardy et al 1989a). Only around one third of patients first seek medical attention for nonaudiologic complaints (Hart et al 1983) and, at the time of presentation, only around 50% of patients will have objective neurological findings other than from the eighth nerve.

Unilateral or asymmetric sensorineural hearing loss is almost always the initial symptom, and has been present usually for a median of 1–3 years at the time of diagnosis (Johnson 1977). If hearing loss is neglected, however, there follows a 'silent' interval, usually of 1–4 years, although it may be much longer, while the tumor expands into the cerebellopontine angle cistern. Symptoms then ensue from compression of the cerebellum, adjacent cranial nerves, or the brainstem. With lesions larger than 4 cm, 58% of patients will exhibit cerebellar dysfunction, and 53% will have corneal or facial hypesthesia (Thomsen et al 1983).

Hearing loss

Patients with unilateral or bilateral asymmetric sensorineural deafness or with unexplained unilateral tinnitus should be investigated to exclude an acoustic neurinoma. Speech discrimination may be affected more than the pure tone loss, and can cause difficulty when using the telephone. Loudness recruitment is uncommon. Although hearing loss is most often progressive it can on occasions be sudden, due perhaps to compromise of the inner ear vasculature. The incidence of sudden hearing loss varies between series, but is around 10–20% (Sataloff et al 1985). Yet, of patients who present with sudden hearing loss, in only around 1% will the cause be found to be an acoustic neurinoma (Shaia & Sheehy 1976). Rarely, hearing loss fluctuates (Pensak et al 1985, Berg et al 1986). Only about 5% of patients with acoustic neurinoma will have normal hearing. This is more likely to occur if the tumor is very small, or if it is confined to the cerebellopontine angle cistern and there is no significant intracanalicular component (Beck et al 1986).

Delayed or missed diagnosis is more likely if the presentation is atypical, or if hearing loss is attributed by the patient to a specific event. It is particularly likely if the patient suffers already from a longstanding ear disorder such as Meniere's disease. The other group likely to be missed are those with normal results in investigations which are almost always abnormal in cases of acoustic neurinoma (pure tone audiometry and auditory evoked brainstem responses; see below). Rarely, a cochlear rather than a retrocochlear pattern of hearing loss develops (Flood & Brightwell 1984).

Dysequilibrium

Because the tumor origin is nearly always from the vestibular nerve, dysequilibrium and vertigo are common. True paroxysmal vertigo is rare (6.3%; Morrison 1975), and is only occasionally accompanied by nausea. The onset is not usually abrupt, as it is in Meniere's disease, although 5% of acoustic neurinoma patients will give a history that would be accepted as typical of that condition. Whilst mild chronic dysequilibrium has often been present for some years before diagnosis, it is unusual for either ataxia or vertigo to be the presenting complaint. The reason why destruction of the vestibular nerve is not often disabling lies with the brainstem and contralateral vestibular apparatus, which compensate for the loss. The elderly, however, appear less well able to adapt to this change.

Clinically, mild abnormalities of balance may be detected by Unterberger's stepping test (Moffat et al 1989a). The patient is asked to stand upright with eyes closed, with the arms outstretched at 90° to the trunk, and then to mark time on the spot (i.e. to raise the legs alternately, bringing the thigh to a horizontal position). The result is positive if the patient deviates more than 50 cm from the spot, or rotates by more than 30° within 50 steps. The presence of severe ataxia is more likely to suggest that the patient has developed compression of the cerebellum, or has obstructive hydrocephalus secondary to distortion of the brainstem. Involvement of the cerebellum causes incoordination, primarily of the lower limbs, and a tendency for the patient to deviate to the side of the tumor. Brainstem compression may also involve the sensory and motor tracts, usually of the contralateral side.

Tinnitus

Tinnitus is the presenting symptom in around 3% of patients (Wiegand & Fickel 1989), and is occasionally the sole manifestation of acoustic neurinoma. Preoperative tinnitus affects 57–83% of patients, but is troublesome in only 13–38% (Brow 1979, Wiegand & Fickel 1989). Symptoms are usually low grade, constant, and confined to the affected ear. There is great variation in the type of sounds experienced.

Raised intracranial pressure

Papilledema is almost exclusive to lesions larger than 3 cm in diameter, and is present in around 7–15% of patients (Hardy et al 1989a, Boesen et al 1992). Large tumors displace the cerebellum and deform the brainstem, compressing the fourth ventricle or aqueduct. Associated features of spontaneous nystagmus, opticokinetic nystagmus, and trigeminal nerve dysfunction are significantly more common in patients with papilledema than in cases in which the tumor is of a comparable size, but where swelling of the optic discs is absent (Boesen et al 1992). Very large tumors may result in herniation of the cerebellar tonsils.

Nystagmus

Nystagmus may be spontaneous, positional (when the neck is hyperextended and the head turned to right or left), or opticokinetic (driven in response to an image slip on the retina from a rotating target). The latter may be evident if there is significant compression of the gaze center in the pons (Thomsen et al 1983). The most common type is unilateral labyrinthine nystagmus, which is evident as fine horizontal beats directed away from the side of the lesion. It is of peripheral vestibular origin, and is enhanced by abolition of ocular fixation using Frenzel's glasses. In about 16% of patients nystagmus will be of Bruns type, which is indicative of a large tumor producing significant brainstem distortion. It comprises bidirectional nystagmus, with a coarse gaze-evoked nystagmus on looking to the ipsilateral side, and a high-frequency small amplitude vestibular nystagmus on looking to the contralateral side (Croxson et al 1988). Electronystagmography will demonstrate impaired vestibular function in over 80% of cases, but is a nonspecific finding and, therefore, of limited diagnostic value.

Cranial nerve palsy

Trigeminal nerve involvement manifests usually as corneal or lower facial hypesthesia. Only rarely is the whole face affected, and the motor division is spared. Facial weakness is uncommon, and is almost exclusive to large tumors (Portmann & Sterkers 1975). Minor degrees of facial weakness can be detected by delay or absence of the blink reflex (Pulec & House 1964), and may be preceded by subtle facial twitching, particularly involving the orbicularis oculi muscle (Jackler & Pitts 1990). Hemifacial spasm is another rare presentation, affecting only 1% of patients. Epidermoid tumor, aneurysm, and facial neurinoma should, in particular, be considered in the differential diagnosis when hemifacial spasm is evident. Altered sensation over the posterior aspect of the external auditory canal, which is innervated by the nervus intermedius, is said to occur in 95% of patients (Hitselberger 1966). Alteration in taste is reported rarely. Facial nerve dys-

Table 31.1 Facial nerve grading system (House & Brackmann 1985)

Grade	Description	Characteristics
I	Normal	Normal facial function in all areas
II	Mild dysfunction	Gross: slight weakness noticeable on close inspection; may have very slight synkinesis At rest: normal symmetry and tone Motion: Forehead: moderate to good function Eye: complete closure with minimum effort Mouth: slight asymmetry
III	Moderate dysfunction	Gross: obvious but not disfiguring difference between two sides; noticeable but not severe synkinesis, contracture, and/or hemifacial spasm At rest: normal symmetry and tone Motion: Forehead: slight to moderate movement Eye: complete closure with effort Mouth: slightly weak with maximum effort
IV	Moderately severe dysfunction	Gross: obvious weakness and/or disfiguring asymmetry At rest: normal symmetry and tone Motion: Forehead: none Eye: incomplete closure Mouth: asymmetric with maximum effort
V	Severe dysfunction	Gross: only barely perceptible motion At rest: asymmetry Motion: Forehead: none Eye: incomplete closure Mouth: slight movement
VI	Total paralysis	No movement

function in the presence of small tumor is much more likely to suggest that the lesion is a facial neurinoma or a meningioma rather than an acoustic neurinoma.

Several classifications have been devised to grade pre- and postoperative facial nerve function. The system of House & Brackmann (1985) has gained wide support, and is shown in Table 31.1.

On occasions very large tumors will compress the nerves in the jugular foramen causing dysphagia, dysphonia, and in late cases, complete bulbar palsy. However, loss of the pharyngeal reflex or the presence of vocal cord palsy may indicate a second neurinoma in the jugular foramen if the patient suffers from neurofibromatosis.

Rarely is the abducent nerve involved directly, except by the largest of lesions. Occasionally an increase in intracranial pressure may displace the brainstem caudally, and thereby cause distortion of the sixth nerve by the anterior inferior cerebellar artery, which overlies it (Bebin 1979).

Other presenting features

Several case reports have documented exceptional presentations, which include subarachnoid hemorrhage (Gleeson et al 1978, Yonemitsu et al 1983), and tumor within the external auditory canal (Tran Ba Huy et al 1987) or middle ear (Amoils et al 1992). Intralabyrinthine schwannomas have also been reported. These may arise from either the cochlear or vestibular nerves. Here tumor is present in the inner ear, but is absent from either the internal auditory canal or the cerebellopontine angle (for review see Amoils et al 1992). Very occasionally, brainstem compression may produce symptoms contralateral to the side of the tumor. This may manifest as contralateral trigeminal nerve dysfunction (Koenig et al 1984), facial pain, or hemifacial spasm (Nishi et al 1987, Snow & Fraser 1987), although such features are much more common with meningiomas than acoustic neurinoma.

Although usually slow-growing, tumors can present with acute neurological deterioration due either to hemorrhage within the tumor (Fig. 31.3), or to rapid expansion of a cyst. Intratumoral hemorrhage is generally confined to lesions larger than 2 cm (Goetting & Swanson 1987). Rapid expansion of a cyst is said to occur in around 2% of patients (Lanser et al 1992). Acute enlargement of a lesion in the cerebellopontine angle may cause multiple cranial nerve palsies, cerebellar dysfunction, and brainstem compromise — symptoms which could be misinterpreted as a vascular event within the posterior fossa (Lanser et al 1992).

IMAGING DIAGNOSIS

Radiology

Plain tomographs of the internal auditory canals will demonstrate enlargement of the porus acousticus in around

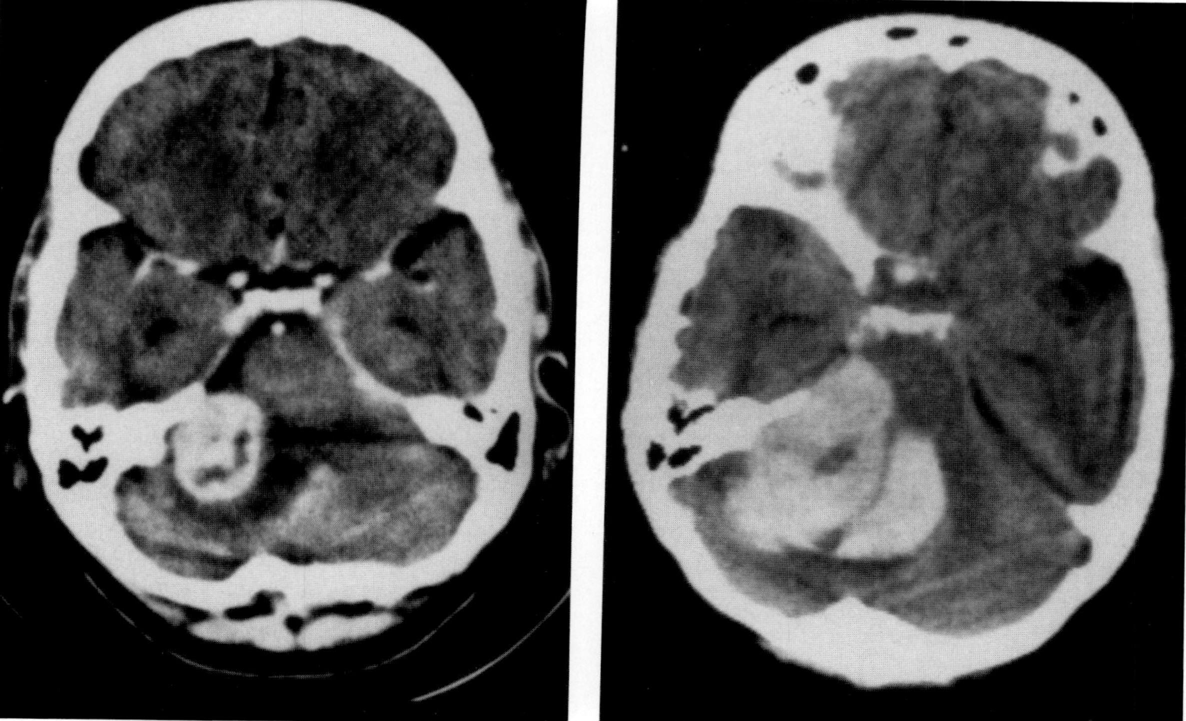

Fig. 31.3 **Left.** Contrast-enhanced CT scan of a large, partially cystic acoustic neurinoma. **Right.** Repeat CT scan following acute deterioration whilst awaiting surgery, showing hemorrhage within the tumor.

80–90% of tumors. Pressure from the tumor causes enlargement of the canal by stimulating osteoclastic activity, although it does not cause necrosis of the dural lining (Pulec & House 1964). A disparity of more than 1–2 mm between the two sides is significant, particularly if it is accompanied by a difference in canal shape, by the presence of bone erosion, or if there is shortening of the posterior canal wall (Fig. 31.4; Valvassori 1984). However, a normal tomograph does not exclude the diagnosis. Pulec et al (1971) found that approximately 10% of tomographs

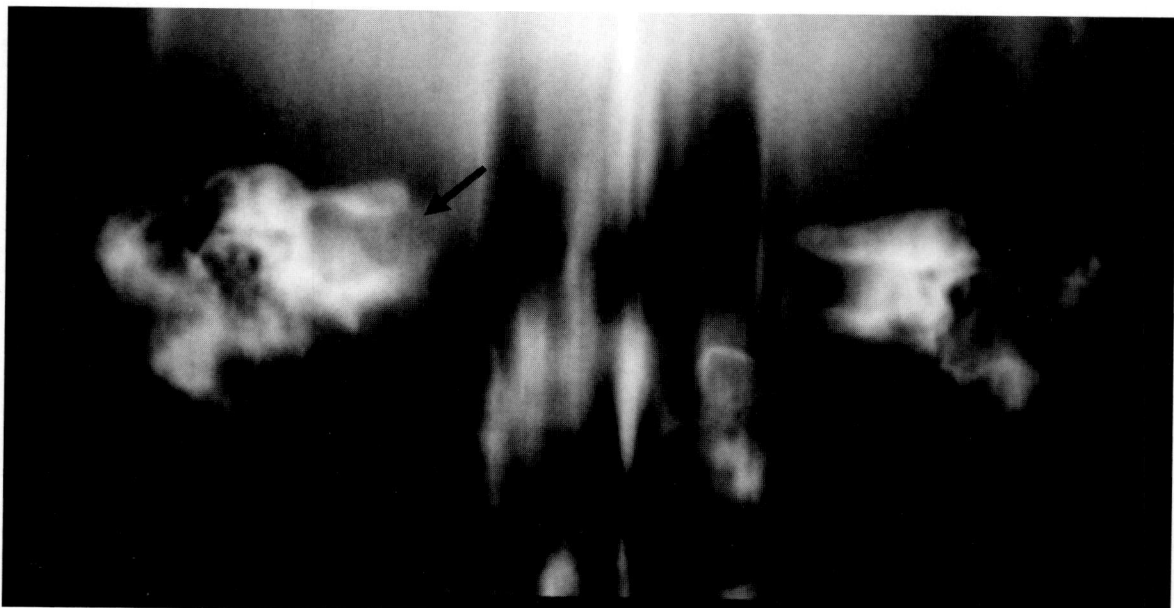

Fig. 31.4 Plain tomograms of the internal auditory meatus showing enlargement of the porus acousticus (arrow), and an alteration in canal shape.

were normal, and Ojemann et al (1972) reported this in 18% of their patients. Positive contrast cistemography has in the past been used as an adjunct for the diagnosis of small tumors, but has now been superseded by computerized axial tomography (CT) and magnetic resonance imaging (MRI).

Computed tomography

Prior to the introduction of MRI, CT was the primary radiologic method for diagnosis (Curtin 1984). Contrast-enhanced CT, with 5 mm axial slices through the skull base, will detect all but the smallest soft tissue masses within the cerebellopontine angle. In one series of 131 cases there were no false negative scans (Harner & Reese 1984), but others have reported a false positive rate of 0.6% (Charabi et al 1992). The center of each internal auditory meatus should be included if a small intrameatal tumor is not to be missed as a result of the partial volume effect. The characteristic CT appearance is of an iso- or hypodense lesion centered upon the internal auditory meatus, with homogeneous enhancement after intravenous contrast (Fig. 31.5). Cerebellopontine angle meningiomas may have similar appearances, but are usually hyperdense prior to contrast injection, and commonly are placed asymmetrically in relation to the porus acousticus. Erosion of the porus is rare in meningioma, but may be seen on the posterior surface of the petrous pyramid — a very uncommon occurrence in all except the largest of acoustic neurinomas. A further feature for differentiating an acoustic neurinoma from a meningioma is the configuration seen at the boundary between tumor and dura. Meningiomas generally have a flat broad-based attachment to the petrous bone, whereas the angle between the tumor and the petrous bone should be acute in cases of acoustic neurinoma (Wu et al 1986). Enhancement of the dural edge adjacent to the main tumor bulk is also highly suggestive of meningioma (Aoki et al 1990), as is the presence of calcification, which will be evident in 25% of cases (Moller et al 1978). Macroscopic calcification is exceptional in acoustic neurinomas (Thomsen et al 1984).

Of the imaging modalities currently available, CT is the most suitable for delineation of the bony anatomy. Bone detail is important for several reasons. Firstly, it may establish the diagnosis. This is true particularly for small tumors which may enhance little, but where expansion of the internal auditory meatus is an early feature (Fig. 31.6). Only on rare occasions is the meatus enlarged by a meningioma, but erosion of the temporal bone by cholesteatoma, facial neurinoma, or carcinoma may be evident, and assist in the differential diagnosis. Secondly, delineation of the anatomy of the temporal bone provides

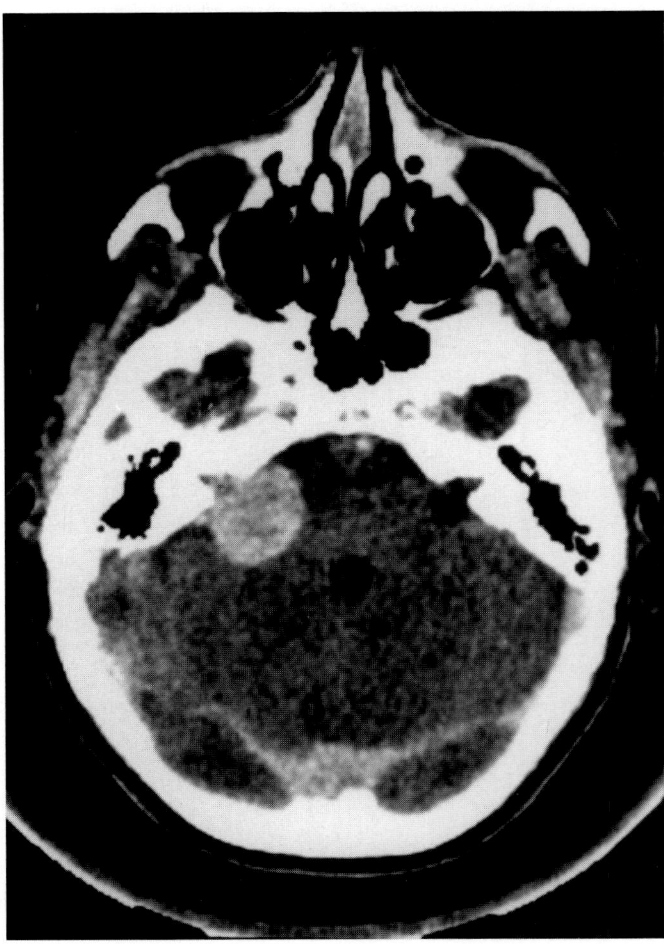

Fig. 31.5 Contrast-enhanced CT scan showing a uniformly enhancing tumor centered on the porus acoustics.

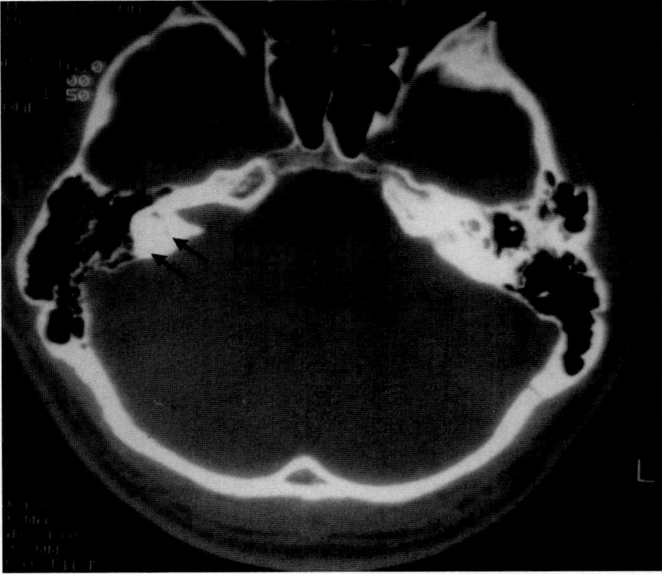

Fig. 31.6 High resolution CT scan of the petrous bones. There is expansion of the internal auditory meatus by an intracanalicular acoustic neurinoma. The mastoid bone is well pneumatized, and the relationship of the posterior semicircular canal (arrows) to the fundus of the internal meatus is evident.

useful information to assist the surgeon. The size of the inferior perimeatal and perilabyrinthine air cells should be noted. A high jugular bulb can be anticipated if the temporal bone is poorly pneumatized (Graham 1975) whereas, if the mastoid is well pneumatized, air cells may extend medially almost to the porus. This increases the likelihood of postoperative CSF leakage when the posterior wall of the internal auditory meatus is removed, and alerts the surgeon to pay particular attention to seal them. High resolution CT may be used also to identify the relationship between the semicircular canals, the vestibule, and the internal auditory meatus (Fig. 31.6). This is important when hearing conservation procedures are contemplated via a suboccipital approach. If the posterior semicircular canal or crus commune lie medial to an imaginary line drawn between the medial aspect of the sigmoid sinus and fundus of the internal auditory canal, they are at risk of injury when the intracanalicular portion of the tumor is exposed (Tatagiba et al 1992). Erosion of bone by tumor in the region of the jugular bulb should also be noted.

A major limiting factor of CT in the posterior fossa is the streak-like beam-hardening (Hounsfield) artefact which originates from the petrous bones, and which tends to interfere with definition in the adjacent soft tissues. The CT detection rate of small lesions can be improved by the introduction of a small amount of air into the cerebellopontine angle cistern (air contrast cisternography, Fig. 31.7), although several authors have warned of the risk of false positive scans. This may arise as a result of a meniscus effect at the gas–CSF interface, an intracanalicular loop of the anterior inferior cerebellar artery, or subdural injection of air (Khangure & Moijtahedi 1983, Barrs et al 1984a, Larsson & Holtas 1986).

MRI

MRI is now the imaging modality of choice, particularly for the detection of intracanalicular tumors (Valvassori 1984, House et al 1986, Stack et al 1988). Most acoustic neurinomas are visible on noncontrasted T1-weighted images (Fig. 31.8), but not on T2-weighted images, where the tumor may be isointense with CSF. Intravenous contrast enhancement with gadolinium-DTPA improves the detection rate of small neurinomas, which may otherwise have a signal intensity similar to that of brain parenchyma (Glasscock et al 1988, Brackmann & Kwartler 1990a). Tumors enhance markedly after gadolinium (Fig. 31.9), with which it becomes possible to detect lesions as small as 2–3 mm (Welling et al 1990). The major advantages of MRI over CT are superior contrast resolution, lack of beam-hardening artefact, the facility to image the tumor in multiple planes, and the ability to identify vascular structures and therefore assess vessel displacement or encasement. However, because cortical bone emits no signal, MRI is inferior to CT for delineation of the anatomy of the petrous temporal bone. False positive MRI has been reported occasionally as a consequence of arachnoiditis or adhesions (Haberman & Kramer 1989, von Glass et al 1991).

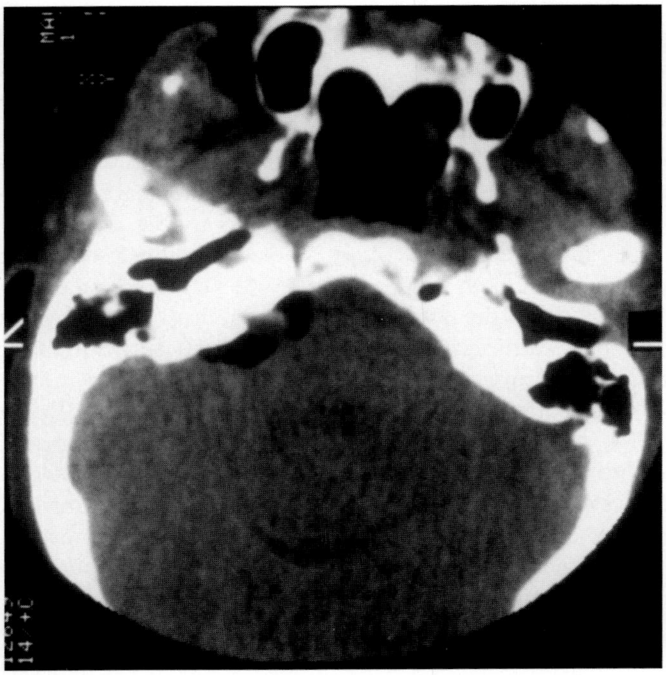

Fig. 31.7 CT air-contrast cisternogram demonstrating a small acoustic neurinoma.

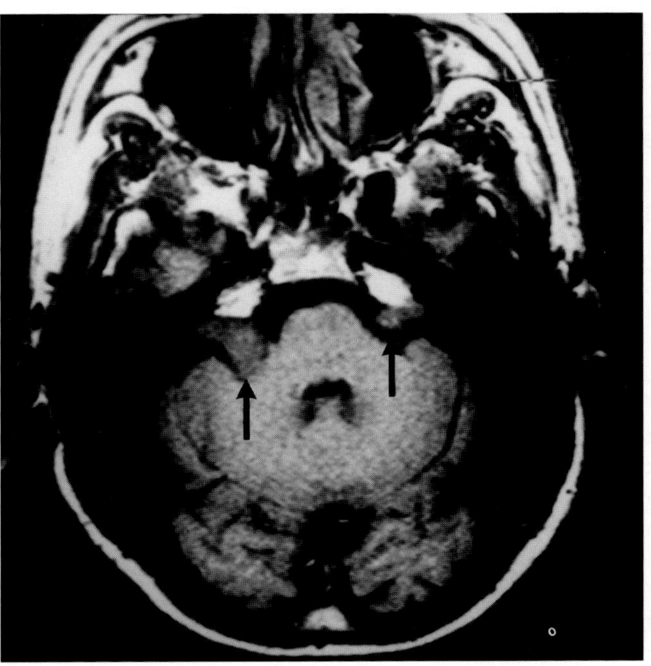

Fig. 31.8 T1-weighted axial MRI scan showing bilateral acoustic neurinomas (arrows).

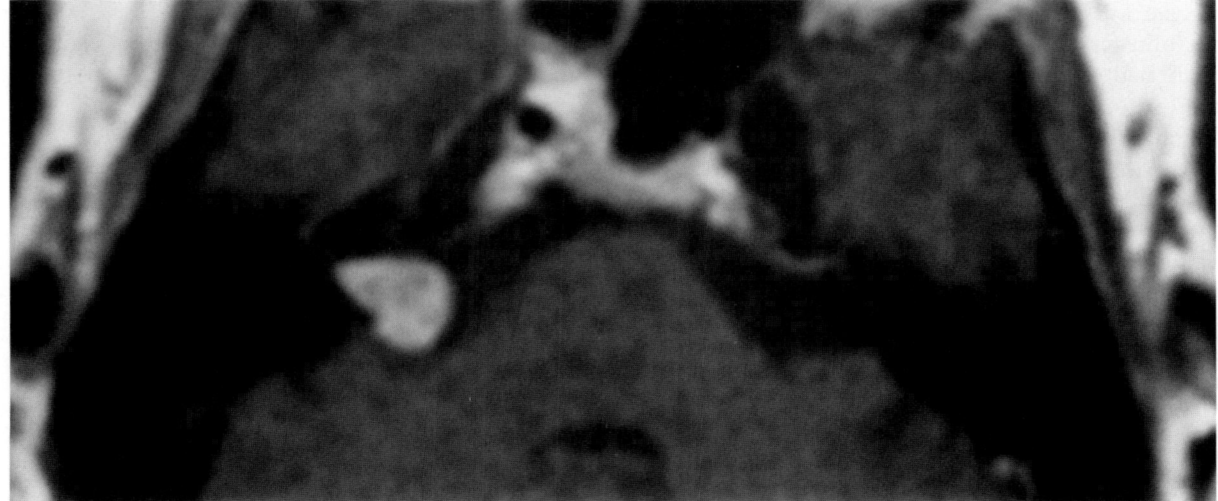

Fig. 31.9 Gadolinium-enhanced axial MRI scan of a small acoustic neurinoma.

Arteriography

The indications for this investigation have diminished considerably with the advent of CT and MRI, but it is necessary if an aneurysm or AVM is suspected in the differential diagnosis (Dalley et al 1986). Some surgeons still advocate angiography to define the vascular anatomy in relation to very large lesions. On occasions it may aid in differentiating a large acoustic neurinoma from a meningioma, particularly if a dilated tentorial artery of Bernasconi is demonstrated in the case of the latter. Angiography has been advocated also for childhood tumors, which may be extremely vascular, and where preoperative embolization is said to be beneficial (Allcutt et al 1991).

Assessment of tumor size

CT and MRI are used routinely to measure tumor size. Unfortunately there are many different classifications in current usage, none of which is accepted universally. Tumors have been classified by Pulec et al (1971) into three groups; small (intracanalicular), medium-sized (extending beyond the internal meatus but by less than 2.5 cm), and large (greater than 2.5 cm). This, and the Koos (1988) classification, are probably used more widely than most. At the recent First International Conference on Acoustic Neuroma, however, Tos & Thomsen (1992) made a plea that the following classification be adopted universally, so that reporting of results can be standardized. They have proposed that the intrameatal component (usually about 1–1.5 cm) not be included in the measurement. Size instead is measured as the largest extrameatal diameter. Tumors are classified as intrameatal, small (1–10 mm), medium (11–25 mm), large (26–40 mm), and extra large (> 40 mm). It remains to be seen whether this becomes the accepted scheme, or just one more to add to the bewildering myriad already in existence. It appears likely that, with the advent of computerized three-dimensional reconstruction imaging, tumor volume rather than maximum diameter will become ultimately the measurement upon which these lesions are graded.

LABORATORY DIAGNOSIS

Audiometry

Air, bone, and speech hearing tests are the mainstay screening procedures for acoustic neurinoma. High frequency hearing loss is the most common abnormality seen on pure tone audiometry (PTA) (Johnson 1977). Only 5% of patients will have normal hearing with good speech discrimination (Beck et al 1986), making PTA an important and reliable test in routine neuro-otological investigation. The pattern of hearing loss is variable. In several large series hearing loss was reported variously as being primarily of a high frequency in 35–66%, low frequency in 4–9%, whilst the audiogram was flat in 13–18% (pure tone pattern differing by not more than 10 dB throughout the speech range), trough-shaped in 4–12%, and in 16–27% of patients the ear was dead (Johnson 1977, Bebin 1979, Hardy et al 1989a). The likelihood of abnormal audiometry correlates with tumor size (Johnson 1977). However, even when the pure tone audiogram is normal, speech discrimination is often impaired, and almost all such patients will exhibit abnormalities also on auditory evoked brainstem response testing (Musiek et al 1986). Tone decay and the absence of recruitment are also characteristic audiological findings (Johnson 1977). Other audiometric parameters include Bekesey audiometry, the SISI test, alternate bilateral loudness balance (ABLB) tests and the acoustic reflex test. A full account can be found in Johnson (1979), although these 'site of lesion' tests are applied only rarely in modern practice.

Speech discrimination

Speech discrimination is not related simply to the degree of pure tone hearing loss. Some patients may have exceptionally poor speech discrimination despite near-normal pure tone audiometry. Speech discrimination scores in a series of 425 cases of acoustic neurinoma were 0% in 35% of patients, very poor (2–30% discrimination score) in 21%, moderate to poor (32–60% discrimination) in 16%, and moderate to good (62–100%) in the remaining 28% of cases (Johnson 1977). In total, only 20% of patients with acoustic neurinoma had good speech discrimination.

The speech discrimination score is an important consideration when contemplating hearing preservation procedures. When hearing is normal in the contralateral ear, residual hearing on the operated side is useful socially only if speech discrimination is good and the pure tone audiogram is within 30 dB of the normal side.

Caloric testing

Over the years, much time and effort has been invested in examination of the vestibular system of patients suspected of harboring an acoustic neurinoma. The object was to find a simple and inexpensive screening test for the condition. Caloric testing was pioneered by Barany, for which he was awarded the Nobel Prize in 1914. In the era before modern neurosurgical imaging the differentiation of labyrinthine from cerebellar ataxia was of considerable importance. Vestibular assessment by caloric testing often reveals an ipsilateral canal paresis in acoustic neurinoma, but this is a nonspecific finding which is often absent in small tumors (Dix 1974). The detection rate for lesions larger than 4.5 cm is considerably better. In this group, Hallpike's caloric test will be normal in less than 4%, diminished in 33%, and absent in the remaining 70% (Boesen et al 1992). Electronystagmography has now superseded bithermal caloric testing in many centers (Linthicum & Churchill 1968).

In a prospective study of 409 patients with asymmetric hearing loss or tinnitus, caloric testing had a sensitivity of 80% for the detection of acoustic neurinoma, but achieved a specificity of only 50% (Swan & Gatehouse 1992). This makes it inappropriate as a screening test, both on the grounds of an unacceptable number of missed tumors, and because of the high false positive rate. Other conditions which may produce abnormal caloric results include vestibular neuronitis and Meniere's disease. One of the reasons for the poor sensitivity of this investigation is that it stimulates primarily the lateral semicircular canal and, therefore, only the superior vestibular nerve.

Auditory evoked brainstem responses

Auditory brainstem evoked responses (ABR) are the most sensitive indicator of a retrocochlear lesion, and have both a higher detection rate and a lower false positive rate than other nonradiological screening tests (Selters & Brackmann 1977). Unlike lesions of the cochlea, compression or stretching of the cochlear nerve produces a delay in the response latency which may be detected even when hearing is normal. The stimulus applied is a click from an earphone, and this elicits an electrical response which is recorded from scalp electrodes sited over the mastoids and vertex. The non-test ear is masked with white noise, and an averaging computer extracts the auditory response from the random signal. Generally, ABR testing is applicable only if hearing is better than 70 dB.

Patients with retrocochlear hearing loss show a consistent interaural difference in the latency of wave V during brainstem auditory evoked responses (Selters & Brackmann 1977). The upper limit of normal is 0.2 ms. Other algorithms used to detect a retrocochlear lesion include the absolute latency of wave V, and the intervals between waves I and V (upper limit of normal = 4.5 ms). ABRs are reported to be abnormal in 95% of patients with acoustic neurinoma (Josey et al 1980), and the false positive rate is said to be about 10% (Brackmann & Kwartler 1990a). Other series, however, have found that ABRs are considerably less specific than this. Weiss et al (1990) reported that the probability of finding a cerebellopontine angle tumor in the presence of an abnormal result was only around 15%. This is perhaps not surprising, because ABR tests the function of the auditory system as a whole. Despite this shortcoming, ABR is still used widely as a screening procedure, even though a negative result does not exclude the diagnosis. Tumor size cannot be predicted from the degree of delay. However, large lesions may cause sufficient brainstem compression to affect contralateral latencies as well (Selters & Brackmann 1977). It is of interest that ABRs are abnormal in more than 30% of patients with NF-1, even though acoustic neurinomas are rare in this group of patients (Schorry et al 1989).

Stapedial reflex testing

This is a further test of retrocochlear pathology, but is less sensitive than ABR. Abnormalities are found in around 80% of patients.

Electrocochleography

Transtympanic electrocochleography (ECoG) is usually nonspecific, although the presence of an action potential complex in the absence of subjective hearing is said to be pathognomonic (Morrison et al 1976). ECoG and ABR may be combined, particularly as the former is more sensitive for the detection of wave I. This increases the number of instances when the wave I–V interval can be measured (Prasher & Gibson 1983).

Electroneuronography

Electroneuronography (ENoG) has been used preoperatively to assess facial nerve involvement in temporal bone tumors. A compound action potential is measured in response to supramaximal bipolar stimulation of the main trunk of the facial nerve, and its amplitude compared to that of the contralateral side. Amplitude reduction is said to relate to tumor size, but cannot predict postoperative facial nerve function (Kartush et al 1987).

Screening tests

Moffat & Hardy (1989) have justified the early diagnosis and treatment of acoustic neurinoma on both economic and humanitarian grounds. Unfortunately MRI, and even CT, are too expensive in most countries to use as a routine screening test for patients with asymmetric hearing loss or other features which may represent a cerebellopontine angle tumor. Over the years many different test results have been proposed as being almost pathognomonic of retrocochlear hearing loss, only to be found wanting on closer examination. Examples include the phenomenon of loudness recruitment, abnormally rapid tone decay, disproportionately poor speech discrimination, and the stapedial reflex threshold.

In order to reduce the financial burden from radiological imaging of large numbers of patients and yet avoid missing a significant number of tumors, several nondiagnostic investigations have been combined to provide a screening battery. The necessary trade-off in every case is between sensitivity and specificity. Of patients with an acoustic neurinoma, over 98% will manifest an abnormality in at least two out of three of the following: caloric testing, ABR, and plain radiology of the internal auditory meatus (Moffat et al 1989b). Other workers have proposed combining pure tone audiometry, ABR, caloric testing, and the stapedial reflex test (Thomsen et al 1992). If the results are abnormal or equivocal, radiological assessment is then undertaken. In a study of 82 cerebellopontine angle tumor suspects, Barrs & Olsson (1987) found that the interaural wave V (IT5) latency difference on ABR testing had a sensitivity of 100% and a specificity of 80%. One tumor was diagnosed for every three abnormal IT5 results. Although the sensitivity from nonradiological screening is high, it is inevitable that a few tumors will be missed using such algorithms. This may have medicolegal implications.

The cost of screening with MRI can be reduced substantially if groups of patients are examined in batches, using T2-weighted fast spin echo series with a 512 matrix and interleaved cuts. In the majority of cases this alone will be adequate, and in only around 12% of patients will it be necessary to repeat the examination after gadolinium enhancement (Uttley, personal communication.)

GROSS MORPHOLOGIC FEATURES

Acoustic neurinomas typically are firm, well circumscribed, and encapsulated. They distort and compress rather than invade brain. The tumor, which is invested in a sheet of arachnoid, is of a yellowish white appearance and has a rubbery consistency. These lesions are relatively avascular except in childhood, or when very large (Kasantikul et al 1980a). The presence of areas of red or brown discoloration indicates old or recent hemorrhage. The surface of large tumors in particular is often irregular and lobulated. Usually the neoplasm is solid, although small thin-walled cysts may be evident. On occasions the majority of the lesion will be found to be cystic. Large tumors compress and deform the cerebellum and the lateral aspect of the pons, the upper medulla, and the brachium pontis. Very large lesions may displace the cerebellum inferiorly, causing tonsillar herniation.

HISTOPATHOLOGY

In 1842, Cruveilhier produced a detailed report of the clinical and pathological features of a 26-year-old patient who died from an acoustic neurinoma. Intracranial schwannomas have a marked preponderance for sensory nerves, particularly the eighth cranial nerve. Although usually confined to the vestibular division, invasion of the cochlear (Neely 1981, Marquet et al 1990) and facial nerves has been described (Luetje et al 1983). Tumors arise at the neurilemmal-glial junction, or anywhere between this and the origin of the nerves within the labyrinth (Stewart et al 1975). There have been no reports of primary tumors occurring in the neuroglial portion of the nerve.

It was Virchow who called these tumors 'neuromas', based upon their macroscopic appearance. Microscopy revealed many parallel fibers, which were mistaken for axons, hence the later term 'neurinoma'. However, Murray & Stout (1940) identified the cell of origin correctly as the Schwann cell, using in vitro tissue culture techniques. Despite this, some controversy still remains as to whether the Schwann cell or related perineural fibroblast is indeed the true source of this neoplasm.

Microscopically, the tumor consists of two distinct patterns of architecture which, in any individual lesion, are intermingled but well demarcated. These are known as Antoni types A and B, and are fundamental to the diagnosis (Antoni 1920). Antoni type A tissue predominates, and consists of groups of spindle-shaped cells with elongated hyperchromatic nuclei. The cytoplasm is pale and has a stringy appearance due to numerous hairlike argyrophilic fibers which lie parallel to the long axis of the cell

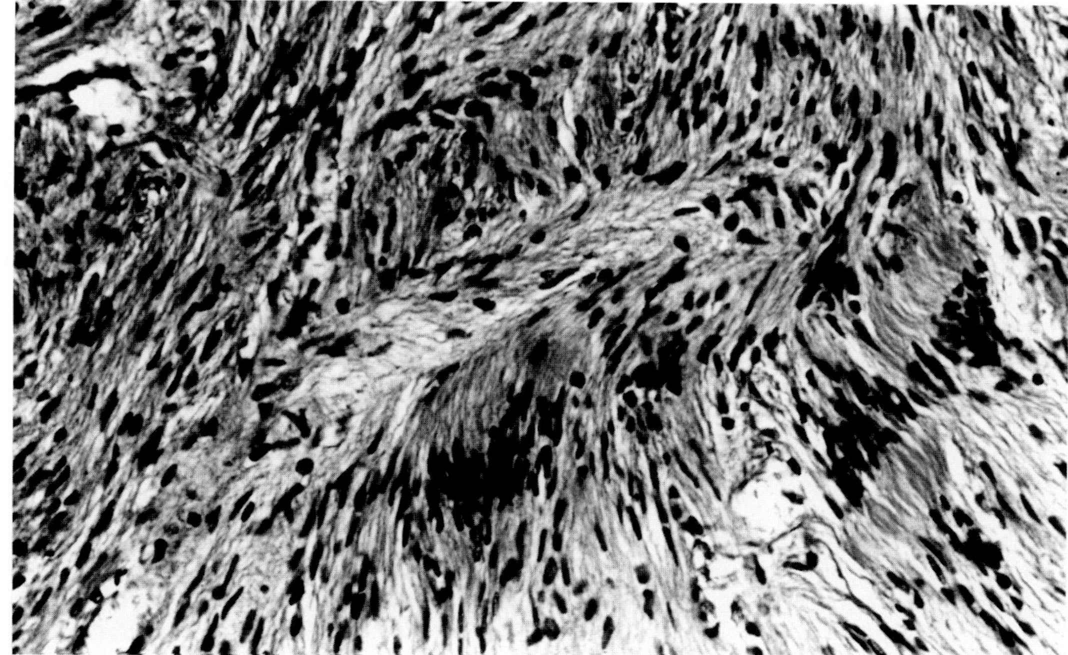

Fig. 31.10 Acoustic neurinoma containing bundles of spindle-shaped cells forming Antoni type A tissue. A Verocay body is present (H&E × 380).

(Fig. 31.10; Russell & Rubinstein 1989). Characteristic of schwannomas in general, although frequently absent in acoustic neurinomas, is the presence of palisading. The cells are grouped together in bundles (Verocay bodies). Within each bundle the cells lie roughly parallel, with their nuclei aligned in rows, separated by clear hyaline bands. The fibers interlace with those of other bundles, which are orientated at different angles.

Antoni type B tissue has a less compact structure. The cells are pleomorphic, vacuolated, and are separated by a loose eosinophilic matrix (Fig. 31.11). Microcystic change is frequent, although Antoni type B tissue does not re-

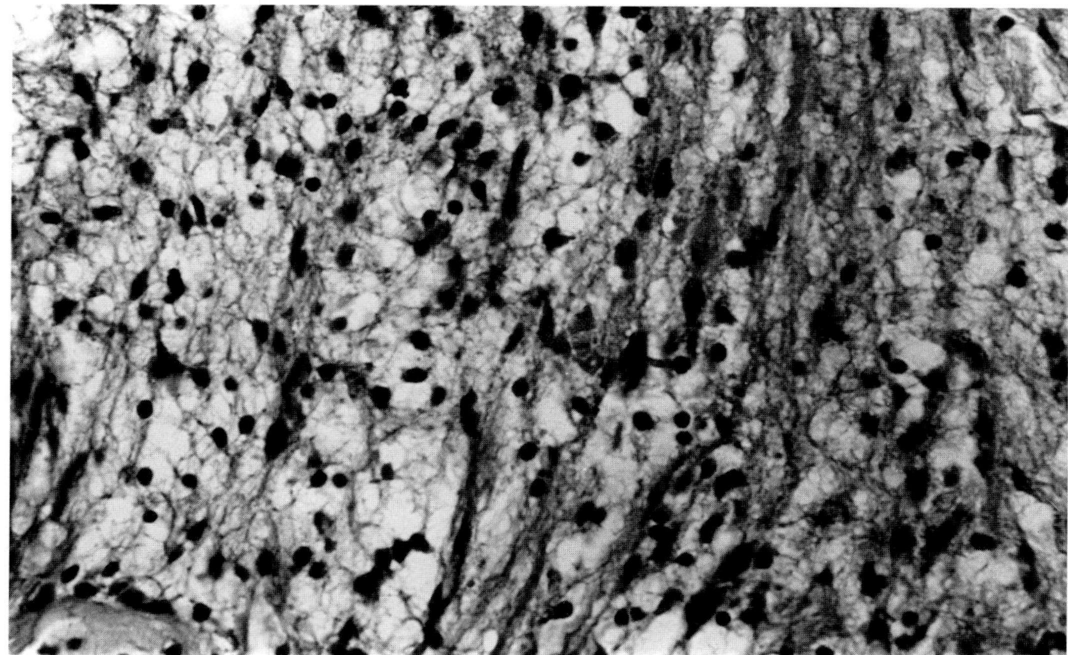

Fig. 31.11 Microscopic appearance of Antoni type B tissue in an acoustic neurinoma. The cells are more pleomorphic than Antoni A, and are separated by a loose eosinophilic matrix (H&E ×380).

present degeneration of type A (Murray & Stout 1940). Confluence of these areas is responsible for the cysts which are sometimes a feature of these tumors. Type B tissue may also become xanthomatous, due to lipid accumulation, which gives rise to a yellowish naked-eye appearance.

The degree of tumor cellularity may be quite variable. Secondary changes occur in some schwannomas. Areas of infarction or hemorrhage may be seen, particularly in tumors with excessive vascularization. On occasions, angiomas may be combined with neurinomas, particularly in women (Kasantikul et al 1980b). Haemosiderin-filled macrophages may be evident within foci of degeneration, and areas of necrosis may be present. Other tumors may contain foci of calcification. The term 'ancient schwannoma' has been given to lesions where the nuclei are atypical, hyperchromatic and enlarged, and the tumor is associated with a dense fibrous stroma. Mitotic activity is not increased in ancient schwannomas, however, and neither this appearance, nor the presence of pleomorphism, by itself signifies malignant change. Other neoplasms have been reported occasionally to metastasize to an acoustic neurinoma (le Blanc 1974), and melanotic acoustic neurinomas have been described on very rare occasions (Russell & Rubinstein 1989).

Benign schwannomas rarely present a diagnostic challenge histologically, although meningiomas may on occasion have similar features, including the presence of Verocay bodies (Sobel & Michaud 1985). Immunohistochemical markers are therefore generally of rather limited value. Acoustic neurinomas stain strongly positive for the S-100 protein (Fig. 31.12). This is a cytoplasmic protein, but it is not specific to this condition. Its uses primarily are for the identification of nerve sheath tumors, amelanotic melanoma, and myoepithelial cells. Meningiomas by contrast stain positively only weakly with S-100, but can be differentiated further by their reaction to HMFG (epithelial membrane antigen; Schnitt & Vogel 1986, Simpson et al 1990). A proportion of acoustic neurinomas will stain positively for glial fibrillary acidic protein (GFAP; Stanton et al 1987).

The bilateral acoustic neurinomas of NF-2 do not differ microscopically from those that occur sporadically. They do, however, show a tendency to be more adherent to adjacent structures (Linthicum & Brackmann 1980). Rarely, meningioma has been observed to be intermixed microscopically with schwannoma (Gruskin & Carberry 1979).

Under the electron microscope, Antoni type A tissue has a lamellar pattern composed of thin elongated cell processes covered by a basal lamina, which are separated by intercellular basement membrane material. Antoni B tissue contains large numbers of organelles and vacuoles, consistent with high metabolic activity (Russell & Rubinstein 1989). Other typical electron microscopic features include long-spaced collagen fibrils, and the development of whorls and lamellae composed of stacks of double membranes grouped tightly together.

MALIGNANCY

Malignancy is far more common in peripheral than in

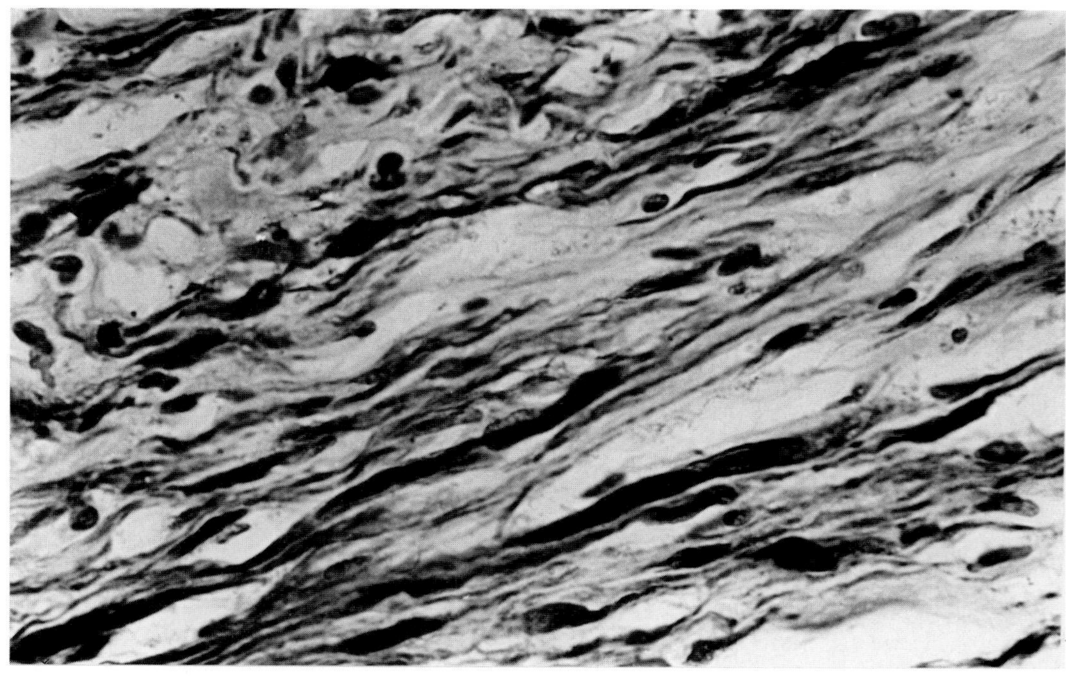

Fig. 31.12 Positivity of an acoustic neurinoma for the S-100 protein (× 620).

cranial neurinomas. The vast majority present de novo rather than as malignant change in a pre-existing benign lesion (Yousem et al 1985). Around 50–70% are associated with von Recklinghausen's disease, and the age at presentation in these cases is considerably younger than for those which occur sporadically (for review see Russell & Rubinstein 1989).

Malignant acoustic neurinomas are exceptionally rare, and only a handful have been reported in the world literature. Russell & Rubinstein (1989) collected a series of only 6, ranging from 26–72 years of age. In one there was considerable bony erosion by tumor, whilst three manifested themselves as recurrence after previous surgical excision. Histologically, the features were similar to neurofibrosarcoma, with increased cellularity and numerous mitoses. Initially the tumors were encapsulated, but later they became locally invasive. Recurrence is common after surgery, and these tumors may become progressively more anaplastic with the passage of time. Because of the risk of recurrence the long-term prognosis is poor, although the rarity of malignant change means that precise details of tumor behavior are lacking. Studies of large numbers of malignant peripheral schwannomas indicate that metastases are uncommon and occur late. The degree of mitotic activity and anaplasia is said not to predict survival (Ducatman et al 1986). Nager (1969) was unable to find any report of malignant degeneration within a pre-existing acoustic neurinoma. Such a case was documented by McLean et al (1990) although, in retrospect, the original specimen did exhibit some atypical features.

A malignant schwannoma with rhabdomyoblastic differentiation is otherwise known as a malignant triton tumor. This very rare soft tissue sarcoma arises almost exclusively from peripheral nerves, usually in patients with von Recklinghausen's disease. Only two acoustic nerve triton tumors have ever been documented (Best 1987, Han et al 1992). Total excision with adjuvant chemotherapy and radiotherapy was advocated, although the prognosis in both cases was poor. The 5-year survival for this tumor in peripheral nerves is 12% (Brooks et al 1985).

GENERAL MANAGEMENT PLAN

Differential diagnosis

Acoustic neurinomas are by far the most common tumors which occur within the cerebellopontine angle. In a review of 205 tumors, Revilla (1948) found that 78% were neurinomas (mostly acoustic), 6% meningioma, 6% cholesteatoma, 6% glioma, and the remaining 4% miscellaneous. The presenting features of meningioma can be similar to acoustic neurinoma but, because the tumor arises frequently from the anterior or superior lip of the internal auditory meatus, there may be early involvement of the facial and trigeminal nerves with relative sparing of hearing (Sekhar & Jannetta 1984). Similarly, inferior extension may involve the cranial nerves at the jugular foramen. The relationship between the cranial nerves and the tumor is much less predictable than with acoustic neurinoma, but the success of hearing preservation is greater, particularly for larger lesions (Maurer & Okawara 1988). Schwannomas of adjacent cranial nerves, in particular of the trigeminal, facial, glossopharyngeal or vagus nerves, can also involve the cerebellopontine angle. Facial neurinomas, which account for about 1% of cerebellopontine angle tumors, may be difficult to differentiate from an acoustic neurinoma preoperatively. However, facial neurinomas sometimes arise from the region of the geniculate ganglion, and may extend into the middle cranial fossa via erosion of the petrous temporal bone (King & Morrison 1990). Very large acoustic neurinomas, by contrast, are more likely to extend into the middle cranial fossa via the tentorial hiatus, although this is uncommon. The presence of contrast enhancement in the region of the geniculate ganglion, despite features otherwise typical of an acoustic neurinoma, can also aid in the differential diagnosis. Facial neurinomas may also evolve from the tympanic or mastoid segments of the nerve. Other schwannomas of the temporal bone include those which arise from the chorda tympani nerve, the auricular branch of the glossopharyngeal (Jacobson's) nerve, and the auricular branch of the vagus (Arnold's) nerve (Amoils et al 1992). At times it may not be possible to ascertain from which nerve a neurinoma of the petrous temporal bone has arisen (Best 1968).

As well as meningioma and neurinomas of adjacent cranial nerves, the differential diagnosis of acoustic neurinoma also includes epidermoid, aneurysm, arteriovenous malformation, glomus jugulare tumor, choroid plexus papilloma, hemangioma, lipoma, lymphoma, medulloblastoma, enterogenous cyst, and metastatic tumor within the temporal bone (Schisano & Olivecrona 1960, Brackmann & Bartels 1980, Robinson & Rudge 1983, Wakahayashi et al 1983, Yoshii et al 1989, Umezu et al 1991, Yamada et al 1993). Differentiation of these lesions is not usually difficult on radiological grounds.

Conservative treatment and the timing of surgery

The question of the timing of acoustic neurinoma surgery remains unresolved and, in many respects, has become less clear with the passage of time. Age by itself is not a contraindication to successful surgery (Samii et al 1992), although an expectant policy with careful follow-up may be a reasonable alternative to surgery when the tumor is small and the patient is infirm or perhaps reluctant to contemplate excision for other reasons.

The difficulty in assessing tumor growth rates in the pre-CT era, and the dramatic reduction in mortality and morbidity from surgery in the 1960s–1980s suggested that all tumors, with a few notable exceptions, should be removed at diagnosis. This view was strengthened by the knowledge that larger tumor size is associated undoubtedly with an increase in morbidity and, in particular, poorer prospects for facial nerve recovery, preservation of residual hearing, and for a good quality of life. Yet despite this, the decision to offer immediate treatment is not always clear cut. Better awareness among clinicians, coupled with improvements in diagnostic screening, has resulted in greater numbers of tumors being diagnosed at an early or even asymptomatic stage. Although the surgical results for facial nerve function and overall morbidity are likely to be excellent under these circumstances, unfortunately this is not yet true for preservation of hearing. With the advent of MRI, and subsequent reports which suggest that up to 50% of untreated patients with small lesions will display no further tumor growth, expectant treatment becomes a viable alternative to surgery in some cases. It can be argued that small tumors should be managed conservatively in the first instance, excision not being contemplated until it has been established that the lesion is actually expanding. In a study of 35 patients, Valvassori & Guzman (1989) determined that any further tumor growth was evident usually within the first 12 months of follow-up. A relatively short observation period may therefore allow patients with indolent forms of the disease to be selected out.

This is not to suggest that delayed treatment is applicable for any but a minority of patients. Conservative management is probably unwise in the younger age groups because the rate of tumor growth is likely to be more rapid. Similarly, an expectant policy is unsuitable for lesions larger than 2.5 cm because any further expansion is liable to have a significant influence upon surgical morbidity. In our experience, the great majority of patients are far more concerned about their facial nerve function and prospects for a good outcome in general than they are about preservation of hearing in the affected ear. Because outcome relates so strongly to tumor size, we believe that early surgery remains the treatment of choice for most patients. If patients are to be managed conservatively in the first instance, repeat MRI at 8 months, 18 months, and subsequently at 2-yearly intervals has been recommended (Valvassori & Guzman 1989), although Laasonen & Troupp (1986) advised annual CT review. The effects of dexamethasone on tumor size, peritumoral edema, and contrast enhancement on serial CT scanning are minimal (Hatam et al 1985).

Neurofibromatosis type 2

This condition is particularly challenging to manage satisfactorily. As well as bilateral acoustic neurinomas other tumors may also occur, notably cranial and spinal neurinomas and meningiomas. Any patient under the age of 30 years who presents with an acoustic neurinoma or meningioma should be suspected of suffering from NF-2. MRI with gadolinium enhancement should be performed to screen both for a small contralateral lesion, and for the presence of other intracranial tumors.

The major objective of treatment is to preserve functional hearing for as long as possible. Unfortunately, auditory symptoms often occur late in the disease (Linthicum & Brackmann 1980, Bess et al 1984). Furthermore, deterioration of hearing in a series of 9 patients with bilateral tumors treated conservatively was rapid in every case, and ranged from 11–16 dB per year (Kitamura et al 1992). However, as with sporadic tumors, the speed of progression does appear to be highly variable (Baldwin et al 1991). The combination of rapid tumor growth and poorer prognosis as the tumor enlarges argues for these lesions being treated promptly. However, examination of the temporal bone in NF-2 patients shows that tumor infiltration of the cochlear nerve and inner ear is more common than with sporadic tumors (Linthicum & Brackmann 1980). The prognosis for hearing preservation is likely therefore to be correspondingly less favorable (Brackmann 1979). The dilemma is whether to offer early treatment, which provides the only hope of preserving long-term hearing, albeit a small one, or to delay surgery until useful hearing has been lost, and to train the patient to cope with impending deafness in the interim. Hearing loss is not the only difficulty when treating this patient subgroup. Involvement of the facial nerve is more common (Martuza & Ojemann 1982, Baldwin et al 1991), and facial nerve preservation rates are correspondingly less good.

A large symptomatic tumor will require treatment, regardless of the risk of total deafness. In every case surgery should aim to conserve residual hearing, unless the tumor is very large. If the tumors are small and hearing is good, the National Institutes of Health consensus document (1988) proposes that an attempt should be made to excise one tumor. The authors' preference is to remove first the tumor on the side of poorer hearing (usually, but not invariably, the larger of the two). In the fortunate circumstance where useful hearing remains intact, the contralateral lesion may be explored later. However, if hearing is lost at the first operation, there are four options. Treatment of the contralateral neurinoma can be delayed until useful hearing is lost, since hearing at even very low levels may assist the patient with lip reading. Alternatively, the remaining tumor can be excised macroscopically or the patient offered stereotactic radiosurgery. The fourth option is to undertake subtotal tumor removal with decompression of the internal auditory canal, which may delay the progression of hearing loss (Miyamoto et al 1991). However, even elective subtotal tumor removal can result in total deafness (Wigand et al 1988, Baldwin et al 1991), and total excision with hearing preservation is very unlikely if the lesion is more than 2 cm in diameter (Hughes et al 1982). Subtotal excision which fails to preserve hearing should be followed shortly by total removal. In a recent report of 19 patients with bilateral tumors, 65% retained facial function after surgery, but the outlook for hearing in both the operated and unoperated groups was dismal (Baldwin et al 1991). Because of the poor results for hearing preservation by both surgery and stereotactic radiosurgery, and the variable course of untreated disease, we do not believe that operation is justified at present on a solitary hearing ear with a small tumor.

If bilateral excision is contemplated, the second operation should, where possible, be delayed until there has been recovery of facial nerve function. Although the likelihood is very small, it should be remembered that surgery carries with it the risk of bilateral rather than just unilateral deafness (Linthicum & Brackmann 1980, Miyamoto et al 1990). Sometimes removal of tumor on one side will result in some improvement in residual hearing in the contralateral ear.

Stereotactic radiosurgery is an alternative to surgery in NF-2 patients. However, this technique also may result in both delayed hearing loss and facial palsy. Progressive hearing deterioration or deafness will ensue in 64% of such patients (Hirsch & Norén 1988).

On rare occasions a cerebellopontine angle tumor in neurofibromatosis will be a facial rather than an acoustic tumor, and theoretically may permit total tumor removal with preservation of hearing (Piffko & Pasztor 1981). King & Morrison (1990) found that 21% of their cases of facial neurinoma developed in patients with NF-2. Unfortunately the translabyrinthine operation, involving destruction of hearing, is often more favorable than a retrosigmoid approach to these tumors because of improved access to the petrous segment of the lesion, and to normal facial nerve beyond it.

Tumor in a solitary hearing ear

Such a patient presents a challenge similar to that faced when dealing with NF-2. Whether or not to operate at the time of diagnosis remains controversial, and is a matter of personal judgement. Some authors advocate early surgery, arguing that the success of hearing preservation will only diminish as the tumor enlarges (Pensak et al 1991). Yet hearing preservation is successful currently in around only one third of patients. We think that the risk of deafness is too high, particularly when the natural history of the condition is uncertain. Initially we favor conservative treatment, unless the tumor is large and exerting mass effect. Large tumors we treat by radical subcapsular excision. At present the results of hearing preservation with stereotactic radiosurgery are insufficient to advocate this form of treatment, although this may change as details of the optimum dose become clearer.

SURGICAL MANAGEMENT

Historical perspective

The first successful operation to remove a cerebellopontine angle tumor is credited to Sir Charles Ballance in 1894. Unfortunately the patient required enucleation of the eye subsequently as a consequence of complications secondary to trigeminal and facial nerve palsy. Krause described the retrosigmoid suboccipital approach in 1903, but mortality at the time was very high, ranging from 67–84% (Dandy 1925). Tumor removal was achieved usually by extraction with a finger inserted into the posterior fossa, a practice which carried with it a high risk of injury to branches of the basilar artery as well as to the cranial nerves and brainstem. As a consequence of the poor results, Cushing proposed subtotal tumor removal. This he achieved by scooping out the center of the lesion, and by the application of Zinker's solution to the cavity for hemostasis. This technique, which was combined with a generous decompressive suboccipital craniectomy and uncapping of the cerebellum, reduced mortality to about 25% by 1917, and 4% by 1931 (Cushing 1917, 1931). However, 40% of patients died within 5 years from tumor recurrence (Cushing 1931). An excellent account summarizing Cushing's techniques and surgical results can be found in German (1961). The first successful attempt at total tumor excision with preservation of the facial nerve was reported by Sir Hugh Cairns in 1932. Recognition that the anterior inferior cerebellar artery was often adherent to the tumor capsule, that changes in vital signs were often related to brainstem ischemia, and that preservation of the arteries within the cerebellopontine angle was essential to a good outcome were further milestones in the surgery of this disease (Adams 1943, Atkinson 1949). Elliott & McKissock (1954) were perhaps the first to report successful preservation of hearing. In 1961, McKissock reported a remarkable series of patients with small tumors undergoing surgery, without the aid of magnification. In each case the facial and cochlear nerves remained intact, and residual hearing was present in some cases.

The translabyrinthine operation was proposed by Panse (1904). A radical mastoidectomy was performed, which included removal of the labyrinth, the cochlea, and the facial nerve. The procedure quickly fell into disrepute because of limited access, subtotal tumor excision, destruction of the facial nerve, hemorrhage from the venous sinuses, cerebrospinal fluid leakage, and the resultant high mortality (Dandy 1925). Later the translabyrinthine and suboccipital approaches were combined, but mortality remained high, mainly because of meningitis secondary to cerebrospinal fluid fistula. The operation was reintroduced by House (1964a), using modern microsurgical techniques. In his monograph, which was to become a landmark in the surgery of acoustic neurinoma, a series of 41 cases was reported in which there were no deaths, and almost all patients achieved some return of facial function. The results from House's group stimulated a great striving for better and better technical excellence. Mortality is now very low, and attention has turned to the preservation of hearing and of normal facial function.

Surgical anatomy

A detailed acount of the surgical anatomy can be found in Rhoton (1986) and Rhoton & Tedeschi (1992). In brief, the cerebellopontine angle cistern is bounded laterally by the petrous face, medially by the pons, and superiorly by the tentorium cerebelli. It contains the trigeminal, facial, and vestibulocochlear nerves, together with the anterior inferior cerebellar artery (AICA), and superior petrosal vein. Although the facial and vestibulocochlear nerves may at first sight appear to pass as a single bundle from the pontomedullary junction to the internal auditory meatus, they are separate. The superior and inferior vestibular nerves lie posteriorly and superiorly, and the cochlear nerve posteriorly and inferiorly. A shallow groove marks the boundary between them. The facial nerve lies anteriorly and slightly superiorly, with the nervus intermedius lying between the facial and vestibular nerves. The labyrinthine artery (and occasionally the main trunk of the anterior inferior cerebellar artery) lies usually between the facial and vestibular nerves. However, in all except the smallest lesions, the neural relationships will be distorted as the tumor enlarges. Because of its position, the facial nerve is usually displaced anteriorly and superiorly, although in around 5% of cases the nerve will lie over the posterior tumor capsule.

The constant landmarks for identification of the neural structures during tumor excision are their medial and lateral extents. Within the internal auditory meatus each of the nerves is separated from the others by two bony septa, the transverse crest, and the vertical crest (Bill's bar, named after William House). Within the porus acousticus the superior and inferior vestibular nerves lie posteriorly, the facial nerve antero-superiorly, and the cochlear nerve antero-inferiorly. Identification of Bill's bar will therefore allow the nerves anterior to it (the facial and cochlear) to be delineated with confidence from those posterior to it (the superior and inferior vestibular).

At the brainstem, the facial, cochlear, and vestibular nerves are more widely separated. The most important structures to identify here are the flocculus and the tuft of choroid plexus which emerges from the foramen of Luschka at the lateral margin of the pontomedullary sulcus. The foramen of Luschka is situated just dorsal to the glossopharyngeal root entry zone (Rhoton 1986). Immediately anterosuperior to the choroid plexus lies the entry of the vestibulocochlear nerve. The facial nerve arises in the pontomedullary sulcus a further 1–2 mm anterior to the vestibulocochlear nerve.

The anterior inferior cerebellar artery may pass around the brainstem either anterior to, ventral to (the most common finding), or between the facial and vestibulocochlear nerves. In only 23% of 132 subjects was AICA not related significantly to the nerves (Sunderland 1945). The degree to which it loops laterally toward the internal auditory meatus is variable. On occasions the artery may actually enter the meatus (around 14%), and it is particularly vulnerable to injury in this instance. In the majority of cases the artery loops laterally almost to the internal meatus (50%), while in 16% of patients there is no loop, and AICA lies close to the brainstem. After passing the nerves, the artery loops back consistently to the surface of the middle cerebellar peduncle above the flocculus (Rhoton 1986). Occasionally AICA may be substituted by a branch of the posterior inferior cerebellar artery. Penetrating branches of AICA enter the pons and upper medulla to supply the facial and vestibular nuclei, the spinal tract of the trigeminal nucleus, part of the medial lemniscus, and much of the middle and inferior cerebellar peduncles.

The superior petrosal vein (vein of Dandy) drains the upper aspect of the cerebellum into the superior petrosal sinus. The vein (or group of veins) may be divided to improve exposure if necessary, or if there is a risk of avulsion during retraction of the cerebellum. It has been suggested, however, that this may on occasions exacerbate postoperative cerebellar swelling, particularly if the suboccipital route has been employed for tumor excision.

Knowledge of the arachnoid is important because it provides the key to dissection of the tumor from the surrounding structures. Within the internal meatus the nerves and internal auditory artery are covered in a sleeve of arachnoid. A tumor arising from the vestibular nerve, therefore, will also be invested in arachnoid. As the lesion grows from the porus acousticus into the cerebellopontine angle, the arachnoid which covers it comes into contact with the arachnoid which overlies the cerebellum and the adjacent nerves and vessels of the angle cistern (Tos et al 1988). The only structures not separated from the tumor by arachnoid are the facial and cochlear nerves, and the brainstem end of vestibulocochlear complex. As a result, when the tumor encroaches on the medially placed structures there is a double layer of arachnoid separating it from the brainstem and cerebellum. This arachnoidal cap provides an important cleavage plane during tumor dissection.

The tumor obtains its blood supply from two sources. The principal supply is via the dura of the petrous pyramid at the margins of the internal auditory meatus. Bleeding in this region may be tedious and troublesome during tumor removal. Medially the tumor is supplied by the labyrinthine artery, and by the other branches of the anterior inferior cerebellar artery.

As well as encroaching upon the cerebellum and brainstem, large tumors may be related to the abducent nerve and basilar artery. The superior pole of large tumors will involve the trigeminal nerve, and may abut on the undersurface of the tentorium cerebelli. It is exceptional for the trochlear nerve to be involved at the incisural notch. Inferiorly, large tumors may become adherent to structures in the region of the jugular foramen.

The height of the jugular bulb is variable, and may on occasions lie above the level of the lower border of the internal auditory canal (Shao et al 1993). This has important consequences during surgery because it limits exposure in the translabyrinthine operation, and there is a risk of injury when the posterior wall of the internal auditory meatus is removed via a suboccipital approach. The relationship between the jugular bulb and the internal meatus should be determined preoperatively by high resolution CT scan of the temporal bones.

Intraoperative monitoring

The facial nerve stimulator is an important if not essential tool during acoustic neurinoma surgery. Electrodes are placed in the ipsilateral orbicularis oculi and orbicularis oris for the detection of muscle action potentials in response to monopolar or bipolar stimulation of the facial nerve. Although objections that the current may harm the nerve have been raised, this is not borne out in clinical practice. The anesthetist can still administer small quantities of paralysing agents to the patient, but must ensure that one twitch is maintained on the 'train-of-four' peripheral nerve stimulator during dissection of the facial nerve.

In a recent study of 108 patients, Dickins & Graham (1991) concluded that facial nerve monitoring does improve functional results. The stimulator is used to identify the anatomic configuration of the facial nerve, to warn the surgeon if the nerve is being traumatized by manipulation or by traction, and to confirm physiologic as well as anatomic integrity at the completion of the procedure. The stimulus intensity should be reduced as much as possible, particularly when a unipolar device is in use (~0.25 mA), or current may leak to the facial nerve when adjacent non-neural tissue is stimulated, and produce a false positive response. Care must be taken also not to confuse a masseter contraction from stimulation of the trigeminal nerve, with movement of the facial musculature. Dissection of the nerve in a medial to lateral direction is likely to maximize the usefulness of monitoring. Clearly, if physiologic function is lost at any stage, the stimulator is of no further use to aid dissection proximal to that point. The region just medial to the porus is usually the most difficult part of the procedure. However, the manner in which the tumor is dissected from the nerve must be tempered by the clinical situation, because a lateral to medial dissection is often easier technically, particularly when the translabyrinthine operation is used.

Intraoperative audiometric monitoring has been employed during hearing preservation procedures (Ojemann et al 1984). The methods available currently are monitoring of the electrocochleogram (ECoG) via a transtympanic electrode placed through the inferior part of the tympanic membrane to rest on the promontory of the medial wall of the middle ear, recording of brainstem auditory evoked potentials (BAEPs) using scalp electrodes, or direct monitoring of the cochlear nerve. ECoG has a larger signal to noise ratio than BAEP, making it more sensitive. A significant reduction in wave V amplitude on BAEP, or a shift in latency, warns the surgeon to moderate dissection, retraction, or the use of bipolar cautery. When wave V is unchanged at the end of surgery useful hearing will be preserved, even if it was lost transiently at some stage (Nadol et al 1992). However the value of such monitoring remains uncertain. In many instances changes are abrupt, dramatic, and irreversible, and reflect compromise to inner ear vascularity or damage to the labyrinth (Ojemann et al 1984). Unlike monitoring of the facial nerve, there is a delay in response because the measurements require averaging. In only a few cases does a change in operative technique, such as modification of cerebellar retraction (Sekiya & Møller 1988) lead to a recovery of monitored potentials. However, identification of the event which caused hearing loss may still be of benefit if it allows the surgeon to modify operative technique in future cases. In a series of 28 patients, Kveton & Book (1992) found no advantage for intraoperative BAEP monitoring in terms of final outcome, although this has not been the experience of other groups (Ebersold et al 1992, Fischer et al 1992).

Instrumentation

In addition to the usual array of microsurgical instruments, a fenestrated sucker of the Brackmann type is a useful aid to dissection, and minimizes risk of injury to the nerves and vessels. It has been suggested that sucker-induced trauma contributes significantly to postoperative facial neurapraxia (Tos et al 1992c). The Cavitron ultrasonic surgical aspirator (CUSA) or House-Urban rotary dissector may be used to debulk large tumors. We have no experience with either the CO_2 or Nd:YAG lasers, which are reported by some authors to be more advantageous still (Takeuchi et al 1982, Cerullo & Mkrdichian 1987). The major benefit is said to be rapid tumor debulking with minimal manipulation of the tumor or neurovascular structures (Gardner et al 1983).

Surgical approach

There are three basic approaches to the cerebellopontine angle: by excision of the labyrinth (translabyrinthine), through a posterior fossa craniectomy (suboccipital/retrosigmoid), or via the middle cranial fossa. On occasions, more than one approach may be combined at the same or separate operations.

No clear consensus has emerged from the literature as to which is the procedure of choice. The route chosen is governed by tumor size, the degree of hearing loss, the hearing level in the contralateral ear, and the surgical preference and expertise of the operator. There have, in particular, been many publications recently which compare and contrast the suboccipital and translabyrinthine operations (Di Tullio et al 1978, Tos & Thomsen 1982, Glasscock et al 1986, Mangham 1988, Hardy et al 1989a). Good results are reported with each method, and a surgeon can expect progressive improvement in results with experience. It has been proposed that a surgeon should perform the operation at least ten times a year to remain proficient.

The major advantage of the translabyrinthine operation is that the facial nerve can be identified lateral to the tumor at an early stage in the dissection, and access to the fundus of the internal auditory meatus is excellent. Furthermore, retraction of the cerebellum is minimal, and the risk of postoperative edema is consequently less. The major disadvantage of this route is that residual hearing is irrevocably destroyed. The approach is unfamiliar to neurosurgeons, and requires the close cooperation of an otologist experienced in dissection of the temporal bone. Access is confined, but even the largest of tumors can be removed safely via this approach.

As a consequence of progressive improvements in operative results, particularly in mortality and facial nerve outcome, attention has turned more recently to the ability to preserve useful hearing. The suboccipital operation provides good access to the cerebellopontine angle but, if hearing is to be conserved, tumor at the fundus of the internal auditory meatus may be difficult to expose under direct vision. This is true particularly when the posterior semicircular canal is medially placed. Theoretically, this may increase the risk of subtotal tumor excision when compared with the translabyrinthine operation. This limitation can be avoided by use of the middle fossa exposure, which unroofs the internal auditory canal from above. However this route provides only very limited access to the cerebellopontine angle, and is therefore restricted to the treatment of small lesions. Few surgeons now advocate this approach, not just because of the confines of the exposure, but because of complications which may result from temporal lobe retraction, the added risk to the facial nerve, and because the outcome is no better than for approaches via the posterior fossa.

The question of hearing conservation deserves careful consideration when selecting the surgical approach. Anatomic preservation of the inner ear and cochlear nerve does not guarantee function, and it is exceptional for hearing to improve on its preoperative level (Telian et al 1988). Whether such hearing is 'useful' depends upon the level of hearing in the contralateral ear. Hearing loss need not be profound before it is socially useless when the other ear is normal. For hearing to be useful socially there must be both good speech discrimination, and a pure tone audiogram within 20–40 dB of the contralateral ear (House & Nelson 1979). Anything less is the equivalent of deafness because there is no balance between the good and impaired ears, directional hearing becomes difficult, and there are problems in coping with noisy environments. In one unselected series only 16% of patients with an intact cochlear nerve were able to use a telephone with the operated side — 4.4% of the entire group who had undergone suboccipital tumor excision (Bentivoglio et al 1988a). As well as the poor success rate for hearing preservation, there is also the issue of whether such attempts compromise the likelihood of complete tumor removal. Neely (1981, 1984) has shown that the cochlear nerve may be involved with tumor, and that attempts to preserve hearing may not be consistent with one of the major goals of surgery, namely macroscopic tumor excision.

We favor the translabyrinthine operation for large tumors, and for medium-sized lesions with poor hearing. It provides a more direct approach to the cerebellopontine angle, and retraction of the cerebellum is negligible. In our hands the morbidity is lower and hospital stay generally a little shorter than after a suboccipital approach. The merits of the different approaches will be considered further in the section dealing with results.

Staged resection

Excision of large lesions is difficult and time-consuming. Although planned two-stage resection was described by Ojemann et al (1972), Ojemann & Crowell (1978), and Sheptak & Jannetta (1979) for dealing with very large tumors (>4 cm), one-stage removal is now the norm. Hitselberger & House (1979) observed that when surgery was abandoned because of persistent vital sign changes, a second operation was often tolerated better than the first. They have proposed that the tumor may disengage itself from the brainstem and major vessels in the interim, and thereby reduce vascular compression. In contrast, Mangham (1988) found that the morbidity of planned two-stage operations was significantly higher than for one-stage resection, particularly in relation to facial nerve function. However, if technical difficulties do force abandonment of the procedure short of total removal a second operation should be undertaken, unless there are strong reasons for not doing so. A second operation is best performed within 2–4 days of the initial exploration, before adhesions start to form and the operative site becomes hyperemic.

Subtotal excision

Elective subtotal removal may be indicated in the elderly, the infirm, or in patients with bilateral tumors in whom the aim is to preserve residual hearing for as long as possible. More contentious is the issue of achieving the twin aims of total tumor excision and hearing preservation, particularly in the light of the histologic study by Neely (1984), in which he showed that microscopic invasion of the cochlear nerve by tumor was common. However, his work has not been confirmed by Perre et al (1990), who found no infiltration of the cochlear nerve by acoustic neurinoma, except in NF-2 patients. Yet recurrence is not an inevitable sequel, even if tumor is left behind at operation. Capsule remnants may be of no clinical significance, and indeed can atrophy. We will return to this issue later.

Suboccipital/retrosigmoid operation

This operative approach is discussed and described in Chapter 33.

Some authors have argued forcefully against attempts at hearing preservation. Marquet et al (1990) could find no connective tissue separating the cochlear nerve from the tumor mass, and observed that tumor tissue was evident frequently between the cochlear nerve fibers. They concluded that hearing preservation was not consistent with total tumor removal. The other major difficulty with the suboccipital approach is that anatomic studies have shown that it is impossible to open the fundus of the internal auditory canal under direct vision without injury to the labyrinth, thereby destroying hearing (Domb & Chole 1980). Although exposure will be adequate in around 80% of cases, the lateral 1–2 mm may give rise to difficulty if the entire canal is filled by tumor (Tatagiba et al 1992). Relatively wide access is provided to the cerebellopontine angle by the lateral suboccipital approach, but a further disadvantage is that the cerebellum and nerves of the jugular foramen must be exposed, and may need to be retracted.

Translabyrinthine operation

The translabyrinthine operation was reintroduced to neurosurgery by William House. The posterior fossa dura is opened in Trautmann's triangle, bounded by the sigmoid sinus, jugular bulb, and superior petrosal sinus. This exposure provides a more direct route to the cerebellopontine angle than does suboccipital craniectomy, and access is at the expense of bone rather than cerebellar retraction. The surgical field is confined, particularly in the region of the inferior pole of large tumors, but the apex of the cerebellopontine angle is more readily exposed than via the suboccipital route. The presence of an anteriorly placed sigmoid sinus or a high jugular bulb may render access slightly more difficult, but rarely does this cause undue problems. A high jugular bulb occurs in around 9–18% of temporal bones, and can be anticipated in petrous bones that are poorly pneumatized (Turgut & Tos 1992, Shao et al 1993). Translabyrinthine exposure can, however, be increased in three ways: (1) superiorly, by opening of the middle fossa dura; (2) posteriorly, with or without division of the sigmoid sinus (venous phase angiography should be undertaken to establish the dominance of the sinus and to assess the size of the torcular herophili if ligation is contemplated); or (3) anteriorly, via a transotic approach.

The transotic approach was proposed by Jenkins and Fisch (1980), as a modification of House & Hitselberger's transcochlear operation (1976). This is essentially a subtotal petrosectomy, but with skeletonization rather than translocation of the facial nerve. Access is thus provided circumferentially around the internal auditory meatus. We have never found this extension to the translabyrinthine approach necessary when dealing with primary tumors.

Sacrifice of residual hearing is the major disadvantage of the operation. However, only 1% of affected ears will have normal hearing after suboccipital surgery (Harner et al 1984), and it is rare for hearing to improve on preoperative levels (Telian et al 1988). The question of hearing preservation will be discussed later. Translabyrinthine surgery is contraindicated in the presence of chronic perforation of the tympanic membrane or acute infection of the middle ear or mastoid, because of the risk of meningitis. The operation requires close cooperation between neurosurgeon and otologist. House (1979) suggests that both should be thoroughly proficient in all phases of the procedure and be able to act interchangeably. We think that this is unnecessary, and that each specialist should utilize the skill in which (s)he has the greater expertise.

Occasionally the preoperative diagnosis of acoustic neurinoma is found at surgery to be incorrect. Although access is more confined via the labyrinth, King & Morrison (1980) removed three jugular neurinomas successfully via this route. Meningiomas with an origin anterior to the porus may however prove more problematic because the angle of approach to the petrous face is less acute than with suboccipital surgery, although access to the petrous apex is unquestionably better. In these cases exposure can be extended by opening the dura over the temporal lobe and dividing the superior petrosal sinus and tentorium. This exposure is best planned in advance, a small temporal craniotomy being used in addition to the usual translabyrinthine exposure. However, it can be done as an ad hoc procedure by extending the mastoid incision upwards onto the temporal squamosa.

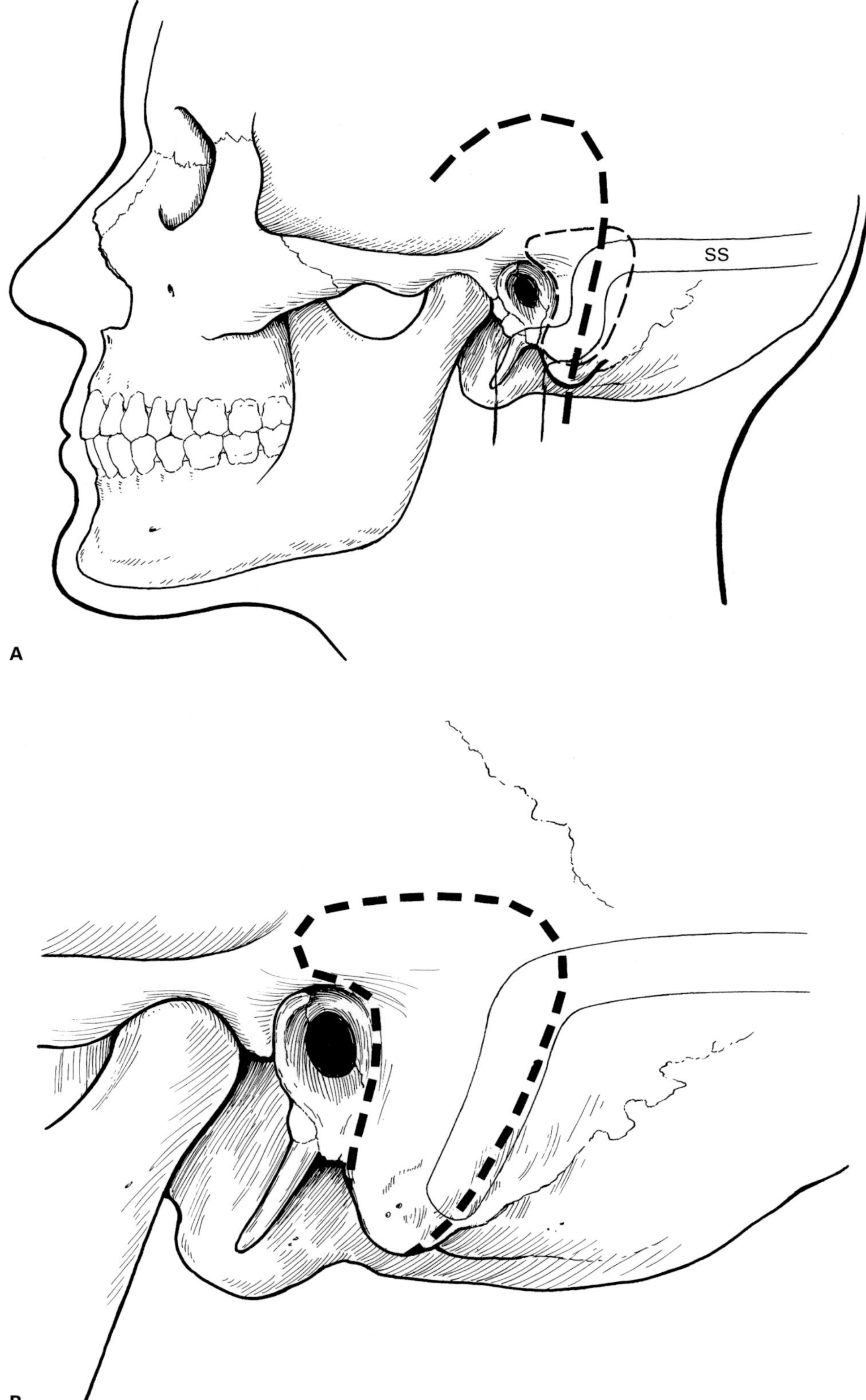

Fig. 31.13 **A.** Skin incision for the translabyrinthine operation. **B.** The superficial extent of bone dissection. SS = sigmoid sinus.

Technique The patient is anesthetized, prepared, and placed in the supine position. The operation is conducted under general anesthesia with endotracheal intubation. Although spontaneous ventilation was at one time popular to identify potential brainstem compromise, mechanical ventilation is now the norm because of the ability to lower intracranial tension. Continuous monitoring of arterial blood pressure, electrocardiogram, and central venous pressure is established, together with adequate venous access. Changes in blood pressure (hypertension) or heart rate (bradycardia or arrhythmia) during tumor dissection warn the surgeon of pressure or traction effects to the brainstem, or impairment of its blood supply. A lumbar drain may be inserted if the tumor is large. The bladder is drained via a urethral catheter. The head is rotated around 45°, avoiding obstruction to the great veins of the neck. Dissection of the petrous bone adds a further 1.5–2 hours to the duration of the procedure, so that attempts to avoid pressure sores and to keep the patient warm are essential. Fat and fascia lata are taken from the lateral aspect of the right thigh and are soaked in antibiotic solution until required. Lumbar drainage is generally unnecessary, although mannitol may be useful if the tumor is large.

An inverted hockey-stick incision commences just below the mastoid tip, runs about 2 cm behind and parallel to the root of the pinna, and curves anteriorly to end about 3 cm above the external auditory meatus (Fig. 31.13A). The exposure from this incision is larger than necessary, but keeps the hemostats away from the operative field. In addition, it allows access to the middle cranial fossa with division of the superior petrosal sinus and tentorium should it be required. This is not necessary for acoustic neurinoma surgery, but may be appropriate when dealing with other lesions of the cerebellopontine angle. The scalp flap is reflected anteriorly. Using cutting diathermy, a pericranial flap is raised in a similar fashion, and turned anteriorly to expose the posterior bony rim of the external meatus.

Next the otologist performs an extensive cortical mastoidectomy using an air drill with a cutting burr. The bone dust is collected for use later. The initial dissection is conducted under direct vision, resorting to the operating microscope as the exposure deepens. The opening is roughly the shape of a large keyhole (Fig. 31.13B). The external opening should be as large as possible, to permit extradural retraction of the cerebellum and temporal lobe if necessary, particularly if the sigmoid sinus is anteriorly placed or the middle fossa dura low. Anteriorly, the posterior wall of the external meatus is thinned. Superiorly, the dissection should expose the edge of the middle fossa dura and superior petrosal sinus. The dissection is carried anteriorly above the external meatus as far as possible. The sigmoid sinus is exposed posteriorly, but a small island of bone may be left over it, allowing the sinus to be depressed without risk of injury (Bill's island; Fig. 31.14). Inferiorly, the mastoid process is hollowed out. It is particularly important to remove sufficient bone posteriorly and superiorly to improve access by retraction of the dura. The margins of the bony defect should be smoothed and beveled to avoid overhanging edges, and perhaps to lessen the risk of postoperative chronic wound pain.

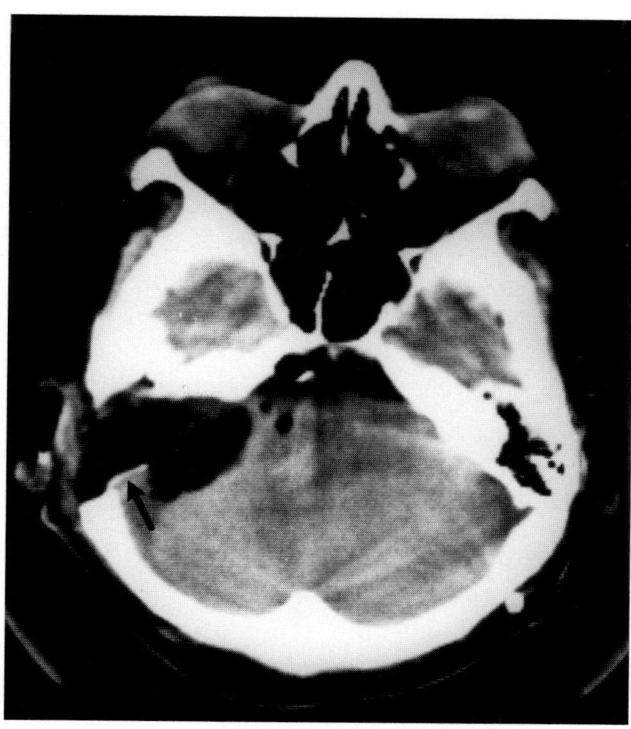

Fig. 31.14 Postoperative CT of the petrous temporal bone after translabyrinthine surgery. Exposure of the cerebellopontine angle and internal meatus is more direct than via a suboccipital route. An island of bone (arrow) is visible protecting the sigmoid sinus from injury (Bill's island). Reproduced from Hardy et al 1989a, with permission.

The dissection is deepened in the space between the middle fossa dura and superior margin of the meatus, to open the mastoid antrum and aditus. The incus and head of the malleus are exposed, and the incus is removed. The lateral semicircular canal is identified on the medial wall of the epitympanic recess. This is the key landmark for the horizontal portion of the facial nerve, which lies below and parallel to its anterior part. Having established the position of the facial nerve, its descending portion can be skeletonized, and this marks the anterior limit of the exposure inferiorly (Fig. 31.15). Even when covered with a thin plate of bone, the stimulator may still be used to identify the location of the intrapetrous portion of the facial nerve, although the stimulus current will have to be increased temporarily.

Dense bone marks the otic capsule surrounding the semicircular canals. The lateral canal is removed first, and

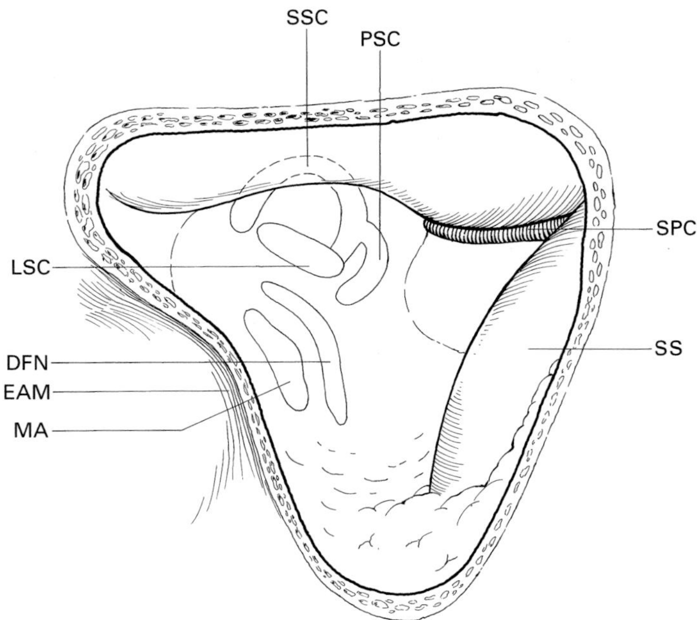

Fig. 31.15 A radical mastoidectomy has been performed. The labyrinthectomy has not yet been carried out, but the semicircular canals have been skeletonized. EAM = external auditory meatus; MA = mastoid antrum; SS = sigmoid sinus; SPS = superior petrosal sinus; DFN = descending portion of facial nerve; SSC, PSC, LSC = superior, posterior, and lateral semicircular canals respectively.

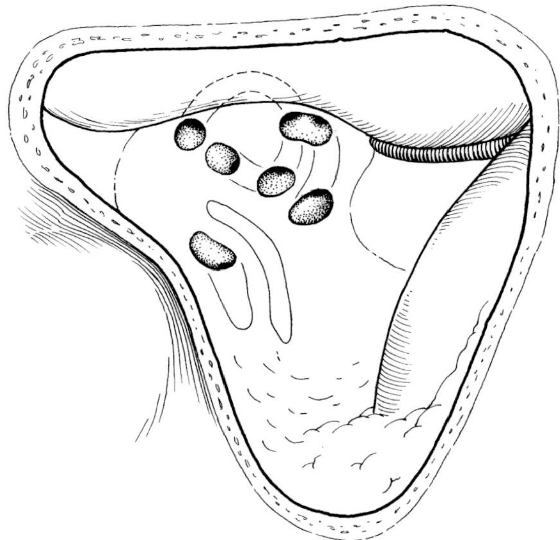

Fig. 31.16 The labyrinthectomy has been completed.

its anterior limb leads into the vestibule. The posterior and superior canals are followed to the crus commune, but the ampullated end of the posterior canal is not removed because it lies deep to the second genu of the facial nerve. The labyrinthine vein traverses the arc of the superior semicircular canal, and is a useful landmark (Fig. 31.16). The posterior fossa dura is skeletonized, and the vestibular aqueduct and endolymphatic sac removed. The jugular bulb is identified. Exposure here must be adequate to allow mobilization of the lower pole of the tumor later. Removal of bone in the angle between the jugular bulb and dura is particularly useful in this regard. The position of the jugular bulb is variable. It may be quite high, on occasions almost reaching the ampulla of the posterior semicircular canal (House 1979). Bleeding from injury to the jugular bulb can be controlled by hemostatic gauze, or with a muscle pack.

The internal auditory meatus lies immediately deep to the vestibule. The most satisfactory way of entering the internal meatus is to remove the utricle and saccule, to identify the stump of the superior vestibular nerve, and to follow it through the thin bone into the internal auditory meatus. Once exposed, the entire posterior wall, and as much of the superior and inferior walls as possible, are removed. A diamond burr is used at this stage. Great care is needed when drilling away the anterior aspect of the superior margin of the meatus, as the facial nerve lies directly beneath the dura. The direction of rotation of the drill should be changed such that, should the drill tip run off, it will be directed away from the nerve. The bone dissection is completed by removing the lateral lip of the porus acousticus. If necessary, the intrapetrous portion of the facial nerve lying between the internal meatus and geniculate ganglion can also be exposed with a diamond burr. In the lateral end of the meatus the facial and superior vestibular nerves are separated by a vertical crest (Bill's bar), which provides a constant landmark for the identification of the facial nerve lateral to the tumor.

The resultant cavity in the temporal bone is roughly pyramidal, bounded posteriorly by the sigmoid sinus and posterior fossa dura, superiorly by the middle fossa dura and superior petrosal sinus, anteriorly by the petrous bone, middle ear cavity and facial nerve, and with the internal auditory meatus as its apex. The otological dissection is completed by using an elevator to remove the remaining bone flakes left behind on the dura.

The neurosurgeon starts the next phase of the procedure by opening the dura, first of the posterior fossa, and then of the meatus. The extent of the dural incision in the posterior fossa is dependent upon the tumor size. For large lesions the incision runs posteriorly from the meatus and divides into upper and lower limbs. The superior limb extends to the junction of the sigmoid and superior petrosal sinuses, and the inferior limb down toward the jugular bulb. Retraction sutures are placed on each of the dural flaps. The incision is then extended into the porus. Here the dura forms a tough fibrous ring, which is often quite vascular. Once divided, the dura is freed from the vestibular nerves using a blunt hook or dissector, and the thin dura of the internal meatus is divided up to the fundus of the canal. The tumor and superior vestibular nerve are

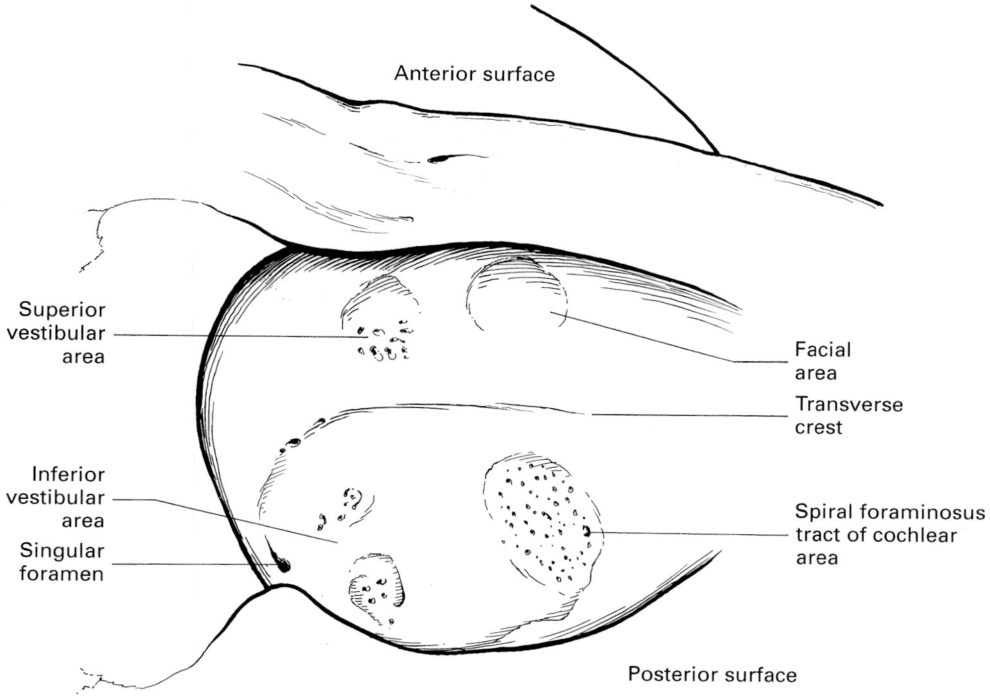

Fig. 31.17 **A.** Anatomic relationships of the posterior aspect of the temporal bone. **B.** The dura of the posterior fossa and internal auditory meatus has been opened to reveal the tumor and the nerves distal to it.

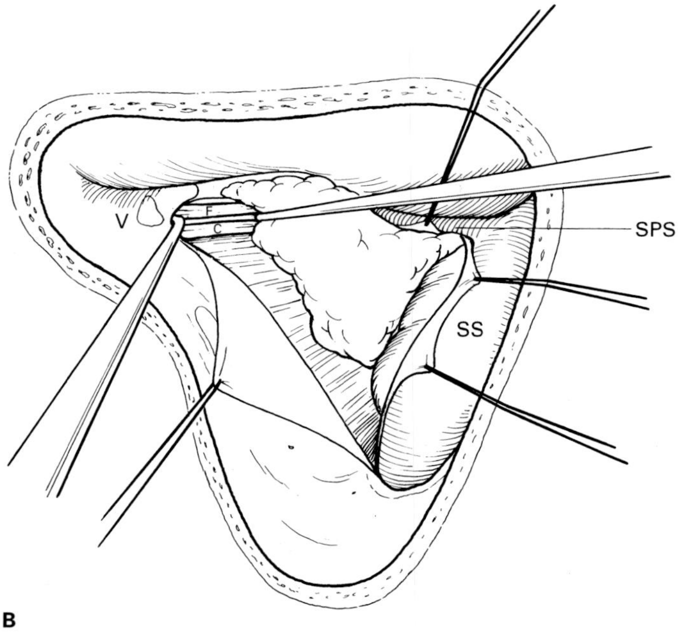

gently displaced inferiorly until the facial nerve is identified anterior to it and Bill's bar, and confirmed with the nerve stimulator. The superior and inferior vestibular nerves are then divided lateral to the tumor. A blunt hook can be passed behind them to assist with division, if required. The apex of the intracanalicular component of the tumor is then displaced posteriorly, and the plane between tumor and facial nerves is developed by sharp dissection. It is necessary to divide the arachnoid lying either side of the facial nerve. Care should be taken not to apply traction to the nerve. The tumor is freed progressively from its attachment to the arachnoid and dura. If the tumor is very small this plane can be continued and the tumor freed from the attachment at the porus, at which point it is always densely adherent to the dura. However, this is not the best strategy for large tumors, for two reasons. Firstly, the facial nerve usually deviates acutely just medial to the porus (almost always either anteriorly or upward), and it is very easy to lose the correct plane and become subcapsular. Secondly, if the attachment of the tumor to the porus is divided completely, the weight of the tumor is suspended from the facial nerve, and may cause a traction neuropraxia. For these reasons, large tumors occupying the cerebellopontine angle should be mobilized and debulked before the dissection is completed at the porus. Particular care should be taken when dissecting along the inferior margin of the porus, as it is here that the anterior inferior cerebellar artery is most likely to be encountered.

The dissection begins in the cerebellopontine angle by incision of the arachnoidal cap between the cerebellum and the posterior tumor capsule. The medullary CSF cistern is opened in the region of the jugular foramen, and the IX–XI nerves are freed from the mass. The anterior inferior cerebellar and vertebral arteries may at times be visible at this point. The plane between tumor and cerebellum is then developed progressively. Only vessels actually entering the lesion can be coagulated. Gentle retraction using a sucker tip held against a pattie will prevent the capsule of more friable tumors from breaking up. Once the limit of mobilization is reached, or when any of the major landmarks are identified, a pattie or small silastic sheet is placed to mark their position, and the point of attack is then shifted to another direction. However, it is a mistake to line the dissection with too much material, and a conscious effort should be made to keep it to a minimum. Larger neurinomas must be debulked to continue the dissection. The cavitron ultrasonic aspirator (CUSA) is ideal for the purpose but curettes and pituitary rongeurs, or a House–Urban rotary dissector, are alternatives. Care must be taken not to breach the tumor capsule or apply excessive movement to it, which might injure the nerves or induce spasm in adjacent arteries. Progressively more of the arachnoidal plane can be developed as the tumor is debulked until, ultimately, the brainstem is exposed. Induced hypotension may be useful if the tumor is excessively vascular, or a small piece of wool soaked in saline or hydrogen peroxide can be left temporarily within the tumor cavity. A systolic blood pressure of 80–100 mmHg can be sustained for long periods without adverse consequences.

The white surface of the brainstem is readily distinguishable from the more yellowish appearance to the cerebellum. The flocculus and the choroid plexus emerging from the foramen of Luschka should be identified, and are important landmarks for the adjacent cranial nerves. With larger tumors, exposure of the facial nerve entry zone is difficult until the vast majority of the tumor has been debulked. Adhesions between tumor and brainstem are rarely dense, but a number of veins are usually encountered here, and bleeding may be troublesome. It is absolutely essential that all arteries are preserved because they may supply not only the tumor, but also the brainstem. Any arterial bleeding should be treated by patient pressure on a piece of hemostatic gauze or muscle. If the anesthetist reports changes in vital signs during this or any other point in the dissection, traction on the tumor should be discontinued. It may be necessary also to remove some of the packing in order to reduce compression of the adjacent vessels. The vestibular and cochlear nerves are divided once they have been differentiated from the facial nerve, remembering that the anterior inferior cerebellar and/or labyrinthine arteries may lie on occcasions directly anterior to the vestibular nerve.

The upper and lower poles of the tumor can be mobilized only when the position of the facial nerve has been established. Usually it is displaced anterior to the tumor mass or, less commonly, over the superior surface. During dissection of the upper pole, the trigeminal nerve is encountered deep down as a white band passing across the subarachnoid space to enter Meckel's cave. The nerve is often adherent to the tumor capsule near the pons, and the basilar artery and abducent nerve may be visible deep to them.

The dissection is completed by working from lateral to, medial to, or above the facial nerve. Sharp dissection is less traumatic to the nerve than blunt, and traction must be avoided. Throughout the dissection the nerve should be irrigated with saline, both to wash away any bleeding which will otherwise obscure the field, and to keep it moist. It is often easier to dissect the facial nerve from the tumor in a lateral to medial direction. However, if the plane has been lost medial to the porus, the facial nerve can usually be identified by displacing the tumor inferiorly with the sucker. The nerve is exposed deep to and slightly above the porus, and is separated from it by sharp dissection. The facial nerve is most vulnerable to injury if it lies on the superior pole or, much more rarely, posteriorly. In either case, the tumor must be dissected deep to the nerve.

Once the tumor has been removed (Fig. 31.18) the facial nerve and porus acousticus should be inspected carefully for capsular remnants or residual neurinoma. If it is necessary to leave tumor fragments behind, bipolar coagulation of the remnants may make regrowth less likely (Lye et al 1992), although care must be taken to avoid heat injury to the structure to which they are adherent. In general, neural integrity should not be jeopardized in an attempt to excise every last vestige of tumor capsule. This occasions some agonizing at operation, and the alternative is resection and nerve grafting. However, the likelihood of symptomatic recurrence from small capsular remnants appears to be slight (Lye et al 1992). The least satisfactory outcome is to leave tumor attached to the nerve, having already damaged it irrevocably in an attempt at total tumor excision.

The physiological integrity of the facial nerve is tested at the conclusion of the procedure. Although nonfunction

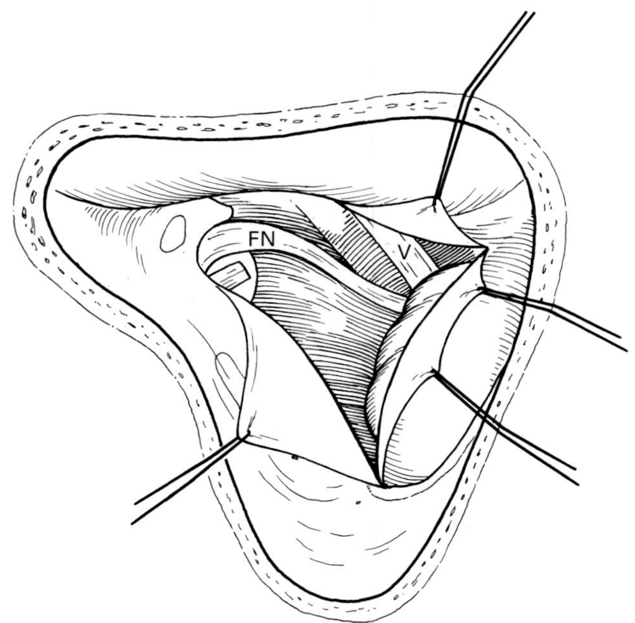

Fig. 31.18 The tumor bed at the completion of the resection. The facial nerve (F) is shown in its most usual position, displaced medially and upward; V = vestibular nerve.

does not preclude a good final outcome, success almost guarantees it. The technique for dealing with a divided facial nerve is given below. All cottonoids and silastic sheeting are then removed from the wound, and any small clots are evacuated. Meticulous hemostasis must be obtained, and the blood pressure should be restored to preoperative levels before the wound is closed. Some surgeons may choose to line the cerebellum and brainstem with hemostatic gauze. This, however, should not be used to excess because it swells over a period of hours by absorption of fluid into the cellulose, and can itself induce pressure effects.

Careful attention is required during wound closure if cerebrospinal fluid leakage, the most common complication of acoustic neurinoma surgery, is to be avoided. The bone dust collected during labyrinthectomy is made into a thick paste (bone pâté) by mixing it with a small amount of autologous blood.

During excision of the labyrinth the incus is removed, and a posterior tympanotomy slot is cut to expose the middle ear cavity and the mesotympanic end of the eustachian tube. Small pieces of fat, each about the size of a grain of wheat, are packed into the eustachian tube and middle ear cavity. Particular attention is paid to the region of the aditus, the head of the malleus, and the stapes footplate. The drilled surface of the petrous bone, posterior canal wall, aditus, and any exposed mastoid air cells are then covered with bone pâté. A patch of fascia lata (~ 2.5 cm × 2 cm) is then applied to the area and sealed with fibrin glue. No attempt is made to close the dural defect. The temporal bone is filled with two or three finger-sized fat strips, which are positioned through the dural defect, just into the cerebellopontine angle. These are sealed laterally with the remaining fibrin glue. The remainder of the wound closure technique is the same as that used for a retrosigmoid approach. If the skin has been elevated from the posterior wall of the external auditory canal, a BIPP pack should be placed in the ear for 7 days.

Middle cranial fossa approach

The middle cranial fossa approach was described by House in 1961. It is unique in allowing access to the labyrinthine segment of the facial nerve without sacrifice of hearing. On its own it has been used for hearing preservation operations on tumors confined to the internal auditory canal, or extending less than 5 mm into the cerebellopontine angle (Glasscock et al 1986). In addition, it may be combined with either the translabyrinthine or suboccipital approaches for the removal of larger lesions (Glasscock et al 1986). It has been criticized on the grounds of its restricted exposure, and because of potential complications which include temporal lobe epilepsy, dysphasia, intracerebral hematoma, and a greater risk to the facial nerve (Gantz et al 1986). Access to the posterior fossa is very limited, and this may give rise to problems in securing adequate hemostasis. With this approach the facial nerve lies superior to the tumor, requiring the surgeon to work around it. Manipulation of the nerve is therefore likely to be greater than with either the suboccipital or translabyrinthine approaches and is reflected in slightly poorer early facial nerve results.

Technique The patient is prepared as described above. The operation is conducted with the patient supine, and with the head rotated into a full lateral position. The surgeon sits at the head of the table. An inverted U-shaped flap is centered just anterior to the external auditory canal, and a small bone flap 3–4 cm in diameter is fashioned two thirds anterior and one third posterior to the external meatus, pedicled on the temporalis muscle. The inferior limb of the bone flap should be as close as possible to the floor of the middle cranial fossa (Fig. 31.19). A House-Urban retractor is attached to the superior margin of the craniotomy. The dura is elevated from the floor of the middle cranial fossa (Fig. 31.20A). Mobilization of the dura should commence posteriorly to avoid elevation of the greater superficial petrosal nerve and, therefore, applying traction to the facial nerve. Care is required in the region of the petrous ridge, which is grooved by the superior petrosal sinus. The middle meningeal artery, greater superficial petrosal nerve, and arcuate eminence (a prominence made by the underlying superior semicircular canal) are identified. If at any stage the dura is torn, the defect should be repaired immediately to prevent herniation of the temporal lobe. Starting at the facial hiatus, a

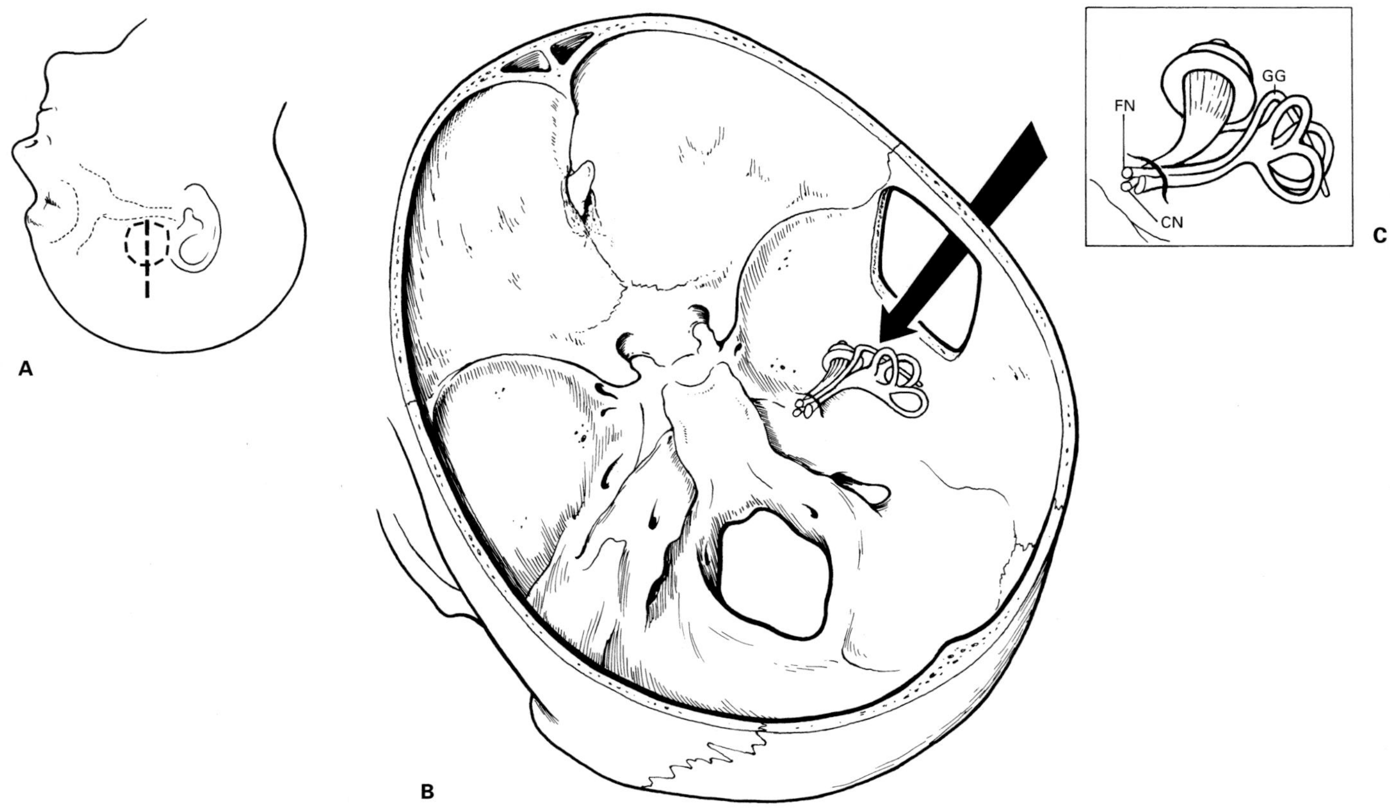

Fig. 31.19 **A.** Skin incision and site of craniotomy for the middle fossa operation. **B.** Surgical approach to the petrous bone via the middle cranial fossa. **C.** Relationship between the facial (FN) and cochlear (CN) nerves, and the inner ear. GG = geniculate ganglion; GSPN = greater superficial petrosal nerve.

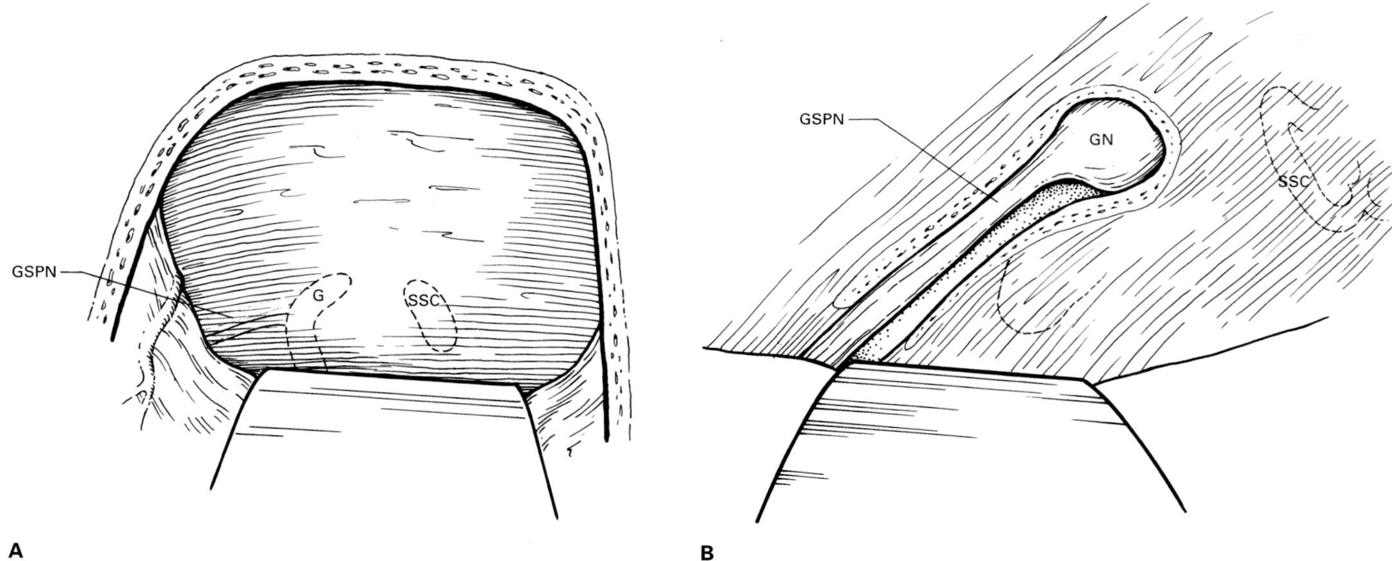

Fig. 31.20 **A.** The dura has been elevated from the floor of the middle cranial fossa to expose the greater superficial petrosal nerve (GSPN). The relationship of the nerve to the cochlea and superior semicircular canal (SSC) is shown. **B.** The facial canal has been unroofed. The relationship to the cochlea and superior semicircular canal (SSC) is again shown.

diamond burr with continuous suction/irrigation is used to unroof the bony canal covering the petrous portion of the greater superficial petrosal nerve and the geniculate ganglion (the nerve and geniculate ganglion are unprotected by bone in 5% of cases; Rhoton et al 1968, Buchheit & Rosenwasser 1988). Bone removal then continues medially to unroof the labyrinthine portion of the facial nerve. The superior surface of the internal auditory canal is then exposed back to the meatus. The ampullated end of the superior semicircular canal lies a few millimeters posterior to the facial nerve, and the cochlea a few millimeters anterior to it at the lateral end of the dissection (Fig. 31.20B). However, these structures diverge from the nerve medially, allowing greater exposure. Bone should be removed from about 75% of the circumference of the internal auditory meatus, leaving the superior petrosal sinus to lie free in the dura. Bill's bar is identified. If necessary the labyrinth and petrous bone posterior to the canal can be removed as far as the jugular bulb and sigmoid sinus by this route, although hearing will be destroyed (House 1964b). The dura is opened to expose the superior vestibular and facial nerves (Fig. 31.21). The vestibular nerves are divided and the tumor is dissected from the facial nerve. The principles of tumor dissection are the same as those outlined above. Particular difficulty may be encountered if the tumor arises from the inferior vestibular nerve. This will necessitate retraction of the facial nerve, and may result in a greater likelihood of subsequent neurapraxia (a normal preoperative caloric response may provide indirect evidence that the tumor arises from the inferior vestibular nerve, and may be considered as a relative contraindication to this approach; House & Luetje 1979). Both vestibular nerves should be sectioned, regardless of the origin of the tumor, to reduce the incidence of postoperative ataxia (Fig. 31.22). Great care is needed when excising the medial aspect of the tumor and freeing it from the margin of the internal meatus because the anterior inferior cerebellar artery may loop up into the porus below the cochlear nerve.

Any exposed air cells are filled with bone pâté, and the bony defect is filled with fat. The bone flap is replaced and the wound closed in layers in the usual fashion. Removal of bone over the superior semicircular canal until it is visible as a blue line, and extending the exposure anterior to the internal auditory canal (taking care anterolaterally to avoid the basal turn of the cochlea) are reported to improve access (Gantz et al 1986).

Combined approaches

Should exposure prove to be inadequate, the translabyrinthine approach may be combined with the transtentorial or suboccipital routes, as may the suboccipital and middle fossa operations. Although we have undertaken combined approaches in the past, and still do so on occasions for other tumors of the cerebellopontine angle, par-

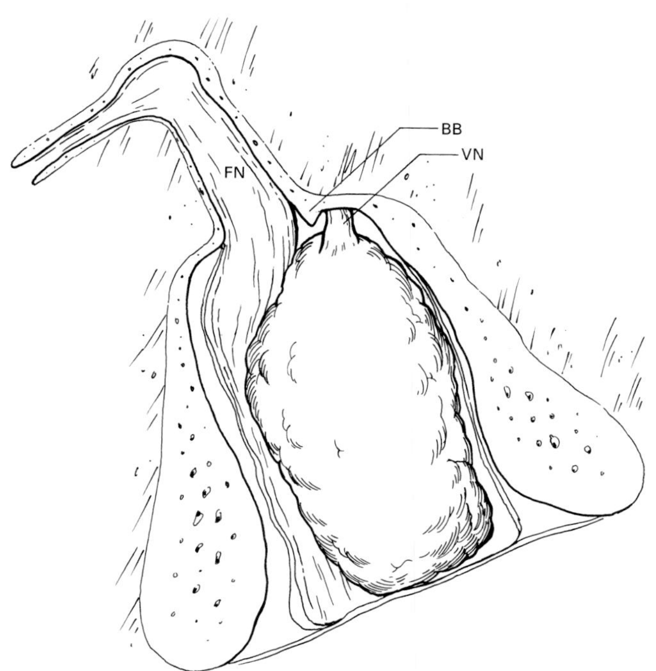

Fig. 31.21 The dura of the internal auditory meatus has been opened to expose the tumor, Bill's bar (BB), and the facial (FN) and superior vestibular (VN) nerves.

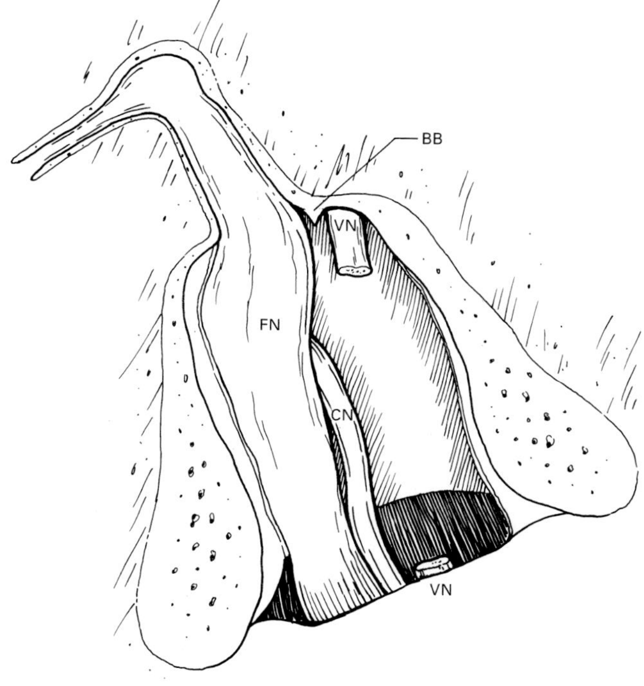

Fig. 31.22 The vestibular nerves (VN) have been divided, and the tumor removed. FN = facial nerve; CN = cochlear nerve; BB = Bill's bar.

ticularly meningiomas, we no longer find them necessary for excision of acoustic neurinomas.

Postoperative care

A brief period of postoperative ventilation may be appropriate after long procedures, particularly if the patient has become hypothermic during surgery. Although this has the advantage that intracranial pressure is kept low, one major disadvantage is that early signs of neurological deterioration from an impending cerebellopontine angle hematoma are masked. The patient should be nursed 15° head-up to reduce venous pressure. A short course of antibiotics should be administered, and dexamethasone may be of limited benefit — not only to reduce postoperative edema in the cerebellum, but to reduce swelling of the facial nerve and resultant delayed facial weakness. If a lumbar drain has not been inserted, lowering of the CSF pressure by daily lumbar puncture may reduce the incidence of cerebrospinal fluid leakage (Hardy et al 1989a).

When large tumors have been excised, the patient should be assessed for bulbar palsy before oral fluids are commenced. The consequences of facial palsy are dealt with below. Vestibular sedatives may be required if dizziness and vomiting are troublesome, but their use should be restricted to a minimum. Scalp sutures and the BIPP ear pack are removed on the seventh day.

Results

Most of the complications which may befall a patient after surgery are common to all three approaches. The exceptions are epilepsy and dysphasia, which are confined to the middle fossa operation, or in the exceptional case when it has been necessary to divide the tentorium. In unselected series mortality figures for the different surgical approaches are almost identical, and range from 0–2% in the hands of experienced surgeons in specialist centers. Almost all fatalities occur in patients with very large tumors. The major causes of death are brainstem infarction and hematoma in the cerebellopontine angle. Most other deaths follow cardiovascular or respiratory complications.

Tumor size is by far the most important single determinant of outcome, both in terms of mortality, facial nerve outcome, and the prospect for a good general recovery (Olivecrona 1967, House & Luetje 1979). Several large series have documented surgical results as they relate to tumor size. Outcome is regarded as excellent if patients are able to resume their previous employment, fair if they remain independent but unable to work, and poor if their independence has been lost. This classification excludes facial nerve function. The results of five series are summarized in Table 31.2.

There has been much discussion in the literature comparing and contrasting the merits and disadvantages of the suboccipital, translabyrinthine, and middle fossa approaches to the cerebellopontine angle. Good results are reported with each method, which indicates that experience, operative microsurgical technique, and postoperative management are more important determinants of outcome than the surgical approach per se. Direct comparisons between large series employing different surgical techniques are often misleading, for two reasons. Firstly, tumor size is the most important predictor of outcome, yet there is no single accepted classification to enable standardization of reporting of results. Secondly, the suboccipital and middle fossa approaches are often selected for hearing preservation procedures. Inevitably these groups

Table 31.2 Surgical results by tumor size

Author	No. cases	Operation	Tumor size**		Mortality	Facial nerve result†	Outcome in survivors		
							Excellent	*Fair*	*Poor*
Yasargil & Fox (1974)	100	SO*	Small	4%	0%	85%	95%	5%	0%
			Medium	19%	0%		82%	13%	5%
			Large	77%	4%		56%	37%	7%
Ojemann et al (1984)	123	SO	Small	15%	0%		100%	0%	0%
			Medium	30%	0%		100%	0%	0%
			Large	55%	1%		91%	7%	2%
King & Morrison (1980)	150	TL*	Small	11%	0%	100%	94%	6%	0%
			Medium	42%	2%	80%	100%	0%	0%
			Large	47%	3%	20%	93%	5%	2%
Bentivoglio et al (1988a)	94	SO	Small	14%	0%	100%	100%	0%	0%
			Medium	28%	0%	85%	92%	4%	4%
			Large	58%	4%	45%	66%	28%	8%
Hardy et al (1989a)	100	TL	Small	4%	0%	82%	100%	0%	0%
			Medium	30%	0%		83%	17%	0%
			Large	66%	4%		66%	29%	5%

Notes: SO = suboccipital; TL = translabyrinthine
* Denotes primary surgical approach, although series mixed.
† Facial nerve figures in some series are anatomic preservation rates, whilst others relate to functional outcome.
** The results of the different series are not strictly comparable as the definitions of tumor size varied. Small, medium, and large approximate to the Pulec classification.

have a higher proportion of small tumors, and therefore a better prognosis than the translabyrinthine operation, which is more appropriate for larger lesions with poor residual hearing. Patients with small or medium-sized tumors also have a significantly shorter mean hospital stay than those with larger lesions (Mangham 1988).

When considering the approach of choice for any one lesion, we agree with Chen & Fisch (1992) that 'most patients are far more concerned about the complete removal of their tumor and their facial function postoperatively than about hearing'. It is primarily for this reason that we favour the translabyrinthine operation for the majority of patients. Postoperative morbidity and hospital stay are generally shorter after translabyrinthine surgery (Tos & Thomsen 1982, Gardner et al 1983, Tator & Nedzelski 1985), although the incidence of postoperative meningitis may be slightly higher because of a more direct route for contamination of the CSF by nasopharyngeal organisms (Mangham 1988). Sterkers et al (1984) initially favored the translabyrinthine operation but used the suboccipital approach subsequently for hearing preservation. They have since reverted to the translabyrinthine operation as a result of higher morbidity and an increased incidence of facial nerve palsy. Although the results reported in the literature are excellent with each of the approaches, it should be remembered that they represent the best in the field. For the less experienced surgeon the translabyrinthine approach is probably more likely to produce a good result. This is because of improved access to the fundus of the tumor, and the ability to identify the facial nerve lateral to it at an early stage of the dissection, but it is unfamiliar to most neurosurgeons, who may be uncomfortable with it, at least to start with.

Facial nerve function. In unselected series, anatomic preservation rates for the facial nerve are generally around 71–90% using the suboccipital route (Yasargil et al 1977, Sugita & Kobayashi 1982, Harner & Ebersold 1985, Bentivoglio et al 1988a), and 80–96% for the translabyrinthine group (House & Luetje 1979, Whittaker & Luetje 1985, Hardy et al 1989a). In neither group was anatomic preservation of the nerve achieved at the expense of subtotal tumor excision, as previously suggested by Di Tullio et al (1978). Success at preservation is highly dependent on tumor size (see Table 31.2). In a series of 444 patients, House & Luetje (1979) reported complete facial paralysis in 0% of patients with small tumors, in 10.4% of those with medium-sized lesions, and in 21.4% of those with large tumors.

In a report of 43 patients with small tumors operated on through the middle fossa, Gantz et al (1986) were able to preserve the facial nerve in all but one case. However, 60% had some facial nerve dysfunction immediately after surgery, and 38% experienced complete paralysis. Ultimately, 86% achieved near-normal function. Shelton et al (1989a) reported their experience of 106 cases operated via the middle fossa, with near-normal facial nerve function in 89% of patients, and with some residual hearing in 59%. The increased trauma to the facial nerve via the middle fossa approach is probably the reason for the higher incidence of early facial weakness. For this reason we favor the suboccipital over the middle fossa approach for hearing conservation surgery.

Anatomic integrity of the nerve does not guarantee facial function, either in the short or long term. If the nerve is intact anatomically but facial paralysis is complete postoperatively, then some return of function can be anticipated in 90% of cases (Hitselberger 1979), although it is unlikely to be complete. The rate at which the nerve recovers also predicts the final outcome. While recovery may continue for up to three years, Hitselberger (1979) found that it was always less than perfect if more than four months had elapsed from the time of surgery. Return of facial function may be heralded by transient facial pain. Facial nerve dysfunction does not usually affect all regions of the face to the same degree. Adequate movement of the oral commissure is more than twice as likely to occur than complete eye closure, and asymmetry of the forehead is particularly common (Wiegand & Fickel 1989). The presence of preoperative facial weakness increases the probability of facial nerve injury at surgery, but does not predict the final outcome if the nerve is spared anatomically (Lye et al 1982). These authors were able to preserve the nerve in 91% of cases with normal preoperative facial nerve function, but in only 67% of patients with preoperative weakness. However, it is not clear whether some of the disparity between the two groups is the result of differences in tumor size.

The degree of facial nerve weakness in the early postoperative period may be predicted at surgery from a comparison of the amplitude of the compound muscle action potential obtained by facial nerve stimulation proximal and distal to the site of tumor excision. If the percentage amplitude is greater than 90% then very good early facial function may be anticipated. If the amplitude lies between 50 and 90% then temporary weakness may occur, but the final outcome is likely to be good. An amplitude of less than 50% suggests that a temporary lateral tarsorrhaphy may be advisable under the same anesthetic, and that some degree of permanent facial weakness is probable (Ebersold et al 1992).

Hearing preservation. In only around 30–50% of hearing preservation operations will functional hearing remain, despite anatomic preservation of the auditory apparatus (Tatagiba et al 1992). In an analysis of the English language literature from 1954–1986, the overall success with hearing preservation was 33% in series with a preponderance of small tumors (Gardner & Robertson 1988). The causes of such high failure rates are thought to be multifactorial. Possible factors include nerve manipulation with disruption of the myelin sheaths (Sekiya &

Møller 1987), impairment to the vasculature of the inner ear or cochlear nerve (Ebersold et al 1992), heat or vibration injury to the nerve and cochlea during removal of the posterior wall of the internal auditory canal, and damage to the labyrinth (Tatagiba et al 1992). From their experience with intraoperative monitoring, Ojemann et al (1984) observed that one of the critical stages in terms of hearing preservation was removal of tumor from the lateral aspect of the internal auditory canal. They proposed that dissection avulses some of the cochlear nerve fibers at the cribriform area, where they enter the modiolus. The most frequently injured labyrinthine structures are the crus commune of the posterior and superior semicircular canals, and the posterior semicircular canal (Tatagiba et al 1992). Hearing loss after labyrinthine injury is ascribed to loss of perilymph from the inner ear, although total deafness is not an inevitable sequel to it (Tatagiba et al 1992).

It is generally accepted that hearing preservation is deemed successful only if that which remains is of serviceable quality. The 50/50 rule is often applied; that there is less than a 50 dB hearing loss in the pure tone range, and that speech discrimination is greater than 50%. Yet this is not sufficient to be useful socially if contralateral hearing is normal. A pure tone average of 30 dB and a speech discrimination score of greater than 70% is required.

As with tumor size and facial nerve function, there is no single accepted classification for the reporting of hearing results. The Shelton-Brackmann classification (Shelton et al 1989b) is, however, gaining support. Hearing is classified as good (PTA < 30 dB; SDS> 70%), serviceable (PTA< 50 dB; SDS> 50%), measurable (any residual hearing), or anacusis. Formal testing is necessary. Great caution must be exercised in believing the patient's evaluation of his/her residual hearing. Some patients have claimed that hearing in the operated ear was unchanged after translabyrinthine surgery. Clearly this is not the case, and that the contralateral ear is responding to the auditory stimulus. For this reason, evaluation must ensure adequate masking of the unoperated ear. Success at preservation varies considerably between series, but Wigand et al (1991) reported recently a success rate of 51% in a series which included tumors as large as 3 cm. Using the middle fossa approach, Gantz et al (1986) retained some measurable hearing in 52% of patients with small tumors. Nadol et al (1992) were able to retain useful hearing in 50% of cases in which the tumor extended less than 5 mm into the cerebellopontine angle, but in only 12% of tumors larger than 25 mm.

It is exceptional for hearing to improve upon the preoperative level. Nadol et al (1992) reported this in only 5% of patients, and Gardner & Robertson (1988) in 6%. This is probably because atrophy of the organ of Corti develops secondary to denervation, because the elevated protein concentration in the perilymph damages the outer hair cells, and because of inner ear ischemia caused by compression of the labyrinthine artery within the porus acousticus. Perlman & Kimura (1955) demonstrated that temporary vascular occlusion of only 30 minutes was sufficient to produce permanent impairment of hearing as a consequence of severe hair cell and spiral ganglion cell loss. Finally, the cochlear nerve itself may be invaded by tumor (Neely 1981). Kveton (1990) hypothesized that improvement in hearing was the result of reversal of conduction block. Small tumor size, good preoperative speech discrimination, and male sex correlate significantly with a good hearing outcome (Nadol et al 1992).

Hearing may worsen or fluctuate months or even years after surgery. The formation of scar tissue around the cochlear nerve as a consequence of packing the drilled surface of the porus may be a contributory factor (Shelton et al 1990). However, because the tumor may on occasions invade the cochlear nerve, delayed hearing loss can represent tumor recurrence (Neely 1984). Delayed edema is a further etiologic factor in early hearing loss, and may respond to corticosteroids (Goel et al 1992). Prophylactic nimodipine administration has been suggested to prevent vasospasm of the internal auditory artery, and also because of its neural protective effects (Nadol et al 1987).

In more than 50% of patients in whom hearing preservation has been successful there will be a significant decline in function as follow-up lengthens, even in the absence of recurrent disease (Shelton et al 1990). In an 8-year follow-up study of 25 patients the unoperated side remained the better hearing ear in all patients over the entire period (Shelton et al 1992). This argues that the philosophy of preserving any measurable hearing in order to safeguard against the possibility of deafness developing in the contralateral ear is unjustified. Taking into account late deterioration, it has been estimated that only 7–9% of the total group who undergo hearing preservation procedures will have useful hearing long term (Whittaker & Luetje 1992).

It may be anticipated that medially placed tumors, that is those which do not occupy the fundus of the internal auditory meatus, might have a better prognosis for both facial nerve function and for hearing preservation than tumors which fill the porus. Although it is much easier to identify the nerves lateral to the tumor, the surgical results are no better in this subgroup of patients, either in terms of facial nerve recovery or hearing preservation. This is because these lesions often present late, and when the tumor is correspondingly of a greater size (Tos et al 1992b).

Complications of surgery

Hematoma in the operative cavity. This is a rare but potentially fatal consequence of surgery. If hemostasis has been meticulous, this complication should occur in less than 2% of cases. Profound unconsciousness, respiratory failure, and pulmonary edema can develop very rapidly, and temperature elevation may be evident. Prompt action is required if the diagnosis is suspected. The patient should be ventilated to protect the airway and, if a frontal burr hole has been placed, intracranial pressure should be lowered by tapping the lateral ventricle. The patient should be transferred with the greatest speed to the operating room although, if the patient's state is parlous, the wound can be opened in the ward. However, this should be avoided if at all possible as the hematoma may lie deep in the cavity, adjacent to the pons. Optimum conditions are required if the clot is to be evacuated without risk to the cranial nerves and brainstem vasculature, and this is unlikely to be achieved without proper illumination, magnification, and instrumentation. Copious irrigation and a fine sucker will help to evacuate the hematoma and lessen the risk of nerve injury. A period of postoperative ventilation is recommended if re-exploration has been necessary.

Brainstem infarction. Devastating neurological sequelae may follow injury to the anterior inferior cerebellar artery. It is a fundamental principle of this type of surgery that arteries of any size within the cerebellopontine angle are preserved, even if they are firmly adherent to the tumor capsule. Only small branches actually entering the substance of the tumor may be cauterized and divided. Larger vessels must be mobilized from the capsule or, if this proves impossible, capsular remnants should be left attached to the vessel. For the same reason, some surgeons have found it necessary on very rare occasions to leave capsular remnants adherent to the brainstem, since subpial dissection in this region may be equally catastrophic. Bleeding from a brainstem vessel should be controlled by gentle pressure on a piece of crushed muscle or hemostatic gauze.

Cerebrospinal fluid leakage. With the exception of facial nerve palsy, cerebrospinal fluid leakage from the wound or middle ear cavity is the most common postoperative complication of acoustic neurinoma surgery (House et al 1982, Tos & Thomsen 1985, Gordon & Kerr 1986, Brackmann & Kwartler 1990a). An incidence of around 10–15% is reported in most major series (Di Tullio et al 1978, King & Morrison 1980, Glasscock et al 1986, Hardy et al 1989a, Ebersold et al 1992). The major contributing factors are poor wound healing, hydrocephalus, and failure to obliterate air cells opened in the porus acousticus or mastoid. After translabyrinthine or suboccipital surgery CSF may leak into the perimeatal or retrofacial air cells, or via the dural defect into the mastoid air cells, and thence gain access to the middle ear cavity and eustachian tube. In addition to CSF leakage, symptomatic aerocele may develop.

Meticulous attention to the technique of wound closure can diminish the incidence of this complication dramatically. Using the method described in the operative section above, Hardy et al (1993) reduced their CSF leakage rate to 1.6% in a recent series of 230 patients. Although some authors have argued that fat should not be used in wound closure because it may make subsequent MRI studies difficult to interpret (Ebersold et al 1992), their CSF leakage rate using bone wax alone is unacceptably high. We have no experience with synthetic bone replacement materials pioneered recently. Ionomeric cement has the ability to adhere even to moist surfaces, and is reported to be a significant advance over other synthetic cements such as polymethyl methacrylate (Ramsden et al 1992).

If CSF leakage does occur, conservative measures such as lumbar drain insertion or the placement of additional sutures in the wound are successful in around 25% of patients (Hardy et al 1989a), but the remainder will require re-exploration. In general, CSF leakage from the wound is much more likely to settle with conservative treatment than is rhinorrhea. The value of prophylactic antibiotics is questionable. The technique used to seal the defect should be the same as described above. Bone pâté is used to fill the exposed air cells, and is reinforced with a fascia lata patch sealed in place with fibrin glue. Fat is used to fill the bony defect, and this too is sealed with fibrin glue. A lumbar drain may be placed for a few days to maintain a low CSF pressure until the wound has had the opportunity to heal.

Meningitis. The risk of postoperative meningitis relates not simply to the development of CSF leakage. The protracted nature of the operation and the communication of the operative site with the eustachian tube are other important factors. Infection rates in the literature are generally around 3–6% (Di Tullio et al 1978, King & Morrison 1980, Bentivoglio et al 1988b, Hardy et al 1989a).

Diplopia. Postoperative unilateral abducent nerve paresis must be differentiated from a gaze palsy secondary to involvement of the lateral gaze center in the pons. The latter usually resolves within a few days of surgery, whereas injury to the abducent nerve may take considerably longer. Diplopia can be treated by an eye patch although, if the patient has a concomitant facial palsy, a more than adequate tarsorrhaphy will achieve the same result. Meningitis should be considered in the differential diagnosis of a delayed sixth nerve palsy.

Hearing loss. It is quite common for hearing to be decreased transiently after any surgery to the posterior fossa. The current hypothesis is that the low CSF pressure is transmitted via the cochlear aqueduct to the perilymph, producing perilymphatic hypotonia (Walstead et al 1991). Hearing loss in the contralateral ear after acoustic neurinoma removal has also been attributed to an autoimmune response (Harris et al 1985). Clemis et al (1982) reported three such patients, all of whom recovered spontaneously.

Special considerations

Tumors in the elderly and infirm. In view of the slow growth rate in the majority of tumors, a conservative approach to management may be appropriate for very elderly or infirm patients. However, an expectant policy in aged but otherwise fit patients is less clear. Nedzelski et al (1986) studied the growth behavior of 50 untreated acoustic neurinomas in elderly patients followed up for between 12 and 144 months. They reported that around 20% of such patients required surgery within a third of their life expectancy. Yet even quite old patients will tolerate surgical excision of tumors. Two recent series, one suboccipital, the other translabyrinthine, have emphasized that age is not a contraindication to successful surgery. House et al (1987) reported a series of 116 patients over the age of 65 years with only one death, and functional preservation of the facial nerve in 91% of cases. Samii et al (1992) recorded 61 patients operated on without mortality, with anatomic preservation of the facial nerve in 95%, and with residual hearing in 41%. In both series the majority of excisions were macroscopic (91% and 97% respectively). As well as tumor size and evidence of mass effect, the presence of disabling symptoms such as vertigo is an indication for early intervention. Predictive factors for a poor outcome are ASA (American Society of Anesthesiologists Grading of Physical Status) of greater than 3, a Karnofsky score of less than 80, and tumor size greater than 3 cm (Samii et al 1992). In the case of surgery for a symptomatic tumor in a frail patient, it may be appropriate to reduce the duration of the operation either by elective subtotal excision, or by macroscopic removal with no attempt at preservation of the facial nerve.

Subtotal excision. This may be a planned procedure in, for example, a patient with a large tumor in a solitary hearing ear, or if facial weakness would be completely unacceptable. On other occasions it may be necessary to leave a rim of capsule adherent to the brainstem or adjacent vessels. Olivecrona (1967) observed that half of his 83 patients remained asymptomatic after partial tumor removal. This was also the experience of Wazen et al (1985): 11 of 13 elderly patients who had residual tumor after surgery showed no significant expansion over an average period of 6 years. In a series of 12 patients who underwent radical intracapsular removal of large tumors, and who were followed for up to 22 years, Lownie & Drake (1991) reported recurrence in only 2 cases, both within 3 years of surgery. However, Hitselberger & House (1979) found that the late recurrence rate necessitating re-exploration in their series was high, and that surgery on the second occasion was more hazardous. Ransohoff et al (1961) noted ultimately that 60% of patients treated in the 1930s by subtotal excision either died from recurrent disease or required a second operation. In Cushing's series of 182 patients, those who underwent subtotal excision but died eventually from tumor recurrence lived for an average of 5 years after the initial operation (German 1961).

With the exception of NF-2 patients, elective subtotal excision is unsatisfactory and illogical for small or medium-sized tumors. If a cure is not to be effected when the tumor is of a favorable size, then treatment should be delayed until symptoms become more serious. A more vexing issue is whether it is preferable to excise every last remnant of tumor at the risk of compromise to neural integrity, or to minimize the possibility of nerve or brainstem injury by leaving capsular or tumor remnants behind. This issue is particularly relevant to attempts at hearing preservation. The success rate is generally poor, and any residual hearing may not be useful socially. In order to answer this question fully it is clear that longitudinal MRI studies are required, given that the growth potential of residual tumor appears at present to be unpredictable. Lye et al (1992) reported recently the results of a follow-up MRI study of 14 patients with capsular remnants left attached to vital structures at the time of otherwise total tumor removal. Over a mean period of 70 months, half the patients had radiologic evidence of persistent neurinoma. Four of these showed signs of progressive enlargement, although none was symptomatic and CT was normal in each. Persistence of tumor was more common if the residual fragments had not been not cauterized at the time of operation (Lye et al 1992).

Facial nerve neurinoma. These neurinomas account for less than 2% of lesions thought preoperatively to be acoustic neurinomas (House & Luetje 1979). The radiologic differential diagnosis has been discussed. At operation the facial nerve fibers are found to enter the tumor, and cannot be separated from it. The lateral extent of the tumor is often considerably greater than tumors of vestibular origin, and may on occasions reach the geniculate ganglion. The basic principles of excision are the same as for removal of an acoustic neurinoma, although the facial nerve will be divided. Direct end-to-end anastomosis may be possible, or a primary graft may be fashioned from the greater auricular or sural nerves.

INDICATIONS FOR AND RESULTS OF RADIATION THERAPY

Conventional external beam radiotherapy has been used as an adjuvant therapy for patients with subtotal tumor resection, or in cases of advanced disease (Cushing 1921). In a series of 31 patients receiving postoperative irradiation, Wallner et al (1987) reported that a dose of 50–55 Gy was well tolerated, and reduced the probability of recurrence from 46% to 6%. Treatment was administered in 1.8 Gy fractions, 5 days per week. However, irradiation did not influence recurrence rates if more than 90% of the tumor had been excised, and radiation therapy for tumor recurrence after a previous surgical resection was associated with a poor prognosis. Irradiation is reported also to reduce tumor vascularity (Wallner et al 1987), and has been used in the preoperative management of highly vascular tumors (Ikeda et al 1988). Sequelae of radiation therapy include multiple cranial nerve palsies, brainstem edema, and brainstem ischemia (Brackmann & Kwartler 1990a).

Stereotactic radiosurgery

Experience of stereotactic radiosurgery using a 201-source ^{60}Co Gamma Knife remains limited, and series with longer follow-up are required. Only lesions less than 3 cm are suitable for this form of treatment. The principle of the technique is that multiple converging gamma beams are collimated to a focus, targeted on the lesion via a stereotactic frame applied to the skull. A dose of 10–15 Gy is delivered to the tumor periphery and a maximum of 15–25 Gy to the center (Norén et al 1992). The entire dose is delivered as a single fraction over 10–20 minutes. The dose gradient of the radiation is extremely steep at the target tissue.

A report on 26 patients followed for up to 19 months after treatment noted a decrease in tumor size in 11 patients, with arrest of growth in the remainder (Linskey et al 1990). Loss of central tumor contrast enhancement was the characteristic CT appearance, and the median onset of tumor shrinkage was one year after therapy. Delayed facial paresis developed in 6 patients (usually around 5 months after treatment), and trigeminal sensory loss in 7. Most facial neuropathies were partial and improved with time, although only 20% ever regained normal facial nerve function (Lunsford et al 1992a). Of patients who had good or serviceable hearing preoperatively, around 50% reported either reduced or total hearing loss within one year. At 1–2 years, only 24% of patients retained useful hearing.

Communicating hydrocephalus has been recorded as a complication of stereotactic radiosurgery (Thomsen et al 1990, Norén et al 1992), even in the absence of further tumor enlargement. This phenomenon is thought to be related to elevation of the CSF protein content. Any evidence of an increase in mass effect after radiosurgery is an indication for surgical decompression. Stereotactic radiosurgery does not preclude future microsurgical excision, although the risk of complete facial palsy may be higher.

At present it is unlikely that stereotactic radiosurgery will replace microsurgery as the treatment of choice for most patients, particularly as it has not been possible to establish a clear-cut dose-volume relationship for the development of complications. However, the technique offers an alternative treatment for the elderly, for patients who are medically unfit, and for those who have tumor in the only hearing ear, are unwilling to submit to surgery, or who develop tumor recurrence following previous excision (Linskey et al 1990, Lunsford et al 1992b). Stereotactic radiosurgery may be an alternative to conventional treatment in cases of NF-2, although the morbidity here is slightly greater than when treating sporadic tumors. Progressive hearing deterioration or deafness may be anticipated in 64% of patients, transient facial palsy in 12%, and progressive tumor growth in 34% (Hirsch & Norén 1988). Brackmann & Kwartler (1990b) do not recommend stereotactic radiosurgery, and have observed symptoms in 3 patients consistent with fibrotic occlusion of the anterior inferior cerebellar artery.

The mechanism by which tumor growth is inhibited remains uncertain. In vitro studies suggest that Schwann cells suffer irreversible damage after single fraction doses of 30 Gy (Anniko et al 1981). Histopathology reveals interstitial fibrosis, tumor necrosis, vascular hyperplasia and hyalinization (Lunsford et al 1992a).

The linear accelerator is a less expensive method of delivering stereotactic radiotherapy than ^{60}Co because dedicated equipment is not required. However, there are as yet no published series which compare the results and complications to those achieved with the Gamma Knife.

INDICATIONS FOR AND RESULTS OF CHEMOTHERAPY

Chemotherapy has little place in the management of this condition, but has been proposed as an alternative treatment for bilateral acoustic neurinomas (Jahrsdoerfer & Benjamin 1988). A course of 6 treatments of cyclophosphamide, doxorubicin, and dacarbazine over a period of 6 months resulted in cessation of tumor growth and stabilization of hearing in 2 patients. Follow-up was for only 15 months, however, and long-term data are lacking.

OTHER ADJUVANT THERAPY

In 1978, Harker et al described in vitro cellular immunity against acoustic neurinoma cells. This has provided a theoretical potential for the development of immunotherapy. The concept of an antitumor cellular immune response has been taken a stage further with a report of the successful treatment of some head and neck cancers using interleukin-2 activated killer cells (Ishikawa et al 1989). However, before such treatment could be considered for the treatment of a benign tumor it will be necessary to identify the antigenic substance involved, and to confirm that it is specific only to acoustic neurinomas.

MANAGEMENT OF ASSOCIATED PHENOMENA

Management of the eye

Incomplete eye closure and reduced lacrimation make the

postoperative patient vulnerable to infection and exposure keratitis, particularly when corneal sensation is also diminished. Poor lid closure, ectropion, inadequate Bell's phenomenon, and/or incomplete blinking may cause drying of the cornea and conjunctiva, leading to corneal epithelial damage. Not only does reduced corneal sensation exacerbate the likelihood of injury, but corneal healing is impaired, and neurotropic keratitis may ensue. The cornea can be protected with artificial tears such as methyl cellulose, but this has the disadvantage of requiring frequent applications. Ointments (e.g. Lacrilube) last much longer, and are useful at night when blurring of vision is not important. Antimicrobial preparations such as chloramphenicol are used if infection develops, while corneal injury may require judicious use of topical steroids and cycloplegics. Although the eye may be protected with a patch at night there is still the risk of dessication and, for this reason, we prefer an eye bubble to retain moisture and prevent contact with the cornea. Protective spectacles may be worn by day.

A lateral tarsorrhaphy should be performed under local anesthetic if eye closure is deficient, and Bell's phenomenon is inadequate to provide corneal cover. The epithelium is denuded over the desired length of the tarsorrhaphy. The lids are sutured through the grey line, using a 5/0 suture over a bolster. The suture is removed at 14 days. With the passage of time there is a tendency for the tarsorrhaphy to open medially, therefore it should be slightly generous in the first instance. If facial weakness persists long term, plastic surgical procedures such as upper lid gold weight and/or wire spring, medial canthoplasty and lower lid shortening may become appropriate.

Management of the facial nerve

Even when the facial nerve has been preserved in anatomic continuity, the inevitable manipulation required to dissect it from the tumor capsule may result in neurapraxia. The lack of protective epineurium in the cerebellopontine angle segment increases the risk of injury (Sunderland 1978). The success with which the nerve can be preserved anatomically, and its ultimate functional outcome, are dependent on tumor size. Of patients with complete clinical paralysis despite anatomic preservation, some improve rapidly within weeks of surgery and the end result is functionally acceptable (Morgon et al 1985). However, 9–18% never recover facial tone or active movement (House & Luetje 1979, Moffat et al 1989c). Patients with Wallerian degeneration have a worse prognosis than those with neurapraxia (Gantz et al 1984). Croxson et al (1989) and Hardy et al (1989b) have reported that postoperative electroneuronography one week after surgery is a good predictor of final outcome in patients with clinically complete paresis. A percentage degeneration is calculated by comparing the amplitude of the ipsilateral compound action potential with that of the normal side. In these two studies all patients with incomplete degeneration attained House grade I–II, whilst those with complete degeneration had a protracted and incomplete recovery in every case. Spontaneous regeneration of an anatomically intact nerve is more likely to provide a good cosmetic result than secondary grafting. If the nerve remains in continuity, facial reanimation should therefore be delayed for around 12 months before any secondary procedures are contemplated. However, if the final outcome is House grade III or worse, there is no significant difference in the cosmetic appearance between regeneration of an intact nerve, primary facial nerve repair, or facial-hypoglossal nerve anastomosis (King et al 1993).

Primary facial nerve repair

If the facial nerve is divided at operation, primary repair is likely to provide the most satisfactory outcome. Although the functional result is probably little different from donor nerve grafting techniques (Stennert 1979), the major advantages are that function in a normal nerve is not sacrificed and a second surgical procedure is not required. A good outcome may be anticipated in around 65% of patients (Barrs et al 1984b), although the final result is unlikely to be known for one year after grafting. The results are considerably poorer in NF-2 patients, possibly because of a more invasive growth pattern (Jaaskelainen et al 1990).

Because the nerve has been stretched by the tumor, direct end-to-end facial nerve anastomosis may be possible. Direct anastomosis without a cable graft was possible in 37% of cases in one suboccipital series (Ebersold et al 1992). If the translabyrinthine approach has been used, an additional 1 cm of length may be gained by mobilization of the nerve from the fallopian canal with detachment of the greater superficial petrosal nerve from the geniculate ganglion (Whittaker & Luetje 1985), although rarely is this of value in practice. If there is insufficient length to allow direct anastomosis of the divided ends, a sural or posterior auricular nerve interposition graft may be used. The anastomosis is either sutured, or wrapped in a tube of fascia lata and sealed with fibrin glue. Fisch et al (1987) have proposed the use of a fenestrated collagen splint for nerve anastomosis.

Primary repair is not always possible, particularly if the nerve has been divided at the brainstem, or if the remnants are severely attenuated. In this instance there are several alternatives. The first involves anastomosis of the distal facial nerve to either the hypoglossal, spinal accessory (Migliavacca 1967), glossopharyngeal (Duel 1934), or phrenic nerves (Conley & Baker 1979), or the performance of a cross-facial anastomosis (Smith 1979). Of these options, the phrenic and glossopharyngeal nerves are unsuitable donors because of the unacceptable consequences of denervation. The spinal accessory nerve, with or without preservation of the branch to trapezius, has been reported by some to give good results (Migliavacca 1967, Ebersold & Quast 1992), but others have found greater success with hypoglossal-facial anastomosis (Mingrino & Zuccarello 1981). This may be because the cortical representation of the tongue is larger and more closely related to the face than is the shoulder. Cross-facial anastomosis is technically more demanding, and involves sural nerve interposition grafts between the two facial nerves. Results are generally poorer than hypoglossal-facial anastomosis, perhaps because of decreased axonal input for reinnervation (Tran Ba Huy et al 1985, Zini et al 1985). For all of these reasons we prefer facial-hypoglossal anastomosis, except if the patient also has a bulbar palsy.

If there has been some return of facial function but the cosmetic result remains unsatisfactory, plastic surgical procedures may be beneficial. An upper lid gold weight can improve eye closure sufficiently for the lateral tarsorrhaphy to be taken down. Facial asymmetry at rest may be restored by a fascia lata sling. If necessary this can be supplemented by a face lift, brow lift, or canthoplasty. These procedures are, however, static, and do not provide active movement. The latter may be achieved to a limited degree by temporalis muscle transfer.

Hypoglossal-facial nerve anastomosis

The first such attempt at facial reanimation is attributed to Korte in 1901 (Pitty & Tator 1992). Many series have been published in the literature, and their results range from poor to good (for review see Pitty & Tator 1992). Results are better in younger patients, and when the interval between nerve division and anastomosis is short, although this latter point has been contested by Hitselberger (1979). In a recent series of 22 cases, good or fair results occurred in 77% of patients. Evidence of reinnervation was seen between 3 and 6 months after surgery in 59%, and in the remainder within 8 months (Pitty & Tator 1992). The result often improves with time, possibly because of the plasticity within the nervous system.

Technique

The operation is conducted with the patient supine, and the head in a neutral position. Rotation of the neck should be avoided as this makes dissection of the hypoglossal nerve more difficult. A facial nerve stimulator is of benefit only if the operation is performed before Wallerian degeneration has occurred in the distal fibers. The skin incision starts anterior to the tragus, curves posteriorly below the pinna, and then forward down into the neck, a fingerbreadth below the angle of the mandible. Where possible, the greater auricular nerve should be preserved.

The facial nerve emerges from the skull through the stylomastoid foramen, anterior and deep to the mastoid tip. Two muscular branches pass posteriorly to supply the occipital belly of occipitofrontalis and the posterior belly of digastric. The main trunk passes forward horizontally, to enter the posteromedial surface of the parotid gland. Here it divides into two branches, the temporozygomatic and the cervicofacial. The facial nerve can be identified at surgery in one of three ways. The plane anterior to the sternomastoid muscle can be developed by sharp dissection, and the posterior belly of digastric exposed near its origin from the digastric notch on the medial aspect of the mastoid tip. The nerve to digastric is then identified, and traced proximally to the main trunk of the facial nerve. The styloid process lies just anterior and slightly deep to the facial nerve, and is a useful landmark. The second option is to use the technique described by Hitselberger (1979). Via a cortical mastoidectomy the descending portion of the facial nerve is identified in the fallopian canal within the mastoid bone. The facial nerve is skeletonized from the midportion of the horizontal segment to the stylomastoid foramen, is divided proximally, and is then delivered down into the neck. The third technique, which we favor, is to expose the tragal cartilage. The facial nerve can be found 1 cm inferior, and 1 cm deep, to the inferior margin of the cartilage (the tragal point; Mattox 1992).

The hypoglossal nerve is readily identified in the anterior triangle of the neck, where it lies above the greater cornu of the hyoid — a useful reference point. The common facial vein is divided between ligatures. The hypoglossal nerve lies on the carotid sheath deep to the internal jugular vein and posterior belly of digastric. It passes in front of the lower branches of the external carotid artery, and divides into several branches shortly before entering the tongue. If the main trunk of the nerve cannot be identified, the descendens hypoglossi (innervation to the infrahyoid muscles) can be exposed on the front of the internal jugular vein and traced proximally.

The entire trunk of the hypoglossal nerve is divided just as it starts to divide at the tongue. It is very important to divide the nerve as distally as possible or there may be insufficient length to reach the facial nerve. An end-to-end anastomosis is fashioned under magnification and without tension between the hypoglossal and distal facial nerves using interrupted 8/0 epineurial sutures. The suture line is then coated with fibrin glue. In an attempt to minimize atrophy of the tongue the descendens hypoglossi nerve may be divided and sutured to the distal hypoglossal nerve stump. Hammershlag et al (1992) reported recently the results of a technique for facial-hypoglossal anastomosis which both avoids wasting of the tongue and reduces facial hypertonus. The hypoglossal nerve is hemi-sectioned obliquely, just distal to the descendens hypoglossi, and a sural or greater auricular nerve graft is interposed between the partially divided nerve and the distal facial nerve.

Results

Pitty & Tator (1992) have summarized the literature on hypoglossal-facial nerve anastomoses over the past 37 years, and summated the results of 562 cases. Good results were achieved in 65% of cases, fair results in 22%, and poor or no recovery in the remaining 13%. Despite reinnervation, incomplete eye closure and mass facial movement may be evident, and require additional cosmetic procedures (see above). Hemiatrophy of the tongue produced only minimal dysfunction (impaired intraoral food manipulation), and anastomosis of the descendens hypoglossi to the distal stump did not influence hemiatrophy (Pitty & Tator 1992). Although results were better if the anastomosis was performed early, it is reported that surgery many years after nerve section may still on occasions produce a satisfactory outcome (McKenzie & Alexander 1950, Hitselberger 1979).

Deafness

Patients with unilateral hearing loss after surgery may benefit from a contralateral routing of offside signals (CROS) hearing aid. Total deafness may face a patient with bilateral acoustic neurinoma, or tumor in a solitary hearing ear. There are two potential surgical options if hearing is lost postoperatively. If the cochlear nerve is physiologically preserved but there is no residual hearing due to impairment of inner ear vasculature or injury to the labyrinth, a response to stimulation of the round window is predictive for likely success with a cochlear implant (Waltzman et al 1990). This is an electronic device placed in the inner ear to stimulate the cochlear nerve. However, if the cochlear nerve is lost, or if the hair cells and spiral ganglion cells have been destroyed, a brainstem auditory stimulator (sometimes called a central electro-auditory prosthesis) is the only other option. This aims to stimulate the cochlear nucleus directly (Hitselberger et al 1984). The optimum electrode placement is thought to be medially in the recess of the fourth ventricle, adjacent to the dorsal cochlear nucleus (Nelson 1992). The number of patients so treated is small, but a significant number are said to receive useful auditory percepts which improve their lip-reading scores (Nelson 1992).

Bulbar palsy

Transient bulbar palsy may develop after removal of large tumors. Provided that the nerves are intact the prognosis for recovery appears good (Hardy et al 1989a). To reduce the risk of aspiration, patients should undergo formal assessment of swallowing to ensure bulbar competence before oral fluids are commenced postoperatively.

PATTERNS OF FAILURE

House (1968) noted that, when tumor regrowth does occur, it does so within four years of the initial resection. Incomplete tumor resection may be a conscious decision at the time of surgery. The most common indications are adherence of the capsule to the brainstem or other vital structures (e.g. AICA), and preservation of good facial nerve function. The behavior of the tumor remnant is unpredictable. Recurrence is not an inevitable sequel, and spontaneous involution of the remnant is well documented (Shea et al 1985). However, in a study of 33 patients with residual tumor followed up for a mean of 5.5 years, 36.5% required surgery for symptomatic recurrent tumor, and 9% died (Shea et al 1985). After 'total' tumor excision, recurrence rates in most large series are less than 1–2%. Inadvertent subtotal excision has been discussed in the preceding sections, but is most likely if visualization of the fundus of the internal auditory canal has been inadequate. Continued tumor expansion can be expected in 5–14% of patients treated with stereotactic radiosurgery.

MANAGEMENT OF RECURRENT DISEASE

The growth rates of recurrent tumors are said to be more rapid than de novo lesions (Sterkers et al 1992). Because of the rarity of recurrence, there are no large series to quantify accurately the risks of reoperation. Many large series include a few recurrent tumors, and the risks of re-exploration and tumor removal may not differ substantially from the treatment of primary tumors (Ebersold et al 1992). Shea et al (1985), however, did note that morbidity for second operations is substantially higher than for primary tumors, and they reported a 25% mortality. Arachnoidal adhesions which result from previous exploration hinder identification of the nerves, and may make the lesion more difficult to free from the brainstem and adjacent vessels. Yet this is not the experience of Hitselberger & House (1979), who have commented that surgical planes are not obscured after a previous translabyrinthine operation. Tos et al (1988) reoperated on 4 patients through the labyrinth between 1 and 6 months after previous translabyrinthine surgery, without apparent difficulty. The interval between operations is likely to have a significant bearing on the density of adhesions.

The treatment options for recurrent disease are similar to those for a primary tumor. If the facial nerve is nonfunctional as a consequence of the first operation, further surgery may be considerably less difficult. The translabyrinthine approach is ideal if the previous exploration was via a retrosigmoid or middle fossa route. The facial nerve can then be identified lateral to the tumor before any scar tissue is encountered. After translabyrinthine surgery a second operation should be via a retrosigmoid or transcochlear approach, so that at least some of the important landmarks may be identified before approaching the area of the tumor, where normal anatomic planes will be obscured by the previous surgery. Hearing preservation is very unlikely in this group, and the results of facial nerve preservation are also likely to be correspondingly less good than for primary tumors.

MANAGEMENT OUTCOME

The results of surgery as they relate to death, facial nerve function, and hearing are discussed in the section dealing with the results of surgery.

Headache

It is our experience, and that of others (Schessel et al 1992), that postoperative headache is much more common with the suboccipital than translabyrinthine operation. Symptoms may last for years after surgery. The etiology remains unclear, but may be related to dissection of the nuchal musculature, scarring around the greater and lesser occipital nerves, or traction on the dura by adherence of the musculature. Replacement of the posterior fossa bone flap and reduction of muscle dissection to a minimum may help to reduce the incidence of this complication. A further factor which merits consideration is that, during the translabyrinthine operation, drilling of the temporal bone is completed before the dura is opened. In contrast, bone dust enters the basal cisterns when the posterior wall of the internal auditory canal is removed during suboccipital surgery, and thereby may precipitate chemical meningitis.

Tinnitus

Tinnitus is thought to be generated by the cochlea (Møller 1984), the cochlear nerve (Shea et al 1981), or the brainstem (Pulec et al 1978). Tinnitus may not be abolished even by section of the cochlear nerve. After tumor removal there is only a 40–60% chance that tinnitus will improve, and a 6–40% likelihood that it will worsen (Silverstein et al 1986, Goel et al 1992). The probability of this is determined in part by the severity of preoperative symptoms. Baguley et al (1992) reported recently the effect of translabyrinthine surgery on tinnitus in a series of 129 patients. If tinnitus was not present preoperatively there was a 27% chance that it would develop after surgery, but it was very unlikely to be troublesome. If mild or moderate tinnitus was present before surgery there was a 25% chance that it would be abolished, and a 37% chance that it would worsen. However, the risk that it would be severe under such circumstances was only around 2.5%. Severe tinnitus was very likely to improve after surgery, and was abolished entirely in a fifth of patients.

Vestibular rehabilitation

Initially, after labyrinthectomy or vestibular nerve section there is ataxia, with the patient veering to the operated ear. Horizontal nystagmus, with the slow phase toward the ablated side, may also be evident. Although it may be anticipated that symptoms and signs are likely to be greatest in patients with small tumors and normal preoperative vestibular function, this is not in fact the case. Jenkins (1985) found that neither age, sex, tumor size nor the presence of brainstem compression altered significantly the rate of postoperative vestibular compensation. In most patients symptoms will be shortlived and, within a few weeks, nystagmus will be abolished and ataxia minimal (Fisch 1973).

Animal studies have shown that early visual and somatosensory stimulation determines both the speed and ultimate recovery after vestibular injury (Igarashi et al 1979). For this reason, vestibular exercises are important in the early postoperative period, and patients with bilateral vestibular nerve loss, impaired vision, or altered proprioception are less likely to make a good recovery. Healthy patients with unilateral vestibular loss should have a structured program of exercise, with emphasis on head movement. Initially the patient will experience feelings of instability, but labyrinthine sedatives should be avoided if possible, as these are likely to delay the compensatory process. An exercise strategy for rehabilitation following vestibular injury can be found in Goebel (1992). However, despite good compensation, all patients will have some chronic disturbance of postural equilibrium after labyrinthectomy, albeit insignificant clinically (House & Nelson 1979).

Quality of life

Figures for quality of life as they relate to tumor size are given in Table 32.2. Although it is customary to exclude facial nerve outcome from this analysis, a poor functional result in this regard may have profound social implications for the patient, because of the disfiguring appearance. In particular, the combination of hearing loss and cosmetic deformity may lead to a reluctance to resume social contacts (Wiegand & Fickel 1989). For others the psychological impact of surgery is less, but the physical aspects are more debilitating, particularly loss of balance. A detailed account of the patient's perspective of his or her illness and recovery can be found in Wiegand & Fickel (1989).

CONCLUSION

The results of treatment have improved dramatically since the early pioneering days of surgery in the early 1900s, and House's landmark monograph of 1964. During that time mortality has fallen from 80% to under 5%, primarily as a result of the introduction of modern anesthesia and the operating microscope. Reduction of morbidity is now the major goal, particularly the preservation of good facial function and the salvage of residual hearing. Incremental modifications of operative technique and the introduction of new technology provide the prospect for further improvements in outcome during the coming decade.

REFERENCES

Adams R D 1943 Occlusion of the anterior inferior cerebellar artery. Archives of Neurology and Psychiatry 49: 765–770

Adeloye A 1979 Neoplasms of the brain in the African. Surgical Neurology 11: 247–255

Allcutt D A, Hoffman H J, Isla A, Becker L E, Humphreys R P 1991 Acoustic schwannomas in children. Neurosurgery 29: 14–18

Allen J, Eldridge R, Koerber T 1974 Acoustic neuroma in the last months of pregnancy. American Journal of Obstetrics and Gynecology 119: 516–520

Amoils C P, Lanser M J, Jackler R K 1992 Acoustic neuroma presenting as a middle ear mass. Otolaryngology — Head and Neck Surgery 107: 478–482

Anniko M, Arndt J, Norén G 1981 The human acoustic neuroma in organ culture. II. Tissue changes after gamma irradiation. Otolaryngology (Stockholm) 91: 223–235

Antoni N 1920 Ueber Ruckenmarkstumoren und Neurofibroma. Bergmann, Munich

Aoki S, Sasaki Y, Machida T, Tanioka H 1990 Contrast-enhanced MR images in patients with meningioma: importance of enhancement of the dura adjacent to the tumor. American Journal of Neuroradiology 11: 935–938

Atkinson W J 1949 The anterior inferior cerebellar artery; its variations, pontine distribution and significance in the surgery of the cerebellopontine angle tumors. Journal of Neurology, Neurosurgery and Psychiatry 12: 137–151

Baguley D M, Moffat D A, Hardy D G 1992 What happens to tinnitus after translabyrinthine acoustic neuroma removal? In: Tos M, Thomsen J (eds) Acoustic neuroma. Kugler, Amsterdam, pp 895–898

Baldwin D, King T T, Chevretton E, Morrison A W 1991 Bilateral cerebellopontine angle tumors in neurofibromatosis type 2. Journal of Neurosurgery 74: 910–915

Ballance CA 1894 Some points in the surgery of the brain and its membranes. Macmillan, London, 1907, p 276

Barker D J P, Weller R O, Garfield J S 1976 Epidemiology of primary tumours of the brain and spinal cord: a regional survey in southern England. Journal of Neurology Neurosurgery and Psychiatry 39: 290–296

Barker D, Wright E, Nguyen K et al 1987 Gene for von Recklinghausen's neurofibromatosis is in the pericentromeric region of chromosome 17. Science 236: 1100–1109

Barrs D M, Olsson J E 1987 The audiologic evaluation of cerebellopontine angle tumor suspects: A review of tumor and non-tumor suspects. Otolaryngology — Head and Neck Surgery 96: 523–532

Barrs D M, Luxford W M, Becker T S, Brackmann D E 1984a Computed tomography with gas cisternography for detection of small acoustic tumors. Archives of Otolaryngology 110: 535–537

Barrs D M, Brackmann D E, Hitselberger D E 1984b Facial nerve anastomosis in the cerebellopontine angle: a review of 24 cases. American Journal of Otology 5: 269–272

Bebin J 1979 Pathophysiology of acoustic tumors. In: House W F, Luetje C M (eds) Acoustic tumors, vol I. University Park Press, Baltimore, pp 45–83

Beck H J, Beatty C W, Harner S G 1986 Acoustic neuromas with normal pure tone hearing levels. Otolaryngology — Head and Neck Surgery 94: 96–103

Bentivoglio P, Cheesman A D, Symon L 1988a Surgical management of acoustic neuromas during the last five years. Part II. Results for facial and cochlear nerve function. Surgical Neurology 29: 205–209

Bentivoglio P, Cheesman A D, Symon L 1988b Surgical management of acoustic neuromas during the last five years. Part I. Surgical Neurology 29: 197–204

Berg H M, Cohen N L, Hammerschlag P E, Waltzman S B 1986 Acoustic neuroma presenting as sudden hearing loss with recovery. Otolaryngology — Head Neck Surgery 94: 15–22

Bess F H, Josey A F, Glasscock M E III, Wilson L K 1984 Audiologic manifestations in bilateral acoustic tumors (von Recklinghausen's disease). Journal of Speech and Hearing Disorders 49: 177–182

Best P V 1968 Erosion of the petrous temporal bone by neurilemmoma. Journal of Neurosurgery 28: 445–451

Best P V 1987 Malignant triton tumor in the cerebellopontine angle. Report of a case. Acta Neuropathologica 74: 92–96

Boesen T, Moller H, Charabi S, Thomsen J, Tos M 1992 Papilledema in patients with acoustic neuromas: vestibular and other oto-neurosurgical findings. In: Tos M, Thomsen J (eds) Acoustic neuroma. Kugler, Amsterdam, pp 235–238

Borck W F, Zulch K J 1951 Ueber die Erbangungshaufigkeit der Geschlechter an Hirngeschwulsten. Zentralbl Neurochir 11: 333–350

Brackmann D E 1979 Middle cranial fossa approach. In: House W F, Luetje C J (eds) Acoustic tumors, vol II. Management. University Park Press, Baltimore, pp 15–41

Brackmann D E, Bartels L J 1980 Rare tumors of the cerebellopontine angle. Otolaryngology — Head and Neck Surgery 88: 555–559

Brackmann D E, Kwartler J A 1990a A review of acoustic tumors: 1983–1988. American Journal of Otology 11: 216–232

Brackmann D E, Kwartler J A 1990b Treatment of acoustic tumors with radiotherapy. Archives of Otolaryngology — Head and Neck Surgery 116: 161–162

Brockes J P, Breakefield X O, Martuza R L 1986 Glial growth factor-like activity in Schwann cell tumors. Annals of Neurology 20: 317–320

Brooks J S J, Freeman M , Enterline H T 1985 Malignant "triton" tumors. Natural history and immunohistochemistry of nine new cases with literature review. Cancer 55: 2543–2549

Brow R E 1979 Pre- and postoperative management of the acoustic tumor patient. In: House W F, Luetje C J (eds) Acoustic tumors, vol II. Management. University Park Press, Baltimore, pp 153–173

Buchheit W A, Rosenwasser R H 1988 Tumors of the cerebellopontine angle: Clinical features and surgical management. In: Schmidek H H, Sweet W H (eds) Operative neurosurgical techniques. Indications, methods, and results, 2nd edn. Grune & Stratton, Orlando, pp 673–683

Cairns H 1932 Acoustic neurinoma of right cerebello-pontine angle. Complete removal. Spontaneous recovery from post-operative facial palsy. Proceedings of the Royal Society of Medicine 25: 35–40

Carney J A, Gordon H, Carpenter P C, Shenoy B V, Go V L W 1985 The complex of myxomas, spotty pigmentation and endocrine overactivity. Medicine 64: 270–283

Carney J A, Hruska L S, Beauchamp G D, Gordon H 1986 Dominant inheritance of the complex of myxomas, spotty pigmentation and endocrine overactivity. Mayo Clinic Proceedings 61: 165–172

Cerullo L J, Mkrdichian E H 1987 Acoustic nerve tumor surgery before and since the laser: comparison of results. Lasers in Surgery and Medicine 7: 224–228

Charabi S, Thomsen J, Tos M, Youssef M 1992 False-positive CT findings in a series of 525 patients with acoustic neuromas. In: Tos M, Thomsen J (eds) Acoustic neuroma. Kugler, Amsterdam, pp 127–130

Chen J M, Fisch U 1992 The transotic approach in acoustic neuroma surgery. In: Tos M, Thomsen J (eds) Acoustic neuroma. Kugler, Amsterdam, pp 317–323

Clemis J D, Mastricola P G, Schuler-Vogler M 1982 Sudden hearing loss in the contralateral ear in postoperative acoustic tumor: three case reports. Laryngoscope 92: 77–79

Clemis J D, Ballad W J, Baggot P J, Lyon S T 1986 Relative frequency of inferior vestibular schwannoma. Archives of Otolaryngology Head and Neck Surgery 112: 190–194

Conley J, Baker D C 1979 Hypoglossal-facial nerve anastomosis for reinnervation of paralyzed face. Plastic and Reconstructive Surgery 63: 63–72

Croxson G R, Moffat D A, Baguley D 1988 Bruns bidirectional nystagmus in cerebellopontine angle tumors. Clinical Otolaryngology 13: 153–157

Croxson G R, Moffat D A, Hardy D G, Baguley D M 1989 Role of post-operative electroneuronography in predicting facial nerve recovery after acoustic neuroma removal: a pilot study. Journal of Laryngology and Otology 103: 60–62

Cruveilhier J 1842 Anatomie pathologique du corps humain II, part 26. Bailliere, Paris, pp 1–8

Curtin H D 1984 CT of acoustic neuroma and other tumors of the ear. Radiological Clinics of North America 22: 77–105

Cushing H 1917 Intracranial tumours. Charles C Thomas, Springfield, Ill
Cushing H 1921 Further concerning the acoustic neuromas. Laryngoscope 31: 209–228
Cushing H 1931 Tumors of the nervus acousticus and the syndrome of the cerebellopontine angle. Saunders, Philadelphia, p 277
Cushing H 1932 Intracranial tumors. Charles C Thomas, Springfield, Ill
Dalley R W, Robertson W D, Nugent R A, Durity F A 1986 Computed tomography of anterior inferior cerebellar artery aneurysm mimicing an acoustic neuroma. Journal of Computer Assisted Tomography 10: 881–884
Dandy W E 1925 An operation for the total removal of cerebellopontine (acoustic) tumors. Surgery, Gynecology and Obstetrics 41: 129–148
Dastur D K, Lalitha V S, Prabhakar V 1968 Pathological analysis of intracranial space-occupying lesions in 1000 cases including children: Part I. Age, sex and pattern; and the tuberculomas. Journal of Neurological Science 6: 575–592
Dickins J, Graham S 1991 A comparison of facial nerve monitoring systems in cerebellopontine angle surgery. American Journal of Otology 12: 1–6
Di Tullio M V, Malkasian D, Rand R W 1978 A critical comparison of neurosurgical and otolaryngological approaches to acoustic neuromas. Journal of Neurosurgery 48: 1–12
Dix M R 1974 The vestibular acoustic system. In: Vinken P J, Bruyn B W (eds) Handbook of clinical neurology. Elsevier, New York, vol 16
Domb G H, Chole R A 1980 Anatomical studies of the posterior petrous apex with regard to hearing preservation in acoustic neuroma removal. Laryngoscope 90: 1769–1776
Ducarman B S, Scheithauer B W, Piepgras D G, Reiman H M, Ilstrup D M 1986 Malignant peripheral nerve sheath tumors. A clinicopathologic study of 120 cases. Cancer 57: 2006–2021
Duel A B 1934 Advanced methods in the surgical treatment of facial paralysis. Annals of Otology, Rhinology and Laryngology 43: 76–88
Ebersold M J, Quast L M 1992 Long-term results of spinal accessory nerve–facial nerve anastomosis. Journal of Neurosurgery 77: 51–54
Ebersold M J, Harner S G, Beatty C W, Harper C M, Quast L M 1992 Current results of the retrosigmoid approach to acoustic neurinomas. Journal of Neurosurgery 76: 901–909
Elderidge R 1981 Central neurofibromatosis with bilateral acoustic neuroma. In: Riccardi V M, Mulvihill J J (eds) Advances in neurology, vol 29: Neurofibromatosis. Raven, New York, pp 57–65
Elliott F A, McKissock W 1954 Acoustic neuroma. Early diagnosis. Lancet ii: 1189–1191
Evans D G R, Huson S M, Donnai D et al 1922a A genetic study of type 2 neurofibromatosis in the United Kingdom. I. Prevalence, mutation rate, fitness, and confirmation of maternal transmission effect on severity. Journal of Medical Genetics 29: 841–846
Evans D G R, Huson S M, Donnai D et al 1992b A genetic study of type II neurofibromatosis in the United Kingdom. II. Guidelines for genetic counselling. Journal of Medical Genetics 29: 847–852
Fabiani A, Croveri G, Torta A 1975 Neurinoma de la fossa posteriore in un bambino di un anno. Acta Neurologica (Napoli) 30: 218–222
Fisch U 1973 The vestibular response following unilateral vestibular neurectomy. Acta Oto-laryngologica (Stockholm) 76: 229–238
Fisch U, Dobie R A, Gmur A, Felix H 1987 Intracranial facial nerve anastomosis. American Journal of Otology 8: 23–29
Fischer G, Fischer C, Rémond J 1992 Hearing preservation in acoustic neuroma surgery. Journal of Neurosurgery 76: 910–917
Flood L M, Brightwell A P 1984 Cochlear deafness in the presentation of a large acoustic neuroma. Journal of Laryngology and Otology 98: 87–92
Gantz B J, Gmuer A A, Holliday M 1984 Electroneurographic evaluation of the facial nerve. Method and technical problems. Annals of Otology, Rhinology and Laryngology 93: 394–398
Gantz B J, Parnes L S, Harker L A, McCabe B F 1986 Middle cranial fossa acoustic neuroma excision: results and complications. Annals of Otology Rhinology and Laryngology 95: 454–459
Gardner G, Robertson J H 1988 Hearing preservation in unilateral acoustic neuroma surgery. Annals of Otology, Rhinology and Laryngology 97: 55–66
Gardner G, Robertson J H, Clark W C 1983 105 patients operated upon for cerebellopontine angle tumors — experience using combined approach and CO_2 laser. Laryngoscope 93: 1049–1055
German W J 1961 Acoustic neurinomas: A follow-up. Clinical Neurosurgery 7: 21–39
Glasscock M E, Kveton J F, Jackson C G, Levine S C, McKennan K X 1986 A systematic approach to the surgical management of acoustic neuroma. Laryngoscope 96: 1088–1094
Glasscock M E III, Levine S C, McKennan K X 1987 The changing characteristics of acoustic neuroma patients over the last ten years. Laryngoscope 97: 1164–1167
Glasscock M E III, McKennan K X, Levine S C 1988 False negative MRI scan in an acoustic neuroma. Otolaryngology — Head and Neck Surgery 98: 612–614
Gleeson R K, Butzer J F, Grin O D Jr 1978 Acoustic neurinoma presenting as subarachnoid hemorrhage. Case report. Journal of Neurosurgery 49: 602–604
Goebel J A 1992 Experimental and practical considerations for rehabilitation following vestibular injury. In: Tos M, Thomsen J (eds) Acoustic neuroma. Kugler, Amsterdam, pp 905–911
Goel A, Sekhar L N, Langheinrich W, Kamerer D, Hirsch B 1992 Late course of preserved hearing and tinnitus after acoustic neurilemoma surgery. Journal of Neurosurgery 77: 685–689
Goetting M G, Swanson S E 1987 Massive hemorrhage into intracranial neurinomas. Surgical Neurology 27: 168–172
Gordon D S, Kerr A G 1986 Cerebrospinal fluid rhinorrhea following surgery for acoustic neuroma. Journal of Neurosurgery 64: 676–678
Graham M D 1975 The jugular bulb: its anatomic and clinical considerations in contemporary otology. Archives of Otolaryngology 101: 560–564
Graham M D, Sataloff R T 1984 Acoustic tumors in the young adult. Archives of Otolaryngology 110: 405–407
Gruskin P, Carberry J N 1979 Pathology of acoustic tumors. In: House W F, Luetje C M (eds) Acoustic tumors. Vol I Diagnosis. University Park Press, Baltimore, pp 85–148
Guyot J-P, Hausler R, Reverdin A, Berney J, Montandon P B 1992 The value of otoneurologic diagnostic procedures compared with radiology and operative findings. In: Tos M, Thomsen J (eds) Acoustic neuroma. Kugler, Amsterdam, pp 31–37
Haberman R S II, Kramer M B 1989 False-positive MRI and CT findings of an acoustic neuroma. American Journal of Otology 10: 301–303
Hammerschlag P E, Cohen N L, Brundy J 1992 Rehabilitation of facial paralysis following acoustic neuroma excision with jump interpositional graft hypoglossal-facial anastomosis and gold weight lid implantation. In: Tos M, Thomsen J (eds) Acoustic neuroma. Kugler, Amsterdam, pp 789–792
Han D H, Kim D G, Chi J E, Park S H, Jung H-W, Kim Y G 1992 Malignant triton tumor of the acoustic nerve. Case report. Journal of Neurosurgery 76: 874–877
Hardy D G, Macfarlane R, Baguley D, Moffat D A 1989a Surgery for acoustic neurinoma. An analysis of 100 translabyrinthine operations. Journal of Neurosurgery 71: 799–804
Hardy D G, Macfarlane R, Baguley D, Moffat D A 1989b Facial nerve recovery following acoustic neuroma surgery. British Journal of Neurosurgery 3: 675–680
Hardy D G, Macfarlane R, Moffat D A 1993 Wound closure after acoustic neuroma surgery. British Journal of Neurosurgery 7: 171–174
Hardy M, Crowe S J 1936 Early asymptomatic acoustic tumors. Archives of Surgery 32: 292–301
Harker L A, Nysather J, Katz A 1978 Immunologic detection of acoustic neuroma: a preliminary report. Laryngoscope 88: 802–807
Harner S G, Ebersold M J 1985 Management of acoustic neuromas, 1978–1983. Journal of Neurosurgery 63: 175–179
Harner S G, Reese D F 1984 Roentgenographic diagnosis of acoustic neurinoma. Laryngoscope 94: 306–309
Harner S G, Laws E R Jr, Onofrio B M 1984 Hearing preservation after removal of acoustic neuroma. Laryngoscope 94: 1431–1434
Harris J P, Low N C, House W F 1985 Contralateral hearing loss following inner ear injury: sympathetic cochleolabyrinthitis? American Journal of Otology 6: 371–377

Hart R G, Gardner D P, Howieson J 1983 Acoustic tumors: atypical features and recent diagnostic tests. Neurology 33: 211–221

Hatam A, Bergstram M, Norén G 1985 Effects of dexamethasone treatment on acoustic neuromas: evaluation by computed tomography. Journal of Computer Assisted Tomography 9: 857–860

Hernanz-Schulman M, Welch K, Strand R, Ordia J I 1986 Acoustic neuromas in children. American Journal of Neuroradiology 7: 519–521

Hirsch A, Norén G 1988 Audiological findings after stereotactic radiosurgery in acoustic neurinomas. Acta Oto-laryngologica (Stockholm) 106: 244–251

Hitselberger W E 1966 External auditory canal hypesthesia. An early sign of acoustic neuroma. American Surgeon 32: 741–743

Hitselberger W E 1979 Hypoglossal-facial anastomosis. In: House W F, Luetje C M (eds) Acoustic tumors. Vol II: Management. University Park Press, Baltimore, pp 97–103

Hitselberger W E, House W F 1979 Partial versus total removal of acoustic tumors. In: House W F, Luetje C M (eds) Acoustic tumors. Vol II: Management. University Park Press, Baltimore, pp 265–268

Hitselberger W, House W, Edgerton B, Whitaker S 1984 Cochlear nucleus implant. Otolaryngology — Head and Neck Surgery 92: 52–54

Holt G 1978 ENT manifestations of von Recklinghausen's disease. Laryngoscope 88: 1617–1632

House J W, Brackmann D E 1985 Facial nerve grading system. Otolaryngology — Head and Neck Surgery 93: 146–147

House J W, Hitselberger W E, House W F 1982 Wound closure and cerebrospinal fluid leak after translabyrinthine surgery. American Journal of Otology 4: 126–128

House J W, Waluch V, Jackler R K 1986 Magnetic resonance imaging in acoustic neuroma diagnosis. Annals of Otology, Rhinology and Laryngology 95: 16–20

House J W, Nissen R L, Hitselberger W E 1987 Acoustic tumor management in senior citizens. Laryngoscope 97: 129–130

House W F 1961 Surgical exposure of the internal auditory canal and its contents through the middle cranial fossa. Laryngoscope 71: 1363–1385

House W F 1964a Evolution of transtemporal bone removal of acoustic tumors. Laryngoscope 94: 731–742

House W F 1964b Transtemporal bone microsurgical removal of acoustic neuromas. Archives of Otolaryngology 80: 597–756

House W F 1968 Partial tumor removal and recurrence in acoustic tumor surgery. Archives of Otolaryngology 88: 644–654

House W F 1979 The translabyrinthine approach. In: House W F, Luetje C M (eds) Acoustic tumors, vol II. University Park Press, Baltimore, pp 43–89

House W F, Hitselberger W E 1976 The transcochlear approach to the skull base. Archives of Otolaryngology 102: 334–342

House W F, Luetje C M 1979 Evaluation and preservation of facial function. In: House W F, Luetje C M (eds) Acoustic tumors. University Park Press, Baltimore, pp 89–94

House W F, Nelson J R 1979 Long-term cochleo-vestibular effects of acoustic tumor surgery. In: House W F, Luetje C M (eds) Acoustic tumors. Vol II: Management. University Park Press, Baltimore, pp 207–234

Huang W-Q, Zheng S-J, Tian Q-S et al 1982 Statistical analysis of central nervous system tumors in China. Journal of Neurosurgery 56: 555–564

Hughes G B, Sismanis A, Glasscock M E III, Hays J W, Jackson C G 1982 Management of bilateral acoustic tumors. Laryngoscope 92: 1351–1359

Huson S M, Harper P S, Compston D A S 1988 Von Recklinghausen neurofibromatosis: a clinical and population study in south east Wales. Brain 111: 355–381

Igarashi M, Levy J K, Takahashi M, Alford B R, Homink J L 1979 Effect of exercise upon locomotor balance modification after peripheral vestibular lesions (unilateral utricular neurotomy) in squirrel monkeys. Advances in Oto-Rhino-Laryngology 25: 82–87

Ikeda K, Ito H, Kashihara K, Fujisawa H, Yamamoto S 1988 Effective preoperative irradiation of highly vascular cerebellopontine angle neurinomas. Neurosurgery 22: 566–573

Ishikawa T, Ikawa T, Eura M, Fukiage T, Masuyama K 1989 Adoptive immunotherapy for head and neck cancer with killer cells induced by stimulation with autologous or allogeneic tumour cells and recombinant interleukin-2. Acta Oto-laryngologica (Stockholm) 107: 346–351

Jaaskelainen J, Pyykko I, Blomstedt G, Porras M, Palva T, Troupp H 1990 Functional results of facial nerve suture after removal of acoustic neurinoma: an analysis of 25 cases. Neurosurgery 27: 408–411

Jackler R K, Pitts L H 1990 Acoustic neuroma. Neurosurgical Clinics of North America 1.1: 199–223

Jahrsdoerfer R A, Benjamin R S 1988 Chemotherapy of bilateral acoustic neuromas. Otolaryngology — Head and Neck Surgery 98: 273–282

Jenkins H A 1985 Long term adaptive changes of the vestibulo ocular reflex in patients following acoustic neuroma surgery. Laryngoscope 95: 1224–1234

Jenkins H A, Fisch U 1980 The transotic approach to resection of difficult acoustic tumors of the cerebellopontine angle. American Journal of Otology 2: 70–76

Johnson E W 1977 Auditory test results in 500 cases of acoustic neuroma. Archives of Otolaryngology 103: 152–158

Johnson E W 1979 Results of audiometry tests in acoustic tumor patients. In: House W F, Luetje C M (eds) Acoustic Tumors. Vol I: Diagnosis. University Park Press, Baltimore, pp 209–224

Josey A F, Jackson C G, Glasscock M E 1980 Brainstem evoked audiometry in confirmed 8th nerve tumors. American Journal of Otolaryngology 1: 285–290

Kanter W R, Eldridge R, Fabricant R et al 1980 Central neurofibromatosis with bilateral acoustic neuroma. Genetic, clinical and biochemical distinctions from peripheral neurofibromatosis. Neurology 30: 851–859

Kaplan J C, Aurias A, Julier C, Prieur M, Szajnert M F 1987 Human chromosome 22. Journal of Medical Genetics 24: 65–78

Karjalainen S, Nuutinen J, Neittaanmaki H, Naukkarinen A, Asikainen R 1984 The incidence of acoustic neuroma in autopsy material. Archives of Otorhinolaryngology 240: 91–93

Kartush J M, Niparko J K, Graham M D, Kemink J L 1987 Electroneuronography: preoperative facial nerve assessment for tumors of the temporal bone. Otolaryngology — Head and Neck Surgery 97: 257–261

Kasantikul V, Netsky M G, Glasscock M E III, Hays J W 1980a Acoustic neurilemmoma: clinicoanatomical study of 103 patients. Journal of Neurosurgery 52: 28–35

Kasantikul V, Netsky M G, Glasscock M E III, Hays J W 1980b Intracanalicular neurilemmomas: clinicopathologic study. Annals of Otology, Rhinology and Laryngology 89: 29–32

Khangure M S, Moijtahedi S 1983 Air CT cisternography of anterior inferior cerebellar artery loop simulating an intracanalicular acoustic neuroma. American Journal of Neuroradiology 4: 994–995

King T T, Morrison A 1980 Translabyrinthine and transtentorial removal of acoustic nerve tumors. Results of 150 cases. Journal of Neurosurgery 52: 210–216

King T T, Morrison A W 1990 Primary facial nerve tumors within the skull. Journal of Neurosurgery 72: 1–8

King T T, Sparrow O C, Arias J M, O'Connor A F 1993 Repair of facial nerve after removal of cerebellopontine angle tumors: a comparative study. Journal of Neurosurgery 78: 720–725

Kitamura K, Kakoi H, Ishida T 1992 Audiological assessment of bilateral acoustic tumors during conservative management. In: Tos M, Thomsen J (eds) Acoustic neuroma. Kugler, Amsterdam, pp 835–838

Koenig M, Kalyan-Raman K, Sureka O N 1984 Contralateral trigeminal nerve dysfunction as a false localizing sign in acoustic neurinoma: a clinical and electrophysiological study. Neurosurgery 14: 335–337

Koos W T 1988 Criteria for preservation of vestibulo-cochlear nerve function during microsurgical removal of acoustic neurinomas. Acta Neurochirurgica 92: 55–66

Korf 1990 The genetic basis of neurofibromatosis. Neurological Forum 2: 2–7

Krause F 1903 Zur Freilegung der hinteren Felsenbeinflache und des Kleinhirns. Beitrage zur Klinischen Chirurgie 37: 728–764

Kurland L T, Schoenberg B S, Annegers J F, Okazaki H, Molgaard C A 1982 The incidence of primary intracranial neoplasms in

Rochester, Minnesota 1935–1977. Annals of the New York Academy of Science 381: 6–16
Kveton J F 1990 Delayed spontaneous return of hearing after acoustic tumor surgery: evidence for cochlear nerve conduction block. Laryngoscope 100: 473–476
Kveton J F, Book J 1992 A comparison of auditory nerve monitoring techniques in acoustic tumor surgery. In: Tos M, Thomsen J (eds) Acoustic Neuroma. Kugler, Amsterdam, pp 537–542
Laasonen E M, Troupp H 1986 Volume growth rate of acoustic neurinomas. Neuroradiology 28: 203–207
Lanser M J 1992 The genetics of acoustic neuromas: a linkage and physical map of chromosome 22. In: Tos M, Thomsen J (eds) Acoustic neuroma. Kugler, Amsterdam, pp 165–171
Lanser M J, Jackler R K, Pitts L H 1992 Intratumoral hemorrhage and cyst expansion as causes of acute neurological deterioration in acoustic neuroma patients. In: Tos M, Thomsen J (eds) Acoustic neuroma. Kugler, Amsterdam, pp 229–234
Larsson E M, Holtas S 1986 False diagnosis of acoustic neuroma due to subdural injection during gas CT cisternogram. Journal of Computer Assisted Tomography 10: 1025–1026
Le Blanc R A 1974 Metastasis of bronchogenic carcinoma to acoustic neurinoma. Case report. Journal of Neurosurgery 41: 614–617
Lee J P, Wang A D 1989 Acoustic neurinoma presenting as intratumoral bleeding. Neurosurgery 24: 764–768
Leonard J R, Talbot M L 1970 Asymptomatic acoustic neurilemmoma. Archives of Otolaryngology 91: 171–224
Levy L F, Auchterlonie W C 1975 Primary cerebral neoplasia in Rhodesia. International Surgeon 60: 286–293
Linskey M E, Lunsford L D, Flickinger J C 1990 Radiosurgery for acoustic neurinomas: early experience. Neurosurgery 26: 736–745
Linthicum F H, Brackmann D E 1980 Bilateral acoustic tumors. A diagnostic and surgical challenge. Archives of Otolaryngology 106: 729–733
Linthicum F H, Churchill D 1968 Vestibular test results in acoustic tumor cases. Archives of Otolaryngology 88: 604–607
Lownie S P, Drake C G 1991 Radical intracapsular removal of acoustic neurinomas. Long-term follow-up of 11 patients. Journal of Neurosurgery 74: 422–425
Luetje C M, Whittaker C K, Callaway L A, Veraga G 1983 Histological acoustic tumor involvement of the VIIth nerve and multicentric origin in the VIIIth nerve. Laryngoscope 93: 1133–1139
Luetje C M, Whittaker C K, Davidson K C, Vergara G G 1988 Spontaneous acoustic tumor involution: a case report. Otolaryngology — Head and Neck Surgery 98: 95–97
Lunsford L D, Linskey M E, Flickinger J C 1992a Stereotactic radiosurgery for acoustic nerve sheath tumors. In: Tos M, Thomsen J (eds) Acoustic neuroma. Kugler, Amsterdam, pp 279–287
Lunsford L D, Kondziolka D, Flickinger J C 1992b Radiosurgery as an alternative to microsurgery of acoustic tumors. Clinical Neurosurgery 38: 619–634
Lye R H, Dutton J, Ramsden R T, Occleshaw J V, Ferguson I T, Taylor I 1982 Facial nerve preservation during surgery for removal of acoustic nerve tumors. Journal of Neurosurgery 57: 739–746
Lye R H, Pace-Balzan A, Ramsden R T, Gillespie J E, Dutton J M 1992 The fate of tumor rests following removal of acoustic neuromas: an MRI Gd-DTPA study. British Journal of Neurosurgery 6: 195–201
McKenzie K G, Alexander E Jr 1950 Restoration of facial function by nerve anastomosis. Annals of Surgery 132: 411–415
McKissock W 1961 Cited by Walsh L 1965. Acoustic tumors. Proceedings of the Royal Society of Medicine 58: 1033–1037
McLean C A, Laidlaw J D, Brownbill D S B, Gonzales M F 1990 Recurrence of acoustic neurilemoma as a malignant spindle-cell neoplasm. Case report. Journal of Neurosurgery 73: 946–950
Mangham C A 1988 Complications of translabyrinthine vs. suboccipital approach for acoustic tumor surgery. Otolarnyngology — Head and Neck Surgery 99: 396–400
Mansell P I, Higgs E, Reckless J P D 1991 A young woman with spotty pigmentation, acromegaly, acoustic neuroma and cardiac myxoma: Carney's complex. Journal of the Royal Society of Medicine 84: 496–497
Markwalder T M, Waelti E, Markwalder R V 1986 Estrogen and progestin receptors in acoustic and spinal neurilemmomas. Clinicopathologic correlations. Surgical Neurology 26: 142–148
Marquet J F E, Forton G E J, Offeciers F E, Moeneclaey L L M 1990 The solitary Schwannoma of the eighth cranial nerve. An immunohistochemical study of the cochlear nerve – tumor interface. Archives of Otolaryngology — Head and Neck Surgery 116: 1023–1025
Martuza R L, Eldridge R 1988 Neurofibromatosis 2 (bilateral acoustic neurofibromatosis). New England Journal of Medicine 318: 684–688
Martuza R L, Ojemann R G 1982 Bilateral acoustic neuroma: clinical aspects, pathogenesis, and treatment. Neurosurgery 10: 1–22
Martuza R L, MacLaughlin D T, Ojemann R G 1981 Specific estradiol binding in Schwannomas, meningiomas, and neurofibromas. Neurosurgery 9: 665–671
Mattox D E 1992 Infratemporal fossa approaches (Fisch) to the clivus. In: Long D M (ed) Surgery for skull base tumors. Blackwell, Oxford, pp 204–210
Maurer P K, Okawara S H 1988 Restoration of hearing after removal of cerebellopontine angle meningioma: diagnostic and therapeutic implications. Neurosurgery 22: 573–575
Migliavacca F 1967 Facial nerve anastomosis for facial paralysis following acoustic neuroma surgery. Acta Neurochirurgica 17: 274–279
Mingrino S, Zuccarello M 1981 Anastomosis of the facial nerve with accessory or hypoglossal nerves. In: Samii M, Jannetta P J (eds) The cranial nerves. Springer-Verlag, Berlin, pp 512–514
Miyamoto R T, Campbell R L, Fritsch M, Lochmueller G 1990 Preservation of hearing in neurofibromatosis-2. Otolaryngology — Head and Neck Surgery 103: 619–624
Miyamoto R T, Roos K L, Campbell R L, Worth R M 1991 Contemporary management of neurofibromatosis. Annals of Otology, Rhinology and Laryngology 100: 38–43
Moffat D A, Hardy D G 1989 Early diagnosis and surgical management of acoustic neuroma: is it cost effective? Journal of the Royal Society of Medicine 82: 329–332
Moffat D A, Harries M L L, Baguley D M, Hardy D G 1989a Unterberger's stepping test in acoustic neuroma. Journal of Laryngology and Otology 103: 839–841
Moffat D A, Hardy D G, Baguley D M 1989b The strategy and benefits of acoustic neuroma searching. Journal of Laryngology and Otology 103: 51–59
Moffat D A, Croxson G R, Baguley D M, Hardy D G 1989c Facial nerve recovery after acoustic neuroma removal. Journal of Laryngology and Otology 103: 169–172
Møller A R 1984 Pathophysiology of tinnitus. Annals of Otology, Rhinology and Laryngology 93: 39–44
Møller A R, Hatam H, Olivecrona H 1978 The differential diagnosis of pontine angle meningioma and acoustic neuroma with computed tomography. Neuroradiology 17: 21–23
Morgon A, Disant F, Fischer G, Dubreuil C 1985 In: Portmann M (ed) Facial nerve. Masson, New York, pp 445–450
Morrison A W 1975 Management of sensorineural deafness. Butterworths, London
Morrison A W, Gibson W P R, Beagley H 1976 Transtympanic electrocochleography in the diagnosis of retrocochlear tumours. Clinical Otolaryngology 1: 153–167
Murray M R, Stout A P 1940 Schwann cell versus fibroblast as origin of specific nerve sheath tumor; observations upon normal nerve sheaths and neurilemomas in vitro. American Journal of Pathology 16: 41–60
Musiek F E, Kibbe-Michal K, Guerkink N A et al 1986 ABR results in patients with posterior fossa tumors and normal pure tone hearing. Otolaryngology — Head and Neck Surgery 94: 568–573
Nadol J B Jr, Levine R A, Ojeman R G et al 1987 Preservation of hearing in surgical removal of acoustic neuromas of the internal auditory canal and cerebellar pontine angle. Laryngoscope 97: 1287–1294
Nadol J B, Chiong C M, Ojemann R G et al 1992 Preservation of hearing and facial nerve function in resection of acoustic neuroma. Laryngoscope 102: 1153–1158
Nager G T 1969 Acoustic neuromas: pathology and differential diagnosis. Archives of Otolaryngology 89: 252–279
National Institutes of Health Consensus Development Conference 1988 Neurofibromatosis. Conference Statement. Archives of Neurology 45: 575–578

Nedzelski J M, Canter R J, Kassel E E, Rowed D W, Tator C H 1986 Is no treatment good treatment in the management of acoustic neuromas in the elderly? Laryngoscope 96: 825–829
Nedzelski J M, Schessel D A, Pfleiderer A, Kassel E E, Rowed D W 1992 The natural history of growth of acoustic neuromas and its role in non-operative management. In: Tos M, Thomsen J (eds) Acoustic neuroma. Kugler, Amsterdam, pp 149–158
Neely J G 1981 Gross and microscopic anatomy of the eighth cranial nerve in relationship to the solitary schwannoma. Laryngoscope 91: 1512–1531
Neely J G 1984 Is it possible to totally resect an acoustic tumor and preserve hearing? Otolaryngology — Head and Neck Surgery 92: 162–167
Neely J G, Hough J 1986 Histologic findings in two very small intracanalicular solitary schwannomas of the eighth nerve. Annals of Otology, Rhinology and Otolaryngology 95: 460–465
Nelson R A 1992 Auditory brainstem implant. In: Tos M, Thomsen J (eds) Acoustic neuroma. Kugler, Amsterdam, pp 869–872
Nishi T, Matsukado Y, Nagahiro S, Fukushima M, Koga K 1987 Hemifacial spasm due to contralateral acoustic neuroma: case report. Neurology 37: 339–342
Norén G, Greitz D 1992 The natural history of acoustic neurinomas. In: Tos M, Thomsen J (eds) Acoustic neuroma. Kugler, Amsterdam, pp 191–192
Norén G, Greitz D, Hirsch A, Lax I 1992 Gamma knife radiosurgery in acoustic neurinomas. In: Tos M, Thomsen J (eds) Acoustic neuroma. Kugler, Amsterdam, pp 289–292
Ojemann R G, Crowell R C 1978 Acoustic neuromas treated by microsurgical suboccipital operations. Progress in Neurological Surgery 9: 337–373
Ojemann R G, Montgomery W W, Weiss A D 1972 Evaluation and surgical treatment of acoustic neuroma. New England Journal of Medicine 287: 895–899
Ojemann R G, Levine R A, Montgomery W M, McGaffigan P 1984 Use of intraoperative auditory evoked potentials to preserve hearing in unilateral acoustic neuroma removal. Journal of Neurosurgery 61: 938–948
Olivecrona H 1967 Acoustic tumors. Journal of Neurosurgery 26: 6–13
Panse R 1904 Ein Gliom des Akustikus. Archiv fur Ohrenheilkunde 61: 251–255
Pensak J L, Glasscock M E III, Josey A F, Jackson C G, Gulya A J 1985 Sudden hearing loss and cerebellopontine angle tumors. Laryngoscope 95: 1188–1193
Pensak M, Tew J, Keith R, van Loveren H R 1991 Management of acoustic neuroma in an only hearing ear. Skull Base Surgery 1: 93–96
Perlman H, Kimura R 1955 Observations of the living blood vessels of the cochlea. Annals of Otology, Rhinology and Laryngology 64: 1176–1192
Perre J, Viala P, Foncin J-F 1990 Involvement of the cochlear nerve in acoustic tumors. Acta Orolaryngologica (Stockholm) 110: 245–252
Piffko P, Pasztor E 1981 Operated bilateral acoustic neuromas with preservation of hearing and facial nerve function. Otology, Rhinology, Laryngology 43: 255–261
Pitty L F, Tator C H 1992 Hypoglossal-facial nerve anastomosis for facial nerve palsy following surgery for cerebellopontine angle tumors. Journal of Neurosurgery 77: 724–731
Portmann M, Sterkers J M 1975 The internal auditory meatus. In: Portmann M, Sterkers J M, Charachon R, Chouard C H (eds) Tumors of the internal auditory meatus and surrounding structures. Churchill Livingstone, Edinburgh, pp 193–232
Prasher D K, Gibson W P 1983 Brainstem auditory-evoked potentials and electrocochleography: comparison of different criteria for detection of acoustic neuroma and other cerebello-pontine angle tumours. British Journal of Audiology 17: 163–174
Pulec J L, House W F 1964 Facial nerve involvement and testing in acoustic neuroma. Archives of Otolaryngology 80: 685–692
Pulec J L, House W F, Britton B H Jr, Hitselberger W E 1971 A system of management of acoustic neuroma based on 364 cases. Transactions of the Academy of American Ophthalmology and Otolaryngology 75: 48–55
Pulec J L, Hodell S F, Anthony P F 1978 Tinnitus: diagnosis and treatment. Annals of Otology, Rhinology and Laryngology 87: 821–833
Ramsden R T, Panizza F, Lye R H 1992 The use of ionomeric bone cement in the prevention of CSF leakage following acoustic neuroma surgery. In: Tos M, Thomsen J (eds) Acoustic neuroma. Kugler, Amsterdam, pp 725–727
Ransohoff J, Potanos J, Boschenstein F, Pool L 1961 Total removal of recurrent acoustic tumor. Journal of Neurosurgery 18: 804–810
Rasmussen N, Tribukait B, Thomsen J, Holm L E, Tos M 1984 Implications of DNA characterization of human acoustic neuromas. Acta Oto-laryngologica (Stockholm) (suppl) 406: 278–281
Revilla A G 1947 Neurinomas of the cerebellopontine angle recess. Clinical study of 160 cases including operative mortality and end results. Bulletin of Johns Hopkins Hospital 80: 254–296
Revilla A G 1948 Differential diagnosis of tumors at the cerebellopontine recess. Bulletin of Johns Hopkins Hospital 83: 187
Rhoton A L 1986 Microsurgical anatomy of the brainstem surface facing an acoustic neuroma. Surgical Neurology 25: 326–339
Rhoton A L, Tedeschi H 1992 Microsurgical anatomy of acoustic neuroma. The Otolaryngologic Clinics of North America 25(2): 257–294
Rhoton A L, Pulec J L, Hall G M, Boyd A S 1968 Absence of bone over the geniculate ganglion. Journal of Neurosurgery 28: 48–53
Riccardi V M, Eichner J E 1986 Neurofibromatosis. Phenotype, natural history, and pathogenesis. Johns Hopkins University Press, Baltimore
Robinson K, Rudge P 1983 The differential diagnosis of cerebellopontine angle lesions. Journal of Neurological Science 60: 1–21
Rubenstein A E 1986 Neurofibromatosis: A review of the clinical problem. Annals of the New York Academy of Science 486: 1–13
Ruberti R F, Poppi M 1971 Tumors of the central nervous system in the African. East African Medical Journal 48: 576–584
Russell D S, Rubinstein L J 1989 Pathology of tumors of the nervous system, 5th edn. Edward Arnold, London, pp 541–545
Rutka J T, Trent J M, Rosenblum M L 1990 Molecular probes in neuro-oncology: a review. Cancer Investigation 8: 419–432
Samii M, Tatagiba M, Matthies C 1992 Acoustic neurinoma in the elderly: factors predictive of postoperative outcome. Neurosurgery 31: 615–620
Sataloff R T, Davies B, Myers D L 1985 Acoustic neuromas presenting as sudden deafness. American Journal of Otology 6: 349–352
Schessel D A, Nedzelski J M, Rowed D W, Feghali J G 1992 Pain after surgery for acoustic neuroma. Otolaryngology — Head and Neck Surgery 107: 424–429
Schisano G, Olivecrona H 1960 Neurinomas of the gasserian ganglion and trigeminal root. Journal of Neurosurgery 17: 306–322
Schnitt S J, Vogel H 1986 Meningiomas: Diagnostic value of immunoperoxidase staining for epithelial membrane antigen. American Journal of Surgical Pathology 10: 640–649
Schorry E K, Stowens D W, Crawford A H, Stowers A P, Schwartz W R, St Dignan P 1989 Summary of patient data from a multidisciplinary neurofibromatosis clinic. Neurofibromatosis 2: 129–134
Seizinger B R, Martuza R L, Gusella J F 1986 Loss of genes on chromosome 22 in tumorigenesis of human acoustic neuroma. Nature 322: 644–647
Sekhar L N, Jannetta P J 1984 Cerebellopontine angle meningiomas. Microsurgical excision and follow-up results. Journal of Neurosurgery 60: 500–505
Sekiya T, Møller A R 1987 Cochlear nerve injuries caused by cerebellopontine angle manipulations. An electrophysiology and morphological study in dogs. Journal of Neurosurgery 67: 244–249
Sekiya T, Møller A R 1988 Effects of cerebellar retractions on the cochlear nerve: an experimental study on rhesus monkeys. Acta Neurochirurgica 90: 45–52
Selters W A, Brackmann D E 1977 Acoustic tumour detection with brainstem evoked electric response audiometry. Archives of Otolaryngology 103: 181–187
Shaia F T, Sheehy J L 1976 Sudden sensorineural hearing impairment; a report of 1220 cases. Laryngoscope 86: 389–398
Shao K-N, Tatagiba M, Sammi M 1993 Surgical management of high jugular bulb in acoustic neurinoma via retrosigmoid approach. Neurosurgery 32: 32–37

Shea J J, Emmett J R, Orchik D J et al 1981 Medical treatment of tinnitus. Annals of Otology, Rhinology and Otolaryngology 90: 601–606
Shea J J, Hitselberger W E, Benecke J E, Brackmann D E 1985 Recurrence rate of partially resected acoustic tumors. American Journal of Otology November suppl: 107–109
Shelton C, Brackmann D E, House W F, Hitselberger W E 1989a Middle fossa acoustic tumor surgery: results in 106 cases. Laryngoscope 99: 405–408
Shelton C, Brackmann D E, House W F, Hitselberger W E 1989 Acoustic tumor surgery: prognostic factors in hearing preservation. Archives of Otolaryngology, Head and Neck Surgery 115: 1213–1216
Shelton C, Hitselberger W E, House W F et al 1990 Hearing preservation after acoustic tumor removal: longterm results. Laryngoscope 100: 115–119
Shelton C, Hitselberger W E, House W F, Brackmann D E 1992 Long-term results of hearing preservation after acoustic tumor removal. In: Tos M, Thomsen J (eds) Acoustic neuroma. Kugler, Amsterdam, pp 661–664
Sheptak P E, Jannetta P J 1979 The two-stage excision of huge acoustic neurinomas. Journal of Neurosurgery 51: 37–41
Shore-Freedman E, Abrahams C, Recant W, Schneider A B 1983 Neurilemomas and salivary gland tumors of the head and neck following childhood irradiation. Cancer 51: 2159–2163
Silverstein H, Haberkamp T, Smouha E 1986 The state of tinnitus after inner ear surgery. Otolaryngology — Head Neck Surgery 99: 438–441
Simpson R H W, Sparrow O C, Duffield M S 1990 Cerebellopontine angle tumors in black South Africans — how rare are acoustic schwannomas? South African Medical Journal 78: 11–14
Smith J W 1979 Treatment of facial palsy by cross-face nerve grafting. In: Buchheit W A, Truex R C Jr (eds) Surgery of the posterior fossa. Raven Press, New York, pp 173–179
Snow R B, Fraser R A 1987 Cerebellopontine angle tumor causing contralateral trigeminal neuralgia: a case report. Neurosurgery 21: 84–86
Sobel R A, Michaud J 1985 Microcystic meningioma of the falx cerebri with numerous palisaded structures: an unusual histological pattern mimicking schwannoma. Acta Neuropathologica (Berlin) 68: 256–258
Sorour O, Rifaat M, Lofti M 1973 The relative frequency of brain tumors in Egypt. African Journal of Medical Science 4: 178–186
Stack J P, Ramsden R T, Antoun N M, Lye R H, Isherwood I, Jenkins J P 1988 Magnetic resonance imaging of acoustic neuromas: the role of gadolinium-DTPA. British Journal of Radiology 61: 800–805
Stanton C, Perentes E, Collins V P, Rubinstein L J 1987 GFA protein reactivity in nerve sheath tumors: a polyvalent and monoclonal antibody study. Journal of Neuropathology and Experimental Neurology 46: 634–643
Stennert E 1979 I. Hypoglossal facial anastomosis: its significance for modern facial surgery. II. Combined approach in extratemporal facial nerve reconstruction. Clinics in Plastic Surgery 6: 471–486
Sterkers J M, Desorges M, Sterkers O, Corlieu P 1984 Our present approach to acoustic neuroma surgery. Advances in Oto-Rhino-Laryngology 34: 160–163
Sterkers O, El Dine M B, Martin N, Viala P, Sterkers J M 1992 Slow versus rapid growing acoustic neuromas. In: Tos M, Thomsen J (eds) Acoustic neuroma. Kugler, Amsterdam pp 145–147
Stewart T J, Liland J, Schuknecht H 1975 Occult schwannomas of the vestibular nerve. Archives of Otolaryngology 101: 91–95
Sugita K, Kobayashi S 1982 Technical and instrumental improvements in the surgical treatment of acoustic neurinomas. Journal of Neurosurgery 57: 747–752
Sunderland S 1945 The arterial relations in the internal auditory meatus. Brain 68: 23–27
Sunderland S 1978 Nerves and nerve injuries, 2nd edn. Churchill Livingstone, London
Swan I R C, Gatehouse S 1992 Screening for acoustic neuromas in routine otolaryngological practice. In: Tos M, Thomsen J (eds) Acoustic neuroma. Kugler, Amsterdam, pp 13–15
Symon L, Bord L T, Compton J S, Sabin I H, Sayin E 1989 Acoustic neuroma: a review of 392 cases. British Journal of Neurosurgery 3: 343–348
Takeuchi J, Handa H, Taki W, Yamagami T 1982 The Nd:YAG laser in neurological surgery. Surgical Neurology 18: 140–142
Tatagiba M, Samii M, Matthies C, Azm M E, Schonmayr R 1992 The significance for postoperative hearing of preserving the labyrinth in acoustic neuroma surgery. Journal of Neurosurgery 77: 677–684
Tator C H, Nedzelski J M 1985 Preservation of hearing in patients undergoing excision of acoustic neuromas and other cerebellopontine angle tumors. Journal of Neurosurgery 63: 168–174
Telian S A, Kemink J L, Kileny P 1988 Hearing recovery following suboccipital excision of acoustic neuroma. Archives of Otolaryngology — Head and Neck Surgery 114: 85–87
Thomsen J, Tos M 1990 Acoustic neuroma: clinical aspects, audiovestibular assessment, diagnostic delay, and growth rate. American Journal of Otology 11: 12–19
Thomsen J, Zilstorff K, Tos M 1983 Acoustic neuromas (diagnostic value of testing the function of the trigeminal nerve, cerebellum and opticokinetic nystagmus). Journal of Laryngology and Otology 97: 801–812
Thomsen J, Klinken L, Tos M 1984 Calcified acoustic neurinoma. Journal of Laryngology and Otology 98: 727–732
Thomsen J, Tos M, Borgesen S 1990 Gamma knife: hydrocephalus as a complication of the stereotactic radiosurgical treatment of acoustic neuroma. American Journal of Otology 11: 330–333
Thomsen J, Tos M, Møller H 1992 Diagnostic strategies in acoustic neuroma surgery: findings in 504 cases. In: Tos M, Thomsen J (eds) Acoustic neuroma. Kugler, Amsterdam, pp 69–72
Tos M, Thomsen J 1982 The price of preservation of hearing in acoustic neuroma surgery. Annals of Otology, Rhinology and Laryngology 91: 240–245
Tos M, Thomsen J 1985 Cerebrospinal fluid leak after translabyrinthine surgery. Laryngoscope 95: 351–354
Tos M, Thomsen J 1992 Proposal of classification of tumor size in acoustic neuroma surgery. In: Tos M, Thomsen J (eds) Acoustic neuroma. Kugler, Amsterdam, pp 133–137
Tos M, Thomsen J, Harmsen A 1988 Results of translabyrinthine removal of 300 acoustic neuromas related to tumor size. Acta Otolaryngologica (Stockholm) suppl 452: 38–51
Tos M, Thomsen J, Charabi S 1992a Epidemiology of acoustic neuromas: has the incidence increased during the last years? In: Tos M, Thomsen J (eds) Acoustic neuroma. Kugler, Amsterdam, pp 3–6
Tos M, Drozdziewicz D, Thomsen J 1992b The medial acoustic neuroma: a new clinical subgroup. In: Tos M, Thomsen J (eds) Acoustic neuroma. Kugler, Amsterdam, pp 211–215
Tos M, Youssef M, Thomsen J, Turgut S 1992c Causes of facial nerve paresis after translabyrinthine surgery for acoustic neuroma. Annals of Otology, Rhinology and Laryngology 101: 821–826
Tran Ba Huy P, Monteil J P, Rey A 1985 Results of twenty cases of transfacio-facial anastomosis as compared with those of XII–VII anastomosis. In: Portmann M (ed) Facial nerve. Masson, New York, pp 85–87
Tran Ba Huy P, Hassan J M, Wassef M, Mikol J, Thurel C 1987 Acoustic schwannoma presenting as a tumor of the external canal. Case report. Annals of Otology, Rhinology and Laryngology 96: 415–418
Turgut S, Tos M 1992 Relation between temporal bone pneumatization and jugular bulb variations. In: Tos M, Thomsen J (eds) Acoustic neuroma. Kugler, Amsterdam, pp 257–261
Umezu N, Aiba T, Unakami M 1991 Enterogenous cyst of the cerebellopontine angle cistern: case report. Neurosurgery 28: 462–466
Valvassori G E 1984 Radiologic evaluation of eighth nerve tumors. American Journal of Otolaryngology 5: 270–280
Valvassori G E, Guzman M 1989 Growth rate of acoustic neuromas. American Journal of Otology 10: 174–176
Valvassori G E, Potter G D 1982 Radiology of the ear, nose and throat. Georg Thieme Verlag, Stuttgart, p 95
von Glass W, Haid C T, Cidlinsky K, Stenglein C, Christ P 1991 False-positive MR imaging in the diagnosis of acoustic neuromas. Otolaryngology — Head and Neck Surgery 103: 583–585
Wakahayashi T, Tamaki N, Satoh H, Matsumoto S 1983 Epidermoid tumor presenting painful tic convulsif. Surgical Neurology 19: 244–246

Wallner K E, Sheline G E, Pitts L H, Wara W M, Davis R L, Boldrey E B 1987 Efficacy of irradiation for incompletely excised acoustic neurilemomas. Journal of Neurosurgery 67: 858–863
Walstead A, Salomon G, Olsen K S 1991 Low frequency hearing loss after spinal anesthesia: perilymphatic hypotonia? Scandinavian Audiology 20: 211–215
Waltzman S B, Cohen N L, Shapiro W H, Hoffman R A 1990 The prognostic value of round window electrical stimulation in cochlear implant patients. Otolaryngology — Head and Neck Surgery 103: 102–106
Wazen J, Silverstein H, Norrell H, Besse B 1985 Preoperative and postoperative growth rates in acoustic neuromas documented with CT scanning. Otolaryngology — Head and Neck Surgery 93: 151–155
Weiss M N, Kisiel D, Bhatia P 1990 Predictive value of brainstem evoked response in the diagnosis of acoustic neuroma. Otolaryngology — Head and Neck Surgery 103: 583–585
Welling D B, Glasscock M E, Woods C I, Jackson C G 1990 Acoustic neuroma: a cost-effective approach. Otolaryngology — Head and Neck Surgery 103: 364–370
Wennerberg J, Mercke U 1989 Growth potential of acoustic neuromas. American Journal of Otology 10: 293–296
Whittaker C K, Luetje C M 1985 Translabyrinthine removal of large acoustic tumours. American Journal of Otology November suppl: 155–160
Whittaker C K, Luetje C M 1992 Vestibular Schwannomas. Journal of Neurosurgery 76: 897–900
Whittle I R, Hawkins R A, Miller J D 1987 Sex hormone receptors in intracranial tumors and normal brain. European Journal of Surgical Oncology 13: 303–307
Wiegand D A, Fickel V 1989 Acoustic neuroma: the patient's perspective: subjective assessment of symptoms, diagnoses, therapy, and outcome in 541 patients. Laryngoscope 99: 179–187
Wigand M E, Goertzen W, Berg M 1988 Transtemporal planned partial resection of bilateral acoustic neurinomas. Acta Neurochirurgica (Wien) 92: 50–54
Wigand M E, Haid T, Berg M 1991 Extended middle cranial fossa approach for acoustic neuroma surgery. Skull Base Surgery 1: 183–187
Wu E H, Tang Y S, Zhang Y T, Bai R J 1986 CT in diagnosis of acoustic neuromas. American Journal of Neuroradiology 7: 645–650
Yamada S, Aiba T, Hara M 1993 Cerebellopontine angle medulloblastoma: case report and literature review. British Journal of Neurosurgery 7: 91–94
Yasargil M G, Fox J L 1974 The microsurgical approach to acoustic neurinomas. Surgical Neurology 2: 393–398
Yasargil M G, Smith R D, Gasser J C 1977 Microsurgical approach to acoustic neuromas. Advances and Technical Standards in Neurosurgery 4: 93–129
Yonemitsu T, Niizuma H, Kodama N, Fujiwara S, Suzuki J 1983 Acoustic neurinoma presenting as subarachnoid hemorrhage. Surgical Neurology 20: 125–130
Yoshii Y, Yamada S, Aibi T, Miyoshi S 1989 Cerebellopontine angle lipoma with abnormal bony structures. Neurologica Medico-Chirurgica (Tokyo) 29: 48–51
Yousem S A, Colby T V, Urich H 1985 Malignant epithelioid schwannoma arising in a benign schwannoma. A case report. Cancer 55: 2799–2803
Zini C, Sanna M, Gandolfi A 1985 Hypoglossal-facial anastomosis in the rehabilitation of irreversible facial nerve palsies. In: Portmann M (ed) Facial nerve. Masson, New York, pp 519–522

32. Acoustic neurinoma (vestibular schwannoma) — the suboccipital approach

Robert G. Ojemann

TERMINOLOGY

In December 1991, the National Institutes of Health held a Consensus Development Conference on acoustic neurinoma (Eldridge & Parry 1992). One of the conclusions was 'that the preferred name for this tumor is vestibular schwannoma because it is composed of Schwann cells and generally arises on the vestibular branch of the eighth cranial nerve'. It is likely that acceptance of the change in terminology will be slow since the term 'acoustic neurinoma' has been used for so many years.

Acoustic neurinomas occur in two different patient groups. Unilateral tumors occur sporadically and are not associated with other central nervous system tumors or abnormalities. Bilateral vestibular schwannomas occur in patients with neurofibromatosis type 2 (NF-2), an autosomal dominant disorder. This may be the only manifestation of the disease or there may be associated intracranial and spinal tumors and central nervous system malformations.

INCIDENCE

It is estimated that between 2000 and 3000 new patients with unilateral acoustic neurinomas are diagnosed in the United States each year (an incidence of about one per 100 000 per year). These neoplasms account for approximately 8–10% of intracranial tumors in adults and 80% of tumors in the cerebellopontine angle (Sobel 1993).

NF-2 affects about one in 50 000 people (Baldwin et al 1991). The frequency of patients with bilateral tumors in reported series of patients with acoustic neurinoma has ranged from 2–10%.

AGE AND SEX DISTRIBUTION

In a review of 341 patients who had surgical pathological specimens analyzed between 1975 and 1991 at the Massachusetts General Hospital, Sobel (1993) reported the age distribution at the time of the first surgery for both unilateral and bilateral acoustic neurinomas (Fig. 32.1). In the 293 patients with unilateral tumors, the age ranged from 15–79 years, with a mean age of 47.4 years, and there were 155 females (53%) and 138 males (Sobel 1993). In this author's surgical series of 461 consecutive patients with unilateral tumors treated between 1979 and 1993 there were 265 females (57%) and 196 males, ranging in age from 18–89. In the series of House & Hitselberger (1985), 49% of patients were female, with an average age of 47.3 years. In the Mayo Clinic series, 58% were female with a median age of 54 years (Harner & Ebersold 1985).

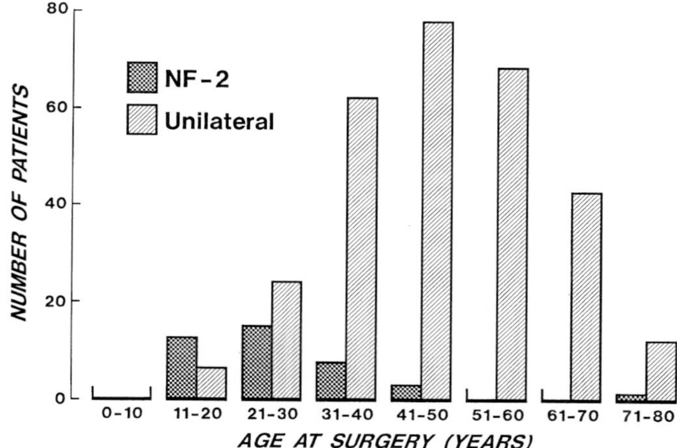

Fig. 32.1 Patients' ages by decades at time of surgery for unilateral and bilateral (NF-2) acoustic neurinomas. Modified from Sobel (1993).

In the 48 patients with NF-2 reviewed by Sobel (1993) the age ranged from 15–74 years but the mean age was 27.1 years, and 35 were under the age of 40 at the time of the first operation. There were 20 males and 19 females. In an early review of 15 of our patients with NF-2, two thirds were 21 years of age or younger when their symptoms were first noted (Martuza & Ojemann 1982).

CLINICAL DIAGNOSIS

In over 95% of patients with an acoustic neurinoma, the first symptom will relate to the auditory-vestibular system (Martuza et al 1985, Ojemann & Martuza 1990). In more than 70% hearing loss is the first symptom. Usually there is a gradual diminution of hearing but a sudden loss can occur and the hearing level may fluctuate. Difficulty in understanding words on the telephone is often an early symptom. Tinnitus, dizziness, unsteadiness, vertigo, and a sensation of fullness in the ear can also occur as an initial symptom or following the onset of hearing loss. As the tumor enlarges it begins to compress the trigeminal nerve, and numbness or altered sensation on the face is the next most common symptom. With large tumors, symptoms may include headache, diplopia, hoarseness, difficulty swallowing, ataxia of gait and incoordination.

Rarely a patient has symptoms and signs of high pressure hydrocephalus (headache and papilledema). Occasionally an elderly patient will present with symptoms of normal pressure hydrocephalus (worsening gait and mild dementia) and enlarged ventricles.

IMAGING DIAGNOSIS

The diagnosis of an acoustic neurinoma is established with magnetic resonance imaging (MRI) after gadolinium enhancement (Fig. 32.2). Usually this is the only test needed. If information is desired about the pneumatization of the petrous bone or there is concern from the MR image that there may be a high jugular bulb, computed tomographic (CT) images including bone windows are obtained. Angiography, even for larger tumors, does not add enough useful information to warrant the use of this study.

LABORATORY DIAGNOSIS

In patients with acoustic neurinoma the characteristic finding is a unilateral sensorineural hearing loss with poorer speech discrimination than would be anticipated from the pure tone findings (Sheehy 1979). From a practical standpoint, pure tone auditometry, speech discrimination and brainstem auditory evoked responses are the only tests that are now done on a regular basis (Martuza et al 1985). On pure tone testing the most common pattern is a high frequency loss with approximately two thirds of patients having this pattern (Johnson 1979). There may, however, be a flat loss, low tone loss, trough-shaped loss or a normal study. Therefore, an asymmetric hearing loss needs careful evaluation irrespective of the pure tone findings.

Speech discrimination is tested by presenting a word list after a speech recognition threshold (SRT) is determined (Johnson 1979). A score of the percentage of words correctly identified is recorded. The discrimination is usually reduced in patients with acoustic neurinoma.

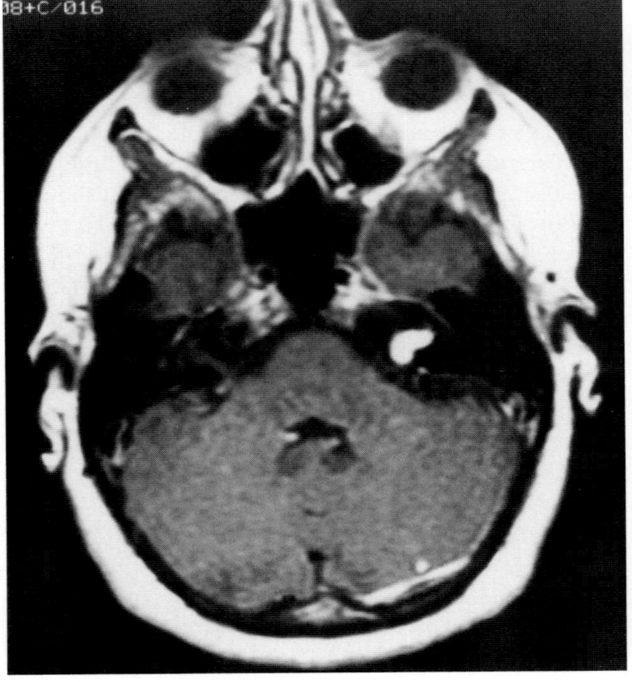

A

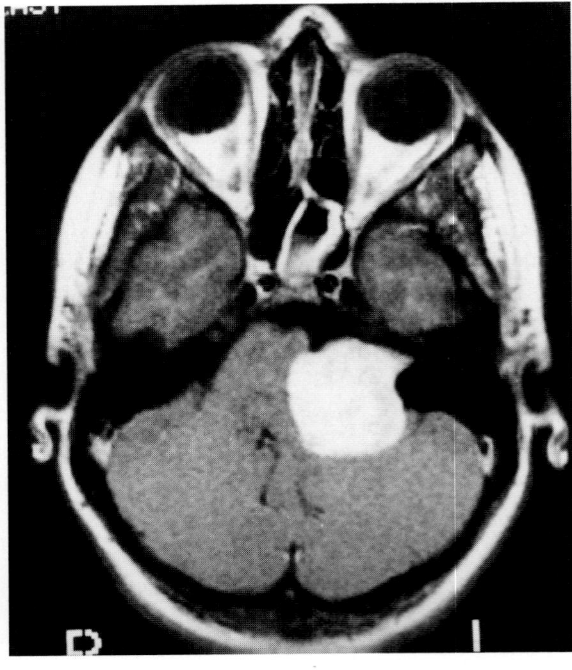

B

Fig. 32.2 Magnetic resonance T1-weighted axial images after gadolinium administration of a small (**A**) and large (**B**) acoustic neurinoma.

Brainstem auditory evoked response testing will be abnormal in 98% of the patients with acoustic neurinoma and has been used as a screening test (Barrs et al 1985). Five waves can usually be detected from scalp electrodes using repetitive click stimuli and computerized averaging methods (Martuza & Rouleau 1990). Wave I is thought to be generated by the auditory nerve next to the cochlea, wave II by the cochlear nucleus in the pons, wave III is from the superior olive, wave IV from the lateral lemniscus in the pons, and wave V is thought to originate from the rostral pons or inferior colliculus. In patients with acoustic neurinoma all or some of the waves may be absent. When wave I is present there will almost always be a delay (increased latency) in the appearance of the remaining waves. While cochlear hearing loss may prolong the absolute latency, it will not affect the interwave latency, which is prolonged when there is compression of the eighth nerve. The most sensitive indicators of involvement of the eighth nerve are prolongation of the I–III or I–V interwave latencies. If wave I cannot be seen, the inter-ear difference and absolute latency of wave V are useful indicators of eighth cranial nerve dysfunction.

PATHOLOGY

Gross morphologic features

The typical acoustic neurinoma has a pale yellow or yellow-tan appearance but the color can vary and some have a reddish-gray appearance (Gruskin & Carberry 1979). Most tumors are well circumscribed with a smooth capsule but occasionally they are lobulated. Except for the smallest tumors, they are adherent to the area of the internal auditory meatus.

The tumor has a firm consistency but there may be areas of soft tissue and in some a cyst within the tumor may be found (Ojemann & Martuza 1990). The cyst size can vary from a few millimeters to one or more centimeters in diameter and on occasion may represent a significant volume of the tumor mass.

Histopathologic features

The histologic criteria for the diagnosis of acoustic neurinoma are the same as those of schwannomas that arise from other nerves (Russell & Rubinstein 1959, Gruskin & Carberry 1979, Sobel 1993). The classic description of a schwannoma is tissue composed of densely packed elongated spindle cells in interlocking fascicles with a tendency to palisading (Antoni type A tissue), often intermingled with loosely textured tissue with extracellular clear spaces sometimes associated with cyst formation (Antoni type B tissue) and, frequently, nuclear atypia (Gruskin & Carberry 1979, Sobel 1993) (Fig. 32.3). Varying patterns can be seen. Other findings may include Verocay bodies, hemosiderin deposition, hyalinized blood vessels, malformation-like vessels, recent and old thromboses, sheets of foam macrophages, foci of high cellularity, whorls and collagenous scarring. In the review by Sobel (1993), lobular growth patterns were found in about 40% and meningioma tissue in 20% of the patients with NF-2.

MANAGEMENT PLAN

Three management options are considered when eva-

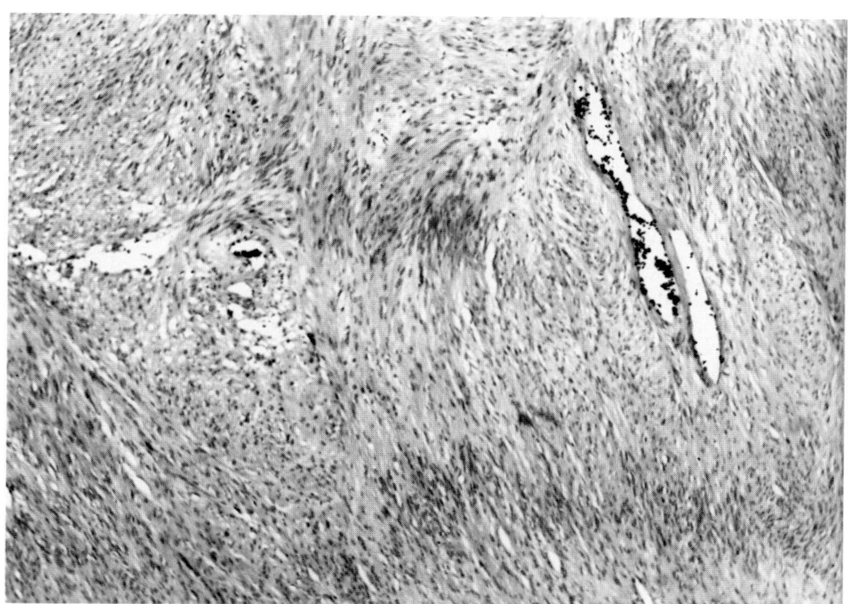

Fig. 32.3 Histopathology. The tissue is composed of denser Antoni A tissue with nuclei arranged in palisades and more loosely textured Antoni B tissue (×100).

luating a patient with an acoustic neurinoma: surgery, radiation therapy and observation. To make the best recommendation on each individual patient the physician needs to: (1) take the history to have a clear idea of the patient's course and of how the symptoms are affecting the patient's life; (2) make an objective assessment of any neurologic deficit; (3) carefully review the radiographic studies to be sure they are adequate; and (4) make a decision as to whether any additional studies are needed. The management options are then evaluated. What will be the impact of the proposed treatment on the patient's daily life? Will the treatment improve or arrest the progression of symptoms? Can further growth or recurrence of the tumor be prevented? What are the risks of the treatment? Do the short and long-term benefits justify these risks? It is important to discuss with the patient his/her hopes and expectations from the treatment. The informational brochures from the Acoustic Neuroma Association have been a great help to many patients and their families.

In some patients there is little doubt as to what should be done. In other patients the decision may be difficult (Ojemann & Black 1988). To arrive at a decision the physician must have up-to-date knowledge about the management alternatives.

Indications for operation are:

1. Recent or worsening symptoms, except in elderly patients with mild symptoms.
2. Enlargement of the tumor in patients who are being followed, except in the elderly patient with a small tumor.
3. Regrowth after subtotal removal in younger patients.
4. Enlargement of a tumor after radiosurgery once the initial swelling reaction has subsided.
5. The patient's decision after discussion of the treatment options.

Indications for radiation therapy are:

1. Enlarging small or medium-sized tumor in an elderly patient with mild symptoms who is being followed.
2. Regrowth after subtotal removal.
3. Major medical illness that significantly increases the risk of operation.
4. The patient's decision after discussion of the treatment options.

Indications for observation are:

1. A long history of auditory symptoms in a patient of any age and with any size tumor.
2. An elderly patient with mild symptoms.
3. An incidental finding of the tumor on a scan done for some other reason.
4. The patient's decision after discussion of the treatment options.

SURGICAL MANAGEMENT

Overview

The history of the development of the surgical removal of acoustic neurinomas has been reviewed (House 1979a,b, Ojemann & Martuza 1990). The contributions of Cushing (1917) and Dandy (1925) were particularly important in improving the surgical techniques.

The microsurgical removal of an acoustic neurinoma can be done using a suboccipital, translabyrinthine or middle fossa approach. Both the suboccipital and translabyrinthine approaches have been used to remove tumors of all sizes. When hearing is to be preserved the suboccipital approach is preferred. Some surgeons use the middle fossa approach for small tumors in the internal auditory canal, particularly at the lateral end when an attempt is being made to preserve hearing. The surgeon must have a thorough understanding of the anatomy of the cerebellopontine angle and petrous bone and the relationship of anatomic structures to the tumor (Rhoton 1986).

The details of the translabyrinthine approach have been described in Chapter 31 and by House and associates (House 1979c, House & Hitselberger 1985), and the middle fossa approach by Brackmann and co-workers (Brackmann 1979, Brackmann et al 1985). Good results from all three approaches have been reported by experienced groups of surgeons (Ojemann & Martuza 1990). For most patients, our preference is the suboccipital (posterior fossa) approach because of the wide visualization it allows, the ability to save hearing in appropriate cases and the good results our group (Ojemann et al 1972, Ojemann 1978, Ojemann & Crowell 1978, Ojemann 1979, 1980, Ojemann et al 1984, Nadol et al 1987, Ojemann & Black 1988, Ojemann 1990, Ojemann & Martuza 1990, Nadol et al 1992, Ojemann 1992, 1993) and others have reported (Koos & Perneczky 1985, Rhoton 1986, Symon et al 1989, Baldwin et al 1990, Harner et al 1990, Klemink et al 1990, Samii et al 1991, Ebersold et al 1992, Fisher et al 1992, Samii et al 1992).

Our operative approach and techniques have been reported and illustrated in detail in previous publications (Ojemann et al 1984, Ojemann & Martuza 1990, Ojemann 1992, 1993). The operation is done in collaboration with an otologic surgeon who exposes the internal auditory canal and dissects the tumor in that area.

Perioperative medical therapy

Steroids are usually started 48 hours prior to operation and a higher dose is given just before operation. The blood sugar is monitored. The high steroid dose is continued every 6 hours during the operation and then is gradually tapered over 5–10 days depending on the size of the tumor and facial nerve function.

An antibiotic is given intravenously starting just before surgery. This is continued for 24 hours after operation.

After anesthesia is induced, an indwelling Foley catheter is inserted and 10–20 mg of furosemide is given intravenously. During the preparation and exposure of the dura a 20% solution of mannitol is given intravenously in a dosage of 1–1.5 g/kg over 20–30 minutes.

Management of preoperative hydrocephalus

Occasionally patients with acoustic neurinomas will have enlarged ventricles with no symptoms of hydrocephalus. No special treatment is needed.

High pressure hydrocephalus is now uncommon in a patient with acoustic neurinoma but if this is present the symptoms will usually improve with steroids. A ventricular drain may be needed at operation and for a few days postoperatively. Rarely does a patient need a ventriculo-peritoneal shunt.

Occasionally, an elderly patient with a large tumor and large ventricles who has symptoms suggesting normal pressure hydrocephalus is seen. If the only symptom is hearing loss, a ventriculo-peritoneal shunt may be the only treatment needed. If there are also symptoms of increasing cranial nerve and/or brainstem compression, treatment has been subtotal removal of the tumor and placement of a ventriculo-peritoneal shunt, usually in the same operation. These patients have generally had good long-term results.

Monitoring

Continuous electrophysiological monitoring of facial nerve function during the operation has become an established procedure (Ojemann & Martuza 1990, Eldridge & Parry 1992). The benefits of this monitoring have been documented (Jellinek et al 1991).

A continuous drip of a muscle relaxant is carefully administered in order to assess facial nerve function. The dosage is monitored by following the twitches elicited with ulnar nerve stimulation. Facial nerve function is monitored by continuous recording of electromyographic activity with two recording electrodes, one in the orbicularis oculi and the other in the orbicularis oris muscles (Fig. 32.4). The muscle contractions, which could occur from stimulation of the facial nerve during coagulation when the electrodes are inactive, are recorded from a motion sensor placed on the cheek. Monopolar stimulation is used to locate the seventh nerve. Fifth nerve function is monitored with electrodes placed in the masseter and temporalis muscles.

When auditory evoked responses are monitored during an attempt to save hearing, we use a system developed by Dr Robert Levine (Levine et al 1978, 1984, Ojemann et al

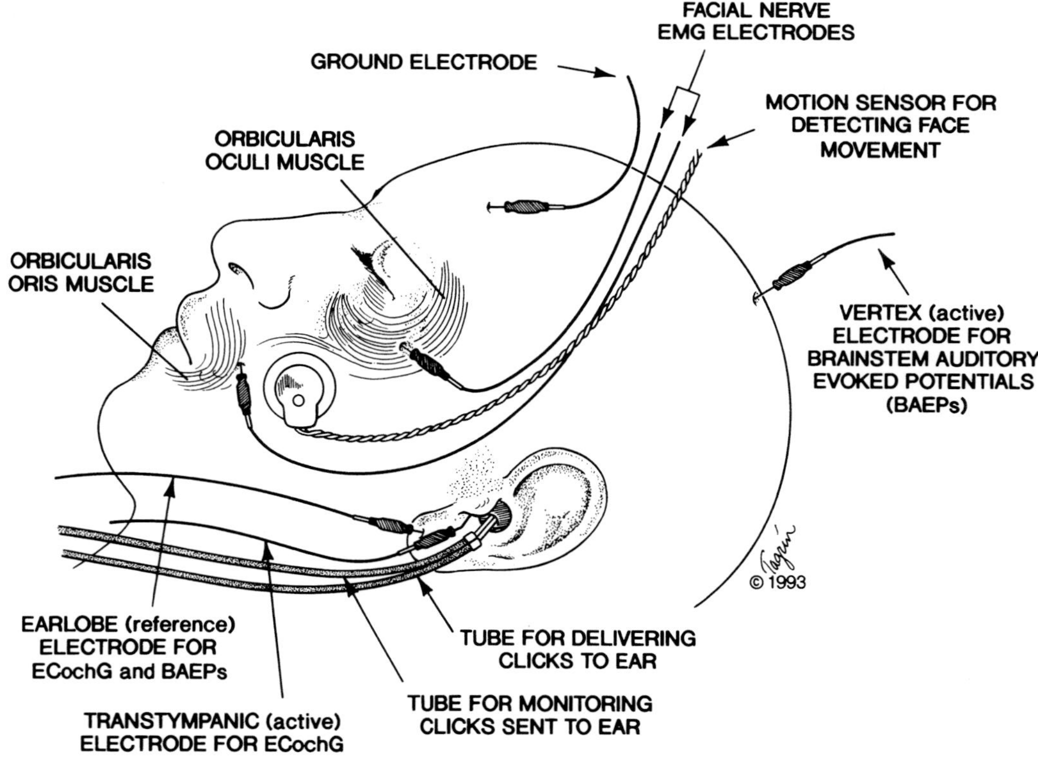

Fig. 32.4 Monitoring of facial and cochlear nerve function during the operation.

1984, Levine 1988, 1990, 1991). A transtympanic electrode is placed for electrocochleography, scalp electrodes are inserted for brainstem auditory evoked potential monitoring, and a microphone system is placed in the external ear canal to provide the sound stimulus (Fig. 32.4).

Position

The semi-sitting, prone, supine-oblique, lateral or park bench, and lateral-oblique positions have been used for removal of acoustic neurinomas (Ojemann & Martuza 1990, Tew & Scodary 1993). The author's experience with the semi-sitting position has been described in previous publications (Ojemann et al 1972, Ojemann 1978, Ojemann & Crowell 1978). There was no major permanent morbidity related to this position, but occasional problems with air embolus and hypotension were encountered. Because of the risk of hypotension in older patients, a supine-oblique position was utilized. In addition to preventing hypotension, other advantages of this position were excellent visualization of the cerebellopontine angle, ease of tumor removal, no concern about air embolus, and comfort of the surgeon. This position is now used for removal of most cerebellopontine angle tumors. If there is severe cervical spondylosis or limitation of neck motion from a previous injury, a lateral position is used. The intermittent pulsation of cerebrospinal fluid into the operative area is not a problem and, in fact, keeps the neural and vascular structures from drying; however, some surgeons prefer continuous drainage of the fluid.

The operating table is turned so that the surgeon can sit behind the head with his/her feet under the table. The patient lies supine with the shoulder that is ipsilateral to the tumor slightly elevated (Fig. 32.5). The head is turned parallel to the floor, elevated, and held with a three-point skeletal fixation headrest. During the operation the line of sight to the brainstem may be altered by rotating the table from side to side. An armrest is placed for the arm nearest the vertex. The other arm rests on the patient.

Incision and exposure

A vertical incision is centered 1–2 cm medial to the mastoid process (Fig. 32.5). Other types of incisions that have been used include an inverted J-shaped incision, an S-shaped incision and a semi-curved incision (Ojemann & Martuza 1990). A graft of pericranial tissue, about 4 cm in diameter, is taken from the occipital region by extending the superior aspect of the incision as needed. This graft is used in closing the cerebellar convexity dura at the end of the operation. The suboccipital muscles and fascia are incised in line with the incision and carefully separated from their attachments to the bone using subperiosteal dissection and electrocautery. Special care is taken to occlude the arterial vessels as they are encountered in the muscle. An emissary vein is usually exposed in the region of the medial mastoid area.

The bone over the lateral two thirds of the cerebellar hemisphere is exposed. It is usually not necessary to visualize the midline bone or rim of the foramen magnum. A burr hole is placed, the dura carefully separated from the overlying bone, and a bone flap cut (Fig. 32.5). This opening exposes the dura over the lateral two thirds of the cerebellar hemisphere and usually exposes the transverse sinus. Further bone is removed as needed to expose the turn from the transverse to the sigmoid sinus and the edge of the petrous bone laterally. This will allow the edge of the sinus to be retracted with the sutures placed to hold

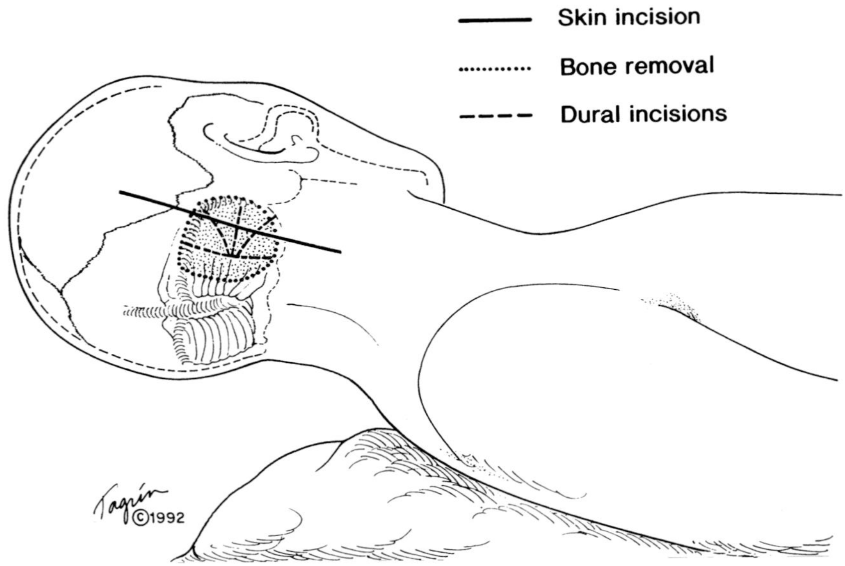

Fig. 32.5 Position, skin incision, craniotomy opening and dural incisions.

the dural flaps and a direct line of sight down the posterior surface of the petrous bone. The mastoid air cells are usually entered and are occluded with bone wax.

The dura is opened vertically, keeping an area of medial dura intact to protect the retracted cerebellum. Stellate dural incisions provide superior, lateral and inferior flaps of dura which are held back with sutures (Figs 32.5 and 32.6).

The cerebellum is then gently elevated, the arachnoid opened and cerebrospinal fluid allowed to drain (Fig. 32.6). This will usually relieve any bulging of the cerebellum and allow exposure of the cerebellopontine angle with minimal retraction. The arachnoid should be opened enough to allow cerebrospinal fluid to continue to drain during the operation. In most tumors the tip of a small catheter (#10 Bardic) is placed in the cistern and sutured to the inferior medial corner of the dural opening to drain cerebrospinal fluid continuously during the operation. In some patients with large tumors, a small portion of the lateral cerebellar hemisphere will be removed to facilitate the exposure. Following placement of the self-retaining Greenberg retractors, the operating microscope is positioned.

Removal of small tumors and hearing preservation

Under the microscope, the arachnoid over the tumor is opened and the petrosal vein coagulated and divided if necessary. The retractors are repositioned. With small tumors the eighth nerve complex will be seen coming into the inferior medial side of the tumor. The next step is usually exposure of the tumor in the internal auditory canal. Dura is removed over the region of the internal auditory canal and bone is carefully removed using an air drill with constant suction-irrigation for cooling. When hearing preservation is a consideration, the bone removal extends for a distance of no more than 10 mm laterally. A more lateral exposure risks entering the labyrinth — an event which is usually associated with loss of hearing (Tatagiba et al 1992). Dissection then depends on an assessment of the relationship of the tumor to the vestibular and cochlear nerves. In some patients the vestibular nerve fibers entering the medial edge of the tumor are divided, the cochlear and facial nerves identified, and the dissection proceeds from medial to lateral. In other patients it may be difficult to define the cochlear nerve medially. The tumor is then carefully rotated near the lateral end of the canal, looking for the seventh nerve anterosuperiorly and the cochlear nerve anteroinferiorly (Fig. 32.7). It is important to avoid stretching or putting tension on the cochlear nerve so the fibers are not avulsed. The position of the seventh nerve is confirmed with stimulation. An internal decompression of the tumor may be done using sharp dissection to facilitate the exposure. Dissection along the facial and cochlear nerves is done with fine straight or curved microdissectors, canal knives and sharp dissection with microscissors. Dissection is alternated from different directions, depending on what seems to give the best exposure, the easiest plane of dissection and the least traction on the nerves. When the cochlear and facial nerves have been clearly defined, the vestibular nerves coming into the tumor are divided on both the medial and lateral aspects of the tumor. In some patients the lateral end of the tumor may not be exposed because of the limitation in bone removal. In these patients the tumor is

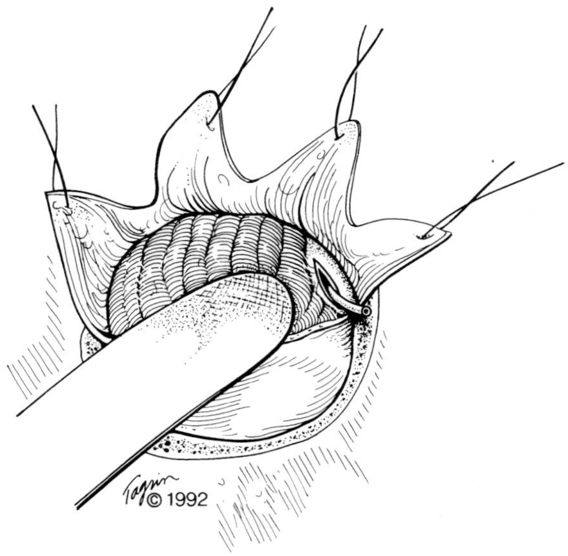

Fig. 32.6 The dural flaps have been retracted with sutures. The cerebellum is elevated and the arachnoid opened to allow drainage of cerebrospinal fluid. In medium and large tumors a catheter is placed in the cistern to drain the fluid during the operation.

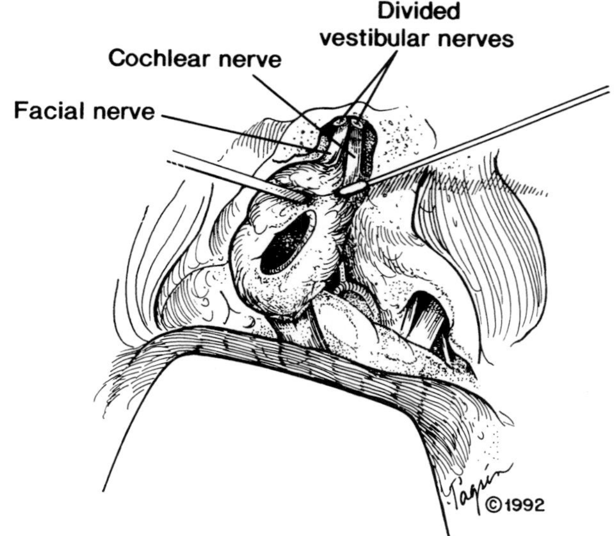

Fig. 32.7 In small tumors where hearing is to be preserved the internal auditory canal is exposed and a decision made how best to proceed with the dissection (see text). With large tumors the vestibular and cochlear nerves are divided and the seventh nerve followed back to the meatus.

transected near the end of the canal and the lateral extent of the tumor removed with a small ring curette.

During the dissection there may be intermittent bleeding along the nerves. A fine suction will keep the field clean and will not damage the nerves. Most of the bleeding will stop spontaneously. When trying to save hearing an attempt is made to preserve any significant arterial vessel entering the internal auditory meatus.

Removal of medium and large tumors

The arachnoid over the posterior capsule of the tumor is opened. A separate cystic collection of cerebrospinal fluid surrounded by thickened arachnoid and containing xanthochromic fluid may occasionally be loculated in relation to the tumor capsule. The petrosal vein, which usually is coming off the cerebellum or middle cerebellar peduncle to the petrosal sinus just above the tumor, is coagulated and divided. In order to complete the initial exposure of the posterior capsule it is often necessary to shrink the cerebellar tissue next to the tumor with bipolar coagulation or to remove a small amount of cerebellar tissue which may obscure the inferior medial pole.

The posterior capsule is stimulated to locate the facial nerve. In the majority of patients the facial nerve will be on the anterior surface of the tumor and there will be no response on this first stimulation. In some patients, however, the nerve is displaced more superiorly, particularly in its lateral course just before it enters the internal auditory canal. In this situation a response may be seen on the initial stimulation. There can also be anterior medial displacement of the facial nerve along the brainstem and over the anterior superior aspect of the tumor. In this circumstance the facial nerve may be displaced against the fifth nerve. On rare occasions the nerve is inferior or across the posterior surface. Only one patient in the author's series of 461 cases had the facial nerve displaced posteriorly.

The ninth, tenth and eleventh cranial nerves are identified and arachnoid adjacent to the cerebellum is carefully dissected to aid exposure of the inferior medial capsule. The arachnoid may need to be opened over these nerves to aid the exposure and prevent traction on the nerves. With larger tumors the ninth and tenth nerves are carefully reflected off the tumor capsule. A small rubber dam is placed over the lower nerves for protection during the rest of the operation.

The next step is internal decompression of the tumor which is done intermittently as needed. This allows all the pressure to be placed on the tumor capsule while separating it from the cranial nerves and brainstem. The ultrasonic aspirator, bipolar coagulation and sharp dissection are used for internal decompression.

Dissection begins inferiorly and medially. In medium-sized tumors, the eighth nerve complex can usually be defined with moderate dissection (Fig. 32.8). In larger

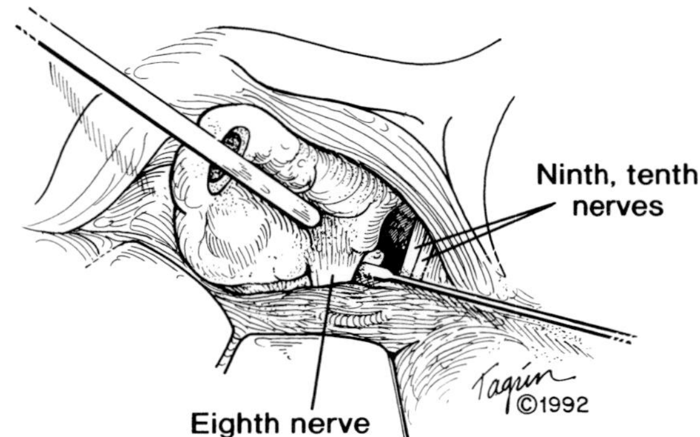

Fig. 32.8 Internal decompression of the tumor has been performed. The tumor capsule is being reflected laterally and superiorly to bring into view the eighth nerve complex.

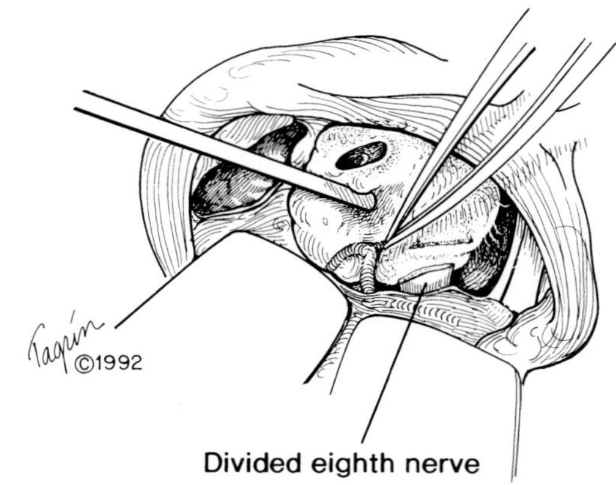

Fig. 32.9 The eighth nerve has been divided. A small arterial branch entering the tumor is being coagulated, preserving the main arterial trunk.

tumors these nerves will usually not be seen initially. After carefully reflecting the capsule laterally and superiorly into the area of decompression, one looks for the eighth nerve complex along the inferior medial capsule. Being a right-handed surgeon, the author prefers a fine suction in the left hand to retract the tumor and keep the area of dissection clean. The vestibular and cochlear nerve fibers entering the tumor are divided using bipolar coagulation and sharp dissection (Fig. 32.9).

Care is taken to look for the facial nerve, which can be just under the eighth nerve complex or may be a few millimeters away. It often can be recognized by its white or gray color, which is different from the adjacent brainstem. If the seventh nerve has not yet been localized, intermittent stimulation is used. In some patients spontaneous electromyographic activity will indicate when one is on or near that nerve. If the facial nerve is not seen anterior to the divided eighth nerve complex, it is usually located by reflecting the inferior and medial tumor capsule further laterally and superiorly (Fig. 32.10). Usually the facial nerve forms a solid band on the tumor capsule but it

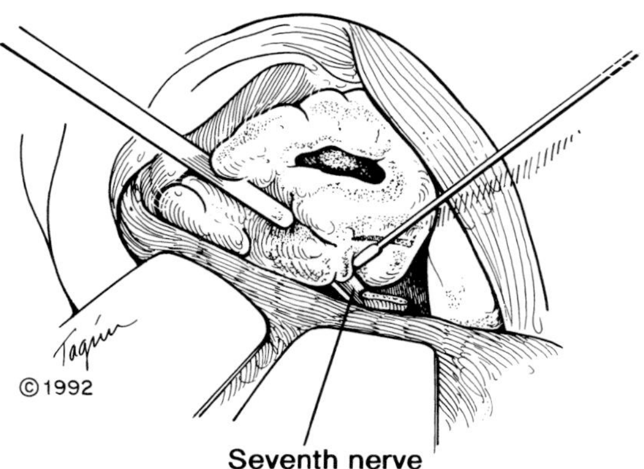

Fig. 32.10 The seventh nerve is identified anterior to the divided eighth nerve as it angles superiorly and laterally.

may be spread out over a wide area and occasionally is surrounded by the tumor.

As the dissection of the capsule progresses not only is further internal decompression done as indicated but sections of the tumor capsule are removed to allow room to reflect the capsule laterally. It may also be advantageous to alternate dissection of the inferior medial capsule with dissection superiorly and medially to define the fifth nerve and brainstem attachments (Fig. 32.11). Arterial vessels adjacent to the tumor are preserved, dividing only branches entering the tumor. There are often vascular attachments in the region of the fifth nerve root entry zone. Small rubber dams may be placed on the brainstem for protection as the dissection progresses.

Dissection extends along the seventh nerve toward the internal auditory meatus. We use fine straight or curved microdissectors, canal knives and sharp dissection with microscissors as needed (Fig. 32.12). When the point is reached where the bone over the internal auditory canal is impeding further dissection or the dissection is difficult, attention is directed to the tumor in the internal auditory

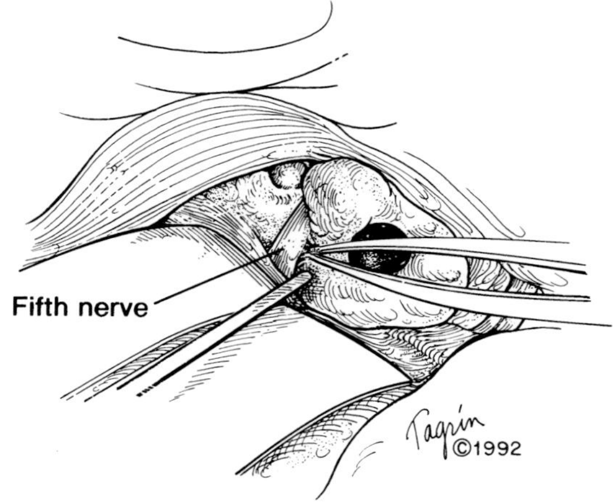

Fig. 32.11 The fifth nerve is visualized with gentle inferior and lateral traction on the tumor capsule.

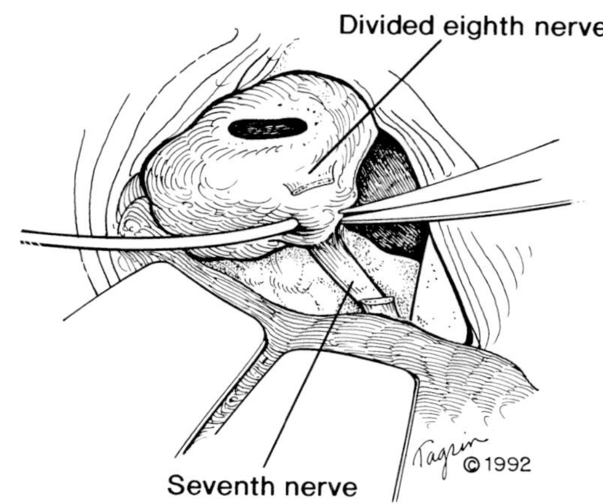

Fig. 32.12 Dissection along the seventh nerve is often facilitated by sharp dissection.

canal. The exposure is the same as that described for small tumors. In some patients the tumor extends quite far laterally in the canal and it is advisable to make the usual exposure, remove a portion of the tumor and then do further drilling within the lateral end of the canal as needed. Occasionally there can be a high jugular bulb which may be exposed.

After separation of the tumor from the facial nerve in the internal auditory canal, the attachments along the edge of the internal auditory meatus are divided. The facial nerve starts to turn anteriorly or anterosuperiorly as the posterior fossa is entered. The surgeon can then decide how best to proceed. The dissection may be continued medially along the brainstem and cerebellar peduncle, dividing arachnoid and vascular attachments as they are encountered and gradually freeing the facial nerve. On occasion a large branch of the anterior inferior cerebellar artery is embedded in the tumor capsule but it can usually be dissected free, dividing the small branches directly supplying the tumor. In large tumors, the trochlear nerve and superior cerebellar artery may be adherent superiorly, the sixth nerve adherent anteriorly and the ninth and tenth nerves adherent inferiorly. The objective is to reduce the bulk and attachments of the tumor so that finally the surgeon is dealing only with dissection from the facial nerve. The facial nerve is usually most adherent to the tumor capsule in the posterior fossa near the internal auditory meatus where the nerve may be splayed over the anterior-superior capsule or may occasionally be surrounded by tumor. The dissection in this area is often complicated by vascular and fibrous attachments. The surgeon must adapt to the characteristics of the tumor and it may be necessary to work alternately from various angles.

In some patients with large tumors the capsule will be so intimately adherent to the brainstem and cranial nerves that a plane cannot be developed. In such cases a thin layer of tumor capsule is left (radical subtotal removal).

Closure

Once the tumor is removed, hemostasis is checked. The area of bone removal over the internal auditory meatus is carefully waxed to occlude air cells. In addition, an adipose tissue graft taken from a superficial incision on the lower abdomen is carefully placed in the area where bone has been removed. Surgicel is used to hold this graft in place and is also used to cover the area of resected or retracted cerebellum.

This author closes the dura in a watertight fashion using the graft of pericranial tissue taken at the beginning of the operation. The dura is covered with Gelfoam. The bone flap is replaced and held with stainless steel wire, which does not interfere with future imaging, and a dural tenting suture. The wound is thoroughly irrigated with antibiotic solution prior to closure.

RADIATION THERAPY MANAGEMENT

In 1971, Leksell reported the first use of stereotactic radiosurgery to treat a patient with an acoustic neurinoma. Subsequently, further experience was reported (Norén et al 1983). Detailed and comprehensive follow-up reports have been published by Lunsford and his group summarizing the experience at the University of Pittsburgh with the first North American 201-source ^{60}Co gamma unit (Linskey et al 1992). Reports from both these groups show a high rate of tumor growth control and an acceptable rate of complications. These facts have established stereotactic radiosurgery as one of the three treatment alternatives to consider in a patient with an acoustic neurinoma.

The treatment results of 74 patients with unilateral acoustic neurinomas were reported by the Pittsburgh group (Linskey et al 1992). There was no mortality and all returned to their previous level of activity in 5–7 days. The follow-up ranged from 3–36 months, and 2 tumors (3%) were larger, 54 (73%) were the same and 18 (24%) were smaller. The measurement error was estimated to be ±1.3 mm and a change of ±2.6 mm was required to categorize the change as smaller or larger. The 2 patients with larger tumors had no new symptoms and are being followed.

In the same report, 70 patients with normal preoperative facial nerve function 24 (34%) developed a delayed facial nerve weakness (Linskey et al 1992). At the time of follow-up, 13 of the 24 had made a good recovery (6 grade 1, 7 grade 2), leaving 11 of the 70 (16%) with grade 3 or worse. The preservation of useful hearing, as defined by this group, of at least 50% discrimination and pure tone average of 50 decibels or less, was 38% at one year. Of 66 patients with normal preoperative trigeminal nerve function, 32% developed delayed trigeminal neuropathy. In those with abnormal function it was 46%. Only 10% had resolved completely at follow-up but most seemed to be improving. A significant correlation between radiation dose and delayed cranial neuropathies could not be demonstrated.

Other persistent problems included worsened balance in 20–30%, and a small percentage of patients had dizziness or vertigo, persistent nausea and worsened headaches. Eight patients developed new parenchymal changes in the middle cerebellar peduncle and pons on MRI scans. No associated symptoms were noted and these changes tended to resolve. Four patients required ventriculo-peritoneal shunt 5–16 months after radiosurgery. The cause of the hydrocephalus was thought possibly to be elevated cerebrospinal fluid protein levels.

Other types of radiation therapy have also been reported to have a beneficial effect on an acoustic neurinoma. These include fractionated conventional therapy, proton beam and radiosurgery using the linear accelerator (Wallner et al 1987, Darrouzet et al 1990).

OBSERVATIONAL MANAGEMENT

Acoustic neurinomas usually enlarge slowly. It has been well documented, however, that some of these tumors stop growing, that occasionally spontaneous regression may occur, and that a rare tumor may unexpectedly grow rapidly (Nedzelski et al 1986, Bederson et al 1991, Valvassori & Shannon 1991). Bederson et al (1991) reported 70 patients who were initially followed because they did not want surgery or did not have progressive symptoms. The average follow-up was 36 months (range 6–84). During the first year 29 patients (41%) had no detectable tumor growth, and of 18 who had a second year scan, only 1 showed detectable growth. In 37 patients (53%), growth ranging from 1–17 mm (average 3.4 ± 0.5 mm) occurred during the first year, and in 23 patients with a second year follow-up scan, 21 showed further growth. In 4 patients (6%) there was regression in tumor size. Rapid growth rate in 7 and clinical deterioration in 2 other patients without change in the size of the tumor led to surgical intervention. There was no relationship of tumor growth to age, duration of symptoms, or initial tumor size. Another study also documented that there was no correlation between tumor growth and the patient's age, and that over a period of 8 months to over 4 years, 50% showed no change (Thedinger et al 1991). The true incidence of cessation of growth is unknown since these were selected patients, many of whom had stable symptoms.

RESULTS OF SUBOCCIPITAL OPERATION FOR UNILATERAL ACOUSTIC NEURINOMA

Summary

Good results using the suboccipital (posterior fossa) approach for removal of acoustic neurinomas have been reported by many surgeons (Koos & Perneczky 1985, Rhoton 1986, Symon et al 1989, Baldwin et al 1990, Harner et al 1990, Klemink et al 1990, Samii et al 1991, Ebersold et al 1992, Fisher et al 1992, Samii et al 1992). A personal series of 461 patients with unilateral acoustic neurinomas operated using a suboccipital approach in conjunction with an otologist has been reviewed. Some of these patients' results were included in previous publications (Ojemann 1978, Ojemann & Crowell 1978, Ojemann 1979, 1980, Ojemann et al 1984, Nadol et al 1987, Ojemann & Black 1988, Ojemann 1990, Ojemann & Martuza 1990, Nadol et al 1992, Ojemann 1992, 1993).

The functional results of the operation are reported as good, fair or poor. The term 'good' was used for those patients who were free of major neurologic deficit and returned to their pre-illness level of activity. Seventh and eighth nerve function was not considered. 'Fair' described patients who were functionally independent but were not able to return to their previous full activity because of a neurologic deficit or who had a significant preoperative neurologic deficit which, while improved, continued to cause disability. Many of these patients returned to work and are leading essentially normal lives. The term 'poor' described those patients who were dependent because of a major new or preoperative neurologic disability. Patients who died as a result of the surgery were considered an operative mortality. In the overall series, 99% were independent in their activities. All patients with tumors up to 1.0 cm had a good result, as did 96% in the 1.0–1.9 cm group and 93% in the 2.0–2.9 cm group. Even patients with large tumors had an 80% chance of having a good outcome. The most common reasons for the fair results were impaired balance, gait or coordination. Dysarthria or diplopia occurred in a few patients. In 6 of the 43 'fair' patients there was a significant preoperative deficit which improved but still limited their activity. In a small percentage of patients a significant headache problem lasted longer than expected and in 2 patients prevented full recovery, placing them into a 'fair' result category.

There were 2 poor results and 2 deaths (operative mortality 0.5%). The poor results were due to a stroke from a middle cerebral embolus and the effects from an intraoperative brainstem hemorrhage. One death was a 69-year-old woman who made a full recovery only to develop a chronic meningitis which progressed over several months with no diagnosis and no response to treatment. The other operative mortality followed a hemorrhage into the cerebellum and brainstem during the removal of a 4 cm tumor.

Extent of tumor removal and recurrence

The goal of the operation is total removal of the tumor. This goal must be tempered, however, by surgical judgement which considers the need to preserve and improve function as well as the long-term results. Personal experience indicates that there is a place for subtotal and radical subtotal removal of acoustic neurinomas because the recurrence rate has been low, and in larger tumors the incidence of postoperative neurologic problems has been low. This has been especially true in elderly patients.

Radical subtotal removal describes those procedures in which a small fragment of tumor is left, usually because it is densely adherent to the facial nerve or brainstem. The term subtotal removal is used to describe those patients in whom an extensive removal of the tumor is done but a portion of the rim of the capsule is left attached to the brainstem and cranial nerves.

The reasons for doing a radical subtotal or subtotal removal include adherence of the tumor to the facial nerve or brainstem, age (70 years or older), treatment of a tumor affecting a solitary hearing ear, and the patient's request. After carefully considering all the treatment options some patients now request a less than total removal to reduce the risk to the facial nerve and neurologic disability.

With the decision to do radical subtotal and subtotal removal the recurrence rate needs careful evaluation. Over the 15 years of this series none of the 43 patients with radical subtotal removals has had a recurrence requiring treatment. These patients have been followed for 1–14 years (average 5.4 years). In 7 of the patients their tumors could not be seen on follow-up scans.

In this series, 9 of 56 (16%) patients with subtotal removal had recurrence requiring treatment (average follow-up 5.2 years). Treatment of the recurrence included total removal of the tumor in 4, radical subtotal removal in 1, radiation therapy in 2, and another subtotal removal in 2. One patient with subtotal removal and the patient with radical subtotal removal have shown no further growth over 4 years. The other patient with a second subtotal removal has had an aggressive regrowth of her tumor and she is considering radiation therapy.

Recurrence can also occur following apparent total removal of the tumor. The known recurrence rate in this series was 0.8% (3 of 360). The first patient was 69 years old. She exhibited a large recurrence over 2 years and had another apparent total removal. Subsequent MRIs over 3 years have shown no recurrence. The second patient had recurrence diagnosed 5 years after surgery. She was given fractionated radiation therapy and, subsequently, there was no change over 4 years. The last patient had a small tumor seen on her first MRI scan 9 years after surgery. Repeat MRI over 2 years has shown no change.

Wazen et al (1985) found that in 9 of 13 patients with subtotal removal (age 66–81 years) there was no growth in the residual tumors in follow-up ranging from 6 months to 15 years. Klemink et al (1991) reported 20 patients who had incomplete removal of the tumor to reduce the operative risks. Two groups were defined — a subtotal group (resection of less than 95% of the tumor) and a near-total group (resection of 95% or more of the tumor). The subtotal group included mostly elderly patients (mean age 68.5) with large tumors. The near-total group consisted of young patients (mean age 45.8 years). The mean length of follow-up was 5 years, and only 1 patient showed regrowth. Lownie and Drake (1991) reported that 9 of 11 patients followed for 10–22 years after radical intracapsular removal did not have recurrence. The two recurrences were at 2 and 3 years postoperatively.

The low incidence of recurrence and the ability to treat recurrence effectively when it does occur suggest that we should consider a radical subtotal or subtotal removal in some patients with large tumors, particularly in the elderly.

Management of postoperative complications

Hematoma and cerebellar infarction

During the initial exposure particular attention is paid to occluding the arterial vessels in the muscles as they are encountered. Then, during the closure, the muscles are again carefully checked for bleeding. A significant epidural hematoma can result from hemorrhage from these blood vessels.

Prior to closure of the dura, the systemic blood pressure is often elevated to approximately 140 mmHg if it is not already at that level. Postoperatively the blood pressure is controlled, beginning in the operating room with an intravenous antihypertensive medication, and is monitored continuously for as long as necessary.

If the cerebellum is unusually full at the end of the operation and there has been good CSF drainage, cerebellar infarction or hematoma should be considered. In this situation a resection of the lateral 1–2 cm of cerebellum may need to be done.

If the patient does not recover promptly from anesthesia, or there is an unexpected significant neurologic deficit or a delayed neurologic deterioration, a CT scan is done immediately to look for cerebellar hematoma or infarction. Prompt removal of a significant hematoma or area of infarction can lead to a dramatic recovery.

In this series there were 5 patients with posterior fossa hemorrhage. One epidural and 1 cerebellar hemorrhage were diagnosed on CT scan when the patients were showing increasing neurologic symptoms. Reoperation was followed by a good recovery. Another patient with an epidural hematoma had the sudden onset of coma. Intubation and opening of the incision in the intensive care unit was followed by a good recovery. Two patients developed a hemorrhage into the cerebellum and brainstem during removal of a large tumor. One did not recover. The other has a severe neurologic disability.

There were 3 patients with cerebellar infarction diagnosed on CT. One had a mild disability and he responded to steroids and intermittent mannitol therapy. The other 2 were not doing as well as expected 12–18 hours after surgery, and resection of the lateral cerebellum was followed by recovery with mild residual deficits.

Cerebrospinal fluid leak

If a cerebrospinal fluid leak should develop, a lumbar drain is placed for 72 hours and this often resolves the problem. When the leak persists, a transmastoid repair using an adipose tissue graft is done.

The incidence of cerebrospinal leak in this series has been 8.5%. In 6% the leak subsided with the use of a lumbar drain for 72 hours. In the other 2.5% a transmastoid obliteration was done and there has not been any recurrence.

Hydrocephalus

In the postoperative period the patient may develop neurologic symptoms that suggest hydrocephalus, or a tense subgaleal fluid collection may be present. Ventricular size is followed by CT scan. Fortunately, persistent hydrocephalus is a rare complication. Most patients recover spontaneously, a few require a temporary lumbar drain, and only occasionally is a ventriculo-peritoneal shunt needed.

In this series 3 patients required a ventriculo-peritoneal shunt for hydrocephalus within a few weeks of the operation. In 2 patients a lumbar drain was used for 72 hours and there was no recurrence of the problem. One other patient developed a pseudomeningocele and a loculated cyst in the cerebellopontine angle and cerebellum causing brainstem compression 4 months after his operation. The symptoms were relieved with a cyst-to-peritoneal shunt.

Meningitis

When there is postoperative fever with headache or stiffness in the neck, the possibility of either bacterial or aseptic meningitis must be considered. CT with contrast is done to look for an area that might suggest a local infection. A lumbar puncture is then done and broad spectrum antibiotics started. Subsequent treatment is guided by the results of the cerebrospinal fluid examination and cultures. If the findings suggest an aseptic meningitis, steroids are used.

Bacterial meningitis occurred in 5 patients in this series (1.1%) including 2 with wound infection. All responded to antibiotic treatment.

A chronic granulomatous meningitis starting one week after operation developed in one patient. All cultures and biopsy were negative. She did not respond to several medical programs of treatment and died several months later.

Two patients had aseptic meningitis. They responded to steroid treatment.

Wound infection

When the infection is superficial and the organism is sensitive to antibiotics it may not be necessary to remove the bone flap. If the infection is extensive, debridement of the wound and removal of the bone flap will be necessary. There were 5 patients with wound infection (1.1%) and all made a good recovery.

Neurological

If there is any significant postoperative disability the patient is seen by physical and occupational therapists. Some patients note mild unsteadiness that clears over several days to several weeks. More severe impairment in walking and difficulties with coordination and dysarthria take longer to recover and there may be some permanent disability.

If there is transient difficulty in focusing the eyes or diplopia it usually clears over days to a few weeks.

Transient vertigo may occur, especially when vestibular function was still present preoperatively. The loss of function in the vestibular nerve is gradually accommodated by central compensation (Jackler & Pitts 1990).

The postoperative neurologic problems causing fair and poor results were discussed. In this series approximately 8% had persistent deficits (usually mild) in coordination or gait. Several patients had increased facial numbness which was not a problem except in the few patients who also had a facial paralysis. Recovery of the facial numbness was variable. Two patients had an isolated eleventh nerve palsy. Three patients noted impaired sensation in the opposite extremities. Difficulty swallowing due to impaired function in the ninth and tenth nerves should be carefully evaluated with a modified barium swallow and followed by a specialist in swallowing disorders. Often the patient can be given instructions that will facilitate swallowing and prevent aspiration. On rare occasion a gastrostomy is needed. Mild trouble swallowing was noted in a few patients but this improved.

Medical

Five patients had deep venous thrombus and 2 had pulmonary emboli. We now use alternating compression thigh-high air boots, beginning when the patient enters the operating room. There were no serious permanent postoperative cardiac problems. ECG changes and any cardiopulmonary symptoms were immediately evaluated by a cardiologist. When there were mild changes on the ECG these tended to resolve in the early postoperative period. One patient had an intraoperative ECG change which led to cessation of the operation and a subtotal removal was done, but the ECG changes resolved postoperatively.

Headache

Persistent headache remains a significant problem in a small percentage of the patients. MRI rarely shows a structural abnormality such as hydrocephalus. In most patients it seems to be a myofascial problem, in a few a neurinoma of the occipital nerve and in some cervical spine degenerative disease. The headache usually improves with time and responds to a program of physical therapy and, in a few patients, to local blocks.

Facial nerve function

The House-Brackmann facial nerve grading system is used to record facial nerve function (House & Brackmann 1985). Grade 1 is normal function, grade 2 is minimal weakness seen only on close inspection, grade 3 is moderate weakness with an obvious but not disfiguring difference, grade 4 is a moderate severe obvious weakness, grade 5 is severe weakness with barely perceptible motion, and grade 6 is complete paralysis. Good facial nerve function is represented by grades 1 and 2. Good facial nerve function at approximately one year or the last time the patient was seen prior to one year postoperatively in this series, in patients who had good preoperative function, was recorded as follows: intracanalicular, 24 patients, 96%, 0.0–0.9 cm, 35 patients, 100%, 1.0–1.9 cm, 121 patients, 96%; 2.0–2.9 cm, 95 patients, 77%, 3.0–3.9 cm, 102 patients, 60%; and over 4.0 cm, 71 patients, 58%.

The facial nerve is so involved with tumor in some patients that it cannot be saved. A decision has to be made whether to leave a small piece of tumor capsule with the nerve (radical subtotal removal) or to divide the nerve and approximate the ends or to do a nerve graft using the great auricular or sural nerve. In personal experience tumor has been left in patients who, in the preoperative discussion, requested this to reduce the risk of facial paralysis knowing that they might need further surgery in the future. The results of long-term follow-up on these patients are encouraging.

When the patient awakens from anesthesia with a facial paralysis or develops a delayed complete facial paralysis, the cornea must be protected. Initially the eyelids may almost close but as muscle tone is lost the opening becomes wider. Beginning immediately after surgery the eyelids are approximated with tape, and artificial tears are used regularly during the day and an ophthalmic ointment at night. The use of a tarsorrhaphy and/or a gold weight in the upper eyelid is essential to the maintenance of a healthy cornea and prevention of visual loss and incapacitating pain. Which oculoplastic procedure is best suited for a particular patient depends upon the patient's age, skin laxity and the presence or absence of corneal anesthesia. These procedures have the advantage of being reversible. When there is loss of corneal sensation, the cornea is at great risk and both a medial and lateral tarsorrhaphy may be necessary for protection. When facial paralysis does not recover, improved results may be obtained using a modification of the classic hypoglossal-facial anastomosis with partial division of the hypoglossal nerve and anastomosis of half of the nerve to the lower branch of the facial nerve combined with one of the eye procedures and a temporalis transposition flap.

Cochlear nerve function

In 1984 our group published the results of a series of 22 patients in whom an attempt was made to save hearing (Ojemann et al 1984). Subsequent publications have updated this series (Nadol et al 1987, Ojemann 1990, Ojemann & Martuza 1990, McKenna et al 1992, Nadol et al 1992, Ojemann 1992, 1993). In 1988 Gardner & Robertson reviewed the reports on hearing preservation published in the English literature from 1954–1986. Several publications have subsequently discussed hearing preservation (Neely 1984, Palva et al 1985, Tator 1985, Wazen et al 1985, Cohen et al 1986, Rosenberg et al 1987, Compton et al 1989, Harner et al 1990, Klemink et al 1990, Shelton et al 1990, Pensak et al 1991, Samii et al 1991, Slavit et al 1991, Cohen 1992, Ebersold et al 1992, Fisher et al 1992, Glasscock et al 1993). In spite of extensive clinical interest in this subject our experience is similar to that of Cohen (1992), who found that the results of attempts at hearing preservation have not improved over the past decade.

The question of what constitutes useful serviceable hearing has been discussed by several authors, with the most common criteria being a speech reception threshold (SRT) less than 50 dB with a speech discrimination score (SDS) of 50% or more (Silverstein et al 1986, Gardner & Robertson 1988, Whittaker & Luetje 1992). On the other hand, Whittaker & Luetje (1992) support the definition of SDS of 70% or better for serviceable hearing while we have used a SDS of 35% or better because for some patients this has been very useful.

Our results show that, for patients with at least a 35% speech discrimination score, the chance of saving useful hearing near the preoperative level is 60% when the tumor extends less than 5 mm into the posterior fossa, and 36% if it extends from 0.6–1.5 cm (Nadol et al 1992). Tumors 2 cm or larger have a low probability of hearing preservation even if there is excellent preoperative hearing. Preservation of hearing has been reported in a few patients following removal of large tumors, including one of my patients (Ojemann 1980).

In an attempt to help preserve hearing during removal of an acoustic neurinoma we have investigated the monitoring of auditory evoked potentials using a system developed by Dr Robert Levine (Levine et al 1978, Levine et al 1984, Ojemann et al 1984, Nadol et al 1987, Levine 1988, 1990, 1991, Nadol et al 1992). Electrocochleography (ECochG) monitors the status of the cochlea and the auditory nerve peripheral to the tumor, and brainstem auditory evoked potential (BAEP) monitors the neural activity central to the tumor. ECochG is a nearfield potential that provides rapid feedback of the compound actin potential of the auditory nerve (NI), probably generated near the cochlea, and cochlear microphonics potentials which are generated by the hair cells of the inner ear. BAEP is a farfield potential which has a slower feedback. In practice, only wave V, which is generated within the brainstem, is monitored because the other potentials are much smaller and often undetectable.

The short-latency ECochG potentials are the most useful for monitoring during operation because they are generally not affected by anesthesia, they are almost always detectable and have immediate feedback (Levine 1990). On the other hand, BAEPs, while useful, are undetectable in some patients even when there is useful hearing and it may take up to a minute or more to obtain satisfactory recordings because of the small amplitude of the potentials.

By monitoring both ECochG and BAEP, the entire portion of the auditory system at risk during an acoustic neurinoma operation can be monitored. The presence or absence of N1 indicates the integrity of the auditory nerve peripheral to the tumor, wave V is an indication of auditory nerve activity central to the tumor, and the cochlear microphonics indicate the status of the cochlea which is at risk from interruption of blood supply or from damage to other structures essential for cochlear function such as the posterior semicircular canals.

When the status of N1 and wave V at the end of the operation are correlated with the hearing outcome it is found that if N1 and wave V are lost there is no hearing (Levine 1990). In our series, if wave V and N1 were present, all but one patient had useful hearing. If N1 was present and wave V lost or never detected, the results were not predictable. A fundamental limitation of the monitoring is related to how the individual nerve fibers react to the injury. They may stop conducting completely, there may be too few fibers left to generate a gross potential that can be detected, or they may conduct a modified or desynchronized impulse.

The hope is that monitoring will give an indication of early hearing compromise that is reversible and allow the surgeon to alter the dissection (Ojemann et al 1984, Ojemann & Martuza 1990, Levine 1991). This has likely been the case in some patients in whom a change occurred which recovered when the dissection was stopped or altered. Monitoring has not made a definite difference in the outcome when there has been abrupt loss of function without warning which does not recover, presumably due to interruption of vascular supply, when gradual loss of function occurs, and when there is no change in any wave form during the operation. We believe, however, that monitoring has helped us to understand better the problems in preserving hearing function. Slavit et al (1991) compared two matched series of patients with and without auditory monitoring and concluded that there is a benefit from intraoperative monitoring, but Compton et al (1989) found it of little help.

The long-term results of hearing preservation have been evaluated. In the report of Shelton et al (1990), 14 of 25 patients (56%) who underwent removal of an acoustic neurinoma by the middle fossa approach suffered a significant loss of hearing in the operated ear over a mean follow-up of 8 years (range 3–20 years). On the other hand, Palva et al (1985) reported a significant loss in only 2 of 13 patients during the first 4 years following suboccipital removal. Rosenberg et al (1987) did not observe a significant decline in 9 patients followed for 1.3–11 years. McKenna et al (1992), reporting our series of 18 patients with follow-up ranging from 3.4–10.4 years (mean 5.4 years), found 4 patients (22%) with a significant decline in hearing. Changes did not correlate with tumor size, preoperative hearing, intraoperative changes in hearing, the interval between initial symptoms and surgery, sex or age.

Concern about recurrence following removal of an acoustic neurinoma with preservation of the cochlear nerve has been discussed in the literature. Thedinger et al (1991) emphasize that inadequate exposure of the lateral end of the internal auditory canal may be associated with leaving a remnant of tumor. Neely (1984) reported that in patients where all of the tumor appeared to have been removed, residual tumor was found in the cochlear nerve and he concluded that, 'histologic data suggests that complete tumor removal in attempts to preserve hearing may be beyond our surgical capabilities'. Samii et al (1991), however, reported no recurrence in 16 patients who had removal of intracanalicular acoustic neurinomas with anatomic preservation of the cochlear and facial nerves who had been followed 1–8 years. In our series, an attempt to preserve hearing was made in 119 patients with tumors less than 2.0 cm. Follow-up CT and MRI have shown no definite recurrence in those in whom the cochlear nerve was kept intact. A few patients have an area of gadolinium enhancement in the internal auditory canal on postoperative MRI. Whether this represents residual tumor or postoperative scar is unknown but follow-up scans have remained unchanged.

Tinnitus may persist in the ear following removal of an acoustic neurinoma. There does not seem to be any difference in the incidence of tinnitus between those patients who had the cochlear nerve preserved to save hearing and those in whom the cochlear nerve was divided to remove the tumor (Goel et al 1992).

Management of tumor in solitary hearing ear with unilateral acoustic neurinoma

The largest experience with acoustic neurinomas involving the solitary hearing ear is in patients with bilateral acoustic neurinomas. Their management is discussed on page 638. This problem will, however, occasionally be encountered in patients with a unilateral tumor when the opposite ear is deaf because of previous infection or trauma. The following guidelines for treatment of these patients are suggested:

1. If hearing is stable, the patient is carefully followed with audiograms and MRI scans.
2. If the tumor is under 1.5 cm and there is progressive hearing loss, the chances of hearing preservation based on the size of the tumor, the patient's age and audiogram findings (see section on cochlear nerve function) are discussed with the patient and a decision is made between total and subtotal removal.
3. If the tumor is over 1.5 cm and there is progressive hearing loss we have recommended an internal auditory canal decompression and subtotal removal of the tumor utilizing intraoperative monitoring.

In this series there were two patients. One patient with a 1.5 cm tumor did not want to risk loss of hearing and had a decompression with subtotal removal. The hearing loss has stabilized. The other patient has been previously reported (Ojemann 1980). The patient had a large tumor where total removal was required to relieve brainstem compression and she did enjoy retention of preoperative hearing.

Pensak et al (1991) reviewed this problem and reported two patients in whom unilateral acoustic neuromas, 1.0 cm and 2.0 cm in the solitary hearing ear, were treated with complete removal and retention of usable hearing.

Management of elderly patients (70 years and older)

Patients 70 years of age and older were considered for surgery if they had a progressive or disabling neurologic deficit or symptoms. In 22 of 29 patients in this series there was a good result, 6 had a fair result, and only 1 had a poor result. Total removal was done in 5 — all of whom had tumors 2.5 cm or less. A radical subtotal removal was done in 5, and 19 had a subtotal removal. No patient has had to stay in a nursing home and even the patients with fair results are able to care for themselves and do many activities. Only 2 required a second operation for recurrence.

House et al (1987) reported a low morbidity and mortality in elderly patients. Samii et al (1992) observed that in the majority of their elderly patients (65 years and older) there was minimal postoperative morbidity even with complete removal of the tumor.

BILATERAL ACOUSTIC NEURINOMA

Neurofibromatosis is an autosomal dominant genetic disorder that occurs as two distinct forms caused by different genes (Martuza & Rouleau 1990): von Recklinghausen's neurofibromatosis (NF-1), and bilateral acoustic neurofibromatosis (NF-2). The criteria for the diagnosis of NF-2 are: evidence on imaging of bilateral tumors consistent with acoustic neurinoma, or a first-degree relative with NF-2 and a unilateral acoustic neurinoma or multiple intracranial tumors. Some patients with bilateral acoustic neurinoma may also have intracranial and spinal tumors and central nervous system malformations. Occasionally, the disorder may occur as a spontaneous mutation with no family history. Deletions in the long arm of chromosome 22 that may involve tumor suppressor genes are found in patients with both unilateral and bilateral vestibular schwannomas but in NF-2 the deletion is in the germ line (Sobel 1993).

Some patients do not meet these criteria, but NF-2 must be suspected in any patient below the age of 30 presenting with an acoustic neurinoma, any young patient with a Schwann cell tumor, and patients with multiple meningiomas. We have reviewed this disorder in previous publications (Martuza & Ojemann 1982, Martuza & Rouleau 1990, Ojemann & Martuza 1990).

Diagnosis

The skin stigmata in patients with bilateral acoustic neurofibromatosis are easily overlooked. Café-au-lait spots, axillary freckles, and multiple typical skin neurofibromas (features of von Recklinghausen's neurofibromatosis) are usually minimal or absent. In contrast, slightly raised skin plaques, often with increased or more prominent hair, are typical of this disorder. Lisch nodules of the iris are not seen in bilateral acoustic neurofibromatosis, but lens opacities at an early age are relatively common. In patients suspected of having NF-2 the skin and eye lesion should be sought, a brainstem auditory evoked response should be performed, and MRI with gadolinium enhancement should be done as indicated.

Early diagnosis provides the best opportunity for treatment choices to be instituted with the lowest morbidity. In contrast to a patient with a unilateral acoustic neurinoma, however, the patient with bilateral acoustic neurinomas provides a set of much more difficult treatment decisions.

Management

Patients with neurofibromatosis often have multiple tumors, and removal of all lesions is not warranted; therefore, the treatment goals must be specified in relation to each lesion and should be discussed with the patient and family. In general, preservation of brainstem and spinal cord function is the first priority, and preserving facial function and hearing for as long as possible are the next goals.

The operation for a bilateral acoustic tumor occurring in patients with little or no expression of neurofibromatosis is similar to that already described for the unilateral tumor. In these patients the bilateral tumor is usually well circumscribed and displaces the facial and often the cochlear nerves. In contrast, the bilateral acoustic neurinoma associated with expansive expression of neurofibromatosis is often multilobulated, suggesting that it may be formed from multiple foci of tumorigenic cells. Between the lobules are poorly formed planes of fibrous tissue and, in some cases, nerves and blood vessels (Ojemann & Martuza 1990). Therefore, once the tumor is exposed, frequent facial nerve stimulation is performed. If multiple lobules are noted, each is internally decompressed separately. The intervening planes are stimulated, looking for the facial nerve. Constant facial nerve monitoring is especially useful in these tumors because this nerve can be trapped within the tumor capsule and can be damaged even during the stage of internal decompression. Constant auditory evoked potential monitoring is done when an attempt is being made to preserve hearing.

Complete removal of an acoustic neurinoma is the recommended procedure whenever possible; however, exploration may disclose multiple tumors involving both the facial and the vestibulocochlear nerves. Complete removal should be attempted if there is already loss of hearing in the involved ear, but the multilobular nature of these lesions may make complete removal difficult without sacrificing the facial or other cranial nerves. At operation, other tumors may be present in the trigeminal, glossopharyngeal, or vagus nerves.

When the patient has bilateral acoustic neurinomas and bilateral useful hearing, complete removal should be considered for a small tumor on one side with an attempt to save hearing if the audiogram shows progressive hearing loss or the radiographic studies show an enlarging tumor. This group of patients is at risk of losing hearing without operation. Thus, although there is the potential for loss of hearing as a result of the operation, the risk is worth taking because the procedure may be the last chance to save hearing in this ear.

In contrast, for patients who show progressive hearing loss in their solitary hearing ear, especially with larger tumors when complete removal would likely be associated with deafness, we have used auditory evoked response monitoring, internal auditory canal decompression, and intracapsular tumor removal to try and preserve hearing for as long as possible. It has been possible to stabilize the hearing in about 50% of these patients. Such patients know that they may need an additional operation in the future, but preservation of hearing for a few years or more is often worthwhile.

Patients whose symptoms are stable and in whom sequential radiographic studies show no increase in tumor size are carefully observed. This decision is made because of the inability to improve their neurologic state and the inability to predict which tumor (if any) will enlarge with time. Careful clinical, audiologic, and radiologic follow-up is essential.

Other lesions

Multiple Schwann cell tumors on peripheral nerves, cranial nerves, and spinal roots are common in bilateral acoustic neurofibromatosis, as are cranial and spinal meningiomas and astrocytomas. In all patients with bilateral acoustic neurofibromatosis, we do cranial and spinal MRI. Asymptomatic spinal neurofibromas are left untreated no matter what the size. Operation is indicated when symptoms develop or if there is enlargement on follow-up image studies. The same rules apply to meningiomas, which are often multiple and asymptomatic in these patients. Deep intrinsic cerebral lesions that are asymptomatic and stable are often managed the same way; however, if there is evidence of increase in size, stereotactic biopsy guided by CT is performed to obtain a tissue diagnosis.

Family screening and genetic counseling

The patient and the family are referred to an appropriate physician for adequate counseling, and screening tests are recommended as indicated. A woman with bilateral acoustic neurofibromatosis has a 50% risk that her children will acquire this disorder, as well as the risk that pregnancy could cause tumor enlargement.

Rehabilitation

Because of the multiple cranial, spinal and peripheral tumors in bilateral acoustic neurofibromatosis, patients may exhibit progressive neurologic deficits at a relatively young age. It is important that an audiologist and a speech therapist are involved as early as possible so that sign language or lip-reading education can start prior to total hearing loss. Physical and occupational therapy are recommended as needed. Finally, there is often a great psychological burden on the patient and the family, and a psychiatrist, psychologist, nurse, social worker and national support groups conversant with these multiple problems are of great benefit to patients with bilateral acoustic neurofibromatosis and their families.

REFERENCES

Baldwin D L, King T T, Morrison A W 1990 Hearing conservation in acoustic neuroma surgery via the posterior fossa. Journal of Laryngology and Otology 104: 463–467

Baldwin D, King T T, Chevetton E, Morrison A W 1991 Bilateral cerebellopontine angle tumors in neurofibromatosis type 2. Journal of Neurosurgery 74: 910–915

Barrs D M, Brackmann D E, Olson J E, House W F 1985 Changing concepts of acoustic neuroma diagnosis. Archives of Otolaryngology 111: 17–21

Bederson J B, von Ammon K, Wichmann W W, Yasargil G 1991 Conservative treatment of patients with acoustic neuroma. Neurosurgery 28: 646–651

Brackmann D E 1979 Middle cranial fossa approach. In: House W F, Luetje C M (eds) Acoustic tumors, vol I. University Park Press, Baltimore, p 15–41

Brackmann D E, Hitselberger W E, Beneke J E, House W F 1985 Acoustic neurinomas: Middle fossa and translabyrinthine removal. In: Rand R W (ed) Microneurosurgery. C V Mosby, St Louis, p 311–334

Cohen N L 1992 Retrosigmoid approach for acoustic tumor removal. Otolaryngology Clinics of North America 25: 295–310

Cohen N L, Berg H, Hammerschlag P, Ransohoff J 1986 Acoustic neuroma surgery: An eclectic approach with emphasis on preservation of hearing. Annals of Otology Rhinology and Laryngology 93: 21–27

Compton J S, Bordi L T, Chesseman A D et al 1989 The small acoustic neuroma; a chance to preserve hearing. Acta Neurochirurgica (Wien) 98: 115–117

Cushing H 1917 Tumors of the nervus acusticus and the syndrome of the cerebellopontine angle. W B Saunders, Philadelphia

Dandy W F 1925 An operation for total removal of cerebellopontine (acoustic) tumors. Surgery, Gynecology, Obstetrics 41: 139–148

Darrouzet V, Maire J P, Flocquet A et al 1990 Irradiation of neurinoma. Why: How? First results. Annals of Laryngology Otology and Rhinology (Bard) 111: 211–215

Ebersold M J, Harner S G, Beatty C W et al 1992 Current results of retrosigmoid approach to acoustic neurinoma. Journal of Neurosurgery 76: 901–909

Eldridge R, Parry D 1992 Summary: Vestibular schwannoma (Acoustic Neuroma) Consensus Development Conference. Neurosurgery 30: 962–964

Fisher G, Fisher C, Remond J 1992 Hearing preservation in acoustic neuroma surgery. Journal of Neurosurgery 76: 910–917

Gardner G, Robertson J H 1988 Hearing preservation in unilateral acoustic neuroma surgery. Annals of Otology Rhinology and Laryngology 97: 55–66

Glasscock M E III, Hays J W, Monor L B et al 1993 Preservation of hearing in surgery for acoustic neuromas. Journal of Neurosurgery 78: 864–870

Goel A, Sekhar L N, Langheinrich W et al 1992 Late course of preserved hearing and tinnitus after acoustic neurilemoma surgery. Journal of Neurosurgery 77: 685–689

Gruskin P, Carberry J N 1979 Pathology of acoustic tumors. In: House W F, Luetje C M (eds) Acoustic tumors, vol I. University Park Press, Baltimore, p 85–148

Harner S G, Ebersold M J 1985 Management of acoustic neuroma 1978–1983. Journal of Neurosurgery 63: 175–179

Harner S G, Beatty C W, Ebersold M J 1990 Retrosigmoid removal of acoustic neuroma. Experience 1978–1988. Otolaryngology Head And Neck Surgery 103: 40–45

House J W, Brackmann D E 1985 Facial nerve grading system. Otolaryngology Head and Neck Surgery 93: 184–193

House J W, Nissen R L, Hitselberger W E 1987 Acoustic tumor management in senior citizens. Laryngoscope 97: 129–130

House W F 1979a A history of acoustic tumor surgery 1900–1917, the Cushing era. In: House W F, Luetje C M (eds) Acoustic tumors, vol I. University Park Press, Baltimore, p 9–23

House W F 1979b A history of acoustic tumor surgery 1917–1961, the Dandy era. In: House W F, Luetje C M (eds) Acoustic tumors, vol I. University Park Press, Baltimore, p 25–32

House W F 1979c Translabyrinthine approach. In: House W F, Luetje C M (eds) Acoustic tumors, vol II. University Park Press, Baltimore, p 43–87

House W F, Hitselberger W E 1985 The neuro-otologist's view of the surgical management of acoustic neuromas. Clinical Neurosurgery 2: 214–222

Jackler R K, Pitts L H 1990 Acoustic neuroma. Neurosurgery Clinics of North America 1: 199–223

Jellinek D A, Tan L C, Symon L 1991 The import of continuous electrophysiological monitoring on preservation of the facial nerve during acoustic neuroma surgery. British Journal of Neurosurgery 5: 19–24

Johnson E W 1979 Results of auditory tests in acoustic tumor patients. In: House W F, Luetje C M (eds) Acoustic tumors, vol I. University Park Press, Baltimore, p 209–227

Klemink J L, LaRouare M J, Kileny P R et al 1990 Hearing preservation following suboccipital removal of acoustic neuromas. Laryngoscope 100: 597–601

Klemink J L, Langman A W, Niparko J K, Graham M D 1991 Operative management of acoustic neuromas: The priority of neurologic function over complete resection. Otolaryngology Head and Neck Surgery 104: 96–99

Koos W T, Perneczky A 1985 Suboccipital approach to acoustic neurinomas with emphasis on preservation of facial nerve and cochlear nerve function. In: Rand R W (ed) Microneurosurgery. C V Mosby, St Louis, p 335–365

Leksell L 1971 A note on the treatment of acoustic tumors. Acta Chirurgica Scandinavica 137: 763–765

Levine R A 1988 Surgical monitoring applications of the brainstem auditory evoked response and electrocochleography. In: Owen J, Donohoe C (eds) Clinical atlas of auditory evoked potentials. Grune & Stratton, New York, p 103–106

Levine R A 1990 Short-latency auditory evoked potentials: Intraoperative applications. International Anesthesiology Clinics 28: 147–153

Levine R A 1991 Monitoring auditory evoked potentials during cerebellopontine angle tumor surgery: Relative value of electrocochleography, brainstem auditory evoked potentials, and cerebellopontine angle recordings. In: Schramm J, Moelle A N (eds) Intraoperative neurophysiologic monitoring. Springer-Verlag, Berlin, p 193–204

Levine R A, Montgomery W W, Ojemann R G, Springer M F B 1978 Evoked potential detection of hearing loss during acoustic neuroma surgery. Neurology 28: 339

Levine R A, Ojemann R G, Montgomery W M, McGaffigan P M 1984 Monitoring auditory evoked potentials during acoustic neuroma surgery: Insights into the mechanism of the hearing loss. Annals of Otology Rhinology and Laryngology 93: 116–123

Linskey M E, Lunsford L D, Flickinger J C, Kondziolka D 1992 Stereotactic radiosurgery for acoustic neuroma. Neurosurgical Clinics of North America 3: 191–205

Lownie S P, Drake C G 1991 Radical intracapsular removal of acoustic neuroma: Long term follow-up review of 11 patients. Journal of Neurosurgery 74: 422–425

McKenna M J, Halpin C, Ojemann R G et al 1992 Long-term hearing results in patients after surgical removal of acoustic tumors with hearing preservation. The American Journal of Otology 13: 134–136

Martuza R L, Ojemann R G 1982 Bilateral acoustic neuromas. Clinical aspects, pathogenesis and treatment. Neurosurgery 10: 1–12

Martuza R L, Rouleau G 1990 Genetic aspects of neurosurgical problems. In: Youmans J R (ed) Neurological surgery, 3rd edn. W B Saunders, Philadelphia, p 1061–1080

Martuza R L, Parker S W, Nadol J B Jr et al 1985 Diagnosis of cerebellopontine angle tumors. Clinical Neurosurgery 32: 177–213

Nadol J B Jr, Levine R A, Ojemann R G et al 1987 Preservation of hearing in surgical removal of acoustic neuromas of the internal auditory canal and cerebellar pontine angle. Laryngoscope 97: 1287–1294

Nadol J B Jr, Chiong C M, Ojemann R G et al 1992 Preservation of hearing and facial nerve function in resection of acoustic neuroma. Laryngoscope 102: 1153–1158

Nedzelski J M, Canter R J, Kassel E E et al 1986 Is no treatment good treatment in the management of acoustic neuromas in the elderly? Laryngoscope 96: 825–829

Neely J G 1984 Is it possible to totally resect an acoustic tumor and conserve hearing? Otolaryngology Head and Neck Surgery 92: 162–167

Norén G, Arndt J, Hindmarsh T 1983 Stereotactic radiosurgery in cases of acoustic neurinoma: Further experiences. Neurosurgery 13: 12–22

Ojemann R G 1978 Microsurgical suboccipital approach to cerebellopontine angle tumors. Clinical Neurosurgery 25: 461–479

Ojemann R G 1979 Acoustic neuroma. Contemporary Neurosurgery 20: 1–6

Ojemann R G 1980 Comments on Fischer G, Costantini J L, Mercier P. Improvement of hearing after microsurgical removal of acoustic neuroma. Neurosurgery 7: 158–159

Ojemann R G 1990 Strategies to preserve hearing during resection of acoustic neuroma. In: Wilkins R H, Rengachary S S (eds) Neurosurgery update I. McGraw-Hill, New York, p 424–427

Ojemann R G 1992 Suboccipital approach to acoustic neuromas. In: Wilson C B (ed) Neurosurgical procedures: personal approaches to classic techniques. Williams & Wilkins, Baltimore, p 78–87

Ojemann R G 1993 Management of acoustic neuroma (vestibular schwannoma). Clinical Neurosurgery 40: 498–535

Ojemann R G, Black P McL 1988 Difficult decisions in managing patients with benign brain tumors. Clinical Neurosurgery 35: 254–284

Ojemann R G, Crowell R M 1978 Acoustic neuromas treated by microsurgical suboccipital operations. In: Progress in neurological surgery, vol 9. Karger, Basel, Switzerland, p 334–373

Ojemann R G, Martuza R L 1990 Acoustic neuroma. In: Youmans J R (ed) Neurological surgery, 3rd edn. W B Saunders, Philadelphia, p 3316–3350

Ojemann R G, Montgomery W W, Weiss A D 1972 Evaluation and surgical treatment of acoustic neuroma. New England Journal of Medicine 287: 895–899

Ojemann R G, Levine R A, Montgomery W M, McGraffigan P 1984 Use of intraoperative auditory evoked potentials to preserve hearing in unilateral acoustic neuroma removal. Journal of Neurosurgery 61: 938–948

Palva T, Troupp H, Jauhiainene T 1985 Hearing preservation in acoustic neurinoma surgery. Acta Otolaryngology (Stockholm) 99: 1–7

Pensak M L, Tew J M Jr, Keith R W, Van Loveren H R 1991 Management of the acoustic neuroma in an only hearing ear. Skull Base Surgery 1: 93–96

Rhoton A L Jr 1986 Microsurgical anatomy of the brain stem surface facing an acoustic neuroma. Surgical Neurology 25: 326–339

Rosenberg R A, Cohen N L, Ransohoff J 1987 Long term hearing preservation after acoustic neuroma surgery. Otolaryngology Head and Neck Surgery 97: 270–274

Russell D S, Rubinstein L J 1959 Pathology of tumors of the nervous system. Edward Arnold, London, p 236–239

Samii M, Matthies C, Tatagiba M 1991 Intracanalicular acoustic neurinomas. Neurosurgery 28: 189–199

Samii M, Tatagiba M, Matthies C 1992 Acoustic neurinoma in the elderly: Factors predictive of postoperative outcome. Neurosurgery 31: 615–620

Sheehy J L 1979 Neuro-otologic evaluation. In: House W F, Luetje C M (eds) Acoustic tumors, vol I. University Park Press, Baltimore, p 199–208

Shelton C, Hitselberger W E, House W F, Brackmann D E 1990 Hearing preservation after acoustic tumor removal: Long term results. Laryngoscope 100: 115–119

Silverstein H, McDaniel A, Norrell H, Haberkamp T 1986 Hearing preservation after acoustic neuroma surgery with intraoperative direct eighth cranial nerve monitoring: A classification of results. Otolaryngology Head and Neck Surgery 95: 285–291

Slavit D H, Harner S C, Harper C M Jr, Beatty C W 1991 Auditory monitoring during acoustic neuroma removal. Archives Otolaryngology Head and Neck Surgery 117: 1153–1157

Sobel R A 1993 Vestibular (acoustic) schwannomas: Histologic features in neurofibromatosis 2 and in unilateral cases. Journal of Neuropathology and Experimental Neurology 52: 106–113

Symon L, Bordi L T, Comptor J J et al 1989 Acoustic neurinoma. A review of 392 cases. British Journal of Neurosurgery 3: 343–347

Tatagiba M, Samii M, Matthies C et al 1992 The significance for postoperative hearing of preserving the labyrinth in acoustic neurinoma surgery. Journal of Neurosurgery 77: 677–684

Tator C H K 1985 Acoustic neuromas: Management of 204 cases. Canadian Journal of Neurologic Science 12: 353–357

Tew J M, Scodary D J 1993 Infratentorial procedures — neoplastic disorders — surgical positioning. In: Apuzzo M L J (ed) Brain surgery complication avoidance and management. Churchill Livingstone, New York, p 1609–1620

Thedinger B S, Whittaker C K, Luetje C M 1991 Recurrent acoustic tumor after a suboccipital removal. Neurosurgery 29: 681–687

Valvassori G E, Shannon M 1991 Natural history of acoustic neuroma. Skull Base Surgery 1: 165–167

Wallner K E, Sheline G E, Pitts L H et al 1987 Efficacy of irradiation for incompletely excised acoustic neurilemomas. Journal of Neurosurgery 67: 858–863

Wazen J, Silverstein H, Norrell H, Besse B 1985 Preoperative and postoperative growth rate in acoustic neuromas documented with CT scanning. Otolaryngology Head and Neck Surgery 93: 151–155

Whittaker C K, Luetje C M 1992 Vestibular schwannomas. Journal of Neurosurgery 76: 897–900

33. Other schwannomas of cranial nerves

Richard Strauss   Kalmon D. Post

INTRODUCTION

Schwannomas are benign neoplasms of the peripheral nerve sheath. They are variously referred to in the literature as 'neuromas', 'neurinomas' (Verocay 1910) and 'neurilemmomas' (Stout 1935). As the name implies, the cell of origin is the Schwann cell, which normally functions to insulate the peripheral axon through its production of myelin. Schwannomas are to be distinguished from traumatic neuromas, which involve a non-neoplastic proliferation of Schwann cells at the site of a partial or complete nerve transection (Burger et al 1991). They are also distinct from neurofibromas, which are infiltrative peripheral nerve sheath tumors whose cell of origin is still not confirmed (Erlandson & Woodruff 1982).

As neoplasms of the peripheral nerve sheath, schwannomas may arise intracranially, intraspinally, or in the periphery. Sensory roots are more often affected than motor or autonomic, and there is a female predilection (Burger et al 1991). They represent approximately 5–10% of all intracranial tumors (Zulch 1962, Rubinstein 1972) and occur predominantly in the third to sixth decades of life (DasGupta et al 1969). The intracranial tumors are usually found along the fascicles of a cranial nerve, but there are several reports of tumors arising within the brain parenchyma or the ventricles (Gibson et al 1966, New 1972, Ghatak et al 1975, Van Rensberg et al 1975, Prakash et al 1980). The vestibular division of the eighth cranial nerve represents by far the most common site for an intracranial schwannoma, followed only distantly by the trigeminal (Pool & Pava 1970). Most are solitary neoplasms and arise de novo. There is, however, a well-described association with type 2 or 'central' neurofibromatosis. In this phakomatosis of autosomal dominant inheritance, there is a predilection for the development of cranial and spinal schwannomas, as well as glial tumors and meningiomas (Rubinstein 1972). The presence of bilateral acoustic schwannomas is considered pathognomonic (Kanter et al 1980). In addition to those arising de novo and in association with neurofibromatosis, there are reports of schwannomas arising after radiation treatment (Salvati et al 1992).

Grossly, schwannomas are typically solitary, discrete, well-encapsulated tumors. They tend to displace the parent nerve eccentrically, as opposed to neurofibromas which cause a fusiform enlargement of the nerve (Fig. 33.1A). They have a smooth, lobulated appearance and vary in color from tan to yellow, although case reports exist of so-called 'melanotic' intracranial schwannomas (Dastur et al 1967).

Microscopically, schwannomas are classically described as being composed of Antoni A and B regions (Fig. 33.1B). The Antoni A regions are well-ordered arrays of elongated, spindle-shaped cells with hyperchromatic, cigar-shaped nuclei and eosinophilic cytoplasm. The nuclei may line up in palisades with intervening nuclear-free zones; these structures are called Verocay bodies (Fig. 33.1C). The Antoni B regions are composed of poorly organized large vacuolated cells, often with pyknotic or irregular nuclei. Cystic changes, as well as hyalinization of blood vessel walls with thrombosis and perivascular hemosiderin deposition, are common. The Antoni B areas may represent degenerative changes. Although the classic histology of these tumors is common in the intraspinal and peripheral tumors, intracranial schwannomas typically lack the prominent palisades and are composed of tissue of intermediate organization.

Attention has been focused on two microscopic variants. The 'ancient' schwannoma is usually a large tumor of longstanding duration which has undergone extensive degenerative changes (Burger et al 1991). Bizarre and pleomorphic nuclei may be common, but do not indicate malignant transformation. No case of an 'ancient' intracranial schwannoma exists in the literature. The 'cellular' schwannoma demonstrates a striking predominance of Antoni A tissue without the nuclear palisading and Verocay bodies (Woodruff et al 1981). Mitoses may be common, but again do not indicate malignancy. Cellular schwannomas have been described on the facial and trigeminal nerves (White et al 1990).

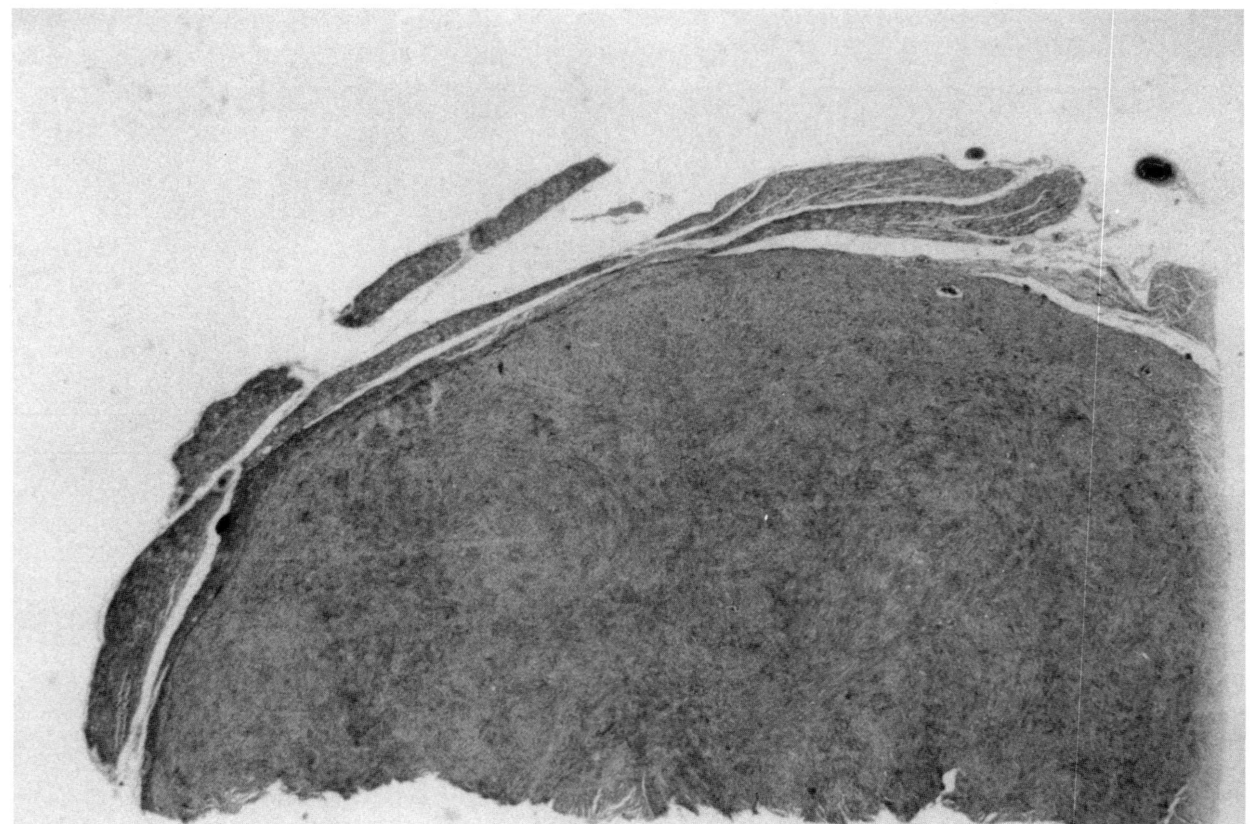

A

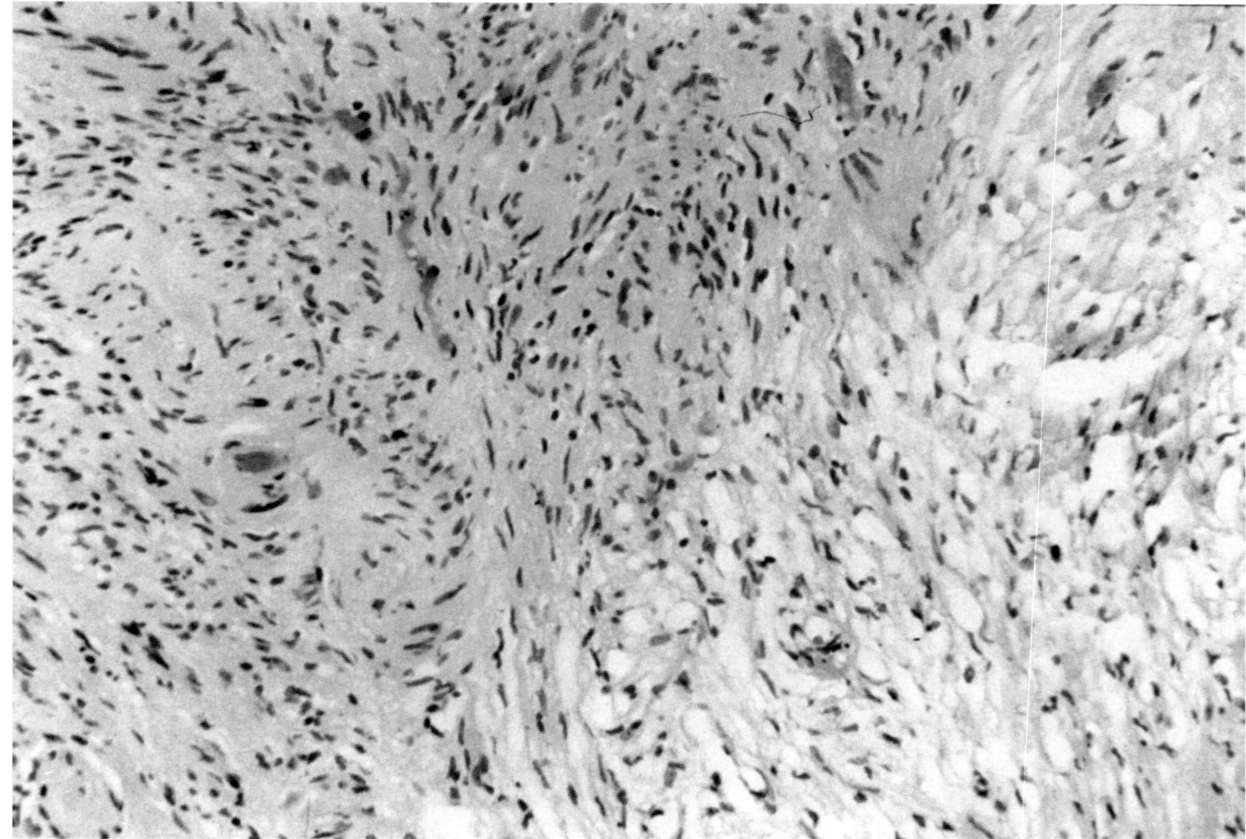

B

Fig. 33.1A & B

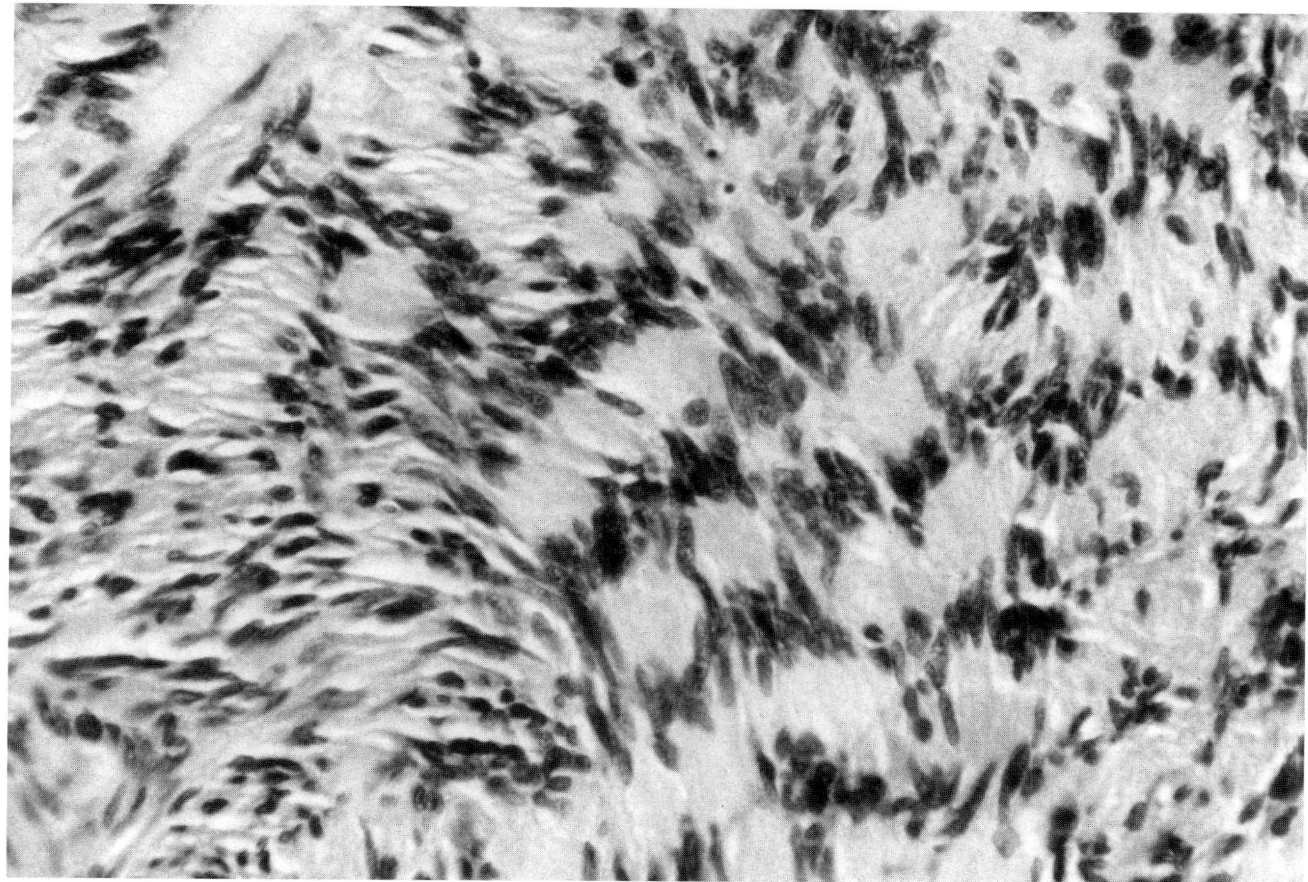

Fig. 33.1 **A.** Low power photomicrograph demonstrates schwannoma compressing peripheral nerve. This contrasts with neurofibroma, which infiltrates nerve fascicles (not shown). (Luxol fast blue stain for myelin). **B.** Photomicrograph demonstrating histology appearance of schwannoma with Antoni A (left) and Antoni B (right) regions. (H&E). **C.** High power photomicrograph demonstrating Verocay bodies, with palisading nuclei and central regions of Schwann cell cytoplasm. (H&E). All photomicrographs compliments of Dr S Morgello.

The characteristic ultrastructure is that of long, complexly entangled cell processes enveloping the intervening stroma in a manner analogous to the normal axon Schwann cell-axon sheathing arrangement (pseudomesaxon). This is in contrast to the neurofibroma, in which true axons are found within the tumor surrounded by Schwann cell processes (mesaxons) (Erlandsson & Woodruff 1982). A well-defined continuous basement membrane separates cell processes from surrounding stroma. Cell–cell junctions and pinocytotic vesicles are rare. These features serve to distinguish the schwannian origin of these tumors from the other cellular components of the peripheral nerve sheath, the perineurial cell and the fibroblast.

Immunohistochemically, the tumors are usually distinctly positive for the S-100 protein (Johnson et al 1988). They may also be positive for myelin-associated glycoprotein (Leu-7) and glial fibrillary acidic protein (GFAP) (Kawahara et al 1988). They are usually negative for myelin basic protein.

Malignant transformation of a schwannoma is an exceedingly rare event. Nine such cases are documented in the literature, and only five of these meet the strict criteria of demonstrating unequivocal malignancy within a typical benign schwannoma (Carstens & Schrodt 1969, Woodruff et al 1981, Hanada et al 1982, Robey et al 1987, McLean et al 1990). One case is that of a gross totally resected acoustic schwannoma which spontaneously recurred 11 months later as a malignant nerve sheath tumor (McLean et al 1990). In general, malignant peripheral nerve sheath tumors arise de novo or in a pre-existing neurofibroma, especially in conjunction with von Recklinghausen's disease. The schwannian origin of these tumors is in doubt, and the term 'malignant schwannoma' should be avoided (Erlandsson & Woodruff 1982).

The clinical and radiographic features of an intracranial schwannoma will vary somewhat according to the parent nerve involved. In general, these tumors present as mass lesions producing neurologic dysfunction by distorting the parent nerve and compressing surrounding cranial nerves, brainstem and cerebellum. Their presence can sometimes be detected on plain film due to widening of bony foramina and scalloping or erosion of bone at the skull base (Fig. 33.2A). As extra-axial masses within the subdural

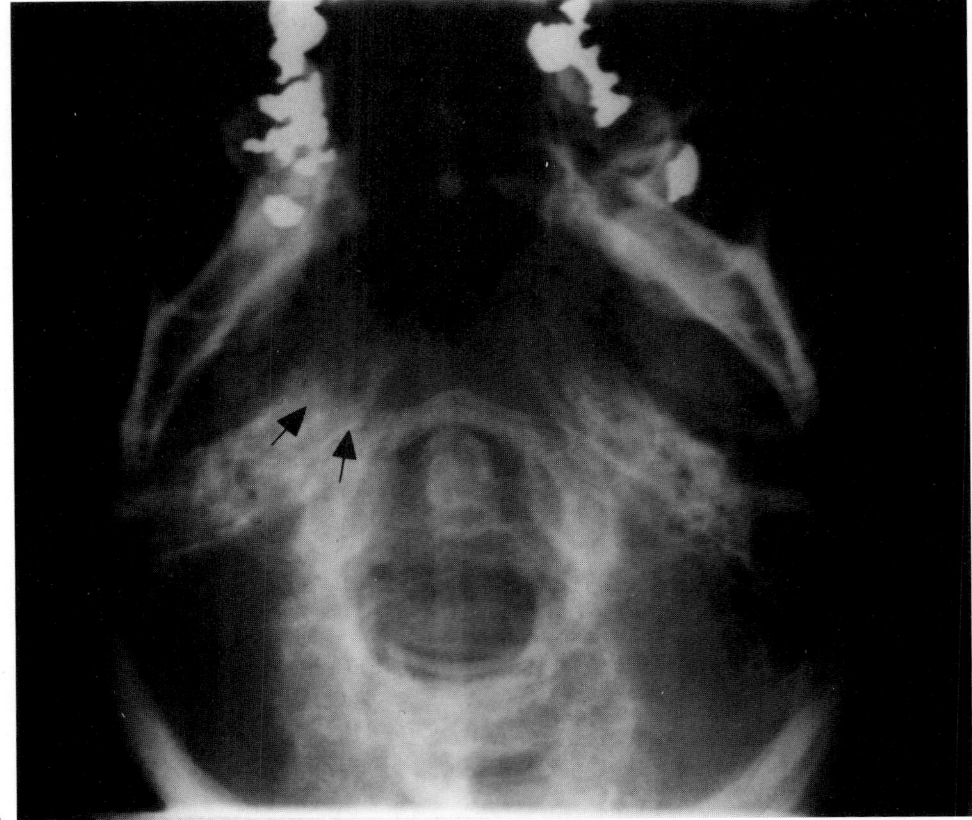

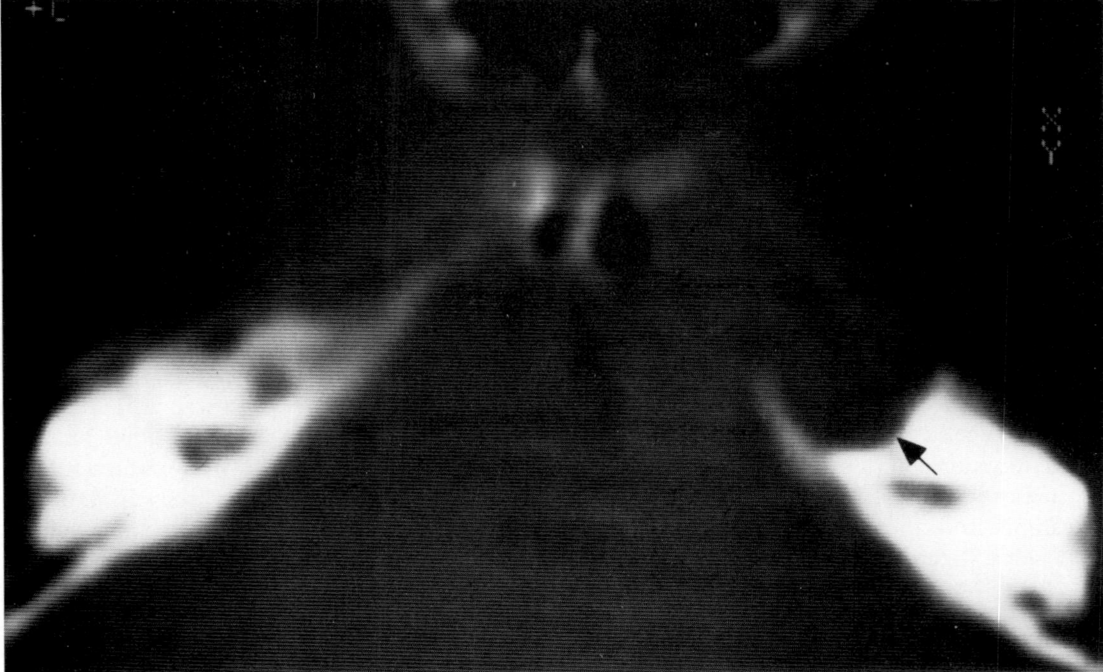

Fig. 33.2 **A.** Skull roentgenogram; base view demonstrates amputation of the right petrous apex (arrows). **B.** Axial CT correlate on a different patient demonstrates similar erosion of the left petrous apex (arrow). **C.** T1-weighted coronal MR image demonstrates an extra-axial mass eroding through the floor of the middle fossa into the pterygoid fossa. The tumor is inhomogeneous in signal intensity and somewhat hypointense with respect to the surrounding brain. **D.** T1-weighted axial MR image demonstrates the relationship of the tumor to the cavernous sinus. Note the integrity of the dura which clearly demarcates the tumor from the cavernous sinus. Note the atrophy of the masticatory muscles innervated by V. **E.** Subtraction film from bilateral carotid artery arteriogram (superimposed) demonstrating medial displacement of the precavernous segment of the right internal carotid artery (arrow).

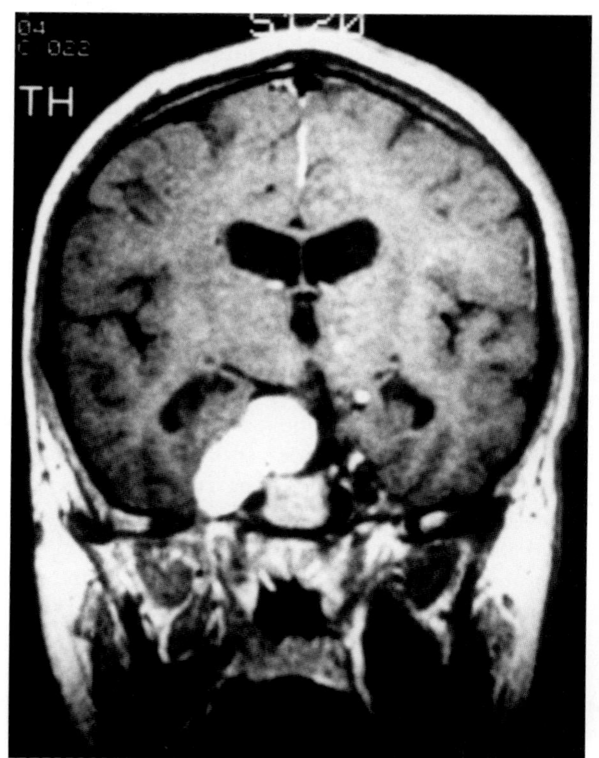

C

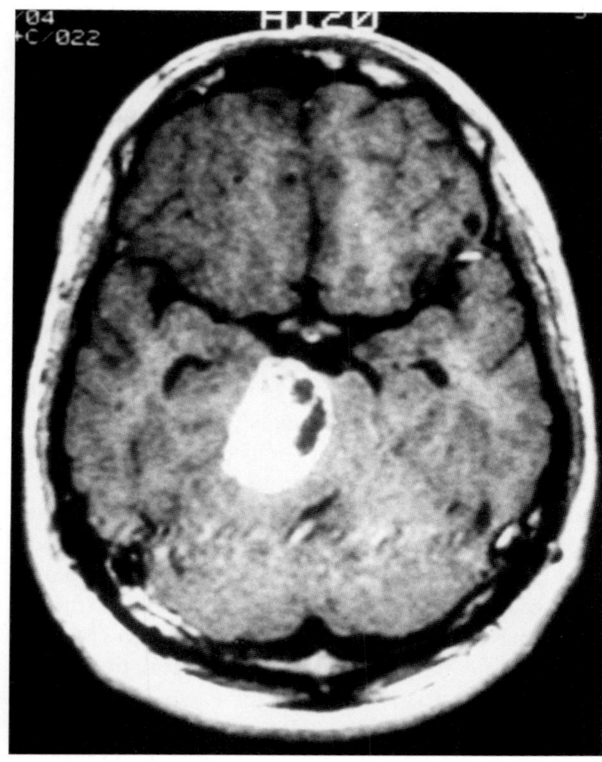

D

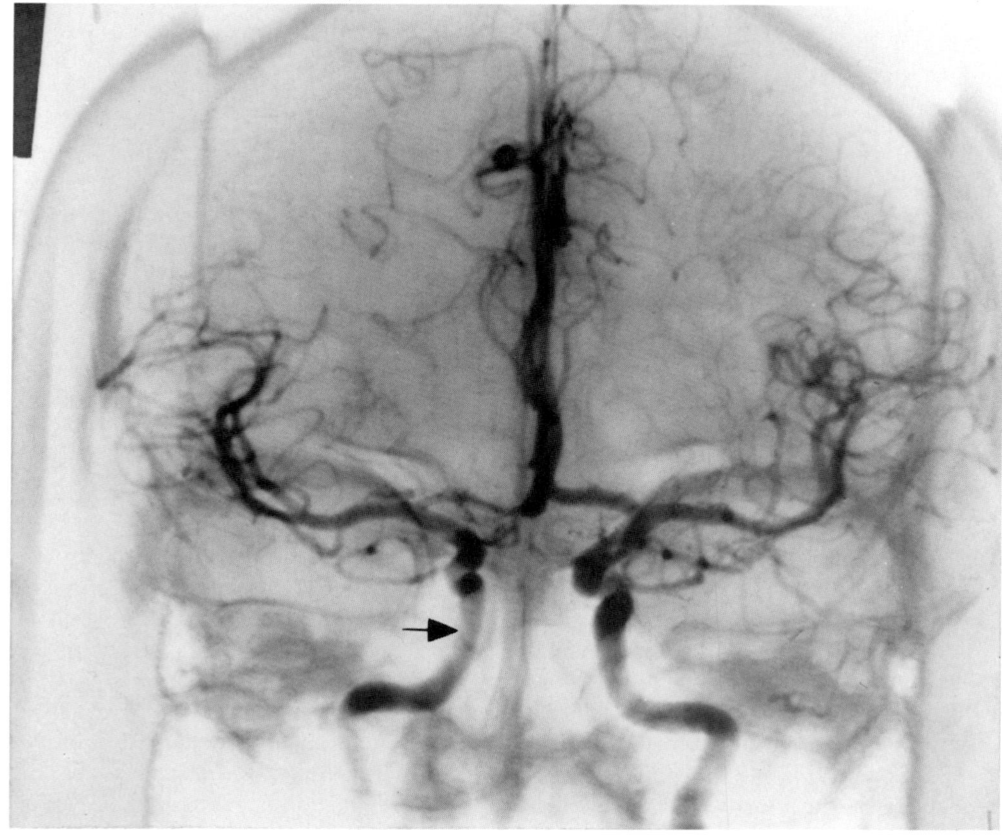

E

Fig. 33.2 C, D & E

space they widen the cisterns within which they are located. This phenomenon is the basis for their recognition on contrast cisternography and pneumoencephalography. On angiogram, they are usually relatively avascular, and derive their blood supply from branches of the external carotid system. On computerized tomography they usually appear as iso- to slightly hyperdense, well-circumscribed lesions which enhance homogeneously and intensely following iodinated contrast administration. As previously described for plain film, they often produce benign-type changes in the skull base on CT bone windows (Fig. 33.2B). With nuclear magnetic resonance, schwannomas tend to be slightly hypointense on T1 and hyperintense on T2-weighted images (Fig. 33.2C). Again, they usually enhance uniformly and intensely following the administration of contrast agents (Fig. 33.2D).

Schwannomas are surgically curable if complete excision is performed. The specific surgical approach and associated complications will vary according to the parent nerve involved and the extension of the tumor. Although there is extensive experience with focused beam radiation as a primary means of treatment for acoustic tumors (Lunsford et al 1990), no such series exists in the literature for schwannomas along the other cranial nerves. Conventional radiation may play a role in reducing the frequency of recurrence after subtotal resection (Wallner et al 1987).

TRIGEMINAL SCHWANNOMAS

Schwannomas arising from the trigeminal nerve, although the second most frequent intracranial site, are very rare tumors. Smith described the first case of a primary tumor of the trigeminal ganglion in 1849 (Peet 1927). Since that time over 250 cases have been reported in the literature (McCormick et al 1988, Bordi et al 1989, Pollack et al 1989). They represent 0.07–0.36% of all intracranial tumors, and 0.8–8% of all intracranial schwannomas (Olive & Svien 1957, Schisano & Olivecrona 1960, Knudson & Kolze 1972, Arseni et al 1975, deBenedittis et al 1977, McCormick et al 1988, Pollack et al 1989). They tend to occur during mid-life, with a peak incidence in the fourth and fifth decades (Olive & Svien 1957, Arseni et al 1975, Nager 1984) and are slightly more common in women (McCormick et al 1988). Frazier (1918) reported the first successful removal of a primary gasserian ganglion tumor.

The trigeminal nerve arises from the lateral aspect of the rostral pons and courses superiorly and anterolaterally through the cerebellopontine angle cistern toward the petrous apex. The root acquires a Schwann cell sheath approximately 2.2 mm from the brainstem (Westberg 1963). The length of the central or glial segment of the trigeminal root is second only to the vestibulocochlear among the true peripheral cranial nerves. The root carries its own sleeve of posterior fossa arachnoid and dura with it into the middle fossa as perineurium and dura propria, respectively. It penetrates the dura of the middle cranial fossa at the porus trigeminus, just inferior to the lateral tentorial attachment. The gasserian ganglion lies in a groove along the anteromedial aspect of the petrous pyramid known as Meckel's cave. The ganglion and third division are extradural in the middle fossa. The first and second divisions pass within the lateral wall of the cavernous sinus. The trochlear nerve lies above the trigeminal root, the seventh and eighth nerves below it, and the oculomotor and sixth nerves lie anteromedial to the ganglion in the cavernous sinus. The posterior cerebral and superior cerebellar arteries pass over the root, while the anterior inferior cerebellar artery passes under. The horizontal portion of the precavernous internal carotid artery, the eustachian tube, and the greater superficial petrosal nerve course below the distal part of the ganglion. There is often a bony defect in the floor of the middle cranial fossa such that a dural membrane alone separates the precavernous carotid from the ganglion. The petrosal vein lies lateral and posterior to the root, which enters the porus trigeminus just below the superior petrosal sinus. The motor fibers are situated medially along the root, but come to lie inferiorly at the level of the ganglion as the sensory fibers rotate anteromedially. The motor fibers pass through the foramen ovale with the mandibular division (Fig. 33.3).

Schwannomas may arise from the ganglion, root, or rarely the divisions of the trigeminal nerve. Jefferson (1955) classified them according to location. Approximately 50% arise predominantly within the middle cranial fossa, 30% within the posterior fossa, and 20% are dumbbell-shaped with significant extension into both cranial fossae. The predominant symptoms and signs, and the surgical approach, will vary somewhat according to the location of the tumor.

The most common complaint at the time of presentation is that of a sensory disturbance in the ipsilateral face (McCormick et al 1988, Bordi et al 1989) (Table 33.1). The duration of symptoms may vary from a few months to more than 15 years (McCormick et al 1988, Bordi et al 1989, Pollack et al 1989). The disturbance is most often described as numbness, but may include pain or paresthesias. It may be confined to the distribution of one division, but more commonly involves all three to a variable degree. Complete anesthesia in all three divisions is distinctly uncommon, and suggests malignant invasion of the gasserian ganglion (Cohen 1933, Jefferson 1955). The pain associated with a schwannoma differs from that seen in trigeminal neuralgia in the duration of the paroxysms (often hours) and the lack of trigger zones. Sensory disturbance is especially common in middle fossa tumors. Tumors in this location can compress adjacent nerves within the

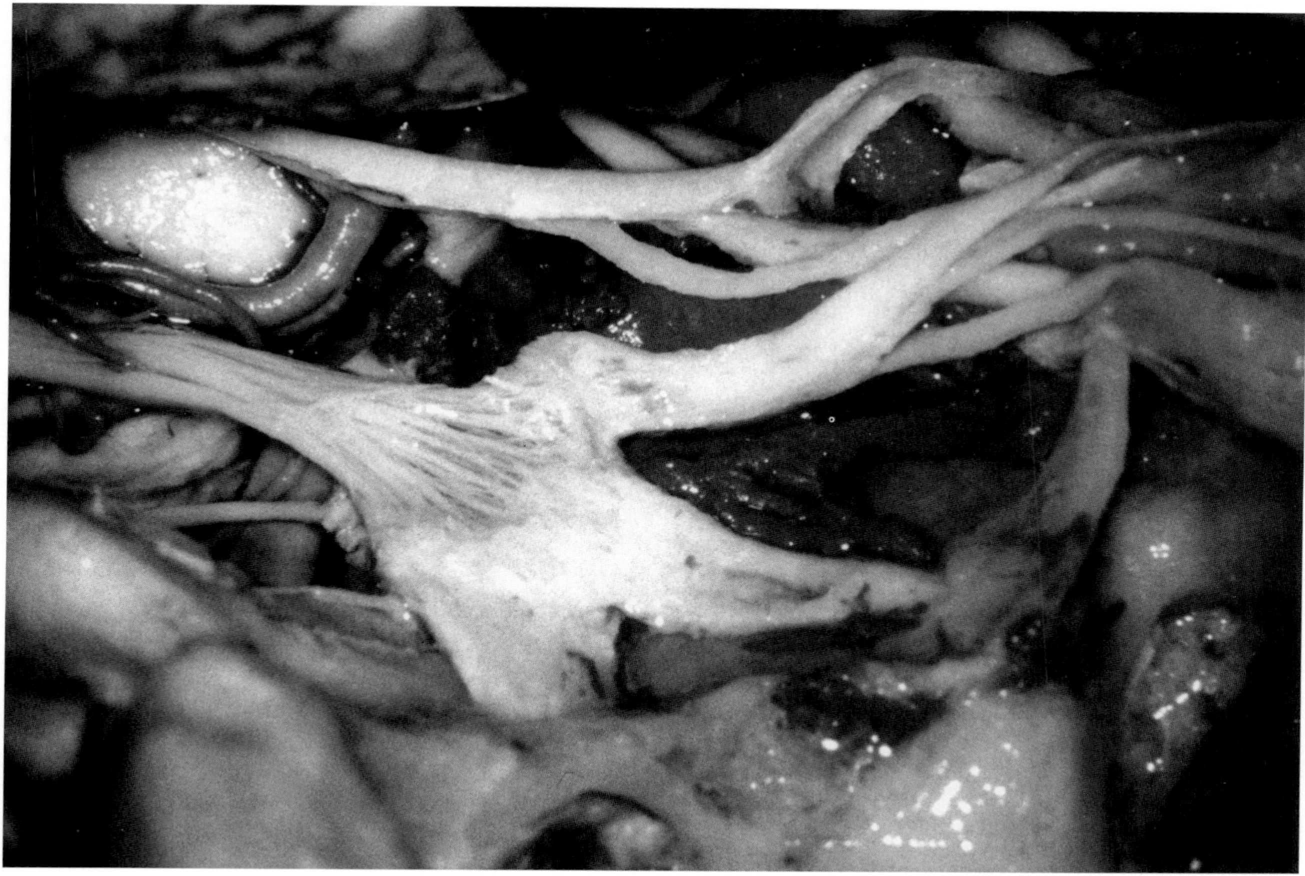

Fig. 33.3 Dissection demonstrating the anatomy about Meckel's cave. The gasserian ganglion is well defined, with the three major sensory branches clearly dissected.

Table 33.1 Initial symptom in 130 patients with trigeminal neuroma

Symptom	No. of cases	Percent
Trigeminal nerve dysfunction	72	55
Numbness	35	27
Pain	30	23
Paresthesias	7	5
Headache	19	15
Diplopia	13	10
Hearing loss/tinnitus	10	8
Visual loss	7	5
Ear pain	4	3
Other*	10	8
Total	132	

*Other symptoms = subarachnoid hemorrhage, vertigo, seizure, exophthalmos, gait difficulty, hemifacial spasm. Two patients had more than one initial symptom.

cavernous sinus, resulting in diplopia. They may extend into the orbital apex producing exophthalmos and visual loss. Tumors located primarily within the posterior fossa more often present with hearing loss, tinnitus or a gait disturbance (Pollack et al 1989). Dumbbell-shaped tumors can present with a combination of middle and posterior fossa-type symptoms. Other complaints, in descending order of relative frequency, include headache, seizure, and hemifacial spasm (McCormick et al 1988).

Objective findings are common and are usually referable to the involved trigeminal nerve. Decreased sensation in one or more dermatomes along with a diminished or absent corneal is seen in 80–90% of patients (Krayenbuhl 1936, Lesois et al 1986). Mild weakness in the muscles of mastication is found in 30–40% (Arseni et al 1975, deBenedittis et al 1977, McCormick et al 1988, Bordi et al 1989). Findings referable to adjacent cranial nerves are found in 75% of cases (McCormick et al 1988). Middle fossa tumors can produce a conductive hearing loss from eustachian tube destruction, and a facial paresis secondary to compression of the nerve in the fallopian canal or traction on the greater superficial petrosal nerve (Jefferson 1955, Nager 1984). Tumors arising in the root usually produce signs of a cerebellopontine angle syndrome. This consists of hearing loss and facial weakness secondary to distortion of cranial nerves VIII and VII, as well as ataxia and spasticity secondary to cerebellar and brainstem compression. Large posterior fossa tumors may extend downward and cause dysfunction of the lower cranial nerves resulting in abnormal phonation, deglutition, and an absent palatal reflex. The large dumbbell-shaped tumors often produce a combination of middle and posterior fossa signs. Although objective findings are common, 10–20% of patients will have a normal neurologic exam (Jefferson 1955, Olive & Svien 1957, Mello & Tanzer 1972, Arseni et al 1975, deBenedittis et al 1977) (Table 33.2).

Plain films will often demonstrate amputation of the petrous apex (Holman et al 1961, Palacios & MacGee 1972). The margins are smooth and without sclerosis, unlike the more common malignant and primary bone lesions in this region (Fig. 33.2A). The middle fossa floor may be eroded, and one or more foramina at the skull base enlarged (Fig. 33.2B). A ganglion tumor which extends anteriorly may erode the lateral aspect and dorsum of the sella or the clinoid processes. It may enlarge the superior orbital fissure or optic foramen. Alternatively, it may extend extracranially and erode the pterygoid plates. Isolated posterior fossa tumors may produce very few bony changes and be impossible to detect on plain films. Conversely, they may erode the anterior lip of the internal acoustic meatus and be mistaken for acoustic tumors. They may also produce nonspecific changes within the sella and calvarium associated with increased intracranial pressure.

Cerebral angiography will most often show inferomedial displacement of the precavernous portion of the petrous carotid (Chase & Taveras 1963) (Fig. 33.2E). This finding is characteristic of middle fossa tumors. Tumors in the posterior fossa will often elevate and medially displace the posterior cerebral and superior cerebellar arteries. The basilar artery may be displaced posteriorly and contralaterally. The petrosal vein may be elevated, or may fail to fill. The tumors are usually relatively avascular, although a blush from feeders off the precavernous carotid or the external circulation is noted in 20–25% (Westberg 1963, Gordy 1965, Mello & Tanzer 1972, Palacios & MacGee 1972, deBenedittis et al 1977, McCormick et al 1988). At the time of angiography a balloon occlusion test of the ipsilateral internal carotid may be performed in order to evaluate the extent of cross-circulation should the carotid have to be sacrificed (Pollack et al 1989).

Table 33.2 Abnormal findings on admission examination in 136 patients with trigeminal neurinoma*

Neurologic abnormality	No. of cases	Percent
Trigeminal nerve		
Decreased sensation	100	74
Diminished or absent corneal reflex	93	68
Pain	52	38
Motor weakness	53	39
Other cranial nerve deficits		
II	14	10
III	19	14
IV	9	7
VI	47	35
VII	31	23
VIII	44	32
IX, X	11	8
XI	2	1
XII	4	3
Cerebellar signs	31	23
Long tract signs	22	16
Papilledema	14	10

*Only 27 patients (21%) had abnormal findings limited to the trigeminal nerve.

The bony changes seen on plain film are exquisitely demonstrated on CT bone windows (Fig. 33.2B). The soft tissue mass itself usually appears iso- to hyperdense relative to surrounding brain (Goldberg et al 1980). Cystic changes within the tumor may be present (Fig. 33.4). Following the administration of iodinated contrast, the tumors usually enhance homogeneously and intensely (Goldberg et al 1980, Nager 1984); however, ringlike or irregular enhancement is not uncommon. With MR imaging, the soft tissue mass usually appears hypointense on T1-weighted images and hyperintense on T2 (Rigamonti et al 1987). The enhancement pattern following the administration of gadolinium is similar to that seen with enhanced CT — usually homogeneous and intense (Fig. 33.2C,D). CT and MR imaging are critical in defining the extent of the tumor and planning the surgical approach (Fig. 33.4).

The clinical and neuroradiologic evaluation should allow accurate preoperative diagnosis in most cases. The differential diagnosis includes skull base metastases, primary bone tumors, meningiomas, epidermoids, and acoustic schwannomas. Metastases and primary bone tumors, such as chondrosarcomas and chordomas, usually produce a pattern of irregular bony destruction rather than a smooth scalloping of bone. Meningiomas more often produce hyperostosis than erosion, and there is often intratumoral calcification, which is uncommon in schwannomas. Epidermoids often show a sclerotic margin in areas of bony erosion not usually seen in schwannomas. Acoustic schwannomas almost always produce a symmetric enlargement of the internal auditory canal. In addition, hearing loss is an earlier and more prominent complaint in the acoustic schwannoma.

The surgical approach is principally dependent on the location and extension of the tumor, hence the need for detailed preoperative neuroradiologic evaluation. Most common is the subtemporal intradural approach through the middle cranial fossa, since the majority of these tumors arise from the ganglion and lie predominantly in the middle cranial fossa. In addition, tumors which straddle the middle and posterior cranial fossae, and do not extend below the internal auditory canal, can be

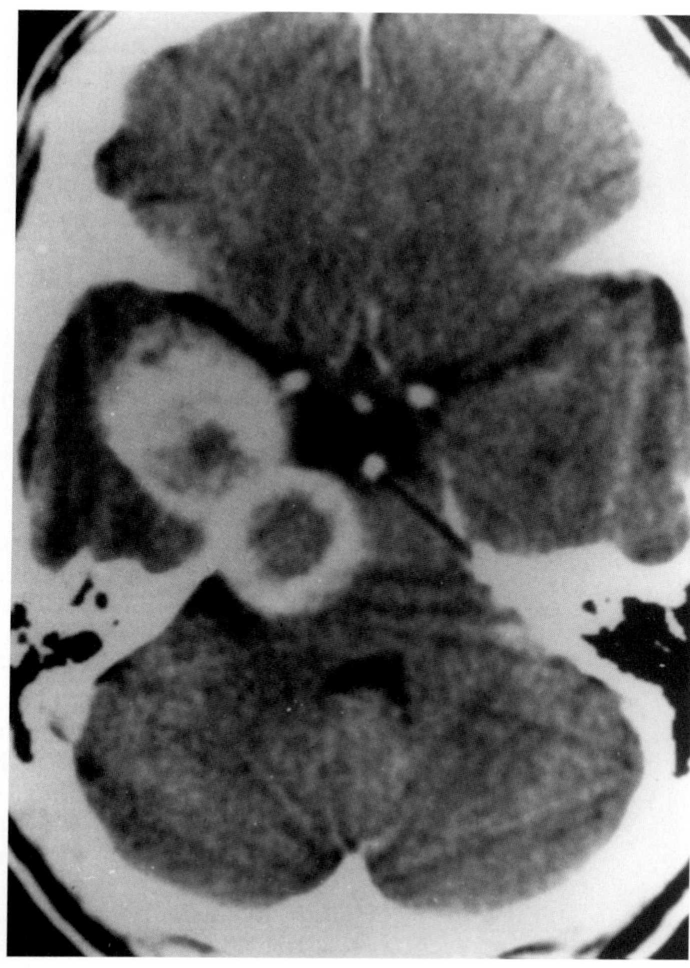

A

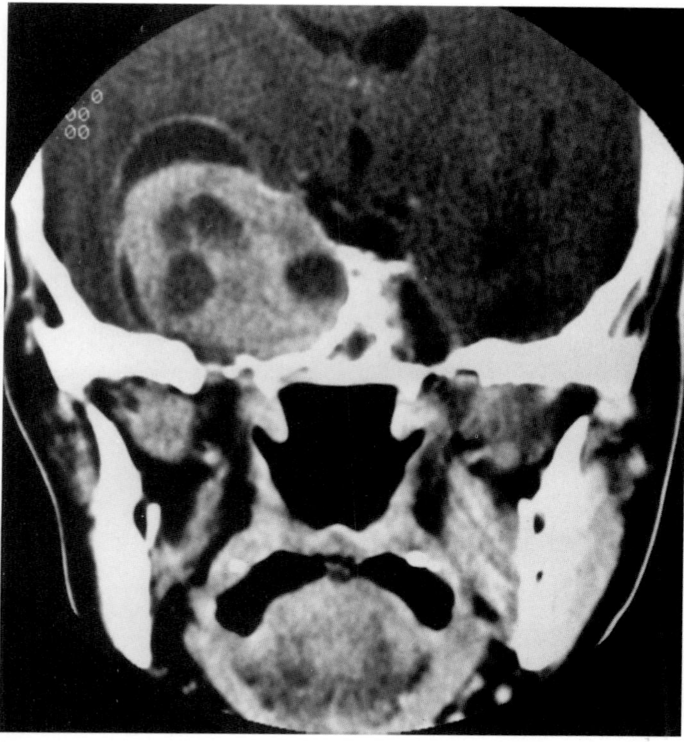

B

Fig. 33.4 **A.** Contrast-enhanced CT scan of a dumbbell-shaped tumor shows areas of decreased attenuation representing either necrosis or cystic degeneration. **B.** Contrast-enhanced coronal CT scan shows a large inhomogeneous mass in the right middle fossa with marked erosion of the dorsum sellae and upper clivus. Note the marked atrophy of the masseter and pterygoid muscles on the right side.

removed through a middle fossa approach (Fig. 33.5A). This is accomplished by incising the free margin of the tentorium and ligating the superior petrosal sinus. In contrast, very little access can be gained to the middle cranial fossa through a standard suboccipital approach. This is therefore confined to those tumors which lie exclusively within the posterior fossa. The combined or petrosal approach is employed for large dumbbell-shaped tumors which extend ventral to the lower brainstem and below the internal acoustic meatus. Newer skull base procedures used for large middle fossa tumors incorporate the use of an orbitozygomatic osteotomy to facilitate exposure of the cavernous sinus and minimize temporal lobe retraction (Sekhar 1987).

The use of mannitol and/or a lumbar subarachnoid drain help to slacken the brain. Intraoperative brainstem auditory and somatosensory evoked potentials are sometimes employed (Findler et al 1983, Takayasu et al 1987).

The tumors are removed through an intracapsular debulking procedure using either the bipolar cautery, the laser, or the ultrasonic aspirator. After debulking, the capsule must be carefully dissected away from surrounding structures. In large tumors, the trochlear nerve will usually be found on the superior pole of the capsule, and the auditory and facial nerves along the inferior pole. The oculomotor and abducens nerves will usually be found medially along with the carotid artery. Part or all of the trigeminal complex may have to be excised because of tumor involvement. In the past, many of these tumors were subtotally resected, as they were adherent to the cavernous sinus, the internal carotid artery, or the brainstem. Long-term results following subtotal resection are controversial. Some authors report an inevitable symptomatic recurrence, usually within 3 years (Pollack et al 1989). Others report a satisfactory clinical outcome with very few symptomatic recurrences (Bordi et al 1989, Pollack et al 1989). With the recent advent of more sophisticated cavernous sinus surgery, it is anticipated that complete removal will be performed more often.

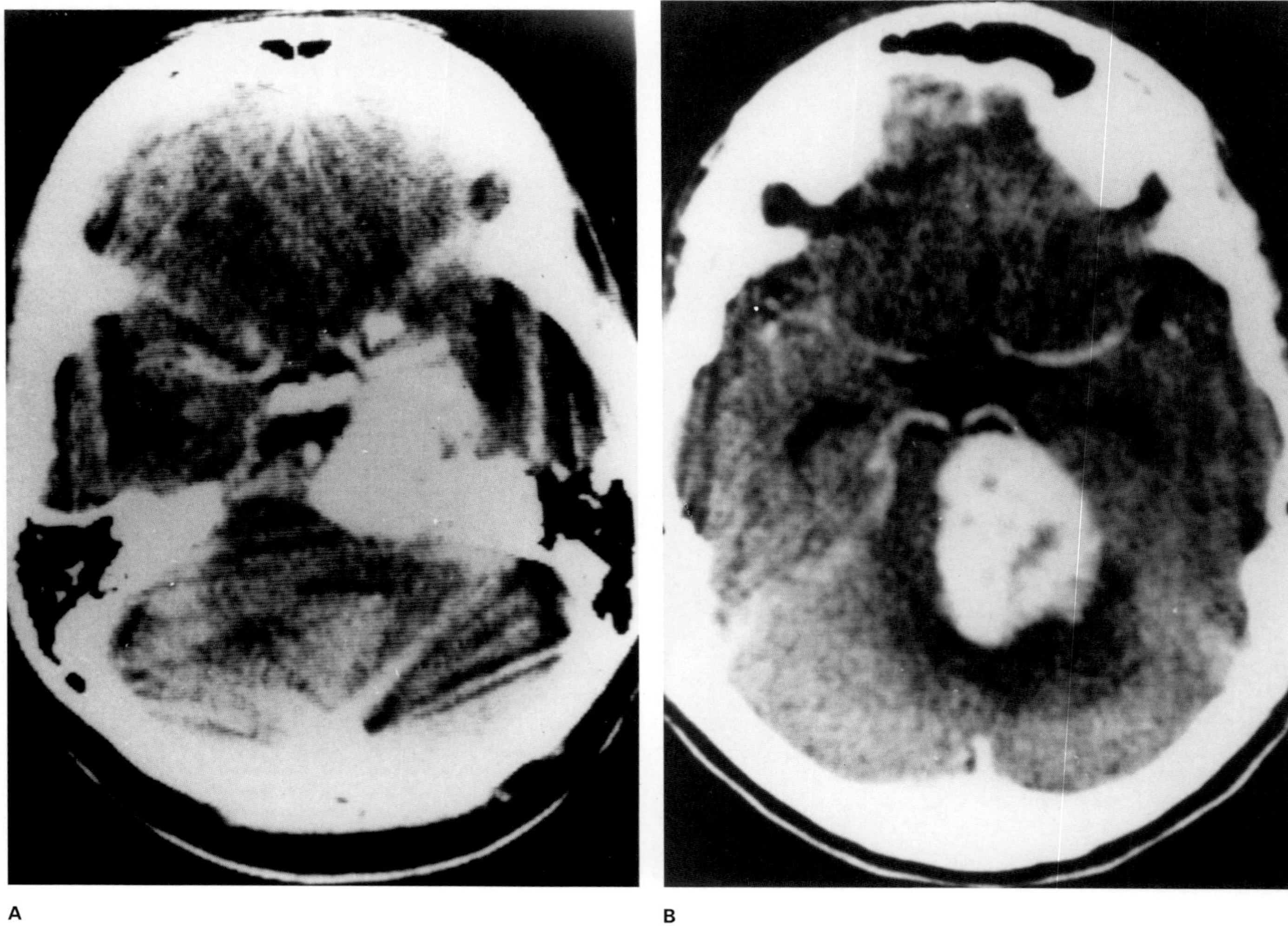

Fig. 33.5 **A.** Axial CT scan demonstrating a dumbbell-shaped tumor. Although the posterior fossa tumor is not large, its wide-based apposition to the posterior aspect of the petrous pyramid makes it unlikely that this tumor can be removed safely through a subtemporal approach. **B.** Axial CT scan shows a large trigeminal root neurinoma totally confined to the posterior fossa.

In the past, the surgical mortality rate was as high as 25% (Arseni et al 1975). With modern microsurgical technique this has been drastically reduced. Three large recent series comprising a total of 41 patients contained only one operative death: a mortality rate of 2.2% (McCormick et al 1988, Bordi et al 1989, Pollack et al 1989). Morbidity includes cranial nerve injury, CSF leak, meningitis, and hydrocephalus. Many patients will be left with some degree of permanent trigeminal dysfunction. This may result in the need for tarsorrhaphy to prevent neurotrophic keratitis. New onset postoperative cranial nerve dysfunction, such as abducens and oculomotor palsies, will usually resolve within 4 months. Some pre-operative neurologic deficits, such as cerebellar and brain-stem compression syndromes, diplopia, facial pain and weakness, and hearing loss may improve postoperatively. CSF leak and/or hydrocephalus may require shunt placement.

FACIAL SCHWANNOMAS

Schwannomas arising from the facial nerve account for approximately 1.9% of all intracranial schwannomas (Symon et al 1993). The first such case was described by Schmidt in 1931. Since then a number of isolated reports and a few large series have been published, totalling more than 180 cases (Neely & Alford 1974, Isamat et al 1975, Murata et al 1985, Rosenblum et al 1987). The incidence of facial schwannoma may actually be much higher, as autopsy reports have found incidental tumors in up to 0.8% of petrous bones (Saito & Baxter 1972). These tumors most commonly present in the fourth and fifth decades of life, although pediatric patients as young as 1 year old have been reported (O'Donoghue et al 1989). There is a distinct female predilection in most of the larger series. From 15–21% of patients have been known to have neurofibromatosis (King & Morrison 1990, Symon et al 1993).

The facial nerve has a rather long and complex course from the brainstem to the stylomastoid foramen. This may be divided on an anatomic and clinical basis into five segments (Schuknecht & Gulya 1986). As it emerges from the lateral aspect of the brainstem just above the pontomedullary junction, it courses superiorly and laterally toward the internal acoustic meatus. Here it is cradled in a groove on the superior surface of the cochlear division of the eighth cranial nerve. This first segment lies within the cerebellopontine angle cistern. The second segment of the nerve travels approximately 7–8 mm within the internal auditory canal, where it occupies the anterosuperior quadrant. At the lateral end of the canal it passes above the transverse crest to enter the fallopian canal within the petrous bone. The third or labyrinthine segment travels anteriorly and laterally, superior to the cochlea and vestibule. This is the shortest segment, only 3–4 mm in length, and perpendicular to the long axis of the petrous pyramid. This segment terminates at the geniculate ganglion, which contains the cell bodies of the parasympathetic fibers of the nervus intermedius. The geniculate ganglion lies just below the middle cranial fossa, from which it is sometimes separated only by dura. The greater superficial petrosal nerve carries some of the autonomic fibers forward into the middle fossa through the facial hiatus on the anterior surface of the petrous pyramid. The remaining facial fibers turn sharply backward and run posterolaterally along the medial wall of the tympanic cavity. This horizontal or tympanic segment of the nerve runs parallel to the long axis of the petrous bone. After crossing the medial wall of the tympanic cavity a second genu is created as the nerve turns sharply downward. In this vertical or mastoid segment the nerve runs along the posterior aspect of the middle ear cavity. Here the parasympathetic fibers of the chorda tympani and the branch to the stapedius muscle are given off. Finally the nerve exits the skull base at the stylomastoid foramen (Fig. 33.6).

The facial nerve acquires a Schwann cell sheath approximately 2 mm after exiting the brainstem (Tarlov 1937). Therefore, tumors of Schwann cell origin may arise anywhere along the aforementioned course. The older literature indicated a predilection for the vertical or mastoid segment of the nerve (Lipkin et al 1987). More recent work, however, implicates the region of the geniculate ganglion as the most common epicenter (Fisch & Ruttner 1977, Horn et al 1981, O'Donoghue et al 1989, Symon

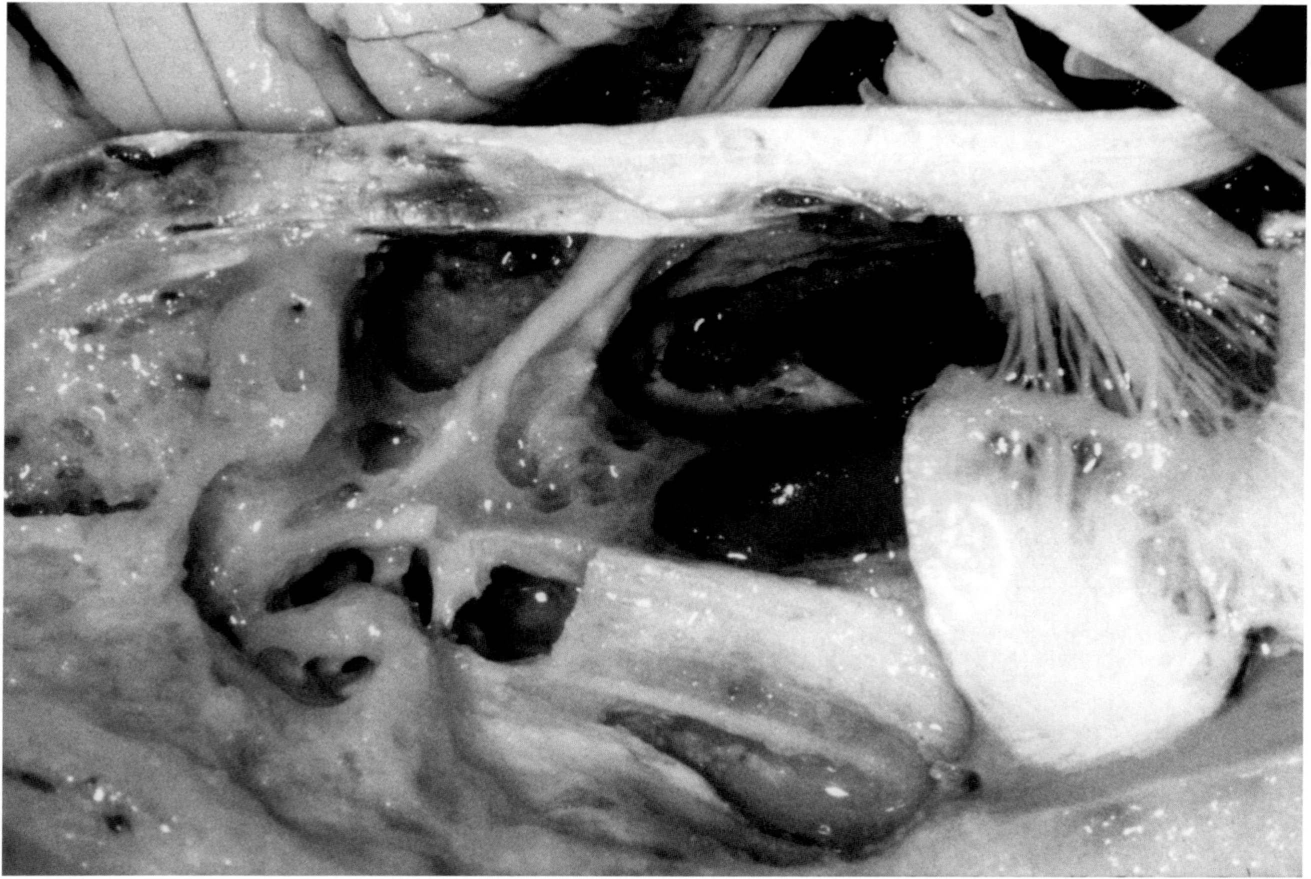

Fig. 33.6 Anatomic dissection demonstrating the course of the facial nerve.

et al 1993). The clinical symptoms and signs will vary according to the site of origin, and the direction and degree of spread to adjacent segments. The majority of tumors will involve two or more segments of the nerve. The earliest symptom is hearing loss, occurring in 41–91% of cases (Tew et al 1983, King & Morrison 1990, Symon et al 1993). The hearing loss is sensorineural if the mass is predominantly in the cisternal or intracanalicular segment of the nerve, and conductive if the tympanic or mastoid segment is involved. Tinnitus occurs in up to 60% of cases and vertigo in as many as 34% (Symon et al 1993). Facial weakness is common at the time of presentation, though it is not usually the first symptom. From 46–90% of patients will have weakness, twitching, or both (O'Donoghue et al 1989, King & Morrison 1990, Symon et al 1993). The facial palsy usually develops slowly and gradually, indicating neoplastic rather than inflammatory involvement; however, up to 20% of patients will develop sudden onset of facial weakness which may be mistaken for a Bell's palsy (Pulec 1969, Fisch & Ruttner 1977). Recurrent attacks of facial weakness with incomplete recovery between episodes may also occur. Although facial weakness is a very frequent finding in this group of patients, only about 5% of cases of peripheral facial palsy are found to be attributable to a schwannoma of the facial nerve (Neely & Alford 1974). Other symptoms and signs include mass in the middle ear cavity, otalgia, otorrhea, facial pain or sensory loss, headache, seizures, ataxia, and dry eye (Symon et al 1993) (Table 33.3).

CT and MR are the most useful preoperative tests. The diagnosis is based on the recognition of one or more enlarged segments of the fallopian canal filled with homogeneously enhancing soft tissue. CT is superior for demonstrating bony changes, while MR is more sensitive in detecting small tumors and defining extension. Tumors which arise primarily in the cisternal or canalicular segment of the nerve may be extremely hard to distinguish from the much more common acoustic schwannoma, and as many as 36% will be misdiagnosed as such (O'Donoghue et al 1989). Large tumors which extend into the middle cranial fossa may be distinguished from acoustic and trigeminal schwannomas based on their pattern of extension. Facial schwannomas extend through the midpetrosal area, whereas trigeminal tumors erode the petrous apex and acoustic tumors extend through the tentorial incisura (Inouye et al 1987). Angiography is usually not required. Preoperative neuro-otologic testing has been largely supplanted by detailed neuroradiologic imaging.

Table 33.3 Signs and symptoms of seventh nerve schwannomas

Hearing loss	41–91%
sensorineural — intracanalicular	
conductive — tympanic or mastoid	
Tinnitus	60%
Vertigo	34%
Facial weakness	46–90%
sudden onset 20%	
Other: mass in middle ear	
otalgia	
otorrhea	
facial pain	
sensory loss	
dry eye	

The approach to these tumors is determined by the location and extent of the mass and the patient's preoperative level of neurologic function. Tumors lying proximal to the geniculate ganglion may be approached through the middle fossa, the posterior fossa, or the labyrinth. If hearing is poor, the translabyrinthine approach allows for excellent visualization and mobilization of the proximal and distal segments of the nerve, as well as access to both the middle and posterior fossae (Fish & Ruttner 1977, House & Brackmann 1985, Lipkin et al 1987, O'Donoghue et al 1989, King & Morrison 1990). If hearing preservation is to be attempted, a subtemporal/middle fossa approach is preferable unless the tumor lies predominantly within the cerebellopontine angle. In these cases a lateral suboccipital approach is employed (Symon et al 1993). Nerve repair is more difficult with either the subtemporal or suboccipital exposure, and the latter has the additional disadvantage of offering minimal access to the middle fossa. Tumors involving the tympanic or mastoid segment of the nerve may be removed via a simple mastoidectomy. Some have advocated a conservative approach in those cases in which facial function remains intact and no intracranial extension exists (King & Morrison 1990). Others have argued that in order to maximize the chances of successful nerve grafting, surgery should be performed before the onset of facial weakness whenever possible (Fisch & Ruttner 1977, Symon et al 1993).

The technique involved in removing these tumors is the same as in the acoustic and trigeminal schwannomas. First, an intracapsular debulking is performed, followed by stripping of the capsule from adjacent neurovascular structures. Sacrifice of the involved facial nerve has been required in 75–100% of cases (O'Donoghue et al 1989, Symon et al 1993). Even in those cases in which more than 50% of the nerve was preserved, postoperative facial function was extremely poor. Consideration must therefore be given to the possibility of an immediate nerve grafting procedure. If the proximal and distal ends of the nerve can be brought into apposition, either in situ or after distal rerouting, a primary anastomosis can be accomplished with suture or fibrin glue. Alternatively, an interpositional graft using the sural or greater auricular nerve can be performed. Both techniques result in similar postoperative facial function. The primary determinant is the duration of preoperative facial paralysis (O'Donoghue et al 1989, Symon et al 1993). When paralysis has been present for more than 2 years, nerve grafting is probably not indicated. Successful grafts can be expected to take

Table 33.4 Facial nerve grading system (House & Brackmann 1985)

Grade	Description	Characteristics
I	Normal	Normal facial function in all areas
II	Mild dysfunction	Gross: slight weakness noticeable on close inspection; may have very slight synkinesis At rest: normal symmetry and tone Motion: Forehead: moderate to good function Eye: complete closure with minimum effort Mouth: Slight asymmetry
III	Moderate dysfunction	Gross: obvious but not disfiguring difference between two sides; noticeable but not severe synkinesis, contracture, and/or hemifacial spasm At rest: normal symmetry and tone Motion: Forehead: slight to moderate movement Eye: complete closure with effort Mouth: slightly weak with maximum effort
IV	Moderately severe dysfunction	Gross: obvious weakness and/or disfiguring asymmetry At rest: normal symmetry and tone Motion: Forehead: none Eye: incomplete closure Mouth: asymmetric with maximum effort
V	Severe dysfunction	Gross: only barely perceptible motion At rest: asymmetry Motion: Forehead: none Eye: incomplete closure Mouth: slight movement
VI	Total paralysis	No movement

from 6 months to a year to function. In those patients without longstanding preoperative facial paralysis in whom immediate nerve grafting was either not possible or successful, a faciohypoglossal anastomosis can be considered. Regardless of the reanimation procedure performed, a House-Brackmann (1985) grade III is the best level of facial function to be expected (Table 33.4). During the period of recovery, care must be taken to protect the involved eye. This may include tarsorrhaphy, gold weight insertion, or the use of an eye bubble.

Facial nerve schwannomas are curable if completely excised. The mortality rate using modern microsurgical technique has been extremely low. Morbidity, other than the expected facial paralysis, includes hearing loss. This occurs in up to 33% of patients, and is permanent in approximately half of these cases (Symon et al 1993). Other complications include CSF leak, meningitis, and/or hydrocephalus. Care must be taken to seal completely the mastoid air cells, the external auditory canal, and the eustachian tube when these structures are opened.

JUGULAR FORAMEN SCHWANNOMAS

Schwannomas have been known to arise from the nerve roots exiting the jugular foramen since the report by Gerhardt in 1878. The first successful surgical removal was described by Cairns in 1935 (Cohen 1937). Since then less than 100 such cases have been reported in the literature (Naunton et al 1969, Arenberg & McCreary 1971, Mountjoy et al 1974, Gacek 1976, Maniglia et al 1979, House et al 1985, Ohl et al 1988, Shiroyama et al 1988, Claesen et al 1989, Suzuki et al 1989). As with most schwannomas, these tumors usually present in the third to fifth decades of life, with a slight female predilection. Most reports do not identify the specific root of origin. The glossopharyngeal nerve appears to be most commonly affected, however, with approximately 28 cases cited (Sweasey et al 1991).

The glossopharyngeal, vagus, and cranial accessory nerves emerge as a series of rootlets from the retro-olivary sulcus of the medulla and pass inferolaterally toward the jugular foramen. A Schwann cell sheath is acquired within 1.1 mm of the root entry zone, with the more caudal rootlets exhibiting the shortest glial segments (Tarlov 1937). The jugular foramen itself is divided into a pars nervosa and a pars vascularis by a fibrous or bony septum (DiChiro et al 1974). The former contains the glossopharyngeal nerve and the inferior petrosal sinus, the latter the vagus and accessory nerves, the jugular vein, and the posterior meningeal artery (Fig. 33.7).

Kaye has classified jugular foramen schwannomas into three types according to their primary location: within the posterior fossa in the cerebellopontine angle cistern, within the skull base, or extending inferiorly from the

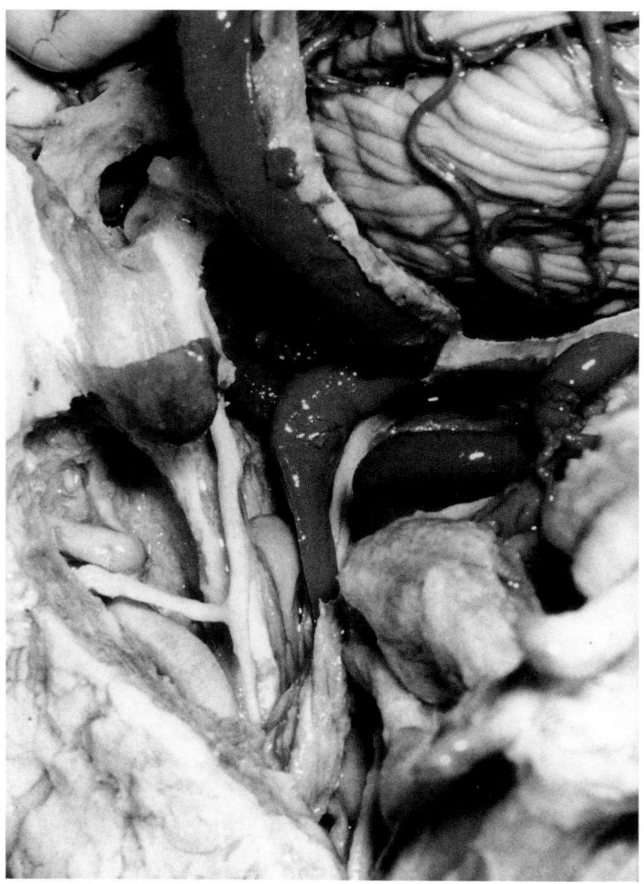

Fig. 33.7 Anatomic dissection of the jugular fossa region.

jugular foramen into the neck (Kaye et al 1984). The clinical presentation will vary somewhat according to this classification scheme. In general, symptoms and signs associated with jugular foramen schwannomas may be present for many years before diagnosis, with an average duration of about 2.7 years (Hakuba et al 1979). Blurred vision was a frequent complaint amongst patients with jugular foramen schwannomas as a whole (Hakuba et al 1979). Tumors confined to the posterior fossa most commonly present with ipsilateral sensorineural hearing loss, sometimes accompanied by tinnitus. This is especially common in glossopharyngeal tumors, in which over 90% of the cases presented in such a fashion (Fink et al 1978, Kaye et al 1984, Tan et al 1990, Sweasey et al 1991). Facial numbness, weakness, or hemifacial spasm may also be present. Large tumors in this location may present with symptoms and signs of brainstem and/or cerebellar compression such as nystagmus and ataxia, along with evidence of raised intracranial pressure such as headache, nausea, vomiting, and papilledema. Palsies of the nerves of the jugular foramen are distinctly uncommon amongst these tumors (Tan et al 1990). Schwannomas confined to the jugular foramen and those with extension into the neck are more likely to present with evidence of lower cranial nerve palsies such as hoarseness, swallowing difficulties and/or weakness and atrophy of the sternomastoid and trapezius muscles. Diminished gag reflex with a unilateral vocal cord paralysis is common. Loss of taste is a notably uncommon complaint and rarely found on examination.

Detailed neuroimaging, including contrast-enhanced MR and CT, is the most important preoperative evaluation. The jugular foramen is usually enlarged, and CT bone windows will show scalloping of the margins. MR is the most sensitive imaging modality for discovering small tumors and demonstrating tumor extension (Fig. 33.8). Angiography will demonstrate an avascular mass which displaces the anterior inferior cerebellar artery superomedially and the posterior inferior cerebellar artery inferomedially (Hakuba et al 1979). The venous phase is especially important for evaluating the jugular bulb and vein, which are often occluded. The differential diagnosis includes acoustic schwannoma, meningioma, metastasis, and glomus jugulare tumor. Acoustic schwannomas will usually enlarge the internal auditory canal rather than the jugular foramen. Meningiomas more often produce hyperostosis than bone erosion or scalloping, and demonstrate a much more prominent blush on angiography. Metastases and glomus jugulare tumors tend to destroy bone irregularly rather than smoothly erode or scallop. In addition, the latter have a very prominent blush on angiography and invade rather than compress the jugular bulb and vein.

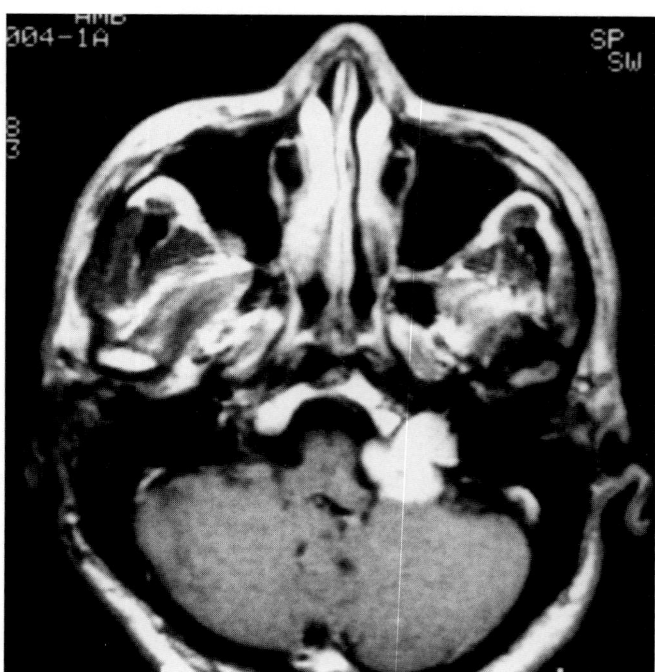

Fig. 33.8 Axial enhanced MRI demonstrating a left ninth nerve schwannoma.

The surgical approach to these lesions is determined by their location and extension. Those tumors confined to the posterior fossa can be removed through a standard lateral suboccipital craniectomy as performed for the more common acoustic schwannoma (Tan et al 1990). For tumors located primarily within the jugular foramen a presigmoid inferolabyrinthine mastoidectomy combined with a retrosigmoid craniectomy allows for ligation of the sigmoid sinus and direct exposure of the lateral margin of the jugular foramen (Hakuba et al 1979, Kaye et al 1984). This exposure minimizes the distance between the surgeon and the tumor. Alternatively, the jugular foramen may be opened intracranially through a standard lateral suboccipital craniectomy by removing a triangular-shaped wedge of bone between the foramen and the internal auditory canal (Hakuba et al 1979). Significant extension into the neck usually requires a combined approach with the aid of an otolaryngologist, either simultaneously or in a staged procedure (Kaye et al 1984). The neck dissection allows for control of the carotid artery, jugular vein, and adjacent lower cranial nerves below the skull base.

As with all intracranial schwannomas, complete surgical excision is curative. In general, tumors which are subtotally resected tend to regrow and produce symptoms (Tan et al 1990, Sweasey et al 1991). There are patients, however, who have been observed for long periods after subtotal resection without neurologic deterioration (Sweasey et al 1991). No reliable information is available on the effectiveness of radiation in reducing the incidence or time to recurrence.

Complications following surgical removal of these tumors might be expected to involve the swallowing mechanism. While this has been noted in some series (Hakuba et al 1979, Kaye et al 1984, Sweasey et al 1991) and early tracheostomy has been recommended by some authors (Pluchino et al 1975), the most recent reports have demonstrated a remarkably low incidence of serious dysphagia and aspiration (Tan et al 1990). Many patients can be managed with temporary nasogastric feedings and meticulous pulmonary toilet. Most will eventually adapt and tolerate a regular diet. Other complications include CSF leak, meningitis, and hydrocephalus.

HYPOGLOSSAL SCHWANNOMAS

In 1933 de Martel et al described the first case of a schwannoma arising from the intracranial portion of the hypoglossal nerve. Since then 35 such cases have been reported in the literature (Odake 1989). As a purely motor nerve, the hypoglossal would be expected to be an unusual site for the development of a schwannoma. Five of the cases cited, or approximately 14%, arose in patients afflicted with central neurofibromatosis (Morelli 1966, Fujiwara et al 1980). The remaining 30 cases involved 23 purely intracranial tumors (Scott & Wycis 1949, Williams & Fox 1962, Ignelzi & Bucy 1967, Arumugasamy et al 1972, Ulso et al 1981, Yajima et al 1981, Berger et al 1982, Tuck et al 1984, Kuramitsu et al 1986) and 7 dumbbell-shaped masses with extracranial extension (Bartal et al 1973, Robinson et al 1979, Dolan et al 1982, Tuck et al 1984, Odake 1989). The age range of the patients was from 17–62 years, with a mean age at diagnosis of 41 years. The female predilection noted in most series of schwannomas is even stronger for the hypoglossal; 23 of the 30 patients without neurofibromatosis were female.

The hypoglossal nerve arises as a series of rootlets from the rostral medulla in the preolivary sulcus between the inferior olive and the pyramid. The rootlets coalesce and usually form two motor roots which acquire a Schwann cell sheath within 0.1 mm of the brainstem (Tarlov 1937). The roots pass anteriorly, inferiorly, and laterally through the cerebellomedullary cistern toward the hypoglossal canal. Within the cisternal segment the nerve passes over the vertebral artery at the level of the origin of the posterior inferior cerebellar artery. The hypoglossal canal lies inferomedial to the jugular foramen within the occipital bone. In addition to the hypoglossal nerve, the canal usually contains a meningeal artery and a venous plexus. The posterolateral aspect of the canal is bordered by the anteromedial aspect of the occipital condyle. This becomes important in the surgical removal of dumbbell-shaped tumors with extracranial extension. After passing through the canal, the nerve lies between the jugular vein and the carotid artery. It is the only cranial nerve which crosses both the internal and external branches of the carotid artery.

Dysfunction of the hypoglossal nerve alone rarely produces symptoms of concern to the patient. Most patients present with symptoms related to raised intracranial pressure, or mass effects on the brainstem, cerebellum or adjacent lower cranial nerves. Thus headache, often suboccipital or nuchal, is the most common presenting complaint, occurring in 73% of cases (Morelli 1966). This may be associated with nausea, vomiting, or papilledema. This clinical description is especially common in the older literature when the tumors often grew to a large size before diagnosis. Dysfunction of the nerves of the adjacent jugular foramen is common (67%) (Odake 1989) resulting in swallowing difficulty, hoarseness, or hypesthesia of the pharynx. There may be ipsilateral palatal deviation and diminished gag reflex. Limb weakness with spasticity resulting from pyramidal tract compression is present in up to 66% (Odake 1989) of patients. Vestibulocerebellar symptoms such as ataxia, dizziness, vertigo and nystagmus are common. Other symptoms can include facial numbness or weakness, sensorineural hearing loss, or weakness and atrophy of the ipsilateral sternomastoid and trapezius muscles (Table 33.5). The classic finding on examination is that of hemiatrophy of the tongue with fasciculations and ipsilateral deviation on protrusion. This

Table 33.5 Signs and symptoms of twelfth nerve schwannomas

Tongue hemiatrophy	
Headache	73%
IX, X, XI nerve dysfunction	67%
Limb weakness (spastic)	66%
Ataxia, vertigo, nystagmus	
Facial weakness, hearing loss	

finding may be present for many years, but as it produces little difficulty for the patient it is often ignored.

Plain skull radiographs are not helpful. Special tomographic projections of the skull base have been largely replaced by the use of computed tomography, which will sometimes demonstrate enlargement of the hypoglossal

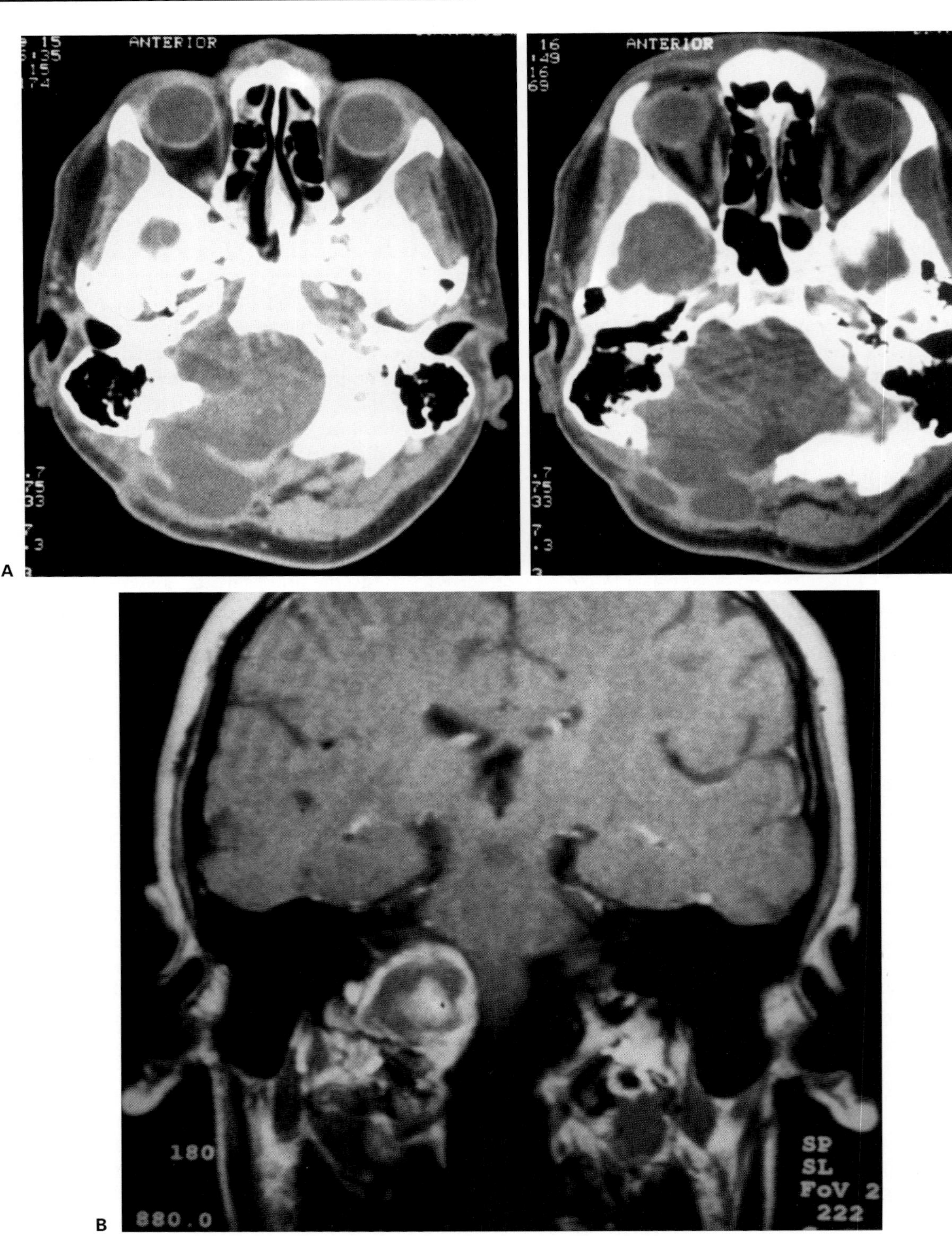

Fig. 33.9A & B

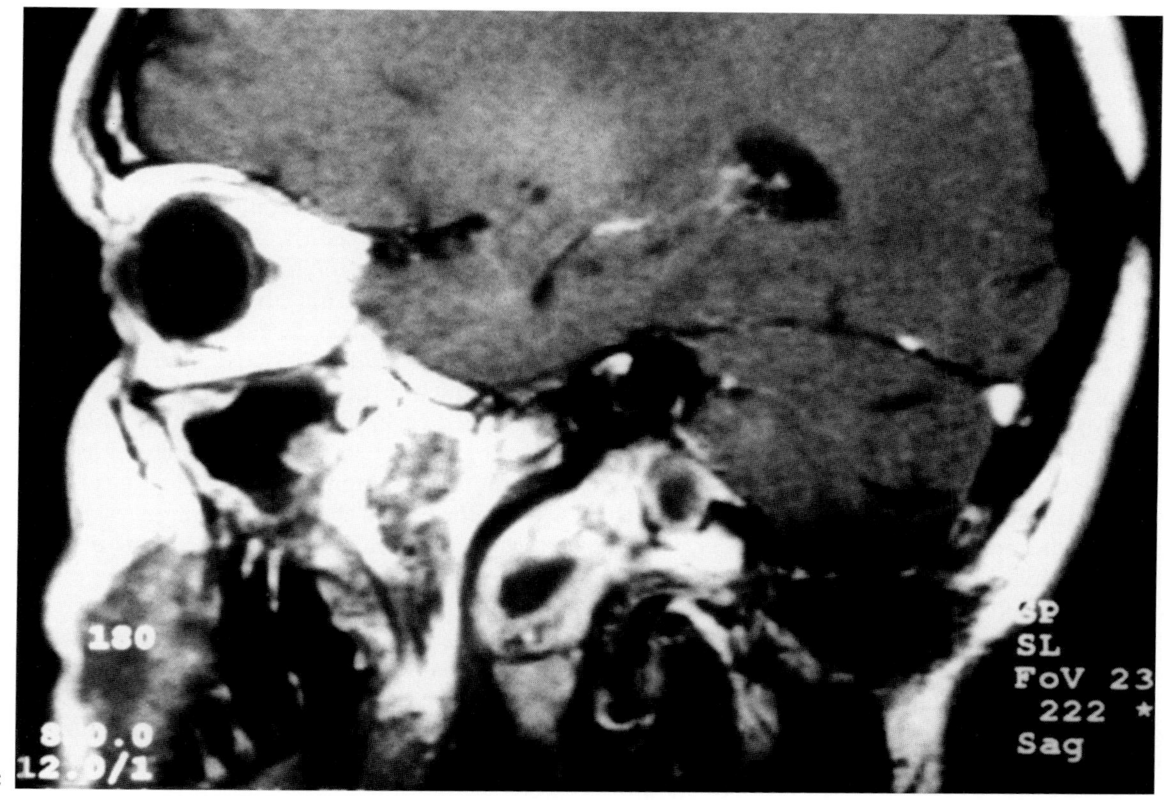

Fig. 33.9 **A.** Axial CT scan demonstrating erosion of the hypoglossal foramen and adjacent skull base secondary to a twelfth nerve schwannoma. **B.** Coronal gadolinium-enhanced MRI demonstrating the same twelfth nerve schwannoma. Note extension through the skull base. **C.** Sagittal gadolinium-enhanced MRI demonstrating the twelfth nerve schwannoma. The extracranial extension is well visualized.

canal; however, the hypoglossal or condylar canal lies in an especially thick region of the occipital bone. Therefore, widening of this skull base foramen is not as common as elsewhere. In some instances the adjacent jugular foramen is eroded, making the differential diagnosis almost impossible (Morelli 1966) (Fig. 33.9A). CT will usually demonstrate an iso- to hyperdense mass ventral to the lower brainstem which enhances homogeneously and intensely following contrast administration. Together with gadolinium-enhanced magnetic resonance, which is the most sensitive means of demonstrating the shape and extent of the soft tissue mass, the surgical approach can be effectively planned (Fig. 33.9A–C). Angiography will demonstrate local vascular displacement, usually elevation of the ipsilateral vertebral artery, by an avascular mass. The jugular bulb and vein are usually not obstructed or infiltrated. This helps to distinguish the hypoglossal from the jugular foramen schwannoma, and from other lesions such as the glomus jugulare tumor.

The surgical approach is dictated largely by the extent of the tumor. Those tumors which appear purely intracranial may be approached through a standard lateral suboccipital craniectomy, as for the acoustic schwannoma (Scott & Wycis 1949, Morelli 1966, Bartal et al 1973). A more direct exposure of the region of the hypoglossal canal can be gained by performing a mastoidectomy and retrolabyrinthine petrosectomy as described by Hakuba et al (1979) for tumors of the jugular foramen (Dolan et al 1982, Odake 1989). Dumbbell-shaped tumors with significant extracranial extension can be removed via an extreme lateral approach, as decribed by Sen & Sekhar (1990). This includes removal of the posterior half of the occipital condyle and lateral mass of C1. Alternatively, dumbbell-shaped tumors can be removed in two stages by combining a standard retrosigmoid craniectomy with a neck dissection. As with schwannomas occurring elsewhere, the tumors are internally debulked prior to any attempt at dissection of the capsule from adjacent neurovascular structures. Most of the cases cited have required the sacrifice of the involved hypoglossal nerve.

Complete surgical extirpation is curative; subtotal resection can be expected to result in recurrence (Odake 1989), although long-term follow-up in many of the cases is lacking. A mortality rate of approximately 7% exists among the reported cases (Odake 1989). Respiratory difficulties with aspiration and pneumonia appeared to be the cause, however, most of these cases preceded the microsurgical era. Morbidity includes CSF leak, meningitis and hydrocephalus. Pre-existing associated lower cranial nerve palsies often do not improve, but brainstem and cerebellar findings can be expected to do so (Odake 1989).

EXTRAOCULAR NERVE SCHWANNOMAS

Schwann cell tumors arising on the intracranial component of the oculomotor, trochlear, or abducens nerve are extremely rare. Approximately 38 cases exist in the literature (Celli et al 1992), consisting of 22 from the oculomotor (Shuangshoti 1975, Hiscott & Symon 1982, Kansu et al 1982, Leunda et al 1982, Okamoto et al 1985, Katsumata et al 1990, Lunardi et al 1990, Mehta et al 1990), 11 from the trochlear (King 1976, Boggan et al 1979, Ho 1981, Garen et al 1987, Yamamoto et al 1987, Maurice-Williams 1989, Celli et al 1992), and 5 from the abducens nerve (Chen 1981, Ginsberg et al 1988). As with schwannomas arising elsewhere, the tumors tend to occur during middle age, with a peak incidence in the fourth and fifth decades. There is a slight female predilection (58% vs 42%) (Celli et al 1992).

The oculomotor nerve arises from the oculomotor sulcus along the medial surface of the cerebral peduncle at the level of the mesencephalon. It passes through the interpeduncular cistern, acquiring a Schwann cell sheath within approximately 0.6 mm of its emergence from the brainstem (Tarlov 1937). It passes inferolaterally, between the posterior cerebral and superior cerebellar arteries toward the cavernous sinus. It enters the roof of the sinus in a triangular-shaped fold of dura formed by the anterior, posterior, and interclinoid ligaments. Passing forward in the superior aspect of the lateral wall of the cavernous sinus, it exits the intracranial cavity through the superior orbital fissure (Fig. 33.3).

The trochlear nerve arises from the dorsal aspect of the brainstem at the level of the pontomesencephalic junction. It emerges from the superior medullary velum just below the inferior colliculus, and acquires a Schwann cell sheath within approximately 0.6 mm (Tarlov 1937). It swings around the brainstem in the ambient cistern, adjacent to the superior cerebellar and cerebral peduncles. Running anteriorly below the free margin of the tentorium, it pierces the dura of the cavernous sinus just behind the posterior clinoid process. It travels forward in the lateral wall of the cavernous sinus below the oculomotor nerve toward the superior orbital fissure.

The abducens nerve emerges from the ventral aspect of the pontomedullary sulcus and heads anteriorly through the prepontine cistern to pierce the dura overlying the dorsum sellae. The glial segment of the nerve is approximately 0.5 mm long (Tarlov 1937). It ascends the rostral clivus between the meningeal and periosteal layers of the dura. It passes through a notch at the base of the posterior clinoid process, below Gruber's ligament, to enter the back of the cavernous sinus. Within the cavernous sinus the nerve lies lateral to the internal carotid artery. It enters the orbit through the superior orbital fissure.

Celli et al (1992) have divided this group of tumors into three categories according to their anatomic extent. This classification scheme is analogous to that devised by Jefferson (1955) for the trigeminal schwannomas. Tumors may be considered cisternal, cavernous, or cisternocavernous (dumbbell-shaped). Unlike schwannomas developing along the other cranial nerves, extraocular schwannomas usually arise far from the glial-Schwann cell junction. Those tumors which lie predominantly in the subarachnoid space around the brainstem are considered cisternal. Those which lie predominantly in the cavernous sinus are considered cavernous. Those tumors which have a significant component in both regions are considered cisternocavernous. Symptoms, signs, and surgical approaches will vary according to the class of tumor.

Oculomotor schwannomas tend to be evenly divided between the cisternal and cavernous types. The majority of oculomotor schwannomas (70%) will present with a third nerve palsy as the initial symptom (Celli et al 1992). When cisternal, they tend to spread upward into the interpeduncular and suprasellar cisterns, resulting in compression of the brainstem, third ventricle and hypothalamus. Patients present with either an isolated parent nerve palsy, or a combination of a parent nerve palsy with signs of brainstem compression. The cavernous variety produces compression of the nerves of the cavernous sinus and occasionally, in addition, the optic nerve, resulting in a cavernous sinus syndrome or orbital apex syndrome, respectively.

Trochlear nerve schwannomas are most often cisternal. They tend to grow upward into the tentorial incisura, or medially into the prepontine or interpeduncular cisterns. Palsy of the parent nerve is an unusually uncommon presenting symptom, occurring in less than half (44%) of patients (Celli et al 1992). Up to one third of patients will actually present with an isolated oculomotor palsy. When the tumors grow to a large size within the ambient cistern, a characteristic clinical syndrome may result which has been called 'ataxic hemiparesis' (Bendheim & Berg 1981). As a consequence of compression of the superior cerebellar and cerebral peduncles, an ipsilateral limb ataxia combined with a contralateral spastic hemiparesis is present.

Abducens schwannomas are most often cisternocavernous. Most will present with a combination of a parent nerve palsy and symptoms/signs of raised intracranial pressure. In addition, there may be a hemiparesis secondary to brainstem compression, or palsies of other nerves within the cavernous sinus. These tumors may be difficult to distinguish from the more common trigeminal schwannoma, which often (20%) presents with a sixth nerve palsy.

Plain film and CT bone windows will demonstrate scalloping of the clinoids, sella, and petrous apex in cisternocavernous tumors. In cavernous lesions there may be widening of the superior orbital fissure or erosion of the middle fossa floor. Cisternal tumors may produce nonspecific changes within the sella if intracranial pressure is elevated. As with schwannomas elsewhere, these tumors tend to enhance following contrast administration. MR imaging may be helpful in distinguishing cisternal schwannomas from intrinsic tumors of the brainstem (Garen et al 1987), and is the most sensitive imaging modality for detecting small lesions.

Cisternal schwannomas of the oculomotor nerve may be approached through a frontotemporal craniotomy as these tumors tend to grow up into the suprasellar cistern. Those of the trochlear nerve may require a subtemporal/transtentorial approach. Occasionally, a cisternal tumor of the trochlear or abducens nerve will lie entirely within the posterior fossa and may be removed via a lateral suboccipital approach. The majority of cisternal tumors can be entirely removed, and the parent nerve clearly identified. Cisternocavernous tumors may be approached either subtemporally or frontotemporally, while cavernous tumors are usually removed via a frontotemporal approach. Newer skull base approaches incorporating an orbitozygomatic osteotomy may prove useful in the management of tumors with a significant cavernous component. To date, only about 50% of these tumors have been completely resected, and the parent nerve has been identified in only half of the cases (Celli et al 1992).

Only one operative mortality has been reported, however, resection nearly always requires sacrifice of the parent nerve, resulting in a permanent extraocular palsy. Despite the large proportion of subtotal resections, there has been only one documented symptomatic recurrence (Vaquero et al 1985). At present, however, insufficient follow-up exists to provide reliable information regarding the incidence or time to recurrence after subtotal resection.

OLFACTORY SCHWANNOMAS

Six case reports of schwannomas arising from the olfactory nerve exist in the literature (Spiller & Hendrickson 1903, Christin & Naville 1920, Molter 1920, Sturm et al 1968, Sehrbundt et al 1973, Ulrich et al 1978). Three of the cases represent solitary schwannomas (Sturm et al 1968, Sehrbundt et al 1973, Ulrich et al 1978) and 3 represent schwannomas arising in conjunction with central neurofibromatosis (Spiller & Hendrickson 1903, Christin & Naville 1920, Molter 1920). The tumors are believed to have arisen on the fila olfactoria, which acquire a Schwann cell sheath approximately 0.5 mm beyond the olfactory bulbs (Tarlov 1937). Very little is known about the epidemiology and clinical manifestations of these tumors. To date, the solitary cases cited have occurred in young males. The tumors have been very large, with anosmia, decreased visual acuity, seizures and evidence of raised intracranial pressure being common findings at the time of presentation. All cases cited precede CT, MRI, and modern microsurgical technique. Given the large size of the tumors at the time of surgery or autopsy, it is difficult to prove an olfactory origin in all the cases cited. A more precise definition of the clinical, radiologic and surgical aspects of these extremely rare tumors awaits further description.

REFERENCES

Abdul-Rahim A S, Savino P J, Zimmerman R A, Sergott R C, Bosley T M 1989 Cryptogenic oculomotor nerve palsy. The need for repeated neuroimaging studies. Archives of Ophthalmology 107: 387–390

Arenberg I K, McCreary H S 1971 Neurilemmoma of the jugular foramen. Laryngoscope 81: 544–577

Arseni C, Dumitrescu L, Constantinescu A 1975 Neurinomas of the trigeminal nerve. Surgical Neurology 4: 497–503

Arumugasamy A, Sarvananthan K, Rudraligam V, Pillary D R P 1972 Intracranial hypoglossal neurinomas: a report of two cases. Journal of Malaya 26: 142–168

Bartal A D, Djaldetti M M, Mandel E M, Lerner H A 1973 Dumbbell neurinoma of the hypoglossal nerve. Journal of Neurology, Neurosurgery, and Psychiatry 36: 592–595

Bendheim P E, Berg B O 1981 Ataxic hemiparesis from a midbrain mass. Annals of Neurology 9: 405–406

Berger M S, Edwards M S B, Bingham W G 1982 Hypoglossal neurinoma: case report and a review of the literature. Neurosurgery 10: 617–620

Boggan J E, Rosenblum M L, Wilson C B 1979 Neurilemmoma of the fourth cranial nerve. Case report. Journal of Neurosurgery 50: 519–521

Bordi L, Compton J, Symon L 1989 Trigeminal neuroma. Surgical Neurology 31: 272–276

Burger P C, Scheithauer B W, Vogel F S 1991 Surgical pathology of the nervous system and its coverings, 3rd edn. Churchill Livingstone, New York

Carstens P H B, Schrodt G R 1969 Malignant transformation of a benign encapsulated neurilemmoma. American Journal of Clinical Pathology. 51: 144–149

Celli P, Ferrante L, Acqui M, Mastronardi L, Fortuna A, Palma L 1992 surgical neurinoma of the third, fourth, and sixth cranial nerves: a survey and report of a new fourth nerve case. Neurology 38: 216–224

Chase N E, Taveras J M 1963 Carotid angiography in the diagnosis of extradural parasellar tumors. Acta Radiologica (Diagn) 1: 214–224

Chen B H 1981 Neurinoma of the abducens nerve. Journal of Nervous and Mental Disease 9: 64–66

Christin E, Naville F 1920 A propos de neurofibromatoses centrales. Leurs formes familiales et hereditaires. Les neurofibromes des nerfs optiques. Cas a evolution atypique. Diversités des structures histologiques (étude clinique et anatomique). Annals of Medicine 8: 30–50

Claesen P, Plets C, Goffin J, Van den Bergh R, Baert A, Wilms G 1989 The glossopharyngeal neurinoma. Clinical Neurology and Neurosurgery 91: 65–69

Cohen H 1937 Glosso-pharyngeal neuralgia. Journal of Laryngology and Otology 52: 527–536

Cohen I 1933 Tumors of the gasserian ganglion. Journal of Nervous and Mental Disease 78: 492–499

Das Gupta T K, Brasfield R D, Strong E W, Hajdu S I 1969 Benign solitary schwannomas (neurilemmomas). Cancer 24: 355–366

Dastur D K, Sinh G, Pandya S K 1967 Melanotic tumor of the acoustic nerve. Journal of Neurosurgery 27: 166–170
de Martel T, Subirana A, Guillaume J 1933 Los tumores de la fossa cerebral posterior: voluminoso neurinoma del hipogloso con desarrollojuxta-bulbo-protuberancial. Operacion-curacion. Ars Medicina 9: 416–419
deBenedittis G, Bernasconi V, Ettore G 1977 Tumors of the fifth cranial nerve. Acta Neurochirurgica 38: 37–64
DiChiro G, Fisher R L, Nelson K B 1964 The jugular foramen. Journal of Neurosurgery 21: 447–460
Dolan E J, Tucker W S, Rotenberg D, Chui M 1982 Intracranial hypoglossal schwannoma as an unusual cause of facial nerve palsy. Journal of Neurosurgery 56: 420–423
Erlandson R A, Woodruff J M 1982 Peripheral nerve-sheath tumors: an electron microscopic study of 43 cases. Cancer 49: 273–287
Findler G, Feinsod M, Sahar A 1983 Trigeminal neurinoma with unusual presentation. Report of a case with trigeminal somatosensory-evoked response. Surgical Neurology 19: 351–353
Fink K H, Early C B, Bryan R N 1978 Glossopharyngeal schwannomas. Surgical Neurology 9: 239–245
Fisch V, Ruttner J 1977 Pathology of intratemporal tumors involving the facial nerve. In: Fisch V (ed) Facial nerve surgery. Aesculapius, Birmingham, pp 448–456
Frazier C H 1918 An operable tumor involving the gasserian ganglion. American Journal of the Medical Sciences 156: 483–490
Fujiwara M, Hachisuga S, Numaguchi Y 1980 Intracranial hypoglossal neurinoma; report of a case. Neuroradiology 20: 87–90
Furlow L T 1960 The neurosurgical aspects of seventh nerve neurilemmoma. Journal of Neurosurgery 17: 721–735
Gacek R R 1976 Schwannoma of the jugular foramen. Annals of Otolaryngology 85: 215–224
Garen P D, Harper C G, Teo C, Johnston I H 1987 Cystic schwannoma of the trochlear nerve mimicking a brain-stem tumor. Case report. Journal of Neurosurgery 67: 928–930
Gerhardt C 1978 Zur Diagnostik multipler Nerombildung. Deutsh Archives Klinical Medecine 21: 268–289
Ghatak N R, Norwood C W, Davis C H 1975 Intracerebral schwannoma. Surgical Neurology 3: 45–47
Gibson A A M, Hendrick E B, Cowen P E 1966 Intracerebral schwannoma: a report of a case. Journal of Neurosurgery 24: 552–557
Ginsberg F, Peyster R G, Rose W S, Drapkin A J 1988 Sixth nerve schwannoma: MR and CT demonstration. Journal of Computer Assisted Tomography 12: 482–484
Goldberg R, Byrd S, Winter J 1980 Varied appearance of trigeminal neuromas on CT. American Journal of Radiology 134: 57–60
Gordy P D 1965 Neurinoma of the gasserian ganglion: report of a case and a review of the literature. Journal of Neurosurgery 22: 90–94
Hakuba A, Hashi K, Fujitani K, Ikuno H, Nakamura T, Inour Y 1979 Jugular foramen neurinomas. Surgical Neurology 11: 83–94
Hanada M, Tanaka T, Kanayama S, Takami M, Kimura M 1982 Malignant transformation of intrathoracic ancient neurilemmoma in a patient without von Recklinghausen's disease. Acta Pathologica Japonica 32: 527–536
Hansman M L, Hoover E D, Peyster R G 1986 Sixth nerve neuroma in the cavernous sinus: CT features. Case report. Journal of Computer Assisted Tomography 10: 1030–1032
Hiscott P, Symon L 1982 An unusual presentation of neurofibroma of the oculomotor nerve. Journal of Neurosurgery 56: 854–856
Ho K L 1981 Schwannoma of the trochlear nerve. Case report. Journal of Neurosurgery 55: 132–135
Holman C B, Olive I, Svien H J 1961 Roentgenologic features of neurofibromas involving the gasserian ganglion. American Journal of Radiology 86: 148–153
Horn K L, Crumley R L, Schindler R A 1981 Facial neurilemmomas. Laryngoscope 91: 1326–1331
House J W, Brackmann D E 1985 Facial nerve grading systems. Otolaryngology Head and Neck Surgery 93: 146–147
House W F, Horn K L, Hitselberger W E 1985 Schwannomas of the jugular foramen. Laryngoscope 95: 761–765
Ignelzi R J, Bucy P C 1967 Intracranial hypoglossal neurofibroma. Journal of Neurosurgery 26: 352–356
Inouye Y, Tabuchi T, Hakuba A et al 1987 Facial nerve neuromas: CT findings. Journal of Computer Assisted Tomography 11: 942–947
Isamat F, Bartumeus F, Mirand A M, Prat J, Pons L C 1975 Neurinomas of the facial nerve: report of three cases. Journal of Neurosurgery 43: 600–613
Jefferson G 1955 The trigeminal neurinomas with some remarks on malignant invasion of the gasserian ganglion. Clinical Neurosurgery 1: 11–54
Johnson M D, Glick A D, Davis B N 1988 Immunohistochemical evaluation of Leu-7, myelin basic-protein, S100-protein, glial fibrillary acidic-protein, and LN3 immunoreactivity in nerve sheath tumors and sarcomas. Archives of Pathology and Laboratory Medicine 112: 155–160
Kansu T, Ozcan O E, Ozdirim E, Onol B, Gurcay O 1982 Neurinoma of the oculomotor nerve. Case report. Journal of Clinical Neurology and Ophthalmology 2: 271–272
Kanter W R, Eldridge R, Fabricant R 1980 Central neurofibromatosis with bilateral acoustic neuroma: genetic, clinical and biochemical distinctions from peripheral neurofibromatosis. Neurology 30: 851–859
Katsumata Y, Maehara T, Noda M, Shirouzu I 1990 Neurinoma of the oculomotor nerve. CT and MR features. Journal of Computer Assisted Tomography 14: 658–661
Kawahara E, Oda Y, Ooi Y, Katsuda S, Nakamishi T, Umeda S 1988 Expression of glial fibrillary acidic protein (GFAP) in peripheral nerve sheath tumors. American Journal of Surgical Pathology 12: 115–120
Kaye A H, Hahn J F, Kinney S E, Hardy R W, Bay J W 1984 Jugular foramen schwannomas. Journal of Neurosurgery 60: 1045–1053
King J S 1976 Trochlear nerve sheath tumor. Case report. Journal of Neurosurgery 44: 245–247
King T T, Morrison A W 1990 Primary facial nerve tumors within the skull. Journal of Neurosurgery 72: 1–8
Knudson V, Kolze V 1972 Neurinoma of the gasserian ganglion and the trigeminal root: report of four cases. Acta Neurochirurgica 26: 159–164
Krayenbuhl H 1936 Primary tumors of the root of the fifth cranial nerve: their distinction from tumors of the gasserian ganglion. Brain 59: 337–352
Kuramitsu T, Seiki Y, Shibata I, Terano H 1986 A case of intracranial hypoglossal neurinoma. No Shinkei Geka 14: 1463–1469
Lesois F, Rousseaux M, Villette 1986 Neurinomas of the trigeminal nerve. Acta Neurochirurgica 82: 118–122
Leunda G, Vaquero J, Cabezudo J, Garcia-Uria J, Bravo G 1982 Schwannoma of the oculomotor nerve. Report of four cases. Journal of Neurosurgery 57: 563–565
Liliequist B, Thulin C A, Tori D, Wilberg A, Ohman J 1972 Neurinoma of the labyrinthine portion of the facial nerve: case report. Journal of Neurosurgery 37: 105–109
Lipkin A F, Coker N J, Jenkins H A, Alford B R 1987 Intracranial and intratemporal facial neuroma. Otolaryngology — Head and Neck Surgery 96: 71–79
Lunardi P, Rocchi G, Rizzo A, Missori P 1990 Neurinoma of the oculomotor nerve. Clinical Neurology and Neurosurgery 92: 333–335
Lunsford L D, Kamerer D B, Flickinger J C 1990 Stereotactic radiosurgery for acoustic neuromas. Archives of Otolaryngology — Head and Neck Surgery 116: 907–909
Maniglia A J, Chandler J R, Goodwin W J Jr, Parker J C 1979 Schwannomas of the parapharyngeal space and jugular foramen. Laryngoscope 89: 1405–1414
Maurice-Williams R S 1989 Isolated schwannoma of the fourth cranial nerve: case report. Journal of Neurology, Neurosurgery and Psychiatry 52: 1442–1443
McCormick P C, Bello J A, Post K D 1988 Trigeminal schwannoma: surgical series of 14 patients and a review of the literature. Journal of Neurosurgery 70: 737–745
McLean C A, Laidlaw J D, Brownbill D S, Gonzales M F 1990 Recurrence of acoustic neurilemmoma as a malignant spindle-cell neoplasm. Journal of Neurosurgery 73: 946–950
Mehta V S, Singh R V P, Misra N K, Choudhary C 1990 Schwannoma of the oculomotor nerve. British Journal of Neurosurgery 4: 69–72

Mello L R, Tanzer A 1972 Some aspects of trigeminal neurinomas. Neuroradiology 4: 215–221

Molter K 1920 Uber gleichzeitige cerebrale, medullare und periphere. Neurofibromatosis (Inauguraldissertation, Universitat zu Jena). Wendt und Klauwell, Jena

Morelli R J 1966 Intracranial neurilemmoma of the hypoglossal nerve: review and case report. Neurology 158: 709–713

Mountjoy J R, Dolan K D, McCabe B F 1974 Neurilemmoma of the ninth nerve masquerading as an acoustic neuroma. Archives of Otolaryngology 100: 65–67

Murata T, Hakuba A, Okumura T et al 1985 Intrapetrous neurinomas of the facial nerve: report of three cases. Journal of Neurosurgery 23: 507–512

Nager G T 1984 Neurinomas of the trigeminal nerve. American Journal of Otolaryngology 5: 301–331

Naunton R F, Proctor L, Elpern B S 1969 The audiologic signs of ninth nerve neurinoma. Archives of Otolaryngology 87: 20–25

Neely J G, Alford B R 1974 Facial nerve neuromas. Archives of Otolaryngology 100: 298–301

New P F J 1972 Intracerebral schwannoma: case report. Journal of Neurosurgery 36: 795–797

O'Donoghue G M, Brackmann D E, House J W, Jackler R K 1989 Neuromas of the facial nerve. The American Journal of Otology 10: 49–54

Odake G 1989 Intracranial hypoglossal neurinoma with extracranial extension: review and case report. Neurosurgery 24: 583–587

Ohl M, Ohara S, Tokita T, Ikeda O, Oyama K 1988 Huge jugular foramen neuroma extending to the pharyngeal region: a case report. No Shinkei Geka 6: 763–767

Okamoto S, Handa H, Yamashita J 1985 Neurinoma of the oculomotor nerve. Surgical Neurology 24: 275–278

Olive I, Svien H J 1957 Neurifibromas of the fifth cranial nerve. Journal of Neurosurgery 14: 484–505

Palacios E, MacGee E E 1972 The radiographic diagnosis of trigeminal neurinomas. Journal of Neurosurgery 36: 153–156

Peet M M 1927 Tumor of the gasserian ganglion. With the report of two cases of extra-cranial carcinoma infiltrating the ganglion by direct extension through the maxillary division. Surgery, Gynecology and Obstetrics 44: 202–207

Pluchino F, Crivelli G, Vaghi M A 1975 Intracranial neurinomas of the nerves of the jugular foramen. Acta Neurochirurgica 31: 201–221

Pollack I F, Sekhar L N, Jannetta P J, Janecka I P 1989 Neurilemmomas of the trigeminal nerve. Journal of Neurosurgery 17: 306–322

Pool J L, Pava A A 1970 Acoustic nerve tumors. Charles C Thomas, Springfield, Ill

Prakash B, Roy S, Tandon P N 1980 Schwannoma of the brain stem. Case report. Journal of Neurosurgery 53: 121–123

Pulec J L 1969 Facial nerve tumors. Annals of Otology, Rhinology, and Laryngology 78: 962–982

Pulec J L 1972 Symposium on ear surgery. II. Facial nerve neuroma. Laryngoscope 82: 1160–1176

Rigamonti D, Spetzler R F, Shetter A, Drayer B P 1987 Magnetic resonance imaging and trigeminal schwannoma. Surgical Neurology 28: 67–70

Robey S S, deMent S H, Eaton K K, Aoun H 1987 Malignant epithelioid peripheral nerve sheath tumor arising in a benign schwannoma. Surgical Neurology 28: 441–446

Robinson J S, Lopes J, Moody R 1979 Intrcranial hypoglossal neurinoma. Surgical Neurology 12: 496–498

Rosenblum B, Davis R, Camins M 1987 Middle fossa facial schwannoma removed via the intracranial extradural approach: case report and review of the literature. Neurosurgery 21: 739–741

Rubinstein L J 1972 Tumors of the central nervous system. Armed Forces Institute of Pathology, Washington

Saito H, Baxter H 1972 Undiagnosed intratemporal facial nerve neurilemmomas. Archives of Otolaryngology 95: 415–419

Salvati M, Ciapetta P, Raco A, Capone R, Artico M, Santoro A 1992 Radiation-induced schwannomas of the neuraxis. Report of three cases. Tumori 78: 143–146

Schisano G, Olivecrona H 1960 Neurinomas of the gasserian ganglion and trigeminal root. Journal of Neurosurgery 17: 306–322

Schmidt C 1931 Neurinom des nervus facialis. Zentralblatt Hals Nas-Ohrenheilk 16: 329

Schuknecht H F, Gulya A J 1986 Anatomy of the temporal bone with surgical implications. Lea & Feiberger, Philadelphia

Scott M, Wycis H 1949 Intracranial neurinoma of the hypoglossal nerve, successful removal, case report. Journal of Neurosurgery 6: 333–336

Sehrbundt V, Pau A, Turtas S 1973 Olfactory groove neurinomas. Journal of Neurosurgical Sciences 17: 193–196

Sekhar L N 1987 Operative management of tumors involving the cavernous sinus. In: Sekhar L N, Schramm V L Jr (eds) Tumors of the cranial base: diagnosis and treatment. Futura Publishing, Mt Kisco, NY, pp 393–419

Sen C N, Sekhar L N 1990 An extreme lateral approach to intradural lesions of the cervical spine and foramen magnum. Neurosurgery 27: 197–204

Shambaugh G E, Arenberg I K, Barney P L, Vasvassori G E 1969 Facial neurinomas: a study of four diverse cases. Archives of Otolaryngology 90: 742–755

Shiroyama Y, Inoue S, Tshua M, Abiko S, Aoki H 1988 Intracranial neurinomas of the jugular foramen and hypoglossal canal. No Shinkei Geka 16: 313–319

Shuangshoti S 1975 Neurilemmoma of the oculomotor nerve. British Journal of Ophthalmology 59: 64–66

Spiller W G, Hendrickson W F 1903 A report of two cases of multiple sarcomatosis of the central nervous system and one case of intramedullary primary sarcoma of the spinal cord. American Journal of the Medical Sciences 126: 10–33

Stout A P 1935 Peripheral manifestations of a specific nerve sheath tumor (neurilemmoma). American Journal of Cancer 24: 751–796

Sturm K, Bohnis G, Kosmaoglu V 1968 Uber ein Neurinom der Lamina cribrosa. Zentralblatt Fur Neurochirurgiebl 29: 217–222

Suzuki F, Hanada J, Todo G 1989 Intracranial glossopharyngeal neurinomas. Report of two cases with special emphasis on computer tomography and magnetic resonance imaging findings. Surgical Neurology 13: 390–394

Sweasey T A, Edelstein S R, Hoff J T 1991 Glossopharyngeal schwannoma: review of five cases and the literature. Surgical Neurology 35: 127–130

Symon L, Cheesman A D, Kawauchi M, Bordi L 1993 Neuromas of the facial nerve: a report of 12 cases. British Journal of Neurosurgery 7: 13–22

Takayasu M, Shibuya M, Suzuki Y 1987 Trigeminal sensory evoked potentials in patients with trigeminal neurinoma: report of two cases. Neurosurgery 20: 453–456

Tan L C, Bordi L, Symon L, Cheesman A D 1990 Jugular foramen neuroma: a review of 14 cases. Surgical Neurology 34: 205–211

Tarlov I M 1937 Structure of the nerve root. II. Differentiation of sensory from motor roots; observations on identification of function in roots of mixed cranial nerves. Archives of Neurology and Psychiatry 37: 1338–1355

Tew J M, Yen H, Miller G W, Shahbabian S 1983 Intratemporal schwannoma of the facial nerve. Neurosurgery 13: 186–188

Tuck R R, Mokri B, Cilluffo J M 1984 Intracranial schwannoma of the hypoglossal nerve. Archives of Neurology 41: 502–505

Ulrich J, Levy A, Pfister C 1978 Schwannoma of the olfactory groove. Case report and review of previous cases. Acta Neurochirurgica 40: 315–321

Ulso C, Sehested J, Overgaard J 1981 Intracranial hypoglossal neurinoma: Diagnosis and post-operative care. Surgical Neurology 16: 65–68

VanRensberg M J, Proctor N S, Danzinger J, Orelowitz M S 1975 Temporal lobe epilepsy due to an intracerebral schwannoma: case report. Journal of Neurology, Neurosurgery and Psychiatry 38: 703–709

Vaquero J, Martinez R, Salazar J 1985 Suprasellar recurrence of a third nerve neurinoma (letter). Journal of Neurosurgery 62: 317

Verocay J 1910 Zur kenntnis der neurofibrome. Beitrage Zur Pathologischen Anatomie Und Zur Allgemeinen Pathologie 48: 1–69

Wallner K E, Sheline G E, Pitts L H, Wara W M, Davis R I, Boldrey E B 1987 Efficacy of irradiation for incompletely excised acoustic neurilemmomas. Journal of Neurosurgery 67: 858–863

Westberg G 1963 Angiographic changes in neurinoma of the trigeminal nerve. Acta Radiologica (Diagn) 1: 513–520

White W, Shiu M H, Roseblum M K, Erlandson R A, Woodruff J M 1990 Cellular schwannoma: a clinicopathologic study of 57 patients and 58 tumors. Cancer 66: 1266–1275
Williams J M, Fox J L 1962 Neurinoma of the intracranial portion of the hypoglossal nerve: review and case report. Journal of Neurosurgery 19: 248–250
Woodruff J M, Godwin T A, Erlandson R A, Susin M, Martini N 1981 Cellular schwannoma. American Journal of Surgical Pathology 5: 733–744
Yajima K, Nakazawa S, Itagaki S 1981 Intracranial hypoglossal neurinoma. No Shinkei Geka 9: 669–680
Yamamoto M, Jimbo M, Ide M, Kubo O 1987 Trochlear neurinoma. Surgical Neurology 28: 287–290
Yousem S A, Colby T V, Urich H 1985 Malignant epithelioid schwannoma arising in a benign schwannoma. Cancer 55: 2799–2803
Zulch K J 1962 Brain tumors: their biology and pathology. Springer-Verlag, New York

34. Brain tumors associated with neurofibromatosis

Vincent M. Riccardi

INTRODUCTION

The neurofibromatoses include both the well-recognized forms, currently designated NF-1 (von Recklinghausen disease) and NF-2 (bilateral acoustic neurinomas), as well as other less well-characterized forms, such as that limited to a single body quadrant (NF-5 or segmental neurofibromatosis) and that with a distinctively late adult onset (NF-7) (Riccardi 1982, Riccardi 1992a). This chapter will deal primarily with NF-1 and NF-2, noting the other forms of neurofibromatosis (NF) only occasionally for making specific points; for additional reading on these alternative forms, the reader is referred elsewhere (Riccardi 1992a). Other forms of familial brain tumors (Ikizler et al 1992) are not considered in this presentation.

NF-1

As adults, virtually 100% of patients with NF-1 have the triad of café-au-lait spots, cutaneous neurofibromata, and iris Lisch nodules. Other features of the disorder include a wide variety of, but nonetheless characteristic, features, such as skeletal dysplasias, vascular dysplasias, learning disabilities, seizures, and other types of neural crest tumors, for example, pheochromocytomas. For children in the first decade of life, particularly the first half, the clinical features are more variable in their frequency. Many of these children may have café-au-lait spots, with or without skin-fold freckling, as the sole feature of the disorder. Conversely, however, many children, as well as adults with NF-1, have multiple features of the disorder that leave little doubt as to diagnosis at the time of initial presentation (Riccardi 1992b).

Central nervous system tumors occur in about 15% of patients with NF-1. Almost all such tumors are intracranial astrocytomas, although spinal cord astrocytomas do occur rarely. While there have been occasional reports of intracranial ependymomas and meningiomas as part of NF-1, these reports are generally unconvincing that the basic diagnosis is actually NF-1; that is, the NF diagnosis is, in such instances, NF-2 or yet another form of NF (Rodriguez & Berthrong 1966). The rare finding of acoustic neurinomas (i.e. vestibular schwannomas) among patients with bona fide NF-1 is a special matter, discussed more completely below. Neurofibrosarcoma, which may complicate the course of NF-1 in 6% or so of patients (Riccardi & Powell 1989), often metastasizes to the brain, however, neurofibrosarcoma will not be considered further in this chapter.

Of the intracranial astrocytomas that characterize NF-1, there are three distinct varieties: optic pathway glioma, posterior fossa glioma, and cerebral hemisphere glioma. The question whether some of these lesions represent not 'tumors' in a strict sense, but rather 'hamartomas', has been a source of controversy for some time (Hoyt & Baghdassarian 1969, Imes & Hoyt 1986). For the most part, this potential distinction revolved around the clinical behavior of the lesion in question: did it behave like a static lesion (hamartoma) or was it a progressive lesion, more typical of an actively growing tumor per se? More recently, however, the finding of hyperintense T2-weighted signals in the basal ganglia, periventricular white matter, brainstem and cerebellum of young patients with NF-1 (Mirowitz et al 1989, Sevick et al 1992) has added another level to the concern about hamartoma as part of this disorder. In their reports of brain MRI studies of young patients with NF-1, many neuroradiologists designate such lesions as representing hamartomas. At the present time, however, there is no basis for referring to this MRI phenomenon as a hamartoma and there is even less cogency for considering it to be a precursor of tumors of any sort. On the other hand, the true nature of these hyperintense T2-weighted signals is not at all clear.

There is no consistent association of NF-1 gliomas with other variable features of the disorder. Likewise, the different types of NF-1 gliomas appear to occur independently of each other. Intracranial astrocytomas are very rarely, if ever, a feature of NF-2.

Molecular biology

The molecular biology of NF-1 has been very exciting, with remarkably rapid developments over the last five years or so. The NF-1 locus has been known since 1987 (Barker et al 1987, Diehl et al 1987) and details of its structure have been known since 1990 (Collins et al 1989, Xu et al 1990, Yagle et al 1990). The gene is large, spanning 350 kilobases or more of DNA (Gutmann & Collins 1992). The resultant protein, *neurofibromin* (Huynh et al 1992, Golubic et al 1992), apparently occurs in two forms (Baizer et al 1992), with differential expression — that is, regulated tissue-specific alternative splicing (Teinturier et al 1992). Expression of the NF-1 gene in brain tumors and surrounding normal brain is different (Mochizuki et al 1992). In NF-1, neurofibromin has been detected immunologically and by Northern blotting in all tumor types except for neurofibrosarcomas. Although there is speculation that the NF-1 gene functions as a tumor suppressor gene, similar, for example, to the NF-2 gene or the p53 gene, proof has been wanting. Loss of heterozygosity for the p53 gene appears to be part of the development and progression of gliomas (El-Azouzi et al 1989, Fults et al 1992), though to what extent this is relevant to the astrocytomas or gliomas of NF-1, and particularly the latter disorder's optic pathway gliomas is not clear (Von Deimling et al 1992).

A gene 'knockout' mouse model (involving a mutation at the mouse locus paralogous to the human NF-1 locus), interestingly, does not manifest brain tumors either in the heterozygote or in the homozygote, although the latter do not survive embryologic development (Jacks et al 1992). On the other hand, mutations at the paralogous *Drosophila melanogaster* locus are said to cause a developmental disorder 'similar' to NF (Hackstein 1992).

Optic pathway glioma

It has been relatively well established for several years that optic pathway gliomas occurred with a frequency of 15% among patients with NF-1, with one third of those tumors being symptomatic one way or another (Lewis et al 1984). Since then, other groups have corroborated these findings (Listernick et al 1989, Lund & Skovby 1991).

As noted above, there has been controversy for many years whether NF-1 optic pathway gliomas were merely hamartomas or true tumors, the latter designation indicating a progressively enlarging lesion, necessarily leading ultimately to symptoms. A hamartoma presumably would be clinically benign, not actually a cause of significant symptoms, if any symptoms at all. Histopathologically, almost all NF-1 optic pathway gliomas are characterized as 'grade II pilocytic astrocytoma' (Daumas-Duport et al 1988, Cutarelli et al 1991, Ito et al 1992, Wang & Ho 1992). This histologic diagnosis is quite distinct from that of other histologic grades or types of astrocytomas. In particular, indolent, slow progression, if any, is expected. The notion that NF-1 optic pathway gliomas may be histologically different from other pilocytic astrocytomas (Stern et al 1980) has not been confirmed (Rush et al 1982). Approximately two thirds of NF-1 optic pathway gliomas are relatively static lesions, with little or no growth, and do not cause symptoms. In those that do cause symptoms, the nature of the symptoms depends primarily on the location of the lesion or lesions along the optic pathway.

All portions of the optic pathway can be involved, from the immediate retrobulbar region of the optic nerve through the chiasm and optic tracts to the farthest reaches of the optic radiations. The lesions may be unilateral or bilateral. Tumors of the optic nerves per se may be asymptomatic or cause varying degrees of visual impairment, from merely restricted visual fields to total blindness in the involved eye. Tumors of the optic chiasm may also be asymptomatic or cause visual compromise, and may be associated as well with hypothalamic-pituitary disturbances, including the Russell diencephalic syndrome or precocious puberty (or, less often, delayed puberty). The true frequency of puberty disturbances in association with chiasmal gliomas is not clear, but this author presumes the risk to be in the range of 5–10% among patients with NF-1 and a chiasmal glioma. It is uncertain whether short stature without an unequivocal growth hormone deficiency is related to optic chiasm gliomas. In the vast majority of instances, the short stature associated with NF-1 has no tumor or other specifiable basis. Tumor involvement of the optic tracts or optic radiations may, again, be asymptomatic or be associated with varying degrees of visual loss. Whether such lesions contribute to the visual-motor deficits that characterize the learning disabilities of patients with NF-1 is unknown. Visual compromise or strabismus in a youngster with NF-1 should prompt a rapid evaluation for an optic pathway glioma, in the hope of identifying a tumor still amenable to treatment. Preferably, presymptomatic screening will increasingly obviate the need to rely on the presence of irreversible compromise as an indicator of the tumor's presence (see below).

Lesions may be identified at any age. The key for clinical management, however, is not merely the presence of the lesion, but, rather, the combination of current symptoms and apparent rate of progression. The point is that treatment other than monitoring is based on progression over time, either in terms of specific symptoms or in terms of neuroimaging.

An adult with NF-1 who is free of an optic pathway glioma will almost certainly remain free of this tumor. If an optic pathway glioma shows up at all, it will do so during childhood. It is not clear at what point in childhood the 'cut-off' period lies. On the other hand, it is now clear that a normal neuroimaging study in early childhood does not preclude subsequent development. From this author's experience, the first birthday may represent a reasonable measuring point (Riccardi 1992a). Thus, if the neuroimaging study is negative after 1 year of age, it is likely to remain so. This estimation obviously involves considerable guesswork, and some investigators prefer to be more conservative and use a 5-year-old cut-off (Listernick et al 1992).

Treatment remains controversial (Easley et al 1988, Sanford et al 1991, Shapiro 1992), but there is no doubt in the author's mind that properly timed treatment can be effective (Wright et al 1989, Bataini et al 1991, Riccardi 1992a). The key is proper timing, specifically prior to the development of irreversible symptoms, such as blindness. The treatment choices include *surgery* (for optic nerve tumors (Wilson 1988) or drainage and marsupialization of cystic enlargements of chiasmal tumors), *chemotherapy* to avoid radiotherapy in a very young child (Rosenstock et al 1985, Kretschmar & Linggood 1991), and *radiotherapy* (Gould et al 1987, Pierce et al 1990).

The combination of the need to treat before symptoms become irreversible and the acknowledged efficacy of all three modes of therapy serves to substantiate the case for screening of all young patients with NF-1 for presymptomatic optic pathway gliomas. The author continues to favor the approach that seeks to minimize the frequency and burden of one of the serious types of handicap that can be caused by NF-1, namely blindness, partial or complete (Riccardi 1988b, Listernick et al 1989, Lund & Skovby 1991, Riccardi 1992a).

Posterior fossa glioma

As part of NF-1, gliomas of the posterior fossa occur in two distinct locations, the brainstem and the cerebellum. In either location the lesions may be of the relatively static type II pilocytic variety or more aggressive tumors, including those of the type IV anaplastic variety. It is these latter types that contribute to untimely deaths among patients with NF-1. There may be an excess of such tumors among women with NF-1 (Sorensen et al 1986). It is estimated that about 1% of all patients with NF-1 have a posterior fossa glioma, about one third to one half of which become symptomatic.

If a posterior fossa tumor is identified on the basis of screening neuroimaging, it is uncertain whether there will be progression and compromise of health. Serial monitoring with clinical neurologic examinations and neuroimaging is appropriate. Conversely, it is uncertain whether a normal neuroimaging study in an older child or adult precludes the subsequent development of a posterior fossa glioma, as might be the case for optic pathway gliomas.

Presentation is usually on the basis of hydrocephalus and its associated findings, headaches, cerebellar ataxia, or a combination of such problems. Treatment, if called for, usually involves both surgery and irradiation.

Cerebral hemisphere glioma

As part of NF-1, gliomas of the cerebral hemispheres occur in 0.5% or less of the patients, and are identified primarily as a coincidental finding on neuroimaging, done on a screening basis or as part of an evaluation for seizures. Although these tumors are not usually treated surgically, one patient's temporal lobe lesion (associated with focal seizures) was considered to be a grade II pilocytic astrocytoma.

One interesting patient was reported because of the de novo development of a temporal lobe astrocytoma subsequent to immunosuppressive therapy following a heart transplant (Wijdicks et al 1990).

NF-2

The defining feature of NF-2 has been bilateral vestibular schwannomas, although other central nervous system tumors have frequently been present as well (Martuza & Eldridge 1988). In the last five years or so, ocular features have assumed special importance, allowing for clinical diagnosis of the condition long before the central nervous tumors might present (Landau et al 1990, Kaye et al 1992). Retinal astrocytomas (Landau et al 1990) and posterior subcapsular and other types of cataracts (Kaiser-Kupfer et al 1989) are seen in well over half, and more probably upwards of 80% or so of patients with NF-2. Although bilateral vestibular schwannomas are a defining feature of NF-2 (National Institutes of Health 1988), tending to homogenize the patients to some degree, and linkage to the 22q locus is consistent (Narod et al 1992), there does appear to be more than one type of NF-2 (Evans et al 1992a,b). More clinical investigation is needed in this regard.

Vestibular schwannoma

The so-called acoustic neurinoma of NF-2 (or that occurring sporadically, for that matter) is actually a vestibular schwannoma. Other designations for such tumors include neurinoma and neurilemmoma, neither of which is as specific as the term schwannoma; these tumors are comprised of densely packed Schwann cells.

Vestibular schwannomas are slowly growing tumors that arise primarily at the internal ostium of the internal auditory canal. They apparently can develop at any age, though their presence in children in their first decade of life is distinctly unusual. Even as part of NF-2, their onset is almost always after the first decade of life, and most often in the second, third and fourth decades (Martuza & Eldridge 1988, Evans et al 1992a,b). Symptoms include hearing deficits, tinnitus, cerebellar ataxia, headache, and ipsilateral facial nerve weakness. Most often the presenting symptoms are unilateral, even if bilateral tumors are present. Pregnancy may aggravate a presymptomatic tumor, leading, for example, to tinnitus, hearing loss, headache, or all of these symptoms. Adverse effects of birth control pills are less well established, but caution is advised.

The preferred diagnostic technique for identifying small tumors is MRI scanning with gadolinium contrast enhancement (Aoki et al 1989, Jackler et al 1990, Duvoisin et al 1991, Kanzaki et al 1991). Hearing assessment with brainstem auditory evoked response (BAER) studies is also useful, primarily for monitoring the functional significance of the respective tumors and thereby for making decisions about the timing of treatment.

The details of treatment are beyond the scope of this chapter. It is clear, however, that surgery appears to be the routine treatment of choice, the specific technique also being a factor in the outcome (Kemink et al 1991, Eldridge & Parry 1992, Harper et al 1992, Nadol et al 1992). Stereotactic radiotherapy is an alternative approach (Steiner et al 1989, Linskey et al 1992). Routine types of radiotherapy or systemic chemotherapy are not ordinary options.

Molecular biology. Since 1986 the locus for NF-2 has been known to be on chromosome 22 (Seizinger et al 1986, Rouleau et al 1987), determined in part from showing loss of heterozygosity for portions of the long arm of that chromosome in vestibular schwannomas that occur sporadically, separate from NF-2, or in such tumors occurring as part of NF-2. The gene for NF-2 was specifically identified and its characterization begun in early 1993 (Bianchi et al 1994). Even before its isolation, the NF-2 gene was considered to be a tumor suppressor gene, largely reflecting the relatively consistent loss of heterozygosity at this locus in schwannomas and other tumors typical of NF-2 (Seizinger et al 1986). This aspect of the NF-2 gene is considered to be a key aspect of devising genetic engineering treatment approaches to the brain tumors characteristic of the disorder (Martuza 1992).

Other cranial nerve schwannomas

After the vestibular nerve, the *trigeminal nerve* is the most likely site for an intracranial schwannoma in NF-2, also at its middle fossa bony ostium. It is of interest that in several animal models of NF in which intracranial schwannomas occur, including the bicolor damselfish (Schmale et al 1983, Riccardi 1992a), HTLV-I *tax* gene transgenic mice (Hinrichs et al 1987), and transplacental exposure to ethylnitrosourea (Riccardi 1988a), the trigeminal nerve is also a consistent site manifesting the disorder. The *facial nerve* may be involved, either by impingement of an adjacent vestibular schwannoma or by a tumor of the nerve itself. The *oculomotor*, *trochlear*, and *abducens nerves* all may be compromised in NF-2, though it is uncertain whether it is always on the basis of a schwannoma per se — as opposed, for example, to a meningioma. The point nonetheless is that cranial nerve involvement in NF-2 extends beyond the vestibular nerve. In particular, several children with NF-2, whose earliest symptoms were due to ocular palsies from tumor involvement of cranial nerves III, IV, VI, or VII, or various combinations thereof, have been treated by the author.

Meningioma

One or multiple meningiomas may be the presenting tumor of NF-2. The meningioma may involve the spinal cord or any portion of the intracranial meninges. Optic nerve meningiomas may compromise vision and otherwise appear to represent optic nerve gliomas (Cunliffe et al 1992). More often, however, NF-2 meningiomas occur over the cerebral hemispheres at just about any site; they may be present at more than one location, either simultaneously or sequentially.

Presentation is often with headache, and, as with vestibular schwannomas, pregnancy may lead to aggravation of an otherwise silent tumor. Birth control pills perhaps are more solidly contraindicated for this tumor of NF-2.

Molecular biology. Loss of heterozygosity for a portion of the long arm of chromosome 22 in meningiomas from patients with NF-2 led to the identification of the site of the NF-2 locus (Seizinger et al 1986, 1987). In addition, there is a second, perhaps meningioma-specific locus near, but not identical with, the NF-2 locus (Dumanski et al 1990, Cogen et al 1991, Sanson et al 1992). The interplay, if any, between these two loci in the initiation and progression is not known.

Ependymoma

Ependymomas may occur within the spinal cord, as well as in the brain of patients with NF-2. When they occur in or about the brainstem they can be particularly troublesome. At least several percent of patients with NF-2 develop ependymomas. The clinical behavior of NF-2 ependymomas is no different from such tumors occurring independently of NF-2.

Spinal cord astrocytoma

Spinal cord astrocytomas are mentioned here for two reasons. One is because this tumor may occur so high in the spinal cord as to be essentially a brainstem tumor, that is, a low posterior fossa tumor. Another reason for focusing on spinal cord astrocytomas is to emphasize that such tumors are distinctly unusual in NF-1.

NF-3

The patterns of tumors described above for NF-1 and NF-2 are more or less mutually exclusive: the presence of a true optic pathway glioma inclines the diagnosis away from NF-2 and toward NF-1; conversely, the presence of unilateral or bilateral vestibular schwannomas — or meningioma, or ependymoma, or spinal cord astrocytoma — inclines the diagnosis away from NF-1 and toward NF-2. Do these patterns of tumors ever occur together? And if they do, what is the diagnosis?

If both patterns of tumors are present simultaneously in a single patient (or perhaps in a single family) the logical nosologic choices are:

a. *NF-1* with one or more features of NF-2;
b. *NF-2* with one or more features of NF-1;
c. *NF-3*, a distinct disorder comprising features of both NF-1 and NF-2 (Riccardi 1982, 1992a); or
d. the *coincidental* presence of both *NF-1 and NF-2*, as has already been reported in at least one instance (Sadeh et al 1989).

For possibility (a), one would have to show that the chromosome 17 long arm locus of NF-1 was mutated — i.e. that the mutation was an allele for NF-1 — while no mutation was detectable at the NF-2 locus. If the vestibular schwannoma was unilateral, it is also possible that it was simply a sporadic vestibular schwannoma merely coincidental to the NF-1. For possibility (b), the obverse would be required: that the chromosome 22 long arm locus NF-2 was mutated — i.e. that the mutation was an allele for NF-2 — while no mutation was detectable at the NF-1 locus. For possibility (c), there would be no detectable mutation at either the NF-1 locus or the NF-2 locus, but rather a third locus would be identified. To my knowledge, no such case has been reported.

Most cases of bone fide NF-1 said to have an acoustic neurinoma turn out not to have the latter tumor at all, but, rather, another type of tumor, including a neurofibroma, in the posterior fossa. Similarly, most cases of bone fide NF-2 said to have an optic pathway glioma have another type of tumor, usually an optic nerve meningioma (Cunliffe et al 1992). On the other hand, there do appear to be several instances of apparent NF-1 with unilateral or bilateral vestibular schwannomas (Michels et al 1989). Resolution of the problem at the molecular level is still pending.

REFERENCES

Aoki S, Barkovich A J, Nishimura K et al 1989 Neurofibromatosis types 1 and 2: Cranial MRI findings. Radiology 172: 527–534

Baizer L, Ciment G S, Stocker K M, Schafer G L 1992 Expression of alternatively sliced forms of neurofibromin mRNA in the chick embryo. Society Neuroscience Abstracts 18 (part 2): 1447 (abstract)

Barker D, Wright E, Nguyen K et al 1987 Gene for von Recklinghausen neurofibromatosis is in the pericentromeric region of chromosome 17. Science 236: 1100–1102

Bataini J P, Delanian S, Ponvert D 1991 Chiasmal gliomas: Results of irradiation management in 57 patients and review of literature. International Journal of Radiation Oncology, Biology, and Physics 21: 615–623

Bianchi A B, Hara T, Ramesh V et al 1994 Mutations in transcript isoforms of the neurofibromatosis 2 gene in multiple human tumor types. Nature Genetics 6: 185–192

Cogen P H, Daneshvar L, Bowcock A M, Metzger A K, Cavalli-Sforza L L 1991 Loss of heterozygosity for chromosome 22 DNA sequences in human meningioma. Cancer Genetics and Cytogenetics 53: 271–277

Collins F S, Ponder B A J, Seizinger B R, Epstein C J 1989 The von Recklinghausen neurofibromatosis region on chromosome 17 — genetic and physical maps come into focus. American Journal of Human Genetics 44: 1–5

Cunliffe I A, Moffat D A, Hardy D G, Moore A T 1992 Bilateral optic nerve sheath meningiomas in a patient with neurofibromatosis type 2. British Journal of Ophthalmology 76: 310–312

Cutarelli P E, Roessmann U R, Miller R H, Specht C S, Grossniklaus H E 1991 Immunohistochemical properties of human optic nerve glioma: Evidence of type 1 astrocyte origin. Investigative Ophthalmology and Visual Sciences 32: 2521–2524

Daumas-Duport C, Scheithauer B W, O'Fallon J, Kelly P 1988 Grading of astrocytomas: a simple and reproducible method. Cancer 62: 2152–2165

Diehl S R, Boehnke M, Erickson R P et al 1987 Linkage analysis of von Recklinghausen neurofibromatosis to DNA markers on chromsosome 17. Genomics 1: 361–363

Dumanski J P, Rouleau G A, Nordenskjöld M, Collins V P 1990 Molecular genetic analysis of chromosome 22 in 81 cases of meningioma. Cancer Research 50: 5863–5867

Duvoisin B, Fernandes J, Doyon D, Denys A, Sterkers J-M, Bobin S 1991 Magnetic resonance findings in 92 acoustic neuromas. European Journal of Radiology 13: 96–102

Easley J D, Scharf L, Chou J L, Riccardi M D 1988 Controversy in the management of optic pathway glioma. 29 patients treated at the Baylor College of Medicine from 1967 through 1987. Neurofibromatosis 1: 248–251

El-Azouzi M, Chung R Y, Farmer G E et al 1989 Loss of distinct regions on the short arm of chromosome 17 associated with tumorigenesis of human astrocytomas. Proceedings of the National Academy of Science USA 86: 7186–7190

Eldridge R, Parry D 1992 Vestibular schwannoma (acoustic neuroma). Consensus Development Conference. Neurosurgery 30: 962–964

Evans D G R, Huson S M, Donnai D et al 1992a A genetic study of type 2 neurofibromatosis in the United Kingdom. II. Guidelines for genetic counselling. Journal of Medical Genetics 29: 847–852

Evans D G R, Huson S M, Donnai D et al 1992b A genetic study of type 2 neurofibromatosis in the United Kingdom. I. Prevalence, mutation rate, fitness, and the confirmation of maternal transmission effect on severity. Journal of Medical Genetics 29: 841–846

Fults D, Brockmeyer D, Tullous M W, Pedone C A, Cawthon R M 1992 p53 Mutation and loss of heterozygosity on chromosomes 17 and 10 during human astrocytoma progression. Cancer Research 52: 674–679

Golubic M, Roudebush M, Dobrowolski S, Wolfman A, Stacey D W 1992 Catalytic properties, tissue and intracellular distribution of neurofibromin. Oncogene 7: 2151–2159

Gould R J, Hilal S K, Chutorian A M 1987 Efficacy of radiotherapy in optic gliomas. Pediatric Neurology 3: 29–32

Gutmann D H, Collins F S 1992 Recent progress toward understanding the molecular biology of Von Recklinghausen neurofibromatosis. Annals of Neurology 31: 555–561

Hackstein J H P 1992 The lethal prune/Killer-of-prune interaction of Drosophila causes a syndrome resembling human neurofibromatosis (NF-1). European Journal of Cell Biology 58: 429–444

Harper C M, Harner S G, Slavit D H et al 1992 Effect of BAEP monitoring on hearing preservation during acoustic neuroma resection. Neurology 42: 1551–1553
Hinrichs S H, Nerenberg M, Reynolds R K, Khoury G, Jay G 1987 A transgeneic mouse model for human neurofibromatosis. Science 237: 1340–1343
Hoyt W F, Baghdassarian S A 1969 Optic glioma of childhood: Natural history and rationale for conservative management. British Journal of Ophthalmology 53: 793–798
Huynh D P, Lin C T, Pulst S M 1992 Expression of neurofibromin, the neurofibromatosis 1 gene product: Studies in human neuroblastoma cells and rat brain. Neuroscience Letters 143: 233–236
Ikizler Y, Van Meyel D J, Ramsay D A et al 1992 Gliomas in families. Canadian Journal of Neurological Sciences 19: 492–497
Imes R K, Hoyt W F 1986 Childhood chiasmal gliomas: update on the fate of patients in the 1969 San Francisco Study. British Journal of Ophthalmology 70: 179–182
Ito S, Hashino T, Shibuya M, Prados M D, Edwards M S B, Davis R L 1992 Proliferative characteristics of juvenile pilocytic astrocytomas determined by bromodeoxyuridine labeling. Neurosurgery 31: 413–419
Jackler R K, Shapiro M S, Dillon W P, Pitts L, Lanser M J 1990 Gadolinium-DTPA enhanced magnetic resonance imaging in acoustic neuroma diagnosis and management. Otolaryngology — Head and Neck Surgery 102: 670–677
Jacks T, Schmitt E, Weinberg W A 1992 Targeted disruption of the NF-1 gene in the mouse. NNFF Consortium for NF-1 and NF-2 Genes — Salt Lake City 1: 12 (abstract)
Kaiser-Kupfer M I, Freidlin V, Datiles M B et al 1989 The association of posterior capsular lens opacity with bilateral acoustic neuromas in patients with neurofibromatosis type. Archives of Ophthalmology 107: 541–544
Kanzaki J, Ogawa K, Tsuchihashi N, Yamamoto M, Ogawa S, O-Uchi T 1991 Diagnostic procedure for acoustic neuroma. Acta Otolaryngology (Stockholm) 111 (supplement 487): 114–119
Kaye L D, Rothner A D, Beauchamp G R, Meyers S M, Estes M L 1992 Ocular findings associated with neurofibromatosis type II. Ophthalmology 99: 1424–1429
Kemink J L, Langman A W, Niparko J K, Graham M D 1991 Operative management of acoustic neuromas: The priority of neurologic function over complete resection. Otolaryngology — Head and Neck Surgery 104: 96–99
Kretschmar C S, Linggood R M 1991 Chemotherapeutic treatment of extensive optic pathway tumors in infants. Journal of Neuro-Oncology 10: 263–270
Landau K, Dossetor F M, Hoyt W F, Muci-Mendoza R 1990 Retinal hamartoma in neurofibromatosis 2. Archives of Ophthalmology 108: 328–329
Lewis R A, Riccardi V M, Gerson L P, Whitford R, Axelson K A 1984 Von Recklinghausen neurofibromatosis: II. Incidence of optic nerve gliomata. Ophthalmology 91: 929–935
Linskey M E, Lunsford L D, Flickinger J C 1992 Tumor control after stereotactic radiosurgery in neurofibromatosis patients with bilateral acoustic tumors. Neurosurgery 31: 829–839
Listernick R, Charrow J, Greenwald M J, Esterly N B 1989 Optic glioma in children with neurofibromatosis type I. Journal of Pediatrics 114: 788–792
Listernick R, Charrow J, Greenwald M 1992 Emergence of optic pathway gliomas in children with neurofibromatosis type 1 after normal neuroimaging results. Journal of Pediatrics 121: 584–587
Lund A M, Skovby F 1991 Optic gliomas in children with neurofibromatosis type 1. European Journal of Pediatrics 150: 835–838
Martuza R L 1992 Molecular neurosurgery for glial and neuronal disorders. Stereotactic and Functional Neurosurgery 59: 92–99
Martuza R L, Eldridge R 1988 Neurofibromatosis 2 (bilateral acoustic neurofibromatosis). New England Journal of Medicine 318: 684–688
Michels V V, Whisant J P, Garrity J A, Miller G M 1989 Neurofibromatosis type 1 with bilateral acoustic neuromas. Neurofibromatosis 2: 213–217
Mirowitz S A, Sartor K, Gado M 1989 High-intensity basal ganglia lesions on T1-weighted MR images in neurofibromatosis. American Journal of Neuroradiology 10: 1159–1163
Mochizuki H, Nishi T, Bruner J M, Lee P S Y, Levin V A, Saya H 1992 Alternative splicing of neurofibromatosis type 1 gene transcript in malignant brain tumors: PCR analysis of frozen-section mRNA. Molecular Carcinogenesis 6: 83–87
Nadol J B Jr, Chiong C M, Ojemann R G et al 1992 Preservation of hearing and facial nerve function in resection of acoustic neuroma. Laryngoscope 102: 1153–1158
Narod S A, Parry D M, Parboosingh J et al 1992 Neurofibromatosis type 2 appears to be a genetically homogeneous disease. American Journal of Human Genetics 51: 486–496
National Institutes of Health 1988 National Institutes of Health Consensus Development Conference statement: Neurofibromatosis. Neurofibromatosis 1: 172–178
Pierce S M, Barnes P D, Loeffler J S, McGinn C, Tarbell N J 1990 Definitive radiation therapy in the management of symptomatic patients with optic glioma: Survival and long-term effects. Cancer 65: 45–57
Riccardi V M 1982 Neurofibromatosis: clinical heterogeneity. Current Problems in Cancer 7(2): 1–34
Riccardi V M 1988a A germline mutation rodent model for neurofibromatosis: neurofibrosarcoma in the untreated offspring of rats exposed in utero to ethylnitrosourea. American Journal of Human Genetics 42: A32
Riccardi V M 1988b Routine cranial neuroimaging of patients with or at risk for neurofibromatosis. Neurofibromatosis 1: 65–68
Riccardi V M 1992a Neurofibromatosis: Phenotype, natural history and pathogenesis, 2nd edn. Johns Hopkins University Press, Baltimore, pp 1–450
Riccardi V M 1992b Type 1 neurofibromatosis and the pediatric patient. Current Problems in Pediatrics 22(2): 66–106
Riccardi V M, Powell P P 1989 Neurofibrosarcoma as a complication of von Recklinghausen neurofibromatosis. Neurofibromatosis 2: 152–165
Rodriguez H A, Berthrong M 1966 Multiple primary intracranial tumors in von Recklinghausen's neurofibromatosis. Archives of Neurology 14: 467–475
Rosenstock J G, Packer R J, Bilaniuk L, Bruce D A, Radcliffe J L, Savino P 1985 Chiasmatic optic glioma treated with chemotherapy. Journal of Neurosurgery 63: 862–869
Rouleau G A, Wertelecki W, Haines J L et al 1987 Genetic linkage of bilateral acoustic neurofibromatosis to a DNA marker on chromosome 22. Nature 329: 246–248
Rush J A, Younge B R, Campbell R J, MacCarty C S 1982 Optic glioma: long-term follow-up of 85 histopathologically verified cases. Ophthalmology 89: 1213–1219
Sadeh M, Martinovits G, Goldhammer Y 1989 Occurrence of both neurofibromatosis 1 and 2 in the same individual with a rapidly progressive course. Neurology 39: 282–283
Sanford R A, Kun L E, Langston J W, Kovnar E H 1991 Pitfalls in the management of low grade gliomas. Concepts in Pediatric Neurosurgery 11: 133–149
Sanson M, Richard S, Delattre O et al 1992 Allelic loss on chromosome 22 correlates with histopathological predictors of recurrence of meningiomas. International Journal of Cancer 50: 391–394
Schmale M C, Hensley G T, Udey L R 1983 Multiple schwannomas in the bicolor damselfish, Pomacentrus partitus: A possible model of von Recklinghausen neurofibromatosis. American Journal of Pathology 112: 238–241
Seizinger B R, Martuza R L, Gusella J F 1986 Loss of genes on chromosome 22 in tumorigenesis of human acoustic neuroma. Nature 322: 644–647
Seizinger B R, de la Monte S, Atkins L, Gusella J F, Martuza R L 1987 Molecular genetic approach to human meningioma: Loss of genes of chromosome 22. Proceedings of the National Academy of Science USA 84: 5419–5423
Sevick R J, Barkovich A J, Edwards M S B, Koch T, Berg B, Lempert T 1992 Evolution of white matter lesions in neurofibromatosis type 1: MR findings. American Journal of Roentgenology 159: 171–175
Shapiro W R 1992 Low-grade gliomas: When to treat. Annals of Neurology 31: 437–438

Sorensen S A, Mulvihill J J, Nielsen A 1986 Nation-wide follow-up of Recklinghausen neurofibromatosis: Survival and malignant neoplasms. New England Journal of Medicine 314: 1010–1015

Steiner L, Linqvist C, Steiner M 1989 Radiosurgery with focused gamma beam irradiation in children. In: Edwards M, Hoffman H (eds) Cerebral vascular disease in children and adolescents. Williams & Wilkins, Baltimore, pp 1–450

Stern J D, Jakobiec F A, Housepian E M 1980 The architecture of optic nerve glioma with and without neurofibromatosis. Archives of Ophthalmology 98: 505–511

Teinturier C, Danglot G, Slim R, Pruliere D, Launay J M, Bernheim A 1992 The neurofibromatosis 1 gene transcripts expressed in peripheral nerve and neurofibromas bear the additional exon located in the GAP domain. Biochemical and Biophysical Research Communications 188: 851–857

Von Deimling A, Eibl R H, Ohgaki H et al 1992 p53 Mutations are associated with 17p allelic loss in grade II and grade III astrocytoma. Cancer Research 52: 2987–2990

Wang H-C, Ho Y-S 1992 Clinicopathological evaluation of 78 astrocytomas in Taiwan with emphasis on a simple grading system. Journal of Neuro-Oncology 13: 265–276

Wijdicks E F M, Jambroes G, Riccardi V M 1990 De novo astrocytoma following immunosuppression in neurofibromatosis. Neurology 40: 1467–1468

Wilson W B 1988 The North American Study Group for Optic Gliomas. Neurofibromatosis 1: 199–200

Wright J E, McNab A A, McDonald W I 1989 Optic nerve glioma and the management of optic nerve tumors in the young. British Journal of Ophthalmology 73: 967–974

Xu G, O'Connell P, Viskochil D et al 1990 The neurofibromatosis type 1 gene encodes a protein related to GAP. Cell 62: 599–608

Yagle M K, Parruti G, Xu W, Ponder B A J, Solomon E 1990 Genetic and physical map of the von Recklinghausen neurofibromatosis (NF-1) region on chromosome 17. Proceedings of the National Academy of Science USA 87: 7255–7259

PART IV

Meningeal tumors

35. Meningiomas

Franco DeMonte Ossama Al-Mefty

INTRODUCTION

Meningiomas are usually benign growths that rarely invade the substance of the brain, thus presenting the potential for curative surgery. Their sometimes difficult location and propensity to recur if not completely excised represent formidable problems for the patient and the neurological surgeon.

In 1922, Cushing coined the term 'meningioma' to refer to a tumor histopathology that was, at the time, the subject of great controversy. He sought to avoid this controversy by conveying the constant proximity of this tumor to the meninges (Cushing 1922). Since then, meningiomas have been recognized as originating from the arachnoidal cap cells that are commonly found associated with the arachnoid villi at the dural venous sinuses and their tributaries, at the cranial nerve foramina, at the cribriform plate and the medial middle fossa. Meningothelial cells, which can be found in the choroid plexus, the tela choroidea, and arachnoid villi at the spinal nerve exit zones are presumed to be the origin of intraventricular, pineal region, and spinal meningiomas.

In 1938, Cushing & Eisenhardt established a landmark categorization of meningiomas, and since that time the common practice has been to classify meningiomas by their site of origin. Of all intracranial meningiomas, 85–90% are located supratentorially, one third to one half of which (30–40% of total) are located along the base of the anterior and middle fossae (Gautier-Smith 1970, Quest 1978, MacCarty & Taylor 1979, Rohinger et al 1989). Children show an increased incidence of intraventricular and posterior fossa meningiomas, as well as meningiomas without dural attachment (Herz et al 1980, Deen et al 1982, Drake et al 1985). Table 35.1 lists the most common sites and their relative incidence.

Table 35.1 Common sites and relative incidences of intracranial meningiomas. Based on data from Cushing & Eisenhardt (1938), Gautier-Smith (1970), Quest (1978), MacCarty & Taylor (1979), Rohinger et al (1989).

Site	Relative incidences
Parasagittal/falcine	25%
Convexity	19%
Sphenoid ridge	17%
Suprasellar (tuberculum)	9%
Posterior fossa	8%
Olfactory groove	8%
Middle fossa/Meckel's cave	4%
Tentorial	3%
Peritorcular	3%
Lateral ventricle	1–2%
Foramen magnum	1–2%
Orbit/optic nerve sheath	1–2%

EPIDEMIOLOGY

The frequency of meningiomas among primary intracranial neoplasms may be derived from either hospital- or community-based studies. A compilation of several large US hospital-based brain tumor series is shown in Table 35.2. The mean incidence of meningioma is approximately 20% (Cushing 1932, Grant 1956, Zimmerman 1969, Walker et al 1985).

Table 35.2 The frequency of meningiomas among primary intracranial neoplasms — hospital-based studies

Authors	Total primary intracranial neoplasms	% intracranial meningiomas
Cushing (1932)	2158	13.4
Grant (1956)	2099	19.4
Zimmerman (1969)	2262	27.3
Walker et al (1985)	13 720	19.5
Total	20 239	Mean 19.9

A comparison of these figures with those derived from population-based surveys (Table 35.3) shows very little difference between the frequency of meningioma among primary intracranial neoplasms in North America (Schoenberg et al 1976, Kurland et al 1982, Preston-Martin et al 1982, Sutherland et al 1987). Although the study by Katsura in Japan (Katsura et al 1959) and

Table 35.3 The frequency of meningiomas among primary intracranial neoplasms — population-based studies

Authors & time period of study	% incidence of intracranial meningioma
Schoenberg et al (1976) 1935–1964	17
Kurland et al (1982) 1935–1977	40 (21)*
Preston-Martin et al (1982) 1972–1977	30
Sutherland et al (1987) 1980–1985	22
Mean	22.5

*21% is the incidence of intracranial meningioma in this population if autopsy data is ignored.

several European studies (Olivecrona 1952, Zulch 1965, Fogelholm et al 1984) show a similar frequency (Table 35.4), reports and surveys from Africa indicate a significantly higher frequency of meningioma among primary intracranial neoplasms in that population (Table 35.5) (Froman & Lipschitz 1970, Giordano & Lamouche 1973, Levy 1973, Manfredonia 1973, Odeku & Adeloye 1973). The incidences in the latter population may be of critical importance from a genetic/molecular biologic perspective, but these statistics should be interpreted cautiously, considering the much lower frequency of primary glial tumors in these peoples.

Reported incidence rates of meningioma per 100 000 population vary from <1 to >6 (Schoenberg et al 1976, Kurland et al 1982). An overall incidence of 2.6/100 000 population is indicated by the combined results of three large recent studies of intracranial neoplasms, all of which support the finding of higher incidence rates in women (Kurland et al 1982, Preston-Martin et al 1982, Sutherland et al 1987). The ratio of male to female incidences range from 1:1.4 to 1:2.8. These differences are less evident in Africans and African Americans, who show equal ratios or a male preponderance (Fan & Pezeshkpour 1992). Likewise, the incidence rates for African Americans have been found to be higher (average 3.1/100 000) than for Caucasian Americans (average 2.3/100 000) in a Los Angeles County population-based survey (Preston-Martin et al 1982).

Table 35.4 The frequency of intracranial meningiomas in European and Japanese studies

Authors	% frequency of intracranial meningioma
Zulch (1965)	21
Olivecrona (1952)	20.6
Fogelholm et al (1984)	27
Katsura et al (1959)	17
Mean	21.4

Table 35.5 The frequency of intracranial meningiomas in African peoples

Authors & geographical area	% frequency of intracranial meningioma
Giordano & Lamouche (1973) Ivory Coast	23.5
Levy (1973) Malawi, Rhodesia, Zambia	28.6
Odeku & Adeloye (1973) Nigeria	29.9
Froman & Lipschitz (1970) Transvaal	30.3
Manfredonia (1973) Ethiopia	38
Mean	30.1

The incidence of intracranial meningioma increases with increasing age (Kurland et al 1982, Preston-Martin et al 1982, Sutherland et al 1987). In a study by Rohinger et al, the incidence for males peaked in the seventh decade at 6.0/100 000 population, whereas that in females peaked at 9.5/100 000 in the 70–79-year age group (Rohinger et al 1989). This and other clinical studies indicate a decline in incidence for both sexes following the seventh decade but inclusion of autopsy data indicates otherwise, suggesting that a less aggressive investigative posture in the elderly accounts for the reported declining rate in incidence past the seventh decade (Kurland et al 1982).

ETIOLOGY

Trauma

Although trauma was suggested by Cushing in the 1930s as a significant etiologic factor in the development of meningiomas (Cushing 1932), there has been little subsequent evidence beyond isolated reports to give firm support to this theory. Preston-Martin, in a large case-control study of 189 women with meningioma (and their neighbors and old friends), found significantly more recall of prior trauma requiring medical attention in the meningioma-bearing group than either control group (Preston-Martin et al 1980). However, case-control studies by Parker & Kernohan (1931) and Choi et al (1970) found no difference between patients with brain tumors and matched controls. Similarly, Annegars et al, in a prospective study of 2953 patients with head injury over 29 859 person-years, found no significant increase in the number of intracranial tumors (or meningiomas, in particular) in these patients, a finding that circumvents the recall bias which might be present in the smaller case-control studies (Annegers et al 1979).

Viruses

It is known that some viruses, when inoculated into laboratory animals, will produce central nervous system (CNS) tumors. All of the polyoma viruses (polyoma, SV-40), a subgroup of papovaviruses, are capable of producing CNS tumors in animals, as are several types of adenoviruses (human, simian, and avian) (Rachlin & Rosenblum 1991). Immunocytochemical techniques have identified papovavirus antigen in human meningiomas (Weiss et al 1975). Likewise, DNA hybridization techniques have found BK viral DNA, SV-40 viral DNA (both papovaviruses), and adenovirus DNA within meningiomas, but the viral DNA material was not integrated into the tumor cell DNA in all cases (Fiori & Di Mayorca 1976, Ibelgaufts & Jones 1982, Ibelgaufts et al 1982, Barbanti-Brodano et al 1987). Southern blot results showed that 2 of 9 meningiomas studied had DNA sequences homologous to SV-40 DNA (Rachlin et al 1984). The presence of viral protein, RNA or DNA, in human meningioma cells suggests a possible role in tumor induction, maintenance of transformation, or both, in which case the implicated viruses may act alone or in a permissive manner with other mutagens. Of course, the presence of viral material is not prima facie evidence that it is causally related to meningioma formation, and the actual role, if any, of viruses in human brain tumor formation is as yet undefined.

Postirradiation

The diagnosis of a radiation-induced neoplasm requires the fulfilment of specific criteria, the most important of which are that the neoplasm must (1) occur in the irradiated field, (2) appear following an appropriate (usually long) period of latency following irradiation, and (3) differ from any pre-existing neoplasms (Fig. 35.1). Numerous reports show that meningiomas have occurred following low levels of irradiation such as those given in the past for tinea capitis (1000 cGy; Modan et al 1974), following the high doses of radiation given for the treatment of primary head and neck malignancies (5500–7500 cGy; Mack & Wilson 1993), and following intermediate levels of radiation (Bogdanowicz et al 1974, Waga & Handa 1976).

Since the cellular DNA is the level at which radiation has its injurious effect, it may be hypothesized that radiation leads to injury to genetic material found within the long arm of chromosome 22, in the locus subtending the 'tumor-suppressor gene' (see below).

Genetics and molecular biology

Reports of familial aggregation of meningiomas and a considerably higher incidence of meningiomas in patients with neurofibromatosis type 2 have prompted cytogenetic studies of meningiomas. These studies have found that up to 70% of meningiomas have monosomy of chromo-

A

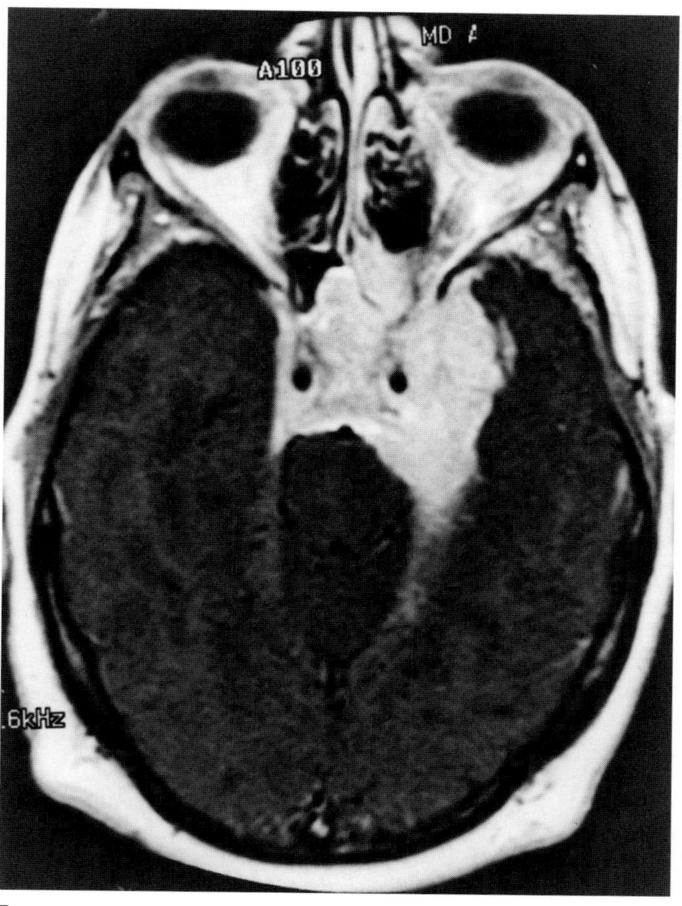

B

Fig. 35.1 **A.** Axial contrast-enhanced CT scan. This scan was performed in 1985 as follow-up for a left optic nerve glioma that was treated with 5470 cGy in 1970. Note the enlarged, nodular left optic nerve. **B.** Axial contrast-enhanced T1-weighted MRI. This MRI scan from the same patient was performed in 1993 due to the new onset of a complex partial seizure disorder. The tumor is within the previously irradiated area, and is in all likelihood a radiation-induced meningioma.

some 22 (Zankl & Zang 1980). With the development of chromosomal mapping techniques using restriction fragment length polymorphisms (RFLP), additional meningiomas, although karyotypically normal, were found to have deletions of the long arm of chromosome 22. As the number of available RFLPs increased, these deletions were identified as being specific to the long arm of chromosome 22q 12.3-qter (Dumanski et al 1987, Seizinger et al 1987). These incidences of monosomies and deletions of chromosome 22 support the thesis that a tumor suppressor gene is present on the long arm of chromosome 22 and that its absence leads to tumor formation (Rouleau et al 1987). According to this theory, the occurrence of a sporadic meningioma would require (1) that a mutation form a recessive oncogene on chromosome 22, and (2) that the dominant allele (tumor suppressor gene) from the second copy of chromosome 22 be lost (Collins et al 1990, Rachlin & Rosenblum 1991). In contrast, in patients with neurofibromatosis type 2 (bilateral acoustic neurofibromatosis), in which the recessive oncogene is probably dominantly inherited, only a single mutation is required — the deletion of the tumor suppressor gene (Collins et al 1990, Rachlin & Rosenblum 1991).

A recent report from Harvard has identified a specific candidate gene for the neurofibromatosis 2 tumor suppressor gene. The product of this gene, which spans a 35–45 kilobase region on the long arm of chromosome 22, is a novel protein related to other cytoskeletal proteins that link the cell membrane to the cytoskeleton (Trofatter et al 1993). The final proof required to confirm the nature of this discovery is the reversal of the tumor phenotype by reintroduction of the gene. It is uncertain whether this gene is involved in meningioma formation.

Gonadal steroid hormones and other receptors

Donnell et al described the presence of an 'estrogen-receptor protein' in 4 of 6 meningiomas in 1979. Since then, numerous reports have described estrogen receptors, progesterone receptors, androgen receptors, and others. Studies from the early- to mid-1980s using traditional receptor-binding assays (competitive binding in a radioreceptor assay with Scatchard plot analysis) yielded variable results, especially regarding the presence and significance of the estrogen receptor (Table 35.6) (Schnegg et al 1981, Poisson et al 1983, Brentani et al 1984, Zava et al 1984, Kornblum et al 1988, Olson et al 1988, Butti et al 1991, Black 1993). These techniques, however, led to the identification of progesterone and androgen receptors. Modern techniques using monoclonal antibodies to specific receptor proteins, in situ hybridization, and Northern blot analyses have more clearly defined the presence and localization of the gonadal steroid receptors, as well as others. Table 35.7 lists the results of several investigators' attempts to define the gonadal steroid receptor immunoreactivity of meningiomas (Lesch et al 1987, Halper et al 1989, Horsfall et al 1989, Waelti & Markwalder 1989, Schrell et al 1990a, Perrot-Applanat et

Table 35.6 Estrogen, progesterone and androgen receptor detection by competitive binding in meningiomas*

Series	Technique	Specimen	Patient	Estrogen receptor	Progesterone receptor	Androgen receptor
Blaauw	Charcoal adsorption	Tissue	67	Few	80%	
Brentani et al (1984)	Density gradient	Meningioma tissue	6	2 (33%)	6 (100%)	6/6
Cahill	Density gradient	Tissue	23	4	8	
Concolino	Density gradient	Spinal meningioma	6	Yes	No	
Hayward	Radioreceptor	Spinal meningioma	22	None	17	
Hinton	Radioreceptor	Spinal meningioma	11	4/11	6/11	
Ironside	Isoelectric focusing	Cryostat section	45	0	24	
Magdelenat	Competitive binding	Meningioma tissue	42	30/38 (79%)	39 (93%)	
Markwalder	Saturation binding	Meningioma tissue	44	Miniscule	34 (77%)	
Martuza	Saturation binding	Meningioma tissue	10	7	Not tested	
Martuza	Saturation binding	Meningioma tissue	42	25 (50%) cytosolic 16/28 (57%) nuclear	16/22	
Schwartz	Competitive binding	Meningioma tissue	26	8	8	
Whittle	Competitive binding	Meningioma tissue	29	0	16/29	
Whittle	Competitive binding	Meningioma tissue	20	0	11	
Yu	Competitive binding	Meningioma tissue	16	15/16 (94%)	9/11	
Zava et al (1984)	Competitive binding	Culture	10	0	7	4/4
Blankenstein	Competitive binding	Culture	20	0	18	
Blankenstein	Competitive binding	Cytosol tissue	45	7	40	
Poisson et al (1983)	Competitive binding	Meningioma tissue	25	?	24/25	23/25
Punnonen	Competitive binding	Cytosol	4	0	3/4	
Kobayashi	Competitive binding	Cytosol	8	3	0	
Courriere	Competitive binding	Cytosol	12	0	10	
Kornblum et al (1988)	Competitive binding	Cytosol	29	0	8	8
Schnegg et al (1981)	Competitive binding	Meningioma tissue	10	0/10	4/10	2/9
Butti et al (1991)	Competitive binding	Cytosol	24	4	21	15
Olson et al (1988)	Competitive binding	Cytosol	8	—	—	8/8

*Table adapted from Black (1993). Please refer to Black for non-referenced studies.

Table 35.7 The gonadal steroid receptor immunoreactivity of meningiomas

Authors	Estrogen receptor immunoreactivity	Progesterone receptor immunoreactivity
Lesch et al (1987)	36/70	—
Waelti & Markwalder (1989)	—	5/6
Horsfall et al (1989)	0/19	6/12
Halper et al (1989)	0/52	46/52
Schrell et al (1990a)	1/50 (cytosolic)* 0/50 (nuclear)*	50/50 (cytosolic) 5/50 (nuclear)
Perrot-Applant et al (1992)	0/36	26/36
Totals	38/227 (17%)	133/156 (85%)

*Refers to cellular localization of receptors, i.e. either in the cytosol or the nucleus

al 1992). To date, the lack of an appropriate monoclonal antibody for the androgen receptor has precluded the reporting of androgen receptor protein immunoreactivity in meningiomas.

The development of molecular biological techniques has allowed the analysis of the expression of gonadal steroid receptor messenger ribonucleic acid (mRNA) and protein product, and in situ hybridization allows for cellular localization of these proteins. Schrell et al were unable to detect mRNA coding for the estrogen receptor in any of 50 meningiomas tested by in situ hybridization using an oligonucleotide probe complementary to a fraction of human receptor mRNA (Schrell et al 1990a), a finding that was confirmed by Maxwell et al, who were unable to detect estrogen receptor expression in any of 9 meningiomas sampled (Maxwell et al 1993). Of the meningiomas analyzed in the latter study, progesterone receptor mRNA and protein, and androgen receptor mRNA and protein, were found in 88% and 66%, respectively.

These more recent studies indicate the general absence of estrogen receptor in meningioma tissue and confirm the generally high levels of progesterone receptor and moderate concentrations of androgen receptor previously described by competitive binding assay techniques.

Reubi, Lamberts and colleagues (Reubi et al 1986) have identified a high incidence of somatostatin receptors in meningioma tissue. In vitro binding assays showed these receptors in all tumors tested, and autoradiography showed them on normal human leptomeninges as well, although receptor density varied greatly (Reubi et al 1986, 1989). Radioactive labeling of somatostatin analogs allowed imaging of somatostatin receptors in 11 of 11 meningiomas in vivo (Lamberts et al 1992a). The functional significance of these receptors is unknown. No effect of the somatostatin analog SMS 201–995 on basal or EGF-stimulated growth of meningiomas in culture could be detected (Reubi et al 1989).

Schrell et al (1990b) have detected dopamine D1 receptor activity by using radioligand assays on meningioma cell membranes following their observation of a decreased meningioma proliferation rate when cell cultures were treated with bromocriptine.

Since abnormal expression of certain proto-oncogenes may lead to neoplastic transformation of normal cells, the epidermal growth factor (EGF) receptors on various tumor cells gained particular attention once it was known that certain receptor subunits for EGF were products of the expression of a particular oncogene (v-erb B) (Downward et al 1984, Westphal & Hermann 1986). Westphal & Hermann (1986) discovered functionally intact EGF receptors in all 12 cultures of human meningiomas in their laboratory. Noting increased DNA synthesis in a dose-dependent manner following EGF treatment of their meningioma cell cultures, Weisman et al (1986, 1987) more fully characterized the EGF receptor in human meningioma and noted a modulatory effect on the receptor by platelet-derived growth factor (PDGF). Earlier studies had revealed near maximal levels of DNA synthesis in meningioma culture when PDGF and EGF were added in combination (Weisman et al 1986). Studies by Reubi et al and Horsfall et al revealed the presence of EGF receptors in 23 of 27 (radioligand receptor binding) and 57 of 57 (immunocytochemical staining) meningiomas, respectively (Horsfall et al 1989, Reubi et al 1989).

The finding of expression of c-*erb*/EGF receptor in meningiomas prompted searches for other oncogene-receptor-mitogen systems. Maxwell et al, using Northern blot analysis, demonstrated that all meningiomas tested (n = 9) expressed both the c-*sis*/PDGF-2 proto-oncogene and the PDGF receptor gene (Maxwell et al 1990). In situ hybridization localized the c-*sis*/PDGF-2 and the PDGF receptor (PDGF-R) mRNAs and their protein products in the tumor cells of the meningiomas. Control pachymeninges expressed only PDGF-R mRNA, but not c-*sis*/PDGF-2 mRNA.

The coexpression of PDGF-2 (a potent mitogen) and PDGF-R suggests an autocrine loop which may contribute to the growth and maintenance of these tumors. Adams et al (1991) supported the presence of autocrine control of meningioma proliferation. In their study, a neutralizing antibody against PDGF abolished the stimulation of meningioma cell culture growth by meningioma-conditioned medium. Gel chromatography of the conditioned media resulted in an elution profile with a major peak corresponding to a molecular weight of 28 kD. This is similar to the molecular weight of the PDGF β chain. This same group has demonstrated inhibition of meningioma cell proliferation pharmacologically by a PDGF antagonist (Todo et al 1993).

PRESENTING FEATURES — SYMPTOMS AND SIGNS

There is no single symptom or sign that alone identifies

which patients harbor an intracranial meningioma. Indeed, some tumors are identified fortuitously in patients who have no symptoms or signs of intracranial disease. Other patients have a variety of presenting features, including headache, paresis, seizures, personality change/ confusion, and visual impairment. Rohinger et al (1989), in a population-based study of 193 patients with intracranial meningioma, found headache and paresis to be the most common symptom and sign, occurring in 36% and 30% of patients respectively, and an increased incidence of abnormal physical findings in those patients with malignant meningiomas.

Meningiomas in specific locations may have, more or less, a typical clinical presentation. Examples include tumors of the olfactory groove, which historically have been associated with anosmia and the Foster-Kennedy syndrome (optic atrophy and scotoma in the ipsilateral eye with papilledema in the other eye); tuberculum sellae meningiomas, which cause early significant visual loss (usually a 'chiasmal syndrome' with ipsilateral optic atrophy and an incongruous bitemporal hemianopsia; Al-Mefty & Smith 1991); cavernous sinus meningiomas, which may result in proptosis, diplopia or primary aberrant oculomotor regeneration (Schatz et al 1977); and foramen magnum tumors, which have associated nuchal and suboccipital pain and stepwise appendicular sensory and motor deficits (Meyer et al 1984). Further examples are given in the surgical approaches and techniques by tumor location section, found later in this chapter.

In contradistinction to the multitude of signs and symptoms which may occur in adults, children may present with signs of increased intracranial pressure without further localizing features.

DIAGNOSTIC IMAGING

Computerized tomography of intracranial meningiomas

Computerized tomographic (CT) scanning can detect the majority of meningiomas and can, in most instances, determine their extent (Latchaw & Hirsch 1991). CT at wide window and level settings optimally identifies bone involvement, either hyperostosis or bone lysis. This ability is especially useful for skull base tumors because it aids in the specificity of diagnosis and in planning the extent of surgical resection required to rid the patient of the meningioma.

On nonenhanced CT scans, the typical meningioma is isodense to slightly hyperdense to brain and of homogeneous density, although calcification may be present and may range from tiny punctate areas to dense calcification of the entire lesion (Latchaw & Hirsch 1991) (Fig. 35.2). Intravenous contrast usually shows intense, homogeneous enhancement, and morphologic features, such as sharp demarcation and a broad base against bone or free dural margins, are easily seen.

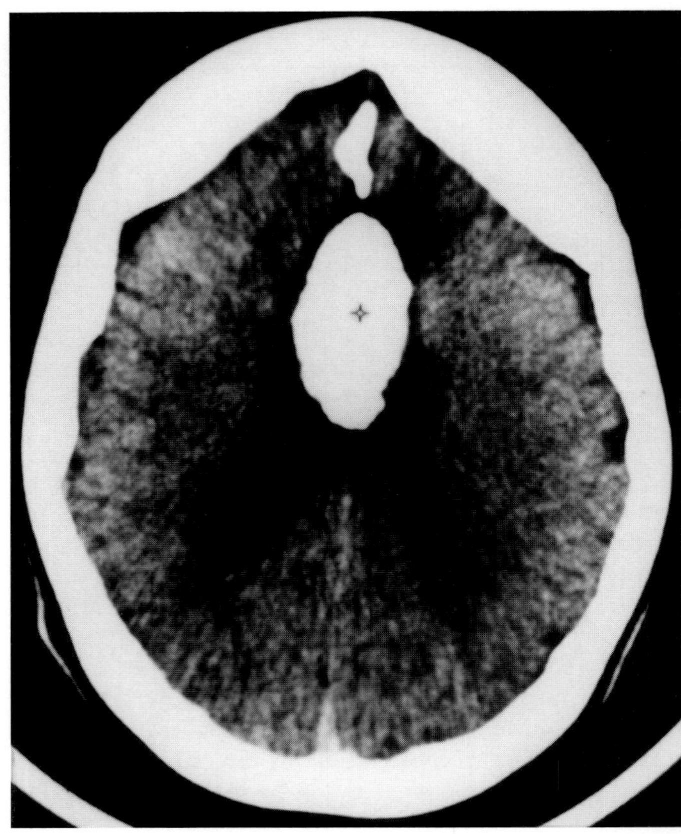

Fig. 35.2 Axial CT scan. A large, densely and completely calcified falcine meningioma is present.

On CT, approximately 15% of benign meningiomas have an unusual appearance (Russell et al 1980). Areas of hyperdensity, hypodensity, and non-uniform enhancement may be seen and may represent hemorrhage, cystic degeneration or necrosis, respectively. Aggressive meningiomas may at times be distinguished by preoperative imaging findings of indistinct or irregular margins or mushroom-like projections from the main tumor mass (Fig. 35.3).

Angiography of intracranial meningiomas

Angiography, which once played a pre-eminent role in the diagnosis of intracranial meningioma, has, to a large extent, been supplanted by high resolution CT, magnetic resonance imaging (MRI), and magnetic resonance angiography (MRA). Indeed, the determination of venous sinus patency, historically the purview of the angiogram, can be well visualized on MRA, thus eliminating this as an indication for angiography. However, angiography remains a vital means by which the feasibility and safety of preoperative embolization can be determined. Furthermore, pertinent collateral circulation can be identified.

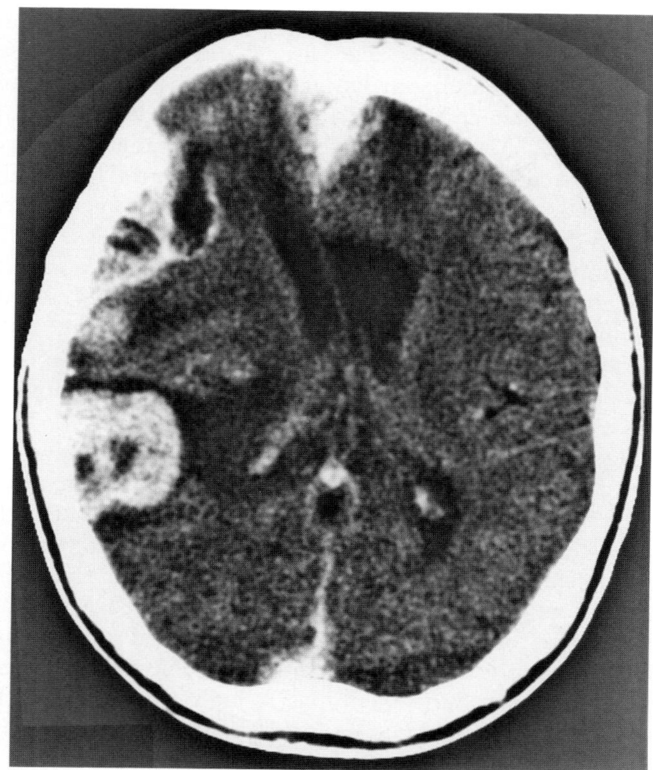

Fig. 35.3 Axial CT scan, post-contrast. This axial contrast-enhanced CT scan of a multiply recurrent malignant meningioma demonstrates the radiologic sign known as mushrooming. Irregular projections from the main mass of the tumor are seen. A previous craniectomy has been performed.

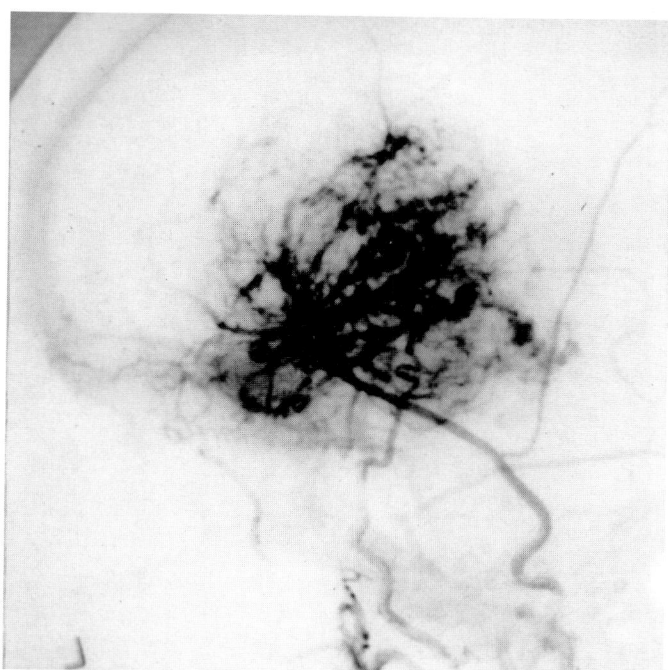

Fig. 35.4 Selective external carotid artery arteriogram (lateral projection). The initial nutrient arteries to this sphenoid wing meningioma can be seen in the center of the tumor. The irregular tortuous radially orientated branches are also seen.

To date, only selective angiography can resolve the generally small communicating branches present between the internal carotid arteries and vertebral arteries and the external carotid arteries, the presence of which to a large extent determines the safety of embolization of intracranial meningiomas.

As they grow, meningiomas first access the adjacent meningeal arterial supply. These initial nutrient arteries remain as the supply to the center of the tumor. From this central site, there is usually a radiant spread of branches toward the periphery of the tumor (Fig. 35.4). As the angiogram extends into the middle to late venous phase, a uniform blush can be seen. Venous drainage tends to occur in the usual temporal sequence typical of the brain. Large meningiomas will also parasitize the pial arterioles, which can be visualized in the arterial phase of the angiogram (Jacobs & Harnsberger 1991).

Magnetic resonance imaging of intracranial meningiomas

The high-field MR imaging characteristics of meningiomas are relatively consistent. On T1-weighted images, 60–90% of meningiomas are isointense, whereas 10–30% are mildly hypointense when compared to gray matter (Spagnoli et al 1986, Elster et al 1989, Demaerel et al 1991a, Zimmerman 1991) (Fig. 35.5). T2-weighted imaging reveals that 30–45% of meningiomas are of increased signal intensity, whereas approximately 50% are isointense to gray matter (Spagnoli et al 1986, Elster et al 1989, Demaerel et al 1991a, Zimmerman 1991).

Vascular distortion or encasement and tumor vascularity are better assessed by MR imaging than by CT scanning. Flow voids produced by flowing blood identify the vasculature local to the tumor.

The ability to decide on an extra-axial localization of a neoplasm is also heightened on MR imaging. Spagnoli et al (1986) identified one or more marginating characteristics in all of their reported cases imaged at 1.5T (Fig. 35.5).

There is increasing interest in using MRI characteristics to tissue-subtype meningiomas preoperatively. The results of these studies have been varied, with studies reporting 75–96% accuracy and others finding no correlation (Spagnoli et al 1986, Elster et al 1989, Demaerel et al 1991a, Kaplan et al 1992). The MRI characteristics which allowed accurate preoperative identification of meningioma subtypes were confined to findings on T2-weighted studies. Specifically, meningothelial and angioblastic variants were found to have a persistently higher signal intensity on T2-weighted sequences than fibroblastic and transitional meningiomas, which demonstrated a higher relative signal intensity on intermediate images.

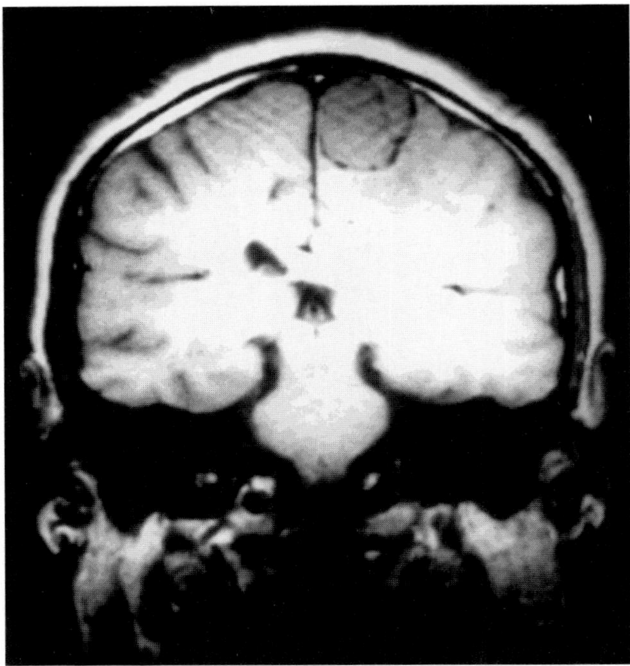

Fig. 35.5 Coronal T1-weighted magnetic resonance image. A parasagittal meningioma is seen. It is isointense to slightly hypointense with respect to the gray matter. Note the low intensity signal surrounding the tumor, thus confirming its extraparenchymal origin.

The amount of cerebral edema present in association with the meningiomas was also found generally to be greater when meningothelial or angioblastic variants were present (Elster et al 1989, Demaerel et al 1991a, Chen et al 1992, Kaplan et al 1992). High signal intensity on T2-weighted images has also been correlated with microscopic hypervascularity and soft tumor consistency (Chen et al 1992).

Contrast-enhanced MRI provides the highest level of detection of meningiomas (Zimmerman 1991). Most meningiomas enhance intensely and homogeneously with intravenous paramagnetic contrast material, and in approximately 10% of cases small additional meningiomas are encountered that are missed on unenhanced MR images (Fig. 35.6). Likewise, contrast enhancement of the dura extending away from the margins of the mass is typical of meningioma, although it can be seen with other dural-based lesions. This 'dural tail' can represent tumor extension and its resection is important to lessen the risk of recurrence. Postoperative enhanced MRI has also been found to be more sensitive and specific in the detection of residual or recurrent meningioma. Thick and nodular enhancement has a high correlation with recurrent or residual neoplasm (Weingarten et al 1992).

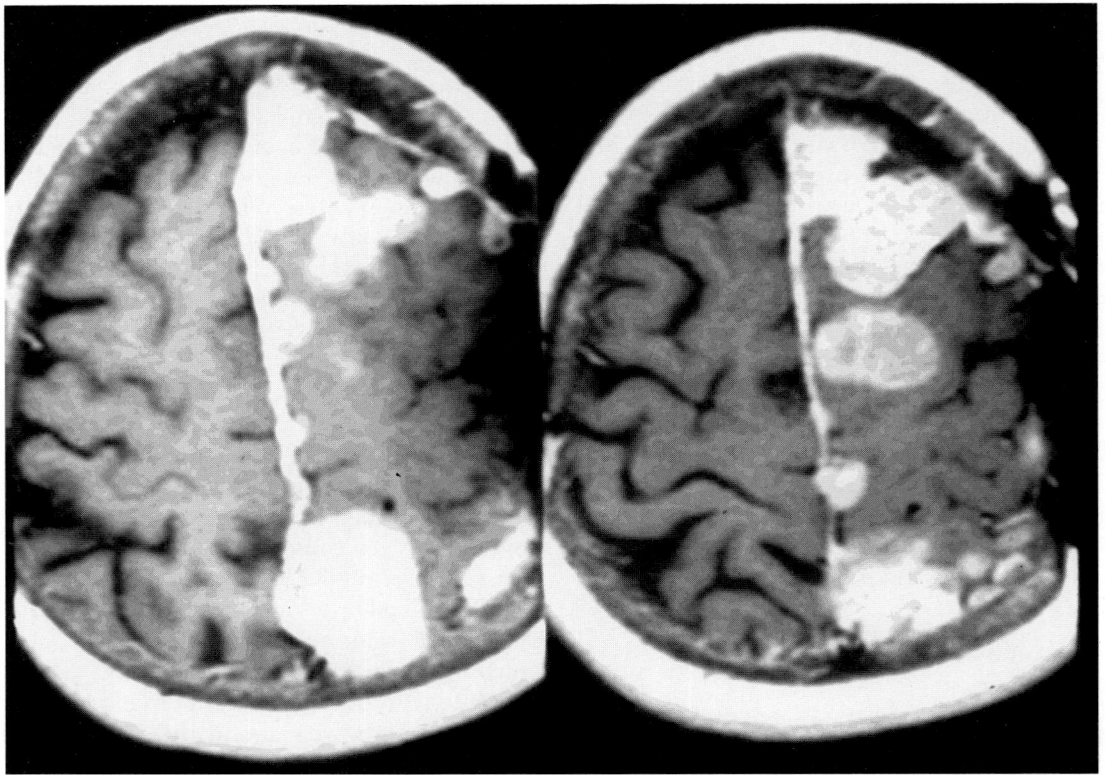

Fig. 35.6 Axial post-gadolinium enhanced T1-weighted magnetic resonance image. Multiple meningiomas are clearly seen. Prior to contrast enhancement the extent and number of meningiomas were grossly underestimated.

Magnetic resonance spectroscopy of intracranial meningiomas

In vivo magnetic resonance spectroscopy (MRS) is an evolving area of study which hopes to increase the preoperative ability to discern differing pathologies. Both hydrogen- (proton) and phosphorus-based in vivo MRS have been reported, although the relatively low sensitivity to phosphorus of the clinically-used MR systems restricts measurements to volumes not less than 30 ml, thus increasing the likelihood of contamination from surrounding edema or nontumor tissue (Kugel et al 1992). It also does not allow the detection of heterogeneity within larger tumors. For these reasons, proton-based MRS systems have been more useful clinically.

The normal ^{1}H MR spectrum for brain tissue is displayed in Figure 35.7. Well-defined peaks occur at 3.2 ppm for choline, 3.0 ppm for phosphocreatine/creatine (PCr/Cr), and 2.0 ppm for N-acetylaspartate (NAA). A less well-defined peak for lactate occurs at 1.3 ppm. A typical proton MR spectrum for meningioma is shown in Figure 35.8. Note the marked increase in choline signal, which may reflect an elevated concentration of mobile membrane precursors. Such an increased pool of membrane components would be necessary during increased cell proliferation, but because the increased choline peak is common to most neoplasms studied, it is not specific for meningioma (Demaerel et al 1991b, Kugel et al 1992).

A marked reduction of both the NAA and PCr/Cr peaks is typically seen in meningioma. As NAA is essentially confined to neurons, this is not a surprising finding. The reason for the marked reduction of the PCr/Cr peak in meningiomas is less clear, although it has been confirmed by in vivo phosphorus MRS and in vitro ^{1}H MRS, as well as biochemically (Lowry et al 1977). This reduction is greater than that seen in astrocytomas (Kugel et al 1992, Peeling & Sutherland 1992). An additional peak seen in some meningiomas at 1.47 ppm has been assigned to alanine (Kugel et al 1992, Ott et al 1993). Although ^{1}H MRS allows in vivo metabolic study of neoplasms, specific features of various tumor types are not, as yet, forthcoming. There is increasing evidence, however, that ^{1}H MRS may be more useful in the grading of tumor aggressiveness and in the differentiation of recurrent tumor growth from treatment effects (Ott et al 1993). Greater pathologic specificity has been claimed for phosphorus MRS (Arnold et al 1991), but until it can sample smaller tissue volumes its clinical usefulness will be limited.

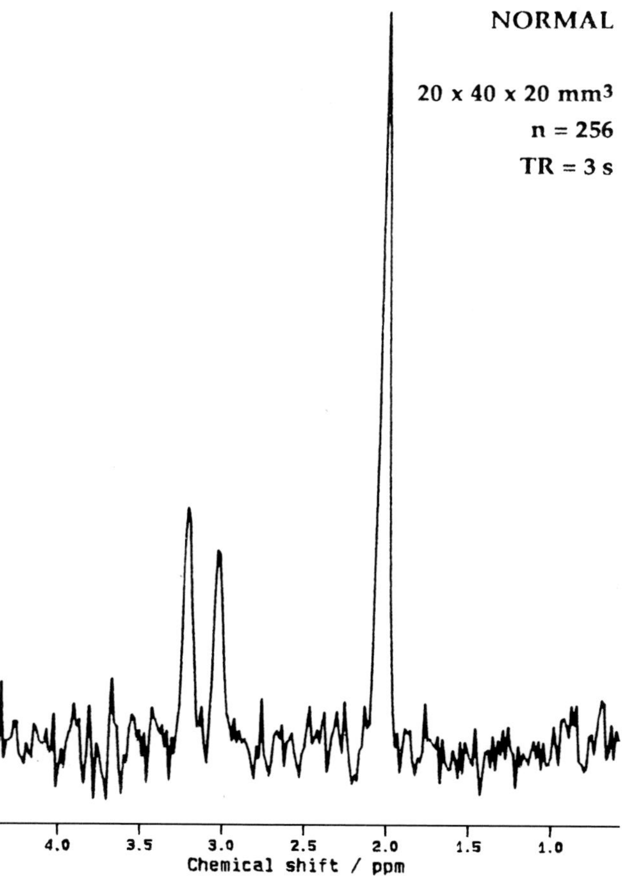

Fig. 35.7 Normal proton MR spectrum for brain tissue. Note the well-defined peaks at 3.2 ppm for choline, 3.0 ppm for phosphocreatine/creatine, and 2.0 ppm for N-acetylaspartate. A less well defined peak for lactate occurs at 1.3 ppm. Reproduced with permission from Demaerel et al 1991b.

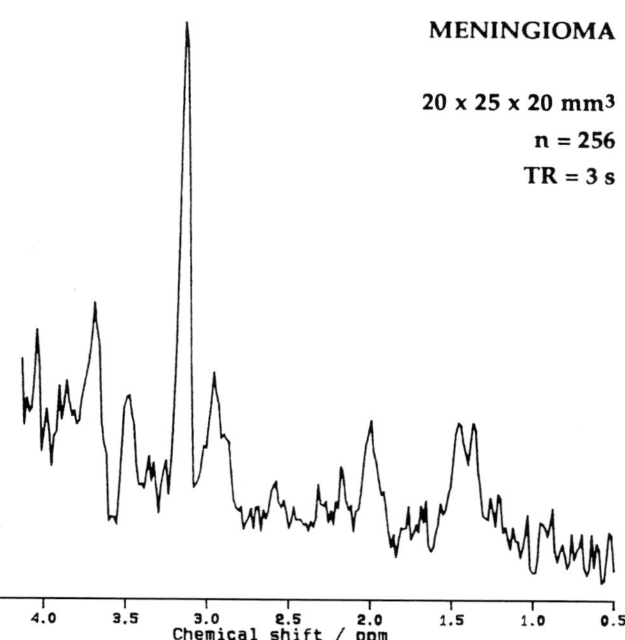

Fig. 35.8 Typical proton MR spectrum for meningioma. Note the marked increase in the choline signal and decreases in both the phosphocreatine/creatine peak and N-acetylaspartate peaks. A fourth peak is seen at just under 1.5 ppm and has been attributed to alanine. Reproduced with permission from Demaerel et al 1991b.

PATHOLOGY

Macroscopically, meningiomas appear smooth and lobulated with a fine vascular pattern on the surface. Meningiomas that are more vascular have a reddish meaty appearance with a fine nodular surface extending to the surrounding arachnoid that gives it a thickened, opaque appearance. Xanthomatous change may impart a yellowish hue to the tumor. Most meningiomas tend to be globular but their locations result in peculiarities of shape, including dumbbell (falcine, Meckel's cave, tentorial), tubular (optic sheath), or flat, diffuse growths (en plaque). Microscopically, meningiomas have a varied but characteristic histopathologic appearance, the diversity of which forms the basis for the pathologic classification of meningiomas (Table 35.8).

Table 35.8 World Health Organization classification of tumors of meningothelial cell origin

1. Meningioma
   a. meningothelial (syncytial)
   b. transitional
   c. fibrous
   d. psammomatous
   e. angiomatous
   f. microcystic
   g. secretory
   h. clear cell
   i. chordoid
   j. lymphoplasmactye-rich
   k. metaplastic variants (xanthomatous, myxoid, osseous, cartilagenous, etc.)
2. Atypical meningioma
3. Anaplastic [malignant] meningioma
   a. variants of 1 a–k (see above)
   b. papillary

Meningothelial (syncytial) meningioma

As the synonym 'syncytial' implies, the cells of the meningothelial meningioma are often poorly defined with indistinct borders. They are polygonal with large, spheroidal, and centrally situated nuclei. A common occurrence in these tumors is nuclear vacuolization, which is due to invagination of cytoplasm seen face on. The cytoplasm may be finely granular or fibrillary. Using other meningothelial cells, collagen fibers, blood vessels, or other structures as their central element, meningothelial cells wrap themselves in a concentric fashion forming whorls (Fig. 35.9). These whorls may become impregnated by amorphous periodic acid-Schiff (PAS) positive material, may have internal structures that become indistinct and

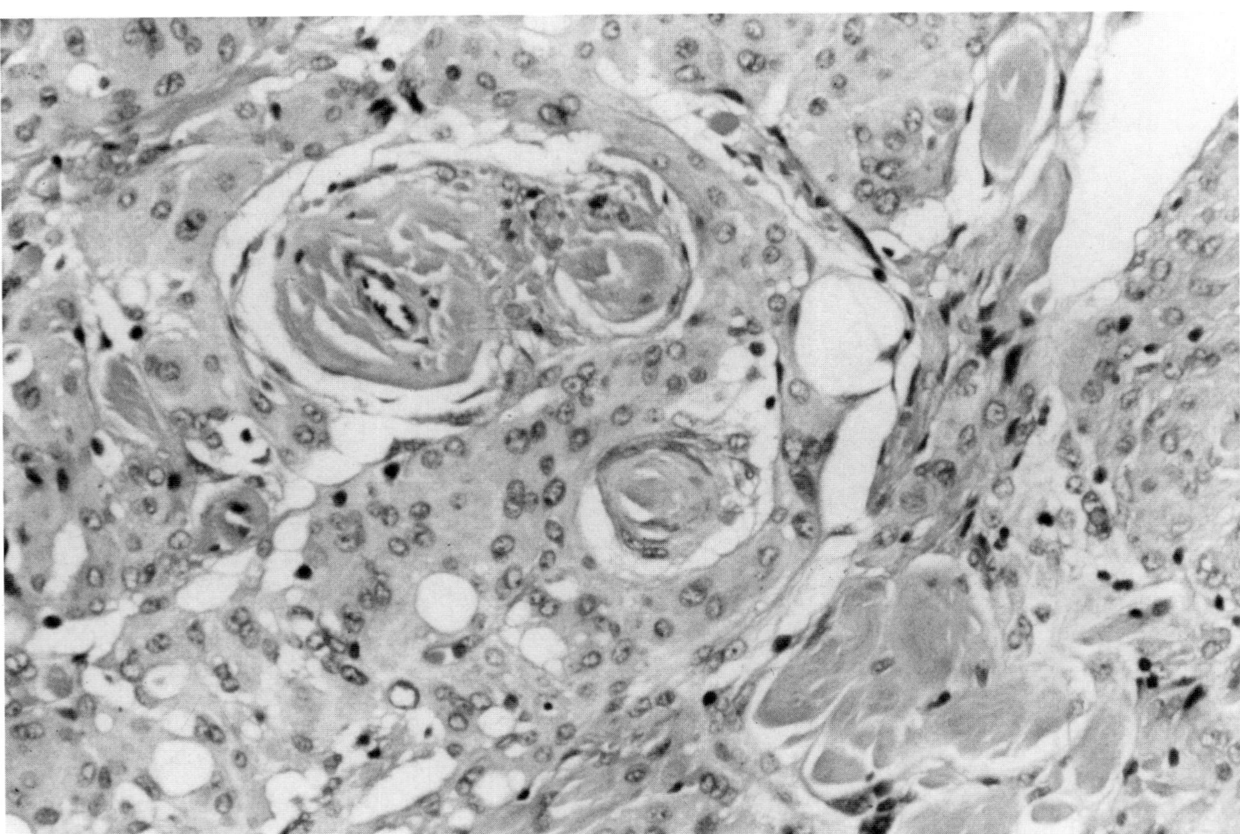

Fig. 35.9 Photomicrograph of a meningioma which had invaded the temporalis muscle. The meningothelial tumor cells are forming whorls around trapped and degenerating muscle fibers. (×200).

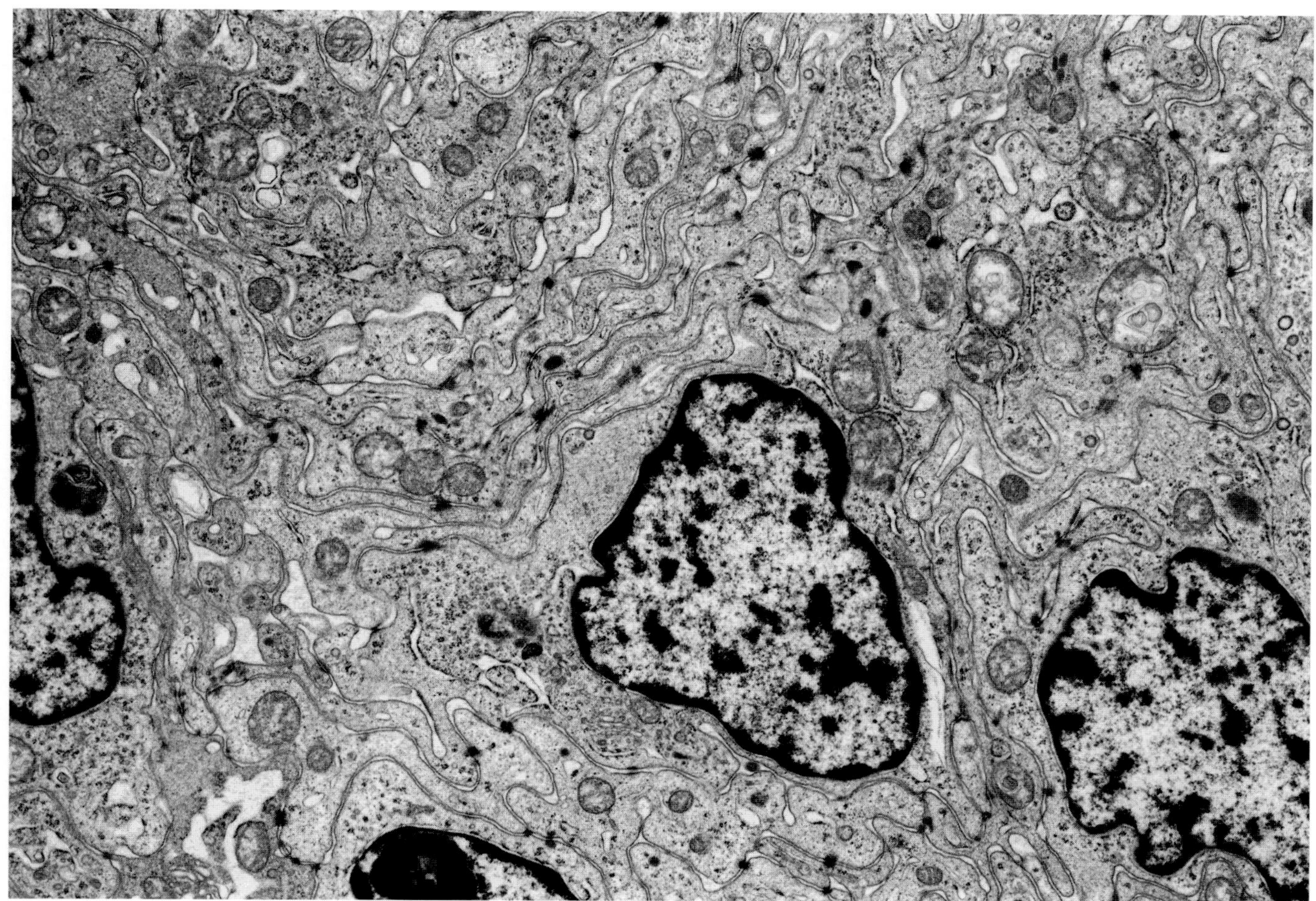

Fig. 35.10 Electron photomicrograph of a meningothelial meningioma. There is marked interdigitation of the cytoplasm. Numerous desmosomes can be seen. These findings are typical of meningioma. (×11 600).

hyalinized, or may become calcified, in which case they are known as psammoma bodies and the meningioma itself is termed psammomatous (Kepes 1982).

Ultrastructurally, extensive cytoplasmic interdigitation exists that cannot be resolved by light microscopy. Intracytoplasmic filaments, desmosomes, and gap junctions are features shared by all histologic variants of meningioma (Fig. 35.10).

Fibrous (fibroblastic) meningioma

In this histologic variety of meningioma, the meningothelial cells are more elongated, may be in sheets and/or fascicles, and have a spindle shape and high chromatic density that give a fibroblastic quality, although the nuclei usually retain a meningothelial appearance (Fig. 35.11). Whorl formation and psammoma bodies may be absent, but more commonly are focally present. Ultrastructurally, there are fewer desmosomes and less intermediate filaments. When meningothelial and fibroblastic areas coexist in the same tumor, the term 'transitional meningioma' is used.

Histologic variants

Numerous histopathologic variants of meningioma exist. None of these has any prognostic significance, but it is important to recognize them as they may at times have striking similarity to other neoplasms (Kepes 1982, Burger et al 1991). In this regard, microcystic meningiomas and 'mucoid' meningiomas must be differentiated from hemangioblastomas and chordomas, respectively. Highly vascularized meningothelial meningiomas, often referred to as 'angiomatous meningiomas', often have dilated blood vessels and may have thickened or hyalinized walls. This tumor must be differentiated from hemangioblastoma and hemangiopericytoma, as it rarely shows atypia or aggressive behavior (Jellinek & Slowik 1975) (Fig. 35.12).

Cystic changes that may be associated with meningiomas are usually found extrinsic to the tumor, between it and the adjacent cortex (Worthington et al 1985, Borovich et al 1988, Fortuna et al 1988, Umansky et al 1988). The cysts are lined by glial tissue and filled with a fluid that is usually clear amber. Less commonly, intratumoral cysts may occur. Intrinsically cystic meningi-

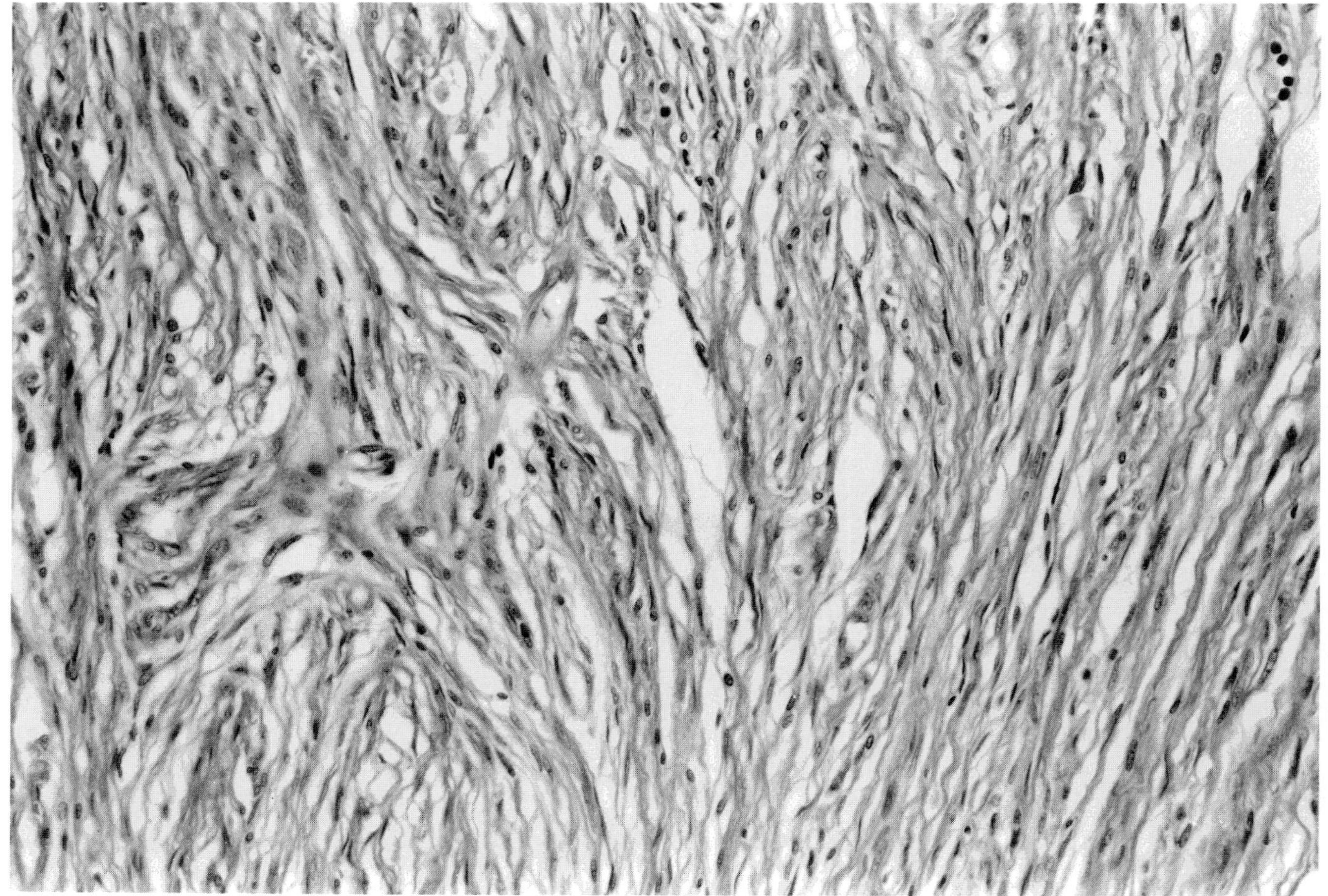

Fig. 35.11 Photomicrograph of a typical fibroblastic meningioma. Note the more elongated cells arranged in fascicles. Although they are spindle shaped and have high chromatic density, careful review reveals numerous cells with the typical cytoplasmic indentation of the nucleus. (Original magnification ×250).

omas occur more commonly in males and in the pediatric population; indeed, a majority of the meningiomas in children who are less than 12 months old are cystic (Bowen et al 1981, Katayama et al 1986). Of importance, surgically and prognostically, is that up to 20% of cystic meningiomas may be aggressive or frankly malignant.

Another characteristic, although not invariable, feature of meningiomas is a change in adjacent bone, namely hyperostosis. Hyperostosis, an osteoblastic process that may simply be a reactive change to the adjacent tumor but more commonly is secondary to invasion of the Haversian canals by the meningioma (Derome & Visot 1991) (Fig. 35.13), is visible on skull X-rays or computerized tomography scans. It not only allows improved diagnostic accuracy, but also has vital implications to the surgeon: if this bone is left behind, recurrence may be expected. The bone is laid down in radiating spicules perpendicular to the skull surface, which gives a stippled appearance to the surface of the bone. Osteolytic changes may occur as well, although rarely (Younis & Sawaya 1992).

Atypical meningioma

Besides brain invasion and metastatic spread, which define malignancy, certain features that may be seen by light microscopy portend an increased tumor aggressiveness and increased likelihood for recurrence. Among these features are loss of architectural pattern, high cellularity, increased mitotic figures, necrosis, prominent nucleoli, and nuclear pleomorphism (de la Monte et al 1986). Hypervascularity and hemosiderin deposition have also been identified as histologic parameters influencing prognosis (de la Monte et al 1986), although these are less widely held convictions (Jellinek & Slowik 1975, Burger et al 1991). If available, a bromodeoxyuridine labeling index > 1% would also categorize meningiomas as atypical (Hoshino et al 1986, Shibuya et al 1992).

Malignant meningioma

The diagnosis of malignant meningioma generally requires histologic evidence of brain invasion or distant metastasis,

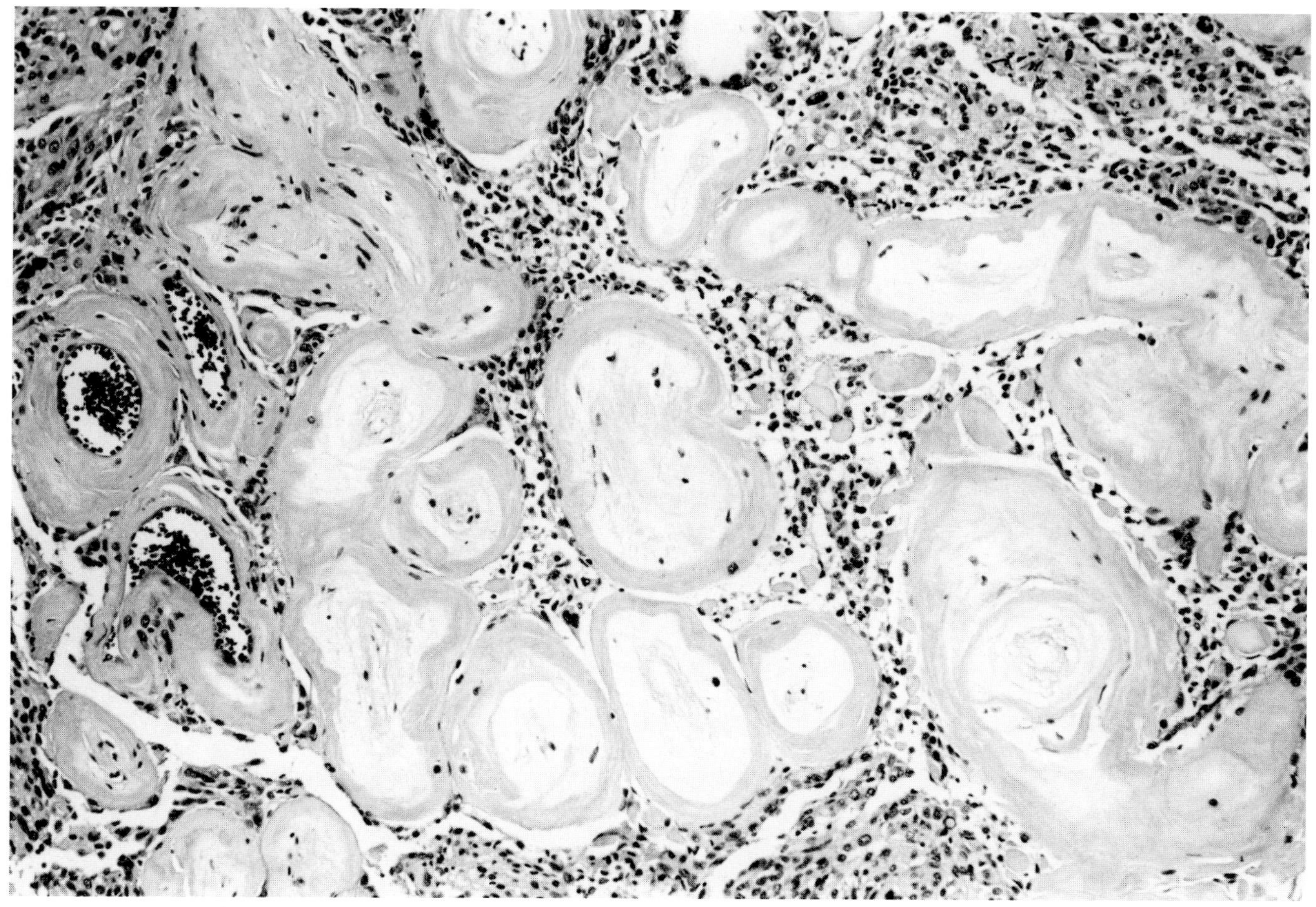

Fig. 35.12 Photomicrograph of an angiomatous meningioma. Note the numerous blood vessels with thickly hyalinated walls. (Original magnification ×125).

which, in most cases, is accompanied by further evidence of aggressiveness such as cellular sheeting, nuclear pleomorphism, increased cellularity and mitoses, and necrosis (Fig. 35.14). An exception to these requirements is the finding of a papillary pattern, which occurs more commonly in children and young adults (Ludwin et al 1975, Deen et al 1982). This pattern, caused by artefactual fragmentation, has been associated with a predictable aggressive behavior, with late distant metastases occurring with significant frequency (Pasquier et al 1986), whereas metastases from intracranial meningiomas rarely occur even though invasion of bone and the dural venous sinuses is common. When dissemination occurs, the more common sites of implantation and growth are the lungs/pleura, abdominal viscera (especially liver), lymph nodes and bones (Stoller et al 1987).

MANAGEMENT

The mainstay of treatment for meningiomas remains surgical resection. Critical parameters that affect the ease of surgical removal include tumor location, size, consistency, vascular and neural involvement, and, in the case of recurrence, prior surgery and/or radiotherapy. New and innovative approaches have been devised to reach and widely expose meningiomas in any location. Furthermore, a greater appreciation of risk factors for, and patterns of, tumor recurrence has changed surgical planning and goals. The necessity of resection of not only all of the neoplasm but also all of the involved dura, soft tissue, and bone in order to decrease the incidence of recurrence is now accepted procedure.

The only validated form of adjuvant therapy for meningiomas remains radiotherapy, although much investigation continues to find an effective chemotherapeutic agent.

Surgery

Preoperative care

The diagnosis of a probable intracranial meningioma on

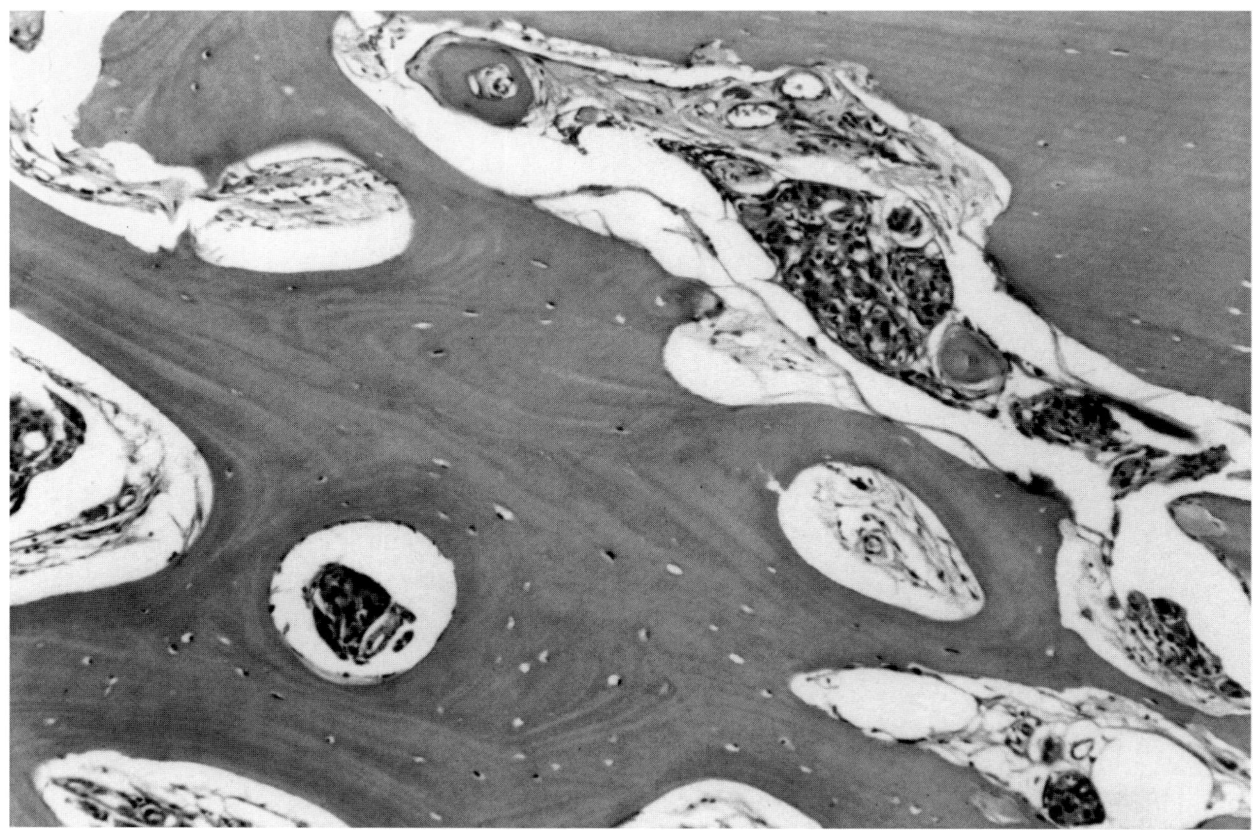

Fig. 35.13 Photomicrograph of the same meningioma shown in Figure 35.9. The tumor had transgressed the greater sphenoid wing. Tumor cells are clearly seen within the bone. (×100).

either CT or MRI requires a decision as to whether or not further invasive investigation is required. In most cases, pertinent intracranial vasculature, both arterial and venous, can be imaged by MRA; conventional arteriography is unnecessary. MRA may also predict for which neoplasm endovascular embolization would be most beneficial.

Conventional arteriography remains necessary, however, as a prelude to embolization and in cases in which arterial occlusion or reconstruction is a possibility. In the latter instances, injections during arterial compression provide valuable information about the patency of the circle of Willis, and temporary balloon occlusion may be performed to assess tolerance to vascular occlusion. To enhance the sensitivity of the balloon occlusion test, examinations with transcranial Doppler (TCD), xenon CT, or single photon emission computed tomography (SPECT) may be added (Erba et al 1988, De Monte et al 1993b).

Prior to surgical resection, endovascular embolization of meningiomas may reduce tumor vascularity and decrease surgical bleeding (Manelfe et al 1986). Surgical resection should be performed soon after to prevent recanalization of embolized vessels and neovascularization. Khayata and colleagues (1993) reported that, although matched embolized and non-embolized tumors showed no difference in the length of surgery or hospitalization, a significant reduction in blood loss and the number of transfusions was found. The greatest contribution of embolization is the preoperative occlusion of tumor vessels which, because of their location, can be reached only late in the resection of the tumor.

For all patients with supratentorial meningiomas, anticonvulsant therapy is initiated if it is not already being used, dexamethasone is administered beginning one to several days prior to the operation, and an H_2 antagonist is coprescribed. Pneumatic compression devices are placed on the legs when the patient is admitted to the hospital and they remain in use for the entire period of hospitalization. Perioperative antibiotics are used prophylactically for staphylococcal organisms in all patients, and a third-generation cephalosporin with activity against pseudomonal organisms and, at times, metronidazole (for anaerobic organisms) are added when surgery in the mouth, paranasal sinuses, ear, or mastoid is planned.

General operative procedures

Positioning of the patient should be done in a fashion

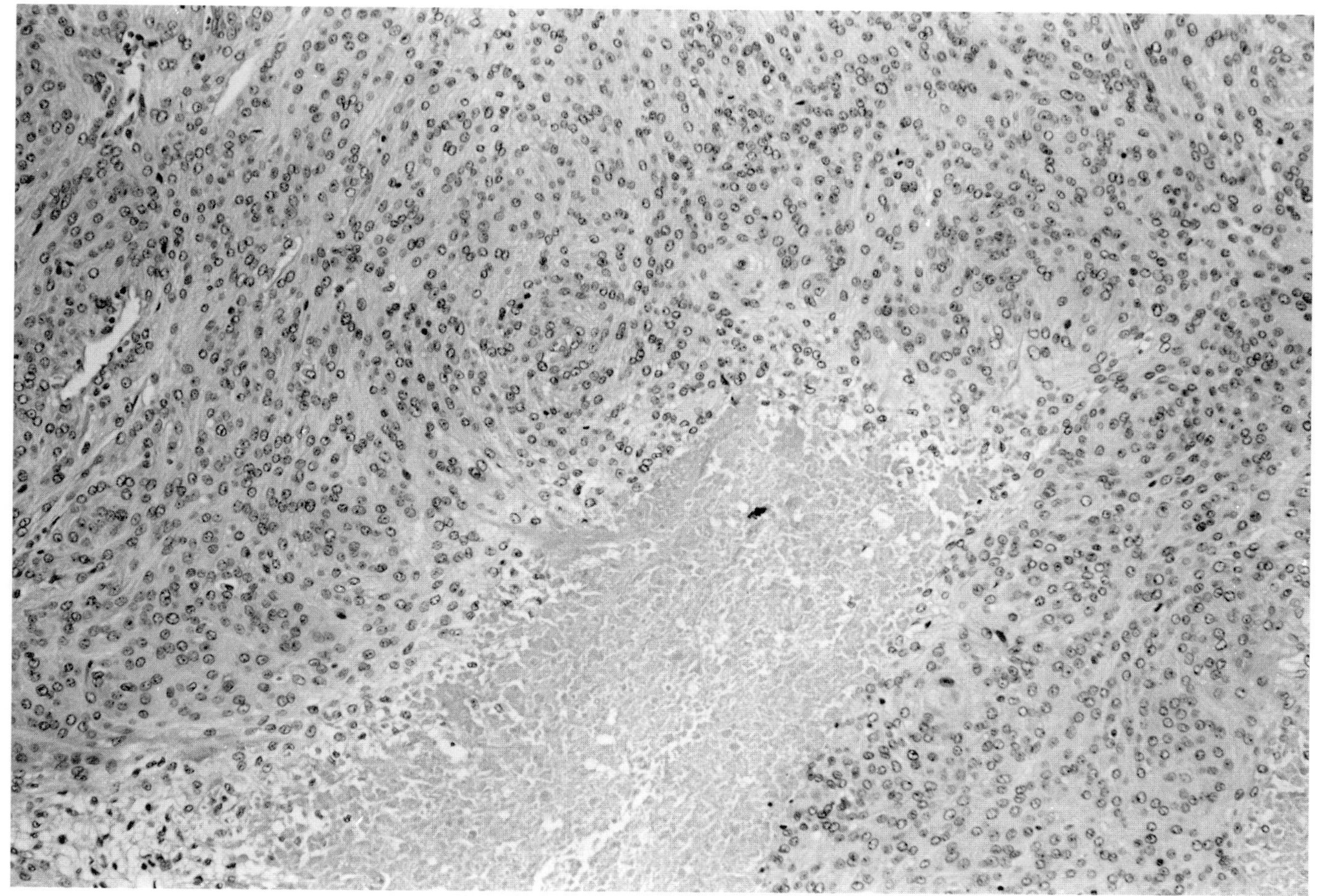

Fig. 35.14 Photomicrograph of a malignant meningioma. Note the area of focal necrosis, the increased cellularity and the cellular sheeting. (Original magnification ×125).

that maximizes the patient's safety, the accessibility of the tumor, the allowance for unimpeded venous drainage, the beneficial effects of gravity, and the surgeon's comfort. Most patients with either supra- or infratentorial meningiomas may be placed in the supine position; since many excellent alternatives exist, the patient should not be subjected to the increased risk nor the surgeon to the increased discomfort of the sitting position. Monitoring for air embolism, that should be used with any position that involves placing the head above the heart level, is particularly important during meningioma surgery since many tumors are closely related to the venous sinuses and their large tributaries.

As well as taking advantage of the effects of gravity, several methods are employed to minimize brain retraction, among which is spinal drainage. However, contraindications such as large tumors or obstructive hydrocephalus should be considered. Hyperventilation to a pCO_2 of 25–30 and a 20% solution of mannitol at a dosage of 0.25 g/kg contribute to the degree of brain relaxation.

The best means of reducing brain retraction, however, is to eliminate the need to do so by using one of the basal approaches. Since these approaches utilize orbital and zygomatic osteotomies and increase removal of the bony skull base, they allow a low flat route to basally located tumors (Jane et al 1982, Al-Mefty et al 1988, Sen & Sekhar 1990, Al-Mefty et al 1991, DeMonte & Al-Mefty 1993a).

Scalp flaps, which should be wide-based to allow for a rich blood supply and designed to facilitate any subsequent reoperation, should be linear, gently curvilinear, or bicoronal incisions (rather than 'horseshoe' flaps).

In the vast majority of first operations for meningiomas, a layer of arachnoid separates the tumor from the brain parenchyma, cranial nerves, and blood vessels. When it does, the chances of neural and/or vascular injury can be greatly reduced by defining and staying within this surgical plane. One maneuver that facilitates the definition of the arachnoidal borders is the extensive debulking of the tumor, thus allowing the tumor capsule to collapse inward. The method used to debulk the tumor, which may be suction, coagulation, sharp excision, or use of the ultrasonic aspirator or the surgical laser, depends on the tumor consistency, vascularity, and location.

Once the mass of the meningioma is resected, careful attention must be given to removing the involved dura and bone. The extent of bone that must be removed can be determined by inspection of the preoperative CT scan's 'bone windows'. All of the hyperostotic bone should be considered contaminated by neoplastic cells: the fear of entering the mastoid air cells, or paranasal sinuses is not a reason for failing to remove this diseased bone. A wide margin of dura should be resected, and the defect should be repaired with pericranium, temporalis fascia or fascia lata.

Surgical approaches and techniques by tumor location

Convexity meningiomas. Meningiomas having the greatest potential for total removal and cure are those that overlie the cerebral convexities, since they allow for excision with a wide dural margin. Even in instances of transdural bone and soft tissue invasion, en bloc removal is still possible in a procedure that is termed a 'grade zero' removal (Kinjo et al 1993).

There is usually a long clinical history in the majority of patients. Depending on the location of the tumor the patient may experience mental deterioration, contralateral limb weakness, sensory aberration, or visual loss, or disturbances of speech when the dominant hemisphere is affected. Seizures are especially frequent when the central or temporal cortices are compressed. Occasionally a bump on the patient's head is the only finding.

Once identified, the arachnoidal dissection plane, the initial vital step for the resection of any meningioma, should be developed circumferentially for convexity meningiomas by using sharp dissection and nonadhering surgical cottonoids inserted between the arachnoid layer and the tumor capsule. Although the initial isolation of the arachnoidal dissection plane is generally difficult superficially, it usually becomes apparent within the first few millimeters from the surface. Recurrent tumors and some aggressive meningiomas do not have the normal anatomic layers and require careful sharp dissection under the operative microscope to minimize cortical injury.

A consideration for convexity meningiomas that overlie the sylvian fissure is the possibility that branches of the middle cerebral artery have adhered to the tumor capsule. The best procedure for freeing these branches is to begin at points where they are uninvolved and follow them through the tumor. The branches can usually be dissected free in a straightforward fashion, unless the surgical plane is incorrect or the case is a reoperation.

Once the meningioma and a wide dural margin have been resected, the dural defect is repaired with pericranium, temporalis fascia, or fascia lata in a watertight fashion. If excision of bone was required, an acrylic cranioplasty may be fashioned.

Parasagittal and falcine meningiomas. The signs and symptoms associated with meningiomas arising from these areas are related to where the tumor mass lies along the anteroposterior plane. Anteriorly situated tumors may cause headache, slowly progressive mental decline, visual deterioration secondary to increased intracranial pressure, or generalized seizures. In contradistinction, focal seizures, at times following a Jacksonian pattern, are more frequently seen in patients with meningiomas localized in the middle third. These seizures, as any motor findings, are generally first evident in the contralateral foot and leg. Symptoms from tumors of the posterior third can, like those in the anterior third, be of insidious onset. Headache, mental symptoms, and intracranial hypertension are common. A distinguishing feature, however, is the finding of visual field loss.

The primary consideration in the removal of parasagittal meningiomas is management of the superior sagittal sinus and the cerebral veins that drain into it. Sagittal sinus involvement anterior to the rolandic veins can be managed by ligation and excision of the sinus. However, since two thirds of parasagittal meningiomas occur posterior to the coronal suture, the management of superior sinus involvement may result in serious complications for the patient. Hakuba et al (1979) and Bonnal & Brotchi (1978) have classified superior sinus involvement by meningiomas into 8 distinct groups (Fig. 35.15). Their surgical approaches and management are based on this classification, and are: (1) simple dissection of the meningioma off the lateral wall of the sinus (for type I involvement), (2) sagittal sinus reconstruction (for type II–VII), and (3) excision of the sinus in the case of a totally occluded sinus (type VIII and some type VII).

During reconstruction of the superior sagittal sinus, the blood flow through the sinus may be maintained by using an intraluminal shunt (Hakuba et al 1979). This may be essential in posterior third involvement, since even temporary occlusion may result in cerebral engorgement and swelling.

The above considerations and the high (25%) incidence of parasagittal meningiomas that are bilateral, require a craniotomy that crosses the midline to allow access to both sides of the sinus (Gautier-Smith 1970). The craniotomy must be raised carefully, as skull changes occur in 25–50% of parasagittal meningiomas (Gautier-Smith 1970) and rough elevation of the bone plate may tear an adherent superior sagittal sinus or important draining veins.

Large parasagittal meningiomas that extend deep into the interhemispheric fissure and, especially, falcine meningiomas often have anterior cerebral artery branches that have adhered to the bottom edge of the tumor near the free edge of the falx.

Meningiomas of the falx cerebri are less common (20–50% less) than parasagittal tumors, more commonly bilateral, and rarely involve the superior sagittal sinus

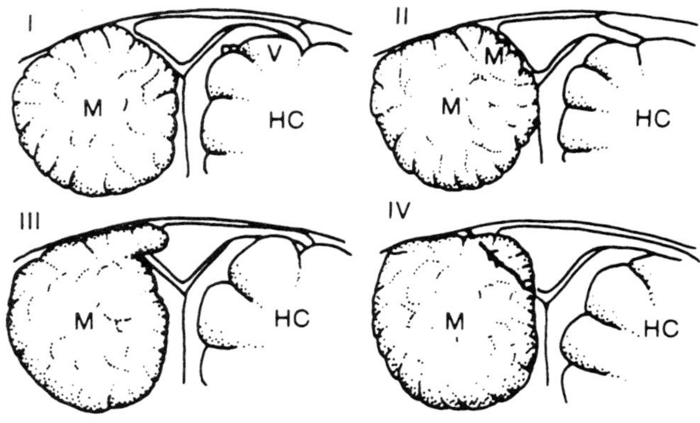

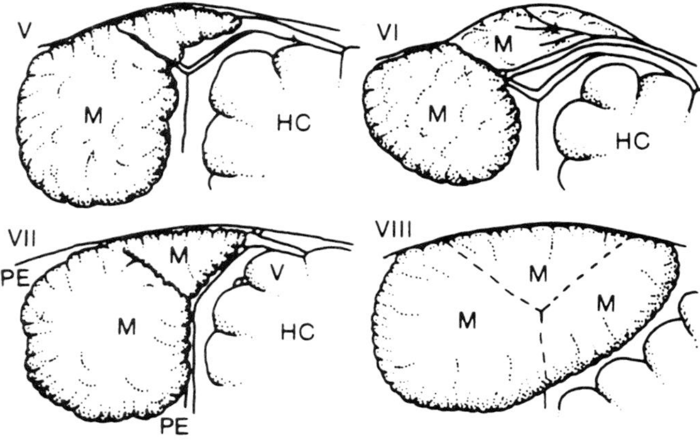

Fig. 35.15 Artist's representation of the classification of superior sagittal sinus involvement by parasagittal meningiomas.

(Gautier-Smith 1970). As in the case of parasagittal meningiomas, extensive central debulking decreases the need for cerebral retraction. Excision of the falx allows complete removal, as well as access to the opposite side for removal of contralateral tumor extension. The inferior sagittal sinus, which is usually involved by the meningioma, can usually be excised with the tumor unless it provides an essential avenue for venous drainage.

Olfactory groove and tuberculum sellae. Surgical approaches to meningiomas arising from the olfactory groove and to those of the tuberculum sellae (TS) are similar in many respects. Since both tumors are midline lesions that, to a variable degree, derive their blood supply from the ethmoidal branches of the ophthalmic artery, the anterior branch of the middle meningeal artery, and the meningeal branches of the ICA, interruption of this transbasal blood supply is the initial step (Al-Mefty & Smith 1991). Following devascularization, the tumor is debulked with the CUSA or laser, and, finally, the capsule is dissected free and removed.

A low basal approach is highly preferred to avoid the brain injury and excessive morbidity that can occur from excessive frontal lobe retraction, especially if it is bilateral. The surgeon's line of vision can be lowered by at least 1.5–2.0 cm when compared with a standard craniotomy by removing the supraorbital rim (Jane et al 1982). A unilateral supraorbital craniotomy is usually sufficient, but it can easily be extended bilaterally if required. The olfactory nerves are dissected free from the frontal lobes and can be functionally preserved in the case of smaller tumors.

Both tuberculum sellae and large olfactory groove meningiomas displace the optic nerves (ON) posterolaterally, at times placing them lateral to the carotid arteries. Since the ONs may be quite attenuated and their distinction from the tumor capsule may be quite difficult, extreme caution and piecemeal removal of the tumor using fine-tipped bipolars and microdissection are required. At times, it may be necessary to start the dissection at the chiasm to locate and dissect an obscure optic nerve on the contralateral side. Also, the optic nerves are fixed at their entrance into the optic canal, and their dissection may begin there. Operative inspection of both optic canals, especially in cases of TS meningiomas, is essential since a tongue of tumor may extend into this area and be missed if efforts are not made to determine its existence.

The anterior cerebral arteries (ACA) and their branches are the vascular structures most at risk during removal of TS or olfactory groove meningiomas. The A1 segments tend to be particularly stretched or adherent (Fig. 35.16).

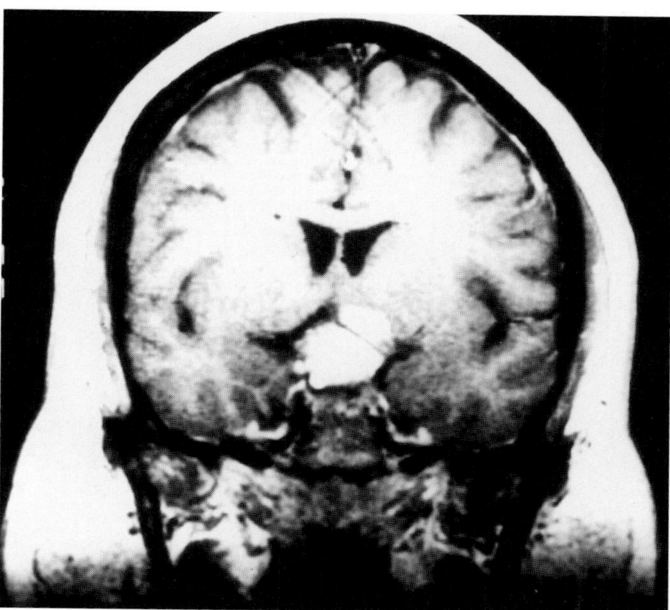

Fig. 35.16 T1-weighted MRI post-gadolinium. The signal void representing the left A1 segment of the anterior cerebral artery can be seen encased by this tuberculum sellae meningioma. Careful dissection is required to preserve perforating arteries arising from this vessel and the anterior communicating complex.

Further, the arterial twigs arising from the ACAs may be a source of vascular supply for the tumor. These vessels should be carefully followed, prior to occlusion, to ascertain that they are not hypothalamic perforators or optic apparatus supply.

The pituitary stalk, which is generally displaced posteriorly and to one side, can be identified by its characteristic vascular pattern and distinctive color.

Liliequist's membrane is virtually always intact in primary operations and, therefore, dissection of a posteriorly extending tumor from the upper basilar artery is usually straightforward.

Once the tumor has been resected intracranially, any extension into the paranasal sinuses can be removed by drilling through the planum sphenoidale or the more anterior cranial base to reach the paranasal sinuses. Thorough dural repair is necessary and can be accomplished with fascia lata, autologous fat graft, and a vascularized pericranial flap.

Sphenoid wing meningiomas. The most common of the basal meningiomas are those that occur along the sphenoid wing (Table 35.1 and Fig. 35.17). These meningiomas are subclassified according to their point of origin along the sphenoid ridge (Table 35.9) (Cushing & Eisenhardt 1938, Bonnal et al 1980, Al-Mefty 1990), and include the meningioma en plaque. Those meningiomas of the latter group have no significant intracranial component and are characterized by marked hyperostosis of the sphenoid bone, a result of diffuse tumor invasion that causes progressive painless proptosis and, occasionally, diverse cranial neuropathies (due to foraminal encroachment). The dural involvement is widespread, affecting the frontal, temporal, orbital, and sphenoidal regions. The surgical approach to this type of pathology is the complete removal of the greater and lesser sphenoid wings (including the anterior clinoid), the opening of the basal foramina, and the removal of the superior and lateral orbital walls, which then facilitates the removal of the involved dura. Resection of the dura of the superior orbital fissure and the lateral wall of the cavernous sinus can be included. Careful dural repair with fascia lata is reinforced with autologous fat and/or pericranium or temporalis muscle and/or fascia, as needed.

Table 35.9 Classification of sphenoid wing meningiomas (Cushing & Eisenhardt 1938, Bonnal et al 1980, Al-Mefty 1990)

1. Clinoidal
   a. group 1
   b. group 2
   c. group 3
2. Alar
3. Pterional
4. En plaque

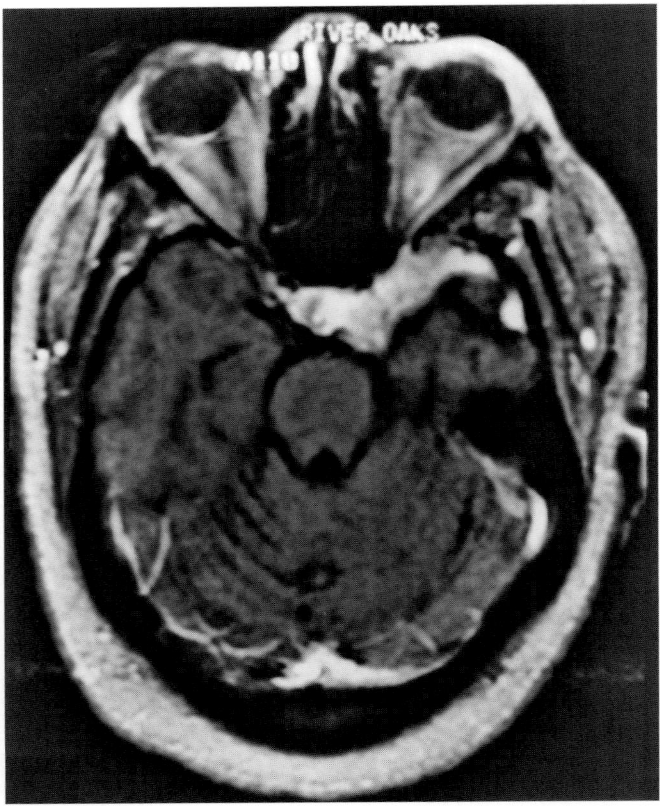

Fig. 35.17 T1-weighted axial MRI following gadolinium contrast administration. This recurrent sphenoid wing meningioma extended from the cavernous sinus to the lateral sphenoid wing. A second small meningioma overlying the temporal convexity is also seen which was not appreciated on the noncontrasted study.

En masse lesions of the pterional third of the sphenoid ridge can be associated with relatively localized head pain and bulging of the frontal and temporal bones. Seizures and contralateral hemiparesis are not uncommon.

These tumors can be resected in a fashion similar to convexity meningiomas once the sphenoid ridge is drilled away to allow for the circumferential dural resection needed to remove the tumor's attachment. Drilling away the sphenoid ridge causes interruption of the blood supply to these tumors, which is from the branches of the internal maxillary artery, and leaves a less vascular tumor, thus aiding its removal and minimizing blood loss. Meningiomas in this location spread the sylvian fissure apart and may adhere to or, at times, encase the MCA branches. An arachnoidal plane is invariably present, however, and, with care, the vessels can be freed.

The extradural removal of the sphenoid ridge devascularizes more medially located meningiomas as well. Furthermore, it allows the optic canal to be opened to decompress the optic nerve. The subclinoid carotid artery can be isolated, which provides distal control of the cavernous carotid artery and facilitates opening and dissecting the tumor from the cavernous sinus. If dissection is planned in the cavernous sinus, proximal ICA control in either the petrous canal or the neck is necessary.

A cranio-orbital-zygomatic approach meets all the requirements for an optimal approach to meningiomas of the sphenoid ridge: (1) it provides the surgeon a low basal approach and multiple avenues for dissection, (2) it allows the resection of hyperostotic bone and interruption of tumor blood supply early in the operation, and (3) it achieves proximal and distal control of the intracavernous carotid artery if required (Fig. 35.18). Furthermore, it can easily be tailored to fit the need of each patient.

During removal of middle and inner third (alar and clinoidal) meningiomas, the internal carotid, the middle and anterior cerebral arteries, and their branches, as well as the optic, oculomotor, and olfactory nerves, are the neurovascular structures at greatest risk. Additionally, anterior clinoidal meningiomas (ACM), which commonly invade the cavernous sinus, put the third, fourth, sixth, and seventh cranial nerves at risk (Bonnal et al 1980, Al-Mefty 1990). Because of their direct adventitial adherence to the supraclinoid carotid, group 1 ACM carry an especial risk of carotid injury.

The surrounding arachnoidal layer allows for these meningiomas to be separated from the neurovascular structures by careful dissection (with the exception of the group 1 ACM — vide supra), although the tumor may cause marked distortion of the normal anatomy. Initially, the distal MCA branches are identified in the sylvian fissure and followed back to the tumor. In a similar fashion, the olfactory nerve is dissected from the inferior frontal lobe and followed back to the optic nerve and carotid artery. Identification of the opposite optic nerve allows identification of the optic chiasm. Following the chiasm will allow the identification of the ipsilateral optic nerve.

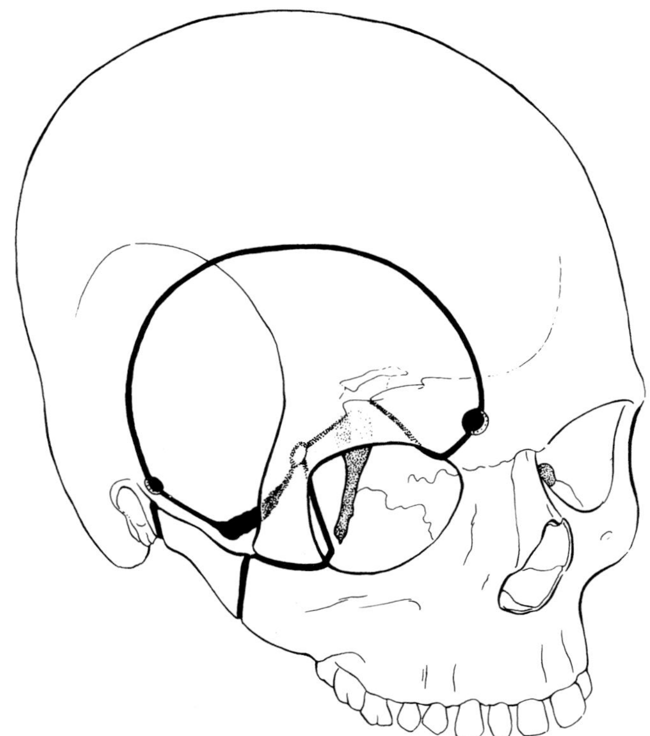

Fig. 35.18 Artist's representation of the osteotomies and areas of bone removal required to perform a cranio-orbital-zygomatic craniotomy.

As in all cases of meningioma surgery, intratumoral debulking facilitates removal, but care must be taken in the optico-carotid triangle and posterior to the carotid bifurcation where injury to perforating arteries may lead to visual loss and hemiparesis, respectively. The location of the ophthalmic artery, which crosses the anterior corner of the optico-carotid triangle, must be anticipated.

Clinoidal meningiomas, which usually present with unilateral loss of vision and optic atrophy, require opening the optic canal and sheath since tumor ingrowth occurs with a high frequency and leaving residual meningioma in this area may contribute to lack of visual improvement postoperatively. As mentioned, clinoidal meningiomas frequently involve the cavernous sinus, which they invade through the superior wall (Bonnal et al 1980, Al-Mefty 1990). Entry through the superior wall may be made via the medial, anteromedial, and paramedial triangles, which thereby exposes the anterior loop of the cavernous ICA to allow dissection of the tumor from this space.

Cavernous sinus meningiomas. Involvement by meningioma of the cavernous sinus does not preclude aggressive tumor removal. Progressive neurologic deficit and/or progressive enlargement of the tumor, as imaged by serial MR images, are indicators for resection of cavernous sinus meningioma (Fig. 35.19). Extensive eva-

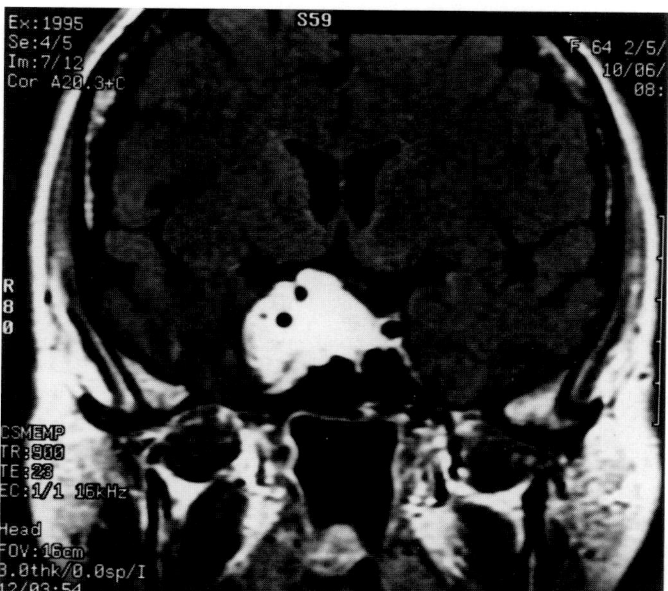

Fig. 35.19 Coronal T1-weighted post-contrast MRI. This large cavernous sinus meningioma was completely asymptomatic in this patient even though there is clear compression of the right optic nerve.

luation of the available anatomic and physiologic collateral circulation should be made prior to surgery in order to predict the potential risk of cerebral ischemia in the event of carotid artery occlusion. Proximal and distal ICA control, which must be established prior to dissection within the cavernous sinus space, may be achieved by exposing the ICA in the cervical or intrapetrous portions. The cervical exposure is associated with less morbidity, as section of the greater superficial petrosal nerve is not required, thereby avoiding a dry-eye syndrome that can be especially troublesome when there is an ipsilateral V1 lesion. Entry into the CS may be either through the medial triangles mentioned above or through the lateral triangles. Dissection of the tumor progresses in a stepwise fashion, beginning by opening of the dura propria of the optic nerve sheath longitudinally along the length of the optic canal (De Monte & Al-Mefty 1993a). The distal dural ring is opened next, with the opening extending posteriorly to the oculomotor trigone, and thereby also opening the proximal dural ring and allowing a wide entry into the anterior and superior CS space. The carotid artery can be mobilized laterally by releasing it from its proximal and distal dural rings, which then allows dissection in the medial CS space. Lateral entry into the cavernous sinus begins by an incision beneath the projected course of the third nerve, allowing elevation of the outer dural layer of the lateral wall of the cavernous sinus, which is peeled away. The ICA can be located by dissection between the third and fourth nerves and the first division of the trigeminal nerve (Parkinson's triangle). The course of the sixth nerve, which runs lateral to the ICA and is usually directly apposed to it, is usually parallel, but deep to V1. The tumor is removed from within the cavernous sinus space by suction, bipolar coagulation, and microdissection. A plane of cleavage along the carotid artery can usually be developed. Venous bleeding, typically not a problem when the tumor fills the sinus, may occur as the venous plexus is decompressed by tumor removal. In that event, hemostasis can be obtained by packing the CS space with oxidized cellulose or another similar hemostatic agent.

In the author's series, total removal of cavernous sinus meningioma has been possible in 76% of patients. The surgical major morbidity and mortality rates were 4.8% and 2.4% respectively. Preoperative CN deficits improved in 14%, remained unchanged in 80%, and permanently worsened in 6%. Seven patients experienced 10 new CN deficits (DeMonte et al 1993b).

Posterior fossa meningiomas. 10% of all intracranial meningiomas, arise in the posterior fossa (Table 35.1). Almost half of these meningiomas are located in the cerebellopontine angle, 40% are tentorial or cerebellar convexity, and 9% and 6% are clival or at the foramen magnum, respectively (Castellano & Ruggiero 1953, Yasargil et al 1980, Martinez et al 1983). Meningiomas arising medial to the trigeminal nerve (petroclival meningiomas) must be differentiated from those arising lateral to it (CPA or posterior petrous pyramid meningiomas) because petroclival meningiomas carry a significantly higher rate of surgical morbidity (Castellano & Ruggiero 1953, Sekhar & Jannetta 1984, Al-Mefty et al 1988).

CPA (posterior petrous pyramid) meningiomas. Cranial nerve findings are quite common with meningiomas in this location. Hearing loss, facial pain or numbness, and facial weakness or spasm are common, as are headache and cerebellar hemispheric signs (De Monte & Al-Mefty 1993b).

The cranial nerves of the posterior fossa have a relatively constant relationship to CPA meningiomas: the trochlear nerve is usually superior and lateral to the tumor, whereas the trigeminal nerve is superior and anterior; the abducens nerve is found anteriorly, whereas the seventh and eighth cranial nerves are posterior and the ninth through eleventh cranial nerves are inferior (De Monte & Al-Mefty 1993b).

A standard retrosigmoid approach usually allows sufficient exposure for removal of these tumors (Sekhar & Jannetta 1984, Samii & Ammirati 1991); exposure of the presigmoid dura is, nevertheless, performed to allow retraction of the sigmoid sinus laterally and thus decrease its obstruction of the surgeon's view. The meningioma's dural attachment to the posterior pyramid, which is progressively coagulated and divided to devascularize the tumor, must be done with care to avoid injury to the exiting cranial nerves. If the size of the tumor precludes safe removal, the tumor capsule should be opened and the tumor centrally debulked. After the tumor has been debulked and devascularized, the capsule is carefully dissected from the surrounding cranial nerves, the brainstem, the superior cerebellar artery (SCA—superior and medial), the anterior inferior cerebellar artery (AICA — medial), and posterior inferior cerebellar artery (PICA — inferior and medial). Once the tumor is removed, the dural attachment should be removed or coagulated (either with the bipolar or laser) and any hyperostotic bone drilled away, keeping in mind the location of the nearby inner ear structures.

Petroclival meningiomas. Like CPA meningiomas, these tumors cause diverse cranial neuropathies. Facial hypesthesia may occur in upwards of 80% of patients, while hearing loss and facial weakness occur in 50% and 40%, respectively. The lower cranial nerves and the ocular motor nerves (usually the abducens nerve) are affected in approximately one third of the patients. Headache and ataxia are common (De Monte & Al-Mefty 1993b).

For petroclival meningiomas (Fig. 35.20), which require a more lateral approach to maximize visualization and decrease the need for cerebellar retraction, the petrosal approach is an ideal choice (Fig. 35.21). The patient

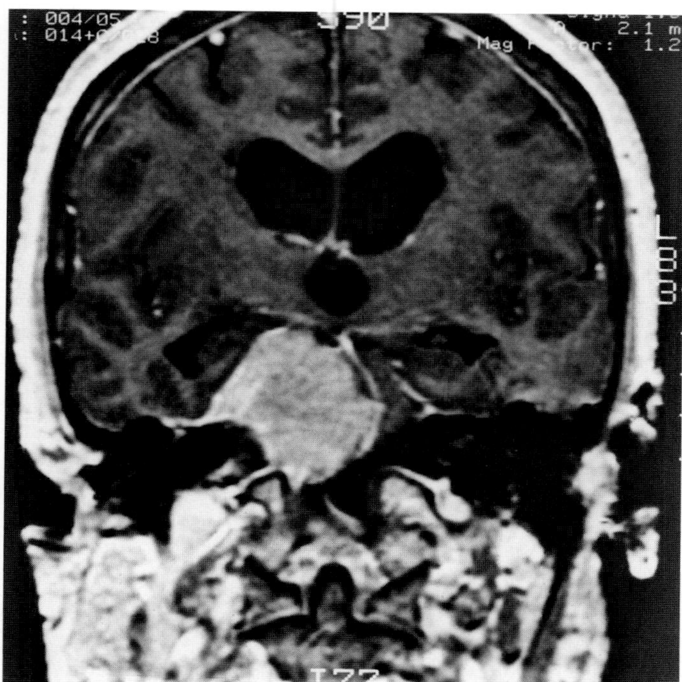

Fig. 35.20 Coronal T1-weighted post-contrast MRI. Obstructive hydrocephalus and hypesthesia in the distribution of the right trigeminal nerve were the only symptoms of this large petroclival meningioma.

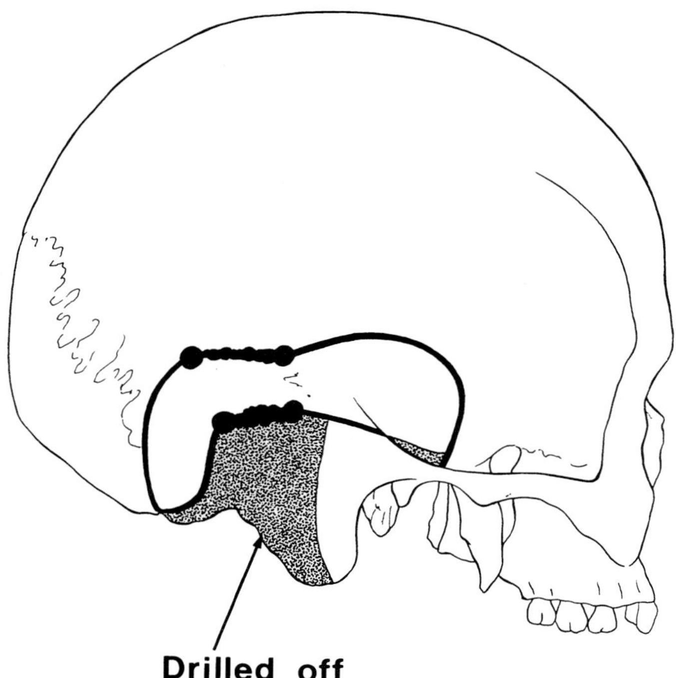

Fig. 35.21 Artist's representation of the osteotomies and areas of bone removal required to perform a petrosal craniotomy.

is placed supine, with the ipsilateral shoulder elevated and the patient's head turned 45° away from the side of the tumor, lowered, and tilted toward the opposite side to bring the base of the petrous pyramid to the highest point of the operative field. A bone flap is carefully elevated, exposing the transverse and sigmoid sinuses (Al-Mefty et al 1991). A mastoidectomy is performed, exposing the sigmoid sinus and the dura anterior to it, the jugular bulb, the lateral and posterior semicircular canals, and the facial nerve in the fallopian canal. Next, the bone overlying the sinodural angle is removed, exposing the superior petrosal sinus. If hearing is absent, a total labyrinthectomy can be performed at this point, thereby increasing the anterolateral exposure of the tumor. After the dura mater is opened along the anterior border of the sigmoid sinus and along the floor of the temporal fossa, the vein of Labbé is identified and protected, the superior petrosal sinus is coagulated and divided, and this division is carried medially through the tentorium, avoiding injury to the trochlear nerve and the superior petrosal vein. Complete sectioning of the tentorium allows the sigmoid sinus, along with the cerebellar hemisphere, to fall back, thus decreasing the need for retraction. Angling the microscope allows the fourth through twelfth cranial nerves, as well as the entire vertebrobasilar system and the anterolateral brainstem, to be visualized.

The relationship of the cranial nerves to petroclival meningiomas is similar to CPA meningiomas except that in the former the sixth cranial nerve is usually anterior and inferior and may be encased by the tumor (De Monte & Al-Mefty 1993b). The basilar artery may be displaced posteriorly or to the opposite side, or it may be encased. The posterior cerebral artery (PCA), the SCA, AICA, and PICA are usually posterior and medial to the tumor, but they, too, may be encased by it.

Tumor removal begins with progressive devascularization of the tumor by coagulating and dividing its vascular supply from the tentorium and from its insertion on the petrous pyramid and clivus. The arachnoid over the tumor is opened to allow entry through the capsule and central debulking. As noted above, neurovascular structures may be embedded in the meningioma, requiring that great care be taken, especially when using tools such as the ultrasonic aspirator or laser. The tumor capsule is then dissected free from the surrounding structures, but this must be done gently to avoid hypotension and bradycardia from vagal stimulation. The need to preserve the small perforating arteries to the brainstem and cranial nerves cannot be overemphasized.

As for CPA meningiomas, the point of dural attachment is vaporized and the hyperostotic bone removed with a high-speed diamond-tipped drill, working under constant irrigation between the cranial nerves. After the dura is closed in a watertight manner, the drilled petrous bone is covered with autologous fat, the temporalis muscle is rotated over the defect and sewn to the sternocleidomastoid muscle, and the soft tissues are closed in multiple layers.

Tentorial and cerebellar convexity meningiomas. Intracranial hypertension, headache and progressive cerebellar signs (dysmetria, ataxia, hypotonia and nystagmus) are the usual clinical features associated with either cerebellar convexity meningiomas or those tentorial meningiomas with a large posterior fossa component. If the supratentorial component of a tentorial meningioma is large, visual field defects may also be present.

In many respects, cerebellar convexity and tentorial meningiomas are quite similar to their supratentorial counterparts, the parasagittal and falcine meningiomas. The major area of concern is the status of the transverse sinus: a totally occluded transverse sinus may be excised with the rest of the meningioma whereas the management of an incompletely occluded transverse sinus is similar to that used for the superior sagittal sinus. When the two transverse sinuses are proven to be interconnected at the torcula, occlusion of the transverse sinus may be accomplished by a temporary vascular clip to measure its filling pressures. If there is no swelling, venous engorgement or rise in filling pressures of >7–10 mmHg, the transverse sinus may be divided if invaded by meningioma (Spetzler et al 1992). If the sinus is not involved, it should not be sacrificed; rather, the surgeon should alternate the field of vision from the supratentorial to the infratentorial compartments. The technique for removing the tumor is the same as that described for supratentorial parasagittal and falcine meningiomas.

Foramen magnum meningiomas. Foramen magnum tumors, the least common of the posterior fossa meningiomas, are located anterior or anterolateral to the cervicomedullary junction, and are usually intimately involved with the lower cranial nerves (IX–XII), the cervicomedullary junction, and the vertebral artery and its branches (especially PICA). The typical clinical syndrome consists of suboccipital and neck pain (usually in the C2 dermatome), ipsilateral upper extremity dysesthesias, contralateral dissociated sensory loss, progressive limb weakness beginning in the ipsilateral upper extremity and progressing in a counterclockwise fashion, and wasting of the intrinsic muscles of the hand (De Monte & Al-Mefty 1993b).

Since the traditional posterior approach to meningiomas in this location does not address the anterior location of the tumors, the transcondylar or far-lateral approach has been devised (Sen & Sekhar 1990, De Monte & Al-Mefty 1993b) (Fig. 35.22). For the transcondylar approach, the patient is placed in the supine position with the ipsilateral shoulder and back elevated 30–45°. A C-shaped incision that begins above the ear is extended caudally along the edge of the sternocleidomastoid muscle to expose the suboccipital area. The scalp flap is elevated in the subcutaneous plane to the level of the external auditory canal and, next, the sternocleidomastoid muscle is detached from the mastoid and retracted inferomedially. Injury to the accessory nerve must be avoided. The lateral mass of C1 is palpated and the muscles are dissected in a subperiosteal plane from the lamina of the first and second vertebrae. Once the inferior oblique muscle is detached, the ventral ramus of the second cervical root is followed medially to the vertebral artery between C1 and C2. The vertebral artery may be transposed medially once the transverse foramen of C1 is opened. A lateral suboccipital craniotomy is fashioned, the sigmoid sinus is skeletonized to the jugular bulb and, if necessary, a C1 and C2 laminectomy is performed. The occipital condyle and the lateral mass of C1 are then drilled. Next, the dura is incised posterior to the sigmoid sinus with the durotomy extending inferiorly to the entry of the vertebral artery. The dural incisions circumscribe the dural entry of the vertebral artery allowing its complete mobilization.

The uppermost dentate ligament and, if necessary, the posterior C2 nerve root are divided. The accessory nerve is located between the dentate ligaments and the posterior spinal nerve rootlets while the hypoglossal nerve may be either anterior or posterior to the tumor, depending on the tumor's point of origin, which if anteriorly placed, may involve both hypoglossal nerves.

The tumor capsule is opened carefully, with particular care given to avoid injury to the cranial nerve or blood vessels, and debulked. It may be detached from its clival base to decrease the vascularity. Careful separation of the tumor from the medulla and upper cervical spinal cord, the lower cranial nerves, and the vertebral artery, may be accomplished by dissection in the arachnoidal plane surrounding the tumor. The area of dural attachment is removed, as is any hyperostotic bone, and the dura is closed in a watertight manner to prevent CSF leakage. If the entire occipital condyle has been removed, an occipital-cervical fusion should be performed. Postoperatively, the patient is managed in either a stiff collar or a halo-thoracic brace, depending on the nature of the fusion construct. Injury to the lower cranial nerves, the major cause of operative morbidity, has led to the routine use, in some centers, of electromyographic monitoring of the muscles supplied by the vagus, accessory, and hypoglossal nerves (De Monte et al 1993a).

As mentioned, dysfunction of the lower cranial nerves is the primary cause of postoperative morbidity. Hence, careful assessment of the patient's ability to protect the airway is mandatory, and, in some cases, early tracheostomy may be warranted to avoid the complication of aspiration pneumonitis.

Intraventricular meningiomas. Meningiomas of the lateral ventricles, which arise from arachnoid cells contained in the choroid plexus and tela choroidea, account for a mere 1% of all intracranial meningiomas. They are

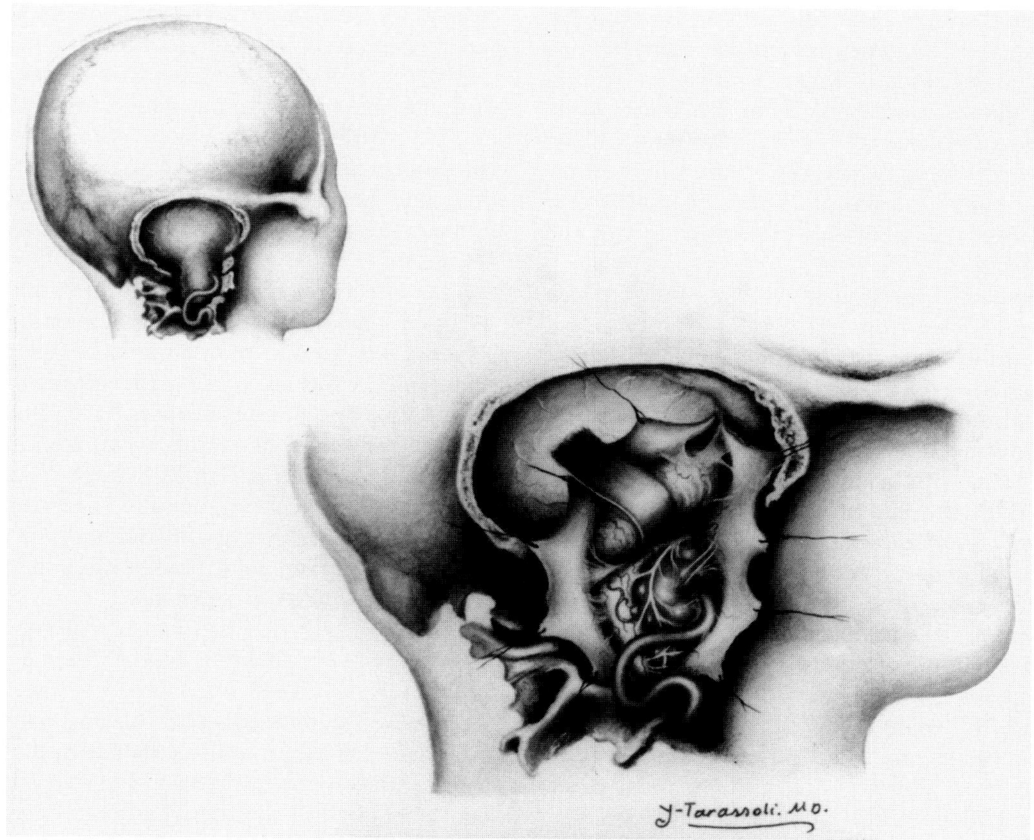

Fig. 35.22 Artist's representation of the transcondylar (far-lateral) approach for a foramen magnum meningioma. Note the complete mobilization of the vertebral artery and the anterolateral approach to the tumor allowing dissection in front of the brainstem. Used with permission from Al-Mefty O: Operative atlas of meningiomas. Raven Press.

almost always (90% of cases) located in the trigone of the lateral ventricle. The vascular supply is from the anterior choroidal artery; in larger lesions, the posterior choroidal artery will also contribute (Konovalov et al 1991).

Numerous approaches to this region have been described and include cortical incisions in the middle temporal gyrus, the posterior paramedian parietal cortex, and the lateral temporal-parietal lobe (Fornari et al 1981, Guidetti et al 1985, Criscuolo & Symon 1986). Access following a temporal or occipital lobectomy has also been proposed (Spencer et al 1991). Since all of these incisions and approaches traverse the cerebral cortex, the possibility of postoperative epilepsy is increased, as is secondary local cortical dysfunction resulting from the vigor of the cerebral retraction required for these routes. Kempe & Blaylock (1976) have described removal of trigonal meningiomas through a midline section of the corpus callosum, which does not require a cortical incision and, with modification, requires little cerebral retraction (Kempe & Blaylock 1976, McComb & Apuzzo 1987). However, it may be contraindicated for patients with a right homonymous hemianopsia since complete splenial section in this circumstance results in alexia without agraphia, a highly morbid condition. This limits the use of this approach as preoperative visual field defects are present in 40–70% of cases (Fornari et al 1981, Konovalov et al 1991). In these patients, and in those with very large tumors a middle temporal gyrus or posterior paramedian parieto-occipital approach may be better.

The preferred approach, however, remains the transcallosal approach. For this approach, the patient is positioned in the lateral, parkbench, or 3/4-prone position, with the side harboring the lateral ventricular meningioma placed inferiorly (McComb & Apuzzo 1987). The head is laterally flexed upward and the table angled such that the falx is placed 30° above the horizontal. A craniotomy straddling the superior sagittal sinus is fashioned, the dura is flapped over the sinus, and any bridging veins are dissected from the cortical surface. The arachnoidal adhesions to the falx are divided, allowing the dependent hemisphere to fall away from the midline, with the rigid falx acting as a retractor and supporting the opposite hemisphere. Once the corpus callosum and the pericallosal arteries are identified, an incision 1.5–2.0 cm in length is made in the corpus callosum between the pericallosal arteries and carried into the tumor-containing lateral ventricle. If the arterial supply to the tumor can be reached, it is divided and then the meningioma is removed in a piecemeal fashion. In cases of large tumors the arterial supply is often inaccessible. The tumor is carefully dissected from the ventricular walls and the choroidal fissure. The internal cerebral veins, which run in the velum interpositum of the transverse cerebral fissure, may adhere to any inferomedial extension of the meningioma into the choroidal fissure.

Pineal region meningiomas. Meningiomas of the pineal region, which arise from either the posterior velum interpositum or more commonly from the dura at the falco-tentorial junction, are quite rare (Tung & Apuzzo 1991). Neuro-ophthalmologic symptoms and signs (impaired upgaze, diminished pupillary reflexes) are less common than seen with other pathologies. Generally, signs of increased intracranial pressure and hydrocephalus bring the patient to medical attention. The two chief approaches for removing these tumors are the supracerebellar-infratentorial route and the supratentorial approaches. The latter is most appropriate for falco-tentorial meningiomas as it allows options for tentorial or falcine incisions to increase exposure or to devascularize the neoplasm (Tung & Apuzzo 1991). The infratentorial approach, on the other hand, has the advantage of being the shortest and most direct route, and, in most cases, of having the internal cerebral veins and vein of Galen anterior and superior to the meningioma.

Radiotherapy

The use of external beam irradiation as part of the management of meningiomas has become commonplace. The controversy during the late 1960s and 1970s concerning its effectiveness has since declined as a result of several well-executed retrospective studies supporting its use (Wara et al 1975, Barbaro et al 1987, Taylor et al 1988, Miralbell et al 1992). The positive results of the modern studies are likely due to the use of increased standard doses of 4500–6000 cGy in contrast to the earlier treatment doses of 3000–4000 cGy. External beam irradiation has been reported to be effective both following subtotal resection at the primary operation and at the time of recurrence, whether or not preceded by reoperation (Wara et al 1975, Barbaro et al 1987, Taylor et al 1988, Miralbell et al 1992). Less conclusive effectiveness has also been reported for meningiomas considered inoperable because of location, poor patient health, or patient refusal of surgery (van Effenterre et al 1979, Bloom 1982, Carella et al 1982, Forbes & Goldberg 1984, Kennerdell et al 1988).

External beam irradiation would seem to be beneficial for aggressive meningiomas (atypical, malignant), but to date very little information exists to support this thesis. Salazar (1988) combined several studies and found a 58% recurrence rate following gross total resection (GTR) and a 90% recurrence rate following subtotal resection (STR) of malignant meningiomas which were decreased to 36% and 41%, respectively, when surgery was followed by external beam irradiation. The recommended radiation dose and target volume for malignant meningiomas are greater, averaging at least 6000 cGy with a 3–4 cm margin (Busse 1991).

The effectiveness of higher radiation doses must be weighed against possible complications, especially when dealing with benign meningiomas (Al-Mefty et al 1990). The optic nerves are particularly sensitive to doses greater than 5500 cGy, but lower doses have also been implicated in the production of radiation-induced optic neuropathy (Harris & Levene 1976, Al-Mefty et al 1990). Other potential complications include the production of pituitary insufficiency, radionecrosis, and, because of the long survival of patients with benign meninigiomas, secondary (radiation-induced) neoplasms.

Stereotactic irradiation

The use of stereotactic radiosurgery to treat intracranial meningiomas began in the 1960s with the Harvard proton beam (Spiegelman & Friedman 1991). Since then, stereotactic irradiation has increasingly been used to treat meningiomas. The first use of the Gamma Knife to treat a patient with a meningioma was in 1970 (Steiner et al 1991). However, the technology required for the successful use of the linear accelerator (Linac) as an energy source for stereotactic radiosurgery delayed the inception of its use until the 1980s. The technique is used with various energy sources, the most common of which are photons from ^{60}Co gamma ray sources (Gamma Knife) or linear accelerators (Linac), and heavy particles (protons, helium ions) from cyclotrons. Irradiation with heavy par-ticles has a distinct radiobiologic advantage, especially for larger lesions, but all forms of radiation beams in use have shown a low incidence of complications, especially for lesions <2.5 cm in size (Luxton et al 1993).

As reported by Spiegelmann & Friedman (1991), Luchin et al (Burdenko Neurosurgical Institute), using the proton-beam, and Kjellberg and Candia (Harvard Cyclotron) showed 84% and 40% local control rates, respectively. The mean length of follow-up for both groups was <5 years. Steiner, in his review of patients treated with the Gamma Knife, found an 88% control rate (Steiner et al 1991). This series also had a mean length of follow-up of <5 years. Kondziolka et al (1991) calculated an actuarial 2-year tumor growth control rate of 96%.

Experience with the Linac is the most limited. In 1990, Engenhart et al reported on 17 patients treated with Linac-generated stereotactic irradiation with a mean dose of 29 Gy. Of 13 patients available for follow-up, none has had recurrence of their meningioma over a median follow-up time of 40 months (Engenhart et al 1990).

Despite the promising results of stereotactic irradiation, numerous limitations and uncertainties remain. For one, tumor size must be limited to a target limit of 35–40 mm, a size that can receive a single dose of appropriate strength with a 1% risk of radiation necrosis (Kjellberg et al 1983). The advent of fractionated delivery of stereotactic irradiation may overcome this size limitation (Souhami et al 1991).

The nature of recurrence and spread of meningiomas along dural margins (dural tails on MRI) pose a significant hindrance to focal therapies, due to the difficulty in targeting extensions of the tumor. Since the basic feature of stereotactic irradiation is the quick drop-off of radiation dose, this may result in these more diffuse margins receiving inadequate doses. Furthermore, little is known about the acute and, especially, the long-term effects on encased or immediately adjacent neurovascular structures. At present, some authors recommend a minimum distance of 5 mm from the optic chiasm as a selection criterion, whereas others limit the dose to the optic apparatus to $\leq$ 10 Gy (Kondziolka et al 1991, Steiner et al 1991). The optimal treatment dose required for meningiomas is also unknown, but some guidelines have been extrapolated from experience with acoustic neurinomas. Doses of 15–20 Gy to the tumor margin are the most commonly employed since higher dosages have been associated with higher rates of morbidity (Engenhart et al 1990). Stereotactic irradiation will likely become increasingly pertinent to the management of meningiomas, but the full extent of its benefits can be determined only with the passage of time.

Brachytherapy

The stereotactic and direct microsurgical implantation of radioactive seeds into meningiomas has been reported by several groups who have found these procedures to be beneficial, but so far the number of patients treated is low and the length of follow-up is short (Gutin et al 1987, Kumar et al 1991). The concern with tumor size is not as great as it is with stereotactic irradiation since the radiation dose is slowly delivered by the decay of the radioisotope (usually ^{125}I).

Accurate and precise planning of dosimetry is crucial. Marked changes in tumor sizes that can be seen with treatment indicate a concern that seed migration and the delivery of unwanted radiation to nearby neurovascular structures might occur (Al-Mefty 1991). If this concern can be successfully dealt with, then brachytherapy may become a very valuable adjunct for treating meninigiomas.

Chemotherapy

Little information is available on the efficacy of the traditional antineoplastic agents against either benign or malignant meningiomas. Adjuvant chemotherapy for malignant meningiomas and for recurrences of benign or atypical meningiomas has been administered to a small number of patients, but chemotherapeutic regimens [using either cis-platinum, intravenous and/or intra-arterial or dacarbazine (DTIC) and adriamycin] have generally been unsuccessful (De Monte & Yung, unpublished data), despite their effectiveness against other soft tissue tumors.

Antagonism of possible mitogenic hormones or factors has also been attempted. Early human trials were conducted on tamoxifen (anti-estrogen) and mifepristone (anti-progesterone). Tamoxifen (40 mg/m^2 b.i.d. for 4 days and 10 mg b.i.d. thereafter) was used to treat 19 patients with unresectable or refractory meningiomas by the Southwest oncology group (Goodwin et al 1993). There was progression of tumor in 10 patients, temporary stabilization of the disease process in 6 patients, and a partial or minor response in 3. In two separate studies of a 200 mg daily dose, mifepristone (RU486) was given for 2–31 months. In the earlier study, 5 of 14 patients experienced objective improvement, namely a minor decrease in the size of the tumor in 4 patients and an improved visual field examination without change in tumor size in the fifth; regrowth subsequently occurred in one of these patients (Grunberg et al 1991). A later study from the Netherlands that included 10 patients showed the tumor progressed in 4, remained stable in 3, and minimally decreased in size in 3 (Lamberts et al 1992b). These agents are currently under investigation in larger trials, but as yet no known role has been determined regarding their use in the treatment of meningiomas.

In vitro studies with bromocriptine and trapidil (a platelet-derived growth factor antagonist) have been promising, and it is likely that human trials will follow (Schrell et al 1990b, Todo et al 1993).

RECURRENCE OF MENINGIOMA

In his 1957 landmark paper, Simpson retrospectively applied a classification system to 265 patients with meningiomas derived from the 'Oxford' and 'London' series (Table 35.10). His system showed that the extent of surgical excision is directly related to the risk of recurrence. Of the 265 patients, 55 experienced recurrences (21%). Patients with a grade I excision had a recurrence rate of 9%; the rates increased to 19% for grade II, 29% for grade III, and 44% for grade IV excisions. The extent of resection has since become strongly confirmed as the primary factor influencing recurrence rate. Melamed et al (1979), who reported a particularly high recurrence

Table 35.10 Simpson's classification of the extent of resection of intracranial meningiomas (Simpson 1957)

Grade I	gross total resection of tumor, dural attachments and abnormal bone
Grade II	gross total resection of tumor, coagulation of dural attachments
Grade III	gross total resection of tumor, without resection or coagulation of dural attachments, or alternatively of its extradural extensions (e.g. invaded sinus or hyperostotic bone)
Grade IV	partial resection of tumor
Grade V	simple decompression (biopsy)

rate of 34%, found that the site of tumor origin and the extent of excision were significant prognostic factors for recurrence. Likewise, Adegbite et al (1983) found a trend of increased recurrence rate with less accessible tumor locations. Chan & Thompson (1984) reported 11% and 22% recurrence rates for Simpson grades I and II excisions respectively, and when complete tumor excision was accomplished the patients had a longer survival time and a higher quality of life.

Mirimanoff et al (1985) reported overall survival rates of 83% at 5 years, 77% at 10 years, and 69% at 15 years, and recurrence-free rates significantly affected by the extent of removal. The recurrence-free survival rates for total resection were 93%, 80%, and 68% respectively, whereas partial resection had recurrence-free survival rates that dropped to 63%, 45% and 9%, respectively. They also noted the first statistics on the incidence of total resection with respect to the location of the meningioma: as expected, the incidence of total resection correlated positively with the accessibility of the tumor (96% for convexity meningiomas, 28% for sphenoid wing meningiomas) and negatively with the 5-year recurrence rate.

The most comprehensive studies to date come from Finland, where the structure of the health care system allows for identification of essentially all cases of meningioma in the population. Jääskeläinen (1986), in his study of patients with benign intracranial meningiomas, found an overall recurrence rate at 20 years to be 19% (life-able analysis). Multivariate analysis showed that strong risk factors for recurrence included coagulation of the dural insertion, invasion of bone, and soft consistency of the tumor. For patients with none of these risk factors, the recurrence rate at 20 years was 11%, whereas the presence of one or two risk factors increased the recurrence rate to 15–24% and 34–56%, respectively. In a second study from the same group, the diagnoses of atypical or anaplastic meningioma carried an increased risk of recurrence of 38% and 78% at 5 years, respectively (Jääskeläinen et al 1986). Finally, a recently published survival study reported that the cumulative relative survival rates (ratio of observed rate to expected survival rate) at 1, 5, 10, and 15 years were found to be 83%, 79%, 74% and 71%, indicating a persisting incidence of increased mortality in patients with meningiomas (Kallio et al 1992).

Böker et al (1985), de la Monte et al (1986), and Marks et al (1986) all found positive correlation between the histopathologic findings of mitoses and focal necrosis and recurrence of meningiomas. Other positively correlated histopathologic features were brain invasion (Böker et al 1985), syncytial tumors (Marks et al 1986), hypervascularity, hemosiderin deposition, tumor cells in sheets, prominent nucleoli, and nuclear pleomorphism (de la Monte et al 1986).

The imprecision and controversy surrounding the histopathologic predictors of aggression and, thus, recurrence, have led to numerous attempts to identify quantitative parameters. In 1979, Zankl & Zang, using chromosome banding techniques, reported a higher degree of hypodiploidy and atypical chromosome loss in 8 of 10 recurrent meningiomas (Zankl & Zang 1980). Using flow cytometry, May et al (1989) had a significantly higher proliferative index (% S phase +% G_2/M phase) in recurring meningiomas and suggested that a proliferative index of ≥ 20%, irrespective of the histopathologic appearance, was strongly suggestive that the tumor would recur.

The determination of the bromodeoxyuridine labelling index (BUdR LI) or of the number of argyrophilic nucleolar organizer regions (AgNOR) has also been used to identify intracranial meningiomas with a higher propensity to recur. Hoshino et al (1986) found that a BUdR LI of ⩾ 1% was indicative of meningiomas with a faster growth rate (higher proliferative potential) and that meningiomas with a BUdR LI ⩾ 5% had a 100% recurrence rate. The recurrence rate dropped to 55.6% for meningiomas with a BUdR of 3–5% and to 30.6% for those with a BUdR of 1–3% (Hoshino et al 1986, Shibuya et al 1992). Chin & Hinton reported that the mean AgNOR counts were statistically different between benign meningiomas (245 ± 156), atypical meningiomas (497 ± 135), and malignant meningiomas (921 ± 59) (Chin & Hinton 1991). They also noted a statistically different AgNOR count for recurrent meningiomas (544 ± 76) when compared to nonrecurrent tumors (329 ± 183).

Finally, positron emission tomography studies of glucose utilization showed it to be lower (1.9 mg/dl/min ± 1.0) in nonrecurring tumors than in those which recurred (4.5 mg/dl/min ± 1.9) (DiChiro et al 1987).

The quantitative methods of predicting meningioma aggressiveness and probability of recurrence will likely experience increased popularity and usage as the techniques used become more widely available, allowing for more rational choices to be made among the various treatment options for patients following the primary meningioma removal and at the time of recurrence.

REFERENCES

Adams E F, Todo T, Schrell U M H et al 1991 Autocrine control of human meningioma proliferation: secretion of platelet-derived growth factor-like molecules. International Journal of Cancer 49: 398–402

Adegbite A B, Khan M I, Paine K W E et al 1983 The recurrence of intracranial meningiomas after surgical treatment. Journal of Neurosurgery 58: 51–56

Al-Mefty O 1990 Clinoidal meningiomas. Journal of Neurosurgery 73: 840–849

Al-Mefty O 1991 Comment on Kumar P P, Patil A A, Liebrock L G et al 1991 Brachytherapy: a viable alternative in the management of basal meningiomas. Neurosurgery 29: 680

Al-Mefty O Operative atlas of meningiomas. Raven Press, New York (in press)

Al-Mefty O, Smith R R 1991 Tuberculum sellae meningiomas. In: Al-Mefty O (ed) Meningiomas. Raven Press, New York, pp 397–398

Al-Mefty O, Fox J L, Smith R R 1988 Petrosal approach for petroclival meningiomas. Neurosurgery 22: 510–5174b

Al-Mefty O, Kersh J E, Routh A et al 1990 The long-term side effects of radiation therapy for benign tumors in adults. Journal of Neurosurgery 73: 502–512

Al-Mefty O, Schenk M P, Smith R R 1991 Petroclival meningiomas. In: Rengachary S S, Wilkins R H (eds) Neurosurgical operative atlas, vol 3. Williams & Wilkins, Baltimore, pp 339–350

Annegers J F, Laws E R, Kurland L T et al 1979 Head trauma and subsequent brain tumors. Neurosurgery 4: 203–206

Arnold D L, Emrich J F, Shoubridge E A et al 1991 Characterization of astrocytomas, meningiomas, and pituitary adenomas by phosphorus magnetic resonance spectroscopy. Journal of Neurosurgery 74: 447–453

Barbanti-Brodano G, Silini E, Mottes M et al 1987 DNA probes to evaluate the possible association of papovaviruses with human tumors. In: Gallo R C et al (eds) Monoclonals and DNA probes in diagnostic and preventive medicine. Raven Press, New York, pp 147–155

Barbaro N M, Gutin P H, Wilson C B et al 1987 Radiation therapy in the treatment of partially resected meningiomas. Neurosurgery 20: 525–528

Black P McL 1993 Meningiomas. Neurosurgery 32: 643–657

Bloom H J G 1983 Intracranial tumors: response and resistance to therapeutic endeavors, 1970–1980. International Journal of Radiation Oncology, Biology and Physics 8: 1083–1113

Bogdanowicz W M, Sachs E et al 1974 The possible role of radiation in oncogenesis of meningioma. Surgical Neurology 2: 379–383

Böker D K, Meurer H, Gullotta F 1985 Recurring intracranial meningiomas. Journal of Neurosurgical Sciences 29: 11–17

Bonnal J, Brotchi J 1978 Surgery of the superior sagittal sinus in parasagittal meningiomas. Journal of Neurosurgery 48: 938–945

Bonnal J, Thibaut A, Brotchi J et al 1980 Invading meningiomas of the sphenoid ridge. Journal of Neurosurgery 53: 587–599

Borovich B, Guilburd J N, Doron Y et al 1988 Cystic meningiomas. Acta Neurochirurgica (Wien) 42 (suppl): 147–151

Bowen J H, Burger P C, Odom G L et al 1981 Meningiomas associated with large cysts with neoplastic cells in the cyst walls. Journal of Neurosurgery 55: 473–478

Brentani M M, Lopes M T P, Martins V R et al 1984 Steroid receptors in intracranial tumors. Clinical Neuropharmacology 7: 347–350

Burger P C, Scheithauer B W, Vogel F S 1991 Surgical pathology of the nervous system and its coverings, 3rd edn. Churchill Livingstone, New York, p 83

Busse P M 1991 Radiation therapy for meningiomas. In: Schmidek H H (ed) Meningiomas and their surgical management. W B Saunders, Philadelphia, p 506

Butti G, Gaetani P, Chiabrando C et al 1991 A study on the biological behaviour of human brain tumors. Journal of Neuro-Oncology 10: 241–246

Carella R J, Ransohoff J, Newall J 1982 Role of radiation therapy in the management of meningioma. Neurosurgery 10: 332–339

Castellano F, Ruggiero G 1953 Meningiomas of the posterior fossa. Acta Radiologica 104 (suppl): 1–177

Chan R C, Thompson G B 1984 Morbidity, mortality, and quality of life following surgery for intracranial meningiomas. Journal of Neurosurgery 60: 52–60

Chen T C, Zee C S, Miller C A et al 1992 Magnetic resonance imaging and pathological correlates of meningiomas. Neurosurgery 31: 1015–1022

Chin L S, Hinton D R 1991 The standardized assessment of argyrophilic nucleolar organizer regions in meningeal tumors. Journal of Neurosurgery 74: 590–596

Choi N W, Schuman L M, Gullen W H 1970 Epidemiology of primary central nervous system neoplasms II. Case-control study. American Journal of Epidemiology 91: 467–485

Collins V P, Nordenskjöld M, Dumanski J P 1990 The molecular genetics of meningiomas. Brain Pathology 1: 19–24

Criscuolo G R, Symon L 1986 Intraventricular meningioma. A review of 10 cases of the National Hospital, Queen Square (1974–1985) with reference to the literature. Acta Neurochirurgica (Wein) 83: 83–91

Cushing H 1922 The meningiomas (dural endotheliomas): Their source, and favoured seats of origin. Brain 45: 282–316

Cushing H 1932 Intracranial tumors. Notes upon a series of two thousand verified cases. Charles C Thomas, Springfield, Ill

Cushing H, Eisenhardt L 1938 Meningiomas: Their classification, regional behaviour, life history, and surgical end results. Charles C Thomas, Springfield, Ill

Deen H G, Scheithauer B W, Ebersold M J 1982 Clinical and pathological study of meningiomas of the first two decades of life. Journal of Neurosurgery 56: 317–322

de la Monte S M, Flickinger J, Linggood R M 1986 Histopathologic features predicting recurrence of meningiomas following subtotal resection. American Journal of Surgical Pathology 10: 836–843

Demaerel P, Wilms G, Lammens M et al 1991a Intracranial meningiomas: correlation between MR imaging and histology in fifty patients. Journal of Computer Assisted Tomography 15: 45–51

Demaerel P, Johannik K, Van Hecke P et al 1991b Localized ^{1}H NMR spectroscopy in fifty cases of newly diagnosed intracranial tumors. Journal of Computer Assisted Tomography 15: 67–76

DeMonte F, Al-Mefty O 1993a Anterior clinoidal meningiomas. In: Rengachary S S, Wilkins RH (eds) Neurosurgical operative atlas, vol 3. Williams & Wilkins, Baltimore, pp 49–61

DeMonte F, Al-Mefty O 1993b Neoplasms and the cranial nerves of the posterior fossa. In: Barrow D L (ed) Surgery of the cranial nerves of the posterior fossa. American Association of Neurological Surgeons, Park Ridge, Ill, pp 253–274

DeMonte F, Warf P, Al-Mefty O 1993a Intraoperative monitoring of the lower cranial nerves during surgery of the jugular foramen and lower clivus. In: Loftus C, Traynelis V (eds) Intraoperative monitoring techniques in neurosurgery. McGraw-Hill, New York, pp 205–212

DeMonte F, Smith H K, Al-Mefty O 1993b Outcome of aggressive removal of cavernous sinus meningiomas. Skull Base Surgery 3(suppl): 11 abstract 1: 30

Derome P J, Visot A 1991 Bony reaction and invasion in meningiomas. In: Al-Mefty O (ed) Meningiomas. Raven Press, New York, p 169

DiChiro G, Hatazawa J, Katz D A et al 1987 Glucose utilization by intracranial meningiomas as an index of tumor aggressiveness and probability of recurrence. Radiology 164: 521–526

Donnell M S, Meyer G A, Donegan W L 1979 Estrogen-receptor protein in intracranial meningiomas. Journal of Neurosurgery 50: 499–502

Downward J, Yarde Y, Mayes E et al 1984 Close similarity of epidermal growth factor receptor and verb-B oncogene protein sequences. Nature 307: 521–527

Drake J M, Hendrick E B, Becker L et al 1985 Intracranial meningiomas in children. Pediatric Neuroscience 12: 134–139

Dumanski J P, Carlbom E, Collins V P et al 1987 Deletion mapping of a locus on human chromosome 22 involved in the oncogenesis of meningioma. Proceedings of the National Academy of Sciences of the USA 84: 9275–9279

Elster A D, Challa V R, Gilbert T H et al 1989 Meningiomas: MR and histopathologic features. Radiology 170: 857–862

Engenhart R, Kimmig B N, Hover K H et al 1990 Stereotactic single dose radiation therapy of benign intracranial meningiomas. International Journal of Radiation Oncology, Biology, and Physics 19: 1021–1026

Erba S M, Horton J A, Latchaw R E et al 1988 Balloon test occlusion of the internal carotid artery with stable Xenon/CT cerebral blood flow imaging. Americal Journal of Neuroradiology 9: 533–538

Fan K J, Pezeshkpour G H 1992 Ethnic distribution of primary central nervous system tumors in Washington, DC, 1971–1985. Journal of the National Medical Association 84: 858–863

Fiori M, Di Mayorca G 1976 Occurrence of BK virus DNA in DNA obtained from certain human tumors. Proceedings of the National Academy of Science of the USA 73: 4662–4666

Fogelholm R, Uutela T, Murros K 1984 Epidemiology of central nervous system neoplasms: A regional survey in central Finland. Acta Neurologica Scandinavia 69: 129

Fornari M, Savoiardo M, Morello G et al 1981 Meningiomas of the lateral ventricles: neuroradiological and surgical considerations in 18 cases. Journal of Neurosurgery 54: 64–74

Forbes A R, Goldberg I D 1984 Radiation therapy in the treatment of meningioma: The joint center for radiation therapy experience, 1970–1982. Journal of Clinical Oncology 2: 1139–1143

Fortuna A, Ferrante L, Acqui M et al 1988 Cystic meningiomas. Acta Neurochirurgica (Wein) 90: 23–30

Froman C, Lipschitz R 1970 Demography of tumors of the central nervous system among the Bantu (African) population of the Transvaal, South Africa. Journal of Neurosurgery 32: 660–664

Gautier-Smith P C 1970 Parasagittal and falx meningiomas. Butterworths, London

Giordano C, Lamouche M 1973 Méningiomes en Côte D'Ivoire. African Journal of Medical Science 4: 249–263

Goodwin J W, Crowley J, Stafford B et al 1993 A phase II evaluation of tamoxifen in unresectable or refractory meningiomas: a southwest oncology group study. Journal of Neuro-Oncology 15: 75–77

Grant F C 1956 A study of the results of surgical treatment in 2326 consecutive patients with brain tumors: The national survey of intracranial neoplasms. Neurology 32: 219–226

Grunberg S M, Weiss M H, Spitz I M et al 1991 Treatment of unresectable meningiomas with the antiprogesterone agent mifepristone. Journal of Neurosurgery 74: 861–866

Guidetti B, Delfini R, Gagliardi F M et al 1985 Meningiomas of the lateral ventricles. Clinical, neuroradiologic and surgical consideration in 19 cases. Surgical Neurology 24: 364–370

Gutin P, Leibel S A, Hosobuchi Y et al 1987 Brachytherapy of recurrent tumors of the skull base and spine with iodine-125 sources. Neurosurgery 20: 938–945

Hakuba A, Huh C W, Tsujikawa S et al 1979 Total removal of a parasagittal meningioma of the posterior third of the sagittal sinus and its repair by autogenous vein graft: case report. Journal of Neurosurgery 51: 379–382

Halper J, Colvard D S, Scheithauer B W et al 1989 Estrogen and progesterone receptors in meningiomas: comparison of nuclear binding, dextran-coated charcoal, and immunoperoxidase staining assays. Neurosurgery 25: 546–553

Harris J R, Levene M B 1976 Visual complications following irradiation for pituitary adenomas and craniopharyngiomas. Radiology 120: 167–171

Herz D A, Shapiro K, Shulman K 1980 Intracranial meningiomas of infancy, childhood and adolescence. Review of the literature and addition of 9 case reports. Child's Brain 7: 43–56

Horsfall D J, Goldsmith K G, Ricciardelli C et al 1989 Steroid hormone and epidermal growth factor receptors in meningiomas. Australian and New Zealand Journal of Surgery 59: 881–888

Hoshino T, Nagashima T, Murovic J A et al 1986 Proliferative potential of human meningiomas of the brain: a cell kinetics study with bromodeoxyuridine. Cancer 58: 1466–1472

Ibelgaufts H, Jones K W 1982 Papovavirus related RNA sequences in human neurogenic tumors. Acta Neuropathologica (Berlin) 56: 118–122

Ibelgaufts H, Jones K W, Maitland N et al 1982 Adenovirus related RNA sequences in human neurogenic tumors. Acta Neuropathologica (Berlin) 56: 113–117

Jääskeläinen J 1986 Seemingly complete removal of histologically benign intracranial meningioma: Late recurrence rate and factors predicting recurrence in 657 patients. Surgical Neurology 25: 461–469

Jääskeläinen J, Haltia M, Servo A 1986 Atypical and anaplastic meningiomas: Radiology, surgery, radiotherapy and outcome. Surgical Neurology 25: 233–242

Jacobs J M, Harnsberger H R 1991 Diagnostic angiography and meningiomas. In: Al-Mefty O (ed) Meningiomas. Raven Press, New York, pp 225–241

Jane J A, Park T S, Pobereskin L H et al 1982 The supraorbital approach: Technical note. Neurosurgery 11: 537–542

Jellinger K, Slowik F 1975 Histological subtypes and prognostic problems in meningiomas. Journal of Neurology 208: 278–298

Kallio M, Sankila R, Hakulinen T et al 1992 Factors affecting operative and excess long-term mortality in 935 patients with intracranial meningioma. Neurosurgery 31: 2–12

Kaplan R D, Coons S, Drayer B P et al 1992 MR characteristics of meningioma subtypes at 1.5 Tesla. Journal of Computer Assisted Tomography 16: 366–371

Katayama Y, Tsubokawa T, Yoshida K 1986 Cystic meningiomas in infancy. Surgical Neurology 25: 43–48

Katsura S, Suzuki J, Wada I 1959 A statistical study of brain tumors in the neurosurgical clinics in Japan. Journal of Neurosurgery 16: 570–580

Kempe L G, Blaylock R 1976 Lateral-trigonal intraventricular tumors: a new operative approach. Acta Neurochirurgica (Wien) 35: 233–242

Kennerdell J S, Maroon J C, Malton M et al 1988 The management of optic nerve sheath meningiomas. American Journal of Ophthalmology 106: 450–457

Kepes J J 1982 Meningiomas: Biology, pathology and differential diagnosis. Masson Publishing, New York

Khayata M H, Dean B, Flom R et al 1993 Comparison between the amount of blood loss, length of stay in embolized versus non-embolized meningioma patients. Skull Base Surgery 3(suppl): 12 (abstract) 3: 40

Kinjo T, Al-Mefty O, Kanaan I 1993 Grade zero removal of supratentorial convexity meningiomas. Neurosurgery 33: 394–399

Kjellberg N R, Hanamura T, Davis K R et al 1983 Bragg-peak proton beam therapy for arteriovenous malformations of the brain. New England Journal of Medicine 309: 269–274

Kondziolka D, Lunsford L D, Coffey R J et al 1991 Stereotactic radiosurgery of meningiomas. Journal of Neurosurgery 74: 552–559

Konovalov A N, Filatov Y M, Belousova O B 1991 Intraventricular meningiomas. In: Schmidek H H (ed) Meningiomas and their surgical management. W B Saunders, Philadelphia, p 364

Kornblum J A, Bay J W, Gupta M K 1988 Steroid recepters in human brain and spinal cord tumors. Neurosurgery 23: 185–188

Kugel H, Heindel W, Ernestus R I et al 1992 Human brain tumors: spectral patterns detected with localized H_1 MR spectroscopy. Radiology 183: 701–709

Kumar P P, Patil A A, Leibrock L G et al 1991 Brachytherapy: a viable alternative in the management of basal meningiomas. Neurosurgery 29: 676–680

Kurland L T, Schoenberg B S, Annegers J F et al 1982 The incidence of primary intracranial neoplasms in Rochester, Minnesota. Annals of the New York Academy of Sciences 381: 6–16

Lamberts S W J, Reubi J C, Krenning E P 1992a Somatostatin receptor imaging in the diagnosis and treatment of neuroendocrine tumors. Journal of Steroid Biochemistry and Molecular Biology 43: 185–188

Lamberts S W J, Tanghe H L J, Avezaat C J J et al 1992b Mifepristone (RU 486) treatment of meningiomas. Journal of Neurology, Neurosurgery, and Psychiatry 55: 486–490

Latchaw R E, Hirsch W L 1991 Computerized tomography of intracranial meningiomas. In: Al-Mefty O (ed) Meningiomas. Raven Press, New York, pp 195–207

Lesch K P, Schott W, Engl H G et al 1987 Gonadal steroid receptors in meningiomas. Journal of Neurology 234: 328–333

Levy L F 1973 Brain tumors in Malawi, Rhodesia and Zambia. African Journal of Medical Science 4: 393–397

Lowry O H, Bergers S J, Chi M et al 1977 Diversity of metabolic patterns in human brain tumors. I. High energy phosphate compounds and basic composition. Journal of Neurochemistry 29: 959–977

Ludwin S K, Rubinstein L J, Russell D S 1975 Papillary meningiomas: a malignant variant of meningioma. Cancer 36: 1363–1373

Luxton G, Petrovich Z, Jozsef G et al 1993 Stereotactic radiosurgery: principles and comparison of treatment methods. Neurosurgery 32: 241–259

MacCarty C S, Taylor W F 1979 Intracranial meningiomas: Experiences at the Mayo Clinic. Neurologica Medico-Chirurgica (Tokyo) 19: 569–574

McComb J G, Apuzzo M L J 1987 Posterior interhemispheric retrocallosal and transcallosal approaches. In: Apuzzo M L J (ed) Surgery of the third ventricle. Williams & Wilkins, Baltimore, pp 623–626

Mack E E, Wilson C B 1993 Meningiomas induced by high-dose cranial irradiation. Journal of Neurosurgery 61: 136–142

Manelfe C, Lasjaunias P, Ruscalleda J 1986 Preoperative embolization of intracranial meningiomas. American Journal of Neuroradiology 7: 963–972

Manfredonia M 1973 Tumors of the nervous system in the African in Eritrea (Ethiopia). African Journal of Medical Science 4: 383–387

Marks S, Whitwell H L, Lye R H 1986 Recurrence of meningiomas after operation. Surgical Neurology 25: 436–440

Martinez R, Vaquero J, Areitio E et al 1983 Meningiomas of the posterior fossa. Surgical Neurology 19: 237–243

Maxwell M, Galanopoulos T, Hedley-Whyte E T et al 1990 Human meningiomas co-express platelet-derived growth factor (PDGF) and PDGF-receptor genes and their protein products. International Journal of Cancer 46: 16–21

Maxwell M, Galanopoulos T, Neville-Golden J et al 1993 Expression of androgen and progesterone receptors in primary human meningiomas. Journal of Neurosurgery 78: 456–462

May P L, Broome J C, Lawry J et al 1989 The prediction of recurrence in meningiomas. A flow cytometric study of paraffin-embedded archival material. Journal of Neurosurgery 71: 347–351

Melamed S, Sahar A, Beller A J 1979 The recurrence of intracranial meningiomas. Neurochirurgia 22: 47–51

Meyer F B, Ebersold M J, Reese D F 1984 Benign tumors of the foramen magnum. Journal of Neurosurgery 61: 136–142

Miralbell R, Linggood R M, de la Monte S et al 1992 The role of radiotherapy in the treatment of subtotally resected benign meningiomas. Journal of Neuro-Oncology 13: 157–164

Mirimanoff R O, Dosoretz D E, Linggood R M et al 1985 Meningioma: Analysis of recurrence and progression following neurosurgical resection. Journal of Neurosurgery 62: 18–24

Modan B, Baidatz D, Mart H 1974 Radiation-induced head and neck tumors. Lancet 1: 277–279

Odeku E L, Adeloye A 1973 Cranial meningiomas in the Nigerian Africans. African Journal of Medical Science 4: 275–287

Olivecrona H 1952 The cerebellar angioreticulomas. Journal of Neurosurgery 9: 317–330

Olson J J, Beck D W, Maclndoe J W et al 1988 Androgen receptors in meningiomas. Cancer 61: 952–955

Ott D, Hennig J, Ernst T 1993 Human brain tumors: assessment with *in vivo* proton MR spectroscopy. Radiology 186: 745–752

Parker H L, Kernohan J W 1931 The relation of injury and glioma of the brain. Journal of the American Medical Association 97: 535–539

Pasquier B, Gasnier F, Pasquier D et al 1986 Papillary meningioma: clinicopathologic study of seven cases and review of the literature. Cancer 58: 299–305

Peeling J, Sutherland G 1992 High-resolution ^{1}H NMR spectroscopy studies of extracts of human cerebral neoplasms. Magnetic Resonance in Medicine 24: 123–136

Perrot-Applanat M, Groyer-Picard MTh, Kujas M 1992 Immunocytochemical study of progesterone receptor in human meningioma. Acta Neurochirurgica (Wein) 115: 20–30

Poisson M, Pertuiset B F, Hauw J J et al 1983 Steroid hormone receptors in human meningiomas, gliomas and brain metastases. Journal of Neuro-Oncology 1: 179–189

Preston-Martin S, Paganini-Hill A, Henderson B E et al 1980 Case control study of intracranial meningiomas in women in Los Angeles County. Journal of the National Cancer Institute 65: 67–73

Preston-Martin S, Henderson B E, Peters J M 1982 Descriptive epidemiology of central nervous system neoplasms in Los Angeles County. Annals of the New York Academy of Science 381: 202–208

Quest D O 1978 Meningiomas: An update. Neurosurgery 3: 219–225

Rachlin J R, Rosenblum M L 1991 Etiology and biology of meningiomas. In: Al-Mefty O (ed) Meningiomas. Raven Press, New York, pp 27–35

Rachlin J R, Wollmann R, Dohrmann G 1984 SV40 viral DNA in human CNS tumors. Journal of Neuropathology and Experimental Neurology 43: 301 abstract

Reubi J C, Maurer R, Klijn J G M et al 1986 High incidence of somatostatin receptors in human meningiomas: biochemical characterization. Journal of Clinical Endocrinology and Metabolism 63: 433–438

Reubi J C, Horisberger U, Lang W et al 1989 Coincidence of EGF receptors and somatostatin receptors in meningiomas but inverse, differentiation-dependent relationship in glial tumors. American Journal of Pathology 134: 337–344

Rohinger M, Sutherland G R, Louw D F et al 1989 Incidence and clinicopathological features of meningioma. Journal of Neurosurgery 71: 665–672

Rouleau G A, Wertelecki W, Haines J L et al 1987 Genetic linkage of bilateral acoustic neurofibromatosis to a DNA marker on chromosome 22. Nature 329: 246–248

Russell E J, George A E, Kricheff I I et al 1980 Atypical computed tomographic features of intracranial meningioma: radiological-pathological correlation in a series of 131 consecutive cases. Radiology 135: 673–682

Salazar O M 1988 Ensuring local control in meningiomas. International Journal of Radiation Oncology, Biology and Physics 15: 501–504

Samii M, Ammirati M 1991 Cerebellopontine angle meningiomas (posterior pyramid meningiomas). In: Al-Mefty O (ed) Meningiomas. Raven Press, New York, pp 508–511

Schatz N J, Savino P J, Corbett J J 1977 Primary aberrant oculomotor regeneration. A sign of intracavernous meningioma. Archives of Neurology 34: 29–32

Schnegg J F, Gomez F, LeMarchand-Beraud T et al 1981 Presence of sex steroid hormone receptors in meningioma tissue. Surgical Neurology 15: 415–418

Schoenberg G S, Christine B W, Whisnant J P 1976 The descriptive epidemiology of primary intracranial neoplasms: The Connecticut experience. American Journal of Epidemiology 104: 499–510

Schrell U M H, Adams E F, Fahlbusch R et al 1990a Hormonal dependency of cerebral meningiomas. Journal of Neurosurgery 73: 743–749

Schrell U M H, Fahlbusch R, Adams E F et al 1990b Growth of cultured human cerebral meningiomas is inhibited by dopaminergic agents. Presence of high affinity Dopamine-D_1 receptors. Journal of Clinical Endocrinology and Metabolism 71: 1669–1671

Seizinger B R, de la Monte S, Atkins L et al 1987 Molecular genetic approach to human meningioma: Loss of genes on chromosome 22. Proceedings of the National Academy of Science of the USA 84: 5419–5423

Sekhar L N, Jannetta P J 1984 Cerebellopontine angle meningiomas. Microsurgical excision and follow-up results. Journal of Neurosurgery 60: 500–505

Sen C N, Sekhar L N 1990 An extreme lateral approach to intradural lesions of the cervical spine and foramen magnum. Neurosurgery 27: 197–204

Shibuya M, Hoshino T, Ito S et al 1992 Meningiomas: clinical implications of a high proliferative potential determined by bromodeoxyuridine labeling. Neurosurgery 30: 494–498

Simpson D 1957 The recurrence of intracranial meningiomas after surgical treatment. Journal of Neurology, Neurosurgery and Psychiatry 20: 22–39

Souhami L, Olivier A, Podgorask E B et al 1991 Fractionated stereotactic radiation therapy for intracranial tumors. Cancer 68: 2101–2108

Spagnoli M V, Goldberg H I, Grossman R I et al 1986 Intracranial meningiomas: high-field MR imaging. Radiology 161: 369–375

Spencer D D, Collins W, Sass K J 1991 Surgical management of lateral intraventricular tumors. In: Schmidek H H (ed) Meningiomas and their surgical management. W B Saunders, Philadelphia, pp 345–348

Spetzler R F, Daspit C P, Pappas C T E 1992 The combined supra- and infratentorial approach for lesions of the petrous and clival regions, experience with 46 cases. Journal of Neurosurgery 76: 588–599

Spiegelmann R, Friedman W 1991 Radiosurgical treatment of meningiomas. In: Schmidek H H (ed) Meningiomas and their surgical management. W B Saunders, Philadelphia, pp 508–514

Steiner L, Lindquist C, Steiner M 1991 Meningiomas and gamma knife radiosurgery. In: Al-Mefty O (ed) Meningiomas. Raven Press, New York, pp 263–272

Stoller J K, Kavuru J, Mehta A C et al 1987 Intracranial meningioma metastatic to the lung. Cleveland Clinic Journal of Medicine 54: 521–527

Sutherland G R, Florell R, Louw D et al 1987 Epidemiology of primary intracranial neoplasms in Manitoba, Canada. Canadian Journal of Neurological Sciences 14: 586–592

Taylor B W, Marcus R B, Friedman W A et al 1988 The meningioma controversy: postoperative radiation therapy. International Journal of Radiation Oncology, Biology and Physics 15: 299–304

Todo T, Adams E F, Fahlbusch R 1993 Inhibitory effect of trapidil on human meningioma cell proliferation via interruption of autocrine growth stimulation. Journal of Neurosurgery 78: 463–469

Trofatter J A, MacCollin M M, Rutter J L et al 1993 A novel moesin-, ezrin-, radixin-like gene is a candidate for the neurofibromatosis 2 tumor suppressor. Cell 72: 791–800

Tung H, Apuzzo M L J 1991 Meningiomas of the third ventricle and pineal region. In: Al-Mefty O (ed) Meningiomas. Raven Press, New York, pp 583–591

Umansky F, Pappo I, Pizov G et al 1988 Cystic changes in intracranial meningiomas. A review. Acta Neurochirurgica (Wien) 95: 13–18

van Effenterre R, Bataini J P, Cabanis E A et al 1979 High-energy radiotherapy in the treatment of meningiomas of the cavernous sinus. Acta Neurochirurgica 28(suppl): 464–467

Waelti E R, Markwalder T M 1989 Immunocytochemical evidence of progesterone receptors in human meningiomas. Surgical Neurology 31: 172–176

Waga S, Handa H 1976 Radiation-induced meningioma with review of the literature. Surgical Neurology 5: 215–219

Walker A E, Robins H, Weinfeld F D 1985 Epidemiology of brain tumors: The national survey of intracranial neoplasms. Neurology 32: 219–226

Wara W M, Sheline G E, Newman H et al 1975 Radiation therapy of meningiomas. American Journal of Radiology 123: 453–458

Weingarten K, Ernst R J, Jahre C et al 1992 Detection of residual or recurrent meningioma after surgery: value of enhanced vs unenhanced MR imaging. American Journal of Radiology 158: 645–650

Weisman A S, Villemure J G, Kelly P A 1986 Regulation of DNA synthesis and growth of cells derived from primary human meningiomas. Cancer Research 46: 2545–2550

Weisman A S, Raguet S S, Kelly P A 1987 Characterization of epidermal growth factor receptor in human meningioma. Cancer Research 47: 2172–2176

Weiss A F, Portmann R, Fischer H et al 1975 Simian virus 40-related antigens in three human meningiomas with defined chromosome loss. Proceedings of the National Academy of Science of the USA 72: 609–613

Westphal M, Hermann H D 1986 Epidermal growth factor-receptors on cultured meningioma cells. Acta Neurochirurgica (Wien) 83: 62–66

Worthington C, Caron J-L, Melanson D et al 1985 Meningioma cysts. Neurology 35: 1720–1724

Yasargil M G, Mortara R W, Curcic M 1980 Meningiomas of basal posterior cranial fossa. Advances and Technical Standards in Neurosurgery 7: 3–115

Younis G, Sawaya R 1992 Intracranial osteolytic malignant meningiomas appearing as extracranial soft tissue masses. Neurosurgery 30: 932–935

Zankl H, Zang K D 1980 Correlations between clinical and cytogenetical data in 180 human meningiomas. Cancer Genetics and Cytogenetics 1: 351–356

Zava D T, Markwalder T M, Markwalder R V 1984 Biological expression of steroid hormone receptors in primary meningioma cells in monolayer culture. Clinical Neuropharmacology 7: 382–388

Zimmerman H M 1969 Brain tumors: their incidence and classification in man and their experimental production. Annals of the New York Academy of Science 159: 337–359

Zimmerman R D 1991 MRI of intracranial meningiomas. In: Al-Mefty O (ed) Meningiomas. Raven Press, New York, pp 209–223

Zulch K J 1965 Brain tumors: Their biology and pathology. Springer, New York, pp 62–69

36. Meningeal hemangiopericytomas

Barton L. Guthrie

Meningeal hemangiopericytoma is a malignant neoplasm with sarcoma-like behavior. It is postulated to arise from meningeal capillary pericytes or precursor cells with angioblastic tendencies (Stout & Murray 1942a, Horten et al 1977). Information about this tumor comes from approximately 250 cases, reported variably as 'angioblastic meningiomas' within large series of meningiomas (Simpson 1957, Skullerud & Loken 1974, Jellinger & Slowik 1975, Kepes 1982, de la Monte et al 1986) and a few series devoted exclusively to meningeal hemangiopericytomas (Pitkethly et al 1970, Goellner et al 1978, Fabiani et al 1980, Thomas et al 1981, Jääskeläinen et al 1985, Kochanek et al 1986, Schroder et al 1986, Guthrie et al 1989).

The classification and nomenclature of this lesion is interesting. Cushing & Eisenhardt, in their 1938 classification of meningiomas, identified a vascular form of the tumor that they called angioblastic meningioma. They recognized three variants of angioblastic meningioma: a vascular, but otherwise ordinary, meningioma (angiomatous meningioma), a tumor occurring primarily in the posterior fossa that is essentially a hemangioblastoma, and a third variety that appeared to have arisen from meningothelial cells with angioblastic features. This latter tumor was noted to behave in a malignant fashion with a tendency for local recurrence despite aggressive resection. It is this tumor to which the term angioblastic is generally applied (Bailey et al 1928, Cushing & Eisenhardt 1938). In 1942, Stout & Murray (1942a) described a malignant and vascular tumor of the soft tissues (thigh, buttock, retroperitoneum) made of cells resembling capillary pericytes. They called it hemangiopericytoma, and it has since become a well-recognized soft tissue sarcoma (Enzinger & Smith 1976). In a later series, they reported a case that involved the meninges (Stout & Murray 1942b) but was felt to have invaded the meninges rather than to have had a primary meningeal origin. Begg & Garret first reported a primary cranial meningeal hemangiopericytoma in 1954. Significantly, they noted that it was histologically identical to both the soft tissue hemangiopericytoma of Stout & Murray (1942a) and the aggressive variant of angioblastic meningioma originally described by Cushing & Eisenhardt in 1938. They proposed that this variant of Cushing & Eisenhardt's angioblastic meningioma was actually a meningeal hemangiopericytoma, which was compatible with the known aggressive behavior of systemic hemangiopericytoma.

Since these early reports, various investigators have argued whether meningeal hemangiopericytoma is a form of meningioma. Popoff et al (1974) found that meningeal hemangiopericytomas were histologically and ultrastructurally identical to the same tumor arising in soft tissues elsewhere and proposed that the meningeal tumor not be classified as a meningioma. On the other hand, Horten et al (1977), reviewing 79 cases of vascular (angioblastic) meningiomas, found areas within these tumors that appeared transitional between hemangiopericytomas and fibrous meningiomas and/or hemangioblastomas. They concluded that these tumors and ordinary meningiomas arise from multipotential precursor cells so that classification of meningeal hemangiopericytomas as angioblastic meningiomas was not inconsistent with their postulated origin from capillary pericyte. The question of categorization aside, it is crucial that the tumor be recognized because of its malignant behavior, which is quite different from that of ordinary meningiomas.

GROSS AND MICROSCOPIC PATHOLOGY

Meningeal hemangiopericytomas are lobulated and vary from pink-gray to red in color. Their texture is usually firm, but they may occasionally be soft in consistency (Fig. 36.1). They are extremely vascular with a distressing tendency to bleed at surgery. They often adhere to the dura but usually do not invade the brain, so that a plane of dissection is evident (Jääskeläinen et al 1985, Guthrie et al 1989). Of note is that they do not spread en plaque and rarely, if ever, do they contain calcification.

Microscopically, the tumors are very cellular, with round to oval cells (Fig. 36.2). The architecture may vary

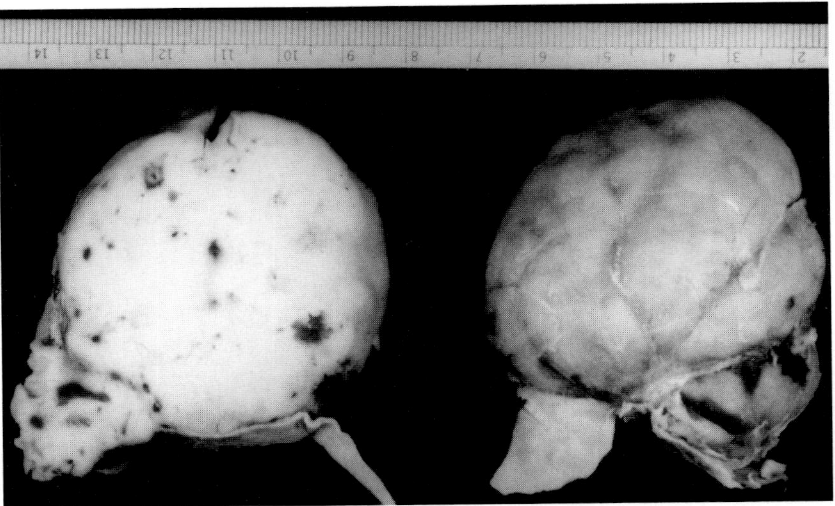

Fig. 36.1 This meningeal hemangiopericytoma was removed in toto. Notice the dural attachment and lobular appearance.

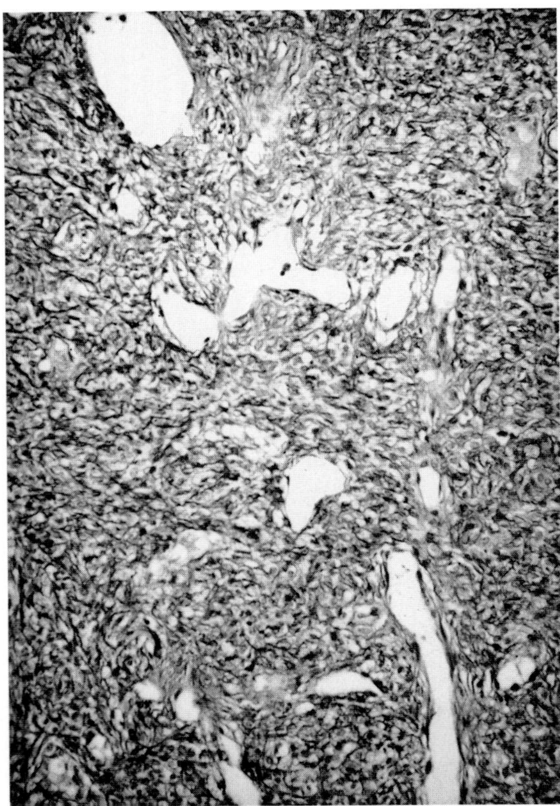

Fig. 36.2 Microscopically, these tumors appear as sheets of cells with numerous vascular spaces which can assume a 'staghorn' configuration.

from field to field and occasionally resemble either meningotheliomatous or fibrous meningiomas (Horten et al 1977, Guthrie et al 1989). Thin-walled 'staghorn' shaped capillaries are a distinguishing feature and can be quite numerous (Rubinstein 1972, Horten et al 1977, Kochanek et al 1986) (Fig. 36.2). Mitoses are frequent and are regionally variable, numbering from one to several per high powered field (Kochanek et al 1986, Guthrie et al 1989). Microcysts, necrosis, and papillary architecture may be seen (Guthrie et al 1989) and have been reported in up to 50% of the tumors (Kochanek et al 1986). Whorls and psammoma bodies are not seen (Kochanek et al 1986, Guthrie et al 1989). Reticulin, which is usually abundant, tends to envelop individual cells, as opposed to meningiomas, which exhibit reticulin enveloping cell groups, giving this typical lobulated appearance of meningiomas. A thorough description of the histology of this tumor can be found in the review by Kochanek et al (1986).

These tumors typically recur after surgical therapy, and the histology does not change from one recurrence to the next (Guthrie et al 1989). Likewise, primary and metastatic hemangiopericytomas are histologically identical (Guthrie et al 1989). Meningeal hemangiopericytomas are distinct from atypical or malignant meningiomas. The latter display a meningothelial architecture not usually present in hemangiopericytomas, but show varying degrees of atypical or anaplastic features such as loss of architecture, increased cellularity, nuclear pleomorphism, mitosis, necrosis, or brain infiltration (Jääskeläinen et al 1986).

INCIDENCE

Meningeal hemangiopericytomas are rare. In large series of meningiomas, their incidence ranges from 2–4% of that of meningiomas, thus comprising far less than 1% of intracranial neoplasms (Simpson 1957, Pitkethly et al 1970, Jellinger & Slowik 1975, Wara et al 1975, Fabiani et al 1980, Chan & Thompson 1985, Jääskeläinen et al

1985, Mirimanoff et al 1985, Guthrie et al 1989). Their rarity undoubtedly accounts for the fact that they are frequently misdiagnosed.

CLINICAL FINDINGS

As opposed to meningioma, the tumor is more common in males (56–75%) than females, even in the spinal location (Goellner et al 1978, Jääskeläinen et al 1985, Schroder et al 1986, Guthrie et al 1989). The average age at diagnosis is 38–42 years (Kochanek et al 1986, Schroder et al 1986, Guthrie et al 1989). The location is similar to meningiomas, with approximately 15% located in the posterior fossa and 15% located in the spine (Cappabianca et al 1981, Schroder et al 1986, Guthrie et al 1989). Of the spinal tumors, about half have been in the cervical region (Schroder et al 1986). While the vast majority of these tumors are based in the meninges, at least two have been reported in the pineal region (Stone et al 1983, Lesion et al 1984). Primary multifocal meningeal hemangiopericytomas have not been reported (Schroder et al 1986, Guthrie et al 1989).

The average patient is symptomatic for less than a year, particularly in the CT era (Guthrie et al 1989). Presenting symptoms are related to tumor location (Jääskeläinen et al 1985, Kochanek et al 1986, Schroder et al 1986, Guthrie et al 1989). Seizures are initially present in only about 16% of patients with supratentorial tumors (Guthrie et al 1989) which is compatible with the fact that they do not infiltrate the brain and grow rather rapidly.

IMAGING

Meningeal hemangiopericytomas resemble meningiomas on imaging studies. Plain films are of interest only in that no hyperostosis has been reported, and, if there is bone change, it is erosion (Osborne et al 1981, Jääskeläinen et al 1985, Guthrie et al 1989). Computerized tomography typically shows broad-based meningeal attachment and may show features suggesting malignancy (macroscopic brain invasion of 'mushrooming' inhomogeneous contrast enhancement or irregular borders) (New et al 1982). The tumors frequently show characteristic arteriographic features including a 'corkscrew' vascular configuration and a longlasting venous stain (Fig. 36.3) (Marc et al 1975). As many as half have a significant internal carotid artery blood supply (Marc et al 1975, Jääskeläinen et al 1985, Guthrie et al 1989), and few show early venous drainage, another factor which distinguishes them from ordinary meningiomas (Jääskeläinen et al 1985, Guthrie et al 1989). Despite these features, Guthrie et al (1989) found that, of 20 angiographic studies, only one was diagnosed preoperatively as a meningeal hemangiopericytoma. Jääskeläinen et al (1985) reported that, in hindsight, with knowledge of the above characteristics, at least 8 of their 17 meningeal hemangiopericytomas could have been diagnosed as such by angiography.

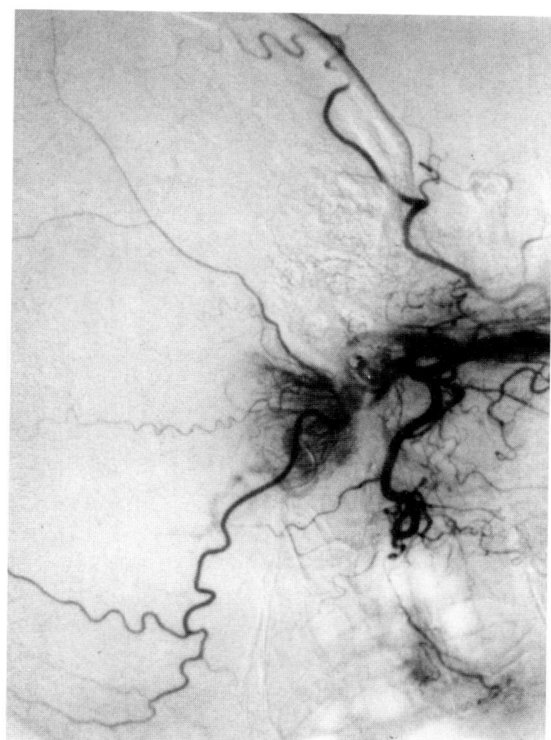

Fig. 36.3 Arteriography of this tuberculum meningeal hemangiopericytoma illustrates the early filling vessels in a corkscrew configuration. Notice also the early draining vein.

Gadolinium-enhanced MRI is helpful in delineating anatomy, but is nonspecific with regard to differentiation from ordinary meningiomas (Guthrie et al 1989). Di Chiro et al (1987) have shown that metabolically active meningiomas, including angioblastic meningiomas (hemangiopericytomas), may be differentiated by hypermetabolic activity on positron emission tomography (PET) and that such 'hot spots' on PET were of prognostic significance.

TREATMENT

Management of patients with meningeal hemangiopericytoma is difficult. At initial presentation these patients are often thought to have meningioma. However, meningeal hemangiopericytoma should be suspected if the history is brief and the lesion appears extremely vascular by CT, MRI or MRA. Surgery, if possible, is the treatment of choice. If hemangiopericytoma is suspected, arteriography should be considered for the possibility of embolization, which can markedly reduce intraoperative bleeding. It should be remembered that these tumors can parasitize cerebral vasculature such that embolization of meningeal feeders may not be as effective in stopping bleeding as it is for ordinary meningioma. Likewise, during surgery, amputation of the meningeal attachment of this tumor may not adequately devascularize a tumor, and significant blood loss may still occur.

Since these tumors have a propensity for recurrence, every attempt should be made to achieve a complete removal at the time of the initial surgery. In large series reporting surgery for these tumors, however, this has been possible in only 50–67% of the cases (Jääskeläinen et al 1985, Schroder et al 1986, Guthrie et al 1989). If complete removal is not possible, adjuvant radiation is recommended. Some authors have suggested preoperative radiation and then waiting several months for a response in order to simplify the surgery (Wara et al 1975, Fuki et al 1980). Given the difficulties of a previously irradiated surgical field, however, radiation should not be routinely used in an attempt to reduce the difficulty of a resection.

Radiosurgery

The availability and attractiveness of radiosurgery have forced consideration of this as a treatment option. Radiosurgery has been reported as probably effective against inoperable meningiomas (Duma et al 1993). Its efficacy for hemangiopericytoma has not been formally delineated. It would seem that this tumor, with its relatively discrete margins and known radiosensitivity, should be susceptible to radiosurgery. This author has experience with only one such patient, for whom the short-term response has been dramatic. However, as with any new treatment modality, recommendation for radiosurgery as a primary treatment must be made with caution and, at the time of writing, probably should be used for patients for whom surgery is not an option.

Surgical mortality

Operative mortality for meningeal hemangiopericytomas has ranged from 9–27%, with many deaths attributable to exsanguination (Jääskeläinen et al 1985, Schroder et al 1986, Guthrie et al 1989). Using current technology, including embolization, Guthrie et al (1989) report no surgical deaths since 1974, and, with care, surgical complications should be minimal. As with most tumors, operation for recurrence is more hazardous both in terms of morbidity and mortality (Guthrie et al 1989).

RECURRENCE

Meningeal hemangiopericytomas have a relentless tendency to recur. The reported recurrence-free interval after the first operation varies due to the variable measures of tumor recurrence. In an exhaustive review of the literature to 1985, Schroder et al (1986) found a median recurrence-free interval of 50 months (range 1 month to 26 years). Jääskeläinen et al (1985) found a mean time to recurrence of 78 months in 18 patients. Guthrie et al (1989), diagnosing recurrence as a progression of symptoms with radiographic or operative confirmation, found a median recurrence-free interval of 40 months (mean 47 months). After reviewing the literature, Schroder et al (1986) found the 5-year recurrence to be around 60%. From an actuarial standpoint, Guthrie et al (1989) calculated a 5-, 10-, and 15-year recurrence rate of 65%, 76% and 87% respectively (Table 36.1) From these data, it is obvious that meningeal hemangiopericytomas are much more aggressive than meningiomas and that recurrence is likely if a patient survives for 5 years, and becomes more likely with extended survival. The fact is that if the patient lives long enough, the tumor will recur.

Table 36.1 Prognosis of patients with meningeal hemangiopericytoma (%). Compiled from Guthrie et al (1989)

	5 years	10 years	15 years
Rate of recurrence	65	76	87
Rate of metastasis	13	33	64
Survival	67	40	23

After the first recurrence, meningeal hemangiopericytomas tend to recur at shorter intervals. Guthrie et al (1989) reported a series of 44 patients operated 79 times, in whom the average interval to subsequent recurrences tended to shorten. The average time to second, third, and fourth operations for recurrence was 38, 35, and 17 months respectively. In addition, these investigators found that 53% of patients improved and 3% worsened after the first operation, whereas only 22% improved and 13% worsened after subsequent operations, suggesting that the time for optimal patient benefit is at the first operation.

METASTASIS

Unlike any other primary intracranial tumor, meningeal hemangiopericytoma frequently metastasizes outside the CNS. The most common sites of metastasis in descending frequency are bone, lung and liver (Simpson 1957, Kruse 1961, Pitkethly et al 1970, Horten et al 1977, Thomas et al 1981, Kepes 1982, Inoue et al 1984, Jääskeläinen et al 1985, Schroder et al 1986, Guthrie et al 1989). The median time to metastasis ranges from 84–99 months, with a range of 1–20 years (Schroder et al 1986, Guthrie et al 1989). The probability of metastasis at 5, 10, and 15 years is 13%, 33%, and 64% respectively (Table 36.1) (Guthrie et al 1989). Realization that distant metastasis can occur after years of apparent tumor-free life is crucial for appropriate long-term management of these patients.

SURVIVAL

Guthrie et al (1989) found that the medial survival after the first operation was 60 months, with actuarial 5-, 10-, and 15-year survival of 67%, 40%, and 23% respectively

(Table 36.1). This is comparable to the cumulative survival of approximately 65%, 45%, and 15% compiled by Schroder et al (1986) from reviewing 118 cases in the literature to 1985.

FACTORS AFFECTING PROGNOSIS

As with any intracranial tumor, there are clinical and pathologic features that are important in predicting a patient's clinical course. In a detailed review of this disease, Guthrie et al (1989) studied the relationship of multiple factors to the long-term prognosis of their 44 patients. Age and sex were not important, nor were the histologic characteristics of the tumor, including mitotic activity. Kochaneck et al (1986), on the other hand, report that tumors with a higher mitotic rate tend to recur faster. It seems reasonable that tumors with a higher mitotic rate should be more aggressive, but actual evidence that this is the case for hemangiopericytoma is lacking. The extent of tumor removal is less clearly correlated with the recurrence of meningeal hemangiopericytomas than it is for meningiomas (Kochanek et al 1986, Guthrie et al 1989). Guthrie et al (1989) found an average survival of 109 months after apparent complete removal versus 65 months after incomplete removal. Oddly enough, the recurrence-free interval was unrelated to the extent of removal, possibly because patients with significant residual tumor tended to be radiated (Jääskeläinen et al 1985, Guthrie et al 1989).

Extraneural metastasis is a devasting occurrence and significantly shortens survival. In the Mayo Clinic series, 10 of 44 patients experienced extraneural metastasis at an average time of 99 months. The average survival after metastasis was 24 months. Five patients alive at 99 months who did not develop metastasis survived an additional 76 months (Guthrie et al 1989).

The treatment variable most strongly related to prognosis is postoperative radiation therapy. Chan & Thompson (1985) found that 12 patients with 'malignant meningiomas' (most likely unrecognized hemangiopericytomas) receiving postoperative radiation therapy survived an average of 4.6 useful years, while those not radiated survived less than a year. Guthrie et al (1989) found that patients radiated after the first operation experienced recurrence at an average of 74 months, with a 5- and 10-year recurrence rate of 38% and 64% respectively. Those patients not radiated suffered recurrence at an average of 29 months, with a 5- and 10-year recurrence of 90% (Guthrie et al 1989 — Table 36.2). These authors found a dose effect in that patients receiving less than 4500 cGy tended to experience recurrence sooner than those receiving 5000 cGy or more. In this same series, patients radiated after the first operation survived an average of 92 months, but those not radiated lived 62 months. This response by a hemangiopericytoma to radiation has been observed by others for intracranial as well as peripheral locations (Friedman & Egan 1960, Lal et al 1976, Mira et al 1977, Fuki et al 1980, Schroder et al 1986).

Table 36.2 Effect of postoperative radiation for meningeal hemangiopericytoma. Compiled from Guthrie et al (1989)

	Probability of recurrence (%)		
	3 years	5 years	10 years
Radiation	30	50	70
No radiation	50	100	100

DISCUSSION

The malignant nature of this tumor has long been recognized and, regardless of whether it is categorized as a meningioma (Rubinstein 1972, Horten et al 1977, Zulch 1979) or not (Popoff et al 1974, Pena 1977, Goellner et al 1978, Fabiani et al 1980, Kochanek et al 1986), the treating physician must realize that its behavior is drastically different than that of meningiomas. Meningiomas afflict females at a ratio of 1.5:1 to 3:1 over males (Cushing & Eisenhardt 1938, Simpson 1957, Jellinger & Slowik 1975, MacCarty & Taylor 1979, Adegbite et al 1983, Chan & Thompson 1985), but meningeal hemangiopericytomas show a slight male predominance. The average age of patients with meningeal hemangiopericytomas is 38–42 years, younger than that of 50 years for patients with meningioma (Skullerud & Loken 1974, Jellinger & Slowik 1975, Yamashita et al 1980, Chan & Thompson 1985, Mirimanoff et al 1985). Most hemangiopericytomas are symptomatic less than a year, while patients with meningiomas may be symptomatic for several years. Patients with meningeal hemangiopericytomas tend not to present with seizures. The two lesions arise at similar foci; however, meningeal hemangiopericytomas are never multifocal, whereas up to 16% of meningiomas may be (Kepes 1982).

Meningeal hemangiopericytomas are much more aggressive than ordinary meningiomas, with a 5- and 10-year recurrence rate of 65% and 76% respectively (Guthrie et al 1989), while that for meningiomas is 20% and 30% respectively (Adegbite et al 1983, Mirimanoff et al 1985). As with many malignant versus benign tumors, meningeal hemangiopericytomas are relatively more responsive to radiation (King et al 1966, Carella et al 1982, Guthrie et al 1989). Perhaps the most striking difference from meningiomas is the tendency for meningeal hemangiopericytomas to metastasize. Kepes (1982), in his thorough monograph on meningiomas, found very few ordinary meningiomas that metastasized. In contrast, the rate of metastasis of meningeal hemangiopericytomas at 5, 10, and 15 years is 13%, 33%, and 64% respectively (Guthrie et al 1989), making metastasis likely with prolonged survival.

Meningeal hemangiopericytomas should not be equated with atypical or malignant meningiomas. The latter tumors show loss of architecture, increased cellularity, nuclear atypia, and mitoses, but remain recognizable as meningiomas. Jääskeläinen et al (1986) studied a series of atypical and anaplastic meningiomas and found them to be more aggressive than meningiomas, but less so than meningeal hemangiopericytomas. In particular, malignant meningiomas have little or no tendency to metastasize.

In summary, a meningeal hemangiopericytoma is an aggressive extra-axial central nervous system tumor that behaves like a soft tissue sarcoma. It has a relentless tendency for local recurrence and, even if local control can be achieved, distant metastasis remains a threat as long as the patient lives. Optimal treatment includes aggressive local excision at the time of the first operation, followed by radiation therapy of at least 5000–5500 cGy. Diligent, long-term observation with periodic chest X-rays and workup of bone pain and abnormal liver function studies to rule out metastasis is required in all patients.

REFERENCES

Adegbite A B, Khan M I, Paine K W E, Tan L K 1983 The recurrence of intracranial meningiomas after surgical treatment. Journal of Neurosurgery 58: 51–56

Bailey P, Cushing H, Eisenhardt L 1928 Angioblastic meningiomas. Archives of Pathology 6: 953–990

Begg C F, Garret R 1954 Hemangiopericytoma occurring in the meninges. Cancer 7: 602–606

Cappabianca P, Mauri F, Pettinato G, Di Prisco B 1981 Hemangiopericytoma of the spinal canal. Surgical Neurology 15: 298–302

Carella R J, Ransohoff J, Newal J 1982 Role of radiation therapy in the management of meningioma. Neurosurgery 10: 332–339

Chan R C, Thompson G B 1985 Morbidity, mortality, and quality of life following surgery for intracranial meningiomas. A retrospective study in 257 cases. Journal of Neurosurgery 62: 18–24

Cushing H, Eisenhardt L 1938 Meningiomas: their classification, regional behavior, life history, and surgical end results. Charles C Thomas, Springfield, Illinois

de la Monte S M, Flickinger J, Linggood R M 1986 Histopathologic features predicting recurrence of meningiomas following sub-total resection. American Journal of Surgery and Pathology 10: 836–843

Di Chiro G, Hatazawa J, Katz D A, Rizzoli H V, De Michele D J 1987 Glucose utilization by intracranial meningiomas as an index of tumor aggressivity and probability of recurrence: a PET study. Radiology 167: 521–526

Duma C M, Lunsford L D, Kondziolka D, Harsh G R, Flickinger J C 1983 Stereotactic radiosurgery of cavernous sinus meningiomas as an addition or alternative to microsurgery. Neurosurgery 32: 699–705

Fabiani A, Favero M, Trebini F 1980 On the primary meningeal tumors with special concern to the hemangiopericytoma pathology and biology. Zentralbl Neurochir 41: 273–284

Friedman M, Egan J W 1960 Irradiation of hemangiopericytoma of Stout. Radiology 74: 721–729

Fuki M, Kitamura K, Nakagaki H et al 1980 Irradiated meningiomas: a clinical evaluation. Acta Neurochirurgica 54: 33–43

Goellner J R, Laws E R Jr, Soule E H, Okazaki H 1978 Hemangiopericytoma of the meninges: Mayo Clinic experience. Journal of Clinical Pathology 70: 375–380

Guthrie B L, Ebersold M J, Scheithauer B W, Shaw E G 1989 Meningeal hemangiopericytoma: histopathological features, treatment, and long-term follow-up of 44 cases. Neurosurgery 25: 514–522

Horten B C, Urich H, Rubinstein L J, Montague S R 1977 The angioblastic meningioma: a reappraisal of a nosological problem. Journal of Neurological Science 31: 387–410

Inoue H, Tamura M, Koizumi H, Nakamura M, Naganuma H, Ohye C 1984 Clinical pathology of malignant meningiomas. Acta Neurochirurgica 73: 179–191

Jääskeläinen J, Servo A, Haltia M, Walhstrom T, Valtonen S 1985 Intracranial hemangiopericytoma: radiology, surgery, radiotherapy, and outcome in 21 patients. Surgical Neurology 23: 227–236

Jääskeläinen J, Haltia M, Servo A 1986 Atypical and anaplastic meningiomas: radiology, surgery, radiotherapy and outcome. Surgical Neurology 25: 233–242

Jellinger K, Slowik F 1975 Histological subtypes and prognostic problems in meningiomas. Journal of Neurology 208: 279–298

Kepes J J 1982 Meningiomas: biology, pathology and differential diagnosis. Masson, New York

King D L, Chang C H, Pook J L 1966 Radiotherapy in the management of meningiomas. Acta Radiol 5: 26–33

Kochanek S, Schroder R, Firsching R 1986 Hemangiopericytoma of the meninges. I. Histopathological variability and differential diagnosis. Zentralbl Neurochir 47: 183–190

Kruse F Jr 1961 Hemangiopericytoma of the meninges (angioblastic meningioma of Cushing and Eisenhardt). Clinicopathologic aspects and follow-up studies in 8 cases. Neurology 11: 771–777

Lal H, Sanyal B, Pant C G, Rastogy B L, Khanna N N, Udupa K N 1976 Hemangipericytoma: report of three cases regarding role of radiation therapy. American Journal of Roentgenology 126: 887–891

Lesion F, Bouchez B, Krivosic I, Delandsheer J M, Jomin M 1984 Hemangiopericytic meningioma of the pineal region. Case report. European Neurology 23: 274–277

MacCarty C S, Taylor W F 1979 Intracranial meningiomas: experiences at the Mayo Clinic. Neurol Med Chir (Tokyo) 19: 569–574

Marc J A, Takei Y, Schecter M M, Hoffman J C 1975 Intracranial hemangiopericytomas: angiography, pathology, and differential diagnosis. American Journal of Roentgenology 125: 823–832

Mira J G, Chu F C H, Fornter J F 1977 The role of radiotherapy in the management of malignant hemangiopericytoma: report of eleven new cases and review of the literature: Cancer 39: 1254–1259

Mirimanoff R O, Dosoretz D E, Linggood R M, Ojemann R G, Martuza R L 1985 Meningioma: analysis of recurrence and progression following neurosurgical resection. Journal of Neurosurgery 62: 18–24

New P F J, Hesselink J R, O'Caroll C P, Kleinman G M 1982 Malignant meningiomas: CT and histologic criteria, including a new CT sign. AJNR 3: 267–276

Osborne D R, Dubois P, Drayer B, Sage M, Burger P, Heinz E R 1981 Primary intracranial meningeal and spinal hemangiopericytoma: radiologic manifestations. AJNR 2: 69–74

Pena C E 1977 Meningioma and intracranial hemangiopericytoma. A comparative electron microscopic study. Acta Neuropathologica (Berlin) 39: 69–74

Pitkethly D T, Hardman J M, Kempe L G, Earle K M 1970 Angioblastic meningiomas. Clinicopathologic study of 81 cases. Journal of Neurosurgery 32: 539–544

Popoff N A, Malinin T, Rosomoff H L 1974 Fine structure of intracranial hemangiopericytoma and angiomatous meningioma. Cancer 34: 1187–1197

Rubinstein L J 1972 Tumors of the central nervous system, 2nd series, fasc 6. Armed Forces Institute of Pathology, Washington, DC

Russell D S, Rubinstein L J 1977 Pathology of tumors of the nervous system, 4th edn. Edward Arnold, London

Schroder R, Firsching R, Kochanek S 1986 Hemangiopericytoma of the meninges. II. General and clinical data. Zentralbal Neurochir 47: 191–199

Simpson D 1957 The recurrence of intracranial meningiomas after surgical treatment. Journal of Neurology, Neurosurgery and Psychiatry 20: 22–39

Skullerud K, Loken A C 1974 The prognosis in meningiomas. Acta Neuropathologica (Berlin) 29: 337–344
Stone J L, Cybulski G R, Rhee H L, Bailiey O T 1983 Excision of a large pineal region hemangiopericytoma (angioblastic meningioma, hemangiopericytoma type). Surgical Neurology 19: 181–189
Stout A P, Murray M R 1942a Hemangiopericytoma: a vascular tumor featuring Zimmermann's pericyte. Annals of Surgery 116: 26–33
Stout A P, Murray M R 1942b Hemangiopericytoma occurring in the meninges. Cancer 2: 1027–1035
Thomas H G, Dolman C L, Berry K 1981 Malignant meningioma: clinical and pathological features. Journal of Neurosurgery 55: 929–934
Wara W M, Sheline G E, Newman H, Townsend J J, Boldrey E B 1975 Radiation therapy of meningiomas. Am J Roentgenol Radium Ther Nucl Med 123: 453–458
Yamashita J, Handa H, Iwaki K, Abe M 1980 Recurrence of intracranial meningiomas, with special reference to radiotherapy. Surgical Neurology 14: 33–40
Zulch K J 1979 Histological typing of tumors of the central nervous system. World Health Organization, Geneva

37. Meningeal sarcoma

Georges F. Haddad Ossama Al-Mefty

Sarcoma, autrement dit fungus, est une excroissance de chair qui vient de l'aliment propre de le partie où elle naist.

Ambroise Paré (Bailey 1929)

The subject of meningeal sarcomas is intricately related to intracranial sarcomas in general. Robbins & Cotran (1979) define sarcomas as malignant tumors arising from mesenchymal tissue. The term *sarcoma* was coined from the Greek word for fleshy — *sar*. These tumors usually have very little connective tissue stroma and appear to be fleshy (Robbins & Cotran 1979). According to Russell & Rubinstein (1989), the sources of mesenchymal cells within the cranial cavity are as follows: dura, leptomeninges, pial or adventitial fibroblasts covering perforating blood vessels deep in the cerebral matter, tela choroidea, and the stroma of the choroid plexus. Thus, primary intracranial sarcomas can be superficial and involve the meninges, and are termed *meningeal sarcomas*. They can also arise within the parenchyma or be intraventricular, arising presumably from the choroid plexus stroma.

We will review the history, etiology, classification and epidemiology of this lesion.

HISTORY

The first systematic classification of cerebral tumors dates back to Virchow (Rubinstein 1971), who used the term *sarcoma* to refer to fleshy malignant neoplasms of the central nervous system. This name was in contradistinction to a more benign type of neoplasm of the central nervous system he had previously named *glioma*. According to Rubinstein (1971), these *sarcomas* most probably represented glioblastoma multiforme. Virchow's inadequate definition and classification explains why older statistics list sarcomas as comprising 30–40% of brain tumors (Zülch 1986).

The first major study of intracranial sarcomas postdating the 1926 monograph of Bailey & Cushing was published by Bailey in 1929. He reported eight sarcomas that he fitted into five categories. Several classification schemes were subsequently devised; some were based on the histologic architecture (perivascular, perithelial, alveolar), others on the site of origin within the cranial vault (dural, leptomeningeal), and still others according to histologic subtype (Rubinstein 1971). This latter classification was adopted by Christensen & Lara (1953), who reviewed 24 cases of primary intracranial fibrosarcomas and classified them as fibrous, spindle cell, and polymorphocellular, in increasing degree of malignancy. Russell & Rubinstein still use these categories in the latest edition of *Pathology of Tumours of the Nervous System* (1989).

Apart from the lack of agreement on any one classification scheme, the study of intracranial sarcomas was hampered by the fact that not all major investigators could agree on which tumors were actually of mesenchymal origin, and thus sarcomas, rather than of neuroectodermal origin and thus gliomas. Examples of these are *monstrocellular sarcomas*, regarded by Zülch (1986) and Kernohan & Uihlein (1962) as true sarcomas, but considered by Rubinstein (1971) and Paulus et al (1991) to be giant cell glioblastoma multiforme. Foerster & Gagel first reported a group of circumscribed cerebellar tumors that they termed circumscribed arachnoidal cerebellar sarcoma; Rubinstein & Northfield (1964), however, believed that this tumor was actually a desmoplastic variant of a medulloblastoma. In 1986, Zülch stated that 'discussion about the nature of the tumor may not yet be over, since many of its characteristics . . . are very *atypical* of medulloblastomas . . .'.

CLASSIFICATION

The latest World Health Organization (WHO) classification of tumors of the central nervous system dates to 1979 (Zülch 1979). A modified classification of meningiomas has been proposed by Scheithauer (1990), who states that 'instead of our historical tendency to focus upon histogenesis and to apply "cell-of-origin" thinking in our efforts at classification, we might be better served to concentrate our diagnostic efforts upon demonstrating specific cellular differentiation'.

Table 37.1 Alternative histologic classification of tumors arising in meningeal and related tissues. After Scheithauer (1990)

1. Meningiomas (tumors arising from or differentiating toward arachnoidal cells)
   a. meningioma with its variants
   b. atypical meningioma
   c. malignant meningioma
2. Mesenchymal neoplasms
   a. benign
   b. malignant
      (i) hemangiopericytoma
      (ii) fibrosarcoma/malignant fibrous histiocytoma
      (iii) mesenchymal chondrosarcoma
      (iv) leiomyosarcoma
      (v) angiosarcoma
      (vi) meningeal sarcomatosis
      (vii) sarcoma, not otherwise specified
      (viii) others
3. Primary melanocytic neoplasms
4. Hemopoietic neoplasms
5. Tumors of uncertain nature including hemangioblastoma
6. Pseudotumors

Speaking about sarcomas, Enzinger & Weiss (1988) say 'earlier classifications have been largely descriptive . . . More recent classifications have been based principally on the line of differentiation of the tumor, that is, the type of tissue formed by the tumor rather than the type of tissue from which the tumor arose'.

The proposed WHO classification of tumors arising in meningeal and related tissues (Scheithauer 1990) follows the scheme of Table 37.1. In the following description, we will briefly review the descriptive classification used by Russell & Rubinstein (1989), recognizing that the immunohistochemical techniques used to pinpoint the WHO classification of tumors are not widely available. We will then describe the different subtypes of meningeal sarcomas according to the WHO classification. We will not deal with sarcogliomas, gliosarcomas, monstrocellular sarcomas, circumscribed arachnoidal sarcomas, or reticulum cell sarcomas, the latter being a hemopoietic neoplasm.

PATHOLOGY

Meningeal sarcomas usually present as a massive growth; tumors that arise from dura are often firmer than those originating from the leptomeninges or within the brain. The tumors are sharply demarcated from the adjacent brain in places but they lack a capsule and often infiltrate the brain. They sometimes spread over the cortex in a sheath, following the gyri and sulci (Russell & Rubinstein 1989).

Under light microscopy, meningeal sarcomas are divided into fibrosarcomas (Fig. 37.1), spindle cell sarcomas and polymorphocellular sarcomas (Fig. 37.2), in increasing degrees of malignancy. Fibrosarcomas are characterized by parallel streams of elongated spindle cells. Mitotic figures are usually evident. The nuclei may be hyperchromatic but multinuclear and giant cells are rare. A rich network of parallel intercellular reticulin fibers is aligned along the long axis of the tumor (Rubinstein 1971).

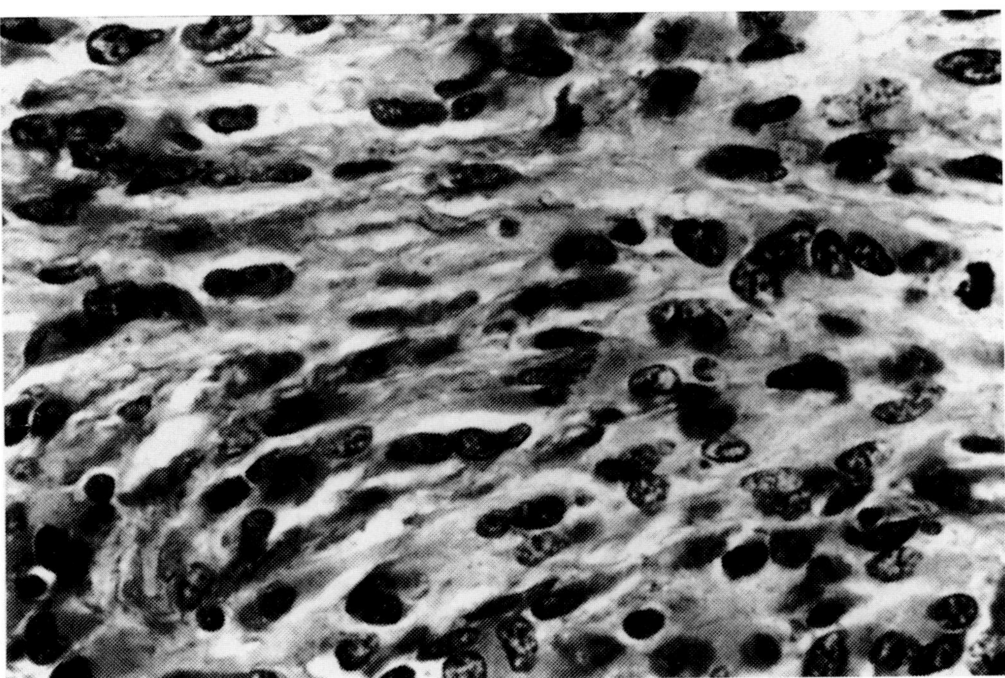

Fig. 37.1 Fibrosarcoma originating from the parietotemporal dura in a 2½-month-old boy. Note the abundant stroma of reticulin fibers aligned along the long axis of the tumor cells (H&E × 360). Reproduced with permission from Russell & Rubinstein (1989).

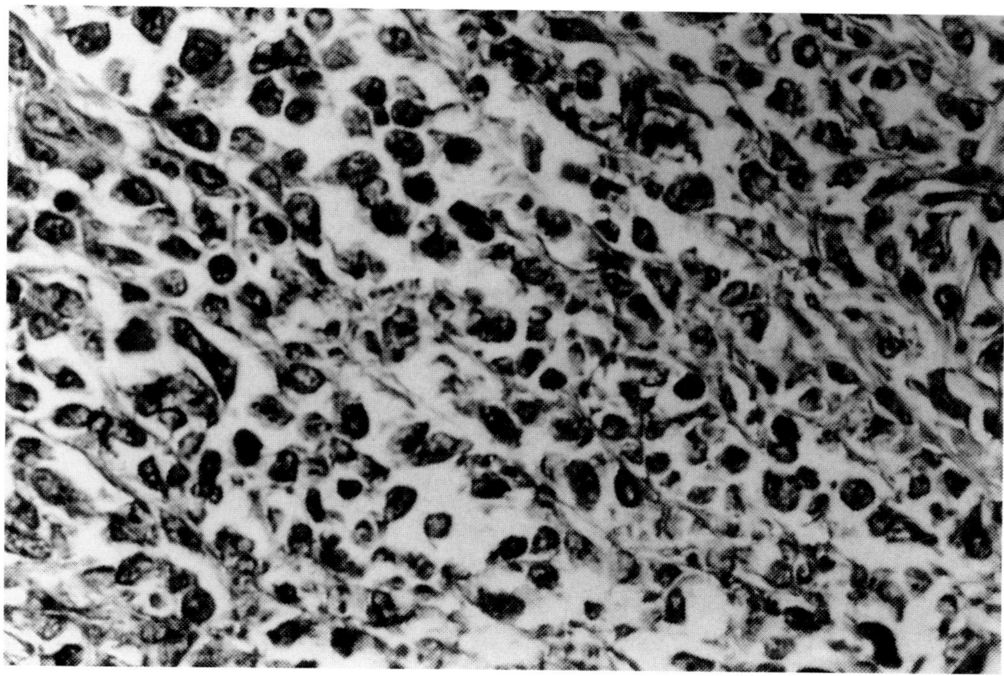

Fig. 37.2 Pleomorphic cell sarcoma originating in the lateral ventricle of an 8-month-old boy. Note the sheets of polygonal cells of varying sizes (PTAH × 300). Reproduced with permission from Russell & Rubinstein (1989).

Spindle cell sarcomas resemble fibrosarcomas except that the cells are usually smaller and plumper, are arranged in more compact masses, and may reveal a greater degree of pleomorphism (Rubinstein 1971).

Polymorphocellular sarcomas are the least differentiated subgroup, and usually occur in infants. There is considerable pleomorphism, including some multinucleated and giant cells. The cytoplasm is ill-defined and the nuclei frequently irregular. The stromal blood vessels are thin-walled in contradistinction to the endothelial proliferation seen in malignant gliomas. Microscopic necrosis may be seen (Rubinstein 1971). Russell & Rubinstein (1989) describe several other variants, namely myxosarcoma, myxochondrosarcomas, chondrosarcomas, osteochondrosarcomas, osteosarcomas, myosarcomas, and angiosarcomas.

Rather than describe every possible differentiation of mesenchymal cells and quote in detail the few reviews and case reports that deal with each subgroup, we will just say that meningeal sarcomas can differentiate according to several lines, thus producing fibrous tissue (fibrosarcoma), cartilage (chondromas, chondrosarcomas, and mesenchymal chondrosarcomas), smooth muscle (leiomyosarcomas), striated muscle (rhabdomyosarcomas), bone (osteosarcomas), or blood vessels (angiosarcomas).

Malignant fibrous histiocytomas are composed of several morphologic cell types: fibroblasts, xanthomatous cells, histiocytic-type cells and multinucleated giant cells (Tomita & Gonzales-Crussi 1984, Ho et al 1992). They accounted for 6 of 19 sarcomas reported by Paulus et al (1991).

Cartilage-producing sarcomas can be chondromas, chondrosarcomas (Fig. 37.3), or mesenchymal chondrosarcomas (Tomita & Gonzales-Crussi 1984, Cybulski et al 1985, Katayama et al 1987) (Fig. 37.4). In chondrosarcomas, only the cartilaginous elements are neoplastic, whereas both cartilaginous and mesenchymal elements are neoplastic in mesenchymal chondrosarcomas (Harsh & Wilson 1984, Shuangshoti & Kasantikul 1989). Some authors have reported positive staining of glial fibrillary acidic protein (GFAP) in malignant chondrocytes (Shuangshoti & Kasantikul 1989).

Every meningeal sarcoma should be subjected to a battery of tests to determine into which subgroup it fits. Some differentiating factors may be apparent on light microscopy (cartilage islands, osseous elements). Others may be seen only on electron microscopy (thick and thin filaments or Z-band material in rhabdomyosarcomas) (Enzinger & Weiss 1988). Special stains may be of use to differentiate subgroups of meningeal sarcomas. For example, the PAS stain for glycogen may be positive in rhabdomyosarcomas but negative in fibrosarcomas (Enzinger & Weiss 1988). The mainstay of diagnosis, however, is immunohistochemistry, which detects specific antigens in pathologic tissues. Table 37.2 provides a quick overview of the different useful antigens. One should keep in mind, however, that antibodies may cross-react with antigens other than the intended one, thus

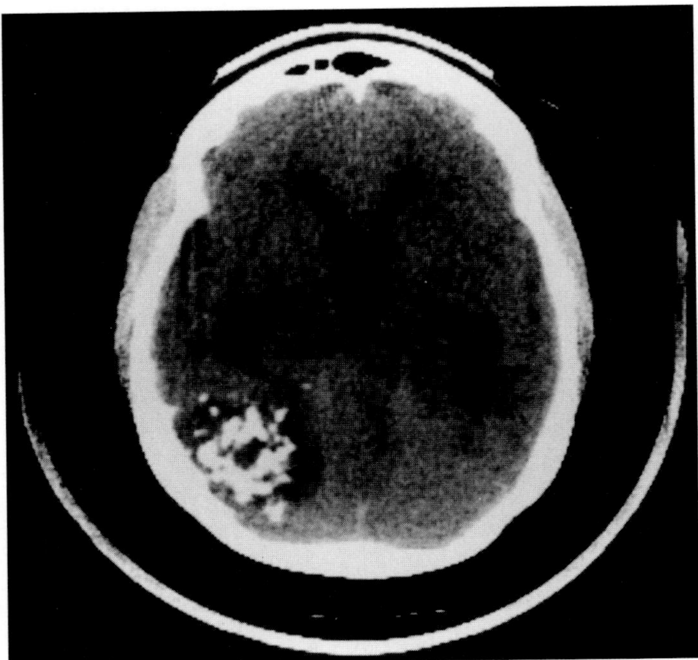

A

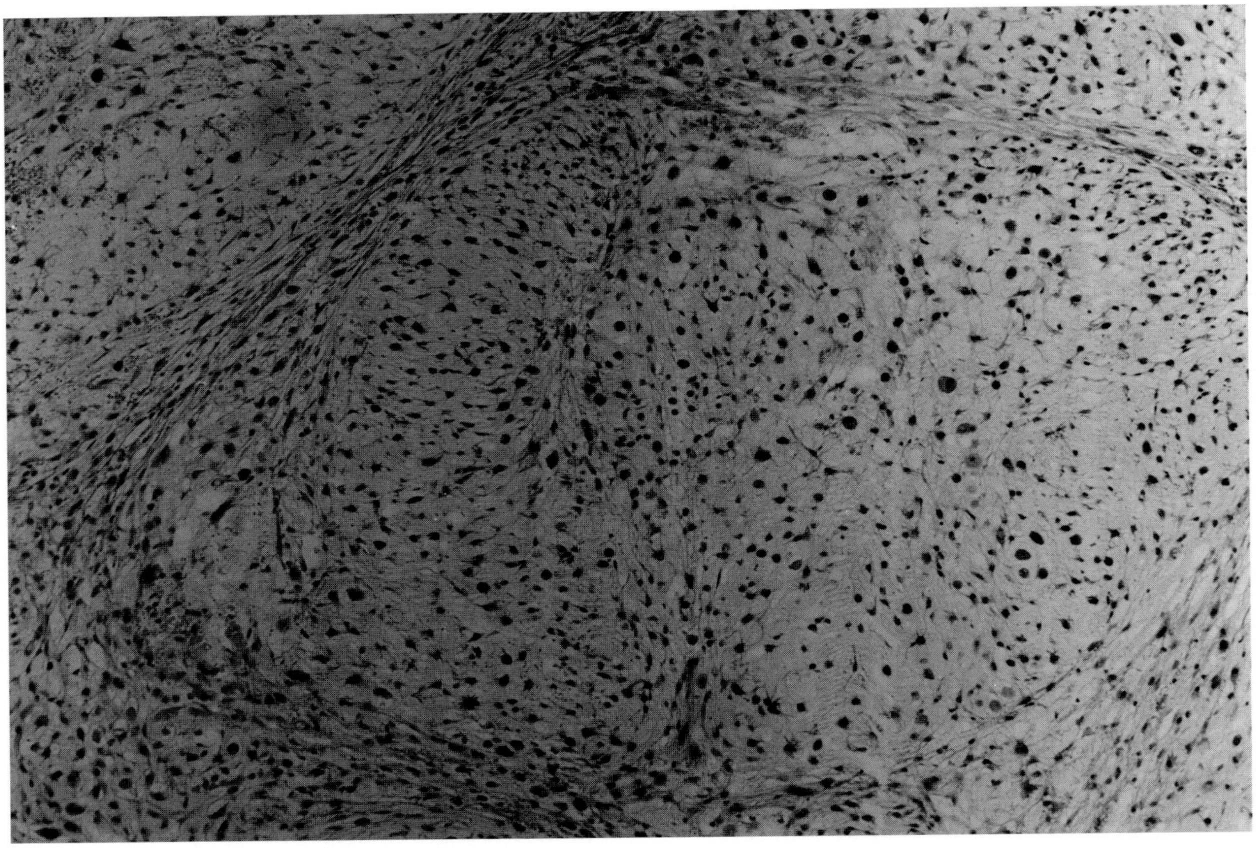

B

Fig. 37.3 A. Plain CT scan of a 33-year-old woman with a chondrosarcoma. Note the hypodense tumor with areas of calcification. The mass was avascular on cerebral angiography. Reproduced with permission from Hassounah et al (1985).
B. Photomicrograph of the neoplasm showing a lobulated pattern. The tumor cells are stellate-shaped and surrounded by abundant mucoid intercellular material (H&E × 150). Reproduced with permission from Hassounah et al (1985).

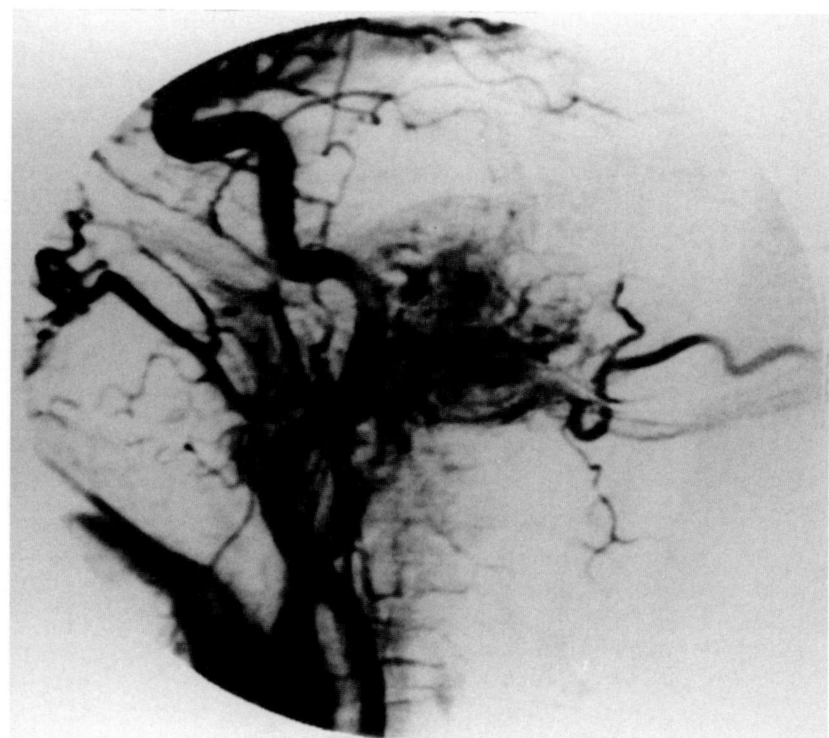

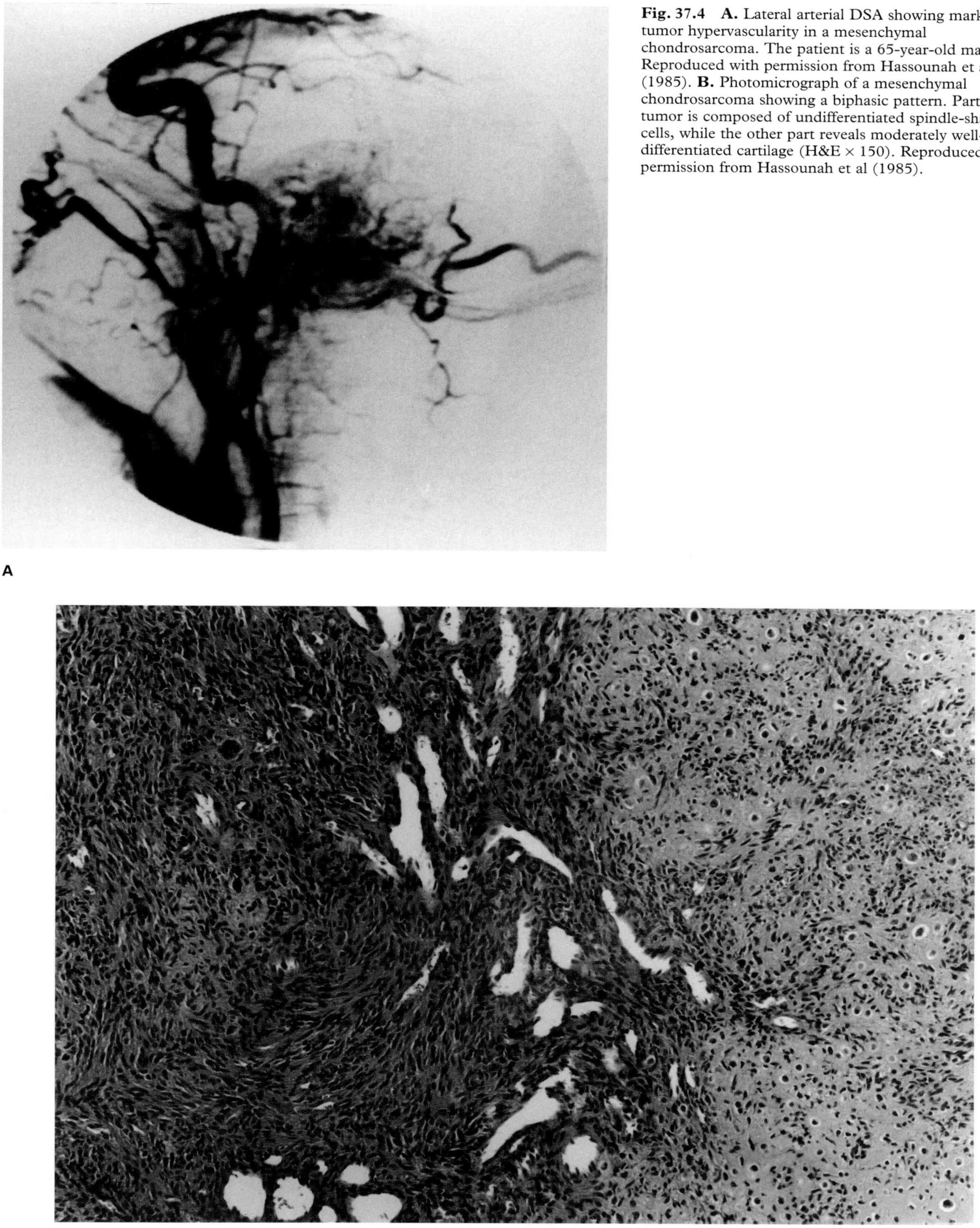

A

B

Fig. 37.4 **A.** Lateral arterial DSA showing marked tumor hypervascularity in a mesenchymal chondrosarcoma. The patient is a 65-year-old man. Reproduced with permission from Hassounah et al (1985). **B.** Photomicrograph of a mesenchymal chondrosarcoma showing a biphasic pattern. Part of the tumor is composed of undifferentiated spindle-shaped cells, while the other part reveals moderately well-differentiated cartilage (H&E × 150). Reproduced with permission from Hassounah et al (1985).

Table 37.2 Distribution of common antigens within soft tissue tumors. Modified from Enzinger & Weiss (1988)

Antigen	Tumor	Comment
Vimentin	Most mesenchymal tumors, some carcinomas	
Cytokeratin	Chordoma	Rarely in other intracranial sarcomas
EMA	Meningiomas	Rarely in other intracranial sarcomas
Desmin	Skeletal and smooth muscle tumors	Staining of leiomyosarcomas highly variable
Myoglobin	Skeletal muscle tumors	Not detected in poorly differentiated rhabdomyosarcomas
Factor VIII-AG	Benign vascular tumors, angiosarcomas (variable)	
S-100 protein	Benign nerve sheath tumors, benign chondroid tumors, granular cell tumor, clear cell sarcoma, melanoma, histiocytosis X, paraganglioma, some malignant schwannomas	Occasional liposarcomas, chondrosarcomas

giving a false positive result. False negatives may occur secondary to breaches in technique when handling and fixing the tissue.

Some distinctive features are sometimes seen in meningeal sarcomas. The edges of the neoplasm encompass, at times, islands of reactive hypertrophied fibrillated glia (Rubinstein 1971, Russell & Rubinstein 1989). These islands stain positive for GFAP. A sarcoglioma is produced if these islands of glial tissue become frankly malignant. Rubinstein (1971) notes that, whereas in glioblastoma multiforme the most malignant cellular elements are centrally located within the tumor, the opposite is true of sarcomas. The central portion of the tumor may be better differentiated and present as a fibrosarcoma with increased reticulin fibers, while the growing edges of the tumor show the least degree of differentiation.

Sarcomas, especially the least differentiated group, may seed the subarachnoid space (Bishop et al 1983, Russell & Rubinstein 1989). Extraneural metastases have also been reported (Bishop et al 1983); Russell & Rubinstein (1989) counted five such cases. Previous surgery or shunting of cerebrospinal fluid may play a role in systemic seeding of these tumors.

Primary meningeal sarcomatosis refers to involvement of the leptomeninges by sarcomatous spread in the absence of a localized tumor. Primary meningeal sarcomatosis is more frequent in infants and children; the cellular features are usually those of a polymorphic cell sarcoma, even though features of a fibrosarcoma may predominate at times (Russell & Rubinstein 1989). The spinal cord may be completely encased by the tumor (Russell & Rubinstein 1989). The protein content of cerebrospinal fluid is usually high, while the glucose concentration is low (Guthrie et al 1990). Cerebrospinal fluid cytology is usually positive for malignant cells. We should also mention that several case reports of primary central nervous system Ewing sarcomas have been reported (Russell & Rubinstein 1989).

The term *meningeal granulocytic sarcoma* refers to infiltration of the dura by granulocytic cells, usually as a late complication of acute myelogenous leukemia (Guthrie et al 1990). This has also been reported in the context of other myeloproliferative disorders (Roy et al 1989). To summarize, we agree with Paulus et al (1991) that 'primary intracranial sarcomas should be classified in a manner similar to their extracranial counterparts'.

INCIDENCE

Zülch believes that the average frequency of intracranial sarcomas may be between 2.5% and 3%. Russell & Rubinstein (1989), adjusting the figures of Kernohan & Uihlein (1962), estimate that the true incidence is around 1.2% of intracranial tumors. Tomita and colleagues found 8 primary sarcomas in a review of 402 children with intracranial tumors, giving a rate of about 2% in a pediatric population (Tomita & Gonzales-Crussi 1984). Paulus et al (1991) reported 19 primary intracranial sarcomas out of 25 000 cases, yielding an incidence of less than 0.1%. These authors, however, did not include meningeal sarcomatosis in their tally.

AGE AND GENDER

Russell & Rubinstein (1989) state that meningeal sarcomas can occur at any age but that the less differentiated polymorphic variety occurs predominantly in infants and children. Paulus et al (1991) report that malignant fibrous histiocytomas and fibrosarcomas occur in adults (Malat et al 1986), whereas sarcomas showing muscle differentiation tend to occur in children. This fact is also confirmed by Russell & Rubinstein (1989). However, a rhabdomyosarcoma was reported in a 61-year-old man (Ferracini et al 1992). No difference in incidence according to gender has been reported (Zülch 1986, Russell & Rubinstein 1989, Paulus et al 1991).

SITE

Meningeal sarcomas have no preferential site of involvement (Zülch 1986, Russell & Rubinstein 1989). The ratio of supratentorial to infratentorial tumors is equal to the ratio of brain mass in these compartments (Zülch 1986). Of 19 cases reported by Paulus et al (1991), 12 involved the meninges; the rest were located exclusively within the brain. Russell & Rubinstein (1989) report that most rhabdomyosarcomas arise in the midline.

ETIOLOGY

Zülch (1986) believes that there is no indication that sarcomas arise as an anaplastic variant of a pre-existing tumor (i.e. meningioma). On the other hand, Russell & Rubinstein (1989) concede that distinctions between secondary sarcomatous changes (in a pre-existing meningioma) and primary sarcomas are not always clear. Several reports have emphasized the finding of meningothelial elements amid the sarcomatous cells (Russell & Rubinstein 1989, Ferracini et al 1992). This may represent the dedifferentiation of meningioma cells into more malignant cells or, possibly, the reaction of mesenchymal tissue into sarcomas secondary to irritation by the meningioma. This latter concept is similar to sarcomas arising secondary to gliomas and thus forming a sarcoglioma.

Trauma has been cited as a possible factor in the development of sarcomas. Zülch (1986) cites a case recorded by Reinhardt in 1928 in which a metal wire was found embedded within 'a sarcomatous meningeal tumor (meningioma?) [sic]'. Kristoferitsch & Jellinger (1986) reported a case of angiosarcoma occurring at the site of a cordotomy performed 5 years earlier. Ho et al (1992) report on an intracerebral malignant fibrous histiocytoma diagnosed at the operative site of a posterior communicating artery aneurysm clipped 3 months earlier.

Several reports have linked meningeal sarcomas to previous irradiation of the brain, either for brain tumors, pituitary adenoma or leukemia (Russell & Rubinstein 1989).

Monosomy 22 has been reported in rhabdoid tumors (Biegel et al 1990), which is interesting especially because monosomy 22 has been implicated in the pathogenesis of meningiomas and schwannomas (Ironside 1991). Familial occurrence of cerebral sarcomas has also been reported (Gainer et al 1975). A higher incidence of fibrosarcomas has been reported in neurofibromatosis (Malat et al 1986).

DIFFERENTIAL DIAGNOSIS

The differential diagnosis of primary intracranial sarcomas is as follows (Paulus et al 1991). One should rule out:

1. An extracranial sarcoma presenting with a cerebral metastasis.
2. An intracranial extension from the skull or other parameningeal sites (rhabdomyosarcoma, chondrosarcoma).
3. A neoplastic mesenchymal component in the context of a neuroectodermal tumor (gliosarcoma; medulloblastoma with rhabdomyoblastic, leiomyoblastic or cartilaginous differentiation; primitive neuroectodermal tumors with rhabdomyoblastic areas and islands of cartilage produced by astrocytoma).
4. A malignant meningioma. Meningiomas would stain positive for epithelial membrane antigen (Russell & Rubinstein 1989).
5. Nonmalignant tumors that may simulate sarcomas because of pleomorphism (pleomorphic xanthoastrocytoma, benign fibrous histiocytoma) or fascicular arrangement of spindle cells with desmoplasia (superficial cerebral astrocytoma).

PRESENTATION

Meningeal sarcomas present as space-occupying lesions (Katayama et al 1987, Reusche et al 1990), with seizures (Cybulski et al 1985), hydrocephalus, or symptoms referable to the spinal cord (Bishop et al 1983).

RADIOLOGY

There is no pathognomonic radiologic picture of meningeal sarcomas. On computed tomography (Fig. 37.5) and magnetic resonance images (Fig. 37.6), they enhance as solitary or multiple lesions. The mass may enhance heterogeneously (Cybulski et al 1985, Katayama et al 1987), or in a ring-like fashion (Lee et al 1988), and the tumor may appear cystic (Reusche et al 1990). On

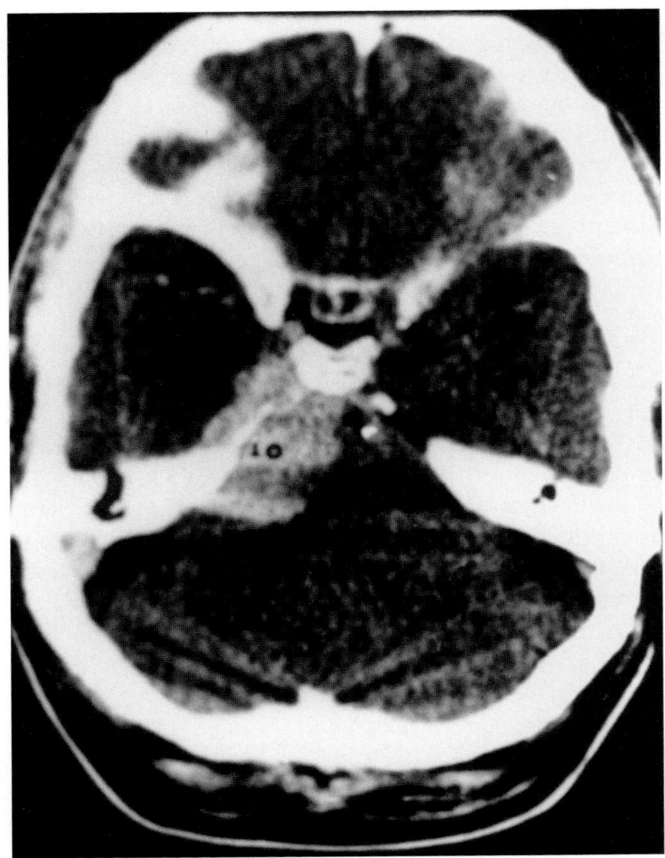

Fig. 37.5 CT scan with enhancement of a meningial sarcoma. Courtesy of Atul Goel.

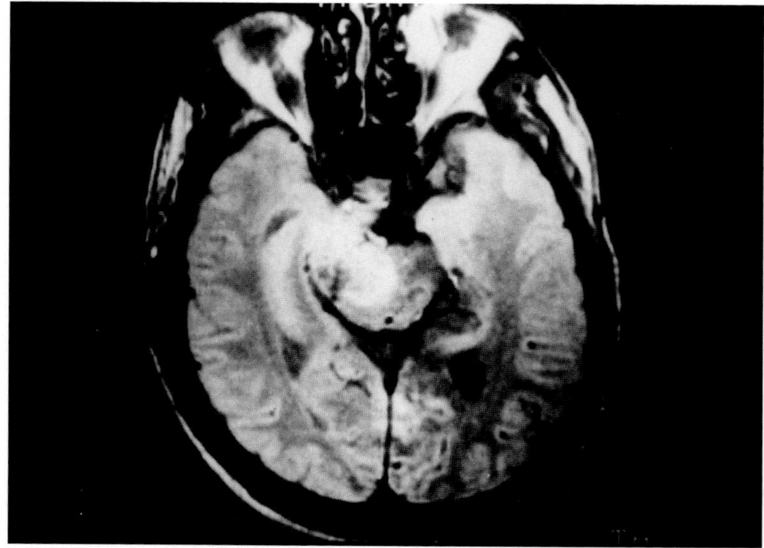

Fig. 37.6 MRI of a meningeal sarcoma shown in Fig. 37.5. Courtesy of Atul Goel.

magnetic resonance, the mass is hypointense on T1 and hyperintense on T2 (Lee et al 1988). Angiography reveals the mass effect of the tumor. The tumor appears as an avascular area (Lee et al 1988) or as a blush (Wang et al 1986) with neovascularity (Guthrie et al 1990). The blood supply may be from either the internal or external carotid artery (Guthrie et al 1990), and the intracranial arteries may be encased by tumor (Tomita & Gonzales-Crussi 1984). Skull erosion is seen in 25% of patients (Guthrie et al 1990), but there is no evidence of hyperostosis. The tumor may elicit severe edema from the adjacent brain (Wang et al 1986) or no parenchymal edema may be seen (Lee et al 1988).

PROGNOSIS

The 5-year postoperative survival rate is quoted at 16%, with an average survival of 32 months (Guthrie et al 1990); however, long-term survival after radical removal has been reported (Christensen & Lara 1953, Rubinstein 1971, Harsh & Wilson 1984, Ferracini et al 1992). Some patients have survived up to 20 years after surgery and radiation therapy (Rubinstein 1971). A favorable outcome is most likely after radical excision of a better-differentiated, well-circumscribed tumor (fibrosarcoma, mesenchymal chondrosarcoma) (Rubinstein 1971).

TREATMENT

Most authors agree that radical resection offers a patient the best chance for long-term survival (Tomita & Gonzales-Crussi 1984). The benefits of radiotherapy and chemotherapy are still not clear (Reynier et al 1984, Tomita & Gonzales-Crussi 1984). Drawing on the results of treatment for patients with extracranial sarcomas (Raney et al 1987, Alert et al 1988), both radio- and chemotherapy appear to have a genuine role, especially for more undifferentiated forms. The benefits of chemotherapy and radiotherapy in the treatment of parameningeal sarcomas seem to be proven (Raney et al 1987, Alert et al 1988), although some authors have questioned the efficacy of radiotherapy (Gasparini et al 1990). One should keep in mind, however, that chemotherapy may precipitate the demise of the patient, as reported in a case of intracranial osteosarcoma treated with intravenous methotrexate (Villareal et al 1990). Massive edema leading to fatal herniation has occurred after chemotherapy (Villareal et al 1990).

REFERENCES

Alert J, Longchong M, Valdés M, Menéndez J 1988 Cranial irradiation of children with soft-tissue sarcomas arising in parameningeal sites. Neoplasma 35: 627–633

Bailey P 1929 Intracranial sarcomatous tumors of leptomeningeal origin. Archives of Surgery 18: 1359–1402

Biegel J A, Rorke L B, Packer R J, Emanuel B S 1990 Monosomy 22 in rhabdoid or atypical tumors of the brain. Journal of Neurosurgery 73: 710–714

Bishop N, Chakrabarti A, Piercy D, Harriman D G F, Pearce J M S 1983 A case of sarcoma of the central nervous stem presenting as a Guillain-Barré syndrome. Journal of Neurology, Neurosurgery and Psychiatry 46: 352–354

Christensen E, Lara D E 1953 Intracranial sarcomas. Journal of Neuropathology and Experimental Neurology 12: 41–56
Cybulski G R, Russell E J, D'Angelo C M, Bailey O T 1985 Falcine chondrosarcoma: case report and literature review. Neurosurgery 16: 412–415
Enzinger F M, Weiss S W 1988 Soft tissue tumors, 2nd edn. CV Mosby, St Louis
Ferracini R, Poggi S, Frank G et al 1992 Meningeal sarcoma with rhabdomyoblastic differentiation: case report. Neurosurgery 30: 782–785
Foerster O, Gagel O 1939 Z. ges. Neurol Psychiat 144: 565
Gainer J V, Chou S M, Chadduck W M 1975 Familial cerebral sarcomas. Archives of Neurology 32: 665–668
Gasparini M, Lombardi F, Gianni M C, Massimino M, Gandola L, Fossati-Bellani F 1990 Questionable role of CNS radioprophylaxis in the therapeutic management of childhood rhabdomyosarcoma with meningeal extension. Journal of Clinical Oncology 8: 1854–1857
Guthrie B L, Ebersold M J, Scheithauer B W 1990 Neoplasms of the intracranial meninges. In: Youmans J R (ed) Neurological surgery, vol 5. 3rd edn. W B Saunders, Philadelphia, pp 3250–3315
Harsh G R IV, Wilson C B 1984 Central nervous system mesenchymal chondrosarcoma: case report. Journal of Neurosurgery 61: 375–381
Hassounah M, Al-Mefty O, Akhtar M, Jinkins J R, Fox J L 1985 Primary cranial and intracranial chondrosarcoma: a survey. Acta Neurochirurgica 87: 123–132
Ho Y-S, Wei C-H, Tsai M-D, Wai Y-Y 1992 Intracerebral malignant fibrous histiocytoma: case report and review of the literature. Neurosurgery 31: 567–571
Ironside J W 1991 Classification of primary intracranial sarcomas and other central nervous system neoplasms. Histopathology 18: 483–486
Katayama Y, Tsubokawa T, Maejima S, Satoh S, Sawada T 1987 Meningeal chondrosarcomatous tumor associated with meningocytic differentiation. Surgical Neurology 28: 375–380
Kernohan J W, Uihlein A 1962 Sarcomas of the brain. Charles C Thomas, Springfield, Ill
Kristoferitsch W, Jellinger K 1986 Multifocal spinal angiosarcoma after chordotomy. Acta Neurochirurgica 79: 145–153
Lee Y-Y, Van Tassel P, Raymond A K 1988 Intracranial dural chondrosarcoma. American Journal of Neuroradiology 9: 1189–1193
Malat J, Virapongse C, Palestro C, Richman A H 1986 Primary intraspinal fibrosarcoma. Neurosurgery 19: 434–436
Paulus W F, Slowik L, Jellinger K 1991 Primary intracranial sarcomas: histopathological features of 19 cases. Histopathology 18: 395–402
Raney R B Jr, Tefft M, Newton W A et al 1987 Improved prognosis with intensive treatment of children with cranial soft tissue sarcomas arising in nonorbital parameningeal sites: a report from the intergroup rhabdomyosarcoma study. Cancer 59: 147–155
Reusche E, Rickels E, Reale E, Stolke D 1990 Primary intracerebral sarcoma in childhood: case report with electron-microscope study. Journal of Neurology 237: 382–384
Reynier Y, Hassoun J, Vittini F, Gambarelli-Dubois D, Vigouroux R P 1984 Meningeal fibrosarcomas. Neurochirurgie 30: 1–10
Robbins S L, Cotran R S 1979 Pathologic basis of disease. W B Saunders, Philadelphia
Roy E P, Rogers J S III, Riggs J E 1989 Intracranial granulocytic sarcoma in postpolycythemia myeloid metaplasia. Southern Medical Journal 82: 1564–1567
Rubinstein L J 1971 Sarcomas of the nervous system. In: Minckler J (ed) Pathology of the nervous system, vol 2. McGraw-Hill, New York, pp 2144–2164
Rubinstein L J, Northfield D W C 1964 The medulloblastoma and the so-called "arachnoidal cerebellar sarcoma": a critical re-examination of a nosological problem. Brain 87: 379–410
Russell D S, Rubinstein L J 1989 Pathology of tumours of the nervous system, 5th edn. Williams & Wilkins, Baltimore
Scheithauer B W 1990 Tumors of the meninges: proposed modifications of the World Health Organization classification. Acta Neuropathologica 80: 343–354
Shuangshoti S, Kasantikul V 1989 View from beneath — pathology in focus. Primary intracranial mesenchymal chondrosarcoma. The Journal of Laryngology and Otology 103: 545–549
Tomita T, Gonzales-Crussi F 1984 Intracranial primary nonlymphomatous sarcomas in children: experience with eight cases and review of the literature. Neurosurgery 14: 529–540
Villareal B, Baum L G, Vinters H V, Feig S A 1990 Transtentorial herniation caused by an intracranial mass lesion following high-dose methotrexate. American Journal of Pediatric Hematology and Oncology 12: 215–219
Wang A-M, Fitzgerald T J, Lichtman A H et al 1986 Neuroradiologic features of primary falx osteosarcoma. American Journal of Neuroradiology 7: 729–732
Zülch K J 1986 Brain tumors: their biology and pathology, 3rd edn. Springer, Berlin, p 383
Zülch K J 1979 Histologic typing of tumours of the central nervous system. WHO, Geneva, pp 53–58

PART V

Pineal region tumors

38. Pineal cell and germ cell tumors

Jeffrey N. Bruce   E. Sander Connolly Jr   Bennett M. Stein

INTRODUCTION

A complete understanding of pineal cell and germ cell tumors is hindered by the often confusing nomenclature associated with them. Although most pineal cell and germ cell tumors occur in the pineal region, tumors of the pineal region can encompass a wide variety of tumor histologies including astrocytomas, meningiomas, ependymomas and metastatic tumors. It is important to recognize that, in references to 'pineal region tumors', not all tumors are of pineal or germ cell origin. Furthermore, although all pineal cell tumors originate within the pineal gland, many intracranial germ cell tumors may originate in areas other than the pineal region, particularly the suprasellar region.

Germ cell tumors refer to a group of pluripotential tumors of germ cell origin spanning a wide range of differentiation and malignant characteristics. At the benign end of the spectrum these include teratomas, dermoid tumors and epidermoid tumors. Endodermal sinus tumors, embryonal cell tumors, and choriocarcinomas are at the malignant end of the spectrum, with germinomas and immature teratomas falling somewhere in between. Although most intracranial germ cell tumors occur in the pineal region, a sizeable number can be found in the suprasellar region as well.

Pineal cell tumors, otherwise known as pineal parenchymal tumors, are derived from pineal parenchymal cells within the pineal gland, and therefore primarily occur in the pineal region. They are categorized as either pineocytomas or pineoblastomas, although mixed tumor forms can occur.

The term 'pinealoma' was originally used by Krabbe in 1923 to refer to pineal parenchymal tumors. Gradually this term adopted a more general meaning and was used to refer to any tumor of the pineal region regardless of its histology. This term is now obsolete and the preferred term is 'pineal region tumor' when referring to tumors of unspecified pathology in the pineal region. Since this term encompasses all tumors of the pineal region, the histology should be specified to avoid confusion (e.g. 'pineal region teratoma').

Similarly, the nomenclature regarding germinomas can be confusing. These particular germ cell tumors are known as seminomas when they occur in the testes or as dysgerminomas when the ovaries are involved. Although histologically identical to their gonadal counterparts, germinoma is the preferred term for intracranial occurrences. Older literature sometimes uses the outdated term 'atypical teratoma'.

INCIDENCE AND PREVALENCE

Estimation of the true incidence and prevalence of pineal cell and germ cell tumors is problematic for several reasons. Historically, many presumed pineal cell tumors and germ cell tumors of the pineal or suprasellar region were treated empirically without definitive histologic confirmation. Furthermore, over the years pathologic terminology has changed, making studies from past eras difficult to analyze. In addition to these problems of inconsistent specification of tumor histology, estimates of proportional representation of a given tumor type are subject to natural bias due to referral patterns of the specialized institutions that often treat these rare tumors. Most case series report the relative frequency of tumors based as a percentage of brain tumors, which does not necessarily reflect the actual incidence within a given population. Although the figures cited in the ensuing sections concerning incidence and prevalence are useful estimates, accurate figures must await prospective population-based studies using modern pathologic classification.

Pineal region tumors

When analyzing epidemiologic data on pineal region tumors, it is important to realize that these tumors encompass a wide variety of histopathology. Since tumors of pineal cell and germ cell origin are not always reported separately, statistics for pineal region tumors cannot always be extrapolated to make generalizations about specific histologic subtypes. Nevertheless, certain trends are apparent from the available epidemiologic data, which has historically been drawn from series of pineal region tumors (Fig. 38.1). Zimmerman & Bilaniuk (1982) have reported the most comprehensive series analyzing pineal region tumor incidence, comparing their brain tumor series (4865 cases) to that of Cushing (2141 cases), Dastar of India (774 cases), Ito of Japan (1365 cases) and Zulch of Germany (5955 cases), and determining the incidence of 'pinealoma' to be 0.6%, 0.7%, 0.9%, 5.9%, and 0.4% respectively. Zulch's and Ito's series also make mention of a separate category of teratoma (0.2% and 1.6%, respectively). While the terms 'pinealoma' and 'teratoma' in these series are never clearly defined, it is likely that pinealoma refers to pineal cell neoplasms whereas teratoma refers to germ cell neoplasms. This interpretation of the terminology is responsible for the traditional teaching that pineal region tumors (including both germ cell and pineal cell tumors) are more common in Japan than elsewhere. The Japanese predilection is supported by both Sano's series, in which pineal tumors accounted for 4% of the overall total (Sano 1984), and the annual report of pathologic autopsy cases in Japan for 1965–1974, which shows 6.23% of 3382 brain tumors to be of the pineal region (Koide et al 1980).

Recently, the validity of this presumed Japanese predilection has been questioned because of possible bias by selective case reporting (Ojeda et al 1987). No statistically significant difference was demonstrated between the number of pineal region tumors seen in Niigata Prefecture, Japan (0.07 per 100 000 person years) and Western Australia (0.06) in a prospective study of actual population-based incidence. Furthermore, other population-based figures from Southern England (0.02—Barker et al 1976), Connecticut (0.03 — Schoenberg et al 1976), and all Japan (0.02 — Araki & Matsumoto 1969), failed to demonstrate an excessively increased incidence in Japan. It should be emphasized once again that these figures refer to pineal region tumors of all histologies, not only pineal cell or germ cell origin.

Germ cell tumors

Intracranial germ cell tumors are a heterogeneous group of tumors which include germinomas, teratomas, embryonal cell tumors, endodermal sinus (yolk sac) tumors, choriocarcinomas, dermoid tumors and epidermoid tumors. Altogether, germ cell tumors account for 0.4–3.4% of the intracranial neoplasms seen each year in both the United States and Europe (Jennings et al 1985). In the USA, this calculates to an average yearly incidence of 0.2/100 000. Considerable geographic variation exists among germ cell tumors, with the highest incidence in Japan, varying between 2.1% and 4.8% (Sano 1976b, Arita et al 1980, Takakura 1985).

Germinomas are the most common intracranial germ cell tumor. Among large series, pure germinomas comprise between 40% and 65% of all germ cell tumors,

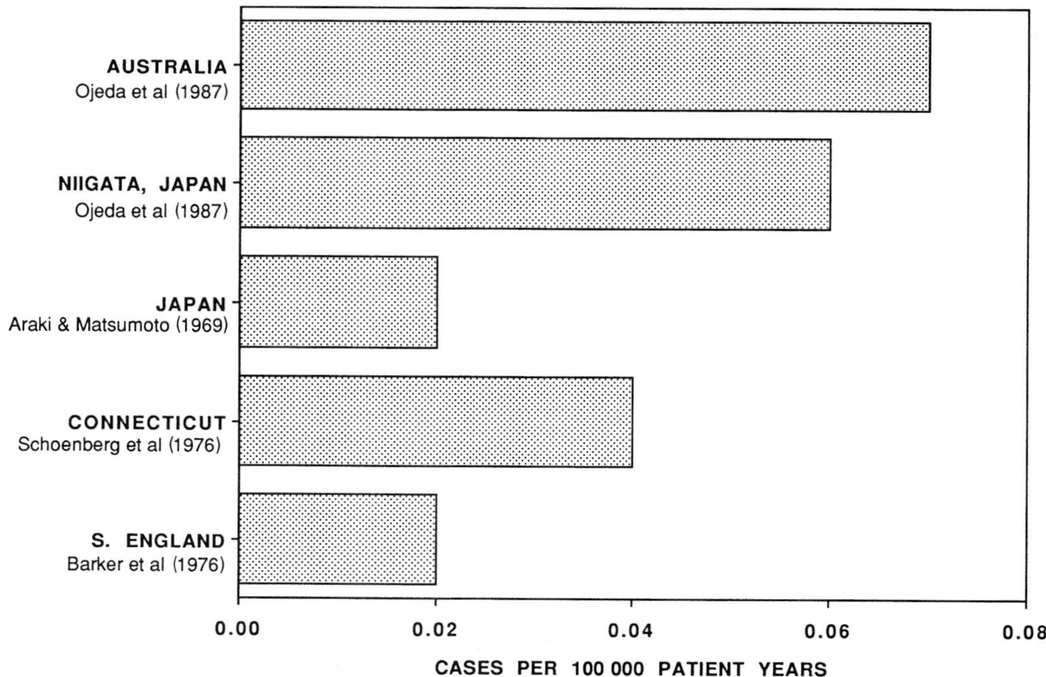

Fig. 38.1 Incidence of pineal region tumors by geographic location.

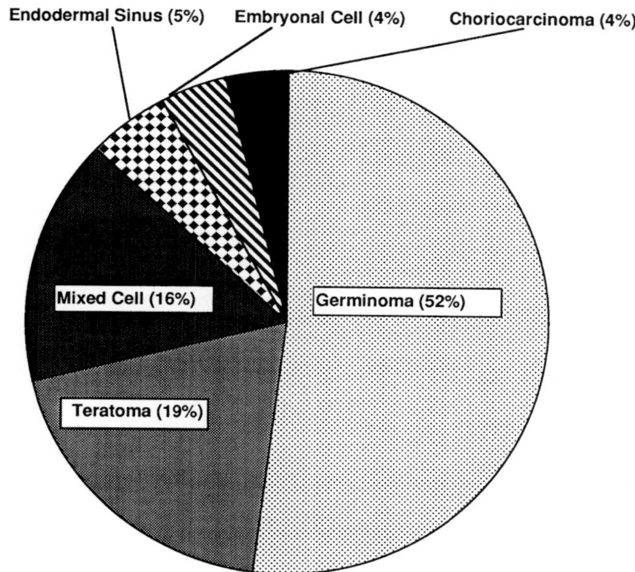

Fig. 38.2 Relative percentages of histologic subtypes among intracranial germ cell tumors (total incidence 0.2/100 000 per year) based on 389 tumors reviewed by Jennings et al (1985).

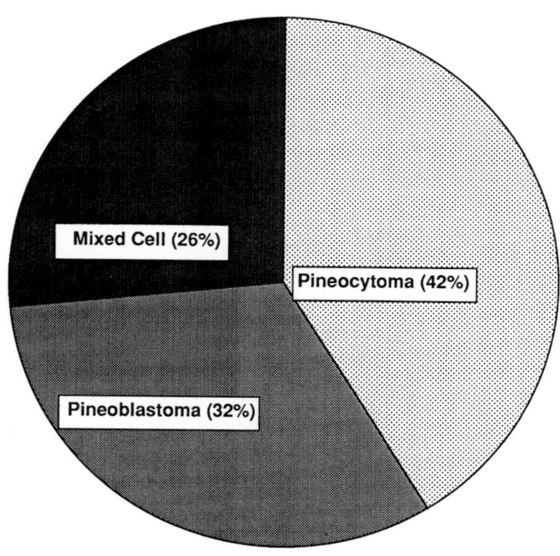

Fig. 38.3 Relative percentages of histologic subtypes among pineal cell tumors in the US (total incidence 0.1/100 000 per year) based on 90 tumors from the series of Herrick & Rubinstein (1979), Bruce (1993), and Schild et al (1993).

giving an average US incidence of 0.1/100 000 (Horowitz & Hall 1991). Teratomas (18–20%), endodermal sinus tumors (4–7%), embryonal cell tumors (3–5%), and choriocarcinomas (3–5%) are correspondingly less frequent (Fig. 38.2) (Jennings et al 1985). Moreover, large series with extensive tissue sampling have shown mixed germ cell tumors to comprise 25% of germ cell tumors (Russell & Rubinstein 1989a, Stein & Bruce 1992). The percentage of pure germinomas among germ cell tumors varies between populations, with the Taiwanese showing 82% germinomas compared to approximately 50% in an unselected Western series, and 16% in a Western pediatric series (Jennings et al 1985, Ho & Liu 1992).

Most germ cell tumors occur before the second decade of life, with regional differences among pediatric populations. In children, germ cell tumors account for between 4.8% and 15% of all brain tumors in Japan (Sano 1976b, Takakura 1985, Matsutani et al 1987). In western countries, the incidence in the pediatric population is between 0.3% and 3.4% (Jenkin et al 1978, Wara et al 1979, Hoffman et al 1984, Jennings et al 1985). Ho & Liu (1992) have also shown increased incidence among the children of Taiwan (11%), but Taiwanese adults seem to be affected no more often than European adults (0.6%).

Pineal cell tumors

The true incidence of pineal cell tumors is unknown, but indirect calculations based on data from Schild et al (1993) estimate it to be 0.01 per 100 000 persons per year in the United States. Schild et al found that pineal region neoplasms, 15–30% of which are of pineal cell origin, account for 0.4–1.0% of the 17 000 cerebral neoplasms diagnosed each year (Schild et al 1993). Thus, in the United States, one would expect to newly diagnose between 10 and 50 pineal cell tumors each year.

Schild's study of 30 pineal parenchymal tumors found approximately 50% to be pineoblastomas, 30% to be pineocytomas and the remaining 20% to be mixed tumors (Fig. 38.3). In the same publication, however, 110 cases reviewed in the literature showed a slightly greater percentage of pineocytomas at 53% compared to 47% pineoblastomas. In Russell and Rubinstein's series of 53 pineal cell tumors, pineocytomas accounted for 57% (Russell & Rubinstein 1989b). In the New York Neurological Institute operative series of 35 cases, 57% were pineocytomas, 23% were pineoblastomas and 20% were mixed tumors.

Although the incidence of pineal region tumors is four to five times higher in Japan than in the United States, pineal cell tumors make up only about 11% of these tumors compared to 30% in the United States. Thus, the overall incidence of pineal cell tumors is about the same as it is in the United States (Koide et al 1980). As mentioned previously, Ojeda's study has shown that, in comparison to Western Australia, Niigata (Japan) has a similar 10-year prevalence (Ojeda et al 1987).

AGE DISTRIBUTION

Germ cell tumors

Intracranial germ cell tumors occur most frequently between ages 10 and 12 (27%), with 70% occurring be-

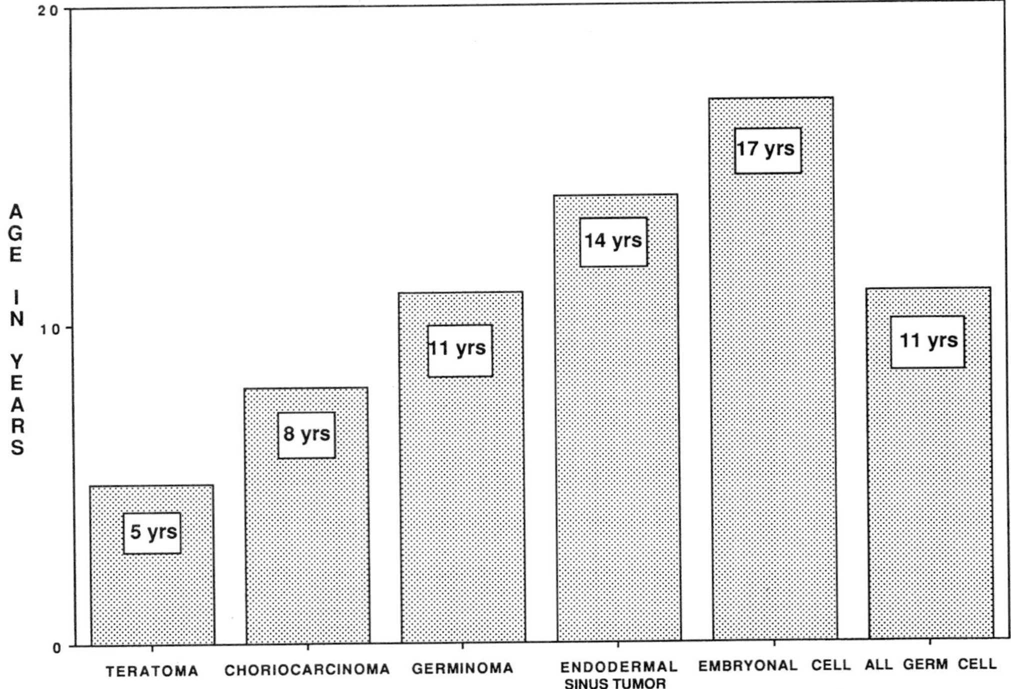

Fig. 38.4 Most common age of onset for intracranial germ cell tumors. From Jennings et al (1985).

tween 10 and 21 years, and 95% before age 33 (Fig. 38.4) (Jennings et al 1985). These rates are similar for both sexes. Germinomas occur with relatively the same frequency by age, with 26% between 10 and 12, 65% between 10 and 21 and 95% before age 27. Only 11% occur before the age of 9, although a 16-month-old boy with germinoma has been reported (Ammar et al 1991). Although it is not statistically significant, women are affected at slightly younger ages than men. Overall the age distribution of nongerminomatous germ cell tumors resembles that seen for germinomas, except that twice as many occur in children of less than 9 years (24%). The large number of cases in very young children is mainly due to teratomas and choriocarcinomas. Both of these tumors have one third of their presentations in early childhood.

Teratomas have two incidence peaks, with the greatest number in children less than 9, but with 20% occurring between ages 16 and 18. Overall, 65% of teratomas occur between 4 and 18, and 95% occur before age 36. Choriocarcinomas also show a proclivity for younger groups: 35% before the age of 9, 25% between 7 and 9, 70% between 7 and 15, and 95% between 1 and 21. By contrast, endodermal sinus tumors and embryonal cell tumors tend to occur in middle and late adolescence, respectively. Of endodermal sinus tumors, 40% occur between 13 and 15, 65% between 10 and 15 and 95% between 4 and 21. Only 12% occur in children less than 9. Of embryonal cell tumors, 30% occur between 16 and 18, 70% between 10 and 18, and 95% between 7 and 27. Only 10% of cases occurred in very young children.

In summary, germ cell tumors occur almost exclusively during the first three decades of life. Germinomas are most common in early adolescence around the time of puberty but may occur any time during youth. Nongerminomatous tumors show a similar pattern, with choriocarcinomas and teratomas especially prevalent in early childhood, and endodermal sinus tumors and embryonal carcinomas more common in late adolescence.

Pineal cell tumors

In Schild's series, the mean age of presentation for all pineal cell tumors was 22, ranging from 11 months to 77 years (Fig. 38.5) (Schild et al 1993). In 35 adult patients with pineal cell tumors at the Neurological Institute, the mean age of presentation was 36 years, with a range from 7–70 years.

The 9 cases of pineocytoma in Schild's study occurred between age 17 and 72, with a mean age of 36. Of Russell and Rubinstein's 30 cases of pineocytoma, 25 occurred in adulthood and only 5 (17%) occurred in children, all in the first decade of life (Russell & Rubinstein 1989b). In 20 adult patients at the Neurological Institute, the mean age of presentation was 40, with a range of 21–57 years.

Of the 15 cases of pineoblastoma reviewed by Schild, all presented between the ages of 11 months and 66 years, with an average age of 18 years (Schild et al 1993). Russell and Rubinstein also found this more malignant variety of pineal cell tumor in a younger population, evidenced by 14 of their 23 cases (61%) occurring in the

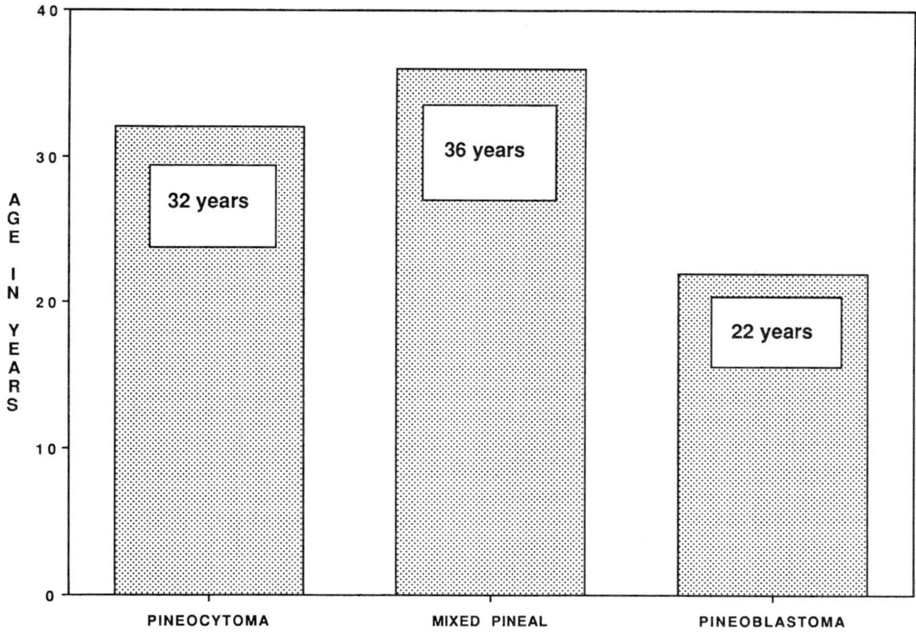

Fig. 38.5 Average age of onset for pineal cell tumors, based on 90 tumors from the series of Herrick & Rubinstein (1979), Bruce (1993b), and Schild et al (1993).

first decade of life and all the remaining cases occurring before the age of 40 (Russell & Rubinstein 1989b). In the 8 adult patients at the Neurological Institute, a mean age of presentation of 33 years was found which dropped to 27 years if the unusual case of a 70-year-old male was ignored.

In summary, pineal cell neoplasms generally occur in the third and fourth decades. Nonetheless, they may occur earlier, especially the more malignant pineoblastoma (61% present in the first decade). Isolated cases may present in old age.

SEX DISTRIBUTION

Germ cell tumors

Intracranial germ cell tumors are overwhelmingly more likely to occur in males. Summing the English language literature, Jennings et al (1985) showed that, for all intracranial germ cell tumors, males are 2.24 times more likely to be affected. A similar male predominance of 1.88:1 exists for pure germinomas but is stronger for nongerminomatous germ cell tumors, which show a slightly stronger male preponderance of 3.25:1. Men were more likely to have pineal involvement (65%) while women were more likely to have suprasellar involvement (75%). Several studies, however, showed equal gender representation for suprasellar germ cell tumors (Takeuchi et al 1978, Jennings et al 1985, Hoffman et al 1991).

Pineal cell tumors

Among large series of pineal cell tumors, there seems to be either no gender preference for these tumors or a very small one in favor of men (Russell & Rubinstein 1989b, Stein & Bruce 1992, Schild et al 1993). A slight male predominance has been shown in the Japanese literature (7:5 male to female — Koide et al 1980).

FAMILY HISTORY AND GENETIC FACTORS

Germ cell tumors

A familial tendency for germ cell tumors has not been found, although one exceptional mixed germ cell tumor in two brothers has been reported (Wakai et al 1980). Hereditary features have been demonstrated in presacral teratomas; however, these are also exceptional (Hunt et al 1977).

Pineal cell tumors

Heritable examples of pineal cell tumors are rare, although the occurrence of pineoblastoma in a 12-year-old girl and her 43-year-old mother has been reported (Lesnick et al 1985). A more striking familial association involves the 30 or so documented cases of the childhood syndrome known as 'trilateral retinoblastoma' consisting of simultaneous pineoblastoma and bilateral retinoblastoma (Bader et al 1982, Russell & Rubinstein 1989a). Retinoblastomas, especially in the bilateral form, are genetically inherited and have been associated with gene deletions (Murphree & Benedict 1984, Russell & Rubinstein 1989b). In trilateral retinoblastoma, the pineoblastoma is thought to represent an additional neoplastic focus originating in the vestigial photoreceptors of the pineal gland. Photoreceptor morphology in the human pineal gland demonstrates a common embryological origin with the retinal photoreceptor, although the function within the pineal gland has been lost through evolution (Bader et al 1982). Studies have demonstrated common immunostaining for neuron-specific enolase, S-antigen and rhodopsin in patients with trilateral retinoblastoma (Rodrigues et al 1987).

SITES OF PREDILECTION

Germ cell tumors

Germ cell tumors may arise in a variety of midline sites, most commonly in the gonads and mediastinum, but also in the sacrococcygeum, retroperitoneum, nasopharynx and orbit (Gonzalez-Crussi 1982). Within the central nervous system, the pineal gland is the main site of predilection, followed by the suprasellar region, with synchronous lesions at both sites also possible (Fig. 38.6) (Jennings et al 1985, Russell & Rubinstein 1989a, Sugiyama et al 1992). Other less common locations involve the central neuraxis in the midline as included in Russell & Rubinstein's review of 120 germ cell tumors: pineal (45 cases), suprasellar (33 cases), intrasellar (3 cases), fourth ventricle (18 cases), spinal (5 cases), massive intracranial (3 cases), and other sites (13 cases) (Russell & Rubinstein 1989a). Bjornsson's series of 41 germinomas consisted of 25 situated anteriorly and 16 posteriorly in the third ventricle (Bjornsson et al 1985). Jennings et al (1985) reviewed 389 intracranial germ cell tumors and found that 95% arose from the midline, with 37% in the suprasellar cistern, 48% in the pineal gland and an additional 6% involving both. In this large series, which may reflect referral bias, germinomas were more likely to arise in the suprasellar region, with nongerminomatous germ cell tumors more likely to involve the pineal gland.

Several other rare sites of intracranial germ cell tumor have been reported including the thalamus, basal ganglia, ventricular system, cerebellum, frontal region, and septum pellucidum (Ogaka et al 1964, Tanaka & Veki 1979, Jennings et al 1985, Masuzawa et al 1986). Germinoma of the infundibulum and of the optic chiasm has also been described (Stefanko et al 1979, Manor et al 1990).

Pineal cell tumors

Pineal cell tumors are derived from the pinealocytes of the pineal gland. Although they may spread anywhere throughout the cerebrospinal pathways, the primary site is always within the pineal gland.

PRESENTING FEATURES

Suprasellar germ cell tumors

The most common presenting features for patients with suprasellar germ cell tumors include diabetes insipidus,

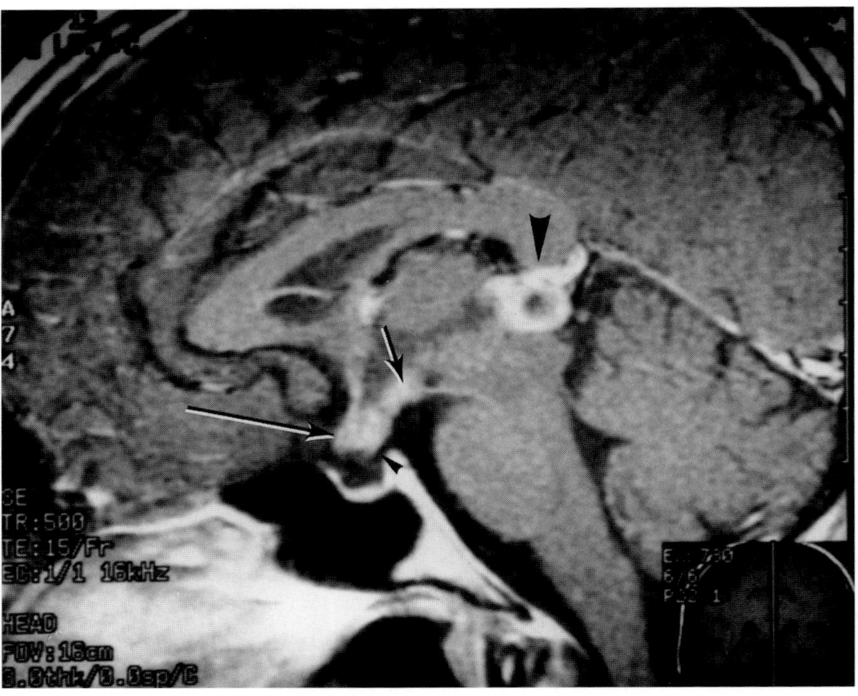

Fig. 38.6 Gadolinium-enhanced MRI of a 33-year-old woman who presented with visual loss, amenorrhea, and diabetes insipidus. MRI shows germinomatous invasion of the pineal gland (large arrowhead), optic chiasm (long arrow), pituitary stalk (small arrowhead) and floor of the third ventricle (short arrow).

visual field defects and other hypothalamic-pituitary abnormalities (Fig. 38.6) (Takeuchi et al 1978, Jennings et al 1985, Sakai et al 1988, Farwell & Flannery 1989, Hoffman et al 1991). Neuroendocrine dysfunction can include hypopituitarism, delayed sexual development, growth failure and precocious puberty. Less commonly, hypothalamic dysfunction can cause obtundation, behavioral disturbance, anorexia and obesity. Tumors of sufficiently large size may present with hydrocephalus.

Pineal region tumors

Tumors in the pineal region, regardless of their histology, may become symptomatic by three possible mechanisms: (a) increased intracranial pressure from hydrocephalus, (b) direct compression of brainstem or cerebellum, or (c) endocrine dysfunction (Sawaya et al 1990, Bruce 1993b). Headache is the most common pre-senting symptom and occurs following obstruction of the third ventricle outflow at the aqueduct of Sylvius. More advanced hydrocephalus can result in nausea, vomiting, papilledema, obtundation and other cognitive deficits.

Direct brainstem compression may lead to disturbances of extraocular movements, classically known as Parinaud's syndrome (Parinaud 1886, Posner & Horrax 1946). This can include paralysis of upgaze or convergence, retractory nystagmus and light-near pupillary dissociation. Compression or infiltration of the dorsal midbrain and periaqueductal area can cause paralysis of downgaze, ptosis and lid retraction. Double vision from fourth nerve palsy is rare but may occur. Eye movement dysfunction may also be caused by hydrocephalus, in which case improvement would be expected following ventricular shunting. Involvement of the superior cerebellar peduncles can lead to ataxia and dysmetria. Hearing disturbances can occasionally occur, probably from compression of the inferior colliculi (DeMonte et al 1993).

Endocrine dysfunction is rare and may be caused by direct tumor involvement in the hypothalamus or from secondary effects of hydrocephalus (Fetell & Stein 1986). In general, diabetes insipidus and other neuroendocrine disturbances are indicative of hypothalamic infiltration by tumor, even when not radio-graphically visualized (Grote et al 1980, Jennings et al 1985). Precocious puberty has been historically associated with pineal region tumors, however true documented cases are rare (Krabbe 1923, Zondek et al 1953, Borit 1981, Fetell & Stein 1986). This syndrome is limited to boys with ectopic β-HCG (β-human chorionic gonadotropin) secretion from choriocarcinomas or germinomas with syncytiotrophoblastic cells (Jennings et al 1985, Fetell & Stein 1986). The β-HCG secondarily stimulates androgen secretion by the Leydig cells of the testes, resulting in the premature sexual maturation characteristics of what is more appropriately termed pseudopuberty.

A rare, but notable presentation is pineal apoplexy from hemorrhage into a pineal tumor (Fig. 38.7) (Steinbok et al

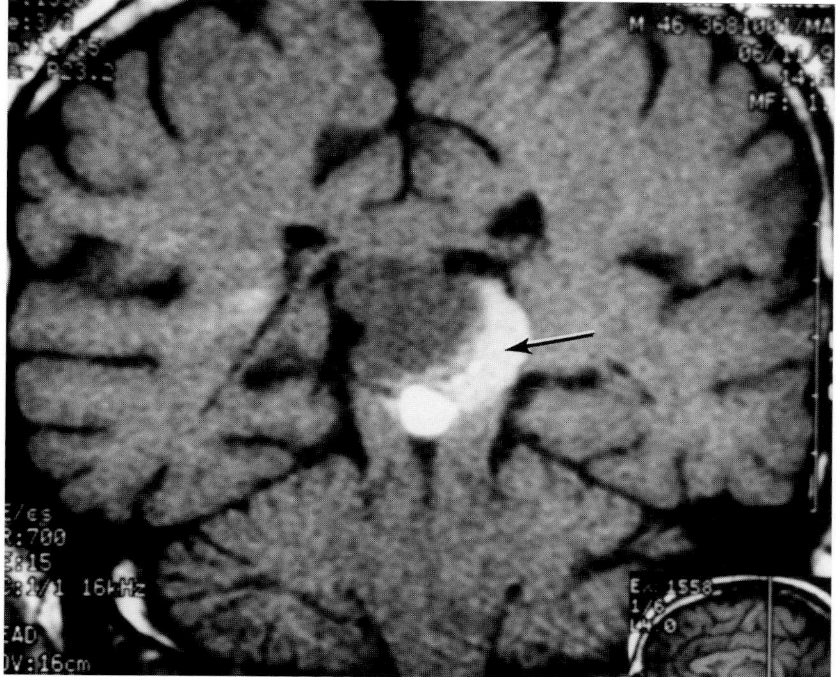

Fig. 38.7 Noncontrast MRI of a pineocytoma in a 40-year-old man presenting with acute hydrocephalus. At surgery the high signal area (arrow) turned out to be acute hemorrhage.

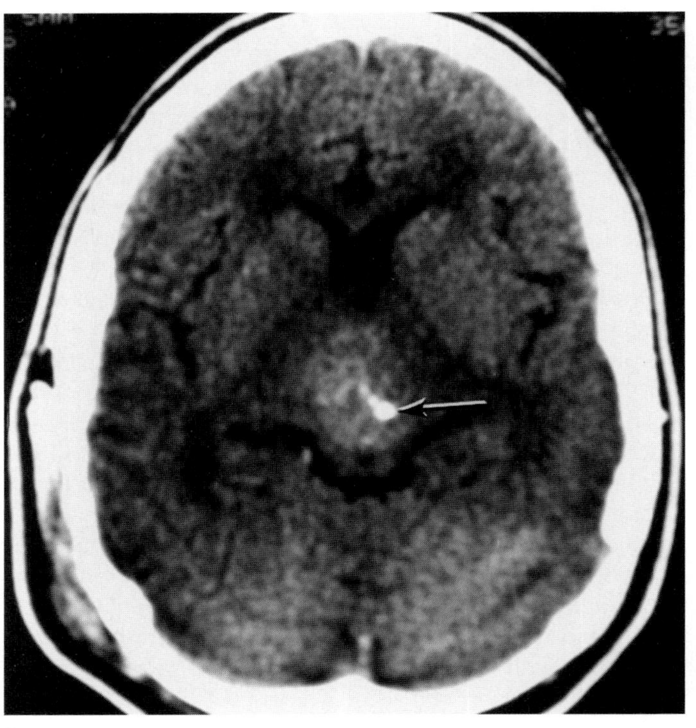

A

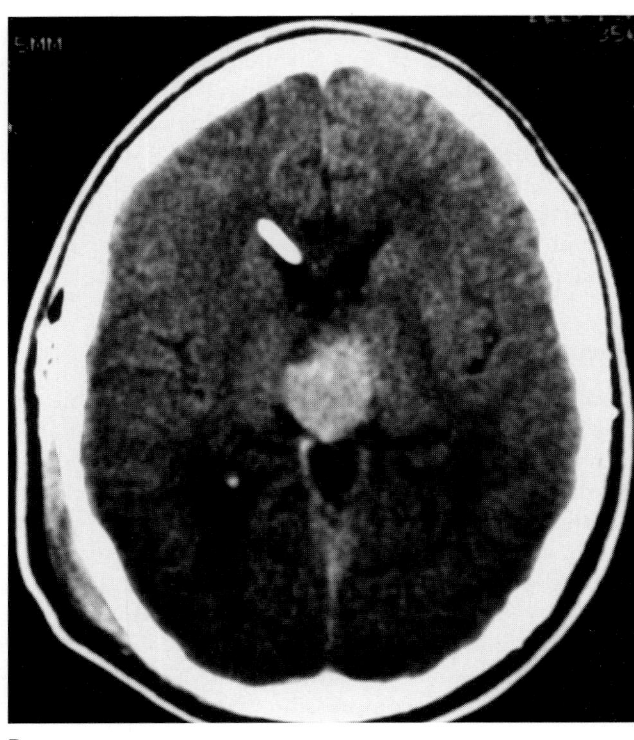

B

Fig. 38.8 Noncontrast (**A**) and contrast enhancing (**B**) CT scan in an 18-year-old man with a germinoma. The tumor can be seen engulfing the calcification (arrow) on the noncontrast scan.

1977, Burres & Hamilton 1979, Herrick & Rubinstein 1979, Higashi et al 1979). Pineal cell tumors in particular, and choriocarcinomas to a lesser extent, are associated with this phenomenon, probably because of their prominent vascularity. These same characteristics may predispose to postoperative hemorrhage as well (Bruce & Stein 1993a).

IMAGING DIAGNOSIS

Despite advances in radiographic imaging, accurate prediction of tumor histology based solely on radiographic characteristics remains unreliable (Zimmerman 1985, Ganti et al 1986, Müller-Forell et al 1988, Tien et al 1990, Bruce 1993b). MRI has replaced CT as the diagnostic method of choice for all pineal tumors. High resolution MRI with gadolinium can visualize the tumor size, vascularity, homogeneity and its relationship with surrounding structures. Besides detecting the presence of hydrocephalus, MRI provides useful anatomic information necessary for planning operative approaches, including the tumor's position within the third ventricle, its extension laterally and supratentorially, its degree of brainstem involvement, and its position relative to the deep venous system. The margination pattern and irregularities of the tumor border depicted on MRI can provide some idea of tumor invasiveness; however, the true degree of encapsulation is best defined at surgery (Stein & Bruce 1992). CT scans may be complementary by providing details of calcification, blood-brain breakdown, and degree of vascularity. Angiograms are generally not helpful unless a vascular anomaly is suspected.

Germ cell tumors

On CT scans, germinomas tend to be homogeneous and either isointense or of slightly higher attenuation than gray matter while exhibiting moderate to marked contrast enhancement. Calcification is likely to occur in both suprasellar and pineal region germinomas, with the tumor tending to surround and engulf the calcification (Fig. 38.8) (Chang et al 1981, Ganti et al 1986, Smirniotopoulos et al 1992). On MRI, germinomas are relatively isointense to normal white matter on T1-weighted image and slightly hyperintense on T2-weighted images (Fig. 38.9). Cystic areas can occasionally be seen (Tien et al 1990, Zee et al 1991). Gadolinium helps to define these tumors well, as they enhance markedly and homogeneously (Fig. 39.9C).

The heterogeneous histologic composition of teratomas is reflected in their radiographic appearance, which is notable for heterogeneity, multilocularity, and irregular

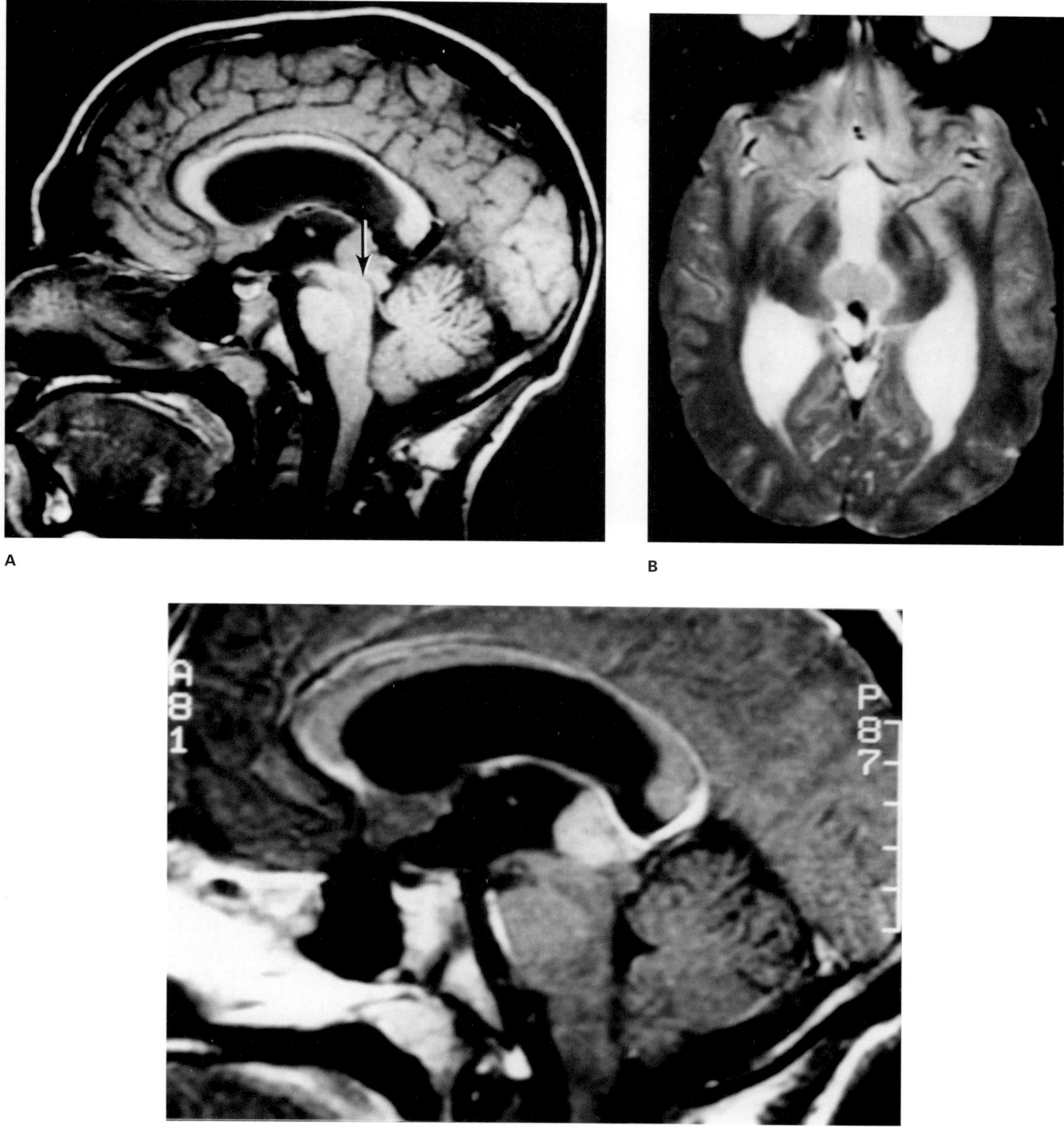

Fig. 38.9 MRI of a 21-year-old man with a germinoma. **A.** T1-weighted noncontrast sagittal scan shows isointense tumor which has obstructed the aqueduct of Sylvius (arrow) to cause hydrocephalus. **B.** T2-weighted noncontrast axial scan tumor hyperintense to brain matter but hypointense to CSF. **C.** Homogeneous gadolinium enhancement of the tumor on T1-weighted sagittal scan.

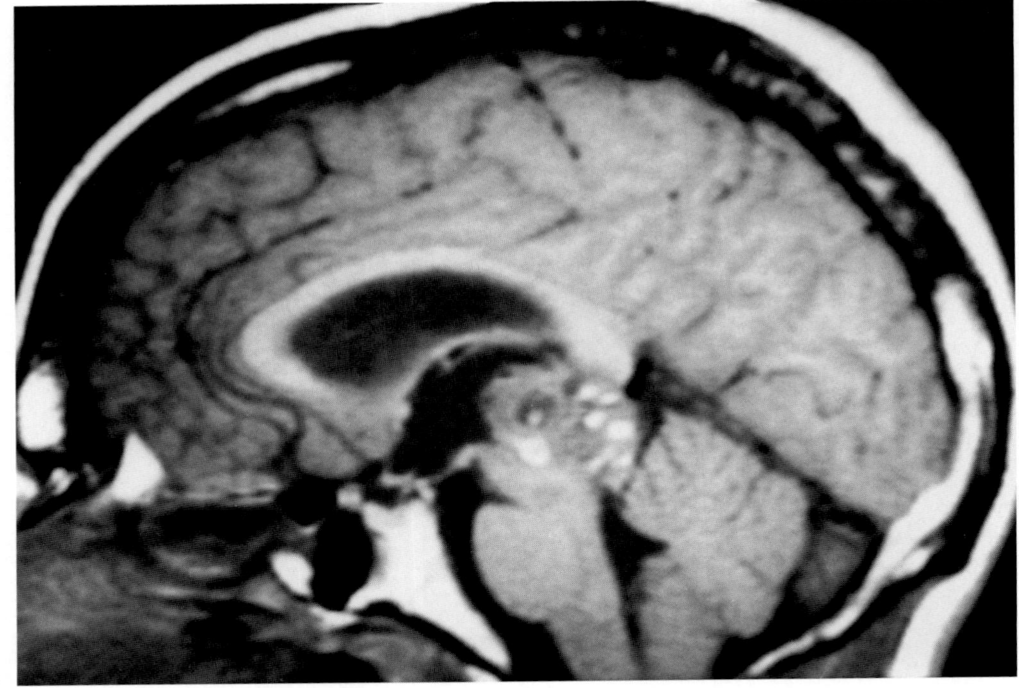

A

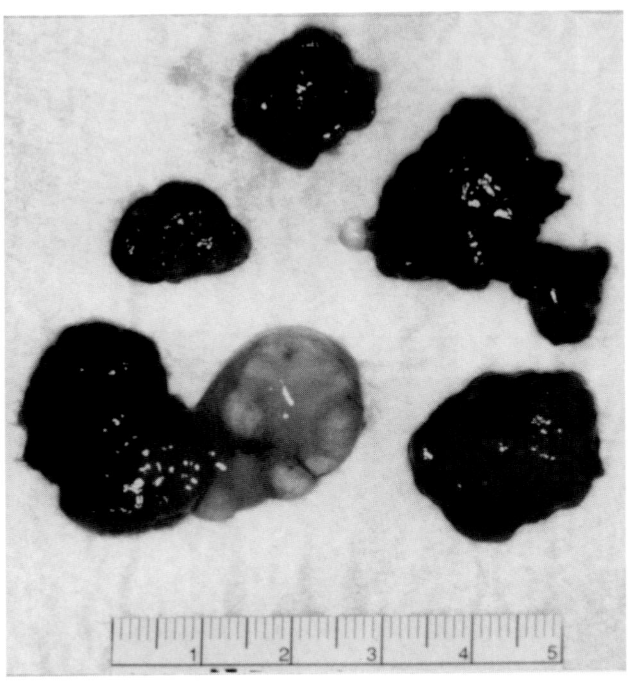

B

Fig. 38.10 **A.** Sagittal MRI of a heterogeneous mixed germ cell tumor of the pineal region in a 21-year-old man who presented with hydrocephalus. After pathologic examination following complete surgical resection, the tumor was found to have multiple components including endodermal sinus tumor, embryonal cell carcinoma, immature teratoma and mature teratoma. **B.** Gross tissue specimens, reflecting heterogeneity of various germ cell components.

enhancement (Fig. 38.10). Various signal characteristics reflect lipid content, soft-tissue components, calcification, and cystic elements. Malignant teratomas have similar characteristics but are distinguished by invasion into surrounding structures (Tien et al 1990). On CT scanning, teratomas are generally well-circumscribed and, unlike most other pineal tumors, contain areas of low attenuation due to their adipose tissue. Contrast enhancement with both CT and MRI can be irregular, heterogeneous, or ring-enhancing.

Accurate description of the radiographic features of malignant nongerminomatous germ cell tumors is difficult because of their rarity in any clinical series. The heterogeneity that is often described may represent mixed germ cell elements. In general, malignant germ cell tumors tend to have infiltrating borders with varying degrees of enhancement. Areas of prior hemorrhage can be seen, particularly with choriocarcinoma.

Epidermoid tumors have decreased signal intensity on T1 and increased signal on T2 (Tien et al 1990). They are distinguished from dermoid tumors which have increased signal on both T1 and T2, although isointensity on T2 has been described (Hudgins et al 1987, Tien et al 1990).

Pineal cell tumors

Both pineocytomas and pineoblastomas tend to be hypo- or isointense on T1-weighted imaging and hyperintense on T2 (Fig. 38.11). In general, pineal cell tumors tend to be homogeneous and have uniform enhancement. Hemorrhage and necrosis are more common in pineoblastomas, while cysts are occasionally seen in pineocytomas (Smirniotopoulos et al 1992). Pineocytomas are not encapsulated, yet tend to be well defined. Calcifications can be present, although usually in a pattern different from germinomas (Fig. 38.11D). With pineal cell tumors, this is usually in the form of intratumoral calcifications, whereas the germinoma often engulfs a calcified pineal gland (Chang et al 1981, Ganti et al 1986, Smirniotopoulos et al 1992).

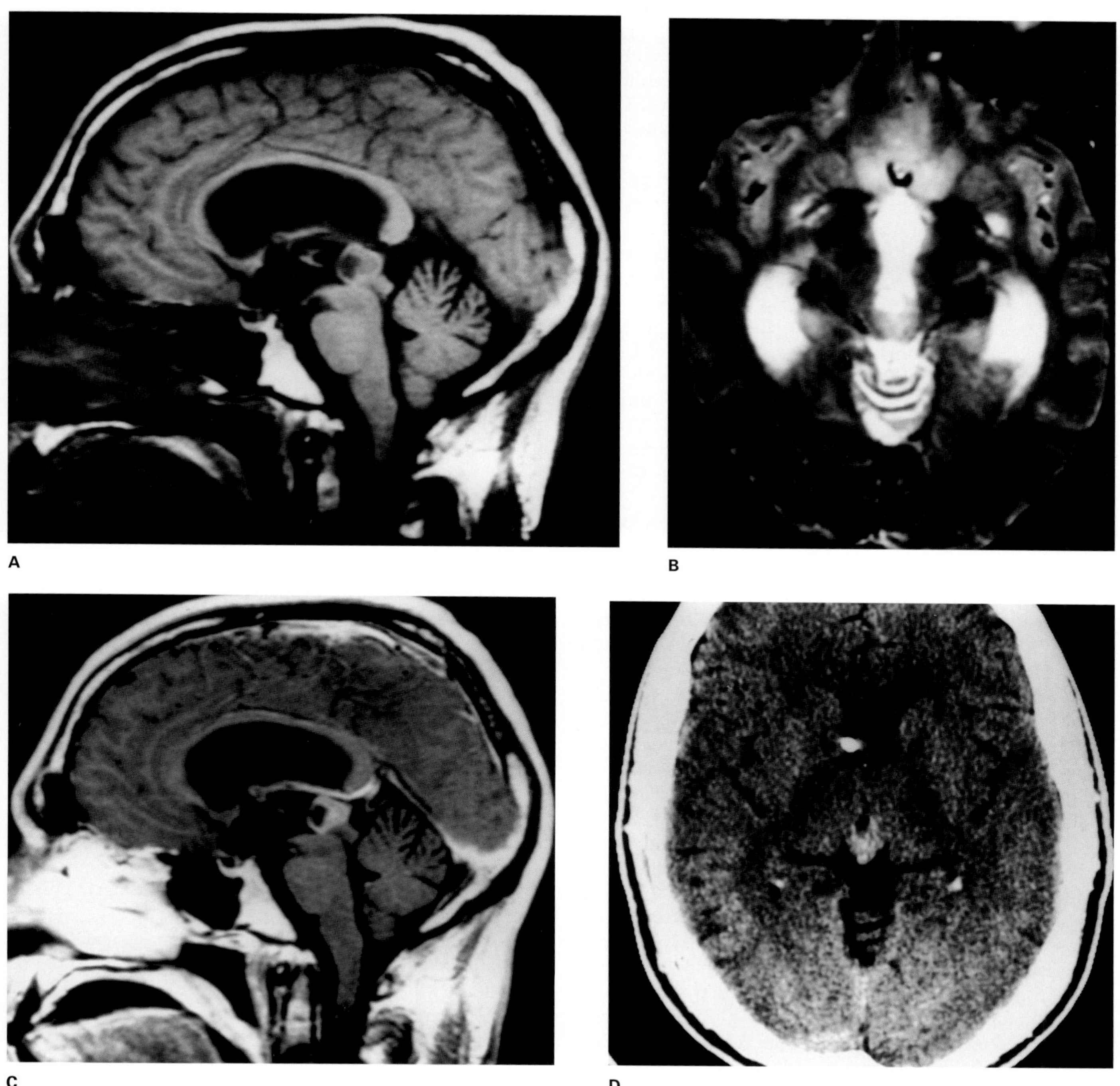

Fig. 38.11 Pineocytoma in a 41-year-old man. **A.** T1-weighted noncontrast MRI shows isointense tumor. A small cyst is seen in the anterior portion of the tumor. **B.** On T2-weighted MRI, the tumor is hyperintense to brain tissue. **C.** Tumor enhances homogeneously with gadolinium except for the cystic portion. **D.** Noncontrast CT scan shows typical calcified pattern in pineocytoma.

LABORATORY DIAGNOSIS

The tumor markers α-fetoprotein (AFP) and β-human chorionic gonadotropin (β-HCG) are specific for malignant germ cell elements and should be measured in all patients with suspected germ cell tumors (Allen et al 1979, Bruce & Stein 1990, Sawaya et al 1990). Measurement of germ cell markers can be helpful not only for diagnostic purposes but also for monitoring response to therapy or as an early sign of tumor recurrence. Marker levels should be measured in both blood and CSF, as CSF measurements are generally more sensitive, although not always consistently (Allen et al 1979, Arita et al 1980, Ono et al 1982, Chan et al 1984, Sano 1984, Sawaya et al 1990).

AFP is a glycoprotein normally produced by fetal yolk sac elements and has a biologic half-life of approximately 5 days (Sawaya et al 1990). AFP is markedly elevated with endodermal sinus tumors, while smaller elevations may occur with embryonal cell carcinomas and immature teratomas (Allen et al 1979, Wilson et al 1979, Arita et al 1980, Jooma & Kendall 1983, Bamberg et al 1984, Allen et al 1985, Jennings et al 1985, Sawaya et al 1990). Although elevated AFP has been reported with germinomas (Arita et al 1980), this may reflect sampling error of what are actually mixed germ cell tumors. Teratomas do not secrete AFP or β-HCG; however, immature teratomas may have slightly elevated AFP levels (Jooma & Kendall 1983, Ho & Liu 1992, Bruce 1993b).

β-HCG is a glycoprotein that is normally secreted by placental trophoblastic tissue and has a biologic half-life of 15–20 hours (Sawaya et al 1990). Markedly elevated levels are found with choriocarcinomas while mild elevations can sometimes be seen with embryonal cell carcinomas and germinomas (Takeuchi et al 1978, Allen et al 1979, Haase & Norgaard-Pederson 1979, Neuwelt et al 1979, Arita et al 1980, Jooma & Kendall 1983, Jennings et al 1985, Page et al 1986, Sawaya et al 1990, Bruce 1993b). Most germinomas are nonsecretory; however, a small percentage will contain low levels of β-HCG if syncytiotrophoblastic giant cells are present (Takeuchi et al 1978, Neuwelt et al 1979, Arita et al 1980, Bloom 1983, Jennings et al 1985, Bruce 1993b). Elevations of β-HCG in germinomas may correlate with a less favorable prognosis (Vematsu et al 1992, Yoshida et al 1993). The absence of AFP or β-HCG elevation should be interpreted with caution since it does not necessarily rule out the presence of a germinoma or embryonal cell carcinoma. Similarly, elevated AFP associated with a germinoma should be cause for suspecting the additional presence of mixed tumor elements containing either embryonal cell carcinoma or endodermal sinus tumor (Russell & Rubinstein 1989a).

Other tumor markers are currently under investigation but are not universally used in clinical situations. Placental alkaline phosphatase has been studied as a tumor marker for germinomas (Shinoda et al 1988) while carcinoembryonic antigen has been reported in association with germinomas, but neither marker has been consistently correlative (Arita et al 1980, Suzuki & Tanaka 1980). Other tumor markers have been studied in extracranial germ cell tumors, such as lactate dehydrogenase and B5 monoclonal antibody; however, correlations for intracranially located tumors are lacking (Metcalfe & Sikora 1985, Sawaya et al 1990).

No reliable markers exist for pineal parenchymal tumors, although several have been investigated. Melatonin, as the primary secretory protein of the pineal gland and the one responsible for its association with circadian rhythm in humans (Erlich & Apuzzo 1985, Bruce et al 1991), has been measured in pineal tumors, usually with inconsistent results (Wurtman & Kammer 1966, Arendt 1978, Barber et al 1978, Miles et al 1985, Vorkapic et al 1987). Curiously, these abnormalities have also been seen in patients with other intracranial or systemic malignancies, but the significance is unknown (Tamarkin et al 1982, Dempsey & Chandler 1984, Vaughan 1984, Erlich & Apuzzo 1985). Similarly, the use of S-antigen has been evaluated as a potential marker for pineal parenchymal tumors and will require further investigation before its clinical usefulness is demonstrated (Korf et al 1986, Perentes et al 1986, Korf et al 1987, 1989).

GROSS MORPHOLOGIC FEATURES

Germ cell tumors

Germinomas are generally soft and grayish-pink in color. Most are friable but they may have a granular consistency. Focal hemorrhages and cysts are not common but may be seen. Germinomas are generally not well-defined and, in the pineal region, infiltrate adjacent structures including the quadrigeminal plate, posterior commissure, thalamus, and roof of the third ventricle (Russell & Rubinstein 1989a). Smaller germinomas may be better defined. Suprasellar germinomas tend to infiltrate the lamina terminalis, optic chiasm, septum pellucidum, and the hypothalamus, sometimes causing a thickening without forming a definite mass. More advanced tumors may project as a lobulated mass from the floor of the third ventricle producing symptomatic compression of the optic chiasm and pituitary stalk.

Embryonal cell carcinomas and endodermal sinus tumors have variable gross appearances depending on the degree of mixed cell types present (Fig. 38.10). Choriocarcinomas are often well demarcated and may show signs of hemorrhage.

Teratomas are well-defined, heterogeneous tumors, with lobulated surfaces. These well-differentiated tumors may contain cartilage, bone, hair, or teeth (Russell & Rubinstein 1989a). Cystic components may be present, containing desquamated debris of a dermoid nature.

Immature teratomas differ by having more invasive characteristics and increased likelihood of hemorrhage or necrosis.

Pineal cell tumors

Pineoblastomas are soft tumors that are pinkish gray in color and may contain hemorrhagic, necrotic or cystic components (Fig. 38.7, 38.11) (Russell & Rubinstein 1989b, Schild et al 1993). They can be relatively well-circumscribed or ill-defined and invasive into local surrounding structures, often destroying the pineal gland with growth. By comparison, pineocytomas are better defined and have a pale gray color and lobulated surface. Like pineoblastomas, pineocytomas generally replace the pineal gland as they grow; however, necrosis and hemorrhage are rare findings.

HISTOPATHOLOGIC FEATURES

Germ cell tumors

Histologically, germinomas are identical to seminomas of the testis and dysgerminomas of the ovary (Fig. 38.12) (Gonzalez-Crussi 1982). Germinomas are distinguished by the presence of two characteristic cell types: large primitive germ cells and lymphocytes (Russell & Rubinstein 1989a, Ho & Liu 1992). When occurring in the pineal region, germ cells can be surrounded by fibrous connective tissue subdividing the tumor into lobules, a finding less common with suprasellar tumors. Germ cells are large, polygonal or spheroidal cells without clear cell boundaries and contain large, round, vesicular nuclei within a large central nucleus. Mitotic figures and karyosomes can be present. The pale, ill-defined cytoplasm may contain vacuolation and glycogen. The second cell population is composed of the comparatively smaller lymphocytes, which monoclonal antibody techniques have defined as T-cells (Neuwelt & Smith 1979). The infiltration of these lymphocytes, predominantly adjacent to blood vessels, is thought to represent a granulomatous reaction, the immunological significance of which is unclear (Marshall & Dayan 1964, Kraichoke et al 1988, Russell & Rubinstein 1989a).

Electron microscopy has verified the ultrastructural similarity between germinomas and testicular seminomas (Cravioto & Dart 1973, Markesbery et al 1976). With electron microscopy, germinomas display the following

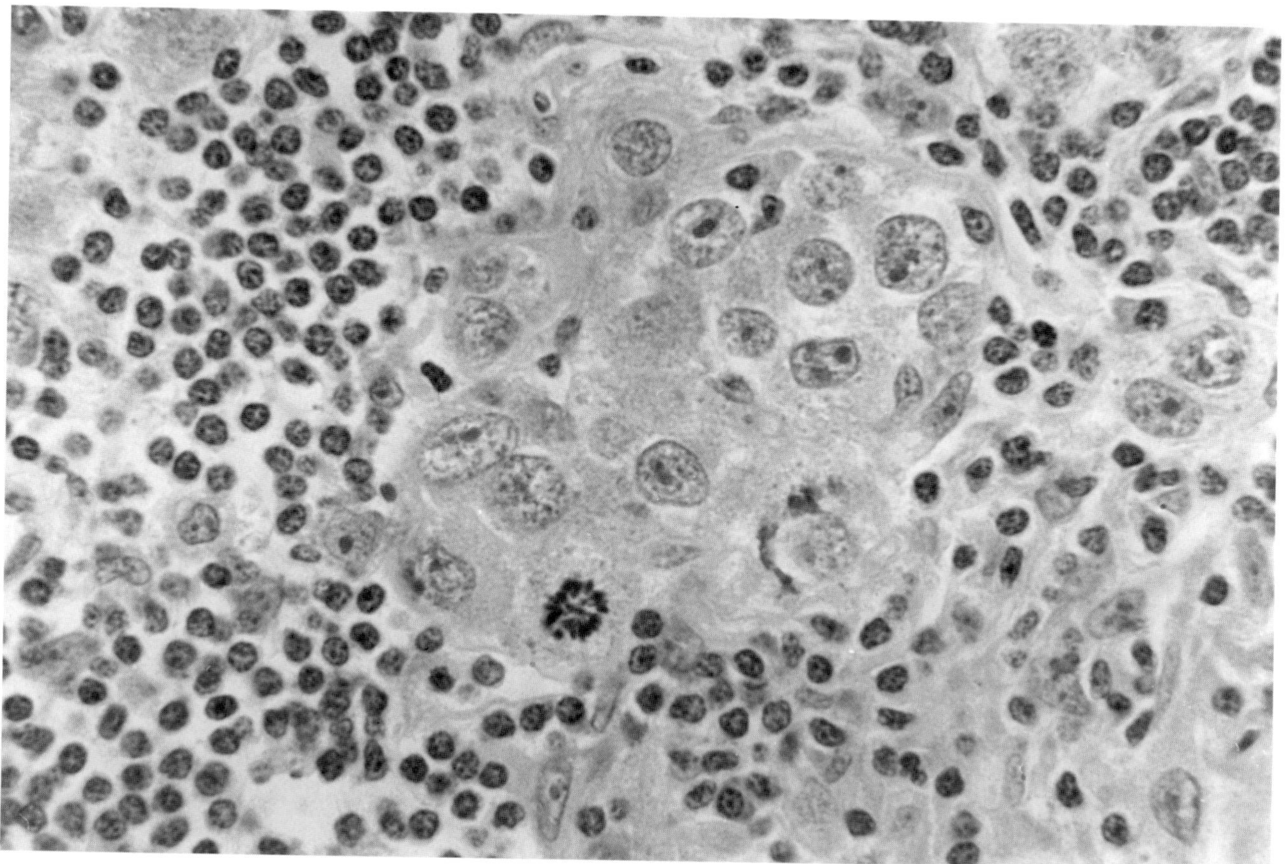

Fig. 38.12 Cytologic features of a typical germinoma. Note the two-cell population consisting of large germ cells and smaller infiltrating lymphocytes. A mitotic figure is seen in the center.

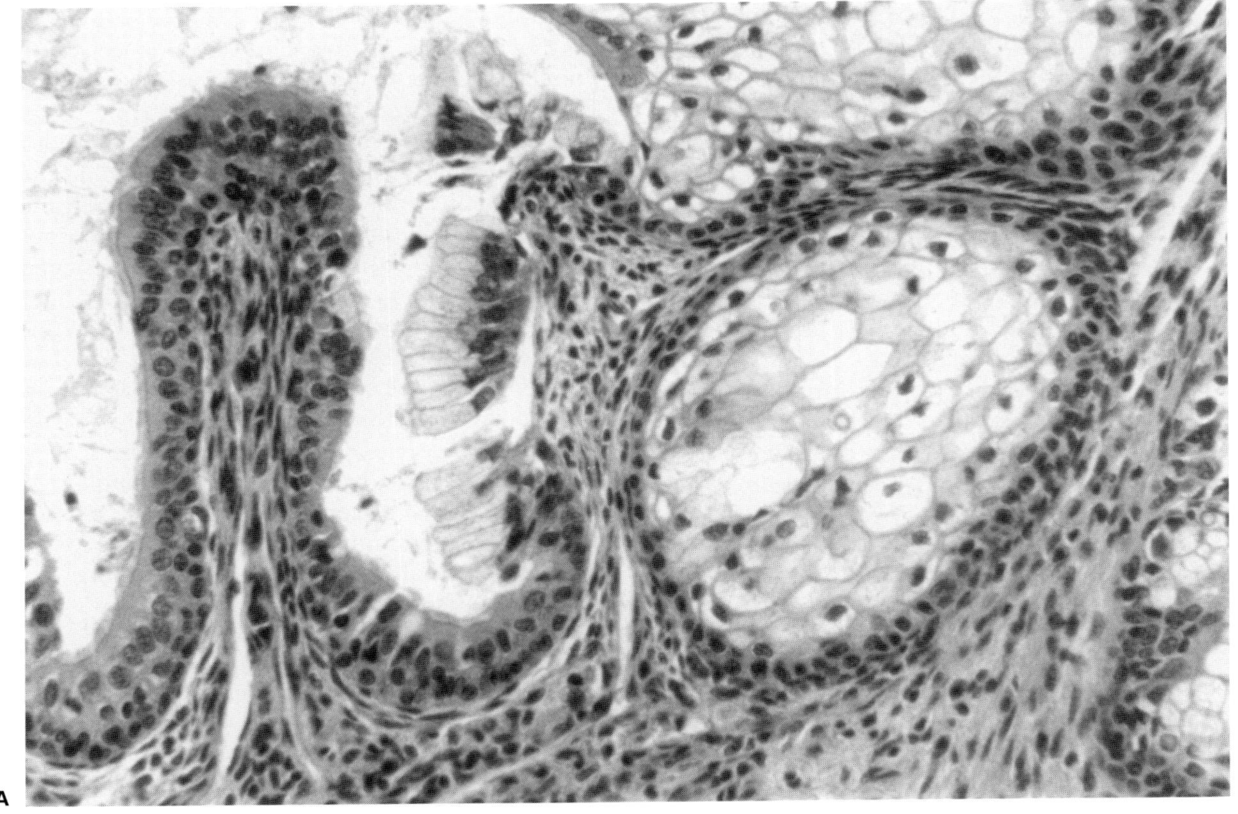
A

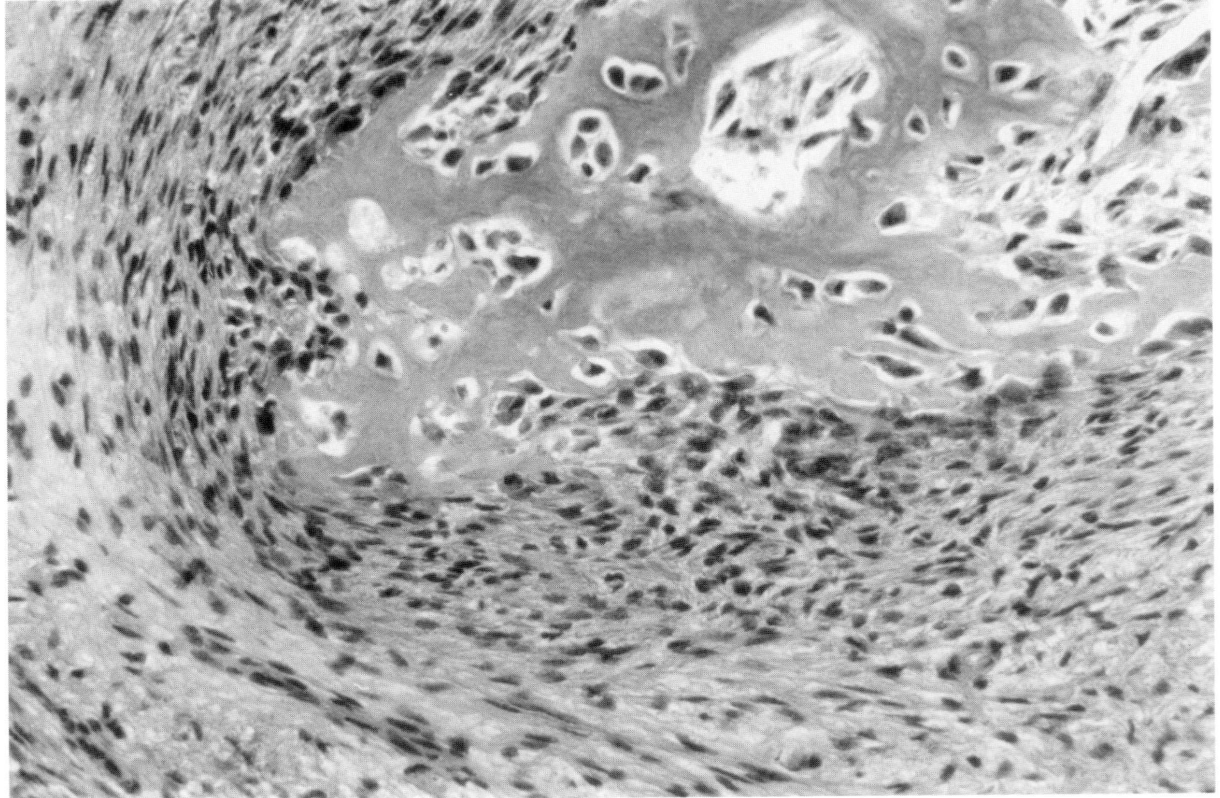
B

Fig. 38.13A & B

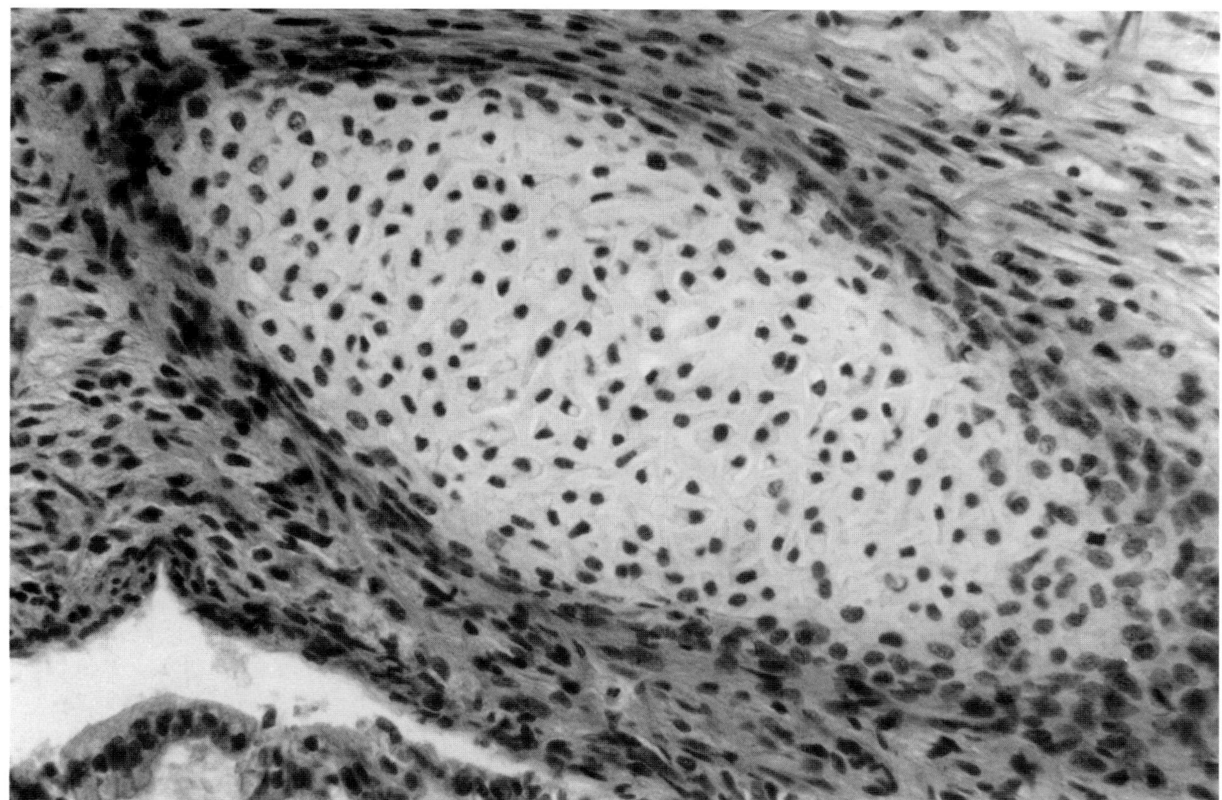

Fig. 38.13 Mature teratoma with heterogenous features consisting of well-differentiated tissue from all three germinal layers: **A.** non-keratinizing squamous cell epithelium alternating with areas of ciliated columnar epithelium; **B.** osteoid bone with surrounding periosteal tissue and mesenchymal stroma; **C.** cartilaginous tissue.

features: glycogen granules, annulate lamellae, prominent Golgi apparatus, stacks of rough endoplasmic reticulum and bundles of intracytoplasmic filaments. When present, syncytiotrophoblastic giant cells may be multinucleated and will stain positively for β-HCG (Bjornsson et al 1985, Shokry et al 1985). Germinoma cells will stain positively for placental alkaline phosphatase, particularly on the cell membranes (Shinoda et al 1988, Ho & Liu 1992). Within a germinoma, cells may show variable positivity for cytokeratins, the epithelial membrane antigen (EMA) or vimentin (Russell & Rubinstein 1989a).

Teratomas are composed of well-differentiated tissues from all three germinal layers: ectoderm, mesoderm, and endoderm (Russell & Rubinstein 1989a). Mature teratomas may contain any of the following features: solid or cystic foci of squamous epithelium, cartilage, glandular or tubular structures lined by columnar mucus-secreting cells or cuboidal undifferentiated epithelium (Fig. 38.13). These tubules may be separated by mesenchymal stroma including bundles of prominent nonstriated muscle. Varying degrees of differentiation may be present.

Immature teratomas are distinguished from their benign counterparts by slightly more primitive features and are likely to contain cells predominantly from only one of the three germinal layers (Fig. 38.14) (Russell & Rubinstein 1989a). Immature teratomas contain poorly differentiated non-neuroepithelial cells in high density, often staining positive for CEA, cytokeratins or epithelial membrane antigen (Bjornsson et al 1985, Ho & Liu 1992). Immature glandular epithelium is often immunopositive for AFP. Primitive rhabdomyoblastic elements may be present (Glass & Culbertson 1946, Preissig et al 1979, Bjornsson et al 1985).

Embryonal cell carcinomas contain poorly-differentiated epithelial cells arranged in solid sheets and ribbons (Fig. 38.15) (Russell & Rubinstein 1989a). Both the cytoplasm and extracellular globules may stain positively for AFP (Naganuma et al 1984, Bjornsson et al 1985, Shokry et al 1985, Russell & Rubinstein 1989a). Multinucleated syncytiotrophoblastic giant cells, when present, will stain for β-HCG. Many embryonal cell carcinomas do not stain for either tumor marker. Limited information is available on electron microscopic characteristics; however, cells are known to contain abundant secretory granules.

Endodermal sinus tumors characteristically form papillary projections constructed of low cuboidal epithelium (Eberts & Ransburg 1979, Russell & Rubinstein 1989a).

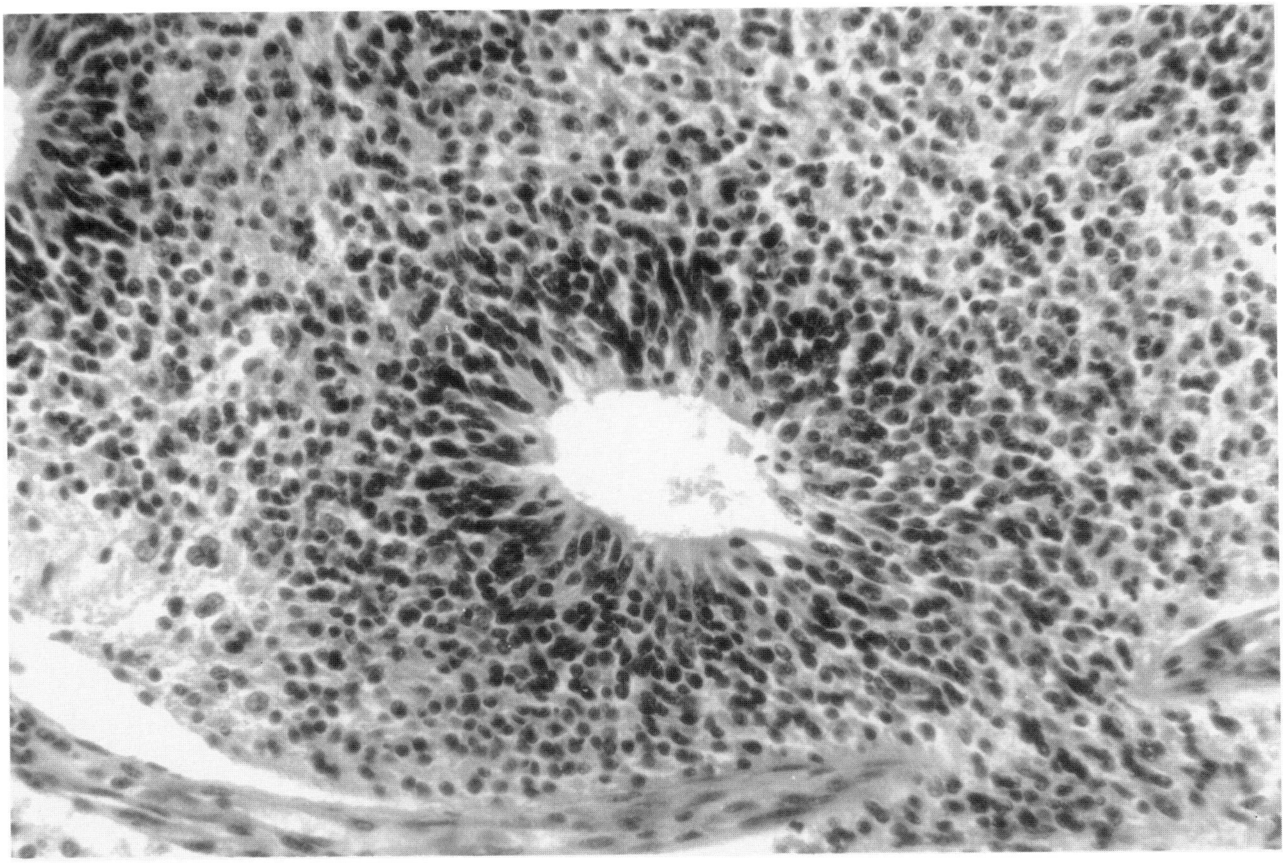

Fig. 38.14 Immature teratoma with highly cellular primitive elements resembling fetal neural tube structure.

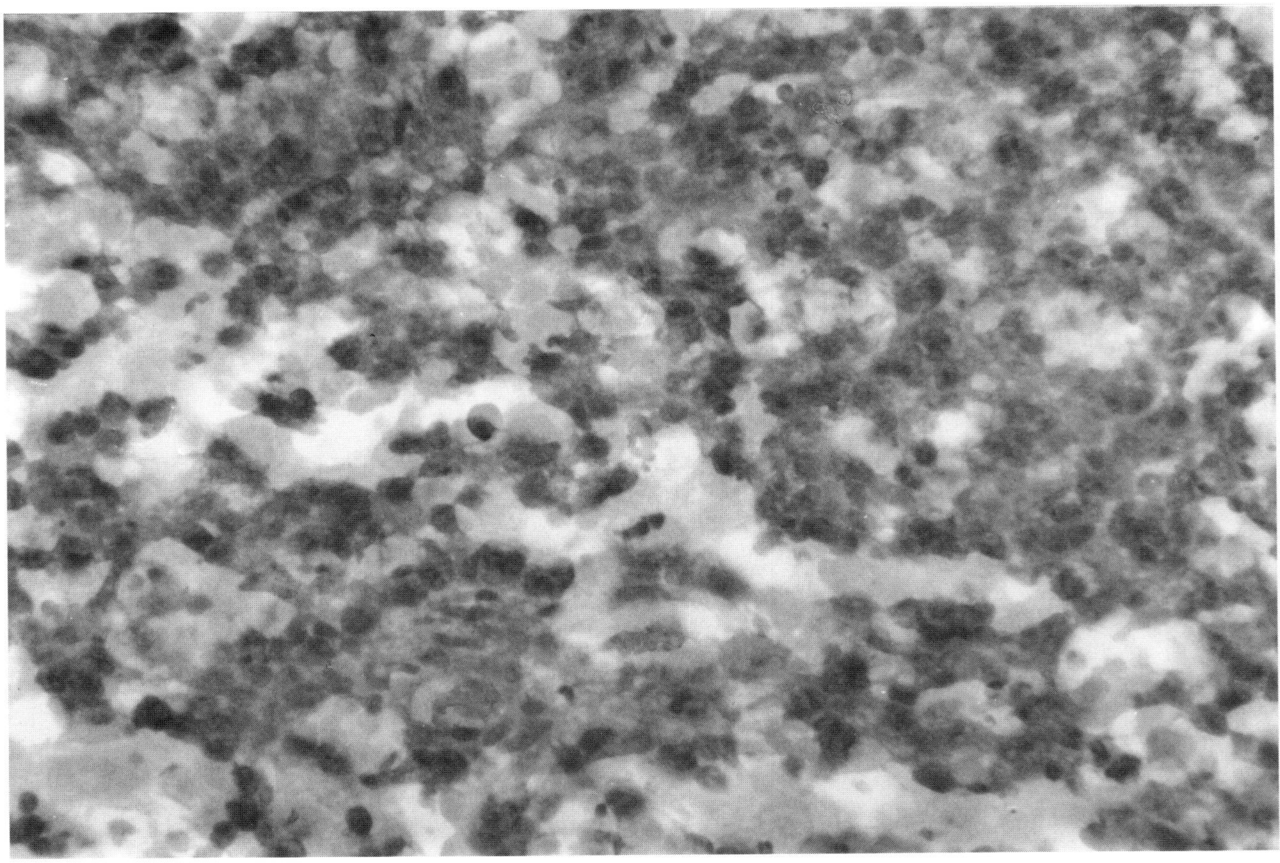

Fig. 38.15 Embryonal carcinoma composed of patternless sheets of primitive cells and frequent mitotic figures.

A delicate connective tissue framework supports these papillary projections which enclose thin-walled capillaries. Embryoid bodies, Schiller-Duval bodies and structures resembling immature placental villi with tubular and acinar-like structures are characteristic features (Fig. 38.16). Globular masses or membrane-bound vesicles immunopositive for AFP may be found intra- or extracellularly. The ultrastructure of endodermal sinus tumor shows prominent microvilli on the apical surfaces of the gland-like spaces formed by the endodermal cells (Stachura & Mendelow 1980, Takei & Pearl 1981, Masuzawa et al 1986). Intracellular junctional complexes including tight junctions and desmosomes may be seen.

Choriocarcinomas are characterized by areas containing multinucleated giant cells, areas of syncytiotrophoblastic differentiation and prominent blood-filled sinuses (Fig. 38.17) (Russell & Rubinstein 1989a). Necrosis and hemorrhage may occur (Ho & Liu 1992). The syncytiotrophoblastic elements are strongly positive for β-HCG, human placental lactogen and the pregnancy specific antigen.

Mixed germ cell tumors account for approximately one fourth of germ cell tumors (Russell & Rubinstein 1989a, Bruce 1993a). Immunohistochemical characterization of tumor markers can be helpful for determining the presence of specific tumor elements. When disparities between tumor marker measurements and the histologic features of the surgical specimen occur, it may be assumed that there has been inadequate tissue sampling.

Pineal cell tumors

The pineal gland develops embryologically by the proliferation of neuroepithelial cells lining the diencephalic roof during the second month of gestation (Russell & Rubinstein 1989b). The normal pineal gland receives innervation via the sympathetic nervous system and is composed primarily of pinealocytes and some surrounding astrocytes forming lobules (Erlich & Apuzzo 1985). Pinealocytes are specialized neuronal cells which contain secretory granules and have argyrophilic cytoplasmic processes surrounding blood vessels. A shared ontogenetic relationship between the pineal gland and photoreceptor cells is reflected in their common positive immunostaining for S-antigen (Perentes et al 1986, Rodrigues et al 1987).

Some of the neuronal, hormonal and secretory properties of normal pinealocytes are retained in pineal parenchymal tumors. Pineal parenchymal tumors exist along a continuum, with pineocytomas being the most

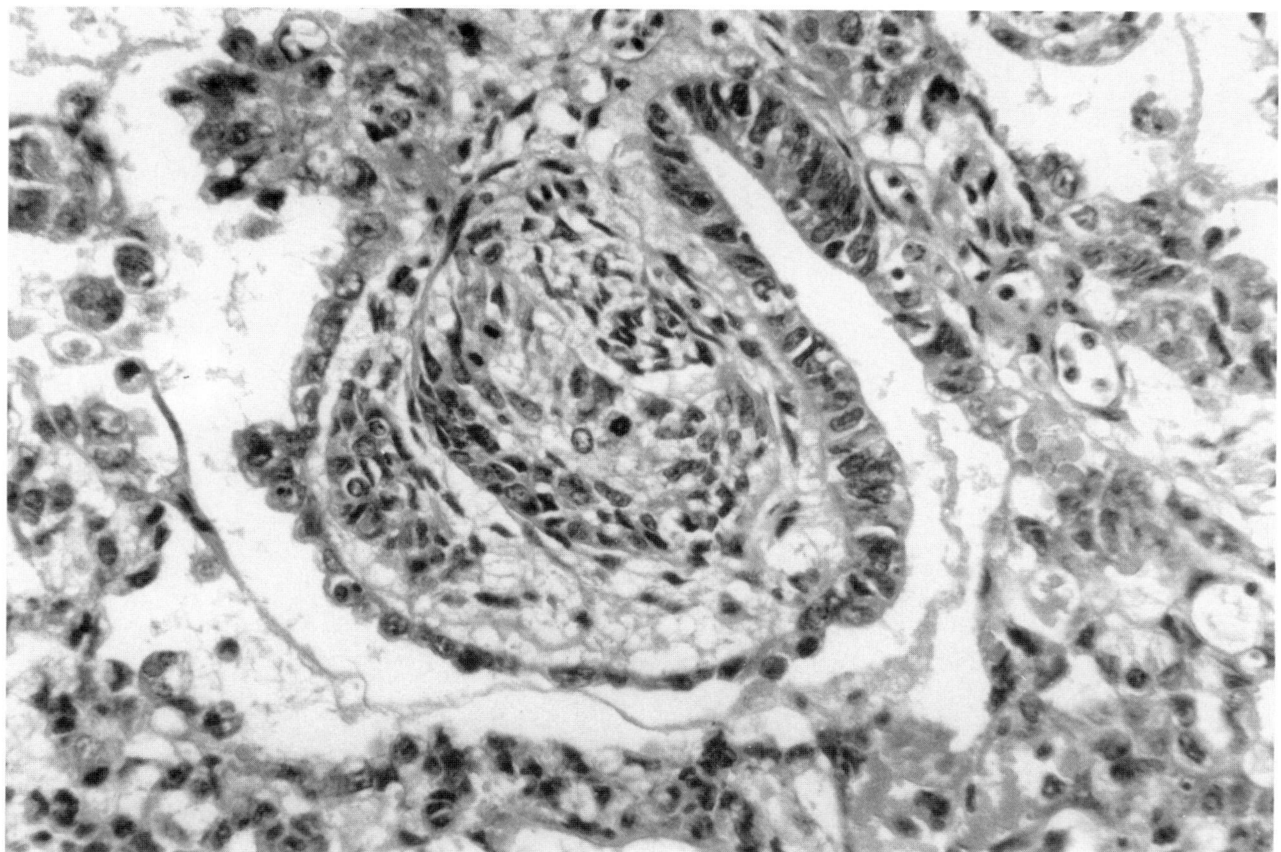

Fig. 38.16 Endodermal sinus tumor with characteristic Schiller-Duval body.

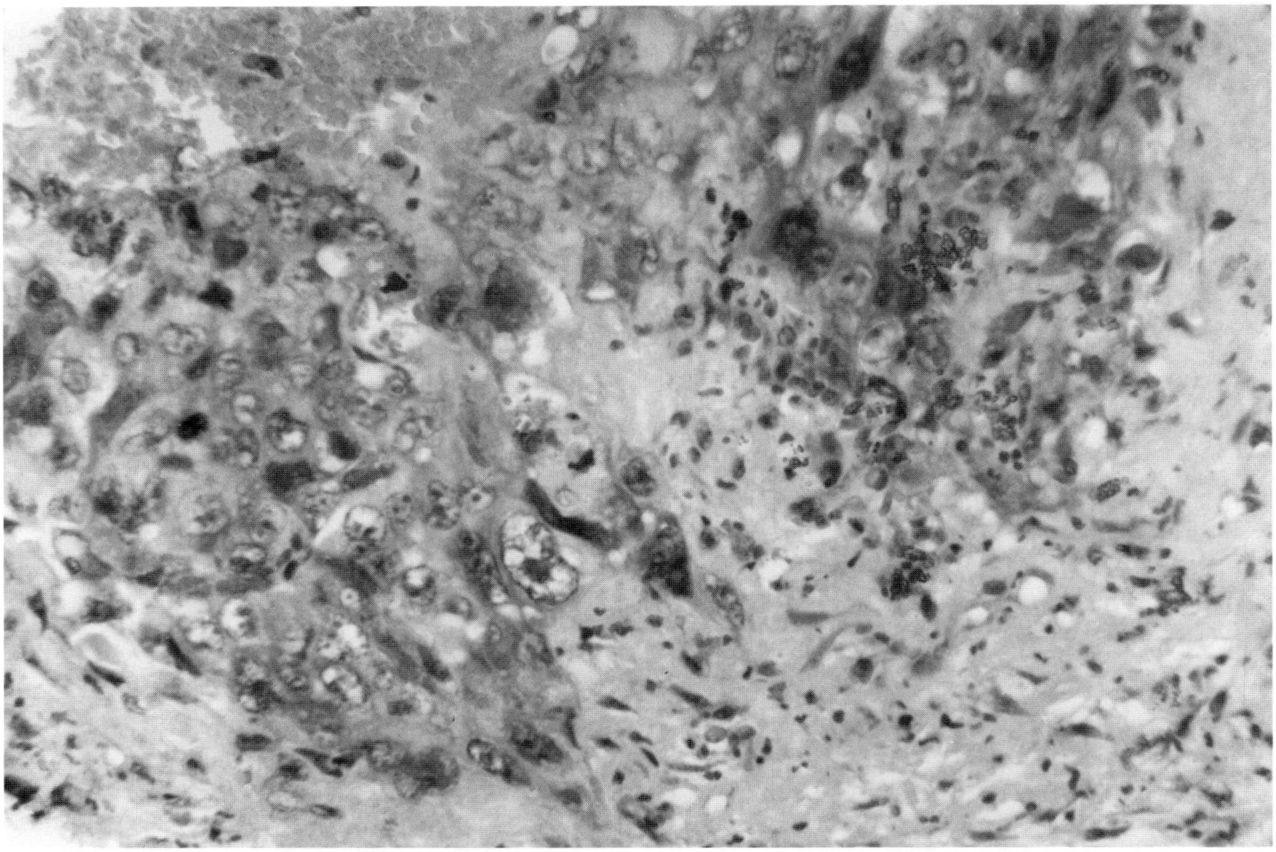

Fig. 38.17 Choriocarcinoma with bizarre, pleiomorphic, syncytiotrophoblastic cells which are immunopositive for β-HCG.

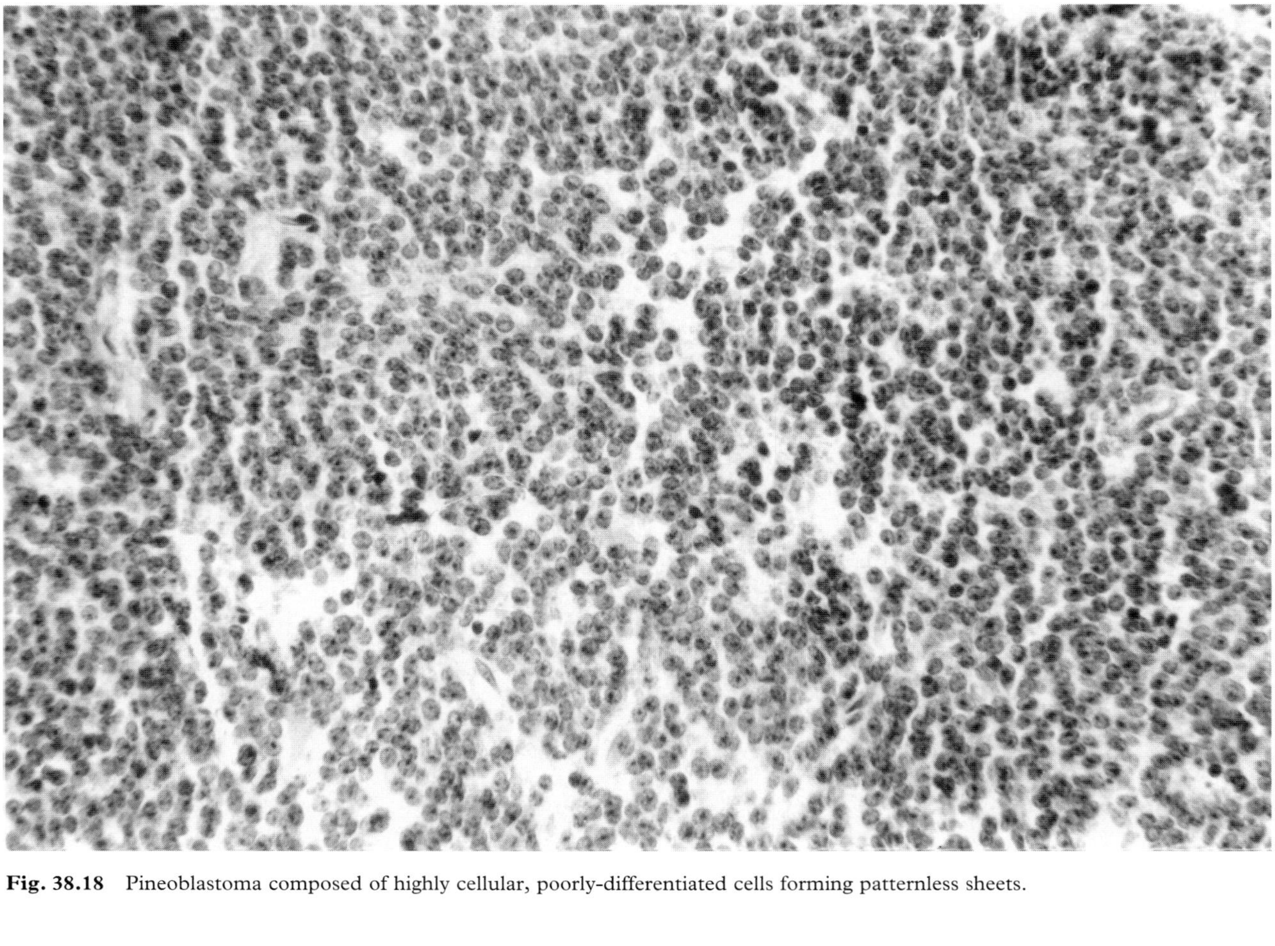

Fig. 38.18 Pineoblastoma composed of highly cellular, poorly-differentiated cells forming patternless sheets.

differentiated and pineoblastomas the least differentiated. Whereas description of the tumors at each end of the spectrum is straightforward, controversy arises when trying to characterize tumors that are of an intermediate classification. Pineoblastomas are highly cellular tumors composed of undifferentiated immature cells with small round nuclei and scant cytoplasm but lacking the extensive cellular processes seen in pineocytomas (Fig. 38.18). The number of mitotic figures can be variable. Tumors may contain Homer-Wright or Flexner-Wintersteiner rosettes, focal hemorrhages, giant cells or necrosis (Borit et al 1980, Schild et al 1993). The high cellularity, lack of differentiation and sheet-like arrangement of cells are reminiscent of medulloblastomas and other primitive neuroectodermal tumors (Herrick & Rubinstein 1979, Borit et al 1980, Becker & Hinton 1983, Rubinstein 1985, Schild et al 1993). Tumors may be immunopositive for the S-antigen (Perentes et al 1986, Rodrigues et al 1987). Rare cases of melanin pigment have been found (Herrick & Rubinstein 1979). The ultrastructure has not been described in a systematic fashion, however reports suggest some commonality between these tumors and the photosensory cells of pineals in lower vertebrates as evidenced by cytoplasmic protrusions resembling the end bulbs of the human fetal gland and giant club-shaped cilia with the 9 + 0 pattern (Markesbery et al 1981, Russell & Rubinstein 1989b).

Pineocytomas can be quite cellular, but are generally less so than pineoblastomas. The tumor cells are benign, mature cells that may be indistinguishable from normal pinealocytes and are arranged in sheets or diffuse lobules (Fig. 38.19). Giant cells may be present, but mitotic figures are not common. Perivascular bulbous cellular terminations can often be seen with Bielschowski stain (Schild et al 1993). Pineocytomas may exhibit neuronal or astrocytomatous differentiation (Borit & Blackwood 1979, Herrick & Rubinstein 1979, Borit et al 1980). Whether these differentiation patterns reflect the multipotentiality of pineal parenchymal tumors or the simultaneous transformation of adjacent astrocytic and neuronal cells is not clear. Neuronal differentiation is often accompanied by the formation of rosettes, the centers of which contain the tangles of small knobbed terminations of delicate argyrophilic processes. A separate designation as 'pineocytomatous rosettes' has been given to distinguish them from the more primitive Homer-Wright rosettes (Borit et al 1980, Schild et al 1993). Synaptophysin may be positive if neuronal differentiation is present (Schild et al 1993). Pineocytomas may stain positive for the S-antigen (Korf et al 1986, Perentes at al 1986, Rodrigues

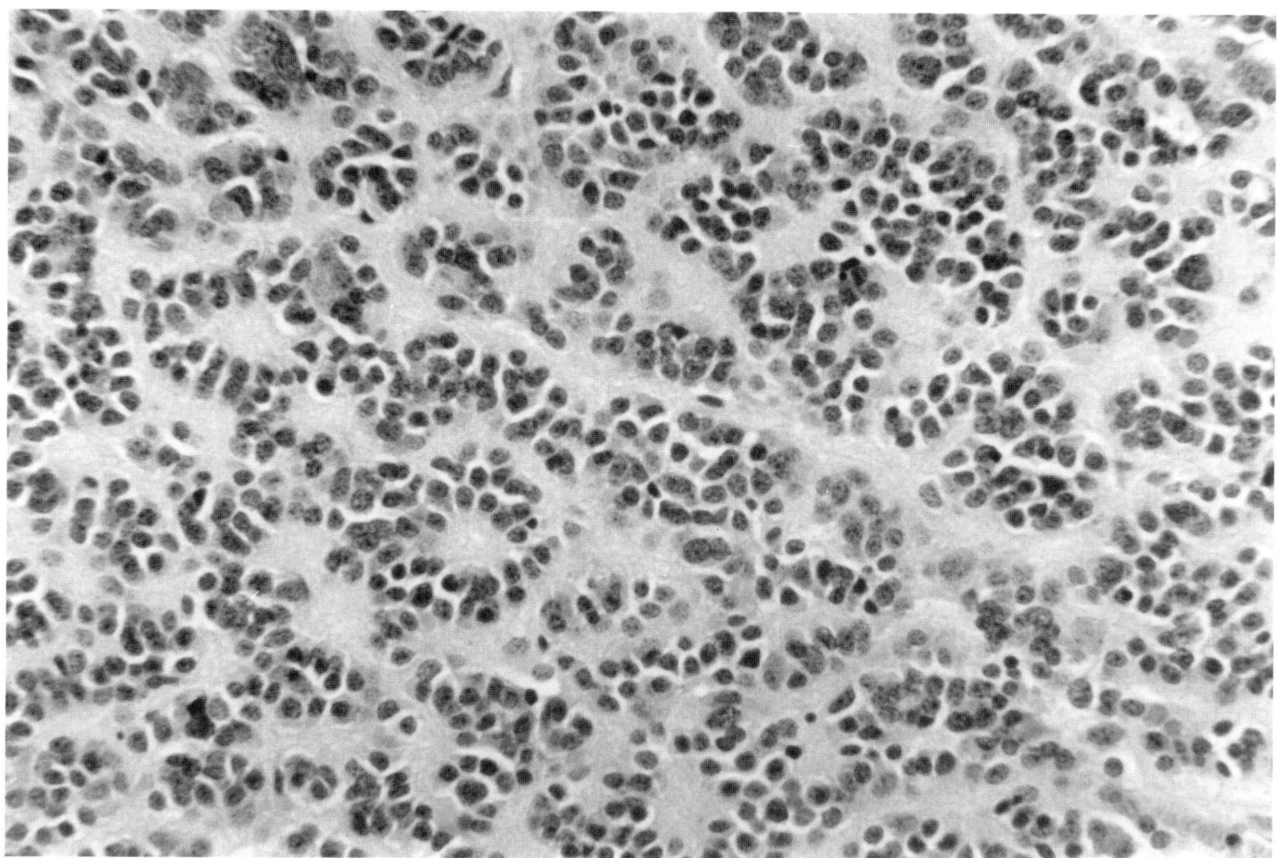

Fig. 38.19 Pineocytoma consisting of benign, well-differentiated cells forming rosettes.

et al 1987). As viewed with electron microscopy, pineocytomas may contain dense-core vesicles in the tumor cell processes, cilia with characteristic 9 + 0 filament complex, synaptic ribbons, bulbous cell process endings with microtubules, and occasional clear-centered vesicles with synapse formation (Herrick & Rubinstein 1979, Markesbery et al 1981, Russell & Rubinstein 1989b). Alternating electron-dense and electron-lucent cells joined by zonulae adherens and a complex system of vacuoles and organelles similar to normal mammalian pinealocytes have also been described (Hassoun et al 1983).

Despite the characteristic appearances of pineocytomas or pineoblastomas, the intermediately differentiated tumors are more variable and therefore more difficult to characterize. Tumors may contain features of both pineocytomas and pineoblastomas, although no consensus exists on where the transition from well-differentiated pineocytoma to undifferentiated pineoblastoma occurs. Mixed tumors have been designated when divergent differentiation exists along neuronal, glial or glioneuronal lines (Borit et al 1980); however, currently the designation is more applicable to tumors showing coexistent pineocytoma and pineoblastoma elements (Schild et al 1993). Such lack of uniformity in defining mixed tumors makes it difficult to correlate clinical behavior among the different reported series of pineal cell tumors.

DEFINITION AND INCIDENCE OF MALIGNANCY

Germ cell tumors

Malignant germ cell tumors are capable of systemic and CSF metastases. Dissemination may occur through a variety of mechanisms including hematogenous spread (Stowell et al 1945, Tompkins et al 1950, Borden et al 1973, Galassi et al 1984), direct paraspinal extension (Dayan et al 1966, Rubery & Wheeler 1980) and via ventriculo-peritoneal shunts (Dayan et al 1966, Neuwelt et al 1979, Salazar et al 1979, Wilson et al 1979, Rubery & Wheeler 1980, Kun et al 1981, Takei & Pearl 1981, Jennings et al 1985). Extraneural metastasis to various sites has been reported in up to 3% of all germ cell tumors, with lung and bone the most common sites, but also kidney, bladder, mediastinum, gastrointestinal tract, breast, and mesentery (Stowell et al 1945, Tompkins et al 1950, Dayan et al 1966, Borden et al 1973, Salazar et al 1979, Rubery & Wheeler 1980, Galassi et al 1984, Jennings et al 1985). Various estimates, ranging from 5–57%, have been given for the incidence of CSF seeding, with large series around 10% (Jenkin et al 1978, Chapman & Linggood 1980, Sano & Matsutani 1981, Jennings et al 1985, Brada & Rajan 1990, Bruce et al 1990). Although positive CSF cytology has been cited as evidence of spinal seeding, this assumption has not been convincingly proven (Jennings et al 1985). Likewise a negative CSF cytology does not preclude leptomeningeal dissemination (Sung et al 1978, Chapman & Linggood 1980, Jooma & Kendall 1983). Surgical intervention does not appear to increase the risk of spinal dissemination (Brada & Rajan 1990).

Germinomas can spread directly along the floor and walls of the third ventricle or alternatively via CSF pathways (Jennings et al 1985). Seeding and infiltration of a germinoma into the optic nerve sheath has also been reported (Stefanko et al 1979, Manor et al 1990). In general, the nongerminomatous malignant germ cell tumors have a higher incidence of metastatic dissemination than germinomas. Jennings et al (1985) have found correlations between: (1) hypothalamic involvement and third ventricle involvement simultaneously; (2) involvement of the third ventricle and dissemination through a noncontiguous site; and (3) the presence of spinal cord extension with additional metastasis in other sites. Spinal cord metastases were more likely to occur with germ cell tumors in the pineal region compared to other locations (Jennings et al 1985).

Pineal cell tumors

Pineal parenchymal tumors are capable of spread along the cerebrospinal fluid pathways (Fig. 38.20) (Herrick & Rubinstein 1979, Borit et al 1980, Schild et al 1993). Remote spread is unusual, although dissemination through a ventriculo-peritoneal shunt is possible (Pfletschinger et al 1986, Lesoin et al 1987). In general, pineoblastomas have more malignant potential and propensity for CSF dissemination compared to pineocytomas (Borit et al 1980, Schild et al 1993). Herrick & Rubinstein (1979) reported evidence of leptomeningeal dissemination at autopsy in all 11 patients with pineoblastoma whereas Hoffman et al (1984) reported metastases in 6 of 13 pineoblastomas. Pineocytomas, despite decreased growth rate and malignant potential, do have the propensity for CSF dissemination, although to a much lesser degree (Herrick & Rubinstein 1979, D'Andrea et al 1987, Disclafani et al 1989, Bruce et al 1990).

Schild et al (1993) reported leptomeningeal failure following radiation therapy in 0 of 4 pineocytomas, 0 of 4 intermediately differentiated pineal parenchymal tumors, 1 of 2 mixed pineal parenchymal tumors, and 4 of 9 pineoblastomas. Leptomeningeal failure occurred only in the presence of persistent primary tumor. In this same series of 21 pineal parenchymal tumors, radiographic seeding at the time of diagnosis was present in only 1 of the 11 patients with pineoblastoma. Malignant cells were present in the CSF in the case of 3 of the 21 tumors (1 intermediately differentiated pineal parenchymal tumor and 2 pineoblastomas); however, it is debatable whether the presence of a positive cytology is associated with

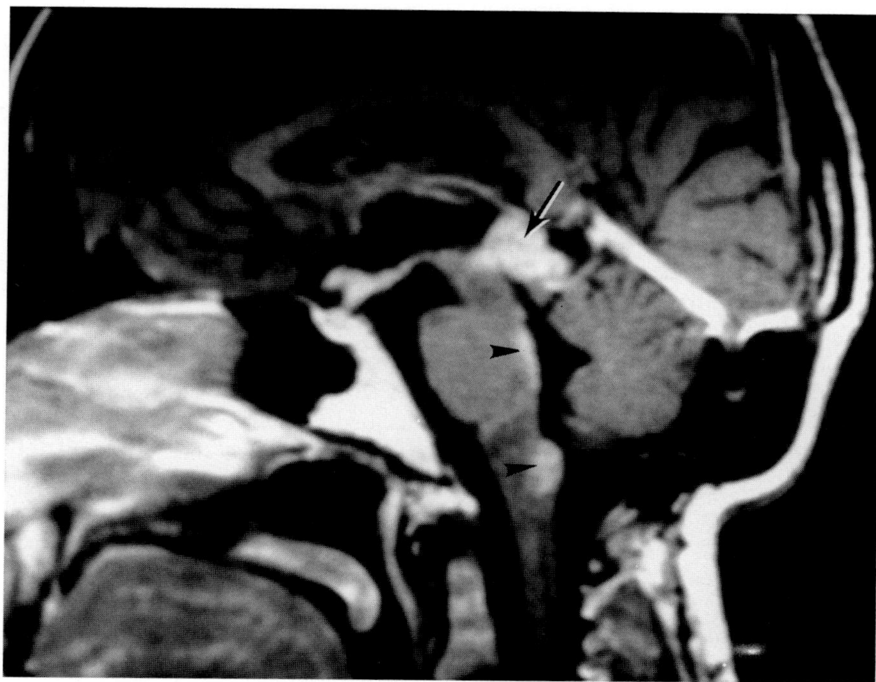

Fig. 38.20 MRI scan of a 44-year-old woman 10 years after resection of a mixed pineal cell tumor. The tumor has recurred in the pineal region (arrow) and has seeded the fourth ventricle (arrowheads).

spinal seeding. Considerable controversy exists regarding the correlation of neuronal differentiation with prognosis and malignant features (Herrick & Rubinstein 1979, Schild et al 1993). Differentiating between pineocytoma and pineoblastoma is more useful for predicting CSF dissemination than local tumor recurrence (Schild et al 1993).

GENERAL MANAGEMENT PLAN

All patients with suspected germ cell or pineal cell tumors should have the following workup:

1. high resolution MRI scan with gadolinium of the head, with particular attention to possible multicentric disease within the CSF pathways
2. measurement of AFP and β-HCG in the serum and CSF to detect malignant germ cell elements
3. cytologic examination of CSF
4. evaluation of pituitary function if endocrine abnormalities are suspected
5. formal visual field examination for suprasellar tumors.

Since most patients will have hydrocephalus, it may be best to wait until shunt placement to obtain CSF for cytology and measurement of tumor markers. Shunt placement is necessary prior to tumor resection in most cases of pineal region tumor.

Following the preoperative workup, a histopathologic diagnosis must be made, preferably by craniotomy, although stereotactic biopsy may be indicated under certain circumstances. Most patients derive benefit from aggressive tumor resection.

Postoperative adjuvant therapy depends upon the tumor histology. Surgical resection is usually curative for benign tumors. Most malignant germ cell or pineal cell tumors will require radiation therapy. Malignant non-germinomatous germ cell tumors will usually require chemotherapy prior to radiation.

SURGICAL MANAGEMENT

Suprasellar germ cell tumors

Suprasellar tumors can usually be approached through a subfrontal or pterional approach (Hoffman 1987, Bruce 1993a). Resection is limited by the extent of invasion of the optic structures and hypothalamus. A subfrontal approach allows access to the third ventricle through the lamina terminalis, depending upon whether the chiasm is prefixed. Pterional approaches provide access to the suprasellar and parasellar region, but exposure of the third ventricle is insufficient unless combined with a subfrontal approach. All approaches to the suprasellar region carry a risk of visual loss from injury to the optic structures; endocrine disturbance, particularly diabetes insipidus, from hypothalamic or pituitary stalk injury; or cognitive deficits and memory loss from damage to the fornices and anterior commissure (Apuzzo & Litofsky

1993). A transcallosal approach may be preferable for large tumors that extend to the foramen of Munro, although direct visualization of the optic structures is limited (Hoffman 1987, Bruce 1993a). Ideally such tumors are removed through a dilated foramen of Monro; however, if exposure is insufficient, an interfornical or subchoroidal transvelum interpositum approach may be used (Cossu et al 1984, Sawaya et al 1990, Apuzzo & Litofsky 1993). The transcallosal approaches carry an increased risk of memory loss, presumably due to fornical damage.

Approaches to the pineal region

Surgery has assumed an increasingly more important role, coinciding with improvements in surgical technique and neuroanesthesia, along with a better appreciation of the value of aggressive resection and accurate diagnosis in the subsequent management of pineal region tumors. In view of the wide variety of tumor subtypes and mixed tumors that occur in the pineal region, the foremost consideration among surgical goals is the accurate establishment of a histologic diagnosis (Suzuki & Iwabuchi 1965, Stein 1971, Chapman & Linggood 1980, Ventureyra 1981, Hoffman et al 1983, 1984, Packer et al 1984a, Rout et al 1984, Neuwelt 1985, Shokry et al 1985, Graziano et al 1987, Edwards et al 1988, Pluchino et al 1989, Bruce & Stein 1990, Casentini et al 1990, Dempsey et al 1992, Stein & Bruce 1992, Fuller et al 1993). The establishment of an accurate histologic diagnosis has implications for the choice of postoperative adjuvant therapy, necessity for metastatic workup, planning of optimal long-term follow-up and prediction of long-term prognosis. Radiographic features, tumor marker measurement and CSF cytologic examination can lead to educated predictions of tumor histology; however, accurate histologic diagnosis can only be established with pathologic examination of a surgical specimen (Wood et al 1981, Zimmerman 1985, Ganti et al 1986, D'Andrea et al 1987, Kersh et al 1988).

The role of surgery extends beyond providing a histologic diagnosis, as there is a growing appreciation of the value of aggressive tumor removal for improving the prognosis of patients. With benign tumors, complete resection is usually curative (Stein & Bruce 1992). With malignant tumors, radical debulking is thought to improve the outcome and response to adjuvant therapy (Sano 1976a, Shokry et al 1985, Lapras et al 1987, Hoffman et al 1991, Stein & Bruce 1992). In some instances complete resection of a malignant tumor may be possible, although it is not necessarily considered curative (Neuwelt 1985, Stein & Bruce 1992).

Pineal region tumors may be approached through one of the several variations of either an infratentorial or supratentorial approach. Supratentorial approaches include the parietal-interhemispheric approach popularized by Dandy (1921) and the occipital-transtentorial approach originally described by Horrax (1937) and later modified by Poppen (1966). The supratentorial approaches are useful for tumors with a significant supratentorial extension or lateral extension to the trigone of the lateral ventricle (Bruce 1993b). Supratentorial approaches offer the advantage of wide exposure but have the disadvantage of encountering the tumor beneath the convergence of the deep venous system which interferes with tumor removal. The transcallosal-interhemispheric approach involves a paramedian trajectory between the falx and the right parietal lobe with partial resection of the corpus callosum (Dandy 1936, Lapras & Patet 1987). Complications may result from parietal lobe retraction or venous infarction from sacrifice of a bridging vein (Bruce & Stein 1993b). The occipital-transtentorial approach involves retraction of the occipital lobe and division of the tentorium for adequate exposure. This provides a good view of the quadrigeminal plate but may result in visual field defects (Reid & Clark 1978, Neuwelt 1985, Nagao et al 1988, Nazarro et al 1992).

The infratentorial-supracerebellar approach provides a midline trajectory between the tentorium and cerebellum (Krause 1926, Stein 1971, Bruce & Stein 1992). The tumor is encountered below the deep venous system where it is less likely to interfere with resection. Gravity works in the surgeon's favor by allowing the cerebellum to fall away to expose the pineal region, by minimizing pooling of venous blood in the operative field, and by assisting with the dissection of the tumor off the deep venous system. Although this can often involve a long reach, tumors extending to the foramen of Monro can be removed.

Various positions have been described for these different approaches. The sitting slouch position is generally used for the infratentorial-supracerebellar and transcallosal-interhemispheric approaches. Potential complications include ventricular and cortical collapse with subdural hematoma, pneumocephalus, and air embolus (Bruce & Stein 1993a,b). Use of this position, however, facilitates surgery by allowing gravity to assist in the tumor dissection from the roof of the third ventricle, and it avoids venous blood pooling. The threequarter prone lateral decubitus position is designed to avoid many of the above complications and is often used for the occipital-transtentorial approach; however, gravity does not work in the surgeon's favor (Ausman et al 1988, McComb & Apuzzo 1988). The Concorde position has been proposed to combine the benefits of both positions while minimizing the risks (Kobayashi et al 1983).

The most common complications following pineal region surgery are: extraocular movement dysfunction, altered mental status and ataxia (Bruce & Stein 1993a,b). Less common complications include shunt malfunction and aseptic meningitis. Many neurologic deficits are present preoperatively and may be temporarily worse following surgery. Most postoperative deficits tend to be transient and improve spontaneously with time. Several factors correlate with a higher incidence and severity of deficits including prior radiation therapy, advanced preoperative symptoms, higher degree of malignant features, and invasive tumor characteristics (Stein 1979, Lapras & Patet 1987, Bruce & Stein 1993a,b). Supratentorial approaches can result in seizures, hemianopsia, or hemiparesis (Hoffman et et al 1984, Nazzaro et al 1992, Bruce & Stein 1993b). The most significant complication of pineal region surgery is hemorrhage into a partially resected tumor bed (Bruce & Stein 1993a,b). Hemorrhage is a common associated phenomenon with pineal region tumors and pineal parenchymal tumors in particular (Fig. 38.7) (Herrick & Rubinstein 1979, Peragut et al 1987, Dempsey et al 1992, Bruce & Stein 1993a,b). Hemorrhage may occur up to several days postoperatively and may be related to tumor vascularity or malignant characteristics. Tumors may also hemorrhage prior to surgery, presenting with pineal apoplexy (Steinbok et al 1977, Burres & Hamilton 1979, Higashi et al 1979).

Most large series in the microsurgical era, reporting on greater than 20 patients and involving all types of pineal region pathology, have an operative mortality from 0–8% and permanent morbidity from 0–12% (Stein 1979, Wood et al 1981, Jooma & Kendall 1983, Rout et al 1984, Neuwelt 1985, Pendl 1985, Lapras et al 1987, Sano 1987, Edwards et al 1988, Pluchino et al 1989, Herrman et al 1992, Stein & Bruce 1992). In the largest reported series of surgery for pineal region tumors, gross total removal was possible in 90% of benign tumors and 25% of malignant tumors (Stein & Bruce 1992).

Long-term outcome for malignant tumors following surgery depends on tumor histology and the effects of adjuvant therapy. Gross total resection of a malignant tumor may be associated with a more favorable prognosis (Lapras et al 1987, Sano 1987, Stein & Bruce 1992). For benign tumors (teratomas, dermoid tumors, epidermoid tumors and lipomas) the long-term prognosis following surgical resection is excellent and usually curative (Bruce & Stein 1990, Stein & Bruce 1992). There is a small subset of pineocytomas (up to 16% of all pineal cell tumors) that are discrete, histologically benign, and fully resectable (Vaquero et al 1990, Stein & Bruce 1992). These patients have an excellent prognosis, are likely to be cured with surgery alone, and are optimally managed by careful monitoring without any adjuvant therapy (Rubinstein 1981).

Stereotactic biopsy

In certain situations, stereotactic biopsy is the procedure of choice for obtaining a tissue specimen (Bruce & Stein 1990, Bruce 1993b). Many series have demonstrated the relative ease and safety of stereotactic biopsy, which may be performed using a precoronal or superior parietal lobule entry point (Canway 1973, Pecker et al 1979, Moser & Backlund 1984, Pluchino et al 1989, Dempsey et al 1992). The pineal region is among the more hazardous areas of the brain to biopsy stereotactically because of the adjacent deep venous system and the periventricular location. This procedure is generally reserved for patients presenting with multiple medical problems, clearly invasive tumors or obvious tumor dissemination at the time of presentation. Although stereotactic biopsy has an overall relative ease and low morbidity, open surgical resection is the preferred procedure for several reasons (Edwards et al 1988, Bruce 1993b). Open surgical resection is advantageous in facilitating removal of most, if not all, of the tumor. This is most crucial for benign pineal tumors (accounting for approximately one third of all pineal tumors), where surgical resection is curative. For malignant tumors, surgical debulking may improve the response to adjuvant therapy (Shokry et al 1985, Lapras & Patet 1987, Sano 1987, Stein & Bruce 1992). Furthermore, because of the wide variety of tumors that occur in the pineal region, as well as the high incidence of mixed tumors, the small samples provided by stereotactic biopsy are more likely to lead to an erroneous diagnosis from sampling error or inherent difficulties in evaluating limited specimens by even experienced neuropathologists (Fig. 38.10) (Edwards et al 1988, Chandrasoma et al 1989, Bruce & Stein 1993b). Germ cell tumors are particularly problematic as they often contain mixed cell types and may be accompanied by granulomatous reactions (Kraichoke et al 1988, Ho & Liu 1992).

In addition to possible diagnostic inaccuracies, stereotactic biopsies carry considerable risk of hemorrhage from either highly vascular tumors such as pineal parenchymal tumors or direct injury to the adjacent deep venous system (Pecker et al 1979, Peragut et al 1987, Edwards et al 1988, Chandrasoma et al 1989, Bruce & Stein 1993b). A rare but notable potential complication of biopsy of a pineoblastoma is implantation metastasis (Rosenfeld et al 1990).

RADIATION THERAPY

All patients with malignant germ cell or pineal cell tumors require radiation therapy consisting of 4000 cGy to the ventricular system with an additional 1500 cGy to the tumor bed. The total radiation dose of 5500 cGy should be given in 180 cGy daily fractions. Recent studies suggest a more limited field of radiation may be as efficacious while avoiding the adverse side effects of ventricular exposure (Dattoli & Newall 1990).

Radiation therapy may be withheld for the rare, histologically benign pineocytoma which has been completely resected (Vaquero et al 1990, Stein & Bruce 1992). Identification of these exceptions is based on intraoperative observation of a well-circumscribed tumor and histologic analysis. These tumors can have good long-term control with surgery alone, although careful follow-up is necessary.

Germinomas are among the most radiosensitive of any malignant brain tumors and a significant majority are cured with radiation. With germinomas, surgery and radiation of 5000–6000 cGy has achieved 5-year survival of above 75% and 10-year survival as high as 69% (Sung et al 1978, Sano & Matsutani 1981, Edwards et al 1988). Dosages of less than 5000 cGy have been correlated with a higher incidence of local failure in both pineal cell tumors (Schild et al 1993) and germ cell tumors (Sung et al 1978, Kersh et al 1988).

Long-term complications from radiation therapy are of particular concern in pineal tumor patients since many of them can expect extended long-term survival and even cure. Delayed complications of cranial radiation therapy include cognitive deficits, hypothalamic and endocrine dysfunction, cerebral necrosis, and de novo tumor formation (Duffner et al 1985, Noell & Herskovic 1985, Edwards et al 1988, Nighoghossian et al 1988, Sakai et al 1988, Hodges et al 1992, Bruce 1993b). Pediatric patients are particularly vulnerable to adverse radiation effects (Rowland et al 1984, Bendersky et al 1988, Donahue 1992). In a series of 27 pediatric pineal germinomas treated with radiation therapy, 26% had no improvement in preoperative diabetes insipidus, 22% developed hypopituitarism, all had minor growth defects and nearly all had some degree of mild cognitive dysfunction (Jenkin et al 1990). In another series, 7 of 26 patients irradiated for germ cell tumors developed intellectual retardation or cerebral dullness (Sakai et al 1988).

All patients with malignant germ cell or pineal cell tumors should have postoperative staging with spinal MRI to look for evidence of tumor seeding (Bruce 1993b). MRI has supplanted CT myelography as the procedure of choice for this screening (Rippe et al 1990, Stein & Bruce 1992). Early studies recommended CSF cytological examination as a diagnostic test for spinal metastases, however the correlation between metastases and CSF cytology is not strong (DeGirolami et al 1973, Waga et al 1979, Veki & Tanaka 1980, Jooma & Kendall 1983, Shibamoto et al 1988, Bruce et al 1990). Definitive documentation of spinal metastases is important since the use of prophylactic spinal radiation is controversial. Previously, craniospinal irradiation was recommended routinely for malignant pineal tumors (Jenkin et al 1978, Sung et al 1978, Griffin et al 1981, Rich et al 1985). Several reports, however, have noted the actual incidence of spinal metastasis to be relatively low and therefore recommend that prophylactic spinal radiation not be given (Wood et al 1981, Edwards et al 1988, Linstadt et al 1988, Disclafani et al 1989, Bruce & Stein 1990, Bruce et al 1990, Dattoli & Newall 1990, Fuller et al 1993). In Jennings' review of intracranial germ cell tumors, the incidence of spinal seeding was 10% (Jennings et al 1985). This study noted higher incidence of spinal cord metastasis with germinomas (11%) and endodermal sinus tumors (23%), and higher incidence among pineal versus suprasellar tumors. Estimates of spinal seeding with pineal cell tumors have been variable and complicated by the difficulty in uniformly distinguishing between pineocytomas and pineoblastomas. Overall estimates are in the range of 10–20%, with markedly increased rates for pineoblastoma compared to pineocytoma (Bruce et al 1990, Schild et al 1993). The prevailing recommendation currently is to give spinal radiation only for documented seeding, using a dose of 3500 cGy (Rao et al 1981, Wood et al 1981, Amendola et al 1984, Edwards et al 1988, Disclafani et al 1989, Bruce & Stein 1990, Bruce et al 1990, Rippe et al 1990).

CHEMOTHERAPY

Germ cell tumors

Among germ cell tumors, chemotherapy has been of greatest value in patients with nongerminomatous malignant germ cell tumors. Although chemotherapy has been effective for many patients with nongerminomatous germ cell tumors in extracranial sites (Einhorn 1981, Hainsworth & Greco 1983, Logothetis et al 1985, Pinkerton et al 1986, McLeod et al 1988), these successes have not been duplicated with intracranial tumors, and survival beyond two years is rare (Jennings et al 1985). Several reports describe sporadic responses for these tumors, however the overall results are pessimistic (Prioleau & Wilson 1976, Haase & Norgaard-Pedersen 1979, Ono et al 1982, Chan et al 1984, Packer et al 1984a,b, Takakura 1985, Page et al 1986, Graziano et al 1987, Edwards et al 1988, Kobayashi et al 1989, Patel et al 1992, Yoshida et al 1993). A wide variety of chemotherapeutic treatments have been tried, with the most successful regimens derived from the treatments for testicular cancer using the Einhorn regimen of cisplatin, vinblastine and bleomycin (Einhorn & Donohue 1977, Sawaya et al 1990). Recently, VP-16 (etoposide) has been substituted for vinblastine and bleomycin to avoid the pulmonary toxicity of bleomycin, and several studies have demonstrated significantly improved response rates (Neuwelt 1985, Kobayashi et al 1989, Patel et al 1992, Yoshida et al 1993). Conventionally, nongerminomatous malignant germ cell tumors are treated with chemotherapy prior to radiation therapy, however optimal timing of adjuvant therapy has not been conclusively determined. Whether the addition of radiotherapy improves survival over chemotherapy alone is unclear, although several studies anecdotally showed increased survival in patients treated aggressively with a combination of chemotherapy, radiation and surgery (Bamberg et al 1984, Chan et al 1984, Takakura 1985). Given the poor prognosis of these tumors, an aggressive therapy seems justified (Jennings et al 1985, Hoffman et al 1991, Bruce 1993b).

Because germinomas are so radiosensitive and often curable with radiation, chemotherapy has been reserved for patients with recurrent or metastatic disease. The most popular regimes have involved variations of the Einhorn regimen of cisplatin, vinblastine and bleomycin, with combinations involving cyclophosphamide or etoposide (Neuwelt et al 1980, Siegal et al 1983, Allen et al 1985, Pinkerton et al 1986, Sawaya et al 1990). More recent studies have demonstrated an impressive response with cisplatin and etoposide alone (Kobayashi et al 1989, Patel et al 1992, Yoshida et al 1993). The success with chemotherapy in germinomas has led to studies evaluating its effectiveness prior to radiation therapy as a means of reducing the dose of radiation (Allen et al 1987). Despite the excellent response to chemotherapy for germinomas, radiation is still recommended (Patel et al 1992, Yoshida et al 1993). Furthermore, the presence of syncytiotrophoblastic giant cells within a germinoma may result in a less favorable chemotherapeutic response (Yoshida et al 1993).

Pineal cell tumors

Chemotherapy for pineal cell tumors has not been studied extensively, although several studies have demonstrated sporadic, anecdotal responses in pineoblastomas (Packer et al 1984a, Sawaya et al 1990, Schild et al 1993). Overall, there is no definitive study demonstrating a significant response, and as such chemotherapy is generally used secondarily for recurrent or disseminated pineal cell tumors. Treatment regimens have included various combinations of vincristine, lomustine, cisplatin, etoposide, cyclophosphamide, actinomycin D, and methotrexate. Because of the limited experience, no dominant chemotherapy regimen has emerged as superior. Chemotherapy has been used for recurrent pineocytomas with little success (D'Andrea et al 1987, Disclafani et al 1989). A recent study, whose design was based on similarities between medulloblastoma and pineoblastoma, utilized melphalan in four patients with pineoblastoma and demonstrated a partial response (Friedman et al 1989).

OTHER ADJUNCTIVE THERAPY

Radiosurgery is a relatively new and promising technique which has gained widespread interest for the treatment of pineal region tumors. 2 patients with pineocytomas treated radiosurgically by Backlund experienced improvement in symptoms and tumor shrinkage (Backlund et al 1974). Casentini et al (1990) were able to reduce the dosage of radiation to healthy brain tissue in 6 patients with germinomas by providing a radiosurgical boost. Nine patients with pineal tumors, including 1 patient with a pineocytoma, were treated without morbidity and with good clinical result at an average follow-up of 21 months in a recent report (Dempsey et al 1992).

The distinct differences and biologic effects between conventional fractionated radiation and radiosurgery must be considered when choosing optimal therapeutic regimens. Due to limited experience and follow-up, the indications for stereotactic radiation have not been definitively established. Radiosurgery is generally limited to tumors that are less than three centimeters in diameter. Germinomas have historically responded well to fractionated radiation and it is unlikely that radiosurgery will improve on these results. The greatest potential value of radiosurgery may lie in its usefulness in providing a local boost to reduce the overall radiation exposure of the entire brain (Casentini et al 1990).

Due to the rarity of germ cell and pineal cell tumors, other adjunctive therapy has not been extensively explored. Coakham et al (1988) reported a 22-month remission in a patient with disseminated pineoblastoma who was treated with intrathecally administered antibody-guided irradiation. Apuzzo et al (1987) have described the use of interstitial radiobrachytherapy for pineal region tumors.

MANAGEMENT OF ASSOCIATED PHENOMENA

Most patients with pineal region tumors present with hydrocephalus (Bruce & Stein 1990, Sawaya et al 1990). Generally a shunt is placed prior to surgery to allow the ventricles an opportunity to decompress gradually (Bruce & Stein 1992). If a total tumor removal is anticipated, a permanent shunt may not be necessary and a ventricular drain can be placed at the time of surgery and subsequently either converted to a shunt or removed on post-operative day 2 or 3, depending on whether it is needed (Edwards et al 1988, Bruce & Stein 1992). An alternative approach is to leave a ventricular catheter connecting the third ventricle and cisterna magna at the time of tumor resection (Stein & Bruce 1992, Bruce & Stein 1993a).

Several reports have documented metastases into the intraperitoneal cavity following shunt placement; however, the incidence is quite low (Wilson et al 1979, Hoffman et al 1983, Edwards et al 1988). Filters are generally not recommended since they will increase the possibility of shunt malfunction (Neuwelt 1985, Edwards et al 1988). A possible option for relieving the obstructive hydrocephalus without the hazards of shunting is stereotactic endoscopic third ventriculostomy (Goodman 1993).

Among other associated phenomena, patients with suprasellar tumors often develop hypopituitarism. Diabetes insipidus is particularly common and may require hormone replacement (Jooma & Kendall 1983, Farwell & Flannery 1989).

PATTERNS OF FAILURE

Germ cell tumors

Germ cell tumors most often fail locally (Sano & Matsutani 1981, Dearnaley et al 1990). Spinal failure generally does not occur without simultaneous local failure (Shokry et al 1985). Systemic metastases are rare but can occur to bone with germinomas or to lung with malignant teratomas (Farwell & Flannery 1989, Dearnaley et al 1990). Recurrence of germinomas outside radiation ports has been described (Vematsu et al 1992).

Pineal cell tumors

Pineal cell tumors are most likely to fail locally, and spinal failures, when they occur, are nearly always in the setting of residual or recurrent local tumor (Schild et al 1993). At autopsy, nearly all fatal pineoblastomas and, to a lesser extent, pineocytomas have evidence of leptomeningeal and ependymal spread (Fig. 38.20) (Herrick & Rubinstein 1979, Borit et al 1980, Packer et al 1984a).

MANAGEMENT OF RECURRENT DISEASE

Because of the scarcity of these tumors, management of recurrences is generally handled on an individual basis. Possible therapeutic options include radiosurgery, chemotherapy, or additional external beam radiation, particularly if not given to its maximum. Reoperation is reserved for patients with relatively slow-growing tumors who are in stable condition with reasonable expectation for longevity and a favorable outcome following prior surgery (Bruce & Stein 1990). Chemotherapy may be useful for germ cell and pineal cell tumors that have recurred following radiation (Einhorn & Donohue 1977, Neuwelt et al 1980, Siegal et al 1983, Allen et al 1985, Edwards et al 1988, Sawaya et al 1990, Schild et al 1993).

MANAGEMENT OUTCOME

Germ cell tumors

Long-term expectations for germ cell tumors are most dependent on tumor histology. Benign germ cell tumors such as teratoma, dermoid, and epidermoid tumors are generally associated with 100% 5- and 10-year survivals following surgical treatment alone (Bjornsson et al 1985, Stein & Bruce 1992).

Among malignant germ cell tumors, an important distinction is made between germinomas and nongerminomatous tumors. The 5-year survival for germinomas is generally in the 75–80% range following surgery and radiation (Jennings et al 1985, Hoffman et al 1991, Bruce 1993b). Whether survival is improved for patients with suprasellar germinomas compared to pineal region germinomas is unclear. Takakura reported survival rates of 65% at both 5 and 10 years in 49 pineal germinomas while corresponding rates were 90% and 84% respectively for 22 suprasellar germinomas (Takakura 1985). Other reports have shown as high as 100% 5-year survival for patients with suprasellar germinomas following surgery and radiation (Sano & Matsutani 1981, Legido et al 1988). Germinomas with syncytiotrophoblastic giant cells may have higher recurrence rates (Vernatsu et al 1992, Yoshida et al 1993). Germinomas in children tend to have a better prognosis than those in adults (Jenkin et al 1978, Sano & Matsutani 1981).

Patients with malignant nongerminomatous germ cell tumors have the worst prognosis and rarely survive beyond 2 years (Tavcar et al 1980, Chan et al 1984, Packer et al 1984b, Jennings et al 1985, Page et al 1987, Edwards et al 1988). Recent improvements in chemotherapy, however, are likely to surpass these results (Neuwelt 1985, Kobayashi et al 1989, Patel et al 1992, Yoshida et al 1993). Among malignant nongerminomatous germ cell tumors, immature teratomas have a slightly better prognosis, with a 5-year survival in the range of 25%. A worse prognosis is associated with the presence of elevated tumor markers in these patients (Takakura 1985).

Pineal cell tumors

It is difficult to establish specific outcome parameters for pineal cell tumors due to small series size, lack of uniform histologic classification, and lack of uniform treatment regimens. The largest series project a 5-year survival between 55% and 62% for tumors treated primarily with surgery and radiation, although a small number included chemotherapy as well (Stein & Bruce 1992, Schild et al 1993). Among pineal cell tumors, there is a small group with discrete, histologically benign, and completely resectable pineocytomas which can be treated with surgery alone and have an excellent prognosis (Vaquero et al 1990, Stein & Bruce 1992).

Acknowledgement

The authors wish to thank Dr Steve Chan, Department of Pathology, College of Physicians and Surgeons of Columbia University, for his helpful assistance.

REFERENCES

Allen J C, Nisselbaum J, Epstein F, Rosen G, Schwartz M K 1979 Alphafetoprotein and human chorionic gonadotropin determination in cerebrospinal fluid. An aid to the diagnosis and management of intracranial germ-cell tumors. Journal of Neurosurgery 51: 368–374

Allen J C, Bosl G, Walker R 1985 Chemotherapy trials in recurrent primary intracranial germ cell tumors. Journal of Neuro-Oncology 3: 147–152

Allen J C, Kim J H, Packer R J 1987 Neoadjuvant chemotherapy for newly diagnosed germ-cell tumors of the central nervous system. Journal of Neurosurgery 67: 65–70

Amendola B, McClatchey K, Amendola M 1984 Pineal region tumors: analysis of treatment results. International Journal of Radiation Oncology Biology Physics 10: 991–997

Ammar A, Al-Majid H, Kutty M 1991 Germinoma in a 16-month old baby: A case report and brief review of the literature. Acta Neurochirurgica (Wien) 110: 189–192

Apuzzo M, Litofsky N 1993 Surgery in and around the anterior third ventricle. In: Apuzzo M (ed) Brain surgery: complication avoidance and management, vol 1. Churchill Livingstone, New York, pp 541–579

Apuzzo M L J, Petrovich Z, Luxton G, Jepson J H, Cohen D, Breeze R E 1987 Interstitial radiobrachytherapy of malignant cerebral neoplasms: rationale, methodology, prospects. Neurological Research 9: 91–100

Araki C, Matsumoto S 1969 Statistical re-evaluation of pinealoma and related tumors in Japan. Progress in Experimental Tumor Research 30: 307–312

Arendt J 1978 Melatonin as a tumor marker in a patient with pineal tumor. British Medical Journal 26 Aug 1978: 635–636

Arita N, Ushio Y, Hayakawa T, Uozumi T, Watanabe M, Mori T, Mogami H 1980 Serum levels of alpha-fetoprotein, human chorionic gonadotropin and carcinoembryonic antigen in patients with primary intracranial germ cell tumors. Oncodev Biol Med (Amsterdam) 1: 235–240

Ausman J I, Malik G M, Dujovny M, Mann R 1988 Three-quarter prone approach to the pineal-tentorial region. Surgical Neurology 29: 298–306

Backlund E-O, Rahn T, Sarby B 1974 Treatment of pinealomas by stereotaxic radiation surgery. Acta Radiol Ther Phy Biol 13: 368–376

Bader J L, Meadows A T, Zimmerman L E, Rorke L B, Voute P A, Champion L A A, Miller R W 1982 Bilateral retinoblastoma with ectopic intracranial retinoblastoma: trilateral retinoblastoma. Cancer Genetics Cytogenetics 5: 201–213

Bamberg M, Metz K, Alberti W, Heckemann R, Schulz U 1984 Endodermal sinus tumor of the pineal region. Metastasis through a ventriculoperitoneal shunt. Cancer 54: 903–906

Barber S, Smith J, Hughes R 1978 Melatonin as a tumor marker in a patient with pineal tumour. Lancet ii: 328

Barker D, Weller R, Garfield J 1976 Epidemiology of primary tumors of the brain and spinal cord: a regional survey in southern England. Journal of Neurology, Neurosurgery and Psychiatry 39: 290–296

Becker L E, Hinton D 1983 Primitive neuroectodermal tumors of the central nervous system. Human Pathology 14: 538–550

Bendersky M, Lewis M, Mandelbaum D E, Stanger C 1988 Serial neuropsychological follow-up of a child following craniospinal irradiation. Developmental Medicine and Child Neurology 30: 808–820

Bjornsson J, Scheithauer B, Okazaki H, Leech R 1985 Intracranial germ cell tumors: Pathobiological and immunohistochemical aspects of 70 cases. Journal of Neuropathology and Experimental Neurology 44: 32–46

Bloom H 1983 Primary intracranial germ cell tumours. Clinical Oncology 2: 233–257

Borden S, Weber A L, Toch R, Wang C C 1973 Pineal germinoma. Long term survival despite hematogenous metastases. Journal of Pathology 114: 9–12

Borit A 1981 History of tumors of the pineal region. American Journal of Surgical Pathology 5: 613–620

Borit A, Blackwood W 1979 Pineocytoma with astrocytomatous differentiation. Journal of Neuropathology and Experimental Neurology 38: 253–258

Borit A, Blackwood W, Mair W G P 1980 The separation of pineocytoma from pineoblastoma. Cancer 45: 1408–1418

Brada M, Rajan B 1990 Spinal seeding in cranial germinoma. British Journal of Cancer 61: 339–340

Bruce J 1993a Intracranial germinomas. Neurosurgical Consultations 4: 1–8

Bruce J N 1993b Management of pineal region tumors. Neurosurgery Quarterly 3: 103–119

Bruce J N, Stein B M 1990 Pineal tumors. In: Rosenblum M (ed) The role of surgery in brain tumor management. Neurosurgery Clinics of North America, vol 1. W B Saunders, Philadelphia, pp 123–138

Bruce J N, Stein B M 1992 Infratentorial approach to pineal tumors. In: Wilson C B (ed) Neurosurgical procedures: personal approaches to classic operations. Williams & Wilkins, Baltimore, pp 63–76

Bruce J, Stein B 1993a Supracerebellar approaches in the pineal region. In: Apuzzo M (ed) Brain surgery: complication avoidance and management. Churchill-Livingstone, New York, pp 511–536

Bruce J N, Stein B M 1993b Complications of surgery for pineal region tumors. In: Post K D, Friedman E D , McCormick P C (eds) Postoperative complications in intracranial neurosurgery. Thieme Medical Publishers, New York, pp 74–86

Bruce J N, Fetell M R, Stein B M 1990 Incidence of spinal metastases in patients with malignant pineal region tumors: Avoidance of prophylactic spinal irradiation. Journal of Neurosurgery 72: 354A

Bruce J, Tamarkin L, Riedel C, Markey S, Oldfield E 1991 Sequential cerebrospinal fluid and plasma sampling in humans: 24-hour melatonin measurements in normal subjects and after peripheral sympathectomy. Journal of Clinical Endocrinology and Metabolism 72: 819–823

Bruce J, Stein B, Fetell M Pineal region tumors. In: Rowland L (ed) Merritt's Textbook of neurology, 9th edn. In press

Burres K P, Hamilton R D 1979 Pineal apoplexy. Neurosurgery 4: 264–268

Casentini L, Colombo F, Pozza F, Benedetti A 1990 Combined radiosurgery and external radiotherapy of intracranial germinomas. Surgical Neurology 34: 79–86

Chan H, Humphreys R, Hendrick E, Chuang S, Fitz C, Becker L 1984 Primary intracranial choriocarcinoma. A report of two cases and a review of the literature. Neurosurgery 15: 540–545

Chandrasoma P T, Smith M M, Apuzzo M L J 1989 Stereotactic biopsy in the diagnosis of brain masses: comparison of results of biopsy and resected surgical specimen. Neurosurgery 24: 160–165

Chang C, Kageyama T, Yoshida J, Negoro M 1981 Pineal tumors: Clinical diagnosis, with special emphasis on the significance of pineal calcification. Neurosurgery 8: 656–668

Chapman P H, Linggood R M 1980 The management of pineal area tumors: a recent reappraisal. Cancer 46: 1253–1257

Coakham H B, Richardson R B, Davies A G, Bourne S P, Eckert H, Kemshead J T 1988 Neoplastic meningitis from a pineal tumor treated by antibody-guided irradiation via the intrathecal route. British Journal of Neurosurgery 2: 199–209

Conway L W 1973 Stereotaxic diagnosis and treatment of intracranial tumors including an initial experience with cryosurgery for pinealomas. Journal of Neurosurgery 38: 453–460

Cossu M, Labinu M, Orunesu M et al 1984 Subchoroidal approach to the third ventricle: Microsurgical anatomy. Surgical Neurology 21: 552–565

Cravioto H, Dart D 1973 The ultrastructure of "pinealoma" (Seminoma-like tumor of the pineal region). Journal of Neuropathology and Experimental Neurology 32: 552–564

D'Andrea D A, Packer R J, Rorke L B, Bilaniuk L T, Sutton L N, Bruce D A, Schut L 1987 Pineocytomas of childhood. A reappraisal of natural history and response to therapy. Cancer 59: 1353–1357

Dandy W E 1921 An operation for the removal of pineal tumors. Surgery, Gynecology and Obstetrics XXXIII: 113–119

Dandy W E 1936 Operative experience in cases of pineal tumor. Archives of Surgery 33: 19–46

Dattoli M J, Newall J 1990 Radiation therapy for intracranial germinoma: the case for limited volume treatment. International Journal of Radiation Oncology Biology Physics 19: 429–433
Dayan A, Marshall A, Miler A, Pick F, Rankin N 1966 Atypical teratomas of the pineal and hypothalamus. Journal of Pathology and Bacteriology 92: 1–25
Dearnaley D P, A'Hern R P, Whittaker S, Bloom H J G 1990 Pineal and CNS germ cell tumors: Royal Marsden Hospital experience 1962–1987. International Journal of Radiation Oncology Biology Physics 18: 773–781
DeGirolami U, Schmidek H 1973 Clinicopathological study of 53 tumors of the pineal region. Journal of Neurosurgery 39: 455–462
DeMonte F, Zelby A, Al-Mefty O 1993 Hearing impairment resulting from a pineal region meningioma. Neurosurgery 32: 665–668
Dempsey P K, Kondziolka D, Lunsford L D 1992 Stereotactic diagnosis and treatment of pineal region tumours and vascular malformations. Acta Neurochirurgica (Wien) 116: 14–22
Dempsey R, Chandler W 1984 Abnormal serum melatonin levels in patients with intrasellar tumors. Neurosurgery 15: 815–819
Disclafani A, Hudgins R J, Edwards S B, Wara W, Wilson C B, Levin V A 1989 Pineocytomas. Cancer 63: 302–304
Donahue B 1992 Short- and long-term complications of radiation therapy for pediatric brain tumors. Pediatric Neurosurgery 18: 207–217
Duffner P, Cohen M, Thomas P, Lansky S 1985 The long-term effects of cranial irradiation on the central nervous system. Cancer 56: 1841–1846
Eberts T J, Ransburg R C 1979 Primary intracranial endodermal sinus tumor. Journal of Neurosurgery 50: 246–252
Edwards M S B, Hudgins R J, Wilson C B, Levin V A, Wara W M 1988 Pineal region tumors in children. Journal of Neurosurgery 66: 689–697
Einhorn L 1981 Testicular cancer as a model for curable neoplasm. Cancer Research 41: 3275–3280
Einhorn L H, Donohue J 1977 Cis-Diaminedichloroplatinum, Vinblastine, and Bleomycin combination therapy in disseminated testicular cancer. Annals of Internal Medicine 87: 293–298
Erlich S, Apuzzo M 1985 The pineal gland: Anatomy, physiology and clinical significance. Journal of Neurosurgery 63: 321–341
Farwell J R, Flannery J T 1989 Pinealomas and germinomas in children. Journal of Neuro-Oncology 7: 13–19
Fetell M R, Stein B M 1986 Neuroendocrine aspects of pineal tumors. In: Zimmeman E A, Abrams G M (eds) Neurologic clinics: neuroendocrinology and brain peptides, vol 4. W B Saunders, Philadelphia, pp 877–905
Friedman H S, Schold S C Jr, Mahaley M S et al 1989 Phase II treatment of medulloblastoma and pineoblastoma with melphalan: clinical therapy based on experimental models of human medulloblastoma. Journal of Clinical Oncology 7: 904–911
Fuller B, Kapp D, Cox R 1993 Radiation therapy of pineal region tumors: 25 new cases and a review of 208 previously reported cases. International Journal of Radiation Oncology Biology Physics 28: 229–245
Galassi E, Tognetti F, Frank F, Gaist G 1984 Extraneural metastases from primary pineal tumors. Review of the literature. Surgical Neurology 21: 497–504
Ganti S R, Hilal S K, Silver A J, Mawad M, Sane P 1986 CT of pineal region tumors. AJNR 7: 97–104
Glass R, Culbertson C 1946 Teratoma of the pineal gland with choriocarcinoma and rhabdomyosarcoma. Archives of Pathology 41: 552–555
Gonzalez-Crussi F 1982 Extragonadal teratomas. Atlas of tumor pathology, series 2, fascicle 18. Armed Forces Institute of Pathology, Washington, DC
Goodman R 1993 Magnetic resonance imaging-directed stereotactic endoscopic third ventriculostomy. Neurosurgery 32: 1043–1047
Graziano S L, Paolozzi F P, Rudolph A R, Stewart W A, Elbadawi A, Comus R L 1987 Mixed germ-cell tumor of the pineal region. Journal of Neurosurgery 66: 300–304
Griffin B, Griffin T, Tong D, Russell A, Kurtz J, Laramore G, Groudine M 1981 Pineal region tumors: results of radiation therapy and indications for elective spinal irradiation. International Journal of Radiation Oncology Biology Physics 66: 300–304
Grote E, Lorenz R, Vuia O 1980 Clinical and endocrinological findings in ectopic pinealoma and spongioblastoma of the hypothalamus. Acta Neurochirurgica 53: 87–98
Haase J, Norgaard-Pedersen B 1979 Alpha-fetoprotein (AFP) and human chorionic gonadotropin (HCG) as biochemical markers of intracranial germ cell tumors. Acta Neurochirurgica 53: 269–274
Hainsworth J, Greco F 1983 Testicular germ cell neoplasms. American Journal of Medicine 75: 817–832
Hassoun J, Gambarelli D, Peragut J C, Toga M 1983 Specific ultrastructural markers of human pinealomas. A study of four cases. Acta Neuropathologica 62: 31–40
Herrick M K, Rubinstein L J 1979 The cytological differentiating potential of pineal parenchymal neoplasms (true pinealomas). A clinicopathological study of 28 tumours. Brain 102: 289–320
Herrmann H-D, Winkler D, Westphal M 1992 Treatment of tumors of the pineal region and posterior part of the third ventricle. Acta Neurochirurgica 116: 137–146
Higashi K, Katayama S, Orita T 1979 Pineal apoplexy. Journal of Neurology, Neurosurgery and Psychiatry 42: 1050–1053
Ho D M, Liu H-C 1992 Primary intracranial germ cell tumor: pathologic study of 51 patients. Cancer 70: 1577–1584
Hodges L C, Smith L J, Garrett A, Tate S 1992 Prevalence of glioblastoma multiforme in subjects prior to therapeutic radiation. J Neurosci Nurs 24: 79–83
Hoffman H 1987 Considerations and techniques in the pediatric age group. In: Apuzzo M (ed) Surgery of the third ventricle. Williams & Wilkins, Baltimore, pp 727–750
Hoffman H, Yoshida M, Becker L, Hendrick E, Humphreys R 1983 Pineal region tumors in childhood. Experience at the Hospital for Sick Children. In: Humphreys R (ed) Concepts in pediatric neurosurgery 4. S. Karger, Basel, pp 360–386
Hoffman H J, Yoshida M, Becker L E, Hendrick E B, Humphreys R P 1984 Experience with pineal region tumors in childhood. Neurology Research 6: 107–112
Hoffman H J, Otsubo H, Bruce E et al 1991 Intracranial germ-cell tumors in children. Journal of Neurosurgery 74: 545–551
Horowitz M B, Hall W A 1991 Central nervous system germinomas. Arch Neurologica 48: 652–657
Horrax G 1937 Extirpation of a huge pinealoma from a patient with pubertas praecox. Archives of Neurology and Psychiatry 37: 385–397
Hudgins R J, Rhyner P A, Edwards M S B 1987 Magnetic resonance imaging and management of pineal region dermoid. Surgical Neurology 27: 558–562
Hunt P, Davidson K, Ashcraft K 1977 Radiography of hereditary presacral teratoma. Radiology 122: 187–191
Jenkin D, Berry M, Chan H et al 1990 Pineal region germinomas in childhood treatment considerations. International Journal of Radiation Oncology Biology Physics 18: 541–545
Jenkin R D T, Simpson W J K, Keen C W 1978 Pineal and suprasellar germinomas. Results of radiation treatment. Journal of Neurosurgery 48: 99–107
Jennings M T, Gelman R, Hochberg F 1985 Intracranial germ-cell tumours: natural history and pathogenesis. Journal of Neurosurgery 63: 155–167
Jooma R, Kendall B E 1983 Diagnosis and management of pineal tumors. Journal of Neurosurgery 58: 654–665
Kersh C R, Constable W C, Eisert D R, Spaulding C A, Hahn S S, Jenrette J M, Marks R D 1988 Primary central nervous system germ cell tumors: effect of histologic confirmation on radiotherapy. Cancer 61: 2148–2152
Kobayashi S, Sugita K, Tanaka Y, Kyoshima K 1993 Infratentorial approach to the pineal region in the prone position: Concorde position. Journal of Neurosurgery 58: 141–143
Kobayashi T, Yoshida J, Ishiyama J, Noda S, Kito A, Kida Y 1989 Combination chemotherapy with cisplatin and etoposide for malignant intracranial germ-cell tumors. An experimental and clinical study. Journal of Neurosurgery 70: 676–681
Koide O, Watanabe Y, Sato K 1980 A pathological survey of intracranial germinoma and pinealoma in Japan. Cancer 45: 2119–2130
Korf H W, Klein D C, Zigler J S, Gery I, Schachenmayr W 1986 S-antigen-like immunoreactivity in a human pineocytoma. Acta Neuropathologica (Berl) 69: 165–167

Korf H W, Czerwionka M, Reiner J, Schachenmayr W, Schalken J J, De Grip W, Gery I 1987 Immunocytochemical evidence of molecular photoreceptor markers in cerebellar medulloblastomas. Cancer 60: 1763–1766

Korf H W, Bruce J A, Vistica B, Rollag M, Stein B M, Klein D C 1989 Immunoreactive S-antigen in cerebrospinal fluid: a marker of pineal parenchymal tumors? Journal of Neurosurgery 70: 682–687

Krabbe K H 1923 The pineal gland, especially in relation to the problem on its supposed significance in sexual development. Endocrinology 7: 379–414

Kraichoke S, Cosgrove M, Chadrasoma P T 1988 Granulomatous inflammation in pineal germinoma. American Journal of Surgical Pathology 12: 655–660

Krause F 1926 Operative Frielegung der Vierhugel, nebst Beobachtungen uber Hirndruck und Dekompression. Zentrabl Chir 53: 2812–2819

Kun L E, Tang T T, Sty J R, Camitta B M 1981 Primary cerebral germinoma and ventriculoperitoneal shunt metastasis. Cancer 48: 213–215

Lapras C, Patet J D 1987 Controversies, techniques and strategies for pineal tumor surgery. In: Apuzzo M L J (ed) Surgery of the third ventricle. Williams & Wilkins, Baltimore, pp 649–662

Lapras C, Patet J D, Mottolese C, Lapras C Jr 1987 Direct surgery of pineal tumors: occipital-transtentorial approach. Progress in Experimental Tumor Research 30: 268–280

Legido A, Packer R J, Sutton L N, D'Angio G, Rorke L B, Bruce D A, Schut L 1988 Suprasellar germinomas in childhood. A reappraisal. Cancer 63: 340–344

Lesnick J E, Chayt K J, Bruce D A, Rorke L B, Trojanowski J, Savino P J, Schatz N J 1985 Familial pineoblastoma. Report of two cases. Journal of Neurosurgery 62: 930–932

Lesoin F, Cama A, Dhellemes P, Nuyts J P, Andreussi L, Jomin M, Vallee L 1987 Extraneural metastasis of a pineal tumor. Report of 3 cases and review of the literature. European Neurology 27: 55–61

Linstadt D, Wara W M, Edwards M S B, Hudgins R J, Sheline G E 1988 Radiotherapy of primary intracranial germinomas: the case against routine craniospinal irradiation. International Journal of Radiation Oncology Biology Physics 15: 291–297

Logothetis C J, Samuels M L, Selig D E, Dexeus F H, Johnson D E, Swanson D A, von Eschenbach A C 1985 Chemotherapy of extragonadal germ cell tumors. Journal of Clinical Oncology 3: 316–325

McComb J G, Apuzzo M L J 1988 The lateral decubitus position for the surgical approach to pineal location tumors. Concepts in Pediatric Neurosurgery 8: 186–199

McLeod D G, Taylor H G, Skoog S J, Knight R D, Dawson N A, Waxman J A 1988 Extragonadal germ cell tumors. Clinicopathologic findings and treatment experience in 12 patients. Cancer 61: 1187–1191

Manor R S, Bar-Ziv J, Tadmor R, Eisbruch A, Rechavi G 1990 Pineal germinoma with unilateral blindness. Seeding of germinoma cells with optic nerve sheath. Journal of Clinical Neurology and Ophthalmology 10: 239–243

Markesbery W R, Brooks W H, Milsow L, Mortara R H 1976 Ultrastructural study of the pineal germinoma in vivo and in vitro. Cancer 37: 327–337

Markesbery W R, Haugh R M, Young A B 1981 Ultrastructure of pineal parenchymal neoplasms. Acta Neuropathologica (Berl) 55: 145–149

Marshall A, Dayan A 1964 An immune reaction against seminomas, dysgerminomas, pinealomas and mediastinal tumours of similar histological appearance. Lancet 2: 1102–1104

Masuzawa T, Shimabukuro H, Nakahara N, Iwasa H, Sato F 1986 Germ cell tumors (germinoma and yolk sac tumor) in unusual sites in the brain. Clinical Neuropathology 5: 190–202

Matsutani M, Takakura K, Sano K 1987 Primary intracranial germ cell tumors: pathology and treatment. Progress in Experimental Tumor Research 30: 307–312

Metcalfe S, Sikora K 1985 A new marker for testicular cancer. British Journal of Cancer 52: 127–129

Miles A, Tidmarsh S, Philbrick D, Shaw D 1985 Diagnostic potential of melatonin analysis in pineal tumors. New England Journal of Medicine 313: 329–330

Moser R, Backlund E 1984 Stereotactic techniques in the diagnosis and treatment of pineal region tumors. In: Neuwelt E (ed) Diagnosis and management of pineal region tumors. Williams & Wilkins, Baltimore, pp 236–253

Müller-Forell W, Schroth G, Egan P J 1988 MR imaging in tumors of the pineal region. Neuroradiology 30: 224–231

Murphree A, Benedict W 1984 Retinoblastoma: Clues to human oncogenesis. Science 223: 1028–1033

Naganuma H, Inoue H, Misumi S, Nakamura M, Tamura M 1984 Intracranial germ-cell tumors. Immunohistochemical study of three autopsy cases. Journal of Neurosurgery 61: 931–937

Nagao S, Kuyama H, Murota T, Suga M, Tanimoto T, Kawauchi M, Nishimoto A 1988 Surgical approaches to pineal tumors: complications and outcome. Neurol Med Chir 28: 779–785

Nazzaro J M, Shults W T, Neuwelt E A 1992 Neuro-ophthalmological function of patients with pineal region tumors approached transtentorially in the semisitting position. Journal of Neurosurgery 76: 746–751

Neuwelt E A 1985 An update on the surgical treatment of malignant pineal region tumors. Clinical Neurosurgery 32: 397–428

Neuwelt E, Smith R 1979 Presence of lymphocyte membrane surface markers on "small cells" in a pineal germinoma. Annals of Neurology 6: 133–136

Neuwelt E A, Glasberg M, Frenkel E, Clark W K 1979 Malignant pineal region tumors. Journal of Neurosurgery 51: 597–607

Neuwelt E, Frenkel E, Smith R 1980 Suprasellar germinomas (ectopic pinealomas): Aspects of immunological characterization and successful chemotherapeutic responses in recurrent disease. Neurosurgery 7: 352–358

Nighoghossian N, Confavreaux C, Sassolas G, Boisson D, Vighetto A, Aimard G, Trillet M 1988 Insuffisance hypothalamique après irradiation démence tardive, subaigue et curable. Rev Neurol (Paris) 144: 215–218

Noell K, Herskovic A 1985 Principles of radiotherapy of CNS tumors. In: Wilkins R, Rengachary S (eds) Neurosurgery, vol 1. McGraw-Hill, New York, pp 1084–1095

Ogata M, Yamashita T, Ishikawa T et al 1964 Report on treatment results on ectopic pinealoma apparently arising from septum pellucidum. No To Shinkei 16: 615–618

Ojeda V J , Ohama E, English D R 1987 Pineal neoplasms and third-ventricular teratomas in Niigata (Japan) and Western Australia. A comparative study of their incidence and clinicopathological features. Medical Journal of Australia (Sydney) 146: 357–359

Ono N, Takeda F, Uki J, Zama A, Hayashi Y, Sampi K 1982 A suprasellar embryonal carcinoma producing alpha-fetoprotein and human chorionic gonadotropin; treated with combined chemotherapy followed by radiotherapy. Surgical Neurology 18: 435–443

Packer R, Sutton L N, Rosenstock J G et al 1984a Pineal region tumors of childhood. Pediatrics 74: 97–101

Packer R J, Sutton L N, Rorke L B et al 1984b Intracranial embryonal cell carcinoma. Cancer 54: 520–524

Page R, Doshi B, Sharr M 1986 Primary intracranial choriocarcinoma. Journal of Neurology, Neurosurgery and Psychiatry 49: 93–95

Parinaud H 1886 Paralysis of the movement of convergence of the eyes. Brain 9: 330–341

Patel S R, Buckner J C, Smithson W A, Scheithauer B W, Groover R V 1992 Cisplatin-based chemotherapy in primary central nervous system germ cell tumors. Journal of Neuro-Oncology 12: 47–52

Pecker J, Scarabin J-M, Vallee B, Brucher J-M 1979 Treatment in tumors of the pineal region: value of stereotaxic biopsy. Surgical Neurology 12: 341–348

Pendl G 1985 Case material. In: Pendl G (ed) Pineal and midbrain lesions. Springer-Verlag, Wien, pp 128–207

Peragut J C, Dupard T, Graziani N, Sedan R 1987 De la prévention des risques de la biopsie stéréotaxique de certaines tumeurs de la région pinéale: a propos de 3 observations. Neurochirurgie 33: 23–27

Perentes E, Rubinstein L J, Herman M D, Donoso L A 1986 S-antigen immunoreactivity in human pineal glands and pineal parenchymal tumors. A monoclonal antibody study. Acta Neuropathologica (Berlin) 71: 224–227

Pfletschinger J, Olive D, Czorny A, Marchal A-L, Hoeffel J-C, Schmitt M, Brasse F 1986 Metastases peritoneales d'un pinealoblastome chez une patiente porteuse d'une derivation ventriculo-peritoneale. Pediatritrie 41: 231–236

Pinkerton C R, Pritchard J, Spitz L 1986 High complete response rate in children with advanced germ cell tumors using cisplatin-containing combination chemotherapy. Journal of Clinical Oncology 4: 194–199

Pluchino F, Broggi G, Fornari M, Franzini A, Solero C L, Allegranza A 1989 Surgical approach to pineal tumors. Acta Neurochirurgica 96: 26–31

Poppen J L 1966 The right occipital approach to a pinealoma. Journal of Neurosurgery 25: 706–710

Posner M, Horrax G 1946 Eye signs in pineal tumors. Journal of Neurosurgery 3: 15–24

Preissig S, Smith M, Huntington H 1979 Rhabdomyosarcoma arising in a pineal teratoma. Cancer 44: 281–284

Prioleau G, Wilson C 1976 Endodermal sinus tumor of the pineal region. Cancer 38: 2489–2493

Rao Y, Medini E, Haselow R, Jones T, Levitt S 1981 Pineal and ectopic pineal tumors: the role of radiation therapy. Cancer 48: 708–713

Reid W S, Clark W K 1978 Comparison of the infratentorial and transtentorial approaches to the pineal region. Neurosurgery 3: 1–8

Rich T, Cassady J, Strand R, Winston K 1985 Radiation therapy for tumors of the pineal region. Cancer 55: 932–940

Rippe J D, Boyko O B, Friedman H S, Oakes W J, Schold S C Jr, DeLong G R, Meisler W J 1990 Gd-DTPA-enhanced MR imaging of leptomeningeal spread of primary intracranial CNS tumor in children. AJNR 11: 329–332

Rodrigues M M, Bardenstein D S, Donoso L A, Rajagopalan S, Brownstein S 1987 An immunohistopathologic study of trilateral retinoblastoma. American Journal of Ophthalmology 103: 776–781

Rosenfeld J V, Murphy M A, Chow C W 1990 Implantation metastasis of pineoblastoma after stereotactic biopsy. Journal of Neurosurgery 73: 287–290

Rout D, Sharma A, Radhakrishnan V V, Rao V R K 1984 Exploration of the pineal region: observations and results. Surgical Neurology 21: 135–140

Rowland J H, Glidewell O J, Sibley R F et al 1984 Effects of different forms of central nervous system prophylaxis on neuropsychologic function in childhood leukemia. Journal of Clinical Oncology 2: 1327–1335

Rubery E, Wheeler T 1980 Metastases outside of the central nervous system from a presumed pineal germinoma. Case report. Journal of Neurosurgery 53: 562–565

Rubinstein L J 1981 Cytogenesis and differentiation of pineal neoplasms. Human Pathology 12: 441–448

Rubinstein L J 1985 Embryonal central neuroepithelial tumors and their differentiating potential. A cytogenetic view of a complex neuro-oncological problem. Journal of Neurosurgery 62: 795–805

Russell D S, Rubinstein L J 1989a Tumors and tumor-like lesions of maldevelopmental origin. In: Russell D S, Rubinstein L J (ed) Pathology of tumors of the nervous system. Williams & Wilkins, Baltimore, pp 664–765

Russell D S, Rubinstein L J 1989b Tumors of specialized tissues of central neuroepithelial origin. In: Russell D S, Rubinstein L J (eds) Pathology of tumors of the nervous system. Williams & Wilkins, Baltimore, pp 351–420

Sakai N, Yamada H, Andoh T, Hirata T, Shimizu K, Shinoda J 1988 Primary intracranial germ-cell tumors. A retrospective analysis with special reference to long-term results of treatments and the behavior of rare types of tumors. Acta Oncologica 27: 43–50

Salazar O M, Castro-Vita H, Bakos R S, Feldstein M L, Keller B, Rubin P 1979 Radiation therapy for tumors of the pineal region. International Journal of Radiation Oncology Biology Physics 5: 491–499

Sano K 1976a Diagnosis and treatment of tumors in the pineal region. Acta Neurochirurgica 34: 153–157

Sano K 1976b Pinealoma in children. Child's Brain 2: 67–72

Sano K 1984 Pineal region tumors: problems in pathology and treatment. Clinical Neurosurgery 30: 59–89

Sano K 1987 Pineal region and posterior third ventricular tumors: a surgical overview. In: Apuzzo M (ed) Surgery of the third ventricle. Williams & Wilkins, Baltimore, pp 663–683

Sano K, Matsutani M 1981 Pinealoma (germinoma) treated by direct surgery and postoperative irradiation. Child's Brain 8: 81–97

Sawaya R, Hawley D K, Tobler W D, Tew J M Jr, Chambers A A 1990 Pineal and third ventricular tumors. In: Youmans J (ed) Neurological surgery. W B Saunders, Philadelphia, pp 3171–3203

Schild S E, Scheithauer B W, Schomberg P J et al 1993 Pineal parenchymal tumors: clinical, pathologic, and therapeutic aspects. Cancer 72: 870–880

Schoenberg B, Christine B, Whisnant J 1976 The descriptive epidemiology of primary intracranial neoplasms: the Connecticut experience. American Journal of Epidemiology 104: 499–510

Shibamoto Y, Abe M, Yamashita J, Takahashi M, Hiraoka M, Ono K, Tsutsui K 1988 Treatment results of intracranial germinoma as a function of irradiated volume. International Journal of Radiation Oncology Biology Physics 15: 285–290

Shinoda J, Yamada H, Sakai N, Ando T, Hirata T, Miwa Y 1988 Placental alkaline phosphatase as a tumor marker for primary intracranial germinoma. Journal of Neurosurgery 68: 710–720

Shokry A, Janzer R C, Von Hochstetter A R, Yasargil M G, Hediger C 1985 Primary intracranial germ-cell tumors. A clinicopathological study of 14 cases. Journal of Neurosurgery 62: 826–830

Siegal T, Pfeffer M R, Catane R, Sulkes A, Gomori M J, Fuks Z 1983 Successful chemotherapy of recurrent intracranial germinoma with spinal metastases. Neurology 33: 631–633

Smirniotopoulos J G, Rushing E J, Mena H 1992 Pineal region masses: differential diagnosis. Radiographics 12: 577–596

Stachura I, Mendelow H 1980 Endodermal sinus tumor originating in the region of the pineal gland. Cancer 45: 2131–2137

Stefanko S Z, Talerman A, Mackay W M, Vuzevski V D 1979 Infundibular germinoma. Acta Neurochirurgica (Wien) 50: 71–78

Stein B M 1971 The infratentorial supracerebellar approach to pineal lesions. Journal of Neurosurgery 35: 197–202

Stein B M 1979 Surgical treatment of pineal region tumors. Clinical Neurosurgery 26: 490–510

Stein B M, Bruce J N 1992 Surgical management of pineal region tumors. Williams & Wilkins, Baltimore, pp 509–532

Steinbok P, Dolmen C, Kaan K 1977 Pineocytomas presenting as subarachnoid hemorrhage. Report of 2 cases. Journal of Neurosurgery 47: 776–780

Stowell R, Sachs E, Russell W 1945 Primary intracranial chorioepithelioma with metastases to lung. American Journal of Pathology 21: 787–801

Sugiyama K, Uozumi T, Kiya K et al 1992 Intracranial germ-cell tumor with synchronous lesions in the pineal and suprasellar regions: report of six cases and review of the literature. Surgical Neurology 38: 114–120

Sung D I, Harisiadis L, Chang C H 1978 Midline pineal tumors and suprasellar germinomas: highly curable by irradiation. Radiology 128: 745–751

Suzuki J, Iwabuchi T 1965 Surgical removal of pineal tumors (pinealomas and teratomas). Experience in a series of 19 cases. Journal of Neurosurgery 23: 565–571

Suzuki Y, Tanaka R 1980 Carcinoembryonic antigen in patients with intracranial tumors. Journal of Neurosurgery 53: 355–360

Takakura K 1985 Intracranial germ cell tumors. Clinical Neurosurgery 32: 429–444

Takei Y, Pearl G S 1981 Ultrastructural study of intracranial yolk sac tumor: with special reference to oncologic phylogeny of germ cell tumors. Cancer 48: 2038–2046

Takeuchi J, Handa H, Nagata I 1978 Suprasellar germinoma. Journal of Neurosurgery 49: 41–48

Tamarkin L, Danforth D, Lichter A 1982 Decreased nocturnal plasma melatonin peak in patients with estrogen positive breast cancer. Science 216: 1003–1005

Tanaka R, Ueki K 1979 Germinomas in the cerebral hemisphere. Surgical Neurology 12: 239–241

Tavcar D, Robboy S J, Chapman P 1980 Endodermal sinus tumor of the pineal region. Cancer 45: 2646–2651

Tien R D, Barkovich A J, Edwards M S B 1990 M.R. Imaging of pineal tumors. AJNR 11: 557–565
Tompkins V, Haymaker W, Campbell E 1950 Metastatic pineal tumors. A clinicopathological report of two cases. Journal of Neurosurgery 7: 159–169
Ueki K, Tanaka R 1980 Treatment and prognoses of pineal tumors — experience of 110 cases. Neurol Med Chir 20: 1–26
Uematsu Y, Tsuura Y, Miyamoto K, Itakura T, Hayashi S, Komai N 1992 The recurrence of primary intracranial germinomas. Special reference to germinoma with STGC (syncytiotrophoblastic giant cell). Journal of Neuro-Oncology 13: 247–256
Vaquero J, Ramiro J, Martinez R, Coca S, Bravo G 1990 Clinicopathological experience with pineocytomas: report of five surgically treated cases. Neurosurgery 27: 612–619
Vaughan G 1984 Melatonin in humans. Pineal Research Review 2: 141–201
Ventureyra E C G 1981 Pineal region: surgical management of tumors and vascular malformations. Surgical Neurology 16: 77–84
Vorkapic P, Waldhauser F, Bruckner R, Biegelmayer C, Schmidbauer M, Pendl G 1987 Serum melatonin levels: a new neurodiagnostic tool in pineal region tumors? Neurosurgery 21: 817–824
Waga S, Handa H, Yamashita J 1979 Intracranial germinomas: treatment and results. Surgical Neurology II: 167–172
Wakai W, Segawa H, Kithara S, Asano T, Sano K, Ogihara R, Tomita S 1980 Teratoma in the pineal region in two brothers. Case reports. Journal of Neurosurgery 53: 239–243
Wara W M, Jenkin R T D, Evans A et al 1979 Tumors of the pineal and suprasellar region: Children's cancer study group treatment results 1960–1975. Cancer 43: 698–701
Wilson E R, Takei Y, Bikoff W T, O'Brien M S, Tindall G T, Boehm W M 1979 Abdominal metastases of primary intracranial yolk sac tumors through ventriculoperitoneal shunts: report of three cases. Neurosurgery 5: 356–364
Wood J H, Zimmerman R A, Bruce D A, Bilaniuk L T, Norris D G, Schut L 1981 Assessment and management of pineal-region and related tumors. Surgical Neurology 16: 192–210
Wurtman R J, Kammer H 1966 Melatonin synthesis by an ectopic pinealoma. New England Journal of Medicine 274: 1233–1237
Yoshida J, Sugita K, Kobayashi T et al 1993 Prognosis of intracranial germ cell tumours: effectiveness of chemotherapy with cisplatin and etoposide (CDDP and VP-16). Acta Neurochirurgica (Wien) 120: 111–117
Zee C-S, Segall H, Apuzzo M, Destian S, Colletti P, Ahmadi J, Clark C 1991 MR imaging of pineal region neoplasms. Journal of Computer Assisted Tomography 15: 56–63
Zimmerman R 1985 Pineal region masses: Radiology. In: Wilkins R, Rengachary S (eds) Neurosurgery, vol 1. McGraw-Hill, New York, pp 680–686
Zimmerman R A, Bilaniuk L T 1982 Age-related incidence of pineal calcification detected by computed tomography. Neuroradiology 142: 659–662
Zondek H, Kaatz A, Unger H 1953 Precocious puberty and choriepithelioma of the pineal gland with report of a case. Journal of Endocrinology 10: 12–16

PART VI

Pituitary tumors

39. Pituitary tumors

Kamal Thapar Edward R. Laws Jr.

THE PITUITARY GLAND: REGIONAL ANATOMY AND PHYSIOLOGY

One of the most clinically satisfying aspects of pituitary oncology relates to the precision with which the symptomatology localizes the lesion and the predictable correlations which exist between endocrinologic function, clinical phenotype, and tumor morphology. Recognition of these neurologic, endocrinologic, and pathologic correlates is predicated on some appreciation of the normal anatomic and physiologic relationships of the pituitary.

The pituitary gland is a composite neuroendocrine structure consisting of two lobes, each differing in embryologic origin, structure, function, and pathologic processes. The larger anterior lobe, or adenohypophysis, is the site of meticulously regulated hormone secretion and synthesis, and is also the primary site of clinically significant pathology. It consists of a somewhat regimented topological arrangement of five distinct cell types, each engaged in the production of a different hormonal product. These five cell types are categorized as being somatotrophs, lactotrophs, corticotrophs, thyrotrophs, and gonadotrophs, and are distinguished functionally in their ability to secrete growth hormone (GH), prolactin (PRL), corticotrophin (ACTH), thyroid-stimulating hormone (TSH), and gonadotropins — luteinizing hormone (LH) and follicle-stimulating hormone (FSH), respectively. The secretory and proliferative capabilities of these cells are governed by a precise balance between hypothalamic trophic influences and negative feedback effects imposed by target organ hormones. Although susceptibilities vary, neoplastic transformation can, in a multistep, multicausal fashion, occur in any one of these cell types. The resulting adenoma retains the secretory capability, morphologic characteristics, and nomenclature of the cell of origin.

In addition to the five distinct hormonally active cell populations described above, a sixth cell type is believed to be randomly dispersed in the normal pituitary. Known as null cells, these are hormonally inactive cells whose functional contribution to the pituitary remains obscure. They too are susceptible to neoplastic transformation, giving rise to a commonly occurring class of pituitary tumors known as null cell adenomas. As null cells do not produce measurable amounts of any known hormonal product, these cells and their respective tumors are designated as nonfunctioning (see Tables 39.1 and 39.2.)

The posterior pituitary (neurohypophysis) is an extension of the CNS, and is composed of interlacing nerve fibers and specialized glial elements known as pituicytes. Vasopressin and oxytocin are the primary hormonal products released by the posterior pituitary. The former is the

Table 39.1 Anterior pituitary cell types: their hormonal, clinical, and neoplastic correlates (After Kovacs & Horvath, 1986)

Cell type	Peptide/hormone product	Clinical syndrome	Tumor type (Ultrastructural diagnosis)
Somatotroph	Growth hormone	Acromegaly/gigantism	Sparsely granulated GH cell adenoma Densely granulated GH cell adenoma
Lactotroph	Prolactin	Amenorrhea/galactorrhea	Sparsely granulated PRL cell adenoma Densely granulated PRL cell adenoma (rare)
Somatotroph/Lactotroph	Growth hormone and prolactin	Acromegaly + hyperprolactinemia Acromegaly + hyperprolactinemia Amenorrhea/galactorrhea ± acromegaly	Mixed GH-PRL adenoma Mammosomatotroph adenoma Acidophil stem cell adenoma
Corticotroph	ACTH, POMC, β-LPH, MSH	Cushing's disease, Nelson's syndrome	Densely granulated ACTH cell adenoma Sparsely granulated ACTH cell adenoma (rare)
Gonadotroph	FSH, LH, α-subunit	Hypopituitarism	Gonadotroph adenoma
Thyrotroph	TSH, α-subunit	Hyperthyroidism, hypopituitarism	Thyrotroph adenoma
Null cell (?)	none	Hypopituitarism	Null cell adenoma Oncocytoma

Table 39.2 Less common pituitary tumor types

Tumor type	Immunocytochemical profile	Clinical syndrome
Plurihormonal adenomas	Any combination of GH, PRL TSH, ACTH, LH, FSH, or α-subunit	Variable: acromegaly or endocrine inactive sellar mass, rarely other hypersecretory states
'Silent' adenomas	ACTH or GH	Endocrine-inactive sellar mass (usually with hypopituitarism)
Pituitary carcinoma	GH, PRL, ACTH, TSH, LH, FSH, or no hormonal product	Hypersecretory state or endocrine-inactive sellar mass (with demonstrated craniospinal and/or systemic metastases)

essential regulator of water and osmolar homeostasis, and the latter is important during labor and lactation. Although the posterior pituitary is occasionally the site of metastatic tumors, it is rarely the site of clinically significant primary tumors.

PITUITARY ADENOMAS: GENERAL FEATURES

Epidemiology

Pituitary adenomas are common lesions, accounting for up to 15% of all primary intracranial neoplasms treated surgically (Cushing 1912). Depending on the population studied, their reported annual incidence ranges from 1–14.7 per 100 000 population (Annegers et al 1978). By this measure, pituitary adenomas represent the third most common primary intracranial neoplasm encountered in neurosurgical practice, following gliomas and meningiomas. It is quite likely that these figures considerably under-represent the true incidence of pituitary adenomas, as their prevalence in several unselected autopsy series approaches 25% (Costello et al 1936). From this perspective, adenomatous transformation in the pituitary appears to be a very common event, although one which does not always become clinically apparent. There is a tendency for pituitary tumors to become more common with age, with the highest incidence occurring between the third and sixth decades. A female preponderance exists in younger patients, with women of childbearing years being at greatest risk for tumor development. The basis for this assessment of increased susceptibility in women is related to the frequency of prolactinoma in women aged 18–35. Attempts to implicate oral contraceptive use as a potential predisposing or causative factor in pituitary tumorigenesis have been largely dismissed by appropriate case-controlled studies (Coulam et al 1981). Some contend that the increased frequency of pituitary tumors in premenopausal women is more apparent than real, as manifestations of pituitary dysfunction are more conspicuous and of greater diagnostic sensitivity in women than in men.

Etiology and pathogenesis

Despite exhaustive laboratory and epidemiologic studies, no definitive environmental, pharmacologic or physiologic agent has been identified as being causative for pituitary tumorigenesis. A single known genetic predisposition for pituitary tumors exists in the form of hereditary multiple endocrine neoplasia type 1 syndrome (MEN I). This is an autosomal dominant condition characterized by the spontaneous and simultaneous development of tumors of the pituitary, pancreas islet cells and parathyroid glands. Pituitary tumors develop in approximately 25% of these MEN I patients, and most commonly occur as macroadenomas associated with GH and/or PRL hypersecretion. The nature of this genetic defect has been recently defined on a molecular basis, and involves allelic loss of a tumor suppressor gene at the 11q13 locus. Subsequent mutation, deactivation or loss of remaining normal alleles initiates a series of tumor promoting events, ultimately leading to the development of the MEN I syndrome.

Only 3% of surgically resected pituitary adenomas have a hereditary basis (in the context of MEN I). The vast majority of pituitary tumors are therefore acquired lesions, and seemingly without well-defined etiologic correlates. Current concepts of pituitary tumorigenesis suggest that most pituitary tumors arise as monoclonal expansions of a single adenohypophyseal cell that has sustained a somatic mutation in a multistep, multicausal fashion (Alexander et al 1990, Jacoby et al 1990). The oncogenic process appears to be divided into an initiation phase and a maintenance phase. A number of oncogenes/proto-oncogenes have been implicated as initiators of this process (*c-myc, v-fos, N-ras,* p53 gene, as well as the *hst* and *gsp* oncogenes). Of these, the *gsp* oncogene has received the greatest attention, as oncogenic versions of this gene are found in up to 40% of GH-secreting adenomas (Landis et al 1990). Once initiated, pituitary tumors are thought to be maintained by dysregulated autocrine and paracrine influences mediated by a number of growth factors and hypothalamic trophic influences.

Clinical presentation

Pituitary tumors are recognized clinically by one or more of three highly predictable presentation patterns: symptoms of pituitary hypersecretion, symptoms of pituitary hyposecretion, or neurologic symptoms of a sellar mass. In about 70% of cases, the clinical picture is dominated by features of anterior pituitary hypersecretion resulting in a characteristic hypersecretory syndrome (Zervas & Martin 1980, Klibanski & Zervas 1991). Acromegaly, Cushing's disease, amenorrhea-galactorrhea syndrome and, rarely, secondary hyperthyroidism represent the classical paradigms of GH, ACTH, PRL, and TSH hypersecretion, respectively. It is important to recognize that hyperprolactinemia is not always a feature specific to PRL-producing adenomas. Moderate hyperprolactinemia (< 150–200 ng per milliliter) can occur with any of a variety of structural lesions involving the sellar region. This phenomenon, frequently referred to as the 'stalk section effect', is the result of compressive or destructive lesions involving the hypothalamus or pituitary stalk. Prolactin secretion is under the inhibitory control of various hypothalamic 'prolactin inhibitory factors' of which dopamine is the most important. Dopamine released from the hypothalamus descends via the portal vessels to the anterior lobe, where it inhibits the release of PRL by normal lactotrophs. Processes which impair the hypothalamic release of dopamine (compressive or destructive hypothalamic lesions), or those impairing its adenohypophyseal transfer (compressive or destructive lesions of the pituitary stalk), place pituitary lactotrophs in a disinhibited state. Moderate degrees of hyperprolactinemia are thus generated. As a rule, PRL levels greater than 150 ng/ml are generally the result of a PRL producing tumor; lesser elevations may also be due to a small PRL producing adenoma, but may also be the result of other types of pituitary adenoma, or any of a variety of other mass, inflammatory, or infiltrative lesions involving the sellar region. Even low grade PRL elevations may be symptomatic, manifesting as hypogonadism and/or galactrorrhea in both women and men. Pituitary tumors can manifest with symptoms of partial or total hypopituitarism (fatigue, weakness, hypogonadism, regression of secondary sexual characteristics, hypothyroidism). This usually occurs insidiously in association with pituitary macroadenomas which have achieved sufficient size to compress and impair the secretory capability of the adjacent nontumorous pituitary. In the face of chronic and progressive compression, the various secretory elements of the pituitary differ in their functional reserve. The gonadotrophs are most vulnerable, and are usually affected first, followed sequentially by thyrotrophs and somatotrophs, with corticotrophs demonstrating the greatest functional resilience. Pituitary insufficiency can also occur acutely in the context of pituitary apoplexy, where sudden intratumoral hemorrhage or infarction can occasionally produce the life-threatening combination of acute hypopituitarism and an expanding intracranial mass (Ebersold et al 1983).

A third pattern of presentation is one dominated by neurologic symptomatology, either in isolation or coexisting with one or more of the endocrinologic perturbations described above. As alluded to earlier, a progressively enlarging pituitary mass will generate a constellation of neurologic signs and symptoms, depending on its growth trajectory and which of the critical neural structures in the vicinity have been compromised. Headache may be an early finding and is attributed to stretching of the enveloping dura or diaphragma sellae. The single most common objective neurologic feature, however, is visual loss, and relates to suprasellar extension of the tumor, with compression of the optic nerves and chiasm. The classic and most common pattern of visual loss is that of a bitemporal hemianopic field deficit, often in association with diminished visual acuity. Large pituitary adenomas can encroach upon the hypothalamus, causing alterations of sleep, alertness, behavior, eating and emotion. These tumors can extend into the region of the third ventricle, where obstruction to effluent CSF flow can result in obstructive hydrocephalus. The tumor extends laterally into the region of the cavernous sinus quite commonly. With progressive cavernous sinus invasion, the cranial nerves transiting the sinus can occasionally become affected. In this regard, the onset of ptosis, facial pain or sensory changes, and diplopia suggests involvement of cranial nerves III, V, and III, IV or VI respectively. Finally, some pituitary adenomas can assume gigantic proportions, extending well into the anterior, middle and occasionally posterior cranial fossae, where they can produce the full spectrum of focal neurologic signs and symptoms. In such circumstances, tumor origin may not be immediately apparent. Large temporal lobe extension may be associated with partial complex seizures.

Classification

Although pituitary tumors have been subject to a variety of classification schemes, only two have proven consistently informative. The first is a radiologic classification, based on tumor size and geometry. The second is a pathologic classification based on the immunohistochemical character, ultrastructural morphology and cytogenesis of the tumor. Each of these classification schemes therefore addresses different, but complementary, aspects of the clinical problem. As both of these classifications furnish practical, pathologic and conceptual data highly relevant to the understanding and management of pituitary tumors, both schemes will be reviewed.

Known as the Hardy classification, the radiologic classification distinguishes tumors on the basis of size and gross pathoanatomic features (Hardy 1969). Tumors are classified according to size, with lesions less than 10 mm recognized as microadenomas, and those greater than 10 mm designated as macroadenomas. On the basis of the sellar radiology, 5 classes of tumors are identified.

Microadenomas are designated as being either grade 0 or grade I tumors, depending on whether the sella appears normal, or whether minor focal sellar changes are present. Macroadenomas causing diffuse sellar enlargement, focal sellar erosion and extensive sellar and skull base destruction are referred to as grade II, grade III, and grade IV respectively. The macroadenomas are further subclassified by the degree of suprasellar extension. The Hardy classification has proven useful in surgical planning, identifying operative risk, and determining the potential for surgical 'cure' (Fig. 39.1).

Regardless of the presence or nature of secretory capabilities, all pituitary tumors are morphologically similar at the light microscopic level. Although they are not truly encapsulated, they are delineated from the surrounding normal adenohypophysis by a reticulin pseudocapsule. Histologically, they lack the septated acinar structure of the normal pituitary, and appear as a uniform population of polygonal cells arranged in sheets, cords or nests.

SELLA TURCICA RADIOLOGICAL CLASSIFICATION
Gr 0 (Normal)
Gr I
Gr II
Gr III
Gr IV
A

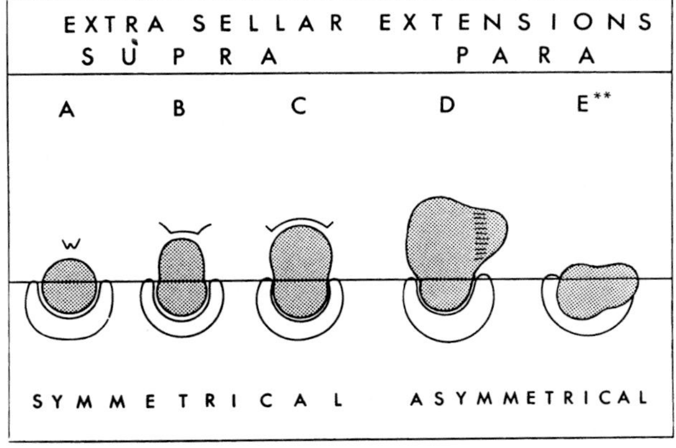

Fig. 39.1 Radiologic classification proposed by Jules Hardy: **A**, grade of sellar involvement; **B**, stage of extrasellar extension. Reproduced from Hardy (1969) with permission.

Nuclear pleomorphism and mitotic figures can be seen to a variable degree. By convention, pituitary tumors have been classified pathologically according to cytoplasmic staining affinities as determined by the application of a few simple histologic stains. Under such a scheme, three traditional morphologic entities emerged: *acidophilic*, *basophilic* and *chromophobic*. The acidophilic adenomas were assumed to be the exclusive pathologic substrate for acromegaly. The basophilic adenomas were thought to be specifically causative of Cushing's disease. The chromophobic category was reserved for those tumors which failed to stain with acidic or basic dyes, and were therefore assumed to be hormonally inactive. Although the simplicity of this method engendered its appeal for many years, the evolution of immunohistochemical and ultrastructural methods have demonstrated that cytoplasmic staining affinities correlate poorly with reliable cell type recognition and secretory activity. The current standard for classifying pituitary tumors relies on immunohistochemistry and electron microscopy to categorize tumors on the basis of hormonal content, ultrastructural morphology and cytogenesis (Kovacs & Horvath 1986, Hsu et al 1993). This functional classification, assembled by Kovacs & Horvath, identifies 10 principal anterior pituitary tumor types, each with its own structural, functional and biologic character (Table 39.1, 39.2).

GENERAL PRINCIPLES OF DIAGNOSIS AND THERAPY FOR PITUITARY TUMORS

Because pituitary tumors are clinically and endocrinologically heterogeneous, diagnostic parameters, therapeutic options and long-term outcome show individual variation amongst each of the major types. These practical differences not withstanding, there are some common diagnostic and therapeutic principles applicable to all pituitary tumors (Abboud & Laws 1979).

Diagnosis

Pituitary tumors represent a clinical problem which stands at the interface of a number of medical and surgical disciplines. The evaluation of patients suspected of having pituitary adenomas therefore rests on a comprehensive interdisciplinary effort. In the patient with endocrinologic and/or neurologic findings suggestive of a pituitary adenoma, the diagnostic process begins with a determination of an endocrinologic diagnosis and an anatomic diagnosis. Guided by findings in the history and physical examination, an endocrine diagnosis is reached by measuring pituitary and/or target organ hormones in basal and provoked states. These are sensitive indicators of disturbed pathophysiologic activity, and allow for differentiation of the various pituitary adenoma subtypes. A useful initial screening should include basal measurements of PRL,

Table 39.3 Relative frequency of different pituitary adenoma types treated by trans-sphenoidal microsurgery (1972–1993)

Tumor type	Number	%
Prolactinoma	771	34.2
Somatotroph adenoma	396	17.6
Corticotroph adenoma		15.4
–Cushing's Disease	289	
–Nelson's Syndrome	57	
Clinically non-functioning adenomas	717	31.8
–(Null cell, oncocytoma, plurihormonal)		
Miscellaneous pituitary adenomas	24	1.0
Total	2254	

GH, plasma cortisol, ACTH, LH/FSH, α-subunit thyroxine and TSH. This initial survey estimates the integrity of the various hypothalamic-pituitary-target organ axes, identifying states of relative excess or deficiency. Further provocative, dynamic and special hormonal assays may be required to precisely define a specific endocrinopathy. The relative incidence of various types of pituitary adenomas in our surgical series is presented in Table 39.3.

Anatomic diagnosis, once based on plain skull radiographs, is now routinely achieved with magnetic resonance imaging (MRI). High resolution MRI with gadolinium enhancement has virtually supplanted computerized tomography (CT) in the diagnosis of pituitary tumors. The superior resolution capabilities of MRI are particularly evident in cases of microadenoma, where lesions as small as 3 mm can be routinely detected. Although diagnostic sensitivity is generally less of an issue for macroadenomas, the merits of MRI for these larger tumors lie in its capacity to identify critical spatial relationships between the tumor and surrounding neurovascular structures. In this regard, the position of the carotid arteries, the status of the optic chiasm, the extent of supra- and parasellar tumor extension are of particular operative concern and are clearly delineated by MRI (Fig. 39.2).

Because visual compromise is a complicating feature of many pituitary tumors, a complete neuro-ophthalmologic evaluation is mandatory in all patients with visual complaints and in all patients with tumors that extend beyond the confines of the sella. Visual field deficits are formally recorded with either manual or automated perimetry. These determinations are frequently performed serially to document disease progression and responses to therapeutic intervention.

Treatment

Once the diagnosis of a pituitary adenoma has been established on clinical, biochemical and radiologic grounds, an assessment of therapeutic options is made. Therapy for pituitary tumors should be directed at the following goals:

1. Reversal of endocrinopathy and restoration of normal pituitary function

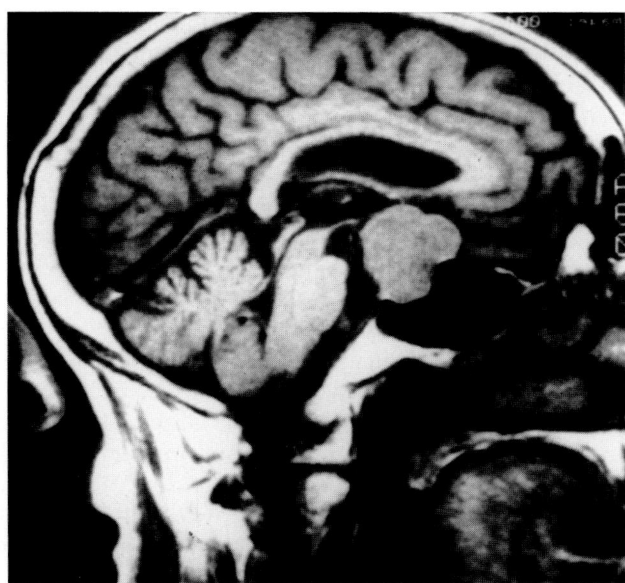

Fig. 39.2 MRI scan, sagittal view. Large, clinically nonfunctioning pituitary macroadenoma.

2. Removal of tumor mass and restoration of normal neurologic function.

Fortunately, absolute realization of these goals has become an increasingly feasible event, attributable to the evolution of microsurgical techniques, the development of receptor-mediated pharmacotherapy, and refinements in the delivery of radiation therapy. Each of these treatment modalities has specific merits and limitations which must be collectively considered and thoughtfully individualized to each pituitary tumor patient, to provide a program of comprehensive management (Wilson 1984).

Trans-sphenoidal microsurgery

Although there is some emerging latitude for the initial use of nonsurgical therapies in selected cases of pituitary adenoma, surgery remains the initial treatment of choice for the overwhelming majority of pituitary tumors. The increased efficacy and safety of pituitary surgery can be ascribed to the development of the trans-septal trans-sphenoidal microsurgical approach, which is the most direct and least traumatic corridor of surgical access to the pituitary (Laws 1977, 1980, Laws et al 1982b, Ciric et al 1983, Laws 1985, Niederhuber 1993). Currently, more than 95% of pituitary tumors are approached trans-sphenoidally, with conventional transcranial approaches reserved for the remaining few cases in which anatomic features of the sella or unusual intracranial tumor extensions limit trans-sphenoidal accessibility (MacCarty et al 1973). For the majority of pituitary microadenomas, and for many macroadenomas, trans-sphenoidal surgery alone is curative, obviating the need for adjuvant pharmacologic or radiation therapy. As precise definitions of 'cure' differ among the various hypersecretory syndromes, details of surgical efficacy are best discussed in the context of the individual tumor types. Complications from transsphenoidal surgery are uncommon (Laws & Kern 1976, Zervas 1984). Operative mortality and morbidity rates, as determined from several cumulative series, are 0.5% and 2.2% respectively. The nature of complications which occur reflect the critical nature of the operative field (Laws et al 1985b). The most devastating of these include traumatic or hemorrhagic hypothalamic injury resulting in coma and death. Equally severe are injuries or lacerations of the carotid arteries, resulting in cerebral hemorrhage or ischemia. Traction injuries, ischemia, or direct trauma to the optic nerve and chiasm can result in blindness. Transgression of the arachnoid membrane can result in cerebrospinal fluid rhinorrhea and predispose to meningitis. Fortunately such complications are rare and their occurrence can be minimized with attention to meticulous surgical technique. A relatively common and usually transient postoperative complication of pituitary surgery is diabetes insipidus (Laws et al 1980). This is the result of damage to the infundibulum or posterior pituitary gland, structures highly susceptible to transient functional injury in response to even the most modest surgical manipulation. The result is a state of relative vasopressin deficiency, characterized by the excretion of large amounts of dilute urine. If unrecognized, dehydration and hypernatremia may become extreme, even life-threatening. Appropriate therapy includes early recognition, careful fluid management, and the judicious use of synthetic vasopressin. The condition is very rarely permanent, and usually resolves by the tenth postoperative day. Some patients develop delayed postoperative hyponatremia, usually on the 5th to 7th postoperative day. This is usually attributed to SIADH, and it responds to fluid restriction and urea therapy when necessary.

Pharmacologic therapy

The observation that secretory activity of neoplastic pituitary cells does not entirely escape physiologic regulatory controls establishes the susceptibility to and therapeutic rationale for pharmacologic manipulation of these regulatory mechanisms as a form of medical therapy for pituitary adenomas. Two classes of pharmacologic agents have emerged as primary or adjuvant therapies for pituitary tumors: dopamine agonists and somatostatin analogs. Bromocriptine is the prototypical and most widely used dopamine agonist, which mediates its clinical effect by amplifying existing inhibitory dopaminergic hypothalamic-pituitary pathways. Dopamine is the native physiologic inhibitor of prolactin secretion. By saturating dopamine receptors on the tumor cell surface, bromocriptine effectively inhibits prolactin secretion. Its ability to normalize prolactin levels and to reduce tumor size has made this agent an effective alternative to surgical therapy for many prolactinomas. Bromocriptine is also effective, although to a lesser degree, in reducing GH levels in tumors associated with acromegaly.

With the discovery that GH secretion is physiologically inhibited by somatostatin, the potential therapeutic value of somatostatin in treating GH-secreting tumors was clearly recognized. Somatostatin analogs, which are biologically more stable than native somatostatin, have an evolving role in the management of tumors associated with acromegaly. Although the effectiveness of somatostatin analogs in reducing GH levels and tumor size has been affirmed, the durability of the response is uncertain. Therefore somatostatin analogs are not currently considered long-term alternatives to surgical therapy. At present, they are best viewed as important adjunctive therapy, reserved for those patients with persistent or recurrent postoperative disease.

Radiation therapy

Radiation therapy has traditionally had a major adjuvant role in the postoperative treatment of pituitary tumors. With the increasing effectiveness of surgical therapy and the increasing feasibility of adjuvant medical therapy, it is becoming increasingly difficult to define precisely the role of radiation in contemporary pituitary tumor management. The goal of radiation therapy is to prevent progression or recurrence of tumor growth. Probably the clearest indication for radiation therapy is the persistence or recurrence of a medically refractory hypersecretory state following surgery. For large nonfunctioning pituitary adenomas, postoperative radiation is also considered in cases of invasive or incompletely resected tumors. Complications of pituitary irradiation include delayed panhypopituitarism, cognitive impairment, optic nerve and temporal lobe radionecrosis, and the possibility of radiation-induced tumors. Conceptual and technical advances in radiation delivery have minimized the frequency of many of these complications; however, delayed panhypopituitarism is still a major concern. The increasing availability and accuracy of radiosurgery with stereotactically focused radiation should assist in the management of many difficult pituitary lesions.

ACROMEGALY AND GH-SECRETING ADENOMAS

Acromegaly is an insidiously progressive, physically disabling systemic affliction having the well-defined metabolic basis of pathologic growth hormone excess (Laws et al 1985c). Should this growth hormone excess manifest at an early age prior to long bone epiphyseal closure, gigantism is the result. So distinctive is the clinical syn-

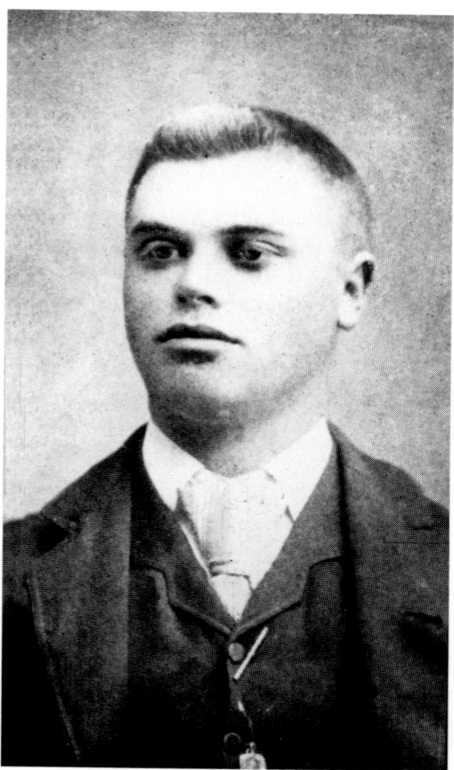

The patient some years before onset of symptoms.

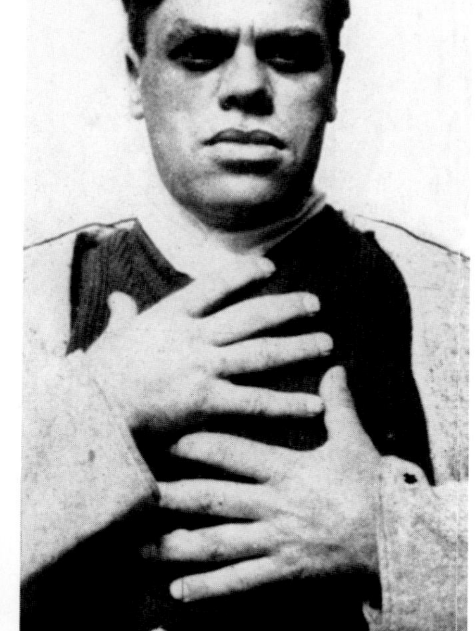

Condition on admission. (For comparison with Fig. 1.)

Fig. 39.3 Acromegaly. The first acromegalic patient operated upon by Harvey Cushing. Reproduced from Cushing (1909) with permission.

drome that acromegalics and related giants have been the subject of mythical reference in folklore and legend as keepers of great strength and power. This was rarely the case, particularly in the later debilitating stages of the disease when these individuals became freakish outcasts, often regarded with horror and ridicule (Fig. 39.3).

Most acromegalic patients reach medical attention between the third and fifth decades, although the disease may have been slowly progressive for many years prior to presentation. Focal enlargement of bones and soft tissues is apparent at characteristic body locations. The facial features become classically coarse, with frontal bossing, prognathism, dental malocclusion and macroglossia. There is broad spade-like enlargement of hands and feet. Bone density increases, and the hypertrophy of joints and cartilage leads to degenerative joint disease and debilitating spinal stenosis. Peripheral neuropathy in the form of carpal tunnel syndrome and other nerve entrapments produces paresthesias, a common presenting feature. Cardiac enlargement leads to congestive heart failure, which is further complicated by the hypertension commonly seen in these patients. Abnormalities of glucose metabolism are common, ranging from impaired glucose tolerance to insulin resistance and frank diabetes mellitus. Finally, depending on the tumor size, local mass effects can produce visual complaints and hypopituitarism (Cushing 1909).

Suspicion of acromegaly on historical and clinical grounds must be carefully validated with endocrine studies. Although elevations of serum GH levels are the hallmark of acromegaly, this study alone does not conclusively secure a diagnosis of acromegaly. Random elevations of GH occur in a variety of conditions including diabetes, renal failure, cirrhosis, malnutrition, and stress. The two most sensitive means to confirm a diagnosis of acromegaly are:

1. Demonstration of lack of suppression of GH levels following a glucose load
2. Elevations of somatomedin-C (IGF-1 levels).

Somatomedin-C, also known as insulin-like growth factor 1, is secreted under the influence of GH and is the principal mediator of the clinical effects seen in acromegaly. It is therefore an excellent indicator of active acromegaly for both initial diagnosis and postoperative surveillance of residual or recurrent disease.

An anatomic diagnosis is established with MRI scanning of the head (Fig. 39.4). This will localize all macroadenomas and approximately 90% of small intrasellar tumors. GH levels generally correlate well with the size,

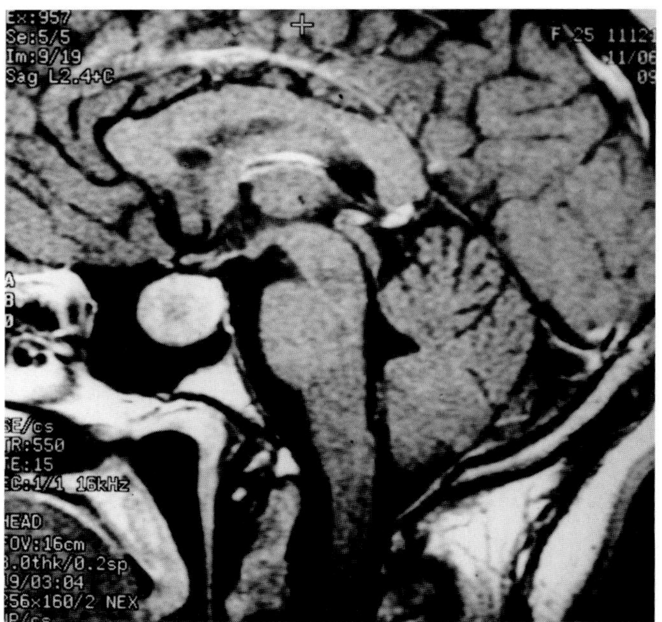

Fig. 39.4 MRI scan, sagittal view. Intrasellar pituitary macroadenoma associated with acromegaly.

invasiveness, and Hardy class of the tumor. With regard to anatomic diagnosis, the rare possibility of extrapituitary causes of acromegaly must always be considered. These include growth-hormone-releasing, hormone-producing adenomas associated with hypothalamic hamartomas, occasional pancreatic tumors, and carcinoid tumors of the lung and intestine. The growth-hormone-releasing hormone produced by these entities may also cause hyperplasia of pituitary somatotrophs with sellar changes mimicking that of a primary pituitary tumor.

Pure growth-hormone-producing tumors occur in two forms: the densely granulated GH adenoma and the sparsely granulated GH adenoma. Both occur with equal frequency, but the sparsely granulated variety is notorious for its larger size, invasive tendency, and overall more aggressive character (Fig. 39.5).

Of the three existing treatment modalities (medical, surgical, and radiation therapy), trans-sphenoidal surgery provides the most satisfactory results and is recommended for virtually all patients with active acromegaly. The other therapeutic options are used adjuvantly. Criteria for successful management or 'cure' include removal of tumor mass, resolution of acromegalic signs and symptoms,

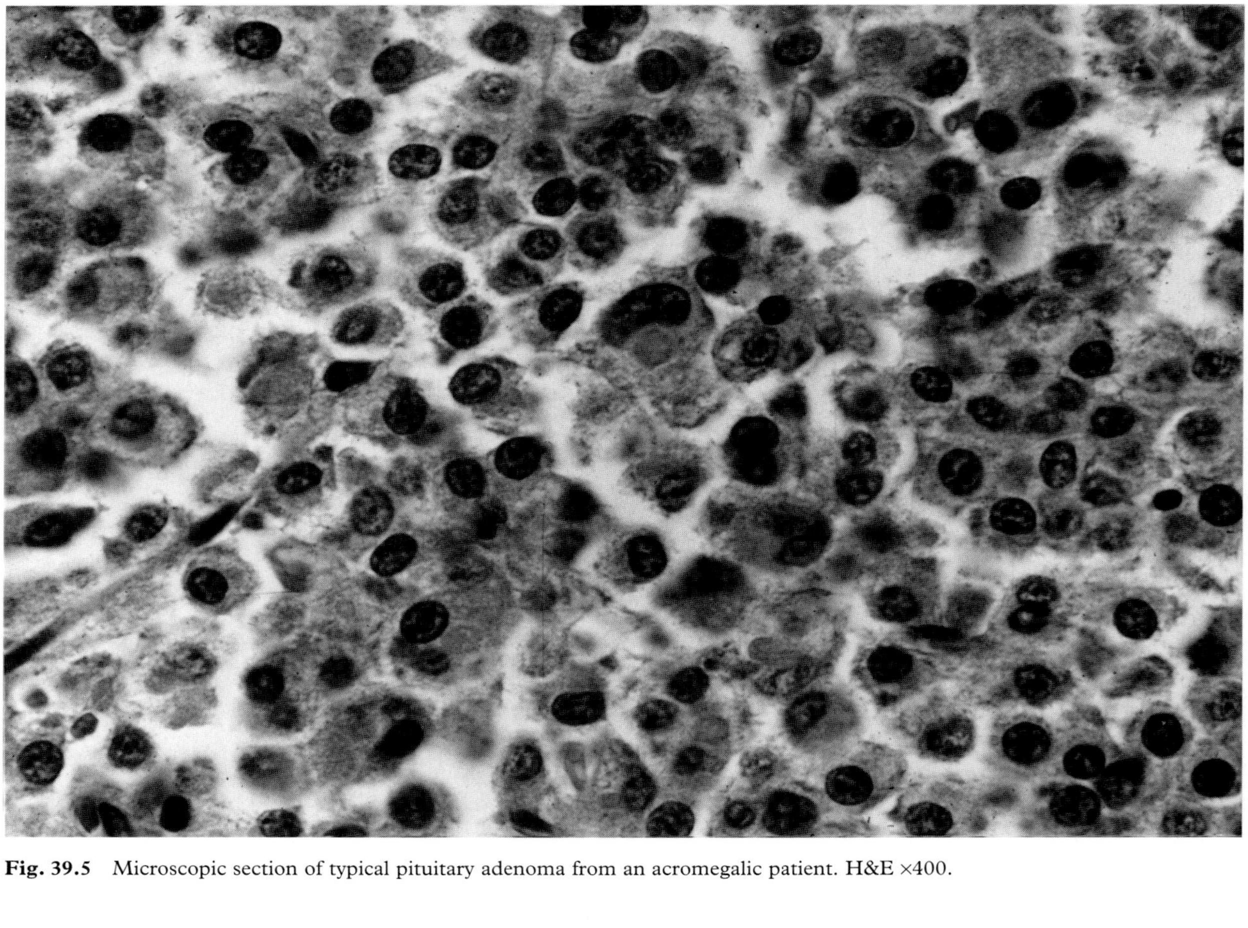

Fig. 39.5 Microscopic section of typical pituitary adenoma from an acromegalic patient. H&E ×400.

and restitution of normal GH dynamics. For practical purposes, basal GH levels should be reduced to less than 5 mg per milliliter and less than 2 mg per milliliter following a glucose tolerance test. Normalization of somatomedin-C levels occurs over a period of weeks and is probably the single best biochemical and physiologic index of cure. In our surgical series of 360 acromegalics, a significant reduction in GH levels occurred in nearly all patients, and more than 90% have shown improvement in acromegalic symptomatology. Based on the numerical criteria above, our surgical results indicate that 74% of patients are 'cured' and 7% of these recurred during a 10-year follow-up period (Laws et al 1979, 1982a). Radiation therapy is considered for those patients in whom endocrinologic cure was not achieved surgically, as determined by persistently elevated GH and somatomedin-C levels.

PROLACTINOMAS

Prolactin-secreting pituitary adenomas are the most common tumors of the pituitary gland, accounting for 30–40% of all pituitary tumors encountered in clinical practice. Prolactinomas occur in both sexes, but there are a number of fundamental differences in epidemiology, clinical presentation, and treatment strategies between tumors of men and women. Women are affected almost four times as frequently as men, as they account for 78% of prolactinomas. Women usually present during the second and third decades, whereas affected males are typically older, presenting in the fourth and fifth decades. Tumors of men are larger, more often invasive, and have usually transgressed sellar confines at the time of diagnosis. Women usually present on an endocrinologic basis with symptoms of amenorrhea and galactorrhea (Forbes-Albright syndrome) as the direct consequence of prolactin excess. Men usually present on a neurologic basis with headache, visual loss, and relative hypopituitarism, features directly attributable to an enlarging sellar mass. Prolactin excess in men produces hypogonadism as in women, but symptoms of impotence and decreased libido are not as conspicuous as the corresponding menstrual disturbances seen in women. This may provide a partial explanation of why tumors of men are so advanced when recognized while those of women are readily detected in the microadenoma stage. Alternatively, tumors of men may be inherently more aggressive.

An endocrine diagnosis is made by confirmation of elevated basal PRL levels. Other conditions causing hyperprolactinemia (drugs, hypothyroidism, cirrhosis, and renal failure) are usually easily excluded. The degree of hyperprolactinemia is a critical determinant of both the nature of the pathologic process and the likelihood of surgical cure. Serum PRL levels are normally less than 21 ng per milliliter. PRL elevations up to 150–200 ng per milliliter are not necessarily due to a prolactin-secreting tumor. Other non-prolactin-producing pituitary tumors as well as other structural lesions in the vicinity of the sella can cause these mild PRL elevations due to the 'stalk section effect'. PRL levels in excess of 200 ng per milliliter are very likely produced by prolactinomas, and levels in excess of 1000 ng per milliliter indicate invasive prolactinomas.

Once the diagnosis of prolactinoma is established on clinical and endocrinologic grounds, an anatomic diagnosis is obtained with MRI imaging. Macroadenomas will always be identified, as will 90% of microadenomas.

Treatment options for prolactinomas consist of pharmacologic control, surgical resection, and radiation therapy. The consistency and efficacy with which bromocriptine normalizes PRL levels, restores reproductive function, and reduces tumor mass add both dimension and controversy to the relative roles of surgery and medical therapy in the treatment of prolactinomas. Surgical therapy provides the opportunity for both endocrinologic and oncologic *'cure'*; however, success rates are limited by the size and invasiveness of the tumor (Tindall et al 1978). Alternatively, bromocriptine provides for endocrinologic and oncologic *control*. It is effective to some degree in the majority of patients but is often associated with intolerable side effects and must be taken indefinitely. Although some latitude exists in the selection of therapeutic approach, treatment strategies must be individualized, with careful consideration of treatment goals, the size and invasiveness of the tumor, the degree of hyperprolactinemia, and the inclinations of the patient.

Microadenomas, the majority of which occur in women, are usually managed with primary bromocriptine therapy. It effectively ameliorates the endocrinopathy in the majority of patients and restores ovulation for those desiring fertility. If pregnancy occurs, bromocriptine should be stopped and resumed following delivery. Although accelerated tumor growth can occur during pregnancy, it rarely occurs in patients with microadenomas. In contrast, patients with bromocriptine-treated PRL-secreting macroadenomas have a small but genuine risk of accelerated tumor growth during pregnancy when bromocriptine is stopped. Many patients with PRL-secreting microadenomas desiring fertility are also treated surgically (Landolt 1981). Curative tumor resection and subsequent pregnancy has been achieved in 83% of our patients harboring PRL microadenomas (Fode et al 1980, Laws et al 1983).

In our clinic, indications for surgical management for PRL-secreting macroadenomas include mass effect (progressive visual loss), apoplexy, bromocriptine resistance, and desire for fertility (Randall et al 1983). 'Cure' rates for macroadenomas are only 53%, which are further reduced to 28% if local invasion is present (Randall et al 1985). Preoperative PRL levels also serve as a prognostic index of surgical success, with tumors having PRL levels less than 200 ng per milliliter being most susceptible to surgical 'cure' (Laws et al 1985a). In patients with larger or invasive tumors, and in those with persistent post-operative hyperprolactinemia, adjunctive therapy with bromocriptine is recommended. Radiation therapy has an adjuvant, though relatively restricted, role in prolactinoma therapy. It is generally recommended for those patients with recurrent or persistent disease, in whom bromocriptine and surgery fail to control tumor growth or PRL levels.

CUSHING'S DISEASE AND NELSON'S SYNDROME: CORTICOTROPH ADENOMAS

Corticotroph adenomas account for 14% of all pituitary tumors. Most are hormonally active lesions, engaged in the deregulated hypersecretion of ACTH, and result in two clinically distinct but pathologically related conditions: Cushing's disease and Nelson's syndrome.

Cushing's disease

Although the term *Cushing's syndrome* represents the general description of any iatrogenic or endogenous hypercortisolemic state, *Cushing's disease* refers specifically to a hypercortisolemic state generated in response to a hypothalamic-pituitary disorder of ACTH hypersecretion. When defined etiologically, 80% of noniatrogenic cases of Cushing's syndrome are in fact cases of Cushing's disease due to an ACTH-producing pituitary tumor. The remaining causes include cortisol-producing adrenal tumors and ectopic sources of ACTH production (bronchogenic carcinoma, carcinoid tumors, pancreatic tumors).

Cushing's disease is a serious endocrinopathy, whose clinical features are attributable to endogenous cortisol excess. Women constitute over 75% of affected patients, with individuals being most commonly afflicted between the ages of 30 and 40 years. The classic features include a characteristic change in body habitus with the development of moon facies, centripetal obesity, 'buffalo hump', and supraclavicular fat deposition. Skin changes include hirsutism, occasional hyperpigmentation, plethora, and vascular fragility leading to ecchymoses and purple abdominal striae (Fig. 39.6). Generalized weakness, fatigue, and myopathy are common. Metabolic effects include hypertension, glucose intolerance, and osteoporosis. Menstrual abnormalities, immunosuppression, and psychiatric symptoms can also occur. In its most florid form, the disorder is easily recognizable; however, subtle and cyclical versions of the condition can occur and may not be immediately obvious. In addition to the genuine hypercortisolemic states listed above, alcoholism, depression, and obesity may all mimic some of the features of Cushing's disease, and must be distinguished. In contrast to the other hypersecretory states (hyperprolactinemia, acromegaly), the endocrinopathy of Cushing's disease is

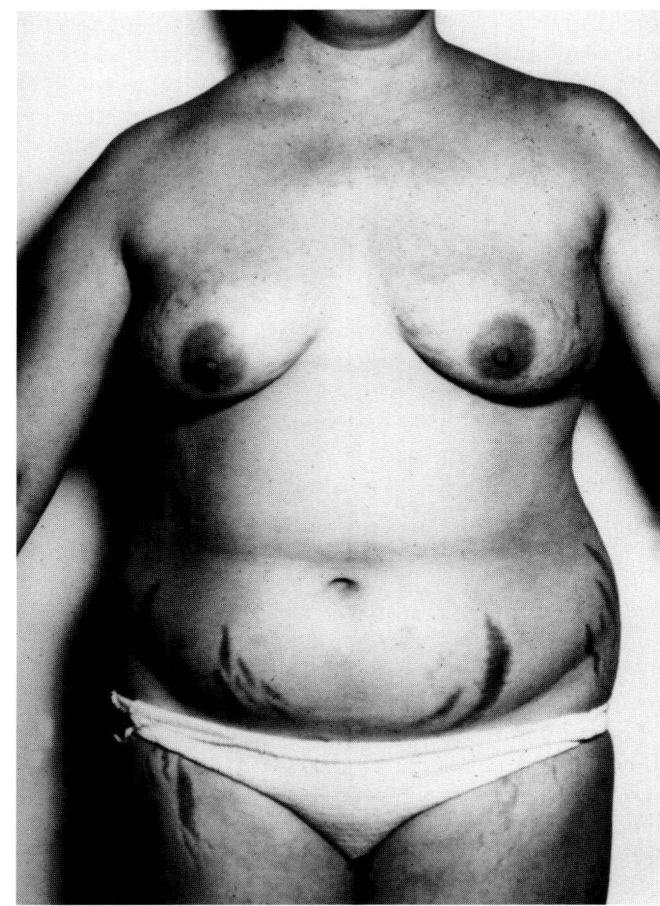

Fig. 39.6 Cushing's disease. Typical body habitus and striae.

life-threatening. Untreated, the disease carries a 5-year mortality rate of 50%. For this reason, Cushing's disease is accompanied by certain therapeutic imperatives, which are much more pressing than those occurring in any other hypersecretory state.

Distinguishing Cushing's disease from other hypercortisolemic states is critical, as appropriate therapy for hypercortisolism is contingent upon precise identification of the pathologic nature and anatomic site of the causative lesion. In this regard, rigorous endocrine diagnosis is most important. Cushing's disease has the following endocrinologic profile:

1. Hypercortisolism: as demonstrated by elevations of serum cortisol and 24-hour urinary free cortisol
2. Loss of serum cortisol diurnal variation
3. Moderately elevated ACTH levels
4. Cortisol suppressibility with high dose dexamethasone testing but no suppression with low dose dexamethasone testing.

In many cases these tests are sufficient to secure an endocrine diagnosis of Cushing's disease, but occasionally atypical results necessitate additional testing. In such circumstances, CRH-stimulated ACTH measurements of effluent blood in the inferior petrosal sinus can help identify whether a pituitary-hypothalamic source is responsible for ACTH excess and, if so, where within the pituitary gland the hypersecreting focus is located (Oldfield et al 1991).

Because the majority of corticotroph adenomas are microadenomas, often less than 5 mm in size, anatomic diagnosis is achieved radiologically in only 40–60% of cases. MRI studies have the highest yield, particularly when gadolinium is used. When pituitary imaging is normal, particularly when endocrine testing is atypical, normal CT or MRI scans of the lungs and adrenals provide indirect evidence of hypothalamic-pituitary source of excess cortisol production. Nevertheless, even if the causative tumor is radiologically occult, a confirmatory preoperative endocrine diagnosis of Cushing's disease ensures a high measure of confidence that a pituitary adenoma is indeed present and can be selectively identified and removed with trans-sphenoidal surgery.

Distinguished by their ultrastructural morphology, corticotroph adenomas are of two pathologic types: densely granulated and sparsely granulated corticotroph adenomas. The former occurs commonly and is well differentiated. The latter is less common, less well differentiated and notorious for its aggressive and invasive tendencies (Scheithauer et al 1986). ACTH immunopositivity is demonstrated in both tumor types. More than 80% of corticotroph adenomas are microadenomas, often only a few millimeters in size, but usually well demarcated from surrounding tissue.

The merits of trans-sphenoidal surgery are exemplified in the treatment of Cushing's disease. Whether the lesion is visible on imaging studies or is radiologically occult, trans-sphenoidal exploration of the pituitary gland enables identification and selective resection of the offending microadenoma while preserving normal pituitary function. Based on our series of 260 patients, curative resection can be achieved in more than 90% of microadenomas and in 65% of macroadenomas and invasive tumors (Salassa et al 1978). Successfully treated patients have an immediate fall in blood cortisol levels and eventual regression of cushingoid features. Recurrence is uncommon, occurring in 8.5% of cases, sometimes many years after successful surgery. In the minority of cases where surgery fails to achieve an immediate endocrinologic cure, medical therapy, radiation therapy and bilateral adrenalectomy are all potential options. Medical therapy consists primarily of agents which pharmacologically block adrenal steroidogenesis (Mitotane, ketoconazole). They effectively reduce cortisol levels, but are often associated with unpleasant side effects. The delayed therapeutic effect of radiation therapy limits its use in Cushing's disease, although it is used for persistent disease (in conjunction with medical therapy) and in cases of invasive tumors. Bilateral adrenalectomy is immediately effective in ameliorating hypercortisolism and is recommended in patients with persistent and debilitating disease that is unresponsive to other therapies.

Nelson's syndrome

Nelson's syndrome refers to the clinical condition which occurs when pituitary corticotroph adenomas become manifest following bilateral adrenalectomy for Cushing's disease. Approximately 15% of patients with Cushing's disease so treated will develop Nelson's syndrome. Although these tumors are morphologically identical to tumors responsible for Cushing's disease, they are characteristically much more aggressive, frequently exhibiting unrelenting invasion of neighboring neural, vascular and bony structures. The enhanced aggressiveness of these tumors has been attributed to loss of negative feedback inhibition consequent to the adrenalectomy. These tumors produce ACTH, but the adrenalectomy prevents the occurrence of hypercortisolemia. Because these tumors also secrete melanocyte-stimulating hormone, patients with Nelson's syndrome are hyperpigmented. The syndrome is easily recognizable, beginning with a history of Cushing's disease in which the pituitary lesion was either unsuspected, undetected, or incompletely resected. Persistent hypercortisolism would subsequently be treated with bilateral adrenalectomy, which effectively ameliorated the hypercortisolemic state. This temporary remission would be followed by later aggressive tumor recurrence with manifestations of hyperpigmentation and extrasellar tumor extension (visual loss, cranial nerve palsies, headache). Serum ACTH levels are often markedly elevated and, depending on the size of the tumor, varying degrees of hypopituitarism will be detected clinically and biochemically.

As a result of their invasive nature, corticotroph adenomas in the setting of Nelson's syndrome are frequent refractory to surgical 'cure'. In our series, normalization of ACTH levels was achieved in only 23% of cases and improvement in hyperpigmentation occurred in only half of all surgical treated patients. In the few patients in whom endocrinologic cure can be achieved, the long term outlook is favorable, however tumor recurrence can still be expected in approximately 15% of cases (Thapar et al 1992).

THYROTROPHIC ADENOMAS

With fewer than 100 cases reported in the world literature, thyrotrophic adenomas are the least common form of pituitary neoplasia, representing only 1% of all pituitary adenomas. The clinical history is most remarkable for some form of thyroid dysfunction, typically hyperthyroidism, although they can arise anywhere along the spectrum of thyroid function, ranging from normal to extremes of hypo- or hyperthyroidism. It was once held that most thyrotrophic adenomas arose in the setting of longstanding hypothyroidism, presumably by way of feedback inhibitory loss, the induction of thyrotrophic hyperplasia, and eventually, adenomatous transformation. As experience with thyrotrophic adenomas has been accumulated, it is now clear that, in the majority of patients, the initial manifestation of thyrotrophic adenomas are hyperthyroidism and goiter, findings wholly compatible with tumoral TSH hypersecretion (McCutcheon et al 1990). In a substantial proportion of cases, particularly those subjected to prior thyroid ablation, these tumors are frequently invasive macroadenomas in whom visual field deficits can often be detected. In the absence of prior thyroid ablation, the endocrine diagnosis of thyrotrophic adenomas requires the presence of an elevated serum thyroxine, usually with clinical evidence of hyperthyroidism and an inappropriately high TSH level. That more than 80% of thyrotrophic adenomas also co-secrete alpha subunit, emphasizes the utility of this marker in the diagnosis of this tumor type. In the appropriate clinical context, an alpha subunit/TSH molar ratio greater than 1.0 is strongly suggestive of a TSH adenoma (Klibanski & Zervas 1991). Not infrequently, thyrotrophic adenomas also co-secrete other anterior pituitary hormones, typically GH and PRL.

Therapy for TSH adenomas is surgical excision. In those cases where the diagnosis is established early in the course of the disease, these tumors can be detected in microadenoma stage, where selective trans-sphenoidal resection of the tumor is curative. When the diagnosis is delayed, however, especially in the context of prior thyroid ablation, these tumors are sufficiently large and invasive that cure rates after trans-sphenoidal surgery are reduced to approximately 40%. Adjuvant radiotherapy is usually recommended in such cases of invasive lesions. Pharmacologic therapy in the form of somatostatin analog has shown some promise in reducing TSH levels, but is generally ineffective in reducing tumor mass.

NONFUNCTIONING PITUITARY ADENOMAS

Nonfunctioning pituitary adenomas are those tumors which do not cause a clinically recognizable endocrinopathy, presenting instead with features of a progressive sellar mass (headache, visual loss and varying degrees of hypo-pituitarism). By virtue of their size, they may also produce mild hyperprolactinemia on the basis of the 'stalk section effect' as described earlier. There are three distinct morphologic entities which constitute this nonfunctioning class of pituitary tumors: null cell adenomas, oncocytomas, and gonadotropin-producing adenomas. The latter is actually a functioning tumor producing the gonadotropic hormones (LH and FSH). Because there is no discernible endocrinopathy attributable to gonadotropin excess, their presentation is like that of the genuine nonfunctioning entities and they are therefore discussed here. Collectively, nonfunctioning adenomas account for 25 % of all pituitary adenomas, and they can reach such a large size at presentation that their management can be a formidable challenge. Nonfunctioning tumors can also secrete the α subunit of the glycoprotein hormones (FSH, LH and TSH). 'Silent' forms of otherwise hormonally active tumors (ACTH, GH) also exist, and have the same clinical features as other nonfunctioning adenomas (Black et al 1987). Null cell adenomas and oncocytomas account for 17% and 6% of all pituitary adenomas respectively. Null cell adenomas are so named because they are unassociated with any distinctive morphologic or immunohistochemical marker referable to any one of the five known adenohypophyseal cell types. Oncocytomas are simply null cell adenomas which exhibit intracellular accumulation of large numbers of dilated mitochondria. This is a descriptive term without biologic or clinical significance, so in practice, both these entities are oncologically equivalent. These tumors typically occur in older patients and are virtually all macroadenomas at presentation. It is likely that the majority of these have limited proliferative potential and have been slowly growing for many years before reaching medical attention. Gross invasion of neighboring anatomic structures is present in approximately 40% of these tumors (Selman et al 1986).

Gonadotroph adenomas arise as a neoplastic derivative of normal pituitary gonadotroph cells, and account for 3–5% of all pituitary adenomas. They most commonly occur in older patients, often in the context of gonadal failure, although they can occasionally be seen in younger patients. They are all macroadenomas at presentation and a fifth are locally invasive. Despite the presence of a distinct endocrinopathy, elevations of FSH, the glycoprotein hormone α subunit, and, rarely, LH can be detected. These elevations serve as useful markers for the initial diagnosis and later postoperative surveillance of residual or recurrent disease.

The diagnosis of nonfunctioning adenoma rests primarily on MRI imaging (Fig. 39.7). As these are usually large lesions, careful consideration must be given to their full extent and their relationships to surrounding neural and vascular structures. These considerations are critical in determining optimal surgical access, potential operative hazards and possibility of cure. Endocrinologic testing is used primarily to exclude a hypersecretory state and to identify the presence and degree of coexisting hypopituitarism. As mentioned, mild elevation of PRL levels is common, and elevated levels of α subunit may be present.

Although each of the hyperfunctioning tumors has a pharmacologic option for treatment, none exists for nonfunctioning adenomas. Therapy is therefore primarily surgical, with judicious adjuvant use of irradiation. Despite their size, the majority of nonfunctioning tumors are accessible trans-sphenoidally. Craniotomy is reserved for

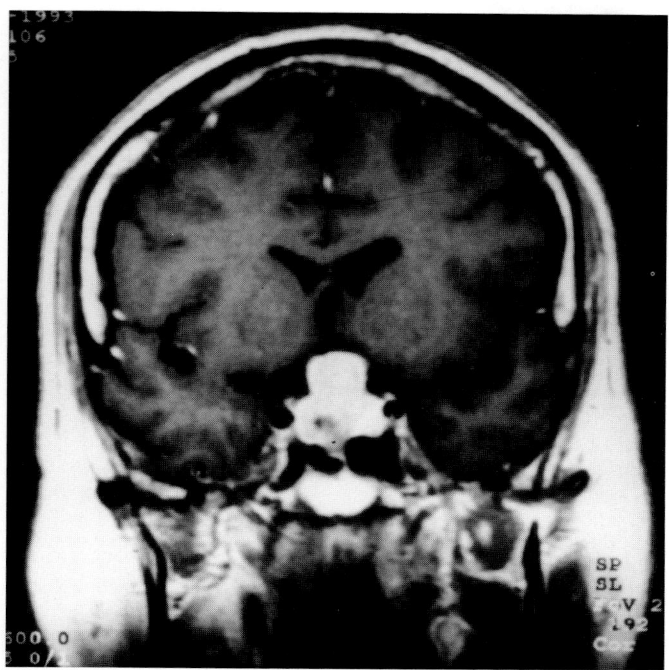

Fig. 39.7 MRI scan, coronal view. Nonfunctioning pituitary macroadenoma with suprasellar extension, chiasmal compression, and visual loss.

the occasional lesion with extreme lateral intracranial extension. Although 'total' surgical removal is the intuitive goal for all pituitary tumors, the fact that most nonfunctioning tumors occur in the elderly and are usually slow growing necessitates that judgment prevail and therapy be individualized. When progressive visual loss occurs in the elderly patient for example, a radical procedure with attempt at 'total' surgical resection may be less prudent than a satisfactory but less radical and less dangerous decompression. Guided by these principles, the surgical outcomes in our series of over 600 nonfunctioning tumors have been quite satisfactory (Ebersold et al 1986). Visual function improves or is stabilized in 94% of patients (Laws et al 1977, Trautmann & Laws 1983), and symptoms of headache and cavernous sinus compression are almost always relieved. Because of their large size and longstanding compression of the normal pituitary, restoration of normal pituitary function, if it was impaired preoperatively, occurs only in a minority of patients. Therefore, recognition of postoperative pituitary deficiency followed by adequate hormone replacement therapy is an important aspect of long-term care (Laws et al 1981). Adjuvant radiation therapy is often recommended in cases of residual or recurrent disease.

PITUITARY CARCINOMA

Primary carcinoma of the pituitary gland has long been an entity enshrouded in controversy, as for some the entity did not exist, and for those who acknowledged its existence, no consensus could be reached on how it should be defined. Earlier literature suggested that tumors exhibiting local invasion were malignant; however, the observation that up to 85% of benign pituitary tumors show histologic invasiveness has rendered this perspective obsolete. The currently accepted criterion for a pituitary carcinoma is that of a pituitary tumor with distant spread, either within or outside of the neuraxis. Using this definition, fewer that 40 well documented cases have been described (Pernicone & Scheithauer, 1993).

Pituitary carcinomas primarily affect adults. All types of hormonally active pituitary carcinomas have been reported; endocrine-inactive carcinomas also occur, but less frequently. In some patients the initial course is indistinguishable from that of a benign pituitary adenoma. Local invasion may or may not be present, and tumor histology may be entirely benign. A protracted course, often punctuated by multiple local recurrences, is then followed by metastatic dissemination. In many such cases, a clear escalation in histologic abnormalities is observed when comparing primary tumors to metastatic deposits. In such cases, the process appears to be one of malignant transformation in a previously benign tumor. Alternatively, the behavior of other pituitary carcinomas suggests de novo malignancy. Such tumors are biologically malignant from the outset, beginning as locally invasive, cytologically atypical or malignant tumors which promptly give way to metastatic dissemination. Metastatic dissemination rather often involves the cerebrospinal fluid axis. A variety of extraneural metastatic sites have also been reported, including bone, liver, lymph nodes, lung, kidney, and heart.

For most patients with pituitary carcinomas, the most symptomatic aspect of their disease is the primary sellar tumor; craniospinal deposits occasionally cause symptoms, however, extraneural metastases seldom do. Therapy is therefore directed at control of the primary tumor, which often necessitates repeat resections, radiotherapy, and pharmacologic therapy as indicated. In most instances, death from pituitary carcinoma results from a failure to effectively control the primary lesion, which, despite therapy, progresses with unrelenting local invasiveness.

TUMORS OF THE POSTERIOR PITUITARY

The posterior pituitary is rarely the site of clinically significant primary tumors. Granular cell tumors (also termed choristomas or granular cell myoblastomas) are the most common primary tumors of the neurohypophysis. Most are only a few millimeters in size and are incidental findings in up to 8% of unselected autopsies. Hamartomas or low grade gliomas arising from the infundibular stalk or extending down from the hypothalamus are additional rarities constituting the remaining neurohypophyseal tumor types. If posterior lobe tumors are symptomatic, diabetes insipidus is the most common symptom. Depending on their size and nature, hyperprolactinemia, hypopituitarism, precocious puberty and acromegaly have all been reported with the various neurohypophyseal entities.

As the posterior pituitary receives more than 10 times the arterial blood supply of the anterior lobe, it is a relatively common site of metastatic dissemination. Again, if symptomatic, diabetes insipidus is the most common presenting feature. Although metastases from a wide range of solid and hematogenous tumors can develop in this area, breast cancers are the most common source of such metastases.

CONCLUSION

Much continues to be learned with regard to the pathogenesis, control mechanisms and molecular biology of pituitary tumors. The current effective levels of disease control should become even more comprehensive as these advances in basic science become translated into clinical practise.

REFERENCES

Abboud C F, Laws E R Jr 1979 Clinical endocrinological approach to hypothalamic-pituitary disease. Journal of Neurosurgery 51: 271–291

Alexander J M, Biller B M K, Bikkal H, Zervas N T, Arnold A, Klibanski A 1990 Clinically non-functioning pituitary tumors are monoclonal in origin. Journal of Clinical Investigation 86: 336–340

Annegers J F, Coulam C B, Abboud C F et al 1978 Pituitary adenoma in Olmsted County, Minnesota, 1935–1977. Mayo Clinic Proceedings 53: 641–643

Black P M, Hsu D W, Klibanski A et al 1987 Hormone production in clinically non-functioning pituitary adenomas. Journal of Neurosurgery 66: 244–250

Ciric I, Mikhael M, Stafford T et al 1983 Transsphenoidal microsurgery of pituitary macroadenomas with long-term follow-up results. Journal of Neurosurgery 59: 395–401

Costello R T 1936 Subclinical adenoma of the pituitary gland. American Journal of Pathology 12: 205–216

Coulam C B, Laws E R Jr, Abboud C F, Randall R V 1981 Primary amenorrhea and pituitary adenomas. Fertility and Sterility 35: 615–619

Cushing H 1909 Partial hypophysectomy for acromegaly. Annals of Surgery 30: 1002–1017

Cushing H 1912 The pituitary body and its disorders. J B Lippincott, Philadelphia, p 297

Hsu D W, Hakim F, Biller B M K, de la Monte S, Zervas N T, Klibanski A, Hedley-White E T 1993 Significance of proliferating cell nuclear antigen index in predicting pituitary adenoma recurrence. Journal of Neurosurgery 78: 753–761

Ebersold M J, Laws E R Jr, Scheithauer B W, Randall R V 1983 Pituitary apoplexy treated by transsphenoidal surgery. A clinicopathological and immunocytochemical study. Journal of Neurosurgery 58: 315–320

Ebersold M D, Quast L M, Laws E R Jr et al 1986 Long-term results in transsphenoidal removal of non-functioning pituitary adenomas. Journal of Neurosurgery 64: 713–719

Fode N C, Laws E R Jr, Abboud C T et al 1980 Prolactin secreting pituitary adenoma: A review and study of their implications for fertility in women. Journal of Neurosurgical Nursing 12: 210–213

Hardy J 1969 Transsphenoidal microsurgery of the normal and pathological pituitary. Clinical Neurosurgery 16: 185–217

Jacoby L B, Hedley-Whyte E T, Pulaski K, Seizinger B R, Martuza R L 1990 Clonal origin of pituitary adenomas. Journal of Neurosurgery 73: 731–735

Klibanski A, Zervas N T 1991 Diagnosis and management of hormone-secreting pituitary adenomas. New England Journal of Medicine 324: 822–831

Kovacs K, Horvath E 1986 Tumors of the pituitary gland. Atlas of tumor pathology, second series, fascicle 21. Armed Forces Institute of Pathology, Washington, DC

Landis C A, Harsh G, Lyons J, Davis R L, McCormick F, Bourne H R 1990 Clinical characteristics of acromegaly patients whose pituitary tumors contain mutant Gs protein. Journal of Clinical Endocrinology and Metabolism 71: 1416–1420

Landolt A M 1981 Surgical treatment of pituitary prolactinomas: Postoperative prolactin and fertility. Fertility and Sterility 35: 620–625

Laws E R Jr 1977 Transsphenoidal approach to lesions in and about the sella turcica. In: Schmidek H H, Sweet W H (eds) Current techniques in operative neurosurgery. Grune & Stratton, New York, pp 161–172

Laws E R Jr 1980 Transsphenoidal microsurgery in the management of acromegaly. In: Smith J L (ed) Neuro-ophthalmology focus. Masson, New York, pp 289–293

Laws E R Jr 1985 Pituitary adenomas. In: Johnson R T (ed) Current therapy in neurologic disease 1985–86. B C Decker, Philadelphia, pp 220–225

Laws E R Jr, Kern E B 1976 Complications of transsphenoidal surgery. Clinical Neurosurgery 23: 401–416

Laws E R Jr, Trautmann J C, Hollenhorst R W Jr 1977 Transsphenoidal decompression of the optic nerve and chiasm: Visual results in 62 patients. Journal of Neurosurgery 46: 717–722

Laws E R Jr, Piepgras D G, Randall R V et al 1979 Neurosurgical management of acromegaly. Results in 82 patients treated between 1972 and 1977. Journal of Neurosurgery 50: 454–461

Laws E R Jr, Abboud C F, Kern E B 1980 Perioperative management of patients with pituitary microadenoma. Neurosurgery 7: 566–570

Laws E R Jr, Abboud C F, Hayles A B 1981 The practical management of pituitary replacement therapy related to sellar and parasellar surgery. Clinical Neurosurgery 28: 108–115

Laws E R Jr, Randall R V, Abboud C F 1982a Surgical treatment of acromegaly: results in 140 patients. In: Givens J (ed) Hormone-secreting pituitary tumors. Year Book, Chicago, pp 225–228

Laws E R Jr, Randall R V, Kern E B, Abboud C F (eds) 1982b Management of pituitary adenomas and related lesions. Appleton-Century-Crofts, New York

Laws E R Jr, Fode N C, Randall R V et al 1983 Pregnancy following transsphenoidal resection of prolactin-secreting pituitary tumors. Journal of Neurosurgery 58: 685–688

Laws E R Jr, Ebersold M J, Piepgras D G et al 1985a The role of surgery in the management of prolactinoma. In: MacLeod R M, Thorner M O, Scapagnini U (eds) Prolactin, basic and clinical correlates. Springer-Verlag, New York, pp 849–853

Laws E R Jr, Fode N C, Redmond M J 1985b Transsphenoidal surgery following unsuccessful prior therapy. Journal of Neurosurgery 68: 823–829

Laws E R Jr, Scheithauer B W, Carpenter S M et al 1985c The pathogenesis of acromegaly. Journal of Neurosurgery 63: 35–38

MacCarty C S, Hanson E J Jr, Randall R V, Scanlon P W 1973 Indications for and results of surgical treatment of pituitary tumors by the transfrontal approach. International Congress Series 303, Diagnosis and treatment of pituitary tumors. Excerpta Medica, Amsterdam

McCutcheon I E, Weintranb B D, Oldfield E H 1990 Surgical treatment of thyrotropin-secreting pituitary adenomas. Journal of Neurosurgery 73: 674–683

Niederhuber J E 1993 Current therapy in oncology. B C Decker, Philadelphia, p 663

Oldfield E H, Doppman J L, Nieman L K et al 1991 Petrosal sinus sampling with and without corticotropin-releasing hormone for the differential diagnosis of Cushing's syndrome. New England Journal of Medicine 325: 897–905

Pernicone P J, Scheithauer B W 1993 Invasive pituitary adenomas and pituitary carcinomas. In: Lloyd R V (ed) Surgical pathology of the pituitary gland. W B Saunders, Philadelphia, pp 121–126

Randall R V, Laws E R Jr, Abboud C F et al 1983 Transsphenoidal microsurgical treatment of prolactin-producing pituitary adenomas: Results in 100 patients. Mayo Clinic Proceedings 58: 108–121

Randall R V, Scheithauer B W, Laws E R Jr et al 1985 Pituitary adenomas associated with hyperprolactinemia: A clinical and immunohistochemical study of 97 patients operated on transsphenoidally. Mayo Clinic Proceedings 60: 753–762

Salassa R M, Laws E R Jr, Carpenter P C, Northcutt R C 1978 Transsphenoidal removal of pituitary microadenoma in Cushing's disease. Mayo Clinic Proceedings 53: 24–28

Scheithauer B W, Kovacs K T, Laws E R Jr, Randall R V 1986 Pathology of invasive pituitary tumors with special reference to functional classification. Journal of Neurosurgery 65: 733–744

Selman W R, Laws E R Jr, Scheithauer B W, Carpenter S M 1986 The occurrence of dural invasion in pituitary adenomas. Journal of Neurosurgery 64: 402–407

Thapar K, Smith M, Elliott E, Kovacs K, Laws E R Jr 1992 Corticotroph adenomas of the pituitary: long term results of operative treatment. Endocrine Pathology 31: 551–553

Tindall G T, McLanahan C S, Christy J H 1978 Transsphenoidal microsurgery for pituitary tumors associated with hyperprolactinemia. Journal of Neurosurgery 48: 849–860

Trautmann J C, Laws E R Jr 1983 Visual status after transsphenoidal surgery at the Mayo Clinic, 1971–1982. American Journal of Ophthalmology 96: 200–208

Wilson C B 1984 A decade of pituitary microsurgery. The Herbert Olivecrona Lecture. Journal of Neurosurgery 61: 814–833

Zervas N T 1984 Surgical results for pituitary adenoma: Results of an international survey. In: Black P, Zervas N, Ridgeway E et al (eds) Secretory tumors of the pituitary gland. Raven Press, New York, pp 377–385

Zervas N T, Martin J B 1980 Management of hormone-secreting pituitary adenomas. New England Journal of Medicine 302: 210–214

PART VII

Skull base tumors

40. Chordomas and chondrosarcomas of the cranial base

Emmanuel Gay Laligam N. Sekhar Donald C. Wright

Since the first description by Luschka in 1856 (Luschka 1864), the management of the treatment of chordomas remains a challenge for neurosurgeons and oncologists.

This embryonal tumor develops from remnants of the notochord (chorda dorsalis), which goes to form the initial axial structures (Heffelfinger et al 1973, Krayenbühl & Yasargil 1975, Zülch 1986, Bouropoulou et al 1989). In vertebrates, the notochord is replaced by a bony structure forming the skull and the spine. The only remnants of the notochord in the normal adult are represented by the nucleus pulposus of intervertebral discs. Chordomas develop from residues of the primitive notochordal cells enclosed in the bony structure. They grow slowly and are locally invasive. Deeply located at the center of the skull base and difficult to remove totally, this infiltrative tumor must be considered a malignant tumor.

The exact origin of chondrosarcomas is still unclear. They may originate from metaplastic change of fibroblasts, from primitive mesenchymal cells, or more likely from embryonal rests of the cartilaginous matrix of the skull (Hassounah et al 1985, Bourgouin et al 1992). Concomitant embryologically derived tumors are occasionally associated with chondrosarcomas, such as multiple enchondromatosis (Ollier's disease), hemangiomatosis (Maffucci's syndrome), and even craniopharyngiomas (Belza 1966, Krayenbühl & Yasargil 1975, Bushe et al 1990).

Chondrosarcomas, at least of low grade, are usually studied with chordomas, even though their origin seems to be different. Their location at the base of the skull, their growth and clinical pattern, allow them to be considered together in most publications.

PATHOLOGY

The slow-growing chordomas and chondrosarcomas are unencapsulated, but a pseudocapsule formed by dura mater is encountered frequently in the intradural part of the tumor. Although these tumors generally start in the extradural space, they may invade the dura late in their course. They may stretch the cranial nerves or displace vascular structures and the brainstem. Usually they are discrete from the brain structures, but are not demarcated from the bone.

Their surface is nodular, the color usually reddish. The tumor is often gelatinous and soft, with a consistency like jelly, but sometimes it is very firm like cartilage. The tumor may contain some hemorrhagic foci and some calcification. Their size is variable. In a recent review of 60 cases of chordomas and chondrosarcomas in our institution, the tumor volume varied from 1 cm^3 to 346 cm^3, with an average volume of 58 cm^3.

Chordomas

A chordoma usually satisfies three histologic criteria: the presence of large vacuolated mucus-containing cells called physaliferous cells, which correspond to the basic architecture of the primitive notochord; the lobular arrangement of these cells; and the abundant extracellular mucus. In some areas, regressive processes can be found with mucoid degeneration, and hemorrhages and calcification can also occur (Dahlin & MacCarty 1952).

In immunochemistry, chordomas show reactivity for epithelial markers (cytokeratin, epithelial membrane antigen) and present a positive reaction with oncofetal antigen antisera (carcinoembryonic antigen, α-fetoprotein). Immunoreactivity for S-100 protein is often seen. Some chordomas stain positive with vimentin antisera, which reflects mesenchymal differentiation (Bouropoulou et al 1989, Walaas & Kindblom 1991).

Chordomas have the common characteristics of a malignant tumor, with local invasiveness, tendency for recurrence, and the potential to metastasize. Metastases are relatively rare with skull base chordomas; only 7–12% of the metastases have primary sites in cranial chordomas (Chambers & Schwinn 1979). Ten percent of chordomas show histologic signs of malignancy, including spindle-shaped elongated cells simulating an anaplastic sarcoma, polymorphism of nuclei and more mitoses. There is a considerable range in the spectrum of histologic pattern in this neoplasm, however, and mitoses and anaplasia can be found in chordomas without effect on length of survival, and without promoting metastases. Therefore there are very few reliable histologic features which may aid in the prediction of a local aggressiveness and a metastatic potential (Dahlin & MacCarty 1952, Krayenbühl & Yasargil 1975, Chambers & Schwinn 1979, Volpe & Mazabraud 1983).

Heffelfinger et al (1973) first described a group of tumors with foci of chordoma amidst a large cartilaginous matrix. These tumors have been termed 'chondroid chordomas'. The authors found a better survival with these tumors and postulated that the malignant potential of chordoma appears to decrease when cartilaginous foci are present. Several authors confirmed these results (Spoden et al 1980, Cummings et al 1983, Raffel et al 1985, Rich et al 1985, Rupa et al 1989, Spaar et al 1990, Muzenrider 1992). Strong controversy still exists concerning the significance of this cartilaginous differentiation of the chondroid chordomas. Based on immunohistochemical findings, others consider this tumor to be a low grade chondrosarcoma rather than a subtype of chordomas (Brooks et al 1987, Bouropoulou et al 1989, Erbengi et al 1991, Bourgouin et al 1992, Tomlinson et al 1992).

Chondrosarcomas

Chondrosarcoma is one of the most difficult of the malignant tumors of bone to diagnose because its histologic appearance lies between the benign chondroma and a malignant sarcoma. The criteria that differentiate a low grade chondrosarcoma from a chondroma or a chordoma are very subtle. The use of immunohistochemical analysis and even electron microscopy is often needed.

Chondrosarcomas have been classified into three categories: classic, mesenchymal, and dedifferentiated (Dahlin & Unni 1986, Meyers et al 1992). Classic chondrosarcomas contain many large cartilaginous cells with large single or multiple nuclei amid a variable abundance of chondroid matrix. This more common subtype is divided into three major grades on the basic of the mitotic rates, the cellularity and the nuclear size of the cells (Finn et al 1984). Grade I lesions resemble benign cartilaginous tumors, grades II and III have more mitoses and less chondroid matrix. Chondrosarcomas of lower grade are less aggressive and tendency to metastasize is minimal (Ariel & Verdu 1975, Evans et al 1977, Hassounah et al 1985, Coltrera et al 1986, Kveton et al 1986, Charabi et al 1989, Bourgouin et al 1992). In immunohistochemistry, they do not express any of the epithelial markers or oncofetal antigens usually shown in chordomas (Brooks et al 1987, Bouropoulou et al 1989, Tomlinson et al 1992).

The dedifferentiated chondrosarcoma has features of an anaplastic sarcoma; the mesenchymal chondrosarcoma is a histologic combination of zones composed of undifferentiated mesenchymal cells and islands of cartilage. These two last subtypes are even more malignant (Dahlin & Unni 1986).

INCIDENCE AND DISTRIBUTION

Chordomas or chondrosarcomas usually originate from the sacrococcygeal region, the spheno-occipital region or the vertebrae. According to most of the series, 40% of the chordomas are primarily intracranial (Heffelfinger et al 1973, Volpe & Mazabraud 1983, O'Neill et al 1985). Both chordomas and chondrosarcomas are rare tumors, representing 0.2% of all intracranial tumors and 6.15% of all primitive skull base lesions (Krayenbühl & Yasargil 1975, Cianfriglia et al 1978, Kveton et al 1986, Zülch 1986). The low grade subtype of chondrosarcomas appears to be more common than the mesenchymal chondrosarcoma (Hassounah et al 1985). In our experience and according to other authors (Charabi et al 1989), the low grade type is common.

Age/sex

Chordomas occur at all ages, but are most common between the third and fifth decades of life. A male predominance is found in some series, with a 2:1 ratio (Dahlin & MacCarty 1952, Heffelfinger et al 1973, Ariel & Verdu 1975, Kendall & Lee 1977). In other series, no sex predominance is described for cranial chordomas (Krayenbühl & Yasargil 1975, O'Neill et al 1985, Sze et al 1988, Muzenrider 1992). With chondrosarcomas, men are involved twice as commonly as women and this tumor occurs frequently during the second and third decades (Kamrin et al 1964, Evans et al 1977, Hassounah et al 1985).

Tumor localization

According to their embryologic origin, chordomas are located in all places where the notochord existed: namely, clivus, sellar and parasellar region, nasopharynx, foramen magnum and C1. Chordomas may invade the dura and infiltrate pia mater, enveloping arteries and brain structures. This invasive tumor usually arises in the vicinity of the clivus but extends widely so that every system of classification is difficult. When planning the surgical approach, however, a classification into three groups has been proposed: a clival group; a parasellar group where tumor invades the cavernous sinus, Meckel's cave and the middle cranial fossa; and the sellar group (Krayenbühl & Yasargil 1975). In the last group, the tumor invades the dorsum sellae with possible extension to the sella and the sphenoid sinus. We prefer to think of them as upper clival, middle clival, lower clival and foramen magnum tumors, with or without invasion of sphenoid, cavernous sinus and petrous bone (Sekhar et al 1993).

Because of their origin, chondrosarcomas are usually petroclival and paramedian, in the parasellar region (51% of the cases—Sindou et al 1989), petrous bone and cerebellopontine angle (Bourgouin et al 1992). They may also invade dura.

CLINICAL PRESENTATION (Dahlin & MacCarty 1952, Kamrin et al 1964, Heffelfinger et al 1973, Kendall & Lee 1977, O'Neill et al 1985, Raffel et al 1985, Rich et al 1985)

Each topographic group may have its own clinical presentation; however, in advanced stages a clinical classification related to the localization of the tumor is difficult. Patients usually complain of headaches (75%) and cranial nerve palsy, especially diplopia (60–90% of the cases). The most common physical findings are a sixth nerve palsy (50–90%) followed by a visual field defect, or loss of visual security. With clivus involvement and cerebellopontine extension, symptoms can be referable to cranial nerves VIII–XII, or to the cerebellum or pons. Motor weakness and endocrine disturbances are less common.

The clinical presentation of the chondrosarcomas is similar to that of chordomas, although their paramedial localization may cause more hearing loss (86%). Both of these tumors can cause symptoms from extension ventrally into nasal cavity, pharynx and the paranasal sinuses.

RADIOLOGIC DIAGNOSIS

CT and MRI scans are most important for diagnosis. Axial and coronal CT before and after administration of intravenous contrast material are necessary to outline the tumor. Without contrast, tumor appears isodense with the brain as a soft tissue mass causing adjacent bony destruction but without changes of the surrounding bony structures. Bone windowed CT scans will show precisely bone destruction margins. Foci of calcification are noted in 30–47% of the cases. Contrast enchancement is always present but to varying degrees (Kamrin et al 1964, Kendall & Lee 1977, Meyer et al 1986, Bourgouin et al 1992).

MRI with sagittal, coronal, axial sections usually shows a well-defined extra-axial tumor (Oot et al 1988, Brown et al 1989, Lee & Tassei 1989, Bourgouin et al 1992). Seventy-five % of chordomas appear isodense, 25% hypointense on T1-weighted images (Sze et al 1988). Chondrosarcomas and chordomas show a variable degree of contrast enhancement with gadolinium (Meyers et al 1992). The hyperintensity in T2 helps to demarcate the tumor from adjacent structures. MRI also has the ability to demonstrate patent major vessels and their relations to the tumor. It may also show some aspects of transdural transgression of the tumor.

Table 40.1 Differential diagnosis of chordomas and chondrosarcomas (differential diagnosis with invasive and calcified tumors).

Chromophobe adenoma
Mucinous adenocarcinoma
Craniopharyngioma
Meningioma
Schwannoma
Nasopharyngeal carcinoma
Salivary gland tumors

Although a chordoma is more likely to be a medial tumor and chondrosarcoma more lateral, there are no imaging features that allow for the accurate differentiation of chordomas and chondrosarcomas (Coltrera et al 1986). In addition, other kinds of tumors may exhibit some common radiologic appearances, making the pathologic examination the key to diagnosis. The differential diagnosis (Table 40.1) is sometimes difficult even if a biopsy is examined (Walaas & Kindblom 1991). Frozen sections give the first approximation during the operative procedure but further analysis with immunohistochemical staining or even electron microscopy will differentiate between the variations of chordomas and chondrosarcomas.

ANGIOGRAPHY AND BALLOON OCCLUSION TEST (Erba et al 1988)

When planning surgery, cerebral angiography is important to evaluate vascular encasement and displacement. A balloon occlusion test of the internal carotid artery may be performed if the vessel is narrowed by the tumor. Evaluation of the venous circulation, including the sigmoid sinuses, is important for tumors near the jugular foramen and in the foramen area.

TREATMENT OPTIONS

Management of chordomas must improve the survival of patients and the recurrence rate. Quality of life is also an important issue with these extensive slow-growing tumors.

In the past, non-treated chordomas had an average survival time between 0.6 and 2 years (Kamrin et al 1964, Heffelfinger et al 1973, Eriksson et al 1981). Heffelfinger et al (1973), in a series of 155 patients demonstrated a 5.2-year average survival time after surgery followed by radiotherapy, 4.8 years after radiotherapy only, and 1.5 years after surgery alone. Most other series demonstrate poor overall survival rates of 51% and 35% at 5 and 10 years respectively after subtotal or partial surgery followed by radiotherapy (Heffelfinger et al 1973, Cummings et al 1983, Forsyth et al 1993). Classic chondrosarcomas are known to have a better prognosis. Depending on the classification, the 5-year survival rates are 90%, 81% and 43% for grade I, II, and III lesions respectively (Evans et al 1977). The mesenchymal subtype of chondrosarcomas has a poorer prognosis.

With these slow-growing tumors, some patients may live for many years while the tumor progresses. It is well known that local recurrence or regrowth is a major cause of failure (Evans et al 1977). Thus, a 'progression-free', 'recurrence-free', or 'disease-free' survival rate is a better criterion of the efficacy of treatment. In this case, the 5-year and 10-year survival rates fall to 33% and 20% (Finn et al 1984, Forsyth et al 1993).

Chemotherapy

Although some authors reported the subjective improvement of a patient after a protocol based on one for soft tissue or osteogenic sarcoma, effective chemotherapy is not yet available (Finn et al 1984, Fuller & Bloom 1988).

Radiotherapy options

Irradiation was first thought not to alter the outcome of the disease (Dahlin & MacCarty 1952); however, further investigations suggested that doses greater than 5000 cGy and as high as 8000 cGy may provide palliation (Pearlman & Friedman 1970, Rich et al 1985, Amendola et al 1986). Some authors, however, found no dose-response relationship or increased survival with higher doses (Belza 1966, Cummings et al 1983).

Radiotherapy is commonly used after surgery, but it seems that conventional external beam radiation therapy after a partial or subtotal resection has no long-term effect on recurrence of tumors (Krayenbühl & Yasargil 1975, Harwood et al 1980, Suit et al 1982, Cummings et al 1983, Rich et al 1985, Fuller & Bloom 1988, Keisch et al 1991). Depending on whether surgery or radiotherapy is the relevant factor, this leads to two controversial hypotheses:

- As tumor is locally invasive and total resection is difficult to achieve, further surgical advances will not increase the survival (Raffel et al 1985); even radiation alone after biopsy has been proposed (Kamrin et al 1964, Rich et al 1985).
- On the contrary, if postoperative radiation has any effect it will be enhanced if the residual tumor volume is as small as possible. Therefore, aggressive and new appropriate approaches should be helpful (Kveton et al 1986, Derome et al 1987, Keisch et al 1991, Meyers et al 1992, Forsyth et al 1993).

A recent report from the Mayo Clinic demonstrated with a large series that conventional postoperative radiotherapy does not improve the survival time but has a significant effect on prolonged disease-free survival (Forsyth et al 1993).

Recently, different potential sources of ultra-high dose radiation have been shown to improve the prognosis of patients.

Radioactive sources (radon, ^{125}I, yttrium) have been implanted stereotactically or microsurgically, but with questionable success (Zoltan & Fenyes 1960, Kumar et al 1988, Kondziolka et al 1991).

Few reports on radiosurgery for chordomas and chondrosarcomas are available at present (Kondziolka et al 1991), but it is clear that radiosurgery as the sole treatment for these tumors is at risk of failure. When small remnants remain after microsurgery, distant from neural structures such as optic nerves, however, control of the tumor may be achieved with few new postoperative deficits.

First described by Suit et al in 1982, proton beam therapy allows the radiotherapist to deliver doses that are superior to high energy X-rays (Suit et al 1982, Berson et al 1988, Austin-Seymour et al 1989, Muzenrider 1992). With such treatment, higher doses can be given to the tumor sites, with acceptable normal tissue doses. Improvement in computerized 3D treatment planning and dose localization has led to better results (Tatsuzaki & Urie 1991). Applied after debulking of the tumor, this treatment leads to an overall local control rate of 76% at 5 years (95% for chondrosarcomas, 62% for chordomas) (Fig. 40.1) (Berson et al 1988, Austin-Seymour et al 1989, Muzenrider 1992). Tissues away from tumor receive a low dose, and it is possible to define a sharp lateral beam edge. Tumor volume is a significant prognostic factor for local failure. Small tumors or small remnants of a previously debulked lesion have a better prognosis. A 34% complication rate, consisting of endocrine, hearing,

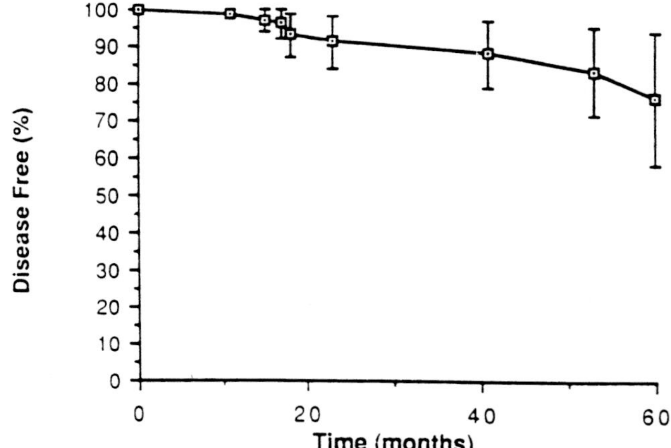

Fig. 40.1 Curve showing the actuarial disease-free survival rate for 68 patients with chordomas and low grade chondrosarcomas of the skull base (76% at 5 years). Based on data from Austin-Seymour et al (1989).

or visual complications, brain injury, seizures or radionecrosis, is described (Muzenrider 1992).

Surgical treatment

Whatever the extent of the resection, most authors agree that surgery is important for a good outcome (Dahlin & MacCarty 1952, Krayenbühl & Yasargil 1975, Hassounah et al 1985, O'Neill et al 1985, Arnold & Herrmann 1986, Kveton et al 1986, Derome et al 1987, Sen et al 1989, Keisch et al 1991, Muzenrider 1992, Forsyth et al 1993). Some authors reported some success in total removal or disease-free control of the tumor, based on postoperative films, with more extensive or combined approaches (Derome & Guiot 1979, Kveton et al 1986, Derome et al 1987, Charabi et al 1989, Sen et al 1989). At present, the best philosophy seems to be to aim at complete surgical removal, even with multiple staged combined approaches. If surgery is incomplete or remnants are still present on postoperative films, operative excision by different approaches or methods of radiation such as proton or helium beam radiation, radiosurgery or even external beam radiation should be discussed. Treatment of recurrences remains the same: reoperation or the options.

In the experience of the senior author at the University of Pittsburgh, about half of the patients referred to us for treatment of chordomas or chondrosarcomas had had previous surgery. We treated such recurrent or residual tumors with combined approaches, frequently in one or two staged procedures. Over a period of 8 years, 88% of patients were free of disease. Radiosurgery or proton beam radiation was used for small remnants or physiologically defined older patients.

SURGICAL PROCEDURE

As these tumors are mainly extradural, an extradural approach should be used. The exception to this rule is the upper clival region where an extradural approach to the tumor is difficult. As a tumor increases in size it will infiltrate the basal dura. Prediction of dural invasion before surgery is difficult, however its treatment is important since dural invasion seems to be a factor indicating a bad prognosis (Derome et al 1987).

Many surgical procedures are used and described: extended maxillotomy and subtotal maxillectomy (Cocke et al 1990), facial translocation (Janecka et al 1990), transsphenoidal approach or transmaxillary-transnasal approach (Rabadan & Conesa 1992), and transoral (Erbengi et al 1991). Some of them are variants of others. We usually used four major approaches that could lead to extensive resection either extradurally and intradurally

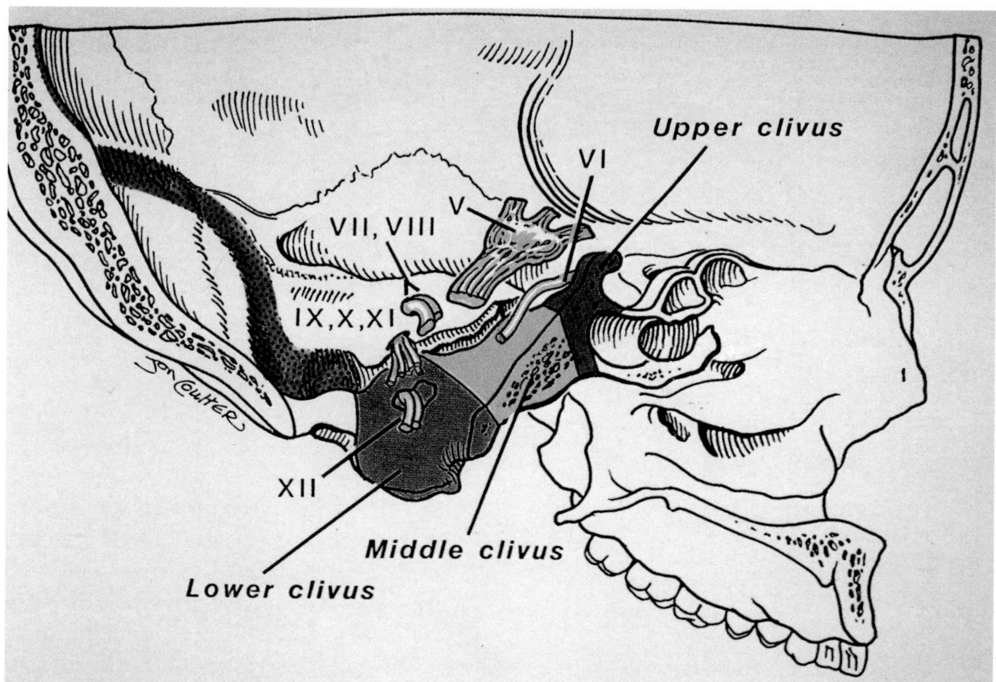

Fig. 40.2 The anatomic divisions of the clivus into upper, mid, and lower regions. Adjacent cranial base structures are shown. (From: Sekhar L N, Janecka I P Surgery of Cranial Base Tumors. Raven Press, New York, with permission).

(Sekhar et al 1987, 1988, Sekhar & Sen 1989, Sen & Sekhar 1990a,b, Sekhar et al 1993). Since chordomas and chondrosarcomas originate from the clivus with local extension, these surgical procedures are usually focused on a direct approach of the clivus.

Approach selections depend on the subregion involved by the tumor extension (Fig. 40.2). For lesions of the upper clivus with extension into the cavernous sinus, the sphenoid region or the petrous apex, the subtemporal, transcavernous, and transpetrous apex approach is used. For lesions of the midclivus laterally extended to the petrous apex, a subtemporal infratemporal approach is preferred. Frequently the entire midclivus is invaded, with the petrous apex and sphenoid areas, and sometimes with bilateral extension. Then a combined surgical approach is used with a subtemporal infratemporal approach in combination with the basal frontal approach. Clival lesions strictly confined to the midline only with invasion of the middle and lower clivus can be removed through a basal frontal approach. When chordomas and chondrosarcomas involve the lower clivus, jugular foramen and condyle area, the extreme lateral transjugular and transcondyle approach is optimal. Large extension of the tumor frequently requires two or more approaches.

The subtemporal, transcavernous, transpetrous apex approach (Fig. 40.3)

This is an intradural approach in which the patient is placed in the supine position with the head slightly extended and turned 60° away from the surgeon. Neurophysiological monitoring of cranial nerves III, VI and VII is employed. A curvilinear incision is made, starting in the temporal region, curving anteriorly above the ear and extending to the preauricular area. After elevation of temporalis muscle, a temporal craniotomy and a zygomatic osteotomy including the condylar fossa are performed. Extradural middle cranial fossa dissection is then guided by important landmarks (middle meningeal artery, arcuate eminence, lesser petrosal nerve, greater superficial petrosal nerve—GSPN, mandibular nerve—V3, and horizontal segment of the petrous internal carotid artery frequently uncovered by bone). Under the surgical microscope, the dura is opened and the temporal lobe retracted after opening the subarachnoid cisterns widely. The tentorium is divided after identification of the fourth cranial nerve and dissection of the vascular contents of the perimesencephalic cistern.

The cavernous sinus is accessed via its lateral wall. The

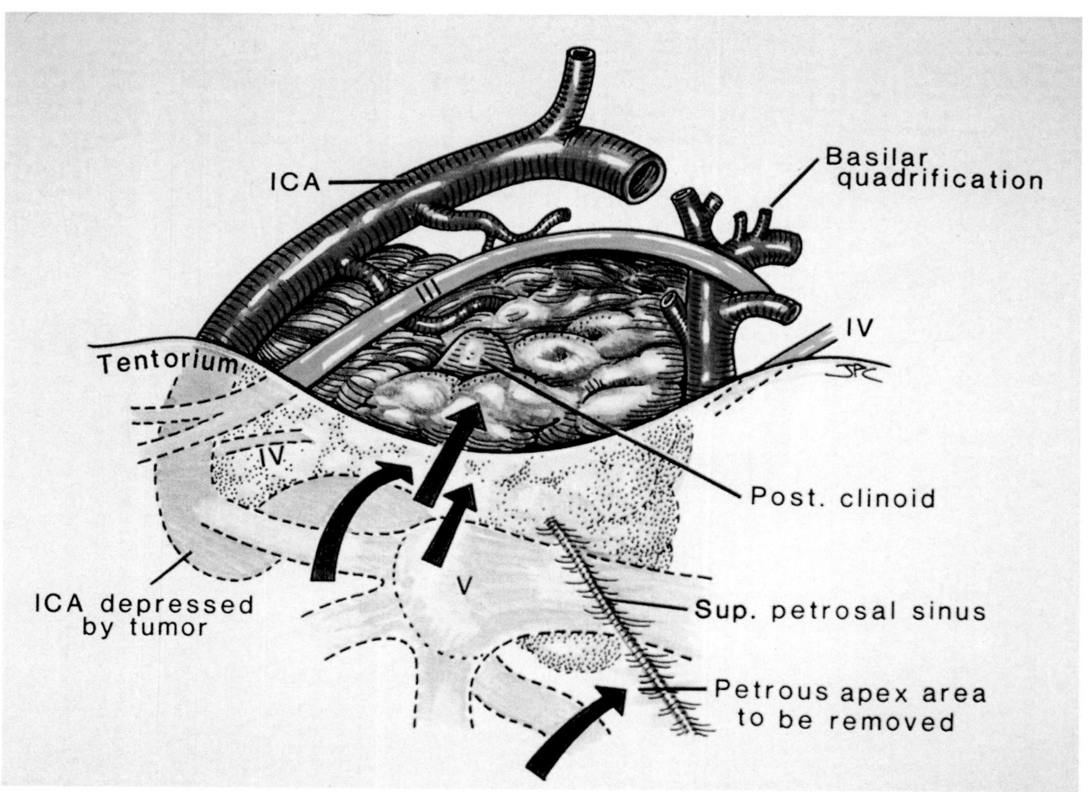

Fig. 40.3 The subtemporal, transcavernous, and transpetrous apex approach. The important anatomic structures encountered during the approach and the tumor are shown. Arrows show the different approaches to the tumor. (From: Sekhar L N, Janecka I P Surgery of Cranial Base Tumors. Raven Press, New York, with permission).

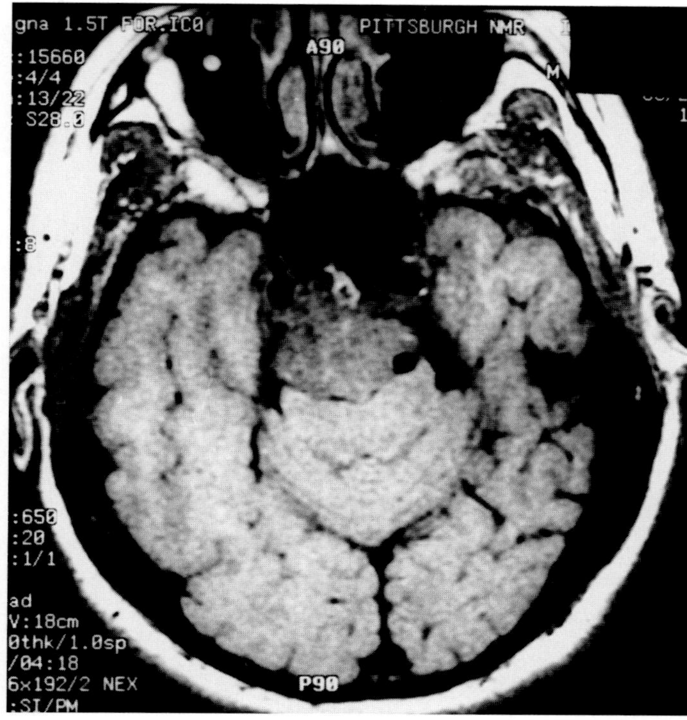

A

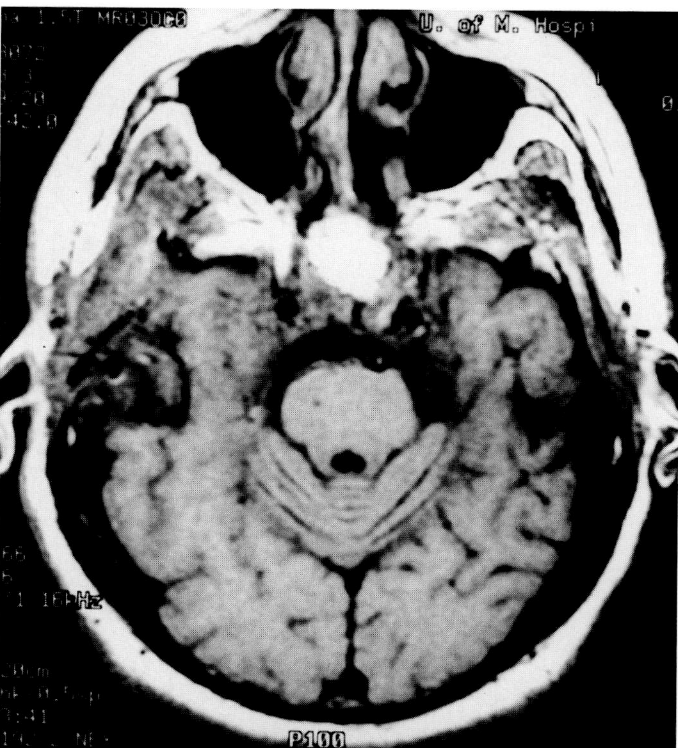

B

Fig. 40.4 This 62 year-old patient complained of headache and double vision with a right sixth nerve palsy. On MR imaging, this large tumor, hypointense on T1-weighted image **A**, was seen to invade the upper region of the clivus with bilateral invasion of the right petrous apex and extension into the right cavernous sinus. A subtemporal, transcavernous, and transpetrous apex approach was performed. The diagnosis of chordoma was histologically confirmed. The tumor was completely removed, as shown on postoperative CT scan, **B** and MRI, **C**.

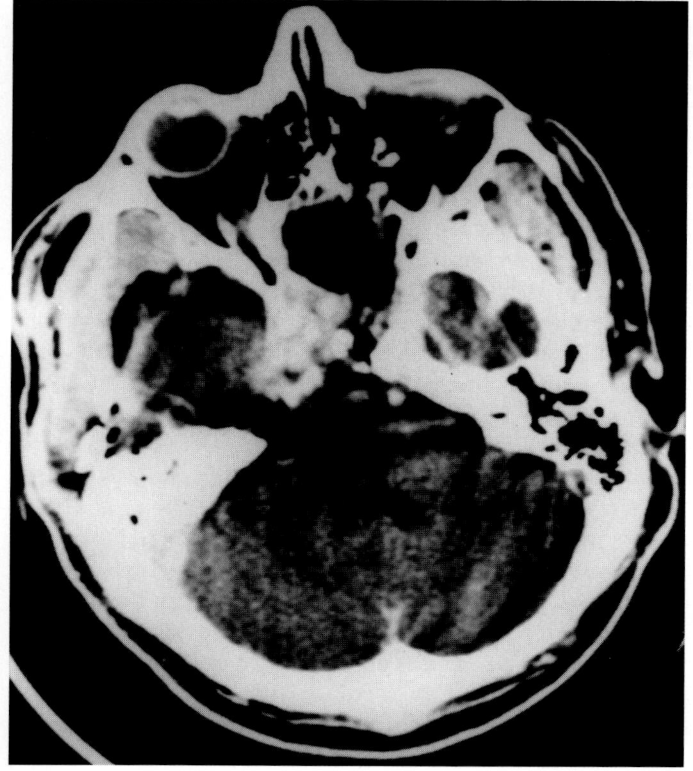

C

surgeon may work between the fourth and fifth nerves, third and fourth nerves, or through the Meckel's cave between rootlets of cranial nerve V. The prepeduncular area and the brainstem may be easily freed of tumor. The petrous apex bone is removed with a drill, working intradurally lateral to the trigeminal root and ganglion, until the horizontal segment of the petrous internal carotid artery is reached. This allows the abducens nerves to be visualized, and the lower pole of the tumor will be seen clearly. With this approach, the surgeon may remove any involved bone of the dorsum sellae, posterior clinoids, floor of the sella turcica and petrous apex (case report — Fig. 40.4).

The subtemporal-infratemporal approach (Figs 40.5, 40.6)

After inserting a spinal drain to relax the brain, the patient

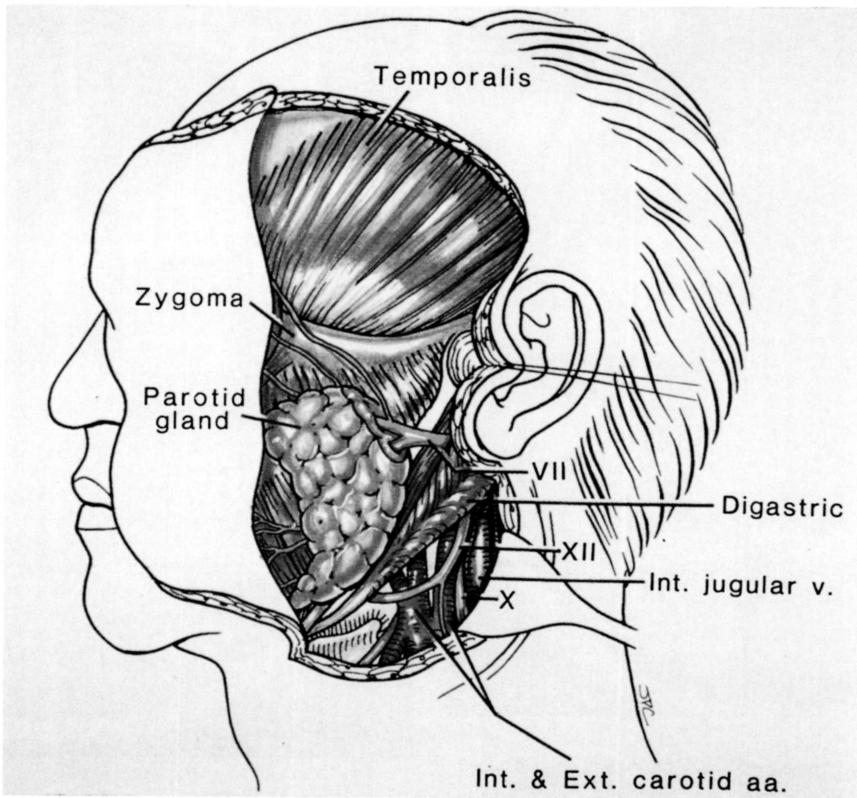

Fig. 40.5 The subtemporal and infratemporal approach: exposure after a temporal incision extended in the preauricular area and the cervical region. The upper branches of the facial nerve and the upper part of the parotid gland have been dissected. The upper cervical vessels and cranial nerves have been exposed. (From: Sekhar L N, Janecka I P Surgery of Cranial Base Tumors. Raven Press, New York, with permission).

is placed in the supine position with head extended and turned about 60° to the opposite side. The skin incision can be bicoronal with extension into the preauricular area, or it can be curvilinear in the temporal region with a preauricular parotidectomy-type extension. The upper part of the parotid gland and upper branches of the facial nerve are elevated from the masseteric fascia. The temporalis muscle is elevated from the temporal fossa, and the masseteric muscle is detached from the zygomatic arch. A temporal craniectomy is performed, followed by a zygomatic osteotomy including the condylar fossa. The condyle of the mandible can usually be displaced inferiorly, without the need for resection. An extradural middle cranial fossa dissection is performed. The upper cervical internal carotid artery is also identified and exposed and the entire petrous internal carotid artery is isolated. The middle meningeal artery and the GSPN are coagulated and divided; V2 and V3 are then unroofed, in order to expose the horizontal segment of the petrous ICA which lies posteromedial to V3 and inferiorly to GSPN. The genu of the petrous ICA is isolated after section of the tensor tympani muscle and the eustachian tube. The lumen of the eustachian tube has to be carefully closed by packing and suturing in order to avoid any postoperative CSF leak. The vertical segment of the petrous ICA is then exposed by drilling away the tympanic bone lying medial to the temporomandibular joint. A dense fibrocartilaginous ring at the entrance to the carotid canal has to be excised to allow further forward mobilization of the ICA.

The petrous ICA is then displaced anteromedially, without any kinking of the artery, and held forward gently with sutures through the periadventitial tissues. Tumor is then removed piecemeal, and abnormal bone is drilled away. Working medial to the vertical segment of the petrous ICA, progressive removal of abnormal bone is performed. The petroclival bone resection can extend to the anterior portion of the occipital condyle if necessary. When V1 is divided, this approach can be extended to the opposite petrous ICA canal and this allows extensive removal of lesions of the lower clivus. By following the ipsilateral ICA medial to V3 the inferior aspect of the cavernous sinus can be dissected free of tumor. If neces-

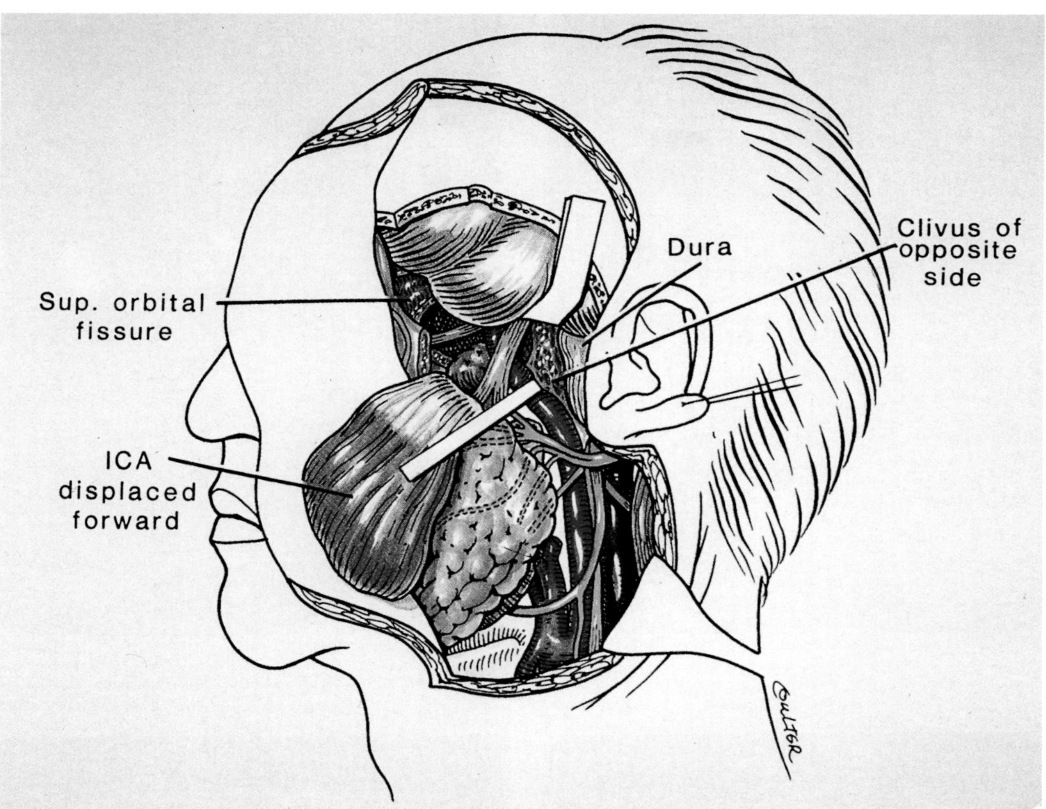

Fig. 40.6 The exposure obtained with the subtemporal and infratemporal approach after the temporal craniotomy and zygomatic osteotomy have been performed. The middle fossa dissection is complete. The petrous internal carotid artery is freed of tumor and mobilized forward to allow extensive drilling and access to the petroclival dura. (From: Sekhar L N, Janecka I P Surgery of Cranial Base Tumors, Raven Press, New York, with permission).

sary, the sphenoid bone and the sphenoid sinus can be accessed, working between V1 and V2 or V2 and V3 (case report — Fig. 40.7).

Extended frontal approach (Figs 40.8, 40.9)

This approach is a modification of the transbasal approach of Derome (Derome & Guiot 1979, Derome et al 1987) with the addition of an orbito-fronto-ethmoidal osteotomy. The main disadvantage of such an approach is the bilateral olfactory denervation. Most recently, we have attempted preservation of olfaction, following the advice of Spetzler et al (1993). The patient lies in the supine position. A bicoronal skin incision is made starting just in front of the ear, extending vertically up to the opposite side. Skin flap and pericranium are reflected forward and exposure of the superior orbital rim is performed bilaterally, taking care of supraorbital nerves and vessels. Frontal craniotomy is performed using two small frontal bone flaps to avoid injury to the sagittal sinus. These craniotomies will include the upper portions of the frontal sinuses. The subfrontal dura is separated from the roof of the orbit bilaterally, and from the planum sphenoidale. An orbito-fronto-ethmoid osteotomy is then performed with mild subfrontal retraction. An extensive ethmoidectomy is performed. The planum sphenoidale is removed with drill and rongeurs, the optic nerves are unroofed bilaterally or unilaterally. Middle and posterior ethmoidal cells are resected to reach the lower aspect of the clivus. Bone of the body of the sphenoid is drilled away and removing it, the sellar dura is unroofed. The anterior bend of the intracavernous carotid artery and medial wall of the cavernous sinus are also unroofed, tracing the ICA back to the posterior vertical segment, and the petrous apex area. Posteriorly, the sphenoclival bone is removed progressively and clival dura can be reached. With this approach, tumor resection can be extended down to the margins of foramen magnum, and to the hypoglossal foramina. The sixth nerve, traveling from the posterior fossa to enter the Dorello's canal in the cavernous sinus, has to be carefully protected during drilling of the clivus. If the dura mater is excised during the tumor resection or because of tumor

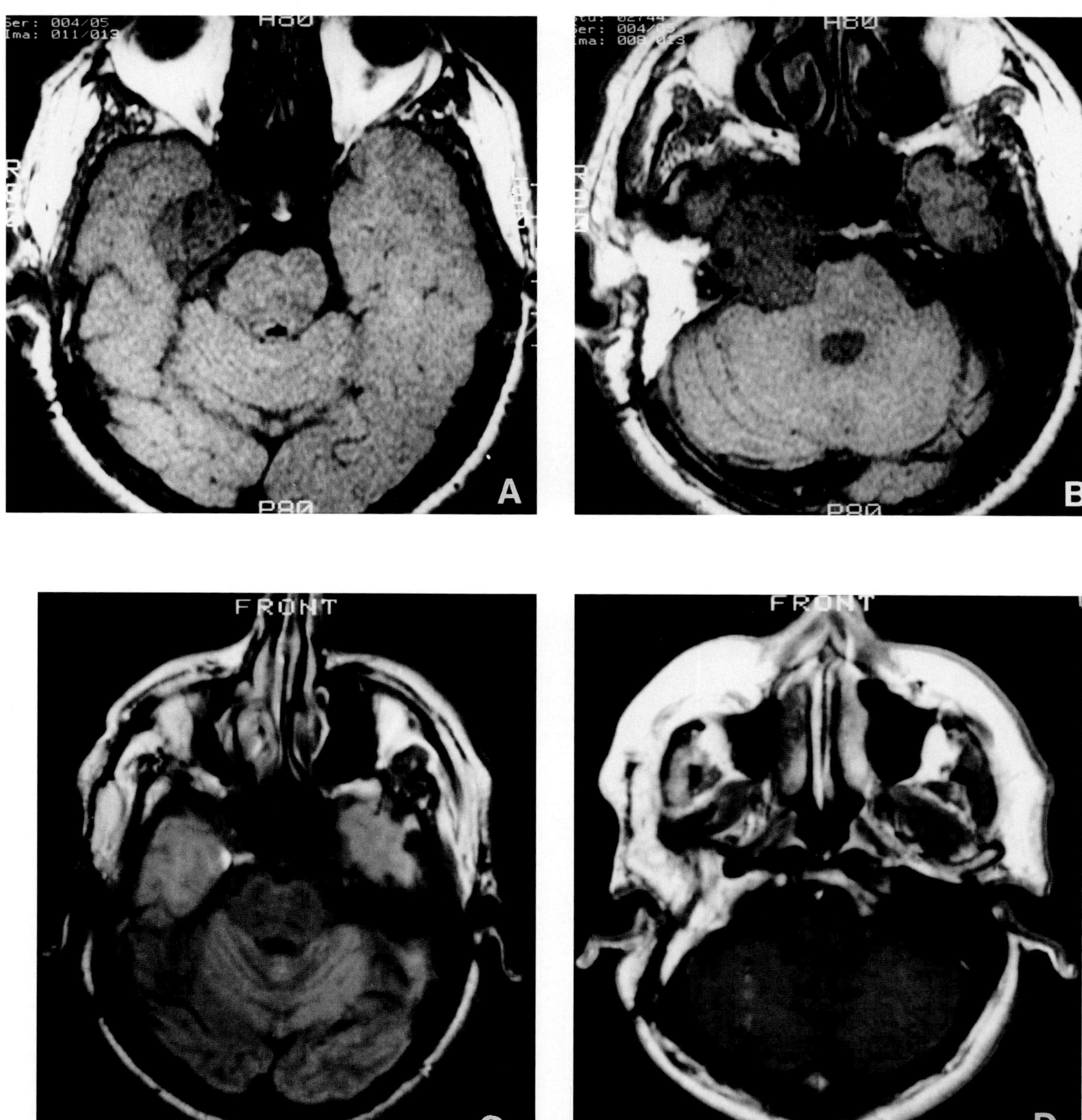

Fig. 40.7 This 48-year-old patient had previously undergone one operation with partial resection of a chondrosarcoma. On admission he complained of diplopia and had a complete right facial palsy. Neurologic deficits of the right fifth and sixth nerves were found. T1-weighted images show a hypointense lesion of the midclivus with invasion of the right cavernous sinus extending into the cerebellopontine angle (**A**, **B**). A subtemporal and infratemporal approach was performed and allowed us to totally remove the tumor (**C**, **D**). A facial nerve graft reconstruction was successfully performed, with a House grade III functional recovery.

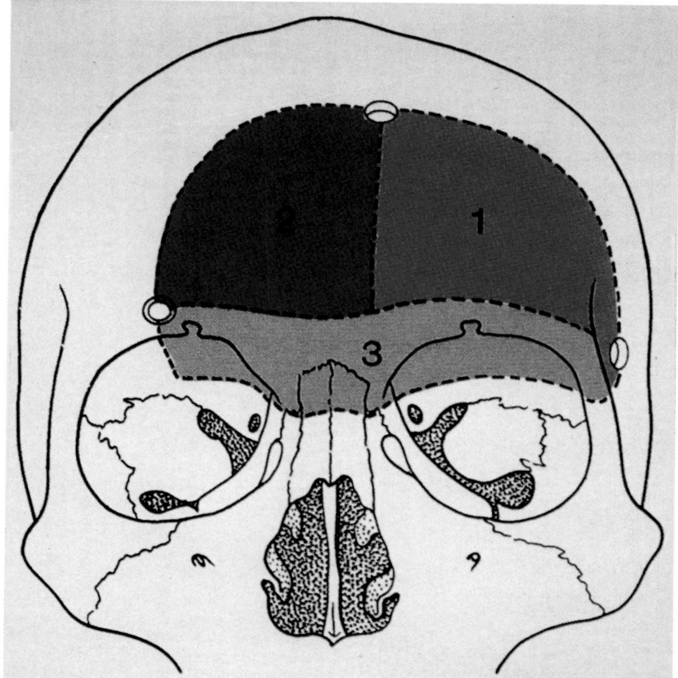

Fig. 40.8 Two frontal craniotomies (1, 2) and an orbito-fronto-ethmoidal osteotomy (3) are performed during the exposure for the extended frontal approach. (From: Sekhar L N, Janecka I P Surgery of Cranial Base Tumors. Raven Press, New York, with permission).

invasion, it can be reconstructed with fascia lata, sutures and fibrin glue. A long pericranial flap and fat grafts are used to obliterate the defect (case report — Fig. 40.10).

Extreme lateral transcondyle and transjugular approach (Figs 40.11, 40.12)

The patient is placed in the lateral position (Sugita position). An L or C shape incision is made behind the ear. The sternocleidomastoid muscle is detached from the mastoid process. The C1 and C2 transverse processes are identified by palpation. The splenius capitis, semispinalis capitis, and recti muscles are detached from the occipital bone and reflected medially. The oblique, recti and levator scapulae muscles are detached from the C1 transverse process and reflected medially. Cranial nerve XI and the jugular bulb must be identified. The suboccipital bone and C1 transverse process are freed of muscles. The vertebral artery is dissected from the foramen transversarium of C1 or C2 to the suboccipital membrane, and displaced inferomedially. The lateral third of the C1 lamina is removed along with the lateral mass, sparing the posterior arch. A laterally placed occipital craniotomy is performed, down to the foramen magnum. A low mastoidectomy

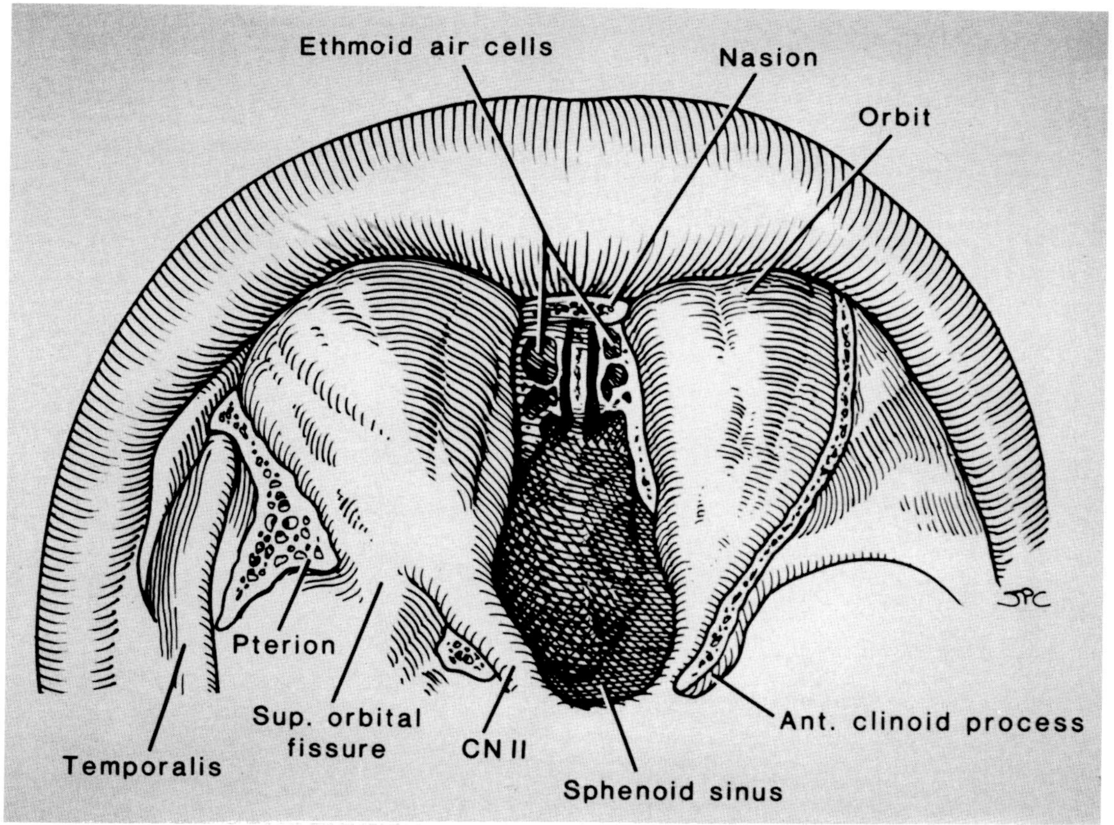

Fig. 40.9 The extended frontal approach: view obtained anteriorly after a fronto-orbital-ethmoidal osteotomy; optic nerve decompression and sphenoidotomy are shown. (From: Sekhar L N, Janecka I P Surgery of Cranial Base Tumors. Raven Press, New York, with permission).

which will unroof the sigmoid sinus and the jugular bulb is also performed. The tumor invading the occipital condyle is resected. When the jugular bulb is invaded, it can be opened after division of the sigmoid sinus if a good demonstration of crossover patency of venous drainage has been demonstrated angiographically. The lower clival bone can be reached; cranial nerves IX–XII should be followed extradurally, and dissected from tumor. When the occipital condyle is completely removed, an occiput to C1, C2, C3 fusion with titanium plates and bone grafts is necessary to prevent the occurrence of a head tilt (case report — Figs 40.13, 40.14).

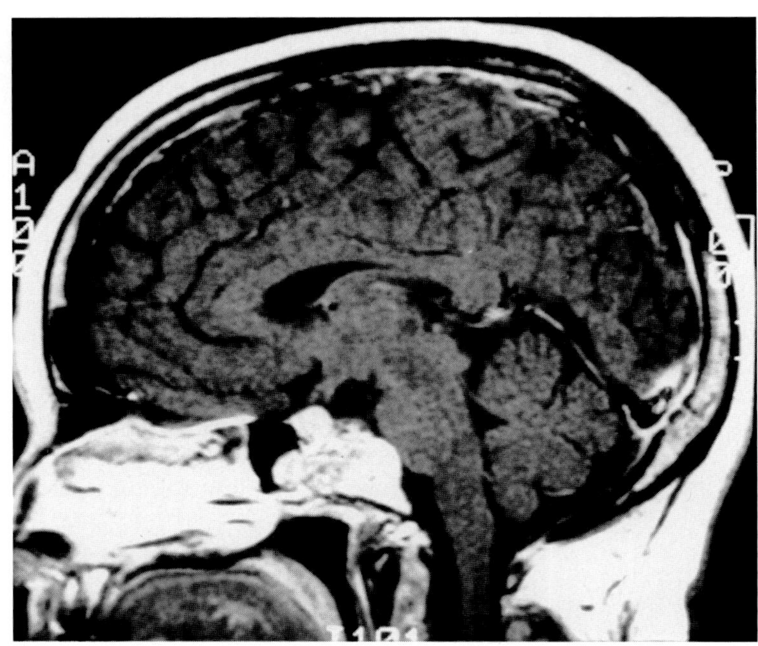

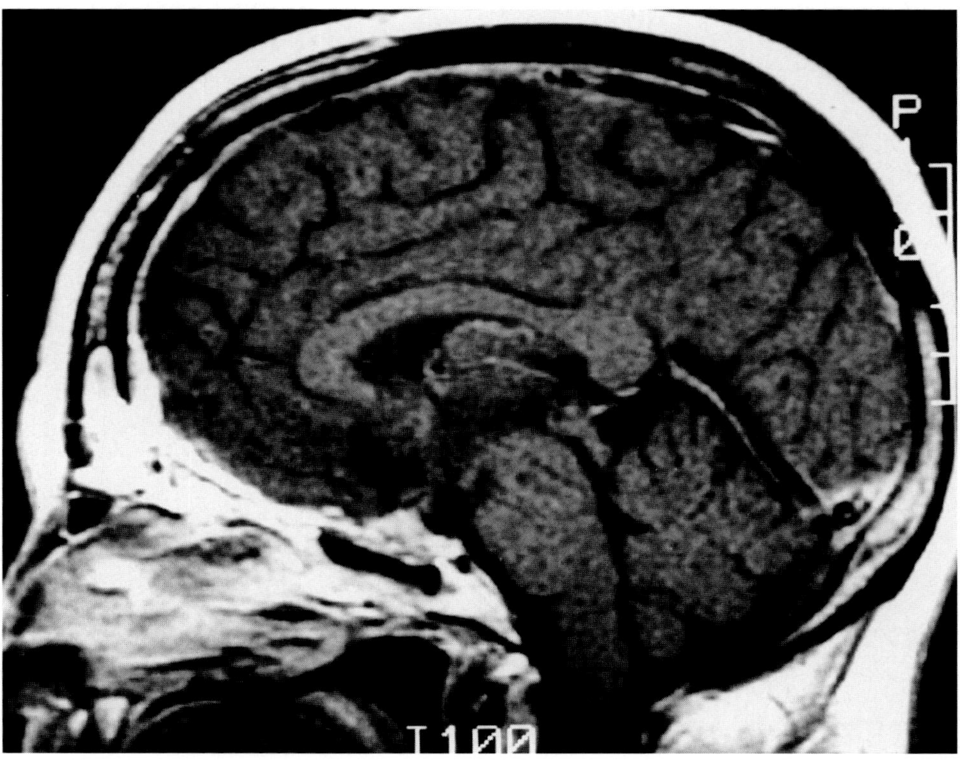

B

Fig. 40.10 This 43-year-old women presented with a right sixth cranial nerve palsy and a severe loss of visual acuity of the right eye. Sagittal post contrast MR shows intense, slightly irregular enhancement of a lesion invading the upper clival bone marrow and protruding into the prepontine cistern (**A**). After an extended frontal approach, this chordoma was removed and the operative cavity was filled in with fat (**B**) (postoperative MR).

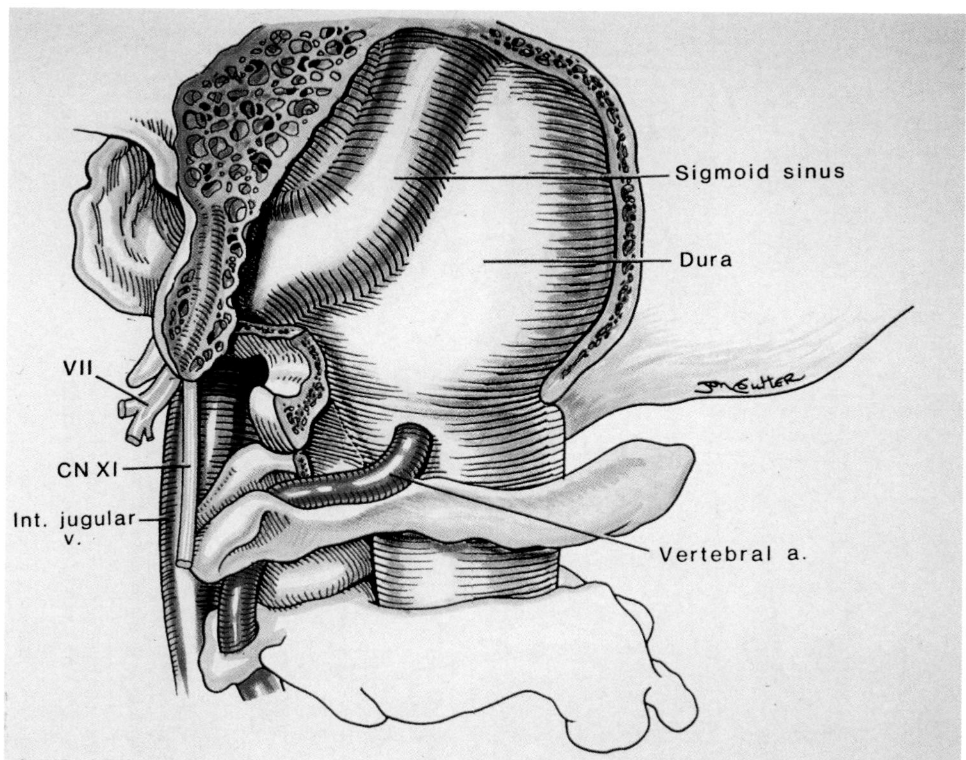

Fig. 40.11 Extreme lateral approach. The vertebral artery has been exposed extradurally. A retrosigmoid craniotomy has been performed with a mastoidectomy. The sigmoid sinus and the jugular bulb have been partially unroofed. The occipital condyle and the articular process of C1 have been partially removed. (From: Sekhar L N, Janecka I D Surgery of Cranial Base Tumors. Raven Press, New York, with permission).

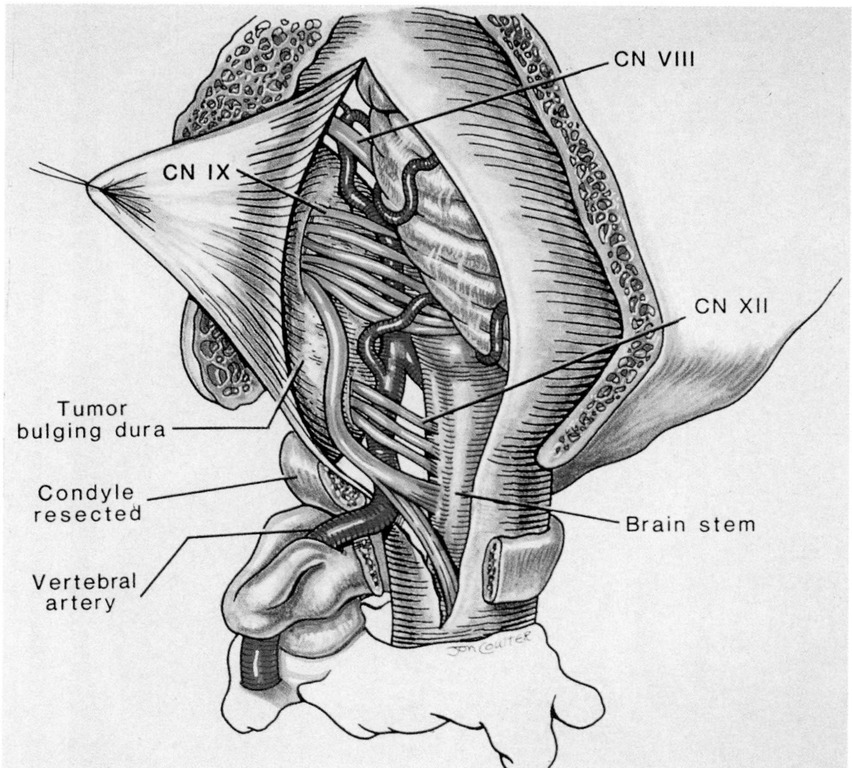

Fig. 40.12 Extreme lateral approach. The dura is opened to remove intradural tumor and to help in the identification of cranial nerves IX–XII extradurally. (From: Sekhar L N, Janecka I D Surgery of Cranial Base Tumors. Raven Press, New York, with permission).

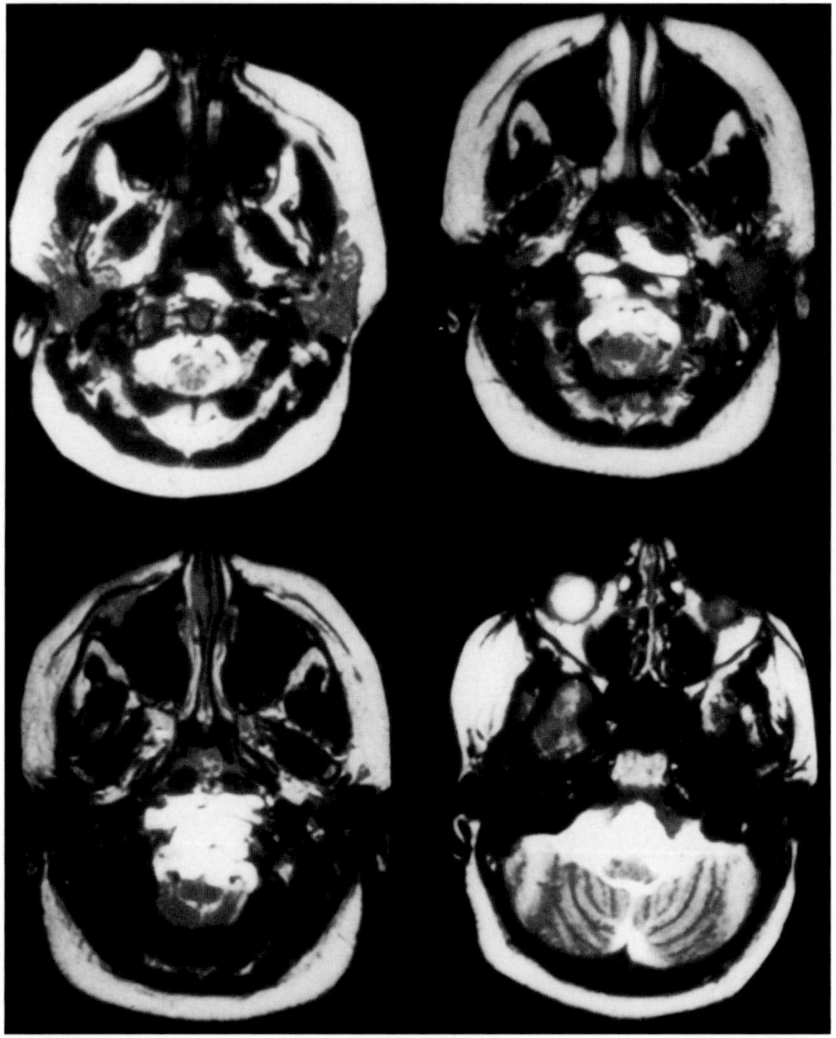

Fig. 40.13 This patient was a 15-year-old girl who complained of neck pain and some disequilibrium. On MR imaging the tumor invaded the lower clivus with extension in the cervico-occipital region. After an extreme lateral approach, this tumor was diagnosed to be a chordoma. The T2-weighted MR sequences show the brightness of the tumor, the encasement of the vertebral arteries, and the severe compression of the brainstem.

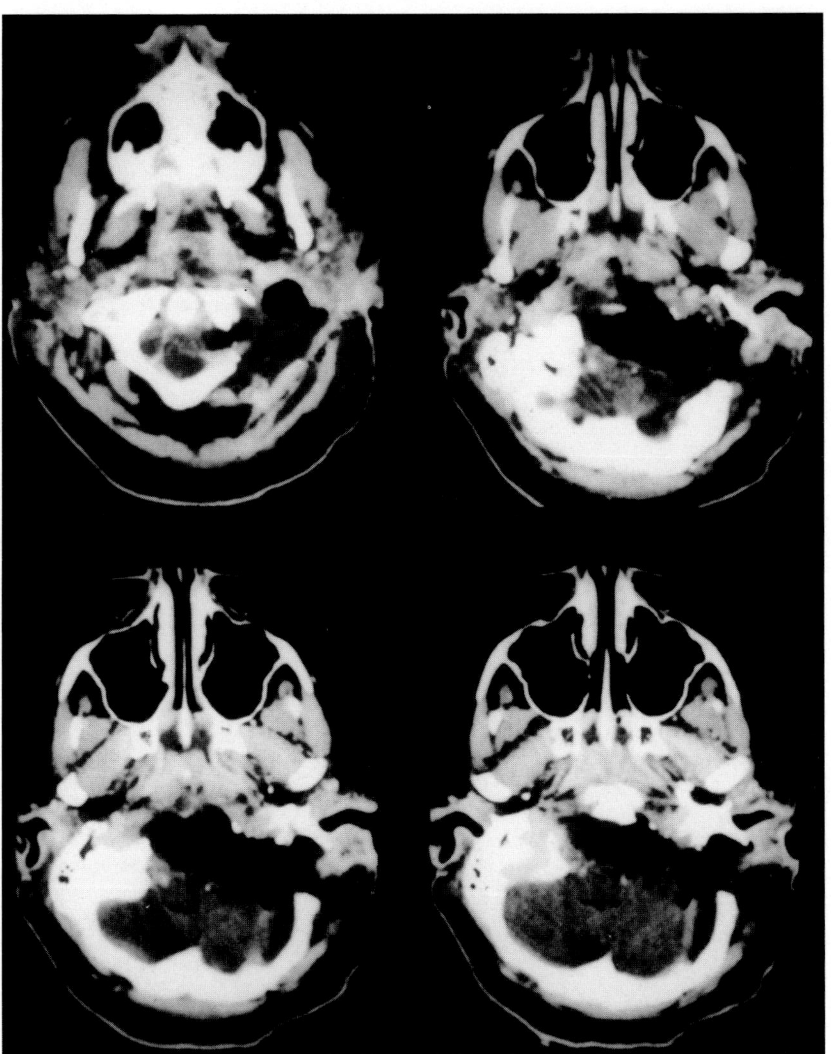

Fig. 40.14 The postoperative CT scans of the patient shown in Fig. 40.13 show the tumor resection, and packing of the cavity with fat.

Reconstruction is performed at the end of the operations with fascia lata patching of dural defects, and autologous fat. A temporalis muscle flap, a vascularized free flap of rectus abdominalis, or latissimus dorsi are frequently employed in conjunction with fat to fill the operative defect (Jones et al 1987, Snyderman et al 1990). Reconstruction after the transbasal approach must be performed using a galeo-pericranial flap before a careful reconstruction of the bone flap.

These approaches are often combined in stages to achieve a total tumor resection. An extreme lateral approach is used to complement the lower reach of the subtemporal infratemporal approach when tumor remains in the occipital condyle or lower clivus. The combined anterior transbasal approach and lateral subtemporal infratemporal approach allow the resection of very extensive clival tumors, involving petrous apex, entire midclivus and sphenoid (Sekhar et al 1988).

Other approaches

The *transoral approach* may be chosen for lesions confined to the middle or the lower third of the clivus and the cranio-cervical junction. After a tracheostomy or positioning of a nasotracheal tube, the patient is placed in the supine or lateral position. A tongue retractor is inserted. The soft and hard palate may be split in order to access lesions above the foramen magnum. The tubercle of the anterior surface of C1 has to be found before infiltration with lidocaine and adrenaline. A midline incision is performed; C1 is freed of muscle and the anterior arch of C1 is drilled out. The odontoid process, the transverse ligament and the posterior longitudinal ligament have to be divided to expose dura in this fashion, allowing extradural tumors to be removed. The pharynx is then closed in two layers. This approach is not recommended for intradural lesions.

The *transmaxillary approach* is suitable for lesions of the upper and middle third of the clivus. An incision is made along the upper alveolar margin. The bone incision is made above the dental roots with an oscillating saw to down fracture the hard palate. After removing the vomer, and reflecting the septum, the sphenoid sinus and the upper portion of the clivus are accessed. Using a high speed drill, the clivus is drilled out, allowing removal of tumor and access to clival dura. Closure is performed as previously described.

The transoral approach is not used by us because of the lateral extensions of the tumor. Transmaxillary and trans-sphenoidal approaches may be applicable to some tumors.

Results of extensive surgical resection

With the general management described before, based on an 'extensive surgical removal', the tumor-free survival time of our patients is around 76% at 5 years (92% and 69% for chondrosarcomas and chordomas — Figs 40.15, 40.16). There were 3 deaths within 3 months postoperatively (due to pulmonary embolism or myocardial infarc-

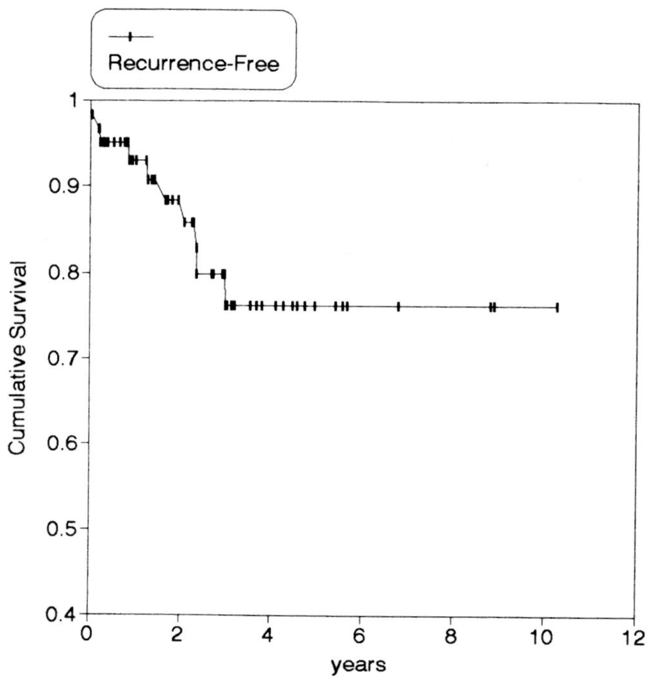

Fig. 40.15 Curve showing the disease-free survival rate for 60 patients with chordomas and chondrosarcomas at the base of the skull.

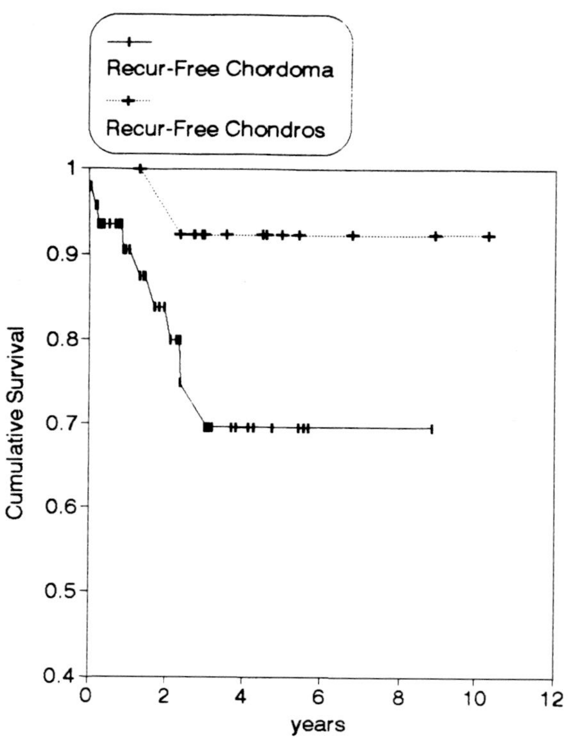

Fig. 40.16 Recurrence-free survival for chordomas (46 patients) and chondrosarcomas (14 patients).

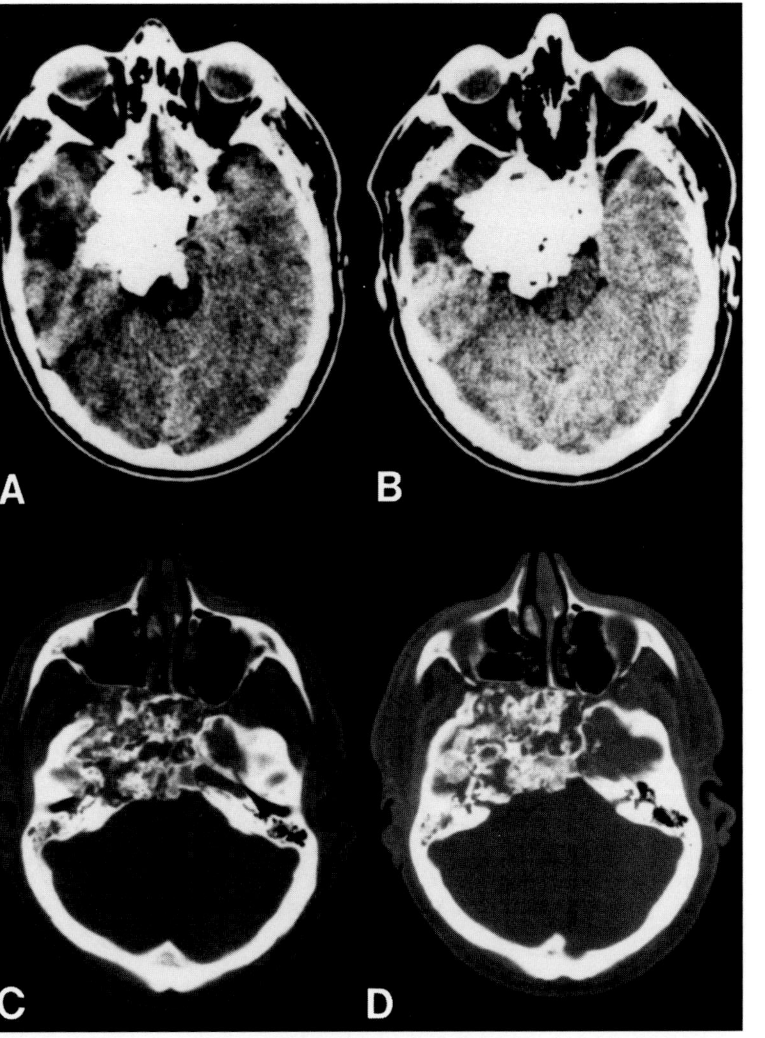

Fig. 40.17 A 41-year-old patient with past medical history significant for two incomplete previous operations for a low grade chondrosarcoma. MRI and CT showed evidence of a large, recurrent, partly calcified mass involving the right petrous apex extending into the middle fossa, the cavernous sinus, the pituitary fossa and the sphenoid sinus, with a contralateral extension in the left cavernous sinus and petrous apex. Marked compression of the brainstem was noted. Bone windowed CT scan shows the destruction of the bone.

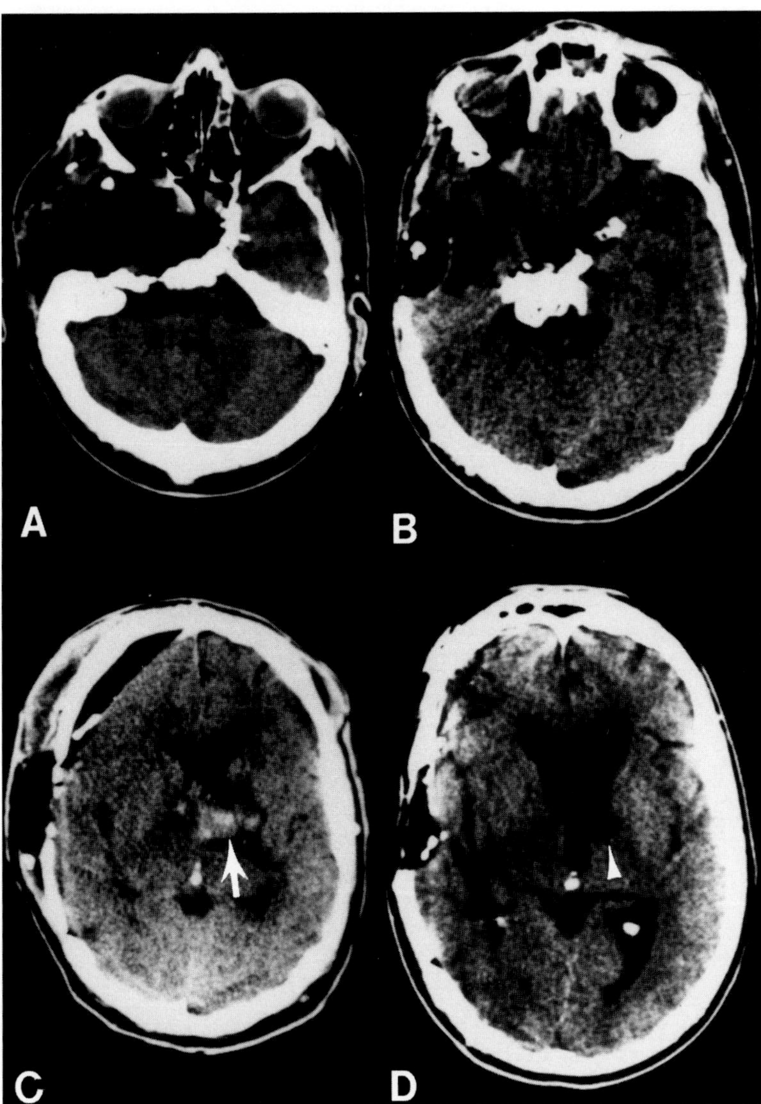

Fig. 40.18 Same patient as in Fig. 40.17. At surgery, a right subtemporal infratemporal approach was performed. A severe intraoperative coagulopathy necessitated premature termination of the procedure. However, the right cavernous sinus was freed of tumor, the petrous internal carotid artery was decompressed, and the contralateral tumor invasion of the petrous apex was removed via the same approach (**A, B**). Postoperatively an area of ischemia was observed in the left basal thalamic region, probably due to injury of perforating vessels of the basilar artery. Hemorrhage into those areas followed a sudden episode of hypertension (**C, D**).

tion), and 7 deaths during the follow-up period because of tumor recurrence, or unrelated causes. We found that the mortality of patients was not related to tumor size or degree of resection, but was strongly related to prior radiotherapy. Incidence of recurrences had no relation to tumor pathology or tumor size, but patients who underwent a total or near-total resection had lower risk of recurrence than patients with a partial or even a subtotal resection.

Quality of life is a difficult problem for patients with chordomas or chondrosarcomas. Multiple surgical approaches for recurrences will add new neurologic problems. Postoperative disability of our patients was mainly related to CSF leakage and infection. Postoperative CSF leak, in approaches where dura has to be opened, has been almost solved by an appropriate dural closure with fascia lata and fibrin glue or free-flap reconstruction, followed by external lumbar spinal drainage; however, a CSF leak was demonstrated as a factor of permanent disability for patients. New surgical technologies will overcome this problem in the future (e.g. hydroxyapatite sealant). New postoperative cranial nerve deficits are seen mostly during the earlier postoperative period. Generally, in 3 or 6 months, or even one year, they improved. One third to one half of preoperative disorders completely resolved after surgery (complications: case report — Figs 40.17, 40.18).

CONCLUSION

Chordomas and chondrosarcomas — thought of in the past as inoperable tumors — seem nowadays to be potentially curable tumors with lower risk of morbidity. Improvement in surgical approaches and in ultra-high dose radiation techniques lead to more hope for patients. Further development in these two fields will prove that those invasive tumors may be controlled safely for extended periods.

REFERENCES

Amendola B E, Amendola A M, Oliver E, McClatchey K D 1986 Chordoma: Role of radiation therapy. Radiology 158: 839–843

Ariel I M, Verdu C 1975 Chordoma: An analysis of twenty cases treated over a twenty-year span. Journal of Surgical Oncology 7: 27–44

Arnold H, Herrmann H D 1986 Skull base chordoma with cavernous sinus involvement. Partial or radical tumour-removal? Acta Neurochirurgica 83: 31–37

Austin-Seymour M, Muzenrider J, Goitein et al 1989 Fractionated proton radiation therapy of chordoma and low-grade chondrosarcoma of the base of the skull. Journal of Neurosurgery 70: 13–17

Belza J 1966 Double middle intracranial tumors of vestigial origin: Contiguous intrasellar chordoma and suprasellar craniopharyngioma. Journal of Neurosurgery 25: 199–204

Berson A M, Castro J R, Petti P et al 1988 Charged particle irradiation of chordoma and chondrosarcoma of the base of skull and cervical spine: The Lawrence Berkeley Laboratory experience. International Journal of Radiation Oncology Biology Physics 15: 559–565

Bourgouin P M, Tampieri D, Robitaille Y et al 1992 Low-grade myxoid chondrosarcoma of the base of the skull: CT, MR, and histopathology. Journal of Computer Assisted Tomography 16: 268–273

Bouropoulou V, Bosse A, Roessner A et al 1989 Immunohistochemical investigation of chordomas: Histogenetic and differential diagnostic aspects. Current Topics in Pathology 80: 183–203

Brooks J J, LiVolsi V A, Trojanowski J Q 1987 Does chondroid chordoma exist? Acta Neuropathologica 72: 229–235

Brown R V, Sage M R, Brophy B P 1989 CT and MR findings in patients with chordomas of the petrous apex. AJNR 11: 121–124

Bushe K A, Naumann M, Warmuth-Metz M, Meixenberger J, Müller J 1990 Maffuci's syndrome with bilateral cartilaginous tumors of the cerebellopontine angle. Neurosurgery 27: 625–628

Chambers P W, Schwinn C P 1979 A clinicopathologic study of metastasis. American Journal of Clinical Pathology 72: 765–776

Charabi S, Engel P, Bonding P 1989 Myxoid tumours in the temporal bone. Journal of Laryngology and Otology 103: 1206–1209

Cianfriglia F, Pompili A, Occhipinti E 1978 Intracranial malignant cartilaginous tumours. Report of two cases and review of literature. Acta Neurochirurgica 45: 163–175

Cocke E W, Robertson J H, Robertson J T, Crook J P 1990 The extended maxillotomy and subtotal maxillectomy for excision of skull base tumours. Archives of Otolaryngology and Head and Neck Surgery 116: 92–104

Coltrera M D, Googe P B, Harrist T J, Hyams V J, Schiller A L, Goodman M L 1986 Diagnosis and treatment of 13 cases and review of the literature. Cancer 58: 2689–2696

Crockard H A 1993 Transoral approach to intra, extra dural tumors and transmaxillary approach to the clivus. In: Sekhar L N, Janecka I P (eds) Surgery of cranial base tumors. Raven Press, New York, pp 225–244

Cummings B J, Ian Hodson D, Bush R S 1983 Chordoma: The results of megavoltage radiation therapy. International Journal of Radiation Oncology Biology Physics 9: 633–642

Dahlin D C, MacCarty C S 1952 Chordoma, a study of fifty-nine cases. Cancer 5: 1170–1178

Dahlin D C, Unni K K 1986 Bone tumors. Thomas, Springfield, pp 244–267

Derome P, Guiot G 1979 Surgical approaches to the sphenoidal and clival areas. Adv tech Stand Neurosurg 6: 101–136

Derome P, Visot A, Monteil J P, Maestro J L 1987 Management of cranial chordomas. In Sekhar L N, Schramm V L (eds) Tumours of the cranial base. Futura, Mount Kisco, pp 607–622

Erba S M, Horton J A, Latchaw R E, Yonas H, Sekhar L N, Schramm V, Penthany S 1988 Balloon test occlusion of the internal carotid artery with Xerion/CT cerebral blood flow imaging. AJNR 9: 533–538

Erbengi A, Tekkok I H, Acikgoz B 1991 Posterior fossa chordomas — with special references to transoral surgery. Neurosurgical Review 14: 23–28

Eriksson B, Gunterberg B, Kindblom L G 1981 Chordoma, a clinicopathologic and prognostic study of a Swedish national series. Acta Orthopedica Scandinavica 52: 49–58

Evans H L, Ayala A G, Romsdahl M M 1977 Prognostic factors in chondrosarcoma of bone. A clinicopathologic analysis with emphasis on histologic grading. Cancer 40: 818–831

Finn D G, Goeffert H G, Batsakis J G 1984 Chondrosarcoma of the head and neck. Laryngoscope 94: 1539–1543

Forsyth P A, Cascino T L, Shaw E G, Scheithauer B W, O'Fallon J R, Dozier J C, Piepgras D G 1993 Intracranial chordomas: a clinicopathological and prognostic study of 51 cases. Journal of Neurosurgery 78: 741–747

Fuller D B, Bloom J G 1988 Radiotherapy for chordoma. International Journal of Radiation Oncology Biology Physics 15: 331–339

Harwood A R, Krajbich J I, Fornasier V L 1980 Radiotherapy of chondrosarcoma of bone. Cancer 45: 2769–2777

Hasssounah M, Al-Mefty O, Akhtar M, Jinkins J R, Fox J L 1985 Primary cranial and intracranial chondrosarcoma. A survey. Acta Neurochirurgica 78: 123–132
Heffelfinger M J, Dahlin D C, MacCarty C S, Beabout J W 1973 Chordomas and cartilaginous tumors at the skull base. Cancer 32: 410–420
Janecka I P, Sen C N, Sekhar L N, Arriaga M 1990 Facial translocation: A new approach to the cranial base. Otology, Laryngology and Head and Neck Surgery 103: 413–419
Jones M F, Schramm V L, Sekhar L N 1987 Reconstruction of the cranial base following tumour resection. British Journal of Plastic Surgery 40: 155–162
Kamrin R P, Potanos J N, Pool J L 1964 An evaluation of the diagnosis and treatment of chordoma. Journal of Neurology Neurosurgery and Psychiatry 27: 157–165
Keisch M E, Garcia D M, Shibuya R B 1991 Retrospective long-term follow-up analysis in 21 patients with chordomas of various sites treated at a single institution. Journal of Neurosurgery 75: 374–377
Kendall B E, Lee B C P 1977 Cranial chordomas. British Journal of Radiology 50: 687–698
Kondziolka D, Lunsford L D, Flickinger J C 1991 The role of radiosurgery in the management of chordoma and chondrosarcoma of the cranial base. Neurosurgery 29: 38–46
Krayenbühl H, Yasargil M G 1975 Cranial chordomas. Progress in Neurological Surgery 6: 380–434
Kumar P P, Good R R, Skultety F M, Leibrock L G 1988 Local control of recurrent clival and sacral chordoma after interstitial irradiation with Iodine-125: New techniques for treatment of recurrent or unresectable chordomas. Neurosurgery 22: 479–483
Kveton J F, Brackmann D E, Glasscock M E, House W F, Hitselberger W E 1986 Chondrosarcoma of the skull base. Ontolaryngology and Head and Neck Surgery 94: 23–32
Lee Y Y, Trassei P V 1989 Craniofacial chondrosarcomas: Imaging findings in 15 untreated cases. AJNR 10: 165–170
Luschka H 1864 Die Altersveranderungen der Zwischen-wirbelknorpel. Virchows Arch Pathol Anat Physiol Klin Med 31: 396–399
Meyer J E, Oot R F, Lindfors K K 1986 CT appearance of clival chordomas. Journal of Computer Assisted Tomography 10: 34–38
Meyers S P, Hirsch W L, Curtin H D, Barnes L, Sekhar L N, Sen C 1992 Chondrosarcomas of the skull base: MR imaging features. Radiology 184: 103–108
Muzenrider J E 1992 Proton beam radiation and chordomas and chondrosarcomas. Proceedings of the 3rd International Conference on head and neck tumors, San Francisco, CA, July 1992
O'Neill P, Bell B A, Miller J D, Jacobson I, Guthrie W 1985 Fifty years of experience with chordomas in Southeast Scotland. Neurosurgery 16: 166–170
Oot R F, Melville G E, New P F et al 1988 The role of MR and CT in evaluating clival chordomas and chondrosarcomas AJR 15: 567–575
Pearlman A W, Friedman M 1970 Radical radiation therapy of chordoma. American Journal of Roentgenology 108: 333–341
Rabadan A, Conesa H 1992 Transmaxillary-transnasal approach to the anterior clivus: A microsurgical anatomical model. Neurosurgery 30: 473–482
Raffel C, Wright D C, Gutin P H, Wilson C B 1985 Cranial chordomas: Clinical presentation and results of operative and radiation therapy in twenty-six patients. Neurosurgery 17: 703–710
Rich T A, Schiller A, Suit H D, Mankin H J 1985 Clinical and pathologic review of 48 cases of chordoma. Cancer 56: 182–187
Rupa V, Rajshekhar V, Bhanu T S, Chandi S M 1989 Primary chondroid chordoma of the base of the petrous temporal bone. Journal of Laryngology and Otology 103: 771–773
Sekhar L N, Sen C N 1989 Anterior and lateral basal approaches to the clivus. Contemporary Neurosurgery 11: 1–8
Sekhar L N, Schramm V L, Jones N F 1987 Subtemporal-preauricular infratemporal fossa approach to large lateral and posterior cranial base neoplasms. Journal of Neurosurgery 67: 488–499
Sekhar L N, Janecka I P, Jones N F 1988 Subtemporal-infratemporal and basal subfrontal approach to extensive cranial base tumours. Acta Neurochirurgica 92: 83–92
Sekhar L N, Sen C N, Snyderman C H, Janecka I P 1993 Anterior, anterolateral and lateral approaches to extradural petroclival tumors. In: Sekhar L N, Janecka I P (eds) Surgery of cranial base tumors. Raven Press, New York, pp 157–223
Sen C N, Sekhar L N 1990a The subtemporal and preauricular infratemporal approach to intradural structures ventral to the brain stem. Journal of Neurosurgery 73: 345–354
Sen C N, Sekhar L N 1990b An extreme lateral approach to intradural lesions of the cervical spine and foramen magnum. Neurosurgery 27: 197–204
Sen C N, Sekhar L N, Schramm V L, Janecka I P 1989 Chordoma and chondrosarcoma of the cranial base: An 8-year experience. Neurosurgery 25: 931–941
Sindou M, Daher A, Vighetto A, Goutelle A 1989 Chondrosarcoma parasellaire: Rapport d'un cas opéré par voie ptériono-temporale et revue de la littérature. Neurochirurgie 35: 186–190
Synderman K H, Janecka I P, Sekhar L N, Sen C N, Eibling D E 1990 Anterior cranial base reconstruction: role of galeal and pericranial flaps. Laryngoscope 100: 607–614
Spaar F W, Spaar U, Markakis E 1990 DNA in chordomas of the clivus Blumenbachi. Neurosurgical Review 13: 219–229
Spetzler R F, Herman J M, Beals S, Joganic E, Milligan J 1993 Preservation of olfaction in anterior craniofacial approaches. Journal of Neurosurgery 19: 48–52
Spoden J E, Bumsted R M, Warner E D 1980 Chondroid chordoma. Case report and literature review. Annals of Otology 89: 279–285
Suit H D, Goitein M, Munzenrider J et al 1982 Definitive radiation therapy for chordoma and chondrosarcoma of base of skull and cervical spine. Journal of Neurosurgery 56: 377–385
Sze G, Uichanco L S, Brant-Zawadzki M N et al 1988 Chordomas: MR imaging. Radiology 166: 187–191
Tatsuzaki H, Urie M M 1991 Importance of precise positioning for proton beam therapy in the base of skull and cervical spine. International Journal of Radiation Oncology Biology Physics 21: 757–765
Tomlinson F H, Scheithauer B W, Forsythe P A, Unni K, Meyer F B 1992 Sarcomatous transformation in cranial chordoma. Neurosurgery 31: 13–18
Volpe R, Mazabraud A 1983 A clinicopathologic review of 25 cases of chordoma. American Journal of Surgical Pathology 7: 161–170
Walass L, Kindblom L G 1991 Fine-needle aspiration biopsy in the preoperative diagnosis of chordoma: A study of 17 cases with application of electron microscopic, histochemical, and immunocytochemical examination. Human Pathology 22: 22–28
Zoltan L, Fenyes I 1960 Stereotactic diagnosis and radioactive treatment in a case of spheno-occipital chordoma. Journal of Neurosurgery 17: 888–900
Zülch K J 1986 Chondrosarcomas, chordomas. Brain tumors. Their biology and pathology. Springer Verlag, Berlin, pp 476–482

41. Glomus jugulare tumors

Michael J. Ebersold   Akio Morita   Kerry D. Olsen   Lynn M. Quast

INTRODUCTION

In 1840, Valentine described the anatomic site and cells of origin of the glomus jugulare tumor. The glomus jugulare was first described by Guild in 1941 as consisting of a collection of neurovascular tissue located in and about the jugular bulb. It was, however, in 1945 that Rosenwasser first recognized the relationship between this unusual vascular tumor of the middle ear and the normally occurring glomus jugulare body.

Glomus jugulare tumors arise in the adventitia of the jugular bulb and along Jacobson's and Arnold's nerves within the tympanic cleft (Glasscock et al 1979).

INCIDENCE AND PREVALENCE

There is marked geographic variation in the incidence of primary brain tumors. The more socio-economically developed countries have higher incidence rates for either sex than less developed nations. Sweden, for example, has the highest rate of approximately 10 per 100 000 primary brain tumors per year, which is closely followed by the United States and Israel. It has been suggested that this difference reflects a difference in the quality of medical practice, availability of diagnostic facilities, and the level of organization of registries for data collection and coding. In addition, many of the primary brain tumors are most common in the elderly, and often longevity is found to be greatest in the more medically developed countries. In the United States, the average annual age-adjusted incidence rate of primary brain tumor is about 10 per 100 000 per year (Radhakrishnan et al 1993). In Rochester, Minnesota, for example, it has been demonstrated that a significant number of brain tumors remain undiagnosed during life. As recently as 1972, Percy et al reported that 37% of brain tumors in the Rochester, Minnesota, series were first diagnosed at autopsy and only one third of these were symptomatic during life. Even in the most sophisticated medical communities, however, the smaller glomus jugulare tumor may escape clinical or radiographic diagnosis or even autopsy detection because of its location.

Glomus jugulare tumors are the most common neoplasms of the middle ear and second only to acoustic tumors as the most common tumors of the temporal bone (Reddy et al 1983, Radhakrishnan et al 1993). Glomus tumors have been said to account for only 0.03% of all neoplasms and approximately 0.6% of head and neck tumors (Boyle et al 1990). Even in most referral centers, glomus jugulare tumors will make up significantly less than 5% of the tumors that require the surgical expertise of a neurosurgeon.

Brown reported a series of 231 cases, of which 198 were females and 33 were males; the age of presentation was from 20–88 years of age, with a mean of 55 years (Brown 1985). In our recent review of 77 patients, 50 were females and 27 were males. The age at presentation was 17–82, with a mean age of 51.66 (Fig. 41.1).

FAMILY HISTORY AND GENETIC FACTORS

Bilateral glomus jugulare tumors are found in 1–2% of cases, glomus jugulare and carotid body tumors in 7% and, overall, multicentricity has been reported in up to 10% of all cases (Spector et al 1979, Jackson et al 1982a, Olsen 1994). Bilateral or multiple tumors are significantly more frequent in familial disease (31.8% of cases) (Grufferman et al 1980, Van Der Mey et al 1992).

The second or third associated tumor may not be apparent at the time of the initial diagnosis. In our recent review, a 33-year-old man underwent surgery to remove a nonhormone-secreting glomus jugulare tumor. Ten years later the patient developed hypertension and at this time was found to have a pheochromocytoma as the cause, therefore patient follow-up is an important aspect of patient care with this entity.

Persons with bilateral or multiple glomus jugulare tumors and persons with a positive family history for such tumors are likely to have a genetic disorder. Genetic evaluation is recommended to outline a plan for screening of at-risk family members and for counseling purposes. The importance of genetic transmission was first noted

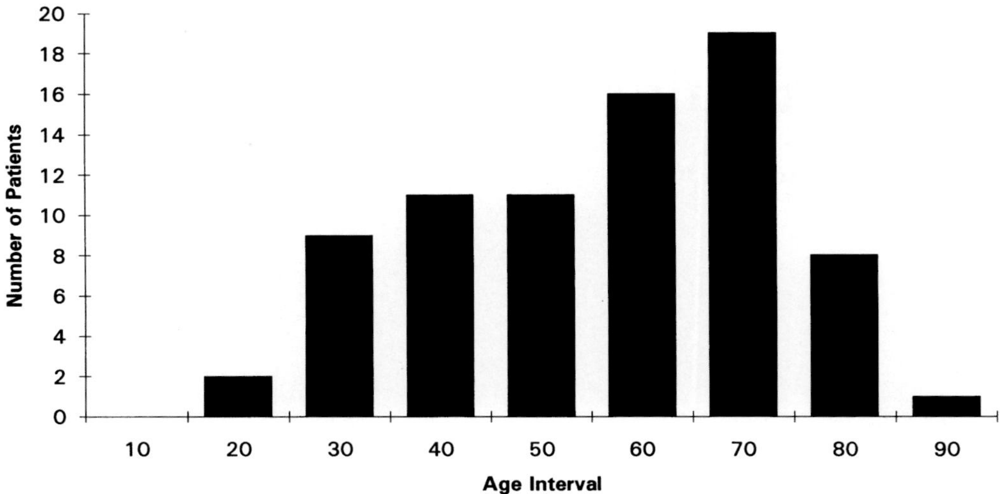

Fig. 41.1 The age of patients at the time of initial evaluation at our institution with diagnosis of glomus jugulare tumor.

by Bartels, in 1949. The predisposition to develop these tumors is inherited as an autosomal trait localized to chromosome 11q23→qter, at least in some cases. This dominant gene is subject to imprinting. Thus, the mutant gene can be transmitted by both males and females. Children of either sex have a 50% risk for inheriting the gene defect, and both men and women can develop the tumors. Unlike traditional autosomal dominant inheritance, however, tumor development depends on the sex of the transmitting parent. If the mutant gene is inherited from the father, tumors are likely to develop. If the abnormal gene is inherited from the mother, tumors do not seem to develop. The gene is believed to be altered (imprinted) during oogenesis, thereby preventing it from playing a role in tumor development in the future person deriving from that egg. This imprint is erased during spermatogenesis, so that future persons derived from the sperm can develop tumors (Van Der Mey et al 1992).

Although the exact molecular defect that causes familial glomus jugulare tumors is unknown, one could speculate that the gene normally acts as a tumor suppressor gene and is normally inactivated during oogenesis. If the mutant gene is inherited from the father and is nonfunctional, tumors could develop. In contrast, when the mutant gene is inherited from the mother and is inactivated, the normal gene from the father prevents development of tumors. The sample pedigree illustrates several of these points (Fig. 41.2).

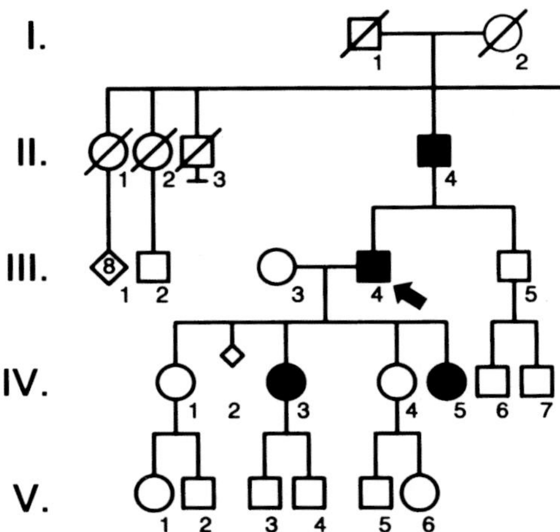

Fig. 41.2 Sample pedigree. Note that all persons with the tumor (blackened symbols) have inherited the gene from their father. Numbers V.3 and V.4, the children of IV.3, are each at 50% risk for having inherited the gene but are not expected to develop tumors. The descendents of V.3 and V.4 may again develop tumors if they inherit the mutant gene.

PRESENTING FEATURES

Tumor within the middle ear often results in conductive hearing loss. Otorrhea, especially with bloody discharge, pain in the ear, and tinnitus are also frequent symptoms of even the smaller tumors. Sometimes the patient may notice a pulsatile sound in the ear, and evaluation may demonstrate a high-pitched bruit over the mastoid. The tympanic membrane is generally abnormal when a glomus jugulare tumor is discovered. The abnormal membrane may demonstrate hypervascularity with dilated vessels or the notation of a dark red mass in the hypotympanum or the presence of a hemorrhagic polyp in the ear canal. Brown's sign is the presence of pulsations in a middle ear mass that is seen when increased pressure is applied to the external ear canal with a pneumatic otoscope. This has been reported to occur in approximately 25% of glomus jugulare tumors.

In general, some of the more common symptoms and findings with glomus jugulare include conductive hearing loss, tinnitus, a retrotympanic mass, the presence of an aural polyp, bleeding, Brown's sign, notation of pain or vertigo, or weakness of the seventh or eighth cranial nerves. A neck mass is rarely apparent. In general, glomus jugulare tumors are benign, slow-growing, and can ultimately cause multiple cranial nerve deficits. Deterioration in hearing, balance, speech and swallowing, and facial deformity and eye problems can occur. The time from the onset of symptoms to the development of multiple cranial nerve deficits may encompass many years. Neurologic deficits found with glomus jugulare lesions include the Vernet syndrome, that is, loss of function of cranial nerves IX, X, and XI, and Billaret's syndrome which is loss of function of cranial nerves IX, X, XI, and XII and generally a partial Horner's syndrome. A partial Horner's syndrome occurs with glomus jugulare tumors because of the anatomy of the sympathetic chain above the superior cervical ganglion. Usually there is absence of facial anhydrosis.

Neurologic deficits or extension of the tumor along adjacent pathways can cause paralysis of the tongue with dysarthria, decreased gag reflex, or dysphonia from involvement of the vagus nerve. Facial nerve paralysis and weakness and atrophy of the trapezius and sternocleidomastoid muscles from accessory nerve involvement can also occur. There may also be a cervical parapharyngeal or nasopharyngeal mass, decreased vision, papilledema, ophthalmoplegia, and absence of the corneal reflex from intracranial extension and loss of the fifth cranial nerve.

The most common clinical findings associated with a glomus jugulare tumor focus on abnormalities in hearing. These lesions initially give a conductive hearing loss and, as they enlarge, may occasionally cause sensorineural loss or vestibular symptoms as well. Pulsatile tinnitus is a common finding. Involvement of the vertical portion of the facial nerve in the temporal bone can also lead to facial nerve paralysis.

In our recent review of patients, the presenting symptoms were: hearing loss (11), ear pain (6), tinnitus (44), hoarseness (10), shoulder weakness (2), and other (4).

Because of the rare possibility of hormonal activity of glomus jugulare tumors as well as the association of some of these tumors with other hormonally active tumors, hormonal assays should be considered. Urine and serum assays for metabolites of catecholamines need to be made.

Glomus jugulare tumors have been reported to be catecholamine-secreting in approximately 1% of all cases (Schwaber et al 1984). A secreting tumor should be especially suspected if a history includes headaches, perspiration, palpitations, nervousness, hypertension, or weight loss. One should screen all patients with glomus jugulare tumors for serum catecholamines, urinary catecholamines, vanillylmandelic acid, and metanephrine. If a catecholamine-secreting tumor is found, the patient should undergo pharmacologic blockade preoperatively, hydration, and the avoidance of catecholamine-potentiating drugs (Levit et al 1969, Farrior et al 1980, Blumenfeld et al 1992).

Advances in neuro-imaging have continued to make the diagnosis of such lesions more certain. Computerized tomography and magnetic resonance imaging are not only excellent means of establishing diagnosis but also of defining the extent of the tumor. Figures 41.3A–C show a typical medium-sized glomus jugulare tumor that has extended intracranially.

Angiography is not only helpful in confirming the diagnosis but also in determining whether selective embolization of feeding vessels may assist with the surgical procedure. The arterial blood supply often arises from the ascending pharyngeal artery through its inferior tympanic branch. The use of preoperative embolization of glomus jugulare tumors has been advocated by a number of authors (Simpson et al 1979, Valvanis et al 1986, Young et al 1988, Murphy & Brackmann 1989, Anand et al 1993). Our own experience is in agreement with Murphy & Brackmann in that embolization has significantly decreased blood loss at operation and the complications of embolization are infrequent (Fig. 41.4).

MORPHOLOGIC FEATURES

These highly vascular tumors are usually red, friable lesions that have no capsule. Early investigators attempted a classification and referred to them as carotid body-like tumors, chemodectomas, and nonparaffin paragangliomas (Lattes & Waltner 1949, Mulligan 1950, Guild 1953, Glasscock et al 1979). The chemodectomas resemble the paragangliomas, which contain chromaffin cells; however, chemodectomas do not contain chromaffin cells (Kempe 1982). The histologic appearance of all glomus tumors is similar and shows a highly vascular stroma containing many clumps of epithelioid cells interspersed within the capillary endothelium and vascular spaces (Hawthorne et al 1988). These clusters of tumor cells (Zellballen) can be nicely demonstrated by silver impregnation of the reticulin fibers (Batsakis 1979, Van Der Mey et al 1992). The histology of the glomus jugulare tumors in general tends to mimic the architecture of a normal carotid body (Spector et al 1974). The chemoreceptor cells for glomera, which are nonchromaffin-staining paraganglion cells, probably develop from the neural crest region during embryogenesis (Lattes & Waltner 1949, Zak 1954, Spector et al 1975, Brown 1985).

CLASSIFICATION

Glomus jugulare tumors can be arbitrarily divided into

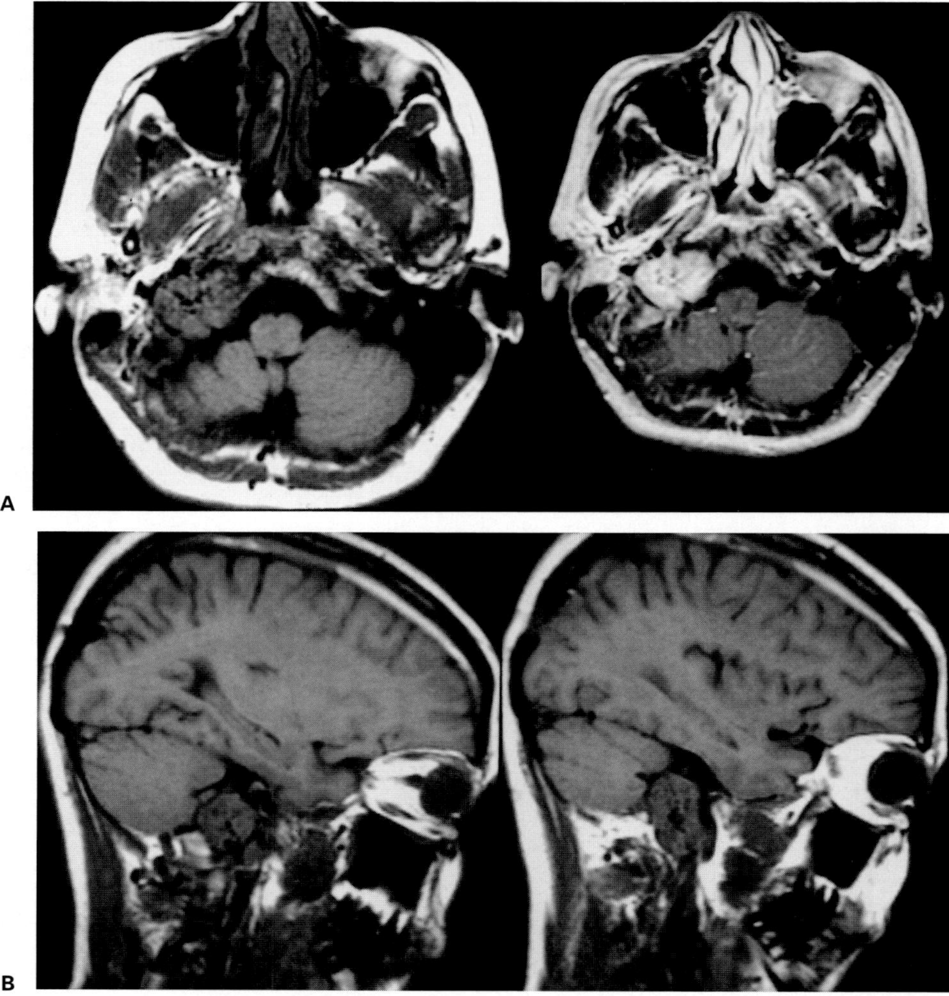

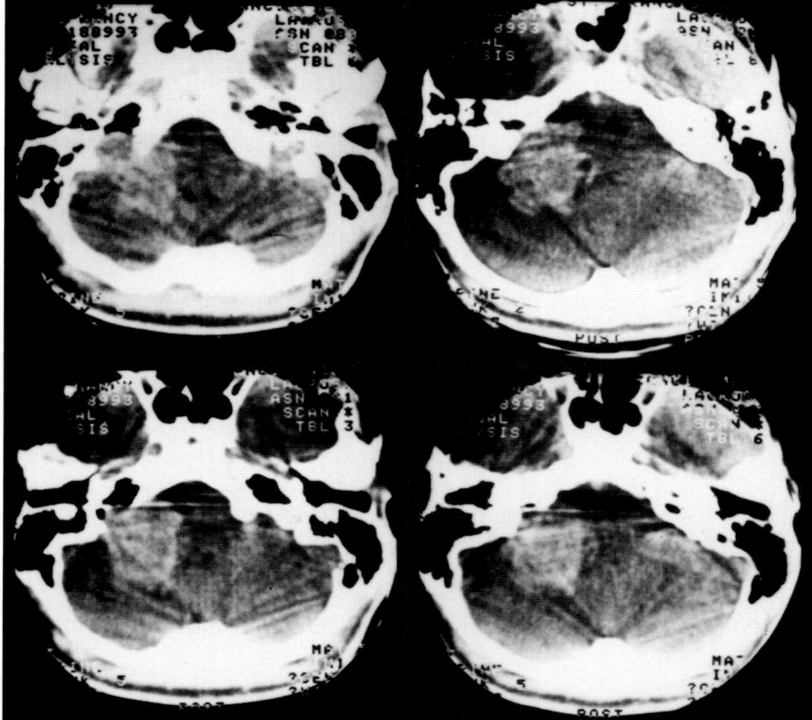

Fig. 41.3 A, B. MRI demonstrating a medium-sized glomus jugulare tumor with minimal intradural extension but rather significant bone destruction. The proximity of the carotid artery to the tumor should be recognized. **C.** CT scan of a glomus jugulare tumor in a 29-year-old woman. Even with this rather large tumor with extensive intradural extension, total tumor removal with a single stage procedure is an achievable goal.

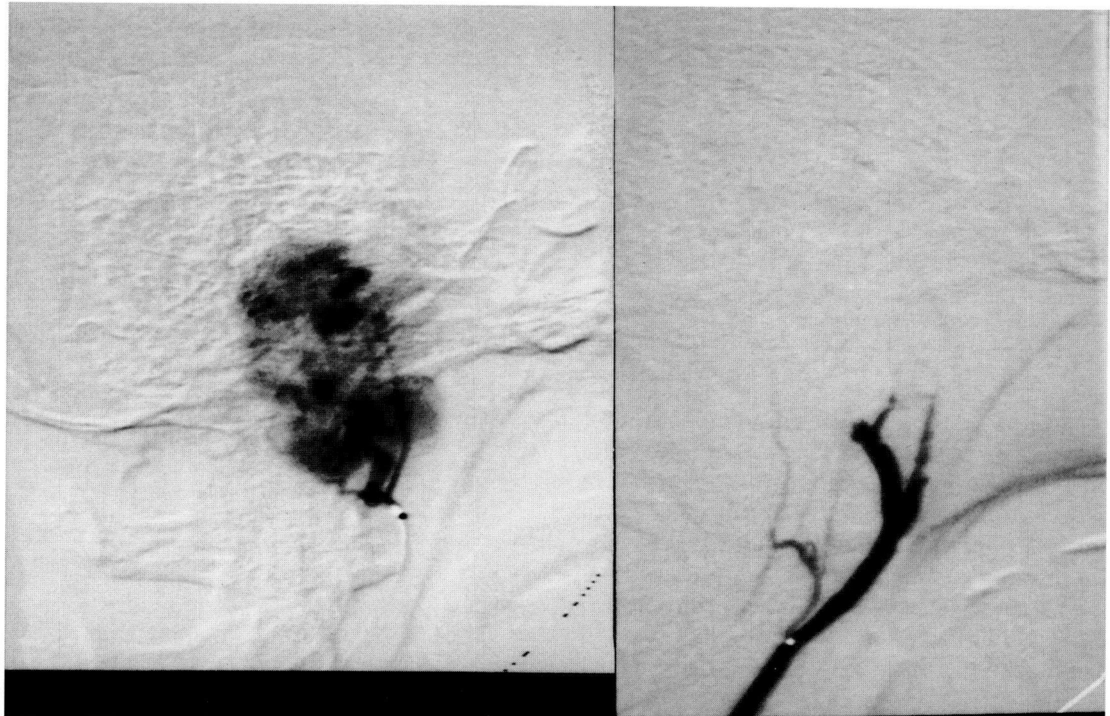

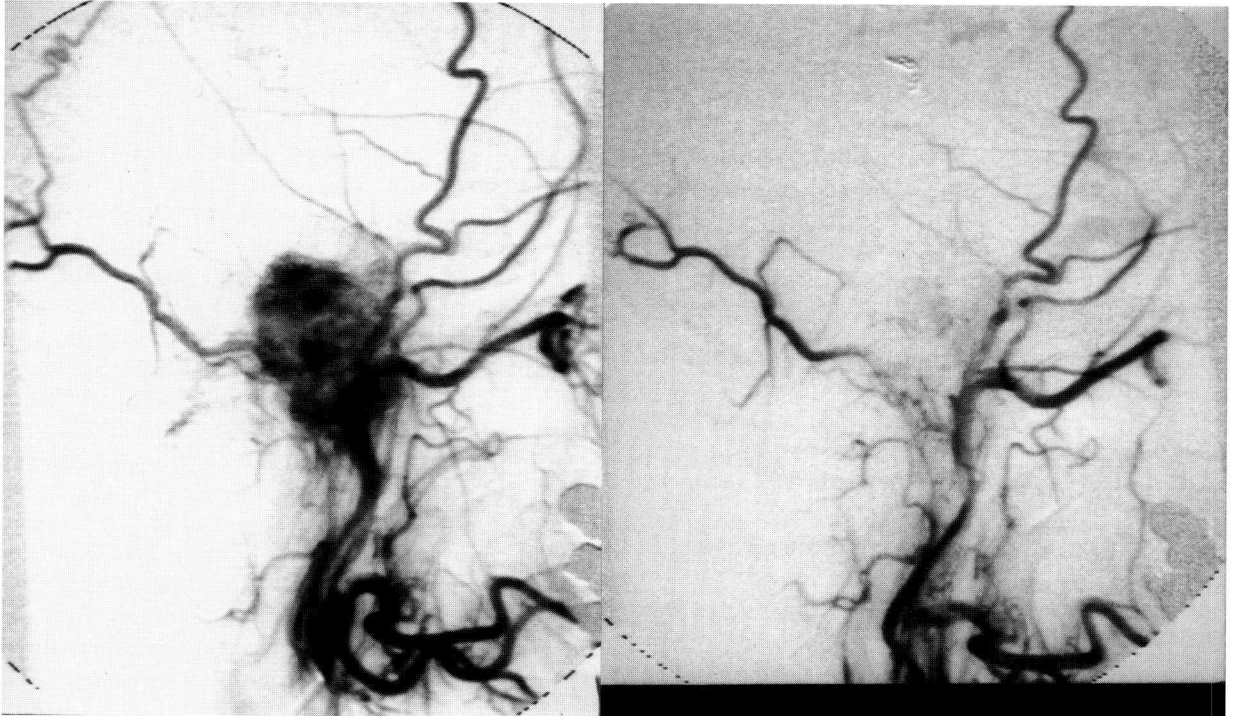

Fig. 41.4 Angiographic evaluation of the ascending pharyngeal arterial injection prior to embolization (**A**) demonstrated significant supply which renders itself to embolization. **B.** Subtraction view of the vascular supply of the external carotid arterial injection pre- and post-embolization.

Table 41.1 Alford & Guilford classification of glomus jugulare tumors. From Brown (1985)

Stage 0:	Tumor confined to the middle ear; symptoms of hearing loss and tinnitus.
Stage 1:	Tumor extending through the ear drum; symptoms of ear discharge, conductive hearing loss and possibly a polypoid mass in the external canal.
Stage 2:	Advanced tumor size with facial paralysis.
Stage 3:	Hearing loss, tinnitus, facial paralysis, possible ear discharge, vertigo, hoarseness (tumor spread beyond confines of the middle ear).
Stage 4:	Multiple cranial nerve involvement with signs and symptoms suggestive of tumor spread beyond temporal bone.

two different groups. The glomus tympanicus tumor arises from the hypotympanum in the neighborhood of the promontory. This lesion often appears to come from the tympanic branch of the ninth nerve and presents with early symptoms of conductive deafness and tinnitus. The second, more common glomus jugulare tumor, seems to arise in the jugular bulb (Lattes & Waltner 1949, Brown 1985). Alford & Guilford (1962) further elaborated on this clinical classification, setting up stages 0 through 4 (Table 41.1).

In 1958, Fisch established his own scheme for classifying these lesions (Fisch 1978). This classification was revised in 1981 to include a D1 and 2 category which was used to describe the intracranial extension (Table 41.2) (Jackson et al 1982b). During this period of time, when advances in CT scanning were improving our ability preoperatively better to define tumor size, Glasscock and Jackson established another classification system (see Table 41.3) which further defines the tumor site and size in an effort to determine extent of disease in patients in their series (Jackson 1981, Jackson et al 1982a).

TREATMENT RECOMMENDATIONS

The management of glomus tumors has long been a frequently debated subject. The role of observation, radiation therapy, surgical management, and more recently Gamma Knife management, each has its proponents and critics (Spector et al 1974, Simko et al 1978, Brackmann

Table 41.2 Fisch classification of glomus tumors of the temporal region. From Jackson C G et al (1982b)

Type A	Tumors limited to the middle ear cleft.
Type B	Tumors limited to the tympanomastoid area with no infralabyrinthine compartment involvement.
Type C	Tumors involving the infralabyrinthine compartment of the temporal bone and extending into the petrous apex.
Type D1	Tumors with an intracranial extension less than 2 cm in diameter.
Type D2	Tumors with an intracranial extension greater than 2 cm in diameter.

Table 41.3 Glasscock & Jackson classification of glomus tumors. From Jackson C G et al (1982b)

Glomus tympanicum	
Type I	Small mass limited to the promontory.
Type II	Tumor completely filling middle ear space.
Type III	Tumor filling middle ear and extending into mastoid.
Type IV	Tumor filling middle ear, extending into mastoid or through tympanic membrane to fill external auditory canal; may also extend anterior to internal carotid artery.
Glomus jugulare	
Type I	Small tumor involving jugular bulb, middle ear, and mastoid.
Type II	Tumor extending under internal auditory canal; may have intracranial extension.
Type III	Tumor extending into petrous apex; may have intracranial extension.
Type IV	Tumor extending beyond petrous apex into clivus or infratemporal fossa; may have intracranial extension.

et al 1972, Wanson & Thomson 1988, Robertson et al 1990, Cece et al 1987, Dawes et al 1987). Most authors agree that surgical resection is a simple and effective treatment for the glomus tympanicum tumor that arises in the middle ear (Cece et al 1987). Although numerous publications advocating the irradiation of glomus jugulare tumors have stated that such treatment is effective in relieving symptoms (Cole 1979, Cummings et al 1984), the surgical literature on this subject has many series of patients who were said to have failed radiation therapy. Undoubtedly some of the series concerning radiation therapy have not involved adequate follow-up time to be certain about the long-term effects or success of such treatment. The often very slow growth rate of such tumors has undoubtedly contributed to some of the success reports of radiation therapy. In a recent series of 231 patients reported by Brown, 4 of 26 patients who had central nervous system involvement with tumor died following radiation therapy alone (Brown 1985). Another 5 of 26 patients died after a combination of surgery and radiation therapy. This certainly suggests that radiation therapy does not by any means cure or control all of these tumors. This series goes on to suggest that slow regression of the tumor may occur. Maruyana et al in 1971 reviewed the angiograms of patients who had an excellent clinical response from radiation therapy and noted that radiographically there was very little change. They suggested that it was better to speak in terms of tumor control rather than cure with radiation therapy. It was their feeling that tumor response in their particular series occurred in 43 of 52 patients (Maruyana et al 1971). To establish a true control rate, extensive follow-ups of even 30 and 40 years would be helpful, but such series are of course not available at present. On the other hand, as with surgery, very significant advances have occurred in the delivery of radiation therapy and, even if long follow-up studies were presently available, we would still really not have such information on patients who have undergone radiation therapy with present day technology. In a recent review by Larner et al (1992), 49 patients underwent radiation therapy for glomus jugulare tumors but 13 of these patients were followed less than 10 years. In spite of this, however, 14% of the patients had clinical or radiologic evidence of disease progression. Only one patient in this series had disease progression when treated with greater than 4000 cGy. Based on these data, 4500–5000 cGy radiation therapy using a wedge pair technique for all but the smallest tumors was recommended (Larner et al 1992). Although much has been written about the alternative treatments, it remains an unresolved issue. The mode of action of radiotherapy is not yet clearly established. Fibrosis has been demonstrated but changes on a cellular level or vascular level seem to be less consistently found. Figure 41.5A demonstrates the rather typical histologic features and Figure 41.5B shows changes produced by radiation therapy. Slow regression of the tumor may occur over time (Brown 1985). The presence of clinically, radiographically, or histologically persistent tumor following radiation therapy has led many to the opinion that radiation has no significant curative effect on glomus tumor (Rosenwasser 1973, Spector et al 1976, Glasscock et al 1979, Cummings et al 1984). Yet, some of these same authors have in the past recommended irradiation for the unresectable or incompletely resected tumors (Rosenwasser 1973, Glasscock et al 1979). Recent advances in surgical technique, however, have certainly improved the likelihood of tumor resectability. Although differences of opinion may exist among surgeons concerning the advisability of preoperative irradiation, we are of the opinion that preoperative irradiation is not advisable electively. It not only increases the difficulty in achieving proper tissue planes but also interferes with wound healing and increases the risk of cerebrospinal fluid leakage. If surgery is being contemplated for the patient who has received prior radiation therapy, it is important for the treating surgeons to be able to deal with skin breakdown or cerebrospinal fluid leak. Muscle flaps, scalp flaps, and more recently the use of vascularized free flaps have markedly decreased the morbidity and even the mortality associated with wound breakdown and cerebrospinal fluid leakage.

RADIOSURGERY FOR GLOMUS TUMORS

As an alternative to conventional surgery, we have employed the Leksell Gamma Unit at the Mayo Clinic to perform radiosurgical treatment on 5 patients with glomus jugulare tumors. Four of the patients were elderly (age, 64–72 years) and had underlying medical conditions that would have increased the risks of anesthesia and open surgery. One 30-year-old patient with a very small glomus tumor entirely within the jugular foramen had already undergone surgical removal of bilateral carotid body tumors. Severe vasomotor instability and lower cranial neuropathies significantly increased the operative and anesthetic risks in this case as well. One patient had undergone two previous attempts at surgical removal of her tumor 11 and 14 years before radiosurgery. All 5 patients had deficits of cranial nerves IX–XI and/or XII on the side of the tumor. At the time of treatment, all patients were living at home and caring for themselves.

We perform radiosurgical treatment during a brief (2 night) inpatient hospital stay. Patients underwent stereotactic headframe application, stereotactic imaging (MRI and/or CT), and radiosurgical treatment during a continuous session that lasted 2–8 hours depending upon the size, shape and complexity of the tumor. The average tumor diameter was 3 cm (range, 2.4–3.6 cm); the average tumor volume was 8.5 cm^3 (range, 4.8–11.5 cm^3). A mean of 5 radiation isocenters (range, 3–10) were required for complete tumor coverage at the 40–50% isodose line. The mean dose to the tumor margin was 15 Gy (range, 12–18 Gy); the mean central dose was 30 Gy (range, 30–36 Gy).

Four patients have been followed longer than 30 months after treatment (mean follow-up, 33.4 months; range, 3–49 months). All patients were alive and neurologically stable at last follow-up. None of the tumors has grown, one is smaller, and four are stable on follow-up imaging studies. In conclusion, in this small series of selected high-risk patients with glomus jugulare tumors, radiosurgery appears to be a safe and effective treatment alternative.

SURGERY

Although much has been written about the surgical technique, it appears that the greatest advances have come from subspecialization, a multidisciplinary approach to surgery especially involving the larger lesions, and of course the use of the operating microscope. There is certainly no substitute for the experience gained by frequent close teamwork of a skull base surgical team, including an otolaryngologist, a neurosurgeon and someone experienced with free vascularized muscle flaps if such should be needed.

Patient selection

The decision regarding treatment of glomus jugulare lesions involves questions related to the patient's age, overall health, the size of the tumor, and the presence of

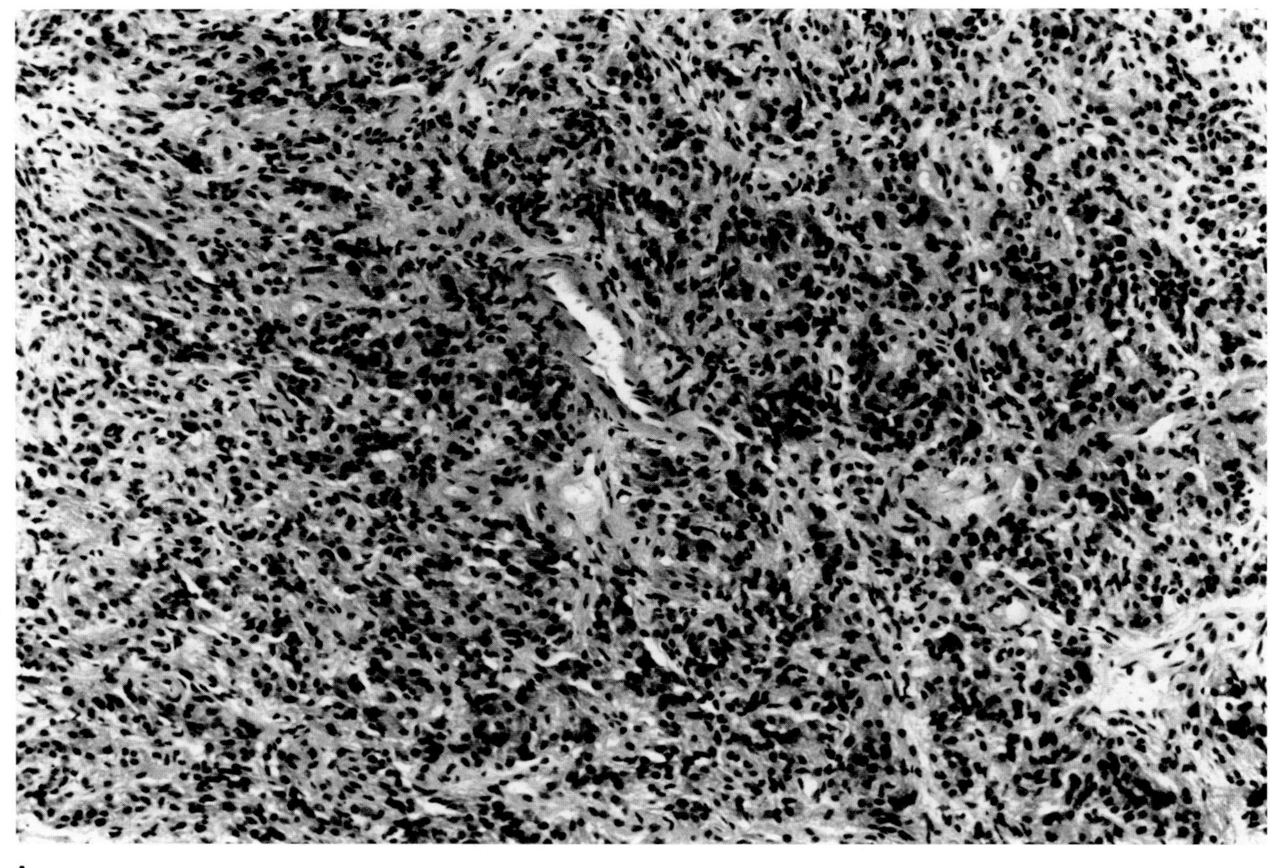

A

Fig. 41.5 **A.** H&E stain of glomus jugulare tumor demonstrating characteristic organoid pattern and high vascularity.

symptoms. Generally, for an individual over the age of 60 with minimal symptoms, observation should be considered. Radiation therapy would need to be considered for the older individual with a symptomatic tumor. Young individuals are generally treated surgically. The dilemma arises with the in-between group of patients, and a decision whether to manage the patient surgically or by radiation therapy is arrived at with full input from the patient and after a discussion regarding expected benefits and risks from the various treatment options.

Surgical technique

The majority of glomus jugulare lesions involve the jugular foramen area, hypotympanum, middle ear, mastoid, or extend into the neck. In these cases, it is generally possible to remove the tumor safely, preserve uninvolved cranial nerves, and preserve hearing and vestibular function. These operations are performed in a combined manner by otolaryngology/head and neck surgeons, and neurosurgeons.

Surgical steps

An incision is made in the postauricular region and connects with a cervical-parotid incision that is made in front of the ear and beneath the mandible into the neck along the sternocleidomastoid muscle. A parotid skin flap is elevated out to the periphery of the parotid gland. A postauricular incision is then made to give complete exposure of the mastoid and suboccipital region (Fig. 41.6). Dissection anteriorly is extended up to the bony ear canal. The parotid gland is then separated from the sternocleidomastoid muscle, from the cartilaginous ear canal, and from the posterior belly of the digastric muscle. The main trunk of the facial nerve is then identified and followed peripherally to the level of the pes. The sternocleidomastoid muscle is then retracted laterally and the internal jugular vein, accessory nerve, hypoglossal nerve, vagus nerve, and internal and external carotid arteries are all isolated; vessel loops are placed around the major vascular structures. The branches of the external carotid artery that are the major source of blood to the tumor as depicted on angiographic studies are now isolated and ligated. This generally includes the postauricular, suboccipital, and the ascending pharyngeal arteries. The sternocleidomastoid muscle is then detached from the mastoid tip and the digastric muscle is also detached from

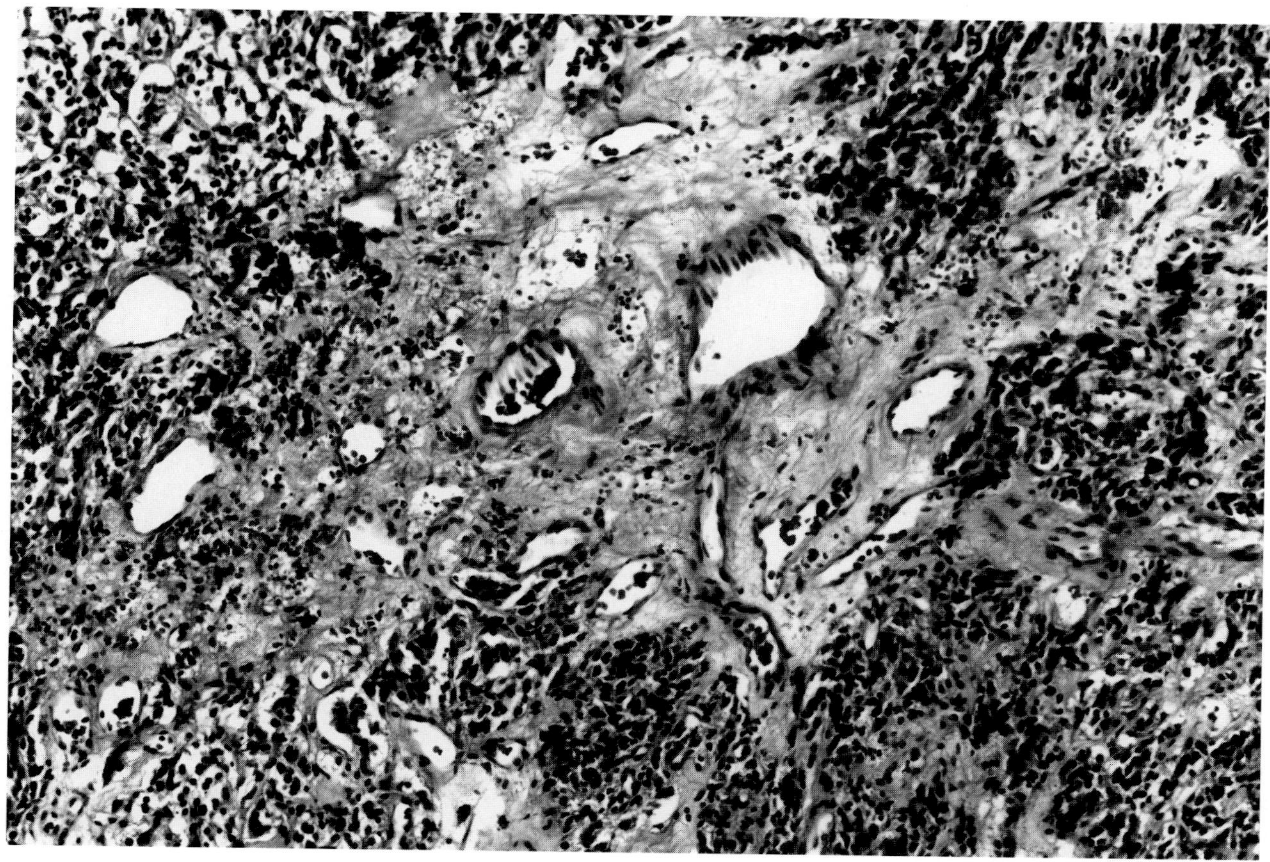

B

Fig. 41.5 B. Following radiation therapy there are persistent tumor cells with increased connective tissue and extensive scarring.

the mastoid bone in the digastric groove and reflected medially. The stylohyoid muscle is generally also reflected medially and the jugular vein isolated up to the jugular foramen, as are the tenth, eleventh, and twelfth cranial nerves. The ninth cranial nerve is often seen at this level above the internal carotid artery, which is followed beneath the styloid process. A complete mastoidectomy is then performed, exposing the sigmoid sinus, antrum, and posterior and horizontal semicircular canals. The extended facial recess is then opened to allow adequate visualization of the middle ear compartment. The bone overlying the facial nerve is then removed using a diamond drill, and the facial nerve is elevated from its canal. The mastoid tip is completely removed using a rongeur, giving adequate exposure of the entire course of the facial nerve and the stylomastoid foramen to avoid excessive trauma in this area. The facial nerve is then elevated out of its canal from the horizontal portion to the pes and brought over the bony ear canal. The bone is then removed over the posterior fossa dura, both anterior and posterior to the sigmoid sinus, and the remaining bone over the tumor in the region of the hypotympanum and deep to the facial nerve is removed using a drill. The bone over the sigmoid sinus is then removed using a drill and curettes, and a combined removal of the tumor then proceeds with the neurosurgeon.

For very large glomus jugulare tumors that extend along the carotid artery into the petrous apex, clival area, or have extensive intracranial extension, it is generally necessary to utilize the infratemporal fossa approach as described by Fisch (1978). In these cases, auditory function is sacrificed.

For these large, rare glomus jugulare tumors, a generous incision is made from the temporal area behind the ear and extended down into the neck along the sternocleidomastoid muscle. This flap is then elevated up to the ear canal where the ear canal is divided at the cartilaginous and bony junction. The ear canal is then oversewn to end in a blind pouch and the ear carried forward onto the parotid gland and temporal fascia and across the neck as a wide, medially based facial, scalp, and neck flap. An identical dissection as for the preceding, smaller glomus jugulare tumors is utilized in the neck. Again, the mastoidectomy is performed and the superior, posterior, and

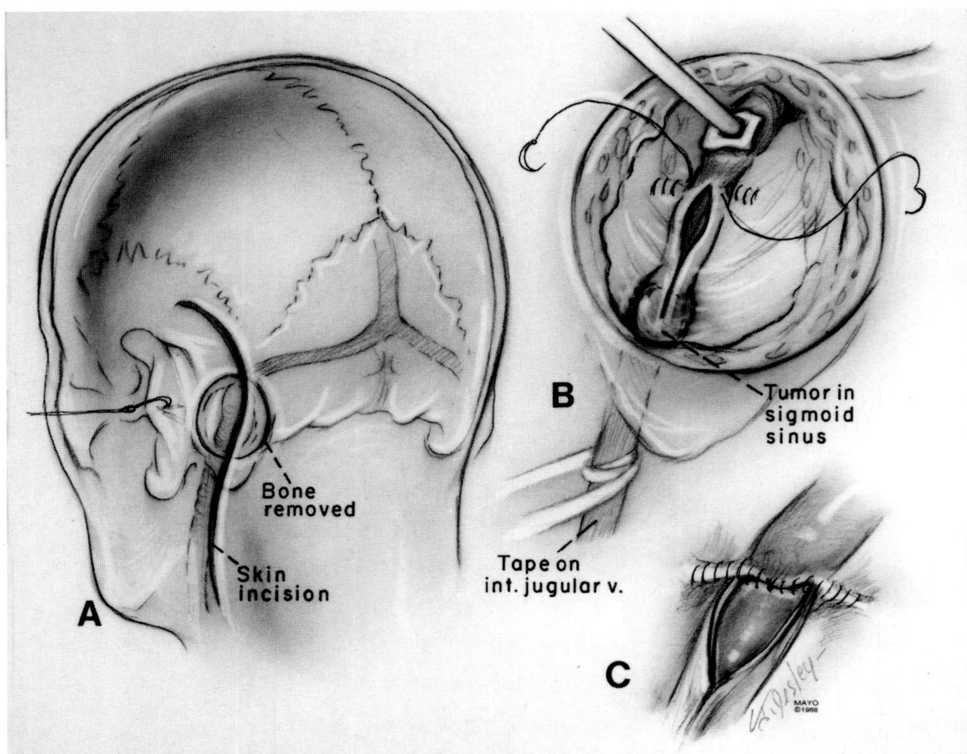

Fig. 41.6 The incision should allow for exposure of at least a small amount of posterior fossa dura so as to accomplish occlusion of the sigmoid sinus. Although a Fogarty catheter can be placed into the opened sinus to control bleeding, direct pressure over the opened sinus also accomplishes control of bleeding while the outer sinus wall is sutured to the inner sinus wall above. The temporary placement of cottonoid patties into the distal sigmoid allows for control of back bleeding from the petrosal sinuses during this portion of the procedure. Following this, the distal sigmoid will be opened along its length, entering sinuses will be packed with Surgicel strips or ligated with figure 8 sutures, and the tumor will be identified and removed in a piecemeal fashion using suction and blunt dissection.

inferior bony ear canals are removed after performing an extended facial recess exposure. The incus, malleus, and the tympanic membrane are likewise removed, and the facial nerve is decompressed and raised from its canal from the geniculate ganglion to the pes. If additional exposure of the course of the temporal portion of the carotid artery is needed, it may be helpful to remove the neck and condyle of the mandible or to attempt retraction and dislocation of the mandible. Often, this exposure places significant traction on the facial nerve, requiring transection of the facial nerve and later anastomosis. This should generally be done beyond the level of the pes to reduce subsequent synkinesis.

Following exposure of the jugular vein and mobilization of the facial nerve, the bone overlying the sigmoid sinus and the distal transverse sinus is thinned with the use of a high speed drill. As the dura is exposed, care is taken to avoid entering venous lakes and sinuses, since such events can result in significant blood loss. It is during this portion of the surgery that the largest blood loss can occur. Sinus bleeding can be difficult to control, especially if it occurs early in the bone removal. Nevertheless, if bleeding does occur, it is venous in origin and can be managed by direct pressure or, for that matter, the placement of a large piece of bone wax on the bone overlying the site of venous bleeding. We have found it helpful to expose the entire sigmoid sinus and even the distal transverse sinus to accomplish good visualization of the tumor site and also to assist us in accomplishing control of bleeding from this structure. Because the sigmoid sinus is not necessarily a tubular structure, but sometimes rather like a cavernous structure between dural layers, it can often be difficult to pass a ligature completely around such a structure, as has been described. In addition, passing a ligature around the structure would require a dural opening on either side of the sigmoid to avoid injury to the underlying brain or vessels with the needle.

We therefore advocate the technique of suturing the external sinus wall to the internal sinus wall. This can be accomplished by starting two running sutures on either side of the sigmoid sinus. The initial stitch secures the suture to the dura on either side of the sigmoid sinus and a running suture is then started on either side of the sigmoid (Fig. 41.6). As the suture line approaches the sinus, the sinus is opened so that the deep wall of the sinus can be identified. Bleeding is controlled by gentle pressure applied by the assistant so as to hold the outer surface of the sinus wall against the deep sinus wall. A cottonoid patty with a suction can be placed immediately over the sinus and a suction tip or a spatula can be used to hold the sinus closed. Following this, the sinus is opened and the front and back walls of the sinus are sutured together with the two running sutures which are then tied in the midline, as shown in Figure 41.6C. The distal sinus can then be packed temporarily with cottonoid patties or cotton balls. Prior to opening the sinus, it is advisable to tighten the previously placed ligature on the internal jugular vein; however, this by no means controls distal back bleeding from the distal sigmoid sinus. Even though the jugular vein is occluded, there is still extensive back bleeding from the petrosal sinuses and veins that enter the sigmoid sinus at the region of the foramen ovale. Other authors, who use a similar technique of suturing the front and back wall of the sinus, have reported using Fogarty catheters placed distally and proximally in the sigmoid sinus, distending the balloon so as to again obstruct blood flow through the sinus, and then in a similar manner opening the sinus between the occluded sites and suturing the front and back walls together. The occlusion of the sigmoid sinus in such a manner does not require exposing the underlying brain or even opening the dura with the loss of cerebrospinal fluid. In many of the smaller tumors, the dura does not even need to be opened, which essentially eliminates the risk of cerebrospinal fluid leakage.

Once the proximal sinus has been occluded by the running suture line extending across the sinus, attention is now devoted to the tumor containing distal sigmoid. The now opened sinus is further opened distally. As the distal sigmoid sinus is opened longitudinally towards the tumor, entering sinuses and veins are entered and controlled by packing them with Surgicel or even small fragments of fascia. Sometimes it is possible to place a figure 8 suture across the orifice of the entering vein, which also controls this back bleeding and achieves hemostasis. As these veins are occluded, the tumor is debulked and removed. Blunt dissection allows the surgeon to strip the tumor off the lower cranial nerves, which sometimes can be preserved even though initially it appears that they run through the tumor. In other cases, the tumor is not significantly adherent to the lower cranial nerves, and the tumor can be removed with minimal trauma to the nerves. Although this portion of the procedure is made more difficult by venous bleeding from the multiple entering channels at the level of the jugular foramen, it is reassuring to know that, once this part of the procedure is complete, the remaining surgical procedure will be much easier. For the small tumor, the procedure can be completed at this stage without opening the dura. The larger tumor, however, often extends intradurally and sometimes it is necessary to further enlarge the dural opening created by the tumor so as to remove the intradural contents. Unlike the acoustic tumor, which is often very adherent to the facial and cochlear nerves as well as to the brainstem, the glomus jugulare tumor is often separated from these structures by an arachnoid layer. The large tumors can also extend rostrally towards the carotid artery, and sometimes can be quite adherent to the carotid artery. Blunt dissection with the use of a spatula or even a bone curette can sometimes be used to strip these tumors from the carotid artery. When the tumor does not strip easily from the carotid artery, it is probably best to leave a small amount of tumor attached, rather than take unnecessary risks of injuring the carotid artery. Since the growth rate of these tumors can be quite slow, small amounts of remaining tumor may not significantly change in size even in many years of follow-up.

Removal of the intradural component of the tumor should, however, be achievable. Following removal of the intradural component of the tumor, a watertight dural closure can often be accomplished using fascia lata or temporalis fascia. In patients who have received radiation therapy or may be receiving radiation therapy, it seems reasonable to make every attempt at accomplishing a watertight dural closure without compromising the more superficial part of the closure by taking fascia from this region. If this cannot be accomplished, obtaining additional fat or muscle and placing this over the defect often seems to result in a very satisfactory seal. In patients who have previously received significant radiation, the skin viability can be considerably compromised. If it appears likely that wound healing is going to be a problem or if in the postoperative course it proves to be a problem, the use of rotational grafts and even vascularized muscle grafts can be life-saving. With such techniques available, the previous morbidity and mortality associated with a persistent cerebrospinal fluid leakage should be essentially eliminated. Spinal drainage is not routinely used following such procedures. If tissue viability is quite poor at the completion of the procedure, however, it may be reasonable to consider this treatment option.

There are a number of excellent reviews on the surgical technique of tumor removal that further describe some of the difficulties and surgical steps associated with tumor removal (Farrior et al 1980, Jackson et al 1982b, Robertson et al 1982, Farrior 1984, 1988).

Results

Much has been written about surgical outcomes (Farrior 1988, Leonetti et al 1989, Lenarz & Plinket 1992). Many advances have been made in recent years, therefore many of the series that include the most modern surgical methods suffer because of lack of follow-up years.

Thirty six patients have undergone a combined intracranial-extracranial tumor removal, as described in this text, between the years 1973 and 1993. One patient, a 17-year-old man with an extensive tumor who had two previous surgical resections elsewhere prior to our treatment, did have symptomatic tumor recurrence requiring further treatment. One 18-year-old woman had initial intracranial-extracranial resection in 1987 and again in 1992 for significant tumor recurrence.

The surgical outcome data of these patients suggest that total tumor removal and therefore cure can be accomplished in essentially all patients, although it does seem prudent to leave a small amount of tumor when this is very adherent to the carotid artery. Sixteen patients developed new permanent neurologic deficits following gross total tumor resection (Table 41.4). There were four patients with tumor recurrence despite apparent gross total resection.

In most cases we now use intraoperative cranial nerve monitoring. Generally, the larger tumors undergo preoperative embolization. Subspecialization has helped us improve our surgical efficiency, and a single stage operative tumor resection is our goal for even the largest tumors. If total tumor removal is not accomplished, which is now extremely rare, it seems reasonable to follow this group closely with serial MRIs since very slow tumor growth may make it unlikely that the small amount of remaining tumor will ever need further treatment. If progressive growth does develop, however, Gamma Knife or radiation therapy should be considered.

Table 41.4 New permanent neurologic deficits following gross total resection of 36 glomus jugulare tumors.

Cranial nerve	VI	VII	IX, X	XI
No. of patients	1	5	8	2

CONCLUSIONS

The evaluation of any treatment result requires prolonged follow-up of at least 15–20 years. At present, surgical excision seems to be the only way to accomplish a cure; however, tumor control in many cases may be a reasonable goal. Treatment mortality, morbidity, and expense, as well as the psychologic effects in patients of knowing there is remaining viable tumor all need to be considered with patient's age, access to follow-up care, and patient's general health when deciding on a treatment for any given patient. The benefits of sophisticated preoperative imaging, preoperative embolization, intraoperative microscopy and monitoring, and in particular an experienced skull base surgical team cannot be overemphasized.

REFERENCES

Alford B R, Guilford F R 1962 A comprehensive study of tumors of the glomus jugulare. Laryngoscope 72: 765–787

Anand V K, Leonetti J P, Al-Mefty O 1993 Neurovascular considerations in surgery of glomus tumors with intracranial extensions. Laryngoscope 103: 722–728

Bartels J 1949 De tumoren van het glomus jugulare (Thesis). University of Groningen, Netherlands

Batsakis J D 1979 Tumors of the head and neck, 2nd edn. Williams & Wilkins, Baltimore, pp 369–380

Blumenfeld J D, Cohen N, Laragh J H et al 1992 Hypertension and catecholamine biosynthesis associated with a glomus jugulare tumor. New England Journal of Medicine 327: 894–895

Boyle J O, Shimm D S, Coulthard S W 1990 Radiation therapy for paragangliomas of the temporal bone. Laryngoscope 100: 896–901

Brackmann D E, House W F, Terry R et al 1972 Glomus jugulare tumors: effect of irradiation. Tr Am Acad Ophth & Otol 76: 1423–1431

Brown J S 1985 Glomus jugulare tumors revisited: A ten-year statistical follow-up of 231 cases. Laryngoscope 95: 284–288

Cece J A, Lawson W, Eden A R et al 1987 Complications in the management of large glomus jugulare tumors. Laryngoscope 97: 152–157

Cole J M 1979 Panel discussion: Glomus jugulare tumors of the temporal bone. Radiation of glomus tumors of the temporal bone. Laryngoscope 89: 1623–1627

Cummings B J, Beale F A, Garrett P G et al 1984 The treatment of glomus tumors in the temporal bone by megavoltage radiation. Cancer 52: 2635–2640

Dawes P J D K, Filippou M, Welch A R et al 1987 The management of glomus jugulare tumours. Clin Otolaryngol 12: 15–24

Farrior J 1984 Infratemporal approach to skull base for glomus tumors: Anatomic considerations. Annals of Otology Rhinology and Laryngology 93: 616–622

Farrior J 1988 Surgical management of glomus tumors: Endocrine-active tumors of the skull base. Southern Medical Journal 81: 1121–1126

Farrior J B III, Hyams V J, Benke R H et al 1980 Carcinoid apudoma arising in a glomus jugulare tumor: review of endocrine activity in glomus jugulare tumors. Laryngoscope 90: 110–119

Fisch U 1978 Infratemporal fossa approach to tumors of the temporal bone and base of the skull. Journal of Laryngology and Otology 92: 949–967

Glasscock M E III, Jackson C G, Dickins J R E et al 1979 Panel discussion: Glomus jugulare tumors of the temporal bone. The surgical management of glomus tumors. Laryngoscope 89: 1640–1651

Grufferman S, Gillman M W, Paternak L R et al 1980 Familial carotid body tumors: Case report and epidemiologic review. Cancer 46: 2116–2122

Guild S R 1941 A hitherto unrecognized structure, the glomus jugularus in man. Anat Rec (suppl) 2; 79: 28 (abstract)

Guild S R 1953 Glomus jugulare, nonchromaffin paraganglioma in man. Annals of Otology Rhinology and Laryngology 62: 1045–1071

Hansen H S, Thomsen K A 1988 Radiotherapy in glomus tumors (paragangliomas). A 24-year review. Acta Otolaryngologica (Stockholm) 449: 151–154

Hawthorne M R, Makek M S, Harris J P et al 1988 The histopathological and clinical features of irradiated and nonirradiated temporal paragangliomas. Laryngoscope 98: 325–331

Jackson C G 1981 Skull base surgery. American Journal of Otology 3: 161–171

Jackson C G, Glasscock M E III, Harris P F 1982a Glomus tumors. Diagnosis, classification, and management of large lesions. Archives of Otolaryngology 108: 401–406

Jackson C G, Glasscock M E III, Nissen A J et al 1982b Glomus tumor surgery: The approach, results, and problems. Otolaryngological Clinics of North America 15: 897–916

Kempe L G 1982 Glomus jugulare tumor. In: Youmans J R (ed) Neurological surgery, 2nd, end, vol 5. W B Saunders, Philadelphia, pp 3285–3298
Larner J M, Hahn S S, Spaulding C A et al 1992 Glomus jugulare tumors. Long-term control by radiation therapy. Cancer 69: 1813–1817
Lattes R, Waltner J G 1949 Non-chromaffin paragangliomas of middle ear. Cancer 2: 447–468
Lenarz Th, Plinket P K 1992 Glomus tumors of the temporal bone: Staging, surgical approach and results. LaryngoRhino-Otol 71: 149–157
Leonetti J P, Brackmann D E, Prass R L 1989 Improved preservation of facial nerve function in the infratemporal approach to the skull base. Otolaryngology — Head and Neck Surgery 101: 74–78
Levit S A, Sheps S G, Espinosa R E et al 1969 Catecholamine secreting paraganglioma of glomus-jugulare region resembling pheochromocytoma. New England Journal of Medicine 281: 805–811
Maruyana Y, Gold L H A, Keiffen S A 1971 Radioactive cobalt treatment of glomus jugulare tumors. Clinical angiographic investigation. Acta Radiologica 10: 239–247
Mulligan R M 1950 Chemodectoma in the dog. American Journal of Pathology 28: 680–681
Murphy T P, Brackmann D E 1989 Effects of preoperative embolization on glomus jugulare tumors. Laryngoscope 99: 1244–1247
Olsen K D 1994 Tumors and surgery of parapharyngeal space. Laryngoscope 104: 1–28
Percy A K, Elveback L R, Okasaki H et al 1972 Neoplasms of the central nervous system: epidemiologic considerations. Neurology 22: 44–48
Radhakrishnan K, Bohnen N I, Kurland L T 1993 Epidemiology of brain tumors. In: Morantz R A, Walsh J W (eds) Brain tumors. A comprehensive text. Marcel Dekker, New York, pp 1–15
Reddy E K, Mansfield C M, Hartman G V 1983 Chemodectoma of the glomus jugulare. Cancer 52: 337–340
Robertson J T, Gardner G, Cocke E W Jr et al 1982 Glomus jugulare tumors. In: Schmidek H H, Sweet W H (eds) Operative neurosurgical techniques. Indications, methods, and results, vol 1. Grune & Stratton, New York, pp 649–670
Robertson J T, Clark W C, Robertson J H et al 1990 Glomus jugulare tumors. In: Youmans J R (ed) Neurological surgery, 3rd edn, vol 5. W B Saunders, Philadelphia, pp 3654–3666
Rosenwasser H 1945 Carotid body tumour of the middle ear and mastoid. Archives of Otolaryngology 41: 64–67
Rosenwasser H 1973 Long-term results of therapy of glomus jugulare tumors. Archives of Otolaryngology 97: 49–54
Schwaber M K, Glasscock M E, Nissen A J et al 1984 Diagnosis and management of catecholamine secreting glomus tumors. Laryngoscope 94: 1008–1015
Simko T G, Griffin T W, Gerdes A J et al 1978 The role of radiation therapy in the treatment of glomus jugulare tumors. Cancer 42: 104–106
Simpson G T II, Konrad H R, Takahashi M et al 1979 Immediate postembolization excision of glomus jugulare tumors. Archives of Otolaryngology 105: 639–643
Spector G J, Maisel R H, Ogura J H 1974 Glomus jugulare tumors. II. A clinicopathologic analysis of the effects of radiotherapy. Annals of Otology 83: 26–32
Spector G J, Ciralsky R, Maisel R H et al 1975 Multiple glomus tumors in the head and neck. Laryngoscope 85: 1066–1075
Spector G J, Fierstein J, Ogura J H 1976 A comparison of therapeutic modalities of glomus tumors in the temporal bone. Laryngoscope 86: 690–696
Spector G J, Sobol S, Thawley S E et al 1979 Glomus jugulare tumors of the temporal bone. Patterns of invasion in the temporal bone. Laryngoscope 89: 1628–1639
Valentine G 1840 Ueber eine gangliöse Anschwellung in der Jacobsenschen Anastomose des Menschen. Arch Anat Physiol Wissensch Med 287–290
Valvanis A 1986 Preoperative embolization of the head and neck: indications, patient selection, goals and precautions. AJNR 7: 927–936
Van Der Mey A G L, Fruns J H M, Van Dulken H et al 1992 Does intervention improve the natural course of glomus tumors? A series of 108 patients seen in a 32-year period. Annals of Otology Rhinology and Laryngology 101: 635–642
Young N, Wiet R, Russell E et al 1988 Superselective embolization of glomus jugulare tumors. Annals of Otology Rhinology and Laryngology 97: 613–620
Zak F G 1954 Expanded concept of tumors of glomic tissue. New York State Journal of Medicine 54: 1153–1165

42. Carcinoma of the paranasal sinuses

R. Andrew Danks   Andrew H. Kaye

INCIDENCE AND PREVALENCE OF TUMOR

Carcinoma of the nasal cavity and paranasal sinuses (PNC) is a comparatively rare group of tumors in Western society. The incidence is 0.3–1 cases per 100 000 people per year in most Western countries (Robin et al 1979, Roush 1979, Muir et al 1987, Olsen 1987, Giles et al 1992). These tumors cause less than 1% of cancer deaths in the United States, and comprise 3% of all head and neck carcinomas in Western series (Roush 1979). The lifetime risk of contracting these cancers is 1 in 1000 men or 1 in 3000 women (Giles et al 1992).

AGE DISTRIBUTION

These tumors are exceedingly rare in childhood, with an incidence of about 0.1 per 100 000 per year or less. The incidence of this disease increases relentlessly with age after the fourth decade to 5–6 per 100 000 per year in the eighth decade (see Fig. 42.1) (Robin et al 1979, Giles et al 1992). The peak age at presentation is 55–65 years for males and 60–80 years for females. The median age at diagnosis is 62 years in men and 72 years in women. There is an apparent decline in incidence after 85 years of age which may be due to under-reporting in the geriatric group.

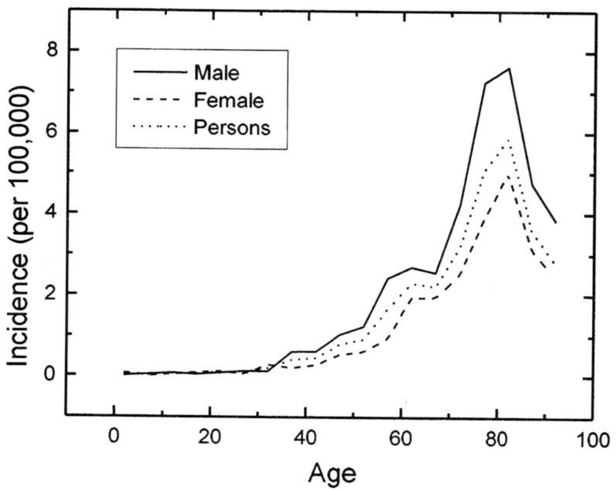

Fig. 42.1 Age- and sex-specific incidence of PNC (Robin et al 1979).

SEX DISTRIBUTION

There is a male preponderance; the male to female ratio varies between 1.5 and 3:1 in all age groups over 35 years of age (Robin et al 1979, Giles et al 1992). The male excess is related to the histology of the tumors. In cases of adenocarcinoma, the overall male to female ratio is 4:1 whilst in squamous carcinomas it is 1.5:1. The probable causes of this male preponderance are occupational factors, which are discussed later.

RACIAL, NATIONAL AND GEOGRAPHIC CONSIDERATIONS

The incidence of these tumors varies about threefold worldwide. Asia, Africa, and South America are three regions of relatively high incidence. In Japan and Colombia, the reported incidence has been between 2 and 3.6 cases per 100 000 people per year (Muir et al 1987). The age-standardized rate in these nations is estimated to be four times that of the American Caucasian population. In Uganda, the rate is also similarly high, but this is due largely to cases of Burkitt's lymphoma occurring in this region (Roush 1979).

FAMILY HISTORY AND GENETIC FACTORS

No familial or genetic tendency has been described in this class of tumors.

SITES OF PREDILECTION

A large English registry-based series reported the site of predilection for PNC to be the maxillary sinus, where 60% of tumors originated. Other paranasal sinuses, principally the ethmoid sinus, comprised 16% of the total, whilst 20% of cases occurred in the nasal cavity and 4% in the nasal vestibule (Robin et al 1979). These figures are similar to hospital-based series from the United States (Roush 1979).

The different histologic types of tumors have differing sites of predilection. Squamous cell carcinoma tends to arise mostly in the maxillary antrum, where it comprises 60% of the tumors. Adenocarcinoma is principally located in the ethmoid sinuses and upper nasal cavity. Transitional cell and anaplastic carcinomas are more evenly distributed amongst the sinuses. In many cases it can be difficult to determine the site of origin because the tumor has invaded far beyond the confines of the sinus of origin (Robin et al 1979, Hyams et al 1988).

EPIDEMIOLOGY

These tumors are rare in the general population. However, local clusters of cases have been recognized and careful epidemiologic studies have been performed to pinpoint various causes. In these studies, the relative risks of those exposed to the occupational hazards described have been as high as 30–1000 times that of the normal population not at risk. Alterations of the working environment to reduce exposure to the hazardous carcinogens have been followed in many situations by a reduction in the incidence of these tumors (Acheson et al 1982, Egedahl et al 1991) (Table 42.1).

The occupational hazard where the association was demonstrated earliest was nickel refining (Doll et al 1970). Workers in this industry in Wales, Norway, USSR and Canada suffered a relative risk of over 100 times that of the normal population. The typical histology of these tumors was anaplastic or squamous cell. There was also an associated large increase in the risk of lung cancer. The carcinogenicity of nickel has been confirmed in multiple animal and in vitro studies (Roush 1979). However, with correct management of the workplace environment, a zero incidence was achievable at one Canadian plant over a 30-year period (Egedahl et al 1991).

Other situations where occupational correlation with this histologic type has been demonstrated are radium usage in watch face painters, mustard gas manufacturing, isopropyl alcohol manufacturing and hydrocarbon exposure (Roush 1979).

Table 42.1 Environmental correlates of PNC

Squamous cell carcinoma	nickel refining mustard gas manufacturing isopropyl alcohol manufacturing watch face painting thorium dioxide contrast medium snuff and tobacco smoking
Adenocarcinoma	hardwood dusts in woodworking footware soles machining flour milling polyaromatic hydrocarbon exposure asbestos inhalation

Snuff taking has been suggested as a risk factor in several studies, but the association was clear only in African studies (Roush 1979), whilst ongoing tobacco smoking has been correlated with a three-fold increase in the risk of squamous cell carcinoma (Fukuda & Shibata 1985, Hayes et al 1987). Other studies have reported no association with cigarette smoking (Olsen 1987, Shimizu et al 1989). An iatrogenic cause of squamous cell carcinoma is the radioactive contrast medium thorium dioxide, retained in the maxillary sinus after radiologic investigations. Tumors have occurred over a period of decades after exposure (Rankow et al 1974).

The high incidence of PNC in Japan is principally due to an elevated incidence of squamous carcinoma of the maxilla. Despite epidemiologic studies demonstrating very modest associations with chronic sinusitis, nasal polyposis, cigarette smoking, and woodworking, this incidence has not been adequately explained (Muir & Nectoux 1980, Fukuda et al 1987, Muir et al 1987, Shimizu et al 1989), but the tumor has become less common over the last decade (Waterhouse et al 1976, Fukuda & Shibata 1985, Muir et al 1987).

Adenocarcinoma of the ethmoid sinus is a very rare tumor in the general population. There is a very strong association, however, between the incidence of this tumor and inhalation of hardwood dusts, particularly from high speed machining. This was first demonstrated convincingly in the Buckinghamshire furniture industry (Acheson et al 1970). The relative risk of those working in this industry was 1000 times that of the general population, making it as common as carcinoma of the lung in that group of workers. By taking detailed occupational histories the authors were able to pinpoint the risk to those workers who were exposed to wood dust during the machining and sanding of furniture, rather than those exposed to varnishes and lacquers during the stage of French polishing. Insecticides and other chemical treatments of the wood were not employed prior to woodworking during the period of risk studied in this paper.

The mean latency period from first exposure to tumor diagnosis was 43 years. As one would expect, there was a strong correlation between the length of exposure and the risk of tumor formation (Acheson et al 1982). The shortest period of exposure in a tumor case was only 5 years. This patient's tumor developed 33 years after leaving the industry.

This association between adenocarcinoma of the ethmoid and exposure to hardwood dusts has been confirmed by reports from Germany, United States, Canada, Denmark, Finland, Sweden, the Netherlands (Hayes et al 1986), France (Luce et al 1991) and Australia (Ironside & Matthews 1975, Franklin 1982, Klintenberg et al 1984). In the Australian reports and in Georgia, USA (Wills 1982), there is a strong association between adenocarcinoma and the processes of timber cutting and machining.

There is also an association with carpentry in the building trade in those countries. In Australia, eucalypt hardwoods are the woods employed in these situations. In England, where softwoods were the material used by workers in such industries, no cases of adenocarcinoma were observed in these occupations (Acheson et al 1968).

In our region of Victoria, Australia, there is a substantial timber industry, and adenocarcinoma comprises 35% of the cases of PNC in registry statistics (Giles et al 1992). In the Royal Melbourne Hospital series of 45 cases of PNC, there were 16 cases of adenocarcinoma and all patients gave a history of prolonged exposure to hardwood dusts. Interestingly, 45% of the 17 cases of squamous cell carcinoma also gave such a history, indicating the possibility of a weaker association with this histologic type (Kaye et al 1994). Some other case series and formal epidemiologic studies have demonstrated a 2–4-fold increase in this type of PNC in woodworkers, but no clear dose-response relation was evident (Hayes et al 1986, Fukuda et al 1987, Mohtashamipur et al 1989).

It would appear that a crucial factor in the risk of this type of cancer is the type of wood dust to which the workers are exposed. At least 48 woods are known to have been used in workshops in which workers have developed these tumors. These woods are derived from both deciduous and evergreen trees and from trees native to both the northern and southern hemispheres. Hardwood species tend to be the wood types most associated with the disease. Since dusts from several different species are generally present in most workplaces, it is difficult to pinpoint the particular species that are the cause (Wills 1982). Nonetheless, there is evidence to implicate beech, oak, walnut and eucalypt woods in particular (Mohtashamipur et al 1989, Ironside & Matthews 1975, Franklin 1982).

Wood dust certainly contains many biologically active chemicals of botanic origin as well as fungal proteins from fungi affecting the wood. The biological chemicals include alkyloids, saponins, aldehydes, quinones, flavinoids, tropalones, oils, cardiotoxic steroids, stilbenes, resins and proteins (Roush 1979). Although extrinsic materials such as pesticides and preservatives may be applied to the wood, the British and Australian data tend to point away from these as the cause for the disease. Such chemicals were not employed in the British furniture industry at the time of greatest risk, which was between the two world wars (Acheson et al 1968, 1982). Nor are they applied prior to machining in the Australian lumber industry.

Surveying workers in the furniture industry, precancerous squamous metaplasia was found in the nasal mucosa of 64% of woodworkers, but in only 18% of other workers in the industry (Hadfield & MacBeth 1971). Impaired mucociliary clearance secondary to the wood dust exposure was found to be associated with these changes. These effects would lead to impaired clearance of the dust from the nose of these workers and thus prolong contact between the carcinogen and the nasal mucosa.

There is some epidemiologic evidence indicating increased incidences of other types of tumors such as gastrointestinal, lung cancers and lymphomas in workers exposed to inhalation of wood dusts, but these data are somewhat conflicting (Mohtashamipur et al 1989).

Organic dusts arising in other situations have also been found to be associated with adenocarcinoma of the ethmoid. Dust arising during the machining of the soles of shoes was found to be associated with a 35-fold increase in the risk of this tumor (Acheson et al 1970). Less well defined associations have been made linking adenocarcinoma with exposure to flour dust, polyaromatic hydrocarbons and asbestos exposure (Roush 1979).

CLINICAL FEATURES

Patients are most commonly in their sixth, seventh or eighth decades at the time of presentation. The common presenting symptoms of these tumors are nasal obstruction, often unilateral, epistaxis and nasal discharge. There is often a preceding history of chronic rhinitis causing similar symptoms, which contributes to the common delay in diagnosis of this tumor. Less frequently, patients present with facial pain, facial sensory disturbance, swelling of the cheek, proptosis, diplopia or visual disturbance (Lund 1983). Presentation with symptoms referable to intracranial involvement is rare. Likewise, lymph node involvement or metastatic disease at presentation is rare. Anosmia, usually unilateral, is a common presenting sign in patients with ethmoid or nasal involvement (Table 42.2).

The diagnosis was delayed by between 3 and 14 months in a recent American series (Sisson et al 1989). The authors recommended vigorous examination in all adults presenting with sinonasal complaints of greater than 6 weeks duration. This should include telescopic endonasal examination and biopsy of all suspicious areas. If the symptoms do not resolve within 2 weeks of vigorous medical therapy a limited CT examination of the sinuses was recommended. Using this regime, the authors were able to reduce the mean diagnostic delay in their practice from 8 months to 4 months, with 33% of the tumors in their series being diagnosed at a relatively early stage (T1 or T2). This is much earlier than in other series, and the

Table 42.2 Clinical features of PNC

Nasal obstruction (often unilateral)
Nasal discharge and epistaxis
Facial pain or sensory disturbance
Proptosis
Facial swelling or invasion
Visual disturbance or diplopia
Anosmia (often unilateral)

authors suggested that this reflected their more vigorous investigation of suspicious presenting complaints.

Cancers of the nasal cavity tend to present earlier due to more pronounced early symptoms and easier diagnosis, and this reflects the better prognosis of these lesions (Hyams et al 1988).

IMAGING DIAGNOSIS

CT scanning and magnetic resonance imaging (MRI) have supplanted plain X-rays as the methods of choice for assessment of these tumors and are the appropriate investigations for patients with suspicious symptoms as described above. Typical CT findings would include a soft tissue density tumor mass with erosion of the bony walls around the sinus of origin, and invasion into adjacent anatomic structures. The tumor enhances non-uniformly with contrast. Multiple fine cuts, using window settings for bone and soft tissue, are required for detailed pre-surgical assessment, allowing assessment of tumor extent and bony erosion. Direct coronal scans are useful and are particularly valuable in assessment of orbital roof, cribriform plate, olfactory groove, and intracranial involvement.

CT assessment of sinus involvement may be misleading, as inspissated mucus in an obstructed sinus may mimic the appearances of tumor. This is particularly crucial when assessing the sphenoid sinus, as tumor involvement there may dictate whether the tumor is resectable in its entirety.

MRI can usually differentiate between tumor and inspissated mucus and may demonstrate invasion of tumor along the perineural space (Pandolfo et al 1989). It may show orbital apex or small intracranial deposits better than CT. Inspissated mucus is variable in its signal intensity, but is often different from the tumor on T1- or T2-weighted images. Most commonly, it is seen as high signal on T2-weighted images, as shown in Figure 42.4.

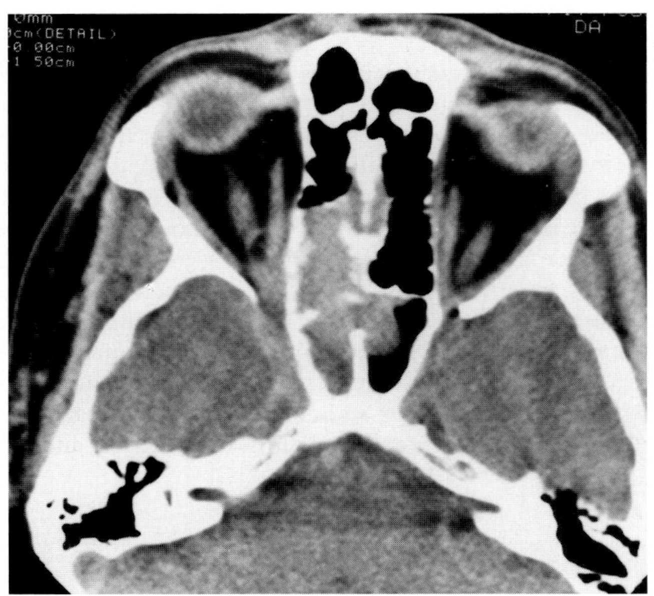

Fig. 42.2 Axial CT scan of patient with adenocarcinoma of the ethmoid, displayed on soft tissue window settings. There is a soft tissue mass in the sphenoid sinus, but one cannot be sure if this is tumor or only mucus trapped there.

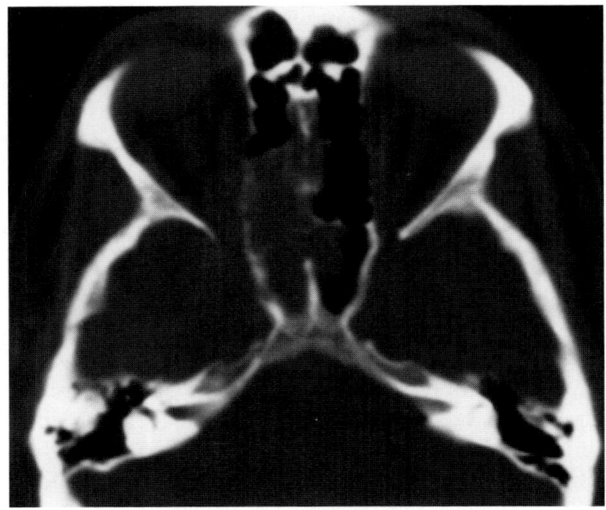

Fig. 42.3 Axial CT scan of the same patient on bone windows to display bony erosion.

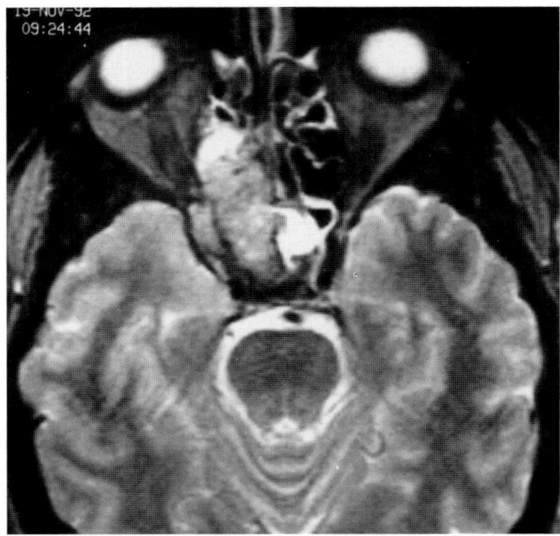

Fig. 42.4 Axial MRI scan of the same patient showing tumor involvement of the right side of the sphenoid sinus, but mucus accumulation on the left, as shown by the high signal there.

Endoscopic or open examination of the nasal cavity and nasal sinuses with biopsy of suspicious areas is the key method of confirming the diagnosis. This is essential before major surgery is undertaken. Cytologic diagnosis of maxillary sinus disease has been suggested by examination

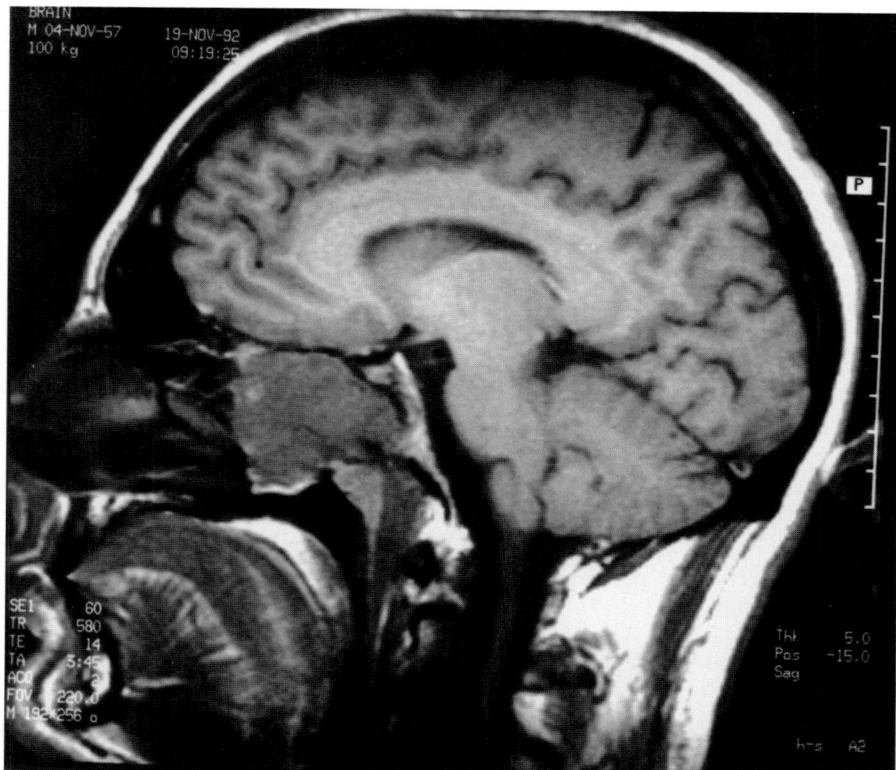

Fig. 42.5 Parasagittal MRI scan of the same patient, slightly to the right of the midline, showing the tumor involvement of the sphenoid sinus. The bony floor of the anterior cranial fossa appears intact as a black line in this section.

of washings of the sinus. Whilst the majority of cancer cases were diagnosed by this method, there were 2 false negative cytology reports amongst the 7 cases of malignant tumor in a recent series (Nishioka et al 1989).

LABORATORY DIAGNOSIS

The transnasal biopsy is of paramount importance in establishing the diagnosis, as discussed above. Other investigations will be required to assess the general condition of the patient. These will vary in each patient. No other specific investigations are required, except that we find it useful to perform preoperative nasal swabs to guide antibiotic prophylaxis during craniofacial resection.

GROSS MORPHOLOGIC FEATURES

These cancers commence in one cavity, but then invade the bony walls to involve adjacent structures. Often tumors grow extraperiosteally before invading further into the invaded cavity. This applies particularly in the orbit, where some surgeons have selectively resected periosteum in an attempt to avoid exenteration (Perry et al 1988). When the tumor arises in or involves the ethmoid, early

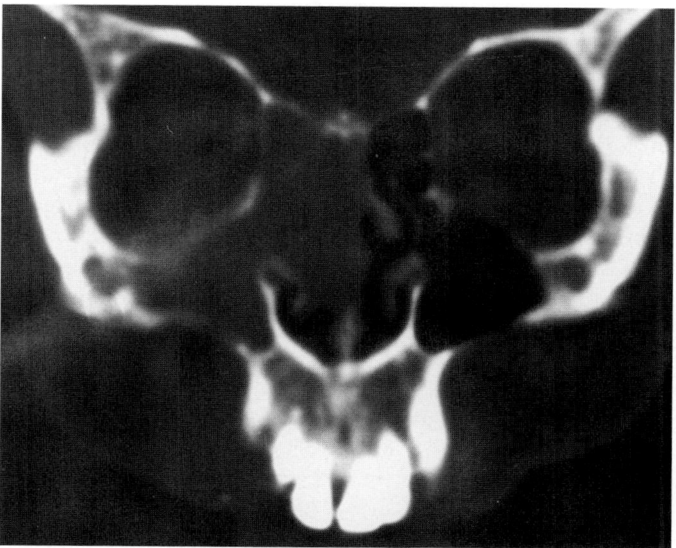

Fig. 42.6 Coronal CT scan of another case, again using bone windows. This displays tumor involvement of the maxilla and ethmoid sinuses, erosion of the orbital wall, and tumor extending right up to the olfactory groove but with no erosion evident there. Nevertheless, microscopic dural involvement was present.

spread to the dura of the olfactory groove is the rule rather than the exception (Kaye et al 1993). Gross intradural disease is less common, presumably reflecting the barrier provided by the dura.

The majority of the tumors are gray to pink or red, friable fungating growths, which are susceptible to bleeding on manipulation (Hyams et al 1988). Some may have a papillomatous appearance or be found in a papilloma after removal. Papillomas are benign but may be bulky and even cause bony erosion by pressure on occasion. They tend to be firm or rubbery in texture.

Maxillary cancers typically invade into the hard palate, the facial skin and the nose, as well as into the ethmoid and sphenoid sinuses, the intracranial cavity, the orbit, and posteriorly into the pterygopalatine fossa.

Adenoid cystic carcinomas are infamous for their diffuse infiltration, which is difficult to demarcate, as well as their tendency to spread along the neural pathways. These features contribute to the very high recurrence rate of this tumor type (Hyams et al 1988).

HISTOPATHOLOGIC FEATURES

There are a number of different tumor types grouped under the generic heading of cancer of the paranasal sinuses (see Table 42.3). Slightly over half of all cases are squamous cell carcinomas. Anaplastic carcinoma, transitional cell carcinoma, and adenocarcinoma each have an incidence of 5–10%. Salivary carcinoma (principally adenoid cystic), lymphoma, melanoma, sarcoma and esthesioneuroblastoma are less common (Robin et al 1979). These are rather more common in the AFIP series, but this may reflect secondary referral bias (Hyams et al 1988).

The relative incidence of the different histologies varies in different regions. For instance, adenocarcinoma makes up 35% of the cases in our state of Victoria, Australia, due to a large hardwood-based woodworking industry (Giles et al 1992). The distribution of histologies in our surgical experience is shown in Table 42.4. Adenocarcinoma is very strongly represented, reflecting both its high incidence in our region, and also a referral bias in patients referred for craniofacial excision.

Table 42.3 Histologic distribution of PNC in a registry series (Robin et al 1979)

Squamous cell carcinoma	51%
Anaplastic carcinoma	10%
Transitional cell carcinoma	8%
Adenocarcinoma	6%
Salivary carcinoma	4%
Lymphoma	5%
Melanoma	3%
Sarcoma	6%
Other	2%

Table 42.4 Histologic distribution of PNC in the RMH series of 45 patients treated by craniofacial resection (Kaye et al 1993)

Squamous cell carcinoma	18 (40%)
Adenocarcinoma	16 (35%)
Adenoid cystic carcinoma	5 (11%)
Esthesioneuroblastoma	1 (2%)
Mixed and other	5 (11%)

Meningioma, hemangiopericytoma and basal cell carcinoma are rare as primary paranasal sinus tumors, but may invade the sinuses by direct spread from adjacent sites and present similar management problems. There are a large number of rare tumor types that may involve the region (Hyams et al 1988).

On microscopic examination, squamous cell carcinoma has the typical appearance of such tumors, with areas of keratin formation either as sheets or as epithelial pearls. Stromal invasion and destruction confirm the malignant nature of the lesion. In the nasal cavity, a well-differentiated tumor may mimic a papilloma because of its regular cellular pattern, exophytic growth and lack of stromal invasion. The diagnosis is made on the basis of cellular abnormalities such as loss of polarity and atypical nuclear changes.

Anaplastic carcinomas have all the features of invasive cancer, but no features typical of a particular type. They have a poor prognosis with a high rate of early metastatic spread.

Transitional cell carcinomas have the appearance of an irregular and excessively thick columnar epithelium, with multiple mitotic figures in the closely packed nuclei. The base is irregular with invasion into surrounding stroma. There is a benign form, the transitional cell papilloma, which may be locally recurrent and progress to carcinoma. Prediction of clinical behavior can be difficult and even the carcinoma has a somewhat better prognosis than other forms of PNC (Robin et al 1979). These tumors are relatively evenly spread amongst the different sinuses and the nasal cavity.

Adenocarcinomas generally arise in the upper nasal cavity or in the ethmoid sinuses. There are papillary and sessile forms. Microscopically, the sessile tumors often bear a strong resemblance to carcinomas of the colon which is accentuated by the presence of goblet cells. The tumors can be graded as low or high grade on histologic appearances, which correlate well with prognosis (Hyams et al 1988).

Adenoid cystic carcinomas arise from the minor salivary glands in the mucosa. They have the characteristic appearance of a mixture of microcystic pseudoluminal spaces and tubular epithelial-lined structures, but may include solid areas. Their biologic behavior is of relentless progression and local recurrence, and late metastasis (Hyams et al 1988).

Esthesioneuroblastoma, or olfactory neuroblastoma, is a variant of neuroblastoma arising from the olfactory apparatus, tending to arise in the upper nasal cavity and ethmoid sinuses. Several patterns have been described. The commonest is that of a cellular tumor comprising uniform small cells with round nuclei, scanty cytoplasm, and a prominent reticular or fibrillary background. Rosettes of the Homer Wright type may be present. Fibrovascular stroma may be abundant. The differential diagnosis may include lymphoma and embryonal rhabdomyosarcoma. Immunohistochemistry is positive for neuron-specific enolase and S-100 (O'Connor et al 1989) and negative for epithelial and lymphoid antigens. Electron microscopy will demonstrate neurofilaments, neurotubules and neurosecretory granules (Rosai 1981). This tumor occurs throughout life, with bimodal peaks of incidence in the second and sixth decades. Grading and staging systems have been proposed and correlate with prognosis (Hyams et al 1988).

Lymphomas in this region tend to be high grade, both histologically and in their clinical behavior. They can be typed by immunohistochemistry for B- and T-cell markers (Ratech et al 1989).

DEFINITION AND INCIDENCE OF MALIGNANCY

These tumors are typically locally malignant on the basis of continuing destructive local invasion, and involvement of vital local structures. Esthetic considerations weigh heavily in the consequences of untreated disease in this area, as well as in the planning of treatment options. Distal spread to regional lymph nodes or other organs is uncommon, but may occur in the more malignant tumors.

Patients with PNC often present at an advanced stage when radical resection is difficult or impossible. The results of treatment are highly dependent on the stage of the disease at presentation. In most series, the 5-year survival for T1 or T2 disease is 3–5 times better than that for T4 disease. Unfortunately, the vast majority of patients present with T3 or T4 disease.

There are at least six classifications currently in use to stage maxillary sinus tumors. The use of different systems in the various series obscures the interpretation of results and makes it difficult to compare different treatment strategies. All systems are based on the TNM system. The T stage is of paramount importance, because nodal and distal spread are relatively uncommon and occur late in this disease. A recent review of 205 patients revealed Harrison's classification to be the most valid of the six classification systems (Willatt et al 1987). This system allowed a balanced distribution of cases with good correlation to treatment and survival in the different stages. Another similar review (Har-El et al 1988) of 70 patients found that Harrison's classification and also that of the Japanese Joint Committee were the most practical and appropriate for staging these tumors. Harrison's classification and those of the American and Japanese Joint Committees are shown in Table 42.5.

There are no widely accepted staging systems for ethmoid carcinoma. Recently, a 3-stage system has been proposed (Parsons et al 1988). Stage 1 tumor is limited to the sinus of origin. Stage 2 includes extension to adjacent areas such as the upper nasal cavity, the orbit, or the sphenoid sinus. Stage 3 includes destruction of the skull base, or the pterygoid plates, or intracranial extension. On the basis of our experience with patients treated by craniofacial resection and radiotherapy, we consider

Table 42.5 Staging of carcinoma of the maxillary sinus

	American Joint Committee	Japanese Joint Committee	Harrison's
T1	Tumor confined to antral mucosa of infrastructure with no bone erosion or destruction	Tumor confined to the maxillary sinus with no evidence of bony involvement	Tumor confined to maxillary sinus with no evidence of bony involvement
T2	Tumor confined to suprastructure without bony destruction or to infrastructure with destruction of medial or inferior walls only	Tumor causing destruction of bony wall with external periosteum remaining intact as the capsule and surrounding tissue not invaded but only compressed. Minimal invasion into the ethmoid cells and the exophytic tumor in the middle nasal meatus included	Bony erosion without evidence of involvement of facial skin, orbit, pterygopalatine fossa or ethmoid labyrinth
T3	More extensive tumor invading skin of cheek, orbit, anterior ethmoid sinuses or pterygoid muscles	Tumor infiltrated deeply into the surrounding tissue by penetration of external periosteum	Involvement of orbit, ethmoid labyrinth or facial skin
T4	Massive tumor with invasion of cribriform plate, posterior ethmoids, sphenoid, nasopharynx, pterygoid plates or base of skull	Tumor extending to the base of skull, nasopharynx, maxilla of opposite side and/or facial skin with ulceration. This includes deep infiltration into the orbit with limited eye movement or visual impairment or extension into the temporal fossa or invasion of the pterygoid muscles	Tumor extension to nasopharynx, sphenoidal sinus, cribriform plate, or pterygopalatine fossa

that sphenoid sinus or orbital apex involvement are the worst prognostic indicators, whilst dural involvement correlated less strongly with worsening of outcome (Kaye et al 1993). Thus we would not entirely concur with this classification.

MANAGEMENT OUTLINE

The ideal management of PNC would incorporate early diagnosis as discussed above, by vigorous investigation of the presenting complaints. However, most cases of carcinoma of the paranasal sinuses are generally far advanced at the time of presentation. The emphasis in this chapter will be on the treatment of advanced PNC, as it is these tumors that usually involve the neurosurgeon.

The results of conventional local removal by transnasal or lateral rhinotomy proved to be very disappointing. Conventional radiotherapy also led to poor results. The 5-year survival rate with either modality alone did not exceed 25%, and was often less (Terz et al 1980). Subsequently, management utilized different combinations of radiotherapy with surgery, generally employing radiotherapy doses above 5000 rads. Ten large mixed series from 1968 to 1983 were reviewed (Knegt et al 1985). The mean 5-year survival rate with these treatments was a disappointing 35%, only a modest improvement on the earlier treatment.

Other authors (Ketcham et al 1973, Millar et al 1973, Terz et al 1980) developed craniofacial resections to adequately excise the tumors, with some apparent improvement in long-term results. Japanese groups developed different approaches using multimodal therapy. They combined chemotherapy and deep X-ray therapy with surgery. Surgery was often less radical than in other series. Chemotherapy was often intra-arterial and also topically applied inside the tumor cavity.

More recent interesting advances include the concurrent use of intravenous infusions of cisplatinum and 5-fluorouracil (5FU) during radiotherapy as radiosensitizers, hyperfractionation of radiotherapy, and the use of three-dimensional computer planning and semi-stereotactic methods of delivering high dose radiotherapy. These modalities will be discussed in detail later in this chapter.

Unfortunately, meaningful comparison between the different published series is extremely difficult for several reasons. Most series are small or extend over many years as these tumors are uncommon. Several series span the period before and after the introduction of CT scanning. Many series are retrospective and draw conclusions between different treatment groups who were selected on various criteria and thus cannot be easily compared. The series all include different mixtures of tumors, histologies, site and stage. They also differ considerably in the ratio of recurrent to previously untreated cases.

Finally, results are reported in different manners in the series. The length of follow-up in many of the series is relatively short for most of the cases in the understandable effort to maximize analysis, and the patient numbers used to calculate 5-year results are often only a modest proportion of the series. In six of the seven series where this was assessable, one third to one quarter of the total 5-year recurrences occurred between 2 and 5 years after treatment. Thus, series which quote follow-up for only 2–3 years do not adequately describe the results of treatment.

Recurrences may occur after 5 years. Of the patients in one large series who died, 8% did so more than 5 years after treatment (Lund 1983). This tendency is especially marked with adenoid cystic carcinoma where the 10-year cure rate may be as low as 7% (Hyams et al 1988). To a lesser degree, this also applies with adenocarcinoma. A patient who survives to 5 years cannot be regarded as cured. Finally, many series do not adequately discuss the treatment morbidity and mortality.

Despite a detailed and exhaustive review of the literature, conclusions as to the relative merits of different modalities of treatment can only be inferential. Many authors conclude by recommending a properly constructed prospective multicenter trial of the different treatment modalities available. Unfortunately, few such studies have been performed to this time.

SURGICAL MANAGEMENT

The goal of surgical management is to achieve a radical tumor resection with a margin of normal tissue. This margin is necessarily limited by the close confines and important relationships of these tumors.

Orbital resection is required where tumor invasion has occurred although this is controversial and will be discussed below. When the tumor involves the ethmoid sinuses, the resection will usually be inadequate unless craniofacial resection is employed to fully resect the roof of the ethmoid sinuses.

Posterior extension into the pterygopalatine fossa or nasopharynx may make radical resection difficult or impossible. In our hands, extensive sphenoid or cavernous sinus involvement has precluded radical curative resection. This may often be suspected on preoperative imaging, but it is often only at surgery that direct inspection and frozen section biopsies can definitively establish resectability. Some authors report radical resection involving the cavernous sinus, but detailed results of this subgroup have not been reported (Perry et al 1988).

On the other hand, a large mass of intracranial disease extending superiorly from the olfactory groove has not precluded successful radical resection. These tumors can be resected by conventional neurosurgical techniques, along with the cranial base, which is then grafted (Sundaresan & Shah 1988, Kaye et al 1993). However, in some cases multiple intradural nodules of tumor spreading over the anterior cranial fossa floor may prevent radical resection.

In the Royal Melbourne Hospital series of 45 cases of PNC treated by craniofacial resection, sphenoid sinus involvement was the major predictor of later tumor recurrence. On the other hand, dural or orbital involvement correlated more weakly with the risk of later recurrence, indicating adequate treatment of these sites by this operative strategy (Kaye et al 1993).

The decision to undertake orbital resection is important and controversial. Certainly this should not be undertaken unless all other disease can be adequately resected. The conventional wisdom is that if there is invasion of the bony walls of the orbit, then orbital exenteration is required. However, in a recent detailed retrospective analysis of a series of 41 patients where there was a strong commitment to preserving the eye (Perry et al 1988), local recurrence did not occur in the orbit. There were 14 cases where there was gross intraorbital tumor invasion without penetration of the periosteum, that were managed by peeling tumor off the periorbita or by local periorbital resection under frozen section control. None of these cases exhibited recurrence in the orbit. However, 10 of these 14 tumors were esthesioneuroblastomas, an otherwise uncommon tumor. Ketcham's experience in a series dominated by advanced squamous cell carcinomas was that there was a 30% survival rate in those who had preservation of the orbital contents, compared with a 50% survival rate in those who had orbital resection (Ketcham & Van 1985).

We preserve the orbit where there is extensive bilateral orbital invasion or other involvement that precludes radical resection. We would prefer to exenterate the orbit if there is breach of the bony orbital walls by tumor in cases where a radical and complete tumor clearance can be achieved. Perhaps the more conservative option would be appropriate in cases of esthesioneuroblastoma.

Craniofacial resection incorporating the anterior cranial fossa floor has in the past been associated with significant morbidity and mortality due to CSF fistula and resultant intracranial infection. However, in the series from the Royal Melbourne Hospital (Kaye et al 1993), there have been no cases of CSF infection, fistula or mortality in 45 cases. We will emphasize certain technical points that have been crucial in achieving these results.

The patient is under the care of the Neurosurgical Department. Preoperative nasal swabs are taken to guide perioperative antibiotics, which are vigorously employed. These include 36 hours of preoperative intranasal soframycin, intraoperative and postoperative intravenous prophylaxis and intraoperative topical antibiotic irrigation.

An intraoperative lumbar drain and neurosurgical anesthetic techniques are employed to ensure adequate brain relaxation. The head is positioned in moderate extension in the 3-point headrest to allow gravity to assist with brain retraction and exposure of the anterior cranial fossa floor. The bicoronal scalp flap is positioned well back to allow a large pericranial flap based upon the supraorbital and supratrochlear vessels of both sides to be reflected inferiorly. A low free bifrontal bone flap is cut just above the supraorbital ridges. We do not employ the approach via a shell-shaped craniotomy through the frontal sinus (Cheeseman et al 1986) nor do we incorporate the superior orbital margin in our craniotomies (Sekhar et al 1992), as we have not encountered complications from brain retraction, which only needs to be light due to the CSF drainage.

The dura is dissected from the anterior cranial floor using magnification and head light for adequate visualization. Involved dura is resected and then grafted with temporalis fascia. All dural tears are meticulously closed with 5–0 nylon. En bloc tumor resection is then performed in conjunction with the lateral nasal approach performed by the ENT surgeon and the tumor is passed out inferiorly via that incision. Frozen section examination of the surgical margins or any suspicious-looking areas is very useful in guiding the extent of resection or in assessing resectability.

After the resection, liberal antibiotic irrigation is employed before and after suturing the pericranial flap to the dura of the anterior cranial fossa floor and to the margin of the bony defect to hold it firmly to the skull base. The edges of this flap are sealed using topical fibrin glue and Surgicel (see Fig. 42.7). No graft is used on the nasal side of this vascularized flap as the nasal epithelium covers this spontaneously over a 3–4-week period. Lumbar CSF drainage is ceased when the pericranial flap is sutured in place.

The pericranial flap technique (Johns et al 1981, Horowitz et al 1984, Kaye et al 1993) is crucial in achieving satisfactory results with low morbidity. This is confirmed by an analysis of the published series of craniofacial resection with and without this technique. There was a 4–10-fold reduction in the rate of CSF fistula, intracranial infection and operative mortality in those series employing this technique over those using other techniques for cranial base reconstruction (see Table 42.6).

In those cases where orbital exenteration is required, the dura of the optic nerve is closed to prevent CSF leak. The eyelids are sutured together and the orbital cavity is filled by transposition of the temporalis muscle. This local flap is more convenient than a microvascular free flap. However, a free flap is required if substantial facial skin needs to be sacrificed due to tumor involvement.

In our series, there have been no significant complications other than 2 cases of nonfatal thromboembolism. Reported complications of craniofacial resection include CSF fistula and infections such as resultant meningitis, intracranial abscess, or bone flap infection. Other compli-

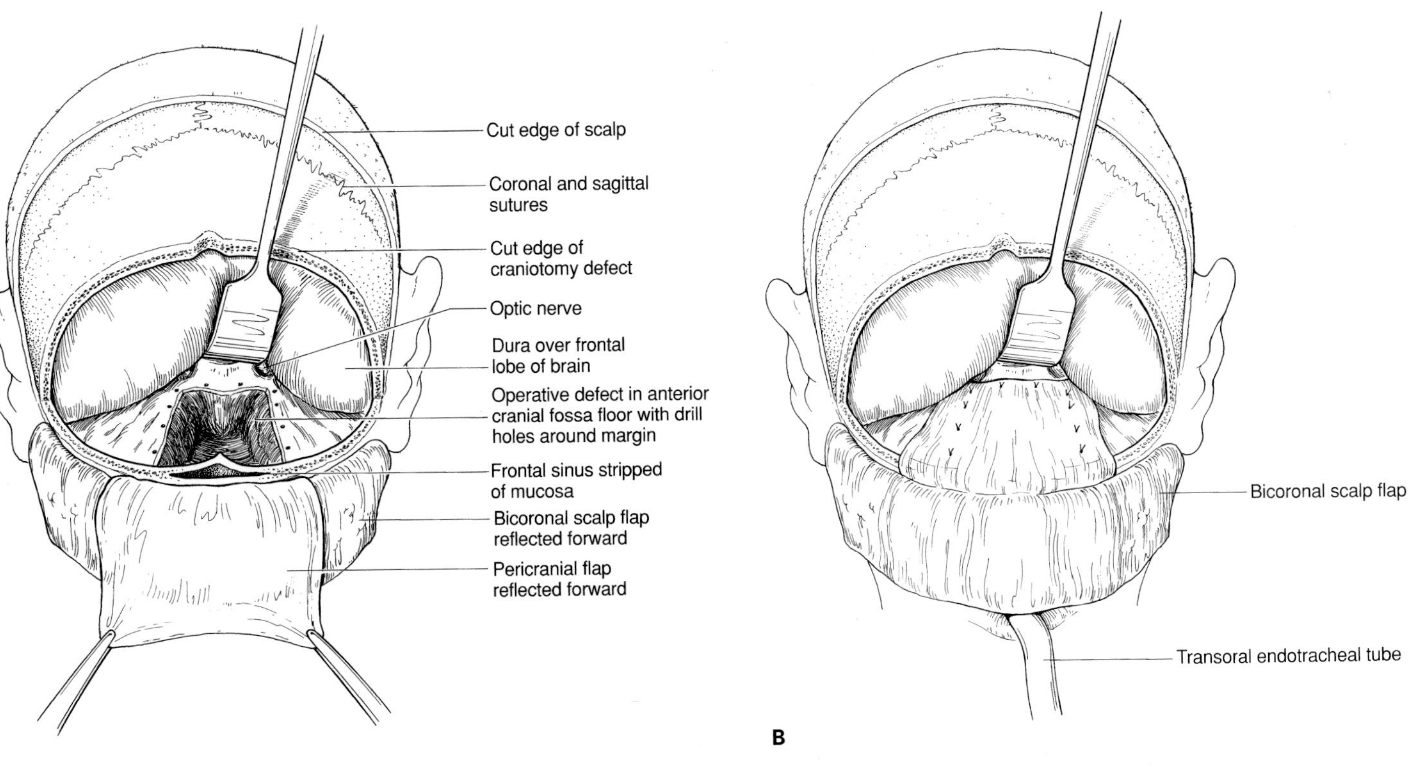

Fig. 42.7 The pericranial flap is designed and positioned to close the defect in the anterior cranial fossa floor. **A.** The defect in the anterior cranial fossa floor following the 'en bloc' removal of the tumor. Fine holes are drilled around the margins of this defect for suturing down the pericranial flap. **B.** Midsagittal section of the operative field showing the pericranial flap being sutured into position around the bony defect. **C.** The pericranial flap in position sutured to the margins of the operative defect, and covering a wide area of the anterior cranial fossa floor beyond that. Fibrin glue is used to seal the edges of the flap.

Table 42.6 Pericranial flaps in craniofacial resection

	Pericranial flap not used[1]	Pericranial flap used[2]	RMH series[3]
No. series	3	5	1
CSF fistula	16%	2%	0
Intracranial infection (early & late)	13%	5%	0
Mortality (all causes)	6%	2%	0

References:[1] Terz et al 1980, Ketcham & Van Buren 1985, Cheeseman et al 1986.
[2] Sundaresan & Shah 1988, Blacklock et al 1989, Snyderman et al 1990, Kaye et al 1993, Sekhar et al 1992.
[3] Kaye et al 1993.

cations may occur due to brain retraction causing frontal lobe edema, hemorrhage or epilepsy, but correct positioning of the head, minimization of brain retraction and careful technique can eliminate these problems. Intracranial aerocele may occur due to excessive lumbar drainage late in the operation and postoperatively.

The eye may be damaged due to exposure to the air or alcoholic skin prep, or by pressure. We use ointment, then suture the eyelids closed before skin preparation, and are vigilant to prevent pressure on the orbital structures during the procedure. Damage to the optic nerve may occur due to dissection at the orbital apex damaging that structure. This may lead to the dreaded complication of bilateral blindness if the other orbit is exenterated.

There are five series assessing the 5-year results of craniofacial resection and radiotherapy in advanced (T4) squamous carcinomas (Terz et al 1980, Ketcham & Van 1985, Sundaresan & Shah 1988, Bridger et al 1991, Kaye & Danks 1993). The 5-year survival was in the range of 50–70%. A similar number of series employing conventional noncraniofacial surgery and radiotherapy for such tumors gave a 5-year survival of 7–25% (Lavertu et al 1989, Sisson et al 1989, Tsujii et al 1989, Anniko et al 1990, Logue & Slevin 1991).

For adenocarcinoma of the ethmoid, the respective results are 78% and 83% for the two series employing craniofacial surgery and radiotherapy (Bridger et al 1991, Kaye et al 1993), as compared with 25–46% for transnasofacial surgery and radiotherapy (Ellingwood & Million 1979, Parsons et al 1988, Sisson et al 1989). In both the above comparisons, there was a much higher ratio of recurrent to untreated tumors in the craniofacial series. Thus the therapeutic advantage from a craniofacial approach is possibly even greater than these figures suggest.

For esthesioneuroblastoma, good results are achievable by radical surgical resection and radiotherapy, with 86–100% 5-year control (O'Connor et al 1989, Beitler et al 1991). This is clearly better than the results with single modality treatment.

RADIOTHERAPY

Radiotherapy is a very important modality for treatment of these tumors. Several studies have compared patient groups treated with surgery alone against similar groups given additional postoperative radiotherapy (Gabriele et al 1986, Kenady 1986, Wustrow et al 1989, Anniko et al 1990). All but one of these series (Wustrow et al 1989) found that additional radiotherapy gave significant improvement in the results. Certainly, it is widely accepted in the literature that postoperative radiotherapy offers additional benefit to the patient after radical tumor resection.

There are several series that have suggested that many of these tumors can be cured by radical high dose radiotherapy, combined with subradical surgery or surgical biopsy only (Ellingwood & Million 1979, Bush & Bagshaw 1982, Parsons et al 1988, Tsujii et al 1989, Karim et al 1990, Haylock et al 1991). There are no series that have compared different radiotherapy dosages in a controlled manner, but comparisons between series suggest that there are better results when doses of 60–80 Gy are delivered to the tumor rather than lower doses. In the three series employing this higher dosage there was a 5-year survival averaging 56% as compared with those series where 45–55 Gy were given where the 5-year survival averaged 37%. One series employing high dose radiotherapy used vigorous orbital shielding to try to limit morbidity due to radiation of the optic apparatus but this group suffered a high rate of orbital relapses, leading to a 5-year survival of 37% (Bush & Bagshaw 1982).

These results indicate that radical radiotherapy can give results similar to those achieved by simple transnasal surgery and radiotherapy combined, but the results are still marginally inferior to those series which employed radical craniofacial surgery to achieve as complete a tumor resection as possible. Furthermore, comparison of two similar groups of patients treated at Toronto by either radiotherapy alone or radiotherapy and surgery revealed better results in the combined therapy group (51% vs 40%) (Beale & Garrett 1983).

Unfortunately many patients suffer significant morbidity following this radical radiotherapy, involving dry eyes, but the most serious morbidity is that of damage to the visual apparatus. Optic nerve or retinal damage to the ipsilateral eye occurs in 25–100% of cases (Midena et al 1987), whilst frank blindness occurs in 7–22%. Several authors stated that blindness is inevitable if the orbit is radically treated, although this may be delayed for up to 2–5 years. This is defended by suggesting that orbital exenteration would otherwise be necessary to control such disease. The dreaded complication of bilateral blindness occurred in 2–8% of cases (Bush & Bagshaw 1982, Parsons et al 1988, Logue & Slevin 1991).

Osteoradionecrosis occurred in a similar number in

these series, but was up to 17% in one series (Bush & Bagshaw 1982). Transient CNS disturbances occurred in up to 10% of cases, but no long-term sequelae were detected.

Two recent series attest that reduction in morbidity can be achieved by the use of immobilizing shells and three-dimensional CT-guided computerized treatment planning systems to deliver precise differential dosimetry to the tumors and surrounding important structures (Tsujii et al 1989, Karim et al 1990). Both these series also claim a modest improvement in disease control attributable to this technique.

A number of papers favored preoperative radiotherapy as a routine (Klintenberg et al 1984, Cheeseman et al 1986) but the results did not differ clearly from those in similar series. However, the authors felt that this technique allowed them to better preserve the orbital contents in some cases. The morbidity of craniofacial resection subsequent to radiotherapy did not appear worse than in other series using similar techniques (Cheeseman et al 1986). Pre- and postoperative radiotherapy was compared at one centre, and no difference in outcome or morbidity was evident (Sisson et al 1989).

Preoperative radiotherapy does allow observation of changes in tumor histology to document the effectiveness of radiotherapy. In 6 of 19 patients with adenocarcinoma treated with preoperative radiotherapy, no tumor could be found at operation 6 weeks later (Klintenberg et al 1984). None of these patients developed recurrence on prolonged follow-up. A substantial number of other tumors in this series exhibited large areas of tumor necrosis. This emphasizes that this tumor type is significantly radiosensitive.

Amongst cases of squamous cell carcinoma, combined preoperative radiation and chemotherapy produced apparent elimination of all viable tumor in 34 of 86 cases on the basis of histopathology of the operative specimen (Konno et al 1980).

To summarize, it is certainly widely accepted that radiotherapy is of major benefit in the treatment of these patients. The most widely accepted view is that radiotherapy should be given after radical surgical resection of the tumor. To achieve maximal effect the radiotherapy needs to be given in high dosage to the tumor, with the whole tumor receiving 60–80 Gy. CT-guided, computer-assisted three-dimensional treatment planning appears to offer benefits in terms of reduced morbidity and possibly increased effectiveness.

CHEMOTHERAPY

Chemotherapy has not been widely used in the primary treatment of these tumors in the English-speaking world. However, regimes containing cisplatinum and 5FU may have a beneficial effect on these tumors. These treatments have been pioneered in Japan, where intra-arterial and topical routes have been combined with intravenous therapy. Treatment regimes have evolved over many years prompted by two factors: the relatively high incidence of this tumor in Japan, and the realization that the mean 5-year survival in paranasal sinus cancer treated by surgery and radiotherapy was a disappointing 35% (Knegt et al 1985). Maximal combination therapy (Sato et al 1970, Konno et al 1980) using preoperative radiotherapy, intra-arterial 5FU and intravenous bromodeoxyuridine combined with surgery achieved results of between 55% and 70% 5-year survival. Subsequently the intra-arterial 5FU therapy was replaced by repeated applications of topical 5FU therapy with maintenance of these good results (Sakai et al 1983, Knegt et al 1985, Inuyama et al 1989).

In another Japanese series, the use of preoperative intra-arterial cisplatinum and pepleomycin was felt to be the major factor in improving the 5-year survival rate from 22% to 55%, despite a reduction in the rate of radical maxillectomy from 50% to 18% (Inuyama et al 1989). Another series (Tsujii et al 1989) found no improvement in patients treated with intra-arterial 5FU. However, the group of patients who received 5FU received lower doses of radiotherapy than the control group. This factor severely confounds the results of this study.

A very careful prospective study was performed in Rotterdam, based on this Japanese work. A vigorous surgical internal decompression of the tumor was performed via an anterior maxillectomy but without removing orbital periosteum or dura, even if involved. The cavity was then packed, internally debrided thrice weekly, and topical therapy of 5FU cream applied to the walls of the cavity before re-packing. This was continued over several weeks depending on the progress and appearance of the cavity. Radiotherapy was commenced preoperatively, giving 4 Gy preoperatively followed by 10 Gy over one week postoperatively.

The 5-year survival in cases of squamous and undifferentiated maxillary sinus carcinoma was 52%. In 20 cases of adenocarcinoma of ethmoid, 100% disease-free 5-year survival was achieved (Knegt et al 1985). This was despite the dura and periorbita being involved, although not penetrated, in many cases. The treatment mortality was 1% due to one case of fatal postoperative pulmonary embolism, but there were no cases of major morbidity. The treatments were well tolerated although the tumor debridement was painful during the first week requiring morphine prior to the procedure. Subsequently analgesia was not required.

Thus the mainstay of their treatment was local 5FU cream and frequent debridement. Their conclusions were appropriately cautious but they suggested that this less aggressive treatment, which did not disturb the patient's appearance, could achieve results equal to or better than conventional combined radical surgery and high dosage radiation. It would certainly be possible to give higher doses of radiotherapy which may permit further improvement in these results.

Recent American series studying the use of chemotherapy have concentrated on salvage treatment of massive recurrent squamous cell carcinomas. Ninety percent of such cases demonstrated significant response to treatment. 45% of tumors resolved completely on radiologic criteria, allowing a mean survival of over 21 months in that group of patients (Rooney et al 1985, LoRusso et al 1988, Lee et al 1989). These authors all employed several courses based on cisplatinum and 5FU. Patients were also given radiotherapy but did not have surgery.

One study tested different protocols and found that a 5-day infusion of 5FU and cisplatinum gave significantly better results than other regimes tested (Rooney et al 1985). This protocol is justified on the basis of theoretical and experimental evidence that only those cells entering cell division during the period of therapy would be killed by such therapy. Thus routines employing short pulses of chemotherapy could only hope to affect a small proportion of the tumor cells, whereas a prolonged treatment would kill a higher number of tumor cells, as the cells entered mitosis in turn.

In transitional cell carcinoma, a dramatic response was reported in one case treated with cisplatinum, methotrexate and bleomycin (Sooriyachi et al 1984). In the rare esthesioneuroblastoma, combination radiotherapy and chemotherapy with cyclophosphamide and vincristine has rendered several advanced tumors operable, and appeared to allow improved disease control (O'Connor et al 1989).

To conclude this discussion on chemotherapy, there is evidence to suggest that regimes based on 5FU and cisplatinum improve the results in the treatment of these tumors. These therapies deserve closer examination than they have hitherto received in the English literature.

OTHER ADJUNCTIVE THERAPIES

There are two recent advances in radiotherapy that have found application in the treatment of these tumors. The use of chemotherapeutic agents as radiosensitizers and hyperfractionated radiotherapy may improve the therapeutic ratio in treating these tumors. This therapy relies on the normal tissue being better able to repair itself after sublethal damage from each treatment, whilst tumor cells typically have defects in their DNA repair mechanisms that render this repair less likely.

Tissue culture and experiments performed in animal models demonstrate that concomitant intravenous infusions of cisplatinum may act as a radiosensitizer to enhance the effect of radiation on tumor cells (Rotman & Aziz 1990). Infusions of 5–7 mg/m^2/24 h of cisplatinum were given in conjunction with hyperfractionated radiotherapy (60–70 Gy, in 60 fractions over 8 weeks). Eleven of 12 patients (92%) with T4 tumors or massive recurrent disease achieved a complete response with this treatment, and 7 of 12 (58%) were alive 3–6 years after treatment (Choi et al 1991). Four of the 12 patients suffered local recurrence. Ophthalmic complications occurred in only 1 of 9 patients receiving radiation to the visual apparatus. These results appear clearly better than in similar patients treated with radiation alone and are supported by other studies in these and other tumor types in a recent review (Rotman & Aziz 1990).

A randomized clinical trial of methotrexate or placebo given synchronously with radiotherapy showed clear improvement in a mixed group of squamous cell carcinomas of the head and neck. The methotrexate was given intravenously on day 0 and day 14 of the 3-week course of radiotherapy in doses of 100 mg/m^2 with folinic acid rescue (Gupta et al 1987).

Techniques based on molecular biology promise improved results in the treatment of many tumor types. One interesting example of this is a case report which described adoptive immunotherapy in combination with deep X-ray therapy causing cellular differentiation of adenoid cystic carcinoma into normal appearing bone (Sato et al 1990). The immunotherapy involved intra-arterial injection of lymphokine-activated killer cells and intravenous recombinant interleukin-2. Gene therapy using many different strategies is currently being trialed in diverse tumor types (Culver et al 1992). It is hoped that practical applications will result from this work to allow better treatment of PNC and other tumor types.

PATTERNS OF FAILURE

Prevention of local recurrence is the major challenge facing those who treat these patients. Traditional limits to resection have been the common sites of recurrence in earlier series. These sites include the floor of the anterior cranial fossa, particularly the olfactory groove, the orbit, and the pterygopalatine fossa. More distant recurrence may occur due to extension of tumor along nerves such as the trigeminal or vidian nerves. This is well documented in adenoid cystic carcinoma in particular (Pandolfo et al 1989).

Spread to local lymph nodes is uncommon at presentation (8% of cases), and occurs in a further 5–10% of cases in long-term follow-up. Generally, this form of recurrence is adequately treated by radical neck dissection and radiotherapy (Konno et al 1980). Distant metastases to bone, lung and liver occur in a similar proportion of patients (5–10% of cases). However, in the subgroup with anaplastic carcinoma, distal metastases occur in up to 50% of cases within one year (Konno et al 1980, Lund 1983). Local radiotherapy to symptomatic metastases and systemic chemotherapy have a role in the management of these problems.

Intracranial metastases are rare although we have noted 2 cases of cerebellar metastasis in our experience of 45 cases (Murphy et al 1991). These were treated by local excision and neuraxis radiotherapy.

TREATMENT OF RECURRENT DISEASE

Recurrent disease can be effectively treated in many cases. Many of the series discussing advanced disease include a high proportion of recurrent cancers.

The patient and the disease state should be assessed fully by clinical examination, CT and MRI, and other tests as appropriate. Interpretation of postoperative scans can be difficult as the healing tissues used in reconstruction may exhibit contrast enhancement that may simulate tumor recurrence (Som et al 1986). Treatment should then be planned accordingly. Details of previous treatment must be gathered. Radical or palliative surgical resection may be appropriate. Craniofacial resection has a major role in cases where there is involvement of the anterior fossa floor. In the larger craniofacial series, including our own, over half of the patients treated with a craniofacial resection had recurrent disease. Despite that, a high proportion (50–70%) have enjoyed long-term disease control and probable cure.

If previous craniofacial resection has been performed, the pericranium may not be available for reconstruction. Frontal galeal flaps (Snyderman et al 1990) or a microvascularized free flap of omentum (Yamaki et al 1991) or other donor material (Sekhar et al 1992) can be used for reconstruction.

Many patients will already have received radiotherapy and may only be able to receive limited further therapy. Chemotherapy with cisplatinum and 5FU-based regimes has a demonstrable effect on these tumors as discussed above. Palliative subtotal surgical resections can be of value in the slower growing tumor types such as adenocarcinoma, adenoid cystic carcinoma and transitional cell carcinoma. Subtotal resection may provide surprisingly long periods of tumor control.

MANAGEMENT OUTCOME

The management outcomes differ widely between series but, as discussed above, it is often difficult to compare series due to many differences in the groups of patients being treated. Nonetheless, on reviewing many series, several broad patterns emerge. These results are discussed in greater detail in the preceding sections.

Treatment by conventional noncraniofacial surgery and radiotherapy gives a 5-year survival of approximately 35% in series including all grades of tumor (Knegt et al 1985). Such treatment yields a 5-year survival of only 7–25% in patients with T4 disease (Lavertu et al 1989, Sisson et al 1989, Tsujii et al 1989, Anniko et al 1990, Logue & Slevin 1991).

In series employing craniofacial resection, about 50–70% of patients with T4 squamous cell carcinoma were alive and disease free at 5 years (Terz et al 1980, Ketcham & Van 1985, Sundaresan & Shah 1988, Bridger et al 1991, Kaye et al 1993). For adenocarcinoma, the figures are somewhat better, with 25–46% 5-year survival for conventional therapy and 78–83% survival for craniofacial series (Bridger et al 1991, Kaye et al 1993). There is a greater tendency for delayed recurrence in this tumor type, resulting in more late recurrences after the 5-year period.

In the case of multimodality therapy employing chemotherapy by various routes, preoperative radiotherapy and noncraniofacial surgery, a number of series report results of approximately 70% 5-year survival for the overall group (Sato et al 1970, Konno et al 1980). This treatment also enjoys the advantage of a lower rate of disfiguring surgery. One group (Knegt et al 1985) achieved the spectacular result of 100% 5-year disease-free survival employing multimodality therapy based on topical 5FU in adenocarcinoma.

Thus, despite the serious nature of these tumors, and the restrictions placed on treatment by the important surrounding structures, at least temporary disease control can be achieved in a majority of patients, and many patients have a long period of relief from the tumor. There remain many challenges in developing more effective therapies and refining their application to improve the results of present therapies.

REFERENCES

Acheson E D, Cowdell R H, Hadfield E, Macbeth R G 1968 Nasal cancer in woodworkers in the furniture industry. British Medical Journal 2: 587

Acheson E D, Cowdell R H, Jolles B 1970 Nasal cancer in the Northamptonshire boot and shoe industry. British Medical Journal 1: 385

Acheson E D, Winter P D, Hadfield E, Macbeth R G 1982 Is nasal adenocarcinoma in the Buckinghamshire furniture industry declining? Nature 299: 263

Anniko M, Franzen L, Lofroth P O 1990 Long-term survival of patients with paranasal sinus carcinoma. Otorhinolaryngology 52: 187

Beale F A, Garrett P G 1983 Cancer of the paranasal sinuses with particular reference to maxillary sinus cancer. Journal of Otolaryngology 12: 377

Beitler J J, Fass D E, Brenner H A et al 1991 Esthesioneuroblastoma: is there a role for elective neck treatment? Head and Neck 13: 321

Blacklock J B, Weber R S, Lee Y Y, Goepfert H 1989 Transcranial resection of tumors of the paranasal sinuses and nasal cavity. Journal of Neurosurgery 71: 10

Bridger G P, Mendelsohn M S, Baldwin M, Smee R 1991 Paranasal sinus cancer. Australian and New Zealand Journal of Surgery 61: 290
Bush S E, Bagshaw M A 1982 Carcinoma of the paranasal sinuses. Cancer 50: 154
Cheeseman A D, Lund V J, Howard D J 1986 Craniofacial resection for tumors of the nasal cavity and paranasal sinuses. Head and Neck Surgery 8: 429
Choi K N, Rotman M, Aziz H, Potters L, Stark R, Rosenthal J C 1991 Locally advanced paranasal sinus and nasopharynx tumors treated with hyperfractionated radiation and concomitant infusion cisplatin. Cancer 67: 2748
Culver K W, Ram Z, Wallbridge S, Ishii H, Oldfield E H, Blaese R M 1992 In vivo gene transfer with retroviral vector-producer cells for treatment of experimental brain tumors. Science 256: 1550
Doll R, Morgan L G, Speizer F E 1970 Cancer of the lung and nasal sinuses in nickel workers. British Journal of Cancer 24: 623
Egedahl R D, Coppock E, Homik R 1991 Mortality experience at a hydrometallurgical nickel refinery in Fort Saskatchewan, Alberta between 1954 and 1984. Journal of Social and Occupational Medicine 41: 29
Ellingwood K E, Million R R 1979 Cancer of the nasal cavity and ethmoid/sphenoid sinuses. Cancer 43: 1517
Franklin C I V 1982 Adenocarcinoma of the paranasal sinuses in Tasmania. Australasian Radiology 26: 49
Fukuda K, Shibata A 1985 Demographic correlation between occupation and maxillary sinus cancer mortality in Japan. Kurume Medical Journal 32: 151
Fukuda K, Shibata A, Harada K 1987 Squamous cell cancer of the maxillary sinus in Hokkaido, Japan: a case-control study. British Journal of Industrial Medicine 44: 263
Gabriele P, Besozzi M C, Pisani P et al 1986 Carcinoma of the paranasal sinuses. Results with radiotherapy alone or with a radio-surgical combination. Radiologica Medica (Torino) 72: 210
Giles G, Farrugia H, Silver B, Staples M 1992 Cancer in Victoria, 1982–1987. Anti-Cancer Council of Victoria, Melbourne, Australia
Gupta N K, Pointon R C S, Wilkinson P M 1987 A randomized clinical trial to contrast radiotherapy with radiotherapy and methotrexate given synchronously in head and neck cancer. Clinical Radiology 38: 575
Hadfield E H, MacBeth R G 1971 Adenocarcinoma of ethmoids in furniture workers. Annals of Otology Rhinology and Laryngology 80: 699
Har-El G, Hadar T, Krespi Y P, Abraham A, Sidi J 1988 An analysis of staging systems for carcinoma of the maxillary sinus. Ear Nose and Throat Journal 67: 511
Hayes R B, Gerin M, Raatgever J W, de Bruyn A 1986 Wood-related occupations, wood dust exposure, and sinonasal cancer. American Journal of Epidemiology 124: 569
Hayes R B, Kardaun J W, de Bruyn A 1987 Tobacco use and sinonasal cancer: a case-control study. British Journal of Cancer 56: 843
Haylock B J, John D G, Paterson I C 1991 The treatment of squamous cell carcinoma of the paranasal sinuses. Clinical Oncology (Royal College of Radiology) 3: 17
Horowitz J D, Persing J A, Nichter L S, Morgan R F, Edgerton M D 1984 Galeal-pericranial flaps in head and neck reconstruction. American Journal of Surgery 148: 489
Hyams V J, Batsakis J G, Micheals L 1988 Tumors of the upper respiratory tract and ear, 2nd edn. Armed Forces Institute of Pathology, Washington, DC
Inuyama Y, Kawaurs M, Toji M, Tanaka K, Ookuma A, Kawasaki K 1989 Intra-arterial chemotherapy of maxillary sinus carcinoma. Gan To Kagaku Ryoho 16: 2688
Ironside P, Matthews J 1975 Adenocarcinoma of the nose and paranasal sinuses in woodworkers in the State of Victoria, Australia. Cancer 36: 1115
Johns M E, Winn H R, McLean W C, Cantrell R W 1981 Pericranial flap for the closure of defects of craniofacial resections. Laryngoscope 91: 952
Karim A B M F, Kralendonk J H, Njo K H, Tabak J M, Elsnaar W H, vanBalen A T M 1990 Ethmoid and upper nasal cavity carcinoma: treatment, results and complications. Radiotherapy and Oncology 19: 109
Kaye A H, Danks R A, Kleide S, Millar H 1994 Cranio-facial resection in the management of cancer of the paranasal sinuses. Journal of Clinical Neuroscience 1: 117
Kenady D E 1986 Cancer of the paranasal sinuses. Surgical Clinics of North America 66: 119
Ketcham A S, Van Buren J 1985 Tumors of the paranasal sinuses: a therapeutic challenge. American Journal of Surgery 150: 406
Ketcham A S, Chretien P B, Van Buren J M, Hoye R C, Beazley J R, Herdt J R 1973 The ethmoid sinuses: a re-evaluation of surgical resection. American Journal of Surgery 126: 469
Klintenberg C, Olofsson J, Hellquist H, Sokjer H 1984 Adenocarcinoma of the ethmoid sinuses. A review of 28 cases with special reference to wood dust exposure. Cancer 54: 482
Knegt P P, de Jong P, van Anfrl J G, de Boer B M, Eykenboom W, van der Shans E 1985 Carcinoma of the paranasal sinuses. Results of a prospective pilot study. Cancer 56: 57
Konno A, Togawa K, Inoue S 1980 Analysis of the results of our combined therapy for maxillary cancer. Acta Oto-Laryngologica (suppl) 372: 2
Lavertu P, Roberts J K, Kraus D H et al 1989 Squamous cell carcinoma of the paranasal sinuses: The Cleveland Clinic Experience 1977–1986. Laryngoscope 99: 1130
Lee Y Y, Dimery I W, Van Tassell P, De Peria C, Blacklock J B, Goepfert H 1989 Superselective intra-arterial chemotherapy of advanced paranasal sinus tumors. Archives of Otolaryngology and Head and Neck Surgery 115: 503
Logue J P, Slevin N J 1991 Carcinoma of the nasal cavity and paranasal sinuses: an analysis of radical radiotherapy. Clinical Oncology 3: 84
LoRusso P, Tapazoglou E, Kish J A et al 1988 Chemotherapy for paranasal sinus carcinoma. A 10-year experience at Wayne State University. Cancer 62: 1
Luce D, Leclerc A, Marne M J, Gerin M, Casal A, Brugere J 1991 Sinonasal cancer and occupation: a multicenter case-control study. Review Epidemiologie Sante Publique 39: 7
Lund V J 1983 Malignant tumors of the nasal cavity and paranasal sinuses. Otolaryngology 45: 1
Midena E, Segato T, Piermarocchi S, Corti L, Zorat P L, Moro F 1987 Retinopathy following radiation therapy of paranasal sinus and nasopharyngeal carcinoma. Retina 7: 142
Millar H S, Petty P G, Hueston J T 1973 A combined intracranial and facial approach for excision and repair of cancer of the ethmoid sinuses. Australian and New Zealand Journal of Surgery 43: 179
Mohtashamipur E, Norpoth K, Luhmann F 1989 Cancer epidemiology of woodworking. Journal of Cancer Research and Clinical Oncology 115: 503
Muir C, Waterhouse J, Mack T, Powell J, Whelan S 1987 Cancer incidence in five continents, 5th edn. IARC, Lyon
Muir C S, Nectoux J 1980 Descriptive epidemiology of malignant neoplasms of nose, nasal cavities, middle ear and accessory sinuses. Clinical Otolaryngology 5: 195
Murphy M A, Kaye A H, Hayes I P 1991 Intracranial metastasis from carcinoma of the paranasal sinus. Neurosurgery 28: 890
Nishioka K, Masuda Y, Yanagi E, Yuen K, Tanaka T, Ogura Y 1989 Cytologic diagnosis of the maxillary sinus re-evaluated. Laryngoscope 99: 842
O'Connor T A, McLean P, Juillard G J, Parker R G 1989 Olfactory neuroblastoma. Cancer 63: 2426
Olsen J H 1987 Epidemiology of sinonasal cancer in Denmark, 1943–1982. Acta Pathologia Microbiologica Immunologica Scandanivica 95: 171
Pandolfo I, Gaeta M, Blandino A, Salvi L, Longo M 1989 MR imaging of perineural metastasis along the vidian nerve. Journal of Computer Assisted Tomography 13: 498
Parsons J T, Mendenhall W M, Mancuso A A, Cassisi N J, Million R R 1988 Malignant tumors of the nasal cavity and ethmoid and sphenoid sinuses. International Journal of Radiation Oncology Biological Physics 14: 11
Perry C, Levine P A, Williamson B R, Cantrell R W 1988 Preservation of the eye in paranasal sinus cancer surgery. Archives of Otolaryngology and Head and Neck Surgery 114: 632
Rankow R M, Conley J, Fodor P 1974 Carcinoma of the maxillary sinus following thorotrast instillation. Journal of Maxillofacial Surgery 2: 119

Ratech H, Burke J S, Blayney D W, Sheibani K, Rappaport H 1989 A clinicopathologic study of malignant lymphomas of the nose, paranasal sinuses, and hard palate, including cases of lethal midline granuloma. Cancer 64: 2525

Robin P E, Powell D J, Stansbie J M 1979 Carcinoma of the nasal cavity and paranasal sinuses: incidence and presentation of different histological types. Clinical Otolaryngology 4: 431

Rooney M, Kish J, Jacobs J et al 1985 Improved complete response rate and survival in advanced head and neck cancer after three-course induction therapy with 120-hour 5-FU infusion and cisplatinum. Cancer 55: 1123

Rosai J 1981 Ackerman's Surgical pathology, 6th edn. C V Mosby, St Louis, Missouri

Rotman M, Aziz H 1990 Concomitant continuous infusion chemotherapy and radiation. Cancer 65: 823

Roush G C 1979 Epidemiology of cancer of the nose and paranasal sinuses: current concepts. Head and Neck Surgery 2: 3

Sakai S, Ebihara T, Ono I, Taketa C 1983 A comparison of AJC and JJC proposals on TNM classification of maxillary sinus carcinoma. Archives of Otorhinolaryngology 237: 139

Sato M, Yoshida H, Kaji R et al 1990 Induction of bone formation in an adenoid cystic carcinoma. Journal of Biological Response Modification 9: 329

Sato Y, Morita M, Takahashi H, Watanabe N, Kirika A 1970 Combined surgery, radiotherapy and regional chemotherapy in carcinoma of the paranasal sinuses. Cancer 25: 571

Sekhar L N, Nanda A, Sen C N, Snyderman C N, Janecka I P 1992 The extended frontal approach to tumors of the anterior, middle and posterior skull base. Journal of Neurosurgery 76: 198

Shimizu H, Hozawa J, Saito H et al 1989 Chronic sinusitis and woodworking as risk factors for cancer of the maxillary sinus in northeast Japan. Laryngoscope 99: 58

Sisson G S, Toriumi D M, Atiyah R A 1989 Paranasal sinus malignancy: a comprehensive update. Laryngoscope 99: 143

Snyderman C H, Janecka I P, Seckhar L N, Sen C N, Eibling D E 1990 Anterior skull base reconstruction: role of galeal and pericranial flaps. Laryngoscope 100: 607

Som P M, Lawson W, Biller H F, Lanzieri C F, Sachdev V D, Rigamonti D 1986 Ethmoid sinus disease: CT evaluation in 400 cases. Radiology 159: 605

Sooriyachi G S, Skuta G L, Busse J M 1984 Transitional cell carcinoma of the nasal passages: dramatic response to chemotherapy. Medical Pediatric Oncology 12: 50

Sundaresan N, Shah J P 1988 Craniofacial resection for anterior skull base tumors. Head and Neck Surgery 10: 219

Terz J J, Young H F, Lawrence W 1980 Combined craniofacial resection for locally advanced carcinoma of the head and neck: carcinoma of the paranasal sinuses. The American Journal of Surgery 140: 618

Tsujii H, Kamada T, Matsuoka Y, Takamura A, Akazawa T, Irie G 1989 The value of treatment planning using CT and an immobilizing shell in radiotherapy for paranasal sinus carcinomas. International Journal of Radiation Oncology and Biological Physics 16: 243

Waterhouse J, Muir C, Correa P, Powell J 1976 Cancer incidence in five continents, 3rd edn. IARC, Lyon

Willatt D J, Morton R P, McCormick M S, Stell P M 1987 Staging of maxillary cancer. Which classification? Annals of Otolology Rhinology and Laryngology

Wills J H 1982 Nasal carcinoma in woodworkers: a review. Journal of Occupational Medicine 24: 526

Wustrow J, Rudert H, Diercks M, Beigel A 1989 Squamous epithelial carcinoma and undifferentiated carcinoma of the inner nose and paranasal sinuses. Strahlentherapia Onkologica 165: 468

Yamaki T, Uede T, Tano-oka A, Asakura K, Tanabe S, Hashi K 1991 Vascularized omentum graft for the reconstruction of the skull base after removal of a nasoethmoidal tumor with intracranial extension: case report. Neurosurgery 28: 877

43. Esthesioneuroblastoma

Michael J. Ebersold Kerry D. Olsen Robert L. Foote Jan C. Buckner Lynn M. Quast

INTRODUCTION

Esthesioneuroblastoma (olfactory neuroblastoma) is an uncommon tumor originating in the upper nasal cavity. This tumor was first reported by Berger & Luc in the French literature in 1924. The recent increase in capabilities with skull base surgery and the advent of nuclear magnetic resonance imaging (MRI) and computed tomography (CT) have resulted in an increased interest in and awareness of this tumor. Since its initial description, however, fewer than 300 cases have been reported in the world literature (Djalilian et al 1977, Chaudhry et al 1979). Because of the rarity of this tumor, few practitioners have had an opportunity to witness the effects of various treatment options for it. A systematic approach to the evaluation of management outcomes is difficult because most series include patients who were entered over a long period, during which diagnostic and therapeutic capabilities varied immensely.

PATHOGENESIS

Although esthesioneuroblastoma is the term used most commonly to describe this tumor, other names, including olfactory neuroblastoma, olfactory neural neoplasm, olfactory esthesioneuroblastoma, and neuroendocrine carcinoma, have been used by various authors (Christiansen et al 1974).

The tumor is thought to arise from olfactory neuroepithelium cells high in the nasal cavity. By the time of detection, these tumors often have attained a large size and resulted in nasal obstruction or epistaxis. Not infrequently, the skull base, cranial vault, and orbit have been invaded by the time of detection. No specific cause for this tumor has yet been identified. In a recent review of 49 patients who received their initial evaluation and treatment at the Mayo Clinic, we found that the ages of the patients at diagnosis ranged from 3–78 years (mean 48 years), and there was a bimodal peak of presentation in the second and fifth decades of life (Morita et al 1993). We found a slight male preponderance (27 male and 22 female patients). In a recent review by Cantrell (1993), the male:female ratio was 1:1.7.

DIAGNOSIS

Most of the patients in our series presented to otolaryngologists because of symptoms suggestive of nasal abnormality or obstruction. The most common symptoms were epistaxis and nasal obstruction. The time from the onset of symptoms to diagnosis can range from months to as long as 10 years. The presenting symptoms at the time of evaluation in our series are included in Table 43.1. Although anosmia is an infrequent presenting complaint, if patients are asked about alterations in smell or lack of smell, they often describe inability to smell or secondary alterations in taste. A physical examination in some of our patients revealed proptosis or signs of obstructive nasal sinuses, but there is no unique history or physical finding specific for this tumor. Evaluation of the nasal cavity often showed a fleshy, lobulated mass, which in some cases was friable and prone to hemorrhage. Such a finding now leads to further evaluation with CT or MRI. Enhancement scanning with contrast material and gadolinium has

Table 43.1 Presenting symptoms of esthesioneuroblastoma in 49 patients. Reproduced from Morita et al (1993) with permission of Congress of Neurological Surgeons.

Symptoms	No. of patients
Nasal obstruction	29
Epistaxis	22
Nasal mass	5
Loss of sense of smell	4
Headache	4
Excessive tearing	2
Nasal discharge	2
Proptosis	2
Mental change	2
Neck mass	2
Face pain	1
Facial mass	1
Diplopia	1

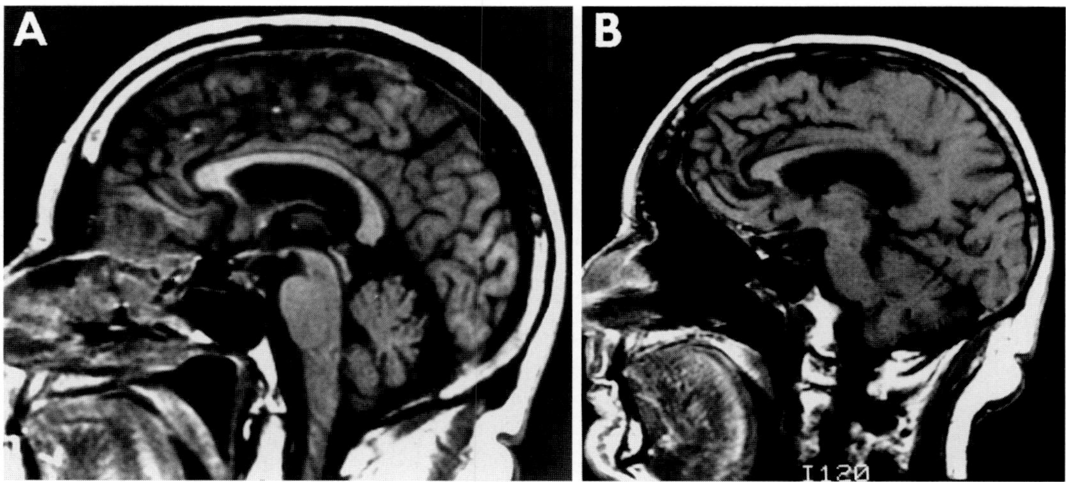

Fig. 43.1 Magnetic resonance imaging scans from a patient with a large esthesioneuroblastoma. **A.** Preoperative scan shows tumor extending through cribriform plate. **B.** Postoperative scan has no evidence of residual tumor.

markedly improved the sensitivity and usefulness of these techniques (Fig. 43.1). After the size and location of the lesion are established, outpatient biopsy is usually performed.

DIAGNOSTIC CRITERIA (PATHOLOGIC FINDINGS)

The diagnosis of this tumor depends on the pathologic findings and the anatomic location of the tumor. The light microscopic features of esthesioneuroblastoma include a lobular architecture, sheets of neoplastic cells, an intercellular neurofibrillary background, round or oval nuclei with poorly-defined cytoplasm, and occasional pseudorosettes or rosettes (Fig. 43.2) (Obert et al 1960). Electron microscopy reveals intracytoplasmic neurosecretory granules and neuritic processes with microtubules and neurofilaments (Fig. 43.3) (Taxy & Hidvegi 1977). Neoplastic cells exhibit positive immunohistochemical staining reactions with antibodies to neuron-specific enolase neurofilaments, chromogranin, synaptophysin, and Leu-7. A distinctive peripheral staining with antibodies to S-100 protein can also be seen in some cases (Taxy & Hidvegi 1977, Hyams et al 1988, Frierson et al 1990, Morita et al 1993).

In an effort to better understand the prognosis and to better individualize treatment, we carefully analyzed the relevance of a staging system proposed by Kadish and others, as outlined in Table 43.2 (Kadish et al 1976). This stage seemed to have less effect on prognosis than histologic appearance.

We agree with Hyams et al (1988) and Taxy et al (1986) and prefer to interpret these neoplasms as constituting a histologic spectrum. The pathologic grade (Hyams system) (Table 43.3) was the most reliable feature for predicting outcome in our recent review.

Specifically, as one might expect, the higher grade tumors also proved to have a higher clinical stage. Nevertheless, when we corrected for grade, stage did not seem, in itself, to alter the duration of survival (Table 43.4). Our data showed that only pathologic differentiation had a statistically significant effect on survival, and it was the most reliable prognostic factor. Although Kadish's clinical staging has been advocated as the most important prognostic indicator by some (Elkon et al 1979, Kadish et al 1976), our data suggested that the pathologic differentiation, as described by others (Fisher 1955, McCormack & Harris 1955, Oberman & Rice 1976, Silva et al 1982, Hyams 1983, Hyams et al 1988), was much more important.

TREATMENT

Because of the rarity of esthesioneuroblastoma, no systematic clinical trial has been evaluated, and controversies remain regarding the optimal treatment plan (Olsen & DeSanto 1983). Skolnik et al (1966) and Elkon et al (1979) reported the largest series of esthesioneuroblastomas, and both concluded that a surgical procedure is an essential part of treatment.

Cantrell, at the University of Virginia, used preoperative radiation therapy for stage A and B disease, and this was followed by craniofacial resection. Stage C disease was treated preoperatively with radiation, and preoperatively and postoperatively with intravenously administered chemotherapy. If a preoperative response to chemotherapy was noted by CT evaluation, additional chemotherapy was given postoperatively. However, the histologic grade

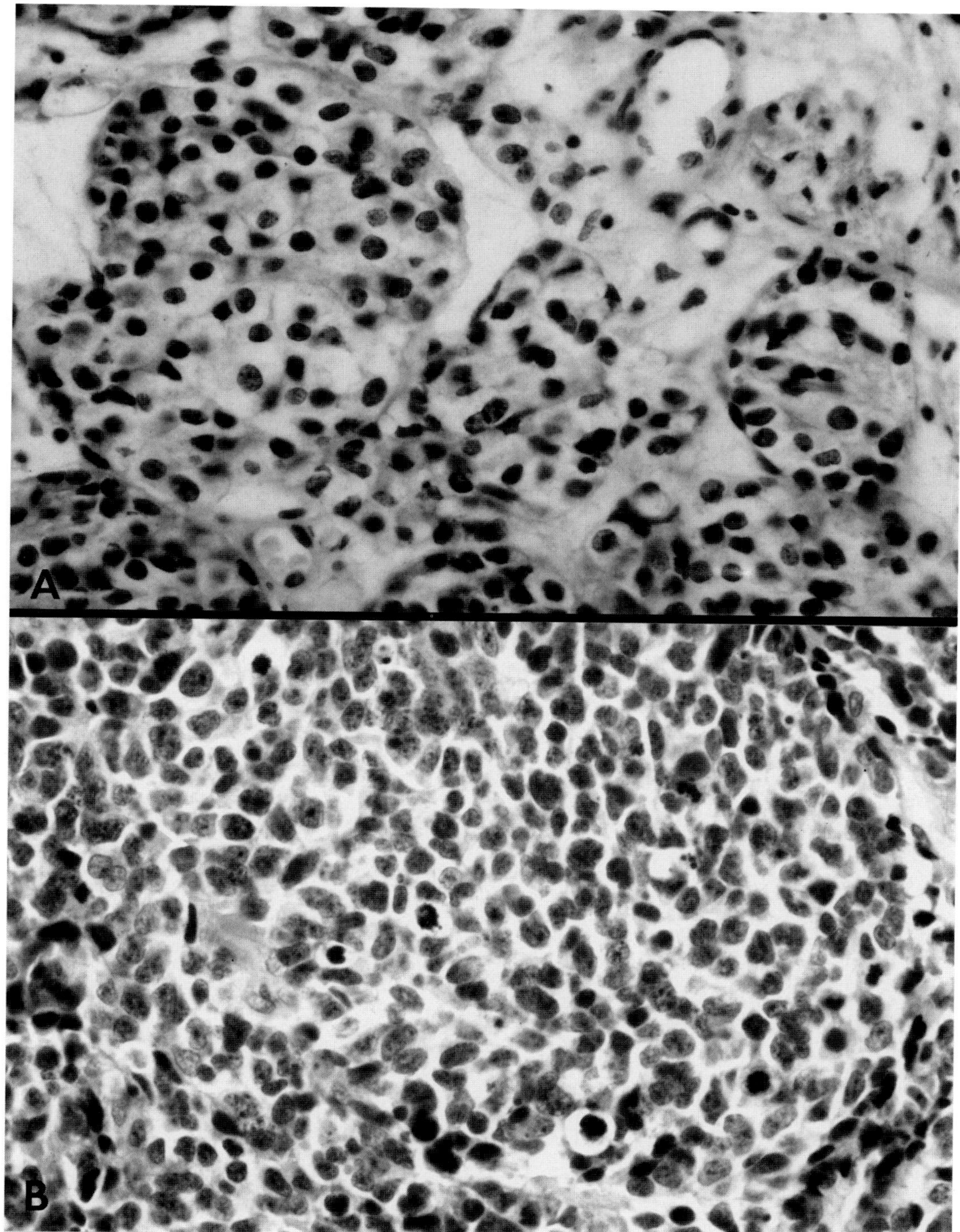

Fig. 43.2 Photomicrograph of representative cases of esthesioneuroblastoma. **A.** Hyams grade 2. Note lobular arrangements of uniform cells with little cytoplasm and occasional Homer Wright rosettes. **B.** Hyams grade 4. Cellular tumor with atypical cells in dense chromatin; no apparent rosette is noted.

rather than stage alone should be considered when deciding on the treatment options.

Our data suggested that radiation therapy, chemotherapy, and surgical treatment need to be considered for high grade tumors. The role of each may vary among various treatment centers; however, our treatment plans are based on the principles that are detailed in the following sections.

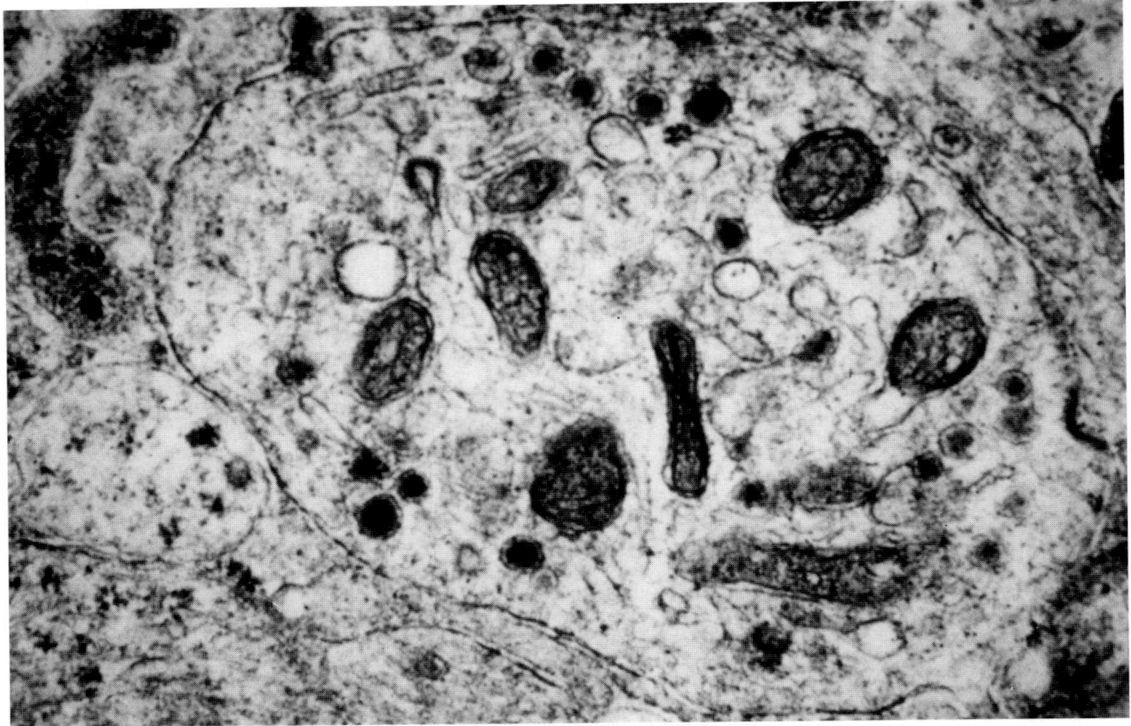

Fig. 43.3 Electron microscopic findings of esthesioneuroblastoma. Dense core vesicles are noted within cytoplasm, and cell processes are noted.

Table 43.2 Modified Kadish staging of esthesioneuroblastoma. Reproduced from Morita et al (1993) with permission of Congress of Neurological Surgeons.

Stage	Finding
A	Tumor confined to nasal cavity
B	Tumor confined to nasal cavity and paranasal sinuses
C	Tumor extent beyond nasal cavity and paranasal sinuses, including involvement of cribriform plate, base of skull, orbit, or intracranial cavity
D	Tumor with metastasis to cervical lymph nodes or distant sites

Table 43.3 Hyams grading system for esthesioneuroblastoma. Reproduced from Morita et al (1993) with permission of Congress of Neurological Surgeons.

	Grade			
Histologic grade	1	2	3	4
Lobular architecture	Present	Present	±	±
Mitotic activity	Absent	Present	Prominent	Marked
Nuclear pleomorphism	Absent	Moderate	Prominent	Marked
Rosettes	H-W ±	H-W ±	Flexner ±	Absent
Necrosis	Absent	Absent	Occasional	Common

Key : H-W = Homer Wright pseudorosette; ± = present or absent.

Table 43.4 Clinical stage, pathologic grade, and outcome in 47 patients* with esthesioneuroblastoma. Reproduced from Morita et al (1993) with permission of Congress of Neurological Surgeons.

	Low grade			High grade				
		5-yr survival†			Survival† 2-yr		Survival† 5-yr	
Stage	No. of patients	%	No. alive/total	No. of patients	%	No. alive/total	%	No. alive/total
A	3	100	3/3	0	—	—	—	—
B	9	75	6/8	3	67	2/3	33	1/3
C	18	82	9/11	11	55	6/11	44	4/9
D	2	100	1/1	1	0	0	0	0

*Pathologic material was not available for review in two patients.
†Some patients did not have 5-year follow-up.

Radiation

Early lesions confined to the nasal cavity or with minimal involvement of the paranasal sinuses can be treated adequately by complete surgical resection or by radiation alone (Obert et al 1960, Djalilian et al 1977, Elkon et al 1979). Elkon et al (1979) reported tumor control in 8 of 10 stage A lesions and 9 of 11 stage B lesions treated with radiation alone. Advanced lesions that are unresectable for cure with acceptable morbidity (invasion of the clivus or internal carotid artery involvement within the cavernous sinus) are referred for radiation therapy or chemotherapy, and success is limited. Patients uncommonly present with very early or far advanced lesions, and most tumors in these cases can be completely resected with the craniofacial approach described previously.

We have found that after complete surgical resection alone, a local recurrence develops within 5 years in 25% of patients with low grade tumors and in 65% of patients with high grade tumors. With the addition of postoperative adjuvant radiation therapy, no local recurrences have developed in 10 patients with low grade tumors, and only 2 local recurrences have been found in 6 patients with high grade tumors. Radiation therapy-associated complications have been acceptable, and no blindness has resulted from retinopathy, optic neuropathy, or keratoconjunctivitis. A review of the literature confirms a recurrence rate of 53% (36 of 68) after complete surgical resection alone, but this can be reduced to 20% (18 of 92) with the addition of postoperative adjuvant radiation therapy. Despite salvage treatments, no differences in disease-free or overall survival rates have been noted. These results need to be interpreted with some caution because the routine addition of postoperative radiation therapy did not begin at our institution until 1981 and thus the duration of follow-up is relatively short.

Some investigators have advocated the use of preoperative radiation therapy (Cantrell 1993). This has the theoretical advantages of improving tumor resectability by shrinkage of the tumor, decreasing local tumor dissemination and distant metastasis at the time of operation by tumor cell sterilization, and reducing the risk of radiation therapy-associated complications by using moderate doses (50 Gy). However, because of the rarity of esthesioneuroblastoma, a prospective, clinically controlled trial comparing preoperative and postoperative radiation therapy is not feasible. We have been concerned about potential wound-healing complications after preoperative radiation therapy. Therefore, we have traditionally favored the use of postoperative radiation therapy and are pleased with the rate of local tumor control (14 of 16 tumors) and the low complication rate in the light of the proportion of patients with high stage (15 of 16 stage C) and high grade (6 of 16) tumors.

When radiation therapy is used, it is important for the patient to be immobilized with some type of face mask and neck rest during treatment to improve reproducibility and accuracy. An oral dental prosthesis can be fabricated to displace the tongue, floor of the mouth, and mandible inferiorly away from the radiation beam and to fill the oral cavity with tissue-equivalent material. CT or MRI should be performed with the patient immobilized in the treatment position. The images can then be utilized for computerized radiation treatment planning and dosimetry. We have found three-dimensional treatment planning to be of value in selected cases. Review of preoperative imaging studies, the operative note, and the pathology report helps to determine the volume to be irradiated. Close communication with the operating surgeons is essential. Our most common radiation field arrangement consists of a three-field technique heavily weighted in favor of an anterior field with opposed lateral fields to supplement the dose posteriorly along the skull base. Wedges, partial transmission blocks, or some other type of compensating system is used for the lateral fields to optimize the dose homogeneity. Isodose lines are calculated every 1–2 cm throughout the treatment volume. Care is taken to limit the dose per fraction to <200 cGy (ideal dose, 180 cGy) to the retina, optic nerve, optic chiasm, and brainstem. The lens and lacrimal glands are blocked whenever possible. We have found the optimal postoperative adjuvant dose to be 55.8 Gy over 6–7 weeks. When treatment involves radiation alone, doses of 65–70 Gy over 7–8 weeks are necessary. When there is parotid or cervical adenopathy, the isocenter is placed at the level of the oral commissure, and the inferior half of the field is blocked and the superior half treats the nasal cavity and paranasal sinuses through the three-field arrangement described above. The upper neck above the larynx is then treated through posterolateral fields, and the superior half of the field is blocked. The lower neck and supraclavicular nodes are then treated through an anterior field. Great detail is given to these matching fields to avoid overlap and cervical myelopathy.

Chemotherapy

The role of chemotherapy in the management of patients with esthesioneuroblastomas continues to evolve. Esthesioneuroblastomas share certain light microscopic and ultrastructural features with other chemosensitive tumors of neural crest origin, such as neuroblastomas, primitive neuroectodermal tumors of the central nervous system, small cell carcinomas of the lung and extrathoracic sites, and high grade neuroendocrine carcinomas. Similarly, chemotherapy regimens effective in these neuroectodermal tumors have also been useful in patients with esthesioneuroblastoma. In 1990, Goldsweig & Sundaresan (1990) reviewed 25 cases from the English literature and reported 1 additional case. In their review, 19 of 20 patients given chemotherapy alone for recurrent or metastatic disease improved. The most commonly reported regimens include cyclophosphamide plus vincristine, often with doxorubicin. Cisplatin-based regimens have also produced tumor regression. We do not have experience with the use of high dose chemotherapy to the extent requiring bone marrow transplantation or the use of intra-arterial chemotherapy for this particular tumor type, although this approach has been discussed by others (O'Conor et al 1985, Watne & Hager 1987). Stewart et al (1989) used high dose chemotherapy with autologous bone marrow transplant to produce transient responses in 3 of 8 heavily pretreated patients. The case reports and small series all point to chemosensitivity of the tumor, but they do not yield definitive conclusions concerning the most appropriate drug regimen, dose intensity, or schedule of drug administration in combination with operation and radiation therapy.

In summary, esthesioneuroblastomas are sensitive to various chemotherapeutic agents. Treatment of metastatic disease is warranted. The optimal regimen has not been identified. The value of adjuvant chemotherapy in conjunction with operation and radiation has not been explored to any significant extent, but multimodality therapy is reasonable in patients with high grade tumors.

Surgery

We also attempted to define the importance of a more radical operation, which even in extensive tumors can often accomplish gross total removal of the tumor. Between 1951 and 1990, 38 (78%) of 49 patients underwent a gross total resection with or without radiation therapy and seemed to have better survival and disease-free survival rates than those who had partial resection or biopsy with radiation therapy alone. This finding, however, needs to be interpreted with some caution because the selection of patients might have biased the outcome; specifically, gross total removal may not have been attempted or accomplished in patients who had extremely extensive tumors. Local recurrence rates were lower in patients treated with total resection and radiation than in those treated with total resection alone. This finding also, however, must be interpreted with some caution because the addition of radiation therapy is a relatively recent change in treatment policy and therefore the duration of follow-up in the irradiated group is relatively short. Radiation therapy alone or partial resection and radiation therapy with the palliative doses (40 Gy) used in our series obtained local control of tumor in only 1 of 9 patients.

We also found that salvage treatment (treatment for recurrent disease) is as effective as initial treatment for 'controlling' tumor. The 5-year survival rate of 82% in our diverse group with local recurrence suggests that patients with tumor recurrence deserve further treatment efforts and cautiously optimistic counseling. The patients who underwent further treatment of local or regional recurrence generally had low grade tumors and, therefore, may have had a more favorable prognosis. For cervical lymph node metastasis, radical neck dissection and radiation therapy offer a reasonable outcome.

Because our recent review demonstrated that prognosis seems to be affected by tumor grade, we believe that treatment options should be decided on the basis of pathologic grade. As demonstrated in Table 43.5, gross total resection without radiation therapy for low grade tumors seems to produce an acceptable outcome. For high grade

Table 43.5 Pathologic grade, treatment, and outcome in 47 patients* with esthesioneuroblastoma. Reproduced from Morita et al (1993) with permission of Congress of Neurological Surgeons.

	Low grade†					High grade†‡				
		5-yr§		5-ydf§			2-yr		2-ydf	
Initial therapy	No. of patients	%	No. alive/ total	%	No. alive/ total	No. of patients	%	No. alive/ total	%	No. alive/ total
Total resection	17	87	13/15	73	11/15	3	67	2/3	33	1/3
Total resection with radiation	10	100	2/2	100	2/2	6	67	4/6	33	2/6
≤ 5000 cGy**						2	0	0/2	0	0/2
> 5000 cGy**						4	100	4/4	50	2/4
Partial resection or biopsy with radiation	5	80	4/5	20	1/5	4	50	2/4	0	0/4
Partial resection						2	0	0/2	0	0/2

*Pathologic material was not available for review in two patients.
†5-yr = 5-year survival; 5-ydf = 5-year disease-free survival; 2-yr = 2-year survival; 2-ydf = 2-year disease-free survival. Percentage survival was based on the number of patients who survived more than 5 (or 2) years/number of patients treated more than 5 (or 2) years earlier.
‡Outcome is based on 2-year survival and 2-year recurrence-free survival in high grade tumor group because prognosis was so poor.
§Some patients did not have 5-year follow-up.
**Radiation dose.

tumors, however, operation alone is inadequate. The patients who had total resection and radiation therapy of more than 5000 cGy had a 2-year survival rate of 100% and a 2-year disease-free survival rate of 50%. Thus, a sound treatment for low grade tumors seems to be combined craniofacial resection alone (without radiation or chemotherapy) if one can be reasonably confident about obtaining tumor-free margins. Radiation therapy can be reserved for local recurrence or for cases in which residual tumor is strongly suspected. For high grade tumors, a combined craniofacial approach followed by high dose radiation therapy (55.8 Gy) seems to be the best initial treatment. The benefits of chemotherapy for high grade tumors need further investigation; however, our experience indicates it is warranted. Because of the rarity of esthesioneuroblastoma, it is impossible to determine whether preoperative chemotherapy or radiation therapy favorably influences outcome in patients with high grade disease. Nevertheless, the bad prognosis for this entity certainly suggests that there is room for improvement.

This tumor has a notorious tendency for not only early but also late local recurrence, even with aggressive treatment. In a review from our institution in which the minimal duration of follow-up was 5 years, metastatic disease occurred in 62% and local recurrence in 57% of all patients with olfactory neuroblastoma (Stewart et al 1989). Therefore, careful follow-up over at least 10 years is indicated in all cases. Figures 43.4 to 43.7 demonstrate how tumor stage, grade, and treatment options influence survival.

Surgical technique

Unlike many of the other skull-base tumors, which require extensive dissection to reach the lesion, tumors in the region of the cribriform plate are easily accessible from both below and above. Extensive flaps and dissections are not required; in fact, general surgical procedures in this region can be quickly and safely done without any major reconstructive procedures.

The patient is placed in the supine position and, under general anesthesia, the forehead, face, and abdomen or

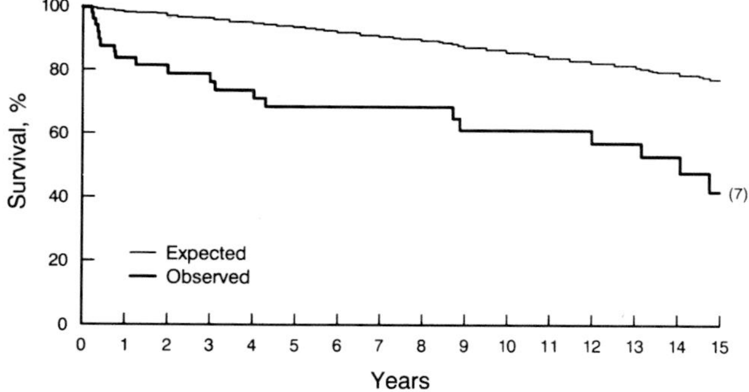

Fig. 43.4 Overall survival rate in 49 patients with esthesioneuroblastoma. Rapid decrease during the first few years was due to death from aggressive tumor. Survival rate at 5 years was 69%. Expected survival curve is that for a population in Minnesota of the same age and sex distribution. Number at end of curve is number of patients still in follow-up. Reproduced from Morita et al (1993) with permission of Congress of Neurological Surgeons.

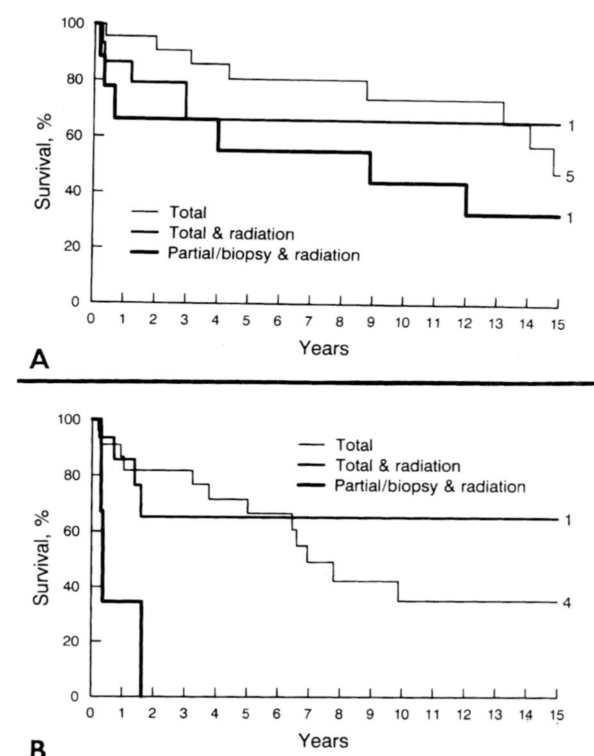

Fig. 43.5 Survival (**A**) and tumor-free survival (**B**) rates after initial treatment, according to the type of treatment. Total = gross total resection; partial = partial resection. Tumor-free survival rate was significantly higher ($p = 0.008$) for patients who had total resection with or without radiation therapy than for those who had biopsy or partial resection with radiation therapy. Numbers at ends of curves are numbers of patients still in follow-up. Reproduced from Morita et al (1993) with permission of Congress of Neurological Surgeons.

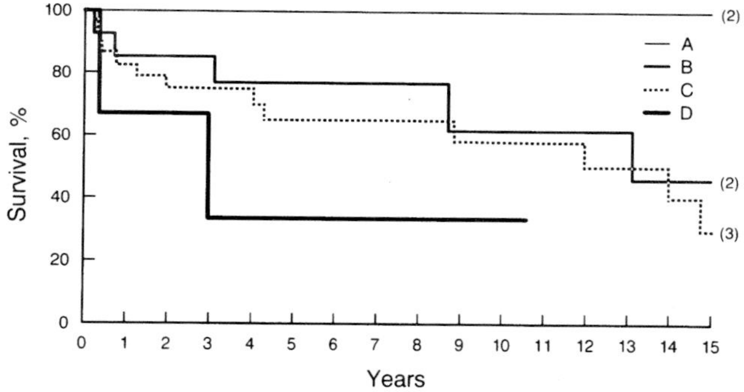

Fig. 43.6 Survival rates according to modified Kadish staging of tumor. The effect of tumor stage on survival is documented. Many of the higher stage tumors, however, were also higher grade. Reproduced from Morita et al (1993) with permission of Congress of Neurological Surgeons.

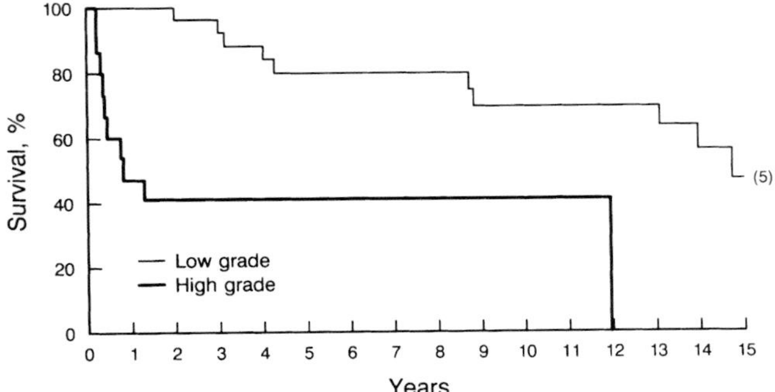

Fig. 43.7 Survival rates according to pathologic differentiation (Hyams grade). The effect of tumor grade on survival, even with more aggressive treatment for higher grade tumors, is demonstrated. The difference is statistically significant ($p = 0.0001$). Reproduced from Morita et al (1993) with permission of Congress of Neurological Surgeons.

thigh are prepared and draped. The abdomen or thigh serves as a site for harvest of a skin graft or, in rare cases, a fascia lata graft. We usually shave the hair of the forehead nearly back to the region of the coronal suture; this approach provides adequate superior exposure even if a hairline skin incision is used. Towels are then used to isolate the surgical field from the endotracheal tube, the ears, and the remaining scalp. We have not found it necessary to suture the eyelids together because a self-adhesive dressing (Steri-Drape) placed over the forehead, eyelids, cheeks, and circumferential towels holds the eyelids closed. This dressing allows complete visibility of the eyes and face throughout the procedure and also helps hold the towels in place. Spinal fluid drainage is not needed because small amounts of spinal fluid are unavoidably drained early in the epidural dissection, and therefore there is ample room for the remaining epidural dissection; also, the likelihood of draining too much spinal fluid during the procedure or from a persistent cerebrospinal fluid leak at the site of the previous spinal catheter is lessened.

We usually start with the incision for the craniotomy, and after completion of the intracranial portion of the procedure the otolaryngologist proceeds with the nasal portion of the operation. We have been very satisfied with the cosmetic results of a coronal incision, a midline incision immediately above the nasion, or a brow incision (Fig. 43.8). In general, however, we do a coronal incision so as to keep the incision site farther from the craniotomy site, thinking that this might decrease the likelihood of skin breakdown after radiation therapy in the post-

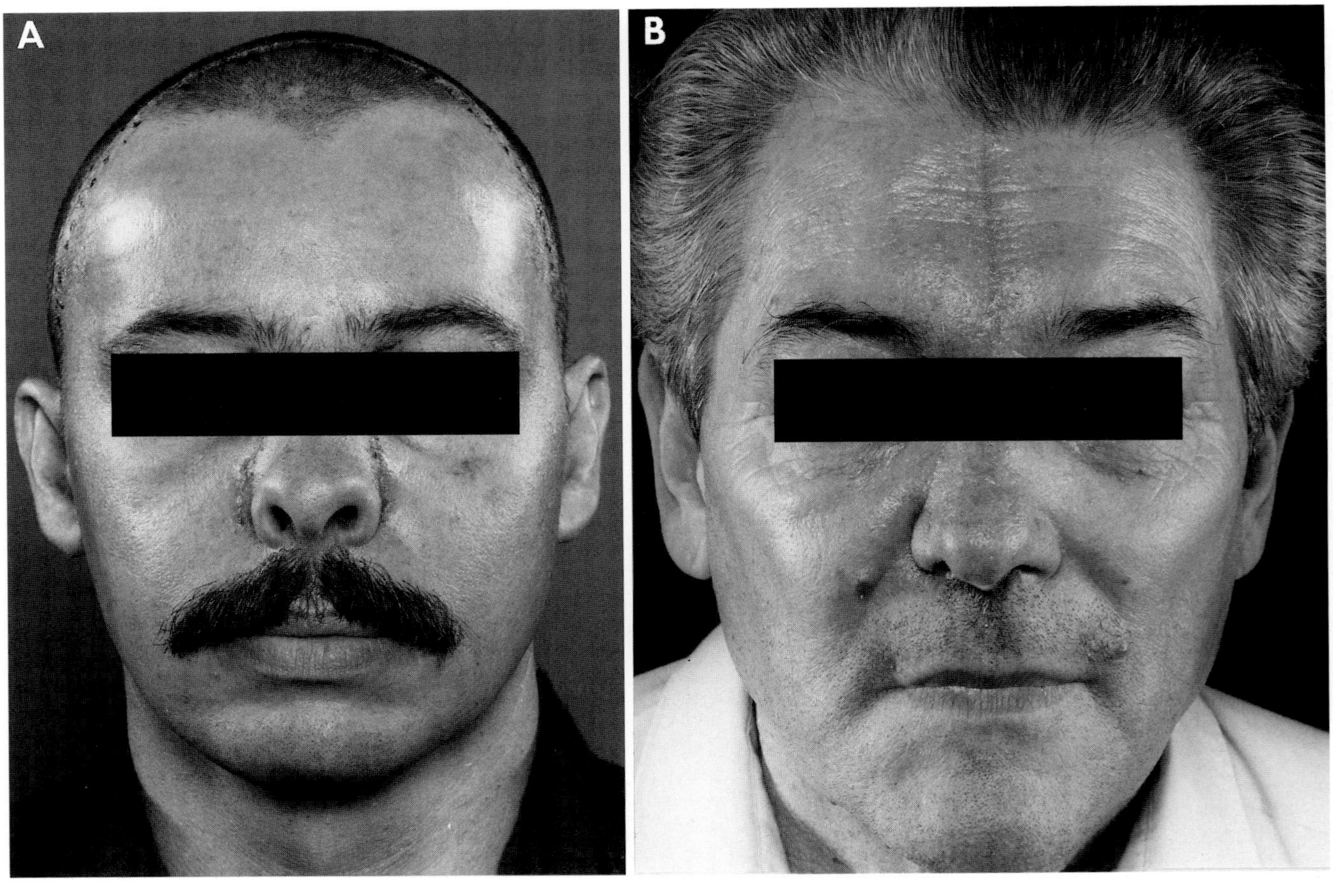

Fig. 43.8 Acceptable cosmetic results of coronal incision (**A**) and of midline vertical skin incision (**B**).

operative period. A skin incision is made, and the scalp is stripped from the bone down to and including the periosteum. Although some surgeons have advocated separating the pericranium from the scalp above and then using this later in the repair, we have found that, in certain cases, this compromises postoperative wound integrity, especially in patients who did or will receive radiation therapy.

After identifying the bone immediately above the nasion and being low enough to palpate the supraorbital rims through the scalp wound, the surgeon proceeds with a 2.5 cm trephine craniotomy as low as possible over the nasion. When there are large pneumatized frontal sinuses, it is also possible to remove the anterior surface of the sinus with a high speed drill so that this bone, like the trephine bone plug, can later be secured in its previous position. We have avoided burr-hole placement in this region because it produces an extra skull defect that requires extra effort to repair. We have not found it necessary to remove the supraorbital rim; in fact, we try to minimize bone removal so that if there is a problem with wound healing or infection, the bone that might be lost would be small and not cause a devastating cosmetic problem. After removal of this bone, the mucous membrane from the frontal sinus is exenterated and the posterior wall of the remaining frontal sinus rostral to the trephine is removed with the rongeur so as to get as low as possible without enlarging the original trephine opening.

The dura is now carefully dissected from the medial orbital roofs bilaterally. This dissection can be accomplished with a large bone curette; as the orbital roofs are exposed medially, the epidural dissection is carried further medially to identify the crista galli, which is then removed (Fig. 43.9). After removal of the crista galli, the olfactory fibers that tether the dura to the cribriform plate are divided as far distally as possible, and the epidural dissection is continued posteriorly to the level of the tuberculum sellae. As this is done, a small amount of spinal fluid drains through the unavoidably opened dural sites along the cribriform plate, and this drainage allows adequate relaxation of the brain anteriorly. We do not remove any more cerebrospinal fluid than what drains through these small openings; in fact, as we dissect posteriorly, we place patties over the dura to minimize cerebrospinal fluid leak and to prevent blood from running intradurally. When tumor extends through the dura, the dissection is carried posteriorly to the tuberculum sellae in much the same way, and in essence the tumor is amputated from its base at the cribriform plate. Although the dura is adherent to the crista galli and cribriform plate region, the epidural dissection becomes much easier as one approaches the tuberculum sella, and the tumor rarely extends through the bone at the tuberculum sellae. In fact, this bone is much thicker and is generally well preserved, even in extensive tumors in this region.

When a large intradural component of the tumor is present, the dura is opened in the region of the cribriform plate, and the tumor is easily dissected from the brain; also, cottonoid patties are placed between the brain and the tumor to prevent blood from running intracranially. After the tumor has been separated from the brain, the

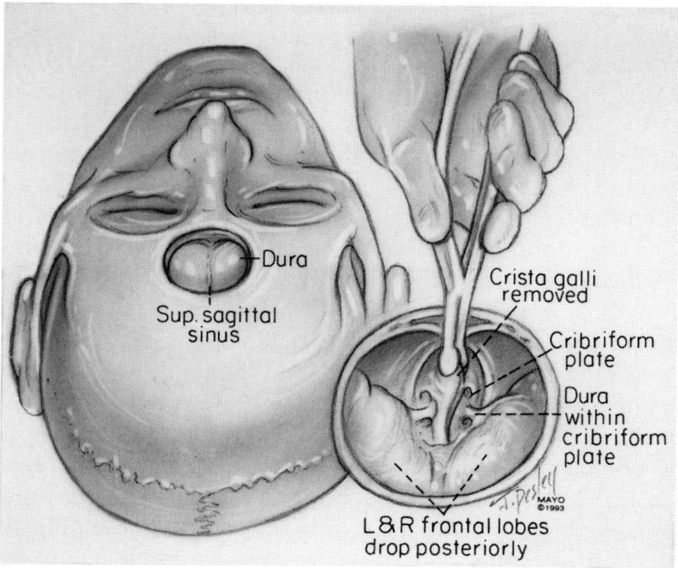

Fig. 43.9 After the trephine craniotomy is completed, the dura is carefully stripped from the orbital roofs. Then the dissection is carried medially, and the dura is freed from the crista galli. After exposure of the crista galli, it is removed to enhance further exposure of the cribriform plate. Reproduced from Morita et al (1993) with permission of Mayo Foundation.

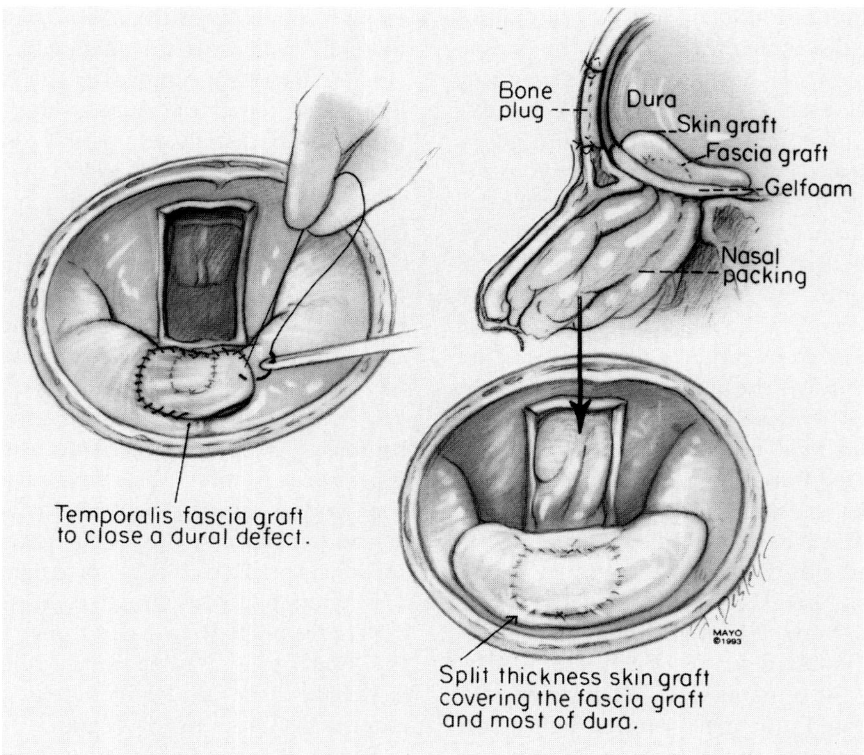

Fig. 43.10 The dural defects that are inevitable after this epidural dissection are repaired primarily when possible. If the tumor extended into the dura, this dura is removed, and temporalis fascia is used for repair. The dotted lines represent sites where primary dural closure might have been accomplished if the lesion had not required dural excision and grafting. It is important for the split-thickness skin graft to cover all of the dura that will be exposed to the nasopharynx. Also, this graft should cover any dural defects, even if they were sutured, so as to avoid cerebrospinal fluid leakage into the nasopharynx. Reproduced with permission of Mayo Foundation.

sites where the tumor is attached to the dura, either intradurally or extradurally, are easily identified, and this dura is removed with the tumor.

After removal of the tumor, a piece of temporalis fascia can then be used to do a watertight dural repair (Fig. 43.10). We have found this process easier when a cottonoid patty is cut approximately the size of the dural defect and placed over the temporalis fascia, and a piece of temporalis fascia is obtained that is circumferentially approximately 5 mm larger than the size of the cottonoid patty. The cottonoid patty and the temporalis fascia are placed together over the dural defect, and a 4–0 polypropylene (Prolene) suture is used to anchor the temporalis fascia to the posterior aspect of the dural opening. The cottonoid template over the temporalis fascia serves to hold the temporalis fascia somewhat in place and allows for relatively easy suturing of the graft circumferentially to the remaining dura. As the two ends of the running 5–0 Prolene suture are used to close this dural defect circumferentially from either side, the underlying brain tissue is irrigated with saline and much of the cerebrospinal fluid previously lost is thereby replaced. Also, any blood that might have entered the intradural space is irrigated free.

Finally, the two ends of the Prolene sutures are tied, and the previously placed cottonoid template that had been over the temporalis fascia is lifted free and removed. At this time, the dural closure is inspected carefully with the aid of the operating microscope to determine whether there are any sites of cerebrospinal fluid leak. If sites of leakage are found, these areas are reinforced with interrupted figure-eight 6–0 Prolene or 5–0 Prolene sutures. Replacement of the cerebrospinal fluid with saline also allows better detection of sites of cerebrospinal fluid leak.

If a tumor does not extend intradurally, use of a temporalis fascia graft is unnecessary; rather, the dura can be closed primarily (Fig. 43.11). This closure is done by starting a double-ended 4–0 Prolene suture at the depth of the wound and by running a suture on either side of the midline to close any small dural openings. Once the sutures are up near the top of the exposure they can be tied, and the operating microscope is used to inspect

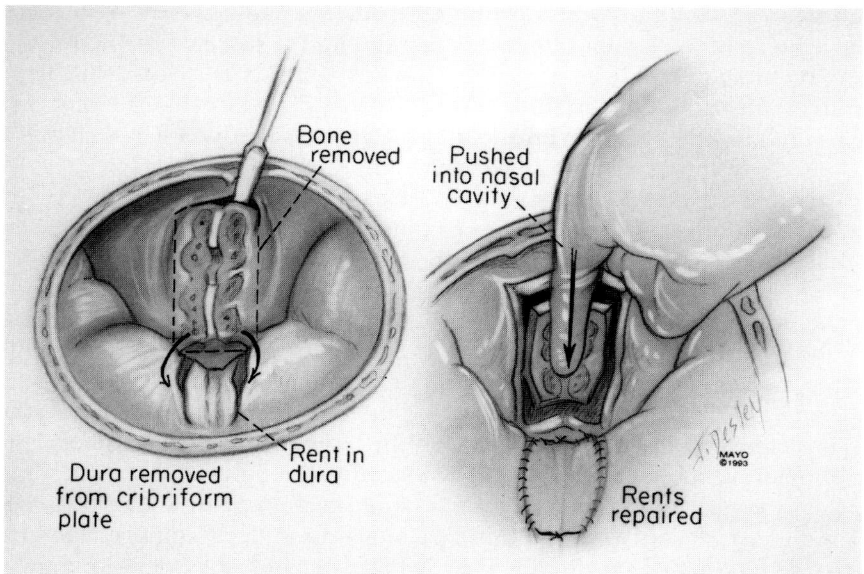

Fig. 43.11 After the dura is dissected free back to the tuberculum sellae, any defect in the dura is closed with primary suture or a patch graft. This closure is started with a suture at the deep extent of the dural opening near the tuberculum sellae and runs along either side of the midline to the top of the defect, where the two sutures are then tied. Reproduced from Morita et al (1993) with permission of Mayo Foundation.

the running closure to determine whether any sites need reinforced closure.

After the dura has been closed, it is reasonable to do the osteotomy around the site of the tumor extending through the cribriform plate (Fig. 43.11). Frequently, a trapdoor is made from above with a high speed drill. Creation of this requires minimal retraction of the now closed dura, and it is generally accomplished quickly and easily with high speed drills and occasionally an osteotome. Generally, the posterior extent of this window is at the anterior edge of the tuberculum sella. At this time, frequently a piece of plastic (similar to the plastic used as the lid of an ice cream container) is cut slightly larger than the original trephine opening and is positioned over the dural closure. This procedure allows for minimal retraction of the dura and serves also to protect the dura and frontal lobes from the dissection that is done inferiorly by the otolaryngologist.

After completion of the initial portion of the craniotomy, a rhinotomy incision is outlined and infiltrated with xylocaine and epinephrine (Mertz et al 1983). The incision is extended down to the underlying bone. The periorbital tissues are separated from the lamina papyracea, and the lacrimal duct is retracted from its fossa. The periorbita and lacrimal system are carefully inspected for evidence of tumor invasion. If the tumor extends inferiorly into the nasal cavity, the lacrimal duct is divided just beyond the sac. If the tumor is confined solely to the superior nasal cavity, the entire lacrimal system is preserved. The periorbita is elevated from the lamina papyracea until the anterior ethmoid artery is identified. Clips are placed on the artery, and the vessel is divided. The location of the anterior ethmoid artery is helpful when working from below because it serves as a marker for the level of the anterior cranial fossa. The soft tissues are then elevated back to the level of the posterior ethmoid artery. Pledgets are placed in the periorbital area for hemostasis.

The soft tissues are elevated from the maxilla up to and beneath the infraorbital nerve. The maxillary sinus is entered after removing the anterior bone with a gouge and Kerrison punch. Preoperative MRI scans should help to determine whether the sinus is involved with tumor or secretions resulting from osteal obstruction. The maxillary sinus is inspected; if there is no evidence of obvious tumor, the lining is removed and sent for pathologic examination.

The rhinotomy incision is then extended around the nasal ala, and the soft tissues are separated from the pyriform aperture with a cautery up to the level of the nasal bone. The attachments of the upper lateral cartilage to the nasal bone are divided to the midline. Generally, it is unnecessary to split the upper lip and elevate the tissues off the maxilla in the labial-gingival sulcus. If the tumor involves the maxilla, however, a partial, total, or extended maxillectomy can be performed after dividing the upper lip through the philtral crest.

The anterior periosteum is separated from the nasal bones up to the midline. Depending on the extent of involvement of the contralateral ethmoid maxillary complex and nasal bone, the elevation can continue across to the opposite side, freeing the orbit from the lamina papyracea through the single rhinotomy incision.

A periosteal elevator frees the nasal tissues from the posterior portion of the frontal process of the maxilla and nasal bone. The frontal process of the maxilla is removed with a rongeur up to the lacrimal bone. A Kerrison punch is used to continue the opening to the inferior portion of the frontal sinus. The nasal soft tissues at the midline of the nose are divided with cautery up to the roof of the nose and across to the ethmoid area. This exposure permits complete inspection of the superior nasal cavity.

The bone connecting the maxillary sinus to the inferior and anterior ethmoid complex is then removed. The amount of bone divided is dictated by the tumor's extent. Generally, this division is made in the medial portion of the infraorbital rim. The soft tissues and bone separating the maxillary sinus from the nasal cavity are removed along the nasal floor back to the posterior antral wall. The soft tissue and bony attachments to the posterior medial antrum are divided, and the inferior turbinate and soft tissues just above the eustachian tube area are progressively separated. The posterior portion of the lamina papyracea is divided beyond the tumor, and the sphenoid sinus is entered.

Tumor involvement of the nasal septum can be determined by direct inspection. The septum is divided anterior or caudally to the tumor and extended posteriorly to the choanae. The remaining posterior septum is now attached in the cribriform area and to the rostrum of the sphenoid. The amount of septum removed is determined by the tumor's extent.

The anterior, posterior, and lateral bone cuts around the tumor are made from above (Fig. 43.11). The orbit is retracted laterally on the ipsilateral side of the tumor, and the optimal location for the lateral cuts can be determined easily from below. After the bone is completely divided, the tumor is delivered into the nasal cavity.

Some tumors also extend into the orbit; if so, an ophthalmic surgeon often continues with the portion of the dissection relative to the orbit or orbital contents. This may involve dissecting tumor from the extraocular muscles or, for some malignant tumors, even exenteration of the orbit.

After completion of the otolaryngologist's portion of the procedure, the remaining cribriform plate is removed with any attached tumor by pushing downward from above and removing it through the nose. At this time, the otolaryngologist, working from below, and the neurosurgeon, working from above, obtain hemostasis, often with the aid of bipolar coagulation. Also at this time, multiple frozen sections are obtained from the margins to determine whether additional tissue should be removed and also to determine the status of the tumor margins.

After hemostasis has been achieved, a split-thickness skin graft is usually obtained from the thigh or the abdomen, and this is placed with its external surface against a piece of absorbable gelatin sponge (Gelfoam) that has been cut slightly larger than the trephine bony opening (Fig. 43.10). The dried piece of Gelfoam serves as a vehicle on which to place the skin graft so it can be more easily managed and placed. Just as the cottonoid patty was used as a template for placement of the temporalis fascia graft, the Gelfoam is used as a vehicle to determine the size of and to help position the skin graft. The excess skin around the Gelfoam template is trimmed so that the skin graft is approximately 5 mm larger than the Gelfoam on all sides. The Gelfoam is then lifted into place by placing it through the trephine craniotomy defect and resting the underlying skin on the dura. It is very important to note that the skin graft has not been folded or is not smaller than the previous dural opening. The skin graft must extend beyond the extent of any previous dural openings; this method ensures a watertight closure even if a tiny dural defect persisted after suture closure of the dura because the skin graft would extend beyond this. The raw surface of the skin graft is placed against the dura and then rolled from the peripheral edges of the Gelfoam over which it was folded so that it extends without tension beyond the limits of the Gelfoam template. Suturing the skin graft in place is unnecessary; rather, a satisfactory approach is to place a small amount of additional Gelfoam or absorbable knitted fabric (Surgicel) superficial to the skin graft and then to pack well-lubricated nasal packing gauze carefully against the Gelfoam, which is holding the skin graft secure to the dura. Usually this packing is brought in through the lateral rhinotomy and placed by the neurosurgeon to ensure that the skin graft is being held tightly against the dura from the level of the tuberculum sellae to the area of exposed dura over the medial orbital roofs and superiorly as far as the dura has been opened.

At this time it is important to ensure that no sharp, bony spicules are protruding from the posterior frontal sinus wall or the trephine bone flap that is to be replaced later — these may snag the nasal pack and prevent its removal from the nose. (In one of our patients we could not remove the nasal pack because it was snagged on a small fragment of bone; the wound had to be reopened from above, and the nasal pack was lifted off a bony spicule.)

At this point in the procedure, the brain generally has already expanded to its normal position because any spinal fluid that may have been lost during the procedure has been mostly replaced by filling the subarachnoid space with saline preceding placement of the final few dural sutures. Also, another hour or two has passed and allowed for some physiologic replacement of any fluid that may not have been replaced with saline. The trephine bone plug is secured in place with usual techniques, and the skin is closed in the usual manner.

The patient receives antibiotics while the nasal packs are in place. The nasal packs usually are removed on the seventh or eighth day after the procedure. By then, the skin graft should have grown to the underlying dura. We have not had problems with spinal fluid leaks when the above-described techniques were followed.

Complications of treatment

In our most recent review of esthesioneuroblastoma, the surgical complication rate was acceptable (Table 43.6). The only spinal fluid leak occurred in a patient who had a very small dural rent over the medial orbital roof. This had been inadvertently made during the epidural dissection. The skin graft that covered the dura did not extend far enough laterally. Meticulous attention must be paid to such detail or reoperation to repair the problem will be necessary.

The most bothersome complication has been skin breakdown after high dose radiation (50.4–57 Gy). Since our original review, one additional patient has had breakdown of the area over the bone flap; this occurred after preoperative radiation therapy (64.0 Gy), which had been performed before our evaluation and treatment. We have not found small plastic procedures helpful to repair these defects because the blood supply to the skin and the underlying tissue is so affected that these procedures seem doomed to failure. In both of our cases of skin breakdown, treatment has been simply having the patient wear an adhesive strip over the area. Anything short of a free flap to this area has a high likelihood of failure, and in our two cases the patients have elected not to proceed with any major procedure. In both cases, the underlying bone of the trephine has been lost; although this loss causes a significant cosmetic deformity, the deformity is acceptable relative to what would be the case if a larger portion of bone had been removed and then lost secondary to inadequate vascularization.

In general, the surgical procedure is tolerated extremely well, and the patient responds postoperatively in much the manner of patients who have a sinus procedure. Usually the patient is alert, awake, and talking by the evening of the day of operation, and the next day the patient is allowed to walk about the hospital room and corridor.

RESULTS

The results of various treatment series are difficult to compare because the numbers of patients are often small and treatment methods have been variable over long periods of time. Because prognosis is affected by tumor grade, we believe that treatment options should be decided on the basis of pathologic grade. A very satisfactory outcome seems to be achieved by total surgical resection alone or by total resection and radiation therapy for low grade tumors (Table 43.5). For high grade tumors, the best option is still unproved because of small numbers of cases. In our series, the group that had total resection and radiation therapy of more than 5000 cGy had a 2-year survival rate of 100% and a 2-year disease-free survival rate of 50%. Radiation therapy is best reserved for local recurrence or residual tumor when the tumor is low grade. However, for high grade tumors, a combined craniofacial approach followed by high dose (55.8 Gy) radiation seems to be the best initial treatment. The literature suggests that preoperative and postoperative chemotherapy also need to be strongly considered for patients with high grade tumors (Figs 43.5–7).

CONCLUSION

Our data and a review of the literature indicate that tumor

Table 43.6 Surgical complications in patients with esthesioneuroblastoma. Reproduced from Morita et al (1993) with permission of Congress of Neurological Surgeons.

	Surgical procedure, no. of patients		
Complication	*Lateral rhinotomy* (n = 29*)	*Craniofacial* (n = 22*)	*Craniotomy* (n = 5*)
Morbidity			
Infection — abscess (intracranial, epidural, subdural, bone flap)	2	5†	1
Cerebrospinal fluid leak	1	0	1
Wound breakdown	0	1	0
Neurologic complication	1 (blindness)	0	1 (semicoma)
Mortality	1 (intracerebral bleeding)	0	0

*n = number of total major surgical procedures, including initial and salvage procedures.
†Four of these patients underwent both operation and radiation therapy. One patient had only aseptic necrosis of the bone flap.

grade is the most important factor for determining prognosis for tumor recurrence and survival in patients with esthesioneuroblastoma. Prolonged follow-up is needed because many tumor recurrences, especially with low grade tumors, can develop after 5 or even 10 years. Patients with recurrent tumor can be helped by additional operation, radiation therapy, and chemotherapy. The decision about additional treatment has to be individualized according to tumor grade, age of the patient, and the extent of the disease. Patients with high grade esthesioneuroblastoma that has metastasized beyond regional cervical lymph nodes likely will not survive more than 1 year even with radiation therapy, chemotherapy, and operation.

In general, radical surgical removal of the tumor is probably adequate treatment for low grade tumors. However, operation alone will be inadequate to control high grade tumors. Aggressive surgical management, radiation therapy, and chemotherapy have, however, impressively improved the quality and the duration of life for many patients with esthesioneuroblastomas.

REFERENCES

Berger L, Luc R 1924 L'Esthésioneuroepithéliome olfactif. Bulletin de l'Association Francaise pour l'étude du Cancer 13: 410–421

Cantrell R W 1993 Esthesioneuroblastoma. In: Sekhar L N, Janecka I P (eds) Surgery of cranial base tumors. Raven Press, New York, pp 471–476

Chaudhry A P, Haar J G, Koul A, Nickerson P A 1979 Olfactory neuroblastoma (esthesioneuroblastoma): a light and ultrastructural study of two cases. Cancer 44: 564–579

Christiansen T A, Duvall A J III, Rosenberg Z, Carley R B 1974 Juvenile nasopharyngeal angiofibroma. Transactions of the American Academy of Ophthalmology and Otolaryngology 78: ORL140–147

Djalilian M, Zujko R D, Weiland L H, Devine K D 1977 Olfactory neuroblastoma. Surgical Clinics of North America 57: 751–762

Elkon D, Hightower S I, Lim M L, Cantrell R W, Constable W C 1979 Esthesioneuroblastoma. Cancer 44: 1087–1094

Fisher E R 1955 Neuroblastoma of the nasal fossa. Archives of Pathology 60: 435–439

Frierson H F Jr, Ross G W, Mills S E, Frankfurter A 1990 Olfactory neuroblastoma: additional immunohistochemical characterization. American Journal of Clinical Pathology 94: 547–553

Goldsweig H G, Sundaresan N 1990 Chemotherapy of recurrent esthesioneuroblastoma: case report and review of the literature. American Journal of Clinical Oncology 13: 139–143

Hyams V J 1983 Olfactory neuroblastoma (case 6). In: Batsakis J G, Hyams V J, Morales A R (eds) Special tumors of the head and neck. American Society of Clinical Pathologists, Chicago, pp 24–29

Hyams V J, Batsakis J G, Michaels L 1988 Tumors of the upper respiratory tract and ear. In: Atlas of tumor pathology, second series, fascicle 25. Armed Forces Institute of Pathology, Washington DC, pp 240–248

Kadish S, Goodman M, Wang C C 1976 Olfactory neuroblastoma: a clinical analysis of 17 cases. Cancer 37: 1571–1576

McCormack L J, Harris H E 1955 Neurogenic tumors of the nasal fossa. Journal of the American Medical Association 157: 318–321

Mertz J S, Pearson B W, Kern E B 1983 Lateral rhinotomy: indications, technique, and review of 226 patients. Archives of Otolaryngology 109: 235–239

Morita A, Ebersold M J, Olsen K D, Foote R L, Lewis J E, Quast L M 1993 Esthesioneuroblastoma: prognosis and management. Neurosurgery 32: 706–715

Oberman H A, Rice D H 1976 Olfactory neuroblastomas: a clinicopathologic study. Cancer 38: 2494–2502

Obert G J, Devine K D, McDonald J R 1960 Olfactory neuroblastomas. Cancer 13: 205–215

O'Conor G T Jr, Drake C R, Johns M E, Cail W S, Winn H R, Niskanen E 1985 Treatment of advanced esthesioneuroblastoma with high-dose chemotherapy and autologous bone marrow transplantation: a case report. Cancer 55: 347–349

Olsen K D, DeSanto L W 1983 Olfactory neuroblastoma: biologic and clinical behavior. Archives of Otolaryngology 109: 797–802

Silva E G, Butler J J, Mackay B, Goepfert H 1982 Neuroblastomas and neuroendocrine carcinomas of the nasal cavity: a proposed new classification. Cancer 50: 2388–2405

Skolnik E M, Massari F S, Tenta L T 1966 Olfactory neuroepithelioma: review of the world literature and presentation of two cases. Archives of Otolaryngology 84: 644–653

Stewart F M, Lazarus H M, Levine P A, Stewart K A, Tabbara I A, Spaulding C A 1989 High-dose chemotherapy and autologous marrow transplantation for esthesioneuroblastoma and sinonasal undifferentiated carcinoma. American Journal of Clinical Oncology 12: 217–221

Taxy J B, Bharani N K, Mills S E, Frierson H F Jr, Gould V E 1986 The spectrum of olfactory neural tumors: a light-microscopic immunohistochemical and ultrastructural analysis. American Journal of Surgical Pathology 10: 687–695

Taxy J B, Hidvegi D F 1977 Olfactory neuroblastoma: an ultrastructural study. Cancer 39: 131–138

Watne K, Hager B 1987 Treatment of recurrent esthesioneuroblastoma with combined intra-arterial chemotherapy: a case report. Journal of Neuro-oncology 5: 47–50

PART VIII

Cerebral lymphoma

44. Cerebral lymphoma

Mark A. Rosenthal   Michael D. Green

INTRODUCTION

The descriptive term 'cerebral lymphoma' encompasses a number of distinct pathologic and clinical entities. Historically the disease has been described under a variety of synonyms including reticulum sarcoma, microgliomatosis, perivascular sarcoma, perithelial sarcoma, adventitial sarcoma and others. Current nomenclature divides 'cerebral lymphoma' into: non-Hodgkin's lymphoma (NHL) or Hodgkin's disease; primary or secondary disease; and patients who are immunocompetent or immunosuppressed. In addition there are a number of rare diseases that may fall under the umbrella of 'cerebral lymphoma'. The categories of cerebral lymphoma are listed below.

1. Non-Hodgkin's lymphoma
   a. Primary cerebral lymphoma
      (i) Immunocompetent
      (ii) Immunosuppressed
         - AIDS related
         - Organ transplant related
         - Congenital
         - Therapeutic
   b. Secondary cerebral lymphoma
2. Hodgkin's disease
   a. Primary cerebral Hodgkin's disease
   b. Secondary cerebral Hodgkin's disease
3. Ocular lymphoma
4. Mycosis fungoides
5. Lymphomatoid granulomatosis
6. Malignant angioendotheliosis

The first formal description of cerebral lymphoma was ascribed to Bailey in 1929 although he suggested that probable cases were reported in the late 19th century (Bailey 1929). Cerebral lymphoma has been the focus of numerous small studies and case reports ever since this initial observation. The disease was seen as a rare and lethal curiosity until the introduction of radiotherapy, when significant gains in survival and symptom relief were obtained. The last decade has seen an unprecedented increase in the number of cases of cerebral lymphoma. Concurrently, our understanding of cerebral lymphoma biology in all its guises has improved dramatically and therapeutic gains have been achieved with the introduction of chemotherapy.

PRIMARY CEREBRAL LYMPHOMA

Incidence and prevalence

Historically, lymphoma involving the central nervous system (CNS) was considered a rare phenomenon, representing less than 3% of all CNS tumors with about half of these lymphomas confined entirely to the CNS. Thus, primary cerebral lymphoma (PCL), that is, lymphoma confined to the CNS, represented approximately 0.85–1.5% of all CNS tumors (Jellinger et al 1975, Zimmerman 1975, Houthoff et al 1978, Freeman et al 1986). In large autopsy series, the diagnosis of PCL in patients dying from all causes was extremely low. In one series of 6000 consecutive autopsies performed between 1960 and 1975 only 9 cases (0.0015%) of PCL were recorded (Reznik 1975). PCL represented between 0.007 and 0.7% of all lymphoma cases and accounted for approximately 0.01% of extranodal lymphomas (Freeman et al 1972, Henry et al 1974, Liang et al 1989, Aozasa et al 1990).

There has, however, been a dramatic re-focus on cerebral lymphoma due to an unprecedented increase in incidence. On the basis of data from the Surveillance, Epidemiology and End Results (SEER) program, a conservative estimate suggests that in 1992 PCL represented up to 8% of all brain neoplasms (Harras 1992 personal communication). The rise in incidence can be directly attributed to at least two known factors: the acquired immune deficiency syndrome (AIDS) epidemic and the extensive use of immunosuppressive therapy.

Perhaps the most perplexing aspect of PCL is an unexplained increase in the incidence of this disease in non-immunosuppressed patients. Eby et al drew attention to this phenomenon in 1988, reporting a threefold increase in the incidence of PCL between the years 1973 and 1975 and 1982 and 1984 (Eby et al 1988). The increase appeared to equally affect males and females, both young and old. At the Massachusetts General Hospital there has been an increase in hospital admissions for PCL compared with admissions for other brain tumors. Prior to 1977, patients with PCL represented 3.3% of the Hospital's primary intracerebral neoplasm cases. In the subsequent years to 1989, this has risen to 6.3% of primary intracerebral neoplasms. The frequency of cases has risen from 2.1 per year (1958–82) to 5 per year (1983–89). There has been no apparent change in median age, sex incidence or tumor location despite this increase in PCL in immunocompetent patients (Hochberg & Miller 1988, Hochberg 1992 personal communication).

Other studies have also suggested an increased incidence of PCL in immunocompetent patients. O'Sullivan et al have documented a rapid rise in the number of PCL cases seen in South-East Scotland, and a similar increase has been suggested in West Scotland and Yorkshire (Murphy et al 1989, Adams & Howatson 1990, O'Sullivan et al 1991). At Memorial Sloane-Kettering Cancer Center, the incidence of PCL in apparently immunocompetent patients as a percentage of all gliomas has risen from 0.9% prior to 1984 to 15.4% since 1985 (DeAngelis 1991a).

There are a number of confounding issues despite this apparent increased incidence. These include population age shifts, observed increases in the incidence of brain tumors (Greig et al 1990) and NHL (DeVita et al 1989), improvements in the accuracy of histologic diagnosis, changes in nosology, improved radiologic diagnostic techniques and increased physician awareness. In addition, immunosuppressive regimens, transplantation and human immunodeficiency virus (HIV) infection may have covertly influenced incidence figures despite the best efforts of investigators to exclude them. While it is difficult to refute some influence, these issues do not fully explain the increase in incidence of PCL in apparently immunocompetent patients (Baumgartner et al 1990, O'Sullivan et al 1991, Desmeules et al 1992).

Age distribution

The median age at presentation in patients with cerebral lymphoma depends on the underlying cause. Primary cerebral lymphoma in immunocompetent patients usually arises in the sixth decade. According to Murray's extensive literature review of 693 PCL cases, the median age at diagnosis was 52 years, with most patients aged between 40 and 75 years (Murray et al 1986). The age range in this series was 2 months to 90 years. More recent series have reported median ages at diagnosis ranging from 48–58 years (Hochberg & Miller 1988, Brada et al 1990, Socie et al 1990, Neuwelt et al 1991, DeAngelis et al 1992a, Rosenthal et al 1993). Reports of PCL in childhood are rare and are usually associated with inherited or acquired immunosuppression (Helle et al 1984, Esptein et al 1988).

In contrast to immunocompetent patients with PCL, the median age at presentation is much lower in patients who are immunosuppressed. The median age at onset in renal transplant patients is approximately 37 years (Schneck & Penn 1971, Morrison et al 1991) and in AIDS patients approximately 39 years (Snider et al 1983, So et al 1986, Beral et al 1991). In AIDS patients the relative frequency of PCL is equal across all age groups (Beral et al 1991). Thus the lower median age at presentation represents the incidence of age-related AIDS cases rather than an intrinsic feature of PCL in AIDS patients.

Sex distribution

The distribution of cerebral lymphoma between the sexes is also dependent on the underlying predisposing disease. Thus for PCL in immunocompetent patients, only a slight male preponderance has been noted in most large series. Murray et al recorded a male:female ratio of 1.5:1 among the 693 cases reviewed. More recent reports of PCL estimate the male:female ratio as ranging between 1:1 and 4:1 (Hochberg & Miller 1988, Brada et al 1990, Socie et al 1990, Neuwelt et al 1991, DeAngelis et al 1992a, Rosenthal et al 1993). This slight male predominance mirrors the male predominance noted in systemic lymphomas (De Vita et al 1989).

As a consequence of the AIDS epidemic, a higher ratio of males is developing cerebral lymphoma. Large series of AIDS-related PCL (AR-PCL) suggest a male:female ratio of approximately 17:1. The relative risk of developing PCL in female AIDS patients appears to be lower than for male AIDS patients, with an estimated risk for females of 0.66 in comparison to males (Beral et al 1991). The reason for this discrepancy has not been elucidated.

Racial, national, and geographic factors

The incidence of PCL in immunocompetent patients is too low to clearly define a particular racial, national or geographic character. Cases of PCL have been reported from centers around the world and the larger series have been reported from most Western countries including USA, United Kingdom, France, Italy, and Australia as well as Japan. In contrast, there is a clear country to country variation in the incidence and character of systemic NHL (DeVita et al 1989). In immunocompetent patients with either PCL or systemic NHL there is no apparent difference in the incidence of disease between whites, blacks or Asians.

Beral et al reviewed 538 cases of AR-PCL and suggested that hispanic and white groups have a higher relative risk of developing the disease compared with blacks.

The relative risks of developing AR-PCL for hispanics, whites and blacks were 1.08, 1.0 and 0.61 respectively ($p < 0.05$) (Beral et al 1991).

The incidence of AR-PCL is directly linked to the prevalence of HIV infection within a community. Thus it is not surprising that the incidence of AR-PCL is highest in major cities in the USA, with the largest single-institution series reporting AR-PCL coming from centers in Los Angeles, San Francisco and New York (So et al 1986, Baumgartner et al 1990, Goldstein et al 1991). Despite this concentration of cases, AR-PCL may arise in any community where HIV infection is present. The relative risk of an AIDS patient developing AR-PCL or for that matter AIDS-related systemic lymphoma is not influenced by state of residence or place of birth (Beral et al 1991).

Family history, genetic factors and predisposition to lymphoma

There are no reported cases of familial PCL among immunocompetent patients. However there are a number of factors that may predispose a person to developing lymphoma and, more specifically, PCL. Some of these factors are listed below.

1. Congenital immunodeficiency syndromes
   a. Wiskott-Aldrich syndrome
   b. Ataxia-telangiectasia
   c. Severe combined immunodeficiency
   d. X-linked lymphoproliferative syndrome
   e. Chediak-Higashi syndrome
   f. Swiss-type agammaglobulinemia
2. Acquired immunodeficiency syndromes
   a. HIV-associated syndromes
   b. Acquired humoral/cellular deficiencies
3. Immunosuppressive therapy
4. Autoimmune disease
   a. Systemic lupus erythematosus
   b. Rheumatoid arthritis
   c. Sjögren's syndrome
   d. Inflammatory bowel disease
   e. Hemolytic anemia
5. Infectious mononucleosis
6. Infections
   a. HTLV-I
   b. Epstein-Barr virus
7. Miscellaneous
   a. Celiac disease
   b. Previous malignancy
   c. Chemotherapy
   d. Radiation

There is strong evidence that patients who are immunodeficient are at higher risk of developing systemic lymphoma. Similarly, the risk of PCL also appears to be increased in immunodeficient patients. In addition, conditions which result in chronic and low grade antigenic stimulation may predispose to the development of lymphoma, and a number of such conditions have been directly linked to the development of both systemic lymphoma and PCL (Riggs & Hagemeister 1988).

It is difficult to be dogmatic about a definite role for these conditions in the development of PCL. However some congenital immunodeficiency syndromes are clearly associated with an increased risk of developing PCL. The Wiskott-Aldrich syndrome, for example, has a strong link with PCL; of 78 cases of cancer in Wiskott-Aldrich syndrome patients reported to the Immunodeficiency Cancer Registry, 17.9% had PCL (Model 1977, Hutter & Jones 1981, Filopovich et al 1987). This represented 24% of the 59 cases of lymphoma reported in these patients. In comparison, there are no reported cases of PCL in patients with ataxia-telangiectasia syndrome, despite 67 cases of systemic lymphoma being recorded in these patients (Filopovich et al 1987).

There is little opportunity to determine the true role that some other conditions play in the pathogenesis of PCL. PCL has been described in association with Sjögren's syndrome (Talal & Bunim 1964), immunoglobulin A deficiency (Gregory & Hughes 1973), hyperimmunoglobulinemia E (Bale et al 1977), rheumatoid arthritis (Good et al 1978), idiopathic thrombocytopenic purpura (Vogel et al 1968), sarcoidosis (Trillet et al 1982), Kleinfelter's syndrome (Liang et al 1990a), and in patients undergoing immunosuppressive therapy for systemic lupus erythematosus (Lipsmeyer 1972, Woolf & Conway 1987) and vasculitis (Jellinger et al 1979). Cases of PCL have also been described in association with progressive multifocal leukoencephalopathy (PML). This rare association may occur in immunosuppressed patients suffering from AIDS, leukemia (GiaRusso & Koeppen 1978) or following renal transplantation (Ho et al 1980). At least one case of PCL in association with PML has been described in an immunocompetent patient (Liberski et al 1982).

PCL has also been reported as a second malignancy occurring many years after therapy for systemic NHL (DeAngelis 1991b), Hodgkin's disease (Yang et al 1986, Miller et al 1989, Davenport et al 1991), systemic small cell lymphocytic lymphoma (Weissman et al 1990), systemic chronic lymphatic leukemia (Richter's syndrome) (O'Neill et al 1989, Ng et al 1991) and cancer of the colon, breast and thyroid respectively (DeAngelis 1991b). PCL has also been described in association with a low grade astrocytoma (Giromini et al 1981), hepatocellular carcinoma and squamous cell carcinoma (Yamasaki et al 1992).

An association may exist between PCL and prior malignancy for three reasons. First there may be an underlying and inherent predisposition to cancer. Second, the lymphoma may have resulted as a complication of chemotherapy or irradiation used as therapy for the initial cancer. Finally, patients may be immunologically compromised in association with tumors such as Hodgkin's disease, thus predisposing them to second malignancies.

Association with Epstein-Barr virus

The role of the Epstein-Barr virus (EBV) in the pathogenesis of PCL in immunocompetent patients has been under increased scrutiny as investigative techniques have improved. Initial reports using the techniques of restriction digests and in situ hybridization record that, in immunocompetent patients, between 5% and 38% of PCL tumors contained EBV (Hochberg et al 1983, Murphy et al 1990, Rouah et al 1990, Bignon et al 1991, MacMahon et al 1991, Geddes et al 1992). Using the more sensitive technique of the polymerase chain reaction, 7 of 13 patients (54%) with PCL had EBV incorporated into the tumor genome (DeAngelis et al 1992b). At least one case of PCL has been reported in a patient who was selectively immunodeficient to the Epstein-Barr virus (Pattengale et al 1979).

The role of Epstein-Barr virus infection in the pathogenesis of AR-PCL has also been explored. In the largest study of its type, in situ hybridization techniques revealed that AR-PCL tumors from 21 patients all expressed the EBV early region protein (EBER) and 45% expressed the latent membrane protein (MacMahon et al 1991). The former is indicative of latent infection and the latter is known to have oncogenic properties (Wang et al 1985). Interestingly, none of 9 AIDS patients with other CNS pathology expressed the early region protein (MacMahon et al 1991). A number of smaller studies have also demonstrated a very high frequency of EBV expression in AR-PCL (Katz et al 1986, Rosenberg et al 1986, Bashir et al 1989, DeAngelis et al 1992b). Also of note is that only about 40% of patients with systemic AR-NHL have evidence of EBER expression (Subar et al 1988, Meeker et al 1991, Levine 1992). The implication from all these studies is that AIDS-related PCL may be directly associated with EBV infection.

Multiple biopsies from different sites in AIDS-related NHL demonstrate an interesting phenomenon. Single clonal EBV genomic terminus fusion configurations can be detected at each individual site, suggesting that all tumor cells at that site were infected with a single form of the EBV genome. However, comparisons of sites demonstrated different configurations, suggesting a multiclonal origin of the lymphoma (Cleary et al 1988). Based on Southern blotting techniques, AR-PCL are usually monoclonal tumors whereas systemic AR-NHL is frequently polyclonal in nature (Meeker et al 1991).

The role of Epstein-Barr virus remains uncertain in the genesis of post-transplant cerebral lymphoma, although at least one case of post-transplant systemic lymphoma was associated with seroconversion for the Epstein-Barr virus capsid antigen and nuclear antigen (Walker et al 1989). As the Epstein-Barr virus appears to have an established role in the pathogenesis of AR-PCL, it would be surprising if the mechanisms were any different for cases of PCL arising from other immunodeficient states such as organ transplantation.

Table 44.1 Site of primary cerebral lymphoma in 434 cases. Adapted from Murray et al (1986).

Location	Number	(%)
Supratentorial		
Frontal	60	(14)
Temporal	34	(8)
Parietal	32	(7.5)
Deep nuclei	30	(7)
Occipital	11	(2)
Pineal	1	(<1)
Site not specified	63	(15)
Infratentorial		
Cerebellum	49	(11)
Brainstem	10	(2)
Spinal cord	2	(<1)
Multiple	142	(33.5)

Sites of predilection

The typical sites of predilection in PCL have been well documented. In Murray's series, there was sufficient information in 434 cases to determine tumor location (Table 44.1). In his analysis the majority of patients develop a solitary supratentorial tumor (52.1%) but a significant minority have multiple tumor sites (33.5%). The most common sites are: frontal lobe, temporal lobe, parietal lobe, deep nuclei, occipital lobe, cerebellum and brainstem (Murray et al 1986). Primary leptomeningeal disease has been reported in approximately 8% of PCL cases (LaChance et al 1991). Rare examples of dural PCL have been described (Jazy et al 1980, Lehrer & McGarry 1968) as has chiasmal PCL (Cantore et al 1989).

Presenting features

There are no pathognomonic presenting symptoms or signs in PCL. Despite this, typical presenting features

Table 44.2 Frequency of symptoms at presentation. Adapted from Hochberg & Miller (1988)

Symptom	% of cases
Personality change	24
Cerebellar signs	21
Headache	15
Seizures	13
Motor dysfunction	11
Visual changes	8

have been well described and these features are simply manifestations of the typical disease sites in PCL (Table 44.2). In particular, the high frequency of frontal lobe involvement results in a common mode of presentation as memory loss, forgetfulness and altered affect. Other typical symptoms include headache, visual disturbance, obtundation and motor or sensory changes. Up to 10% of patients with PCL present with a seizure (Hochberg & Miller 1988).

Similarly, the signs associated with the presentation of PCL can be related to the anatomic site of disease. Thus the most common signs include: motor and sensory deficits, altered visual acuity, diminished visual fields, papilledema and confusion. Careful analysis of cognitive function frequently reveals significant deficits (Neuwelt et al 1986). In view of the incidence of multiple lesions, it is not surprising that many patients present with a constellation of symptoms and signs. The symptoms and signs at presentation in AR-PCL and PCL arising in immunodeficient patients do not appear to be different from those in immunocompetent patients with PCL. The median time from commencement of symptoms to diagnosis is about 2–3 months although in some cases the time to diagnosis may be as long as two years. Some studies have reported a prodrome of respiratory or gastrointestinal illness although this may be incidental (Hochberg & Miller 1988).

Despite the usual manner of presentation, PCL initially may manifest itself as an unusual symptom or sign. Within the literature there are reports of PCL presenting as pure optic ataxia (Ando & Moritake 1990), steroid responsive optic neuropathy (Purvin & van Dyk 1984), diabetes insipidus (Patrick et al 1989), chronic subdural hematoma (Reyes et al 1990), benign intracranial hypertension (Kori et al 1983), narcolepsy (Onofrj et al 1992), parkinsonism and trigeminal neuropathy (Kuntzer et al 1992). We have seen one patient admitted to a psychiatric ward with a paranoid psychosis before a diagnosis of PCL was suggested by a routine CT scan and confirmed at biopsy.

PCL has been suggested as the most common cause of the rare phenomenon of tumor-induced central neurogenic hyperventilation. The mechanism of action in such cases may be anatomic or humoral. Importantly, patients may respond to therapy, including those patients being mechanically ventilated at the time of diagnosis (Pauzner et al 1989).

The differential diagnosis of PCL is extensive. It includes all possible causes of solitary and multiple cerebral mass lesions in immunocompetent and immunosuppressed patients. These include other primary brain tumors, secondary carcinomas and infections. PCL may mimic multiple sclerosis, particularly in patients with nonspecific radiologic findings who have a prolonged response to corticosteroid administration. However the prolonged dependence on these corticosteroids should encourage consideration of PCL as the diagnosis (Ruff et al 1979, DeAngelis 1990).

Imaging diagnosis

Contrast-enhanced computed tomographic (CT) of the brain has been the standard radiologic technique in the imaging of PCL in immunocompetent patients. Although typical appearances have been well described (Enzmann et al 1979, Spillane et al 1982, Thomas & MacPherson 1982, Mendenhall et al 1983, Jack et al 1988, Zimmerman 1990), a definitive diagnosis cannot be made from the scan alone. In one study where experienced radiologists were asked to diagnose a number of solitary brain lesions as seen on CT scan, the diagnosis of PCL was correctly made in only 16.7% of cases (Heimans et al 1990).

Characteristically, there is a hyperdense or isodense mass in the cerebrum with associated mild to moderate edema. Multifocal disease is observed in 30–45% of CT scans. The sensitivity of CT scans in PCL is very high, with less than 5% of scans being falsely negative. The site of the lesion is also typical but not diagnostic, with most PCL tumors arising in the periventricular region particularly involving the corpus callosum, thalamus and basal ganglia. This is in contrast with secondary cerebral NHL which has a propensity to involve subdural, subarachnoid and epidural spaces as well as the spinal cord (Brandt-Zawadski & Enzmann 1979, Thomas & MacPherson 1982, Zimmerman 1990). There is an excellent correlation between radiologic appearance and pathologic findings with respect to site and extent of macroscopic disease (Thomas & MacPherson 1982, Lee et al 1986, Jack et al 1988).

PCL in immunocompetent patients may be confused radiologically with other disease processes. Even the 'typical' appearance may be misdiagnosed as a meningioma, particularly if the lymphoma arises in an unusual site such as the cranial vault (Thomson & Brownell 1981, Agbi et al 1983). PCL may also be confused with any other intracranial pathology that produces solitary or multiple enhancing lesions on CT scanning. However, other pathology — such as metastatic carcinoma, gliomas or intracerebral infections — is suggested by the presence of hypodense lesions, ring enhancement, calcification, hemorrhage or cyst formation.

Magnetic resonance (MR) imaging is now the radiologic investigation of choice for PCL (Figs 44.1A–C). Despite typical appearances, the findings cannot be construed as diagnostic. The lesions are usually hypointense to isointense on T1-weighted imaging and isointense to hyperintense on T2-weighted images (Schwaighofer et al 1989, Zimmerman 1990, Roman-Goldstein et al 1992). A higher signal intensity can be achieved following an intravenous injection of gadolinium-DTPA (Zimmerman

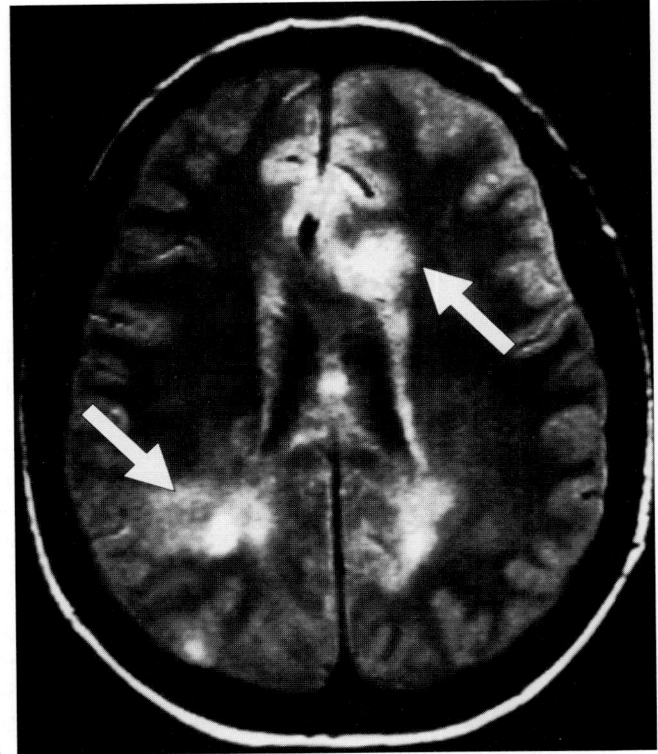

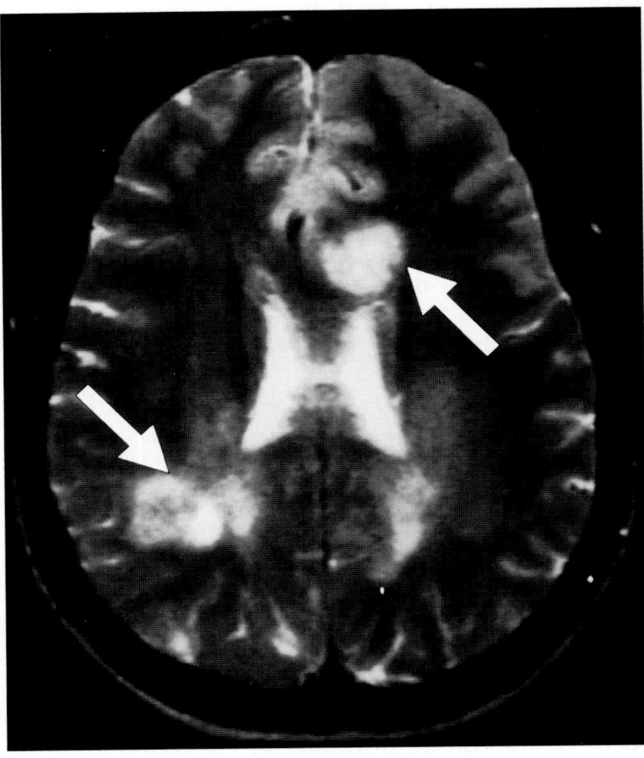

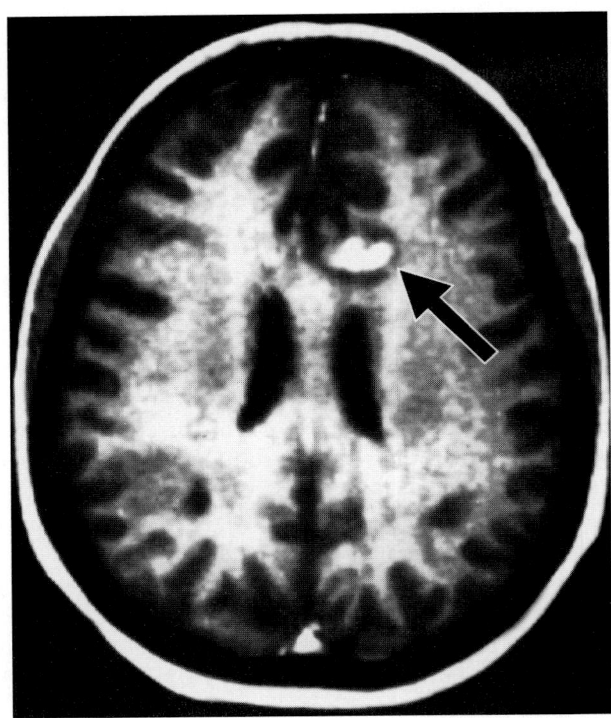

Fig. 44.1 **A.** Proton density-weighted cerebral MR scan demonstrating multifocal PCL. **B.** T2-weighted cerebral MR scan of the same patient. **C.** Gadolinium-enhanced cerebral MR scan of the same patient.

1990). The lesions may be multiple and are generally sharply demarcated with a small rim of surrounding edema. The lesions are frequently large, with more than 75% being greater than 2 cm in diameter but, surprisingly for the size of the lesions, the mass effect may be relatively small (Schwaighofer et al 1989). MR imaging adds little to contrast-enhanced CT scans apart from the rare occasions when it may detect subarachnoid or spinal disease and identify additional intracerebral sites of disease (Zimmerman 1990).

CT and MR scans are sensitive indicators of the disease. The response to treatment is rapid in PCL and, as a consequence, the CT and MR scan appearances may resolve rapidly once therapy is instituted (Schwaighofer et al 1989). Similarly CT and MR scanning may detect relapse early, even prior to a recrudescence of symptoms.

Cerebral angiography has little if any role to play in the diagnosis of PCL. Historically, angiography was frequently used as a method of investigation, however the findings in PCL were nonspecific. Some studies described avascular masses (Cassady & Wilner 1967, Enzmann et al 1979, Ashby et al 1988a), others described increased capillary circulation (Enzmann et al 1979, Spillane et al 1982) or vessel irregularity (Leeds et al 1971), while others still described no abnormal vascularity (Tallroth et al 1981). No angiographic study demonstrated consistent findings that would suggest a diagnosis of PCL. Less invasive modalities such as CT and MR offer more information in PCL without the attendant risks of cerebral angiography.

Other imaging techniques remain experimental. ^{123}I-IMP single-photon emission computerized tomography (SPECT) has had a limited role in the diagnosis of brain tumors as sensitivity does not surpass that of CT and MR scans. Usually brain tumors appear as low density defects, however in 3 patients with PCL there was high uptake in the delayed image (Ohkawa et al 1989, Kitanaka et al 1992). This result points toward a degree of specificity that may assist in the diagnosis of intracerebral lymphoma.

The role of positron emission tomography (PET) in the evaluation of intracerebral lymphoma requires further study. In a study of 10 patients with PCL, PET scanning revealed marked uptake of [^{18}F] fluoro-2-deoxyglucose in a manner similar to anaplastic gliomas and more prominent than for low grade astrocytomas (Rosenfeld et al 1992). High uptake of [^{18}F] fluoro-2-deoxyglucose and 11C-methyl-L-methionine have been previously reported in at least two other studies of PCL (Kuwabara et al 1988, Sawataishi et al 1992) but information regarding this investigative modality is scarce in the realm of PCL.

Despite gallium-67 citrate scanning being frequently used in the investigation of systemic lymphoma, its role in the diagnosis and management of PCL has not been addressed. Although nuclear scanning in PCL may not add to the diagnostic work-up, it may be able to fulfil a prognostic role. In systemic lymphomas, comparison of pre- and post-treatment gallium scans may be a good predictor of clinical outcome with respect to long-term survival (Front et al 1992). Whether these findings can be extrapolated to cerebral lymphoma requires further study.

Laboratory diagnosis

CSF

A careful analysis of the cerebrospinal fluid (CSF) may be diagnostic of intracerebral lymphoma (Matsuda et al 1981, Schmitt-Graff & Pfitzer 1983, Lai et al 1991). However concerns regarding raised intracranial pressure prevent lumbar puncture being performed in the majority of patients (Murray et al 1986). In those for whom lumbar puncture is not contraindicated, cytocentrifugation techniques may increase the cellular yield 60-fold (Hansen et al 1974).

The main abnormality in the CSF of patients with PCL is a monomorphic population of abnormal lymphocytes consistent with the International Working Formulation descriptions of intermediate and high grade lymphomas (Rosenberg et al 1982). Immunohistochemistry may assist in the diagnosis by the demonstration of monoclonality. The CSF protein is usually markedly elevated, the CSF glucose is low, and a pleocytosis is found in about 40% of patients (Matsuda et al 1981, Lai et al 1991).

Murray et al collated information from 12 studies and found that 10% of patients undergoing lumbar puncture had positive CSF cytology at initial presentation (Murray et al 1986). Rarely, the initial diagnosis of PCL has been made on the basis of CSF cytology alone without cerebral CT scan changes (Schmitt-Graff & Pfitzer 1983, Lai et al 1991).

There are no other serum or CSF markers of disease specific for patients with PCL. The serum level of lactate dehydrogenase (LDH) has been shown to predict outcome in patients with systemic NHL (Ship et al 1992), however there are no reports in the literature as to whether this enzyme may be predictive in PCL. Similarly, CSF β_2-microglobulin may be a useful marker of occult CNS disease in patients with systemic NHL (Hansen et al 1992) but its role in the management of PCL remains to be elucidated.

CSF platinum has been shown to be depleted in PCL although this is not specific to this disease. In contrast to leukemia involving the CNS, lymphoma does not result in depletion of CSF manganese (El-Yazigi et al 1990).

Gross morphologic features

Primary cerebral lymphoma has pathologic features comparable with the spectrum of systemic lymphoma. However, the macroscopic appearance of PCL may vary considerably between patients. Most commonly, PCL appears as a solitary, bulky and irregular mass merging into the surrounding edematous brain tissue (Fig. 44.2). The cut surface is yellow-white and granular, and the tumor soft. There may be areas of focal necrosis or hemorrhage but cystic change is rare (O'Neill et al 1987). Multiple lesions occur in up to 30% of patients. On other occasions there may only be poorly defined expansion of tissue with loss of intrinsic markings (Adams & Howakson 1990).

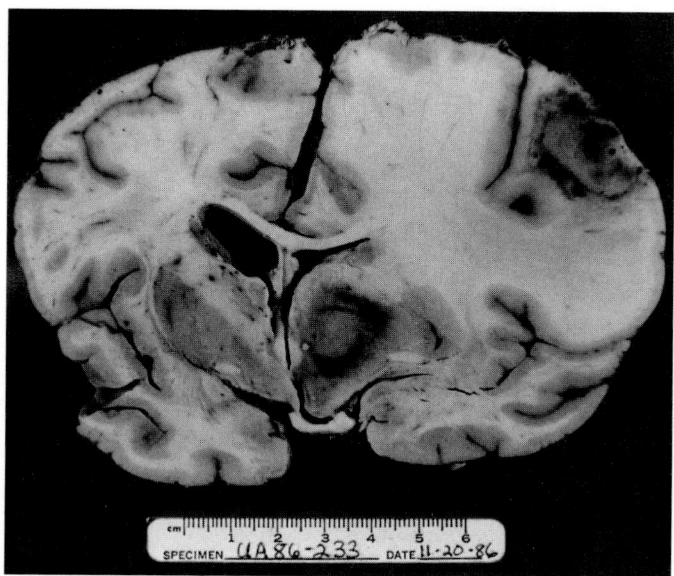

Fig. 44.2 Coronal section of brain demonstrating multifocal primary cerebral lymphoma with associated mass effect.

Histopathologic features

Microscopic examination usually demonstrates tumor infiltration well beyond the macroscopic margin. The tumor invades along perivascular spaces with perivascular cuffing and vessel wall infiltration. This cuffing is most prominent at the tumor margin and for a distance beyond (Ashby et al 1988a, Murphy et al 1989). In advanced tumors there may be a loss of the perivascular relationship (O'Neill et al 1987). There may be an associated astrocytic reaction accompanied by the presence of body macrophages (Ashby et al 1988a). In contrast to gliomas and metastatic tumors, PCL does not produce a significant degree of endothelial proliferation in the tumor or adjacent brain. Multiplication of involved blood vessel basement membranes may be observed (Henry et al 1974). The periphery of the tumor is typically composed of a T-lymphocyte infiltrate with some occasional T-cells seen throughout the tumor itself (Murphy et al 1989). The presence of reactive astrocytes has been described and may mimic a low grade astrocytoma (Kepes 1987, Adams & Howatson 1990). Demyelinative leukoencephalopathy in association with PCL has been noted to occur (Lach et al 1985). This is manifested by large areas of severe myelin loss in proximity to the tumor.

The tumor itself is described and classified according to the International Working Formulation criteria (Rosenberg et al 1982) (Table 44.3). The most common histologic subtypes are diffuse large cell lymphoma and diffuse immunoblastic lymphoma. Higher grade lymphomas, including Burkitt's lymphoma, have frequently been described but there are no reported cases of follicular subtypes in PCL. Many authors have noted the pleomorphic histologic appearance of PCL (Taylor et al 1978, Murphy et al 1989). Table 44.4 shows histopathologic subtypes of PCL arising in immunocompetent patients from a single institution (Hochberg & Miller 1988).

Table 44.3 Histopathologic classification of NHL according to Working Formulation

Grade	Histologic subtype
Low grade	
	A. Small lymphocytic, consistent with chronic lymphocytic leukemia; plasmacytoid.
	B. Follicular, predominantly small cleaved cell; diffuse areas, sclerosis.
	C. Follicular, mixed, small cleaved and large cell; diffuse areas, sclerosis.
Intermediate grade	
	D. Follicular predominantly large cell; diffuse areas; sclerosis.
	E. Diffuse small cleaved cell.
	F. Diffuse mixed small and large cell; sclerosis; epithelioid component.
	G. Diffuse large cell; cleaved cell, noncleaved cell, sclerosis.
High grade	
	H. Large cell, immunoblastic; plasmacytoid, clear cell, polymorphous, epithelioid component.
	I. Lymphoblastic; convoluted cell, nonconvoluted cell.
	J. Small noncleaved; Burkitt's follicular area.

Table 44.4 Frequency of PCL histopathologic subtypes (61 cases). Adapted from Hochberg & Miller (1988)

Histologic subtype	No. of patients	(%)
Large cell immunoblastic	24	(39.3)
Diffuse large cell	15	(24.7)
Small cleaved cell	11	(18)
Large cell (not specified)	6	(9.8)
Small noncleaved	5	(8.2)

Diffuse large cell lymphoma is characterized by large lymphoid cells containing abundant cytoplasm, prominent nucleoli and dense nuclear chromatin (Fig. 44.3) while the small noncleaved cell Burkitt's lymphomas are characterized by uniform cells of moderate size with round to oval nuclei. The nuclei contain numerous and prominent nucleoli and a coarse chromatin pattern; mitoses are frequently seen. The classic 'starry-sky' appearance is notable but not pathognomonic. In comparison, cells of non-Burkitt's small noncleaved cell lymphoma are typically smaller in size and are more pleomorphic with occasional giant forms and bizarre cell types. Similarly, the prominence and number of nucleoli and the pattern of nuclear chromatin are more varied (De Vita et al 1989).

EM appearance

The electron microscopic appearance of PCL is no different from the appearances described for the subtypes of systemic NHL. The most notable features are tumor cells containing few organelles, abundant free ribosomes, large nucleoli and scant cytoplasm. There is an absence of junctional devices (Hirano 1975, Ishida 1975, Houthoff et al 1978).

Immunological markers

When immunohistochemical techniques became available for application in the investigation of systemic NHL, they were also used in PCL. Sophisticated analysis of tumor cell surface immunoglobulins in PCL was initiated in the late 1970s and rapidly found a place in assisting the histopathologist (Taylor et al 1978). Staining for monoclonal B- and T-cell antigens has been performed on frozen and paraffin sections, confirming that almost all cases of PCL are of B-cell origin and only rare cases of T-cell lymphoma have been described (Marsh et al 1983, Murphy et al 1989, Aozasa et al 1990, Grant & von Deimling 1990).

B-cell PCL frequently has immunoglobulin heavy chain rearrangements similar to those of systemic B-cell lym-

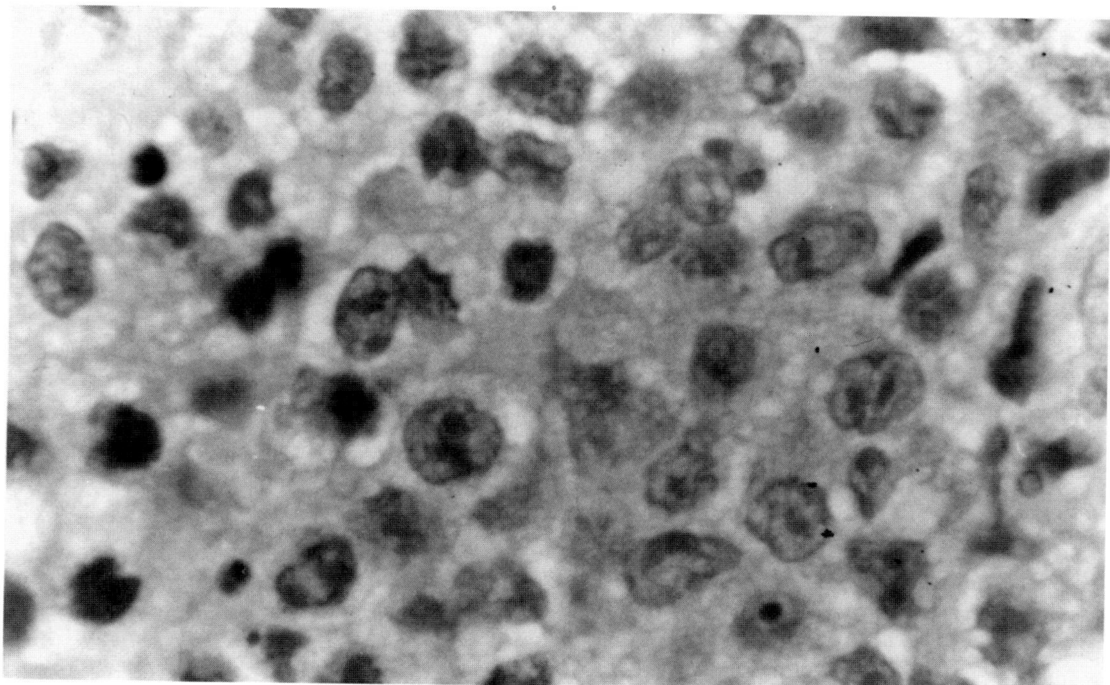

Fig. 44.3 High power photomicrograph demonstrating the typical histologic appearance of primary cerebral lymphoma (large cell type).

phomas. In a number of studies, PCL were demonstrably B-cell tumors with typical immunoglobulin rearrangements suggesting monoclonality (Smith et al 1988, Albrecht et al 1992). These findings are consistent with those seen in systemic B-cell lymphomas.

Oncogenes and tumor suppressor genes such as p53 are currently under investigation in an attempt to define their role in systemic NHL (Rodriguez et al 1991). There are no reports specific to PCL. The expression of adhesion molecules including LFA-1 and ICAM-1 may play a role in organ-specific lymphoid binding, especially between lymphoma cells and cerebral blood vessels (Bashir et al 1992).

General management plan

The principles concerning the management of PCL revolve around obtaining a histologic diagnosis, ensuring that the disease is confined to the brain, excluding an underlying predisposing illness and instituting definitive therapy.

In order to identify the extent of local disease and to exclude systemic NHL, patients with cerebral lymphoma require appropriate 'staging' investigations. The usual sequence of events is a CT or MR scan followed by a biopsy proving intracerebral lymphoma. Having identified the presence of intracerebral lymphoma, the delineation of local disease extent requires an examination of the vitreous and the CSF. Thus slit lamp examination of the eye and CSF analysis (unless contraindicated) should be performed.

The need to exclude systemic disease is debated by some authors. Hochberg & Miller argue that none of 66 cases of PCL in their institution had systemic disease and therefore further investigations are unnecessary and costly (Hochberg & Miller 1988). However, concurrent cerebral and systemic lymphoma has been described, and cases have been reported where the cerebral component predates the systemic component in disseminated NHL (Johnson et al 1984, Haerni-Simon et al 1987, Liang et al 1989). Whether this represents distant relapse of the cerebral tumor or progression of concurrent, albeit covert, systemic disease is difficult to prove. Despite this, most centers at present would perform routine staging investigations in order to exclude systemic disease.

Routine staging includes: a full clinical examination, complete blood count with white cell differentiation and platelet count, serum creatinine, urea and electrolytes, liver function tests, erythrocyte sedimentation rate and lactate dehydrogenase. In addition, the patient should undergo a unilateral bone marrow aspirate and trephine, chest X-ray, and chest and abdominal computerized tomographic scans. Testing for evidence of HIV infection is highly recommended.

Although a number of reports have documented the rare phenomenon of spontaneous regression (Weingarten et al 1983, Sugita et al 1988, Weissman et al 1990), cerebral lymphoma has a rapid, relentless and ultimately fatal course if left untreated. Current therapeutic options include surgery, corticosteroids, radiotherapy and chemotherapy.

If PCL is suspected, then the institution of corticosteroid therapy should be delayed until a definitive biopsy has been performed unless cerebral herniation is imminent. The immediate introduction of corticosteroids prior to diagnosis is tempting in the face of symptoms and focal intracerebral lesions. However, the early use of corticosteroids may make histologic assessment difficult due to the exquisite sensitivity of PCL to the drug. In fact, radiologic disappearance of the tumor can occur rapidly after the commencement of corticosteroids (Singh et al 1982, Vaquero et al 1984, Hochberg & Miller 1988, DeAngelis 1990). The response is due to tumor cell lysis rather than the resolution of cerebral edema (Baxter et al 1971, Gametchu 1987). As a consequence of this rapid lysis, cerebral biopsies may be nondiagnostic and may delay or misdirect definitive therapy (Singh et al 1982, Vaquero et al 1984, DeAngelis 1991a). Once the diagnosis has been established, initial therapy with corticosteroids usually consists of dexamethasone in the dose 16–24 g/day.

Surgical management

It is clear that a definitive diagnosis of PCL can only be made from histologic examination. The method of biopsy needs to consider both operative risk and the success for obtaining satisfactory specimens allowing accurate diagnosis. The goal of surgery in PCL is to obtain tissue for diagnosis with minimum morbidity.

In past years, the diagnostic approach to PCL was one of craniotomy with tumor excision or debulking. However, when Murray et al reviewed the outcome of the 85 patients who underwent surgery alone as reported in the literature to 1986, there was no difference in median survival time as defined by the extent of surgical resection. Moreover, the median survival time for the surgically debulked patients was only 1 month, with only 1 patient surviving beyond 3 years (Murray et al 1986). The recognition that extensive surgery had a very limited role in PCL prompted the use of stereotactic biopsy as a means of obtaining tissue for diagnosis.

Stereotactic biopsy of intracranial lesions has an established role in obtaining an accurate histologic diagnosis without the attendant risks of craniotomy (Apuzzo et al 1987, O'Neill et al 1987, Namiki et al 1988, Feiden et al 1990, Sherman et al 1991). Feiden et al have demonstrated that stereotactic brain biopsy is an excellent means of obtaining tissue in order to establish the diagnosis of PCL. In 34 patients undergoing stereotactic biopsy, 25 had a clear-cut histologic diagnosis of PCL, with the remaining 9 having appearances highly suggestive of PCL (Feiden et al 1990). In a study by Sherman et al, all but 1 of 15 patients with intracerebral lymphoma were diagnosed with tissue obtained from CT-guided stereotactic brain biopsy. In 12 of the 14 patients, sufficient material was obtained to classify the lymphoma according to the Working Formulation (Sherman et al 1991).

The approach toward establishing the diagnosis of PCL may soon incorporate recent advances in surgical techniques. These include the use of intraoperative ultrasound to localize the tumor, intraoperative monitoring of evoked responses, and operating under local anesthesia in order to obtain tumor with precision and safety (Black 1991).

Radiotherapy

PCL is a radiosensitive tumor with clinical response rates of up to 80%. Not surprisingly, this high response rate translates into increased median survival times in PCL patients receiving radiotherapy compared with patients who receive no therapy or surgery alone. In 1974, Henry et al reviewed the survival of 83 patients with PCL and reported a median survival time of 3.3 months in untreated patients, 4.6 months in patients treated with surgical excision alone, and, in 21 patients receiving irradiation, a median survival of 15.2 months (Henry et al 1974).

Subsequent reports of radiation therapy confirmed these findings. Berry & Simpson reported a median survival of 10 months in 21 patients receiving cranial irradiation. Importantly, they documented rapid and sustained clinical improvement in 14 patients (Berry & Simpson 1981). Other studies document median survival times between 14.5 and 40.8 months in those patients receiving cranial irradiation alone for PCL (Leibel & Sheline 1987).

Cranial radiotherapy alone as treatment for PCL rarely produces long-term survivors despite the high response rate and apparent improvement in median survival time. Only a few examples of long-term survival have been documented following cranial radiotherapy (Sagerman et al 1967, Littman & Wang 1975, Leibel & Sheline 1987). When the results of eight separate series reporting radiotherapy alone in patients with PCL are combined, the 1-year survival is 66% and the 2-year survival is 43%, with a 5-year survival of only 7% (Leibel & Sheline 1987).

The dose and volume of irradiation required for disease control have not been clearly defined. Murray et al reviewed dose response in 198 cases to 1986. Dose to the primary tumor was: < 40 Gy (14.0%), 40–50 Gy (23.1%), > 50 Gy (14.3%), and in 38.6% the dose was not recorded. The median survival of the 54 patients receiving doses of 50 Gy or more to the primary tumor was 17 months compared with a median survival of 15 months in the 144 patients who received less than 50 Gy. Actuarial 5-year survival was 42.3% and 12.8% respectively, a statistically significant p value of < 0.05. The conclusion from this study was that there was a demonstrable dose-response relationship, resulting in improved longer-term survival in those patients receiving 50 Gy or more to the primary tumor (Murray et al 1986).

Other studies have suggested a similar trend, with increasing doses of radiotherapy associated with delayed time to local failure (Berry & Simpson 1981, Michalski et al 1990). More recently, a RTOG study attempted to optimize irradiation by delivering 40 Gy to the whole brain with a 20 Gy boost to the tumor plus a 2 cm margin. The results were disappointing, with a median survival from diagnosis of only 12.2 months for the 41 patients enrolled (Nelson et al 1992).

The most appropriate volume of irradiation, like dosage, remains disputed and undefined. Older series point to the incidence of spinal relapse as reason to irradiate the entire neuraxis (Sagerman et al 1967, Rampen et al 1980, Mendenhall et al 1983). The incidence of spinal relapse as the first site of progression has been estimated in older studies to be between 4 and 25% of cases.

Murray et al estimated that between 1967 and 1985, 6.5% of patients relapsed with positive CSF cytology or overt spinal cord disease. He assessed the radiation volume for 308 patients who were part of his large 1986 review. The volume irradiated included whole brain in 124 patients (40.3%), local tumor in 16 patients (5.2%), and the entire neuraxis in 16 patients (5.2%). Treatment volume was not specified in 152 cases (49.3%). There was no clear relationship between the volume irradiated and survival outcome (Murray et al 1986).

Invariably, patients with spinal relapse also develop cerebral relapse and it is this that creates the most significant problems rather than the spinal disease. Even if one still contends that preventing spinal relapse warrants spinal irradiation, it is clear that the current regimens of intrathecal or intravenous chemotherapy may be adequate therapy in themselves for prophylaxis against occult spinal disease. Other arguments against spinal irradiation include the extension of radiation toxicities to other sites and the possibility that spinal irradiation may compromise spinal and pelvic marrow reserve, thus making chemotherapy less tolerable. It is therefore not surprising that the notion of prophylactic spinal irradiation has diminished with time.

While many authors have advocated larger volumes of irradiation, one review, combining data from 7 studies, suggested an improved survival time in those patients who received less radiotherapy. Those patients who received radiotherapy to the primary tumor alone had a median survival of 39.4 months compared to 25.3 months in those patients who received whole brain irradiation. As the study rightly points out, this finding may simply represent a bias in patient selection, with those receiving smaller fields representing patients with less extensive tumors (Leibel & Sheline 1987).

Delineation of the current trends in radiotherapy is complicated by the incorporation of chemotherapy into treatment regimens. The dose, volume and timing of radiotherapy vary between studies. Table 44.5 shows current radiotherapy policy for a number of recent reports. In general, most centers irradiate the whole brain to a dose of at least 50 Gy, including a boost to the tumor site, and do not routinely include spinal irradiation. Despite such recommendations, there is no scientific basis for a dogmatic approach when it comes to radiation dose and volume in the therapy of PCL.

New techniques in delivering cranial irradiation remain experimental. These include: interstitial implants, stereotactic radiosurgery, neutron capture therapy, hyperthermia, radiosensitizers and altered fractionation schedules (Woo & Maor 1990). The aim of such therapies is to improve efficacy and reduce the long-term morbidity associated with cranial irradiation. The role that such methods may play in PCL remains speculative.

Complications of radiotherapy

The complications of cranial irradiation in general have been well described and include acute toxicities such as nausea and vomiting, headache, and local skin reactions. Chronic complications include cerebral necrosis, cataract formation, and cognitive impairment (Leibel & Sheline 1987, Johnson et al 1990). There are no complications of cranial irradiation that are typical or specific to PCL. Acute exacerbations of symptoms or signs due to edema associated with the initiation of irradiation have not been described in PCL. Radiation necrosis may be indistinguishable from recurrent tumor due to its predilection for the sites commonly involved in PCL such as the corpus callosum, basal ganglia, thalamus and deep white matter. As a consequence, focal necrosis may require biopsy for definitive diagnosis (Merchut et al 1985).

Chemotherapy

The most contentious issue in the management of PCL is the role of chemotherapy. There are no studies that clearly define optimal therapy and although current standard management practice includes the use of chemotherapy, no randomized trials yet exist to confirm its value. This is hardly surprising because of small numbers and patient heterogeneity. Patients with PCL have usually been excluded from randomized studies of chemotherapy for systemic lymphoma.

Early reports documented the use of intrathecal or intravenous methotrexate as therapy for disease that had recurred following radiotherapy (Herbst et al 1976, Ervin & Canellos 1980) or in patients with systemic disease with intracranial involvement (Pitman & Frei 1977, Skarin et al 1977). Durable complete responses were noted.

Table 44.5 Chemotherapy (CT) and radiotherapy (RT) regimens

Name	Year	Blood brain-barrier disruption	Chemotherapy regimen	Timing of CT in relation to RT	RT regimen + dose		Median survival (months)	
							RT alone (historical/concurrent controls)	RT + CT
Rosenthal et al	1993	No	CHOP ×6	Post RT	Whole brain Boost	45 Gy 10 Gy	18	25+
DeAngelis et al	1992(a)	No	MTX IV ×2 MTX IT ×6 Ara C ×2	Pre RT Post RT	Whole brain Boost	40 Gy 14.4 Gy	21.7	42.5
Neuwelt et al	1991	Yes	CMPD (1 year)	—	Nil		17.5	44.5
Chamberlain & Levin	1990	No	Hydroxyurea PCV (1 year)	During RT Post RT	Whole brain	55–61 Gy	13	30
Brada et al	1990	No	MACOP B (6–12 weeks)	Pre RT	Whole brain Spine Boost	30–40 Gy 30 Gy 15–25 Gy	16	14
Shibamoto et al	1990	No	VEPA ×4–6	Post RT	Whole brain Boost	30–40 Gy 20–30 Gy	7.5	28.5
Gabbai et al	1989	No	HDMTX IV ×3	Pre RT	Whole brain	30–44 Gy	—	9.5

Note: CHOP = Three weekly: cyclophosphamide 750 mg/m^2 IV Day 1, adriamycin 50 mg/m^2 IV D1, vincristine 1.4 mg/m^2 IV D1, prednisolone 100 mg po D1–5
VEPA = Two weekly: vincristine 1 mg/m^2 IV Day 1, cyclophosphamide 350 mg/m^2 IV D1, doxorubicin 30 mg/m^2 IV D1, prednisolone 30 mg/m^2 po D1–3, then 8 mg/m^2 D4–5
MACOP B = Weekly: cyclophosphamide 350 mg/m^2 IV, adriamycin 50 mg/m^2 IV, oral prednisolone with alternating methotrexate 400 mg/m^2 IV [+ folinic acid rescue] and vincristine 1.4 mg/m^2 IV or bleomycin 10 mg/m^2 IV and vincristine 1.4 mg/m^2 IV
CMPD = Monthly: cyclophosphamide 15 mg/kg IV, methotrexate 2.5 g IA, [+ folinic acid rescue], procarbazine 100 mg po D1–14, dexamethasone 24 g po D1–14
MTX = Methotrexate 1 g/m^2 IV D1,8
MTX IT = methotrexate 12 mg intrathecal
HDMTX = Three weekly: high dose methotrexate 3.5 g/m^2 IV [+ folinic acid rescue]
Ara C = Three weekly: cytarabine 3 g/m^2 IV D1,2
PCV = Second monthly: procarbazine 60 mg/m^2 po D8–21, CCNU 110 mg/m^2 po D1, vincristine 1.4 mg/m^2 IV D8,29
HDR = Hydroxyurea 300 mg/m^2 po QID ×3 per week during RT

Subsequently there have been a number of single institution reports of empiric protocols compared with internal historical controls. Clearly there is no obvious preference for a particular regimen when one considers the conflicting recommendations for therapy. The approach toward chemotherapy in PCL needs to consider the following factors: timing in relation to radiotherapy, radiosensitization, route of administration, use of blood-brain barrier disruption techniques, drug choice, tumor resistance, and treatment toxicity. Table 44.5 shows chemotherapy protocols described in recent reports.

The chemotherapeutic options are almost limitless. Chemotherapy can be given prior to radiotherapy, synchronously with radiotherapy, after radiotherapy or in the absence of radiotherapy. Choices can also be made regarding the route of administration, and the use of either single agent or combination regimens. In addition, the putative role of the blood-brain barrier and its influence on drug choice and method of drug delivery needs to be considered. None of these options have been tested against each other and so empiric decisions are made on the basis of local experience and expertise rather than documented superior efficacy. However at least two observations can be made. First, these studies do suggest that overall survival is improved by the addition of some form of chemotherapy, and second, it is also clear that post-radiotherapy methotrexate increases the risk of multifocal leukoencephalopathy.

Response rates to chemotherapy are very high, with most series documenting complete response rates of between 60 and 100%, and the majority achieving response rates higher than 80%. The choice of chemotherapy does not appear to dramatically influence complete response rates although the lowest complete response rate occurred in the series of patients treated with single agent high dose methotrexate (Gabbai et al 1989). It may be that combination or sequential multi-agent regimens produce a higher percentage of complete responses and possibly an improved median survival.

The reported median survival times following chemotherapy for PCL range from 9.5–44.5 months. This compares to the well-documented survival time of between 14.5 and 40.8 months following radiotherapy alone. A number of institutions have reported their own internal comparisons between patients with PCL receiving chemotherapy in addition to radiotherapy and historical or concurrent controls receiving radiotherapy alone. In most studies the comparison of median survival has favored the group of patients who received chemotherapy (Table 44.5) (Shibamato et al 1990, Chamberlain & Levin 1990, Neuwelt et al 1991, DeAngelis et al 1992a, Rosenthal et al 1993).

In at least two recent series, however, the median survival of patients receiving chemotherapy was not substantially different from 'controls'. One study reported that patients receiving chemotherapy had a median survival of only 14 months compared to 16 months for historical controls receiving radiotherapy alone (Brada et al 1990) while another demonstrated a median survival of only 16.5 months for those patients who received combination systemic chemotherapy (Berube et al 1991). It is not clear why these two studies had such low median survivals in comparison with the majority of recent series.

It is self-evident that the chemotherapeutic agents used in the treatment of PCL should have demonstrable intrinsic activity in systemic NHL, either in combination or as single agents. Thus the most commonly used drugs are those used in the therapy of systemic NHL and include methotrexate, corticosteroids, anthracyclines, vinca-alkaloids, cytosine arabinoside and alkylating agents. Adequate CNS parenchymal penetration of these drugs must also be considered. The use of systemic therapy is based on pharmacokinetic studies demonstrating that intravenous administration of high dose methotrexate and cytosine arabinoside resulted in CSF levels similar to those achieved via the intrathecal route (Pitman & Frei 1977, Gabbai et al 1989, DeAngelis et al 1990). However, penetration of such drugs into cerebral parenchyma and the intracerebral tumors themselves may not be as efficient (Ott et al 1991).

A novel chemotherapeutic approach in the treatment of PCL is blood brain barrier (BBB) disruption. The aim of such therapy is to improve tumor penetration by chemotherapeutic drugs and as a consequence improve their efficacy. In the setting of PCL, BBB permeability may only be modest and nonuniform (Neuwelt et al 1982, Rapoport 1988, Blasberg et al 1990). In addition, as the tumor responds to chemotherapy, the integrity of the BBB may be restored and, as a consequence, the access of systemically delivered drugs to the tumor may be diminished. In animal studies, BBB disruption prior to systemic drug infusion results in higher drug concentrations in both the cerebral tumor itself and in the surrounding brain parenchyma (Neuwelt et al 1985). Studies in humans have documented the efficacy and low toxicity of this approach in the treatment of a variety of brain tumors (Neuwelt et al 1986).

More recently, PET scanning has been used to measure changes in regional BBB permeability in patients undergoing therapy for PCL and other tumors (Ott et al 1991). This initial report suggests that significant changes in permeability can be demonstrated within the tumor following chemotherapy. There was no effect on BBB permeability within the normal brain during chemotherapy or following radiotherapy. Perhaps the most important observation was that, within 5 weeks of the commencement of treatment, permeability values within the tumor fell to levels seen in normal brain tissue.

If these findings can be confirmed, the implications are substantial. The report suggests that repair of the blood-brain barrier is rapid and that the continuation of systemic therapy beyond four to five weeks may result in a significant reduction in drug bioavailability with a consequent reduction in efficacy. In addition, systemic therapy may only poorly penetrate into islands of tumor that may be present in regions of the brain that ostensibly have relatively normal permeability. These areas may be represented on CT scan as nonenhancing regions and as sites of normal permeability based on PET scan.

Neuwelt et al utilized intra-arterial mannitol to disrupt the BBB in patients with PCL and followed this with a year-long protocol consisting of methotrexate, cyclophosphamide, procarbazine and dexamethasone (Neuwelt et al 1991). Patients did not receive cranial radiotherapy as part of their primary therapy. The median survival of 44.5 months for the 17 patients undergoing this therapy compared very favorably with a concurrent cohort of 11 patients who underwent RT alone and who had a median survival of 17.8 months ($p = 0.039$). Further investigation is required in order to determine whether BBB disruption assumes the mantle of standard therapy in PCL.

Toxicity of chemotherapy

The acute and chronic toxicities of chemotherapeutic agents have been well documented (Pinedo et al 1992). The type and severity of toxicity is dependent on the drug regimen, and most side effects can be predicted. Acute side effects include myelosuppression, mucositis, alopecia, nausea and vomiting. These toxicities are usually self-limiting and are rarely severe in the context of treating PCL.

Long-term side effects have been more keenly considered in view of the advances in treating PCL with the resultant improvements in disease-free and overall survival. Chronic side effects may impinge significantly on a patient's quality of life. Long-term sequelae of chemotherapy include secondary malignancy (secondary to alkylating agents), anthracycline-induced cardiomyopathy, pulmonary fibrosis, and infertility in younger patients (Pinedo et al 1992).

In treating PCL, a major concern is the effect of therapy on cognitive function. Cranial irradiation may result in major or minor deteriorations in cognitive function, and post-irradiation intrathecal methotrexate results in a higher incidence of leukoencephalopathy with consequent neuropsychological impairment (Allen et al 1980, Sheline et al 1980, Crossen et al 1992). To a lesser degree, mental state deterioration may occur with other single agent or combination regimens in conjunction with radiotherapy (Turrisi 1980, Johnson et al 1990).

There is little information available regarding the effect of chemotherapy alone in treating PCL. At least one study suggests that chemotherapy and BBB disruption alone does not cause any overt or subtle deterioration in cognitive function (Crossen et al 1992). Small numbers and a selected study population make the interpretation of this series difficult, however, these findings are promising. The toxicity associated with BBB disruption therapy also includes that of the chemotherapy agents themselves plus the additional hazards associated with the BBB disruption. In the study of Neuwelt et al (1991), seizures occurred in 47% of patients (7% of all procedures). The seizures were reported as typically short, focal motor in nature and occurred while the patient was under anesthesia. Procedural complications (pseudoaneurysm, arterial injury, deep vein thrombosis, pulmonary embolus, pneumothorax, and cerebral infarction) were also reported.

The incidence of thromboembolism may be increased in PCL. A retrospective review of 55 patients recorded 10 cases (18%) of thromboembolic complications including 2 instances of pulmonary embolism (Thorin & DeAngelis 1991). In our own series of 12 patients we saw 1 fatal case of pulmonary embolism. The cause of thrombotic disease in these patients is no doubt multifactorial and stems particularly from typical postoperative risks, the hypercoagulable state associated with malignancy and the prothrombotic effects of some chemotherapeutic agents (Luzzatto & Schafer 1990).

This is a worrying complication for the clinician due to the risk of intracerebral bleeding occurring with anticoagulant therapy. This risk may be increased in patients with PCL due to the highly vascular and vasocentric characteristics of this tumor. Despite this theoretical risk, no intracerebral bleeding complications appear to have occurred in those patients treated for thrombotic disease (Thorin & DeAngelis 1991).

Advances in chemotherapy and supportive care

Advances in the treatment of systemic NHL may, in the future, be translated into therapies for PCL. It has become commonplace in the therapy of systemic NHL to treat patients with high dose chemotherapy accompanied by either allogeneic or autologous bone marrow transplantation. The efficacy of this approach still requires formal assessment through well-conducted randomized trials however, recent advances have significantly reduced the toxicity associated with these proceedures. Peripheral blood progenitor cell infusions and post-transplant colony-stimulating factors such as granulocyte colony stimulating factors (G-CSF) used as supportive therapies have managed to dramatically reduce hemopoietic toxicity (Sheridan et al 1992).

Colony stimulating factors such as G-CSF and granulocyte-macrophage colony stimulating factor (GM-CSF) have also been used as supportive therapy in the treatment of standard dose combination chemotherapy regimens for systemic lymphoma. A randomized trial demonstrated that adjunctive G-CSF resulted in significantly fewer episodes of severe neutropenia, fever, and perhaps most importantly, enabled a greater dose intensity than in control patients (Pettengell et al 1992). In other cancers, colony stimulating factors have been shown to abrogate chemotherapy-induced neutropenia, reduce infections and ameliorate stomatitis (Lieschke & Burgess 1992). There are no reports, as yet, of these methods being incorporated into the management of PCL. However, with the increasing use of systemic chemotherapy in the treatment of PCL, colony stimulating factors may play an important role in supportive care. For PCL, the role for high dose chemotherapy with marrow or progenitor cell rescue remains unanswered.

Attempts are also being made to identify agents that may reduce the toxicity of therapy and potentially allow dose escalation. Cardioprotective agents such as ICRF-187 appear to reduce the cardiotoxicity of anthracyclines and may enable higher doses of these drugs to be introduced into treatment regimens (Basser & Green 1993) while new antiemetic drugs such as the 5HT antagonists significantly reduce chemotherapy-induced nausea and vomiting.

Adjunctive therapies

The use of biological agents such as the interleukins, interferons, monoclonal antibodies and tumor vaccines has not been reported in the setting of PCL. One can only speculate on the role that such agents may play in the treatment of PCL. On the horizon, the introduction of 'gene therapies' may also influence therapeutic strategies in the treatment of both PCL and AR-PCL.

Other advances may impinge upon the treatment of PCL. Phase II studies of new combination chemotherapy regimens being undertaken include an escalating dose schedule of intravenous carboplatin and etoposide in conjunction with blood-brain barrier disruption (Williams et al 1992). The role of p-glycoprotein-related multidrug resistance has been raised, with the recognition that cerebral capillary endothelial cells express physiologically active p-glycoprotein in vitro (Tatsuta et al 1992). Thus it may be appropriate and worthwhile to use adjunctive agents that circumvent multidrug resistance (Ma & Bell 1989). Other avenues of improving bioavailability may be the use of lipophilic agents or the packaging of systemic chemotherapeutic agents in liposomes in order to provide better CNS penetration.

Management of associated phenomena

One of the striking radiologic features of PCL is the relative lack of edema and mass effect despite large tumor masses. Thus associated phenomena such as raised intracranial pressure and hydrocephalus are uncommon. Even if present, rapid resolution of such complications occurs due to the exquisite sensitivity of PCL to steroids, chemotherapy and radiotherapy.

In the uncommon circumstance where the histologic diagnosis is known and associated complications mandate urgent intervention, definitive therapy should be introduced immediately. The choice of irradiation or chemotherapy in such circumstances should be predicated by availability, experience and personal prejudice rather than documented superior efficacy of one modality over the other in this situation. Corticosteroids will add to the acute resolution of symptoms.

In the very rare circumstance where a histologic diagnosis has not been made and associated complications mandate urgent intervention, the introduction of parenteral corticosteroids results in rapid tumor lysis and may negate the need for any further acute treatment. A biopsy of the lesion should be performed as soon as possible following recovery in order to obtain a histologic diagnosis.

Patterns of failure

The majority of patients with PCL eventually relapse. In a review of older series, the reported relapse rates ranged from between 60 and 80% (Loeffler et al 1985). With the advent of chemotherapy as part of primary therapy, more recent series have documented a lower relapse rate of between 0 and 50% but with considerably shorter follow-up (Gabbai et al 1989, Shibamato et al 1989, Socie et al 1990, Neuwelt et al 1991, DeAngelis et al 1992a, Rosenthal et al 1993). Relapse can be divided into four typical sites: intracerebral, spinal, ocular and systemic. Many authors would argue that the patterns of relapse are, to an extent, determined by the type of initial therapy. Thus patients receiving whole brain irradiation alone may be more susceptible to spinal and systemic relapse than those who receive adjunctive spinal irradiation or chemotherapy. However, the incidence of spinal and systemic relapse is so low when compared with intracerebral failure that such assertions remain unproven in the face of such small patient numbers.

Reviews of large series of patients prior to the routine introduction of chemotherapy document the main site of relapse as intracerebral. Up to 90% of relapses are confined to the brain. Nelson et al combined data from a number of series and noted that spinal cord relapse occurred in only 4% of 254 patients, and the incidence of distant systemic relapse was 7% (Nelson et al 1992).

A number of distant sites of relapse have been reported. These include the mediastinum, lung, kidney, testis and myocardium (Benjamin & Case 1980, Loeffler et al 1985). Systemic 'relapse' may in truth represent progression of what was always systemic disease rather than distant relapse of PCL. Older studies did not have the luxury of CT or MR scans in order to detect small volume systemic disease; as a consequence, what was called PCL with systemic relapse may have been systemic NHL with intracerebral disease as its initial manifestation. Despite this semantic concern, it should be possible to document the sequence of PCL followed by systemic relapse through thorough staging at initial diagnosis.

There are no clearly documented variables that significantly alter prognosis in PCL. Pollack et al have performed a multivariate analysis for prognostic factors on a series of PCL patients. Their findings suggested that prolonged survival was associated with age < 60 years, good performance status, presence of hemispheric tumor alone, therapy that included cranial radiotherapy to a dose of at least 40 Gy and the addition of chemotherapy (Pollack et al 1989). These data must be seen in the light of being based on only 27 patients and over a 10-year period. On the other hand, when Neuwelt et al analyzed their survival data, the only significant variable appeared to be performance status (Neuwelt et al 1991) while others have suggested that histologic grade influences outcome (Hochberg 1992 personal communication). More recently a multivariate analysis was performed in order to assess prognostic factors influencing the survival of 53 immunocompetent patients with PCL. The findings suggested that the following features resulted in a longer survival: CSF protein < 0.6 g/l, good performance status and treatment with high dose methotrexate (Blay et al 1992).

Data from studies of other intracerebral tumors and systemic NHL may lead to intuitive assumptions as to the outlook for a particular patient with PCL. In patients with systemic NHL, bad prognostic features include increasing age, poor performance status, elevated LDH, aggressive histologic subtypes, disease extent, and failure to achieve a complete response following primary therapy (Ship et al 1992). One may reasonably consider that these criteria are likely to influence prognosis in patients with PCL, however it remains unresolved whether these criteria can truly be applied to PCL.

Management of recurrent disease

There are no clear guidelines as to second line therapy, either for relapsed or resistant disease. In earlier times, patients would be treated with cranial irradiation primarily and if disease recurred or persisted, chemotherapy could be instituted as second line therapy. However, as most patients now receive chemotherapy primarily, the options for second line therapy are reduced in the setting of relapsed disease. Chemotherapy principles recommend non-cross-resistant therapy in this circumstance. Lessons gained from the treatment of systemic NHL would suggest that second line therapies may result in objective responses in PCL, however few studies have addressed this issue. Treatment is generally considered palliative rather than curative, particularly in the face of aggressive histology, poor performance status and advanced age. In younger patients with a relatively good performance status, a trial of aggressive second line chemotherapy may be warranted. One may also speculate on the role of surgical resection when confronted by a patient with local relapse at a solitary site.

Management outcome

Long-term survivors of PCL were rare prior to the advent of routine chemotherapy treatment. In 1986, Murray et al documented 56 of 693 cases (8%) who had survived longer than 3 years; of these only 21 (3%) had survived for more than 5 years. The longest survival time was 16.5 years in an infant diagnosed at age 2 months.

Since the introduction of chemotherapy, the long-term outlook for patients with PCL has improved. Recent chemotherapy series record disease-free survival of between 40 and 100% over periods of time ranging from 4 months to 5 years (Gabbai et al 1989, Shibamoto et al 1989, Brada et al 1990, Socie et al 1990, Neuwelt et al 1991, DeAngelis et al 1992a, Rosenthal et al 1993). In most of these studies the median survival is at least 2 years, with one study documenting a 3-year survival of 53% (DeAngelis et al 1992a).

Although these recent findings are promising, nearly 50% of long-term survivors relapse between 5 and 12.5 years after diagnosis (Murray et al 1986). Thus the frequency of late relapse in PCL dictates that care must be taken before an individual is pronounced cured or a particular regimen is said to be curative.

AIDS-RELATED CEREBRAL LYMPHOMA

In the early 1980s an increase in aggressive NHL was linked to risk groups for AIDS (Zeigler et al 1982, 1984, Ross et al 1985). Shortly after, a definitive relationship between AIDS and NHL was established and, in 1985, disseminated high grade lymphoma and PCL were included in the Centers for Disease Control (CDC) definition of AIDS (Centers for Disease Control 1985). Currently NHL accounts for approximately 3% of new AIDS cases and represents the second most common malignancy in AIDS patients following Kaposi's sarcoma. The relative risk of developing NHL in AIDS patients is 60 times greater than in the normal population and, in patients under 20 years, the relative risk rises to a 360-fold increase (Beral et al 1991, DeWeese et al 1991, Rabkin et al 1991).

AIDS-related NHL (AR-NHL) has a typical but not pathognomonic clinicopathological pattern. These typical features of AR-NHL differ from NHL in the general population on a number of accounts including the frequency of presentations with disseminated or extranodal disease and the markedly increased proportion of high grade NHL. Concurrent CNS involvement is more common in AR-NHL and has been described in up to 50% of AIDS patients with NHL. Finally, there is a significant increase of PCL in AIDS patients (Snider et al 1983, Ziegler et al 1984, Gill et al 1985, Monfardini et al 1990, Beral et al 1991, Hamilton-Dutoit et al 1991).

AIDS-related primary cerebral lymphoma (AR-PCL) has rapidly become a significant clinical problem. In 1988, Levy reviewed 1286 adults with AIDS and found that PCL was the presenting diagnosis in 0.6% of these patients and a further 1.9% eventually developed PCL (Levy et al 1985). Baumgartner et al estimated that, by 1986, AR-PCL had become more common than PCL in immunocompetent patients and that, by 1991, AR-PCL would be more common than low grade astrocytomas and almost as common as meningiomas (Baumgartner et al 1990). The number of AIDS patients who develop intracerebral NHL may in fact be much higher. A number of cases occur after the initial diagnosis of AIDS and as a consequence may not be reported to centers collating epidemiologic data such as the Centers for Disease Control. In addition, up to 84% of AR-PCL are only diagnosed at autopsy (MacMahon et al 1991).

Of 2824 cases of AR-NHL diagnosed among the 97 258 cases of AIDS who were reported to the Centers for Disease Control prior to July 1989, 548 were PCL (19.4%) (Beral et al 1991). The relative risk of developing PCL in AIDS patients was at least 1000 times greater than in the normal population. Other centers have reported similar findings, reporting that PCL represented between 18 and 42% of all NHL cases in their own series of HIV-infected patients (Ziegler et al 1982, Monfardini et al 1988, Formenti et al 1989, Ioachim et al 1991).

Gail et al have predicted that between 8 and 27% of US lymphoma cases in 1992 would occur as a result of HIV infection (Gail et al 1991). The reasons for this are two-fold. First the absolute number of HIV-infected patients continues to increase and, second, prolonged survival with the use of antiviral agents and better control of opportunistic infections renders an HIV-infected patient more likely to develop lymphoma.

A number of studies suggest that the risk of developing NHL increases with time. Pluda et al assessed the risk of developing NHL in patients receiving zidovudine antiviral therapy. After 24 months of therapy, the probability of developing lymphoma was 12% while at 3 years the actuarial probability was 29% (Pluda et al 1990, 1991). In comparison, a study of 1030 patients treated with zidovudine noted a much smaller rise in the risk of developing NHL (3.2% at 2 years) (Moore et al 1991). Although the absolute risk of developing lymphoma is difficult to ascertain there appears no doubt that the longer an HIV infected patient lives, the more likely he or she is to develop NHL. One can only speculate as to whether a comparable increase will occur in the incidence of AR-PCL.

AIDS-related PCL presentation

The clinical features of AR-PCL closely resemble those of PCL in immunocompetent patients (Gill et al 1985, So et al 1986, Formenti et al 1989, Baumgartner et al 1990, Goldstein et al 1991). The most striking differences include the much younger age at presentation and the poor outcome in AR-PCL. Other features that may distinguish the two entities are the higher incidence of B symptoms and poorer performance status in those with AR-PCL (Diamond et al 1990, Remick et al 1990). The incubation period between HIV infection and development of lymphoma is approximately 50 months, a similar period to the AIDS-defining opportunistic infections (Beral et al 1991). The means of acquiring HIV infection does not appear to influence the risk of developing AR-PCL (Beral et al 1991).

The frequent presence of concurrent or alternative intracerebral pathology makes diagnosis difficult. Central nervous system disease is a frequent manifestation of AIDS, with significant neurologic symptoms developing in 40% of AIDS patients at some point in their disease. Up to 10% of AIDS patients present with a neurologic disorder as the initial manifestation of their disease (Snider et al 1983, Moskovitz et al 1984, Levy et al 1985) and autopsy studies reveal the presence of CNS pathology in 55–95% of AIDS patients (Moskowitz et al 1984, Levy et al 1985).

AIDS-related PCL radiology

The CT scan appearance of AR-PCL may be quite different to that of PCL occurring in non-immunosuppressed patients. Typically, the lesions are large and centrally hypodense with ring or target enhancement and have associated edema with mild mass effect (Sze et al 1987, Poon et al 1989). Lee et al demonstrated a consistent correlation between the ring enhancement and central hypodensity with the pathologic appearance of central necrosis and preservation of viable tumor cells at the periphery (Lee et al 1986). In 30–40% of cases, the disease is multicentric, with multiple lesions seen on CT or MR scans (Lee et al 1986, Sze et al 1987, Poon et al 1989). One study suggests that a focal enhancing mass with subependymal spread and hyperattenuation on nonenhanced CT scan were the most reliable features in distinguishing AR-PCL and toxoplasmosis (Dina 1991). Despite such observations and the dramatic appearances on CT scan, AR-PCL cannot be confidently diagnosed by scan alone.

The use of CT scans in the imaging of AR-PCL is associated with a small but significant incidence of false negative findings. A number of studies have reported normal CT scans in patients who have demonstrable disease on MR imaging or at autopsy (So et al 1986, Levy et al 1985, Sze et al 1987). In one study, 7% of AR-PCL not seen on CT scans were diagnosed at autopsy shortly afterwards (Ciricillo & Rosenblum 1990).

The MR scan appearance in patients with AR-PCL is also nonspecific. Typical findings are poorly defined regions of reduced intensity on T1-weighted images which become high intensity on T2-weighted images (Sze et al 1987). Magnetic resonance imaging is more sensitive than CT scanning in locating intracranial lesions later identified at autopsy (Jarvik et al 1988, Ramsay & Geremia 1988, Ciricillo & Rosenblum 1990, Kupfer et al 1990). Despite its apparent increased sensitivity, MR imaging may still provide rare false negative results (Kupfer et al 1990).

The ability to diagnose AR-PCL by CT or MR scans is complicated by the presence of concurrent intracranial pathology. Intracranial toxoplasmosis, for example, also appears on CT and MR scans as multiple, bilateral ring or nodular enhancing lesions with mild to moderate edema and mass effect. These lesions are frequently located at the corticomedullary junction and basal ganglia, as are the lesions of AR-PCL (Lee et al 1986, Poon et al 1989, Kupfer et al 1990). Although CT and MR scans are regarded as nonspecific, solitary lesions are more likely to represent AR-PCL while multiple lesions are more typical of toxoplasmosis. In one study of 17 solitary lesions on MR scan, 12 (71%) were PCL compared to 34% of multiple lesions (Ciricillo & Rosenblum 1990). Confusingly, multiple lesions may represent dual pathology (Levy et al 1985) and most authors caution against making scan-based diagnoses and encourage biopsy of the lesion if the clinical situation warrants such a procedure.

Thus the CT and MR scan appearances of AR-PCL are not only at variance with the appearances of PCL in nonimmunosuppressed patients but also are essentially indistinguishable from toxoplasmosis and in some circumstances other intracranial pathology.

When AIDS-related systemic lymphoma spreads to the CNS, it predominantly involves meningeal invasion rather than parenchymal disease. In these circumstances CT and MR scans are usually unhelpful. On the rare occasions when systemic disease also involves the cerebral parenchyma, the CT and MR scan appearances are the same as for AR-PCL (Sze et al 1987). Other sites of disease have been recorded including epidural lesions resulting in cord compression (Snider et al 1983, Zeigler et al 1984).

AIDS-related PCL laboratory diagnosis

CSF analysis is rarely helpful in the diagnosis of AR-PCL. Many studies report nonspecific findings such as an elevated protein level, pleocytosis and hypoglycorrhachia.

However it is rare to demonstrate diagnostic cytological abnormalities, despite cytocentrification and immunohistochemical techniques (So et al 1986).

AIDS-related PCL pathology

HIV infection itself may be considered as a prelymphomatous state. HIV infection causes B-cell activation resulting in elevated levels of serum immunoglobulins and circulating immune complexes (Schnittman et al 1986). B-cell proliferation occurs as a response to the mitogenic properties of HIV with or without the release of cytokines such as interleukin 6 and 10 or in an antigen-specific manner (Benjamin et al 1991, Pluda et al 1991, Bower 1992, Roithman & Andrieu 1992). Other factors may also be involved in the pathogenesis of AIDS-related NHL including p53 mutations (Gaidano et al 1991) and secondary nonrandom chromosomal abnormalities of band 13q34 (Berger et al 1989). There is no evidence to suggest that HIV itself may be directly responsible for the malignant transformation of B lymphocytes. The molecular components of HIV have not been demonstrated in AIDS-related NHL, either by Southern blot analysis or polymerase chain reaction (Levine 1992).

AR-PCL may involve any region of the brain. Most commonly the disease involves the cerebral hemispheres, cerebellum and brainstem. Concurrent leptomeningeal involvement has been frequently described, in contrast with non AR-PCL where meningeal involvement is rare (Gill et al 1985, So et al 1986). The macroscopic appearance of the disease is indistinguishable from non-AR-PCL, however the tumor is more commonly multicentric and frequently larger in size, with lesions greater than 3 cm in diameter being recorded (Gill et al 1985, MacMahon et al 1991).

In AR-PCL, the most common pathologic subtypes are immunoblastic and diffuse large cell lymphomas, with a smaller percentage of Burkitt's lymphomas (Gill et al 1985, So et al 1986, Baumgartner et al 1990, Goldstein et al 1991, MacMahon et al 1991, Raphael et al 1991, Levine 1992). Some authors have noted the pleomorphic nature of these tumors, with a spectrum of cell type varying between small cleaved cells to large immunoblasts (So et al 1986). As a consequence, it may not be possible to accurately define the Working Formulation Classification for a particular tumor.

The spectrum of pathologic subtypes in AR-PCL distinguishes it from systemic AR-NHL, in which 80–90% of tumors are high grade with almost 30% being Burkitt's lymphoma (Kaplan et al 1989, Hamilton-Dutoit et al 1991, Roithman & Andrieu 1992). This compares to an expected incidence of high grade tumors in non-AIDS systemic NHL of 10–15% (Rosenberg et al 1982). In systemic AR-NHL, tumors are uncommonly of intermediate grade and only rare examples of low grade tumors have been reported (Ioachim et al 1991, Levine 1992).

Immunohistochemical studies have demonstrated that AR-PCL are B-cell-derived tumors (So et al 1986, Roithman & Andrieu 1992). T-cell systemic NHL have been described in AIDS patients but their incidence does not appear to be increased beyond the expected values for non-AIDS populations. Similarly there have been occasional cases reported of mycosis fungoides, lymphoblastic lymphoma, HTLV-1-associated T-cell leukemia and T-cell lymphoma but there is no apparent increase in incidence in AIDS patients (Levine 1992). There is no evidence that these uncommon tumors are disproportionately represented in AR-PCL.

Burkitt's lymphoma accounts for a third of AIDS-related systemic NHL (Ziegler et al 1984, Bower 1992, Roithman & Andrieu 1992) and between 20 and 50% of AR-PCL (So et al 1986, Baumgartner et al 1990). It differs from the other AR-NHL subtypes in two ways. First, it may arise at all stages of the disease, including patients with normal levels of helper lymphocytes (CD4 cells). In one study the median CD4 cell count at diagnosis was 266/μl (range 28–1198) compared to other AIDS-related NHLs such as diffuse large cell lymphoma, where the median figure was significantly less at 112 μl (range 0–1125) (Roithmann et al 1991). Second, Burkitt's lymphoma in AIDS patients more commonly arises as the first manifestation of the AIDS syndrome than other classifications of NHL (Boyle et al 1990, Roithmann et al 1991).

The typical chromosomal translocation t(8,14) is present in almost all AIDS-related Burkitt's lymphomas although the less common translocations of t(2,8) and t(8,22) have also been described (Whang-Peng et al 1984, Roithman & Andrieu 1992). Further analysis of translocation breakpoints demonstrates that in most cases of AIDS-related NHL, the breakpoints occur within the first exon of the *myc* gene on chromosome 8 and the switch region lying between joining regions of the immunoglobulin H gene on chromosome 14. These molecular findings define AIDS-related Burkitt's lymphoma as typical of the sporadic form of this disease rather than the endemic form found in Africa (Subar et al 1988, Shirimazu et al 1991).

AIDS-related PCL management plan

The management of AR-PCL requires an acknowledgement that therapy is palliative, not curative. It is therefore paramount to carefully consider the patient's performance status and likely outcome from any concurrent AIDS-related illness. The aims of therapy should be to alleviate symptoms. As a consequence of therapy, some patients may live longer. Extending survival should not be at the expense of a patient's quality of life although there are no clear-cut guidelines to distinguish the patients who should be treated aggressively from those in whom such treatment is inappropriate. Despite these caveats it is clear that a patient presenting with PCL, a normal CD4 count and an otherwise excellent performance status needs to be approached differently from a moribund patient with PCL and end-stage concurrent opportunistic infections.

Current therapies for AR-PCL include corticosteroids, cranial irradiation and chemotherapy. Oral or intravenous administration of steroids can produce transitory clinical and radiologic improvement, however the duration of response is generally brief, in the order of weeks.

AIDS-related PCL radiotherapy

Radiotherapy as treatment for AR-PCL has been addressed by a number of studies (Table 44.6). Cranial irradiation regularly provides clinical and radiologic responses in these patients, however, response duration is brief, with a median survival less than 5 months overall and in some studies less than 3 months (Rosenblum et al 1988, Formenti et al 1989, Baumgartner et al 1990, DeWeese et al 1991, Goldstein et al 1991).

No adequate dose-response studies have been performed, thus the dose administered varies between studies and remains speculative. Some studies have attempted to assess the efficacy of different doses of radiotherapy in the setting of AR-PCL but the findings are inconsistent. In some studies, higher doses of irradiation resulted in an apparent prolongation of survival (Donahue et al 1989, Formenti et al 1989). Other studies have suggested that survival was dependent on performance status at presentation and that patients with good performance status were selected to receive higher doses of radiotherapy (Goldstein et al 1991).

In view of the palliative nature of this therapy, irradiation should be given over as short a period as possible. Thus some authors have reasonably recommended that patients with poor performance status should receive 30 Gy over 2 weeks (Cooper 1989) or even a more rapid fractionation of 20–25 Gy over one week (Goldstein et al 1991). In patients with excellent performance status and no concurrent opportunistic infections it may be reasonable to treat with higher doses in more protracted fractionation regimens.

Table 44.6 Radiotherapy in AIDS-related PCL. Adapted from DeWeese et al (1991)

Name	Year	No. of patients	Dose (rads)	Volume	Median survival (months)
Goldstein et al	1991	17	3500	Whole brain	2.4
DeWeese et al	1991	7	3000	Whole brain	2.2
Baumgartner et al	1990	55	4000	Whole brain	3.9
Formenti et al	1989	10	4200	Whole brain	5.5
Rosenblum et al	1988	7	4057	Whole brain	3.1

Comparisons between AR-PCL and PCL in non-immunocompromised patients suggest that the AIDS patients have fewer responses to irradiation, less satisfactory symptom relief and significantly shorter survival times (Formenti et al 1989, DeWeese et al 1991). Some authors have even questioned the benefit of such time-consuming and ineffective therapy in patients with such a poor prognosis (DeWeese et al 1991).

AIDS-related PCL chemotherapy

Chemotherapy has rarely been used in the treatment of AR-PCL. Although the addition of systemic or intrathecal chemotherapy may complement cranial irradiation, there is no evidence for its efficacy in this disease. In the face of severe immunodeficiency associated with AIDS, the additional immunodeficiency burden created by chemotherapy may limit its use. Chemotherapy may be indicated in the subset of patients with excellent performance status, relatively normal levels of helper T cells and those who have no evidence of concurrent opportunistic infections.

AIDS-related PCL survival

Despite attempts to treat these patients, the prognosis is very poor. In one review of 247 patients with AR-PCL, the median survival was less than 3 months, with a longest reported survival time of 28 months (Remick et al 1990). Patients die from either uncontrollable progression of lymphoma or as a consequence of other AIDS-related illnesses such as opportunistic infections (So et al 1986, Formenti et al 1989).

OTHER CATEGORIES OF CEREBRAL LYMPHOMA

1. Transplantation-related PCL

The association between immunosuppression and the development of non-Hodgkin's lymphoma was first recognized in renal transplant patients (Schneck & Penn 1971, Penn & Starzl 1972, Hoover & Fraumeni 1973, Barnett & Schwartz 1974). Systemic NHL is the most common post-transplant malignancy excluding non-melanoma skin cancers and carcinoma in situ of the cervix and has been described in all manner of organ transplantations (Hanto et al 1981, Penn 1987, Nalesnik et al 1988). In renal transplantation series, there is a 28–50-fold increase in expected cases of systemic NHL when compared with populations matched for age and sex (Hoover & Fraumeni 1973, Kinlen et al 1979, Riggs & Hagemeister 1988) while in cardiac transplantation series, the incidence of systemic NHL post transplant has been estimated at between 3.5 and 4.6% (Weintraub & Warnke 1982, Gratten et al 1990). The frequency of post-transplant NHL relates to the organ type and the degree of immunosuppression required to prevent rejection (Aisenberg 1991). Reports have noted the peculiarities of these lymphomas — in particular the frequency of PCL, the monotonous appearance of high and intermediate grade lymphomas and the rarity of Hodgkin's lymphoma.

Historically, PCL constituted approximately 25% of all transplant-related lymphomas and, in a further 10% of patients, the CNS was involved as part of a systemic lymphomatous process, usually as leptomeningeal disease (Riggs & Hagemeister 1988). Some studies recorded even higher percentages of PCL, with nearly 50% of post-transplant lymphomas being of cerebral origin (Schneck & Penn 1971, Hoover & Fraumeni 1973). This represented a marked increase in the risk of developing PCL in transplant patients compared with the normal population. One estimate put this as a 350-fold increase in risk (Penn 1981). For PCL, the median time from transplantation to the diagnosis of lymphoma ranged from 5.5–46 months (Schneck & Penn 1971, Hoover & Fraumeni 1973, Hochberg & Miller 1988). In one series the time to develop PCL was shorter than for systemic lymphoma, with median times of 16.5 months and 30.4 months respectively (Schneck & Penn 1971).

The introduction of cyclosporin A into standard post-transplant immunosuppressive regimens has resulted in significant changes to the pattern of post-transplant lymphomas. First, the incidence of extranodal disease has dropped and, furthermore, cerebral involvement is markedly reduced compared to the incidence seen with older immunosuppressive regimens. In Penn's study of transplant recipients receiving cyclosporin A immunosuppressive therapy, only 3% of the post-transplant lymphomas were confined to the brain. Some authors have postulated that the incidence of post-transplant lymphomas following immunosuppression with cyclosporin A is dose-dependent and the reason for the apparent fall in incidence is a result of using lower 'standard' doses of cyclosporin A and improved monitoring of plasma levels (Gratten et al 1990).

The second feature of cyclosporin A immunosuppression is the shorter time to the development of lymphoma than occurred with older regimens. In one such study the median time to the development of lymphoma was only 12 months compared to 44 months in those treated without cyclosporin A (Penn 1987).

Most reported post-transplant lymphomas are of B-cell origin although the lymphomas are frequently multiclonal and polymorphic (Hanto et al 1981, Weintraub & Warnke 1982, Nalesnik et al 1988) and while the true method of tumor evolution has not been elucidated, a common theory suggests that multiple malignant monoclonal lymphomas develop from an initial polyclonal proliferation of B-cells (Penn 1981, Cleary et al 1988, Riggs & Hagemeister 1988, Aisenberg 1991). On the other hand, some authors have suggested that these tumors can be divided into polymorphic diffuse B-cell hyperplasias and polymorphic diffuse B-cell lymphomas (Frizzera et al 1981, Hanto et al 1981, 1982).

There has been much speculation about which factors contribute to the development of lymphoma and, more specifically, PCL in transplant patients. There is no clear pathogenic mechanism, however it appears that a combination of decreased immune surveillance and chronic antigenic stimulation may play a role. Other factors may have an influence including the prolonged use of azathioprine and the cause of end-organ failure, at least in cardiac transplantation (Anderson et al 1978, Weintraub & Warnke 1982, Riggs & Hagemeister 1988). The incidence of post-transplant systemic lymphoma does not appear to be influenced by the sex of the donor or recipient, the use of antilymphocyte globulin, number of rejection crises, donor-host histocompatibility or in cases of renal transplantation, the cause of end-organ failure (Riggs & Hagemeister 1988). It is difficult to know how one may best apply these findings to aid in the identification of risk factors for the development of post-transplant PCL.

Treatment of transplantation-related PCL

It is not clear what constitutes the best therapeutic approach to transplant-related PCL. Historically, this disease had a very poor outlook, with almost all patients dying of progressive lymphoma within a few months (Schneck & Penn 1971). In accordance with the approach to systemic transplant-related lymphoma, therapeutic options include radiotherapy and chemotherapy, a reduction in immunosuppression and the introduction of antiviral agents (Hanto et al 1982, Starzl et al 1984, Nalesnik et al 1988, Locker & Nalesnik 1989). Logically, therapy should at least be comparable with current treatments for PCL in nonimmunosuppressed patients with the addition of a reduction in immunosuppressive therapy. The efficacy of treatment regimens in patients with transplant-related PCL is not well documented and as a result no regimen can be considered superior.

2. Secondary cerebral lymphoma

Cerebral lymphoma may be secondary to systemic lymphoma. Large studies of patients with systemic lymphoma reveal that between 7 and 29% of patients develop clinical or pathologic evidence of cerebral involvement (Haerni-Simon et al 1987, Liang et al 1989, Haddy et al 1991). Almost all cases are associated with relapsed or progressive systemic disease; isolated CNS relapse is not only very rare but is usually followed soon after by systemic relapse (Johnson et al 1984, Haerni-Simon et al 1987, Liang et al 1989).

Based on data from retrospective multivariate analyses, a number of factors have been suggested to predict a higher incidence of CNS relapse. These include unfavorable histology (Burkitt's and lymphoblastic NHL), elevated LDH, stage IV disease, and the presence of 'B' symptoms (fever, weight loss, sweats). Specific sites of systemic involvement may also be associated with an increased risk of developing cerebral disease. These sites include testis, bone marrow, bone, orbit, peripheral blood and paranasal sinuses (Johnson et al 1984, Perez-Soler et al 1986, Haerni-Simon et al 1987, Liang et al 1989, 1990b).

The site of disease in secondary cerebral lymphoma is almost invariably the meninges of the brain or spinal cord, with involvement of the cerebral parenchyma less common. As a consequence, the presenting symptoms and signs of secondary cerebral lymphoma reflect this feature. Thus patients develop headache, meningism, cranial nerve palsies, mental state alterations, sensory and motor deficits and nerve root palsies (Haerni-Simon et al 1987, Liang et al 1989, Zimmerman 1990).

The radiologic appearances of secondary cerebral lymphoma are identical to those of PCL except for sites of disease. MR scanning, with or without gadolinium contrast enhancement, may provide improved resolution with respect to meningeal disease and should be considered in the evaluation of a patient with suspected secondary cerebral or spinal lymphoma, particularly if the CT scan is unrewarding. Other investigative modalities such as myelography are not as sensitive as MR scanning in the detection of meningeal disease (Zimmerman 1990).

The majority of cases of secondary cerebral NHL are high grade lymphomas or diffuse large cell lymphoma according to the Working Formulation criteria. Secondary involvement of the brain occurs in less than 2% of low grade lymphomas. Up to 50% of patients have positive CSF cytology due to the propensity of secondary cerebral lymphoma to involve the meninges (Young et al 1979, Haerni-Simon et al 1987, Liang et al 1989).

The management of secondary cerebral NHL requires the consideration of both cerebral and systemic components of the relapsed disease. There are no studies that adequately define optimal therapy, and treatment should be individualized according to the clinical situation. For a patient with a good performance status and in whom an aggressive treatment approach may be warranted therapy should at least include combination systemic chemotherapy and some form of therapy to treat the cerebral disease. While it would be reasonable to base the therapy of the cerebral component on that used for PCL within a particular institution, consideration of the frequency of meningeal involvement suggests that intrathecal chemotherapy may be the best alternative.

The role of CNS prophylaxis in patients at high risk of developing secondary cerebral NHL is less well defined than for acute lymphocytic leukemia, which also has a propensity to intracerebral involvement. Standard management practice in high grade systemic NHL is to include some form of CNS prophylaxis such as intrathecal methotrexate. In retrospective studies, the use of CNS prophylaxis appears to have significantly reduced the incidence of CNS relapse when compared to groups of historical controls (Perez-Soler et al 1986, Haddy et al 1991).

Overall survival in patients with secondary cerebral lymphoma appears to be less than for PCL. Less than 15% of patients survive 1 year after the diagnosis of secondary cerebral NHL (Young et al 1979, Haerni-Simon et al 1987, Liang et al 1989). These authors have also recognized the fact that many of the former die of progressive systemic disease rather than from their CNS disease. It may be that CNS disease per se simply represents extensive systemic disease and that this is responsible for the poor prognosis rather than an intrinsic feature of secondary cerebral NHL (Haddy et al 1991).

3. Hodgkin's disease

Intracerebral Hodgkin's disease (HD) remains a very rare entity. Unlike non-Hodgkin's lymphoma, there is no apparent increase in its incidence. Reflecting the rarity of the disease, the medical literature contains only a limited number of small series and single case reports.

Almost all cases of intracranial HD are associated with relapsing systemic disease. Large historical series of HD patients document the rarity of intracerebral involvement. A review from the Christie Hospital reported only 2 definite cases of cerebral disease in 1339 HD patients (Todd 1967). On available evidence, the incidence of intracranial HD accompanying systemic disease ranges from 0.2–0.5% (Todd 1967, Cuttner et al 1979, Sapozink & Kaplan 1983, Blake et al 1986, Hair et al 1991). In the setting of systemic disease, intracranial disease stems either from hematogenous metastases or direct meningeal infiltration.

Primary intracranial HD has been sporadically reported (Schricker & Smith 1955, Ashby et al 1988b, Clark et al 1992). Isolated intracranial HD is so rare that less than 20 cases have been published in the literature. Many of the cases were reported prior to improved staging and immunohistochemical techniques and as a result may have had unrecognized systemic disease or alternate histologies such as NHL.

The paucity of data predicates against clear definitions of epidemiologic factors, specific sites of predilection, histologic subtypes and approaches to management. The histologic subtype varies according to reports. All subtypes are represented, although nodular sclerosing HD has been most frequently reported in the recent literature

(Sapozink & Kaplan 1983, Ashby et al 1988, Clark et al 1992). Symptoms and signs of intracranial HD represent local tumor effects, commonly expressed as cranial nerve palsies, headache and long tract motor disturbances. There have been no reported cases of the classic 'B' symptoms — fever, sweats or loss of weight — in primary intracerebral HD.

The diagnosis of primary intracerebral HD cannot be made by CT or MR scan. Although the CT scan usually demonstrates a solitary lesion the appearance may be confused with other intracranial lesions including gliomas, metastases and meningiomas. Examination of CSF should be routine despite the limitations of diagnosing HD by cytologic methods. Diagnostic Reed-Sternberg cells have been recognized in the CSF of some patients with intracerebral HD (Billingham et al 1975, Cuttner et al 1979).

The most likely scenario in the diagnosis of intracranial HD is as an unexpected finding at craniotomy or stereotactic brain biopsy. The surgeon may be alerted by the well-circumscribed and homogeneous appearance of the tumor. Fresh tissue should accompany formalin-fixed specimens so as to provide adequate tissue for immunohistochemical studies. Once the diagnosis of intracerebral HD has been made, the most important aspect of management is the need to exclude systemic disease. Routine staging should include the investigations listed previously for cerebral non-Hodgkin's lymphoma.

Intracerebral HD has been described in at least one patient who was seropositive for the human immunodeficiency virus (Hair et al 1991). HD is not currently recognized as an AIDS-defining illness, however an increasing number of HIV-associated HD cases have been reported, particularly in intravenous drug users, and sero-testing should be considered in 'at risk' patients (Roithmann et al 1990, Ames et al 1991, Ree et al 1991).

The treatment of patients with intracerebral HD accompanying systemic relapse should include therapy for both intracranial and systemic components. Treatment decisions must necessarily be individualized according to the clinical situation. Empirically, however, treatment should include irradiation of intracranial disease in addition to definitive systemic chemotherapy.

In view of its rarity, the standard and optimal therapy of primary intracerebral HD has not been defined. Surgical excision, radiotherapy and chemotherapy have been used in isolation or in combination as treatment for this disease (Ashby et al 1988b, Clark et al 1992). In primary disease with a solitary focus, the most common approach has been surgical excision followed by cranial irradiation. Descriptive accounts of surgery in these patients suggests that the tumor mass is well encapsulated and can be removed in its entirety. Post-operative whole brain irradiation with a tumor dose to 40–45 Gy has been recommended and may confer an added survival benefit. There is no evidence that systemic or intrathecal chemotherapy adds to surgery or radiotherapy in the treatment of primary intracerebral HD.

Long-term outcome for patients with intracranial HD is difficult to determine from reported cases. Amongst the rare cases of primary intracranial HD, complete responses and long-term survival have been described (Ashby et al 1988b, Clark et al 1992). Similarly, in those patients with concurrent intracerebral and systemic disease, aggressive combination therapy may result in complete responses and long-term survival.

4. Intraocular lymphoma

Intraocular lymphoma is a rare condition affecting those in their sixth or seventh decades. Typically the disease presents with a painless reduction in acuity in one or both eyes, and the disease may affect the vitreous, retina or subretinal space. The ocular findings include retinal and subretinal infiltrates, vitreous cells and retinal detachments. The majority of patients have bilateral ocular disease (Margolis et al 1980, Rockwood et al 1984, Strauchen et al 1989, Maiuri 1990).

The diagnosis is established by vitreous aspiration or biopsy (Strauchen et al 1989) with subsequent cytologic or histologic assessment. Most reported cases are large cell NHL of B-cell origin (Kaplan et al 1980). Up to 70% of patients with ocular lymphoma have concurrent cerebral lymphoma whilst less than 25% have associated systemic disease (Vogel et al 1968, Margolis et al 1980, Rockwood et al 1984). In general, the ocular symptoms precede symptoms attributable to the cerebral disease (Maiuri 1990).

In contrast to PCL, ocular lymphoma may not respond to steroids (Margolis et al 1980). Treatment often incorporates binocular irradiation, prophylactic cranial irradiation and, more recently, adjunctive intravenous single agent or combination chemotherapy (Strauchen et al 1989). Therapeutic levels of cytosine arabinoside (Ara-C) have been recorded within the vitreous following intravenous and subconjunctival administration (Rootman et al 1983, Baumann et al 1986, Strauchen et al 1989). This therapeutic approach frequently results in complete or partial responses, however most patients eventually relapse and die. Over 50% of relapses occur within the central nervous system, with rare cases of systemic relapse being reported (Baumann et al 1986).

5. Mycosis fungoides

Mycosis fungoides, a cutaneous T-lymphocyte lymphoma, may disseminate to the CNS as well as to other internal organs. This rare complication is associated with advanced disease and may be diagnosed by stereotactic biopsy or by the presence of typical tumor cells in the CSF. Treatment with cranial irradiation and chemotherapy may have a palliative effect and prolong survival, however long-term survival has not been reported (Zackheim et al 1983, Hallahan et al 1986, Lindae et al 1990).

6. Lymphomatoid granulomatosis

Lymphomatoid granulomatosis (LG) is now recognized as an angiocentric, angiodestructive lymphoproliferative disorder that frequently progresses to lymphoma. Investigators have documented T-cell clonality and, in some cases, an association with Epstein-Barr virus (Jaffe 1984, Donner et al 1990, Mittal et al 1990). Although the disease commonly involves the lungs and skin, the CNS is involved in up to 20% of cases (Hogan et al 1981) and there are a few reported cases of LG isolated to the CNS (Kokmen et al 1977, Schmidt et al 1984, Kleinschmidt-De Masters et al 1992). CNS involvement with LG has been reported in patients with HIV infection (Anders et al 1989, Ioachim 1989).

The sites of CNS involvement appear random and, as a consequence, presenting symptoms and signs vary. Focal neurologic deficits result from solitary lesions whilst multifocal disease may present with a constellation of CNS features. There have also been rare descriptions of diffusely infiltrating disease resulting in dementia (Kleinschmidt-De Masters et al 1992).

Historically, LG was considered as a relatively benign tumor and therapy consisted of low doses of cyclophosphamide and prednisolone. However, increasingly it appears that the disease may run an aggressive course and many authors now advocate an aggressive approach towards therapy utilizing combination chemotherapy regimens and irradiation (Lipford et al 1988, Jenkins & Zaloznik 1989, Nair et al 1989).

7. Malignant angioendotheliosis (intravascular lymphomatosis)

Malignant angioendotheliosis is an unusual intravascular lymphoma that has a predilection for the CNS. The derivation of the neoplastic cells has been questioned since the first description of the disease in 1959 (Pfleger & Tappeiner 1959). There appears no doubt that the cell of origin is a lymphocyte, based on recent immunocytochemical, histologic and molecular evidence (Otrakji et al 1988, Clark et al 1991, Fredericks et al 1991).

More than 60 cases have been described within the literature and a pattern of the disease is apparent. Most patients are elderly and present with cerebral disease manifested by a progressive cognitive decline as a consequence of small vessel occlusion. Focal neurologic deficits may occur in tandem with a global decline or as an isolated feature. The diagnosis of malignant angioendotheliosis may be suggested by the clinical presentation and the MR scan appearance, however the majority of cases are only diagnosed at autopsy (Fredericks et al 1991, Smadja et al 1991).

Untreated, the disease progresses inexorably over weeks or months, with a median survival of only 9.5 months (Smadja et al 1991). The recognition that malignant angioendotheliosis is a lymphoma has prompted the use of cranial irradiation and combined chemotherapy regimens with some success (Fredericks et al 1991, Smadja et al 1991).

REFERENCES

Adams J, Howatson A G 1990 Cerebral lymphomas: review of 70 cases. Journal of Clinical Pathology 43: 544–547

Agbi C B, Bannister C M, Turnbull I W 1983 Primary cranial vault lymphoma mimicking a meningioma. Neurochirurgia 26: 130–132

Aisenberg A C 1991 Malignant lymphoma. Biology, natural history and treatment. Lea & Febiger, Philadelphia

Albrecht S, Bruner J B, SeGall G K 1992 Immunoglobulin heavy chain rearrangements in primary brain lymphomas. Proceedings of the American Association for Cancer Research 33 Abstract 1493

Allen J C, Rosen G, Mehta B M, Horten B 1980 Leukoencephalopathy following high-dose IV methotrexate chemotherapy with leucovorin rescue. Cancer Treatment Reports 64: 1261–1273

Ames E D, Conjalka M S, Goldberg A F et al 1991 Hodgkin's disease and AIDS: Twenty-three new cases and a review of the literature. Hematology and Oncology Clinics of North America 5: 343–356

Anders K H, Latta H, Chang B S 1989 Lymphomatoid granulomatosis and malignant lymphoma of the central nervous system in the acquired immunodeficiency syndrome. Human Pathology 20: 326–334

Anderson J L, Fowles R E, Bieber C P, Stinson E B 1978 Idiopathic cardiomyopathy, age, and suppressor-cell dysfunction as risk determinants of lymphoma after cardiac transplantation. Lancet ii: 1174–1177

Ando S, Moritake K 1990 Pure optic ataxia associated with a right parieto-occipital tumour. Journal of Neurology Neurosurgery and Psychiatry 53: 805–806

Aozasa K, Ohsawa M, Yamabe H et al 1990 Malignant lymphoma of the central nervous system in Japan: Histologic and immunohistologic studies. International Journal of Cancer 45: 632–636

Apuzzo M L, Chandrasoma P T, Cohen D, Zee C S, Zelman V 1987 Computed imaging stereotaxy: experience and perspective related to 500 procedures applied to brain masses. Journal of Neurosurgery 20: 930–937

Ashby M A, Bowen D, Bleehen N M, Barber P C, Freer C E L 1988a Primary lymphoma of the central nervous system: experience at Addenbrooke's Hospital, Cambridge. Clinical Radiology 39: 173–181

Ashby M A, Barber P C, Holmes A E, Freer C E L, Collins R D 1988b Primary intracranial Hodgkin's Disease. A case report and discussion. American Journal of Surgical Pathology 12: 294–299

Bailey P 1929 Intracranial sarcomatous tumors of leptomeningeal origin. Archives of Surgery 18: 1359–1402

Bale J F, Wilson J F, Hill H R 1977 Fatal histiocytic lymphoma of the brain associated with hyperimmunoglobulinemia-E and recurrent infections. Cancer 39: 2386–2390

Barnett L B, Schwartz E 1974 Cerebral reticulum cell sarcoma after multiple renal transplants. Journal of Neurology Neurosurgery and Psychiatry 37: 966–970

Bashir R M, Harris N L, Hochberg F H, Singer R M 1989 Detection of Epstein-Barr virus in CNS lymphoma by in-situ hybridisation. Neurology 39: 813–817

Bashir R, Coakham H, Hochberg F 1992 Expression of LFA-1/ICAM-1 in CNS lymphomas: possible mechanism for lymphoma homing into the brain. Journal of Neuro-Oncology 12: 103–110

Basser R L, Green M D 1993 Strategies for prevention of anthracycline cardiotoxicity. Cancer Treatment Reviews 19: 57–77

Baumann M A, Ritch P S, Hande K R, Williams G A, Topping T M, Anderson T 1986 Treatment of intraocular lymphoma with high dose Ara C. Cancer 57: 1273–1275

Baumgartner J E, Rachlin J R, Beckstead J H et al 1990 Primary central nervous system lymphomas: natural history and response to radiation therapy in 55 patients with acquired immunodeficiency syndrome. Journal of Neurosurgery 73: 206–211

Baxter J D, Harris A W, Tomkins G M, Cohen M 1971 Glucocorticoid receptors in lymphoma cells in culture: relationship of glucocorticoid killing activity. Science 171: 189–191

Benjamin D, Knobloch T J, Abrams J, Dayton M A 1991 Human B cell IL-10: B cell lines derived from patients with AIDS and Burkitt's lymphoma constitutively secrete large quantities of IL-10. Blood 78: abstract 384a

Benjamin I, Case M E S 1980 Primary reticulum-cell sarcoma (microglioma) of the brain with massive cardiac metastasis. Journal of Neurosurgery 53: 714–716

Beral V, Peterman T, Berkelman R, Jaffe H 1991 AIDS-associated non-Hodgkin lymphoma. Lancet 337: 805–809

Berger R, Le Coniat M, Devve J, Vecchione D, Chen S J 1989 Secondary non-random chromosomal abnormalities of band 13q34 in Burkitt's lymphoma-leukaemia. Genes, Chromosomes and Cancer 1: 115–118

Berry M P, Simpson W J 1981 Radiation therapy in the management of primary malignant lymphoma of the brain. International Journal of Radiation, Oncology, Biology and Physics 7: 55–59

Berube C, O'Reilly, Voss N, Fairey R, Connors J M 1991 Primary brain lymphoma in British Columbia from 1980–1990. Proceedings of the American Society of Clinical Oncology 10: abstract 996

Bignon Y J, Clavelou P, Ramos F et al 1991 Detection of Epstein-Barr virus sequences in primary brain lymphoma without immunodeficiency. Neurology 41: 1152–1153

Billingham M E, Rawlinson D G, Berry P F, Kempson R L 1975 The cytodiagnosis of malignant lymphomas and Hodgkin's Disease in cerebrospinal, pleural and ascitic fluids. Acta Cytologica 19: 547–556

Black P McL 1991 Brain tumors. New England Journal of Medicine 324: 1471–1476

Blake P R, Carr D H, Goolden A W G 1986 Intracranial Hodgkin's disease. British Journal of Radiology 59: 414–416

Blasberg R G, Groothuis D, Molnar P 1990 A review of hyperosmotic blood-brain barrier disruption in seven experimental tumor models. In: Johansson B B, Widner C O H (eds) Pathophysiology of the blood-brain-barrier. Elsevier, New York, pp 197–220

Blay J Y, Lasset C, Carrie et al 1992 Multivariate analysis of prognostic factors for survival in non immunodeficient patients with primary cerebral lymphoma. Proceedings of the American Society of Clinical Oncology abstract 1078

Bower M 1992 The biology of HIV-associated lymphomas. British Journal of Cancer 66: 421–423

Boyle M J, Swanson C E, Turner J J et al 1990 Definition of two distinct types of AIDS-associated non-Hodgkin's lymphoma. British Journal of Haematology 76: 506–512

Brada M, Dearnaley D, Horwich A, Bloom H J G 1990 Management of primary cerebral lymphoma with initial chemotherapy: preliminary results and comparison with patients treated with radiotherapy alone. International Journal of Radiation, Oncology, Biology and Physics 18: 787–792

Brant-Zawadzki M, Enzmann D R 1978 Computed tomographic brain scanning in patients with lymphoma. Radiology 129: 67–71

Cantore G P, Raco A, Artico M, Ciappetta P, Delfini R 1989 Primary chiasmatic lymphoma. Clinical Neurology and Neurosurgery 91: 71–74

Cassady J R, Wilner H I 1967 The angiographic appearance of intracranial sarcomas. Radiology 88: 258–263

Centers for Disease Control 1985 Revision of the case definition of acquired immunodeficiency syndrome for national reporting — United States. MMWR 34: 373–375

Chamberlain M C, Levin V A 1990 Adjuvant chemotherapy for primary lymphoma of the central nervous system. Archives of Neurology 47: 1113–1116

Ciricillo S F, Rosenblum M L 1990 Use of CT and MR imaging to distinguish intracranial lesions and to define the need for biopsy in AIDS patients. Journal of Neurosurgery 73: 720–724

Clark W C, Dohan F C, Moss T, Schweitzer J B 1991 Immunocytochemical evidence of lymphocytic derivation of neoplastic cells in malignant angioendotheliomatosis. Journal of Neurosurgery 74: 757–762

Clark W C, Callihan T, Schwartzberg L, Fontanesi J 1992 Primary intracranial Hodgkin's lymphoma without dural attachment. Case report. Journal of Neurosurgery 76: 692–695

Cleary M L, Nalesnik M A, Shearer W T, Sklar J 1988 Clonal analysis of transplant-associated lymphoproliferations based on the structure of the genomic termini of the Epstein-Barr Virus. Blood 72: 349–352

Cooper J S 1989 Radiation therapy and the treatment of patients with AIDS. In: Radiation oncology: rationale, techniques, results. C V Mosby, Baltimore, Md, pp 762–776

Crossen J R, Goldman D L, Dahlborg S A, Neuwelt E A 1992 Neuropsychological assessment outcomes of nonacquired immunodeficiency syndrome patients with primary central nervous system lymphoma before and after blood-brain barrier disruption chemotherapy. Neurosurgery 30: 23–29

Cuttner J, Meyer R, Huang Y P 1979 Intracerebral involvement in Hodgkin's Disease. A report of 6 cases and review of the literature. Cancer 43: 1497–1506

Davenport R D, O'Donnell L R, Schnitzer B, McKeever P E 1991 Non-Hodgkin's lymphoma of the brain after Hodgkin's disease. Cancer 67: 440–443

DeAngelis L M 1990 Primary central nervous system lymphoma imitates multiple sclerosis. Journal of Neuro-Oncology 9: 177–181

DeAngelis L M 1991a Primary central nervous system lymphoma: A new clinical challenge. Neurology 41: 619–621

DeAngelis L M 1991b Primary central nervous system lymphoma as a secondary malignancy. Cancer 67: 1431–1435

DeAngelis L M, Kreis W, Chan K, Akerman S 1990 Plasma (PL) and CSF pharmacokinetics of Ara-C and Ara-U of patients treated with high dose Ara-C (HDARA-C) for primary CNS lymphoma (PCNSL). Proceedings of the American Society of Clinical Oncology 9: abstract 372

DeAngelis L M, Yahalom J, Thaler H T, Kher U 1992a Combined modality therapy for primary CNS lymphoma. Journal of Clinical Oncology 10: 635–643

DeAngelis L M, Wong E, Rosenblum M, Furneaux H 1992b Epstein-Barr virus in Acquired Immune Deficiency Syndrome (AIDS) and non-AIDS primary central nervous system lymphoma. Cancer 70: 1607–1611

Desmeules M, Mikkelsen T, Mao Y 1992 Increasing incidence of primary malignant brain tumors: influence of diagnostic methods. Journal of the National Cancer Institute 84: 442–445

DeVita V T, Jaffe E S, Mauch P, Longo D L 1989 Lymphocytic lymphomas. In: DeVita V T, Hellman S, Rosenberg S A (eds) Cancer principles and practices of oncology. Lippincott, Philadelphia, pp 1741–1798

De Weese T L, Hazuka M B, Hommel D J, Kinzie J J, Daniel W E 1991 AIDS-related non-Hodgkin's lymphoma: the outcome and efficacy of radiation therapy. International Journal of Radiation, Oncology, Biology and Physics 20: 803–808

Diamond C, Remick S, Migliozzi J et al 1990 Primary central nervous system lymphoma (PCL) in patients with and without acquired immunodeficiency syndrome (AIDS). Proceedings of the American Society of Clinical Oncology 9: abstract 367

Dina T S 1991 Primary central nervous system lymphoma versus toxoplasmosis in AIDS. Radiology 179: 823–828

Donahue B, Cooper J S, Rush 1989 Results of empiric radiotherapy for HIV associated primary CNS lymphomas. International Journal of Radiation, Oncology, Biology and Physics 17: (suppl 1) abstract 223

Donner L R, Dobin S, Harrington D, Bassion S, Rappaport E S, Peterson R F 1990 Angiocentric immunoproliferative lesion (lymphomatoid granulomatosis). A cytogenetic, immunophenotypic, and genotypic study. Cancer 65: 249–254

Eby N L, Grufferman S, Flannelly C M, Schold S C, Vogel F S, Burger P C 1988 Increasing incidence of primary brain lymphoma in the US. Cancer 62: 2461–2465

El-Yazigi A, Kanaan I, Martin C R, Siqueira E B 1990 Cerebrospinal fluid content of manganese, platinum, and strontium in patients with cerebral tumors, leukemia and other noncerebral neoplasms. Oncology 47: 385–388

Enzmann D R, Krikorian J, Norman D, Kramer R, Pollock J, Faer M 1979 Computed tomography in primary reticulum cell sarcoma of the brain. Radiology 130: 165–170

Ervin T, Canellos G P 1980 Successful treatment of recurrent primary central nervous system lymphoma with high-dose methotrexate. Cancer 45: 1556–1557

Epstein L G, DiCarlo F J, Joshi V V et al 1988 Primary lymphoma of the central nervous system in children with Acquired Immunodeficiency Syndrome. Pediatrics 82: 355–363

Feiden W, Bise K, Steude U 1990 Diagnosis of primary cerebral lymphoma with particular reference to CT-guided stereotactic biopsy. Virchows Archives. A, Pathological Anatomy and Histopathology 417: 21–28

Filopovich A H, Heinitz K J, Robison L L et al 1987 The Immunodeficiency Cancer Registry. A research source. American Journal of Pediatric Hematology and Oncology 9: 183–184

Formenti S C, Gill P S, Lean E et al 1989 Primary central nervous system lymphoma in AIDS. Results of radiation therapy. Cancer 63: 1101–1107

Fredericks R K, Walker F O, Elster A, Challa V 1991 Angiotropic intravascular large-cell lymphoma (malignant angioendotheliomatosis): report of a case and review of the literature. Surgical Neurology 35: 218–223

Freeman C, Berg J W, Cutler S 1972 Occurrence and prognosis of extranodal lymphomas. Cancer 29: 252–260

Freeman C R, Shustik C, Brisson M, Meagher-Villemure K, Dylewski I 1986 Primary malignant lymphoma of the central nervous system. Cancer 58: 1106–1111

Frizzera G, Hanto D W, Gajl-Peczalska K J et al 1981 Polymorphic diffuse B-cell hyperplasias and lymphomas in renal transplant recipients. Cancer Research 41: 4262–4279

Front D, Ben-haim S, Israel O et al 1992 Lymphoma: predictive value of Ga-67 scintigraphy after treatment. Radiology 182: 359–363

Gabbai A A, Hochberg F H, Linggood R M, Bashir R, Hotleman K 1989 High-dose methotrexate for non-AIDS primary central nervous system lymphoma. Journal of Neurosurgery 70: 190–194

Gaidano G, Ballerini P, Gong J Z et al 1991 P53 mutations in human lymphoid malignancies: association with Burkitt lymphoma and chronic lymphocytic leukemia. Proceedings of the National Academy of Science 88: 5413–5417

Gail M H, Pluda J M, Rabkin C S et al 1991 Projections of the incidence of non-Hodgkin's lymphoma related to Acquired Immunodeficiency Syndrome. Journal of the National Cancer Institute 83: 695–701

Gametchu B 1987 Glucocorticoid receptor-like antigen in lymphoma cell membranes: correlation to cell lysis. Science 236: 456–461

Geddes J F, Bhattacharjee M B, Savage K, Scaravilli F, McLaughlin J E 1992 Primary cerebral lymphoma: a study of 47 cases probed for Epstein-Barr virus genome. Journal of Clinical Pathology 45: 587–590

GiaRusso M H, Koeppen A H 1978 Atypical progressive multifocal leukoencephalopathy and primary cerebral malignant lymphoma. Journal of the Neurological Sciences 35: 391–398

Gill P S, Levine A M, Meyer P R et al 1985 Primary central nervous system lymphoma in homosexual men. Clinical, immunologic, and pathologic features. The American Journal of Medicine 78: 742–748

Giromini D, Peiffer J, Tzonos T 1981 Occurrence of a primary Burkitt-type lymphoma of the central nervous system in an astrocytoma patient. Acta Neuropathologica 54: 165–167

Goldstein J D, Dickson D W, Moser F G et al 1991 Primary central nervous system lymphoma in Acquired Immune Deficiency Syndrome. A clinical and pathological study with results of treatment with radiation. Cancer 67: 2756–2765

Good A E, Russo R H, Schnitzer B, Weatherbee L 1978 Intracranial histiocytic lymphoma with rheumatoid arthritis. The Journal of Rheumatology 5: 75–78

Grant J W, von Deimling A 1990 Primary T-cell lymphoma of the central nervous system. Archives of Pathology and Laboratory Medicine 114: 24–27

Gratten M T, Moreno-Cabral C E, Starnes V A, Oyer P E, Stinson E B, Shumway N E 1990 Eight-year results of cyclosporine-treated patients with cardiac transplants. Journal of Thoracic and Cardiovascular Surgery 99: 500–509

Gregory M C, Hughes J T 1973 Intracranial reticulum cell sarcoma associated with Immunoglobulin A deficiency. Journal of Neurology Neurosurgery and Psychiatry 36: 769–776

Greig N H, Ries L G, Yancik R, Rapoport S I 1990 Increasing annual incidence of primary malignant brain tumors in the elderly. Journal of the National Cancer Institute 82: 1621–1624

Haddy T B, Adde M A, Magrath I T 1991 CNS involvement in small noncleaved-cell lymphoma: is CNS disease per se a poor prognostic sign. Journal of Clinical Oncology 9: 1973–1982

Haerni-Simon G, Suchaud J P, Eghbali H, Coindre J M, Haerni B 1987 Secondary involvement of the central nervous system in malignant non-Hodgkin's lymphoma. Oncology 44: 98–101

Hair L S, Rogers J D, Chadburn A, Sisti M B J, Knowles D M, Powers J M 1991 Intracerebral Hodgkin's disease in a Human Immunodeficiency Virus-seropositive patient. Cancer 67: 2931–2934

Hallahan D, Greim M, Greim S et al 1986 Mycosis fungoides involving the central nervous system. Journal of Clinical Oncology 4: 1638–1644

Hamilton-Dutoit S J, Pallesen G, Franzmann M B et al 1991 AIDS-related lymphoma. Histopathology, immunophenotype and association with Epstein-Barr virus as demonstrated by in situ nucleic acid hybridisation. American Journal of Pathology 138: 149–163

Hansen H H, Bender R A, Shelton B J 1974 Use of the cytocentrifuge and CSF. Acta Cytologica 18: 251–262

Hansen P B, Kjeldsen L, Dalhoff K, Olesen B 1992 Cerebrospinal fluid beta-2-microglobulin in adult patients with acute leukemia or lymphoma: a useful marker in early diagnosis and monitoring of CNS-involvement. Acta Neurologica Scandinavia 85: 224–227

Hanto D W, Frizzera G, Purtilo D T et al 1981 Clinical spectrum of lymphoproliferative disorders in renal transplant recipients and evidence for the role of Epstein-Barr Virus. Cancer Research 41: 4253–4261

Hanto D W, Frizzera G, Gajl-Peczalska K J et al 1982 Epstein-Barr virus-induced B-cell lymphoma after renal transplantation. New England Journal of Medicine 306: 913–918

Heimans J J, De Visser M, Polman C H, Nauta J, Kamphorst W, Troost D 1990 Accuracy and interobserver variation in the interpretation of computed tomography in solitary brain lesions. Archives of Neurology 47: 520–523

Helle T L, Britt R H, Colby T V 1984 Primary malignant lymphomas of the central nervous system. Clinicopathological study of experience at Stanford. Journal of Neurosurgery 60: 94–103

Henry J M, Heffner R R, Dillard S H, Earle K M, Davis R L 1974 Primary malignant lymphomas of the central nervous system. Cancer 34: 1293–1302

Herbst K D, Corder M P, Justice G R 1976 Successful therapy with methotrexate of a multicentric lymphoma of the central nervous system. Cancer 38: 1476–1478

Hirano A 1975 A comparison of the fine structure of malignant lymphoma and other neoplasms in the brain. Acta Neuropathologica (suppl 6): 141–145

Ho K, Garancis J C, Paegle R D, Gerber M A, Borkowski W J 1980 Progressive multifocal leukoencephalopathy and malignant lymphoma of the brain in a patient with immunosuppressive therapy. Acta Neuropathologica 52: 81–83

Hochberg F H, Miller D C 1988 Primary central nervous system lymphoma. Journal of Neurosurgery 68: 835–853

Hochberg F H, Miller G, Schooley R T, Hirsch M S, Feorino P, Henle W 1983 Central-nervous-system lymphoma related to Epstein-Barr virus. New England Journal of Medicine 309: 745–748

Hogan P J, Greenberg M K, McCarty G E 1981 Neurological complications of lymphomatoid granulomatosis. Neurology 31: 619–620

Hoover R, Fraumeni J F 1973 Risk of cancer in renal-transplant recipients. Lancet July 14: 55–57

Houthoff H J, Poppema S, Ebels E J, Elema J D 1978 Intracranial malignant lymphomas. A morphologic and immunocytologic study of twenty cases. Acta Neuropathologica 44: 203–210

Hutter J J, Jones J F 1981 Results of thymic epithelial transplant in a child with Wiskott-Aldrich syndrome and central nervous system lymphoma. Clinical Immunology and Immunopathology 18: 121–125

Ioachim H L 1989 Lymphomatoid granulomatosis versus lymphoma of the brain and central nervous system in the acquired immunodeficiency syndrome. Human Pathology 20: 1222–1224

Ioachim H L, Dorsett B, Cronin W, Maya M, Wahl S 1991 Acquired immunodeficiency syndrome associated lymphomas: Clinical, pathological, immunologic and viral characteristics of 111 cases. Human Pathology 22: 659–673

Isheda Y 1975 Fine structure of primary reticulum cell sarcoma of the brain. Acta Neuropathologica (suppl 6): 147–153

Jack C R, O'Neill B P, Banks P M, Reese D F 1988 Central nervous system lymphoma: histologic types and CT appearance. Radiology 167: 211–215

Jaffe E S 1984 Pathologic and clinical spectrum of post-thymic T-cell malignancies. Cancer Investigation 2: 413–426

Jarvik J G, Hesselink J R, Kennedy C et al 1988 Acquired immunodeficiency syndrome. Magnetic resonance patterns of brain involvement with pathologic correlation. Archives of Neurology 45: 731–736

Jazy F K, Shehata W M, Tew J M, Meyer R L, Boss H H 1980 Primary intracranial lymphoma of the dura. Archives of Neurology 37: 528–529

Jellinger K, Radaskiewicz T H, Slowik F 1975 Primary malignant lymphomas of the central nervous system in man. Acta Neuropathologica (suppl 6): 95–102

Jellinger K, Kothbauer P, Weiss R et al 1979 Primary malignant lymphoma of the CNS and polyneuropathy in a patient with necrotising vasculitis treated with immunosuppression. Journal of Neurology 220: 259–268

Jenkins T R, Zalosnik A J 1989 Lymphomatoid granulomatosis. A case for aggressive therapy. Cancer 64: 1362–1365

Johnson B E, Patronas N, Hayes W et al 1990 Neurologic, computed cranial tomographic, and magnetic resonance imaging abnormalities in patients with small-cell lung cancer. Further follow-up of 6- to 13-year survivors. Journal of Clinical Oncology 8: 48–56

Johnson G J, Oken M M, Anderson J R, O'Connell M J, Glick J H 1984 Central nervous system relapse in unfavourable-histology non-Hodgkin's lymphoma: is prophylaxis indicated? Lancet Sept 22: 685–687

Kaplan J J, Meredith T A, Aaberg M, Keller R H 1980 Reclassification of intraocular reticulum cell sarcoma (histiocytic lymphoma); immunologic characterization of vitreous cells. Archives of Ophthalmology 89: 707–710

Kaplan L D, Abrams D I, Feigel E et al 1989 AIDS-associated non-Hodgkin's lymphoma in San Francisco. Journal of the American Medical Association 261: 719–727

Katz B Z, Andiman W A, Eastman R, Martin K, Miller G 1986 Infection with two genotypes of Epstein-Barr virus in an infant with AIDS and lymphoma of the central nervous system. Journal of Infectious Diseases 153: 601–604

Kepes J J 1987 Astrocytomas: Old and newly recognised variants, their spectrum and morphology and antigen expression. Canadian Journal of Neurological Sciences 14: 109–121

Kinlen L J, Sheil A G R, Peto J, Doll R 1979 Collaborative United Kingdom-Australasian study of cancer in patients treated with immunosuppressive drugs. British Medical Journal 2: 1461–1466

Kitanaka C, Eguchi T, Kokubo T 1992 Secondary malignant lymphoma of the central nervous system with delayed high uptake on ^{123}I-IMP single-photon emission computerized tomography. Journal of Neurosurgery 76: 871–873

Kleinschmidt-De Masters B K, Filley C M, Bitter M A 1992 Central nervous system angiocentric, angiodestructive T-cell lymphoma (lymphomatoid granulomatosis). Surgical Neurology 37: 130–137

Kokmen E, Billman J K, Abell M R 1977 Lymphomatoid granulomatosis clinically confined to the CNS. Archives of Neurology 34: 782–784

Kori S H, Devereaux M, Roessmann U 1983 Unusual presentations of CNS lymphoma. Neurology 33 (suppl 2): abstract 127

Kuntzer T, Bogousslavsky J, Rilliet B, Uldry P A, de Tribolet N, Regli F 1992 Herald facial numbness. European Journal of Neurology 32: 297–301

Kupfer M C, Zee C, Colletti P M, Boswell W D, Rhodes R 1990 MRI evaluation of AIDS-related encephalopathy: Toxoplasmosis vs lymphoma. Magnetic Resonance Imaging 8: 51–57

Kuwabara Y, Ichiya Y, Otsuka M et al 1988 High [^{18}F] FDG uptake in primary cerebral lymphoma: A PET study. Journal of Computer Assisted Tomography 12: 47–48

Lach B, Atack E, Hylton D 1985 Clinical and pathological analysis of primary lymphomas of the brain: association of tumors with demyelinative leukoencephalopathy. Journal of Neuropathology and Experimental Neurology 44: 309

LaChance D H, O'Neill B P, Macdonald D R et al 1991 Primary leptomeningeal lymphoma: report of 9 cases, diagnosis with immunocytochemical analysis, and review of the literature. Neurology 41: 95–100

Lai A P, Wierzbicki A S, Norman P M 1991 Immunocytological diagnosis of primary cerebral non-Hodgkin's lymphoma. Journal of Clinical Pathology 44: 251–253

Lee Y, Bruner J M, van Tassel P, Libshitz H I 1986 Primary central nervous system lymphoma: CT and pathologic correlation. American Journal of Radiology 147: 747–752

Leeds N E, Rosenblatt R, Zimmerman H M 1971 Focal angiographic changes of cerebral lymphoma with pathologic correlation. Radiology 99: 595–599

Lehrer H, McGarry P 1968 Meningeal lymphosarcoma as a primary intracranial lesion. Southern Medical Journal 61: 115–159

Leibel S A, Sheline G E 1987 Radiation therapy for neoplasms of the brain. Journal of Neurosurgery 66: 1–22

Levine A M 1992 Acquired Immunodeficiency Syndrome-related lymphoma. Blood 80: 8–20

Levy R M, Bredesen D E, Rosenblum M L 1985 Neurological manifestations of the acquired immunodeficiency syndrome (AIDS): experience at UCSF and review of the literature. Journal of Neurosurgery 62: 475–495

Liang R H S, Woo E K W, Yu Y et al 1989 Central nervous system involvement in non-Hodgkin's lymphoma. European Journal of Clinical Oncology 25: 703–710

Liang R, Woo E, Ho F, Collins R, Choy D, Ma J 1990a Klinefelter's syndrome and primary central nervous system lymphoma. Medical and Pediatric Oncology 18: 236–239

Liang R, Chiu E, Loke S L 1990b Secondary central nervous system involvement by non-Hodgkin's lymphoma: the risk factors. Hematological Oncology 8: 141–145

Liberski P P, Alwasiak J, Wegrzyn Z 1982 Atypical progressive multifocal leucoencephalopathy and primary cerebral lymphoma. Neuropatologica Polska 20: 413–419

Lieschke G J, Burgess A W 1992 Granulocyte-colony stimulating factor and granulocyte-macrophage colony-stimulating factor. New England Journal of Medicine 327: 99–106

Lindae M L, Luy J, Abel E A, Kaplan R 1990 Mycosis fungoides with CNS involvement: neuropsychiatric manifestations and complications of treatment with intrathecal methotrexate and whole-brain irradiation. Journal of Dermatology and Surgical Oncology 16: 550–553

Lipford E H, Margolick J B, Longo D L, Fauci A S, Jaffe E S 1988 Angiocentric immunoproliferative lesions: a clinicopathologic spectrum of post-thymic T-cell proliferations. Blood 72: 1674–1681

Lipsmeyer E A 1972 Development of cerebral lymphoma in a patient with systemic lupus erythematosus treated with immunosuppression. Arthritis and Rheumatism 15: 183–186

Littman P, Wang C C 1975 Reticulum sarcoma of the brain. A review of the literature and a study of 19 cases. Cancer 35: 1412–1420

Locker J, Nalesnik M 1989 Molecular genetic analysis of lymphoid tumors arising after organ transplantation. American Journal of Pathology 135: 977–987

Loeffler J S, Ervin T J, Mauch P et al 1985 Primary lymphomas of the central nervous system: patterns of failure and factors that influence survival. Journal of Clinical Oncology 3: 490–494

Luzzato G, Schafer A I 1990 The prethrombotic state in cancer. Seminars in Oncology 17: 147–149
Ma D D F, Bell D R 1989 Multidrug resistance and p-glycoprotein expression in human cancer. Australian and New Zealand Journal of Medicine 19: 736–743
MacMahon E M E, Glass J D, Hayward S D et al 1991 Epstein-Barr virus in AIDS-related primary central nervous system lymphoma. Lancet 338: 969–973
Maiuri F 1990 Visual involvement in primary non-Hodgkin's lymphomas. Clinical Neurology and Neurosurgery 92: 119–124
Margolis L, Fraser R, Lichter A, Char C H 1980 The role of radiation therapy in the management of ocular reticulum cell sarcoma. Cancer 45: 688–692
Marsh W L, Stevenson D R, Long H J 1983 Primary leptomeningeal presentation of T-cell lymphoma. Report of a patient and review of the literature. Cancer 51: 1125–1131
Matsuda M, McMurria H, VanHale P, Miller C A 1981 CSF findings in primary lymphoma of the CNS. Archives of Neurology 38: 397
Meeker T C, Shiramizu B, Kaplan L et al 1991 Evidence for molecular subtypes of HIV-associated lymphoma: division into peripheral monoclonal, polyclonal and central nervous system lymphoma. AIDS 5: 669–674
Mendenhall N P, Thar T L, Agee O F, Harty-Golder B, Ballinger W E, Million R R 1983 Primary lymphoma of the central nervous system. Computerized tomography scan characteristics and treatment results for 12 cases. Cancer 52: 1993–2000
Merchut M P, Haberland C, Naheedy M H, Rubino F A 1985 Long survival of primary cerebral lymphoma with progressive radiation necrosis. Neurology 35: 552–556
Michalski J M, Garcia D M, Kase E, Grigsby P W, Simpson J R 1990 Primary central nervous system lymphoma: analysis of prognostic variables and patterns of treatment failure. Radiology 176: 855–860
Miller D C, Knee R, Schoenfeld S, Wasserstom W R, Karp G 1989 Non-Hodgkin's lymphoma of the central nervous system after treatment of Hodgkin's disease. American Journal of Clinical Pathology 91: 481–485
Mittal K, Neri A, Feiner H, Schinella R, Alfonso F 1990 Lymphomatoid granulomatosis in the acquired immunodeficiency syndrome. Evidence of Epstein-Barr virus infection and B-cell clonal selection without myc rearrangement. Cancer 65: 1345–1349
Model L M 1977 Primary reticulum cell sarcoma of the brain in Wiskott-Aldrich Syndrome. Archives of Neurology 34: 633–635
Monfardini S, Tirelli U, Vaccher E et al 1988 Malignant lymphomas in patients with or at risk for AIDS in Italy. Journal of the National Cancer Institute 80: 855–860
Monfardini S, Vaccher E, Foa R et al 1990 AIDS-associated non-Hodgkin's lymphoma in Italy: intravenous drug users versus homosexual men. Annals of Oncology 1: 203–211
Moore R D, Kessler H, Richman D D, Flexner C, Chaisson R E 1991 Non-Hodgkin's lymphoma in patients with advanced HIV infection treated with Zidovudine. Journal of the American Medical Association 265: 2208–2211
Morrison V, Gruber S, Perterson B 1991 Therapy and outcome of post-transplant lymphomas. Proceedings of the American Association of Cancer Research 32: abstract 1137
Moskowitz L B, Hensley G T, Chan J C, Gregorios J, Conley F K 1984 The neuropathology of Acquired Immune Deficiency Syndrome. Archives of Pathology and Laboratory Medicine 108: 867–872
Murphy J K, O'Brien C J, Ironside J W 1989 Morphologic and immunophenotypic characterisation of primary brain lymphomas using paraffin-embedded tissue. Histopathology 15: 449–460
Murphy J K, Young L S, Bevan I S et al 1990 Demonstration of Epstein-Barr virus in primary brain lymphoma by in situ DNA hybridisation in paraffin wax embedded tissue. Journal of Clinical Pathology 43: 220–223
Murray K, Kun L, Cox J 1986 Primary malignant lymphoma of the central nervous system. Results of treatment of 11 cases and review of the literature. Journal of Neurosurgery 65: 600–607
Nair S D, Joseph M G, Catton G E, Lach B 1989 Radiation therapy in lymphomatoid granulomatosis. Cancer 64: 821–824
Nalesnik M A, Jaffe R, Starzl T E et al 1988 The pathology of post-transplant lymphoproliferative disorders occurring in the setting of Cyclosporin A-prednisolone immunosuppression. American Journal of Pathology 133: 173–192
Namiki T S, Nichols P, Young T, Martin S, Chandrasoma P 1988 Stereotaxic biopsy diagnosis of central nervous system lymphoma. American Journal of Clinical Pathology 90: 40–45
Nelson D F, Martz K L, Bonner H et al 1992 Non-Hodgkin's lymphoma of the brain: Can high dose, large volume radiation therapy improve survival? Report on a prospective trial by the Radiation Oncology Group (RTOG): RTOG 8315. International Journal of Radiation, Oncology, Biology and Physics 23: 9–17
Neuwelt E A, Barnett P A, Bigner D D et al 1982 Effects of adrenal cortical steroids and osmotic blood-brain opening on methotrexate delivery to gliomas in the rodent: the factor of the blood-brain barrier. Proceedings of the National Academy of Science (USA) 79: 4420–4423
Neuwelt E A, Frenkel E P, D'Agostino A N 1985 Growth of human lung tumor in the brain of the nude rat as a model to evaluate antitumor agent delivery across the blood-brain barrier. Cancer Research 45: 2827–2833
Neuwelt E A, Howieson J, Frenkel E P et al 1986 Therapeutic efficacy of multiagent chemotherapy with drug delivery enhancement by blood-brain barrier modification in glioblastoma. Neurosurgery 19: 573–582
Neuwelt E A, Goldman D L, Dahlborg S A et al 1991 Primary CNS lymphoma treated with osmotic blood-brain barrier disruption: prolonged survival and preservation of cognitive function. Journal of Clinical Oncology 9: 1580–1590
Ng K, Nash J, Woodcock B E 1991 High grade lymphoma of the cerebellum: a rare complication of chronic lymphatic leukaemia. Clinics in Laboratory Haematology 13: 93–97
Ohkawa S, Yamadori A, Mori E et al 1989 A case of primary malignant lymphoma of the brain with high uptake of ^{123}I-IMP. Neuroradiology 31: 270–272
O'Neill B P, Kelly P J, Earle J D, Scheithauer B, Banks P M 1987 Computer-assisted stereotaxic biopsy for the diagnosis of primary central nervous system lymphoma. Neurology 37: 1160–1164
O'Neill B P, Haberman T M, Banks P M et al 1989 Primary central nervous system lymphoma as a variant of Richter's syndrome in two patients with chronic lymphocytic leukemia. Cancer 64: 1296–1300
Onofrj M, Curatola L, Ferracci F, Fulgente T 1992 Narcolepsy associated with primary temporal lobe B-cell lymphoma in a HLA DR2 negative subject. Journal of Neurology Neurosurgery and Psychiatry 55: 852–853
O'Sullivan M G, Whittle I R, Gregor A, Ironside J W 1991 Increasing incidence of CNS primary lymphoma in south-east Scotland. Lancet 338: 895–896
Otrakji C L, Voigt W, Amador A, Nadji M, Gregorios J B 1988 Malignant angioendotheliosis — a true lymphoma: a case of intravascular malignant lymphomatosis studied by Southern BWT hybridisation analysis. Human Pathology 19: 475–478
Ott R J, Brada M, Flower M A, Babich J W, Cherry S R, Deehan B J 1991 Measurements of blood-brain barrier permeability in patients undergoing radiotherapy and chemotherapy for primary cerebral lymphoma. European Journal of Cancer 27: 1356–1361
Patrick A W, Campbell I W, Ashworth B, Gordon A 1989 Primary cerebral lymphoma presenting with cranial diabetes insipidus. Postgraduate Medical Journal 65: 771–772
Pattengale P K, Taylor C R, Panke T et al 1979 Selective immunodeficiency and malignant lymphoma of the central nervous system. Possible relationship to the Epstein-Barr virus. Acta Neuropathologica 48: 165–169
Pauzner R, Mouallem M, Sadeh M, Tadmor R, Farfel Z 1989 High incidence of primary cerebral lymphoma in tumor-induced central neurogenic hyperventilation. Archives of Neurology 46: 510–512
Penn I 1981 Depressed immunity and the development of cancer. Clinical and Experimental Immunology 46: 459–474
Penn I 1987 Cancers following cyclosporine therapy. Transplantation 43: 32–35
Penn I, Starzl T E 1972 Malignant tumors arising de novo in immunosuppressed organ transplant patients. Transplantation 14: 407–417
Perez-Soler R, Smith T L, Cabanillas F 1986 Central nervous system prophylaxis with combined intravenous and intrathecal methotrexate

in diffuse lymphoma of aggressive histologic type. Cancer 57: 971–977

Pettengell R, Gurney H, Radford J A et al 1992 Granulocyte colony-stimulating factor to prevent dose-limiting neutropenia in non-Hodgkin's lymphoma: a randomized controlled trial. Blood 80: 1430–1436

Pfleger L, Tappeiner J 1959 Zur Kenntnis der systemisierten Endotheliomatose der cutanen Blutgefasse (reticuloendotheliose?). Hautarzt 10: 359–363

Pinedo H M, Longo D L, Chabner B A (eds) 1992 Cancer chemotherapy and biological response modifiers Annual 13. Elsevier, Amsterdam

Pitman S W, Frei E 1977 Weekly methotrexate-calcium leucovorin rescue: effect of alkalinization on nephrotoxicity; pharmacokinetics in the CNS; and use in CNS non-Hodgkin's lymphoma. Cancer Treatment Reports 61: 695–701

Pluda J M, Yarchoan R, Jaffe E S et al 1990 Development of non-Hodgkin lymphoma in a cohort of patients with severe Human Immunodeficiency Virus (HIV) infection on long-term antiretroviral therapy. Annals of Internal Medicine 113: 276–282

Pluda K M, Venzon D, Tosato G et al 1991 Factors which predict for the development of non-Hodgkin's lymphoma (NHL) in patients with HIV infection receiving antiviral therapy. Blood 78 (no. 10) abstract 1129

Pollack I F, Lunsford L D, Flickinger J C, Dameshek H L 1989 Prognostic factors in the diagnosis and treatment of primary central nervous system lymphoma. Cancer 63: 939–947

Poon T, Matoso I, Tchertkoff V, Weitzner I, Gade M 1989 CT features of primary cerebral lymphoma in AIDS and non-AIDS patients. Journal of Computer Assisted Tomography 13: 6–9

Purvin V, Van Dyk H J 1984 Primary reticulum cell sarcoma of the brain presenting as steroid-responsive optic neuropathy. Journal of Clinical Neurology and Ophthalmology 4: 15–23

Rabkin C S, Biggar R J, Horm J W 1991 Increasing incidence of cancers associated with the Human Immunodeficiency virus epidemic. International Journal of Cancer 47: 692–696

Rampen F H J, van Andel J G, Sizoo W, van Unnik J A M 1980 Radiation therapy in primary non-Hodgkin's lymphomas of the CNS. European Journal of Cancer 16: 177–184

Ramsay R G, Geremia G K 1988 CNS complications of AIDS: CT and MR findings. American Journal of Radiology 151: 449–454

Raphael J, Gentilhomme O, Tulliez M et al 1991 Histopathologic features of high grade non-Hodgkin's lymphomas in acquired immunodeficiency syndrome. Archives of Pathology and Laboratory Medicine 115: 15–20

Rapoport S I 1988 Osmotic opening of the blood-brain barrier. Annals of Neurology 24: 677–684

Ree H J, Strauchen J A, Khan A A et al 1991 Human Immunodeficiency Virus-associated Hodgkin's disease. Cancer 67: 1614–1621

Remick S C, Diamond C, Migliozzi J A et al 1990 Primary central nervous system lymphoma in patients with and without the Acquired Immune Deficiency Syndrome. A retrospective analysis and review of the literature. Medicine 69: 345–360

Reyes M G, Homsi M F, Mangkornkanong M, Stone J, Glick R P 1990 Malignant lymphoma presenting as a chronic subdural hematoma. Surgical Neurology 33: 35–36

Reznik M 1975 Pathology of primary reticulum cell sarcoma of the human central nervous system. Acta Neuropathologica (suppl 6): 91–94

Riggs S, Hagemeister F B 1988 Immunodeficiency states: A predisposition to lymphoma. In: Fuller L M, Sullivan M P, Hagemeister F B, Velasquez W S (eds) Hodgkin's disease and non-Hodgkin's lymphomas in adults and children. Raven Press, New York, pp 451–478

Rockwood E J, Zakov Z N, Bay J W 1984 Combined malignant lymphoma of the eye and CNS (reticulum-cell sarcoma). Report of three cases. Journal of Neurosurgery 61: 369–374

Rodriguez M A, Ford R J, Goodacre A, Selvanayagam P, Cabaillas F, Deisseroth A B 1991 Chromosome 17p and p53 changes in lymphoma. British Journal of Haematology 79: 575–582

Roithmann S, Andrieu J M 1992 Clinical and biological characteristics of malignant lymphomas in HIV-infected patients. European Journal of Cancer 28: 1501–1508

Roithmann S, Tourani J M, Andrieu J M 1990 Hodgkin's Disease in HIV-infected intravenous drug abusers. New England Journal of Medicine 323: 275–276

Roithmann S, Toledano M, Tourani J M et al 1991 HIV-associated non-Hodgkin's lymphomas: Clinical characteristics and outcome. The experience of the French Registry of HIV-associated tumors. Annals of Oncology 2: 289–295

Roman-Goldstein S M, Golgman D L, Howieson J, Neuwelt E A 1992 MR of primary CNS lymphoma in immunologically normal patients. American Journal of Neuroradiology 13: 1207–1213

Rootman J, Gudauskas G, Kumi C 1983 Subconjunctival versus intravenous cytosine arabinoside: effect of route of administration and ocular toxicity. Investigative Ophthalmology and Visual Science 24: 1607–1611

Rosenberg N L, Hochberg F H, Miller G, Kleinschmidt-DeMasters B K 1986 Primary central nervous system lymphoma related to Epstein-Barr virus in a patient with Acquired Immune Deficiency Syndrome. Annals of Neurology 20: 98–102

Rosenberg S A, Berard C W, Byron W et al 1982 National Cancer Institute sponsored study of classifications of non-Hodgkin's lymphomas. Summary and description of a working formulation for clinical usage. Cancer 49: 2112–2135

Rosenblum M L, Levy M R, Bredesen D E, Wara W, So Y T, Ziegler J L 1988 Primary central nervous system lymphomas in patients with AIDS. Annals of Neurology 23 (suppl): 13–16

Rosenfeld S S, Hoffman J M, Coleman R E, Glantz M J, Hanson M W, Schold S C 1992 Studies of primary central nervous system lymphoma with Fluorine-18-Fluorodeoxyglucose Positron Emission Tomography. Journal of Nuclear Medicine 33: 532–536

Rosenthal M A, Sheridan W P, Green M D, Liew K, Fox R M 1993 Primary cerebral lymphoma: an argument for the use of adjunctive systemic chemotherapy. Australian and New Zealand Journal of Surgery 63: 30–32

Ross R, Dworsky R, Paganini-Hill A, Levine A, Mack T 1985 Non-Hodgkin's lymphomas in never married men in Los Angeles. British Journal of Cancer 52: 785–787

Rouah E, Rogers B B, Wilson D R, Kirkpatrick J B, Buffone G J 1990 Demonstration of Epstein-Barr virus in primary central nervous system lymphomas by the polymerase chain reaction and in situ hybridisation. Human Pathology 21: 545–550

Ruff R L, Petito C K, Rawlinson D G 1979 Primary cerebral lymphoma mimicking multiple sclerosis. Archives of Neurology 36: 598

Sagerman R H, Cassady J R, Chang C H 1967 Radiation therapy for intracranial lymphoma. Radiology 88: 552–554

Sapozink M D, Kaplan H S 1983 Intracranial Hodgkin's Disease. A report of 12 cases and review of the literature. Cancer 1301–1307

Sawataishi J, Mineura K, Sasajima T, Kowada M, Sugawara A, Shishido F 1992 Effects of radiotherapy determined by 11C-methyl-L-methionine positron emission tomography in patients with primary cerebral malignant lymphoma. Neuroradiology 34: 517–519

Schmidt B J, Meagher-Villemure K, Del Carpio J 1984 Lymphomatoid granulomatosis with isolated involvement of the brain. Annals of Neurology 15: 478–481

Schmitt-Graff A, Pfitzer P 1983 Cytology of the cerebrospinal fluid in primary malignant lymphomas of the central nervous system. Acta Cytologica 27: 267–272

Schneck S A, Penn I 1971 De-novo brain tumours in renal-transplant recipients. Lancet i: 983–986

Schnittman S M, Lane H C, Higgins S E, Folks T, Fauci A S 1986 Direct polyclonal activation of human B lymphocytes by the Acquired Immune Deficiency Syndrome virus. Science 233: 1084–1086

Schricker J L, Smith D E 1955 Primary intracerebral Hodgkin's Disease. Cancer 8: 629–633

Schwaighofer B W, Hesselink J R, Press G A, Wolf R L, Healy M E, Berthoty D P 1989 Primary intracranial CNS lymphoma: MR manifestations. American Journal of Neuroradiology 10: 725–729

Sheline G E, Wara W M, Smith V 1980 Therapeutic irradiation and brain injury. International Journal of Radiation, Oncology, Biology and Physics 6: 1215–1228

Sheridan W P, Begley C G, Juttner C A et al 1992 Effect of peripheral-blood progenitor cells mobilised by filgastrin (G-CSF) on platelet recovery after high-dose chemotherapy. Lancet March 14: 640–644

Sherman M E, Erozan Y S, Mann R B et al 1991 Stereotactic brain biopsy in the diagnosis of malignant lymphoma. American Journal of Clinical Pathology 95: 878–883
Shibamoto Y, Tsutsui K, Dodo Y, Yamabe H, Shima N, Abe M 1990 Improved survival rate in primary intracranial lymphoma treated by high-dose radiation and systemic vincristine-doxorubicin-cyclophosphamide-prednisolone chemotherapy. Cancer 65: 1907–1912
Ship M, Harington D, Anderson J et al 1992 Development of a predictive model for aggressive lymphoma: The International NHL Prognostic Factors Project. Proceedings of the American Society of Clinical Oncology abstract 1084
Shiramizu B, Barriga F, Neequaye J et al 1991 Patterns of chromosomal breakpoint locations in Burkitt's lymphoma: relevance to geography and Epstein-Barr virus association. Blood 7: 1516–1526
Singh A, Strobos R J, Singh B M et al 1982 Steroid-induced remissions in CNS lymphoma. Neurology 32: 1267–1271
Skarin A T, Zuckerman K S, Pitman S W et al 1977 High-dose methotrexate with folinic acid rescue in the treatment of advanced non-Hodgkin lymphoma including CNS involvement. Blood 50: 1039–1047
Smadja D, Mas J, Fallet-Bianco C et al 1991 Intravascular lymphomatosis (neoplastic angioendotheliosis) of the central nervous system: case report and literature review. Journal of Neuro-Oncology 11: 171–180
Smith W J, Garson J A, Bourne S P, Kemshead J T, Coakham H B 1988 Immunoglobulin gene rearrangement and antigenic profile confirm B cell origin of primary cerebral lymphoma and indicate a mature phenotype. Journal of Clinical Pathology 41: 128–132
Snider W D, Simpson D M, Aronyk K E, Nielson S L 1983 Primary lymphoma of the nervous system associated with Acquired Immune-deficiency Syndrome. New England Journal of Medicine 308: 45
So Y T, Beckstead J H, Davis R L 1986 Primary central nervous system lymphoma in Acquired Immune Deficiency Syndrome: A clinical and pathological study. Annals of Neurology 20: 566–572
Socie G, Piprot-Chauffat C, Schlienger M et al 1990 Primary lymphoma of the central nervous system. An unresolved therapeutic problem. Cancer 65: 322–326
Spillane J A, Kendall B E, Moseley I F 1982 Cerebral lymphoma: clinical radiological correlation. Journal of Neurology Neurosurgery and Psychiatry 45: 199–208
Starzl T E, Nalesnik M A, Porter K A et al 1984 Reversibility of lymphomas and lymphoproliferative lesions developing under cyclosporin-steroid therapy. Lancet 1: 583–587
Strauchen J A, Dalton J, Friedman A H 1989 Chemotherapy in the management of intraocular lymphoma. Cancer 63: 1918–1921
Subar M, Neri A, Inghirami G, Knowles D M, Dalla-Favera R 1988 Frequent c-myc oncogene activation and infrequent presence of Epstein-Barr Virus genome in AIDS-associated lymphoma. Blood 72: 667–671
Sugita Y, Shigemori M, Yuge T, Iryo D, Kuramoto S, Nakamura Y, Morimatsu M 1988 Spontaneous regression of primary malignant intracranial lymphoma. Surgical Neurology 30: 148–152
Sze G, Brant-Zawadzki M N, Norman D, Newton T H 1987 The neuroradiology of AIDS. Seminars in Roentgenology 1: 42–53
Talal M, Bunim J J 1964 The development of malignant lymphoma in the course of Sjogren's syndrome. American Journal of Medicine 36: 529–540
Tallroth K, Katevuo K, Holsti L, Andersson U 1981 Angiography and computed tomography in the diagnosis of primary lymphoma of the brain. Clinical Radiology 32: 383–388
Tatsuta T, Naito M, Oh-hara T, Tsuruo T 1992 Physiological function of p-glycoprotein in brain capillary endothelial cells. Proceedings of the American Association for Cancer Research 33: abstract 2789
Taylor C R, Russell R, Lukes R J, Davis R L 1978 An immunohistological study of immunoglobulin content of primary central nervous system lymphomas. Cancer 41: 2197–2205
Thomas M, Macpherson P 1982 Computed tomography of intracranial lymphoma. Clinical Radiology 33: 331–336
Thomson J L G, Brownnell B 1981 Computed tomographic appearances in microgliomatosis. Clinical Radiology 32: 367–374
Thorin L, DeAngelis L M 1991 Thromboembolism in primary central nervous system lymphoma (PCNSL). Proceedings of the American Society of Clinical Oncology 10: abstract 381
Todd D H 1967 Intracranial lesions in Hodgkin's disease. Proceedings of the Royal Society of Medicine 60: 734–736
Trillet M, Pialet J, Chazot G, Bourrat C, Schott B 1982 Lymphome non Hodgkin 'primitif' de l'encephale. Sarcoidose. Cancer thyroidien. Deficit immunitaire cellulaire. Revue Neurologique 138: 241–248
Turrisi A T 1980 Brain irradiation and systemic chemotherapy for small-cell lung cancer: dangerous liaisons? Journal of Clinical Oncology 8: 196–199
Vaquero J, Martinez R, Rossi E, Lopez R 1984 Primary cerebral lymphoma: the 'ghost tumor'. Journal of Neurosurgery 60: 174–176
Vogel M H, Font R L, Zimmerman L E et al 1968 Reticulum cell sarcoma of the retina and uvea. Report of six cases and review of the literature. American Journal of Ophthalmology 66: 205–215
Walker R J, Tiller D J, Horvath J S, Duggin G G 1989 Malignant lymphoma in a renal transplant patient on Cyclosporin A therapy. Australian and New Zealand Journal of Medicine 19: 154–155
Wang D, Liebowitz D, Kieff E 1985 An EBV membrane protein expressed in immortalized lymphocytes transforms established rodent cells. Cell 43: 831–840
Weingarten K L, Zimmerman R D, Leeds N E 1983 Spontaneous regression of intracerebral lymphoma. Radiology 149: 721–724
Weintraub J, Warnke R A 1982 Lymphoma in cardiac allotransplant recipients. Transplantation 33: 347–351
Weissman D E, Kueck B D, Merkow A B 1990 A case of large cell CNS lymphoma associated with a systemic small cell lymphocytic lymphoma. Journal of Neuro-Oncology 9: 171–175
Whang-Peng J, Lee E C, Sieverts H, Magrath I T 1984 Burkitt's lymphoma in AIDS: cytogenetic study. Blood 63: 818–822
Williams P C, Neuwelt E A, Hogan R L, Dana B W, Roman-Goldstein S 1992 Toxicity and efficacy of carboplatin and etoposide in conjunction with blood-brain barrier modification in the treatment of intracranial neoplasms. Proceedings of the American Association for Cancer Research 33: abstract 1527
Woo S Y, Maor M H 1990 Improving radiotherapy for brain tumors. Oncology 4: 41–45
Woolf A S, Conway G 1987 Systemic lupus erythematosus and primary cerebral lymphoma. Postgraduate Medical Journal 63: 569–571
Yamasaki T, Kikuchi H, Oda Y, Moritake K, Miura H, Shimada T 1992 Primary intracerebral malignant lymphoma associated with different histological types of carcinoma: report of two cases. Surgical Neurology 37: 464–471
Yang P J, Burt T B, Stricof D D, Seeger J F 1986 Intracranial non-Hodgkin's lymphoma occurring after treatment of Hodgkin Disease. Radiology 161: 541–543
Young R C, Howser D M, Anderson T, Fisher R I, Jaffe E, DeVita V T 1979 Central nervous system complications of non-Hodgkin's lymphoma. The potential role for prophylactic therapy. American Journal of Medicine 66: 435–443
Zackheim H, Lebo C, Wasserstein P et al 1983 Mycosis fungoides of the mastoid, middle ear and central nervous system: Literature review of MF of the CNS. Archives of Dermatology 119: 311–318
Ziegler J L, Miner R C, Rosenbaum E et al 1982 Outbreak of Burkitt's-like lymphoma in homosexual men. Lancet Sept 18: 631–633
Ziegler J L, Beckstead J A, Volberding P A et al 1984 Non-Hodgkin's lymphoma in 90 homosexual men. Relation to generalized lymphadenopathy and the Acquired Immunodeficiency Syndrome. New England Journal of Medicine 311: 565–570
Zimmerman H M 1975 Malignant lymphomas of the nervous system. Acta Neuropathologica suppl 6: 69–74
Zimmerman R A 1990 Central nervous system lymphoma. Radiologic Clinics of North America 28: 697–721

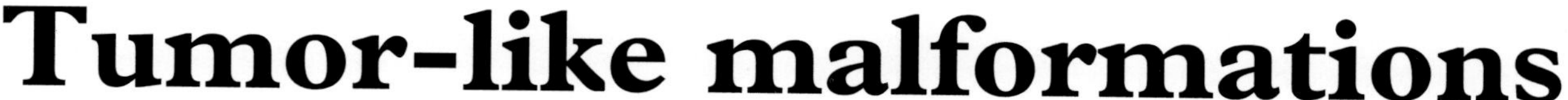

PART IX

Tumor-like malformations

45. Craniopharyngioma

Madjid Samii Marcos Tatagiba

For about a century the craniopharyngioma has been considered by a number of investigators to be one of the most intriguing tumors involving the brain. Since the first detailed description of craniopharyngioma by Erdheim in 1904 many controversies have emerged concerning its genesis, biological behavior, and treatment of choice.

HISTORICAL REVIEW AND DEFINITION

The term *craniopharyngioma* was introduced by Cushing in 1932. At the end of the 19th century Mott & Barrett (1899), two pathologists who studied an unusual group of epithelial tumors of the sella region, postulated that these tumors might arise from the hypophyseal duct or Rathke's pouch. Babinski in 1900 and Fröhlich in 1901 reported tumors of the suprasellar region 'without acromegaly'. Erdheim in 1904 contributed the first correct histologic interpretation and adequate description of these tumors. He postulated that the tumors originated from embryonic squamous cell rests of an incompletely involuted hypophyseal-pharyngeal duct. This idea is still held today although it is not completely established.

In 1909, Halstead (1910) performed the first successful removal of a craniopharyngioma by the transsphenoidal approach. This case was reported by Lewis in 1910 (Choux et al 1991). In 1923, Cushing operated on a child with craniopharyngioma who survived more than 50 years after the surgical intervention, considered the longest survival known (Raimondi 1987). McKenzie & Sosman (1924) called these tumors 'craniopharyngeal pouch tumors' in English literature, and McLean (1930) called them 'craniopharyngealtasche Tumoren' in German literature. It was, however, not until 1932 that Cushing introduced the name 'craniopharyngioma' (Gambarelli & Perez-Castillo 1991).

Some authors have considered the name craniopharyngioma to be inaccurate (Russell & Rubinstein 1989), because the Rathke's pouch is not a evagination of the pharynx but of the primitive stomodeum (Snell 1983). However, the term craniopharyngioma is so widely accepted and used that it would be difficult to change the nomenclature at this time.

ORIGIN

Craniopharyngioma is thought to arise from small ectodermal cellular nests that are usually found in the transition area of the pituitary stalk with the pars distalis of adenohypophysis, and sometimes extending to the pars tuberalis at higher levels of the stalk. Two main hypotheses about the origin of craniopharyngioma exist in the literature, both linking the origin of the tumor with these small nests of ectoderm.

The first hypothesis relates the development of craniopharyngioma to embryogenesis of the adenohypophysis. By the 4th week of embryonic life, the roof of the primitive oral cavity, or stomodeum, forms an upward invagination lined by epithelial cells of ectodermal origin, anterior to the buccopharyngeal membrane. This invagination is called Rathke's pouch. At the same time, the infundibulum forms as a downward growth of neuroepithelium from the floor of the diencephalon (Fig. 45.1). During the second month of development, Rathke's pouch comes into contact with the infundibulum. The neck of the pouch elongates, narrows, and finally separates from the oral epithelium. Rathke's pouch now is a vesicle that flattens itself around the anterior and lateral surfaces of the infundibulum. The cells of the anterior wall of the vesicle proliferate and form the *pars anterior (pars distalis)* of the hypophysis. The cell extension of the vesicle's upper part grows superiorly and around the stalk of the infundibulum, forming the *pars tuberalis.* The cells of the posterior wall of the vesicle form the *pars intermedia.* The cavity of the vesicle is reduced to a narrow cleft (Rathke's cleft) which may disappear completely. The path between primitive adenohypophysis and stomodeum along the migration of Rathke's pouch corresponds to the *craniopharyngeal duct.* Ectoblastic epithelial rests have

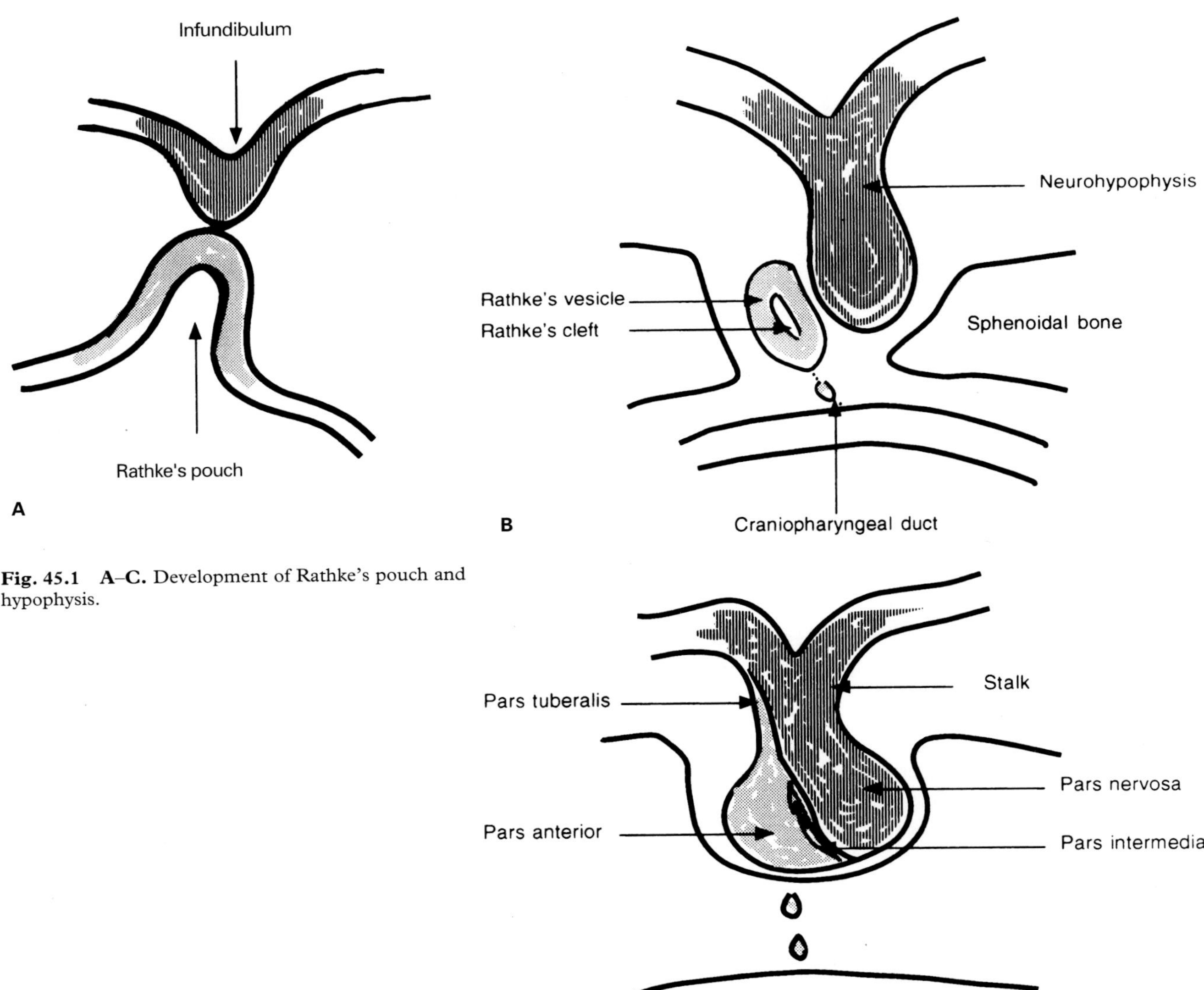

Fig. 45.1 A–C. Development of Rathke's pouch and hypophysis.

been found in the craniopharyngeal duct, and in the pars distalis and tuberalis. Erdheim (1904) proposed the origin of craniopharyngioma from these ectoblastic remnants of primitive craniopharyngeal duct and adenohypophysis. This idea has persisted to the present, and recent studies still support the hypothesis (Zumkeller et al 1991).

The second hypothesis concerning the pathogenesis of craniopharyngioma proposes that the residual squamous epithelium found in the adenohypophysis and anterior infundibulum undergoes metaplasia. Since squamous cell rests were rarely found in children, but were more likely with increasing frequency in each succeeding decade of life, it was suggested that the craniopharyngioma originates from metaplasia of mature cells of the anterior pituitary rather than from embryonic remnants.

Although the origin of craniopharyngioma is still controversial, some authors believe that craniopharyngiomas have dual origins (Kahn & Cosby 1972, Giangaspero et al 1984, Adamson et al 1990). They attribute the so-called childhood (adamantinous) craniopharyngioma to embryonic remnants, and the adult (squamous papillary) craniopharyngioma to metaplastic foci of adenohypophysis cells. This attractive idea may be supported by the fact that the adult type of craniopharyngioma is almost never found in children. Some investigators disagree however; because of the frequent association of both tumor types in histologic examinations, it has been suggested that craniopharyngioma represents a single group of tumors, ranging from the purely childhood type through a mixed variety to the adult type (Petito et al 1976, Russell & Rubinstein 1989).

Relationship between craniopharyngiomas and Rathke's cleft cysts

Rathke's cleft cysts and craniopharyngiomas are both considered to arise from embryonic rests of Rathke's pouch. By the 6th week of embryonic life, the residual lumen of the Rathke's pouch is reduced to a narrow cleft that generally regresses. The persistence and enlargement of this cleft are said to be the cause of Rathke's cleft cysts. Rathke's cleft cysts are epithelium-lined intrasellar cysts containing mucoid material (Voelker et al 1991). Rathke's cleft cysts and craniopharyngiomas are closely related and seem to share a common cellular origin from Rathke's pouch. Histologically, they are considered to constitute a spectrum of disorders ranging from the simplest form, the Rathke's cleft cyst, through transitional forms to the most complex form, the craniopharyngioma.

INCIDENCE AND PREVALENCE OF TUMOR

Craniopharyngiomas account for approximately 1.2–4% of all intracranial tumors (Zülch 1986, Russell & Rubinstein 1989, Choux et al 1991). They formed 4.6% of Cushing's series (1932) of 2000 intracranial tumors, and 1.2% of Zülch's pathological series (1986) of 9000 tumors. In the authors' series, craniopharyngiomas accounted for 1.3% of 3000 intracranial tumors, and for 13% of sellar and suprasellar tumors in all ages. In children, craniopharyngiomas represent approximately 5–10% of all tumors (Zülch 1986), or 56% of sellar and suprasellar tumors (Choux et al 1991). The annual incidence of craniopharyngiomas ranges from 0.5–2 new cases per year per 1 million population (Banna 1973, Sorva & Heiskanen 1986).

AGE AND SEX DISTRIBUTION

Although craniopharyngiomas account for a relatively great percentage of the intracranial tumors of childhood, they are less frequent in children and adolescents than in adults (Carmel 1990, Choux et al 1991), and should no longer be considered as a tumor of childhood and adolescence. Recent evaluation of 30 series with more than 3200 cases shows that approximately 60% of all craniopharyngiomas are seen in patients older than 16, and about 40% in patients 16 years old or younger (Choux et al 1991). The age distribution has a bimodal pattern, with a first high peak at 5–10 years and a second lower peak between 50 and 60 years, but all ages can be affected (Fig. 45.2). Craniopharyngiomas may develop in fetal life; large tumors have occasionally been found in the newborn (Tabbador et al 1974, Weber & Mori 1976, Hurst et al 1988) and even before birth (Snyder et al 1986). On the other hand, patients of 70 years or older have been described (Carmel 1990, van Effenterre et al 1991).

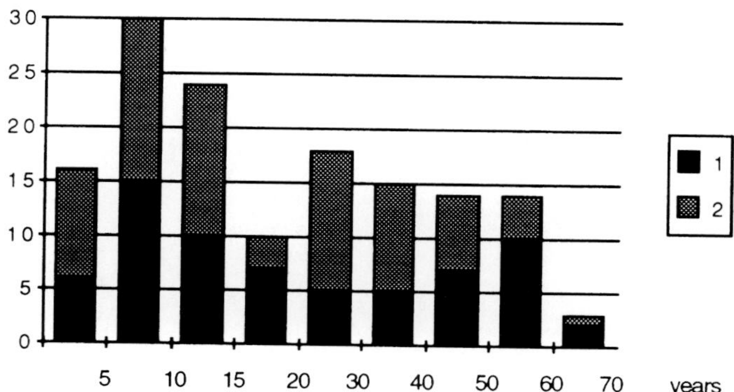

Fig. 45.2 Histogram of age and sex distribution in a series of 144 patients with craniopharyngioma. Data from Yasargil et al (1990). 1 = female, 2 = male.

Recent large series show a slight male predominance (55%) in contrast to female (45%) in all ages (Choux et al 1991).

RACIAL, NATIONAL, AND GEOGRAPHIC CONSIDERATIONS

Craniopharyngiomas represent 5–10% of intracranial tumors in children in most series, but higher frequency rates have been described in Africa (18%), and in the Far East (16%) (Zülch 1986, Choux et al 1991). The Brain Tumor Registry of Japan, however, indicates a frequency of 10.5% (Mori & Kurisaka 1986).

FAMILY HISTORY AND GENETIC FACTORS

Two cases of craniopharyngiomas in siblings have been reported (Vargas et al 1981, Combelles et al 1984). Thomsett et al (1980) described craniopharyngiomas in two cousins, and Wald et al (1982) described a 7-year-old boy with craniopharyngioma in a family in which three further members had different CNS tumors. Despite these few reports, the familial incidence is exceptional and no definitive genetic relationship has been reported in the pathogenesis of craniopharyngiomas. Rarely, craniopharyngiomas have been reported in association with other CNS processes, such as prolactinoma, angioma, pinealoma, germinoma, meningioma, and astrocytoma (Choux et al 1991). Craniopharyngiomas have also been reported in association with congenital malformations including precocious pseudopuberty, polydactyly, and low ear implantation (Drazin et al 1980, Wakai et al 1984).

SITES OF PREDILECTION

Craniopharyngioma arises typically in the infundibulo-hypophyseal axis in the sella and suprasellar area, frequently occupying the suprasellar cisterns, but may grow

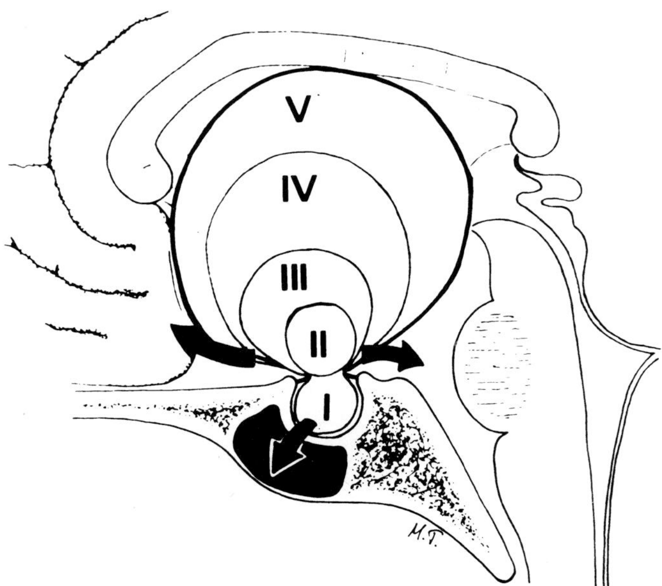

Fig. 45.3 Grade of vertical tumor extension related to sella and third ventricle.

in any direction. Rougerie & Fardeau (1962) first proposed a classification of 92 craniopharyngiomas by recognizing the following locations: intrasellar (11%), intra- and suprasellar with anterior extension (51%), intra- and suprasellar with posterior extension (36%), giant craniopharyngioma (2%), and atypical locations. With the development of MRI, a better topographic classification of craniopharyngioma could be made, recognizing four major types: intrasellar, infundibulum-tuberian, intraventricular, and dumbbell-shaped craniopharyngiomas (Raybaud et al 1991). Taking the optic chiasm as a reference point, approximately one third of cases are retrochiasmatic, one third are subchiasmatic, 20% are prechiasmatic, and 10–15% are intrasellar (Pang 1993).

The degree of *vertical* extension of tumor (Fig. 45.3) can be classified into five grades from grade I to grade V (Table 45.1). In a *horizontal* sense, craniopharyngioma may grow anteriorly into the prechiasmatic cistern and subfrontal space, laterally into the subtemporal space, and posteriorly into the interpeduncular and prepontine cisterns, cerebellopontine angle and foramen magnum.

Table 45.1 Classification of craniopharyngioma according to size of vertical tumor extension. (Samii, unpublished data)

Grade	Description
I	Intrasellar tumor
II	Intracisternal tumor with or without intrasellar component
III	Intracisternal tumor extending into the lower half of the third ventricle
IV	Intracisternal tumor extending into the upper half of the third ventricle
V	Intracisternal tumor extending to the septum pellucidum or into the lateral ventricles

In rare instances the tumor is located extradural and extracranial (nasopharyngeal) (Mukada et al 1984), or primarily in the posterior fossa (Gökalp et al 1991). The primary location of the tumor and its extension will tremendously influence the choice of surgical approach.

Surgical anatomy

Purely intrasellar craniopharyngiomas are uncommon. Intrasellar craniopharyngiomas may expand within the sella and compress the pituitary gland, producing endocrinopathies before the optic nerve is compressed. More frequently, however, the tumor grows pushing the diaphragma upward, breaking through it, and extending in any direction. In relation to the optic chiasm, the tumor may extend anteriorly (prechiasmatic craniopharyngioma) in the direction of the subfrontal spaces. These are frequently cystic tumors and achieve large sizes before being diagnosed. When the tumor grows posterior to the chiasm (retrochiasmatic craniopharyngioma) it displaces the pituitary stalk forward, and the chiasm forward and upward, making the optic nerve appear falsely prefixed (pseudoprefixity of the optic chiasm). Cystic retrochiasmatic craniopharyngioma may reach enormous sizes by expanding into the posterior fossa along the retroclival area.

Tumor extension up to the cervical spine has been described (Baba et al 1978). The tumor may also displace the chiasm upward (subchiasmatic craniopharyngioma), and the pituitary stalk backward. Both retrochiasmatic and subchiasmatic craniopharyngiomas are frequently solid tumors, and usually grow against the third ventricle, causing compression of the hypothalamus and obstruction of the foramen of Monro. By being pushed up by the tumor the ventricular floor may become paper-thin and tear, so that the tumor protrudes directly into the ventricle. The craniopharyngioma may also grow laterally in the subtemporal spaces, producing compression of the temporal lobe.

The craniopharyngioma may arise directly on the floor of the third ventricle. This is an essentially retrochiasmatic tumor, but it may extend anteriorly to the prechiasmatic space, superiorly to the lumen of the third ventricle, posteriorly to interpeduncular and prepontine cisterns, and laterally to the basal ganglia and temporal lobe.

Although large craniopharyngiomas frequently grow into the third ventricle, purely intraventricular craniopharyngioma is rare (Fukushima et al 1990). A recent review of the literature revealed only 24 cases (Iwasaki et al 1992). The pathogenesis of intraventricular craniopharyngiomas has been explained by the hypothesis that the pars tuberalis containing squamous epithelial rests of remnants of Rathke's pouch could rarely grow forward and backward along the pituitary stalk, extending to the infundibulum or tuber cinereum in the floor of the third ventricle (Arwell 1926, Urasaki et al 1988, Iwasaki et al

1992). At clinical examination, most of the patients present with symptoms and signs of obstructive hydrocephalus.

Craniopharyngioma is usually adherent to major arteries at the base of the skull, small perforating arteries coming from the anterior communicating vessels, the posterior communicating artery, and branches from the anterior choroidal artery and thalamoperforating vessels (Symon & Sprich 1985, Samii & Bini 1991). Tumor adhesion to vessels is one of the most important causes of incomplete tumor removal. Attempted radical dissection of tumor capsule from the arterial wall has been associated with weakening of adventitia by injuring the vasa vasorum, which caused fusiform dilatations of the carotid artery (Sutton et al 1991).

The blood supply for the anterior part of the tumor consists of perforators from the anterior communicating artery and the proximal anterior cerebral artery. The lateral part of the tumor receives branches from the posterior communicating artery, and the intrasellar part of the tumor is usually supplied from intracavernous meningohypophyseal arteries. Of great surgical significance is that craniopharyngiomas never receive blood supply from the posterior cerebral and basilar arteries unless the anterior blood supply for the lower hypothalamus and floor of the third ventricle is absent.

PRESENTING FEATURES

Since craniopharyngiomas are slow-growing tumors, they may reach large sizes before they become symptomatic. In the majority of cases the time interval between onset of symptoms and diagnosis of tumor ranges from 1–2 years. The three major clinical syndromes are related to increased intracranial pressure, endocrine dysfunction, and visual problems. Increased intracranial pressure results from an enlarging intracranial mass or obstructive hydrocephalus. Visual deficits may result both from direct compression of the optic pathways by the tumor and secondarily from intracranial hypertension. Endocrine changes are caused by compression of the hypothalamic-hypophyseal axis by the tumor.

Children frequently present with symptoms of increased intracranial pressure (65–75%) such as headaches and vomiting due to an enlarging intracranial mass. About 20% of children have papilledema. Obstructive hydrocephalus is present in about one third of the cases.

Visual deficits are commonly well tolerated by children. Only 20–30% of them complain of visual problems, usually when almost complete visual loss has taken place. Suspicion is raised when deterioration in school performance and the child's insistence on sitting closer and closer to the television are noted (Pang 1993).

Endocrine dysfunctions are present in one half of the children, and frequently manifest as short stature and diabetes insipidus. One third of children with craniopharyngioma have growth failure at the time of diagnosis. Delayed puberty is present in one half of the adolescents, and polydipsia and polyuria due to diabetes insipidus in 20% of cases (Mancini et al 1991).

The hypothalamic-pituitary complex is essential for endocrine, autonomic, and behavioral performance (Plum & van Uitert 1978, Carmel 1979). Disturbance of hypothalamic connections to the thalamus, frontal lobes, and other cortical areas have been related to some of the psychological and social problems seen among affected children (Galatzer et al 1981, Fischer et al 1990, Palm et al 1992). Hypothalamic dysfunction may be manifested as hyperphagia and obesity (25%), but personality changes are often overlooked. Children with craniopharyngioma frequently show psychomotor retardation, emotional immaturity, apathy (abulia minor), and short-term memory deficits. Pang (1993) describes the typical child with a craniopharyngioma as being short, obese, dull, half-blind, and with a poor school record.

Visual deficits and endocrine dysfunction are the most frequent clinical findings in adults. Endocrine dysfunction in adults appears in men as decreased sexual drive (88%) and in women as amenorrhea (82%) (Carmel 1990). Adults are more sensitive to visual deficits than children, and 80% of them complain of visual loss at the time of diagnosis. Signs of increased intracranial pressure are less common than in children. Headaches related to hydrocephalus are present in about half of the patients. Large subfrontal masses may cause neuropsychological symptoms, mentation deficits and memory loss, as well as incontinence, apathy, and Korsakoff's syndrome (Kahn & Crosby 1972). Large subtemporal masses extending laterally to the sylvian fissure may produce complex psychomotor seizures.

In rare instances, craniopharyngioma may spontaneously rupture, producing aseptic meningitis (Ravindram et al 1980, Okamoto et al 1985), intracranial hemorrhage (Kubota et al 1980, Yamamoto et al 1989), or tumor drainage through the nasopharynx (Maier 1985).

IMAGING DIAGNOSIS

Computed tomography (CT) and magnetic resonance imaging (MRI) have become standard evaluation tools in the diagnostic work-up for craniopharyngiomas. However, skull X-ray films are still useful as the first radiologic step, and the large majority of patients have an abnormal skull X-ray. About two thirds of adults and over 90% of children have pathologic changes demonstrable on plain skull films. Major findings include suprasellar calcification, and enlargement of the sella with erosion of anterior clinoids and dorsum sellae. Calcification is seen in 85% of children and 40% of adults with craniopharyngioma.

The development of high-resolution CT provides better delineation of soft tissue after contrast medium injection,

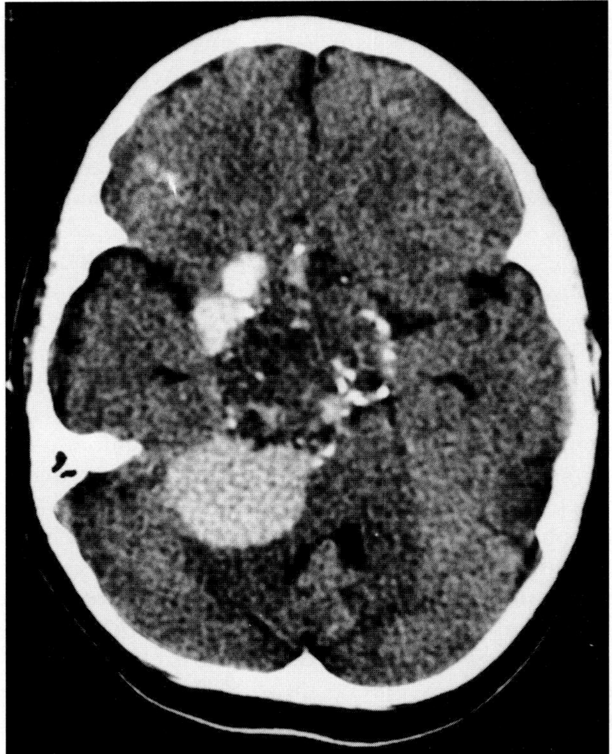

Fig. 45.4 Axial section of CT scan showing a suprasellar calcified mass with cystic portion in the posterior fossa.

identification of cystic parts of tumor and visualization of calcification areas (Fig. 45.4). Cyst content is usually as hypodense as cerebrospinal fluid, but it may appear hyperdense if enough calcification is present. The tumor capsule frequently shows enhancement following injection of contrast agent. Thin slice CT (1.5 mm thickness) with bone algorithm provides an excellent demonstration of calcium deposits in the tumor and erosion of skull base by the tumor.

More recently, MRI has been widely used for demonstrating craniopharyngiomas (Fig. 45.5). MRI does not replace CT, but is an important complementary investigation method. MRI is better than CT in identifying the soft tissue involvement around the tumor, and the displacement of complex anatomic structures of the diencephalon and skull base. The relaxation times of the cysts may be shortened, depending on the cholesterol content or recent hemorrhage. The cysts frequently produce a high, uniform signal on T1-weighted images, which is usually seen even when the lesions appear isodense or hypodense on CT scan (Huk et al 1990). Cysts with a low cholesterol content have a low signal on T1-weighted images. MRI demonstrates cystic spread into the bone and pneumatized spaces of the skull base better than CT. Calcifications produce low signal on MRI. Solid tumor parts tend to be homogeneous and have a marked increase of signal intensity on T1-weighted images after injection of Gd-DTPA (Huk et al 1990) that differentiates craniopharyn-

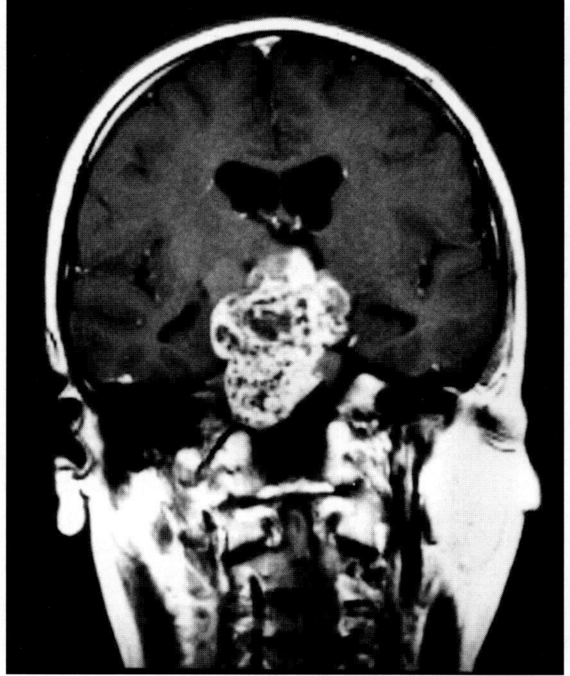

A

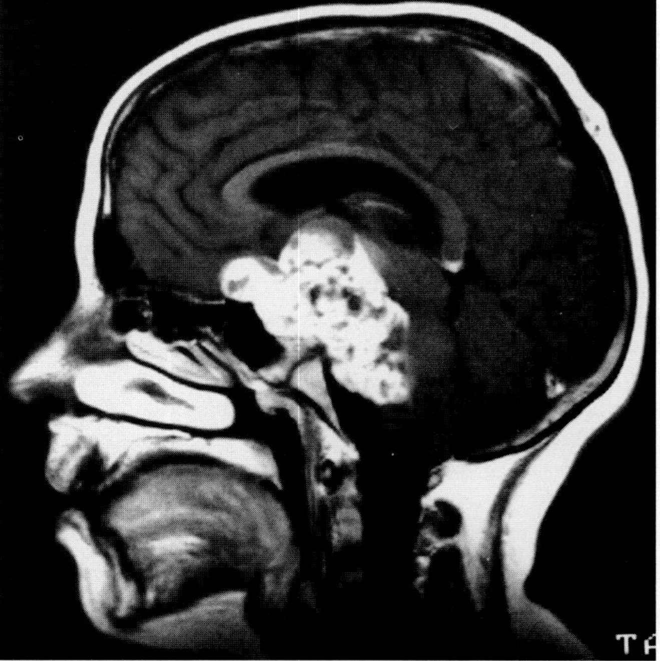

B

Fig. 45.5 Coronal (**A**) and sagittal (**B**) MRI section (T1) after contrast medium showing a large hyperintense mass that extends into the anterior and posterior fossa and into the third ventricle.

Table 45.2 MRI findings in craniopharyngiomas (Raybaud et al 1991)

Tumor type	T1	T2	Tumor contents
Cystic tumor	↓	↑	Cholesterol
	↑	↑	Hemorrhage
	↓	↓	Keratin
Solid tumor	↓	↑	Usual finding
	↑	↑	Hemorrhage or cholesterol
	↑	↓	Cholesterol

↑ = hyperintense; ↓ = hypointense

gioma from other suprasellar cysts (Hua et al 1992). MRI has, in addition, the advantage of providing sagittal and coronal sections of high quality, which are of tremendous importance for planning the surgical approach. Table 45.2 summarizes the MRI findings in craniopharyngioma.

As CT better demonstrates calcifications, and the bone anatomy of the skull base, both CT and MRI should be used as complementary tools in radiologic evaluation for craniopharyngioma.

Cerebral angiography is considered helpful in delineating the position of major vessels and their displacement by the tumor. The small vessels supplying the tumor are usually very difficult to identify at angiography (Carmel 1990). In recent years, the development of MRI-angiography has allowed for the demonstration of major cerebral vessels and their relation to the tumor, reducing the necessity for invasive angiographic studies (Samii & Bini 1991). Thus, angiography is no longer included as a diagnostic tool for craniopharyngiomas. Demonstration of cerebral vessels is of great significance for surgical planning in recurrent craniopharyngioma. Fusiform dilatations of major vessels have been described following primary tumor removal (Sutton et al 1991).

Ventriculography and pneumoencephalography were widely used in the past and are now regarded as historical concerns (Pertuiset 1975).

Ultrasound investigation has been used recently at and before birth for diagnosis of intracranial tumors. Snyder et al reported in 1986 a case of intrauterine detection of craniopharyngioma. Ultrasound in newborn and small children frequently shows enlargement of cranial perimetry up to more than 40 cm. Very large tumors have been described, sometimes occupying 70% of intracranial volume (Helmke et al 1984). Calcifications are visible in 90% of cases.

LABORATORY INVESTIGATION

The marked increase in the availability of laboratory tests has resulted in increasing knowledge of altered physiology and biochemistry of tumors affecting the hypothalamic-pituitary axis. It is essential, however, to bear in mind the limitations of such tests. Correct interpretation of laboratory data is of crucial significance. What is more important, the most sophisticated laboratory investigation cannot replace an accurate physical examination, or relieve the physician from the responsibility of careful observation of the patient. Laboratory investigations are essential in adequate preparation of patients for the surgical stress, and for managing postoperative hypothalamic-pituitary disturbances.

Laboratory tests include evaluation of pituitary function. Craniopharyngiomas frequently compress and displace sellar and diencephalic structures. The hypothalamic-pituitary complex is essential for endocrine performance (Erzin & Weiss 1990). The supraoptic and paraventricular nuclei of the endocrine hypothalamus produce vasopressin and oxytocin. These hormones travel within the axons of the hypothalamic-neurohypophyseal tract to the neurohypophysis, where they are stored for release in response to appropriate stimuli. Small nerve cells of the lower part of the hypothalamus produce anterior pituitary-regulating hormones. Fibers of these cells travel in a tuberopituitary tract to the median eminence of the neurohypophysis. The releasing and inhibiting substances are secreted into capillaries that form a short portal system surrounding the pituitary stalk conducting blood to the anterior pituitary. In the pituitary portal system a link occurs between the hypothalamus-neurohypophysis and adenohypophysis. Thus, the hypothalamic-pituitary complex regulates the secretion of somatotropin, thyrotropin, corticotropin, gonadotropin, vasopressin, prolactin, and several peptides and neurotransmitters (Erzin & Weiss 1990).

Lesions of very small size may easily interrupt this delicately balanced neural-hormonal tissue. The resulting syndromes include endocrine disorders, and disturbances of thirst and osmolarity balance (Carmel 1979, Streeten et al 1987). Although endocrine disorders are very frequent in patients with craniopharyngioma they often are not the reason for initial medical evaluation. A more accurate endocrine exploration will show endocrine dysfunction in the large majority of patients. The most frequent endocrine manifestations are diabetes insipidus and short

Table 45.3 Preoperative endocrine investigation (Mancini et al 1991)

Function	Minimal investigation	Extensive investigation (in addition)
Growth	Weight, size, osseous age, growth rate	—
ADH	24-h diuresis, urine and blood osmolarity	Restriction water test
STH	Somatomedin C	Stimulation test (insulin, glucagon, etc.)
PRL	Prolactin level	Test to TRH
TSH	T3 and T4 (free and total)	Test to TRH
ACTH	Levels of ACTH, cortisol, urine cortisol	Hypoglycemic test
LH-FSH	Testosterone and estrogen	Test to LH RH

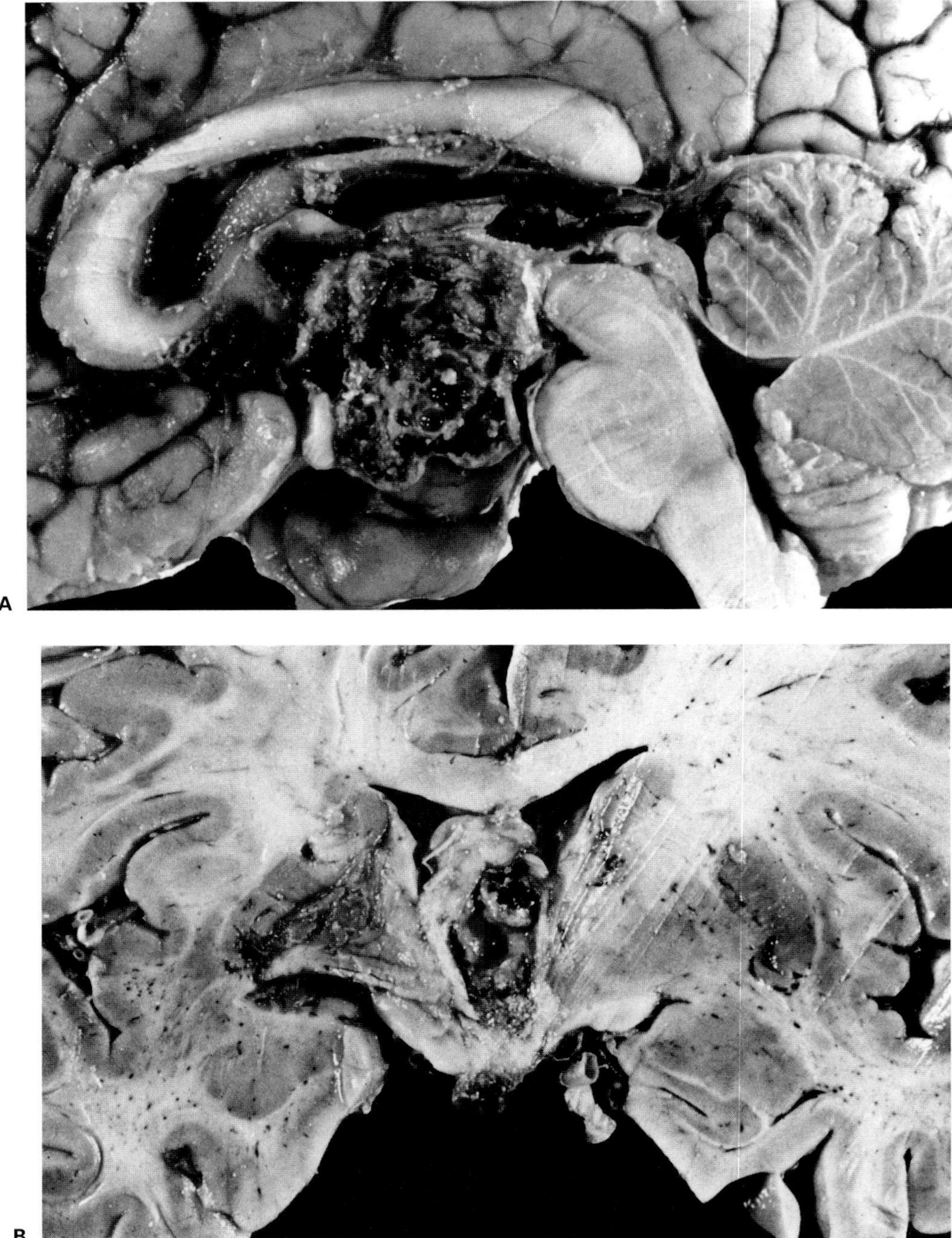

Fig. 45.6 **A.** Sagittal section of a large craniopharyngioma extending into the third ventricle. **B.** Coronal section of a calcified craniopharyngioma of the third ventricle. Courtesy of Prof Walter, Neuropathology, Hannover Medical School.

stature in children, delayed sexual development in adolescents, and gonadal failure in adults presenting as amenorrhea in women and loss of libido in men.

Blood analysis with simple biochemical measurements, and urinalysis often provide the major clue to the presence of more complex disturbances. An attempt should be made to determine the peripheral blood level of adenohypophyseal hormones before operative intervention. The use of hypothalamic releasing hormones allows for distinction between endocrine disorders of pituitary or of hypothalamic origin. The completeness of endocrine exploration depends on certain factors, such as the patient's clinical state and the urgency of neurologic and/or ophthalmologic treatment. Endocrine investigation may be cut to a minimum in cases of increased intracranial pressure or rapidly worsening visual acuity. If no emergency is present, endocrine investigation may be extended to a complete investigation (Table 45.3). For treatment planning, two major endocrine deficits are of essential significance. Hypoadrenalism and diabetes insipidus may contribute to increased operative morbidity and must be corrected before operative intervention.

Preoperative neuro-ophthalmologic evaluation is essential to follow up the patient's visual status after surgical and radiation treatment. Finally, disturbed affective behavior and memory are assessed by neuropsychological tests that will identify cognitive deficits and provide necessary information for postoperative therapy planning.

GROSS MORPHOLOGIC FEATURES

Craniopharyngiomas are considered to be maldevelopmental, histologically benign, well-encapsulated tumors that are structurally similar to suprasellar epidermoid cysts (Zülch 1986, Russell & Rubinstein 1989). Grossly, craniopharyngiomas show three different patterns: cystic, solid and mixed cystic-solid (Fig. 45.6). The tumor may vary greatly in size and extent. Small intrasellar craniopharyngiomas in adults with associated hyperprolactinemia may resemble a pituitary adenoma. Large craniopharyngiomas may reach several centimeters in size and produce compressive neurologic syndromes and obstructive hydrocephalus.

Almost all craniopharyngiomas have solid, cystic and calcified parts, although the relative proportion of these parts may vary greatly. Pediatric craniopharyngiomas are more frequently cystic (40%) and mixed (50%), and in few cases solid (10%). In adults, there are relatively more solid than cystic tumors. The tumor surface is smooth and lobulated, and the thickness of the capsule may vary from thin translucent membrane to grayish opacity. The cut surface in solid parts appears granular and pale. In cystic parts it is spongy and porous with numerous cavities. Fluid within cystic tumors frequently appears dark brownish or black like 'motor oil', containing abundant cholesterol crystals. Degeneration of epithelial cells and central stroma leads to liquefaction of cells, deposition of keratin-like material and cyst formation. These masses of keratin become confluent and undergo calcification. Calcification is seen in almost all childhood craniopharyngiomas and about half of adult craniopharyngiomas.

Areas of actual deposited lamellar bone may be found. Some authors described numerous teeth within the tumor (Seemayer et al 1972, Alvarez-Garijo et al 1981)—although such tumors are to be differentiated from the calcifying odontogenic cyst, which may closely mimic craniopharyngioma. Intratumoral bone formation should not be misinterpreted as a link between craniopharyngioma and teratoma, because bone formation is a secondary, degenerative feature in craniopharyngioma. Neither should bone formation be considered a sign of tumor 'inactivity'. Calcified areas grow by regressive changes of epithelial cells, which may be found between thick lamellae of bone. Indeed, reappearance of calcified areas after tumor removal is considered a reliable sign of tumor recurrence (Pang 1993).

Craniopharyngioma has well-defined outlines relative to the brain. However, it has a tendency locally to infiltrate the surrounding neural tissue, which shows dense productive gliosis. The clinical and surgical significance of these findings is discussed below.

HISTOPATHOLOGIC FEATURES

Light microscopy

Microscopically, solid parts of craniopharyngiomas usually show an external layer of high columnar epithelium, followed by a variable amount of polygonal cells, and a central system of epithelial bands and bridges, which are supported by a vascularized connective tissue stroma (Zülch 1986, Russell & Rubinstein 1989, Adamson et al 1990) (Fig. 45.7). Cystic parts of craniopharyngioma are composed of a simple stratified squamous epithelium. A collagenous basement membrane frequently forms the boundary between the tumor and the surrounding meninges or brain.

The surrounding brain often undergoes intense glial reaction, particularly in the floor of the third ventricle. Small papillary tumor projections into the glial undersurface of hypothalamus appear on histologic slices as detached islands of tumoral epithelium. Cytologic studies of these small islands do not support the interpretation of malignancy (Russell & Rubinstein 1989), and should not be interpreted as actual tumor invasion. It is a strictly localized process that may even provide a dissection plane to remove the craniopharyngioma from surrounding brain without damaging the hypothalamus (Sweet 1980).

Some evidence supports the existence of two distinct craniopharyngioma variants (Kahn et al 1973, Giangaspero et al 1984, Adamson et al 1990). The *adamantinous type*, or so-called childhood craniopharyngioma, resembles histologically the adamantinoma of the jaw, a tumor of odontogenic origin. This type is encountered in virtually all children and in about two thirds of adults. The *papillary type*, so-called adult craniopharyngioma, occurs in about one third of adults and is very rare in children. Only one case of a child with papillary craniopharyngioma has been described (Kahn et al 1973).

Both adamantinous and papillary craniopharyngioma represent benign lesions. However, significant diversity has been emphasized in their histopathologic features and clinical aspects (Kahn et al 1973, Giangaspero et al 1984, Adamson et al 1990). The adamantinous type is histologically characterized by a sparsely cellular stroma surrounded by a single layer of pseudostratified columnar

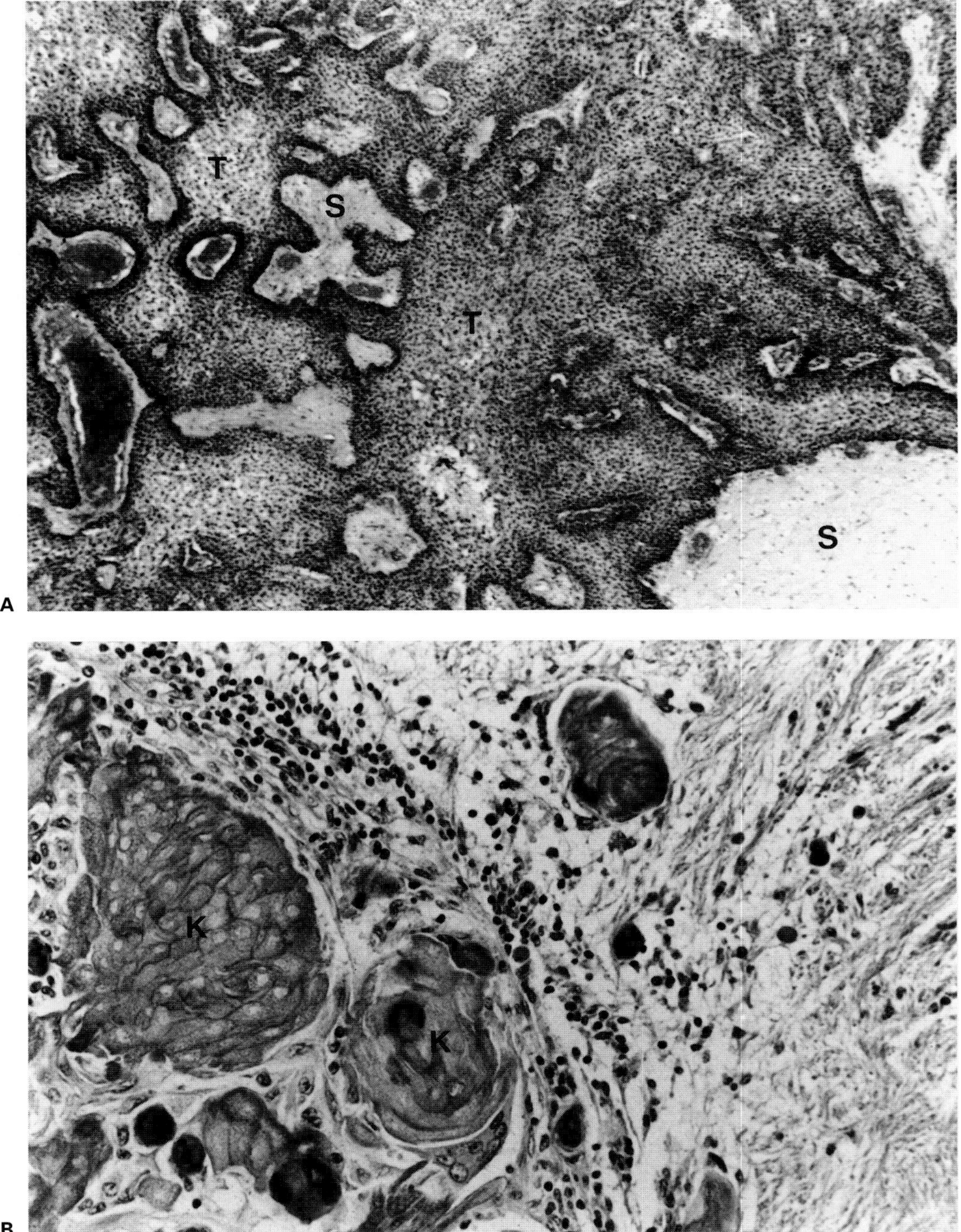

Fig. 45.7 **A.** Light microscopy of adamantinous craniopharyngioma, showing tumor cells (T) surrounded by stroma of connective tissue (S). H&E ×20. **B.** Microscopic appearance of a craniopharyngioma, showing areas of keratin formation (K) surrounded by inflammatory reaction. H&E ×150. Courtesy of Prof Walter, Neuropathology, Hannover Medical School.

epithelium resting on a single basement membrane, calcifications and keratin formation. It represents the classic cystic and calcified craniopharyngioma found in children and most adults. The squamous papillary type is characterized by nests of squamous cells embedded in a connective tissue stroma. It is predominantly solid, noncalcified tumor.

Some authors have questioned the validity of such a distinction between both types of craniopharyngioma (Petito et al 1976, Russell & Rubinstein 1989). Petito et al (1976) described transitional forms of craniopharyngiomas and suggested that craniopharyngiomas represent a single group of tumors, with a range of characteristics from the purely adamantinous type through mixed varied to the squamous papillary type. However, diversity in clinical behavior and outcome between the tumor types has recently been pointed out by Adamson et al (1990). The clinical outcome for the squamous papillary type was much better than for the adamantinous type, and the recurrence rate in the squamous papillary type was much lower than in the adamantinous type. The appearance of small islets of tumor cells in brain tissue seen in adamantinous tumors were not detectable in all 15 squamous papillary craniopharyngiomas examined by Adamson et al (1990).

Moreover, distinct origins have been postulated for childhood and adult craniopharyngiomas (Kahn et al 1973). According to the most popular hypothesis, the adamantinous craniopharyngioma originates from embryonic cell rests of Rathke's pouch, and the squamous papillary craniopharyngioma arises from metaplastic transformation of epithelium found in the adenohypophysis and anterior infundibulum (Goldberg & Eshbaugh 1960). This might explain why adamantinous craniopharyngiomas are more frequently seen in children, while the frequency of squamous papillary craniopharyngiomas increases with age and this type is almost never found in young children. Secretory components of squamous papillary craniopharyngioma have recently been demonstrated by Szeifert et al (1991) in an electron microscopic and mucino-histochemical study. Similar secretory characteristics have been observed in metaplastic adenohypophysis (Adamson et al 1990), and might therefore support the origin of adult craniopharyngioma from metaplastic epithelium of adenohypophysis.

Immunohistochemistry

Immunohistochemical study of cyst fluid production has revealed that the pattern of mucus in cystic craniopharyngioma is quite similar to that produced by the oropharyngeal mucosa (Szeifert et al 1991). Insulin-like growth factor II and its binding proteins have been demonstrated in the cyst fluid of craniopharyngiomas by means of gel chromatography (Zumkeller et al 1991). Since, in the fetal rat, the most intense CNS expression of insulin-like growth factor was found in the epithelium of Rathke's pouch (Ayer-Le Lievre et al 1991), Zumkeller's findings supply additional evidence for the origin of craniopharyngioma from Rathke's pouch.

Shibuya et al (1993) have recently studied the proliferative potential of 7 craniopharyngiomas by means of monoclonal antibodies Ki-67 and anti-DNA polymerase α, bromodeoxyuridine labeling, and nucleolar organizer region counts. Six of the 7 craniopharyngiomas showed a low proliferation cell index, but one tumor revealed a high proliferation index. Although no further information regarding patients' clinical and surgical data is provided, the pattern of proliferative cell activity found in Shibuya's study reflects the variable biological behavior expressed by craniopharyngiomas. This valuable contribution may explain in part the diversity of recurrence rate and heterogeneous response to radiotherapy observed in these tumors.

Electron microscopy

Electron microscopy has added only little to the pool of information obtained with other methods. Although tumor cells vary greatly in size and form, they usually show a relatively uniform pattern with desmosomes, tonofilaments and microvilli. A basal membrane of 45 μm thickness separates aggregates of cells from stroma. The maturation phases to keratin formation have been described, resembling the normal epidermis (Zülch 1986). Hirano et al (1973) described fenestrated capillaries, which are thought to take part in fluid production of cysts. Keratin formation and calcification were studied by Sato et al (1986), who attributed the initial phase of calcification and deposit of hydroxyapatite crystals to small membrane-bound vesicles and tonofibrils. Szeifert et al (1991) have recently studied the pathology of cyst formation. The authors described zymogen granules in the cytoplasm of numerous epithelial cells, and demonstrated secretory activity in microcysts and some epithelial cells. These findings added substantially to the initial idea that cyst formation occurs by purely degenerative changes in the stroma and fenestrated capillaries (Hirano et al 1973, Petito et al 1976). According to the authors, actual mucus secretion also participates in fluid production of cystic craniopharyngiomas.

Tissue culture

Great difficulty in maintaining craniopharyngioma cells in vitro has been the reason for frequent failure of tissue culture in craniopharyngioma. Tissue culture of craniopharyngioma was first successfully described by Cobb & Wright, in 1959, who observed a single layer of epithelium surrounding the implanted cells, and rare mitoses. Characteristics of more aggressive growth expressed in vitro were identified by Liszczak et al (1978). The authors found numerous microvilli on the cell's surface, intense basophilia of the cytoplasm, increase in size and number of nuclei, and retraction of cytoplasm.

Tissue culture has been used for testing tumor sensitivity to colloidal chromic phosphate (32P), which has been employed in vivo as injection into cystic craniopharyngioma (Young et al 1976, van den Berge et al 1992). Kubo et al (1974) tested in tissue culture the sensitivity of craniopharyngioma to bleomycin, a chemotherapeutic agent used against epithelial cancer, with encouraging results.

Cytogenetic study

Very few studies have been done to determine chromosomal patterns of patients with craniopharyngioma (Vagner-Capodano 1991). Vagner-Capodano et al described in 1988 loss of chromosome Y and aneuploidy in three children. Specific chromosomal changes in craniopharyngioma have not yet been defined, and studies with large numbers of cases are lacking. Nonetheless, cytogenetic investigations may present an important key for understanding the pathogenesis of craniopharyngioma.

INCIDENCE OF MALIGNANCY

Craniopharyngiomas grow very slowly and are histologically essentially benign tumors (Russell & Rubinstein 1989). Malignant degeneration is extremely rare (Nelson et al 1988) and metastasis is unknown (Zülch 1986). In the case described by Nelson et al (1988) postoperative radiation therapy was suggested to have induced the craniopharyngioma to malignant transformation (Hoffman 1988).

Characteristics of aggressive tumor growth as demonstrated in vitro (Liszczak et al 1978) may reflect in vivo the tendency of craniopharyngioma to infiltrate the surrounding neural structures. Craniopharyngioma frequently recurs, even after a presumed complete tumor resection. Tumor recurrence usually occurs at the primary site or in contiguous areas. Tumor recurrence along the operative track has been reported (Barloon et al 1988, Ragoowansi & Piepgras 1991) but primary CSF seeding or distal metastasis is unknown.

MANAGEMENT

Management of craniopharyngiomas starts immediately after the diagnostic procedures have been accomplished. Obstructive hydrocephalus and endocrine dysfunction are associated with high peri- and postoperative morbidity, and therefore must be treated before definitive tumor therapy is attempted (Tomita 1988).

Several treatment modalities have been proposed for craniopharyngiomas. There is general agreement on the fact that surgery plays a significant role in the treatment of these tumors (Samii & Bini 1991). Recurrence rates are much lower after total resection than after subtotal resection even when combined with radiation therapy. Management of craniopharyngioma is nevertheless controversial; indications for radiotherapy or a combination of surgery and radiotherapy remain matters of great disagreement among the investigators (Raimondi 1993). Surgical mortality and morbidity have been reduced since the perioperative use of hydrocortisone (Matson & Crigler 1969) and the introduction of microsurgical techniques (Yasargil et al 1990). But there have also been an increasing number of reports of equally successful irradiation of these tumors (Manaka et al 1985, Regine & Kramer 1992, van den Berge et al 1992).

The selection of the most appropriate treatment modality should consider the following aspects: age and general condition of patient, size and growth characteristics of the tumor, experience of the surgeon, and accessibility to radiotherapy. Solid tumors have been treated by radical resection (Samii & Draf 1989, Yasargil et al 1990, Hoffman et al 1992, Wen et al 1992), partial resection with radiation (Regine & Kramer 1992), or primary radiosurgery (Manaka et al 1985). Cystic tumors can be surgically removed (Ammirati et al 1990, Hoffman et al 1992), or stereotactically punctured to reduce the size and permit instillation of radionuclide (van den Berge et al 1992). The value of chemotherapy and the combination of treatment modalities warrant further evaluation.

Management of hydrocephalus

Children usually present preoperatively with symptoms and signs of increased intracranial pressure (70%), and obstructive hydrocephalus is present in about one third of them. Presence of hydrocephalus preoperatively was found to have a negative impact on postoperative outcome and mean survival rate (Wen et al 1989). Ventricular decompression is recommended if the presenting symptoms are mainly related to hydrocephalus. This allows for brain relaxation, after which a definitive tumor approach is carried out.

Disagreement exists whether obstructive hydrocephalus must be treated by external ventricular drainage or shunting. Some authors prefer a shunting procedure in those cases of obstructive hydrocephalus in which the symptoms of high intracranial pressure are disabling (Carmel 1990). If the foramen of Monro is obstructed by a large tumor, bilateral ventricular catheters connected to a single shunting system has been advocated. Others prefer external ventricular drainage at the time of surgery (Pang 1993). Still others prefer a direct tumor approach without ventricle decompression (Choux et al 1991). In the case of chronic hydrocephalus without symptoms of increased intracranial pressure, external ventricular drainage at the time of surgery rather than shunting is preferred to assist in brain relaxation.

Since the majority of cases of hydrocephalus resolve with tumor removal, external ventricular drainage can be closed or elevated (chamber test) postoperatively, and a CT scan evaluation is made. If there is no deterioration of neurologic status or suspicion of enlarging ventricles at CT, the external ventricular drainage is removed. Otherwise, shunting is performed.

Management of endocrine disturbances

Endocrine dysfunction is present in about one half of children and 80% of adults with craniopharyngioma. Growth failure and diabetes insipidus in children, and gonadal failure in adults are the most frequent findings. Hypoadrenalism and hypothyroidism are less common, but when present they lead to intra- and postoperative morbidity unless promptly corrected (Carmel 1990). High stress doses of corticosteroid before surgery replace corticosteroid requirement rapidly. Usually, doses equivalent to three times the physiologic daily cortisone requirement are given in the form of hydrocortisone. In cases of large tumors with brain edema, doses of dexamethasone given for brain stabilization will cover the cortisone lack.

Hypothyroidism takes several days to correct, and therapy should be started promptly. A normal metabolic state must be restored gradually, especially in the elderly or patients with heart disease. L-thyroxine is preferable as a single daily dose, and the dose necessary to sustain a normal metabolic state is usually about 150 μg per day in adults (Ingbar 1987). Infants and children require doses that are disproportionately large in relation to body size. However, in pituitary or hypothalamic hypothyroidism, as occurs in craniopharyngioma, thyroid replacement should never be instituted until treatment with hydrocortisone has been initiated, since acute adrenocortical insufficiency may be precipitated by an increase in metabolic rate (Ingbar 1987).

Diabetes insipidus is frequently present in patients with craniopharyngioma. Children in particular may present with severe alteration of fluid and eletrolytes due to diabetes insipidus. Accurate replacement of deficits along with intravenous or intranasal doses of antidiuretic hormone (desmopressin) will be necessary. Since diabetes insipidus frequently persists after surgery, therapy with desmopressin will usually have to be continued at postoperative care.

Surgical treatment

Since craniopharyngioma is a benign tumor, its total surgical removal is the treatment of choice to achieve cure and prevent recurrence (Pertuiset 1975, Raimondi & Rougerie 1983). If part of the tumor is left in place, it is more likely to recur. The development and refinement of microsurgical techniques have tremendously improved the patient's postoperative outcome.

Surgical approaches

Several surgical approaches have been proposed for removal of craniopharyngiomas (Konovalov 1987, Apuzzo et al 1991) (Fig. 45.8). They range from more 'gentle' procedures such as stereotactic endoscopic intervention for tumor biopsy (Fukushima 1978, Hellwig et al 1991) to more 'aggressive' procedures such as craniofacial splitting for tumor removal (Fujitsu et al 1992). Although craniopharyngioma is considered a midline-located tumor, different patterns of tumor extension, size, consistency, etc.,

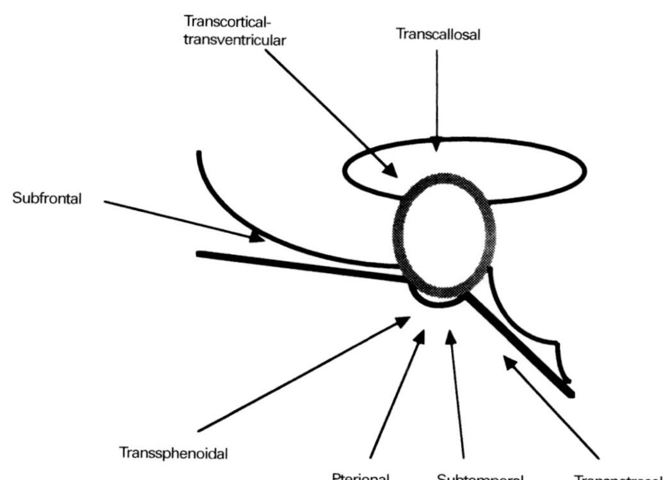

Fig. 45.8 Some of the most usual approaches for craniopharyngioma.

may play a role in choosing the most appropriate approach. For choice of optimal surgical approach four main criteria must be taken into consideration: the shortest route to the tumor, minimal trauma to surrounding structures, the necessary overview, and the flexibility of approach to reach in different directions.

Intrasellar or intra- and suprasellar subdiaphragmatic tumors (grade I–II) can best be operated via a transsphenoidal approach. In the authors' experience, a subfrontal approach is the method of choice for primarily suprasellar tumors (grade III–V). Purely intraventricular craniopharyngiomas can be removed by a transcallosal transventricular approach. Small retrochiasmatic tumors may be operated by a subtemporal route, and large retrochiasmatic tumors extending into the posterior fossa down the clivus may be operated by a transpetrosal-transtentorial approach.

Subfrontal approach. This is the most widely used approach for removal of craniopharyngiomas (Choux et al 1991). We personally prefer this approach because craniopharyngioma is an extra-axial midline lesion whose growth displaces the structures from the midline in any direction. Craniopharyngioma frequently displaces the hypothalamus and optic chiasm upward, creating a large space for dissecting important neurovascular structures. After tumor enucleation, a good view of all important structures is achieved. Large retrochiasmatic tumors with extension forward may convert the lamina terminalis into a paper-thin membrane that can be opened to achieve a view into the third ventricle.

Due to its embryological relationship with the anterior diencephalon, craniopharyngioma does not receive a blood supply from the posterior cerebral or basilar artery; instead it is usually well separated from the posterior vessels and the midbrain by Lilliequist's membrane. During tumor removal, the pituitary stalk can be well recognized under the microscope by its particular striate pattern,

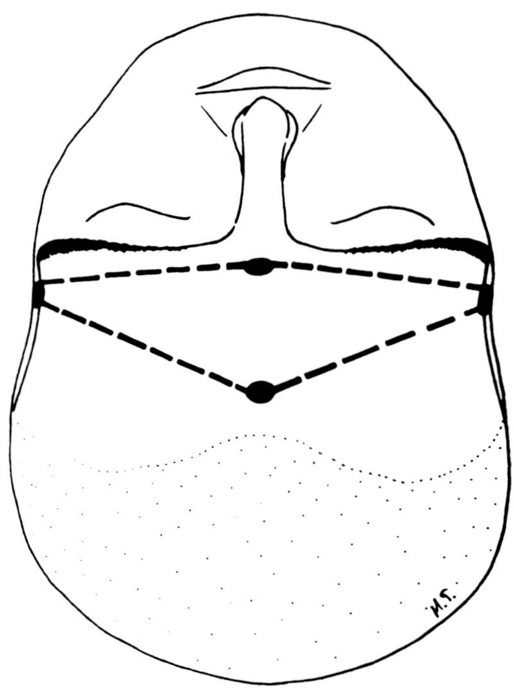

Fig. 45.9 Bilateral subfrontal approach.

determined by long portal veins running along the stalk surface from the inferior hypothalamus to the diaphragma region.

The subfrontal approach starts with a bitemporal coronal incision. For cosmetic reasons we prefer this to a circumscribed flap incision on the forehead. The tumor size and lateral extension will determine whether a unilateral or bilateral exposure is carried out. For a unilateral exposure, three burr holes are made. The lateral burr hole is placed at the root of the zygomatic process of the frontal bone. A small slit can be made in the aponeurosis of the temporal muscle to expose the bony ledge at the temporal fossa. The burr hole is placed directly on that ridge, close to the floor of the anterior cranial fossa. This will avoid a troublesome bony overlapping later on. As the hole is drilled, care is taken not to enter the bony orbit and injure Tenon's capsule. The medial burr hole is placed at the midline, as low as possible. If the frontal sinus is entered, its mucosal lining is stripped away and displaced downward so that the drill can be advanced through the posterior wall of the sinus without damaging the mucosa. This technique helps to prevent spread of pathogenic organisms from the paranasal sinuses into the cranial cavity. If the mucosa is damaged, the frontal sinus is carefully cleaned of mucosa and packed with antibiotic-embedded gauze until the surgical intervention is finished. The third burr hole is placed about 3 cm above and midway between the medial and lateral burr holes. For a bifrontal approach, burr holes are placed bilaterally as the lateral burr hole above, a third burr hole is placed low in the midline, and the fourth about 3–4 cm above the glabella overlying the sagittal sinus (Fig. 45.9).

After turning the craniotomy flap, the dura is opened in

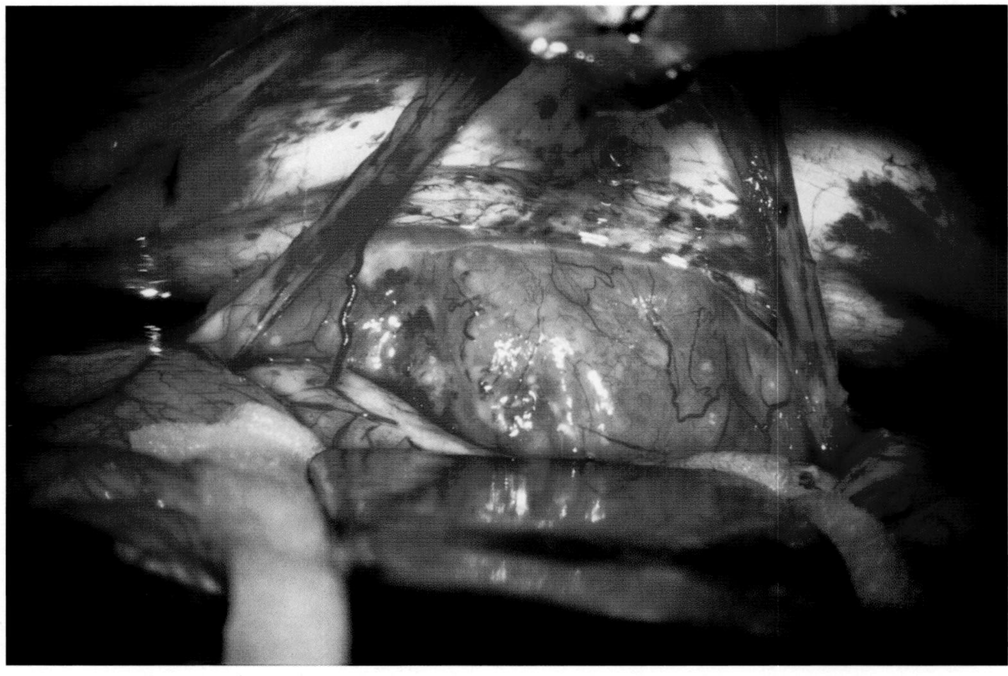

Fig. 45.10 Intraoperative photograph of a craniopharyngioma by subfrontal approach. Both olfactory nerves are preserved after careful microsurgical dissection (note the small artery on the left side running to the nerve). The optic nerves and chiasm are just behind the tumor.

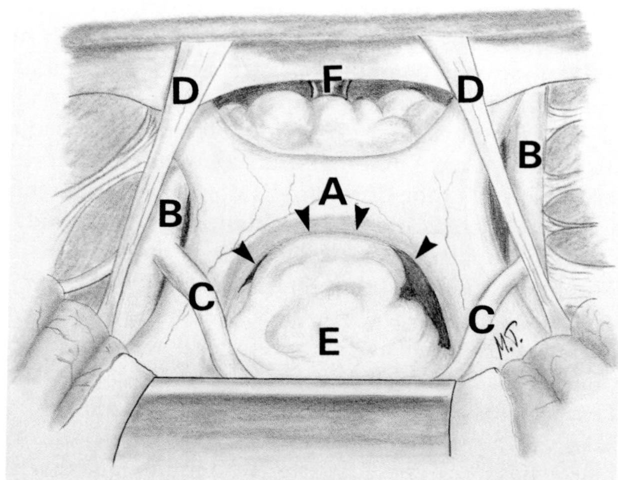

Fig. 45.11 Drawing of the translamina terminalis approach. The lamina terminalis was opened (arrowheads) to expose the intraventricular portion of the tumor (E). A= optic chiasm; B = internal carotid artery; C = anterior cerebral artery; D = olfactory nerve; F = infundibulum.

the unilateral approach with a frontobasal incision lateral to the superior sagittal sinus. The arachnoid cisterns are opened progressively as the frontal lobe is gently retracted. It has proved useful to expose the anterior skull base more from the lateral side, using the lesser sphenoid wing as a landmark. The olfactory nerves are preserved by carefully dissecting them away from the cortical surface (Fig. 45.10). Both optic nerves are exposed. The basal cisterns are then opened to expose the chiasm and to drain CSF, allowing further exposure. In the case of a postfixed chiasm, the tumor removal is first performed between the optic nerves. After tumor debulking, the optic pathway is decompressed, and the pituitary stalk comes into view. The pituitary stalk can be identified by its striate appearance. If there is no tumor infiltration the pituitary stalk should be preserved.

In cases of large retrochiasmatic tumor, giving the chiasm an appearance of prefixity, or in true prefixed chiasm, the approach is through the lamina terminalis (Fig. 45.11). This approach provides access to the inferior part of the third ventricle. By debulking the tumor through the lamina terminalis more space is obtained between the chiasm and the carotid arteries to allow a frontolateral approach for removal of remaining tumor. Tumor with lateral extension beyond the carotid is usually soft and can be removed from a frontolateral approach.

Due to the multidirectional vantage of the bifrontal approach, even large craniopharyngiomas with adherent areas to the hypothalamus can be dissected away and removed (Fig. 45.12). Tumor manipulation can be done not only anteriorly to the chiasm and through the lamina terminalis but also laterally through the optico-carotid space of both sides. During tumor dissection care must be taken to stay within the arachnoid planes. Dissection of the tumor from arterial wall may weaken the adventitia and cause dilatation of major vessels. Tumor dissection on the floor of the hypothalamus should be carried out carefully, so as not to injure functioning nerve tissue.

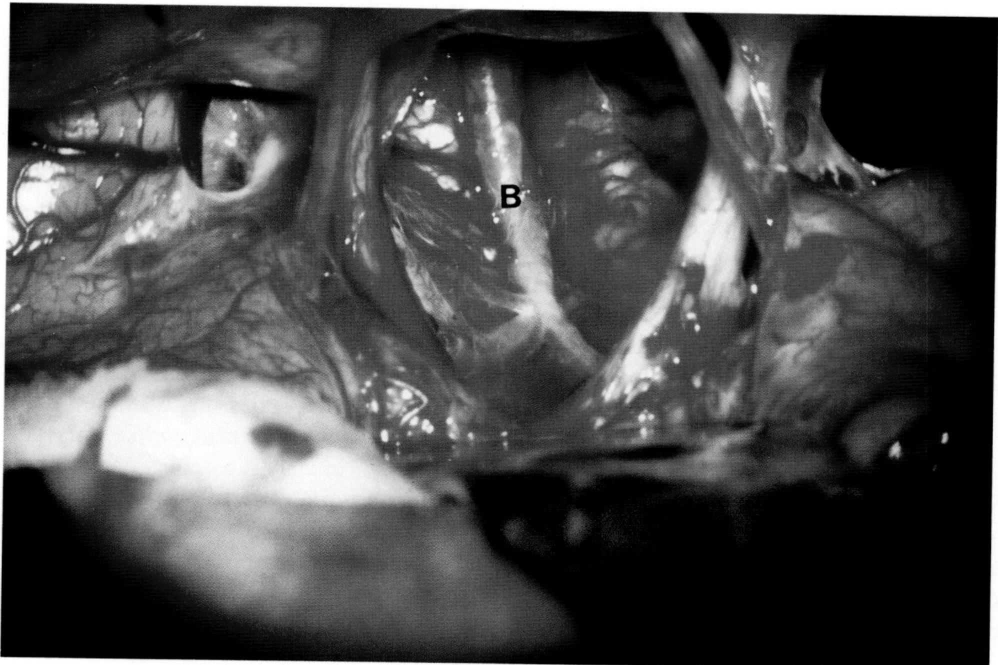

Fig. 45.12 Intraoperative photograph after complete removal of craniopharyngioma by subfrontal approach. The basilar artery (B) is demonstrated between both optic nerves and olfactory nerves.

No attempt is made to remove calcified parts of tumor that are attached to the optic nerves or chiasm until the tumor mass has been enucleated. After thorough enucleation, calcified portions fall away from the optic nerves enough to allow complete removal. When the pituitary stalk is involved it is preferable to free it by section than to pull it with attached tumor because of the risk of damage to the hypothalamus. Sectioning the pituitary stalk must be done as far distally as possible because a remnant of the stalk may recover production of antidiuretic hormone.

When the tumor extends downward in the sella and even in the sphenoid sinus, it can not be removed safely through the standard subfrontal approach. Direct access can be gained by drilling the tuberculum sellae (subfrontal transsphenoidal approach). This provides a good view into the sella, which allows for further tumor excision. If the pituitary stalk is already cut, the sella can be completely curetted. The opening of the sphenoid sinus does not represent a problem; it can be packed with muscle pieces and covered with the same galeal-periosteal flap that is used for closing the frontal sinuses.

Transsphenoidal approach. Primary transsphenoidal surgery is the optimal procedure for intrasellar and suprasellar infradiaphragmatic craniopharyngiomas (grade I–II). This approach involves the nasoseptal or sublabial paraseptal route and opening of the sphenoid sinus (Hardy & Vezina 1976, Laws 1980, Honegger et al 1992). An enlarged pituitary fossa facilitates, but is not a prerequisite for transsphenoidal surgery. Usually, a ballooning of the floor of the sella is found which is extensively removed to amplify the exposure.

When opening the dura, care must be taken not to enter the cavernous sinuses. Anterior compression of the anterior pituitary is a frequent finding and splitting the pituitary is usually necessary to provide access to tumor. The tumor capsule can usually be dissected free from the dura. Removal of the superior portion of the tumor often involves resection of diaphragma that is usually attached to tumor. The pituitary stalk can be preserved in most of the cases.

With the aid of endoscopic technique, parts of tumor beyond the sella can also be visualized (Halves & Sörensen 1982). However, if suprasellar calcifications are found, complete tumor removal is unlikely, and a subfrontal approach will be necessary to accomplish complete excision. Great caution must be used to avoid trauma to the optic nerves and chiasm. Craniopharyngioma with suprasellar extension and attachments to optic chiasm, hypothalamus or vascular structures should not be removed by the transsphenoidal approach. For infradiaphragmatic tumors, however, it is the approach of choice. Low surgical morbidity, and improvement of hyperprolactinemia and preoperative visual deficits have been reported (Honegger et al 1992).

Pterional approach. The frontotemporal (pterional) approach has been employed as the approach of choice by some authors (Yasargil et al 1990, Derome 1991). It may be used alone or in combination with a transsphenoidal or transcallosal approach to access large craniopharyngiomas. This approach allows for a more lateral view than the subfrontal approach although it does not offer a primarily anterior view. Tumor dissection is done in the parachiasmal spaces, such as the prechiasmatic, optico-carotid, or carotido-tentorial spaces, in the triangle superior to the carotid bifurcation, and through the opening of the lamina terminalis (Yasargil et al 1990). The technique of tumor removal is the same as that performed through a subfrontal approach.

Transcallosal approach. This approach is used for primarily intraventricular craniopharyngiomas, although primarily basal craniopharyngioma extending into the third ventricle is better approached by a subfrontal translamina terminalis route as described above.

The transcallosal approach is carried out through a small paramedian frontal craniotomy whose posterior margin is just behind the coronal suture line. The dural flap is turned over the superior sagittal sinus and the exposure is made along the falx with minimal retraction of the frontal lobe away from the falx. The corpus callosum is exposed, which is usually very thin due to obstructive hydrocephalus. A transcallosal incision about 2 cm long is made between or just right lateral to the pericallosal arteries over the location of the foramen of Monro, that is about 1 cm anterior to the interauricular line. This approach provides access into the lateral ventricles just at the dilated foramen of Monro. The tumor capsule is easily visualized. Internal decompression by aspiration of cystic parts and piecemeal removal of solid calcified parts is carried out. Attempts must be made not to damage the fornix, the anterior commissure, the choroid plexus, the choroidal arteries, and the veins of the wall and floor of the third ventricle.

Transcortical approach. The transcortical-transventricular approach was first performed by Busch in 1944 and has been reserved for those cases with large ventricles and tumor extending to the dorsal surface of the frontal lobe (Yasargil et al 1990). This approach is in decreasing use because of difficult ipsilateral dissection, and increased postoperative morbidity such as injury to the floor of the third ventricle, epilepsy, and porencephalic cysts.

Subtemporal approach. This approach has been used for primarily retrochiasmatic and predominantly unilateral tumors. A temporal flap is elevated and extended to the base of the skull. The temporal lobe is retracted and the cisterns are emptied. The tentorium may be divided to access posterior portions of the tumor. Care must be taken not to damage the fourth nerve running at the tentorium surface. If the tumor extends to the posterior fossa along the clivus the subtemporal approach may be combined with a transpetrosal approach (Hakuba et al

1985). The authors believe, however, that such an extensive approach is rarely necessary for craniopharyngioma because the dorsal part of the tumor is usually soft and there are no feeding vessels coming from the basilar artery; the tumor can be debulked, pulled in and freed from surrounding structures from above in most of the cases.

Other approaches. A transfacial approach involving a cranio-nasal median splitting has been described for radical removal of craniopharyngiomas (Fujitsu et al 1992). Standard approaches can sometimes be combined with each other to improve tumor removal. The subtemporal-transpetrosal approach is mentioned above. The pterional approach can be combined with the transcallosal approach for removal of adherent and calcified tumor parts within the third ventricle. The subfrontal approach combined with the pterional approach provides good access to lateral parts of tumor within or beyond the sylvian fissure.

Aspiration and drainage of cystic craniopharyngioma

Different techniques for aspiration and drainage of cystic craniopharyngiomas have been employed since Scarff performed the first cystic drainage in 1941 (Choux et al 1991). Stereotactic aspiration of cystic craniopharyngiomas has been used recently, either before radiotherapy, or for isotope instillation into the cyst cavity (van den Berge et al 1992). Cyst drainage is usually done by inserting a catheter connected to a subcutaneous Ommaya reservoir into the cyst to facilitate repeated aspirations. In children, cyst puncture has sometimes been used to gain time until the child's development is complete and radiotherapy can be performed. Shunting procedures to the ventricles and atrium have been described (Economos 1979).

Surgical results

Total surgical resection of craniopharyngioma is closely related to tumor size, surgical approach, surgeon's experience, and, obviously, attempts to perform a radical resection. A review of the literature revealed rates of total removal using the subfrontal approach of 60%, compared with 53% using the pterional approach (Choux et al 1991). More recent series show total removal rates as high as 90% or higher for craniopharyngioma of all sizes using mainly the subfrontal and pterional approaches (Yasargil 1990, Samii & Bini 1991, Hoffman et al 1992). Purely intrasellar craniopharyngiomas can be totally removed by a transsphenoidal approach in almost all cases (Honegger et al 1992).

Surgical complications and management

Surgical mortality following attempts at radical removal of craniopharyngioma has been reported to be as high as 6%, varying in most large series from 0–15% (Choux et al 1991). Surgical morbidity is still high in most series, mainly due to endocrine, ophthalmologic, and neuropsychological disturbances.

During tumor resection, the pituitary stalk is frequently cut or is so far damaged that endocrinopathy is almost always present after surgery. The most frequent endocrine disorder is diabetes insipidus. The sequence of antidiuretic hormone release after surgery shows three phases. The initial phase with excessive diuresis occurs on the first day, after initial cessation of secretion due to disruption of the pituitary stalk. Between the second and fourth day, distal axons within the pituitary undergo degeneration and release antidiuretic hormone in large amounts. Diuresis reduces and water is retained. The third phase occurs usually after the fourth postoperative day; the stored antidiuretic hormone ceases and excessive diuresis returns.

Fluid balance and electrolyte evaluation twice daily have proved to be essential for therapy. Care must be taken not to give too much fluid during the 'second phase', otherwise water intoxication is likely to occur, aggravating postoperative edema. A short-acting vasopressin preparation is preferred to long-acting preparations because of the rebound effect. Desmopressin is given at first intravenously, and later by nasal spray. Sometimes partial or complete recovery of hypothalamic endocrine function may be observed a long time after surgery.

All patients undergoing craniopharyngioma surgery must be regarded as having hypoadrenalism postoperatively. High doses of hydrocortisone are given for the first few days and then gradually reduced to physiologic daily requirement. Most of the patients have hypothyroidism after surgery, and doses of levothyroxine are started in the second week. Further endocrine dysfunction is evaluated one to two weeks after surgery, and hormone replacement given according to physiologic requirements. Gonadal hormones are usually present in low amounts due to pituitary stalk injury. Male adults usually require testosterone to maintain potency, and females may need to receive FSH and LH preparations for ovulation. Children will not experience puberty unless gonadal hormone replacement is given. Due to growth failure, children may receive growth hormone, starting 6 months after surgery.

Although improvement of preoperative visual deficits has been described after radical tumor resection, the grade and duration of visual loss before surgery are the most significant prognostic factors of postoperative visual status. Severe visual deficits lasting for several days are unlikely to recover after surgery.

With the development of refined microsurgical technique severe hypothalamic trauma during surgery has become unlikely. More often, however, minor surgical trauma to the hypothalamus may result in hypothalamic dysfunctions such as sleep disorders, memory deficits, apathy, and appetite changes (Fischer et al 1990), all having a significant impact on the psychosocial situation of children postoperatively (Palm et al 1992).

Radiation therapy

Before the advent of microsurgery, failure to remove the tumor totally and high postoperative mortality and morbidity rates were the usual picture in surgery for craniopharyngioma. Good operative results presented single reports (Matson & Crigler 1969). Radiotherapy then became widely advocated for the treatment of craniopharyngiomas. With the development of modern neuroimaging tools and microsurgical technique an increasing number of surgeons were re-encouraged to operate on these tumors. Total resection rates higher than 90% and low postoperative mortality and morbidity have become a reality. Today, under the premise that tumor recurrence is lower when total resection is carried out, and because of the potential complications of radiation therapy, some authors have recommended all attempts to achieve total surgical resection of craniopharyngiomas.

However, the role of radiation therapy after subtotal tumor removal of craniopharyngiomas has been advocated by a number of authors (Manaka et al 1985, Fischer et al 1990, Regine & Kramer 1992). Long-term results of combined treatment with surgery and radiation demonstrate that survival rates for patients treated with subtotal removal and irradiation are better than for those with subtotal removal alone (Regine & Kramer 1992). In surgically difficult cases, a conservative surgical procedure combined with radiation therapy has been recommended due to the high risk of surgical complications (Fischer et al 1990). Some authors dare to affirm that the long-term results of combined surgery and radiation are better than results with total resection alone (Fischer et al 1990). Still other authors maintain that the proper treatment of primarily cystic tumors in children is drainage and intracavitary injection of radioactive isotopes (van den Berge et al 1992).

External fractionated radiation

Survival rates for patients treated with surgery and radiotherapy are better than for those treated with surgery alone (Choux et al 1991). Besides, excellent long-term results and good quality of life have been reported with postoperative radiation therapy (Fischer et al 1990). The complications of radiation therapy, however, must not be overlooked, such as radiation necrosis, endocrine deficiency, optic neuritis, and dementia (Carmel 1990). In children in particular, radiation may induce tumors, including meningiomas, sarcomas and gliomas, and reduce intellectual performance (Carmel 1990). Radiation doses usually range from 5000–6500 cGy; doses lower than 5400 cGy have been related to significantly higher tumor recurrence rates (Regine & Kramer 1992). After subtotal tumor removal and radiation therapy, the overall 20-year survival is about 60%, ranging from 78% for patients treated for primary disease to 25% for those treated for recurrence (Regine & Kramer 1992).

Intracavitary irradiation (brachytherapy)

Stereotactic interstitial implantation of radionuclides (brachytherapy) was first described by Leksell & Linden in 1952. It consists of stereotactic aspiration of the cyst followed by implantation of a beta-emitting isotope (Leksell 1971, Backlund 1987). Four different isotopes have been employed: phosphate-32, yttrium-90, rhenium-186, and gold-198, although ^{90}Yt is the most widely used. Brachytherapy has been recommended for solitary cystic craniopharyngiomas (Sturm et al 1988, Backlund et al 1989, Lunsford 1991, Steiner 1991, van den Berge et al 1992). The target radiation dose aimed at the inner surface of the cyst wall is about 200–250 Gy (Lunsford 1991, van den Berge et al 1992). Brachytherapy results in stabilization or reduction in the cyst size in approximately 91% of patients (van den Berge et al 1992). For treatment of residual solid tumor, combination therapy with stereotactic radiosurgery has been used (Lunsford 1991). A major complication is visual impairment; serious deterioration of visual function has been described in about one third of patients (van den Berge et al 1992).

Radiosurgery

Backlund (1973) first used radiosurgery for treatment of craniopharyngiomas. Primary stereotactic radiosurgery has been employed for small solid craniopharyngiomas (size <25 mm). In larger cystic craniopharyngiomas, radiosurgery may follow cyst aspiration and instillation of radioactive material (Backlund et al 1989). Long-term results (3–18 years) of 88 cases were reported by Backlund in 1987; good results were achieved in 55 cases (63%), and 16% of patients died of tumor. The most common adverse effects are sudden impairment of visual fields, described in just under 10% of cases. A target distance from optic pathways of at least 3–5 mm has therefore been recommended (Lunsford 1991).

Summary

The use of radiation therapy for treating craniopharyngiomas is one of the main controversies in neuro-oncology. Indeed, if on one hand an increasing number of data supporting the efficacy of radiation therapy have appeared, on the other hand the adverse effects of radiation, particularly in children, are well known. Results concerning survival rates, recurrences, and morbidity are much better in series of all ages, but this is not always true in pediatric series

(Choux et al 1991). If total surgical resection is likely to be achieved, radiation therapy is not recommended. But if residual tumor is left, radiotherapy may be indicated. Primarily cystic craniopharyngioma may be treated by brachytherapy. Obviously, each case must be considered individually.

Chemotherapy

Intracavitary application of bleomycin in cystic craniopharyngiomas has recently been reported, with encouraging results (Takahashi et al 1985, Broggi et al 1989). Bleomycin is a chemotherapeutic agent used against epithelial tumors. Since craniopharyngioma is a tumor thought to be of epithelial origin, some authors had the idea of testing bleomycin in tissue culture of craniopharyngioma (Kubo et al 1974). The results seemed to be so promising that bleomycin came to be used in cystic recurrence of craniopharyngiomas (Kubo et al 1974, Takahashi et al 1985, Broggi et al 1989). Broggi et al (1989) treated 18 patients with stereotactic intracavitary bleomycin application, and described disappearance of cysts in 13 patients. Transient toxicity from bleomycin, such as fever, nausea, and vomiting may occur, but delayed toxicity including pulmonary fibrosis, rash, stomatitis, and alopecia has not yet been observed.

RECURRENT CRANIOPHARYNGIOMA

A large data collection on craniopharyngioma reveals that the long-term overall recurrence rate of craniopharyngiomas is about 28% (Choux et al 1991). Adults have a lower recurrence rate (20%) than children (30%). Tumors thought to have been totally resected show a recurrence rate of 19%, while those subtotally resected have a recurrence rate of 57%. Postoperative radiation therapy reduces the tumor recurrence rate to 29%, which, however, is higher than the recurrence rate of tumors resected totally. Most recurrences occur during the first 3 years after treatment.

Pathogenesis of recurrence

Tumor regrowth after subtotal resection is an obvious phenomenon. The pathogenesis of tumor recurrence after 'total' tumor resection, however, is not completely understood. Most investigators believe that tumor rests unintentionally left at the floor of the hypothalamus may be the main cause of tumor reappearance. Recurrence rates in children were described to be higher than in adults. Childhood (adamantinous) craniopharyngiomas usually show finger-like projections to the floor of the hypothalamus, which are demonstrated on histologic sections as islets of tumor surrounded by neural tissue; such tumor infiltration into the hypothalamus could not be demonstrated in adult (papillary) craniopharyngiomas (Adamson et al 1990).

Craniopharyngioma recurrence may be related, at least in part, to a tendency of the tumor to 'seed' (Malik et al 1992). Some reports have described tumor recurrence along the line of surgical approach to the parasellar area (Ragoowansi & Piepgras 1991), in the epidural space (Malik et al 1992), or along the line of needle tracks after repeated cyst aspiration (Barloon et al 1988). Malik et al (1992) suggest that craniopharyngioma may behave in a fashion biologically analogous to skin inclusions or seedings of basal cell carcinoma associated with intraoperative tumor manipulation. It is difficult to prove that recurrence of craniopharyngioma may in part be secondary to 'seeding' as proposed in those reports, but this idea represents at least an interesting hypothesis.

Treatment of recurrence

Different treatment modalities are available for recurrences of craniopharyngioma, such as radical tumor resection, subtotal resection combined with radiation therapy, radiation only, brachytherapy, and intracavitary chemotherapy. Reoperation after tumor recurrence or after radiation therapy is considerably more difficult than primary operation, and carries a higher morbidity. Scarring from first operations and irradiated areas may create a monumental task for total tumor resection. However, surgery still has been recommended in recurrent craniopharyngioma if gross total removal seems possible. Regrowth of solid components of tumor in particular may be surgically approached again. Radiation therapy is reserved for those cases in which it is thought that the tumor can not be removed completely by surgery.

OUTCOME

Before the patient is discharged from the hospital, postoperative CT must be obtained to exclude surgical complications such as bleeding, hydrocephalus, and subdural hygroma. CT scan will eventually show small rests of tumor or calcifications, which must be followed up by further investigations, or sent for radiation therapy. The next CT (and MRI) are obtained in about 6 months. If no tumor regrowth is seen, further investigations are done yearly. Endocrine evaluation is performed 2 months after surgery by an endocrinologist. Ophthalmologic tests are done according to postoperative visual status, but at least yearly.

The general survival rate of craniopharyngioma after 10 years is approximately 90% (Choux et al 1991). Survival rate after total tumor removal is a little better than after subtotal removal, but this difference is compensated for if radiation therapy is performed (Choux et al 1991).

Developments in diagnostic tools and treatment modalities have substantially improved the outcome of patients with craniopharyngioma by reducing the frequency of neurologic, endocrine and ophthalmologic complications. However, neuropsychological disorders have still been reported in 30–60% of patients (Choux et al 1991). Children in particular can usually compensate for neurologic and endocrine deficits, but not for psychosocial deficits, which may result in limited quality of life as patients grow into adulthood (Bloom et al 1990, Fischer et al 1990).

Neuropsychological deficits, including intellectual and memory dysfunction, affective immaturity, and hyperphagia, are complex disorders that require a specialized therapy program. Only an interdisciplinary approach employing diagnosticians and therapists from different areas, as well as the patient's social background, will translate the results of improved quantity of life achieved hitherto to an improved quality of life.

REFERENCES

Adamson T E, Wiestler O D, Kleihues P, Yasargil M G 1990 Correlation of clinical and pathological features in surgically treated craniopharyngiomas. Journal of Neurosurgery 73: 12–17

Alvarez-Garijo J A, Froufe A, Taboada D, Vila M 1981 Successful surgical treatment of an odontogenic ossified craniopharyngioma. Case report. Journal of Neurosurgery 55: 832–835

Ammirati M, Samii M, Sepehrnia A 1990 Surgery of large retrochiasmatic craniopharyngioma in children. Child's Nervous System 6: 13–17

Apuzzo M L J, Levy M L, Tung H 1991 Surgical strategies and technical methodologies in optimal management of craniopharyngioma and masses affecting the third ventricular chamber. Acta Neurochirurgica 53 (suppl): 77–88

Arwell W J 1926 The development of the hypophysis cerebri in man, with special reference to the pars tuberalis. American Journal of Anatomy 37: 159–193

Ayer-Le Lievre C, Stålbom P A, Sara V R 1991 Expression of IGF-I and II mRNA in the brain and cranio-facial region of the rat fetus. Development 111: 105–115

Baba M, Iwayama S, Jimbo M, Kitamura K 1978 Cystic craniopharyngioma extending down into the upper cervical spinal canal. No Shinkei Geka 6: 687–693

Babinski J 1900 Tumeur du corps pituitaire sans acromegalie et avec arret de developement des organes genitaux. Revue Neurologique (Paris) 8: 531–533

Backlund E O 1973 Studies on craniopharyngiomas. IV. Stereotaxic treatment with radiosurgery. Acta Chirurgica Scandinavica 139: 344–351

Backlund E O 1987 Role of stereotaxis in the management of midline cerebral lesions. In: Apuzzo M L J (ed) Surgery of the third ventricle. Williams & Wilkins, Baltimore, pp 802–805

Backlund E O, Axelsson B, Bergstrand C G et al 1989 Treatment of craniopharyngiomas — the stereotactic approach in a ten to twenty-three years' perspective. I. Surgical, radiological and ophthalmological aspects. Acta Neurochirurgica 99: 11–19

Banna M 1973 Craniopharyngioma in adults. Surgical Neurology 1: 202–204

Barloon T J, Yuh W T, Sato Y, Sickels W J 1988 Frontal lobe implantation of craniopharyngioma by repeated needle aspirations. American Journal of Neuroradiology 9: 406–407

Bloom H L G, Glees J, Bell J 1990 The treatment and long-term prognosis of children with intracranial tumors. A study of 610 cases, 1950–1981. International Journal of Radiation, Oncology, Biology and Physics 18: 723–745

Broggi G, Giorgi C, Franzini A, Servello D, Sorelo C L 1989 Preliminary results of intracavitary treatment of craniopharyngioma with bleomycin. Journal of Neurosurgical Sciences 33: 145–148

Busch E 1944 A new approach for the removal of tumors of the third ventricle. Acta Psychiatrica 19: 57–60

Carmel P W 1979 Surgical syndromes of the hypothalamus. Clinical Neurosurgery 27: 133–159

Carmel P W 1990 Brain tumors of disordered embryogenesis. In: Youmans J R (ed) Neurological surgery, 3rd edn, vol 5. W B Saunders, Philadelphia, pp 3223–3249

Choux M, Lena G, Genitori L 1991 Le craniopharyngiome de l'enfant. Neurochirurgie (Paris) 37 (suppl 1): 12–165

Cobb J P, Wright J C 1959 Studies of a craniopharyngioma in tissue culture. I. Growth characteristics and alterations produced following exposure to two radiometric agents. Journal of Neuropathology and Experimental Neurology 18: 563–568

Combelles G, Ythier H, Wemeau J L, Cappoen J P, Delandsheer J M, Christiaens J L 1984 Craniopharyngiome dans une même fratrie. Neurochirurgie 30: 347–349

Cushing H 1932 The craniopharyngiomas. In: Intracranial tumors. Notes upon a series of two thousand verified cases with surgical-mortality percentages pertaining thereto. Charles C Thomas, Springfield, IL, pp 93–98

Derome P 1991 Opinions. In: Choux M, Lena G, Genitori L (eds) Le craniopharyngiome de l'enfant. Neurochirurgie (Paris) 37 (suppl 1): 167

Drazin M B, Stelling M W, Johanson A J 1980 Silver-Russel syndrome and craniopharyngioma. Journal of Pediatrics 96: 887–889

Economos D 1979 Systemic shunting of residual intraparenchymatous cystic craniopharyngioma. Acta Neurochirurgica (suppl) 28: 363–366

Erdheim J 1904 Über Hypophysenganggeschwülste und Hirncholesteatome. Sitzungsbericht der Kaiserlichen Akademie der Wissenschaften. Mathematisch-naturwissenschaftliche Classe (Wien) 113 (sect 3): 537–726

Ezrin C, Weiss M 1990 Neuroendocrinology. In: Youmans J R (ed) Neurological surgery, 3rd edn. W B Saunders, Philadelphia PA, pp 741–751

Fischer E G, Welch K, Shillito J, Winston K R, Tarbell N J 1990 Craniopharyngiomas in children. Long-term effects of conservative surgical procedures combined with radiation therapy. Journal of Neurosurgery 73: 534–540

Fröhlich A 1901 Ein Fall von Tumor der Hypophysis cerebri ohne Akromegalie. Wiener Klinische Rundschau 15: 883–906

Fujitsu K, Saijo M, Aoki F, Fuji S, Mochimatsu Y, Gondo G 1992 Cranio-nasal median splitting for radical resection of craniopharyngiomas. Neurological Research 14: 345–351

Fukushima T 1978 Endoscopic biopsy of intraventricular tumors with the use of a ventriculofiberoscope. Neurosurgery 2: 110–113

Fukushima T, Hirakawa K, Kimura M, Tomonaga M 1990 Intraventricular craniopharyngioma: Its characteristics in magnetic resonance imaging and successful total removal. Surgical Neurology 33: 22–27

Galatzer A, Nofar E, Beit-Halachmi N et al 1981 Intellectual and psychosocial functions of children, adolescents and young adults before and after operation for craniopharyngioma. Child's Care, Health and Development 7: 307–316

Gambarelli D, Perez-Castillo M 1991 Histogenèse et anatomopathologie. In: Choux M, Lena G, Genitori L (eds) Le craniopharyngiome de l'enfant. Neurochirurgie (Paris) 37 (suppl 1): 21–28

Giangaspero F, Burger P C, Osborne D R, Stein R B 1984 Suprasellar papillary squamous epithelioma ("papillary craniopharyngioma"). American Journal of Surgical Pathology 8: 57–64

Gökalp H Z, Egemen N, Ildan F, Bacaci K 1991 Craniopharyngioma of the posterior fossa. Neurosurgery 29: 446–448

Goldberg G M, Eshbaugh D E 1960 Squamous cell nests of the pituitary gland as related to the origin of craniopharyngioma. A study of their presence in the newborn and infants up to age four. Archives of Pathology 70: 293–299

Hakuba A, Nishimura S, Inoue Y 1985 Transpetrosal-transtentorial approach and its application in the therapy of retrochiasmatic craniopharyngiomas. Surgical Neurology 24: 405–415

Halstead A E 1910 Remarks on an operative treatment of tumors of the hypophysis. Surgery, Gynecology and Obstetrics 10: 494–502

Halves E, Sörensen 1982 Indications for the trans-sphenoidal approach to craniopharyngioma operations in youth and childhood. In: Voth D, Gutjahr P, Langmaid C (eds) Tumors of the central nervous system in infancy and childhood. Springer, Berlin, pp 270–275

Hardy J, Vezina J L 1976 Transsphenoidal neurosurgery of intracranial neoplasm. Advances in Neurology 15: 261–274

Hellwig D, Bauer B L, List-Hellwig E, Mennel H D 1991 Stereotactic-endoscopic procedures on processes of the cranial midline. Acta Neurochirurgica 53 (suppl): 23–32

Helmke K, Hausdorf G, Moehrs D, Laas R 1984 CCT and sonographic findings in congenital craniopharyngioma. Neuroradiology 26: 523–526

Hirano A, Ghatak N R, Zimmerman H M 1973 Fenestrated blood vessels in craniopharyngioma. Acta Neuropathologica 26: 171–177

Hoffman H J 1988 Comment. In: Nelson G A, Bastian F O, Schlitt M, White R L. Malignant transformation in craniopharyngioma. Neurosurgery 22: 429

Hoffman H J, De Silva M, Humphreys R P, Drake J M, Smith M L, Blaser S I 1992 Aggressive surgical management of craniopharyngiomas in children. Journal of Neurosurgery 76: 47–52

Honegger J, Buchfelder M, Fahlbusch R, Däubler B, Dörr H 1992 Transsphenoidal microsurgery for craniopharyngioma. Surgical Neurology 37: 189–196

Hua F, Asato R, Miki Y et al 1992 Differentiation of suprasellar nonneoplastic cysts from cystic neoplasms by Gd-DTPA MRI. Journal of Computed Assisted Tomography 16: 744–749

Huk W J, Gademann G, Friedmann G 1990 MRI of central nervous system diseases. Springer, Berlin, pp 268–270

Hurst R W, McLlhenny J, Park T S, Thomas W O 1988 Neonatal craniopharyngioma. CT and ultrasonographic features. Journal of Computed Assisted Tomography 12: 858–861

Ingbar S H 1987 Diseases of the thyroid. In: Braunwald E, Isselbacher K J, Petersdorf R G, Wilson J D, Martin J B, Fauci A S (eds) Harrison's Principles of internal medicine, 11th edn, vol 2. McGraw-Hill, New York, pp 1732–1752

Iwasaki K, Kondo A, Takahashi J B 1992 Intraventricular craniopharyngioma: report of two cases and review of the literature. Surgical Neurology 38: 294–301

Kahn E A, Crosby E C 1972 Korsakoff's syndrome associated with surgical lesions involving the mammilary bodies. Neurology 22: 117–125

Kahn E A, Gosch H H, Seeger J F, Hicks S P 1973 Forty-five years' experience with the craniopharyngiomas. Surgical Neurology 1: 5–12

Konovalov A N 1987 Technique and strategies of direct surgical management of craniopharyngioma. In: Apuzzo M L J (ed) Surgery of the third ventricle. Williams & Wilkins, Baltimore, pp 542–553

Kubo O, Takakura K, Miki Y, Okino T, Kitamura K 1974 Intracystic therapy of bleomycin for craniopharyngioma — effect of bleomycin for cultured craniopharyngioma cells and intracystic concentration of bleomycin. No Shinkei Geka 2: 683–688

Kubota T, Fuji H, Ikeda K, Ito H, Yamamoto S, Nakanishi I 1980 A case of intraventricular craniopharyngioma with subarachnoid hemorrhage. No Shinkei Geka 8: 495–501

Laws E R Jr 1980 Transsphenoidal microsurgery in the management of craniopharyngioma. Journal of Neurosurgery 52: 661–666

Leksell L 1971 Stereotaxis and radiosurgery: An operative system. Charles C Thomas, Springfield, Ill

Leksell L, Linden K 1952 Radioisotope techniques. Medical and physiological applications. HM Stationery Office, Oxford, Vol 1, pp 1–4

Lewis D D 1910 A contribution to the subject of tumors of the hypophysis. Journal of American Medical Association 55: 1002–1008

Liszczak T, Richardson E P Jr, Phillips J P, Jacobson S, Kornblith P L 1978 Morphological, biochemical, ultrastructural, tissue culture and clinical observations of typical and aggressive craniopharyngiomas. Acta Neuropathologica (Berlin) 43: 191–203

Lunsford L D 1991 Opinions. In: Choux M, Lena G, Genitori L (eds) Le craniopharyngiome de l'enfant. Neurochirurgie (Paris) 37 (suppl 1): 170–171

McLean D J 1930 Die craniopharyngealtaschen Tumoren (Embryologie, Histologie, Diagnose und Therapie). Zeitschrift der Gesellschaft für Neurologie und Psychiatrie CXXVI: 639–682

McKenzie K G, Sosman M C 1924 The roentgenological diagnosis of craniopharyngeal pouch tumors. American Journal of Roentgenology XI: 171–176

Maier H C 1985 Craniopharyngioma with erosion and drainage into the nasopharynx. An autobiographical case report. Journal of Neurosurgery 62: 132–134

Malik J M, Cosgrove F R, VandenBerg S R 1992 Remote occurence of craniopharyngioma in the epidural space. Journal of Neurosurgery 77: 804–807

Manaka S, Terramoto A, Takakura K 1985 The efficacy of radiotherapy for craniopharyngioma. Journal of Neurosurgery 62: 648–656

Mancini J, Simonin G, Chabrol B 1991 Signes initiaux. In: Choux M, Lena G, Genitori L (eds) Le craniopharyngiome de l'enfant. Neurochirurgie (Paris) 37 (suppl 1): 31–43

Matson D D, Crigler J F Jr 1969 Management of craniopharyngioma in childhood. Journal of Neurosurgery 30: 377–390

Mori K, Kurisaka M 1986 Brain tumors in childhood: statistical analysis of cases from the Brain Tumor Registry of Japan. Child's Nervous System 2: 233–237

Mott F W, Barrett J O W 1899 Three cases of tumor of the third ventricle. Archives of Neurology (Chicago) 1: 417–440

Mukada K, Mori S, Matsumura S, Uozumi T, Goishi J 1984 Infrasellar craniopharyngioma. Surgical Neurology 21: 565–571

Nelson G A, Bastian F O, Schlitt M, White R L 1988 Malignant transformation in craniopharyngioma. Neurosurgery 22: 427–429

Okamoto H, Harada K, Uozumi T, Goishi J 1985 Spontaneous rupture of a craniopharyngioma cyst. Surgical Neurology 24: 507–510

Palm L, Nordin V, Elmqvist D, Blennow G, Persson E, Westgren U 1992 Sleep and wakefulness after treatment for craniopharyngioma in childhood; influence on the quality and maturation of sleep. Neuropediatrics 23: 39–45

Pang D 1993 Surgical management of craniopharyngioma. In: Sekhar L N, Janecka I P (eds) Surgery of cranial base tumors. Raven Press, New York, pp 787–807

Pertuiset B 1975 Craniopharyngiomas. In: Vinken P J, Bryun G W (eds) Handbook of clinical neurology, vol 18. Tumors of the brain and skull, part III. North-Holland, Amsterdam, pp 531–572

Petito C K, De Girolami U, Earle K M 1976 Craniopharyngiomas: A clinical and pathological review. Cancer 37: 1944–1952

Plum F, van Uitert R 1978 Nonendocrine diseases and disorders of the hypothalamus. In: Reichlin S (ed) The hypothalamus. Raven Press, New York, p 415

Ragoowansi A T, Piepgras D G 1991 Postoperative ectopic craniopharyngioma. Case report. Journal of Neurosurgery 74: 653–655

Raimondi A J 1987 Parasellar tumors. In: Pediatric neurosurgery. Theoretical principles, art of surgical techniques. Springer, Berlin, pp 276–291

Raimondi A J 1993 Craniopharyngioma: complications and treatment failures. Weaken case for aggressive surgery. Critical Reviews in Neurosurgery 3: 7–24

Raimondi A J, Rougerie J 1983 A critical review of personal experiences with craniopharyngiomas: clinical history, surgical techniques, and operative results. In: Concepts in pediatric neurosurgery. Karger, Basel, pp 1–34

Ravindram M, Radhakrishnan V V, Rao V R 1980 Communicating cystic craniopharyngioma. Surgical Neurology 14: 230–232

Raybaud C, Rabehanta P, Girard N 1991 Aspects radiologiques des craniopharyngiomes. In: Choux M, Lena G, Genitori L (eds) Le craniopharyngiome de l'enfant. Neurochirurgie (Paris) 37 (suppl 1): 44–58

Regine W F, Kramer S 1992 Pediatric craniopharyngiomas: long term results of combined treatment with surgery and radiation. International Journal of Radiation, Oncology, Biology and Physics 24: 611–617

Rougerie J, Fardeau M 1962 Les cranio-pharyngeomes. Masson, Paris, pp 1–217

Russell D S, Rubinstein L J 1989 Pathology of tumors of the nervous system, 5th edn. Williams & Wilkins, Baltimore, pp 695–704

Samii M, Bini W 1991 Surgical treatment of craniopharyngiomas. Zentrallblatt für Neurochirurgie 52: 17–23
Samii M, Draf W 1989 Surgery of the skull base. An interdisciplinary approach. Springer, Berlin
Sato K, Kubota T, Yamamoto S, Ishikura A 1986 An ultrastructural study of mineralization in craniopharyngiomas. Journal of Neuropathology and Experimental Neurology 45: 463–467
Seemeyer T A, Blundell J S, Wiglesworth F W 1972 Pituitary craniopharyngioma with tooth formation. Cancer 29: 423–430
Shibuya M, Ito S, Miwa T, Davis R L, Wilson C B, Hoshino T 1993 Proliferative potential of brain tumors. Analyses with Ki-67 and anti-DNA polymerase alpha monoclonal antibodies, bromodeoxyuridine labeling, and nucleolar organizer region counts. Cancer 71: 199–206
Snell R S 1983 Clinical embryology for medical students, 3rd edn. Little, Brown and Co, Boston, p 261
Snyder J R, Lustig-Gillman I, Milio L, Morris M, Pardes J G, Young B K 1986 Antenatal ultrasound diagnosis of an intracranial neoplasm (craniopharyngioma). Journal of Clinical Ultrasound 14: 304–306
Sorva R, Heiskanen O 1986 Craniopharyngioma in Finland. A study of 123 cases. Acta Neurochirurgica 81: 85–89
Steiner 1991 Opinions. In: Choux M, Lena G, Genitori L (eds) Le craniopharyngiome de l'enfant. Neurochirurgie (Paris) 37 (suppl 1): 172
Streeten D H P, Moses A M, Miller M 1987 Disorders of the neurohypophysis. In: Braunwald E, Isselbacher K J, Petersdorf R G, Wilson J D, Martin J B, Fauci A S (eds) Harrison's Principles of internal medicine, 11th edn, vol 2. McGraw-Hill, New York, pp 1722–1732
Sturm V, Wowra B, Clorius J et al 1988 Intracavitary irradiation of cystic craniopharyngiomas. In: Lunsford L D (ed) Modern stereotactic neurosurgery. Martinus Nijhoff, Boston, pp 229–233
Sutton L N, Gusnard D, Bruce D A, Fried A, Packer R J, Zimmermann R A 1991 Fusiform dilatations of the carotid artery following radical surgery of childhood craniopharyngiomas. Journal of Neurosurgery 74: 695–700
Sweet W H 1980 Recurrent craniopharyngiomas: Therapeutic alternatives. Clinical Neurosurgery 27: 206–229
Symon L, Sprich W 1985 Radical excision of craniopharyngioma. Results in 20 patients. Journal of Neurosurgery 62: 174–181
Szeifert G T, Julow J, Szabolcs M, Slowik F, Bálint K, Pásztor E 1991 Secretory component of cystic craniopharyngiomas: A mucino-histochemical and electron-microscopic study. Surgical Neurology 36: 286–293
Tabaddor K, Shulman K, Dal Canto M C 1974 Neonatal craniopharyngioma. American Journal of Diseases of Children 128: 381–383
Takahashi H, Nakazawa S, Shimura T 1985 Evaluation of postoperative intratumoral injection of bleomycin for craniopharyngioma in children. Journal of Neurosurgery 62: 120–127
Thomsett M J , Conte F A, Kaplan S L, Grumbach M M 1980 Endocrine and neurological outcome in childhood craniopharyngioma: Review of effect of treatment in 42 patients. Journal of Pediatrics 97: 728–735
Tomita T 1988 Management of craniopharyngiomas in children. Pediatric Neurosciences 14: 204–211
Urasaki E, Fukurama A, Itho Y et al 1988 Craniopharyngioma in the third ventricle. No Shinkei Geka 16: 1399–1404
Vagner-Capodano A M 1991 Étude cytogénétique. In: Choux M, Lena G, Genitori L (eds) Le craniopharyngiome de l'enfant. Neurochirurgie (Paris) 37 (suppl 1): 29–30
Vagner-Capodano A M, Gentet J C, Choux M et al 1988 Chromosome abnormalities in sixteen pediatric brain tumors. Pediatric Neurosciences 14: 113
Van den Berge J H, Blaauw G, Breeman W A P, Rahmy A, Wijngaarde R 1992 Intracavitary brachytherapy of cystic craniopharyngiomas. Journal of Neurosurgery 77: 545–550
Van Effenterre R, van Effenterre G, Cabanis E A, Zizen M T I 1991 Tumeurs suprasellaires chez les sujets agés de plus de 70 ans. Intérêt d'une crâniectomie fronto-temporale limitée. Résultats visuels. A propos de 5 cas. Neurochirurgie 37: 330–337
Vargas J R, Pino J A, Murad T M 1981 Craniopharyngiomas in two siblings. Journal of American Medical Association 16: 1807–1808
Voelker J L, Campbell R L, Muller J 1991 Clinical, radiographic, and pathological features of symptomatic Rathke's cleft cysts. Journal of Neurosurgery 74: 535–544
Wakai S, Arai T, Nagai M 1984 Congenital brain tumor. Surgical Neurology 21: 597–609
Wald S L, Liwnicz B H, Truman T A, Khobadad G 1982 Familial primary nervous system neoplasms in three generations. Neurosurgery 11: 12–15
Weber F, Mori Y 1976 Congenital craniopharyngioma. Helvetica Paediatrica Acta 31: 261–270
Wen B C, Hussey D H, Staples J et al 1989 A comparison of the roles of surgery and radiation therapy in the management of craniopharyngiomas. International Journal of Radiation, Oncology, Biology and Physics 16: 17–24
Wen D Y, Seljeskog E L, Haines S J 1992 Microsurgical management of craniopharyngioma. British Journal of Neurosurgery 6: 467–474
Yamamoto T, Yoneda S, Funatsu N 1989 Spontaneous haemorrhage in craniopharyngioma (letter). Journal of Neurology, Neurosurgery and Psychiatry 52: 803–804
Yasargil M G, Curcic M, Kis M, Siegenthaler G, Teddy P J, Roth P 1990 Total removal of craniopharyngiomas. Approaches and long-term results in 144 patients. Journal of Neurosurgery 73: 3–11
Young H F, Fu Y S, Fratkin M 1976 Organ culture of craniopharyngioma and its cellular effects induced by colloidal chromic phosphate. Journal of Neuropathology and Experimental Neurology 35: 404–412
Zülch K J 1986 Brain tumors. Their biology and pathology, 3rd edn. Springer, New York, pp 426–433
Zumkeller W, Sääf M, Rähn T, Hall K 1991 Demonstration of insulin-like growth factors I, II and heterogeneous insulin-like growth factor binding proteins in the cyst fluid of patients with craniopharyngioma. Neuroendocrinology 54: 196–201

46. Dermoid, epidermoid and neurenteric cysts

Francis G. Johnston   H. Alan Crockard

INTRODUCTION

In contradistinction to some of the lesions described in this volume, the lesions to be described in this chapter are so rare that they may only occasionally present within a general neurosurgical practice. Even in a specialist unit the numbers are relatively few, yet they obtain a fascination well in excess of the morbidity they produce. While within the strict Latin meaning these lesions are *tumors* they do not fall within Willis' definition (Willis 1967) of malignancy but produce morbidity by virtue of their slow expansion or because of associated congenital malformations.

INCIDENCE AND PREVALENCE OF TUMORS

Dermoid and epidermoid cysts

Cruveilhier (1829) provided the first description of a hitherto unrecognized lesion of the central nervous system, an epidermoid tumor, and coined the term 'tumeur perlée'. Although this original description was of an epidermoid lesion, the macroscopic similarity between dermoid and epidermoid tumors led to the assimilation of both under the name of 'pearly tumours' (Tytus & Pennybacker 1956).

The incidence of dermoid and epidermoid tumors is variously reported between 0.2 and 1.8% of all brain tumors (Mahoney 1936, Sweet 1940, Grant & Austin 1950, Berger & Wilson 1985), and the latter outnumber the former in a ratio of 4:1 (Yasargil et al 1989).

Neurenteric cysts

Originally, the term enterogenous cyst was first applied by Harriman (1958) to an anterior intradural cyst bearing a respiratory-type epithelium. Puusepp (1934) described one of these extremely rare lesions as a teratoma but subsequent review demonstrated its true nature and the term neurenteric cyst was used for such lesions (Agnoli et al 1984). Only 64 histologically verified cases had been described, representing 0.01% of central nervous system tumors (Itakura et al 1986, Chang et al 1992) although it is likely that others are now detected but not reported in the literature.

AGE DISTRIBUTION

Dermoid and epidermoid cysts

Dermoids were originally thought to occur in the pediatric age group, while epidermoids are detected in the third to fifth decades although age at presentation varied from birth to 80 years of age (Mahoney 1936). Love & Kernohan (1936) found that the mean age of presentation was 22 years, but this was in the pre-CT scan era.

In Yasargil's series (1989) the mean ages at presentation for dermoids and epidermoids were 36 and 37 years respectively, again with a wide age scatter.

Neurenteric cysts

In a review of 23 cases reported in the literature in which sufficient clinical information was supplied (French 1990) 50% presented between birth and 5 years, 30% between 10 and 20 years, and 20% over 20 years of age. By contrast, a more contemporary series and literature review (Agnoli et al 1984) revealed presentations between 0 and 10 years in 21%, 10 and 20 years in 21%, and the remaining 58% at greater than 20 years of age. Thus, we conclude that there is really no firm age of presentation with this extremely rare lesion.

SEX DISTRIBUTION

Dermoid and epidermoid cysts

The sex distribution of these lesions varies in the literature between no sex predilection and a slight male preponderance (Yasargil et al 1989, Lunardi et al 1989).

Neurenteric cysts

According to Agnoli et al (1984), there are 2 males to every female affected (Fig. 46.1).

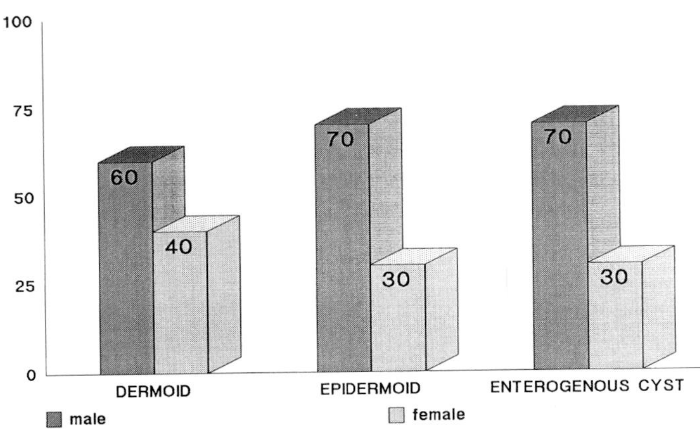

Fig. 46.1 Histogram showing the sex distribution of dermoids, epidermoids and neurenteric cysts.

RACIAL, NATIONAL, GEOGRAPHIC CONSIDERATIONS

To our knowledge there is no literature from which to draw conclusions.

FAMILY HISTORY AND GENETIC FACTORS

Dermoid and epidermoid cysts

Plewes & Jacobson (1971) described the familial clustering in four cases of dermoid cysts. They noted the occurrence of dermoids in relation to the embryologic frontonasal process, at the glabella, the bridge and tip of the nose, and the deep septal region. Apart from these rare cases there is no familial tendency to develop these lesions.

SITES OF PREDILECTION

Dermoids

Dermoid cysts have a greater tendency than epidermoids to occupy midline positions within the neuraxis: in the cerebellar vermis, cauda equina, scalp, orbit and paranasal region (Baxter & Netsky 1985). In the cerebellar midline, the tumors may be related to a dermal sinus, predisposing the patient to pyogenic meningitis (Tytus & Pennybacker 1956). In the cauda equina likewise, lesions within the conus may be related to a sinus with similar consequences; most, however, occur as lesions isolated from the skin. Spinal dermoid tumors, although rare, account for 17% of primary spinal tumors in the first year of life (Takeuchi et al 1978), reducing to 13% for the next 15 years (Matson 1969). List (1941) found dermoids more commonly than epidermoids within the spinal canal at all ages, the reverse of the situation intracranially where epidermoids predominate. Intracranial lesions as a whole are six times more common than their spinal counterparts (Lunardi et al 1989).

In the scalp, dermoid tumors occur anywhere but, in infants, cluster around the anterior fontanelle as the congenital subgaleal dermoid (Martinez-Lage et al 1985). 'External angular dermoids' in children are usually scalp lesions with no deep extension although the diploe may be involved. True dermoids, orbital and paranasal, are relatively rare, epidermoid lesions in this location being more common.

Epidermoids

Epidermoids tend to occupy lateral positions, and Mahoney (1936) noted that most occurred in the cerebellopontine angle (37%), parapituitary region (31%), diploe (16%), rhomboid fossa (11%), and spinal canal (5%). They may also arise in the petrous bone (Pennybacker 1944, King et al 1989), giving rise to progressive deafness and facial palsy (Jefferson & Smalley 1938) (Fig. 46.2).

Lesions of the diploe often involve the frontal and parietal bones; cysts in relation to the anterior fontanelle occur less frequently than their dermoid counterparts (Martinez-Lage et al 1985); giant examples in these locations are rare but reported (Dias et al 1989). The parapituitary group usually abut the medial temporal lobe and middle fossa, although examples occur close to the anterior central skull base and jugum sphenoidale (Fig. 46.3). Occasionally supratentorial epidermoids spread along the ventricular ependyma and may rupture into the ventricle or subarachnoid space. Brainstem epidermoids are rare, only 9 cases being described to date (Obana & Wilson 1991).

In the spine, epidermoids are rarer than dermoids and tend to occur at thoracic levels, with the same tendency to be associated with midline fusion defects. Both dermoids and epidermoids are associated with spina bifida (Bailey 1970, Lunardi et al 1989), dermal sinus (List 1941), myelomeningocele (Martinez-Lage et al 1985), diastematomyelia (Manno et al 1962), and hemivertebra (Pear 1970). Since the introduction of stylets to lumbar puncture needles, implantation lesions have become a rarity (Choremis et al 1956).

Neurenteric cysts

Neurenteric cysts most commonly occur in the cervicodorsal region from C3 to T12 (Agnoli et al 1984) but have been described in various intracranial locations and at the craniovertebral junction (Fabinyi & Adams 1979, Markwalder & Zimmerman 1979, Harai et al 1981, Anderes 1984, Yoshida et al 1986, Koksel et al 1990, Scaravilli et al 1992). They are usually situated anterior to the neuraxis and may communicate with a posterior mediastinal cyst in up to 50% of cases through a vertebral body defect. The incidence of communications and vertebral

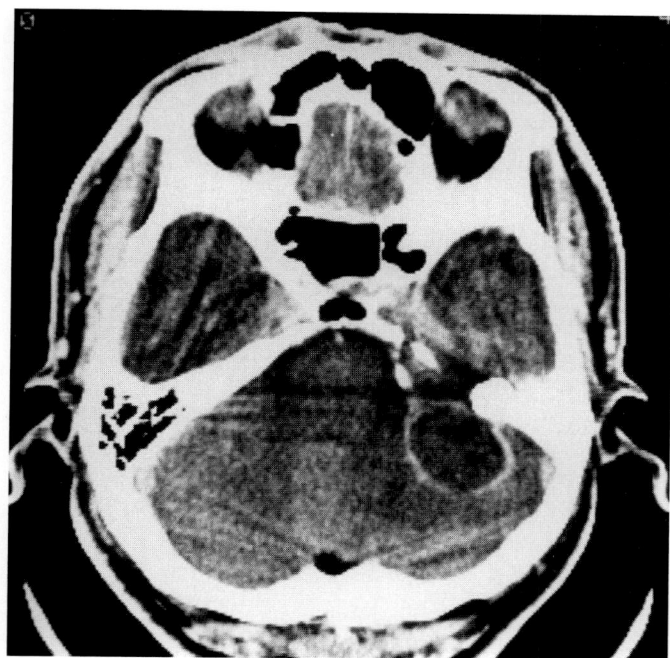

A

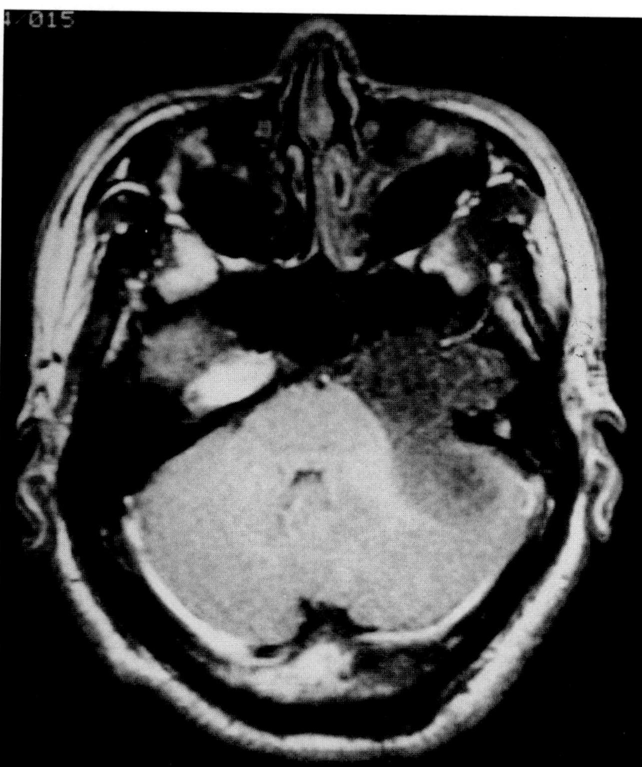

B

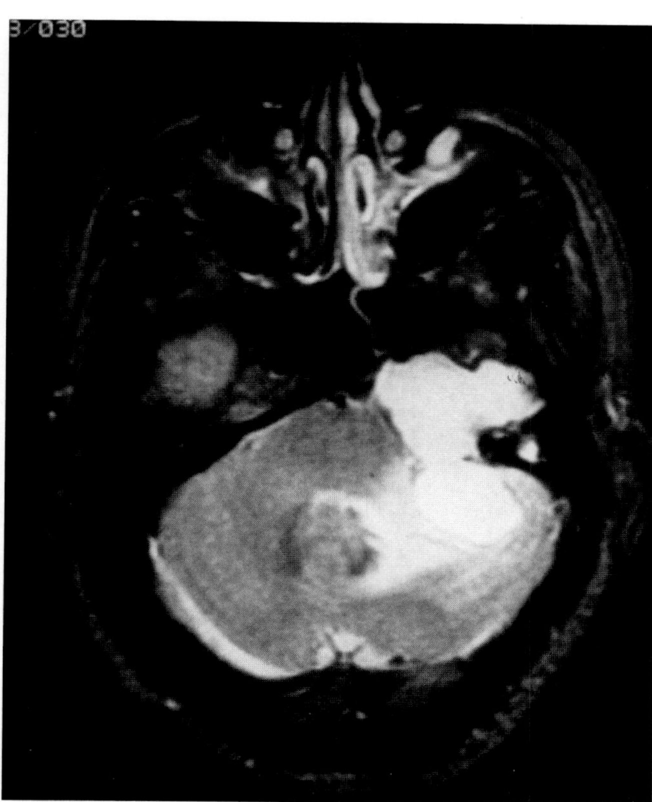

C

Fig. 46.2 Petrous epidermoid. **A.** Enhanced CT scan through the posterior fossa showing a petrous apical epidermoid. Note the osteolysis at the petrous apex and the capsular enhancement. **B.** T1-weighted MR scan of the same lesion. A low intensity lesion extends from the petrous apex into the region of the lateral recess. **C.** T2-weighted image showing the high intensity signal consistent with fat, along with vasogenic edema in the cerebellum.

body defects may be as high as 80% in patients presenting under 10 years of age, compared with 25% in those over that age (French 1990).

PRESENTING FEATURES

Dermoid and epidermoid cysts

In common with location comes diversity in presentation, but there are a few common principles worthy of note. These lesions are congenital and give rise to symptoms by virtue of their slow inexorable growth by desquamation and secretion. They possess a unique capacity to 'flow' into any available space and tend to dissect along naturally occurring planes, usually without neural strangulation until a late phase. By the time of presentation, therefore, these lesions are often extensive, extra-axially enveloping the cranial nerves and blood vessels. They grow so slowly that local mass effect is far less than might be seen with a true tumor in the same area. Cerebrospinal fluid flow is affected late, if at all, and cranial nerve or neuraxial symptomatology is often irritative rather than dysfunctional.

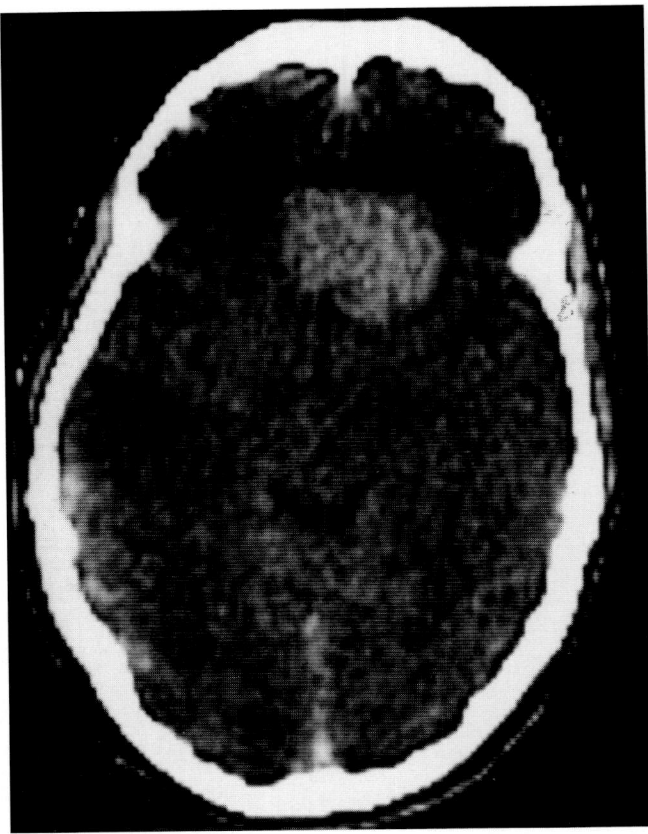

A

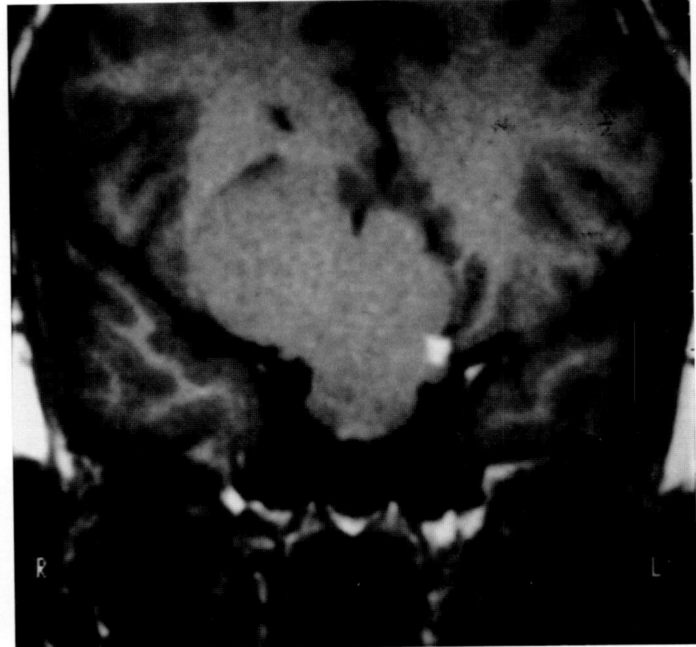

B

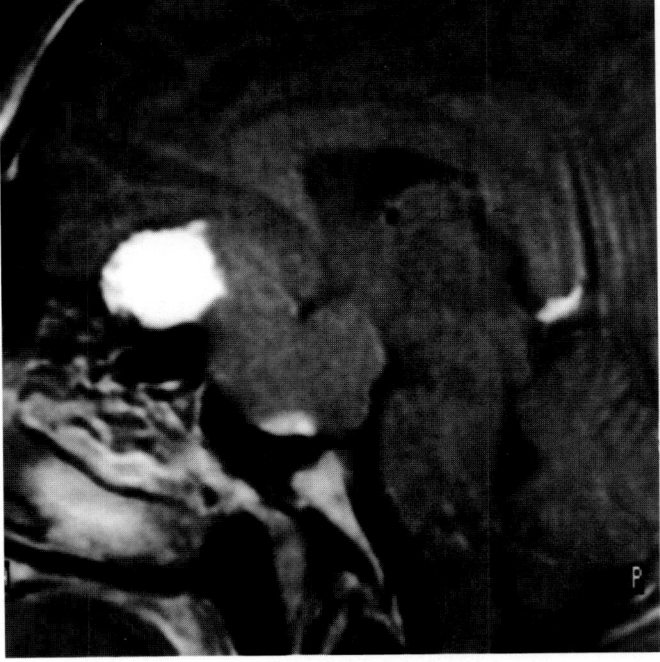

C

Fig. 46.3 Sellar-jugum epidermoid. **A.** Plain axial CT scan showing 'fat-fluid level' in a cystic epidermoid. **B.** T1-weighted coronal MR scan of the same patient. Note the low signal sellar and suprasellar component. **C.** T1-weighted sagittal MR scan showing varying signal intensity within the same lesion. The higher signal anteriorly corresponds to proteinaceous fluid in the cystic component.

Scalp cysts are painless, rubbery, mobile swellings in the region of the anterior fontanelle or midline in children, or in relation to frontal and parietal bones in adults. The lesions are not attached to the skull and are mobile, lying within the dermis. Midline cysts of the scalp in children are associated with midline fusion defects in 25% of cases (spina bifida, myelomeningocele, failure of vertebral segmentation and cleft palate). Associated tracts passing through the bone down to and through the dura must be excluded preoperatively.

Diploic lesions are painless masses with characteristic radiologic features (Cushing 1922); they are commonly frontoparietal, but when in relation to the lateral orbital wall displace the globe downward and medially without neurologic compromise (Ulrich 1964). Petrous lesions cause deafness and facial weakness (Jefferson & Smalley 1938, King et al 1989).

Intracranial lesions arise most commonly in the basal cisterns and Yasargil et al (1989) noted that the clinical history was characteristically protracted with a mean duration of symptoms of 6.8 (dermoid) and 8.2 years (epidermoid). In only 14% of 43 patients was the history less than one year, and in 28% it exceeded a decade. The

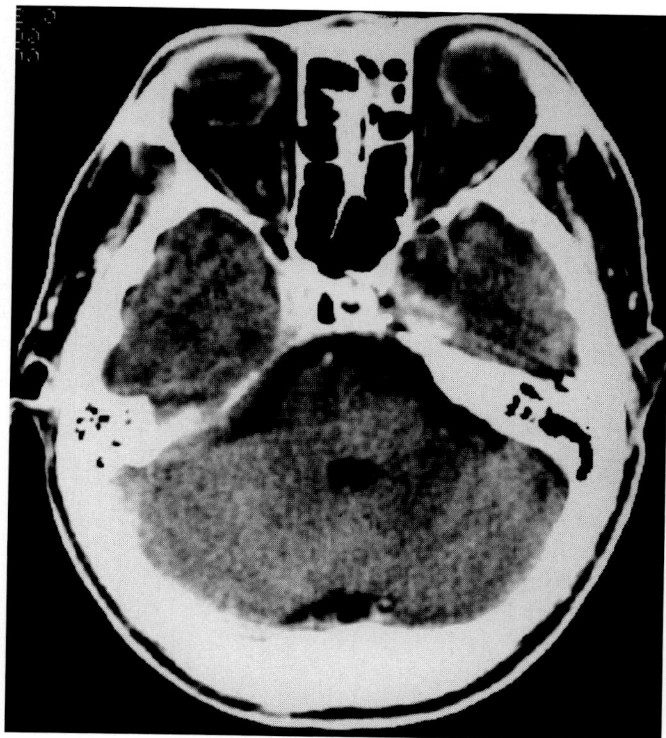

A

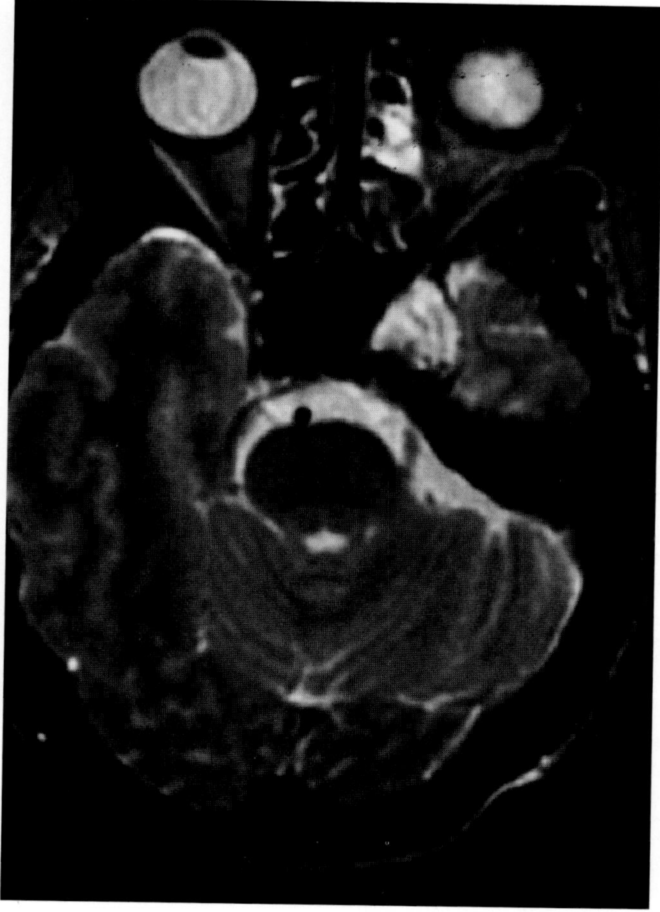

B

Fig. 46.4 Parasellar epidermoid. **A.** Enhanced axial CT scan through the parasellar region showing a low density area in relation to the left cavernous sinus and Meckel's cave. **B.** Axial T2-weighted MR scan of the same patient showing high signal in the parasellar region with displacement of the medial temporal lobe.

17 supratentorial lesions in this series most commonly presented with headache (47%) and epilepsy (53%), hemiparesis and cranial nerve palsies being relatively uncommon. Of the 26 infratentorial lesions, cerebellar impairment (42%) and cranial nerve palsies were common, and facial analgesia or trigeminal neuralgia and vestibulocochlear involvement occurred in 27% and 50% respectively. 12% of patients in this series had no abnormal neurology.

Intracranial lesions occurred in five areas (Conley 1985); suprasellar/chiasmatic lesions produced impairment of visual acuity and hemianopic defects, although pituitary dysfunction and occasionally diabetes insipidus were seen (Tan 1972). Parasellar lesions produced seizures and trigeminal sensory loss (Fig. 46.4). Retrosellar lesions caused trigeminal neuralgia or hemifacial spasm, along with ataxia, nystagmus and hemiparesis. Basilar region cysts usually presented with lower cranial nerve palsies alone, whilst intraventricular lesions exhibited a variable clinical course, with frequent occurrence of dementia or psychiatric disturbance, and this is often attributed to demyelination (Bailey 1920). Hydrocephalus, even with tumors filling the aqueduct, is unusual (Rosario et al 1981).

Spinal dermoids show a caudal predilection maximal at the conus if the extramedullary lesions caused by multiple lumbar punctures with needles lacking stylets are excluded (Choremis et al 1956, Tan 1972). The symptoms are characteristically intermittent, spanning a long period of time. Lunardi et al (1989) noted in their 16 patients with spinal dermoid and epidermoid tumors that 25% presented with localized vertebral pain, and all patients with conus lesions had radicular pain. Motor deficits, usually upper but occasionally lower motor neuron in type, were present in all patients, and 63% had sphincter disturbances. Some lesions (31%) were associated with midline fusion defects such as sinuses, diastematomyelia or angioma planum with a hairy patch and 31% had a subjective sensory loss.

Neurenteric cysts

Spinal neurenteric cysts usually produce cervical cord syndromes ranging from the central cord and Brown-Séquard syndromes to the more common 'numb clumsy hands and spastic paraparesis'. Motor symptoms are often intermittent and have frequently been misdiagnosed as demyelination (Agnoli et al 1984). In this large review of cases available until 1984, Puusepp's (1934) first histologically verified case exhibited chronicity of symptoms for 17 years. Although a large proportion of these patients have radiologic evidence of midline fusion defects, only one patient presented with scoliosis and mild motor neurology.

IMAGING DIAGNOSIS

Dermoid and epidermoid cysts

Cushing (1922) provided the first radiologic description of an epidermoid with a discrete sharply demarcated area of bony destruction with raised edges of increased density.

Computerized tomographic (CT) scanning, particularly with bone windows, will define the relationship of the lesion to bone and show any discrete osteolysis (Fig. 46.5).

Both types present with low attenuation (–22 to +32 Hounsfield units), the range reflecting the content of low density lipid and high density keratin within the lesion, contrast enhancement not usually occurring with either histology. Dermoids show a greater tendency to calcify and display a greater range of X-ray attenuation (Osborne 1985). Characteristically, due to their slow growth, the ventricular system is usually patent and hydrocephalus occurs rarely or very late. In rare cases of malignant change enhancement may be seen (Dubois et al 1981).

MR has superceded CT for accurate preoperative evaluation and planning, especially in posterior fossa lesions. Epidermoid lesions produce increased T1 and T2 relaxation times manifesting as low signal on T1 and high signal on T2 images (Steffey et al 1988). Depending on lipid content, variable signal intensities within the same lesion may be seen (Fig. 46.3).

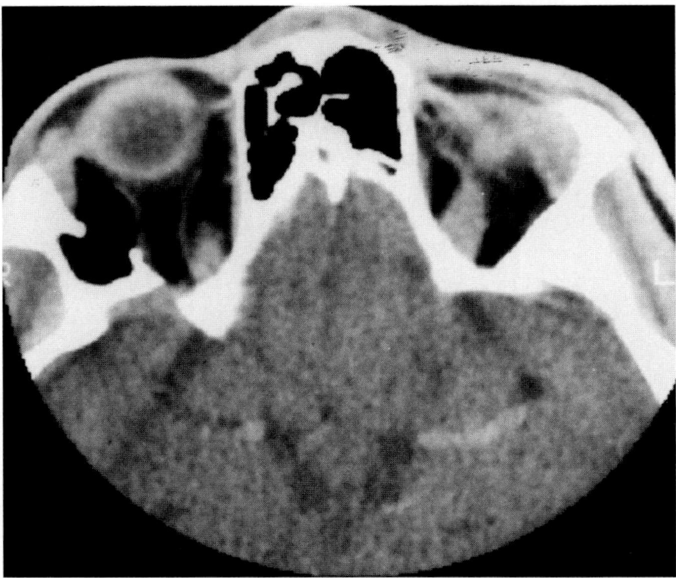

Fig. 46.5 Orbital dermoid. Plain CT scan showing an extraconal lesion of fatty attenuation in the right orbit which has eroded through a bony defect into the infratemporal fossa.

Neurenteric cysts

Plain radiography may reveal associated vertebral defects, and myelography may demonstrate a smooth well-defined lesion usually lying in an intradural extramedullary location. MR scanning has of course now superceded myelography (Fig. 46.6).

LABORATORY DIAGNOSIS

The laboratory has relatively little place in the diagnosis of all lesions excepting histopathologic studies (vide infra). Cerebrospinal fluid analysis in cases of epidermoid cyst rupture has shown cholesterol crystals in the cerebrospinal fluid together with a mild nonspecific lymphocytosis and raised protein .

GROSS MORPHOLOGIC FEATURES

Dermoid lesions are well-defined, opaque, oval or rounded multilobular masses and in general demarcated

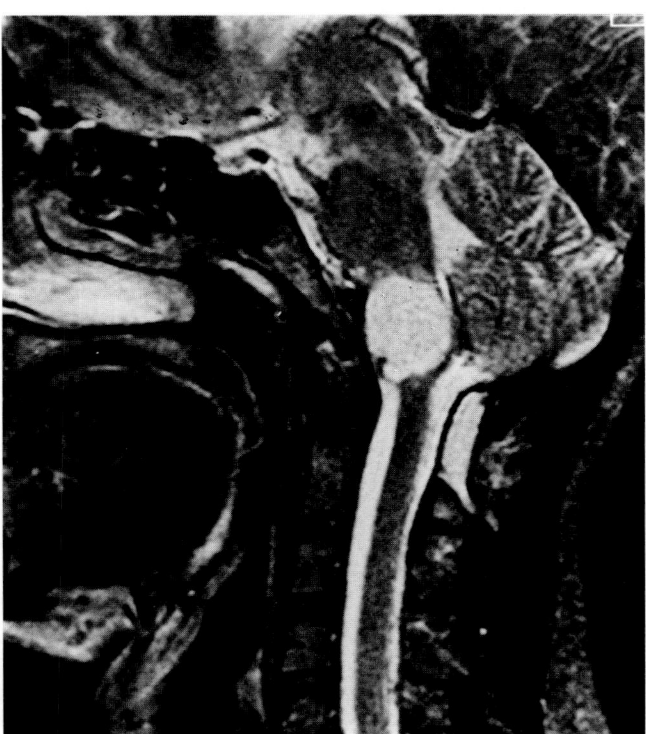

Fig. 46.6 Neurenteric cyst. T2-weighted sagittal MR scan of the craniovertebral junction showing a neurenteric cyst lying within the craniospinal neuraxis which was treated by transoral decompression.

from surrounding structures by a wall which varies considerably in its thickness and adherence and bearing on the internal surface papillary projections to which skin appendages may be related. Calcification may be found in the wall. The contents of the cyst are classically thick, buttery and xanthomatous due to the secretion of sebaceous material and epithelial desquamation, but alternatively may be brown and mucoid. Hairs may be found mixed within this material but teeth are rare (Russell & Rubinstein 1989). It may be related externally to a dermal sinus overlying the lesion, especially in the spinal canal or posterior fossa (Tytus & Pennybacker 1956); this disposes to pyogenic sepsis.

Epidermoid cysts are similar to dermoids but are consistently circumscribed with an irregular nodular surface which may have the mother-of-pearl sheen which gained it the title of 'pearly tumour' (Cruveilhier 1829). Calcification is more commonly found in the capsule than with dermoids (Peyton & Baker 1942). The interior is consistently filled with a white soft material more waxy than with dermoids and which may be rich in cholesterol crystals. It often forms lamellations, but alternatively the contents may be thick, brown and viscid.

Neurenteric cysts macroscopically are smooth lesions bounded by a thin translucent membrane containing fluid varying from clear and colorless through xanthochromic to chocolate color and viscid. There may be mediastinal enteric cysts and ileal duplications; most patients with the former have a direct communication through a defect in a vertebral body to the spinal cyst itself. The incidence of communications as well as vertebral body defects likewise is greater in younger patients, with 80% of the under-10-year group having mediastinal cysts compared to 25% of older patients.

HISTOPATHOLOGIC FEATURES

The lining of ***dermoid cysts*** is usually simple squamous epithelium; however, in some areas this is more differentiated to resemble skin, and in other areas one may see hair follicles along with sebaceous and sweat glands (Fig. 46.7). Upon rupture of a cyst, localized granulomas or granulomatous meningitis with giant cell foreign body reaction to cellular debris, especially cholesterol, is seen.

Epidermoid lesions have a simple stratified squamous epithelium with an external collagen support. Progressive exfoliation produces the lamellar appearance of the lesion (Fig. 46.8). As with dermoid cysts, rupture may lead to a granulomatous response but cholesterol crystals are rare (Love & Kernohan 1936).

Neurenteric cysts bear a simple low or high columnar epithelium (Fig. 46.9) which upon electron microscopy is seen to be ciliated (Hirano et al 1971). Occasionally squamous metaplasia is seen but this is comparatively rare.

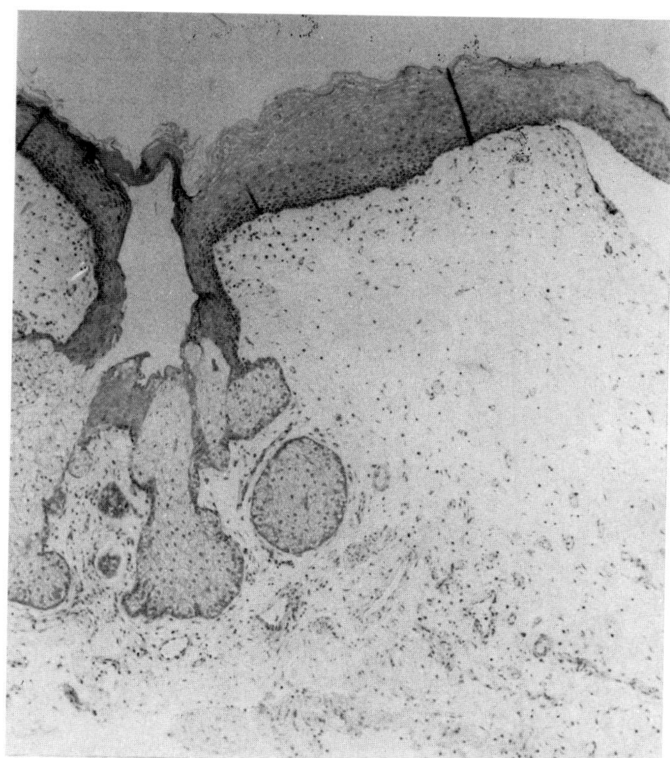

Fig. 46.7 Dermoid cyst. A section from an intramedullary cyst lined by stratified squamous epithelium with sebaceous glands in the wall. H&E ×95. Courtesy of Dr N Alsanjari.

DEFINITION AND INCIDENCE OF MALIGNANCY

Only 13 cases of malignant change in ***dermoid and epidermoid cyst*** have been described (Garcia et al 1981, Lewis et al 1983). Most patients died within one year, a sharp contrast to the usual clinical course. In two cases (Landers and Danielski 1960, Kompf & Menges 1977) there were carcinomatous meningitides. Goldman & Gandy (1987) reported malignant change and development of a squamous carcinoma 33 years after successful surgical resection of a benign intraventricular supratentorial epidermoid cyst. A small number of apparently primary carcinomas occurring in the cerebellopontine angle in patients with 10-year clinical histories implies the occurrence of malignant change in a pre-existing unsuspected cerebellopontine angle epidermoid (Nosaka et al 1979, Garcia et al 1981).

Alvord (1977) has shown that the growth potential of epidermoid tumors is linear and similar to that of normal skin. Hence, if resection leaves a very small microfragment of residual tumor the time for clinical recurrence with the production of a lesion equal in size to that at original presentation is equivalent to the first time plus 9 months. In clinical terms this means an effective clinical cure for the majority of patients, who show no recurrence

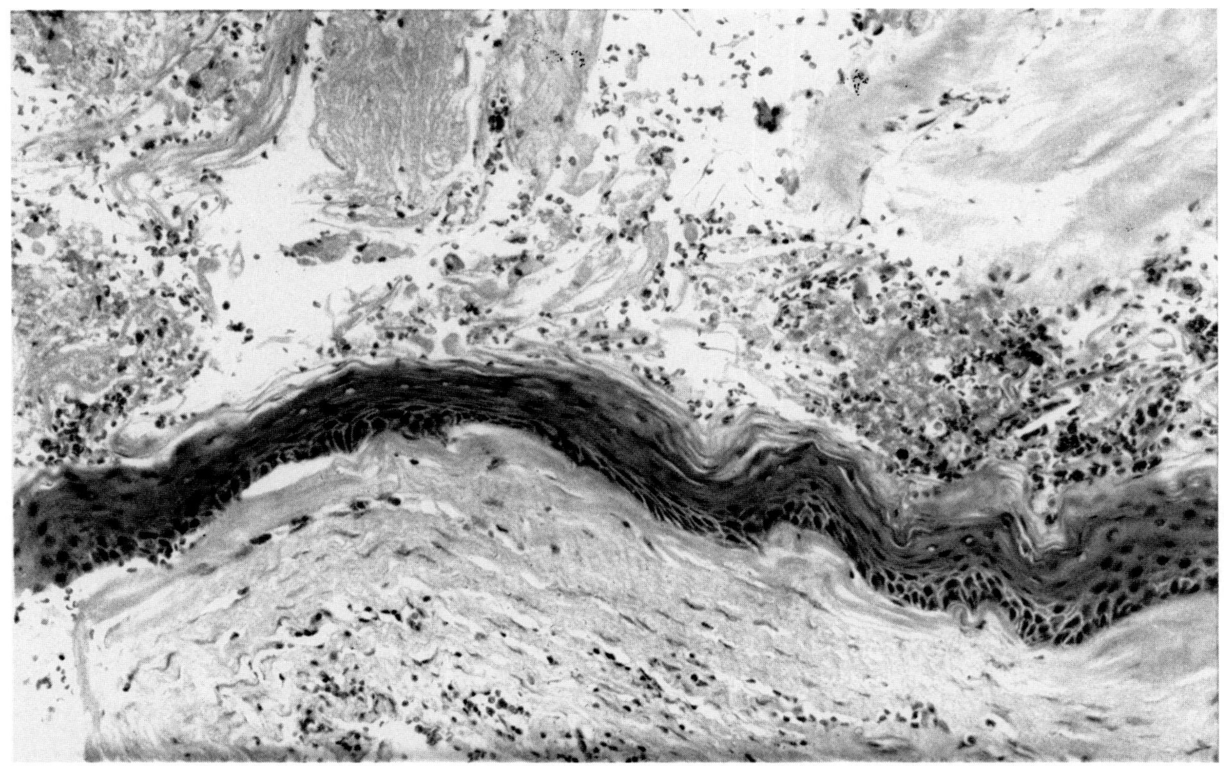

Fig. 46.8 Epidermoid cyst. A cyst lined by cornified stratified squamous epithelium. The lumen is filled with keratin flakes with some inflammatory cells. H&E ×120. Courtesy of Dr N Alsanjari.

over a long follow-up period (Yasargil et al 1989). These tumors never spread by transcranial extension but CSF dissemination in cases of rupture is known (Manno et al 1962, Maravilla 1977).

Neurenteric cysts are histologically entirely benign lesions and no case of malignant change is on record.

GENERAL MANAGEMENT PLAN

The aim of management in these slowly growing lesions is to palliate the patient's symptomatology whilst aiming at a total macroscopic resection, if possible, with minimal neurologic disability. It is to be remembered that patients presenting with lower cranial nerve palsies are unlikely to improve. Lesions found coincidentally may well be observed, as the natural history of the tumor is known according to Alvord (1977).

The ***preoperative assessment*** of the patient's physical status should be full, paying particular attention to cardiovascular and respiratory status. Routine hematological and biochemical investigations, along with a chest X-ray, are mandatory.

In patients presenting with lower cranial nerve palsies, nutritional status requires careful assessment. Hence, in addition to chest radiology and electrocardiology, routine hematological and biochemical analysis should be supplemented by hepatic function tests along with albumin estimation; any malnutrition should be corrected by preoperative nasogastric feeding. Chronic subclinical aspiration may embarass pulmonary function. There is a very strong argument for a temporary tracheostomy and gastrostomy in those patients presenting with lower cranial nerve palsies, poor nutrition and chest problems.

SURGICAL MANAGEMENT

In ***dermoid and epidermoid cysts*** a gross total resection of both cyst contents and lining wall is the gold standard, but is possible only in certain specific sites. These lesions seldom present a clean plane of dissection but encircle cranial nerves and blood vessels and are frequently adherent to vital neurologic structures. The surgical principle is to empty the cyst contents and remove as much cyst wall as is practical without damaging nerves or the microvasculature. The growth rate of these lesions should be taken into account in the extent of surgery or reoperation.

Scalp lesions may be excised completely with the cyst wall intact, and recurrence will be exceptional. Any connection to the dura should be likewise excised. *Diploic* lesions may be either curetted clear and the cyst wall removed along with adjacent bone using an air drill or excised en bloc with a craniotome, depending on the location and size of the lesion. Lesions over venous sinuses in

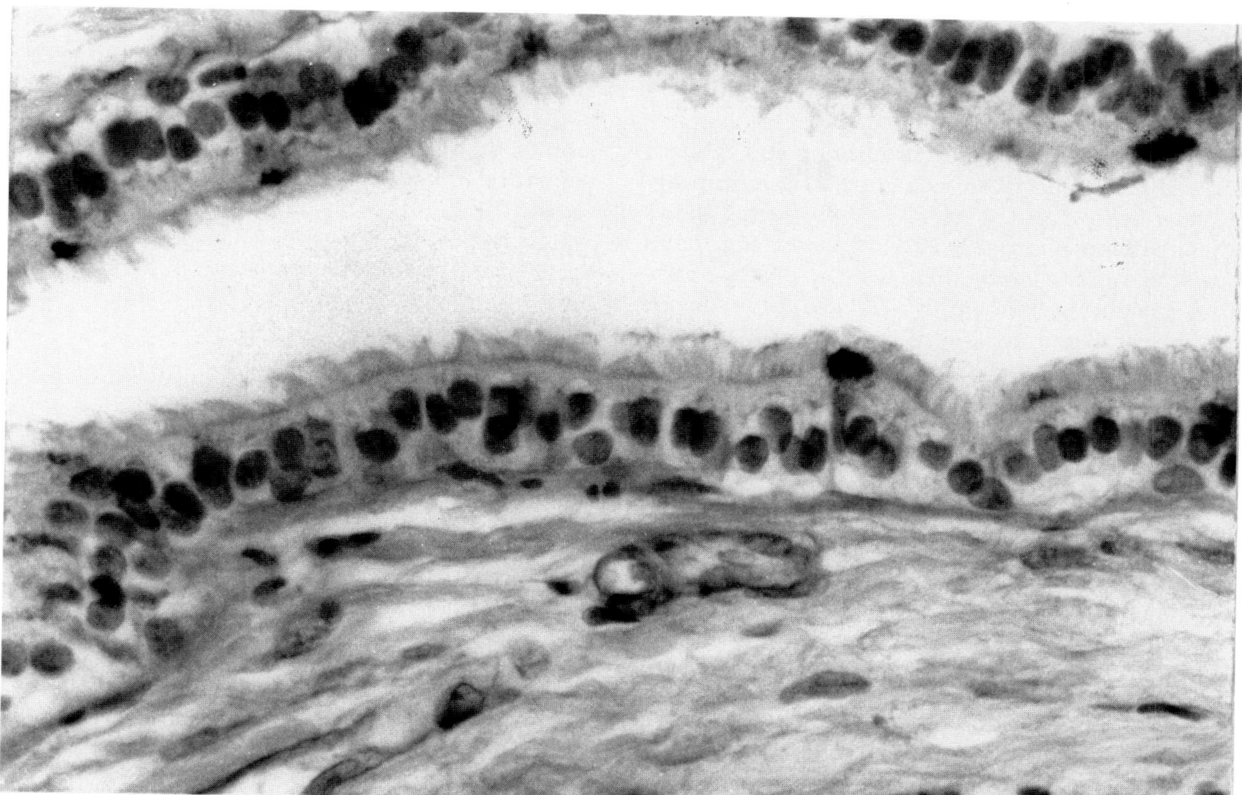

Fig. 46.9 Neurenteric cyst. A cyst lined by ciliated respiratory type of epithelium with goblet cells, the mucin staining black. PAS-diastase ×120. Courtesy of Dr N Alsanjari.

particular cause concern as these may require patch dural repair (Rengachary et al 1978). Cranioplasty, if necessary, may be performed at the same procedure with acrylic, rib or titanium, or at a later stage with a computer-generated titanium plate for large defects. The possibility of sepsis contraindicating primary cranioplasty should be remembered in the presence of midline cutaneous abnormalities. With the *intracranial* and *spinal* lesions the key to success is to gain access to the cyst early and debulk it internally. In this respect the ultrasonic surgical aspirator has been invaluable, as the waxy cyst contents usually emulsify easily. Retraction is minimized and the cyst wall is exposed; dissection of the wall is possible in a large number of cases (Yasargil 1988).

Standard surgical approaches may be used to gain access to intracranial lesions. Suprasellar/chiasmatic and many parasellar lesions are best accessed by a pterional craniotomy, as described for anterior circulation aneurysms (Yasargil et al 1978). Lesions of the cerebellopontine angle and basilar region are approached by lateral retromastoid suboccipital craniectomy whilst midline lesions in relation to the fourth ventricle may be reached by midline suboccipital craniectomy and tonsillar elevation with or without splitting the inferior vermis. The rare pineal/mesencephalic lesion can be approached by the supracerebellar or suboccipital transtentorial routes. Spinal lesions are approached by laminectomy, which should ideally be performed using somatosensory evoked potential monitoring. After myelotomy the lesion is debulked; if the cyst wall separates easily this should be removed, although 44% of Lunardi et al's (1989) series had incomplete resection of spinal lesions.

Neurenteric cysts are usually approached through a laterally placed laminectomy or costotransversectomy with drainage and excision of the cyst wall or marsupialization into the subarachnoid space (Agnoli et al 1984). In cases communicating with posterior mediastinal cysts a later thoracotomy with isolation of the communication may be required.

Results

The operative mortality for ***intracranial dermoids and epidermoids*** has fallen considerably. Before 1936 the mortality was 70% but this rate fell to 10% by 1977 (Giudetti & Gagliardi 1977). More recently, far lower mortality rates have been reported for intracranial dermoids and epidermoids — doubtless due to advances in anesthesia and microsurgical technique. Yasargil et al's recent series (1989), in showing that 86% of patients improved after surgery with only 9% neurologic morbidity and 5% mortality, shows the excellence of surgical results achievable with a follow-up of 5.2 years (range one month to 20 years). Further specific complications with modern techniques include a 19% rate of septic meningitis and hydrocephalus in 19% (Yasargil et al 1989).

With improved diagnosis by neuromaging and modern microsurgical techniques there is a good long-term prognosis. Follow-up in Lunardi et al's (1989) series shows that 69% of patients improved, 19% were unchanged and 12% were worse after surgery; there were no postoperative mortalities but during follow-up (5–30 years) two deaths occurred, one at 6 months due to a pulmonary embolus and one at 15 years due to an unrelated cause. The majority of patients were walking and working.

Neurenteric cysts should be resected if possible; marsupialization or shunting in recurrent lesions shows good results in Agnoli et al's review (1984) of 31 cases. However the younger age group presented with complex anomalies and this was the cause of two out of their three deaths. In these 31 patients the mortality was 9%, whilst 91% were either improved or cured.

INDICATIONS FOR ADJUNCTIVE THERAPIES

The standard adjuncts to surgical treatment so important in the management of other brain tumors are inappropriate with these lesions. It is of interest however that one of the functions of the skin — namely to produce sebaceous material, the main mechanism involved in expansion of these lesions — is amenable to pharmacologic modification by *isotretinoin*. This drug, used in the treatment of acne vulgaris, causes atrophy and involution of sebaceous glands and its use may prove of benefit.

MANAGEMENT OF ASSOCIATED PHENOMENA

Dermoid and epidermoid cysts rarely cause increased intracranial pressure or significant edema. Hydrocephalus used to complicate up to 40% of cases of intracranial dermoids (Conley 1985) but this has fallen to around 20% (Yasargil et al 1989).

RECURRENCE

Local recurrence

While a large number of ***dermoids and epidermoids*** may be completely excised, a subtotal resection may be all that is possible. As the cysts tend to present in the middle decades of life, clinical recurrence is rare. Yasargil et al (1989) noted no cases of clinical or radiologic recurrence in their series, with follow-up of up to 20 years. For spinal lesions, despite a subtotal resection rate of 56%, only one patient (6%) had recurrence at 12 years in Lunardi et al's series (1989).

Recurrence, in the true sense of the word, does not occur with ***neurenteric cysts*** but if the cyst wall is left it may reform and expand.

Multifocal spread by CSF dissemination

Rupture of ***epidermoids*** into the subarachnoid space is a well-recognized pattern of dissemination and many secondary satellites may be seen scattered throughout that space (Maravilla 1977). The presentation is usually with a meningitic syndrome but has even been described manifesting as focal cerebral ischemia (Ford et al 1981).

MANAGEMENT OF RECURRENT DISEASE

Dermoid and epidermoid cysts. Recurrent disease, in the face of adequate primary treatment along the paths described, should be rare.

Further resection of ***neurenteric cysts*** may be possible, but marsupialization into the subarachnoid space or shunting of the cyst into the pleural cavity are the usual methods employed in managing recurrent disease.

MANAGEMENT OUTCOME

The management outcome for such rare benign lesions is governed by the points already covered. The incidental finding of one of these lesions in the asymptomatic middle-aged patient should not necessarily lead to surgery; with their slow growth one might estimate 10-year unoperated survival. By contrast, the outcome of a complex lesion with midline bony defects in an infant with sphincter disturbances will depend on the survival after a series of complex operative procedures. Even in such an example the management mortality is essentially an operative mortality; thus it is imperative that all who embark on surgery for these lesions should be experienced. This is no territory for the occasional operator.

REFERENCES

Agnoli A L, Laun A, Schönmayr R 1984 Enterogenous intraspinal cysts. Journal of Neurosurgery 61: 824–840

Alvord E D Jr 1977 Birthrates of epidermoid tumors. Annals of Surgery 2: 367–370

Anderes J P 1984 Neurenteric cysts of the spinal cord and brain stem. MD Thesis, Lausanne

Bailey J C 1970 Dermoid tumors of the spinal cord. Journal of Neurosurgery 33: 676–681

Bailey P 1920 Cruveilhier's "tumeurs perlées". Surgery, Gynaecology and Obstetrics 31: 390–401

Baxter J W, Netsky M G 1985 Epidermoid and dermoid tumors: pathology. In: Wilkins R H, Rengachary S S (eds) Neurosurgery. McGraw-Hill, New York, pp 655–661

Berger M S, Wilson C B 1985 Epidermoid cysts of the posterior fossa. Journal of Neurosurgery 62: 214–219

Chang W H, Kak V K, Radotra B D, Jena A 1992 Enterogenous cyst

in the thoracic spinal canal in association with a syringomeningomyocele. Childs Nervous System 8: 105–107
Choremis C, Economos D, Papadatos C, Gargoulas A 1956 Intraspinal epidermoid tumors (cholesteatomas) in patients treated for tuberculous meningitis. Lancet 2: 437
Conley F K 1985 Epidermoid and dermoid tumors: clinical features and surgical management. In: Wilkins R H, Rengachary S S (eds) Neurosurgery, vol 1. McGraw-Hill, New York, pp 668–673
Cruveilhier J 1829 Anatomie pathologique de corps humain, vol 1, book 2. Ballière 341
Cushing H 1922 A large epidermoid cholesteatoma of the parietotemporal region deforming the left hemisphere without cerebral symptoms. Surgery, Gynaecology and Obstetrics 34: 557–566
Dias P S, May P L, Jakubowski J 1989 Giant epidermoid cysts of the skull. British Journal of Neurosurgery 3: 51–58
Dubois P J, Sage M, Luther J S, Burger P C, Heinz E R, Drayer B P 1981 Malignant change in an intracranial epidermoid cyst. Journal of Computer Assisted Tomography 5: 433
Fabinyi G C A, Adams J E 1979 High cervical spinal cord compression by an enterogenous cyst. Case report. Journal of Neurosurgery 51: 556–559
Ford K, Drayer B, Osborne D, Dubois P 1981 Case report. Transient cerebral ischaemia as a manifestation of ruptured intracranial dermoid cysts. Journal of Computer Assisted Tomography 5: 895–897
French B N 1990 A complete reference guide to the diagnosis and management of neurosurgical problems. In: Youmans J R (ed) Neurosurgery. W B Saunders, pp 1081–1236
Garcia C A, McGary P A, Rodriguez F 1981 Primary intracranial squamous cell carcinoma of the right cerebellopontine angle. Journal of Neurosurgery 34: 824
Giudetti B, Gagliardi F M 1977 Epidermoid and dermoid cysts: clinical evaluation and late surgical results. Journal of Neurosurgery 47: 12–18
Goldman S A, Gandy S E 1987 Squamous cell carcinoma. The late complication of intracerebroventricular epidermoid cyst. Journal of Neurosurgery 66: 618
Grant F C, Austin G M 1950 Epidermoids: clinical evaluation and surgical results. Journal of Neurosurgery 7: 190
Harai O, Kawamura J, Kukumitsu T 1981 Prepontine epithelium lined cysts. Journal of Neurosurgery 55: 312–317
Harriman D G F 1958 An intraspinal enterogenous cyst. Journal of Pathology and Bacteriology 75: 413
Hirano A, Ghatak N R, Wisoff H S 1971 An epithelial cyst of the spinal cord. An electron microscopic study. Acta Neuropathologica 181: 214–223
Itakura T, Kusumoto S, Yematsu Y 1986 Enterogenous cyst of the cervical spinal cord in a child — case report. Neurology, Medicine, Chirurgie 26: 49–53
Jefferson G, Smalley A A 1938 Progressive facial palsy produced by intratemporal epidermoids. Journal of Laryngology and Otology 53: 417–443
King T T, Benjamin J C, Morrison A W 1989 Epidermoid and cholesterol cysts in the apex of the petrous bone. British Journal of Neurosurgery 3: 451–462
Koksel T, Revesz T, Crockard H A 1990 Craniospinal neurenteric cyst. British Journal of Neurosurgery 4: 425–428
Kompf D, Menges H W 1977 Maligna entartung eines parapontinem epidermoids. Akutes conus-cauda syndrome infolge meningealer aussaat. Acta Neurochirurgica 39: 81
Landers J W, Danielski J J 1960 Malignant intracranial epidermoid cysts. Archives of Pathology 30: 419
Lewis A J, Cooper P W, Kassel E E, Swartz M L 1983 Squamous cell carcinoma arising from a suprasellar epidermoid cyst. Journal of Neurosurgery 59: 538
List C F 1941 Intraspinal epidermoids, dermoids and dermal sinuses. Surgery, Gynaecology and Obstetrics 73: 525
Love J G, Kernohan J W 1936 Dermoid and epidermoid tumours (cholesteatomas) of central nervous system. Journal of the American Medical Association 107: 1876
Lunardi P, Missori P, Gagliardi F M, Fortuna A 1989 Long term results of the surgical treatment of spinal dermoids and epidermoid tumours. Neurosurgery 25: 860–864
Mahoney W 1936 De epidermoide des Zentralnerven zystems. Zeitschrift für die Gesante neurologie und psychiatrie 115: 416
Manno N J, Uihlein A, Kernohan J W 1962 Intraspinal epidermoids. Journal of Neurosurgery 19: 754–765
Maravilla K R 1977 Intraventricular fat — fluid level secondary to rupture of an intracranial dermoid cyst. American Journal of Radiology 128: 500–501
Markwalder T M, Zimmerman A 1979 Intracerebral ciliated epithelial cysts. Surgical Neurology 11: 195–198
Martinez-Lage J F, Quiñonez M A, Pozo M, Puchet A, Casas C, Rodriguez-Costas T 1985 Congenital epidermoid cysts of the anterior fontanelle. Child's Nervous System 1: 319
Matson D D 1969 Neurosurgery of infancy and childhood, 2nd edn. Charles C Thomas, Springfield
Nosaka Y, Nagao S, Tabuchi K, Nashimoto A 1979 Primary intracranial epidermoid carcinoma. Journal of Neurosurgery 50: 830
Obana W G, Wilson C B 1991 Epidermoid cysts of the brain stem: report of three cases. Journal of Neurosurgery 74: 123–128
Osborne D R 1985 Epidermoid and dermoid tumors: Radiology. In: Wilkins R H, Rengachary S S (eds) Neurosurgery, vol 1. McGraw-Hill, New York, pp 662–667
Pear B L 1970 Epidermoid and dermoid sequestrations of the cyst. American Journal of Radiology 1: 148–155
Pennybacker J 1944 Cholesteatoma of the petrous bone. British Journal of Surgery 32: 75
Peyton W T, Baker A B 1942 Epidermoid, dermoid and teratomatous tumors of the central nervous system. Archives of Neurology and Psychiatry 47: 890
Plewes J L, Jacobson I 1971 Familial frontonasal dermoid cysts: report of four cases. Journal of Neurosurgery 34: 683–686
Puusepp M 1934 Variété rare de tératome sous-dural de la regioné cervical (intestinome). Quadriplegie. Extirpation. Guérison complete. Reviews in Neurology 2: 879–886
Rengachary S S, Kishore P R S, Watanabe I 1978 Intradiploic epidermoid cysts of the occipital bone with torcular obstruction: a case report. Journal of Neurosurgery 48: 475–478
Rosario M, Becker D H, Conley F K 1981 Epidermoid tumors involving the fourth ventricle. Neurosurgery 9: 9–13
Russell D S, Rubinstein L J 1989 Pathology of tumors of the nervous system, 5th edn. Williams & Wilkins, Baltimore pp 663–695
Scaravilli F, Lidov H, Spalton D J, Symon L 1992 Neurenteric cyst of the optic nerve: case report with immunohistochemical study. Journal of Neurology, Neurosurgery and Psychiatry 55: 1197–1199
Steffey D J, de Filipp G J, Spera T, Gabrielson T O 1988 MR imaging of primary epidermoid tumors. Journal of Computer Assisted Tomography 12: 438–440
Sweet W 1940 A review of dermoid, teratoid and teratomatous intracranial tumors. Diseases of the Nervous System 1: 228
Takeuchi J, Ohta T, Kajikawa H 1978 Congenital tumors of the spinal cord. In: Vinken P J, Bruyn G W (eds) Handbook of clinical neurology, vol 32. North Holland Publishing Co, Amsterdam, pp 355–392
Tan T I 1972 Epidermoids and dermoids of the central nervous system. Acta Neurochirurgica (Wien) 26: 13–24
Tytus J S, Pennybacker J 1956 Pearly tumors in relation to the central nervous system. Journal of Neurology, Neurosurgery and Psychiatry 90: 241
Ulrich J 1964 Intracranial epidermoids: a study on their distribution and spread. Journal of Neurosurgery 21: 1051–1058
Willis R A 1967 Pathology of tumours, 4th edn. Butterworths, London
Yasargil M G 1988 Microneurosurgery, vols 1–3B. Georg Thieme Verlag, Stuttgart
Yasargil M G, Smith R D, Gosser J R 1978 Microsurgery of aneurysms of the internal carotid artery and its branches. Progress in Neurological Surgery 9: 58–121
Yasargil M G, Abernathey C D, Sarioglu A C 1989 Microneurosurgical treatment of intracranial dermoid and epidermoid tumors. Neurosurgery 24: 5617
Yoshida T, Hakatani S, Shimazu K, Yamada K, Yukitak U, Heitaro M 1986 Huge epithelium lined cysts: report of two cases. Journal of Neurology, Neurosurgery and Psychiatry 49: 1458–1459

47. Colloid cysts

John Laidlaw   Andrew H. Kaye

INTRODUCTION

Although uncommon, colloid cysts attract a particular amount of interest in that they are benign tumors which can be surgically cured but, if untreated, put the patient at risk of sudden neurologic deterioration and death. They occur almost exclusively within the third ventricle, and are the most common tumor occurring at this site.

Wallmann reported the first case in 1858 (Wallmann 1858, Little & MacCarty 1974). The term 'colloid', derived from the description of the cyst contents (glue like), was first used to describe these cysts in the late nineteenth century (Kondziolka & Bilbao 1989). The terms 'paraphysial cyst' and 'neuroepithelial cyst' have also been applied to these structures. However, there have been very few reports of these structures occurring in sites other than the third ventricle and there is still disagreement regarding the embryologic origin of these cysts. Therefore, the original term, colloid cyst, is now considered the most appropriate.

INCIDENCE AND PREVALENCE OF TUMOR

Colloid cysts of the third ventricle are uncommon, representing 0.3–2% of all brain tumors (Ferry & Kemp 1968, Kahn et al 1969, Batnitzky et al 1974, Little & MacCarty 1974, Antunes et al 1980a, Chan & Thompson 1983, Hall & Lunsford 1987). Although a review of the literature indicates that colloid cysts account for less than 1% of symptomatic brain tumors, it has been recently recognized that the widespread availability of CT scanning and MRI scanning for the investigation of patients with headache and dementia has resulted in an increase in frequency of diagnosis of asymptomatic colloid cysts (Antunes et al 1980b, Ganti et al 1981, Hall & Lunsford 1987, Mohadjer et al 1987).

AGE DISTRIBUTION

Colloid cysts are considered to be congenital lesions, and as such can present at any age. However, although the youngest reported case was aged 2 months (Gemperlein 1960, Batnitzky et al 1974), they have only rarely been described as presenting in childhood or early adolescence (Yenerman et al 1958, Buchsbaum & Colton 1967, Batnitzky et al 1974). Symptomatic colloid cysts are most commonly reported between the ages of 20 and 50 years (Mohadjer et al 1987), although in recent times the introduction of noninvasive cerebral imaging has resulted in an increased frequency of diagnosis, particularly in the elderly (Antunes et al 1980a, Ganti et al 1981, Rivas & Lobarto 1985, Hall & Lunsford 1987, Mohadjer et al 1987).

SEX DISTRIBUTION

Colloid cysts of the third ventricle are usually considered to affect both sexes equally (Yenerman et al 1958, Hall & Lunsford 1987). It should be noted, however, that most surgical series of colloid cysts reported in the literature show a slight male predominance (Little & MacCarty 1974, Ganti et al 1981, Hall & Lunsford 1987, Ostertag 1990, Symon & Pell 1990, Yasargil et al 1990).

RACIAL, NATIONAL & GEOGRAPHIC CONSIDERATIONS

Although there have been no reported racial or geographic variations in the distribution of colloid cysts, it must be considered that at present these questions are unresolved. The reported incidence of colloid cysts correlates closely to the local availability of cerebral imaging resources, and consequently most reported cases are from technologically advanced countries.

FAMILY HISTORY AND GENETIC FACTORS

There have been no reports of a hereditary predisposition to colloid cysts, nor has any association with a clinical syndrome been clearly demonstrated.

SITES OF PREDILECTION

More than 99% of reported cases of colloid cysts have occurred within the third ventricle, almost all in the anterior half. The cyst typically has an attachment to the roof of the third ventricle immediately dorsal to the foramen of Monro, although adhesions to the lateral walls of the third ventricle and the floor of the third ventricle are not infrequent.

Rare cases of colloid cysts occurring in the posterior third ventricle have been reported (Shuangshoti & Netsky 1966, Kondziolka & Bilbao 1989), and there have been individual case reports of colloid cyst in the septum pellucidum (Ciric & Zivin 1975) and in the fourth ventricle (Parkinson & Childe 1952, Kchir et al 1992).

A single case of an intracerebral cystic lesion in the right frontoparietal region which had histopathologic features of a colloid cyst has been reported (Campbell & Varma 1991). A case has also been reported of an intrasellar cystic lesion with radiographic and histologic features of a colloid cyst (Sener & Jinkins 1991).

PRESENTING FEATURES

A classic clinical presentation for colloid cyst has long been described, and is characterized by paroxysmal headache associated with changes in head position (Bull & Sutton 1949, Kelly 1951, Yenermen et al 1968, Palacios et al 1976). It was generally considered that such symptoms were due to a pedunculated midline cyst within the third ventricle which was capable of altering position with head movement, and therefore intermittently obstructing either the foramen of Monro or the aqueduct of Sylvius. However, such presentations are not common, nor is the corresponding pathologic entity of a highly mobile cyst (Bull & Sutton 1949, Kelly 1951, Yenermen et al 1958, Little & MacCarty 1974, Palacios et al 1976). Kelly (1951) has made the point that, as well as being rare, the classic presentation is by no means pathognomonic of colloid cysts, and he found that patients presenting in this manner were in fact more likely to have other tumor types. He also found that in his series of cases the most frequent presenting symptom apart from headache was sudden weakness in the lower limbs, causing falling without unconsciousness (Kelly 1951). The association of obstruction of the third ventricle with these sudden drop attacks, although recognized in the more recent literature, has been reported relatively infrequently.

Progressive headache associated with raised intracranial pressure is a common presentation (Little & MacCarty 1974). Little & MacCarty (1974) noted that in these patients the relatively long history of the headaches suggested a benign lesion, although acute presentation with raised intracranial pressure is not uncommon. The presentation of a colloid cyst with headache and papilledema, but no localizing neurologic signs, was well recognized by Dandy (1933).

As would be expected, patients presenting with the symptom of headache not infrequently exhibit the other manifestations of raised intracranial pressure, such as vomiting, altered conscious state, and papilledema. Patients presenting with paroxysmal headaches not uncommonly have associated transient diplopia and blurred vision (Batnitzky et al 1974). It should be noted that these presentations, due to acute hydrocephalus, are in no way different from the presentation for any other cause of acute hydrocephalus.

Patients with colloid cysts can also present with a progressive or fluctuating dementia, often in the absence of headaches or papilledema. This was first described by Riddoch (1936) and has been since confirmed by other authors (Grossiord 1941, Kelly 1951, Yenerman et al 1958, Ojemann 1971, Little & MacCarty 1974). The progressive dementia is frequently associated with gait disturbance and urinary incontinence, and thus has the same clinical presenting features as 'normal pressure hydrocephalus' (Adams et al 1965, Ojemann 1971, Little & MacCarty 1974). Indeed, three of the cases in the original series describing normal pressure hydrocephalus had lesions in the anterior part of the third ventricle (Adams et al 1965). It is necessary to consider third ventricular lesions in patients presenting with the clinical syndrome of normal pressure hydrocephalus, as those patients with third ventricular lesions have a risk of sudden neurologic deterioration, particularly following lumbar puncture (Little & MacCarty 1974).

As has been mentioned, many colloid cysts are asymptomatic and are diagnosed at the time of CT or MR scanning for an unrelated condition.

The most catastrophic event associated with colloid cysts of the third ventricle is sudden death. This has been well recognized in the literature (Grossiord 1941, Cairns & Mosberg 1951, Kelly 1951, Little & MacCarty 1974, Ryder et al 1986). Ryder et al (1986) analyzed 52 cases of colloid cyst reported in the literature as having suffered sudden death, and found that neither the tumor size, the degree of ventricular dilatation as assessed on CT scan, nor the duration of symptoms prior to the patient's collapse could be reliably used to indicate the risk of sudden neurologic deterioration or death. That review noted that while many of the cases of sudden death could be attributed to acute hydrocephalus, this was not always present. They postulated that reflex effects involving cardiovascular centers near the third ventricle may also have played a role in these patients (Ryder et al 1986). The actual incidence of sudden death with asymptomatic colloid cysts is unknown, but with the absence of predicting factors there is generally a marked neurosurgical reluctance not to recommend treatment.

IMAGING DIAGNOSIS

Walter Dandy (1922, 1933) first indicated that it was

impossible to diagnose colloid cysts on clinical grounds alone, and introduced ventriculography for their accurate diagnosis. The pathognomonic ventriculographic findings associated with colloid cysts were described at length by Bull & Sutton (1949); as late as 1974, Little & McCarty considered ventriculography to be still the most reliable diagnostic study for the demonstration of third ventricular lesions. Pneumoencephalography could also be used for the diagnosis of third ventricle lesions, but could not be considered the procedure of choice as it was less accurate than ventriculography (Taveras & Wood 1964, Batnitzky et al 1974, Little & MacCarty 1974) and also had a significant risk of neurologic deterioration in patients with raised intracranial pressure (Bull & Sutton 1949, Batnitzky et al 1974).

Plain X-rays of the skull are of no particular value in the diagnosis of colloid cyst, although they may show non-specific signs of chronically raised intracranial pressure, as was found in 17 of the 25 cases studied by Batnitzky et al (1974) and in 7 of the 38 cases reported by Little & MacCarty (1974). There is only one reported example of a colloid cyst with calcifications visible on skull X-rays (Palacios et al 1976), and calcification seen in the region of the third ventricle would suggest a diagnosis other than colloid cyst (Taveras & Wood 1964, Batnitzky et al 1974). The plain skull X-rays may also show posterior inferior displacement of the calcified pineal, and although this is well recognized it is by no means pathognomonic or common (Davidoff & Dyck 1935, Bull & Sutton 1949, Yenermen et al 1958, Little & MacCarty 1974).

Radionucleotide brain scanning, other than possibly showing some evidence of hydrocephalus, will not aid in the diagnosis of colloid cysts. This study is usually normal (Batnitzky et al 1974, Little & MacCarty 1974).

Cerebral angiography, although not providing a definitive diagnosis, may give useful indications as to the possibility of colloid cyst (Batnitzky et al 1974, Little & MacCarty 1974). Hydrocephalus may be recognized on angiography by outward bowing of the thalamostriate veins in the frontal venous phase and also the increased sweep of the pericallosal artery in the lateral arterial phase. In the presence of a colloid cyst the internal cerebral vein has been commonly described as showing an anterior hump, with flattening and depression in its posterior two thirds (Batnitzky et al 1974, Little & MacCarty 1974). Since the introduction of high resolution CT scanning, the most valuable role of angiography in the study of a third ventricular lesion is the exclusion of a cerebral aneurysm.

With current CT and MRI technology the previously mentioned radiographic investigations are now largely obsolete in the investigation of colloid cysts.

The characteristic CT appearance of a colloid cyst is of a rounded or ovoid lesion, typically 5–25 mm in diameter, lying in the region of the anterior third ventricle adjacent to and just behind the foramen of Monro (Lee et al 1979, Ganti et al 1981). The lesions are usually homogeneous, although occasionally a central lucency has been demonstrated (Ganti et al 1981). Most commonly the colloid cyst is hyperdense on pre-contrast CT scanning. Review of the reported series of colloid cysts investigated with CT scan reveals a total of 144 cases, 100 of which were hyperdense on CT scan (69.4%), 34 isodense

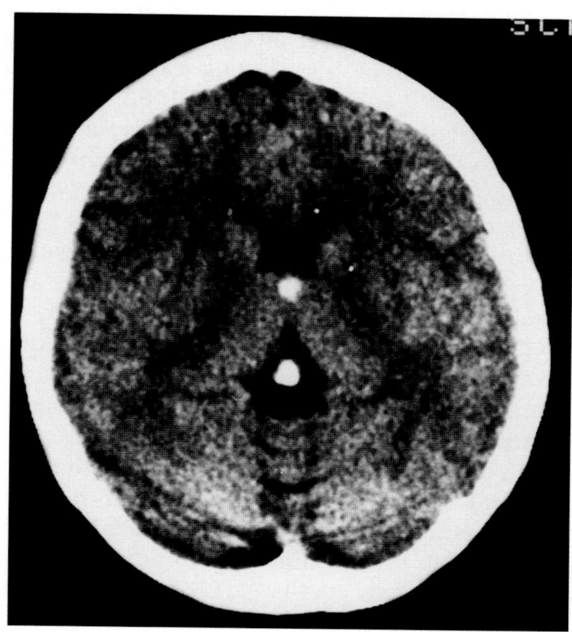

Fig. 47.1 Hyperdense colloid cyst; axial CT scan.

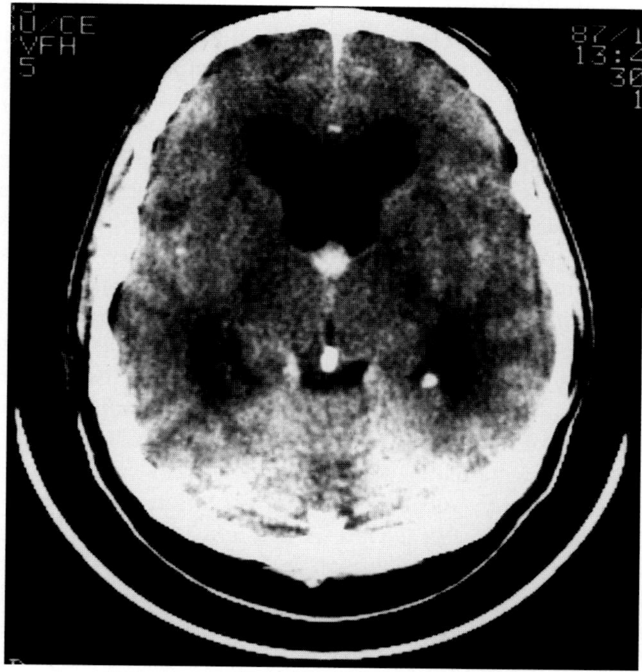

Fig. 47.2 Hyperdense colloid cyst causing obstructive hydrocephalus; axial CT scan.

(23.6%), and 10 (6.9%) hypodense (Sackett et al 1975, Guner et al 1976, Osborn & Wing 1977, Ganti et al 1981, Zilkha 1981, Powell & Torrens 1983, Rivas & Lobarto 1985, Donauer et al 1986, Hall & Lunsford 1987, Mohadjer et al 1987, Abernathey et al 1989, Kondziolka & Bilbao 1989, Musolino et al 1989).

The cyst wall sometimes enhances following intravenous contrast injection, occurring in 2 of the 17 cases reported by Hall & Lunsford (1987) and 8 of the 14 cases reported by Ganti et al (1981). There is one reported case of a colloid cyst having a CT appearance of a ring-enhancing lesion (Bullard et al 1982).

The high density on pre-contrast CT scan is thought to be due to the proteinaceous contents of the cyst, and possibly also due to hemosiderin (Ganti et al 1981). The CT appearance of a hyperdense colloid cyst has also been correlated with the degree of calcium within the colloid cyst content (Sackett et al 1975, Ganti et al 1981, Kondziolka & Lunsford 1991). Donaldson & Simon (1980) determined the elemental composition of the contents of a hyperdense colloid cyst with atomic emission spectometry, and found calcium, sodium and magnesium to be the predominant radiodense ions. Microscopic calcification in the cyst wall is a not infrequent histopathologic finding, and may contribute to increased radiodensity on CT scanning. Actual calcification demonstrated on any radiographic investigation is uncommon (Taveras & Wood 1964, Batnitzky et al 1974, Ganti et al 1981), being noted in 2 of the 17 CT scans reported by Hall & Lunsford (1987).

The radiodensity of the colloid cyst on CT scan has been shown to correlate with the viscosity of the cyst contents, with the hypodense and isodense cysts being less viscous, and relatively more liquid (Powell & Torrens 1983, Rivas & Lobarto 1985, Kondziolka & Lunsford 1991).

Multiplanar MR scanning clearly demonstrates the anatomic location of the rounded cyst in the anterior aspect of the third ventricle adjacent to the foramen of Monro. MRI is also able to differentiate between the colloid cyst and an aneurysm of the basilar tip, which may occasionally be indistinguishable on CT scan. Earlier reports have incorrectly stated that the colloid cyst has a high signal on both T1- and T2-weighted images (Kjos et al 1985, Hall & Lunsford 1987, Symon & Pell 1990). Of the 8 cases of colloid cysts imaged with MRI scan reported by Kondziolka & Lunsford (1991), at a short relaxation time 2 had a low signal, 3 were isointense, and 3 had a high signal intensity, and on the long relaxation time 2 had a low signal intensity, 2 were isointense, and 4 had a high signal intensity. Kondziolka & Lunsford (1991) found that the MRI scanning technique failed to predict the viscosity of the cyst contents, and in this respect CT scan was superior.

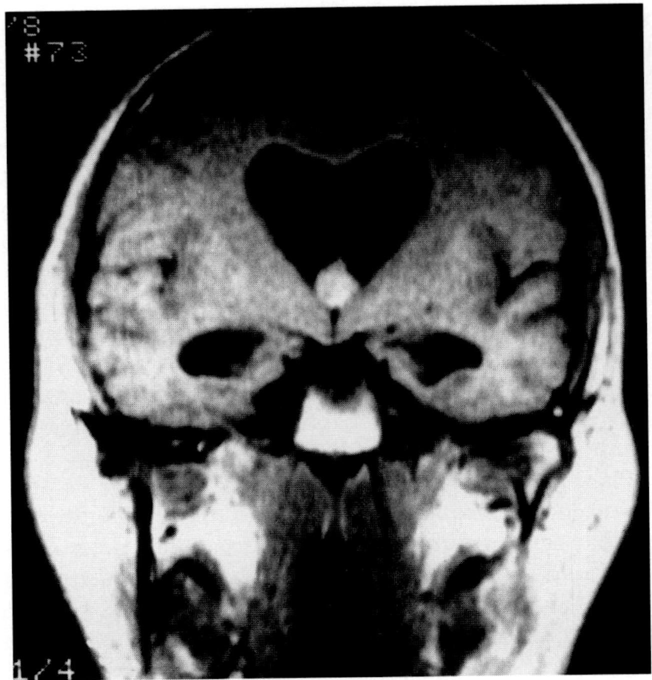

Fig. 47.3 High signal colloid cyst on coronal T1-weighted MR scan (TR 500).

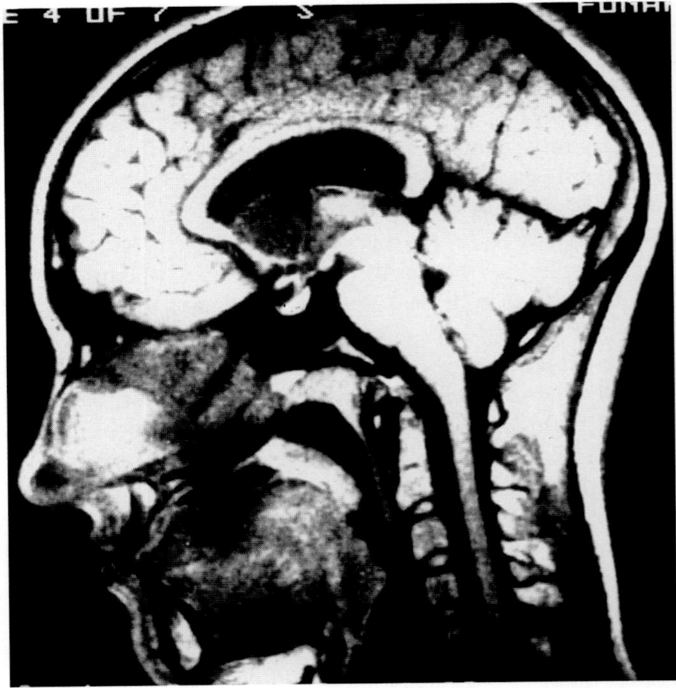

Fig. 47.4 Low signal colloid cyst on sagittal T1-weighted MR scan (TR 500).

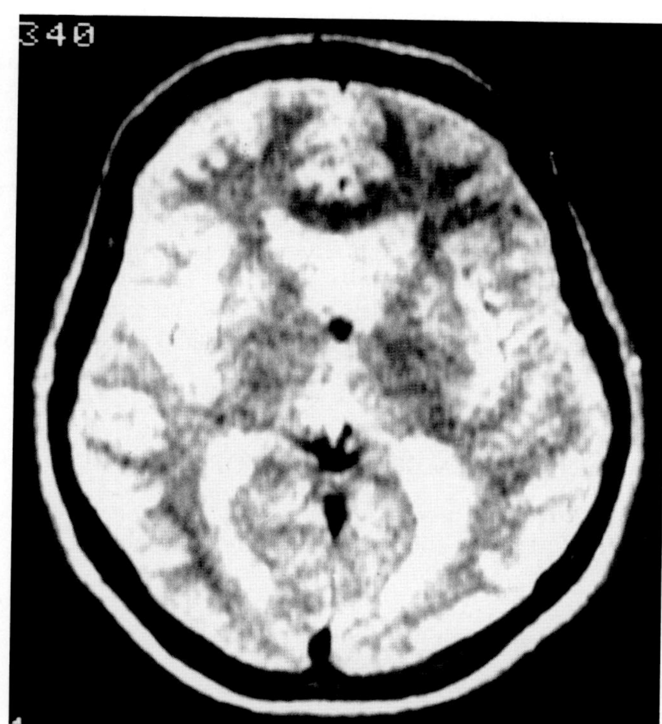

Fig. 47.5 Low signal colloid cyst on axial T2-weighted MR scan (TR 2000).

LABORATORY DIAGNOSIS

Hematologic and biochemical analysis of blood, CSF analysis, and other laboratory tests are of no diagnostic value in patients with colloid cysts. Lumbar puncture poses a significant risk to any patient with a third ventricular lesion, and is absolutely contraindicated in the presence of obstructive hydrocephalus.

GROSS MORPHOLOGIC FEATURES

Colloid cysts range in size, and have been reported from a few millimeters to 9 cm in diameter (Ganti et al 1981). The cyst itself is smooth and spherical or ovoid, and has a semitranslucent wall, the cyst contents often giving it a greenish appearance. The cyst has a variable attachment to the roof of the third ventricle immediately posterior to the foramen of Monro. This attachment ranges from a narrow pedicle to a broad sessile base (McKissock 1951), and very fine vessels traverse it and ramify over the wall of the cyst (Symon & Pell 1990). Typically the colloid cyst can be viewed through the foramen of Monro from the lateral ventricle. From this position, which is the usual surgical approach, the choroid plexus passing through the foramen of Monro is seen to be draped over the wall of the colloid cyst. The choroid plexus is occasionally somewhat adherent to the cyst wall, and there may be other adhesions between the wall of the lateral ventricle and

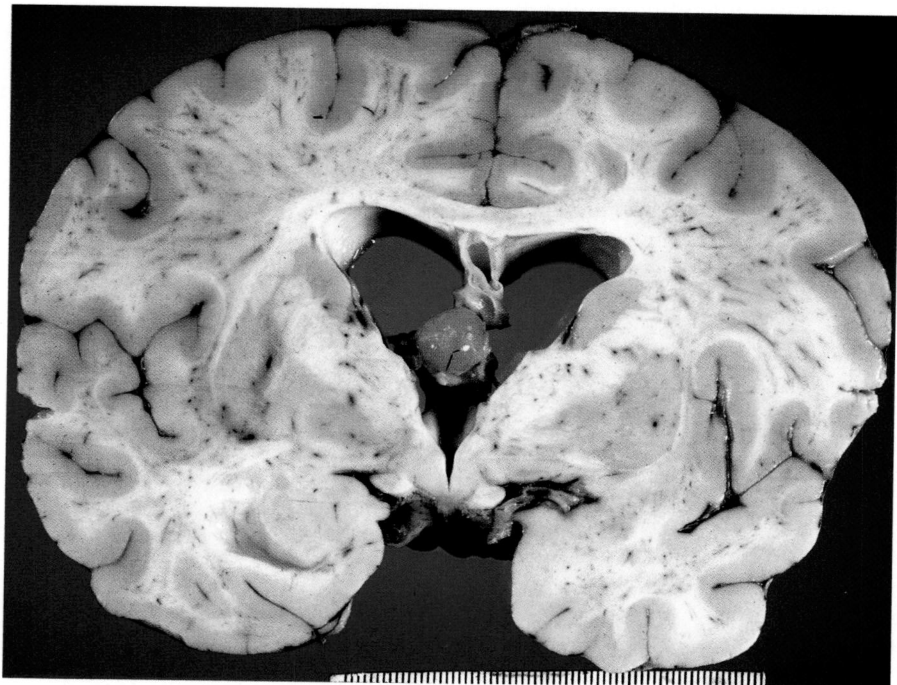

Fig. 47.6 Photograph of colloid cyst; post-mortem coronal brain section.

the cyst wall. These are fibrinous adhesions, and are nonvascular.

Colloid cysts larger than 1 cm in diameter commonly fill the foramen of Monro, and may protrude through this into the lateral ventricle. Fibrinous adhesions may then also develop with the anatomic structures at the foramen of Monro, particularly the fornix and the convergence of the choroid plexus, the thalamostriate vein and the septal veins.

The contents of the cyst vary, sometimes being pale, viscous semiliquid, or more commonly dark and semigelatinous, and may even be granular, semisolid and caseous (Ganti et al 1981, Yasargil et al 1990, Symon & Pell 1990).

HISTOPATHOLOGIC FEATURES

Microscopically the cyst wall consists of an outer fibrous layer, and an inner epithelial layer, which is usually cuboidal or low columnar and which often has ciliated cells and may even have a pseudostratified appearance (Ferrand et al 1971, Ganti et al 1981, Kondziolka & Bilbao 1989). Routine histologic staining shows the presence of cilia in almost all cases (Kondziolka & Bilbao 1989), and mucin-secreting cells are also commonly found (Mosberg & Blackwood 1954, Kondziolka & Bilbao 1989).

The wall of the cyst has been demonstrated to be collagenous on trichrome staining (Kondziolka & Bilbao 1989). PAS positivity was found in the cyst epithelium in 11 of the 12 specimens studied by Kondziolka & Bilbao (1989), and all had no reaction to vimentin, neurofilament, or Bodian's silver stain. It is of interest to note that, whereas the colloid cyst epithelium is uniformly negative to vimentin, the stromal wall is uniformly positive (Kondziolka & Bilbao 1989). The colloid cyst epithelium showed no reaction to GFAP but typically reacts to the polyclonal antibody to S-100 protein, and inconsistently with neuron-specific enolase (Kondziolka & Bilbao 1989). Cytokeratin monoclonal antibody reactions have been noted with many colloid cysts, and the Mallory keratin polyclonal antibody (with a broad spectrum of reactivity) has been found to react positively with most colloid cyst walls (Mietinnen et al 1986, Kondziolka & Bilbao 1989). No reaction to the monoclonal antibody HNK-1 (anti-Leu-7) has been reported, and the cysts also react negatively to leukocyte common antigen monoclonal antibody (Kondziolka & Bilbao 1989). Positivity to the epithelial membrane antigen had been noted in two separate studies (Perentes & Rubinstein 1987, Kondziolka & Bilbao 1989).

THEORIES OF EMBRYOLOGIC ORIGIN

The embryologic derivation of colloid cysts is far from certain. The major theories will be briefly discussed.

Paraphysis/ventricular roof structures

In 1910 Sjovall proposed that these cysts were embryonic remnants derived from the paraphysis (Sjovall 1909, Little & MacCarty 1974), although at that time this embryonal neuroectodermal structure had only been described in lower vertebrates. In 1916 Bailey described the paraphysis in human embryos, and for over 50 years following this description the term 'paraphysial cysts' was commonly used (Bailey 1916, Parkinson & Childe 1952, Shuangshoti & Netsky 1966, Ciric & Zivin 1975, Kondziolka & Bilbao 1989).

The paraphysis has been described by Kappers (1955) to exist transiently in the human embryo (between a crown–rump length of 17 and 100 mm; approximately 7–14 weeks), having normally completely regressed by the 145 mm stage (Kappers 1955, Palacios et al 1976). It is a midline structure within the diencephalic roof immediately rostral to the telencephalic border, and consists

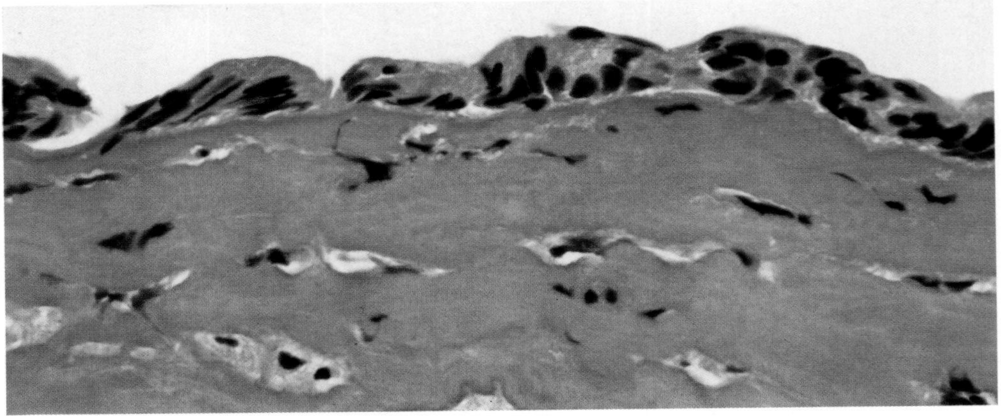

Fig. 47.7 Lining of colloid cyst of third ventricle consisting of columnar and cuboidal cells supported by a fibrous connective tissue layer. H&E ×400.

microscopically of low columnar epithelium which differs from the surrounding epithelium by the absence of cilia and blepharoplasts.

The descriptions of colloid cysts in the posterior third ventricle, the fourth ventricle, and within leaves of the septum pellucidum (Parkinson & Childe 1952, Shuangshoti & Netsky 1966, Ciric & Zivin 1975, Kondziolka & Bilbao 1989) cast doubt on the paraphysial theory and opened debate as to their histologic origin.

Shuangshoti et al (1965, 1966) have presented a theory that the paraphysis itself represents extraventricular choroid plexus, and that colloid cysts arose either from choroid plexus, ependyma or paraphysis, which were all products of neuroepithelium. Electron microscopic examination of the colloid cyst epithelium has demonstrated both normal and abnormal cilia, and Coxe & Luse (1964) considered this appearance to be suggestive of an ependymal origin. Kappers (1955) proposed that the more likely origin of colloid cysts is from diencephalic roof ependymal recesses, which pinch off into closed vesicles. Ciric & Zivin (1975) supported the hypothesis of cyst formation by invagination of neuroepithelium from the diencephalic roof. These theories could account for the occurrence of these cysts at sites closely related to the ventricular system other than within the anterior third ventricle.

Respiratory/enterogenous origin

A comparison between the epithelium found in colloid cysts and the pseudostratified epithelium found in Rathke's cysts has been made, and Leech & Oliveson (1977) have suggested that the colloid cyst may be derived from respiratory epithelium. Respiratory-type epithelium was also described in one of the 21 cases of colloid cysts examined by Loizou et al (1986), and another case was considered to have the appearance of foregut-type epithelium (Loizou et al 1986). More recently, Ho & Garcia (1992) have reported the ultrastructural features of four cases of colloid cysts, and demonstrated ciliated cells, nonciliated cells with microvilli, goblet cells, basal cells, and also junctional complexes between some of the cell types. They considered this to be very similar to normal respiratory epithelium, and also to the lining of intraspinal bronchogenic cysts, and felt that these features were consistent with the hypothesis of an endodermal respiratory origin (Ho & Garcia 1992). Histologic and immunohistochemical similarities between 5 colloid cysts and 2 spinal enterogenous cysts have also been demonstrated by Mackenzie & Gilbert (1991), also supporting an endodermal origin hypothesis.

Another ultrastructural study of 13 colloid cysts has been reported which confirms the ultrastructural similarity between the colloid cyst epithelium and the epithelium from Rathke's cleft cysts and enterogenous cysts and also follicular cysts from the normal pituitary gland. This study also supported the enterogenous origin of colloid cysts (Lach & Scheithauer 1992).

Theories based on immunohistochemical markers

Mucin-secreting cells have been commonly demonstrated in the cyst epithelium (Mosberg & Blackwood 1954, Kondziolka & Bilbao 1989). There is disagreement as to whether or not mucin-containing cells are found in the choroid plexus ependyma, being demonstrated by Shuangshoti & Netsky (1966) but not by Kondziolka & Bilbao (1989).

PAS-positive material was found in the cyst epithelium in 11 of the 12 specimens studied by Kondziolka & Bilbao (1989), but was not found by them in choroid plexus. They also reported that, unlike choroid plexus (Kasper et al 1986), the colloid cyst epithelium had no reaction to intermediate filament antibodies to vimentin and neurofilament, or to Bodian's silver preparation (Kondziolka & Bilbao 1989). Positivity to the epithelial membrane antigen had been noted in two separate studies (Perentes & Rubinstein 1987, Kondziolka & Bilbao 1989) and has not been demonstrated in choroid plexus epithelium (Kondziolka & Bilbao 1989). Negativity of the colloid cyst epithelium for vimentin is in contrast to immature glial tissue, and GFAP negativity is in contrast to mature glial tissue. Kondziolka & Bilbao (1989) considered that these immunohistochemical findings were consistent with the theory that the colloid cyst was derived from primitive neuroectoderm involved in the formation of the tela choroidea, and was inconsistent with the derivation of colloid cyst from either choroid plexus or ependyma.

Immunohistochemical studies of 11 colloid cysts performed by Kuchelmeister & Bergmann (1992) have confirmed the different profiles of colloid cyst epithelium, choroid plexus epithelium and ependyma. However, their conclusion was that the most likely derivation was of a non-neuroepithelial origin.

DEFINITION AND INCIDENCE OF 'MALIGNANCY'

Colloid cysts are considered to be completely benign noninvasive congenital lesions. Studies following simple aspiration suggest that they enlarge very slowly (Bosch et al 1978, Rivas & Lobarto 1985, Donauer et al 1986, Hall & Lunsford 1987, Mohadjer et al 1987, Musolino et al 1989, Kondziolka & Lunsford 1991). There have been no reported cases of malignant transformation, nor have there been cases of seeding in the CSF pathways.

GENERAL MANAGEMENT PLAN

Patients presenting in an obtunded state with acute hydrocephalus must have urgent ventricular drainage.

It should be noted that as the site of obstruction is commonly at the foramen of Monro, bilateral drainage of the lateral ventricles will be necessary.

Alert patients presenting with headache or dementia will need CSF pathways re-established or shunting instituted. Although this can be achieved with bilateral shunting procedures, there is a concern that the patient is still at risk of acute deterioration in the future in the event of shunt dysfunction. It is also considered that a patient with a colloid cyst may be at risk of acute deterioration not only from acute hydrocephalus but also possibly as a result of effects of pressure or venous obstruction on the hypothalamic cardiovascular regulatory centers (Ryder et al 1986), and patients treated with CSF diversion alone may therefore still be at risk of sudden neurologic deterioration and death. In general, therefore, it is considered that surgical decompression of the colloid cyst itself should be performed. As we are currently unable to predict those patients who will deteriorate, even asymptomatic colloid cysts should be surgically treated (Little & MacCarty 1974, Ryder et al 1986, Hall & Lunsford 1987). The question whether direct surgical exposure and excision of the colloid cyst is superior treatment to aspiration of the colloid cyst is as yet unresolved, and the potential advantages and disadvantages of each type of surgical procedure will be discussed.

Excision of the colloid cyst has the surgical objectives of removing the mass lesion from within the third ventricle and re-establishing the normal CSF pathways. However, it should be noted that even after complete surgical removal of the cyst, hydrocephalus may occasionally persist (Little & MacCarty 1974, Ganti et al 1981). This can be explained by obstruction of the ventricular system by cyst contents or blood spilled at the time of surgery, but also air studies and ventriculographic studies have demonstrated that a secondary aqueductal stenosis may be associated with or caused by the colloid cyst (Brun & Egund 1973, Ganti et al 1981).

SURGICAL MANAGEMENT

As discussed, the goals of surgical management of colloid cysts are to relieve hydrocephalus, and remove the risk of sudden deterioration and/or death, this deterioration being due to either the effect of acute hydrocephalus or the third ventricular cyst itself causing a mass effect.

CSF diversion

Urgent bilateral ventricular CSF diversion for the obtunded patient has been discussed.

If an open or ventriculoscopic procedure is planned to remove the cyst, ventricular drainage should be delayed if the patient's condition allows as ventricular dilation technically facilitates these procedures.

After removal of the colloid cyst or decompression of the cyst by aspiration, ventricular shunting is not routinely recommended, and is performed only if clinically and radiologically indicated. In these cases, particularly if the septum pellucidum has been opened at the time of the initial surgery, unilateral shunting of the lateral ventricle is often adequate.

Bilateral shunting of the lateral ventricles has been previously suggested as being indicated as the sole treatment for elderly patients or those whose medical condition constitutes a substantial anesthetic risk. However, with the advent of stereotactic aspiration of the cyst, there is little to recommend this approach.

Open surgical excision of the colloid cyst

At present, only open operative techniques offer the opportunity to remove the cyst wall as well as the cyst contents.

Walter Dandy performed the first successful removal of a colloid cyst from the third ventricle in 1921, and in 1933 published a monograph on benign tumors of the third ventricle in which he had included five colloid cysts, which he had excised with one death (Dandy 1922, 1933). A variety of open surgical approaches to these tumors was developed, with most utilizing a frontal transcerebral approach to the frontal horn of the lateral ventricle. Greenwood (1949) employed a transcallosal interhemispheric approach to remove two colloid cysts and in 1949 advocated this method in preference to the transcortical route. These operations were attended with considerable morbidity and mortality (Gardner & Turner 1937, Greenwood 1949, McKissock 1951, Yenermen et al 1958), both being dramatically reduced with the advent of the operating microscope and modern neurosurgical microdissection techniques (Little & MacCarty 1974, Antunes et al 1980, Symon & Pell 1990, Yasargil et al 1990). As both the transcortical and transcallosal approaches are both currently practised, they will be both described. Of the two approaches, the transcallosal approach has recently become the more widely used.

Transcortical approach

This procedure employs a right frontal craniotomy and a small cerebrotomy through the middle frontal gyrus to approach the frontal horn of the lateral ventricle. McKissock (1951) recommended excision of a conical block of cortex and underlying white matter to expose the frontal horn; however, most surgeons would now employ a smaller linear cerebrotomy (Symon & Pell 1990). The foramen of Monro is located at the point where the septal veins, thalamostriate vein, and choroid plexus converge. The fornix is seen to arch over the superior and anterior margins of the foramen. Symon & Pell (1990) make the

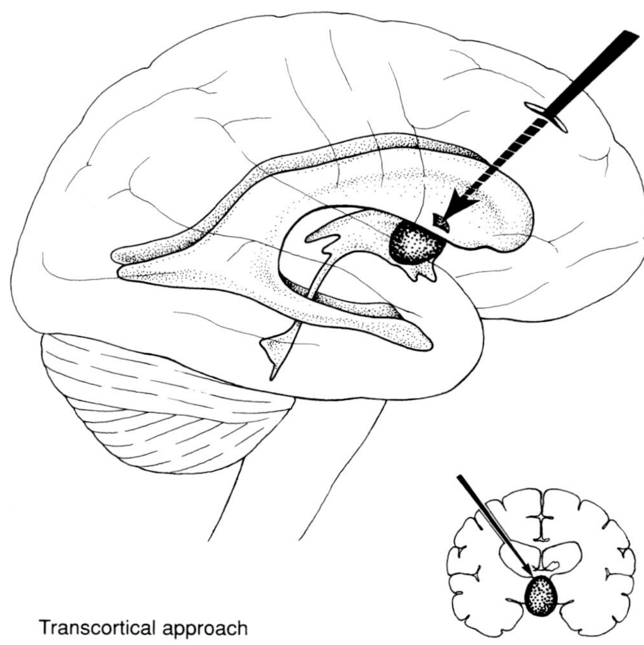

Fig. 47.8 The transcortical approach.

point that the brain retractors should not be advanced such that they lie within the lateral ventricle, as the genu of the internal capsule lies in the immediate subependymal plane in the groove between the head of the caudate nucleus and the thalamus, and retraction or damage to this region is likely to result in motor loss. The colloid cyst is then seen through the foramen of Monro, which is often dilated by the cyst. The cyst is then punctured and aspirated, and after internal decompression the walls of the cyst are delivered through the foramen of Monro using microsurgical dissection techniques.

Sectioning of the fornix to provide better access to the cyst within the third ventricle had been reported without causing clinically overt memory problems (Dott 1938, Cairns & Mosberg 1951, Little & MacCarty 1974). However this is usually not necessary, and should be assiduously avoided as amnesia following unilateral forniceal damage has been reported (Cameron & Archibald 1981, Carmel 1985, Hodges & Carpenter 1991). Similarly, drowsiness, hemiplegia, mutism and hemorrhagic infarction of the basal ganglia have been reported following damage to the thalamostriate and other veins which converge on the foramen of Monro (Hirsch et al 1979, Symon & Pell 1990).

Symon & Pell (1990) have reported 26 cases operated by this approach with the operating microscope (since 1976) with no operative mortality and only one poor result due to persisting memory deficit (this patient presenting in coma). Obvious neuropsychological consequences of a small right frontal cerebrotomy (uncomplicated) have not been reported. The main concern with this approach is the risk of epilepsy, which is in the order of 5% (McKissock 1951, Little & MacCarty 1974, Hall & Lunsford 1987). The major technical disadvantage of this procedure is that it is difficult to perform in the absence of hydrocephalus, some dilatation of the lateral ventricle allowing for improved access, and it is only possible to approach the cyst through one foramen of Monro. For improved access to the third ventricle where the foramen of Monro is small, a subchoroidal trans-velum interpositum approach has been proposed (Lavyne & Patterson 1983), although this is rarely necessary in the case of a colloid cyst (Symon & Pell 1990).

Transcallosal approach

This technique usually employs a small right frontal craniotomy centered just anterior to the coronal suture, extending across the midline and exposing the superior sagittal sinus (Yasargil et al 1990). Large veins draining to the superior sagittal sinus should be protected. Using the operating microscope, the right frontal lobe is gently retracted away from the falx, and the plane between the two frontal lobes is developed until the corpus callosum is exposed. Minimal retraction of the frontal lobe is necessary, and Yasargil et al (1990) have advocated the avoidance of fixed retraction. The pericallosal arteries are protected. A 1 cm incision is made in the corpus callosum, giving access to the lateral ventricle (usually the right). The foramen of Monro is approached and the colloid cyst delivered in the same manner as the transcortical approach. By dividing the septum pellucidum the opposite lateral ventricle may be entered and the colloid cyst also exposed through the other foramen of Monro.

The major advantages of the transcallosal approach are that it is technically more advantageous than the transcortical approach in the absence of hydrocephalus, and it gives ready access to either foramen of Monro (Yasargil et al 1990). It also allows an interforniceal approach for lesions situated more posteriorly in the third ventricle, although this is rarely necessary for colloid cysts (Hall & Lunsford 1987, Yasargil et al 1990). Significant neuropsychological deficits have not been reported in the uncomplicated cases of transcallosal approach to third ventricular tumors (Jeeves et al 1979, Winston et al 1979, Hall & Lunsford 1987), although careful neuropsychometric testing may reveal some deficit (EANS 1990). The transcallosal approach is considered to entail less risk of epilepsy than the transcortical approach (Jeeves et al 1979, Hall & Lunsford 1987), although actual statistical evidence for this is lacking (EANS 1990).

The transcallosal approach does carry a risk of venous infarction, which has been associated with prolonged cortical retraction (Shucart & Stein 1978, Hall & Lunsford 1987) and division of large bridging cortical veins running

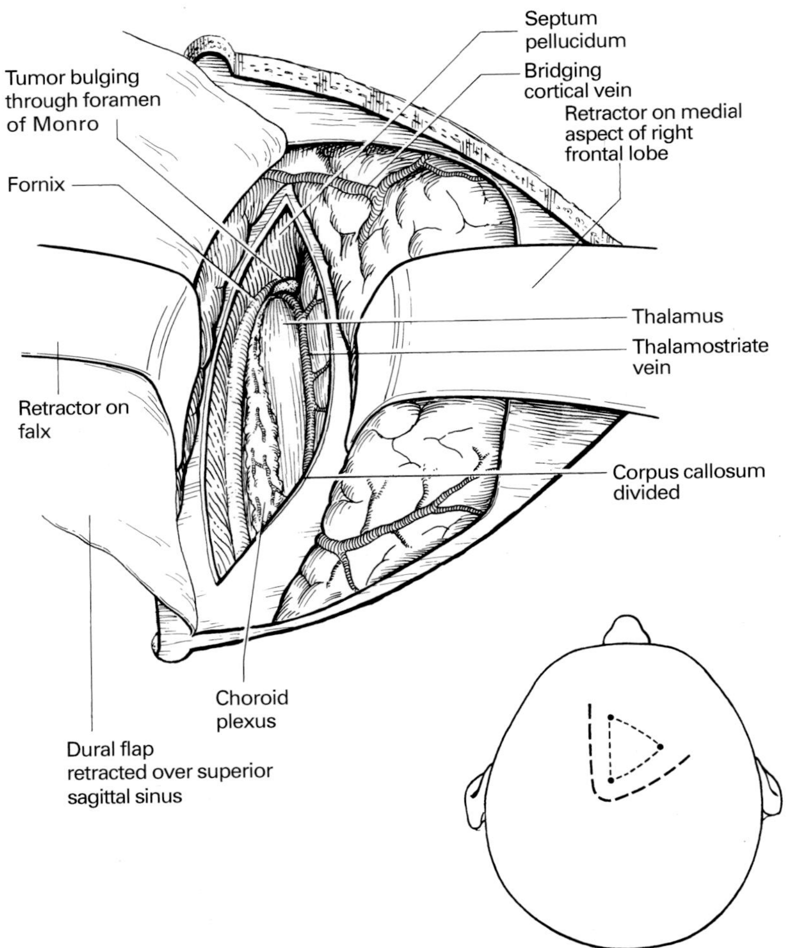

Fig. 47.9 The transcallosal approach.

into the superior sagittal sinus. Cortical retraction may also cause contralateral leg weakness, and the pericallosal arteries are at risk of damage with this procedure. However, with good microsurgical technique the risk of these complications should be minimal. Yasargil et al (1990) have reported a series of 18 cases with 17 good results, 1 fair result, and no specific postoperative technical complications. There was one death two weeks postoperatively from a pulmonary embolus.

Endoscopic aspiration

Endoscopic aspiration follows the same transcortical path to the foramen of Monro as does the open transcortical operation. It has the major advantages that it can be performed through a small burr hole, and requires a much smaller cortical incision. In the case of the patient without hydrocephalus, stereotactic endoscopy may also be performed (Apuzzo et al 1988, Caemart & Calliauw 1990).

Using the endoscope, the colloid cyst may be directly punctured and aspirated, and part of the wall may be removed by diathermy or laser technique. The procedure may be performed under local anesthetic (Powell & Torrens 1983, Auer et al 1988, Caemart & Calliauw 1990, Ostertag 1990). The major disadvantage is that at present the whole wall of the colloid cyst cannot be safely removed without applying traction (and therefore risking hemorrhage). The major advantage of endoscopic treatment is that part of the wall may be removed, and the cyst can be punctured under direct vision, avoiding the small risk of vascular damage which attends blind stereotactic cyst puncture (Ostertag 1990).

Of the series of 15 cases reported by Ostertag (1990), 12 could be completely aspirated. In 3 cases only partial aspiration was possible due to the viscosity of the contents, but in each case the patient's symptoms were relieved. The only complication in the 15 cases was one case of meningitis. None of the cysts have re-collected, although the follow-up period was relatively short (less than 5 years). Of the 7 patients who were not shunted prior to the procedure, none required postoperative shunts (Ostertag 1990).

Stereotactic aspiration of colloid cysts

Gutierrez-Lara et al (1975) first described aspiration of colloid cysts without resection using a free-hand method in 1975. Application of stereotactic localization for aspiration of 4 colloid cysts was then reported by Bosch et al (1978).

Because of the simplicity, relatively low risk, and wide availability of stereotaxy, stereotactic (CT-guided) aspiration of colloid cysts has been recently widely advocated (Bosch et al 1978, Rivas & Lobarto 1985, Donauer et al 1986, Hall & Lunsford 1987, Mohadjer et al 1987, Musolino et al 1989, Kondziolka & Lunsford 1991). The success of the stereotactic aspiration relates largely to the viscosity of the cyst contents, and this has been found to have some correlation with the radiodensity of the cyst on CT scan (Kondziolka & Lunsford 1991). Kondziolka & Lunsford (1991) have reported 22 patients treated with stereotactic aspiration of the colloid cyst as the primary treatment. Of those, 11 patients had a satisfactory result: the cyst was not apparent on postoperative imaging studies in 3 cases, 7 had a small residual cyst, and 1 had more than 30% of the original cyst volume but had relief of CSF obstruction. Eleven (50%) of the patients required further procedures (endoscopic aspiration, shunting procedures or open operation). There was no significant morbidity or mortality from the stereotactic aspiration, regardless of whether this was considered successful or not (Kondziolka & Lunsford 1991). Similarly, Hall & Lunsford (1987) reported 5 cases of CT-guided stereotactic aspiration, with 6 of these having ventricular patency as shown on post-aspiration ventriculography, and one failed aspiration requiring open resection of the tumor. They also found no complications related to stereotactic aspiration. Large size of the cyst does not contraindicate stereotactic aspiration, and Kondziolka & Lunsford (1991) found that size of the cyst related to successful aspiration only insofar as very small cysts were more difficult to puncture.

There have not been reported cases of cyst re-collection, although as yet long-term follow-up data are not available (Rivas & Lobato 1985, Hall & Lunsford 1987, Mohadjer et al 1987, Kondziolka & Lunsford 1991).

ADJUVANT THERAPY

As colloid cysts are benign lesions and produce symptoms by virtue of their mass, surgical therapy (aspiration, excision and/or CSF diversion) is the only recognized form of effective treatment at present. There is no place for radiotherapy or other adjuvant therapy in the treatment of these cysts.

LONG-TERM PROGNOSIS

Following the successful outcome of microscopic resection of a colloid cyst the patient should be considered cured, although in a small number of these cases the patient may still require CSF diversion. Cases of recurrence have not been reported following successful simple aspiration of the cyst, although at present the long-term follow-up data are not available.

REFERENCES

Abernathey C D, Davis D H, Kelly P J 1989 Treatment of colloid cysts of the third ventricle by stereotaxic microsurgical laser craniotomy. Journal of Neurosurgery 70: 195–200

Adams R D, Fisher C M, Hakim S et al 1965 Symptomatic occult hydrocephalus with "normal" cerebrospinal-fluid pressure: a treatable syndrome. New England Journal of Medicine 273: 117–126

Antunes J L, Louis K M, Ganti S R 1980 Colloid cysts of the third ventricle. Neurosurgery 7: 450–455

Apuzzo M L J, Chi-Shing Zee, Breeze R E 1987 Anterior and mid-third ventricular lesions: a surgical overview. In: Apuzzo M L J (ed) Surgery of the third ventricle. Williams & Wilkins, Baltimore, pp 520–522

Auer L, Holzer P, Ascher P W, Heppner F 1988 Endoscopic neurosurgery. Acta Neurochirurgica (Wien) 90: 1–14

Bailey P 1916 Morphology of the roof plate of the fore-brain and the lateral choroid plexuses in the human embryo. Journal of Comparative Neurology 26: 79–120

Batnitzky S, Sarwar M, Leeds N E, Schechter M M, Azar-Kia B 1974 Colloid cysts of third ventricle. Radiology 112: 327–341

Bosch D A, Rahn T, Backlund E O 1978 Treatment of colloid cysts of the third ventricle by stereotaxic aspiration. Surgical Neurology 9: 15–18

Brun A, Egund N 1973 The pathogenesis of cerebral symptoms in colloid cysts of the third ventricle: a clinical and pathoanatomical study. Acta Neurologica Scandinavica 49: 525–535

Buchsbaum H W, Colton R P 1967 Anterior third ventricular cysts in infancy. Case report. Journal of Neurosurgery 26: 264–266

Bull J W D, Sutton D 1949 The diagnosis of paraphysial cysts. Brain 72: 487–518

Bullard D E, Osbourne D, Cook W A 1982 Colloid cyst of the third ventricle presenting as a ring-enhancing lesion on computed tomography. Neurosurgery 11: 790–791

Caemart J, Calliauw L 1990 A note on the use of a modern endoscope. In: Symon L, Calliauw L, Cohadon F et al (eds) Advances and technical standards in neurosurgery, vol 17. Surgical techniques in the management of colloid cysts of the third ventricle. Springer-Verlag, Wien, pp 149–153

Cairns H, Mosberg W H Jr 1951 Colloid cysts of the third ventricle. Surgery, Gynecology and Obstetrics 92: 545–570

Cameron A S, Archibald Y M 1981 Verbal memory deficit after left fornix removal: A case report. International Journal of Neuroscience 12: 201

Campbell D A, Varma T R 1991 An extraventricular colloid cyst: Case report. British Journal of Neurosurgery 5: 519–522

Carmel P W 1985 Tumors of the third ventricle. Acta Neurochirurgica 75: 136–146

Chan R C, Thompson G B 1983 Third ventricular colloid cysts presenting with acute neurological deterioration. Surgical Neurology 19: 258–362

Ciric I, Zivin I 1975 Neuroepithelial (colloid) cysts of the septum pellucidum. Journal of Neurosurgery 43: 69–73

Coxe W S, Luse S A 1964 Colloid cyst of the third ventricle. An electron microscope study. Journal of Neuropathology and Experimental Neurology 23: 431–445

Dandy W E 1922 Diagnosis, localization and removal of tumors of

the third ventricle. Bulletin of the Johns Hopkins Hospital 33: 188–189
Dandy W E 1933 Benign tumors of the third ventricle of the brain: Diagnosis and treatment. Charles C Thomas, Springfield, Ill
Davidoff L M, Dyck C M 1935 Congenital tumors of the third ventricle, their diagnosis by encephalography and ventriculography. Bulletin of the Neurological Institute of New York 4: 221–263
Donaldson J O, Simon R H 1980 Radiodense ions within a third ventricular colloid cyst. Archives of Neurology 37: 246
Donauer E, Moringlane J R, Ostertag C B 1986 Colloid cysts of the third ventricle. Open operative approach or stereotactic aspiration. Acta Neurochirurgica (Wien) 83: 24–30
Dott N M 1938 Surgical aspects of the hypothalamus. In: Clark W E L, Beattie J, Riddoch G, Dott N M (eds). The hypothalamus: morphological, functional, clinical and surgical aspects. Oliver & Boyd, Edinburgh, pp 131–185
European Association Neurosurgical Societies 1990 A short critique of the variety of approaches to handle colloid cysts. In: Symon L, Calliauw L, Cohadon F et al (eds) Advances and technical standards in neurosurgery, vol 17. Surgical techniques in the management of colloid cysts of the third ventricle. Springer-Verlag, Wien, pp 153–155
Ferrand B, Pecker J, Javalet A et al 1971 Le kyste colloide du troisième ventricule. Étude anatomo-pathologique et pathogenique. Annals of Anatomy and Pathology 16: 429–450
Ferry D J, Kemp L G 1968 Colloid cyst of the third ventricle. Military Medicine 773: 734–737
Ganti S R, Antunes J L, Louis K M, Hilai S K 1981 Computed tomography in the diagnosis of colloid cysts of the third ventricle. Radiology 138: 385–391
Gardner W J, Turner M 1937 Neuroepithelial cysts of the third ventricle. Archives of Neurology and Psychiatry 38: 1055–1061
Gemperlein J 1960 Paraphyseal cysts of the third ventricle. Report of two cases in infants. Journal of Neuropathology and Experimental Neurology 19: 133–134
Greenwood J Jr 1949 Paraphysial cysts of the third ventricle with report of 8 cases. Journal of Neurosurgery 6: 153–159
Grossiord A A L A 1941 Le kyste colloide du troisième ventricle. These de Paris. No 216
Gutierrez-Lara F, Patino R, Hakim S 1975 Treatment of tumors of the third ventricle. A new and simple technique. Surgical Neurology 3: 323–325
Guner M, Shaw M D M, Turner J W, Steven J L 1976 Computed tomography in the diagnosis of colloid cysts. Surgical Neurology 6: 345–348
Hall W A, Lunsford L D 1987 Changing concepts in the treatment of colloid cysts. An 11-year experience in the CT era. Journal of Neurosurgery 66: 186–191
Hirsch J F, Zavouri A, Renier D, Pierre-Khan A 1979 A new surgical approach to the third ventricle with interruption of the striathalamic vein. Acta Neurochirurgica (Wien) 47: 137–147
Ho K L, Garcia J H 1992 Colloid cyst of the third ventricle: ultrastructural features are compatible with endodermal derivation. Acta Neuropathologica Berlin 83: 605–612
Hodges J R, Carpenter K 1991 Anterograde amnesia with fornix damage following removal of IIIrd ventricle colloid cyst. Journal of Neurology Neurosurgery and Psychiatry 54: 633–638
Jeeves M A, Simpson D A, Geffen G 1979 Functional consequences of the transcallosal removal of intraventricular tumors. Journal of Neurology Neurosurgery and Psychiatry 42: 134–142
Kahn E A, Crosby E C, De Jonge B R 1969 Tumors of the diencephalon. In: Khan E A, Crosby E C, Schneider R C et al (eds) Correlative neurosurgery, 2nd edn. Charles C Thomas, Springfield, Ill, pp 131–137
Kappers J A 1955 The development of the paraphysis cerebri in man with comments on its relationship to the intercolumnar tubercle and its significance for the origin of cystic tumors in the third ventricle. Journal of Comparative Neurology 102: 425–510
Kasper M, Goertchen R, Stosiek P et al 1986 Coexistence of cytokeratin vimentin and neurofilament protein in human choroid plexus. An immunohistochemical study of intermediate filaments in neuroepithelial tissues. Virchows Arch A 410: 173–177
Kchir N, Haouett S, Chatti S, Voudaouara M A, Chadly A, Boubaker S, Khaldi M, Zitouna M M 1992 Colloid cyst of the fourth ventricle. Apropos of a case. Archives of Anatomy Cytology and Pathology 40(1–2): 36–38 (English abstract).
Kelly R 1951 Colloid cysts of the third ventricle. Analysis of twenty-nine cases. Brain 74: 23–65
Kjos B O, Brant-Zawadzki M, Kuchareczyk W et al 1985 Cystic intracranial lesions: magnetic resonance imaging. Radiology 155: 363–369
Kondziolka D, Bilbao J M 1989 An immunohistochemical study of neuroepithelial (colloid) cysts. Journal of Neurosurgery 71: 91–97
Kondziolka D, Lunsford L D 1991 Stereotactic management of colloid cysts: factors predicting success. Journal of Neurosurgery 75: 45–51
Kuchelmeister K, Bergmann M 1992 Colloid cysts of the third ventricle: an immunohistochemical study. Histopathology 21: 35–42
Lach B, Scheithauer B W 1992 Colloid cysts of the third ventricle: a comparative ultrastructural study of neuraxis cysts and choroid plexus epithelium. Ultrastructural Pathology 16: 331–349
Lavyne M H, Patterson R H Jr 1983 Subchoroidal trans-velum interpositum approach to mid-third ventricular tumors. Neurosurgery 12: 86–94
Lee Y Y, Lin S R, Horner F A 1979 Third ventricle meningioma mimicking a colloid cyst in a child. AJR 132: 699–671
Leech R W, Olafson R A 1977 Epithelial cysts of the neuraxis. Presentation of three cases and a review of the origins and classifications. Archives of Pathology and Laboratory Medicine 101: 196–202
Little J R, MacCarty C S 1974 Colloid cysts of the third ventricle. Journal of Neurosurgery 40: 230–235
Loizou L A, Tsementzis S, Hamilton J G 1986 Colloid cysts of the third ventricle. International Congress on Neuropathology 10: 438 (abstract)
Mackenzie I R, Gilbert J J 1991 Cysts of the neuraxis of endodermal origin. Journal of Neurology Neurosurgery and Psychiatry 54: 572–575
McKissock W 1951 The surgical treatment of colloid cysts of the third ventricle. A report based upon 21 personal cases. Brain 74: 1–9
Mietinnen M, Clark R, Virtanen I 1986 Intermediate filament proteins in choroid plexus and ependyma and their tumors. American Journal of Pathology 123: 231–240
Mohadjer M, Teshmar E, Mundinger F 1987 CT-stereotaxic drainage of colloid cysts in the foramen of Monro and the third ventricle. Journal of Neurosurgery 67: 220–223
Mosberg W H, Blackwood W 1954 Mucus-secreting cells in colloid cysts of the third ventricle. Journal of Neuropathology and Experimental Neurology 13: 417–422
Musolino A, Fosse S, Munari C et al 1989 Diagnosis and treatment of colloid cysts of the third ventricle by stereotactic drainage. Report on eleven cases. Surgical Neurology 32: 294–299
Nitta M, Symon L 1985 Colloid cysts of the third ventricle, a review of 36 cases. Acta Neurochirurgica (Wien) 76: 99–105
Ojemann R G 1971 Normal pressure hydrocephalus. Clinical Neurosurgery 18: 337–370
Osborn A G, Wing S D 1977 Thin-section computed tomography in the evaluation of third ventricular colloid cysts. Radiology 124: 257–258
Ostertag Ch B 1990 The stereotaxic endoscopic approach. In: Symon L, Calliauw L, Cohadon F et al (eds) Advances and technical standards in neurosurgery, vol 17. Surgical techniques in the management of colloid cysts of the third ventricle. Springer-Verlag, Wien, pp 122–133
Palacios E, Azar-Kia B, Shannon M, Messina A V 1976 Neuroepithelial (colloid) cysts. Pathogenesis and unusual features. AJR 126: 56–62
Parkinson D, Childe A E 1952 Colloid cysts of the fourth ventricle. Report of a case of two colloid cysts of the fourth ventricle. Journal of Neurosurgery 9: 404–409
Pasztor E, Pertuiset B, Pickard J D, Yasargil M G (eds) 1990 Advances and technical standards in neurosurgery, vol 17. Surgical techniques in the management of colloid cysts of the third ventricle. Springer-Verlag, Wien, pp 143–149

Perentes E, Rubinstein L J 1987 Recent applications of immunoperoxidase histochemistry in human neuro-oncology. An update. Archives of Pathology and Laboratory Medicine 111: 796–812

Powell M P, Torrens M J 1983 Isodense colloid cysts of the third ventricle. A diagnostic and therapeutic problem resolved by ventriculoscopy. Neurosurgery 13: 234–237

Riddoch G 1936 Progressive dementia, without headache or changes in the optic discs, due to tumors of the third ventricle. Brain 59: 225–233

Rivas J J, Lobato R D 1985 CT-assisted stereotaxic aspiration of colloid cysts of the third ventricle. Journal of Neurosurgery 62: 238–242

Ryder J W, Kleinschmidt D E, Masters B K, Keller T S 1986 Sudden deterioration and death in patients with benign tumors of the third ventricle area. Journal of Neurosurgery 64: 216–223

Sackett J F, Messina A V, Petito C K 1975 Computed tomography and magnification vertebral angiotomography in the diagnosis of colloid cysts of the third ventricle. Radiology 116: 95–100

Sener R N, Jinkins J R 1991 CT of intrasellar colloid cyst. Journal of Computer Assisted Tomography 15: 671–672

Shuangshoti S, Netsky M G 1966 Neuroepithelial (colloid) cysts of the nervous system. Further observations on pathogenesis, location, incidence, and histochemistry. Neurology 16: 887–903

Shuangshoti S, Roberts M P, Netsky M G 1965 Neuroepithelial (colloid) cysts: pathogenesis and relation to choroid plexus and ependyma. Archives of Pathology (Chicago) 80: 214–224

Shucart W A, Stein B M 1978 Transcallosal approach to the anterior ventricular system. Neurosurgery 3: 339–343

Sjovall E 1909 Uber eine ependumcyste embryonalen charakters (paraphyse) im dritten Kirnventrikel mit todlichem Ausgang: Zugleich ein beobacktung wahrer lipochromer Veranderungen mit auftreten con “halbmondkorperchen”. Beitr Path Anat 47: 248–269

Symon L, Pell M 1990 The transcortical approach. In: Symon L, Calliauw L, Cohadon F et al (eds) Advances and technical standards in neurosurgery, vol 17. Surgical techniques in the management of colloid cysts of the third ventricle. Springer-Verlag, Wien, pp 122–133

Taveras J M, Wood E H 1964 Diagnostic neuroradiology. Williams & Wilkins, Baltimore, pp 1376–1378

Wallmann H 1858 Eine Colloidcyste im dritten Hirnventrikl und ein Lipom im Plexus chorioides. Virchow Archives 11: 385–388

Winston K R, Cavazzuti V, Arkins T 1979 Absence of neurological and behavioural abnormalities after anterior transcallosal operation for third ventricular lesions. Neurosurgery 4: 386–393

Yasargil M G, Sarioglu A C, Adamson T E, Roth P 1990 The interhemispheric-transcallosal approach. In: Symon L, Calliauw L, Cohadon F et al (eds) Advances and technical standards in neurosurgery, vol 17. Surgical techniques in the management of colloid cysts of the third ventricle. Springer-Verlag, Wien, pp 122–133

Yenermen M H, Bowerman C I, Haymaker W 1958 Colloid cyst of the third ventricle: a clinical study of 54 cases in the light of previous publications. Acta Neuroveg 17: 211–277

Zilkha A 1981 Computed tomography of colloid cysts of the third ventricle. Clinical Radiology 32: 397–401

PART X

Metastatic brain tumors

48. Metastatic brain tumors

Raymond Sawaya   Rajesh K. Bindal

Brain metastasis is a common complication of systemic cancer and is an important cause of morbidity and mortality in cancer patients. It is the most common type of intracranial tumor and its incidence may be rising. This chapter deals with epidemiology, pathology, clinical features and diagnostic techniques, and methods of treatment of brain (parenchymal) metastases.

EPIDEMIOLOGY

The frequency with which various cancers metastasize to the brain varies dramatically from one type of cancer to another. Generalizations on the overall incidence of brain metastasis in cancer patients are not very useful. Instead, it is important to examine each type of primary cancer separately. Autopsy data are the best source of information regarding the frequency of brain metastasis in patients with various types of cancer; however, published reports sometimes indicate very different rates of brain metastasis, even for the same type of primary cancer. Multiple large autopsy series from different institutions should be examined and evaluated to obtain the best picture of overall rate of metastasis. Lung, breast, melanoma, renal, and colon cancers are by far the most common primary tumors for brain metastases. Table 48.1 presents the frequency of brain metastasis found at autopsy in patients dying of these cancers. It is important to note that in patients with lung primaries, the actual tissue histology is very important in determining metastatic frequency, as adenocarcinoma and small cell cancers metastasize to the brain quite commonly whereas squamous cell carcinomas do so more rarely (Cox & Komaki 1986). Metastases to the brain are more rarely found from other types of cancers such as sarcoma, ovarian, prostate and bladder primaries (Castaldo et al 1983, Taylor et al 1984, Stein et al 1986, Bloch et al 1987, Dauplat et al 1987, Steinfeld & Zelefsky 1987, Lewis 1988, Anderson et al 1992). It must be noted that the rate of total central nervous system metastasis is higher than indicated on this table due to dural, leptomeningeal, and spinal metastases, which are excluded from the above figures.

Table 48.1 Autopsy data on frequency of brain metastases in patients dying of cancer

Study	Year	Histology of primary cancer	Number of autopsies	% with brain metastasis
Galluzzi & Payne	1956	Lung	647	26
Newman & Hansen	1974	Lung	247	23
Takakura et al	1982	Lung	747	36
Sorensen et al	1988	Adeno	87	44
Burgess et al	1979	SCLC	177	40
Hirsch et al	1982	SCLC	87	50
Cox & Komaki	1986	Squamous	123	13
		Adeno	129	54
		SCLC	82	45
		Large	54	52
All lung			2380	33
Takakura et al	1982	Breast	526	21
Tsukada et al	1983	Breast	1044	18
Lee*	1983	Breast	3846	22
All breast			5416	21
Takakura et al	1982	Melanoma	49	49
Amer et al	1978	Melanoma	53	68
de la Monte et al	1983	Melanoma	56	64
Lee*	1980	Melanoma	553	46
All melanoma			711	48
Takakura et al	1982	GI	773	6
Saitoh et al	1982	Renal	1828	10
Takakura et al	1982	Renal	199	17
All renal			2027	11

* Literature review
Adeno = lung adenocarcinoma; SCLC = small cell lung carcinoma; Squamous = squamous cell lung carcinoma; Large = large cell lung carcinoma.

In Table 48.2, the total number of patients developing brain metastases annually is estimated. Cancer mortality statistics were obtained from data compiled by the National Cancer Institute (Boring et al 1991). The frequency of brain metastasis from lung, breast, skin, colon, and kidney cancers is estimated from Table 48.1 while the

Table 48.2 Estimated number of patients developing brain metastases each year in the United States

Primary site	Number of deaths	Frequency of brain metastasis (%)	Number of patients with brain metastasis
Lung	142 000	32	45 400
Breast	44 300	21	9300
Skin	8800	48	4200
Colon	53 300	6	3200
Kidney	10 300	11	1100
Liver and pancreas	36 900	5	1800
Prostate	30 000	6	1800
Leukemia	18 100	8	1400
Sarcoma	4200	15	600
Female genital	23 500	2	500
Lymphoma	19 800	5	1000
Thyroid	1025	17	200
Others	143 600	19	27 300
Total	535 825	19	97 800

frequency of brain metastasis from other types of tumor is estimated from a large autopsy series by Takakura et al (1982). Brain metastasis is by far the most common type of intracranial tumor, and the total number of metastatic brain tumors diagnosed annually outnumbers the total number of all other intracranial tumors combined. Evidence indicates that the overall incidence of brain metastasis is rising due to improved cancer therapy for the systemic (extracranial) disease (Posner & Chernik 1978). As cancer patients live longer, the probability of developing brain metastases at some time in the course of the disease may be increased. Therefore, it is possible that the true incidence of brain metastasis is somewhat higher than that presented in the above table.

Figure 48.1 represents a histogram of the incidence of brain metastases based on age. The incidence of brain metastases based on age is similar to that of primary systemic tumors. It has been reported by many investigators, however, that younger cancer patients with a given type of cancer are more likely than older patients to develop brain metastases (Aaronson et al 1964, Takakura et al 1982, de la Monte et al 1988, Sorensen et al 1988). This tendency is irrespective of length of survival and may represent a biological difference in the aggressiveness of neoplastic cells of younger cancer patients.

Lung cancer is the most common source of brain metastasis in males whereas breast cancer is the most common source in females (Takakura et al 1982). This difference is largely a result of the different incidences of these primary cancers in the sexes. With the increasing frequency of lung cancer in females, it is likely that lung cancer will very soon become the most common primary site for women as well, if it has not already done so. The incidence of brain metastasis from a given primary is the same regardless of the sex of the patient, except in patients with melanoma. Males with melanoma are more likely to develop brain metastasis than are females (Fell et al 1980, Takakura et al 1982). It has been suggested that this difference is because melanoma in males is more likely to develop on the head, neck or trunk. Melanoma primaries in these locations are more likely to spread to the brain (Amer et al 1978, Robinson et al 1987).

PATHOLOGY

Despite their varied sites of origin, the macroscopic appearance of brain metastases have many similarities (Russell & Rubinstein 1971). Tumors are generally spheroid and well demarcated from brain tissue (Fig. 48.2). Cut surfaces tend to be pinkish-gray, granular and soft. Tumors are often surrounded by an extensive zone of edema. The extent of this edema is irrespective of the size

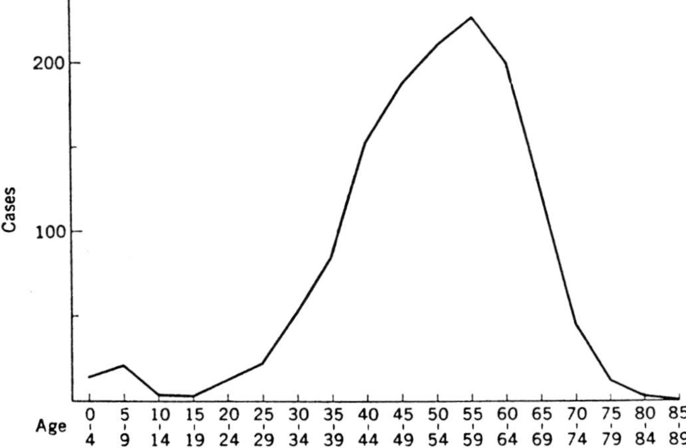

Fig. 48.1 Histogram of the incidence of brain metastasis based on age. Reproduced with permission from Takakura et al (1982).

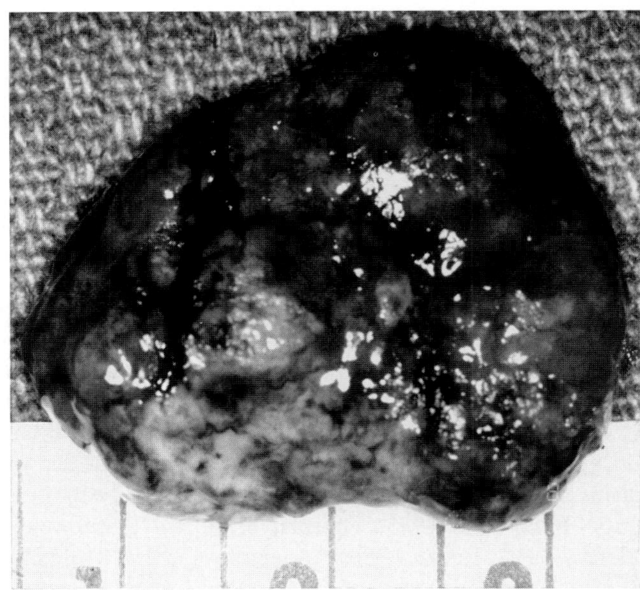

Fig. 48.2 Gross pathologic specimen of a metastatic lung carcinoma to the brain.

of the tumor nodule. Large tumors very often have a central region of necrosis resulting in a softened or even liquified, pus-like core. They also tend to be flattened along the brain surface or even elongated along white-matter fiber tracts. Metastases are most often located at the junction of the gray and white matter of the brain, where the tumor emboli are trapped in the cerebral vasculature. The histologic appearance of these metastases is similar to that of other systemic metastases. It is interesting to note that, although most metastases appear well demarcated from surrounding brain tissue on gross examination, microscopically these tumors may have a somewhat infiltrative appearance (Stortebecker 1954, Henson & Urich 1982). This has been noted for tumors of various histologic types, such as small cell (Takakura et al 1982) and epidermoid lung cancer, (Paillas & Pellet 1975, Sundaresan & Galicich 1985) melanoma (Kaye 1992), and colon carcinoma (Sundaresan & Galicich 1985). This infiltration is not as extensive as that of malignant gliomas, but it still may play an important role in recurrence after surgical excision. Why some metastases may appear infiltrative whereas others do not, and why malignant primary brain tumors are far more infiltrative than metastatic tumors is poorly understood.

Blood-brain barrier

The nature of the blood-brain barrier is changed in metastatic brain tumors. It is well known that blood vessels formed by neoplasms are often defective, even in systemic tumors. In the brain, tumor-induced blood vessels have increased permeability and an imperfect blood-brain barrier. Capillary endothelial cells in metastatic brain tumors display characteristics found in blood vessels of systemic neoplasms, including gap junctions and membrane fenestration, with these characteristics being most common in the center of the tumor (Long 1979). This breakdown in the blood-brain barrier results in an increased capillary permeability to serum proteins and other large molecular weight compounds in the blood. Experimental evidence suggests that tumor angiogenesis and increased permeability begins when a tumor exceeds 1 mm in size (Hasegawa et al 1983). This fact is taken advantage of in contrast-enhanced CT and MRI studies. Tumors show enhancement on radiographs due to their preferential uptake of contrast agents as a result of a defective blood-brain barrier.

This disruption of the blood-brain barrier results in the often extensive edema surrounding metastases. With a disruption, fluids and proteins leak out of blood vessels into brain tissue, causing what is termed vasogenic edema. This edema is largely confined to the extracellular spaces of the white matter of the brain. Interestingly, the size of the lesion itself often does not correlate with the extent of peritumoral edema. The exact relationship between tumors and extent of edema is poorly characterized. The disrupted blood-brain barrier in metastases also has important implications for chemotherapy, which will be discussed in the corresponding section.

Localization and number

The cerebrum is the site of localization of 80–85% of all brain metastases, the cerebellum is the site of 10–15%, and the brainstem is the site of 3–5% (Haar & Patterson 1972, Takakura et al 1982, Delattre et al 1988). There is a rough tendency for the overall distribution of brain metastases to correspond to the relative size and blood flow of regions in the brain; however, there are exceptions to this. Cerebral metastases have an increased tendency to be found at the temporo-parieto-occipital junction, where the terminal branches of the middle cerebral artery are located (Kindt 1964, Delattre et al 1988). It is estimated that the weight of the cerebrum is 9 times that of the cerebellum (Ask-Upmark 1956); however, the relative frequency of metastasis to the cerebellum and brainstem is higher than predicted by their relative weights. The reasons for this are unclear. The relative distribution of metastasis may also vary by the tumor histology (Graf et al 1988), but this phenomenon is poorly characterized. Some reports suggest that the rate of posterior fossa metastasis may be higher in pelvic and gastrointestinal tumors (Takakura et al 1982, Cascino et al 1983a, Delattre et al 1988), a phenomenon which may be the result of spread via Batson's venous plexus (Batson 1941).

The relative frequency of single or multiple metastases varies with the type of primary tumor. Melanoma has the highest tendency to produce multiple lesions, followed by lung and breast primaries. Metastases from colon primaries present with multiple tumors 50% of the time (Cascino et al 1983a), whereas renal metastases usually present with only one lesion (Decker et al 1984, Gay et al 1987). Table 48.3 shows the percentage of patients with multiple brain metastases in various studies. Overall, autopsy studies show that 60–85% of all patients dying

Table 48.3 Studies on tumor multiplicity

Study (autopsy unless otherwise stated)	Tumor histology	% with multiple lesions	Number of patients evaluated
Ask-Upmark (1956)	Mixed	65	696
Chason et al (1963)	Mixed	86	137
Graf et al (1988)	Mixed	58	230
Delattre et al* (1988)	Lung	54	140
Galluzzi & Payne (1956)	Lung	64	166
Tsukada et al (1983)	Breast	58	193
Patel et al (1978)	Melanoma	75	106
Madajewicz et al (1984)	Melanoma	73	64
Cascino et al* (1983a)	Colon	50	40
Decker et al* (1984)	Renal	21	34

*Nonautopsy studies

of cancer harbor multiple brain metastases (Galluzzi & Payne 1956, Chason et al 1963, Amer et al 1978, Takakura et al 1982). However, it is probable that patients diagnosed during life are less likely to present with multiple lesions. Indeed, CT studies show that 37–50% of patients present with a single metastasis (Takakura et al 1982, Delattre et al 1988). Studies comparing contrast-enhanced CT with contrast-enhanced MRI, however, have indicated that patients demonstrating a single lesion on CT may demonstrate multiple lesions on MRI (Davis et al 1991, Sze et al 1991). Thus, the percentage of patients with multiple lesions as demonstrated on MRI is likely to be higher than indicated on CT.

Interval between initial diagnosis and brain metastases

Different primary tumors spread to the brain at different times in the disease course. As most tumors spread to the brain by arterial blood flow via the lungs, lung cancer has the shortest latent interval between initial diagnosis of cancer and diagnosis of brain metastases. Patients who develop brain metastasis from lung cancer do so a median of 6–9 months after the initial diagnosis (Magilligan et al 1986, Mandell et al 1986, Hardy et al 1990). In these patients, brain metastases are also sometimes present during the initial diagnosis of lung cancer, and may be the initial presenting sign of systemic disease (Trillet et al 1991). In fact, in one study of patients with lung cancer but without any symptoms of brain metastases, 6% had CT evidence of brain metastasis (Jacobs et al 1977). Patients with breast cancer who develop brain metastasis have a median interval of 2–3 years between initial diagnosis and diagnosis of brain metastasis (DiStefano et al 1979, Kamby & Soerensen 1988). Melanoma also spreads to the brain a median of 2–3 years after the initial diagnosis (Allan & Cornbleet 1990, Stevens et al 1992). Colon cancer has been reported to spread to the brain a median of 2 years after initial diagnosis (Cascino et al 1983). Renal cancer has a median interval of spread of approximately one year (Decker et al 1984, Gay et al 1987, Badalament et al 1990, Marshall et al 1990). It must be remembered that these time intervals are only medians. Large variations from the median may be observed in individual patients.

BIOLOGY OF METASTATIC BRAIN TUMORS

Great strides have been made in recent years in understanding the process of cancer metastasis (Liotta & Stetler-Stevenson 1989). Neoplasms contain heterogeneous cells, differing in characteristics such as immunogenicity, growth rates, and propensity to invade and metastasize. It is thought that the most aggressive subpopulation is selected out during the formation of metastases.

The process of metastasis involves a cascade of linked sequential steps involving tumor and host organ interactions (Nicolson 1988). Tumor cells must enter the circulation, survive in the circulation, arrest at a distant vascular bed, extravasate into the organ interstitium and parenchyma, and multiply to initiate a metastatic colony. Growth of a neoplastic lesion also involves angiogenesis. These blood vessels are often defective and are more easily invaded by tumor cells than are normal blood vessels; however, invasion in normal blood vessels may also occur. As tumors rarely develop their own lymphatic system, entry of tumor cells into the lymphatic system generally occurs at the periphery of the tumor. Although lymph nodes were thought to present a mechanical barrier or filter for neoplastic cells, it is now known that cells can pass through lymph nodes in up to an hour's time, subsequently entering the venous drainage. Neoplastic cells are discharged into the circulation either individually or in clumps. It has been estimated that a rapidly growing tumor 1 cm in size can shed millions of tumor cells into the circulation each day. Naturally, very few of these cells actually produce metastases.

As the brain has no lymphatic system, all tumors metastasizing to the brain do so by spread through the blood stream. There are two modes of entry into the brain: (1) via the internal carotid and vertebro-basilar arteries and (2) via Batson's venous plexus. The arterial circulation is by far the most important route for metastasis to the brain. Because all arterial blood must pass through the lungs before entering the brain, and tumor cells are filtered out in capillaries, tumor emboli travelling to the brain via the arteries originate from the lungs from either a primary or metastatic site. This hypothesis is supported by the fact that the great majority of patients developing brain metastasis have evidence of tumor in the lungs and that lung cancer tends to travel to the brain faster than other cancers. If there is no evidence of lung metastasis, it is likely that a microscopic lesion exists, or spread may have occurred via Batson's venous plexus. Spread via Batson's venous plexus would be expected to result in increased spinal involvement for cancers from these sites. Some authors have rejected the role of Batson's venous plexus as a route of metastasis by indicating that this increased spinal involvement is not seen (Delattre et al 1988). Some large autopsy studies indicate, however, that patients with brain metastases from gastro-pelvic cancer do indeed have increased spinal involvement (Weiss et al 1986).

DIAGNOSIS

Clinical signs and symptoms

Up to two-thirds of all brain metastases are symptomatic at some time during life (Cairncross et al 1979, Hirsch et al 1982). Clinical evidence of neurologic signs and symptoms is the first indicator of brain metastases in most patients. The signs and symptoms of metastatic tumors are very similar to signs and symptoms of other expanding intracranial mass lesions. Symptoms have two main etiologies: (1) increased intracranial pressure (ICP), and (2) focal irritation or destruction of neurons.

Increased intracranial pressure can be caused by direct mass effect of the tumor, by edematous expansion of the surrounding white matter, by obstructive hydrocephalus or, most commonly, by a combination of these effects. Except in pediatric patients, the skull is a rigid container of fixed volume. Therefore, any increase in intracranial volume from edema or expanding tumor mass must be compensated for in some manner. Initially, the volume of blood in vessels and cerebrospinal fluid (CSF) in ventricles and cisterns is reduced, while ICP is kept constant; however, when this compensatory mechanism is exhausted, ICP rises. Cerebellar lesions often cause increased ICP by compressing the aqueduct of Sylvius and fourth ventricle, resulting in obstructive hydrocephalus. Symptoms of increased intracranial pressure include headache, nausea, vomiting, confusion, and lethargy. These signs and symptoms rarely have any localizing value. Increased ICP can also cause herniation of brain tissue into adjacent compartments, damaging both the herniating tissue and the herniated tissue. This can give rise to false localizing signs since specific areas of the brain distant to the tumor site are affected.

Focal irritation or destruction of surrounding brain tissue can result from direct compression of neurons, effects of peritumoral edema, or hemorrhage. These events often result in focal signs and symptoms that have very important localizing value, including hemiparesis, visual field defects, aphasia, focal seizures, and ataxia.

The presenting signs and symptoms of patients in five representative studies are shown in Table 48.4. The most common symptoms are headache, focal weakness, and mental and behavioral disturbances. Symptoms of brain metastases generally have a gradual onset, but acute onset may occur and is often precipitated by hemorrhage into the tumor. Choriocarcinoma and melanoma have the greatest propensity to present as hemorrhagic lesions (Leeds et al 1992, Nutt & Patchell 1992, Salcman 1992). Up to 80% of brain metastases from melanoma have radiographic evidence of hemorrhage, although the bleeding is often clinically silent (Salcman 1992). Macroscopic evidence of hemorrhage is found at autopsy in 60% of germ cell, 30% of melanoma, 5% of lung, and 1% of breast metastases (Graus et al 1985). Acute stroke-like onset of symptoms occurs in 43% of these patients (Graus et al 1985). Overall, 14% of brain metastases are hemorrhagic (Mandybur 1977). Even though a relatively small percentage of bronchogenic metastases are hemorrhagic, these lesions represent the most common source of hemorrhagic lesions as a direct result of their much greater absolute number (Salcman 1992).

Radiologic appearance

Contrast-enhanced MRI is the single best tool for radiographic evaluation of patients with suspected brain metastasis. It has been proven by numerous studies to be more sensitive and specific than any other imaging technique in determining presence or absence, location, and number of metastases (Healy et al 1987, Russell et al 1987, Davis et al 1991, Sze et al 1991). Both T1- and T2-weighted images play a role in detecting metastases. Multiplicity, marked vasogenic edema, and mass effect are considered the hallmarks of brain metastases (Modic & Beale 1990). Lesions tend to be spheroid and peripherally located, often at a gray-white matter junction. On T1 imaging, metastases appear as loci of increased signal intensity. Larger tumors often appear to have peripheral enhancement with a nonenhancing core, representing central necrosis. Peritumoral edema appears on T1 as a region of decreased signal intensity. In T2 images, tumors often have decreased intensity whereas edema appears with increased intensity. Presence and extent of edema are far better appreciated on T2 than on T1 (Fig. 48.3).

Table 48.4 Study of symptoms in patients with brain metastasis

Symptom	Study (number of patients)					
	Paillas & Pellet 1975 (178) %	Hildebrand 1973 (50) %	Posner 1974 (162) %	Gamache et al 1979 (94) %	Takakura et al 1982 (204) %	Nisce et al 1971 (560) %
Headache	44	26	53	43	57	33
Focal weakness	18	30	40	34	39	75
Mental and behavioral disturbances	22	30	31	34	22	41
Seizure	19	6	15	21	19	18
Ataxia	NS	NS	20	NS	5	NS
Aphasia	1	4	10	NS	10	14
Visual field defect	1	6	NS	13	21	15
Sensory change	10	2	NS	NS	NS	28

NS = not stated

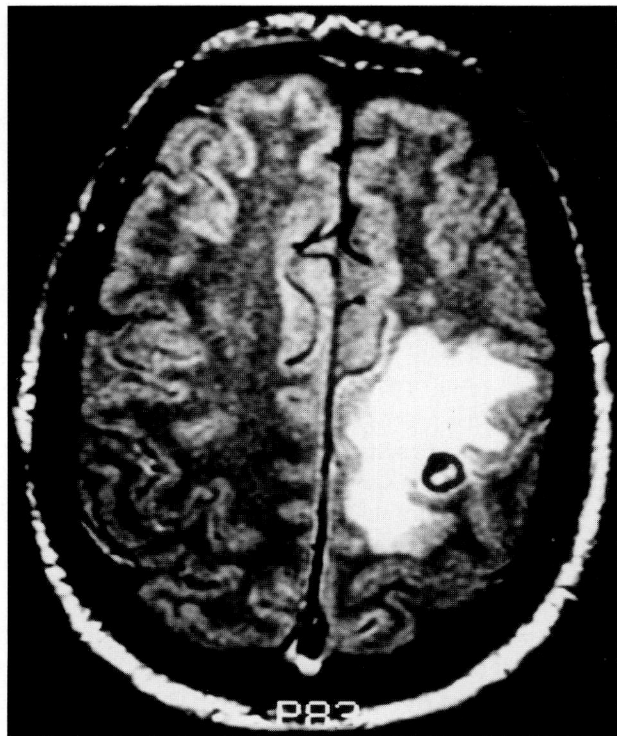

Fig. 48.3 A T2-weighted image of a 1 cm left parietal renal carcinoma metastasis (dark ring) surrounded by an extensive zone of edema (white area).

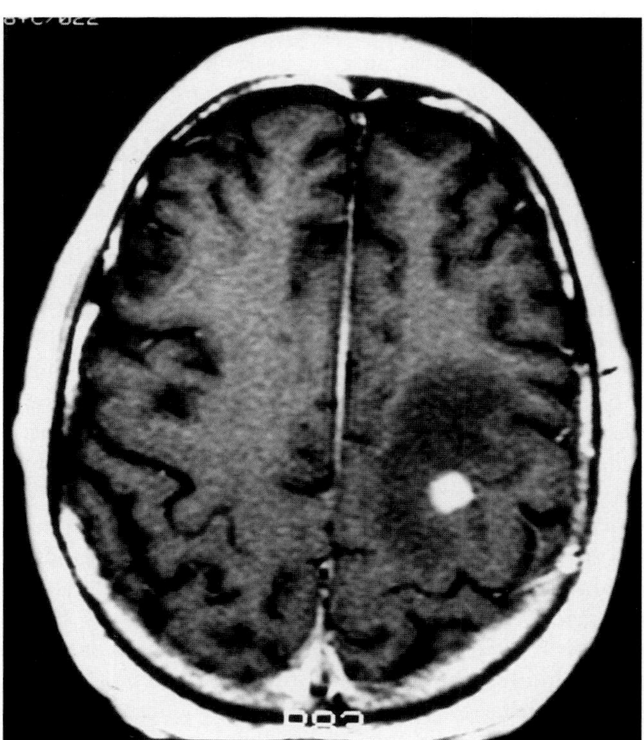

Fig. 48.4 A gadolinium-enhanced image of the patient scan in Fig. 48.3. The metastatic tumor is densely enhancing and is surrounded by a hypointense zone of edema (dark area).

The contrast agent used with MRI is gadolinium diethylenetriaminepenta-acetic acid (Gd-DTPA). Use of contrast makes MR imaging more sensitive; lesions which are not evident on nonenhanced scans often appear with the use of contrast (Fig. 48.4). Although Gd-DTPA is currently the only approved contrast agent for MRI, other compounds such as Gadoteridol, a nonionic, hydrophilic gadolinium chelate, are currently being tested.

Differential diagnosis

In patients with known systemic cancer, the appearance of clinical symptoms and a radiologically evident lesion consistent with brain metastasis are virtually diagnostic. Studies indicate that 89–93% of patients with a history of cancer who present with a single supratentorial lesion have brain metastasis (Voorhies et al 1980, Patchell et al 1990). Patients with multiple lesions are even more likely to have metastatic disease. Even so, the physician must always be aware of other disease states which can produce similar signs, such as primary brain tumor or a cerebrovascular disorder.

Many patients present with clinical and radiographic signs consistent with brain metastasis but without a previous history of cancer. Such patients with multiple intracranial lesions should be strongly suspected of having metastases. Patients with a single brain lesion and no history of cancer are much less likely to have metastasis, but the possibility must be considered. One study indicated that 15% of such patients had eventual histologic diagnosis of brain metastasis (Voorhies et al 1980). Search for a primary site or other sites of metastasis is very important. A number of tests should be performed. History and physical examination are extremely important. Chest radiographs, preferably CT scans and not X-rays, must also be performed. These can be used to find lung primaries or metastases, both of which are very common in patients with brain metastasis. Bronchoscopy can be used to confirm the diagnosis in these patients. Abdomen CT is useful in visualizing colon or kidney primaries and liver metastases. Sputum cytology, stool guaiac, intravenous pyelogram, and blood tests for tumor markers such as carcinoembryonic antigen (Eden et al 1980, Flaschka & Desoye 1987) or fetal antigen 2 (Rasmussen et al 1991) may also prove helpful. A biopsy is, of course, the very best test for diagnosis.

Patients presenting with brain metastases as the first sign of cancer are found to have lung primaries 53–68% of the time (Dhopesh & Yagnik 1985, Merchut 1989, Debevec 1990). Breast primaries are relatively rare in these patients, probably owing to the relative ease of early detection of the primary lesion.

MANAGEMENT AND CLINICAL DECISION MAKING

The management of patients with brain metastasis has been a topic of considerable debate for decades (Black 1979, Cairncross & Posner 1983). One of the few consensus opinions is that these patients have a poor prognosis. The purpose of any therapy is to improve quality and length of life. Management options have been evolving over the years and currently a number of therapeutic techniques and options are available for treatment of these patients. The most important are corticosteroids, radiotherapy, surgery, and stereotactic radiosurgery. Chemotherapy may be useful for some patients, and interstitial brachytherapy may also play a role in the management of these patients. Often, a combination of these treatment modalities is used. Determination of which modality of treatment is best for a patient depends on a large number of factors that are specific to each individual case. The important treatment modalities are discussed below (pp 931–942).

Patients occasionally present in acute emergency situations such as hemorrhage into a suspected metastasis, herniation of brain from greatly increased ICP, or other emergency such as pulmonary embolism. For such patients, complete work-up is not indicated as the results are unlikely to affect decision making. Patients presenting with symptoms consistent with brain herniation from increased ICP should be treated with a high dose bolus of corticosteroids. Intravenous mannitol should also be commenced. Both therapies reduce ICP by reducing brain and CSF volume. Surgical excision of the offending lesion generally follows.

In most instances, however, therapeutic decisions are based on a detailed analysis and informative discussion with the patient. Figure 48.5 represents a management tree that can be used for therapeutic decision making. A detailed discussion of the steps involved in decision making follows; however, the need to tailor the treatment decision to the individual patient cannot be overemphasized.

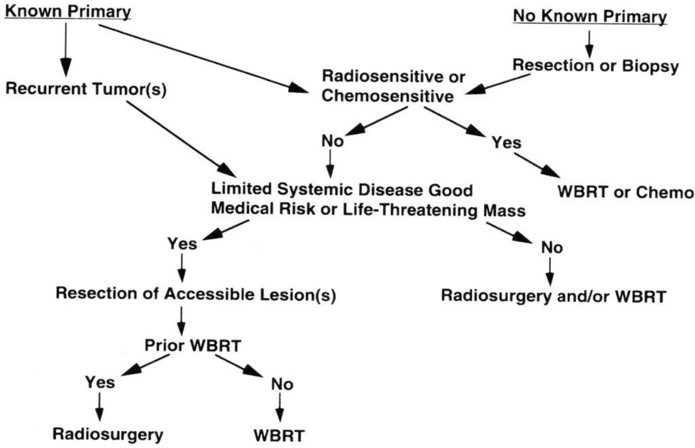

Fig. 48.5 Management tree summarizing the various steps in therapeutic decision making. WBRT = whole brain radiation therapy.

Patients with no known cancer

Patients diagnosed with probable brain metastasis for the first time may or may not have a known primary. Perhaps one-third of all patients developing brain metastasis do not have a previous cancer history (Dhopesh & Yagnik 1985). A diagnosis of brain metastasis cannot be made with certainty unless the primary tumor or other systemic metastasis is found and histologically confirmed or a biopsy of the brain lesion is performed. Procedures useful in searching for systemic cancer have already been described. In patients in whom systemic disease is found, some diagnostic tissue should be obtained from either a systemic or brain site to confirm the diagnosis of cancer. In 16–35% of patients with brain metastasis as the first sign of cancer, however, no systemic cancer is ever found (Dhopesh & Yognik 1985, Debevec 1990, Rasmussen et al 1991). For these patients, the diagnosis of brain metastasis remains uncertain. Obtaining diagnostic tissue is important in determining treatment strategy. If only one lesion is present and it is in an accessible location, surgical excision must be strongly contemplated. Even if the location is inaccessible, stereotactic biopsy should be performed; however, studies indicate that over two-thirds of lesions from unknown primaries are multiple (Delattre et al 1988). For these patients, treatment decisions are more subjective. Surgical excision should be performed if one lesion is particularly large, surrounded by much edema, symptomatic, and accessible. This may relieve symptoms in addition to establishing a diagnosis. Otherwise, biopsy of one lesion should be performed. Even if no primary is ever found, if a tissue specimen is removed and determined to be neoplastic, the patient can be further evaluated under the known or newly diagnosed cancer category.

Patients with known or newly diagnosed cancer

Patients with previously known or newly diagnosed cancer represent the majority of patients with brain metastasis. The first evaluation to be made in these patients is the specific radio- or chemosensitivity of the tumor. Those patients with especially radio- or chemosensitive tumors are generally treated by the respective modality. Metastases from small cell lung cancer, lymphoma, and germ cell tumors generally fall into this category. For these patients treatment with whole brain radiation therapy (WBRT) and/or chemotherapy generally gives very good results. Surgical excision of a brain metastasis of these types should still be performed if there is reason to believe the lesion may not respond to WBRT or chemotherapy or for recurrent lesions previously treated with these modalities.

Unfortunately, most patients with brain metastasis do not have an especially radiosensitive or chemosensitive tumor. In these patients, the status of the systemic disease is crucial in determining appropriate therapy. The majority of patients with brain metastasis have advanced, widespread, and uncontrolled systemic cancer. For example, a patient may have additional lung, liver, and bone metastases that are growing and continuing to spread. These patients have a limited life expectancy, and the goal of treatment is short-term palliation. They should be treated with WBRT and corticosteroids, which usually provide adequate relief from symptoms.

The definition of controlled or limited disease is somewhat subjective. Patients with stable cancer, even with distant metastases to organs such as the lungs, should often be placed into this category. Patients with cancers that are responding well to systemic chemotherapy or radiation are also generally placed into this category. As a general rule, patients who are not expected to expire within 3–4 months from their systemic disease are evaluated for more aggressive therapy because, in such individuals, treatment with WBRT and corticosteroids alone is unlikely to provide adequate palliation for the duration of the patient's life, and more aggressive therapy may also be able to prolong life significantly.

Patients with absent, controlled, or limited systemic cancer are carefully evaluated with the specific goal of surgical excision in mind. The majority of patients with limited, controlled, or absent systemic disease are surgical candidates. The exact number and location of brain lesions are the most important factors in making this determination. As previously discussed, contrast MRI is the best available tool for such an evaluation. All patients who are considered surgical candidates should have a contrast MRI if at all possible; otherwise, double dose contrast CT should be performed. Patients with a single, accessible lesion are definite surgical candidates. A large body of evidence supports the use of surgery for these patients. A recent randomized study by Patchell et al, comparing surgical treatment followed by WBRT to WBRT alone, further supports the benefits of surgery in improving length and quality of life in these patients (Patchell et al 1990). In some patients with a single lesion, the metastasis may not be surgically accessible. These patients should be evaluated for treatment with stereotactic radiosurgery. If multiple lesions are present, more careful evaluation is required. Patients with two or three lesions that can all be removed in one or more craniotomies are still considered surgical candidates (Anderson et al 1992). Patients with two or three lesions may have one or more of these lesions in inaccessible locations. In these patients, the resectable lesions should be surgically removed, and the remaining tumors should be considered for stereotactic radiosurgery. Patients may also present with too many lesions to be surgically removed. These individuals should usually be treated with WBRT alone, but may be surgical candidates in some circumstances. If one or two large, edematous, and highly symptomatic lesions are present and all other lesions are relatively small, the large lesions should be removed if possible. Treatment with WBRT should follow, with the possibility of eradicating all or most of the smaller lesions. A lesion which is immediately life-threatening and accessible should also be removed. Patients who do not fall into any of the above categories should be treated with WBRT alone. Postoperative WBRT is often given as adjuvant therapy to surgically treated patients.

Recurrent metastases

Recurrent metastases are lesions that appear in patients after previous treatment with surgery or WBRT. Any newly detected lesion in a previously treated patient or an old lesion which either reappears after surgery or continues to expand after WBRT is termed recurrent. Since patients treated with WBRT usually have advanced systemic disease and their lesions are not expected to resolve with this treatment alone, these patients generally do not undergo treatment for recurrence. Therefore, most patients considered for treatment of recurrent tumors are those who were previously treated with surgery. These tumors often recur in the brain, either at the location of previous resection or at a new, distant site. The problem of recurrent metastases is growing in significance as surgically treated patients are continuing to live longer than in the past, thus having a greater chance of developing recurrent brain metastasis. The treatment of recurrent metastases is more complex than the treatment of newly diagnosed metastases.

As with patients newly developing brain metastases, the first determination that must be made is the extent of the systemic disease. Patients with advanced disease may be treated with WBRT (Shehata et al 1974, Kurup et al 1980), although if they were previously treated by this modality the indications and potential benefits of retreatment are less clear. Patients with absent, controlled, or limited systemic disease are evaluated for more aggressive treatment. One potential pitfall must be considered at this point. In patients previously treated by adjuvant WBRT, the possibility exists that a presumed recurrent lesion actually represents radiation necrosis. It is often difficult to distinguish a metastatic lesion from radiation necrosis as their CT and MRI appearances are very similar. Radiation necrosis also presents with many of the same signs and symptoms as would a metastatic lesion located in the same area of the brain. Use of positron emission tomography (PET) can be very helpful in making the distinction (Breneman & Sawaya 1991). The best method of confirming whether a patient indeed has a recurrent tumor or radiation necrosis is biopsy. Radiation necrosis should be treated with surgery, corticosteroids, or possibly anticoagulation therapy (Breneman & Sawaya 1991).

If the recurrent lesion is at the same site as a previously treated lesion, the recurrence is termed 'local'. If the recurrence is at a location other than the site of a previously treated lesion, the recurrence is termed 'distant'. Patients may also have both local and distant recurrences. Those individuals developing local recurrence with no other detectable brain metastases must have careful examination of the radiographic appearance of the recurrent tumor. If the lesion appears to be infiltrative and to have recurred in most of the margin surrounding the resection bed, radical surgical resection of the lesion and surrounding brain tissue must be performed to reduce the possibility of re-recurrence. If such a lesion is located close to vital brain tissue, such as the internal capsule motor cortex, or major blood vessels, however, radical resection may not be possible. For these patients, radiosurgery of the lesion is recommended. If a local recurrence appears to be a well-demarcated, nodular mass, surgery is indicated and the lesion should be excised in a manner similar to that of a newly diagnosed lesion. Patients who develop distant metastases should be evaluated in a manner similar to patients with newly diagnosed lesions. Patients with recurrences at multiple sites concurrently should be evaluated using similar guidelines to patients with newly diagnosed multiple lesions, with added consideration of the factors specific to recurrent tumors. Only one study has ever examined the results of surgery for patients with recurrent brain metastasis, but no prognostic factors were determined (Sundaresan et al 1988).

Radiosurgery has been used extensively to treat recurrent lesions, with encouraging results. Brachytherapy, involving direct implantation of a radioactive substance such as ^{125}I, has also been used in a much more limited number of patients with encouraging preliminary results. Unfortunately, many patients suffering from tumor recurrence have been previously treated with WBRT, and reirradiation is generally less effective than the initial treatment. Additionally, if a reirradiated patient survives for a prolonged period of time, the possibility of radiation damage is greatly increased.

SPECIFIC TREATMENT MODALITIES

Corticosteroids

Corticosteroids play an important adjunctive role in the management of patients with brain metastases (Selker 1983). Although survival can not be significantly extended by the use of corticosteroids alone, they play an important part in reducing the often debilitating symptoms of brain metastasis. The first study examining the role of corticosteroids in the palliation of patients with brain metastases was published by Kofman et al in 1957. Steroids have been used since then to control neurologic symptoms of primary and metastatic brain tumors. Patients are generally started on corticosteroids immediately upon diagnosis of brain metastasis. Corticosteroids are produced naturally by the adrenal glands as cortisol and are administered synthetically as dexamethasone or prednisone. Some reports have indicated that corticosteroids may have a direct oncolytic effect on certain brain tumors.

Although corticosteroids provide immediate and dramatic relief of symptoms, their long-term side effects cannot be ignored. Cushing's disease, peripheral myopathies, hypertension, and hyperglycemia are the most important manifestations of chronic high dose administration of corticosteroids. It must be stressed, however, that the benefit a patient receives from relief of symptoms with corticosteroid administration almost always outweighs the potential side effects.

Radiation

Use of whole brain radiation therapy (WBRT) for the treatment of brain metastasis was first reported by Chao et al in 1954. Since then, numerous studies have analyzed its role in the palliation of brain metastasis. It rapidly gained favor as a very simple, noninvasive method of treating brain metastases, providing palliation and some lengthening of life. It is the most widely used method of treating brain metastasis and the only method of choice for patients with advanced systemic disease. These patients represent the majority of patients with metastatic brain tumor. Even patients with controlled or limited systemic disease are usually given WBRT as primary treatment if the tumor is considered especially radiosensitive or if the patient has a large number of metastatic foci in the brain. Many centers treat all patients with multiple metastases solely with WBRT. Even patients treated with surgery or stereotactic radiosurgery are often given WBRT afterwards as adjunctive therapy in an attempt to reduce the possibility of recurrence.

As indicated in Table 48.5, studies have shown that patients treated with WBRT alone have an expected survival of 3–6 months. This survival depends on many factors, such as extent of systemic disease, general performance status at time of treatment, and the radiosensitivity of the tumor (Borgelt et al 1980, Gelber et al 1981, Kurtz et al 1981). Many patients developing brain metastases have widely disseminated and advancing systemic cancer. For these patients, the goal of radiotherapy is solely to palliate symptoms for the short remaining life time. These patients die early, but often not because of failure of radiation to treat the brain lesions. Also, the reduced ability of radiation to affect large lesions limits

Table 48.5 Results of radiation treatment for brain metastases

Study	Year	Number of patients	Tumor histology	Length of survival	1-year survival (%)
Order et al	1986	108*	Mixed	3–6 mos	9
Deeley & Edwards	1968	61*	Lung	<6 mos	14
Nisce et al	1971	560*	Mixed	6 mos	16
Montana et al	1972	62*	Lung	3 mos	10
Young et al	1974	83*	Mixed	2–4 mos	NS
Deutsh et al	1974	88*	Mixed	3–6 mos	10
Hendrickson	1975	993	Mixed	18 wks	NS
Hendrickson	1977	1001	Mixed	15 wks	15
Markesbery et al	1978	129	Mixed	15 wks	12
Brady & Bajpai	1980	343	Mixed	5 mos	NS
Gilbert et al	1980	55	Lung	3–6 mos	NS
		21	Breast	3–7 mos	NS
		14	Other	4–5 mos	NS
DiStefano et al	1979	87	Breast	4 mos	NS
Cairncross	1980	183	Mixed	12 wks	8
Zimm et al	1981	156	Mixed	3.3 mos	12
Kurtz et al	1981	255*	Mixed	18 wks	NS
West & Moshe	1980	350*	Mixed	<6 mos	NS
Borgelt et al	1980	1812	Mixed	15–18 wks	NS
Giannone et al	1987	43	SCLC	5–11 mos	NS
Komarnicky et al	1991	779	Mixed	3.9 mos	15
Gottleib et al	1972	41*	Melanoma	12 wks	5
Carella et al	1980	60	Melanoma	10–14 wks	NS
Byrne et al	1983	63	Melanoma	9–11 wks	NS
Madajewicz et al	1984	23	Melanoma	9 wks	5
Stridsklev et al	1984	39	Melanoma	2 mos	NS
Choi et al	1985	194*	Melanoma	3 mos	9–22
Retsas & Gershuny	1988	100	Melanoma	2.5 mos	8
Maor et al	1988	46*	Renal	8 wks	15
Cascino et al	1983a	32	Colon	9 wks	NS

*Series includes surgically treated patients
SCLC = small cell lung carcinoma; NS = not stated.

the value of this modality for patients with large metastases. Patients with large lesions often have poor performance status, and this is one reason why poor performance status is an indicator of poor prognosis. The radiosensitivity of the tumor can also play a prognostic role. Lymphomas often respond completely to radiation therapy alone. Patients with metastatic small cell lung tumors may survive from 9–11 months with radiotherapy alone, if systemic disease is limited (Giannone et al 1987). Unfortunately, most tumors that metastasize to the brain, such as non-small-cell lung, renal, and colon carcinomas, are considered radioresistant. Melanoma, renal and colon tumors are considered especially radioresistant. As indicated in Table 48.5, the evidence does suggest that patients with brain metastases from these tumors do, indeed, have a poorer prognosis than patients with brain metastases from adenocarcinoma of the lung or breast.

The percentage of patients responding to WBRT varies greatly from study to study. Generally, studies report response rates of 50–70%. Given the somewhat subjective nature of evaluating improvement of symptoms, it is difficult to compare results from different studies. Some evidence indicates, however, that metastases from melanoma respond more poorly than metastases from other primary sites. This is in accordance with the low radiosensitivity of melanoma.

The use of radiosensitizers might be expected to increase the response of brain metastases to WBRT; however, no study examining radiosensitizers has ever indicated that they are effective in improving response rates (Aiken et al 1984, DeAngelis et al 1989c, Komarnicky et al 1991, Buckner 1992).

Dose fractionation

Various dose fraction variations have been examined in the literature. The criteria for defining the best dose fraction regimen include: (1) high initial response rate, (2) short hospital stay, (3) long duration of response, and (4) minimal radiation-induced complications. The best fractionation regimen gives optimal results for all four criteria. Survival is at best a crude measure of the effectiveness of WBRT because 50–75% of patients die of systemic diseases and not of the brain metastases. The Radiation Therapy Oncology Group (RTOG) has performed many studies to determine the effectiveness of various treatment schedules. These studies indicated that 30 Gy delivered in 10 fractions over 2 weeks resulted in a rate and length of palliation equivalent to more protracted and higher dose schedules (Borgelt et al 1980, Gelber et al 1981, Kurtz et al 1981). Use of ultra-rapid fractionation, with 10–12 Gy delivered in 1 or 2 doses, gave an equivalent rate of initial improvement, but this palliation lasted for a shorter length of time (Borgelt et al 1981). Thus, in most centers delivery of 30 Gy in 10 fractions has become the standard treatment schedule for patients with brain metastases.

Prophylactic cranial irradiation

As previously discussed, lung cancer of adenocarcinoma and small cell histologies tends to metastasize to the brain quite often and quite early in the disease course. Because patients developing clinically evident brain metastases undoubtedly had the first seeding occur some time before, it has been proposed that many patients may already have had early seeding of the brain at the time of detection of the primary cancer. Micrometastatic seeds of a size less than 1–3 mm are not detectable by CT or MRI. Additionally, radiation therapy is most effective against smaller tumors. These facts have been used to justify the use of prophylactic cranial irradiation (PCI), in which the brain is irradiated soon after the initial diagnosis of lung cancer, before any evidence of brain metastasis develops. PCI has most commonly been used for small cell cancer, but it has also been used for adenocarcinoma. In theory, small undetectable lesions are destroyed and the patient is spared the pain and short life expectancy accompanying the development of brain metastasis. Both quality and length of life should be increased. In practice, however, the results are mixed. Numerous studies have examined the role of PCI in patients with lung cancer. Many of these studies have shown that the incidence of brain metastases is indeed lower with the use of PCI (Cox & Komaki 1986, Jacobs et al 1987, Kristjansen & Pedersen 1989, Rusch et al 1989, Lishner et al 1990, Russell et al 1991, Rosenstein et al 1992). Only one study, however, has ever demonstrated a statistically significant increase in life-span with PCI (Rosenstein et al 1992). Significant neurotoxicity has been reported in patients receiving PCI (Laukkanen et al 1988, Fleck et al 1990, Johnson et al 1990). The concurrent use of chemotherapy with PCI is likely to result in substantially increased neurotoxicity (Turrisi 1990); however, delaying PCI until after delivery of systemic chemotherapy may reduce its effectiveness (Lee et al 1987). The only study reporting a survival advantage with the use of PCI examined a patient group with only limited stage small cell lung cancer. In this group of patients, prevention of brain metastasis would be expected to play a more important role than in patients with advanced stage disease. A prospective, randomized study of PCI on a group of patients with limited stage small cell lung cancer who achieve complete response of the lung primary after chemotherapy and radiation should be performed. Only if this study indicates a survival benefit with PCI should its use be continued. If PCI is determined to be effective, the optimum dose/fraction schedule that results in minimum long-term morbidity and neurotoxicity must then be determined.

Complications

Despite its noninvasive character, WBRT is not a treatment modality that is completely free of morbidity. Complications from radiation therapy are classified as acute or late, depending on onset interval from therapy. These complications are generally a function of the total dose used, the size of fractions, and the total time over which radiation is given.

Side effects occurring immediately are referred to as acute and include dry desquamation, hair loss, headaches, nausea, lethargy, otitis media, and brain edema leading to increased ICP. A 'somnolence syndrome' of increased fatigue can also appear 1–4 months after treatment. These symptoms are generally transient; however, complications such as dermatitis, alopecia, and otitis media have been known to persist for months after irradiation.

Late effects can be far more serious than acute complications. During the last decade, numerous reports of serious, debilitating side effects have surfaced, including radiation necrosis, atrophy, leukoencephalopathy, and neurologic deterioration with dementia (Sundaresan et al 1981, Sundaresan & Galicich 1985, Lee et al 1986, DeAngelis et al 1989a,b). One report indicated that 11% of 1-year survivors developed severe radiation-induced dementia (De Angelis et al 1989b), while another indicated that 50% of 2-year survivors were so affected (Sundaresan & Galicich 1985). Since very few patients treated with WBRT alone survive longer than one year, long-term radiation effects are not a very important consideration for them; however, patients undergoing surgery for brain metastases often survive significantly more than one year. If these patients are given adjuvant WBRT, radiation-induced dementia could be more significant.

Certain factors such as increased dose per fraction, increased total dose, re-irradiation and concurrent use of chemotherapy are associated with increased development of the late radiation-induced complications. Many patients developing late complications received dose fractions greater than the 30 Gy of radiation in 10 fractions over two weeks that is often given to patients today. Even in patients treated with this fractionation scheme, however, treatment-related white matter changes have been noted (Lee et al 1986). For surgically treated patients with a good prognosis, a more protracted course using smaller doses per fraction is indicated, if WBRT is to be given at all.

Surgery

Surgical excision has been performed in patients with brain metastases since the turn of the century. Results were often discouraging due to the crude techniques available at the time for localization and surgical removal. Some early neurosurgeons, such as Grant, felt that surgery was not warranted in patients with brain metastases because of extensive operative mortality and morbidity and poor postoperative survival (Grant 1926). With improvement in imaging and localization techniques and operative procedures, complication rates have fallen dramatically and survival times have risen. Currently, surgery is accepted as an important part of the management of select patients with brain metastases. Results of studies on surgically treated patients are presented in Table 48.6. Recent series examining heterogeneous groups of patients report survival times of 10–14 months (Sundaresan & Galicich 1985, Ferrara et al 1990, Patchell et al 1990, Bindal et al 1993).

The rationale behind surgical excision is simple. Complete excision of a tumor immediately eliminates the effects of increased ICP and the direct irritation that these tumors cause, providing a large degree of palliation. If all tumor cells can be removed in a patient with a solitary brain metastasis, the possibility of a complete cure exists. This is admittedly a rare occurrence as microscopic metastases are often present, either systemically or in the brain. Even so, in a patient with limited systemic disease, elimination of the brain metastasis can significantly prolong survival. Diagnostic tissue is also obtained to confirm the diagnosis of metastasis. This is important because some patients with a clinical diagnosis of metastasis may in fact have nonmetastatic lesions.

Determination of whether or not a patient is a surgical candidate has already been discussed. It is obvious that a lesion in an inaccessible location cannot be surgically removed. What makes a lesion unresectable is, however, somewhat ill-defined. Lesions located in the brainstem fall into this category; however, cases of successful operation on select patients with such lesions have appeared in the literature (Tobler et al 1986). Lesions located deep within the brain parenchyma have also traditionally been considered unresectable, but with the use of intraoperative ultrasound and stereotactic approaches, these lesions are now accessible (Kelly et al 1988, Rubin & Chandler 1990) (Fig. 48.6). Other lesions considered inaccessible include those located in the internal capsule, thalamus, and basal

Table 48.6 Results of surgical treatment of brain metastases

Investigator	Year	Tumor histology	Number of patients	Postoperative mortality (%)	Survival *Median* (months)	Survival *1-year* (%)
Stortebecker	1954	Mixed	125	25	3–6	<25
Simionescu	1958	Mixed	172	38	<6	3
Richards & McKissok	1963	Mixed	108	32	<5	17
Lang & Slater	1964	Mixed	208	22	4	20
Vieth & Odom	1965	Mixed	155	15	<6	14
Raskind et al	1971	Mixed	51	12	<6	30
Haar & Patterson	1972	Mixed	167	11	<6	22
Ransohoff	1975	Mixed	100	10	<6	38
White et al	1981	Mixed	122	6	7	30
Sundaresan & Galicich	1985	Mixed	125	6	12	50
Ferrara et al	1990	Mixed	100	6	13	>50
Bindal et al	1993	Mixed	30[1]	3	6	23
			26[2]	4	14	55
Salerno et al	1978	Lung	23	9	<6	48
Mandell et al	1986	Lung	35	3	16	NS
Magilligan et al	1986	Lung	41	NS	13	55
Hankins et al	1988	Lung	19	NS	20	65
Catinella et al	1989	Lung	12	0	>48	90
Burt et al	1992	Lung	185	3	14	55
Hafstrom et al	1980	Melanoma	25	12	5	22
Fell et al	1980	Melanoma	42	10	5	21
Madajewicz et al	1984	Melanoma	20	NS	6	15
Hagen et al	1990	Melanoma	19	NS	6.4	NS
Oredsson et al	1990	Melanoma	40	18	8	NS
Brega et al	1990	Melanoma	13	0	11	33
Stevens et al	1992	Melanoma	45	NS	9	NS
Decker et al	1984	Renal	9	NS	14	NS
Badalament et al	1990	Renal	22	9	21	NS
Cascino et al	1983a	Colon	7	NS	8.5	NS

[1]Patients had multiple brain metastases, some lesions remaining after surgery (see text).
[2]Patients had multiple brain metastases, all lesions surgically removed.
NS = not stated.

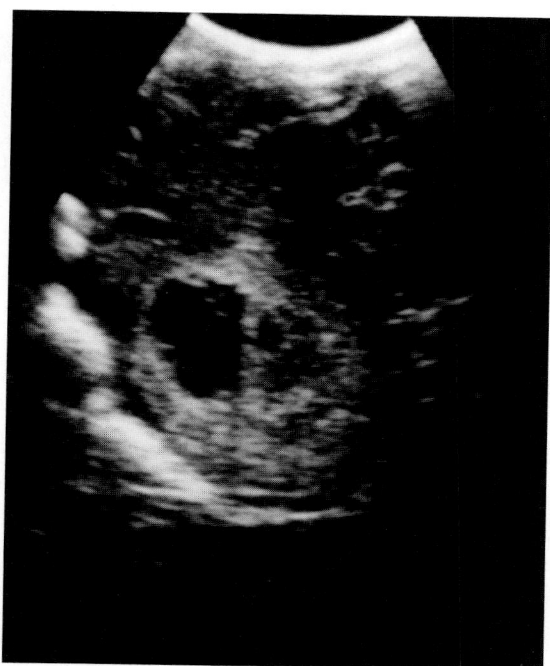

Fig. 48.6 Intraoperative ultrasound image of a large metastatic lung carcinoma located 3 cm below the surface of the brain.

ganglia; however, each lesion must be considered individually, and few generalizations can be made. Ultimately, the level of risk of postoperative morbidity a patient is willing to accept is of utmost importance in determining resectability. The location of an accessible lesion is important regarding potential postoperative deficits or complications. Lesions located in or near the motor cortex and Broca's area require particular care for obvious reasons. Lesions located in the visual cortex can produce temporary or permanent visual deficits. For all of these lesions, careful pre- and intraoperative localization is vital; techniques such as cortical mapping can be useful to minimize damage to vital areas (Landy & Egnor 1991).

Many authors have indicated that the presence of multiple lesions is a strong contraindication to surgery. This is despite the fact that no study has ever specifically analyzed the role of surgery in the management of these patients. We recently evaluated the results of surgery in patients with multiple lesions (Bindal et al 1993). This review indicated that surgery can play a very important role in managing these patients. In our study, 56 patients who underwent surgery for multiple brain metastases were analyzed. These patients were divided into two groups: those who had one or more lesions remaining after surgery (Group A, N = 30), and those who had all lesions removed (Group B, N = 26). Those patients having all lesions removed were matched to a group of patients undergoing surgery for a single lesion (Group C, N = 26). Type of primary tumor, presence or absence of systemic disease, and time from first diagnosis of cancer to diagnosis of brain metastases were matched. Median survival was for those in Group A, 6 months, for those in Group B, 14 months, and for those in Group C, 14 months. There was a significant difference in survival between both Groups A and B and Groups A and C. Additionally, no difference was detected in recurrence or neurologic improvement rates between Groups B and C. This study indicates that surgery for patients with multiple metastatic lesions is just as effective as surgery for a single lesion if all metastases can be removed. (Figs 48.7A–D) Patients in whom all lesions cannot be surgically excised may also be surgical candidates in some circumstances. If a patient has one or two highly symptomatic, debilitating, or life-threatening lesions, resection of these lesions can produce greater and more rapid palliation of symptoms than might be achieved by radiation alone and can possibly extend survival.

Prognostic factors

Certain prognostic factors have been identified in patients who are surgical candidates. These factors can be used to determine which patients might have a better or worse life expectancy after surgery. It must be stressed that patients who are otherwise considered surgical candidates usually will still survive longer than nonsurgical candidates, regardless of unfavorable prognostic factors. Therefore, patients who are otherwise considered surgical candidates should not be denied surgery for these reasons. Prognostic factors include status of systemic disease, extent of neurologic deficit, length of time between the first diagnosis of cancer and the diagnosis of brain metastasis, location of the lesion, and type of primary tumor (Galicich et al 1980, Winston et al 1980, White et al 1981, Yardeni et al 1984, Sundaresan & Galicich 1985, Burt et al 1992). Of these, status of systemic disease and extent of neurologic impairment are the most important factors influencing survival.

The status of the systemic disease is important because most patients undergoing surgery for brain metastasis eventually succumb to the systemic disease, often without any recurrence of the brain metastasis. For this reason, patients with no systemic disease at the time of surgery are expected to survive considerably longer than patients with detectable cancer. Of course, even these patients often have microscopic systemic cancer which only becomes clinically evident at a later time. Those patients with limited or no systemic cancer in whom the brain metastasis can be effectively controlled have a chance of becoming long-term survivors.

Extent of neurologic deficit is also a strong indicator of postoperative survival. Studies which stratify patients in terms of extent of neurologic deficit consistently show that increased neurologic deficit is strongly associated with decreased postoperative survival. The most important goal of surgery in patients with severe neurologic deficits

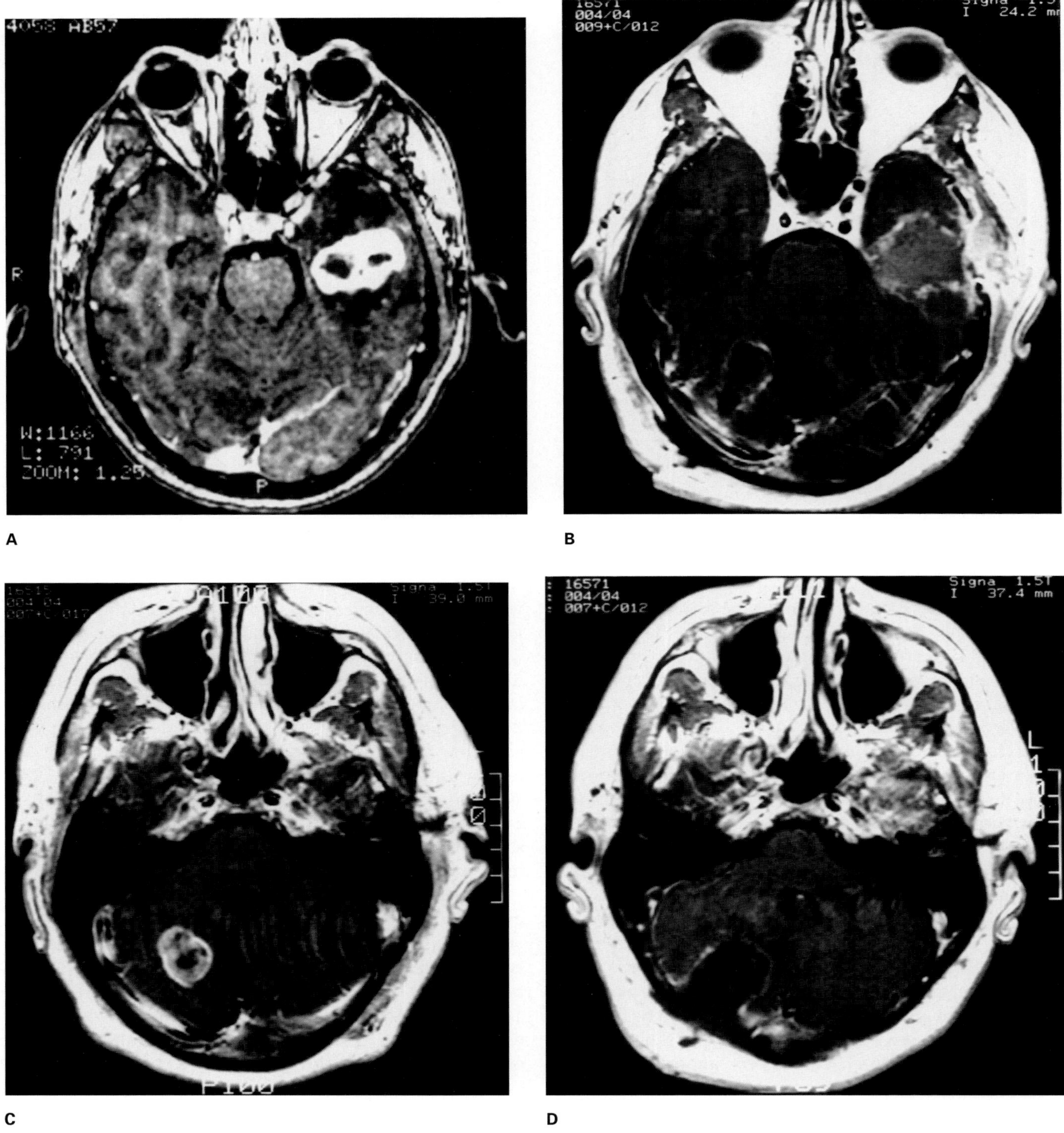

Fig. 48.7 **A** and **C.** Preoperative gadolinium-enhanced MRI images showing a left temporal and a right cerebellar metastatic melanoma. The tumors were resected in two consecutive craniotomies. **B** and **D.** Postoperative gadolinium-enhanced MRI images of the same patient showing a gross total resection of both tumors.

is palliation. Often, excision of a lesion can dramatically reduce symptoms and greatly improve the quality of life for these patients.

The time from first diagnosis of cancer to diagnosis of brain metastasis is also considered to be an important prognostic indicator. A short time interval may be considered a rough indicator of the biological aggressiveness of the neoplastic cells. These tumors may have a greater predilection for overall metastasis or, perhaps, a greater affinity for the brain itself. Regardless of which factor is responsible, the prognosis is poorer than that of patients who have a longer time interval. This indicator is not as important as the previous two factors, however. This indicator is most valuable when compared within a given histologic category. When comparing latent interval and survival between patients with varying primaries, the effect of tissue histology on survival can obscure results. For example, although melanoma has, on average, the longest time interval between diagnosis of the primary and diagnosis of brain metastasis, patients with brain metastases from melanoma often have the poorest median expected survival.

The location of the brain metastasis is also a potential prognostic indicator. Studies of large patient series sometimes give survival breakdowns between patients with supratentorial and infratentorial lesions. Patients with infratentorial lesions often have a lower survival than those with supratentorial lesions. The reasons for this are not clear. Patients with cerebellar lesions are at increased risk for development of leptomeningeal carcinomatosis, and this may contribute to the poorer prognosis (DeAngelis et al 1989a, Kitaoka et al 1990).

The type of primary tumor is also considered an indicator of survival. As Table 48.6 suggests, patients with melanoma have consistently poorer survival after surgery than do patients with other types of cancer. The fact that melanoma appears to have a very high propensity to spread to the brain may mean that these patients have a greater chance of harboring small, undetectable lesions at the time of surgery. These lesions may become evident later, giving the appearance of a recurrence at a site distant to the site of surgery. The relative radioresistance of melanoma would make microscopic lesions less likely to be eradicated by postoperative WBRT. The very unpredictable course of melanoma also may result in a patient with apparently limited systemic disease developing widespread metastases soon after craniotomy. The few studies that report survival after surgical excision for brain metastases from kidney cancers suggest that the prognosis is relatively good for these patients. The importance of the primary tumor on survival is poorly defined, however, as very few studies contain sufficient numbers of patients to statistically examine differences in prognosis due to this factor. No study has ever attempted to compare survival times of similar patients with different primary tumors.

Recurrence

Failure of surgical therapy of a brain metastasis presents in three different ways. The tumor may reappear in the site of a previous resection (local), new metastases may appear at a different site (distant), or patients may have both local and distant recurrences. Recent studies have reported that recurrence occurs in 30–40% of all patients undergoing surgery. Local recurrence occurs in 5–15% of patients, distant recurrence occurs in 10–20%, and 5–10% have both local and distant recurrence (Sundaresan & Galicich 1985, Patchell et al 1990, Bindal et al 1993). Local recurrence is usually caused by incomplete removal of all neoplastic cells during operation. Although the goal of almost all modern operations is gross total removal of tumor, sometimes residual tumor is left in the tumor bed due to invasiveness of the tumor or close proximity to vital tissue such as eloquent brain or major blood vessels. This tumor may be detectable on immediate postoperative contrast CT or MRI; however, even if no visible tissue is left and the postoperative scan appears to indicate complete resection, microscopic amounts of tumor may remain. The use of postoperative radiation or chemotherapy may not eradicate these cells, which will survive and multiply to form a detectable local recurrence. Distant recurrences are caused by new seeding of the brain from the systemic neoplasm, from the release of neoplastic cells into the blood stream during surgical excision, or from pre-existing undetected microscopic lesions that grow to detectable size.

Postoperative WBRT

The role of postoperative WBRT as adjuvant treatment has not yet been clearly defined. Theoretically, postoperative WBRT is expected to destroy microscopic residual cancer cells at the site of resection and at other locations in the brain if they exist. This should reduce the recurrence rate, prolonging survival and sparing the patient the anguish of reoperation. Although most authors recommend postoperative WBRT, only four retrospective studies have specifically examined this question (Dorsoretz et al 1980, Smalley et al 1987, DeAngelis et al 1989a, Hagen et al 1990). Three of these studies have demonstrated that recurrence rate is, indeed, reduced by adjuvant WBRT (Smalley et al 1987, DeAngelis et al 1989a, Hagen et al 1990). Only one of these studies indicated that survival was also significantly extended for patients receiving WBRT (Smalley et al 1987). The patients in this study were operated on between 1972 and 1982, and it is unclear whether all patients were evaluated with CT scan. Without such evaluation, it is obvious that many patients suspected of having had single metastasis would, in fact, harbor multiple lesions. In such patients there would be an obvious advantage to receiving adjuvant WBRT. The other three studies showed no increase in survival. It is likely that adjuvant WBRT does, indeed, reduce the incidence of brain recurrence. Survival is not necessarily extended, however, because the status of the systemic disease is the most important indicator of survival in surgically treated patients. It is interesting to note that the only study which failed to detect any beneficial effect of

WBRT (Dorsoretz et al 1980), either in reducing recurrence or extending survival, also examined patients with no evidence of systemic disease at the time of craniotomy. The most important argument against the routine use of postoperative WBRT involves the significant risk of radiation-induced dementia and other long-term neurotoxicity as discussed in the section on complications from radiation therapy. One of the most important benefits of surgical excision of brain metastasis is the significant chance some patients have of becoming long-term survivors. If these patients are rendered neurologically crippled by WBRT given at the time of craniotomy, the value of surgery is greatly diminished. A randomized trial examining the effects of WBRT must be performed to define its advantages and drawbacks. Until then, if adjuvant WBRT is to be given, a dose/fraction schedule should be utilized which specifically minimizes the risk of long-term complications.

Complications

Operative complications must always be considered in a discussion of surgical therapy. Operative mortality is most often defined as death within 30 days of operation. Causes of death in this time period are often related to: (1) herniation due to edema and increased intracranial pressure, (2) hemorrhage in the operative site or in other metastatic foci, (3) uncontrolled systemic cancer, or (4) thromboembolic phenomena such as pulmonary embolism. Because death from uncontrolled systemic cancer is not related to the brain, the rate of postoperative mortality is not entirely due to the neurosurgical operation. Other, generally nonfatal, complications include hematomas, wound infection, pseudomeningocele formation and surgery-induced neurologic impairment. Although these can potentially be quite serious, often they are transient events without long-term importance. Complications such as hematomas, infections, and pseudomeningocele formation occur in 8–9% of all craniotomies for brain metastasis (Bindal et al 1993). An estimated 10% of patients will develop clinically evident thromboembolic complications such as deep vein thrombosis or pulmonary embolism (Constantini et al 1991, Sawaya et al 1992).

Early neurosurgical studies conducted around the middle of the century reported very high rates of complication. The unsophisticated radiographic methods available and the limited ability to control brain herniation resulted in a high operative mortality and morbidity rates which were a hallmark of surgery in that period. Mortality was generally in the 15–50% range (Horwitz & Rizzoli 1982). With the gradual introduction of advances such as the use of corticosteroids and modern anesthesia, the advent of CT and MRI, the use of the microscope, and the development of intraoperative ultrasound, stereotactic localization, and cortical mapping, operative mortalities and morbidities have steadily declined. Almost all studies of patients treated after the mid 1970s show an operative mortality of less than 10%. Recent studies report an operative mortality rate often 3% or less. Surgical mortality has been reported to vary with the extent of removal of the brain metastasis. Investigators comparing results of gross total removal and partial removal of brain metastases have reported that gross total removal of a metastasis gives the lowest rate of operative mortality. Patients undergoing partial resection may have a doubled 30-day mortality risk (Haar & Patterson 1972). Therefore, the goal of any operation should be gross total tumor removal whenever possible. Surgical morbidity is more difficult to quantify due to the somewhat subjective nature of determination. Morbidity is defined as increased postoperative neurologic deficits. Recent reports indicate that morbidity is generally 5% or lower (Sundaresan & Galicich 1985, Brega et al 1990, Patchell et al 1990, Bindal et al 1993). It is important to distinguish between transient and permanent morbidity. While transient morbidity can be considered to be a relatively unimportant factor, the same cannot be said of severe, permanent surgically induced deficits.

Stereotactic radiosurgery

The technique of stereotactic radiosurgery was first developed in Sweden in 1951 by Leksell. It was originally used primarily to treat functional disorders of the brain by ablating specific sites. Since then, many other potential uses have been developed, especially for arteriovenous malformations, acoustic neurinomas, and Cushing's disease. Other applications being developed for stereotactic radiosurgery include primary and metastatic brain tumors. The radiosurgical system developed by Leksell has become known as the Gamma Knife. Since then, other radiosurgical systems have been developed, requiring a modification of the linear accelerator (Linac).

Stereotactic radiosurgery refers to the use of small, well-collimated beams of ionizing radiation to ablate intracranial lesions. All stereotactic systems have the ability to: (1) accurately locate and immobilize an intracranial target in three-dimensional space, (2) produce sharply collimated beams of radiation with a steep dose gradient at the beam edge, and (3) target the beams accurately, minimizing radiation exposure to surrounding brain tissue. The radiation dose is usually delivered in a single fraction. Hypofractionation has a more lethal effect on tissue than is possible by delivery of the same dose of radiation in many fractions. The use of numerous beams of radiation converging on the target site results in a high dose of radiation delivery to the tumor site. This dose rapidly falls off distant to the target in a ratio dependent on the size of the target. With a small target, surrounding brain tissue receives a smaller radiation dose than with a large target.

The main advantage of stereotactic radiosurgery with

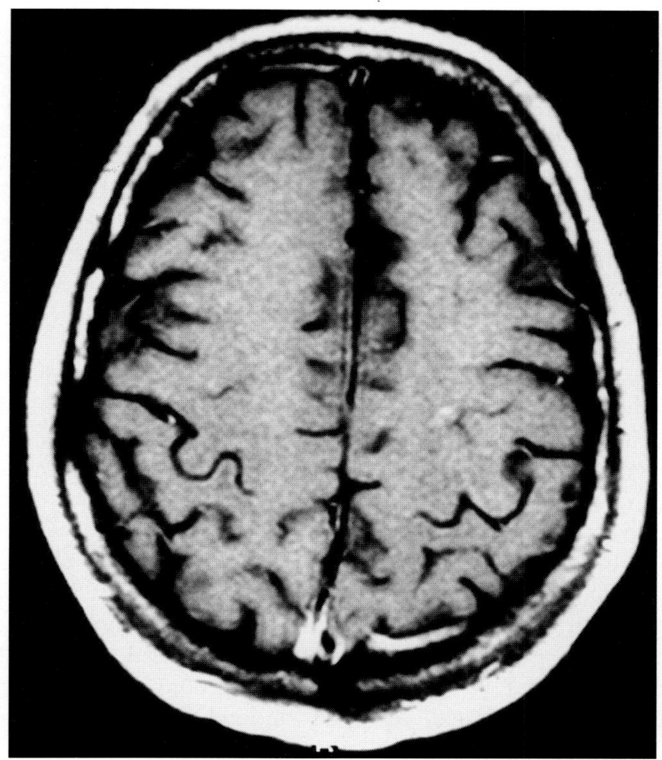

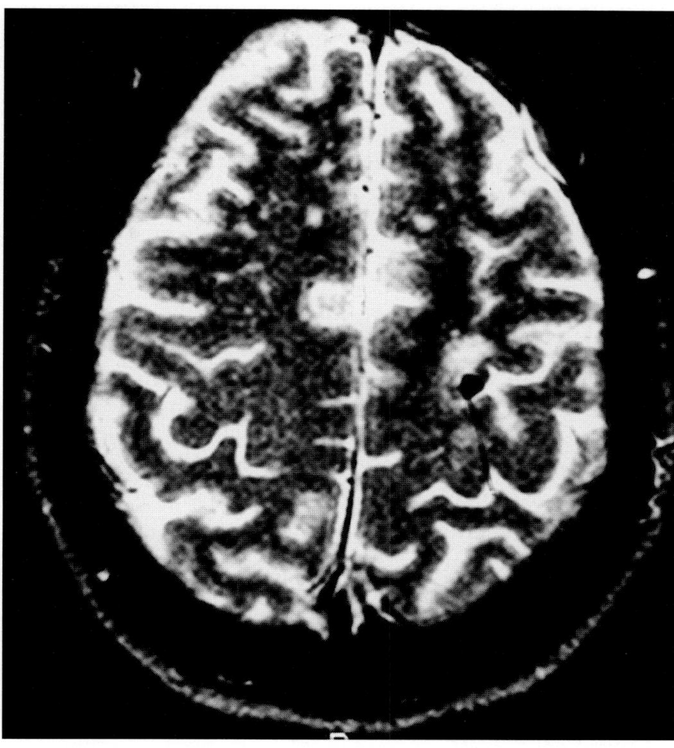

A B

Fig. 48.8 **A.** A gadolinium-enhanced MRI image of patient shown in Fig. 48.4, indicating a near complete eradication of the tumor two months after stereotactic radiosurgery. **B.** A T2-weighted MRI image of patient shown in Fig. 48.3, indicating the virtual disappearance of the zone of edema.

regard to brain metastasis lies primarily in its ability to treat lesions which are not amenable to surgical resection and secondarily in its noninvasive nature, with fewer attendant risks and a shorter hospital stay. Brain metastases are particularly well suited for treatment by stereotactic radiosurgery because: (1) metastases are often spherical with enhancing margins on MRI or CT, (2) they generally are small (< 3 cm) when first detected, (3) normal brain parenchyma is circumferentially displaced by the lesion, reducing the chance of damaging normal brain tissue, and (4) brain metastases tend to be well demarcated and minimally invasive (Alexander & Loeffler 1992). Even so, due to the developing nature of radiosurgery, lesions that would otherwise be surgically resected are only rarely treated by this modality. Recurrent brain metastases and lesions located in unreachable regions of the brain are the ones that are often selected for radiosurgical procedures (Figs 48.8 A, B).

Results of radiosurgery on metastatic tumors are shown in Table 48.7. Median survival is sometimes not reported due to the relatively short follow-up time in many studies. The survival results that are presented indicate that stereotactic radiosurgery gives results that are definitely superior to WBRT alone. It is difficult to compare the results of

Table 48.7 Stereotactic radiosurgery

Investigator	Radiation source	Number of lesions treated	Local control (%)	Median follow-up (months)	Median survival (months)
Alexander & Loeffler (1992)	LINAC	83	94	7.5	9
Adler et al (1992)	LINAC	52	90	5.5	NS
Fuller et al (1992)	LINAC	47	85	5.0	7.5
Engenhart et al (1989)	LINAC	37	95	6.8	NS
Coffey et al (1991)	GU	34	87	10	10
Sturm et al (1991)	LINAC	30	93	NS	6.5*
Kihlström et al (1991)	GU	26	94	9	NS

LINAC = modified linear accelerator; GU = gamma unit; NS = not stated.
*Mean survival.

radiosurgery to surgery because of the retrospective nature of the studies. No investigator has ever attempted to compare the results of radiosurgery to surgery, even in a matched retrospective study. Although radiosurgery appears to give very encouraging results, until a randomized study comparing radiosurgery to surgery is performed, no conclusions on which therapy is superior can be reached.

Prognostic factors

Tissue histology, lesion size, and invasiveness are the most important factors in determining the success of radiotherapy in controlling the treated lesion. Histology is important in that the radiosensitivity of a tumor is of central importance in determining the effectiveness of radiosurgery. Studies indicate that the response of a lesion to radiosurgery is dependent on the radiosensitivity of the tumor, with melanoma responding least well and germ cell tumors demonstrating excellent response (Alexander & Loeffler 1992). Size is important in that tumors of large size cannot be treated very safely because a greater zone of normal brain tissue surrounding the lesion will receive a potentially toxic amount of radiation. Generally, lesions less than or equal to 3 cm in size are considered the best radiosurgical targets. Invasiveness of tumors is important because tumor cells located beyond the sphere of treatment will receive a significantly lower dose of radiation and may survive. These cells might continue to grow into a new lesion located just peripherally to the site of treatment. This has been reported in some studies (Alexander & Loeffler 1992). Improvement in technique will likely reduce the rate of peritumoral growth.

Recurrence

Radiosurgical studies generally report a rate of local control of 85–95%, a level that exceeds the 80% local control expected with surgical excision. In truth, these figures are difficult to compare because recurrence is a function of the length of follow-up of a patient. Many radiosurgery studies have very limited follow-up times. Most studies report that the majority of deaths in these patients are the result of systemic disease or distant brain recurrence and not due to local failure of treatment. It is important to remember that local control for radiosurgery is defined as complete elimination, shrinkage, or stabilization of a tumor, whereas for surgery, local control is defined as complete elimination without local recurrence of any kind at any time in the patient's life. For radiosurgery, failure of local control is defined as continued growth of a lesion at any time in the patient's life (Figs 48.9 A–D). Often, tumor shrinkage continues over a period of months after the treatment date as dead tumor cells continue to be removed from the treated lesion.

Complications

Due to the developing nature of this treatment modality and the relatively small numbers of patients reported on in any given study, little is known regarding complications associated with radiosurgery for brain metastasis. A recent study by Nedzi et al (1991) on this topic identifies variables associated with the development of significant complications. Forty primary and 24 metastatic tumors were treated, and complications were associated with increases in the following five variables: (1) tumor dose inhomogeneity, (2) maximum tumor dose, (3) number of isocenters, (4) maximum normal tissue dose, and (5) tumor volume. It is interesting to note, however, that not a single patient with metastatic tumor developed significant complications. This is probably because metastatic tumors generally are small and homogeneously treated with only one isocenter per lesion.

Complications from radiosurgery stem from the delivery of a high single fraction dose of radiation. By design, the large number of converging radiation beams result in normal brain tissue receiving only a limited amount of radiation that is well within the tolerable range. Brain parenchyma immediately surrounding the tumor, however, may receive an excessive amount of radiation, resulting in necrosis. Radiation necrosis has been estimated to occur in 3% of patients. The percentage of patients developing necrosis may be underestimated because such necrosis is easily mistaken for recurrent tumor on CT or MRI scans. The risk of developing radiation necrosis is increased in patients with large metastases (>3 cm) and in patients who previously received extensive WBRT (>40 Gy) (Adler et al 1992). An additional complication of nausea and vomiting has been noted in patients receiving a dose of over 275 cGy to the area postrema, and these patients should be treated with prophylactic antiemetics (Alexander et al 1989).

Chemotherapy

There are obvious theoretical advantages in the use of chemotherapy to treat patients with brain metastases. Chemotherapy can treat the whole brain, unlike surgery or radiosurgery, which provide only focal treatment. Additionally, systemic sites of cancer can be concurrently treated. Unfortunately its value in the management of these patients is limited. Many reasons have been proposed to explain the apparent ineffectiveness of chemotherapy for brain metastases. These reasons include: (1) the blood-brain barrier, (2) the relative drug resistance of cancers which metastasize to the brain, (3) the fact that brain metastases often occur in patients who failed chemotherapy, and (4) the fact that suboptimal agents were often used in past trials (Greig 1984, Buckner 1991, Siegers 1990).

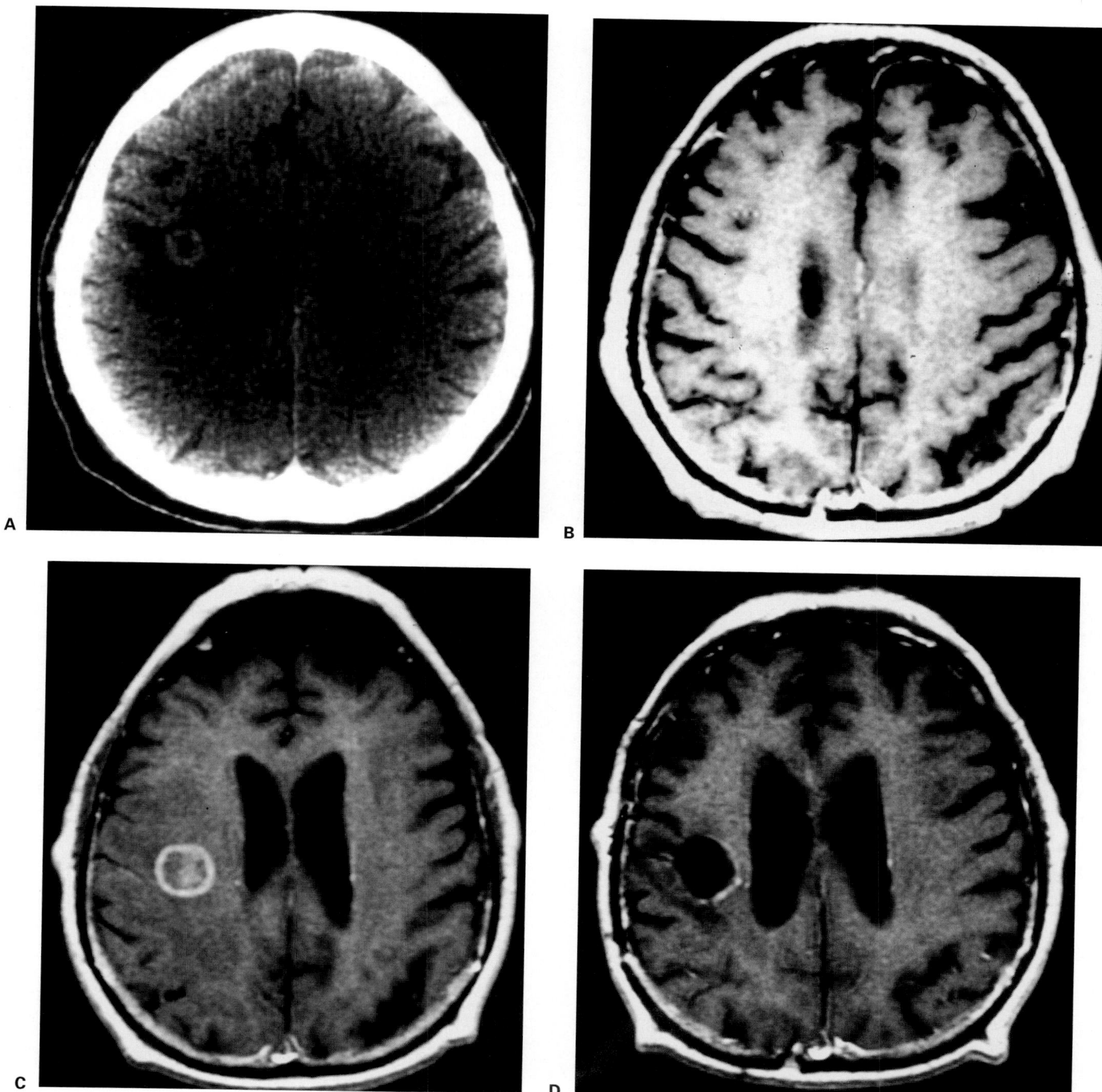

Fig. 48.9 **A.** A CT scan of the head showing a right subcortical metastatic lung carcinoma in a patient previously treated with whole brain radiation therapy. **B.** A gadolinium-enhanced MRI image obtained three months after stereotactic radiosurgery showing marked reduction in the size of the tumor. **C.** A gadolinium-enhanced MRI image taken five months after radiosurgery shows significant regrowth of the tumor. **D.** A gadolinium-enhanced MRI image taken five months after resection of the recurrent metastatic tumor shows no further recurrence.

Most tumors with a known propensity to metastasize to the brain are not considered chemosensitive. The results of chemotherapy in these patients have been mixed (Cascino et al 1983b, Lange et al 1990, Ushio et al 1991). Of all primary tumors known to metastasize to the brain in significant numbers, small cell lung, breast, and germ cell tumors are the only ones considered relatively chemosensitive. There is evidence that chemotherapy, indeed, does have significant effects on brain metastases from these cancers. Chemotherapy for brain metastases from germ cell tumors is considered standard therapy. Its effectiveness, either in conjunction with surgery and WBRT or as sole treatment, has been well documented (Spears et al 1992). The effectiveness of chemotherapy on metastases of small cell lung and breast cancer is less well defined. Reports indicate that chemotherapy in these patients gives response rates for brain metastases that are very similar to response rates for systemic cancer in these patients (Rosner et al 1983, Lange et al 1990, Twelves et al 1990, Boogerd et al 1992). This seems to indicate that the blood–brain barrier has minimal effect in complicating chemotherapy for brain metastasis. It has even been suggested that chemotherapy should be made standard treatment for patients developing brain metastases from small cell lung cancer (Twelves & Souhami 1991). It is unknown whether or not chemotherapy gives better results than could be obtained by WBRT alone or whether the use of chemotherapy as an adjunct to WBRT could be useful. Until a controlled randomized trial is performed, the role of chemotherapy will remain undefined and its use in patients with brain metastases from cancers other than small cell lung and germ cell tumors must remain experimental.

Brachytherapy

Enthusiasm for the use of brachytherapy in the treatment of brain tumors has increased in recent years. The main focus has been primary brain tumors, however. Data on the use of brachytherapy for metastatic tumors are very limited. The theoretical advantages to the interstitial implantation of a radiation source such as ^{125}I directly into a tumor are similar to the advantages of stereotactic radiosurgery. Local control may be increased with brachytherapy, and some lesions that are surgically unresectable may be able to be treated in this manner. The few reports examining the results of brachytherapy in the treatment of metastatic brain tumors suggest that this treatment modality has promise (Heros et al 1988, Prados et al 1989, Bernstein et al 1990, Lucas et al 1991). Unfortunately, significant complications such as radiation necrosis are commonly reported (Heros et al 1988, Prados et al 1989, Bernstein et al 1990, Lucas et al 1991). The role of brachytherapy in the management of brain metastasis is poorly defined and it is unclear which patients are best treated with this modality instead of the previously discussed, better analyzed ones. Perhaps with more experience the risk of complications can be reduced and the specific role of brachytherapy in the management of metastatic brain tumors will be elucidated.

CONCLUSION

Brain metastasis represents by far the most common type of intracranial tumor. Most patients develop such metastases in the setting of advanced systemic disease and require only palliative care. The need to treat brain metastases effectively is becoming increasingly important, however, as advances in the treatment of systemic disease result in an increasing number of patients developing brain metastases in the setting of limited systemic disease. For many such patients, surgery or stereotactic radiosurgery provide the best therapy, but results are still not encouraging as even patients with the best prognostic indicators often die within 18–24 months. Unfortunately, few therapies with more promise appear on the horizon. Until superior treatment modalities are developed, the judicious use of available techniques for treatment of patients with limited systemic disease provides the best opportunities for palliation and extended survival.

REFERENCES

Aronson S, Garcia J, Aronson B 1964 Metastatic neoplasms of the brain: their frequency in relation to age. Cancer 17: 558–563

Adler J, Cox R, Kaplan I et al 1992 Stereotactic radiosurgical treatment of brain metastases. Journal of Neurosurgery 76: 444–449

Aiken R, Leavengood J, Jae-Ho K et al 1984 Metronidazole in the treatment of metastatic brain tumors. Journal of Neurology and Oncology 2: 105–111

Alexander E, Loeffler J 1992 Radiosurgery using a modified linear accelerator. Neurosurgical Clinics of North America 3: 167–190

Alexander E, Siddon R, Loeffler J 1989 The acute onset of nausea and vomiting following stereotactic radiosurgery: Correlation with total dose to area postrema. Surgical Neurology 32: 40–44

Allan S, Cornbleet M 1990 Brain metastases in melanoma. In: Rumke P (ed) Therapy of advanced melanoma. Karger, Basel, pp 36–52

Amer M, Al-Sharraf M, Baker L et al 1978 Malignant melanoma and central nervous system metastases: Incidence, diagnosis, treatment and survival. Cancer 42: 660–668

Anderson R, El-Mahdi A, Kuban D et al 1992 Brain metastases from transitional cell carcinoma of urinary bladder. Urology 39: 17–20

Ask-Upmark E 1956 Metastatic tumors of the brain and their localization. Acta Medica Scandinavica 154: 1–9

Badalament R, Gluck R, Wong G et al 1990 Surgical treatment of brain metastases from renal cell carcinoma. Urology 36: 112–117

Batson O 1941 The role of the vertebral veins in metastatic processes. Annals of Internal Medicine 16: 38–45

Bernstein M, Laperriere N, Leung P et al 1990 Interstitial brachytherapy for malignant brain tumors: preliminary results. Neurosurgery 26: 371–380

Bindal R, Sawaya R, Leavens M et al 1993 Surgical treatment of multiple brain metastases. Journal of Neurosurgery 79: 210–216

Black P 1979 Brain metastasis: Current status and recommended guidelines for management. Neurosurgery 5: 617–631

Bloch J, Nieh P, Walzak M 1987 Brain metastases from transitional cell carcinoma. Journal of Urology 137: 97–99

Boogerd W, Dalesio O, Bais E et al 1992 Response of brain metastases from breast cancer to systemic chemotherapy. Cancer 69: 972–980

Borgelt B, Gelber R, Kramer S et al 1980 The palliation of brain metastases: final results of the first two studies by the Radiation Therapy Oncology Group. International Journal of Radiation Oncology Biology and Physics 6: 1–9

Borgelt B, Gelber R, Larson M et al 1981 Ultra-rapid high dose irradiation schedules for the palliation of brain metastases: Final results of the first two studies by the radiation therapy oncology group. International Journal of Radiation Oncology Biology and Physics 7: 1633–1638

Boring C, Squires T, Tong T 1991 Cancer statistics, 1991. CA 41: 19–37

Brady L, Bajpai D 1980 Intracranial metastatic malignancy: a review of 343 cases. In: Weiss L, Gilbert H, Posner J (eds) Brain metastases. G K Hall, Boston, pp 269–278

Brega K, Robinson W, Winston K et al 1990 Surgical treatment of brain metastases in malignant melanoma. Cancer 66: 2105–2120

Breneman J, Sawaya R 1991 Cerebral radiation necrosis. In: Barrow D (ed) Perspectives in neurological surgery. QMP, St Louis, pp 127–140

Buckner C 1991 The role of chemotherapy in the treatment of patients with brain metastases from solid tumors. Cancer Metastasis Review 10: 335–345

Buckner C 1992 Surgery, radiation therapy, and chemotherapy for metastatic tumors to the brain. Current Opinion in Oncology 4: 518–524

Burgess R, Burgess V, Dibella N 1979 Brain metastases in small cell carcinoma of the lung. Journal of the American Medical Association 242: 2084–2086

Burt M, Wronski M, Arbit E et al 1992 Resection of brain metastases from non-small-cell lung carcinoma. Journal of Thoracic and Cardiovascular Surgery 103: 339–411

Byrne T, Cascino T, Posner J 1983 Brain metastasis from melanoma. Journal of Neurology and Oncology 1: 313–317

Cairncross G, Posner J 1983 The management of brain metastases. In: Walker M (ed) Oncology of the nervous system. Martinus Nejhoff, Boston, pp 341–377

Cairncross J, Jae-Ho K, Posner J 1979 Radiation therapy for brain metastases. Annals of Neurology 7: 529–541

Carella R, Gelber R, Hendrickson F et al 1980 Value of radiation therapy in the management of cerebral metastases from malignant melanoma. Cancer 45: 679–683

Cascino T, Leavengood M, Kemeny N et al 1983a Brain metastases from colon cancer. Journal of Neurology and Oncology 1: 203–209

Cascino T, Byrne M, Deck H et al 1983b Intra-arterial BCNU in the treatment of metastatic brain tumors. Journal of Neurology and Oncology 1: 211–218

Castaldo J, Bernat J, Meier F et al 1983 Intracranial metastases due to prostatic carcinoma. Cancer 52: 1739–1747

Catinella F, Kittle F, Faber L, Milloy F et al 1989 Surgical treatment of primary lung cancer and solitary intracranial metastasis. Chest 95: 972–975

Chao J, Phillips R, Nickson J 1954 Roentgen-ray therapy of cerebral metastases. Cancer 7: 682–689

Chason J, Walker F, Landers J 1963 Metastatic carcinoma in the central nervous system and dorsal root ganglia. Cancer 16: 781–787

Choi K, Withers R, Rothman M 1985 Intracranial metastases from melanoma: clinical features and treatment by accelerated fractionation. Cancer 56: 1–9

Coffey R, Flickinger J, Lunsford L D et al 1991 Solitary brain metastasis: radiosurgery in lieu of microsurgery in 32 patients. Acta Neurochirurgica Suppl 52: 90–92

Constantini S, Kornowski R, Pomeranz S et al 1991 Thromboembolic phenomena in neurosurgical patients operated upon for primary and metastatic brain tumours. Acta Neurochirurgica 109: 93–97

Cox J, Komaki R 1986 Prophylactic cranial irradiation for squamous cell carcinoma, large cell carcinoma, and adenocarcinoma of the lung: indications and techniques. Annual Clinical Conference on Cancer, vol 28. The University of Texas System Cancer Center, Houston, pp 233–237

Dauplat J, Niebert R, Hacker N 1987 Central nervous system metastases in epithelial ovarian carcinoma. Cancer 60: 2559–2562

Davis P, Hudgins P, Peterman S et al 1991 Diagnosis of cerebral metastases: double-dose delayed CT vs contrast-enhanced MR imaging. AJNR 12: 293–300

DeAngelis L, Mandell L, Thaler H et al 1989a The role of postoperative radiotherapy after resection of single brain metastases. Neurosurgery 24: 798–805

DeAngelis L, Delattre J, Posner J 1989b Radiation-induced dementia in patients cured of brain metastases. Neurology 39: 789–796

DeAngelis L, Currie V, Jae-Ho K et al 1989c The combined use of radiation therapy and lonidamine in the treatment of brain metastases. Journal of Neurology and Oncology 7: 241–247

Debevec M 1990 Management of patients with brain metastases of unknown origin. Neoplasma 37: 601–606

Decker D, Decker V, Herskovic A et al 1984 Brain metastases in patients with renal cell carcinoma: prognosis and treatment. Journal of Clinical Oncology 2: 169–173

Deeley T, Edwards J 1968 Radiotherapy in the management of cerebral secondaries from bronchial carcinoma. Lancet 1: 1209–1213

de la Monte S, Morre G, Hutchins G 1983 Patterned distribution of metastases from malignant melanoma in humans. Cancer Research 43: 3427–3433

de la Monte S, Hutchins G, Moore W 1988 Influence of age on metastatic behavior of breast carcinoma. Human Pathology 19: 529–534

Delattre J, Krol G, Thaler H et al 1988 Distribution of brain metastases. Archives of Neurology 45: 741–744

Deutsh M, Parsons J, Mercado R 1974 Radiotherapy for intracranial metastases. Cancer 34: 1607–1611

Dhopesh V, Yagnik P 1985 Brain metastasis: Analysis of patients without known cancer. Southern Medical Journal 78: 171–172

DiStefano A, Yap Y, Hortobagyi G et al 1979 The natural history of breast cancer patients with brain metastases. Cancer 44: 1913–1918

Dorsoretz D, Blitzer P, Russell P et al 1980 Management of solitary metastasis to the brain: the role of elective brain irradiation following complete surgical resection. International Journal of Radiation Oncology Biology and Physics 6: 1727–1730

Eden E, Muggia J, Hiesiger E et al 1980 Plasma carcinoembryonic antigen as an indicator of cerebral metastases. Journal of Neurology and Oncology 8: 281–287

Engenhart R, Kimmig B, Sturm V 1989 Stereotactically guided convergent beam irradiation of solitary brain metastases and cerebral arteriovenous malformation. In: Dyck P, Bouzaglou A (eds) Brachytherapy of brain tumors and related stereotactic treatment. Hanley & Belfus, Philadelphia, pp 119–132

Fell D, Leavens M, McBridge C 1980 Surgical versus nonsurgical management of metastatic melanoma of the brain. Neurosurgery 7: 238–247

Ferrara M, Bizzozzero F, Talamonti G et al 1990 Surgical treatment of 100 single brain metastases. Journal of Neurosurgical Science 34: 303–308

Flaschka G, Desoye G 1987 CEA plasma levels in patients with intracranial tumours. Neurochirurgica 30: 5–7

Fleck J, Einchorn L, Lauer R et al 1990 Is prophylactic cranial irradiation indicated in small-cell lung cancer? Journal of Clinical Oncology 8: 209–214

Fuller B, Kaplan I, Adler J et al 1992 Stereotaxic radiosurgery for brain metastases: The importance of adjuvant whole brain irradiation. International Journal of Radiation Oncology Biology and Physics 23: 413–418

Galicich J, Sundaresan N, Arbit E et al 1980 Surgical treatment of single brain metastasis: factors associated with survival. Cancer 45: 381–386

Galluzzi S, Payne P 1956 Brain metastases from primary brachial carcinoma: a statistical study of 741 necropsies. Cancer 10: 408–414

Gamache F, Posner J, Patterson R 1979 Involvement of the central nervous system by metastatic tumor. In: Youmans J (ed) Neurological surgery, 2nd edn. W B Saunders, Philadelphia

Gay P, Litchy W, Cascino T 1987 Brain metastasis in hypernephroma. Journal of Neurology and Oncology 5: 51–56

Gelber R, Larson M, Borgerlt B et al 1981 Equivalence of radiation schedules for the palliative treatment of brain metastases in patients with favorable prognosis. Cancer 48: 1749–1753

Giannone L, Johnson D, Hande K et al 1987 Favorable prognosis of brain metastases in small cell lung cancer. Annals of Internal Medicine 106: 386–389

Gilbert H, Kagan A, Wagner J et al 1980 The functional results of treating brain metastases with radiation therapy. In: Weiss L, Gilbert H, Posner J (eds) Brain metastasis. G Hall, Boston, pp 269–278

Gottleib J, Frei E, Luce J 1972 An evaluation of the management of patients with cerebral metastases from malignant melanoma. Cancer 29: 701–705

Graf A, Buchberger W, Langmayr H et al 1988 Site preference of metastatic tumours of the brain. Virchows Archives of Anatomy and Histopathology 412: 493–498

Grant F 1926 Concerning intracranial malignant metastases. Their frequency and the value of surgery in their treatment. Annals of Surgery 84: 635–646

Graus F, Rogers L, Posner J 1985 Cerebrovascular complications in patients with cancer. Medicine 64: 16–35

Greig N 1984 Chemotherapy of brain metastases: current status. Cancer Treatment Review 11: 157–186

Haar F, Patterson R H 1972 Surgery for metastatic intracranial neoplasms. Cancer 30: 1241–1245

Hafstrom L, Johnsson P, Strombald L 1980 Intracranial metastases of malignant melanoma treated by surgery. Cancer 46: 2088–2090

Hagen N, Cirrincione C, Thaler H et al 1990 The role of radiation therapy following resection of single brain metastasis from melanoma. Neurology 40: 158–160

Hankins J, Miller J, Salcman M et al 1988 Surgical management of lung cancer with solitary cerebral metastasis. Annals of Thoracic Surgery 46: 24–28

Hardy J, Smith I, Cherryman G et al 1990 The value of computed tomographic (CT) scan surveillance in the detection and management of brain metastases in patients with small cell lung cancer. British Journal of Cancer 62: 684–686

Hasegawa H, Ushio Y, Hayakawa T et al 1983 Changes of the blood-brain barrier in experimental metastatic brain tumors. Journal of Neurosurgery 59: 304–310

Healy M, Hesselink J, Press G et al 1987 Increased detection of intracranial metastases with intravenous Gd-DTPA. Radiology 165: 619–624

Hendrickson F 1975 Radiation therapy of metastatic tumors. Seminars in Oncology 2: 43–46

Hendrickson F 1977 The optimum schedule for palliative radiotherapy of metastatic brain cancer. International Journal of Radiation Oncology Biology and Physics 2: 165–168

Henson R, Urich H 1982 Cancer and the nervous system. Blackwell, London, 1982

Heros D, Kasdon D, Chun M 1988 Brachytherapy in the treatment of recurrent solitary brain metastases. Neurosurgery 23: 733–737

Hildebrand J 1973 Early diagnosis of brain metastases in an unselected population of cancerous patients. European Journal of Cancer 9: 621–626

Hirsch F, Paulson O, Hansen H et al 1982 Intracranial metastases in small cell carcinoma of the lung: correlation of clinical and autopsy findings. Cancer 50: 2433–2437

Horwitz N, Rizzoli H 1982 Postoperative complications of intracranial neurological surgery. Williams & Wilkins, Baltimore

Jacobs L, Kinel W, Vincent R 1977 Silent brain metastasis from lung carcinoma determined by computerized tomography. Archives of Neurology 34: 690–693

Jacobs R, Awan A, Bitran et al 1987 Prophylactic cranial irradiation in adenocarcinoma of the lung. Cancer 59: 2016–2019

Johnson B, Patronas N, Hayes W 1990 Neurologic, computed cranial tomographic, and magnetic resonance imaging abnormalities in patients with small-cell lung cancer: further follow-up of 6- to 13-year survivors. Journal of Clinical Oncology 8: 48–56

Kamby C, Soerensen P 1988 Characteristics of patients with short and long survivals after detection of intracranial metastases from breast cancer. Journal of Neurology and Oncology 6: 37–45

Kaye A 1992 Malignant brain tumors. In: Little J, Awad I (eds) Reoperative neurosurgery. Williams & Wilkins, Baltimore, pp 49–76

Kelly P, Kall B, Goerss S 1988 Results of computed tomography-based computer-assisted stereotactic resection of metastatic intracranial tumors. Neurosurgery 22: 7–17

Kindt G 1964 The pattern of location of cerebral metastatic tumors. Journal of Neurosurgery 21: 54–57

Kitaoka K, Abe H, Aida T et al 1990 Follow-up study on metastatic cerebellar tumor surgery: Characteristic problems of surgical treatment. Neuro Med Chir 30: 591–598

Kihlström L, Karlsson B, Lindquist Ch et al 1991 Gamma knife surgery for cerebral metastasis. Acta Neurochirurgica Suppl 52: 87–89

Kofman S, Garvin J, Nagamani D et al 1957 Treatment of cerebral metastases from breast carcinoma with prednisolone. Journal of the American Medical Association 163: 1473–1476

Komarnicky L, Phillips T, Martz K et al 1991 A randomized phase III protocol for the evaluation of misonidazole combined with radiation in the treatment of patients with brain metastases. International Journal of Radiation Oncology Biology and Physics 20: 53–58

Kristjansen P, Pedersen A 1989 CNS therapy in small-cell lung cancer. In: Hansen H (ed) Basic and clinical concepts of lung cancer. Kluwer Academic Publishers, Boston, pp 275–298

Kurtz J, Gelber R, Brady L et al 1981 The palliation of brain metastases in a favorable patient population: a randomized clinical trial by the Radiation Therapy Oncology Group. International Journal of Radiation Oncology Biology and Physics 7: 891–895

Kurup P, Reddy S, Hendrickson F 1980 Results of re-irradiation for cerebral metastases. Cancer 46: 2587–2589

Landy H, Egnor M 1991 Intraoperative ultrasonography and cortical mapping for removal of deep cerebral tumors. Southern Medical Journal 84: 1323–1326

Lang E, Slater J 1964 Metastatic brain tumors: results of surgical and nonsurgical treatment. Surgical Clinics of North America 44: 865–872

Lange O, Scheef W, Haase K 1990 Palliative radio-chemotherapy with ifosfamide and BCNU for breast cancer patients with cerebral metastases: a 5-year experience. Cancer Chemotherapy Pharmacology 26 (suppl): 78–80

Laukkanen E, Klonoff H, Allan B et al 1988 The role of prophylactic brain irradiation in limited stage small cell lung cancer: clinical, neuropsychologic, and CT sequelae. International Journal of Radiation Oncology Biology and Physics 14: 1109–1117

Lee J, Umsawasdi T, Barkley H 1987 Timing of elective brain irradiation: a critical factor for brain metastasis-free survival in small cell lung cancer. International Journal of Radiation Oncology Biology and Physics 13: 697–704

Lee Y 1980 Malignant melanoma: pattern of metastasis. CA 30: 137–142

Lee Y 1983 Breast carcinoma: pattern of metastastic spread at autopsy. Journal of Surgical Oncology 23: 175–180

Lee Y, Naubert C, Glass P 1986 Treatment related white matter changes in cancer patients. Cancer 57: 1473–1482

Leeds, Sawaya R, Tassel P et al 1992 Intracranial hemorrhage in the oncologic patient. Neuroimaging Clinics of North America 2: 119–136

Leksell L 1951 The stereotaxic method and radiosurgery of the brain. Acta Chirurgica Scandinavica 102: 316

Lewis A 1988 Sarcoma metastatic to the brain. Cancer 61: 593–601

Liotta L, Stetler-Stevenson W 1989 Principles of molecular cell biology of cancer: cancer metastasis In: DeVita V, Hellman S, Rosenberg S (eds) Cancer: Principles and practice of oncology. J B Lippincott, Philadelphia, pp 98–115

Lishner M, Feld R, Payne D et al 1990 Late neurological complications after prophylactic cranial irradiation in patients with small-cell lung cancer: the Toronto experience. Journal of Clinical Oncology 8: 215–221

Long D 1979 Capillary ultrastructure in human metastatic brain tumors. Journal of Neurosurgery 51: 53–58

Lucas G, Luxton G, Cohen D 1991 Treatment results of stereotactic interstitial brachytherapy for primary and metastatic brain tumors. International Journal of Radiation Oncology Biology and Physics 21: 715–721

Madajewicz S, Karakousis C, West C et al 1984 Malignant melanoma brain metastases. Review of Roswell Park Memorial Institute experience. Cancer 53: 2550–2552

Magilligan D, Duvernoy C, Malik G et al 1986 Surgical approach to lung cancer with solitary cerebral metastasis: twenty-five years' experience. Annals of Thoracic Surgery 42: 360–364

Mandell L, Hilaris B, Sullivan M et al 1986 The treatment of single brain metastases from non-oat cell lung carcinoma. Cancer 58: 641–649

Mandybur T 1977 Intracranial hemorrhage caused by metastatic tumors. Neurology 27: 650–655

Maor M, Frias A, Oswald J 1988 Palliative radiotherapy for brain metastases in renal carcinoma. Cancer 62: 1912–1917

Markesbery W, Brooks W, Gupta G et al 1978 Treatment for patients with cerebral metastases. Archives of Neurology 35: 754–756

Marshall E, Pearson T, Simpson W et al 1990 Low incidence of asymptomatic brain metastases in patients with renal cell carcinoma. Urology 36: 300–302

Merchut M 1989 Brain metastases from undiagnosed systemic neoplasms. Archives of Internal Medicine 149: 1046–1080

Modic M, Beale S 1990 Magnetic resonance imaging of supratentorial neoplasms. In: Wilkins R, Rengachary S (eds) Neurosurgery update I: Diagnosis, operative technique, and neuro-oncology. McGraw-Hill, New York, pp 12–29

Montana G, Meacham W, Caldwell W 1972 Brain irradiation for metastatic disease of lung origin. Cancer 29: 1477–1480

Nedzi L, Kooy H, Alexander E et al 1991 Variables associated with the development of complications from radiosurgery of intracranial tumors. International Journal of Radiation Oncology Biology and Physics 21: 591–599

Newman S, Hansen H 1974 Frequency, diagnosis, and treatment of brain metastases in 247 consecutive patients with bronchogenic carcinoma. Cancer 33: 492–496

Nicolson G 1988 Cancer metastasis: tumor cell and host organ properties important in metastasis to specific secondary sites. Biochim Biophys Acta 948: 175–224

Nisce L, Hilaris B, Chu F 1971 A review of experience with irradiation of brain metastasis. American Journal of Roentgenology Radium Therapy and Nuclear Medicine 3: 329–333

Nutt S, Patchell R 1992 Intracranial hemorrhage associated with primary and secondary tumors. Neurosurgical Clinics of North America 3: 591–599

Order S, Hellman S, Von Essen C et al 1968 Improvement in quality of survival following whole-brain irradiation for brain metastases. Radiology 91: 149–153

Oredsson S, Ingvar C, Strombald L et al 1990 Palliative surgery for brain metastases of malignant melanoma. European Journal of Surgical Oncology 16: 451–456

Paillas J, Pellet W 1975 Brain metastases. In: Vinken P J, Bruyn G U (eds) Handbook of clinical neurology, vol 18. North-Holland Publishing, Amsterdam

Patchell R, Tibbs P, Walsh J et al 1990 A randomized trial of surgery in the treatment of single metastases. New England Journal of Medicine 322: 494–545

Patel J, Didolkar M, Pickren J et al 1978 Metastatic pattern of malignant melanoma. A study of 216 autopsy cases. American Journal of Surgery 135: 807–810

Posner J 1974 Diagnosis and treatment of metastases to the brain. Clinical Bulletins 4: 47–57

Posner J, Chernik N 1978 Intracranial metastases from systemic cancer. Advances in Neurology 19: 579–592

Prados M, Liebel S, Barnett C et al 1989 Interstitial brachytherapy for metastatic brain tumors. Cancer 63: 657–660

Ransohoff J 1975 Surgical management of metastatic tumors. Seminars in Oncology 2: 21–28

Raskind R, Weiss S, Manning J et al 1971 Survival after surgical excision of single metastatic brain tumors. American Journal of Roetgenology Radium Therapy and Nuclear Medicine 111: 323–328

Rasmussen B, Teisner B, Schroder H et al 1991 Fetal antigen 2 in primary and secondary brain tumors. Tumor Biology 12: 330–338

Retsas S, Gershuny A 1988 Central nervous system involvement in malignant melanoma. Cancer 61: 1926–1934

Richards P, McKissok W 1963 Intracranial metastases. British Medical Journal 1: 15–18

Robinson W, Jobe K, Stevens R 1987 Central nervous system metastases in malignant melanoma. In: Nathanson L (ed) Basic and clinical aspects of malignant melanoma. Nijhoff, Boston, pp 155–163

Rosenstein M, Armstrong J, Kris M et al 1992 A reappraisal of the role of prophylactic cranial irradiation in limited small cell lung cancer. International Journal of Radiation Oncology Biology and Physics 24: 43–48

Rosner D, Nemoto T, Lane W 1983 Management of brain metastases from breast cancer by combination chemotherapy. Journal of Neurology and Oncology 1: 131–137

Rubin J, Chandler W 1990 Ultrasound in neurosurgery. Raven Press, New York

Rusch V, Griffin B, Livingston R 1989 The role of prophylactic cranial irradiation in regionally advanced non-small cell lung cancer. Journal of Thoracic and Cardiovascular Surgery 98: 335–339

Russell A, Pajak T, Selim H et al 1991 Prophylactic cranial irradiation for lung cancer patients at high risk for development of cerebral metastasis: results of a prospective randomized trial conducted by the Radiation Therapy Oncology Group. International Journal of Radiation Oncology Biology and Physics 21: 637–643

Russell D, Rubinsten L 1971 Pathology of the nervous system. Williams & Wilkins, Baltimore

Russell E, Geremia G, Johnson C 1987 Multiple cerebral metastases: detectability with Gd-DTPA-enhanced MR imaging. Radiology 165: 609–617

Saitoh H, Shimbo T, Tasaka T et al 1982 Brain metastasis of renal adenocarcinoma. Tokai Journal of Experimental and Clinical Medicine 7: 337–343

Salcman M 1992 Intracranial hemorrhage caused by brain tumor. In: Kaufman H (ed) Intracerebral hematomas. Raven Press, New York, pp 95–106

Salerno T, Munro D, Little J 1978 Surgical treatment of bronchogenic carcinoma with a brain metastasis. Journal of Neurosurgery 48: 350–354

Sawaya R, Zuccarello M, Elkalliny M et al 1992 Postoperative venous thromboembolism and brain tumors: part I. Clinical profile. Journal of Neuro-Oncology 14: 119–125

Selker R 1983 Corticosteroids: their effect on primary and metastatic brain tumors. In: Walker M (ed) Oncology of the nervous system. Martinus Nijhoff, Boston, pp 167–191

Shehata W, Hendrickson R, Walid A et al 1974 Rapid fractionation technique and re-treatment of cerebral metastases by irradiation. Cancer 34: 257–261

Siegers H 1990 Chemotherapy for brain metastases: recent developments and clinical considerations. Cancer Treatment Reviews 17: 63–76

Simionescu M 1958 Metastatic tumors of the brain: a follow-up study of 195 patients with neurosurgical considerations. Journal of Neurosurgery 17: 361–373

Smalley S, Schray M, Laws E et al 1987 Adjuvant radiation therapy after surgical resection of solitary brain metastasis: association with pattern of failure and survival. International Journal of Radiation Oncology Biology and Physics 13: 1611–1616

Sorensen J, Hansen H, Hansen M et al 1988 Brain metastases in adenocarcinoma of the lung: frequency, risk groups, and prognosis. Journal of Clinical Oncology 9: 1474–1480

Spears W, Morphis J, Lester S et al 1992 Brain metastases and testicular tumors: long-term survival. International Journal of Radiation Oncology Biology and Physics 22: 17–22

Stein M, Steiner M, Klein B et al 1986 Involvement of the central nervous system by ovarian carcinoma. Cancer 58: 2066–2069

Steinfeld A, Zelefsky M 1987 Brain metastases from carcinoma of bladder. Urology 29: 375–376

Stevens G, Firth I, Alan C 1992 Cerebral metastases from malignant melanoma. Radiotherapy and Oncology 23: 185–191

Störtebecker T 1954 Metastatic tumors of the brain from a neurosurgical point of view: a follow-up of 158 cases. Journal of Neurosurgery 11: 84–111

Stridsklev I, Hagen S, Klepp O 1984 Radiation therapy for brain metastases from malignant melanoma. Acta Radiol Oncol 23: 231–235

Sturm V, Kimmig B, Engenhardt R et al 1991 Radiosurgical treatment of cerebral metastases. Stereotactic Functional Neurosurgery 57: 7–10

Sturm V, Kimmig B, Wowra B et al 1992 Radiosurgery in malignant intracranial tumors. In: Steiner L et al (eds) Radiosurgery: Baseline and trends. Raven Press, New York, pp 155–160

Sundaresan N, Galicich J 1985 Surgical treatment of brain metastases: clinical and computerized tomography evaluation of the results of treatment. Cancer 55: 1382–1388

Sundaresan N, Galicich J, Deck M et al 1981 Radiation necrosis after treatment of solitary intracranial metastases. Neurosurgery 8: 329–333

Sundaresan N, Sachdev V, DiGiacinto G 1988 Reoperation for brain metastases. Journal of Clinical Oncology 6: 1625–1629

Sze G, Shin J, Krol G et al 1988 Intraparenchymal brain metastases: MR imaging versus contrast-enhanced CT. Radiology 168: 187–194

Sze G, Milano E, Johnson C et al 1991 Detection of brain metastases: comparison of contrast-enchanced MR with unhanced MR and enchanced CT. AJNR 11: 785–791

Takakura K, Sano K, Hojo S et al 1982 Metastatic tumors of the nervous system. Igaku-Shoin, New York

Taylor H, Lefkowitz M, Skoog S et al 1984 Intracranial metastases in prostate cancer. Cancer 53: 2728–2730

Tobler W, Sawaya R, Tew J 1986 Successful laser-assisted excision of a metastatic midbrain tumor. Neurosurgery 18: 795–797

Trillet V, Catajar J, Croisile B et al 1991 Cerebral metastases as first symptom of bronchogenic carcinoma. Cancer 67: 2935–2940

Tsukada Y, Fouad A, Pickren J 1983 Central nervous system metastasis from breast carcinoma. Cancer 52: 2349–2354

Turrisi A 1990 Brain irradiation and systemic chemotherapy for small-cell lung cancer: dangerous liaisons? Journal of Clinical Oncology 8: 196–199

Twelves C, Souhami R 1991 Should cerebral metastases be treated by chemotherapy alone? Annals of Oncology 2: 15–17

Twelves C, Souhami R, Harper P et al 1990 The response of cerebral metastases in small lung cancer to systemic chemotherapy. British Journal of Cancer 61: 147–150

Ushio Y, Norio A, Hayakawa T et al 1991 Chemotherapy of brain metastases from lung carcinoma: a controlled randomized study. Neurosurgery 28: 201–205

Vieth R, Odom G 1965 Intracranial metastases and their neurosurgical treatment. Journal of Neurosurgery 23: 375–383

Voorhies R, Sundaresan N, Thaler T 1980 The single supratentorial lesion: an evaluation of preroperative diagnostic tests. Journal of Neurosurgery 53: 364–368

Weiss L, Grundmann E, Torhorst J et al 1986 Haematogenous metastastic patterns in colonic carcinoma: an analysis of 1541 necropsies. Journal of Pathology 150: 195–203

West J, Moshe M 1980 Intracranial metastases: behavioral patterns related to primary site and results of treatment by whole brain irradiation. International Journal of Radiation Oncology Biology and Physics 6: 11–15

White K, Fleming T, Laws E 1981 Single metastasis to the brain. Surgical treatment in 122 consecutive patients. Mayo Clinic Proceedings 56: 424–428

Winston K, Walsh J, Fischer E 1980 Results of operative treatment of intracranial metastatic tumors. Cancer 45: 2639–2645

Yardeni D, Reichenthal E, Zucker G 1984 Neurosurgical management of single brain metastasis. Surgical Neurology 21: 377–384

Young D, Posner J, Chu F et al 1974 Rapid-course radiation therapy of cerebral metastases: results and complications. Cancer 34: 1069–1076

Zimm S, Wampler G, Stablein D et al 1981 Intracerebral metastases in solid-tumor patients: natural history and results of treatment. Cancer 48: 384–394

American Joint Committee on Cancer TNM/UICC Brain tumors

American Joint Committee on cancer TNM/UICC brain tumors

INTRODUCTION

The most critical feature in the classification of brain tumors is histopathology. Accurate pathologic criteria and classification are essential to an understanding of the clinical and biologic behavior of the gliomas in particular, and of most other tumors as well. The anatomic location and extent of tumors within the brain are also of clinical and prognostic significance. Neuroradiologic-diagnostic procedures have become increasingly more accurate and reliable in providing topographic and morphologic information on tumors of the brain and are useful at various points in diagnosis and management. The recommendations in this chapter refer to primary tumors of the brain. A system for staging metastatic tumors of the brain is under development and is currently being tested.

ANATOMY

Primary Site. Various tissues within the brain can give rise to neoplasms, including astrocytes and other glial cells, meninges, blood vessels, pituitary and pineal cells, and neural elements proper. The major structural sites involved include the various lobes of the cerebral hemispheres; the midline structures, including the midbrain, pons, and medulla; and the posterior fossa.

Regional Lymph Nodes. There are no lymphatic structures draining the brain.

Metastatic Sites. Certain brain tumors can seed into the subarachnoid space. Hematogenous spread is very uncommon but on rare occasions has occurred in bone and other sites.

RULES FOR CLASSIFICATION

Clinical Staging. This staging is based on neurologic signs and symptoms and on neurologic diagnostic tests, including skull radiography, electroencephalography, isotopic brain scans, cerebral angiography, pneumoencephalography, computed tomography, and magnetic resonance imaging. All diagnostic information available prior to first definitve treatment may be used.

Pathologic Staging. This staging is based on histopathology, grade, and microscopic evidence of completeness of resected tumor removal.

DEFINITION OF TNM

Primary Tumor (T)

TX Primary tumor cannot be assessed
T0 No evidence of primary tumor

Supratentorial Tumor

T1 Tumor 5 cm or less in greatest dimension; limited to one side
T2 Tumor more than 5 cm in greatest dimension; limited to one side
T3 Tumor invades or encroaches on the ventricular system
T4 Tumor crosses the midline, invades the opposite hemisphere, or invades infratentorially

Infratentorial Tumor

T1 Tumor 3 cm or less in greatest dimension; limited to one side
T2 Tumor more than 3 cm in greatest dimension; limited to one side
T3 Tumor invades or encroaches on the ventricular system
T4 Tumor crosses the midline, invades the opposite hemisphere, or invades supratentorially

Regional Lymph Nodes (N)

This category does not apply to this site.

Distant Metastasis (M)

MX Presence of distant metastasis cannot be assessed
M0 No distant metastasis
M1 Distant metastasis

HISTOPATHOLOGIC GRADE (G)

GX Grade cannot be assessed
G1 Well differentiated
G2 Moderately differentiated
G3 Poorly differentiated
G4 Undifferentiated

STAGE GROUPING

Stage IA	G1	T1	M0
Stage IB	G1	T2	M0
	G1	T3	M0
Stage IIA	G2	T1	M0
Stage IIB	G2	T2	M0
	G2	T3	M0
Stage IIIA	G3	T1	M0
Stage IIIB	G3	T2	M0
	G3	T3	M0
Stage IV	G1	T4	M0
	G2	T4	M0
	G3	T4	M0
	G4	Any T	M0
	Any G	Any T	M1

HISTOPATHOLOGIC TYPE

Tumors included in analysis and evaluation are:

Astrocytomas
Oligodendrogliomas
Ependymal and choroid plexus tumors
Glioblastomas
Medulloblastomas
Meningiomas, malignant
Neurilemmomas (neurinomas, schwannomas), malignant
Hemangioblastomas
Neurosarcomas
Other sarcomas

Histologic grade usually correlates with biologic activity of the tumor. This is particularly the case with malignant astrocytomas, the most common form of glioma. The age of the patient at the time of diagnosis is also of major importance for prognosis.

APPENDIX

Histologic grading of tumors of the central nervous system

Criteria for the Diagnosis of Malignancy in Tumors of the Central Nervous System and Allied Structures

For tumors of the central nervous system and allied structures, the uncritical application of criteria for histologic and biologic malignancy that generally pertain to other neoplasms is inadequate for the following reasons:

1. Irrespective of the histologic malignancy of the tumor, its unimpeded growth within the confines of the skull as a space-occupying and expanding lesion inevitably leads to a fatal termination, which by definition is equated with clinical malignancy.
2. Similarly, the local pressure caused by an intracranial tumor on vital neural structures may result in the clinical effects of malignancy, irrespective of the histologic type of tumor.
3. The obstructive effect of a growing tumor leads to the production of secondary occlusive hydrocephalus.
4. Certain criteria of malignancy of neoplasms that in other body systems pertain to their growth and spread (especially the characteristic of infiltrative growth and the capacity to metastasize, either within or outside the central nervous system) do not necessarily pertain to, or have to be modified to, the evaluation of the malignant behavior of central nervous system tumors.

Thus, tumors of the central nervous system and allied structures, in addition to their intrinsic benign or malignant histologic character that to a considerable extent determines their biologic behavior, may by their specific localization acquire certain characteristics that collectively will add up to a picture regarded as benign, semi-benign, relatively malignant, or highly malignant.

The numerical grading used in this classification is based on histologic criteria of malignancy and should be considered an estimate of the usual behavior of each type of tumor. Numerical grade 1 is considered the least malignant; grades 2, 3, and 4 indicate increasing degrees of malignancy.

In this general evaluation, the pathologist confronted with the problem of malignancy and prognosis is faced with two sets of data. In the first analysis, the evaluation of malignancy must clearly be based on retrospective assessment of the postoperative prognosis and survival rates of other known similar examples, leading to a final and reasonably accurate clinicopathologic correlation that both reinforces the purely histopathologic evaluation of malignancy and is reinforced by it.

Second, the pathologist deduces malignancy from a number of purely histologic and cytologic data. These include increase of cellularity, presence and rate of mitotic figures, presence of atypical mitotic figures, pleomorphism of tumor cells, pleomorphism of tissue architecture (particularly necroses, abnormally prominent stromal reaction, disorderly stromal reaction, and overgrowth), and the formation of pathologic blood vessels (corresponding to the angiographic appearance of arteriovenous fistulas).

On the other hand, other features usually regarded as indicative of or synonymous with malignancy need not necessarily be recognized in the case of tumors of the central nervous system, especially those of neuroectodermal origin. For instance, lack of circumscription and focal parenchymatous invasion is not a necessary accompaniment of cellular anaplasia or ultimate clinical malignancy. Also, the actual presence of mitotic figures (as in oligodendroglioma) does not necessarily imply a particularly malignant behavior; the overall number of mitoses and the presence of abnormal mitotic figures are more important in evaluation. Similarly, local invasion of the leptomeninges is often clearly dissociated from either of the two features just quoted. This is the case, for example, in the pilocytic astrocytoma that involves the wall of the third ventricle, the optic nerve, the cerebellum, and so on.

Although distant meningeal and ventricular metastases are often characteristic of highly malignant tumors such as medulloblastoma, this phenomenon again is not always to be correlated with the highest degrees of cytologic malignancy, as seen in some oligodendrogliomas.

The question of grading

Following Broder's classification of epithelial tumors elsewhere in the body, an attempt has been made by Kernohan and his school to apply a system of grading by ascending degrees of malignancy, numbered 1 to 4, to certain tumors of neuroectodermal origin—namely astrocytoma, oligodendroglioma, ependymoma, and neuroastrocytoma. This attempt stemmed both from a desire to simplify the then current classification of tumors of the central nervous system and from a need to offer to the neurosurgeon a prognostic evaluation of the tumor removed at surgery, based on certain definite histologic and cytologic criteria. Attractive though this attempt at simplification might be, however, it has to meet with a number of objections:

1. The sample of tissue so analyzed may from surgical necessity not be representative of the tumor as a whole.
2. The specific evolution of the particular tumor in terms of its anaplastic potentialities is not fully expressed by such a scheme of grading. For example, a cerebellar pilocytic astrocytoma graded 1 does not have the same anaplastic potential as a cerebral astrocytoma or some other tumors also graded 1.
3. The pleomorphism of cell and tissue structures so frequently inherent in primary neuroectodermal tumors poses additional difficulties to the application of a simplified system of grading.
4. This cytologic grading makes it extremely difficult to place tumors with mixed cell populations into an already predetermined tumor category.

Nevertheless, the above remarks should not be regarded as basically antagonistic to some attempts at expressing the degree of malignancy of a particular tumor of the central nervous system. Indeed, from the clinical and therapeutic points of view, no classification based on purely histologic entities is satisfactory unless adequate cognizance is taken of, and information provided on, the degree of malignancy of a particular tumor submitted for examination. Thus, it is the duty and prerogative of the pathologist to provide his clinical colleagues with an informed opinion on the likely evolution of a particular tumor, and to some extent this prognostic opinion is embodied in the recognition of specific clinicopathologic neuro-oncologic entities. As an illustration, it might be pointed out that two tumors of similar cellularity, isomorphous appearance, and mitotic rate—such as the medulloblastomas and some oligodendrogliomas—usually do not exhibit the same biologic behavior. This acquired body of knowledge is clearly the result of previous collaboration among clinicians and pathologists in the field of neuro-oncology.

BIBLIOGRAPHY

1. Jelsma R, Bucy P C 1969 Glioblastoma multiforme: Its treatment and some factors affecting survival. Archives of Neurology 20: 161–171
2. Salcman M 1980 Survival in glioblastoma: Historical perspective. Neurosurgery 7: 435–439
3. Scanlon P W, Taylor W F 1979 Radiotherapy of intracranial astrocytomas: Analysis of 417 cases treated from 1960 through 1969. Neurosurgery 5: 301–308
4. Walker M D, Alexander E Jr, Hunt W E et al 1978 Evaluation of BCNU and/or radiotherapy in the treatment of anaplastic gliomas: A cooperative clinical trial. Journal of Neurosurgery 49: 333–343
5. Wilson C B, Gutin P, Boldrey E B et al 1976 Single-agent chemotherapy of brain tumors: A five-year review. Archives of Neurology 33: 739–744
6. Zulch K J 1979 Histologic typing of tumors of the central nervous system. WHO International Histological Classification of Tumors, No. 21. Geneva, WHO

BRAIN

Data Form for Cancer Staging

Patient identification ______________________

Name ______________________

Address ______________________

Hospital or clinic number ______________________

Age __________ Sex __________ Race __________

Institution identification

Hospital or clinic ______________________

Address ______________________

Oncology Record

Anatomic site of cancer ______________________

Histologic type ______________________

Grade (G) ______________________

Date of classification ______________________

Chronology of classification

[ ] Clinical (use all data prior to first treatment)

[ ] Pathologic (if definitively resected specimen available)

Clin	Path	DEFINITIONS	
		Primary Tumor (T)	
[ ]	[ ]	TX	Primary tumor cannot be assessed
[ ]	[ ]	T0	No evidence of primary tumor
		Supratentorial tumor	
[ ]	[ ]	T1	Tumor 5 cm or less in greatest dimension; limited to one side
[ ]	[ ]	T2	Tumor more than 5 cm in greatest dimension; limited to one side
[ ]	[ ]	T3	Tumor invades or encroaches upon the ventricular system
[ ]	[ ]	T4	Tumor crosses the midline, invades the opposite hemisphere, or extends infratentorially
		Infratentorial tumor	
[ ]	[ ]	T1	Tumor 3 cm or less in greatest dimension; limited to one side
[ ]	[ ]	T2	Tumor more than 3 cm in greatest dimension; limited to one side
[ ]	[ ]	T3	Tumor invades or encroaches upon the ventricular system
[ ]	[ ]	T4	Tumor crosses the midline, invades the opposite hemisphere, or invades supratentorially
		Lymph Node (N)	
		This category does not apply to this site.	
		Distant Metastasis (M)	
[ ]	[ ]	MX	Presence of distant metastasis cannot be assessed
[ ]	[ ]	M0	No distant metastasis
[ ]	[ ]	M1	Distant metastasis
		Histopathologic Grade (G)	
[ ]	[ ]	GX	Grade cannot be assessed
[ ]	[ ]	G1	Well differentiated
[ ]	[ ]	G2	Moderately differentiated
[ ]	[ ]	G3	Poorly differentiated
[ ]	[ ]	G4	Undifferentiated

Clin	Path	Stage Grouping			
[ ]	[ ]	IA	G1	T1	M0
[ ]	[ ]	IB	G1	T2	M0
			G1	T3	M0
[ ]	[ ]	IIA	G2	T1	M0
[ ]	[ ]	IIB	G2	T2	M0
			G2	T3	M0
[ ]	[ ]	IIIA	G3	T1	M0
[ ]	[ ]	IIIB	G3	T2	M0
			G3	T3	M0
[ ]	[ ]	IV	G1	T4	M0
			G2	T4	M0
			G3	T4	M0
			G4	Any T	M0
			Any G	Any T	M1

Staged by ______________________ M.D.

______________________ Registrar

Date ______________________

(continued on next page)

American Joint Committee on Cancer—1992

Histopathologic Type

Tumors that are included in the analysis and evaluation are as follows:
Astrocytomas
Oligodendroglioma
Ependymal and choroid plexus tumors
Glioblastoma
Medulloblastoma
Meningiomas, malignant
Neurilemmomas (neurinomas, schwannomas), malignant
Hemangioblastoma
Neurosarcomas
Other sarcomas

Illustrations

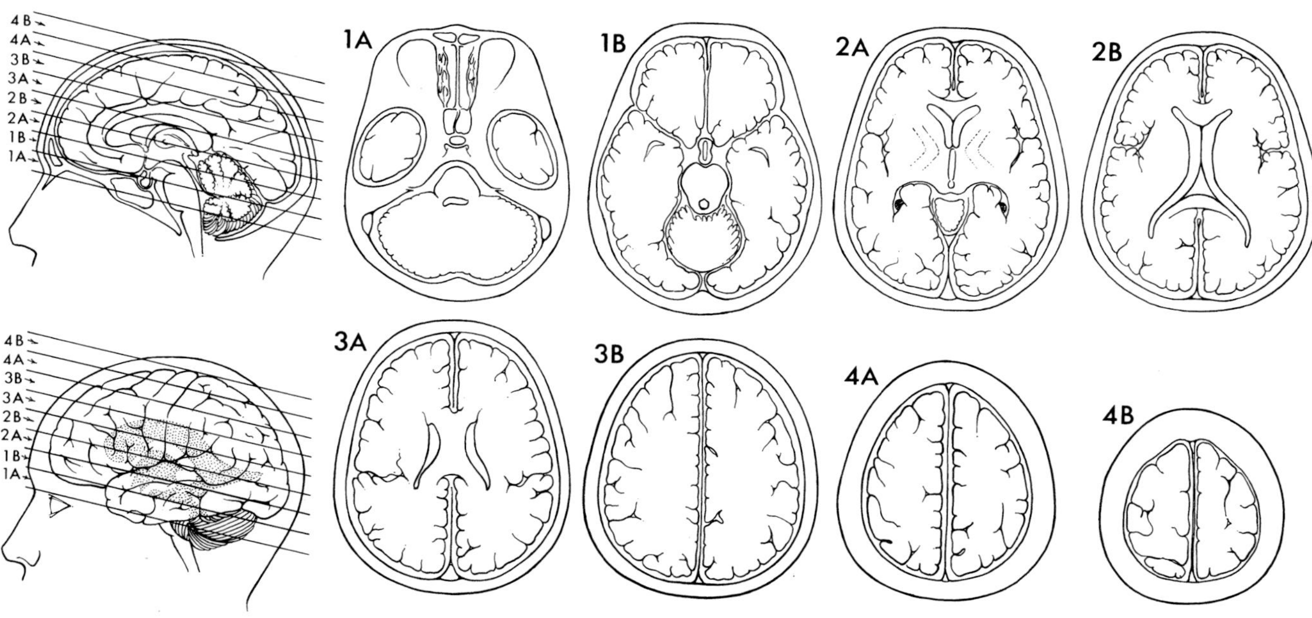

Size: ________ cm
Weight: ________ g

Indicate on diagrams the exact location and characteristics of tumor.

AANS/CNS JOINT TUMOR SECTION STAGING FORM

DATA FORM FOR CANCER STAGING: CNS TUMORS

ASTROCYTOMA, EPENDYMOMA, OLIGODENDROGLIOMA

Primary tumor T stage

		Supratentorial
pre-operative size	Tx	primary tumor cannot be assessed
	T0	not applicable
	T1	tumor less than 5 cm
	T2	tumor greater than 5 cm
	T3	tumor crosses midline, any size (contiguous lesion)
	T4	multifocal tumor, any size (non-contiguous lesion)

		Infratentorial
pre-operative size	Tx	primary tumor cannot be assessed
	T0	not applicable
	T1	tumor less than 3 cm
	T2	tumor greater than 3 cm
	T3	tumor crosses midline, and size (contiguous lesion)
	T4	multifocal tumor, any size (non-contiguous lesion)
	T5	spinal cord tumor, any size

surgical procedure	sT0	not done
	sT1	complete surgical resection (>90%)
	sT2	partial surgical resection (>50% but <90%)
	sT3	partial surgical resection (>5% but <50%)
	sT4	biopsy only (<5% removal)
	sT5	Shunting procedure only

Note: if a shunting procedure was performed with any of the surgical procedures above, add a subcategory "a", e.g. sT1a would indicate a complete surgical resection and a shunting procedure.

post-operative size (applies to discrete or unifocal supratentorial or infratentorial lesions)

pT0	no surgery done, or not applicable
pT1	no visible tumor remains
pT2	<1.5 cm remains
pT3	1.5–5.0 cm remains
pT4	>5.0 cm remains

Note: if the primary tumor were multifocal, the post-operative size applies only to the lesion where a resection was accomplished.

Note: Tumor size is measured by the product of the largest perpendicular cross-sectional diameters, using the contrast-enhancing tumor margins. If a tumor does not enhance, the size will be measured using the margins of the low density lesion on CT, or the T-2 weighted images on MRI. Surgical procedures apply to both supratentorial and infratentorial lesions.

Nodal Status Does not apply

Metastasis

Mx	not assessed
M0	no metastases
M1	positive CSF cytology
M2	spinal metastasis (discrete, may be single or multiple) M2a: without leptomeningeal spread M2b: with leptomeningeal spread
M3	intracranial metastasis (discrete, single or multiple) M3a: without leptomeningeal spread M3b: with leptomeningeal spread
M4	Extracranial metastasis Specify site(s) Skin Nodal Lung Bone Bone Marrow Peritoneum Other (specify ______________)

Histopathological Type (note: Histopathological grade does not apply to CNS tumors)

Juvenile Pilocytic Astrocytoma
Fibrillary or Protoplasmic Astrocytoma
Astrocytoma
Pleomorphic Xanthoastrocytoma
Subependymal Giant Cell Astrocytoma
Ependymoma, non-anaplastic
Oligodendroglioma, non-anaplastic
Mixed oligoastrocytoma, non-anaplastic
Other mixed tumors, non-anaplastic (specify components ______________)
Anaplastic astrocytoma
Anaplastic oligodendroglioma
Anaplastic ependymoma
Anaplastic mixed oligoastrocytoma
Other anaplastic mixed tumors (specify components ______________)
Glioblastoma multiforme
Gliosarcoma

Group Staging Does not apply to CNS tumors

American Joint Committee on Cancer: Staging of tumors metastatic to the brain

BRAIN METASTASIS

AMERICAN JOINT COMMITTEE ON CANCER
Staging of Tumors Metastatic to the Brain

DATAFORM

REGISTRATION DATA

ID # ____________ Social Security # ____________ Date of Birth ____________ Sex ______

Name (Last, First, M.I.) ____________________ Handedness ______ Age ______

Physician/Surgeon ____________________ Hospital ____________________

PRIMARY CANCER

Site of primary cancer ____________________ Date of original diagnosis ____________

Histology ____________________ Grade (when appropriate) ____________

TNM Stage at Initial Diagnosis of Primary Cancer ____________

Therapy of primary cancer (indicate all treatments and dates)

- ☐ biopsy — date ____________
- ☐ incomplete resection — date ____________
- ☐ "complete" resection — date ____________
- ☐ radiation therapy — date(s) ____________ dose ____________
- ☐ chemotherapy — agents ____________ date(s) ____________
- ☐ immunotherapy — agents ____________ date(s) ____________
- ☐ other adjuvant therapy ____________ date(s) ____________

BRAIN METASTASIS

Date of initial diagnosis ____________ Interval from diagnosis of primary cancer (months) ____________

Location of brain metastases at initial diagnosis ____________________

☐ Meningeal carcinomatosis ____________________

Number of metastases at initial diagnosis ____________ Size of largest metastatic lesion (cm) ____________

Assessment: ☐ CT ☐ MRI ☐ CSF cytology ☐ Other ____________

Histology of brain metastasis (when available) ____________________ Grade ____________

Therapy of brain metastases (indicate all treatments and dates)

- ☐ none
- ☐ corticosteroids — dose(s) ____________________ date(s) ____________
- ☐ biopsy — date ____________
- ☐ subtotal resection — date ____________
- ☐ "total" resection (all known brain metastases) — date ____________
- ☐ radiation therapy (conventional, external beam) — dose ____________ date ____________
- ☐ stereotactic external radiation therapy — dose ____________ date ____________
  (gamma knife or linear accelerator)
- ☐ radiation implants — type & tumor dose ____________ date(s) ____________
- ☐ chemotherapy — agents ____________ date(s) ____________
- ☐ immunotherapy ____________ date(s) ____________
- ☐ other ____________ date(s) ____________

AJCC form
PRIMARY CANCER
Page 2

Extent of primary cancer at diagnosis of brain metastasis

- ☐ No evidence of disease
- ☐ Local disease only
- ☐ remote metastasis (other than brain)
- ☐ disseminated disease

Performance Status (Karnofsky Rating)

________________ At diagnosis of primary cancer
________________ At diagnosis of brain metastasis
________________ After treatment of brain metastasis
________________ At most recent follow-up, date ________

Prognostic Markers

________________ At diagnosis of primary cancer
________________ At diagnosis of brain metastasis
________________ At most recent follow-up, date ________

Initial response to therapy of brain metastasis

- ☐ complete response
- ☐ partial response
- ☐ no change
- ☐ complication of therapy
- ☐ death

Date of last contact ________

State at last contact

- ☐ living and well
- ☐ living with disease
- ☐ disabled from disease
- ☐ disabled, other causes
- ☐ dead, other causes
- ☐ dead of disease
- ☐ unknown

If dead of disease —

- ☐ recurrence or progression of brain metastases
- ☐ disseminated cancer

Family history of cancer? ☐ Yes ☐ No

Specify ____
____
____
____
____
____
____

NEUROLOGIC TOPOGRAPHICAL CORRELATION SHEET

NO. ____________________

DATE ____________________

NAME ____________________

SEX ____________________

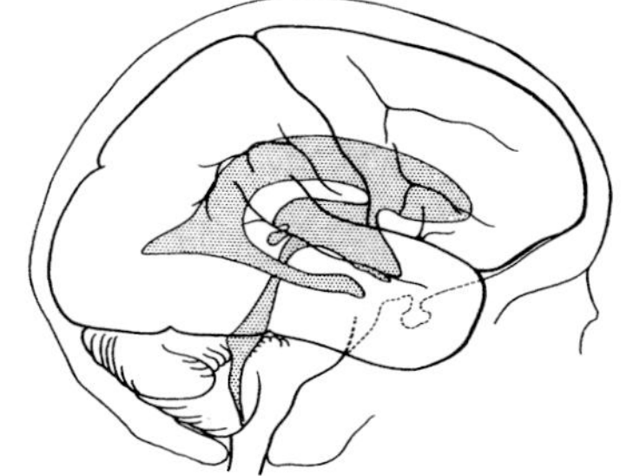

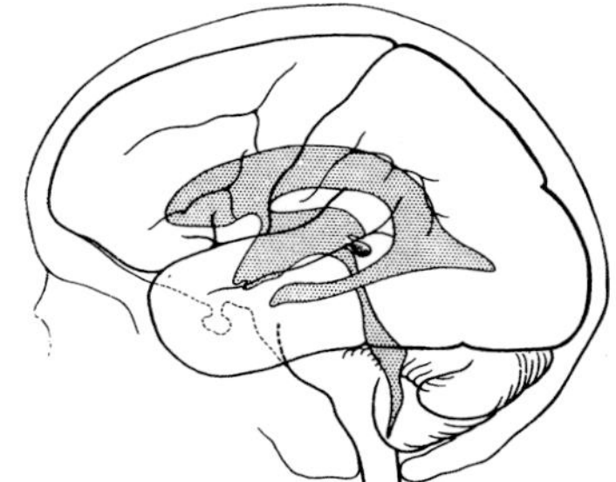

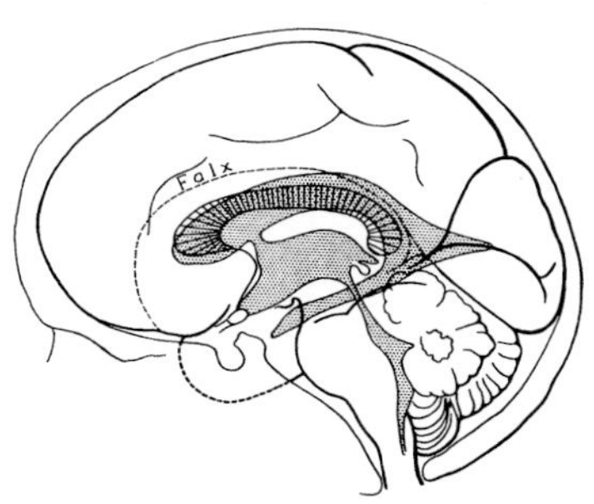

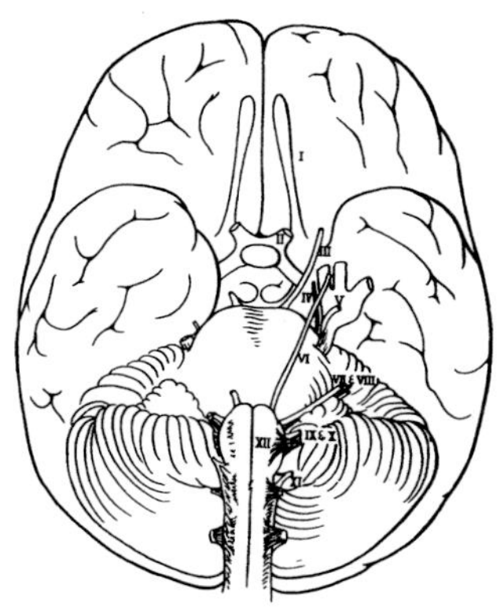

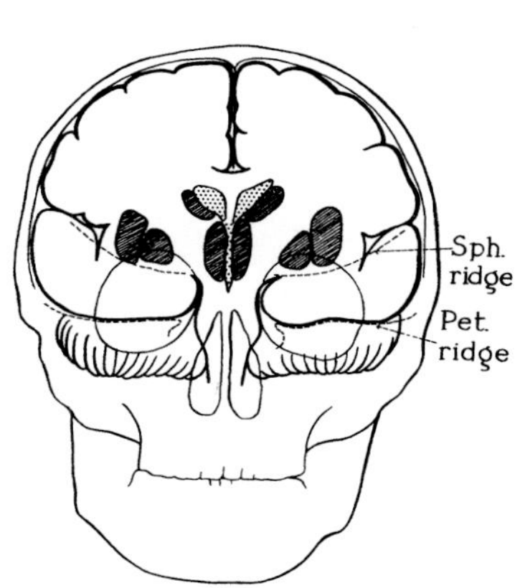

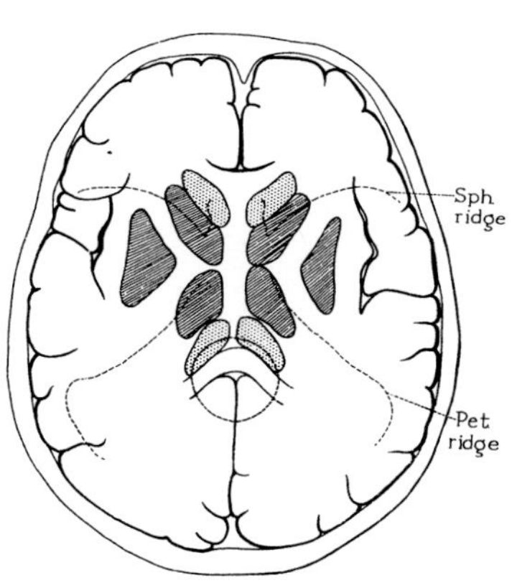

Label metastases and give size in cm

A. ____________________

B. ____________________

C. ____________________

WHO classification of brain tumors

WHO classification of brain tumors

Tumors of Neuroepithelial tissue

Astrocytic tumors

1. Astrocytoma
   Variants: fibrillary, protoplasmic, gemistocytic, or mixed
2. Anaplastic (malignant) astrocytoma
3. Glioblastomas
   variants: giant cell glioblastoma, gliosarcoma
4. Pilocytic astrocytoma
5. Pleomorphic xanthoastrocytoma
6. Subependymal giant cell astrocytoma (usually in association with tuberous sclerosis)

Oligodendroglial tumors

1. Oligodendroglioma
2. Anaplastic (malignant) oligodendroglioma

Ependymal tumors

1. Ependymoma
   variants: cellular, papillary, epithelial, clear cell, mixed
2. Anaplastic (malignant) ependymoma
3. Myxopapillary ependymoma
4. Subependymoma

Mixed gliomas

1. Mixed oligoastrocytoma
2. Anaplastic (malignant) oligoastrocytoma
3. Others

Choroid plexus tumors

1. Choroid plexus papilloma
2. Choroid plexus carcinoma

Neuroepithelial tumors of uncertain origin

1. Astroblastomas
2. Polar spongioblastoma
3. Gliomatosis cerebri

Neuronal and mixed neuronal-glial tumors

1. Gangliocytoma
2. Dysplastic gangliocytoma of cerebellum (Lhermitte-Duclos)
3. Desmoplastic infantile ganglioglioma
4. Dysembryoplastic neuroepithelial tumor
5. Ganglioglioma
6. Anaplastic (malignant) ganglioglioma
7. Central neurocytoma
8. Olfactory neuroblastoma (Esthesioneuroblastoma)
   variant: olfactory neuroepithelioma

Pineal tumors

1. Pineocytoma
2. Pineoblastoma
3. Mixed pineocytoma/pineoblastoma

Embryonal tumors

1. Medulloepithelioma
2. Neuroblastoma
   variant: ganglioneuroblastoma
3. Ependymoblastoma
4. Retinoblastoma
5. Primitive neuroectodermal tumors (PNETs) with multipotent differentiation:
   neuronal, astrocytic, ependymal, muscle, melanotic, etc.
   a. Medulloblastoma
      Variants: medullomyoblastoma, melonocytic medulloblastoma
   b. Cerebral or spinal PNETs

Tumors of Cranial and Spinal Nerves

1. Schwannoma (neurilemoma, neurinoma)
   variants: cellular, plexiform, melanotic
2. Neurofibroma
   variants: circumscribed, plexiform
3. Malignant peripheral nerve sheath tumor (MPNST)
   (neurogenic sarcoma, anaplastic neurofibroma, "malignant schwannoma")
   variants: epithelioid, MPNST with divergent mesenchymal and/or epithelial differentiation, melanotic

Tumors of the Meninges

Tumors of meningothelial cells

1. Meningioma
   histologic types:
   a. meningothelial (syncytial)
   b. transitional/mixed
   c. fibrous (fibroblastic)
   d. psammomamatous
   e. angiomatous
   f. microcystic
   g. secretory
   h. clear cell
   i. chordoid
   j. lymphoplasmacyte-rich
   k. metaplastic variants (xanthomatous, myxoid, osseous, cartilagenous etc.)
2. Atypical meningioma
3. Anaplastic (malignant) meningioma
   a. variants of 1 a-k (see above)
   b. papillary

Non-meningothelial tumors of the meninges

1. Mesenchymal tumors
   Benign neoplasms
   a. Osteocartilagenous tumors
   b. Lipoma
   c. Fibrous histiocytoma
   Malignant neoplasms
   a. Hemangiopericytoma
   b. Chondrosarcoma
   c. Mesenchymal chondrosarcoma
   d. Malignant fibrous histiocytoma
   e. Rhabdomyosarcoma
   f. Meningeal sarcomatosis
2. Tumors of uncertain origin
   a. Hemangioblastoma (capillary hemangioblastoma)

Hematopoietic Tumors

1. Primary malignant lymphomas
2. Plasmocytoma
3. Granulocytic sarcoma
4. Others

Germ Cell Tumors

1. Germinoma
2. Embryonal carcinoma
3. Yolk sac tumor (endodermal sinus tumor)
4. Choriocarcinoma
5. Teratoma
   variants: mature, immature, malignant
6. Mixed germ cell tumors

Classification of Brain Tumors in Children

I. Tumors of neuroepithelial tissue
   A. Glial tumors
      1. Astrocytic tumors
         a. Astrocytoma (fibrillary, protoplasmic, gemistocytic, pilocytic and xanthomatous)
         b. Anaplastic astrocytoma
         c. Subependymal giant cell tumors (tuberous sclerosis)
         d. Gigantocellular glioma
      2. Oligodendroglial tumors
         a. Oligodendroglioma
         b. Anaplastic oligodendroglioma
      3. Ependymal tumors
         a. Ependymoma
         b. Anaplastic ependymoma
         c. Myxopapillary ependymoma
      4. Choroid plexus tumors
         a. Choroid plexus papilloma
         b. Anaplastic choroid plexus tumor (carcinoma)
      5. Mixed gliomas
         a. Oligoastrocytoma
            1. Anaplastic oligoastrocytoma
         b. Astroependymoma
            1. Anaplastic ependymoastrocytoma
         c. Oligoastroependymoma
            1. Anaplastic oligoastroependymoma
         d. Oligoependymoma
            1. Anaplastic oligoependymoma
         e. Subependymoma-subependymal glomerate astrocytoma
         f. Gliofibroma
      6. Glioblastomatous tumors
         a. Glioblastoma multiforme
         b. Giant cell glioblastoma
         c. Gliosarcoma
      7. Gliomatosis cerebri
   B. Neuronal tumors
      1. Gangliocytoma

2. Anaplastic gangliocytoma
3 Ganglioglioma
4. Anaplastic ganglioglioma
C. 'Primitive' Neuroepithelial tumors
1. 'Primitive' neuroectodermal tumor, not otherwise specified (NOS)
2. 'Primitive' Neuroectodermal tumor, with
a. Astrocytes
b. Oligodendrocytes
c. Ependymal cells
d. Neuronal cells
e. Other (melanocytic, mesenchymal)
f. Mixed cellular elements
3. Medulloepithelioma
a. Medulloepithelioma, NOS
b. Medulloepithelioma with:
1. Astrocytes
2. Oligodendrocytes
3. Ependymal cells
4. Neuronal cells
5. Other (melanocytic, mesenchymal)
6. Mixed cellular elements
D. Pineal cell tumors
1. Primitive neuroectodermal tumor (See C above) (pineoblastoma)
2. Pineocytoma
II. Tumors of meningeal and related tissues
A. Meningiomas
1. Meningioma, NOS
2. Papillary meningioma
3. Anaplastic meningioma
B. Meningeal sarcomatous tumors
1. Meningeal sarcoma, NOS
2. Rhabdomyosarcoma or leiomyosarcoma
3. Mesenchymal chondrosarcoma
4. Fibrosarcoma
5. Others
C. Primary melanocytic tumors
1. Malignant melanoma
2. Melanomatosis
3. Melanocytic tumors, miscellaneous
III. Tumors of nerve sheath cells
A. Neurilemmoma (schwannoma, neurinoma)
B. Anaplastic neurilemmoma (schwannoma, neurinoma)
C. Neurofibroma
D. Anaplastic neurofibroma (neurofibrosarcoma, neurogenic sarcoma)
IV. Primary malignant lymphomas
Classify according to local current standards
V. Tumors of blood vessel origin
A. Hemangioblastoma
B. Hemangiopericytoma
C. Neoplastic Angioendotheliosis-angiosarcoma
VI. Germ cell tumors
A. Germinoma
B. Embryonal carcinoma
C. Choriocarcinoma
D. Endodermal sinus tumor
E. Teratomatous tumors
1. Immature teratoma
2. Mature teratoma
3. Teratocarcinoma
F. Mixed
VII. Malformative tumors
A. Craniopharyngioma
B. Rathke's cleft cyst
C. Epidermal cyst
D. Dermoid cyst
E. Colloid cyst or third ventricle
F. Enterogenous or bronchial cyst
G. Cyst, NOS
H. Lipoma
I. Granular cell tumor (choristoma)
J. Hamartoma
1. Neuronal
2. Glial
3. Neuronoglial
4. Meningioangioneurinomatosis
VIII. Tumors of neuroendocrine origin
A. Tumors of anterior pituitary
1. Adenoma
2. Pituitary carcinoma
B. Paraganglioma
IX. Local extensions from regional tumors
Type to be specified according to primary diagnosis
X. Metastatic tumors
XI. Unclassified tumors

From: Rorke, L B et al, Cancer 56: 1869–1886, 1985

Index

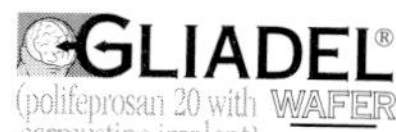

GLIADEL®
(polifeprosan 20 with carmustine implant) WAFER

DESCRIPTION

GLIADEL® Wafer (polifeprosan 20 with carmustine implant) is a sterile, off-white to pale yellow wafer approximately 1.45 cm in diameter and 1 mm thick. Each wafer contains 192.3 mg of a biodegradable polyanhydride copolymer and 7.7 mg of carmustine [1,3-bis (2-chloroethyl)-1-nitrosourea, or BCNU]. Carmustine is a nitrosourea oncolytic agent. The copolymer, polifeprosan 20, consists of poly[bis(p-carboxyphenoxy) propane: sebacic acid] in a 20:80 molar ratio and is used to control the local delivery of carmustine. Carmustine is homogeneously distributed in the copolymer matrix.

The structural formula for polifeprosan 20 is:

$$\left[-\overset{O}{\overset{\|}{C}}-C_6H_4-O(CH_2)_3O-C_6H_4-\overset{O}{\overset{\|}{C}}-O- \right]_m \left[-\overset{O}{\overset{\|}{C}}-CH_2(CH_2)_6CH_2-\overset{O}{\overset{\|}{C}}-O- \right]_n$$

Ratio m:n = 20:80; random copolymer

The structural formula for carmustine is:

$$Cl-CH_2-CH_2-\underset{NO}{\underset{|}{N}}-\overset{O}{\overset{\|}{C}}-NHCH_2-CH_2-Cl$$

CLINICAL PHARMACOLOGY

GLIADEL is designed to deliver carmustine directly into the surgical cavity created when a brain tumor is resected. On exposure to the aqueous environment of the resection cavity, the anhydride bonds in the copolymer are hydrolyzed, releasing carmustine, carboxyphenoxypropane, and sebacic acid. The carmustine released from GLIADEL diffuses into the surrounding brain tissue and produces an antineoplastic effect by alkylating DNA and RNA.

Carmustine has been shown to degrade both spontaneously and metabolically. The production of an alkylating moiety, hypothesized to be chloroethyl carbonium ion, leads to the formation of DNA cross-links.

The tumoricidal activity of GLIADEL is dependent on release of carmustine to the tumor cavity in concentrations sufficient for effective cytotoxicity.

More than 70% of the copolymer degrades by three weeks. The metabolic disposition and excretion of the monomers differ. Carboxyphenoxypropane is eliminated by the kidney and sebacic acid, an endogenous fatty acid, is metabolized by the liver and expired as CO_2 in animals.

The absorption, distribution, metabolism, and excretion of the copolymer in humans is unknown. Carmustine concentrations delivered by GLIADEL in human brain tissue have not been determined. Plasma levels of carmustine after GLIADEL wafer implant were not determined. In rabbits implanted with wafers containing 3.85% carmustine, no detectible levels of carmustine were found in the plasma or cerebrospinal fluid.

Following an intravenous infusion of carmustine at doses ranging from 30 to 170 mg/m^2, the average terminal half-life, clearance, and steady-state volume of distribution were 22 minutes, 56 mL/min/kg, and 3.25 L/kg, respectively. Approximately 60% of the intravenous 200 mg/m^2 dose of ^{14}C-carmustine was excreted in the urine over 96 hours and 6% was expired as CO_2.

GLIADEL wafers are biodegradable in human brain when implanted into the cavity after tumor resection. The rate of biodegradation is variable from patient to patient. During the biodegradation process, a wafer remnant may be observed on brain imaging scans or at re-operation even though extensive degradation of all components has occurred. Data obtained from review of CT scans obtained 49 days after implantation of GLIADEL demonstrated that images consistent with wafers were visible to varying degrees in the scans of 11 of 18 patients. Data obtained at re-operation and autopsies have demonstrated wafer remnants up to 232 days after GLIADEL implantation.

Wafer remnants removed at re-operation from two patients with recurrent malignant glioma, one at 64 days and the second at 92 days after implantation, were analyzed for content. The following table presents the results of analyses completed on these remnants.

COMPOSITION OF WAFER REMNANTS REMOVED FROM TWO PATIENTS ON RE-OPERATION

Component	Patient A	Patient B
Days After GLIADEL Implantation	64	92
Anhydride Bonds	None detected	None detected
Water Content (% of wafer remnant weight)	95-97%	74-86%
Carmustine Content (% of initial)	<0.0004%	0.034%
Carboxyphenoxypropane Content (% of initial)	9%	14%
Sebacic Acid Content (% of initial)	4%	3%

The wafer remnants consisted mostly of water and monomeric components with minimal detectable carmustine present.

CLINICAL STUDIES

In a randomized, double-blind, placebo-controlled clinical trial in adults with recurrent malignant glioma, GLIADEL prolonged survival in patients with glioblastoma multiforme (GBM). Ninety-five percent of the patients treated with GLIADEL had 7-8 wafers implanted.

In 222 patients with recurrent malignant glioma who had failed initial surgery and radiation therapy, the six-month survival rate after surgery increased from 47% (53/112) for patients receiving placebo to 60% (66/110) for patients treated with GLIADEL. Median survival increased by 33%, from 24 weeks with placebo to 32 weeks with GLIADEL treatment. In patients with GBM, the six-month survival rate increased from 36% (26/73) with placebo to 56% (40/72) with GLIADEL treatment. Median survival of GBM patients increased by 41% from 20 weeks with placebo to 28 weeks with GLIADEL treatment. In patients with pathologic diagnoses other than GBM at the time of surgery for tumor recurrence, GLIADEL produced no survival prolongation.

6-MONTH KAPLAN-MEIER SURVIVAL CURVES FOR PATIENTS UNDERGOING SURGERY FOR RECURRENT GBM

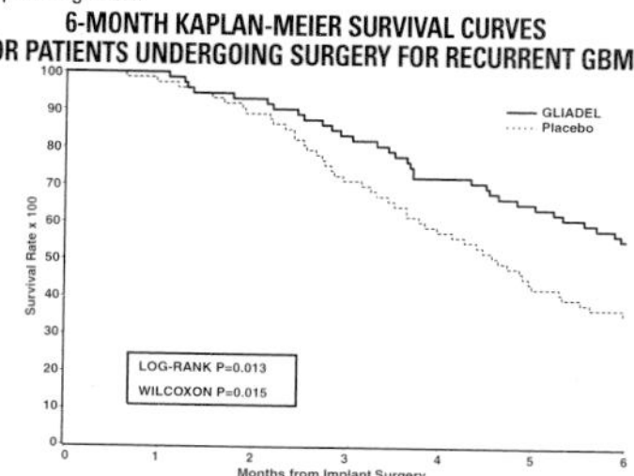

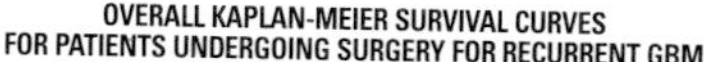

OVERALL KAPLAN-MEIER SURVIVAL CURVES FOR PATIENTS UNDERGOING SURGERY FOR RECURRENT GBM

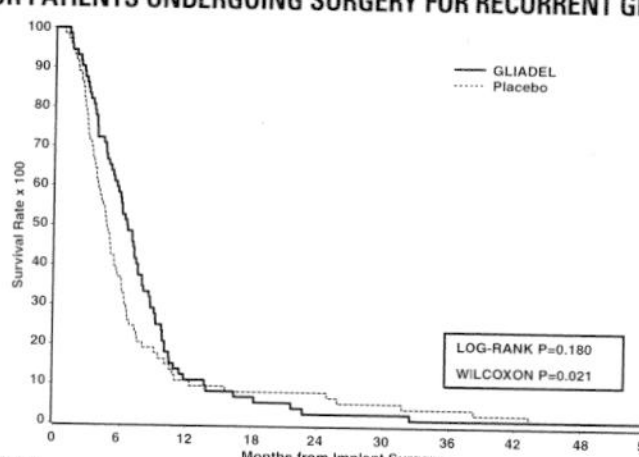

INDICATIONS AND USAGE

GLIADEL is indicated for use as an adjunct to surgery to prolong survival in patients with recurrent glioblastoma multiforme for whom surgical resection is indicated.

CONTRAINDICATIONS

GLIADEL contains carmustine. GLIADEL should not be given to individuals who have demonstrated a previous hypersensitivity to carmustine or any of the components of GLIADEL.

WARNINGS

Patients undergoing craniotomy for malignant glioma and implantation of GLIADEL should be monitored closely for known complications of craniotomy, including seizures, intracranial infections, abnormal wound healing, and brain edema. Cases of intracerebral mass effect unresponsive to corticosteroids have been described in patients treated with GLIADEL, including one case leading to brain herniation.

Pregnancy: There are no studies assessing the reproductive toxicity of GLIADEL. Carmustine, the active component of GLIADEL, can cause fetal harm when administered to a pregnant woman. Carmustine has been shown to be embryotoxic and teratogenic in rats at i.p. doses of 0.5, 1, 2, 4, or 8 mg/kg/day when given on gestation days 6 through 15. Carmustine caused fetal malformations (anophthalmia, micrognathia, omphalocele) at 1.0 mg/kg/day (about 1/6 the recommended human dose (eight wafers of 7.7 mg carmustine/wafer) on a mg/m^2 basis). Carmustine was embryotoxic in rabbits at i.v. doses of 4.0 mg/kg/day (about 1.2 times the recommended human dose on a mg/m^2 basis). Embryotoxicity was characterized by increased embryo-fetal deaths, reduced numbers of litters, and reduced litter sizes.

There are no studies of GLIADEL in pregnant women. If GLIADEL is used during pregnancy, or if the patient becomes pregnant after GLIADEL implantation, the patient must be warned of the potential hazard to the fetus.

PRECAUTIONS

General: Communication between the surgical resection cavity and the ventricular system should be avoided to prevent the wafers from migrating into the ventricular system and causing obstructive hydrocephalus. If a communication exists, it should be closed prior to wafer implantation.

Imaging Studies: Computed tomography and magnetic resonance imaging of the head may demonstrate enhancement in the brain tissue surrounding the resection cavity after implantation of GLIADEL wafers. This enhancement may represent edema and inflammation caused by GLIADEL or tumor progression.

Therapeutic Interactions: Interactions of GLIADEL with other drugs or radiotherapy have not been formally evaluated. In clinical trials, few patients have received systemic chemotherapy within 30 days of GLIADEL (6) or external beam radiation therapy (36). Chemotherapy was withheld at least four weeks (six weeks for nitrosoureas) prior to and two weeks after surgery in patients undergoing re-operation for malignant glioma. External beam radiation therapy was initiated no sooner than three weeks after GLIADEL implantation. Of the 36 patients who received GLIADEL at initial surgery for newly diagnosed, malignant glioma followed by external beam radiation therapy, 3/15 (20%) in one study and 11/21 (52%) in the other study experienced new or worsened seizures. Patients were followed for a maximum of 24 months. The short and long-term toxicity profiles of GLIADEL when given in conjunction with radiation or chemotherapy have not been fully explored.

Carcinogenesis, Mutagenesis, Impairment of Fertility: No carcinogenicity, mutagenicity or impairment of fertility studies have been conducted with GLIADEL. Carcinogenicity, mutagenicity and impairment of fertility studies have been conducted with carmustine, the active component of GLIADEL. Carmustine was given three times a week for six months, followed by 12 months observation, to Swiss mice at i.p. doses of 2.5 and 5.0 mg/kg (about 1/5 and 1/3 the recommended human dose (eight wafers of 7.7 mg carmustine/wafer) on a mg/m^2 basis) and to SD rats at i.p. dose of 1.5 mg/kg (about 1/4 the recommended human dose on a mg/m^2 basis). There were increases in tumor incidence in all treated animals, predominantly subcutaneous and lung neoplasms. *Mutagenesis:* Carmustine was mutagenic *in vitro* (Ames assay, human lymphoblast HGPRT assay) and clastogenic both *in vitro* (V79 hamster cell micronucleus assay) and *in vivo* (SCE assay in rodent brain tumors, mouse bone marrow micronucleus assay). *Impairment of Fertility:* Carmustine caused testicular degeneration at i.p. doses of 8 mg/kg/week for eight weeks (about 1.3 times the recommended human dose on a mg/m^2 basis) in male rats.

Pregnancy: Pregnancy Category D: see **WARNINGS.**

Nursing Mothers: It is not known if either carmustine, carboxyphenoxypropane, or sebacic acid is excreted in human milk. Because many drugs are excreted in human milk and because of the potential for serious adverse reactions from carmustine in nursing infants, it is recommended that patients receiving GLIADEL discontinue nursing.

Pediatric Use: The safety and effectiveness of GLIADEL in pediatric patients have not been established.

ADVERSE REACTIONS

Data in the following table are based on the experience of 222 patients with recurrent malignant glioma randomized to GLIADEL or placebo (wafer without carmustine).

The spectrum of adverse events observed in patients who received GLIADEL or placebo in clinical studies was consistent with that encountered in patients undergoing craniotomy for malignant gliomas.

GLIADEL was not reported to be the cause of death in any of the GLIADEL clinical trials.

The following post-operative adverse events were observed in 4% or more of the patients receiving GLIADEL in the placebo-controlled clinical trial. Except for nervous system effects, where there is a possibility that the placebo wafers could have been responsible, only events more common in the GLIADEL group are listed. These adverse events were either not present pre-operatively or worsened post-operatively during the follow-up period. The follow-up period in the randomized trial was up to 71 months.

COMMON ADVERSE EVENTS OBSERVED IN ≥4% OF PATIENTS IN THE RANDOMIZED TRIAL

Body System Adverse Event	GLIADEL Wafer with Carmustine [N=110] n (%)	PLACEBO Wafer without Carmustine [N=112] n (%)	Body System Adverse Event	GLIADEL Wafer with Carmustine [N=110] n (%)	PLACEBO Wafer without Carmustine [N=112] n (%)
Body as a Whole			**Nervous System (cont'd)**		
Fever	13 (12)	9 (8)	Headache	16 (15)	14 (13)
Pain*	8 (7)	1 (1)	Hemiplegia	21 (19)	22 (20)
Digestive System			Intracranial Hypertension	4 (4)	7 (6)
Nausea and Vomiting	9 (8)	7 (6)	Meningitis or Abscess	4 (4)	1 (1)
Metabolic and Nutritional Disorders			Somnolence	15 (14)	12 (11)
Healing Abnormal*	15 (14)	6 (5)	Stupor	7 (6)	7 (6)
Nervous System			**Skin and Appendages**		
Aphasia	10 (9)	12 (11)	Rash	6 (5)	4 (4)
Brain Edema	4 (4)	1 (1)	**Urogenital System**		
Confusion	11 (10)	9 (8)	Urinary Tract		
Convulsion	21 (19)	21 (19)	Infection	23 (21)	19 (17)

*$p < 0.05$ for comparison of GLIADEL versus placebo groups in the randomized trial (two-sided Fisher's Exact Test)

The following adverse events were also reported in 4-9% of GLIADEL patients but were at least as frequent in the placebo group as in GLIADEL-treated patients: infection, deep thrombophlebitis, pulmonary embolism, nausea, oral moniliasis, anemia, hyponatremia, pneumonia.

The following four categories of adverse events are possibly related to treatment with GLIADEL. The frequency with which they occurred in the randomized trial along with descriptive detail are provided below.

1. Seizures: In the randomized study, the majority of seizures in the placebo and GLIADEL groups were mild or moderate in severity. The incidence of new or worsened seizures was 19% in patients treated with GLIADEL and 19% in patients receiving placebo. Of the patients with new or worsened seizures post-operatively, 12/22 (54%) of patients treated with GLIADEL and 2/22 (9%) of placebo patients experienced the first new or worsened seizure within the first five post-operative days. The median time to onset of the first new or worsened post-operative seizure was 3.5 days in patients treated with GLIADEL and 61 days in placebo patients. The occurrence of seizures did not reduce the survival benefit of GLIADEL.

2. Brain Edema: In the randomized trial, brain edema was noted in 4% of patients treated with GLIADEL and in 1% of patients treated with placebo. Development of brain edema with mass effect (due to tumor recurrence, intracranial infection, or necrosis) may necessitate re-operation and, in some cases, removal of wafer or its remnants.

3. Healing Abnormalities: The majority of these events were mild to moderate in severity. Healing abnormalities occurred in 14% of GLIADEL-treated patients compared to 5% of placebo recipients. These events included cerebrospinal fluid leaks, subdural fluid collections, subgaleal or wound effusions, and wound breakdown.

4. Intracranial Infection: In the randomized trial, intracranial infection (meningitis or abscess) occurred in 4% of patients treated with GLIADEL and in 1% of patients receiving placebo. In GLIADEL-treated patients, there were two cases of bacterial meningitis, one case of chemical meningitis, and one case of meningitis which was not further specified. A brain abscess developed in one placebo-treated patient. The rate of deep wound infection (infection of subgaleal space, bone, meninges, or neural parenchyma) was 6% in both GLIADEL and placebo treated patients.

The following adverse events, not listed in the table above, were reported in less than 4% but at least 1% of patients treated with GLIADEL in all studies (n=273). The events listed were either not present pre-operatively or worsened post-operatively. Whether GLIADEL caused these events cannot be determined.

Body as a Whole: peripheral edema (2%); neck pain (2%); accidental injury (1%); back pain (1%); allergic reaction (1%); asthenia (1%); chest pain (1%); sepsis (1%)

Cardiovascular System: hypertension (3%); hypotension (1%)

Digestive System: diarrhea (2%); constipation (2%); dysphagia (1%); gastrointestinal hemorrhage (1%); fecal incontinence (1%)

Hemic and Lymphatic System: thrombocytopenia (1%); leukocytosis (1%)

Metabolic and Nutritional Disorders: hyponatremia (3%); hyperglycemia (3%); hypokalemia (1%)

Musculoskeletal System: infection (1%)

Nervous System: hydrocephalus (3%); depression (3%); abnormal thinking (2%); ataxia (2%); dizziness (2%); insomnia (2%); monoplegia (2%); coma (1%); amnesia (1%); diplopia (1%); paranoid reaction (1%). In addition, cerebral hemorrhage and cerebral infarct were each reported in less than 1% of patients treated with GLIADEL.

Respiratory System: infection (2%); aspiration pneumonia (1%)

Skin and Appendages: rash (2%)

Special Senses: visual field defect (2%); eye pain (1%)

Urogenital System: urinary incontinence (2%)

OVERDOSAGE

There is no clinical experience with use of more than eight GLIADEL wafers per surgical procedure.

DOSAGE AND ADMINISTRATION

Each GLIADEL wafer contains 7.7 mg of carmustine, resulting in a dose of 61.6 mg when eight wafers are implanted. It is recommended that eight wafers be placed in the resection cavity if the size and shape of it allows. Should the size and shape not accommodate eight wafers, the maximum number of wafers as allowed should be placed. Since there is no clinical experience, no more than eight wafers should be used per surgical procedure.

Handling and Disposal[1-7]: Wafers should only be handled by personnel wearing surgical gloves because exposure to carmustine can cause severe burning and hyperpigmentation of the skin. Use of double gloves is recommended and the outer gloves should be discarded into a biohazard waste container after use. A surgical instrument dedicated to the handling of the wafers should be used for wafer implantation. If repeat neurosurgical intervention is indicated, any wafer or wafer remnant should be handled as a potentially cytotoxic agent.

GLIADEL wafers should be handled with care. The aluminum foil laminate pouches containing GLIADEL should be delivered to the operating room and remain unopened until ready to implant the wafers. **The outside surface of the outer foil pouch is not sterile.**

Instructions for Opening Pouch Containing GLIADEL

Figure 1: To remove the sterile inner pouch from the outer pouch, locate the folded corner and slowly pull in an outward motion.

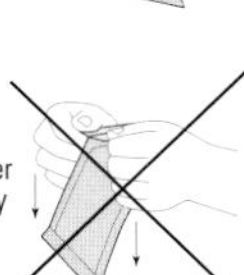

Figure 2: Do NOT pull in a downward motion rolling knuckles over the pouch. This may exert pressure on the wafer and cause it to break.

Figure 3: Remove the inner pouch by grabbing hold of the **crimped** edge and pulling upward.

Figure 4: To open the inner pouch, gently hold the crimped edge and cut in an arc-like fashion around the wafer.

Figure 5: To remove the GLIADEL wafer, gently grasp the wafer with the aid of forceps and place it onto a designated sterile field.

Once the tumor is resected, tumor pathology is confirmed, and hemostasis is obtained, up to eight GLIADEL® Wafers (polifeprosan 20 with carmustine implant) may be placed to cover as much of the resection cavity as possible. Slight overlapping of the wafers is acceptable. Wafers broken in half may be used, but wafers broken in more than two pieces should be discarded in a biohazard container. Oxidized regenerated cellulose (Surgicel®) may be placed over the wafers to secure them against the cavity surface. After placement of the wafers, the resection cavity should be irrigated and the dura closed in a water tight fashion.

Unopened foil pouches may be kept at ambient room temperature for a maximum of six hours at a time.

HOW SUPPLIED

GLIADEL is available in a single dose treatment box containing eight individually pouched wafers. Each wafer contains 7.7 mg of carmustine and is packaged in two aluminum foil laminate pouches. The inner pouch is sterile and is designed to maintain product sterility and protect the product from moisture. The outer pouch is a peelable overwrap. **The outside surface of the outer pouch is not sterile.**

GLIADEL must be stored at or below -20°C (-4°F).

REFERENCES

1. Recommendations for the Safe Handling of Parenteral Antineoplastic Drugs, NIH Publication No. 83-2621. For sale by the Superintendent of Documents, U.S. Government Printing Office, Washington, DC 20402.
2. AMA Council Report, Guidelines for Handling Parenteral Antineoplastics. JAMA, 1985; 253(11):1590-1592.
3. National Study Commission on Cytotoxic Exposure — Recommendations for Handling Cytotoxic Agents. Available from Louis P. Jeffrey, ScD., Chairman, National Study Commission on Cytotoxic Exposure, Massachusetts College of Pharmacy and Allied Health Sciences, 179 Longwood Avenue, Boston, Massachusetts 02115.
4. Clinical Oncological Society of Australia, Guidelines and Recommendations for Safe Handling of Antineoplastic Agents. Med J Australia, 1983; 1:426-428.
5. Jones RB, et al: Safe Handling of Chemotherapeutic Agents: A Report from the Mount Sinai Medical Center. CA — A Cancer Journal for Clinicians, 1983; (Sept/Oct) 258-263.
6. American Society of Hospital Pharmacists Technical Assistance Bulletin on Handling Cytotoxic and Hazardous Drugs. Am J. Hosp Pharm, 1990; 47:1033-1049.
7. OSHA Work-Practice Guidelines for Personnel Dealing with Cytotoxic (Antineoplastic) Drugs. Am J Hosp Pharm, 1986; 43:1193-1204.

NDC: 0075-9995-08

CAUTION: FEDERAL LAW PROHIBITS DISPENSING WITHOUT PRESCRIPTION.

U.S. Patent Nos. 4,789,724 and 5,179,189.

Manufactured for
Rhône-Poulenc Rorer Pharmaceuticals Inc.
Collegeville, PA 19426

By
Guilford Pharmaceuticals Inc.
Baltimore, MD 21224

Rev. 10/96

IN-2250